Pediatric Nursing

Caring for Children and Their Families

Third Edition

Nicki L. Potts, RN, PhD
Former Instructor, College of Nursing
University of New Mexico
Albuquerque, New Mexico
and
Former Assistant Professor, School of Nursing
University of Texas at Austin
Austin, Texas

Barbara L. Mandleco, RN, PhD
Professor, College of Nursing
Brigham Young University
Provo, Utah

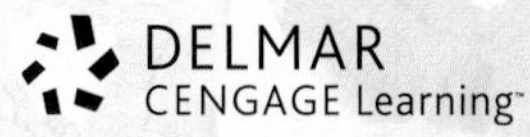

Australia • Brazil • Japan • Korea • Mexico • Singapore • Spain • United Kingdom • United States

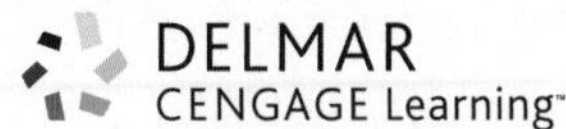

Pediatric Nursing: Caring for Children and Their Families, Third Edition

Nicki L. Potts and Barbara L. Mandleco

Vice President, Career and Professional Editorial: Dave Garza

Director of Learning Solutions: Matthew Kane

Senior Acquisitions Editor: Maureen Rosener

Managing Editor: Marah Bellegarde

Senior Product Manager: Elisabeth F. Williams

Editorial Assistant: Samantha Miller

Vice President, Career and Professional Marketing: Jennifer Baker

Marketing Director: Wendy Mapstone

Senior Marketing Manager: Michele McTighe

Marketing Coordinator: Scott Chrysler

Production Director: Carolyn Miller

Production Manager: Andrew Crouth

Content Project Manager: Anne Sherman

Senior Art Director: Jack Pendleton

Technology Project Manager: Patricia Allen

Library of Congress Control Number: 2010925842

ISBN-13: 978-1-4354-8672-0

ISBN-10: 1-4354-8672-2

Delmar
5 Maxwell Drive
Clifton Park, NY 12065-2919
USA

Cengage Learning is a leading provider of customized learning solutions with office locations around the globe, including Singapore, the United Kingdom, Australia, Mexico, Brazil, and Japan. Locate your local office at: **international.cengage.com/region**

Cengage Learning products are represented in Canada by Nelson Education, Ltd.

To learn more about Delmar, visit **www.cengage.com/delmar**

Purchase any of our products at your local college store or at our preferred online store **www.CengageBrain.com**

Printed in the United States of America
1 2 3 4 5 6 7 15 14 13 12 11

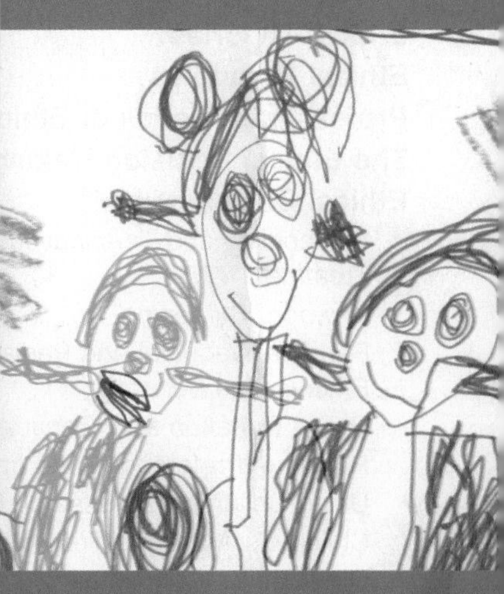

TABLE OF CONTENTS

CHAPTER 3

THE CHILD IN CONTEXT OF THE FAMILY / 57

CHAPTER 4

COMMUNITY AND HOME HEALTH NURSING / 95

CHAPTER 5

SCHOOL NURSING / 119

UNIT 2

Growth and Development of Children / 155

CHAPTER 6

THEORETICAL APPROACHES TO THE GROWTH AND DEVELOPMENT OF CHILDREN / 157

CHAPTER 7

GROWTH AND DEVELOPMENT OF THE NEWBORN / 191

CHAPTER 8

GROWTH AND DEVELOPMENT OF THE INFANT / 227

CHAPTER 9

GROWTH AND DEVELOPMENT OF THE TODDLER / 273

CHAPTER 10

GROWTH AND DEVELOPMENT OF THE PRESCHOOLER / 307

CHAPTER 14

PEDIATRIC ASSESSMENT / 433

CHAPTER 15

INFECTIOUS DISEASES / 469

CHAPTER 16

CARE OF CHILDREN WHO ARE HOSPITALIZED / 507

CHAPTER 17

CHRONIC CONDITIONS / 555

CHAPTER 18

PAIN MANAGEMENT / 581

CHAPTER 19

MEDICATION ADMINISTRATION / 607

CHAPTER 20

LOSS AND BEREAVEMENT / 629

UNIT 4

Alterations in Nutrition and Elimination / 653

CHAPTER 21

FLUID AND ELECTROLYTE ALTERATIONS / 655

CHAPTER 22

GENITOURINARY ALTERATIONS / 697

CHAPTER 23

GASTROINTESTINAL ALTERATIONS / 739

UNIT 5

Alterations in Oxygen Transport / 789

CHAPTER 24

RESPIRATORY ALTERATIONS / 791

CHAPTER 25

CARDIOVASCULAR ALTERATIONS / 845

CHAPTER 26

HEMATOLOGICAL ALTERATIONS / 911

UNIT 6

Alterations in Protective Mechanisms / 949

CHAPTER 27

IMMUNOLOGIC ALTERATIONS / 951

CHAPTER 28

ENDOCRINE ALTERATIONS / 983

CHAPTER 29

CELLULAR ALTERATIONS / 1023

CHAPTER 30

INTEGUMENTARY ALTERATIONS / 1079

UNIT 7

Alterations in Sensorimotor Function / 1147

CHAPTER 31

SENSORY ALTERATIONS / 1149

CHAPTER 32

NEUROLOGICAL ALTERATIONS / 1193

CHAPTER 33

COGNITIVE ALTERATIONS / 1261

CHAPTER 34

MUSCULOSKELETAL ALTERATIONS / 1293

UNIT 8

Other Alterations to Children's Health / 1343

CHAPTER 35

PSYCHOSOCIAL ALTERATIONS / 1345

CHAPTER 36

CHILD ABUSE AND NEGLECT / 1379

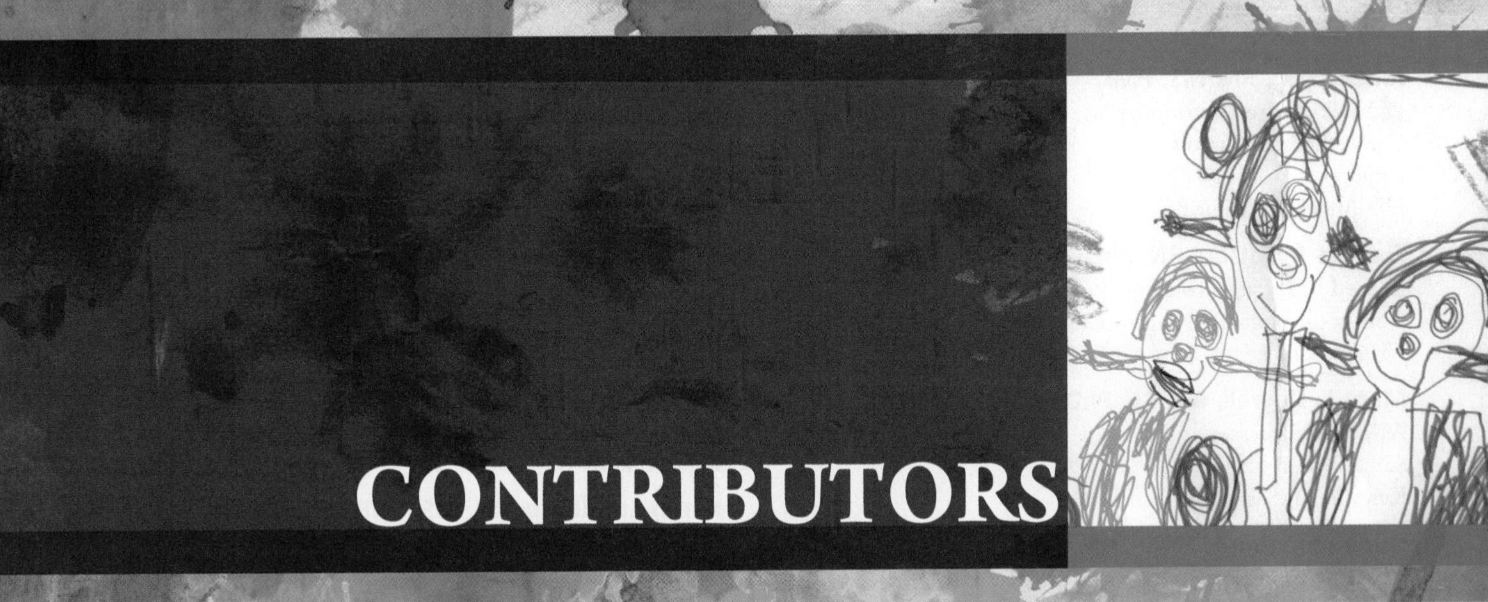

CONTRIBUTORS

Edited by Nicki Lee Potts and Barbara Mandleco

Stephanie Rockwern Amlung, RN, PhD
Research Director
Parexel International
Waltham, Massachusetts

Vicki Ann Andreoni, RN, MSN, CPNP
Visiting Clinical Instructor
Department of Women, Children and Family Health Science
UIC College of Nursing
Chicago, Illinois

Natalie J. Annen, RN, BS
NICU Policy and Procedure Support
Primary Children's Medical Center
Salt Lake City, Utah

Jennifer Beier, RN, MSN, APN-CPNP
Pediatric Nurse Practitioner
Department of Pulmonary Medicine
Children's Memorial Hospital
Chicago, Illinois

Courtney Browning, RN, MSN, CPN
Clinical Faculty
Department of Baccalaureate and Graduate Nursing
Eastern Kentucky University
Richmond, Kentucky

Becky Bunn, RNC, MSN
Assistant Professor
College of Nursing
University of Mary Hardin Baylor
Belton, Texas

Barbara A. Caldwell, APRN-BC, PhD
Associate Professor and Program Director
Joint PhD Program in Urban Systems
UMDNJ-School of Nursing
Newark, New Jersey

Lynn Clark Callister, RN, PhD, FAAN
Professor
College of Nursing
Brigham Young University
Provo, Utah

Kathleen Cervasio, RN, ACNS-BC, CCRN, PhD
Assistant Professor
Long Island University
Brooklyn Campus
Brooklyn, New York

Mary H. Chandler, MSN
Clinic Nurse Manager
Center for Cancer and Blood Disorders of Northern Virginia
Children's National Medical Center
Washington, D.C.

Susan Chasson, MSN, JD, CNM, FNP-BC
Lecturer
College of Nursing
Assistant Lecturer
J. Reuben Clark School of Law
Brigham Young University
Provo, Utah

Bonnie Clay, RN, MS, CCRN, PNP
Pediatric Nurse Practitioner
Department of Pediatric Cardiothoracic Surgery
Primary Children's Hospital
Salt Lake City, Utah

Janet Craig, RN, MS, PNP
Pediatric Nurse Practitioner
Cardiothoracic Surgery
Children's Hospital
Los Angeles, California

Frances J. Dotton, RN, PhD
Retired Associate Professor
College of Nursing, Niagara University
Niagara University, New York

Mary L. Dowell, RN, BC, PhD
Associate Professor
San Antonio College
Kerrville, Texas

Donna Freeborn, FNP, CNM, PhD
Assistant Professor
Brigham Young University
Provo, Utah

Shirley Goodman, RN, BSN, CDE
Diabetes Nurse Educator
Endocrine Nurse Clinician
Children's Memorial Hospital
Chicago, Illinois

Elaine Graf, RN, PNP, NE-BC, PhD
Research and Funding Coordinator
Clinical & Organizational Development
Children's Memorial Medical Center
Chicago, Illinois

Sharon Horner, RN, PhD
Associate Professor
School of Nursing
The University of Texas at Austin
Austin, Texas

Barbara Keating, RN, MSN
Pediatric Clinical Educator
Children's Memorial Medical Center
Chicago, Illinois

Carole Kenner, RNC-NIC, FAAN, DNS
Dean/Professor
University of Oklahoma College of Nursing
Oklahoma City, Oklahoma

Barbara S. Kiernan, APRN, BC, PhD
Associate Professor
Department of Biobehavioral Nursing
Medical College of Georgia
Augusta, Georgia

Patricia King, RN, FNP, MS
Primecare Physicians
Goldsburo, North Carolina

Jane K. Lassetter, RN, PhD
Assistant Professor
College of Nursing
Brigham Young University
Provo, Utah

Christina P. Linton, FNP-BC, PhD
Nurse Practitioner
Department of Dermatology
Central Utah Clinic
Provo, Utah

Maureen L. Lue, RN, MS, CSN
School Nurse
Timber Trails School
School District U46
Elgin, Illinois

Karen Lundberg, RN, MS, CNE
Assistant Teaching Professor
College of Nursing
Brigham Young University
Provo, Utah

Karlen E. Luthy, RN, DNP
Assistant Professor
Brigham Young University
Provo, Utah

Amy Ma, APRN, FNP-BC, DNP
Assistant Professor
Clinical Coordinator of the Nurse Practitioner Program
Long Island University
Brooklyn, New York

J. Kelly McCoy, PhD
Brigham Young University Idaho
Rexburg, Idaho

Debra Ann Mills, RN, MS
Associate Teaching Professor
College of Nursing
Brigham Young University
Provo, Utah

Maribeth Moran, RN, MSN, CPN, CNE
Associate Professor
University of Oklahoma College of Nursing
Oklahoma City, Oklahoma

Kathy Murphy, RN, MSN, CS
Clinical Nurse Specialist/Pediatric Nurse Practitioner
Children's Healthcare of Atlanta-Egleston, Sibley Heart Center
Atlanta, Georgia

Jennifer Obrecht, RN, MS, ARPN
Director of Pediatric/Perinatal CNS Programs
College of Nursing
University of Illinois at Chicago
Chicago, Illinois

Susan O'Connor-Von, RN, PhD
Associate Professor
School of Nursing
University of Minnesota
Minneapolis, Minnesota

Amanda Orme, RN, MS, FNP
Pediatric Emergency Department Nurse Practitioner
Primary Children's Medical Center
Salt Lake City, Utah

Karen D. Peterson, RN, MSN, CPNP
Pediatric Nurse Practitioner
Division of Endocrinology, Formerly of Immunology/Rheumatology
Children's Memorial Medical Center
Chicago, Illinois

Carolyn C. Reynolds, APRN, MS
Operations Director
Pediatric Clinical Program
Intermountain Healthcare
Salt Lake City, Utah

Maria G. Rosario-Sim, RNC, EdD, PNP, BC
Associate Professor
Long Island University
Brooklyn, New York

Sheila Rucki, RN, PCNS, BC, PhD
Associate Director MSN Program
American International College
Springfield, Massachusetts

Hazel M. Sanderson-Marcoux, RN, EdD
Associate Professor and Associate Dean
School of Nursing, RN-BS Program Coordinator
Long Island University, Brooklyn Campus
Brooklyn, New York

Kathleen A. Scarbalis, PA-C
Certified Physician Assistant
Center for Cancer and Blood Disorders of Northern Virginia
Children's National Medical Center
Washington, D.C.

Pam Schlomann, RN, PhD
Professor
Department of Baccalaureate and Graduate Nursing
Eastern Kentucky University
Richmond, Kentucky

Joan Schmitke, ARNP, FNP, BC, DSN
Professor Emerita
Department of Baccalaureate and Graduate Nursing
Eastern Kentucky University
Richmond, Kentucky

E. Ann Sheridan, RN, MS, EdD
Professor Emerita
University of Massachusetts, Amherst
Amherst, Massachusetts

Suzanne Sutherland, RN, PhD
Professor, Division of Nursing
California State University
Sacramento, California
Staff Nurse, Burn Unit
University of California Davis Medical Center
Sacramento, California

Mary Tiedeman, RN, PhD
Associate Professor Emeritus
College of Nursing
Brigham Young University
Provo, Utah

Stacy VandenBranden, RN, MS, APN-CPNP, AE-C
Pediatric Nurse Practitioner
Department of Pulmonary Medicine
Children's Memorial Hospital
Chicago, Illinois

Janice L. Vincent, CRNP, DSN
Assistant Professor
University of Alabama School of Nursing
University of Alabama at Birmingham
Birmingham, Alabama

Barbara C. Woodring, RN, EdD
Professor and Dean
Georgia State University
Atlanta, Georgia

Mary Narvaez Yeaney, MSN, CPNP
Pediatric Nurse Practitioner
Center for Cancer and Blood Disorders of Northern Virginia
Children's National Medical Center
Washington, D.C.

Kerry Fitzgerald Zebold, RN, MSN, CPNP
Urology Nurse Practitioner
Children's Memorial Medical Center
Chicago, Illinois

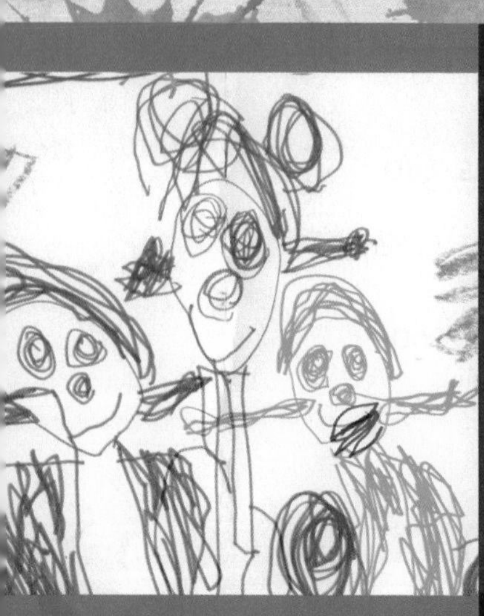

REVIEWERS

Marty Bachman, RN, PhD, CNS, CNE
Nursing Program Director/Department Chair
Front Range Community College, Larimer Campus
Fort Collins, Colorado

Christine R. Bachman, RN, MSN, Ed
Coordinator Evening AD Program
Harrisburg Area Community College, Lancaster Campus
Lancaster, Pennsylvania

Charlene Bell, RN, MSN, CNE, NCSN
Nursing Faculty
Southwest Texas Junior College
Uvalde, Texas

Elizabeth A. Berro, MA, PNP
Clinical Instructor
Pace University
Pleasantville, New York

Amy D. Boitnott, RN, DNP, FNP-BC
Nursing Instructor
University of Virginia
School of Nursing
Charlottesville, Virginia

Sharen Brady, RN, MSN
Associate Professor of Nursing
Weber State University
Ogden, Utah

Jacqueline Brandwein, RN, MA, CPNP
Clinical Faculty
Adelphi University School of Nursing
Garden City, New York

Dotty Cales, RN
Instructor
Northcoast Medical Training Academy
Kent, Ohio

Karen W. Clark, RN, MSN
Nursing Faculty
Western Piedmont Community College
Morganton, North Carolina

Cally M. Claussen, RN, MSN
Pediatric Nursing Instructor
Stephen F. Austin State University
Nacogdoches, Texas

Sherri Comfort, RN
Practical Nursing Department Chair
Holmes Community College
Goodman, Mississippi

Kim Cooper, RN, MSN
Assistant Professor, Nursing Department Chair
Ivy Tech Community College
Terre Haute, Indiana

Patricia Boyle Egland, RN, MSN, CPNP-PC
Certified Pediatric Nurse Practitioner, Pediatric Primary Care
Assistant Professor of Pediatric Nursing
The City University of New York
Borough of Manhattan Community College
New York, New York

Andra Fjone, MN, CPNP
Clinical Assistant Professor
University of Minnesota
Minneapolis, Minnesota

Karla Huntsman, RN, MSN
Instructor
AmeriTech College
Draper, Utah

Jaclynn A. Johnson, RNC-OB, MSN
Nursing Instructor
Otero Junior College
La Junta, Colorado

Nancy L. Kashlak, MS, MSN, CRNP, CPNP
Instructor and Course Coordinator, Pediatric Nursing
Pennsylvania State University
School of Nursing
Hershey, Pennsylvania

Susan Kennel, RN, PhD, ARNP
Assistant Professor
University of South Florida
College of Nursing
Tampa, Florida

Sherry Knoppers, RN, MSN, PhD
Nursing Instructor
Grand Rapids Community College
Grand Rapids, Michigan

Wendy S. Looman, RN, PhD, CNP
Associate Professor
University of Minnesota
School of Nursing
Minneapolis, Minnesota

Diane O. Moss, RN, MSN
Assistant Professor of Nursing
Nursing Care of Children, Lead Instructor
Salt Lake Community College
Salt Lake City, Utah

Patricia A. Pfeiffer, RNC-OB, MSN, MSA
Nursing Department Chair
Wayne Community College
Goldsboro, North Carolina

Barbara A. Sbarra, RN, MSN
Director of the Practical Nursing Program
Eastwick College
Ramsey, New Jersey

Patricia Sunderhaus, RN, MSN
Instructor
Brown Mackie College
Cincinnati, Ohio

Lori L. Van Aken, RN, BSN
Coordinator, Health Careers
Wayne-Finger Lakes BOCES
Newark, New York

Shari L. Washington, RN, MSN
Nursing Faculty
Bowie State University
Bowie, Maryland

Julie A. Will, RN, MSN
Dean, School of Health Sciences
Ivy Tech Community College of Indiana
Terre Haute, Indiana

Juvann M. Wolff, ARNP, MN
Director, Center for Excellence in Nursing Education
School of Nursing
University of Washington
Seattle, Washington

Michele Woodbeck, RN, MS
Nursing Professor
Hudson Valley Community College
Troy, New York

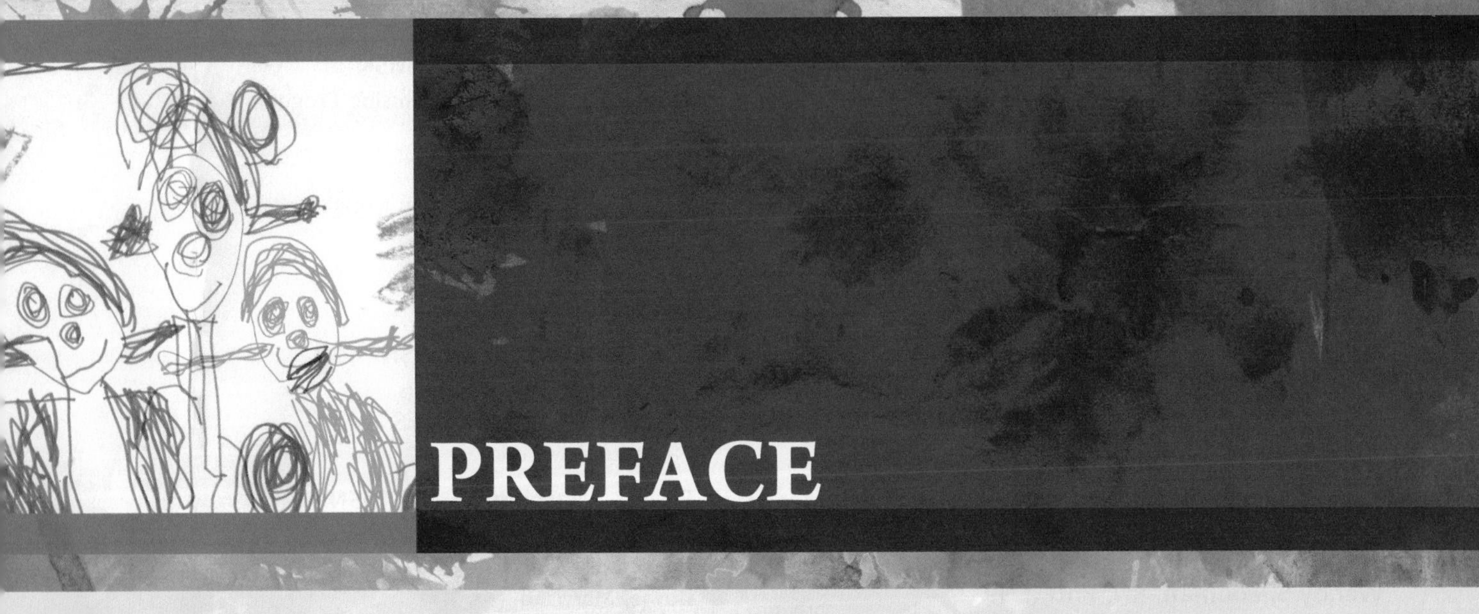

PREFACE

Pediatric Nursing: Caring for Children and Their Families, third edition, is a comprehensive presentation of children's health care from a holistic and family-centered perspective. It provides a learner-oriented, visually attractive approach to understanding and retaining the vast amount of information required to become a safe and caring practitioner and to begin work as a registered nurse.

Caring for children and their families has always been a challenging and rewarding endeavor. Technological advances, health care reform, and cost control measures greatly influence the landscape in which pediatric nursing care is provided. Hospital stays have shortened, acuity levels have increased, and more children are treated and cared for in settings other than acute care. Increasing numbers of families are caring for children with complex health problems in their homes. Many children and their families are feeling the impact of poverty; drug abuse; the cycle of physical, emotional, and sexual abuse; and violence. Nurses must be prepared to help children and their families manage these complex situations to foster optimal health.

We live in turbulent times, both economic and political. All nations in the world are undergoing rapid change. Global threats of pandemics, climate change, and natural disasters provoke anxiety and fear among all peoples of the earth. Mankind has survived these challenges time and time again by adapting to change, and no doubt will continue to rise to meet the new day.

The future will be in the hands of today's and tomorrow's children, and the focus of this textbook is the present. *Pediatric Nursing: Caring for Children and Their Families,* third edition, addresses these changes and realities with a perspective of children as evolving human beings in their family, home, school, community, country, and world. The contemporary social and cultural influences on children and their families are emphasized in addition to the more traditional areas of assessment, disease processes, and health promotion. Providing nursing care to children will be more effective when nursing students are aware of the pressures and problems confronting children and their families.

CONCEPTUAL APPROACH

As the title suggests, this text focuses on children in the context of their families. While discussing and educating about this important yet sometimes vulnerable population, our goal is to present the material in a depth and breadth that is engaging and user-friendly. The book uses simple-to-understand language and full-color pages with visual features that emphasize important points and create a reader-friendly approach that has become the hallmark of this text.

The nursing process provides the organizational framework for the discussion of nursing care. Applicable nursing research has also been incorporated throughout the text to reflect the latest in evidence-based practice. The enhancement of critical thinking skills is encouraged throughout. Emphasis on health and health promotion is reflected in comprehensive growth and development sections and in the alteration chapters. Anticipatory guidance is emphasized throughout the text in teaching boxes and tips. And most importantly, the child is always viewed within the context of the family.

ORGANIZATION

Pediatric Nursing: Caring for Children and Their Families, third edition, consists of 36 chapters, organized into 8 units.

Unit 1: Pediatric Nursing in a Changing Society
(Chapters 1 through 5) These five chapters introduce the student to pediatric nursing and set the stage for the

remainder of the book. The first chapter discusses societal trends affecting children, their health, and their families, as well as *Healthy People 2010/2020*. The various roles a nurse might accept as well as the diverse settings he or she might practice in relative to children and families are also covered. Chapter 2 describes legal and ethical issues nurses working with children and their families might face, including confidentiality. The third chapter provides information about the family and describes its significance to children. Family theories, assessment models, types, and forms are discussed in relation to their impact on individual members. The fourth and fifth chapters describe the pediatric nurse's role in the community, home, and school.

Unit 2: Growth and Development of Children (Chapters 6 through 12) These seven chapters review theories of human development (Chapter 6) and discuss the major developmental milestones and characteristics of the newborn, infant, toddler, preschooler, school-age child, and adolescent. Each of these chapters has a summary table of important developmental indicators, as well as a discussion of the physiological, psychosexual, cognitive, psychosocial, and moral development occurring during that particular stage. Health promotion strategies are also presented relative to nutrition, sleep, rest, activity, dental health, safety, and injury prevention. Recommended health screenings for each age group are also outlined.

Unit 3: Unique Considerations in Children (Chapters 13 through 20) These eight chapters focus on characteristics of children which distinguish them from adults, centering on information needed to appropriately care for children and their families in a variety of settings. To provide a high level of care, the nurse needs to know how to communicate effectively with children and families (Chapter 13). Following communication are assessment strategies with normal and abnormal findings (Chapter 14), infectious diseases (Chapter 15), interaction with children who are ill or hospitalized (Chapter 16), and caring for children with chronic conditions (Chapter 17). Managing pain (Chapter 18) and administering medication (Chapter 19) are presented next. Caring for children experiencing loss or bereavement (Chapter 20) completes the unit.

Unit 4: Alterations in Nutrition and Elimination (Chapters 21 through 23) The body system alteration chapters in this unit as well as in the units to follow have a similar format. They open with a description of the anatomy and physiology of the child's body system. The disorders discussed in each chapter are those that commonly occur or are frequently seen in the pediatric population. Although some alterations may also be seen in adults, the material is centered on information relevant to the child. For each disorder, incidence, etiology, pathophysiology, clinical manifestations, diagnosis, treatment, nursing management, and family teaching are clearly presented. Nursing management for the most common disorders in each body system follows the five steps in the nursing process. All body system alteration chapters also have a case study scenario that introduces the reader to real-life elements of the particular disorder, followed by the nursing process in care plan format, including assessment, nursing diagnosis, expected outcomes, interventions with rationales, and evaluation.

The chapters in this unit describe common pediatric physiological alterations related to nutrition and elimination. Chapter 21 presents fluid and electrolyte alterations, whereas Chapters 22 and 23 discuss genitourinary and gastrointestinal alterations, respectively. The unit organization is logically presented; one needs to have information about fluid and electrolyte imbalances and know what those imbalances mean before entertaining possible causes such as genitourinary (glomerulonephritis, nephrotic syndrome, renal failure) and gastrointestinal (gastroenteritis, pyloric stenosis, gastroesophageal reflux) alterations.

Unit 5: Alterations in Oxygen Transport (Chapters 24 through 26) These three chapters cover respiratory, cardiovascular, and hematological alterations frequently identified in children. Although presented separately, the three body systems are interrelated and dependent upon one another for oxygen transport. Alterations discussed include asthma, bronchiolitis, otitis (respiratory system); congenital cardiac anomalies, rheumatic fever, shock (cardiovascular system); and anemia and sickle cell disease (hematological system).

Unit 6: Alterations in Protective Mechanisms (Chapters 27 through 30) These four chapters discuss alterations related to the immune system (HIV, rheumatoid arthritis, systemic lupus erythematosus), endocrine system (growth hormone deficiency, thyroid disorders, diabetes), and integumentary system (impetigo, tinea infections, pediculosis) that serve to protect the body from illness, as well as cellular alterations (childhood cancer) that may occur when there are problems in the body's ability to protect itself from illness or injury.

Unit 7: Alterations in Sensorimotor Function (Chapters 31 through 34) These four chapters discuss alterations related to the sensory system (hearing, sight), the neurological system (neural tube defects, meningitis, hydrocephalus, cerebral palsy), cognition (mental retardation, autism), and the musculoskeletal system (fractures, congenital hip dysplasia, scoliosis, muscular dystrophy).

Unit 8: Other Alterations to Children's Health (Chapters 35 and 36) These final two chapters explain psychosocial alterations (attention-deficit hyperactivity disorder, depression, eating disorders) and child abuse and neglect (physical, psychological, and sexual abuse; abandonment).

Appendices: Eight appendices augment *Pediatric Nursing: Caring for Children and Their Families,* third edition. They include a family assessment measure, growth charts, the recommended childhood immunization schedule, sexual maturity ratings, common laboratory tests and normal values, temperature and weight conversions, NANDA diagnoses, and abbreviations.

SPECIAL FEATURES

Fundamental themes and critical nursing care points are highlighted through special features.

- *Short vignettes,* written by a child or family member, open each chapter and promote thoughts from the client's perspective.
- *Family Teaching* sections, specific to each chapter, highlight the significance of keeping family members involved in the caring process and offer them the tools to continue the caring at home.
- *Nursing Management* sections provide the reader with the information needed to successfully help the family manage a health alteration.
- *Case Study and Care Plans* are provided throughout the book to provide readers a glimpse of clinical situations and to walk them through a nursing plan of care. Nursing Outcome Classification (NOC) and Nursing Intervention Classification (NIC) labels are provided for each nursing diagnosis.
- *Evidence-Based Practice* boxes underscore the nurse's need to substantiate and document care practices consistent with established research; these will train readers to seek the best practice solutions to care situations.
- *Cultural Considerations* boxes highlight the multicultural and ever-changing makeup of our society, and encourage readers to develop cultural and ethnic sensitivity.
- *Nursing Tips* help the reader apply basic knowledge to practice by offering hints and shortcuts useful to both new and experienced nurses.
- *Nursing Alerts* highlight serious or life-threatening information that the nurse needs to master.
- *Kids Want to Know* presents children's questions and suggested nursing responses to help the reader consider children's needs, concerns, and fears.
- *Eye On* presents content in areas including complementary and alternative therapies; international and spiritual perspectives; and new and controversial treatments related to chapter content.
- *Reflective Thinking* boxes encourage reflection on issues from a personal context, raise awareness of the diversity of opinions, and foster empowerment.
- *Critical Thinking* boxes stimulate the thought process, as readers digest material related to the technical or clinical aspects of the chapter content.
- *Research Highlights* outline current research pertinent to pediatric clients and their families and stress the significance of evidence-based action by linking theory to practice.
- *Reflections from Families* are writings by the child or family member that encourage the nurse's understanding and sensitivity to the feelings of the clients in their care.
- *In the Real World* is found at the end of each chapter. Perspectives on nursing care from the viewpoint of a student or experienced practicing nurse are presented.
- *Review Activities* provide readers with a way to self-assess their comprehension and retention of chapter material.

NEW TO THIS EDITION

Numerous additions and enhancements were made to the textbook and supplements package to increase your understanding and broaden your learning experience. Many new practice guidelines, photographs, and illustrations appear throughout, and each chapter now includes ten new Study Questions in NCLEX style for student review and test preparation. The expanded Resources section includes resource descriptions as well as URLs. Additional selected enhancements include:

Unit 1

- Updated statistics and trends covering poverty, homelessness, migrant farm workers, violence, infant mortality, and DNR orders for children in schools
- Updates for *Healthy People 2020*
- New research on lead toxicity and diabetes
- Expanded discussion of ethical theories including updated guidelines for minor's consent for organ donation, and consent for genetic testing
- New information on immigrant families, families of multiples, families who adopt, and foster families

Unit 2

- Expanded discussion on circumcision and barriers to immunizations
- Added content on baby-friendly hospitals, chest growth during infancy, infant sleeping times, and home care following immunizations
- New discussion on the Millennium Development Goals
- Expanded coverage related to children's healthy eating including calculation of infant's caloric and fluid needs, finger foods, cholesterol testing, vegetarian diets, and childhood obesity

Unit 3

- New research covering the link between the MMR vaccine and autism
- New discussion on siblings of hospitalized children
- Expanded coverage of pertussis, cystic fibrosis, asthma, chronic illness, effects of hospitalization, and administering inhalation medications
- Expanded discussion of cultural considerations related to racial disparity in hospice care

Unit 4
- Expanded coverage of dehydration, water intoxication, rehydration, and oral rehydration solutions
- Updated content on scald burns, virtual reality pain control during wound debridement in hydrotank, and firework danger
- New information on nephrotic syndrome, anemia, pyloric stenosis, nasogastric (NG) tube placement verification, ulcerative colitis, and Crohn's Disease

Unit 5
- Updated guidelines from The National Asthma Education and Prevention Program
- Increased coverage of rheumatic fever, heart transplant, ventricular tachycardia, implantable defibrillator therapy, and surgical treatment of hypoplastic left heart syndrome

Unit 6
- Additional information on diabetes, insulin analogs, insulin pumps, and continuous glucose monitoring
- New discussion on chemotherapy, side effects, and decision making in light of effects on fertility
- Added discussion of molluscum contagiosum, pediculosis capitis, acne, atopic dermatitis, and chronic illness
- Expanded coverage of steroids, UV protection/sunburn, insect repellants, and staging of pediatric tumors

Unit 7
- Revised discussion of bacterial meningitis and autistic spectrum disorders
- Expanded discussion of sports and recreation injuries, slings, braces, splints, and external and internal fixation ("portable traction")
- Expanded discussion on infectious disorders such as osteomyelitis, septic arthritis, and transient synovitis

Unit 8
- Updated research on attention-deficit hyperactivity disorder, depressive disorder, and drug use
- Expanded coverage of depression, sleep hygiene, suicide prevention, and OCD behaviors

LEARNING PACKAGE FOR THE STUDENT

The Premium Website can be accessed at www.CengageBrain.com. Enter your passcode, found in the front of the book, and the Premium Website will be added to your bookshelf. Here you can access the **Online StudyWARE™** which contains: (1) interactive exercises for readers to self-evaluate their mastery of terms; (2) commonly performed pediatric skills, with step-by-step instructions and rationales; (3) checklists to accompany each pediatric skill; (4) NCLEX-style questions with rationales; (5) six case studies of various-age pediatric clients; (6) answers to the text Study Questions; (7) a comprehensive pediatric/maternity audio glossary; and (8) video clips. **ISBN-13: 978-11115-41880**

Student Study Guide provides multiple choice, true-false, and fill-in questions, as well as case studies with critical thinking scenarios (answers appear at the end of the book). **ISBN-13: 978-14354-86706**

Course Cartridges offer must-have classroom management tools such as chats and calendars, as well as additional content resources including frequently asked questions, class notes, overviews, and more. **ISBN-13: 978-14354-86690 (WebCT) and 978-14354-86683 (Blackboard)**

CourseMate, accessed at www.cengage.com/coursemate, helps you make the most of your study time by offering access to everything you need to succeed in one place. Pediatric Nursing CourseMate includes an interactive eBook with highlighting and note taking ability, and an interactive glossary. Interactive learning tools include quizzes, flashcards, videos, and more!
ISBN-13: 978-11115-41842 (printed access code)
ISBN-13: 978-11115-41835 (individual access code)

TEACHING PACKAGE FOR THE INSTRUCTOR

Instructor Resource CD-ROM includes everything an instructor needs to organize and run a class on pediatrics. The **Instructor's Manual** offers chapter competencies, key terms, instructional strategies for classroom use, and suggested answers to critical thinking and review questions found in the text. The **Computerized Testbank** contains 1,700 multiple choice questions with answers, rationales, cognitive level, and text reference. **Lecture Slides in PowerPoint ™** parallel the content found in each chapter of the book and serve as a foundation from which instructors may customize their own unique presentations. **Image Library** is a digital resource of approximately 400 illustrations and photographs from the text.
ISBN-13: 978-14354-86713

CourseMate, accessed at www.cengage.com/coursemate, as described above, includes Engagement Tracker, a first-of-its-kind tool that allows you to monitor student engagement in the course.

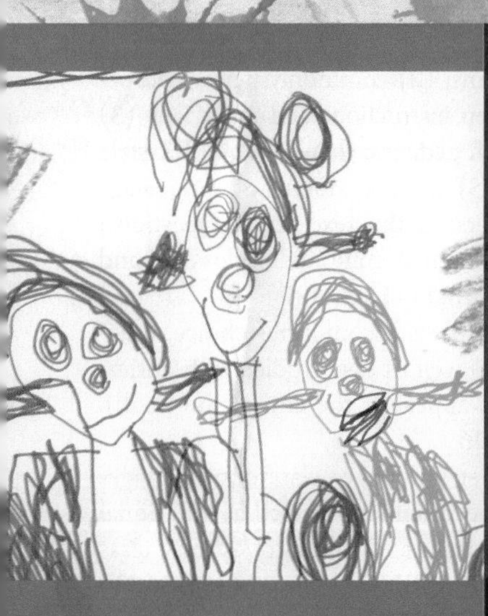

ACKNOWLEDGMENTS

The creation of this textbook represents the efforts of many knowledgeable, hard-working, and dedicated individuals who have supported us for over a decade. First and foremost, I (*Nicki Potts*) want to thank my husband, Stan, and my daughter, Jennifer, for their encouragement and support. Stan stood by me and never failed in his loyalty and dedication; thanks for always being there. Jennifer, thanks for your perpetual encouragement and inspiration. You are the light of my life.

—Nicki

Many individuals are responsible for the completion of this book. Initially, I (*Barbara Mandleco*) express deep appreciation and gratitude to the Brigham Young University College of Nursing administration that provided me with the support and assistance needed to pursue this project, and motivated and encouraged my efforts. I also thank my faculty colleagues, who were a frequent source of help, and the secretarial staff. Most importantly, I wish to express sincere thanks and gratitude to my husband, Carl, our children, Luke and Sarah, their spouses, Christine and Chad, and my grandchildren, Noah, Jonah, Henry, and Madison. Without their patience, understanding, love, and support, I would not have been able to complete this project.

—Barbara

Cengage Learning has provided us with its best in Beth Williams, our developmental editor. Beth helped us crystallize our ideas and clarify the chapter format. Her knowledge, attention to details, and resources were invaluable through two editions. With her help, we were able to get this project up and running and ultimately completed. Without her the book would not be the high quality product that it is.

We acknowledge and thank Primary Children's Medical Center in Salt Lake City, Utah, for allowing us to take photographs of children receiving care. We are grateful to Bonnie Midget, from PCMC Public Relations, for arranging for and coordinating these photo sessions, and also to the children and families who participated in the photo shoots.

A textbook of this magnitude, depth, and breadth would not be possible without the expertise of contributing authors. They have shared their ideas and expert knowledge. We especially thank them for their perseverance and willingness to revise chapters when more work and rewriting was required as the book evolved. Their professional experience and standards of excellence are reflected in the chapters they researched, wrote, and revised.

—Nicki and Barbara

ABOUT THE AUTHORS

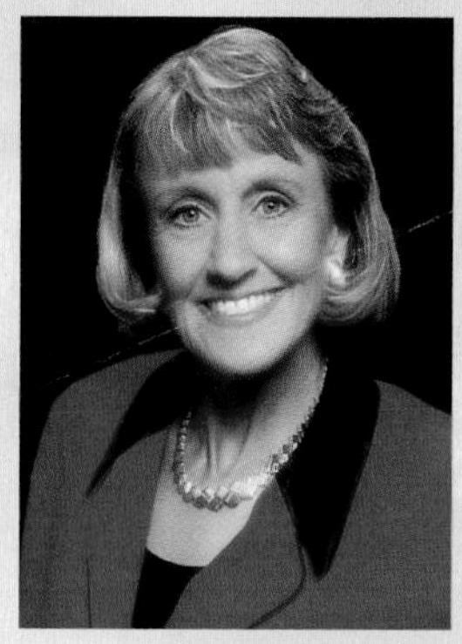

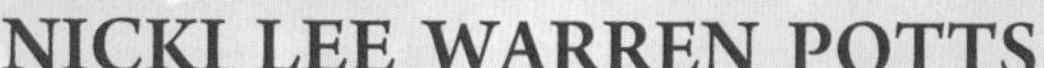

NICKI LEE WARREN POTTS

Nicki Lee Warren Potts is a second-generation registered nurse who earned her Bachelor of Science in Nursing from Texas Christian University, Fort Worth, Texas. She first practiced her profession as an assistant head nurse in medical surgical nursing and public health nursing, and she discovered her true passion in nursing education in Nashville at Tennessee State University. She continued her preparation for a career in education by obtaining a Master of Science in Nursing from the University of Texas at Austin's College of Nursing. Texas Woman's University College of Nursing conferred her Doctor of Philosophy in Nursing Research and Theory.

With over 35 years as a clinician and academician, Dr. Potts has taught psychiatric and mental health nursing and pediatric nursing in associate degree and baccalaureate schools of nursing. The majority of her teaching career has been at Texas Woman's University in Houston, Texas; the University of Texas in Arlington, Texas; and the University of Texas in Austin, Texas. Other areas of professional experience include Assistant Director for Education, Texas Nurse's Association, and Nursing Consultant for Advanced Practice at the Board of Nurse Examiners for the State of Texas.

Dr. Potts' professional development and contributions are well documented at the local and national levels. She has delivered numerous presentations throughout the country based on her special interest and research in females with eating disorders. She is a member of Sigma Theta Tau, Society of Pediatric Nurses, and the American Nurses Association. Dr. Potts has numerous journal, textbook, and abstract publications to her credit.

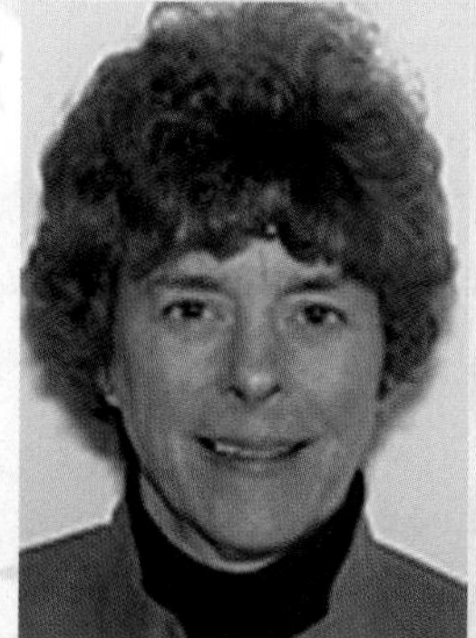

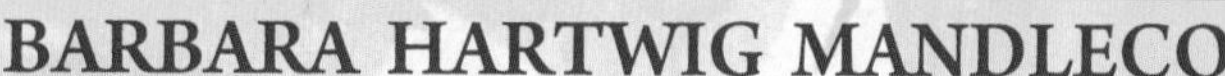

BARBARA HARTWIG MANDLECO

Barbara Hartwig Mandleco received her Bachelor of Science in Nursing from the University of Wisconsin–Madison, her Master of Science in Pediatric Nursing from the University of Florida–Gainesville, and her Doctor of Philosophy in Family Sciences with an emphasis in human development from Brigham Young University. She has been a staff nurse on pediatric and adult medical surgical nursing units and a nursing educator for over 35 years. She has taught advanced human development and pediatric nursing, fundamentals of nursing, nursing research, and management of family issues to undergraduate and graduate students at the University of Utah and Brigham Young University Colleges of Nursing. Currently, Dr. Mandleco is a professor at the Brigham Young University College of Nursing.

Dr. Mandleco is a member of Sigma Theta Tau International, the Utah Nurses Association, the American Nurses Association, the Society of Pediatric Nurses, the Western Institute of Nursing, the Western Academy of Nursing, Phi Kappa Phi, Sigma Xi, and the National Council on Family Relations. She has served as an officer locally and nationally in Sigma Theta Tau International, and the National Council on Family Relations. She currently serves as abstract and collateral reviewer (grants, scientific sessions, podium presentations) for Sigma Theta Tau International, the National Council on Family Relations, the Society of Pediatric Nurses, and the Western Institute of Nursing, and as a manuscript reviewer for *Nursing Research*, *MCN (Maternal Child Nursing)*, the *Journal of Family Nursing*, *Qualitative Health Research*, the *Journal of Pediatric Nursing*, and the *Journal of Nursing Scholarship*. She is a program evaluator for the CCNE and a reviewer for HRSA grants and projects.

Dr. Mandleco has given numerous professional presentations at the local, regional, national, and international levels, and published in several peer-reviewed journals. She also has written several book chapters, was co-author of a pediatric nursing student study guide published in the 1980s, and is the author of *Pediatric Nursing Skills & Procedures,* and *Growth and Development Handbook,* also published by Delmar Cengage Learning. Her research interests include families adapting to a child with a special need or chronic illness, and innovative methods of teaching.

HOW TO USE THIS TEXT

The following are suggestions on how you can use the features of this text to gain competence and confidence in caring for pediatric clients and their families.

Short Vignettes

Read these short stories before you begin to read a chapter to gain perspective of the feelings of the child and family. Once you have completed the chapter, go back and re-read the story. Ask yourself if you have a better comprehension and sensitivity of how the child and family feel.

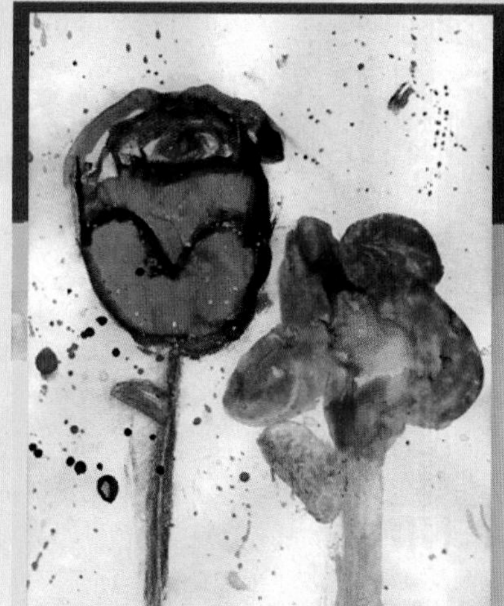

My name is Jennifer Hill and I'm 15 years old. I was diagnosed with type 1 diabetes three years ago. I am on the dance team in my high school, which keeps me very busy the entire school year. I have had an insulin pump for a year, and it has made it easier to manage my diabetes and keep my glucose at normal levels. I used to give myself four insulin injections a day. Now all I have to do is insert a new needle in my abdomen every few days. I still have to count carbohydrates in my diet and test my blood glucose several times a day, but I feel so much better when I monitor what I eat and keep my blood sugar as close to normal as possible.

Cultural Consideration

Pause to read these boxes as you work through each chapter. Familiarize yourself with the impact certain cultural practices or ethnic variations can have on your clients and on the way you competently perform your nursing care.

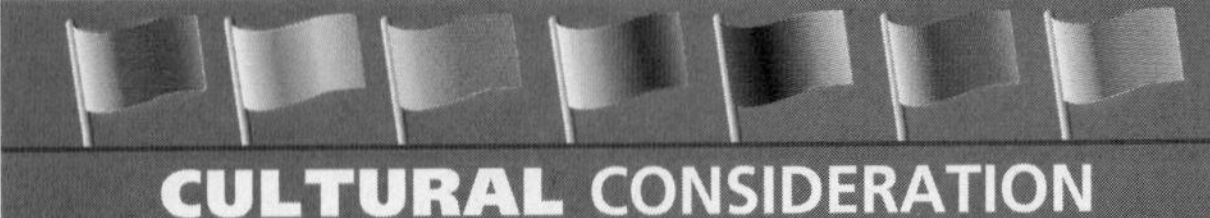

CULTURAL CONSIDERATION

Communication Patterns

It is often difficult to identify communication impairment in children from other cultures, particularly children who have recently arrived in the United States. Nurses should be mindful of how communication may differ, pay particular attention to developmental milestones (they may vary from the established "norm"), observe communication patterns between family members, and consider possible environmental factors. What information would you need to gather from parents or family members to help you in identifying a risk for a communication impairment? How can you develop a cultural perspective with regards to possible communication impairment?

Critical Thinking

This feature is designed to guide you to think analytically in clinical situations and be active in problem solving. As you go through the chapters, consider the questions posed and provide answers. Discuss your answers with other students to promote the exchange of ideas.

CRITICAL THINKING

Identification of Infection in the Neutropenic Child

You are caring for a 4-year-old boy who has an ANC of 300. He was admitted the previous evening with a fever of 102.3°F (39.1°C). He is receiving intravenous antibiotics. While you are bathing him, he complains of pain in the perianal area. You do not note any redness or inflammation in the area. You suspect the source of infection is a rectal abscess. What would you do?

Family Teaching

Family members will look to your expertise for guidelines on caring for their child, especially when making the transition from a care facility to the home or school environment. Read these boxes to ensure that your knowledge is accurate and comprehensive.

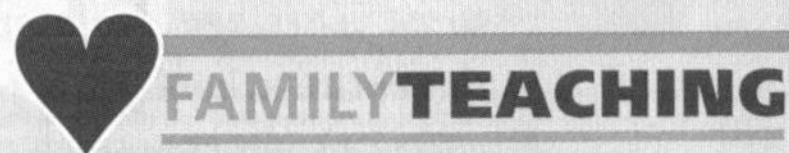

FAMILY TEACHING

Principles of Development

- Teach caregivers that development, although orderly and sequential, may vary in individual children, so that some preschoolers may have advanced language skills and others may not.
- Remind caregivers of the importance of connections that exist among physiological, psychosocial, and cognitive development. Therefore, children need to know what it feels like to have a wet diaper and to be able to tell the caregiver that they are wet before they can be successfully toilet trained.

Kids Want to Know

This feature is designed to enhance the communication between you and the pediatric client, since responses to children's questions about care may differ from those given to adults. Read the questions that have been posed by children and think about what your response would be. Then go ahead and read the suggested nursing responses. Ask yourself, "How do mine compare with the suggested answers?" Would you alter your response based on the suggested responses? Was your response developmentally appropriate for the child?

KIDS WANT TO KNOW

Getting glasses

"My mom said I need to get glasses. It's been hard to see the chalkboard for awhile, but I was afraid to tell her. I don't want to get glasses. What if the kids laugh at me and call me names? I don't want to be different."

To help the child with this transition you can explain, in developmentally appropriate terms, why the child is getting glasses and how they will help him or her; point out other children and adults in the child's life who have glasses; encourage the parents to allow the child some choice in selecting the glasses, as appropriate; and supply developmentally appropriate books and videos to the student's family and teacher such as *Blueberry Eyes,* by M. Driscoll Beatty (1996); *Glasses for D.W.,* by M. Brown (1996);. *Glasses, glasses. What Do I See* by K. Smith Stair (2004) and *Magenta Gets Glasses* (Blues Clues #10) by Reber and Dujas (2008).

Nursing Tip

In any profession there are many helpful hints that can assist you in performing more efficiently. In nursing, you need to be able to practice sensitivity in the process. The wide variety of hints, tips, and strategies presented here help as you work toward professional advancement. Study, share, and discuss with your fellow students.

NURSING TIP

Histrelin Implant is a new treatment for the continuous, slow release of GnRH agonist histrelin. A small 50 mg histrelin implant (a thin, flexible tube) is inserted subcutaneously in the inner, upper arm while the child is under anesthesia (local, twilight, or general). The implant of histrelin achieves and maintains suppression of LH and the sex steroids (estrogen and testosterone) in children with central precocious puberty for one year. The most common side effect, different from other GnRH agonists, is a skin reaction where the implant was placed.

Case Study and Care Plan

Walk through the process of assessment, nursing diagnosis, planning, intervention, and evaluation, to determine the success of the course of care. These features are helpful in strengthening the understanding of the nursing process through a case study approach and in exercising critical thinking skills. Be sure to note the intervention (NIC) and outcome (NOC) termininology.

CASE STUDY / CARE PLAN

THE CHILD WITH TYPE 1 DIABETES MELLITUS

Brian is a 12-year-old African-American boy diagnosed 2 months ago with type 1 diabetes. He was started on an insulin regimen of glargine (Lantus) once a day in the evening and lispro (Humalog) at meals to cover his carbohydrates at a dose of 1 unit for every 15 grams of carbohydrate he is eating. His correction dose is 1 unit of Humalog for every 60 mg/dL he wants to reduce his glucose, to a goal of 120. He was instructed to monitor his blood glucose levels prior to meals and to follow a carbohydrate-counting meal plan, usually eating three meals and one to two snacks.

Brian has been noticing that some of his blood glucose levels are below his target and that he has had repeated episodes of symptoms of hypoglycemia over the last 2 weeks. He often treats his low symptoms without testing, especially when he is in school. He wasn't sure ifi t is better to have lower glucose levels than higher ones, nor is he sure that he's actually low as often as he is having symptoms. He wasn't really worried until he started having several episodes with significant, more severe symptoms of hypoglycemia. He is now so afraid of having a severe low glucose level at school that he is eating extra food between classes.

NURSING CARE PLAN

ASSESSMENT

At time of diagnosis with type 1 diabetes, approximately 90% of the beta cells in the pancreas have been damaged and destroyed. As blood glucose levels rise, glucose toxicity at the cellular level results and can cause the remaining functioning beta cells to not respond to glucose by making insulin. After diagnosis and the initiation ofi nsulin treatment, as glucose levels decline, those beta cells not yet destroyed begin to be able to make insulin. This period is called the honeymoon or remission stage of diabetes. During the honeymoon, insulin needs can decrease because of beta cells' production of endogenous insulin. Doses of insulin that achieved the glucose target shortly after diagnosis may be higher than necessary to achieve the same glucose target during the honeymoon phase. While this honeymoon phase can last anywhere from a few weeks to a few years, typically it is gone by the first anniversary of diagnosis. The honeymoon phase may explain why Brian's glucose levels are suddenly lower than they were shortly after diagnosis. Brian's management plan is not achieving its goals, and he has not made appropriate changes to the plan to achieve his goals more successfully.

NURSING DIAGNOSIS 1

Risk for injury related to hypoglycemia.

EXPECTED OUTCOMES

1. Child will not experience an injury related to a hypoglycemic event.
2. Child and caregivers will identify safety plan to avoid injury.

NOC: Risk Detection
NIC: Surveillance

INTERVENTIONS/*RATIONALES*

1. Child will have access to blood glucose monitoring supplies at all times. *Ability to monitor glucose levels and the easy accessibility to testing equipment will encourage the child and caregivers to test glucose frequently. Symptoms of hypoglycemia, such as headaches and hunger, can be caused by events other than hypoglycemia, and should not be treated in the same manner.*
2. Child will wear medical identification. *Should an injury or accident occur and the child is unable to communicate, the presence of medical identification jewelry will provide diagnosis information for emergency personnel.*

(Continues)

Evidence-Based Practice

Challenge yourself to be up-to-date on new practice guidelines. Read what the experts say regarding research-based care and how to implement new strategies into your professional actions.

EVIDENCE-BASED PRACTICE

Universal Newborn Hearing Screening: Parental Reflections on Very Early Audiological Management

CLINICAL PROBLEM

The implementation of universal newborn hearing screening (UNHS) presents several challenges for both parents and health care professionals. A major challenge is home audiological management of very young infants with hearing loss that promotes maximum achievement of developmental skills and abilities.

BEST CLINICAL PRACTICE

Early identification of hearing impairment/loss is critical to promote the infant's or child's optimum physical, cognitive, psychosocial, and emotional development.

NURSING IMPLICATIONS

- Nurses must be observant of newborn and older infants' responses to sounds.
- Nurses must be alert to assessing hearing at each well child visit in the primary health care setting.
- Nurses need to ask parents if they have any concerns regarding their child's hearing. Nurses need to be alert to parents concern about their infant's or child's hearing.
- Nurses need to activate an interdisciplinary approach, involving pediatricians, audiologists, otolaryngologists, speech-language pathologists, teachers, and social workers.

Reference: McCracken, W., Young, A., & Tattersall, H. (2008). Universal newborn hearing screening: Parental reflections on very early audiological management. *Ear and Hearing, 29*, 54–64.

NURSING ALERT

Early Identification of Communication Disorder

Early identification and intervention of a child with a communication disorder can prevent long-term detrimental effects on learning, development, and self-image. It is essential to conduct a thorough assessment and physical examination, make appropriate referrals, and encourage caregivers to follow through on therapy.

Nursing Alert

As a professional, you will need to be able to react immediately in some situations to ensure the health and safety of your clients. Pay careful attention to this feature, as it helps you to begin to identify and effectively respond to critical situations on your own.

Eye On

Throughout your nursing practice, you are going to be exposed to a myriad of cultures, beliefs, and value systems. Read the information found in this feature to get extra information on various issues. Those presented will include complementary and alternative therapies; cultural, spiritual, and international perspectives; and new and controversial treatments. After you have completed the readings, consider how you feel about the topic discussed. How can you incorporate this information into your nursing care?

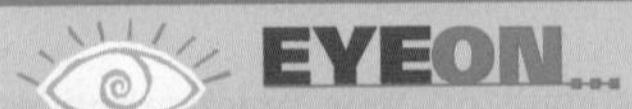

The Use of Herbal Therapies

In schools across the United States, children with a variety of diagnosed conditions are receiving prescription medications at school. Caregivers who worry about their child receiving Ritalin or psychotropic drugs are exploring the possibility of alternative treatments such as herbal therapies. Most school districts still require caregiver and physician permission for the use of herbal therapies at school even if they can be purchased over the counter. For the safety of students, you must remain current on popular herbal preparations and their side effects and contraindications.

REFLECTIVE THINKING

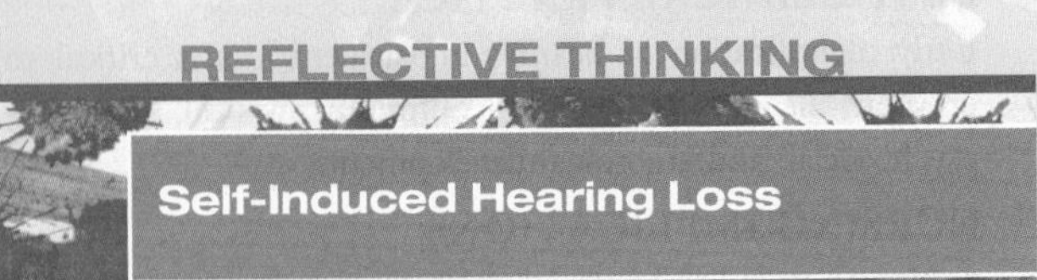

In recent years there is increasing concern over sensorineural deafness induced by frequent exposure to loud music. Studies have discovered sound levels over 80 dB can produce hearing loss in adults. The sound from rock concerts, car stereos, and home speakers can easily exceed the 80 dB level. Availability of high-intensity speakers and personal earphones have put adolescents at risk because adolescents consider loud music part of their lifestyle. The absorption in loud music is an escape from daily living, and is consistent with the normal developmental task of adolescents of achieving independence and developing identity. What can the nurse do to change this behavior? What can caregivers do to change this behavior?

Reflective Thinking

This feature can help you to develop or enhance sensitivity to ethical and moral issues. You may choose to read through each one and explore issues before reading the chapter. After reading through the chapter, re-address each Reflective Thinking item and evaluate your original thoughts. If you choose to read them as you go through the chapter, perhaps write your thoughts down to look at them at a later time.

Research Highlight

This feature emphasizes the importance of clinical research in nursing by linking findings to practice. This useful learning tool focuses attention on current issues and trends in nursing, stresses the significance of evidence-based practice, and illustrates the correct way to write an abstract for a research project.

RESEARCH

Normalization Strategies Used by Children Who Have Asthma

STUDY PURPOSE

To gain an understanding of how children with asthma develop strategies to normalize their lives.

METHODS

Using a qualitative design, 22 children, 11-years-old, were interviewed. Themes were derived from the transcribed interviews. Findings were related to the research question and literature.

FINDINGS

Children used the following strategies to normalize their lives: minimizing the health impact, stressing normality, emphasizing abilities, making adaptations, and managing symptoms.

IMPLICATIONS

Assisting youth to utilize the identified strategies to normalize life may enhance holistic care to this population.

REFERENCE

Protudjer, J., Kozyrskyz, A., Becker, A., & Marchessault, G. (2009). Normalization strategies of children with asthma. *Qualitative Health Research*, *19*, 94–104.

Reflections From Families

Read these as glimpses into a family's mindset and feelings about the loved one in your care before reading the chapter. After you have finished the chapter, go back and revisit your own feelings. Consider if your feelings have changed and examine why.

Reflections from Families

When I received a phone call from the nurse at my son's pediatrician's office a few days after he was born to tell me his newborn blood tests indicated a problem, I was shocked. He looked so healthy, right from the time he was born. His APGAR was perfect. I didn't even know that they had done blood tests before I took him home from the hospital. (I'd wished someone had told me about this while I was pregnant.) When I was told that his thyroid gland didn't seem to be working, I was sure I did something to cause it. While the nurse assured me that this was unrelated to anything I had done during pregnancy, it frightened me when she insisted that I bring him in immediately to confirm the diagnosis and start treatment. I had a million questions. Would he be slow? Would he look different? At our appointment, I was relieved that this could be managed but I worry about how I will give him his medicines so that he's getting the right amount.

IN THE REAL WORLD

My experiences with Helen helped me realize each client requires critical thinking on my part to recognize his or her needs and individualize his or her care. Nurses must gather information about client history, diagnosis, and present illness and then incorporate (organize, analyze) it into meaningful care. Because of her extensive medical experience, Lydia (mother) required far less general teaching and far more precise information. As nurses then, we need to adapt to schedules already established rather than trying to create our own for them. We need to be flexible and creative and help make the hospital environment as normal as possible for the child and family. (Written in response to caring for a child diagnosed at an early age with sensorineural blindness and hearing loss who had been admitted to the hospital frequently for treatment and surgery.)

In the Real World

These short musings from the student or professional nurse are intended to provide a snapshot of actual practice. They are included as a reality check as you read through the text. It may be helpful for you to keep a running journal of your own experiences—Did a certain child and family affect you in some way? Did you work with a practicing pediatric nurse who is a wonderful mentor? Journal writing is a good way to begin to examine your own responses and provide other aspiring nurses the wisdom of your experiences.

Study Questions

Ten new study questions have been added to the end of each chapter. As you finish studying the material, test yourself by completing these questions, then check your answers in the online StudyWARE student tutorial.

STUDY QUESTIONS

1. Which of the following statements accurately describes a physiological change during the school-age period?
   a. The child will grow in height an average of 2.5 inches per year.
   b. The child's weight will triple during the school-age period.
   c. The child's hair color and texture will change.
   d. The child's vision will improve every year.
2. Freud described the school-age years as which period of psychosexual development?
   a. anal
   b. latency
   c. oedipal
   d. oral
3. What is the psychosocial developmental goal for the school-age child according to Erikson?
   a. trust
   b. initiative
   c. guilt
   d. industry
4. According to Piaget, the expanded cognitive abilities of the school-age child include which of the following?
   a. animism
   b. rationalization
   c. inferiority
   d. reversibility
5. According to Kohlberg, the school-age child is at the conventional level of moral development. Which of the following statements accurately represents this level?
   a. Children do not seek the approval of others.
   b. Children show no respect for authority figures.
   c. The child's morality is based on the approval of younger siblings.
   d. The child's conscience develops an internal set of rules.
6. Children who come home alone after school and are without adult supervision are called:
   a. latchkey children.
   b. juvenile delinquents.
   c. foster children.
   d. truants.
7. Javan is a 10-year-old boy who has seen the school nurse multiple times for vague complaints. He tells the nurse he is being bullied by some of the older boys in the school. Which of the following signs or symptoms are often reported by children in response to fear of being bullied?
   a. sleep problems
   b. fever
   c. ear infection
   d. sprained ankle
8. When providing a talk to caregivers of school-age children concerning motor vehicle safety, the nurse includes which of the following statements?
   a. Children age 8 years and older should sit in the front seat of the vehicle.
   b. Children can sit in the cargo area of pickup trucks.
   c. Correct seat belt fit is usually not achieved until the child is 9 years old.
   d. Seat belts fit correctly when the lap portion of the belt rides across the stomach.
9. The leading cause of death for school-age children in the United States is:
   a. cancer.
   b. malnutrition.
   c. accidents.
   d. AIDS.
10. Tymm, age 8 years, is scheduled to have a tonsillectomy. The best time for Tymm to receive preoperative preparation is:
    a. two hours before surgery.
    b. two days before surgery.
    c. one week before surgery.
    d. one month before surgery.

Electronic Resources

This new edition of *Pediatric Nursing* has a wealth of exciting electronic resources to enhance your learning experience. As you study each chapter, be sure to also work with the electronic student tutorial, which helps you verify your understanding of key terminology, learn important pediatric skills, and prepare for the NCLEX examination. The Online Student Tutorial (StudyWARE) and **Course Cartridge** components offer worthwhile course content, exercises, skills checklists, class notes, web links, and more.

COMPETENCIES

Upon completion of this chapter, the reader will be able to:

- Describe the endocrine glands, their hormones, and functions.
- Explain the principle of negative feedback.
- Describe the etiology, clinical manifestations, treatment, and nursing management of common endocrine alterations.
- Discuss the management goals for the child with type 1 and type 2 diabetes mellitus.
- Develop a teaching plan for a child with newly diagnosed type 1 diabetes.
- Compare the causes, clinical manifestations, and treatment of hypoglycemia and hyperglycemia.

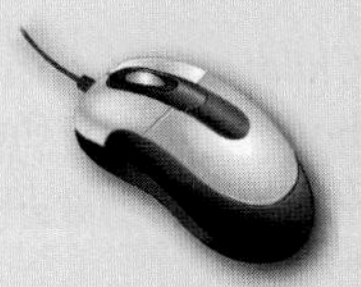

- Successfully complete the games and activities in the online student StudyWARE.

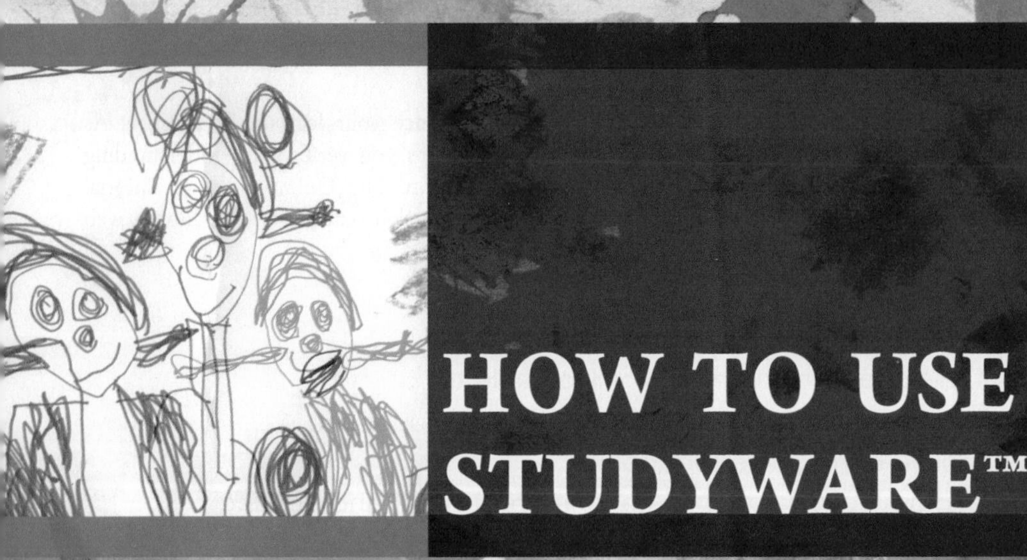

HOW TO USE STUDYWARE™

The online student StudyWARE™ tutorial helps you learn terms and concepts in *Pediatric Nursing: Caring for Children and Their Families,* third edition. As you study each chapter in the text, be sure to explore the activities in the corresponding chapter in the online tutorial. Use StudyWARE™ as your own private tutor to help you learn the material in *Pediatric Nursing: Caring for Children and Their Families,* third edition.

Getting started is easy. Visit the online tutorial website at: **http://www.CengageBrain.com**. When you open the software, enter your name so the software can store your quiz results. Then choose a chapter from the menu to take a quiz or explore some of the activities such as flash card or hangman. Review pediatric procedures to see the step-by-step instructions for completing each skill, then test your competence against the skills checklists. Practice NCLEX-style questions, review case studies, watch pediatric videos, and listen to the audio glossary.

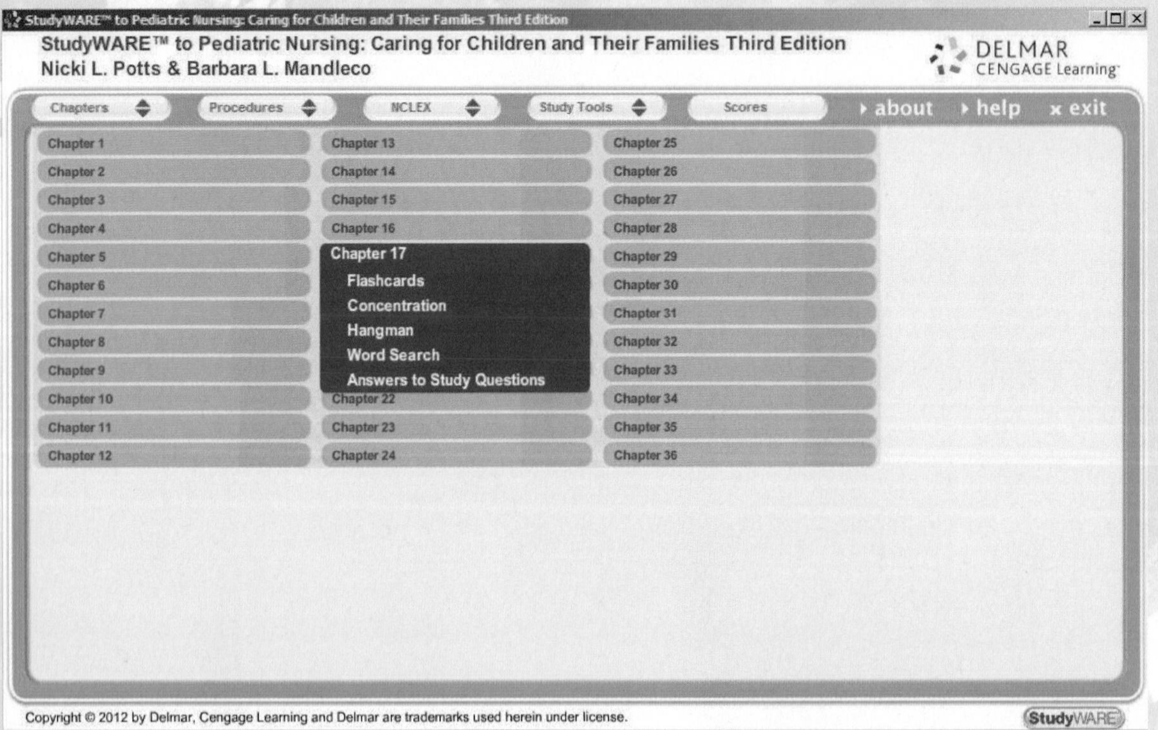

Have fun while increasing your knowledge!

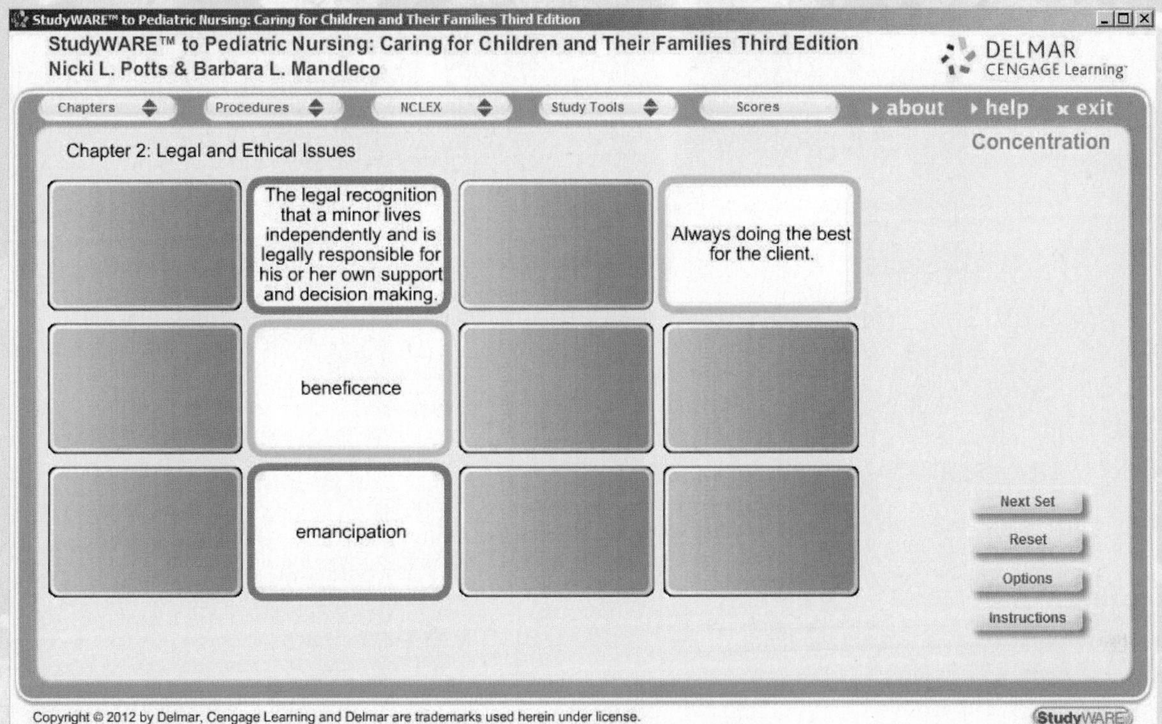

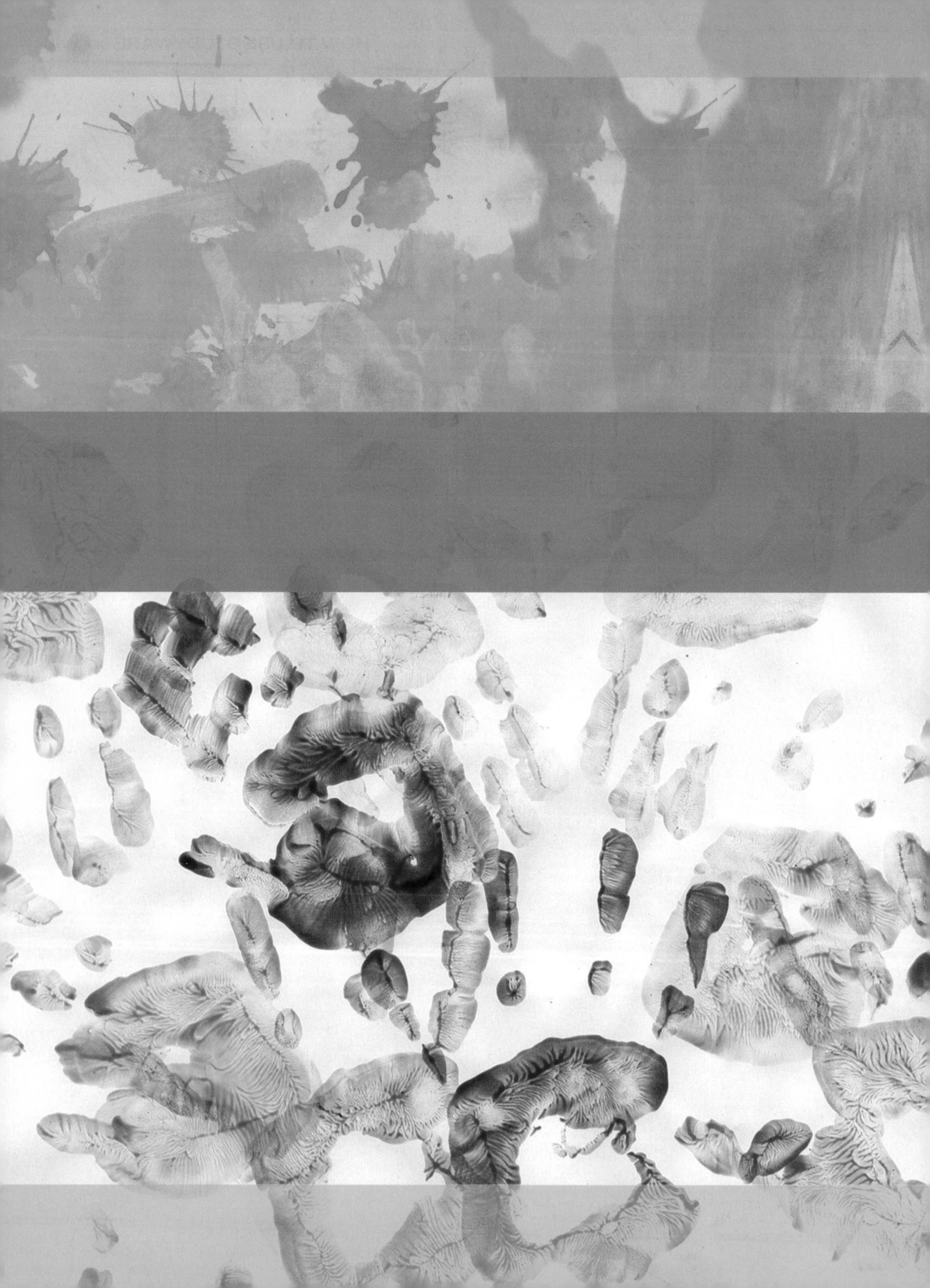

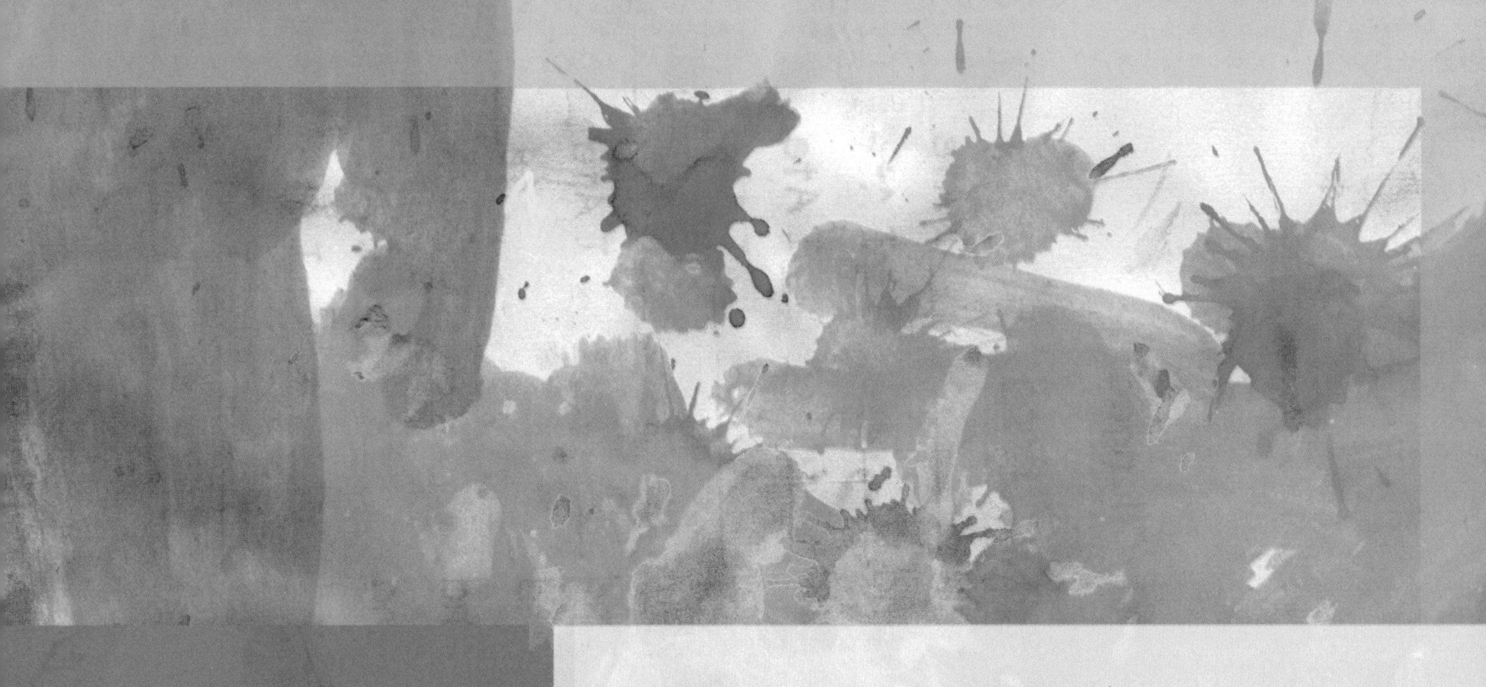

UNIT 1 Pediatric Nursing in a Changing Society

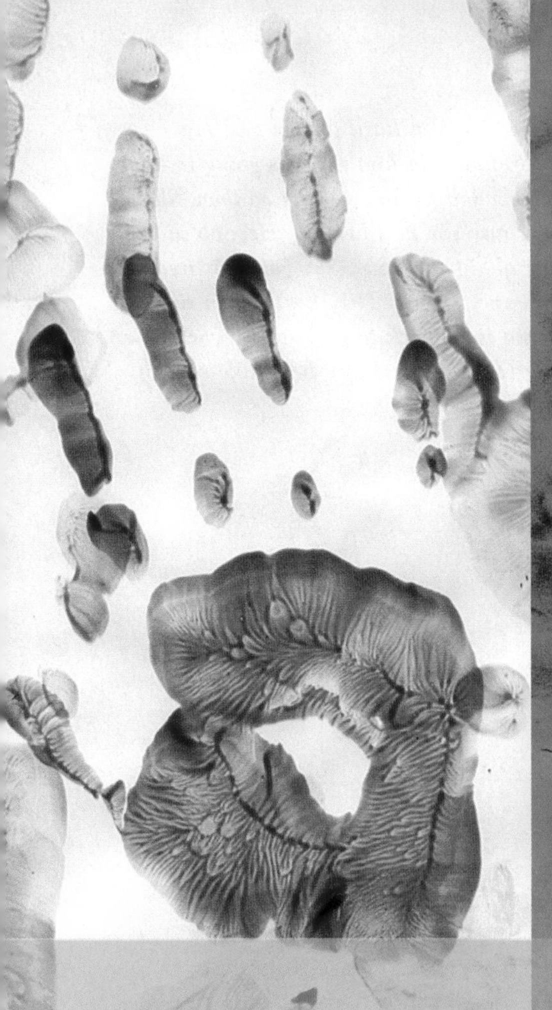

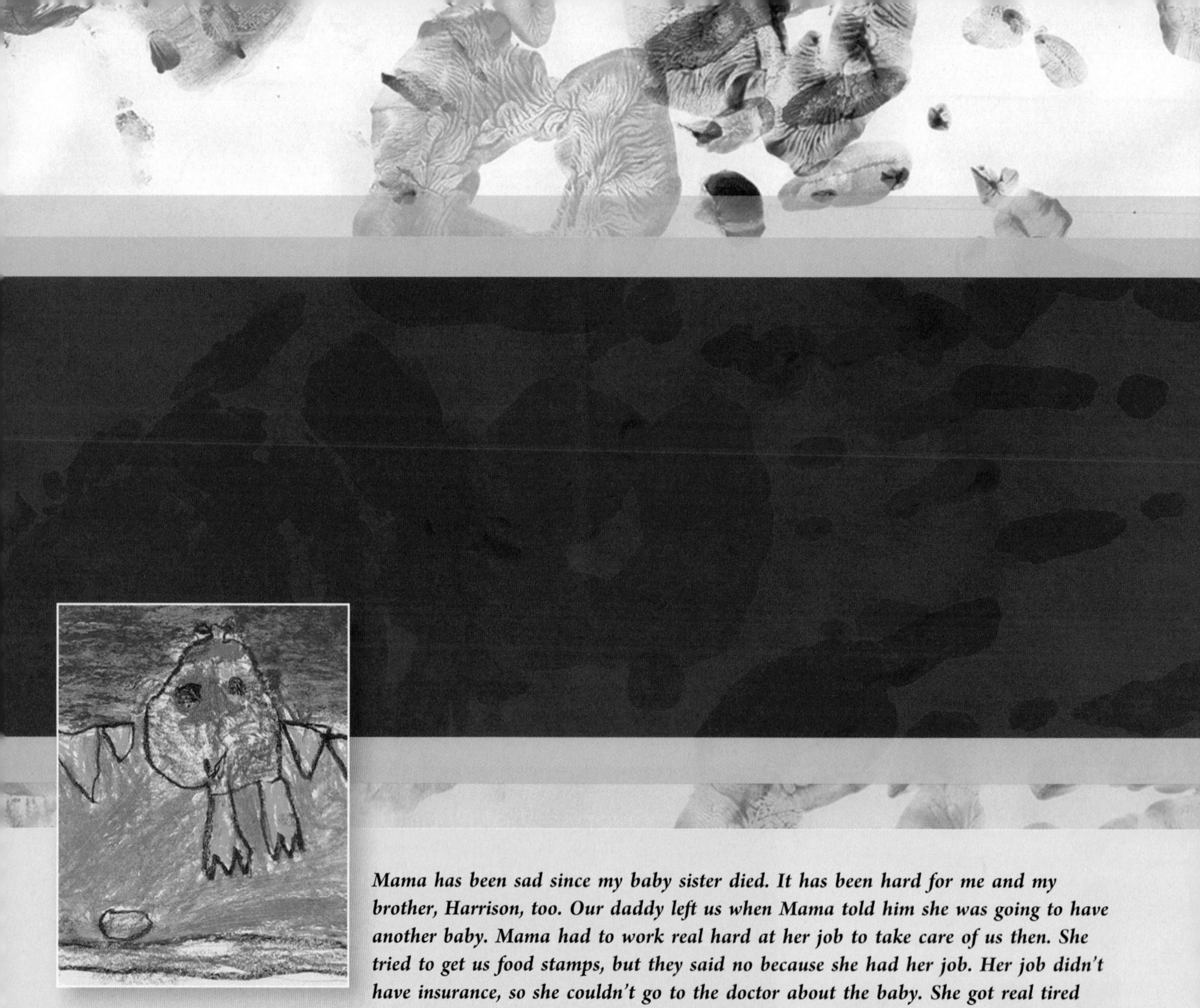

Mama has been sad since my baby sister died. It has been hard for me and my brother, Harrison, too. Our daddy left us when Mama told him she was going to have another baby. Mama had to work real hard at her job to take care of us then. She tried to get us food stamps, but they said no because she had her job. Her job didn't have insurance, so she couldn't go to the doctor about the baby. She got real tired and sick a lot. When my baby sister came, she was very small and wasn't very strong. They kept her in the baby intensive care at the hospital for two weeks, but then she died. Mama is too sick to go back to work now, and she thinks it is her fault the baby died. When I grow up, I am going to be a nurse and help take care of mamas and their babies, so they can get stronger. I miss my baby sister so much too.

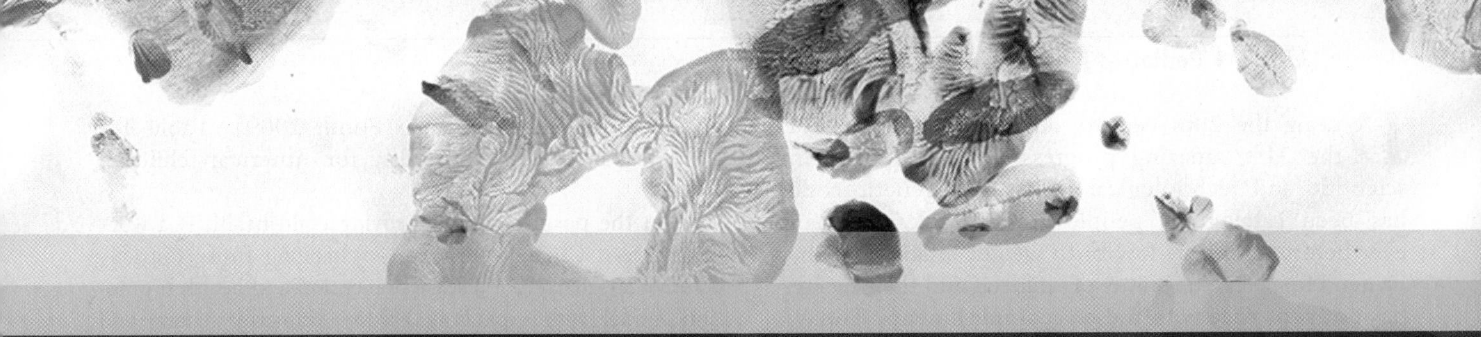

CHAPTER 1
Overview of Pediatric Nursing

BARBARA L. MANDLECO, RN, PhD
NICKI L. POTTS, RN, PhD

COMPETENCIES

Upon completion of this chapter, the reader will be able to:

- Discuss current societal trends and describe their influence on children in the United States.
- Describe some of the effects of immigration, poverty, homelessness, migrant farm work, and violence on children and their health.
- Discuss the current status of children's physical and social health.
- Identify five strategies to prevent unintentional childhood injuries.
- Discuss the effects of problems with access to health care and lack of health insurance on children's health status.
- Identify elements of family-centered care.
- Discuss the influence of professional standards on pediatric nursing.
- Describe and discuss the importance of each role of the pediatric nurse.
- Successfully complete the games and activities in the online student StudyWARE.

During the 20th century and the first decade of the 21st, amazing progress has been made in scientific and technological fields. The genetic code has been catalogued, people are living longer than ever before, and very low birth weight infants are surviving. However, the status of children and their health has not kept pace with these accomplishments. Today, more than 1 in 6 children in the United States is poor, and almost 1 in 13 lives in extreme poverty; 1 in 9 children is uninsured, and most of these are from ethnic minority races (Black, Hispanic, Asian, American Indian). In addition, about 1 in 12 newborns is of low birth weight; about 1 in 15 teens between 16 and 19 years of age have dropped out of school; two-thirds of public school fourth graders cannot read or do math at their grade level; and only about 3% of those infants and preschool children eligible for Head Start programs are enrolled in those programs. Finally, two-thirds of two-year-olds are not immunized, two out of three mothers of preschool children and three out of four mothers of school aged children are working, more than 2.5 million grandparents are raising their grandchildren, and the birth rate for teens is higher in the United States than in any other industrialized nation (Children's Defense Fund, 2009). Table 1-1 provides a view of the reality for American children today.

On the positive side, improving child health is a work in progress. Child health care is changing from a strictly curative approach to a disease prevention and health promotion model with expanding access (primarily federal and state efforts via State Children's Health Insurance Program, or SCHIP, legislation). The role of the pediatric nurse has expanded from child caretaker to child advocate. Today, pediatric nursing focuses on preventing acute and chronic illness while promoting normal growth and development. This focus requires a broad knowledge base consisting of an understanding of the culture at large, a host of health and illness issues, and a wide range of clinical competencies.

Today, more than ever, every nurse must be familiar and knowledgeable with pediatric nursing. In 2008, there were nearly 74 million children ages 0–17 in the United States, about 1 of every 4 persons. Demographic projections suggest this ratio will remain stable through 2021. Hence, given increasing access for children, more than one of four patient encounters will be with an infant, child, or adolescent (Federal Interagency Forum on Child and Family Statistics, 2009).

TABLE 1-1 Moments in America for All Children

- Every second a public school student is suspended.*
- Every 11 seconds a high school student drops out.*
- Every 19 seconds a child is arrested.
- Every 19 seconds a baby is born to an unmarried mother.
- Every 20 seconds a public school student is corporally punished.*
- Every 32 seconds a baby is born into poverty.
- Every 41 seconds a child is confirmed as abused or neglected.
- Every 42 seconds a baby is born without health insurance.
- Every minute a baby is born to a teen mother.
- Every minute a baby is born at low birth weight.
- Every 4 minutes a child is arrested for a drug offense.
- Every 7 minutes a child is arrested for a violent crime.
- Every 18 minutes a baby dies before his or her first birthday.
- Every 45 minutes a child or teen dies from an accident.
- Every 3 hours a child or teen is killed by a firearm.
- Every 5 hours a child or teen commits suicide.
- Every 6 hours a child is killed by abuse or neglect.
- Every 15 hours a woman dies from complications of childbirth or pregnancy.

*Based on calculations per school day (180 days of seven hours each).

Used with permission of the Children's Defense Fund. (2009). "Moments in America for All Children" (Washington, DC: CDF, December 2009). Retrieved January 5, 2010, from http://www.childrensdefense.org/

This chapter begins with an overview of social changes as they affect children. It describes the status of children's health, their health problems, and their care. The focus of the chapter then turns to a discussion of the roles of pediatric nurses and concludes with a discussion of differentiated practice roles and advanced practice.

SOCIETAL TRENDS IMPACTING CHILDREN

Children are members of families, communities, populations, and overall society, which shape the context, experiences, and opportunities of their lives. Their well-being is inextricably linked to the well-being of their families, communities, and the society in which they live. In a world that is continually changing, emergent societal trends have profound effects on the environment surrounding children and their families, and now pose formidable challenges to children, their families, and their health.

During the first decade of the 21st century, notable trends are emerging that may provide further impediments to the well-being of children and their families in the United States of America:

1. a concentration of wealth last seen prior to the advent of the Great Depression of 1929 (Economic Policy Institute, 2009);
2. a weakened middle class that has faced upwardly spiraling costs while wages have stagnated (Economist, 2009);
3. deepened and broadened poverty affecting 40 million Americans (Economist, 2009);
4. increased obesity (up 37% over the decade) leading to an epidemic in diabetes (24 million) and pre-diabetes (57 million more) (CDC, 2008);
5. weakened environmental protections resulting in polluted air and unsafe levels of mercury in our lakes, rivers, and streams (Scudder et al, 2010);
6. consumer safety regulations and enforcement may not be protecting our children from unsafe chemicals used for food packaging and baby bottles, or defective products including toys, and even may include our food supply.

While the most recent data suggests improvements since 2000 in the infant mortality rate, the child death rate, the teen death rate, and the high school dropout rate, four other measures of life quality have worsened: (1) low birth weight babies; (2) children living with jobless or underemployed parents; (3) children living in poverty; and (4) children living in single-parent families (Annie E. Casey Foundation, 2009).

While these emerging trends are troubling, others remain among the most stubborn in the history of the United States of America. This chapter discusses in detail the issues of immigration, poverty, homelessness, migrant farm workers, and violence.

IMMIGRATION

Currently, 20% of children in the United States live with at least one foreign-born parent. In addition, children in these families are less likely to be enrolled in preschool programs, which puts them at risk for being ready for school and able to speak English fluently (Hernandez, Denton, & Macartney, 2007). However, they may face many challenges related to health status and education because they often have difficulty speaking English. This lack of skill in English has a direct impact upon their educational attainment, economic viability, and ability to enter the mainstream of U.S. society. In fact, many of their parents are not high school graduates and consequently less likely to help with their homework. In addition, the majority live in households where a language other than English is spoken and many live in households where no one older than adolescence speaks English well (Behrman, 2004).

With each new wave of immigrants comes debate about whether they contribute to the economy or create a drain on public and private resources. Concerns also include perceived threats to the public health and order from infectious diseases, increased crime, and diverse social mores. These debates have raised the issue of eligibility of immigrants for health, educational, and social services. Some have argued that this group should not be entitled to any local, state, or federal benefits. States that have a large number of immigrants (California, Texas, and Florida) have proposed removing eligibility for these services. Opponents of these efforts counter that denying children access to services is unwise public policy. For example, in health care, denial of preventive services such as prenatal and dental care and immunizations eventually results in spiraling costs for emergency medical services (for which immigrants are eligible).

The health status of immigrant children can be compromised due to conditions originating in their country of origin, and it is also at risk because of significant language, cultural, financial, and legal barriers to receiving health care. Their families often delay seeking care for minor conditions until they become more serious. Another factor affecting their underutilization of health services is the possibility that family members may have different immigration statuses. When one member is an illegal (undocumented) immigrant, the entire family may limit access to care for fear of an investigation.

The immigrant population's access to health care services also affects their psychological well-being. For many children and their families, the immigration process poses unique stresses. Individuals may be torn by conflicting social and cultural demands while trying to adapt to an unfamiliar environment. Other stresses include differences between social and economic status in their country of origin and the United States, separation from support systems, and, for illegal immigrants, fear of deportation.

However, we need to be aware that these families also have several strengths. For example, most families are healthy, two-parent, traditional families, and have lower infant mortality rates. In addition, almost 40% of the families live with nonrelatives or relatives compared with less than 25% of U.S.-born families, and they are strongly connected and live close geographically to their ethnic community. They also have a strong work ethic and aspirations, with parents working hard and expecting the same from their children. Children tend to have a strong sense of ethnic pride and obligation toward their family. Even though they may have difficulty with English, the children often have high educational goals and drop out of school less frequently and spend more time doing homework than their U.S.-born counterparts (Behrman, 2004).

POVERTY

In 2008, the poverty rate for children under 18 years of age was 19% (up from 18% in 2007), and even though children represent just under 25% of the entire population, they made up over 35% of those living in poverty. In addition, 6.3 million children under 18 years old lived in families with an income below 50% of their poverty thresholds, and almost 10% of children under 18 years of age were without health insurance, the lowest since 1987, the first year data was collected. However, children 12–17 years of age were less likely to be insured than children less than 12 years of age (DeNavas-Walt, Proctor, & Smith, 2009).

The incidence of poverty may actually be higher than the official statistics (cited above) as published by the government of the United States. The Annie E. Casey Foundation in their annual publication, *2009 Kids Count Data Book,* urges the government to overhaul its formula for measuring poverty. The method for measuring poverty used by the government was developed in the 1960s. Then, food represented almost a third of the family budget as compared to one seventh today. The 1960s formula does not account for the increased costs of childcare, transportation, health insurance, or taxes; nor does it account for the value of food stamps, rent subsidies, or tax credits. Some argue these inaccuracies should reduce the poverty rate (Economist, 2009), others argue that these inaccuracies understate the poverty rate by 16 million persons (over 6 million of them children) (Economic Policy Institute, 2009). Using the official United States government statistics, as compared to our peers on the world stage (OECD, Organization for Economic Cooperation and Development, the top 20 economies in the world), the United States has the highest rate of poverty of all with a child poverty rate over twice as high as the average of the other 19 nations (Economic Policy Institute, 2009).

Family structure has an important bearing on child poverty. Poverty rates for children in married-couple families are much lower than for those in families headed by a single parent. The explanation for this fact is that when both spouses are present, there are two potential (and, frequently, actual) breadwinners. The risk of poverty in these single-parent households is high for several reasons, including low wages for women, the low educational attainment of many single mothers, and low rates and levels of child support from fathers.

Several factors are at the root of child poverty. Slow growth in wages, the rising inequality in earnings, significant loss of low-skill, high-wage jobs due to a decline in manufacturing industries, and workers' lack of education and skills account for much of child poverty in recent years. Educational level of adults in the family is another factor related to poverty. As education rises, the number of adults who are not in the labor force and who experience a period of unemployment during the year declines dramatically.

Family income also has significant effects on the well-being of children and adolescents. Poor children are at greatest risk for the physical, social, and emotional effects of living in poverty. Compared with non-poor children, poor children experience diminished physical health. They have higher than average rates of death and illness from almost all causes except suicide and motor vehicle accidents, which are most common among white, non-poor children. They also have a higher prevalence of illnesses such as asthma, respiratory infections, anemia, and gastrointestinal infections. Infant mortality rate is closely linked to poverty, and children born to poor families are at great risk of infant death. Deficits in children's nutritional status are associated with poverty. Stunted growth (low height for age), a measure of nutritional status, is more prevalent among poor than non-poor children.

Poverty also affects children's cognitive abilities and achievement. A child's poverty status at 3 years of age predicts the child's IQ at age 5, and persistent poverty has more adverse effects on a child's cognitive functioning than transitory poverty. In addition, children from lower socioeconomic status perform less well than non-poor children and middle-class children on test scores, grade retention, high school graduation rates, and the completed numbers of years of schooling; they also have higher rates of high school drop out, course failure, and placement in special education. School achievement also declines with the time spent in poverty, and the chance a child will be retained in a grade or placed in special education increases 2% to 3% for every year that the child lives in poverty. In fact, long-term poverty is associated with deficits in verbal, mathematical, and reading skills that are two to three times greater than those associated with current poverty status. Poverty also affects a child depending on when, during the child's life, poverty is experienced; poverty during the first five years of life will affect the completed years of schooling more than if poverty occurs during middle childhood and adolescence.

There is a higher prevalence of emotional and behavioral problems (e.g., externalizing, internalizing) among poor and low socioeconomic status children and adolescents than among children from families where there is higher income. The externalizing behavior problems include disobedience, fighting, difficulty getting along with others, and impulsivity, which become more prevalent the longer the children live in poverty. The internalizing behavior problems include anxiety, sadness, depression, and dependency.

HOMELESSNESS

An increasing number of children and families in all communities in the United States are homeless (Institute for Children and Poverty, 2010). Traditionally, the homeless population has been composed of single adults, mostly men. However, families raising young children now make up 40% of the nation's homeless population and over the course of any calendar year, more than 1.3 million children are homeless. In fact, the number of homeless families with children has increased significantly over the past decade, and families with children are among the fastest growing subdivision of the homeless population (National Coalition for the Homeless, 2008).

Homelessness was initially a phenomenon of large urban areas but more recently has swept across the nation, affecting midsize cities as well as suburban and rural areas. Contributing to the rise of homelessness in midsize cities is the migration of disadvantaged families from large urban settings to smaller towns and cities in search of a safer environment and a better life for their children. The homeless population is disproportionately represented by African Americans.

Several societal problems contribute to the increasing rate of homelessness among American families, including the following:

- Increases in poverty
- Lack of affordable housing
- Decreases in availability of rent subsidies
- Unemployment and underemployment, especially among those who have held only marginal jobs
- Personal crises such as divorce, domestic violence, and substance abuse
- Cutbacks in public welfare programs
- Deinstitutionalization of the mentally ill

Having been abused or neglected by a household member as a child is a risk factor for homelessness. Another factor is living in a foster home, a group home, or other out-of-home placement as a child, such as a residential treatment center or juvenile detention.

Homeless children experience the specific health effects directly related to homelessness, as well as the effects of poverty, the umbrella issue of homelessness. The most common physical health problems include upper respiratory, ear, and skin infections; gastrointestinal disorders (diarrhea); and infestations (scabies, lice). Compared with housed children, homeless youth have a higher incidence of chronic health problems such as asthma, anemia, visual and neurological deficits, eczema, and trauma-related injuries. The conditions in many private and public shelters place children at risk of lead poisoning and other environmental hazards. Many health problems may predate shelter entry, including crowding in doubled-up housing situations, or exposure to the elements and lack of sanitary facilities in public places. Access to health care, especially preventive care (immunizations, well-child services), is impaired for homeless families. Because caregivers are struggling to meet the family's basic demands for food and shelter, health becomes a lower priority. When they do seek health care, they are more likely to use emergency services for preventive and sick care than housed families.

To date, the struggle to provide adequate food and nutrition to homeless families has proven to be an overwhelming task. Homeless families have little access to cooking facilities, and families living in shelters report having less access to food than they previously had, with more children going hungry or eating once per day. The children are especially at risk for malnutrition. Inadequate benefits and difficulties in accessing food and entitlements are the major mediators of hunger and poor nutrition in the homeless. The vast majority of homeless families are headed by women who rely on Aid to Families with Dependent

RESEARCH Highlight

Children in Poverty

STUDY PURPOSE

To examine racial and ethnic disparities in medical and dental health, access to care, and use of services in a national sample of US children.

METHODS

A random sample of parents/guardians of 102,353 white, African American, Latino, Asian/Pacific Islander, Native American, and multiracial children/adolescents completed the National Survey of Children's Health to determine which health disparities occurred in these groups.

FINDINGS

Lack of insurance was highest for Latinos and Native Americans. In addition, health disparities were found for ethnic minorities including poorer overall health, being overweight and less active, having dental problems, asthma, behavior/speech problems, and emotional problems, and not having a source of usual health care nor receiving prescribed medications. In addition ethnic minorities had transportation difficulties that were barriers to them receiving care.

IMPLICATIONS

It would be important to provide services to ethnic minority children that meet their unmet needs related to care and access to care as well as to tailor preventative and routine care that reduces disparities according to ethnic or racial group.

REFERENCE

Flores, G., Tomany-Korman, S. (2008). Racial and ethnic disparities in medical and dental health, access to care, and use of services in U.S. children. *Pediatrics, 121*(2), E286–E298.

Children (AFDC) as their primary source of income, and problems are often compounded by failure to receive benefits to which they are entitled, erroneous case closings, and benefit reductions. Loss of these benefits has been shown to have directly contributed to loss of housing. In addition, the children of these women who are eligible to receive benefits under the federally funded Special Supplemental Food Program for Women, Infants, and Children (WIC) often do not receive benefits. Families with limited resources are often left with no other alternative than emergency food assistance facilities, and in many cities, such facilities have reported having to turn away people in need because of lack of resources.

Psychological problems identified most often among homeless children include depression, anxiety, and behavioral problems. Homeless children are more likely to exhibit poor attention span, trouble sleeping, delayed speech, aggressive behaviors, shyness, and withdrawal. Poor school attendance resulting from family transience is also a serious concern. Enrollment in school may be delayed for weeks because of lack of immunizations and records.

Poor school attendance and success in academics resulting from family transience is also a serious concern (Institute for Children and Poverty, 2009). For example, these children are more likely than other children to be held back a grade, and have higher rates of school mobility and grade retention than low-income housed children. In fact, frequent school transfers are the most significant barrier to their academic success.

Nurses, together with other service providers such as physicians, psychologists, and teachers, can increase the local and national awareness of the effects of homelessness on children and bring political attention to the underlying causes of widespread poverty. Nurses are also in a unique position to advocate for homeless children within the social services system concerning access to health care, mental health care, and essential housing, nutritional, and educational needs. Nurses can also advocate for making prenatal care available to homeless mothers. Lack of such care places unborn homeless children at risk of low birth weight, subsequent health problems, chronic diseases, and cognitive and developmental problems. In addition, health problems are associated with psychological problems, classroom performance, and dropout rates, all of which, if unaddressed, can seriously compromise the future of homeless children.

MIGRANT FARM WORKERS

Migrant and seasonal farm workers constitute a major portion of the labor force in the U.S. agricultural industry, and children make up almost one-fourth of all farm labor. The majority of adult workers are married and have children. Children of migrant workers constitute a population at high risk for many health problems because of their living conditions

RESEARCH

Homeless Adolescents

STUDY PURPOSE

To better understand health care experiences and perceptions of homeless adolescents in order to provide more effective approaches to health care, since they experience a number of health-related issues including physical, sexual, or emotional abuse, suicide ideation, depression, and other psychiatric disorders, substance abuse, increased rate of acute and chronic respiratory diseases, and high-risk sexual activity.

METHODS

A critical narrative was used to examine perceptions thirteen homeless adolescents (six female, seven male) between 14 and 19 years of age had about their health care experiences and barriers to receiving health care by asking them questions in a tape recorded semi-structured interview. The interviews were then transcribed verbatim and analyzed according to qualitative methods.

FINDINGS

Many of these interviewed adolescents had feelings of "being stuck" in their situation. They also did not feel safe and had similar backgrounds: grew up in a family where they experienced violence and poverty, and had parents with problems including mental health issues and drug abuse. The female participants experienced more violence than the male participants, and both genders believed health care and support was difficult to obtain because of the energy expended to get services. Finally, most did not have enough education to get meaningful work, leading them to maintain their homeless lifestyle.

IMPLICATIONS

It is important for health care providers to work collaboratively with homeless young people in order to provide sensitive health care based on their needs. Since female homeless adolescents are likely to be exposed to various forms of violence, it would also be important to offer these adolescents a safe haven where they can talk with each other and supportive health care providers about challenges faced as they live on the streets.

REFERENCE

Haldenby, A., Berman, H., & Forchuk, C. (2007). Homelessness and health in adolescents. *Qualitative Health Research, 17*(9), 1232–1244.

and limited access to health care. They suffer from many of the problems seen in homeless children: gastroenteritis, dental caries, inadequate immunizations, intestinal parasites, infestations, skin infections, pesticide exposure, and infectious diseases (Wilson, Wold, Spencer, & Pittman, 2000).

Agriculture surpasses mining and construction as the most hazardous occupation in the United States. Children of migrant families often are involved in farm work and, being physically weaker and less experienced with farm operations and machinery than their adult counterparts, are more at risk for injury. Each year some 24,000 children working in agriculture experience nonfatal trauma, and nearly 300 children die, primarily as a result of accidents involving farm machinery. Children are also at risk for pesticide exposure both in the fields where they work and play, and at home, where they can be exposed through pesticide drift. Although research on childhood exposures is limited, it is believed that children are at greater risk than adults for pesticide-related illnesses because of their higher metabolism, increased body surface area, and potential for long-term chemical exposure. Long-term exposure to pesticides has been implicated in several types of cancer, birth defects, sterility, spontaneous abortion, and cognitive deficits.

The conditions of migrant life place families, and especially children, at increased risk for contracting a variety of viral, bacterial, and fungal infections, including rabies, anthrax, Rocky Mountain spotted fever, tetanus, plague, typhoid, tuberculosis, HIV, and hepatitis. Crowded, unsanitary living conditions create the opportunity for rapid disease spread. Lack of access to health care services results in a high incidence of preventable disease in the migrant population. The high incidence of tuberculosis in this population has been linked with high rates of infection in migrants' countries of origin, substandard housing and overcrowding, poor baseline health status, malnutrition, and lack of access to preventive health care services. There are high rates of HIV infection in the migrant population. Specifically, the number of women with HIV is rising, putting children at risk for contracting the virus *in utero* or at birth. Migrant women are particularly at risk because of their lack of access to educational counseling, prevention, and treatment services.

Migrant children are frequently at risk nutritionally. Migrant communities often have limited choices for the purchase of food, and their low incomes may preclude them from receiving adequate amounts of nourishment. Furthermore, they often lack the means for properly storing or preparing foods (e.g., lack of refrigeration or potable water). Though many are eligible for supplementation through programs such as WIC and food stamps, many do not participate because of multiple barriers to these services. Iron-deficiency anemia is a common diagnosis reported by clinics serving migrant children. Child obesity is also raised as a major clinical concern given the link of obesity to diabetes and hypertension in adults.

The health status of these children is further threatened because of barriers to health care such as family mobility, financial constraints, and legal (fear of immigration penalties), language, and cultural barriers. The mobility of the families impedes adequate follow-up and referral for health problems for the children. Financial constraints stemming from being in a low-wage work group, being paid according to how much is harvested, and lack of health insurance hinder migrant farm workers from seeking health care for their children. Language is a major cultural barrier for Hispanic workers who speak little English and for health care providers who do not speak Spanish.

There is a critical need for nurses working with migrants to advocate for the health of migrant children. Nurses must not only act as health educators for migrant families, but they must also aid them in negotiating a complex and dynamic health care system that is unfamiliar. It is equally important that those familiar with the lives of migrant families educate the public and its leaders about the significant contributions of these workers to the economy. Further, the research literature on migrant children has many critical gaps. Basic information on the number and distribution of migrant children in the United States, prevalence rates for common causes of morbidity and mortality in this group, and measures of the impact of the migrant health system on child health status are lacking. Nurses and other clinicians are in key positions to fill these gaps and thus expand the knowledge base from which further target interventions may be developed.

VIOLENCE

As the 20th century ended, violence by and against children declined. Yet it still occurs. Today children and adolescents are more likely to be the victims of violent crime than the offenders. In fact, in 2007, the rate at which youth were victims of serious violent crimes (homicide, rape, aggravated assault, and robbery) was 10 crimes per 1,000 youth ages 12–17. However, rates are still significantly lower than in 1993 when they peaked (the serious violent crime victimization rate was 44 per 1,000

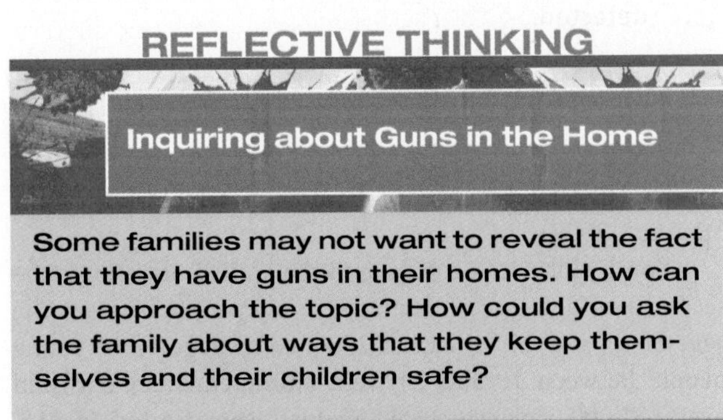

Some families may not want to reveal the fact that they have guns in their homes. How can you approach the topic? How could you ask the family about ways that they keep themselves and their children safe?

Reflections from Families

My family has been devastated ever since my 12-year-old son, Henry, was shot in our home. But we were more fortunate than most. He survived. Henry was seriously injured when his best friend Jonah, also age 12, and he were playing and found my husband's loaded revolver on the shelf of our closet. They began playing with it, and the gun went off in Jonah's hand, hitting Henry in the shoulder at close range. Henry's doctors say the outlook is good and that he will regain full use of his arm, though he will require extensive medical care and long-term physical therapy. But the trauma of that night will never leave us. My husband and I blame ourselves for the shooting and want to do something to prevent other families from going through what we have. We have started working with the schools to help teach gun safety to parents and children. We could have lost our son simply because we didn't take responsibility for owning and keeping a gun in our home. No parent should ever have to find out what that feels like, especially too late.

KIDS WANT TO KNOW

I'm afraid that someone will bring a gun to school.

What should I do if I know someone has brought a gun to school?

- Report any guns brought by classmates to a principal, teacher, or a school nurse.
- When you report guns brought by classmates, your identity does not need to be revealed.
- Many schools have metal detectors so that guns cannot be brought to school without being detected.

youth) (Federal Interagency Forum on Child and Family Statistics, 2009).

Youth violence is common in the United States; it is the second leading cause of death for young people between the ages of 10 and 24. In fact in 2006, an average of 16 young people between 10 and 24 were murdered every day, and over 631,000 violence-related injuries were treated in U.S. emergency rooms during 2007 among youth of this same age (CDC, 2009a). Among homicide victims ages 10- to 24-years-old, 84% were killed with a firearm (CDC, 2009b). Juveniles accounted for 16% of all violent crime arrests and 26% of all property crime arrests in 2007. Specifically, 1,350 juveniles were arrested for murder, 3,580 for forcible rape, and 57,650 for aggravated assault (Puzzanchera, 2009). Risk factors for such violent behaviors in this age group include poor family functioning and grades in school, poverty, drug, alcohol, or tobacco use, history of violence, and associating with delinquent peers (CDC, 2009a).

Although in recent years a great deal of attention has understandably been focused on tragic school shootings and homicides, serious school violence rates have declined over the last few years (CDC, 2010). However, even though violent crimes in schools have decreased, physical fights, thefts, weapon carrying, teacher victimization, and fear of school environments continue to be an issue for some children and adolescents. The most effective strategies for reducing violence in schools involve reducing risk factors including a history of early aggressive behavior, associating with delinquent peers, being involved in gangs, poor academic performance, low commitment to school or school failure, antisocial beliefs and attitudes, poor behavioral control, experiencing rejection by peers, exposure to family violence/conflict, low parental involvement, and poor family functioning and comonitoring/supervision of children (CDC, 2010) as well as coordinating interventions by education, law enforcement, social service, and mental health systems.

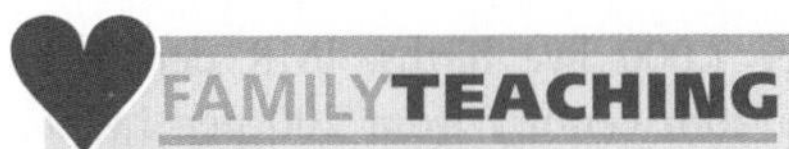

Firearm Injury Prevention

Home

1. Communicate the risks of keeping a firearm in the home.
2. Advise that it's safest not to keep a firearm in the home.
3. Review safe methods of storage.
4. Educate caregivers to teach children not to touch or handle firearms.
5. Explain that handguns and semiautomatic weapons pose the greatest risk of intentional and unintentional injury for children because they are often stored unsafely.
6. Explain to caregivers that it is easier to keep guns away from adolescents than to keep adolescents away from guns, which are often glamorized in the media. Caregivers should watch for signs of depression or changes in behavior since teens feeling this way are at increased risk for suicide.

School

1. Incorporate violence prevention programs in school curricula at an early age, including firearm violence. Examples of such programs include conflict resolution, alternatives to violence, anger management, risk awareness, and coping skills.
2. Have after-school programs for youths, and obtain community support for such programs.

Community

1. In an effort to reduce the romanticization of guns in the popular media, urge the development of violence-free programming among child health and education advocates and the television and motion picture industries.
2. Support legislation that regulates the manufacture and importation of classes of guns, such as handguns and assault weapons, and that requires background checks for weapons purchased at gun shows.
3. Improve playgrounds and parks to make safe play areas for children.

CURRENT STATUS OF CHILDREN'S HEALTH

Beginning in 1979, *Healthy People* has set and monitored national health goals and objectives to meet a wide range of health needs, engage people across the nation to work together, guide individuals toward making informed health decisions, and measure the impact of prevention activity. *Healthy People* embodies science-based, 10-year national objectives for promoting health and preventing disease (USDHHS, 2010). In January 2000, the U.S. Department of Health and Human Services (USDHHS) launched *Healthy People 2010: National Health Promotion and Disease Prevention Objectives,* a comprehensive, nationwide health promotion and disease prevention agenda. The document contains 28 focus areas and 467 objectives designed to serve as a guide for improving the health of all people in the United States during the first decade of the 21st century (USDHHS, 2000). Most of the objectives target the lifestyle choices and environmental conditions that cause 70% of premature deaths in this country. The overarching goals are to increase the quality and years of healthy life and eliminate health disparities between ethnic groups. The *Healthy People* framework allows governments to focus resources in the right place. A variety of indicators reflect the health status of Americans. Health status can be measured by birth and death rates, life expectancy, morbidity from specific diseases, and many other factors (see Box 1-1).

BOX 1-1

***HEALTHY PEOPLE* LEADING HEALTH INDICATORS**

- Physical activity
- Overweight and obesity
- Tobacco use
- Substance abuse
- Responsible sexual behavior
- Mental health
- Injury and violence
- Environmental quality
- Immunizations
- Access to health care

Healthy People 2020 continues the progress from *Healthy People 2010*. Advisory committees met during 2008 and 2009, and public comment has been solicited. By 2010, the goals, objectives, and action plans for *Healthy People 2020* will be launched (USDHHS, 2010). The *Healthy People 2020* vision, mission statement, and overarching goals are included in Box 1-2.

Because *Healthy People* has emphasized health promotion and prevention, almost all of it pertains to nursing.

BOX 1-2
***HEALTHY PEOPLE 2020* FRAMEWORK**

Vision

A society in which all people live long, healthy lives.

Mission Statement

Healthy People 2020 strives to:

- Identify nationwide health improvement priorities;
- Increase public awareness and understanding of the determinants of health, disease, and disability and the opportunities for progress;
- Provide measurable objectives and goals that are applicable at the national, state, and local levels;
- Engage multiple sectors to take actions to strengthen policies and improve practices that are driven by the best available evidence and knowledge;
- Identify critical research, evaluation, and data collections needs.

Overarching Goals

- Attain high quality, longer lives free of preventable disease, disability, injury, and premature death.
- Achieve health equity, eliminate disparities, and improve the health of all groups.
- Create social and physical environments that promote good health for all.
- Promote quality of life, healthy development, and healthy behaviors across all life stages.

U.S. Department of Health and Human Services, Office of Disease Prevention and Health Promotion, Healthy People 2020. Available at http://www.healthypeople.gov/hp2020/ accessed April 11, 2010.

Health promotion and education are central to nursing practice; therefore, nurses need to develop an awareness of the *Healthy People 2020* program and incorporate it as a benchmark for their interventions. Nurses are well educated and prepared to work with individuals, families, and communities to meet the special needs of vulnerable populations and to eliminate health disparities. The public, by and large, trusts nurses and is receptive to their teaching and intervention. Nurses can use their unique position to help meet the goals of *Healthy People 2020* and, in doing so, can improve the health of all Americans: adults, children, and adolescents.

INFANT MORTALITY

Infant mortality is an important measure of a nation's health and a worldwide indicator of health status. The **infant mortality rate** (IMR) is the number of infant deaths during the first year of life per 1,000 live births. IMR declined exponentially during the 20th century from 200 per 1,000 live births in 1900 to a record low of 7.2 per 1,000 live births in 1998. By 2006, the rate fell to 6.7 per 1,000 live births, an average that varies widely based upon ethnicity, race, and state in the United States. For instance, Black/African American infants suffer an IMR of 13.3 as compared to a low of 3.6 among Asian or Pacific Islander babies. Infants born in Washington State have an IMR of 4.7 and infants born in Mississippi are more than twice as likely to die before their first birthday (Annie E. Casey Foundation, 2009).

Compared to our international peers, the United States IMR rate ranked 30th in 2005. Chile ranked 32nd, Cuba ranks 26th, Canada ranks 25th, Singapore ranks 1st and Sweden ranks 2nd (CDC, 2008). One explanation for the low ranking of the United States may be that most countries with lower IMR have national health programs.

The ratio of low birth weight births in this country also continues to be a reason for its unenviable IMR, and the proportion of the smallest and most vulnerable infants increased during the 1990s. The IMR target goal for the year 2010 was 4.5 deaths per 1,000 live births, and continues to be an unmet goal for the United States. It has been reasoned that to achieve further reductions in infant mortality, the public health community, health care providers, and individuals must focus on modifying the behaviors, lifestyles, and conditions that affect birth outcomes. These include smoking, substance abuse, poor nutrition, lack of prenatal care, medical problems, chronic illness, and other psychosocial problems (e.g., stress, domestic violence). However, given the inability to improve access for prenatal care by health care providers and expand education efforts, any new approach must be more focused upon the financial, educational, social, and logistic barriers to receiving prenatal care in the first trimester for all women.

CHILD MORTALITY

Another indicator of children's health status is child mortality. Child mortality decreased by approximately half between 1980 and 2002 among children ages 1 to 4 (from 64 to 31 deaths per 100,000 children) and among children ages 5 to 14 (from 31 to 17 deaths per 100,000 children) (Federal Interagency Forum on Child and Family Statistics, 2005). In 2006, child mortality (deaths per 100,000 children ages 1 to 4 years) has improved more, falling to 28.4. The rate for children ages 5 to 14 has also continued a downward trend, falling to 15.2 in 2006 (CDC, 2008).

At the beginning of the 20th century the major cause of child mortality for 1- to 19-year-olds was infectious diseases. However, the mortality and morbidity from all of these diseases are dwarfed by the numbers of children who die or who are disabled as the result of unintentional injuries. Until recently, injuries were commonly termed *accidents,* suggesting that they were unpredictable and unavoidable events affecting unlucky children. Today, the term *injury* is favored because it more accurately suggests that the problem can be averted and prevented.

CRITICAL THINKING

Healthy People 2020

From the ten leading health indicators found in Box 1-1, choose four that you think would have objectives pertaining to children ages 1 to 18 years and list them. For each one of the four you have chosen, write down an idea for the specific area that the objective should address. For example, if you were to choose priority areas for adults, one area would be cancer, and the specific area the objective could address is to increase the number of adults who receive a colorectal screening exam each year.

Injury is defined as damage or harm to an individual resulting in destruction of health, disability, or death. An injury is classified as intentional or unintentional, denoting whether or not it was meant to harm the victim.

Among children ages 1 to 4, unintentional injuries (9.9%) are responsible for more deaths each year than homicide (2.2%), congenital anomalies (3.2%), cancer (2.3%), heart disease (1%), respiratory illness, and HIV combined in 2006 (CDC, 2008). Although unintentional injuries are the leading cause of death for all children over 1 year of age, the incidence varies by age. More than half of all unintentional injury-related deaths occur in the 15- to 19-year-old group due to motor vehicle-related injuries. Common subcategories of motor vehicle injuries include (1) occupant (drivers and passengers), (2) bicycle-related, (3) motorcycle, and (4) pedestrian injuries.

There is considerable variation in injury rates among children depending on their age group. Among children under 1 year of age, suffocation is the leading cause of unintentional injury-related death, followed by motor vehicle occupant injury, choking, drowning, and fires or burns. Some suffocation deaths in infants are due to entrapment of the head and neck in cribs. Another cause is choking on food or an object, leading to airway obstruction. For children ages 1 to 4 years, drowning is no longer the leading cause of injury death. Drowning now is equal to motor vehicle occupant injury (each at 2.9%), followed by fires or burns (1.3%) and airway obstruction (1%) (CDC, 2008). Infants often drown in bathtubs, usually as a result of poor supervision or neglect, whereas toddlers and young children fall into a body of water such as a swimming pool, lake, or river, usually while unsupervised. Among children ages 5 to 14, motor vehicle traffic-related injury is the leading cause of death (3.0%), followed by firearms (0.9%), suffocation (0.8%), drowning (0.7%), and fires and burns (0.5%) (CDC, 2008). Pedestrian injury often occurs when a child darts out between parked cars or into the street to get a ball or another object. During adolescence (14–19 years), motor vehicle occupant injuries are the primary cause of injury-related deaths. Driver inexperience and alcohol use are key contributors to the high rate of fatal crashes involving adolescents.

Rates of unintentional injury deaths among children have declined by 43% over the past several decades. Decreases in injury deaths have been observed for every age group and for nearly all causes. Reductions have been most evident among adolescents and for poisoning deaths. Additionally, most unintentional injury deaths to children can be prevented. Simple proven interventions include: (1) using child car seats and bicycle helmets; (2) requiring that prescription medications have child-resistant caps: (3) installing smoke detectors in homes; (4) requiring that children's sleep wear be flame retardant; and (5) enclosing swimming pools with fences.

CULTURAL CONSIDERATION

Infant Mortality Rate and Race Ethnicity

Racial and ethnic disparities persist for infant mortality, with whites having the lowest rate. The IMR for African Americans is twice the rate for whites. However, the gap between whites and nonwhites (excluding African Americans) is narrowing. For Hispanics and Asian Pacific Islanders, the IMR has decreased dramatically over the last 20 years (CDC, Health, United States, 2008). One reason for this disparity in IMR is the high rate of **low birth weight** (LBW) infants born to minority mothers, which suggests a decrease in the overall health status or health care access of these women. In 2007, low birth weight (LBW) babies (weighing less than 2500g or 5 lb 8 oz) represented 8.2% of all live births in the United States (Federal Interagency Forum on Child and Family Statistics, 2009).

During 2010, the World Health Organization began an ambitious country-by-country count for preterm birth rates (prematurity is currently considered as any live birth earlier than 37 weeks of gestation). Evidence suggests that worldwide one in every 10 of the world's babies is born preterm (March of Dimes, 2009). The United States has the highest percentage of premature births in the world, with the rate increasing 36% over the last quarter century (March of Dimes, 2009). Data suggests that more than 1 in 4 (28%) of premature babies will not survive (Lawn, Cousens & Zupan, 2006). Premature babies who survive have higher rates of learning disabilities, cerebral palsy, sensory deficits, and respiratory illnesses as compared to babies carried to term (IOM, 2007).

REFLECTIVE THINKING

The Cost of Keeping LBW Infants Alive

Hospitals and health care delivery systems have poured substantial amounts of money into neonatal intensive care units to care for LBW infants. These babies are usually technology dependent and often require extensive medical equipment and nursing care in their homes. How do you feel about this emphasis on high-tech solutions versus allocating some resources to preventive services?

These common sense tactics have annually saved the lives of thousands of children.

The key approaches to injury prevention are education, changes in the environment and in products, and legislation or regulation. Education to promote changes in individuals' behaviors has reduced the risk of childhood injuries. Education by health care professionals has increased individual safety behaviors, including seat belt and car seat use, smoke detector ownership, and safe hot water temperature. Nurses and other health care providers should incorporate education about safety practices into routine health visits. Pediatric nurses can play an important educational role by teaching caregivers about expected behaviors for their child's upcoming developmental stage. This alerts them to the types of injuries common to that age group and to potential environmental hazards. Nurses can initiate safety programs in schools, neighborhoods, and cities (Figure 1-1).

Changes in the environment and in products can make children's physical surroundings, toys, and clothing safer. Strategies that make children's environments safer such as traffic calming to reduce or slow the speed of traffic in neighborhoods and fencing to enclose swimming pools on all sides should be implemented in all communities and be mandated by law. Legislation and regulation are among the most effective tools to reduce injuries, and most environment and product modifications require legal action. However, some laws have not been adopted in every state; for example, 14 of 50 states (Arkansas, Colorado, Idaho, Indiana, Iowa, Minnesota, Mississippi, Nebraska, North and South Dakota, South Carolina, Utah, Vermont, and Wyoming) lack bicycle helmet laws (Bicycle Helmet Safety Institute, 2009). Most states do not require appropriate protection in automobiles for children between the ages of 4 and 8. For maximum effectiveness, laws, regulations, and policies must be supported by the public and enforced at the community level. A major challenge is to coordinate all groups involved in unintentional injury prevention to create a critical mass for action.

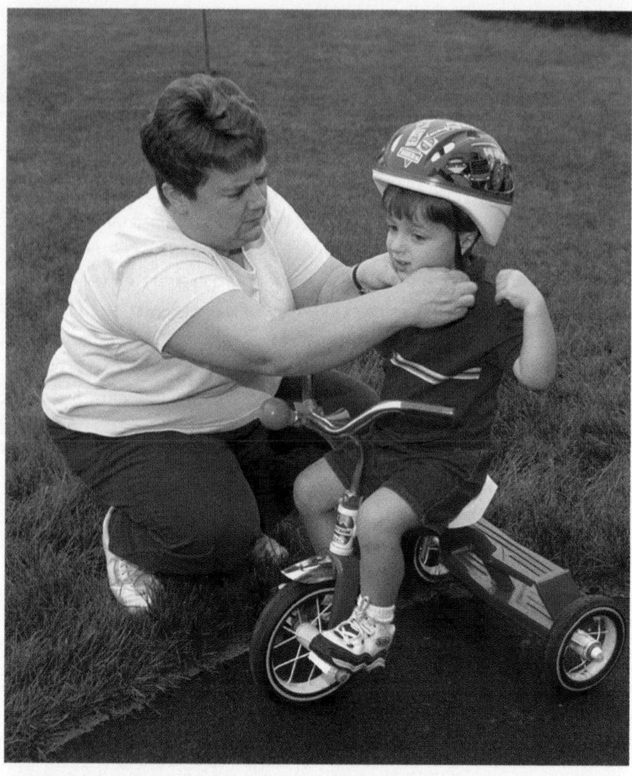

FIGURE 1-1 The use of safety equipment such as helmets helps protect children from injury. What other measures can nurses suggest to parents that might protect children from injury? DELMAR CENGAGE LEARNING.

ACCESS TO HEALTH CARE

For a growing number of children, access to health care is hampered by lack of health insurance. Children without health insurance are less likely to receive health services (CDC, 2008). In 2007, 89% of children (i.e., 8.1 million) had health insurance coverage at some point during the year. While government insurance coverage has continued its upward trend since 1999, the proportion of children covered by private insurance has dropped since 2000 (Federal Interagency Forum on Child and Family Statistics, 2009). Ethnic minority children are overrepresented among the uninsured, as they account for more than half of uninsured children. Three-quarters of uninsured children are among the working poor, that is, in families in which the head of the household is employed full time for all or part of the year. One unintended consequence it that only 77% of children age 19–35 months received a combined vaccination series protecting them against several childhood infectious diseases during 2006, thereby affecting public health in the United States (CDC, 2008).

Socioeconomic status largely dictates the source of children's health insurance. Those from higher income families are more likely to have private health insurance (90%) than are children from lower income families (40%). Uninsured children in low-income families experience substantial

Reflections from Families

Whenever I heard people say that the leading cause of death in teenagers is car accidents, I never thought it would happen to me. I am only 17, but I feel that my life is over since the day my best friend, Kamdin, was killed in the car I was driving. I was driving too fast, and we had the music on real high. We had just left a friend's house, where we had been drinking beer. We were just having fun, we thought, but suddenly when a car turned in front of us too fast, I lost control of my car, and we ended up rolled over in a ditch. Kamdin is gone, and her family will never be the same. Neither will mine. I just keep wishing I had one more chance to go back to that day and do it over again.

difficulties in accessing health care. They tend to lack: (1) the usual sources of routine and sick care, (2) a primary care provider, and (3) recent visits to health care providers.

Beyond the barriers created by lack of health insurance, other factors involved in access to and use of care include demographic factors such as family income, race or ethnicity, place of residence, and type of insurance. Institutional factors such as gate keeping by health plans, distance from families' homes to health site, availability of transportation, and waiting times are other factors. Nurses need to assess barriers for families in accessing health care beyond their insurance status in order to ensure that children will receive needed health care.

PERSPECTIVES ON PEDIATRIC NURSING

FAMILY-CENTERED CARE

All health care professionals recognize that quality health care of children must extend to the entire family. Thus, the focus of pediatric nursing must be on the child as well as the family. The term **family-centered care** describes a philosophy of care that recognizes the centrality of the family in the child's life and inclusion of the family's contribution and involvement in the plan for care and its delivery. It is a health care delivery model that seeks to fully involve families in the care of children. Family-centered care evolved in response to the critical need to maintain the relationship between hospitalized children and their families. Previously this relationship had been neglected or disrupted because of forced separation by the health care system.

In 1987, a revolutionary document that defined the elements of family-centered care was published by the Association for the Care of Children's Health (ACCH). Family-centered care was defined by this group as including eight equally important elements (see Box 1-3). Meeting the ever-changing needs of *all* family members, not just those of the child, is paramount to the concept of family-centered care. When families are incorporated into the care of their children, the physical and psychosocial health of the child improves and accelerated rates of progress have been seen. Additionally, these families have demonstrated enhanced learning, less stress, and more satisfaction with care.

The elements of family-centered care are based on principles that are designed to promote greater family self-determination, decision-making capabilities, control, and self-efficacy. Collectively, these attributes are said to reflect a sense of empowerment. In contrast, the medical model directs health care professionals to assume the roles of evaluator and controller of treatment interventions. This approach results in child and caregiver dependence on the health care providers. This position is in direct conflict with the conditions necessary for more active involvement of caregivers in the care of their health-impaired children.

Many health care providers respect and support the idea of family-centered care; however, the practice of this type of care has not been fully actualized. This discrepancy between their support and actual practice of family-centered care may be attributed in part to the model they employ (family empowerment versus medical approach). Additionally, professionals often inadvertently foster family dependency, alienation, and helplessness by taking control and administering care without family input for the convenience and expediency of the staff and the institution. However, in order to facilitate family-centered care, health care providers must seek caregiver input, suggestions, and advice; incorporate this information into the plan of care; and teach the family the appropriate health care interventions. By providing education and knowledge to the family, caregivers can be empowered to make informed decisions about their child's care. Other strategies that enhance family-centered care include removing limits on the ages or number of visitors (unless directed otherwise by the family); providing adequate sleeping facilities for caregivers in the child's room; offering meals or discounts in cafeterias and free parking or a discount for caregivers; and requesting family

BOX 1-3
KEY ELEMENTS OF FAMILY-CENTERED CARE

1. Incorporating into policy and practice the recognition that the *family is the constant* in a child's life, whereas the service systems and support personnel fluctuate.
2. Facilitating *family/professional collaboration* at all levels of hospital, home, and community care: care of an individual child; program development, implementation, and evaluation; and policy formation.
3. *Exchanging complete and unbiased information* between families and professionals in a supportive manner at all times.
4. Incorporating into policy and practice the recognition and *honoring of cultural diversity,* strengths, and individuality within and across all families, including *ethnic, racial, spiritual, social, economic, educational,* and *geographic diversity.*
5. Recognizing and respecting *different methods of family coping* and implementing comprehensive policies and programs that provide *developmental, educational, emotional, environmental,* and *financial supports* to meet the diverse needs of families.
6. Encouraging and facilitating *family-to-family support* and networking.
7. Ensuring that *hospital, home, and community services and support systems* for children needing specialized health and developmental care and their families are *flexible, accessible, and comprehensive* in responding to diverse family-identified needs.
8. *Appreciating families as families* and children as children, recognizing that they possess a wide range of strengths, concerns, emotions, and aspirations beyond their need for specialized health and developmental services and support.

attendance at interdisciplinary conferences regarding the child's care.

ATRAUMATIC CARE

Atraumatic care is a philosophy of providing care that minimizes or eliminates physical and psychological distress for children and their families in the health care environment. In pediatric care, many interventions are traumatic, stressful, and painful; therefore, it is important for nurses to be cognizant of these situations and provide care that minimizes distress. Three principles provide the basis for atraumatic care: (1) identifying stressors for the child and family, (2) minimizing separation of the child from caregivers, and (3) minimizing or preventing pain. Examples of atraumatic interventions include:

- Preparing the child prior to every procedure using age-appropriate explanations
- For the child scheduled for surgery, preparing her or him prior to hospital admission (encourage child and caregivers to visit the hospital, allow the child to play with equipment and items such as a stethoscope, blood pressure cuff, IV equipment, masks, and gowns)
- Allowing caregivers to be involved and physically present as much as possible to provide support and comfort for the child
- Controlling pain by administering analgesics freely
- Using a euteric mixture of local anesthetics (EMLA) cream at least 1 hour prior to blood draws, insertion of IV needles, and injections

ROLES OF THE PEDIATRIC NURSE

The professional pediatric nurse has the responsibility to provide high-quality care no matter the setting nor the role practiced. Settings where pediatric nurses are involved in caring for children include schools (see Chapter 5), acute care settings, clinics, physicians' offices, home health agencies, rehabilitation centers, hospice programs, day care centers, psychiatric centers, and summer camps. Nurses may also work as administrators or nurse executives. Although each setting may have separate roles and responsibilities, the roles that nurses take are universal. Specifically, the primary roles include caregiver, advocate, educator, researcher, and manager or leader. Secondary roles include behaviors related to coordinating, collaborating, communicating, and consulting, and are embedded within the primary roles. Other roles seen in the acute care setting involve **differentiated practice** (a philosophy that delineates a nurse's role and functions according to experience, competence, and education) and include the clinical care coordinator, care manager, and clinical nurse. In addition to these, nurses function in expanded roles as pediatric nurse practitioners, clinical nurse specialists, and case managers. For the most part, these expanded roles require advanced preparation. See Box 1-4 for a list of the various roles of the nurse in pediatric practice. A discussion of the roles follows.

The roles that the nurse takes in these settings are based on the level of performance expected by practice authorities.

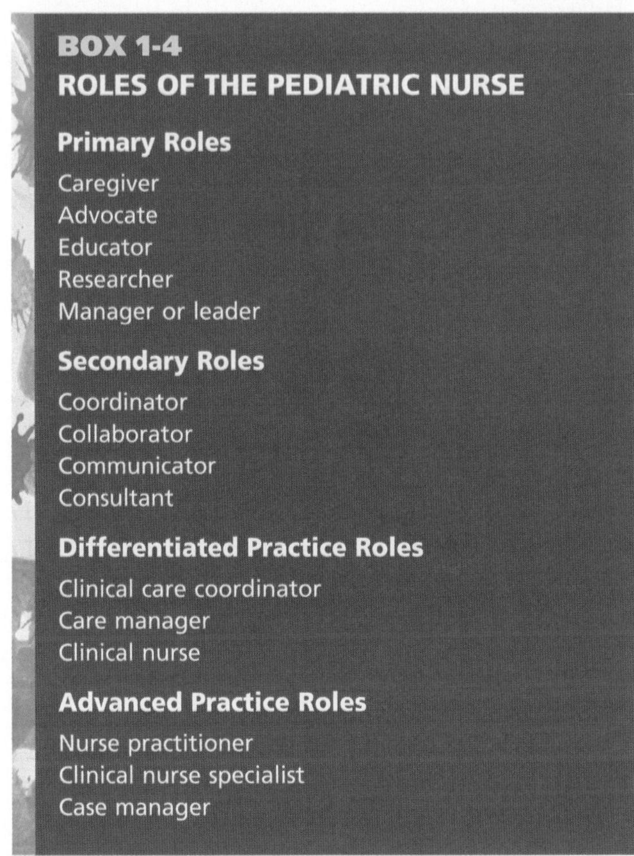

BOX 1-4
ROLES OF THE PEDIATRIC NURSE

Primary Roles

Caregiver
Advocate
Educator
Researcher
Manager or leader

Secondary Roles

Coordinator
Collaborator
Communicator
Consultant

Differentiated Practice Roles

Clinical care coordinator
Care manager
Clinical nurse

Advanced Practice Roles

Nurse practitioner
Clinical nurse specialist
Case manager

The Standards of Maternal and Child Health Nursing Practice as developed by the American Nurses Association describe these standards and set expectations for the general behaviors of pediatric nurses while caring for children and their families. These standards were developed in 1983 and are out of print; therefore, they are not included in this textbook.

Caregiver

Patricia Benner (1984) identified several domains of nursing practice that are inherent in the **caregiver** role. They include helping, patient diagnosing and monitoring, administering and monitoring therapeutic interventions and regimens, monitoring and ensuring the quality of health care practices, organizational and work role competencies, and effectively managing rapidly changing situations. More specifically, the caregiver delivers direct nursing care to children and their families based on the nursing process that considers the child's developmental level, meets the child's emotional and physical needs, and encourages the child to participate in self-care as appropriate. Caregivers also provide family-centered care that embraces diverse cultures and family structures, empowers and encourages families to participate in the care their child needs, and supports families at home, in the acute care setting or in other settings. This requires skills in critical thinking, coordinating, collaborating, and consulting, as well as the ability to incorporate and integrate knowledge of pathophysiology, pediatric illness, human growth and development, and the biological sciences, and findings from the physical, cultural, and spiritual assessment into a plan that accurately reflects child and family needs. Care provided also should demonstrate knowledge of pediatric pharmacology, including methods of administration, dosage, and side effects, and the ability to accurately administer medication by various routes to children of all ages.

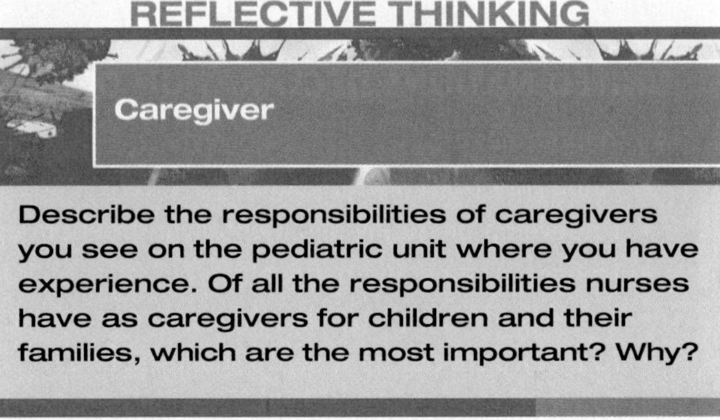

REFLECTIVE THINKING

Caregiver

Describe the responsibilities of caregivers you see on the pediatric unit where you have experience. Of all the responsibilities nurses have as caregivers for children and their families, which are the most important? Why?

Advocate

The **advocate** pleads causes for and assists others in making informed decisions that are in the child and family's best interest. Generally, pediatric nurses acting as advocates inform clients and families of their rights and options as well as the consequences of those options. Pediatric nurse advocates allow clients and families to make their own informed decisions and then support those decisions. Even though advocates do not need to approve the decision, they do need to respect that decision and the right to make that decision. In fact, advocates shouldn't make decisions for clients, but rather facilitate decision making.

Typically, advocates in pediatrics are concerned with informing children and their families about their health care decisions, and providing information about research, experimental protocols, and alternative treatments. They also provide complete, clear, concise, understandable, and accurate information concerning treatment, procedures, and inherent risks; provide for privacy and respect; and allow clients and families to refuse a drug, treatment, test, or procedure. Advocates also need to be careful not to impose their own personal values and standards, but rather allow the child and family to make autonomous decisions.

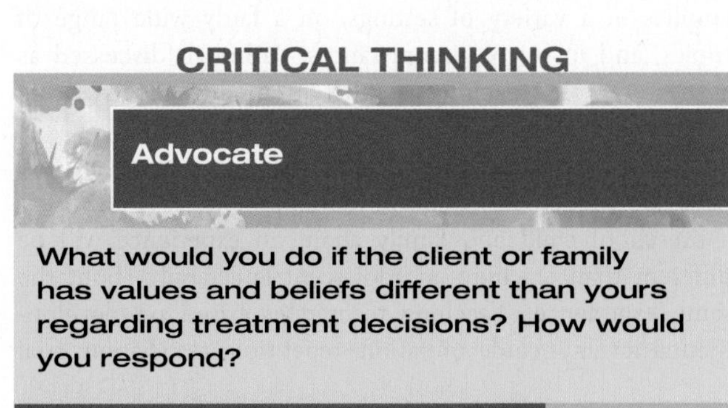

CRITICAL THINKING

Advocate

What would you do if the client or family has values and beliefs different than yours regarding treatment decisions? How would you respond?

BOX 1-5
UNITED NATIONS DECLARATION OF THE RIGHTS OF THE CHILD

All children need:

- To be free from discrimination
- To develop physically and mentally in freedom and dignity
- To have a name and nationality
- To have adequate nutrition, housing, recreation, and medical services
- To receive special treatment if handicapped
- To receive love, understanding, and material security
- To receive an education and develop his or her abilities
- To be the first to receive protection in disaster
- To be protected from neglect, cruelty, and exploitation
- To be brought up in a spirit of friendship among people

Used with permission from Office of the United Nations High Commissioner for Human Rights (http://www.ohchr.org) (1959). *Declaration of the Rights of the Child.* Proclaimed by General Assembly Resolution 1386 (XIV) of November 20, 1959.

Nurses also advocate for clients and families who are vulnerable or cannot speak for themselves; for those who do not know how to speak for themselves because of lack of knowledge, difficulty articulating needs and ideas, physical or mental disability, or perceived lack of power; and for those who are afraid to speak out. The more dependent the client is on the system, the more diligent the advocate should be on his or her behalf. Effective advocates should be assertive, attentive, knowledgeable, and trustworthy, and have the ability to openly communicate with members of the health care team, as well as remain educated about current legal and ethical trends. Finally, the advocate should be aware of the United Nations Declaration of the Rights of the Child (refer to Box 1-5), which ensures children receive optimal care by providing nursing practice guidelines.

EDUCATOR

One of the most important roles the pediatric nurse assumes is that of **educator**, or teacher, because education is one of the major avenues that the nurse uses to enable clients and families to make informed decisions. In fact, Florence Nightingale emphasized the role of the nurse as an educator, and today, nurses spend most of their time teaching, informally and formally. Nurses teach children and their families in a variety of settings, on a fairly wide range of topics, and in many circumstances. Although discussed as a separate role, teaching is inherent in the caregiver role (Figure 1-2).

To be an effective educator, the nurse must initially have knowledge of cognitive development since teaching a preschool child and family about an experience will be different than teaching an adolescent and family about the same experience. Teaching techniques based on developmental levels include imitation, repetition, association, trial and error, conditioning, and concept development, and each developmental level requires particular strategies. For example, infants and toddlers are best taught by their caregiver, and prefer to explore their environment or handle equipment. If toddlers are not interested in learning, it would be better to just delay the session. Most preschool children want to learn, and even though they might have limited verbal abilities, they do like to practice and manipulate equipment. Preschoolers will ask many questions, and answers should be short, at an understandable level, and not imply punishment. Since young children often imitate others, imitation would be an appropriate method of teaching this age group. School-age children have a short attention span and learn best in brief stages and at frequent intervals where they can handle objects, draw pictures, and color in books. Since the school-age child asks many "why"

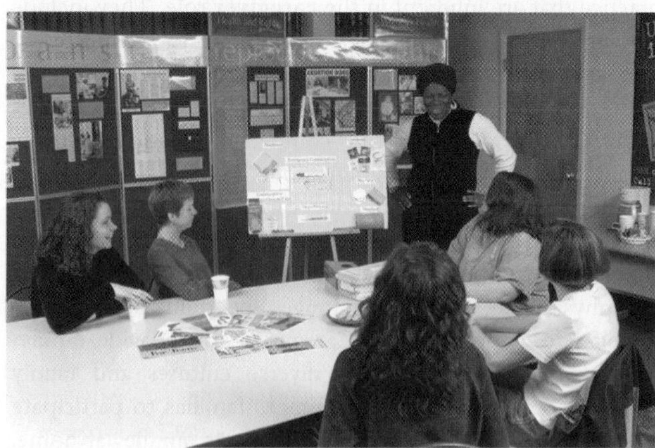

FIGURE 1-2 Pediatric nurses have a number of opportunities to teach, including teaching adolescents about contraception or risky behaviors that should be avoided. DELMAR CENGAGE LEARNING

questions, explanations should meet their needs and use words they understand. Adolescents often learn by associating new information with what they already know and may not want parents present during educational sessions. Adolescents also learn best when they see an immediate personal benefit. For example, if they understand taking medicine regularly will permit continuation of current activities, they often will comply.

Typically, nurses working with children and families will act in the educator role as they prepare children and families for procedures, surgery, or the hospitalization experience itself. Educators will also answer questions about experiences and treatments, help interpret and integrate information received from the health care team, and help parents learn how to care for their child. They also may provide information related to child rearing; answer questions about human development; discuss injury and illness prevention, health promotion and maintenance, and immunization schedules; clarify diagnoses or treatment plans; supply children and their families with appropriate literature; and refer to helpful lay or professional groups.

Since learning takes place in three domains—cognitive, affective, and psychomotor—the nurse educator must integrate all domains into teaching if it is to be effective. **Cognitive learning** is concerned with intellectual activities, can be compared to thinking, and involves describing or explaining something, or answering questions. **Affective learning** is learning that takes place in relation to feelings and emotions; as, for example, in role-playing, modeling, or one-to-one discussion where learners are asked to share their feelings and ideas about the information taught. **Psychomotor learning** is concerned with physical skills; as when the opportunity to actually practice what is being taught is offered. Often psychomotor learning is accompanied by explanation, demonstration and then practice with hands-on experiences, repetition, and immediate feedback.

An example of these types of learning could be applied to learning how to use an inhaler. Cognitive learning would include information about when to use the inhaler, how much medicine to use in the inhaler, and how to evaluate the effectiveness of the treatment. Affective learning occurs when the child recalls feelings before and after the treatment and the effects of using the inhaler. Psychomotor skills are needed to correctly administer the inhaler therapy and encouraged by allowing practice in front of the nurse.

Nurses may also be responsible for teaching their colleagues. For example, they may need to teach other nurses or health care providers about new information relative to a specific disease or condition, treatment, or intervention, or how to improve their skills and troubleshoot when things go wrong. Finally, the physical environment, the child or family's previous experiences, the culture, and the teacher's skill and organizational ability need to be considered if the nurse is to be an effective educator. The place where the teaching occurs should be carefully chosen so there is sufficient lighting, comfortable seating, an appropriate room temperature, and opportunities for either privacy or group discussion as needed. If children or families already know about the topic, the information should be tailored to their needs and not be redundant. If children and their family are from a culture with specific beliefs that impact the information presented, those beliefs need to be incorporated into the presentation. Finally, if the presentation is disorganized or the presenter is not skilled in teaching, the material may not be easily understood by the audience.

CRITICAL THINKING

Teaching a 4-Year-Old

A 4-year-old boy has been admitted to the same day surgery department for a tonsillectomy and adenoidectomy. How would you prepare him for the experience both prior to surgery and after surgery?

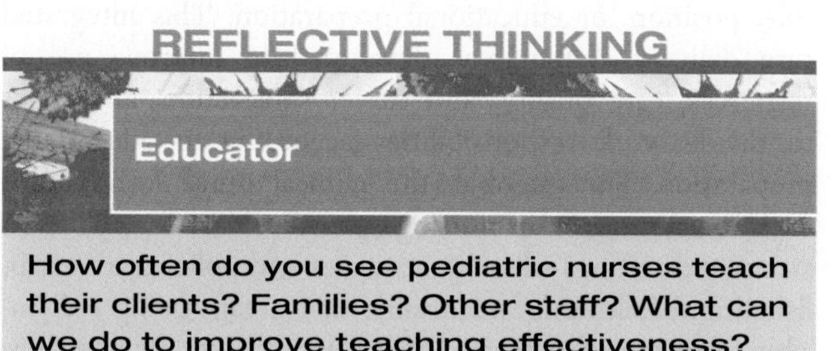

REFLECTIVE THINKING

Educator

How often do you see pediatric nurses teach their clients? Families? Other staff? What can we do to improve teaching effectiveness? What needs to be done to increase client and family teaching opportunities?

Researcher

One criterion for a profession is the existence of a body of knowledge that is distinct from other disciplines. Nursing has traditionally borrowed from the natural and social sciences, and has only recently begun to concentrate on establishing a unique body of knowledge allowing clear identification as a distinct profession. Scientific research is a valid way to develop this knowledge, and pediatric nurses are in an important position to improve this knowledge. Nurses have a responsibility to identify problems that warrant scientific investigation and provide evidence-based practice. In fact, professional accountability demands nurses determine the usefulness of this evidence before integrating it into practice. Pediatric nurses are also called upon to evaluate the methods used to carry out research projects and estimate how confident they are in the results.

There is now an emphasis in health care on determining whether interventions are cost effective and provide positive client outcomes. The evidence-based practice movement,

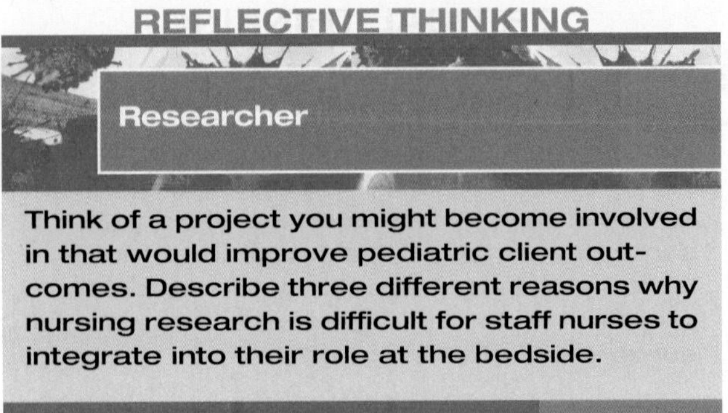

Think of a project you might become involved in that would improve pediatric client outcomes. Describe three different reasons why nursing research is difficult for staff nurses to integrate into their role at the bedside.

one outcome of this emphasis, involves not only identifying clinical questions needing to be answered, but also analyzing published research on interventions and then using his/her knowledge and integrating patient/family preferences and values into practice. The pediatric nurse, therefore, needs to always be aware of or identify clinical practice questions needing answers, examine the literature for answers to these questions, and then determine whether those answers (interventions) are appropriate for practice.

The ANA has differentiated the investigative function of nurses at various educational levels, from the associate degree through the doctorate. Although certain responsibilities have been spelled out specifically, it is not uncommon for nurses at all levels to work together on teams investigating a particular practice problem. In fact, involving all levels of education improves the project since each nurse brings different knowledge and skills to the team. More specifically, nurses can be principal investigators on a research project (although special preparation is often necessary, usually a doctorate) or a member of a research team. As team members they could be involved as a data collector; be responsible for administering a new nursing intervention; create, manage, and analyze data files; develop questionnaires; interview and observe subjects; transcribe and analyze audio tapes and interviews; analyze diaries, journals, photographs, and drawings; conduct literature searches; synthesize and critique articles; or assist in writing proposals and editing manuscripts. Being a member of a team may also raise interest and enthusiasm for nurses to conduct their own research (Polit & Beck, 2010) and should be encouraged.

Manager/Leader

Another role discussed is **manager**, which includes management of one's own clients if caring for more than one client, as well as managing staff. Typically, managing requires prioritizing, planning, and organizing comprehensive and accountable nursing care for a group of clients. It also requires one to differentiate care that is important from care that is urgent, so children and their families have needs met in a timely fashion.

Managing also means delegating aspects of care to others on the nursing staff, consistent with their level of expertise and education. However, the nurse is always held accountable for delegated tasks to be sure that there is adherence to ethical and legal standards. Since managing also requires that one assume a leadership role in health care management, effective pediatric nurse managers need to have knowledge of the care requirements of children and their families even though they may not be personally delivering the care in order to efficiently and effectively supervise the care others give. Effective nurse managers interact with clients and their families both directly and indirectly by visiting clients on rounds, reviewing records, receiving reports on client status, and answering questions from staff and requests from clients and families.

Nurse managers are also responsible for representing the institution to the client and family and the client and family to the institution, and must also work within the bureaucratic environment, which sometimes means subordinating the needs of individuals to the needs of the institution. This may cause serious conflicts for professionals attempting to give individualized care and may require the manager to step in to help staff handle the conflict. Finally, nurse managers determine the character of the unit, attitudes and behavior of staff, and relationships with other professionals at the agency. For example, if the managers' interactions with other health care providers and housekeeping are professional, the relationships these departments have with the staff will also be professional. The atmosphere of the unit also mirrors the manager's. That is, if the manager is quiet and efficient, those feelings will be communicated to children and their families; if the manager is stressed and seemingly unorganized, this too will be communicated.

DIFFERENTIATED PRACTICE ROLES

Differentiated practice, a nursing practice model implemented in some care settings, refers to a philosophy that delineates a nurse's role and functions according to experience, competence, and education (Boston, 1990). It also promotes contributions, and recognizes and values all nursing personnel delivering care to clients regardless of their role, position, or educational preparation. This integrated care delivery system was developed to improve use of resources, care quality, and career satisfaction, and seeks to divide work responsibilities according to educational preparation. For example, the clinical nurse (who holds an associate degree in nursing) provides care for clients in structured settings where procedures and policies are established and followed. Specifically, that means being responsible for managing the care of pediatric clients for one shift; monitoring, evaluating, and documenting responses to treatments and the plan of care; performing nursing skills within the scope of practice; delegating aspects of care to other team members according to their role and responsibilities;

actually implementing the individualized plan of care; assessing clients to determine needs and learning readiness; and networking with team members to enhance continuity of care.

The care manager (who holds a baccalaureate degree in nursing) is responsible for integrating client care from preadmission to post discharge and uses independent nursing judgment. This nurse may or may not work in a structured environment, where there may or may not be established procedures and policies. Specifically, this means assessing and developing a plan of care reflecting client discharge needs; designing, implementing, and evaluating teaching plans that restore, maintain, and promote health; determining long-term goals for clients in collaboration with the family; collaborating with health care team members to implement care plans both within and outside the acute care setting; assuming responsibility for care plan outcomes; completing discharge planning assessment; and collaborating with other disciplines as needed to facilitate referrals to other agencies within the community.

The clinical care coordinator (who holds a master's degree in nursing) provides leadership; functions in a variety of settings; uses independent nursing judgment based on specialized knowledge, research, and theory; and promotes health care outcomes for clients. Specifically, this means assessing nursing resources and staffing needs and then implementing a staffing plan reflective of this assessment; facilitating communication within the health care team; serving as a resource to clients, families, and the health care team; fostering development and education of students and staff; using unit resources effectively; and providing administrative and clinical assistance as needed.

ADVANCED PRACTICE ROLES

Advanced practice or expanded roles include the pediatric nurse practitioner, clinical nurse specialist, and case manager. For the most part, these roles require a master's degree and additional skills in assessing and managing children.

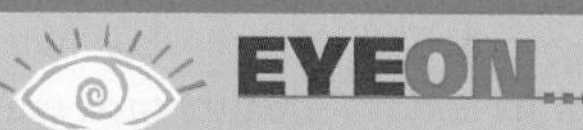

Alternative Treatment Modalities

Many pediatric nurse practitioners use alternative or complementary modalities, either by themselves or in conjunction with conventional medical therapies. One example is herbal therapy, which uses plant extracts for therapeutic outcomes. In pediatrics, infants who are teething may experience pain, fever, diarrhea, and inflamed gums. Traditional medical treatment involves medications such as analgesics, sedatives, or local anesthetics. Many PNPs utilize herbs such as chamomile in conjunction with medications and have found this therapy effective.

Pediatric Nurse Practitioner

The **pediatric nurse practitioner** (PNP) role evolved to meet the need in the 1960s and 1970s for primary care providers of routine health maintenance and preventative services in ambulatory settings. The PNP usually is a registered nurse who has received advanced education (often a master's degree) and graduated from a nurse practitioner program. In the past, the PNP traditionally worked in ambulatory or clinic settings and focused on disease prevention, minor disease management, and well children and families. Today, the PNP may be employed in acute care settings and focus on management of particular disease entities, or partner with physician groups, HMOs, or other types of managed care organizations.

Practitioners are independent, autonomous, and highly skilled at performing nursing assessments and physical examination, counseling, treating minor health problems, and teaching. The PNP also is able to order, carry out, and evaluate laboratory studies; discriminate between normal and abnormal findings that require treatment, referral, or collaboration with other health care professionals; serve as a consultant to other health care professionals; and identify topics, interpret results, and implement evidence-based findings into practice.

Clinical Nurse Specialist

The **clinical nurse specialist** (CNS) "provides an expert approach to health focused on a refined body of knowledge and specialized practice competencies" (ANA, 1980) and usually has a master's degree in nursing. When initially developed, the CNS role was seen as a way for the nurse who wanted to maintain direct client contact to remain at the bedside and still advance in the profession. The CNS provides expert physical, social, and psychological support and care, consults with nursing staff and other health care personnel, educates clients and families in health care management, conducts practice outcome research, serves as a role model for staff, and validates the nursing observations and interventions that staff make. It is not unusual for the CNS to be competent in providing care during all stages of an illness and function in any setting where clients are found, such as clinics, community agencies, or long-term care facilities. Many work in acute care facilities and have prescriptive practice privileges. Others are used as staff educators or consultants to the health care team, managers, expert clinicians, or researchers. They may also specialize in oncology, neurology, cardiology, or orthopedics.

Case Manager

Case management is a practice model initially developed to minimize fragmentation of services and maximize individualization of care. Both quality and cost outcomes are important in case management, which promotes continuity of care by using an interdisciplinary team (nurses, physicians, physical and occupational therapists, social workers). The case manager, often the nurse, coordinates the interdisciplinary care plan which is based on evidence-based research and past medical decisions, so the most effective practices, considering the client's condition, are used. Typically, the case manager obtains services the client needs, and then monitors the effectiveness of the services provided. Case management uses a systematic approach that ensures optimal outcomes for clients, including decreasing length of acute care stay, by developing clinical pathways which are designed to achieve specific client outcomes in a defined time frame. These critical pathways guide the team through the client's course of therapy, indicating key events that must occur each day in order to achieve an appropriate length of stay. Case management also allocates and coordinates services for individuals who cannot manage their own care or cannot negotiate the health system.

STANDARDS OF CARE AND STANDARDS OF PROFESSIONAL PERFORMANCE

Professional nurses, as well as all health care professionals, are being held more accountable for their actions. This change is translating into more emphasis on adherence to standards of care. The **standard of care** is the accepted action expected of an individual of a certain skill or knowledge level. It is considered the minimal level of functioning and what a reasonable and prudent person would do in a similar situation. Standards are a tool for determining if the care provided was adequate or negligent (less than adequate). Professional standards are derived from regulatory agencies, nursing practice acts, professional nursing organizations, and state or federal laws. Additionally, they come from scientific literature, which is typically research-based or evidence-based, and from health care institutions' policies and procedures. Standards are used not only to evaluate the effectiveness of nursing care provided, but also are used in litigation as a legal yardstick to determine if care can be considered acceptable nursing practice.

Specific standards of care and professional performance have been developed for pediatric clinical nursing practice by the American Nurses Association (ANA) and the Society of Pediatric Nurses (SPN). Other standards of practice have been developed by pediatric nursing specialty groups, such as oncology and emergency nursing.

MEETING THE CHALLENGES OF THE 21ST CENTURY

Child health care has changed considerably over the past 20 years. Health care systems were previously focused on the treatment of disease. Health care personnel placed a greater emphasis on treating disease while neglecting early detection and treatment of illness as well as health promotion and maintenance. Disease treatment usually involved invasive procedures through medical technology in acute care settings, a costly approach. Financing and reorganization of services has changed to a managed care system. With managed care, the traditional physician-oriented focus has shifted to a payer-oriented focus emphasizing health promotion, disease prevention, and cost containment. Cost cutting in health care institutions is currently pervasive in the market-driven system of the United States, resulting in a move from inpatient acute care to more ambulatory and community-based care. Health promotion has always been an area of strength for nursing practice. Nurses are in an excellent position to be leaders in today's health care market. Additional major shifts have occurred in providing health care, including:

- Children in inpatient facilities having conditions that are more acute
- Shorter length of stay in these facilities
- Increased incidence of chronic illnesses
- Constraints on delivery of care, including reduced human and material resources
- Advances in telecommunications and information technology

These changes in the health care delivery system have resulted in unprecedented challenges for nurses who care for children and their families.

IN THE REAL WORLD

I have been so impressed with the attention paid to the prevention of disease and the promotion of health here at the hospital even though many children have an already existing disease like diabetes. I also have begun to realize that when working with children who have a disease like diabetes, as much if not more attention is directed toward teaching and advocating for the patient and family than toward administering medications and performing other nursing activities. Yes, I know that medical expertise is important, but the teaching from nursing staff and the encouraging of the family to ask questions of the staff and give input regarding what will work for them in managing the disease is so important. Physicians and nurses must realize that patients (and their families) who do not understand how to control their disease will have problems and may return to the hospital for care. Taking the time to answer questions over and over again is so important. Indeed, being an educator and an advocate are important roles for the nurse when working with children and their families.

Broad access to the Internet has made available vast amounts of health information for health care providers as well as for caregivers. The public is becoming so well informed about its health problems that the mystique and, therefore, the power of medical providers is diminishing. Clients are challenging clinicians with information obtained on the Web, and the increasing available health information is changing the nurse's role from health expert to information broker. Pharmaceutical manufacturers are widely advertising benefits of their latest medication, generating additional questions. Yet this information is of variable quality. Nurses caring for children will need to be able to use critical appraisal skills to evaluate health information and to help caregivers interpret it. They can direct families to valid websites, identify reliable sources of information, and teach evaluation skills.

KEY CONCEPTS

- Current societal trends affecting children, their health, and their families include many challenges; among the most persistent in the United States are immigration, poverty, homelessness, migrant farm work, and violence.
- *Healthy People 2010 and 2020* sets forth national health goals and objectives for adults and children, and focuses on disease prevention and health promotion.
- The aggregate health status of infants, children, and adolescents is determined statistically by keeping records of indicators such as infant mortality rate, low birth weight, child mortality rate, and immunization rate.
- The infant mortality rate remains stubbornly high in the United States, and low birth weight is considered the leading cause of infant mortality.
- The leading cause of death in children 1 to 19 years of age is unintentional injuries, with the majority of deaths resulting from motor vehicle occupant injury.
- Family-centered care is based on principles that are designed to promote greater family self-determination, decision-making capabilities, control, and self-efficacy.
- The primary roles of pediatric nurses include caregiver, advocate, educator, researcher, and manager or leader.
- Diversity of pediatric health care settings and a shift in focus of health care from treatment of disease to promotion of health have led to nurses functioning in advanced practice or expanded roles such as pediatric nurse practitioners, clinical nurse specialists, and case managers.

REVIEW ACTIVITIES

1. Describe how poverty affects children.
2. Define infant mortality and child mortality.
3. What can nurses do to prevent firearm-related injuries and deaths in the home, school, and community?
4. Which of the following is the leading cause of death in children under 19 years of age?
   a. Cancer
   b. Heart disease
   c. Congenital anomalies
   d. Unintentional injuries
5. Name a few major health protection measures that have reduced the incidence of childhood mortality.
6. What strategies can nurses include in their practice that relate to family-centered care?
7. Describe each of the roles that nurses take when interacting with children and their families, and explain how they are connected to one another.
8. Define differentiated practice, and describe why it was developed.
9. Discuss the differences between the pediatric nurse practitioner and the pediatric clinical specialist.
10. Describe case management, and discuss why it was developed.

STUDY QUESTIONS

1. Parents and children from immigrant families face several challenges. Which of the statements below related to these children and families is true?
   a. These parents are able to help their children with homework.
   b. These parents have an excellent understanding of the English language.
   c. These children often are not enrolled in preschool programs that prepare them for school.
   d. These children rarely face challenges related to their health status.
2. Children growing up in poverty are affected by their situation in a number of ways. Which one of the following statements is correct?
   a. Children living in a two-parent home are more likely to live in poverty than children growing up in a single-parent home.
   b. Compared with non-poor children, poor children experience diminished physical health, and suffer such ailments as asthma, respiratory infections, and anemia.
   c. Stunted growth (low height for age), a measure of nutritional status, is more prevalent among non-poor than poor children.
   d. A child's poverty status at 3 years of age is not related to the child's IQ at age 5, and transitory poverty has more adverse effects on a child's cognitive functioning than persistent poverty.
3. An increasing number of children and families in all communities in the United States are homeless. Which one of the following statements is true?
   a. Families with children are among the fastest growing subdivision of the homeless population.
   b. Homelessness is rarely seen in suburban and rural areas.
   c. Compared with housed children, homeless youth have a lower incidence of chronic health problems.
   d. Homeless families rarely have difficulty accessing health care and most homeless children receive adequate preventive care including immunizations and well-child services.
4. Which of the following is a true statement related to violence?
   a. Schools need to have violence prevention programs in schools starting at the middle school level, since if presented earlier the children do not have the cognitive ability to understand the message.
   b. Physical fights, thefts, weapon carrying, teacher victimization, and fear of school environments are no longer the issues they once were for children and adolescents.
   c. Risk factors for violence include history of early aggressive behavior, associating with delinquent peers, involvement in gangs, poor academic performance, low commitment to school, or school failure.
   d. It is easier to keep adolescents away from guns than to keep guns away from adolescents.
5. There are several roles pediatric nurses can take in practice. Which of the following statements is true?
   a. Researchers inform clients and families of their rights and options as well as the consequences of those options.
   b. Nurses working with children and families in the advocate role will prepare children and families for procedures, surgery, or the hospitalization experience itself.
   c. Educators identify clinical practice questions needing answers, examine the literature for answers to these questions, and then determine whether or not those answers (interventions) are appropriate for practice.
   d. Caregivers diagnose and monitor patients, administer therapeutic interventions and regimens, ensure quality health care practices, and effectively manage rapidly changing situations.
6. A pediatric nurse fulfills one or several different roles in practice. These roles are described as primary or secondary. Select the secondary role.
   a. advocate
   b. educator
   c. coordinator
   d. caregiver
7. The terminology "accident" has been replaced with "injury, intentional or unintentional" for the purposes of gathering statistics. Select the one answer below which is the primary reason for this change.
   a. "Injury" is easier to chart than "accident."
   b. "Accidents" are the leading cause for mortality or morbidity among the pediatric population.
   c. "Accident" suggests a lack of predictability or avoidability, whereas intentional or unintentional injury suggests avoidance or prevention is possible.
   d. Infectious disease, not accident, is the leading cause of mortality among children today.
8. Several key tactics have been credited as critical in reducing the incidence of unintentional injuries of

children. Which of the following is NOT one of these tactics?
a. using child car seats and bicycle helmets
b. requiring child-resistant caps for prescription medications
c. suggesting that all guns be stored unloaded with bullets in a separate place
d. enclosing swimming pools with fences

9. The health status of children in the United States can be assessed using statistics gathered by public health agencies and organizations around the world. When compared to the developed economies of the world, the United States:
a. has the lowest percentage of children living in poverty.
b. has the lowest infant mortality rate (IMR).
c. has the highest percentage of premature births in the world.
d. has a lower infant mortality rate than Canada or Cuba.

10. In the prevention of unintentional injuries among children, several key strategies have been identified as very important for parent education. Which of the following is NOT one of these strategies?
a. Nurses need to educate caregivers to promote safe behaviors for themselves and their children.
b. Nurses need to educate caregivers about expected behaviors for the child's current developmental stage and the upcoming developmental stage (anticipatory guidance).
c. Nurses need to educate caregivers about making the home environment safer for the child.
d. Nurses need to educate caregivers about making the school environment safer for the child.

REFERENCES

American Nurses Association. (1980). *Nursing: A social policy statement.* Kansas City: Author.

Annie E. Casey Foundation. (2009). *2009 KIDS COUNT Data Book*, Baltimore, MD. Retrieved from http://www.aecf.org.

Behrman, R. (2004). Children of immigrant families. *The Future of Children, 14*(2). Retrieved from http://www.futureofchildren.org/futureofchildren/publications/journals/journal_details/index.xml?journalid=39.

Benner, P. (1984). *From novice to expert: Excellence and power in clinical nursing practice.* Menlo Park: Addison-Wesley.

Bicycle Helmet Safety Institute. (2009). *Mandatory helmet laws: A summary.* Retrieved September 15, 2009, from http://www.helmets.org.

Boston, C. (1990). Introduction. In C. Boston (Ed.). *Current issues and perspectives on differentiated practice.* Chicago: American Organization of Nurse Executives.

Centers for Disease Control and Prevention. (2008). *Health, United States, 2008.* Hyattsville, MD: National Center for Health Statistics.

Centers for Disease Control and Prevention. (2009a). Understanding Youth Violence Fact Sheet 2009. Retrieved September 15, 2009, from http://www.cdc.gov/ViolencePrevention/pdf/YV-FactSheet-a.pdf.

Centers for Disease Control and Prevention. (2009b). Youth Violence Fact at a Glance Summer 2009. Retrieved September 15, 2009, from http://www.cdc.gov/ViolencePrevention/pdf/YV-DataSheet-a.pdf.

Centers for Disease Control and Prevention. (2010). Understanding School Violence Fact Sheet 2010. Retrieved April 11, 2010 from http://www.cdc.gov/ViolencePrevention/pdf/SchoolViolence_FactSheet-a.pdf.

Children's Defense Fund. (2009). The state of America's children December 2009. Washington, DC: Author. Retrieved January 5, 2010, from http://www.childrensdefense.org/.

DeNavas-Walt, C., Proctor, B., & Smith, J. (2009). U.S. Census Bureau, Current Population Reports, P60-236, *Income, Poverty, and Health Insurance Coverage in the United States: 2008*, U.S. Government Printing Office, Washington, DC.

Economic Policy Institute. (2009). "The promises and pitfalls of the new economy": The state of working America. Retrieved November 19, 2009, from http://www.stateofworkingamerica.org.

Economist United States. (2009). Poorer, but at least not sicker. Sep 17, 2009. Retrieved November 19, 2009, from http://www.economist.com/world/unitedstates/PrinterFriendly.cfm?story_id=14460209.

Federal Interagency Forum on Child and Family Statistics. (2005). America's Children: Key National Indicators of Well-Being, 2005.

Federal Interagency Forum on Child and Family Statistics. (2009). America's Children: Key National Indicators of Well-Being, 2009. Retrieved September 15, 2009, from http://www.childstats.gov/pdf/ac2009/ac_09.pdf.

Flores, G., & Tomany-Korman, S. (2008). Racial and ethnic disparities in medical and dental health, access to care, and use of services in US children. *Pediatrics, 121*(2), E286–E298.

Haldenby, A., Berman, H., & Forchuk, C. (2007). Homelessness and health in adolescents. *Qualitative Health Research, 17*(9), 1232–1244.

Hernandez, D., Denton, N., & Macartney, S. (2007). Children in immigrant families firmly rooted in America; Three out of four speak English fluently. Retrieved April 11, 2010, from http://www.childtrends.org/_pressrelease_page.cfm?LID=FCC35EFD-8F63-475D-86871DB5535AA710.

Institute for Children and Poverty. (2010). National data on family homelessness. Retrieved April 11, 2010, from http://www.icpny.org/index.asp?CID=7.

Institute of Medicine. (2007). Preterm birth: Causes, consequences and prevention. Washington, DC: National Academies Press.

Lawn, J., Cousens, S., & Zupan, J. (2005). 4 million neonatal deaths: When? Where? Why? *Lancet, 365*, 891–900.

March of Dimes Foundation. (2009). White paper on preterm birth. White Plains, NY. Retrieved April 11, 2010, from http://marchofdimes.com.

National Coalition for the Homeless. (2008). Who is homeless? NCH Fact Sheet #3. Retrieved April 11, 2010, from http://www.nationalhomeless.org/factsheets/who.html.

Polit, D., & Beck, C. (2010). *Essentials of nursing research: Appraising evidence for nursing practice* (7th ed.). Philadelphia, PA: Lippincott Williams & Wilkins.

Puzzanchera C. (2009). Juvenile Arrests 2007: Juvenile Justice Bulletin. Washington, DC: Office of Juvenile Justice and Delinquency Prevention. Retrieved September 15, 2009, from http://www.ncjrs.gov/pdffiles1/ojjdp/225344.pdf.

Scudder, B. C., Chaser, L. C., Wentz, D. A., Bauch, N. J., Brigham, M. E., Moran, P. W., & Krabbenhoft, D. P. (2010). Mercury in fish, bed sediment, and water from streams across the United States, 1998–2005: U.S. Geological Survey Scientific Investigations Report 2009-5109. Retrieved April 11, 2010, from http://pubs.usgs.gov/sir/2009/5109.

Shelton, T. L., & Stepanek, J. S. (1994). *Family-centered care for children needing specialized health and developmental services.* Bethesda, MD: Association for the Care of Children's Health.

United Nations High Commissioner for Human Rights. (1959). *Declaration of the Rights of the Child.* Proclaimed by General Assembly Resolution 1386 (XIV) of November 20, 1959. Retrieved August 8, 2005, from http://www.kidsrights.org/UNDeclaration.htm.

U.S. Department of Health and Human Services. (2010). *Healthy People 2020: The Road Ahead.* Washington DC: Author. Retrieved April 11, 2010, from http://www.healthypeople.gov/hp2020/.

U.S. Department of Health and Human Services. (2000). *Healthy People 2010: National health promotion and disease prevention objectives.* Washington DC: Author.

Wilson, A., Wold, J., Spencer, L., & Pittman, K. (2000). Primary health care for Hispanic children of migrant farm workers. *Journal of Pediatric Health Care, 14,* 209–215.

SUGGESTED READINGS

Alfaro-Lefevre, R. (2004). *Critical thinking and clinical judgment* (3rd ed.). Philadelphia: WB Saunders.

American Association of Colleges of Nursing (AACN), American Organization of Nurse Executives. (1995). *A model for differentiated nursing practice.* Washington, DC: AACN.

Chistopherson, T., & Jordan-Marsh, M. (2004). Culture and risk taking in adolescents' behavior. *Journal of Maternal and Child Nursing, 29*(2), 100–105.

Melnyk, B., Fineout-Overholt, E., Stone, P., & Ackerman, M. (2000). Evidence-based practice: The past, the present, and recommendations for the millennium. *Pediatric Nursing, 26*(1), 77–80.

Velsor-Friedrich, B. (2000). *Healthy People 2000/2010*: Health appraisal of the nation and future objectives. *Journal of Pediatric Nursing, 15*(1), 47–48.

RESOURCES

Refer to the online student StudyWARE for Potts & Mandleco at http://www.CengageBrain.com for additional content and study aids.

Organization: **Agency for Health Care Research and Quality**
Description: The federal agency charged with improving the quality, safety, efficiency, and effectiveness of health care for all Americans; offers information on current research, approved surveys/data collection methods, and customer/patient safety policies.
Website/Resource: http://www.ahrq.gov

Organization: **American Academy of Nurse Practitioners**
Description: The only full-service national professional membership organization for NPs; continually advocates at local, state, and federal levels for the recognition of NPs as providers of high-quality, cost-effective, and personalized health care.
Website/Resource: http://www.aanp.org

Organization: **American Academy of Pediatrics**
Description: Offers general information related to child health, specific guidelines concerning many pediatric issues, information regarding AAP programs, activities, policies, guidelines, publications, and other child health resources.
Website/Resource: http://www.aap.org

Organization: **American Nurses Association**
Description: Offers access to information regarding registered nurse career updates, professional nursing practice guidelines, nursing ethnics, current health care policies, government affairs, and occupational environment information.
Website/Resource: http://www.ana.org

Organization: **Annie E. Casey Foundation**
Description: Dedicated to helping build better futures for disadvantaged children, this website offers information regarding Foundation initiatives, child and family services, and publications.
Website/Resource: http://www.aecf.org

Organization: **Case Management Society of America**
Description: Offers information regarding individual/employer/partner case management options; information regarding current policy and local outreach efforts pertaining to case management.
Website/Resource: http://www.cmsa.org

Organization: **Centers for Disease Control and Prevention (CDC)**
Description: Offers information regarding current disease conditions, emergency preparedness/response, life stages/populations, healthy living, workplace environment/health.
Website/Resource: http://www.cdc.gov

Organization: **Children's Defense Fund (CDF)**
Description: A nonprofit child advocacy organization; website offers information regarding CDF's policies and mission, child advocacy resources, and child research data.
Website/Resource: http://www.childrensdefense.org

Organization: **Maternal and Child Health Bureau (MCHB)**
Description: Offers information regarding current MCHB programs, funding opportunities, reports and resources/publications.
Website/Resource: http://mchb.hrsa.gov

Organization: **National Association of Pediatric Nurse Associates and Practitioners (NAPNAP)**
Description: Offers information regarding NAPNAP's mission/efforts, upcoming events, associated programs and access to NAPNAP's online store.
Website/Resource: http://www.napnap.org

Organization: **National Safety Council**
Description: Offers information regarding safe practices at work, home and on the road as well as information concerning current safety news/resources and safety products.
Website/Resource: http://www.nsc.org

Organization: **Office of Juvenile Justice and Delinquency Prevention (OJJDP)**
Description: Offers information regarding OJJDP partnerships/programs, statistics, publications, funding, and events.
Website/Resource: http://ojjdp.ncjrs.org

Organization: **Society of Pediatric Nurses (SPN)**
Description: Offers access to information regarding SPN committees, conventions, chapters, awards/scholarships, and much more.
Website/Resource: http://www.pedsnurses.org

Organization: **The Brady Center to Prevent Handgun Violence**
Description: Offers blogging opportunities as well as general facts and legislation regarding gun violence.
Website/Resource: http://www.bradycenter.org

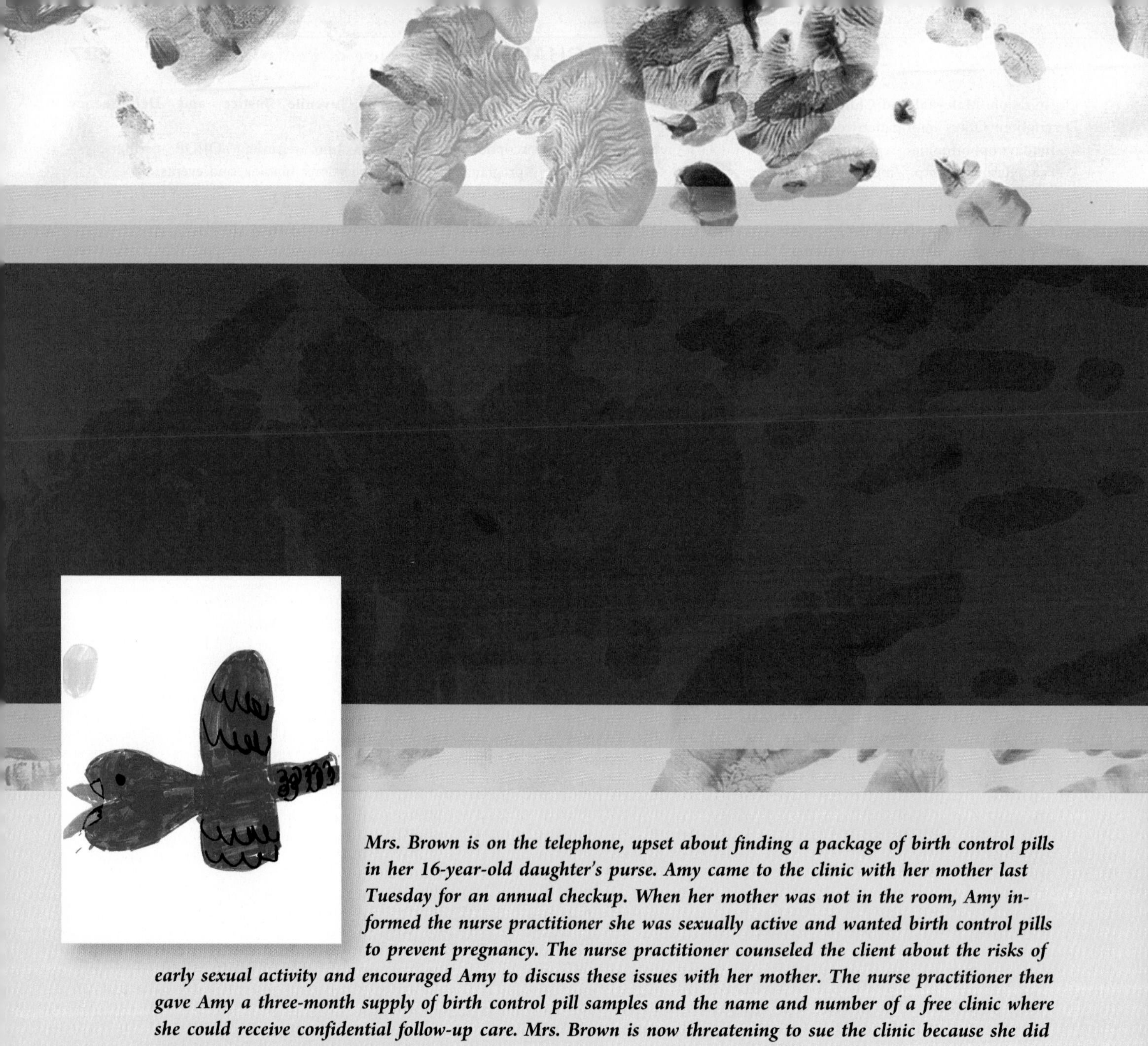

Mrs. Brown is on the telephone, upset about finding a package of birth control pills in her 16-year-old daughter's purse. Amy came to the clinic with her mother last Tuesday for an annual checkup. When her mother was not in the room, Amy informed the nurse practitioner she was sexually active and wanted birth control pills to prevent pregnancy. The nurse practitioner counseled the client about the risks of early sexual activity and encouraged Amy to discuss these issues with her mother. The nurse practitioner then gave Amy a three-month supply of birth control pill samples and the name and number of a free clinic where she could receive confidential follow-up care. Mrs. Brown is now threatening to sue the clinic because she did not give permission for Amy to receive birth control pills.

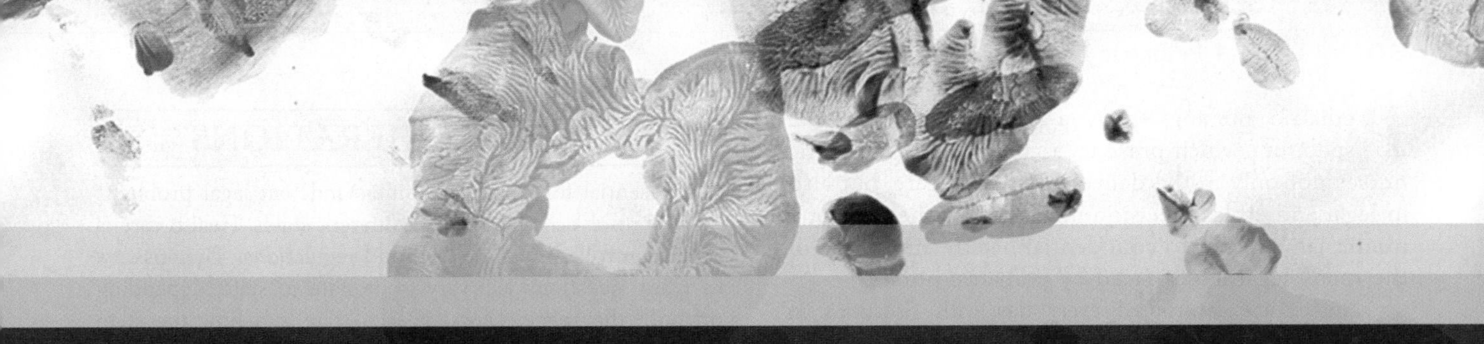

CHAPTER 2

Legal and Ethical Issues

Lynn Clark Callister, RN, PhD, FAAN
Susan Chasson, MSN, JD, CNM, FNP-BC

COMPETENCIES

Upon completion of this chapter, the reader will be able to:

- List state, federal, and judicial sources of law.
- Identify the elements of informed consent.
- Describe a situation in which a minor can consent to or refuse health care.
- Identify situations in which a nurse can breach confidentiality.
- List the elements of negligence, and describe nursing practices that can reduce the risk of malpractice claims.
- Identify major ethical theories and principles.
- Describe the process of ethical decision making.
- Discuss several ethical dilemmas and how these influence children, their caregivers and families, and health care professionals.
- Describe the role of ethics councils in nursing practice.
- Successfully complete the games and activities in the online student StudyWARE.

Pediatric nursing spans a broad developmental spectrum which presents a challenge for pediatric nurses not only in the delivery of health care, but also in legal and ethical decision making. Whether or not a minor can consent to confidential health care is one of the many legal issues faced by pediatric nurses.

Nurses are confronted every day with situations in which difficult decisions must be made based on the determination of right and wrong. Technological advances have created unprecedented choices for nurses as well as children and their families. Pediatric critical care nurses encounter ethical dilemmas such as whether or not to resuscitate a dying child whose quality of life may be tenuous, or which treatment option will provide the most benefit with the least harm for a child. Nurses experience moral distress which occurs when poor quality or futile care is provided, when nurses have not been successful in being patient advocates, or when unrealistic hope has been provided to children and their families (Schulter, Winch, Holzhauser, & Henderson, 2008). It is essential for nurses to have a basic understanding of the laws that affect their practice and the ethical guidelines that can be used to resolve dilemmas. This chapter explores pediatric legal topics, along with the concept of ethics, ethical theories and principles, and the process of ethical decision making.

LEGAL CONSIDERATIONS

It is essential for nurses to understand that legal problems may be resolved differently in different states. Health care is often controlled by state laws and regulations. The answers to many questions will vary from state to state, depending on both the specific laws of each state and how the state courts interpret those laws. If a nurse needs a legal opinion about an issue or concern, a licensed attorney who is familiar with the specific area of law should be consulted. Table 2-1 lists the different sources of law.

INFORMED CONSENT AND ASSENT FOR HEALTH CARE

In 1914, Justice Benjamin Cardozo stated, "Every human being of adult years and sound mind has a right to determine what shall be done with his own body ..." (*Schloendorff v. Society of N.Y. Hospital*, 1914). This landmark court case provided the legal foundation for requiring informed consent prior to receipt of health care. **Informed consent** is the duty of a health care provider to discuss the risk/benefits of a treatment/procedure with an individual prior to giving care. Informed consent includes the nature of the procedure, and

TABLE 2-1 Sources of Law

SOURCES OF LAW	EXAMPLES
Constitutional law (uphold Constitution, Bill of Rights, and other 16 Constitutional amendments)	The U.S. Supreme Court has interpreted the Constitution to include the right of privacy. The right of privacy is fundamental to the Supreme Court's decisions involving the right to die and access to contraception and abortion.
Federal laws and regulations (congressional laws or federal statutes, Health Care Financing Administration [HCFA], Occupational Safety and Health Administration [OSHA], Food and Drug Administration [FDA])	Law: Emergency Medical Treatment and Active Labor Act require all hospitals that accept payment for Medicaid and Medicare to follow specified procedures before transferring a client from an emergency room to another hospital. Regulations: OSHA-developed regulations.
State laws and regulations	Laws: Nurse Practice Acts; Good Samaritan Acts; Mandatory Reporting Laws (child or elder abuse). Regulations: Nurse Practice Acts can state a nurse needs to graduate from an approved nursing program, yet board of nursing will determine by regulation what is an approved nursing program.
Case law (laws that result from judicial decision)	Judicial interpretation of Americans with Disabilities Act (ADA) of 1990 (federal law). The act states that "reasonable accommodation" must be made for handicapped employees. The ADA does not define reasonable accommodation. In the case of *Howell v. Michelin Tire Corp.* (1994), the court decided that it would be "reasonable accommodation" to reassign an employee with a disability to an existing light-duty job that was vacant. Once a case is decided by a judge, attorneys use these legal decisions to help their clients understand how to interpret and follow the law.

the risks, alternatives, and benefits of treatment. After receiving informed consent, an individual has the right to accept or refuse any health care. A health care facility or health care provider that treats an individual without proper consent may be charged with assault and held liable for any damages. While children and adolescents are entitled to informed **assent**, it is usually the role of the child's parent or legal guardian to give informed consent. In most cases, a child is asked to give assent prior to receiving a treatment or a procedure. Assent means the pediatric client has been informed about what will happen during the treatment or procedure, and is willing to permit a health care provider to perform the care.

For example, a 10-year-old boy comes into the office to have stitches placed in his right hand. The health care provider asks the child's parent for informed consent after the parent has been provided information about the risks and benefits of local anesthesia and the placement of sutures. Alternatives to suturing and the risks of leaving the wound open are discussed. Once the parent provides informed consent, the boy is asked to assent to the procedure. The boy is told that a tiny needle will be used to put a little numbing medication in the skin. When the skin is numb, the health care provider will place some stitches to close the cut. If the child agrees to have stitches, he has given assent to the procedure. While assent from the minor is not legally required when giving needed health care, federal law requires that all children age seven and older give assent before participating in medical research (Unguru, Coppes, & Kamani, 2008). Assent from the child may maximize success of the procedure and minimize trauma to the child.

WHEN INFORMED CONSENT IS NOT REQUIRED

Most health care facilities will provide care to a minor or an adult in an emergency situation if informed consent cannot be obtained. A **minor** is defined as a person (18 years or younger, by the laws of most states) who has not yet obtained the age at which she or he is considered to have the rights and responsibilities of an adult. When consent is not obtained for an adult, it is usually because the individual is unconscious or physically unable to consent. The care given under these circumstances is usually an emergency lifesaving procedure. Health care providers may provide emergency care to a child if they have made a reasonable attempt to contact the child's parent or legal guardian. When that person cannot be located, especially in the case of an adolescent, it is prudent to obtain informed consent from the child (Roberson, 2007). Many states allow the evaluation and treatment of a child for suspected physical or sexual abuse without the informed consent of a parent or guardian. In Utah, physicians can take photographs or x-rays of a child without parental consent if they suspect child abuse (Utah Code Annotated 62A-4a-406).

Legally, it may not be necessary to obtain parental consent prior to performing a forensic examination such as for evidence of sexual assault, but it is important to have the assent of the child or adolescent prior to starting an examination. A **medical forensic examination** is performed for the dual purpose of the "provision of medical care for victims ... (and) collection of evidence from victims, which may aid investigation and prosecution" (U.S. Department of Justice Office of Violence Against Women, 2004, p.13). In cases of sexual assault or abuse, a child should never be forcibly restrained for an examination. If there is a medical reason to obtain an examination, such as vaginal bleeding, anesthesia may be considered (Bernard, Peters, & Makoroff, 2006). Forcing a child to participate in a forensic examination may damage the child's ability to testify in a criminal case, especially if the child perceives the medical examination as another episode of abuse (Figure 2-1).

WHEN A MINOR CAN CONSENT FOR CARE

In all but three states a minor is a person under the age of 18. In Alabama and Nebraska the age of majority is 19 and in Mississippi the age of majority is 21. The **age of majority** is the age at which a person is considered to have all the legal rights and responsibilities of an adult. One of the rights given to adults is the legal right to give consent for health care. There are exceptions for when a minor can consent to health care. In many states a child under the age of 18 can consent to care involving pregnancy, contraception, or treatment of sexually transmitted infections, without consent from or notification of a parent or guardian. In many states, a child under the age of 18 can consent to specialized types of care without the notification or consent of parents. Children may also seek drug and alcohol treatment without the consent of a caregiver. The purpose of these laws is to encourage children to seek help in situations in which they might avoid care if they were required to inform their caregivers (Baren, 2006). Some states allow minors to make

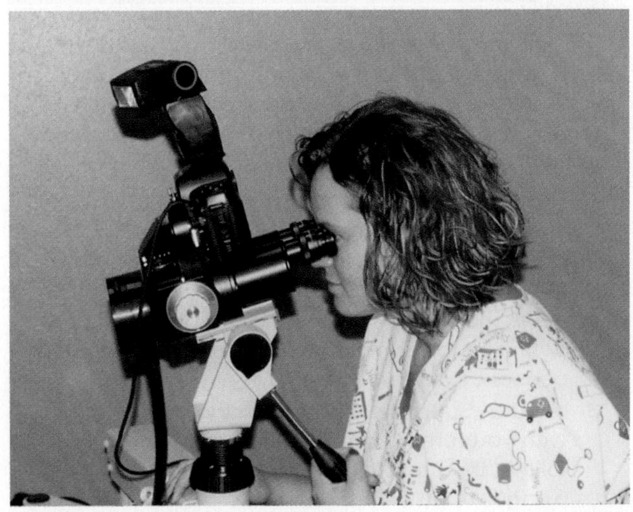

FIGURE 2-1 Sexual Abuse Examination. DELMAR CENGAGE LEARNING.

health care decisions if, under the laws of the state, the minor is considered to be emancipated. **Emancipation** is the legal recognition that a minor lives independently and is legally responsible for his or her own support and decision making. Emancipation can occur through an official court proceeding. During the proceeding, the judge will establish whether the minor is living on his or her own and no longer requires the financial support of parents. In some states, a minor may become automatically emancipated by marrying, joining the military, or becoming a parent before the age of majority. Emancipation laws vary from state to state, and some states do not officially recognize any form of emancipation.

A minor who has not achieved emancipation may be able to consent to health care in some states following the **mature minor doctrine**, under which a minor can consent to care as long as the individual demonstrates the maturity to understand the risks and benefits of the treatment. The mature minor doctrine is another example of how the courts create laws through decisions made by judges. Unless the definition of a mature minor is defined by a law or statute, appellate courts in each state have the ability to define the legal requirements for a mature minor. This definition can be created only when a case that disputes the ability of a child to make a health care decision is brought to court. In 1989, the Illinois Supreme Court decided, "To permit a minor to make her own health care decisions a court must find, by clear and convincing evidence, that a minor is mature enough to appreciate consequences of actions and mature enough to exercise the judgment of an adult ..." (*E.G. v. E.G.*, 1989). In Tennessee, "Whether a minor has capacity to consent to medical treatment depends upon age, ability, experience, education, degree of maturity or judgment obtained by the minor ..." (*Caldwell v. Bechtol*, 1987).

CRITICAL THINKING

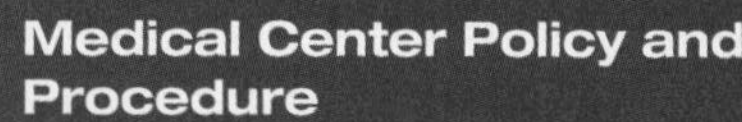

Medical Center Policy and Procedure

You are the nurse risk manager for a hospital in a state where there are no statutes or court decisions determining when a minor can consent for health care. It is your job to create a hospital policy defining when a child can consent for care.

1. Does the Illinois Supreme Court provide a definition that would allow your hospital to create precise guidelines for when a minor can consent to care? Why?
2. Does the Tennessee court provide a better definition for deciding when a minor can give consent for health care? Why?
3. If a U.S. Supreme Court decision conflicts with your state statute, which rule would you follow, the state law or the Supreme Court ruling?

PARENTAL CONSENT AFTER DIVORCE

After divorce, the ability to consent for health care rests with the parent who has been granted legal custody by the **divorce decree** (the legal document approved by the court that grants divorce, divides marital property, and specifies child custody). In order to serve the best interests of the child, the court will often grant both parents legal custody of the child. This means that both parents will be able to give consent for medical care. Even when one parent has legal custody, the parent who has physical custody of the child may be able to give informed consent for emergency care (Elrod, 2001). For example, if a child is visiting the parent who does not have legal custody, the one who is physically present with the child may be able to consent for emergency care. If parents have joint legal custody and disagree on whether or not a child needs medical care, it may be necessary to obtain a court order before providing care.

REFUSAL OF HEALTH CARE BY PARENT OR CHILD

What are the rights of the child when a parent refuses health care that could benefit the child? In most instances, a parent will seek appropriate health care for an ill child. However, there are cases in which an individual refuses to give consent for potentially lifesaving health care when it conflicts with her or his religious beliefs. If a parent refuses to act in the best interests of the child, the state may step in and make legal decisions for the child. Under the theory of parens patrie, the state has an overriding interest in the health and welfare of a child. **Parens patrie** is a legal rule that allows the state to make decisions in place of parents when they are unable or unwilling to provide for the best interests of the child.

In certain situations, adolescents have been able to refuse health care without notifying or obtaining consent from their parents. Using the mature minor doctrine, some courts have allowed older adolescents to refuse lifesaving medical treatment or to refuse health care that prolongs a terminal illness (Slonina, 2007).

Some states use child abuse statutes that make medical neglect a form of abuse as legal justification to take custody of a child who needs medical care. While many of these abuse statutes include an exemption for religious practices, the court will still take custody of an endangered child. The religious exemption clause only prevents the parents from being prosecuted for medical neglect. However, religious exemptions do not protect parents when medical neglect has resulted in the death of a child (Chen, 2007). The ability of the state to take legal custody or guardianship of a child is usually limited to circumstances in which the life of a child is endangered.

OBTAINING INFORMED CONSENT UNDER SPECIAL CIRCUMSTANCES

Advances in medical and nursing science create both new opportunities and new legal conflicts. Often the legal implications of new technologies are not anticipated until a conflict occurs. Legislation is often created after a problem is given a legal interpretation by the courts.

CONSENT FOR DONATION OF TISSUE OR ORGANS

The improved availability of transplant technology has increased the demand for suitable donors of tissue and organs. An organ or tissue from a living child may be the only hope of survival for a terminally ill sibling or other family member. When a child is too young to give informed consent for organ or tissue donation, the parent or legal guardian may consent for the child. Usually a court hearing will be required to establish whether the individual providing consent is acting in the best interests of the child who is donating the tissue or organ. In the case of *Curran v. Bosze* (1990), the Supreme Court of Illinois decided that for a minor child to donate tissue, three requirements must be met. First, the parent who is consenting must be aware of the risks and benefits. Second, the child's primary caregiver must be able to provide emotional support for the child. Third, there must be a close relationship between the donor and the recipient. The American Academy of Pediatrics feels it is permissible for minors to donate organs if the following conditions are met: both the potential donor and recipient will benefit, the surgical risk to the donor is low, no other options for transplantation from an adult donor exists, the minor is able to freely consent without coercion, and emotional and psychological risks to the donor are minimized (Ross, Thistlethwaite, & the Committee on Bioethics, 2008). It is important to realize that other state courts may require different standards to be met before allowing a minor to participate in tissue or organ donation.

CONSENT FOR GENETIC TESTING

Another dilemma created by new technology is genetic testing of children. While a parent or guardian can consent to genetic testing for the child, as in the case of all diagnostic tests, the benefits and the risks should be discussed with the child when appropriate. Since most genetic testing requires only a blood sample, there is usually no physical risk to the child. There are numerous guidelines for the genetic testing of children for adult onset diseases. Also, many others recommend testing only when there is medical benefit to the child and medical interventions exist to treat the condition (Stultiens, Nys, Cassiman, & Dierickx, 2006).

REFLECTIVE THINKING

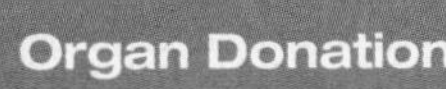

Organ Donation

You are a registered nurse and your 17-year-old son is the star quarterback for his high school football team. A football scholarship may be his only hope for a college education. Your 13-year-old daughter is in renal failure and her only chance for long-term survival is a kidney transplant. Her brother is a perfect match for a transplant. If your son donates a kidney, he will be advised not to participate in contact sports, including football, due to the possibility of injuring his one remaining kidney. How would you approach your children and talk to them about choices that will determine their futures?

Overall, the best interests of the child should be evaluated before any genetic testing is ordered. A health care facility that offers genetic testing should be able to provide appropriate counseling both before testing and after results are received. The facility should also establish policies for advocating for the best interests of the child. When possible, informed consent should be obtained from the parent and assent obtained from the child. Finally, there needs to be a process by which a mature adolescent can receive test results without the consent or notification of the parent (American Academy of Pediatrics, 2008a).

CHILDREN AND MEDICAL EXPERIMENTATION

Medical research is an important part of improving health care. Since there are many diseases and physical conditions that have an impact on the lives of children, there is often a need for them to participate in research studies. Most researchers try to use children as research subjects only when the research will benefit the child, or poses little or no risk to the subject. All research facilities that receive federal funds must comply with federal regulations that require review of all experimental protocols by an Institutional Review Board (IRB) (U.S. Dept. of Health & Human Services, 1994). An IRB is a group of professionals that reviews research proposals for an institution to evaluate potential harm to subjects. The IRB also makes sure that all state and federal regulations are followed by researchers at the institution. Federal regulations require the consent of one or both parents and the assent of the child, depending on the amount of the potential risk and benefit associated with the treatment or procedure. As client advocates, nurses who are involved in pediatric experimental protocols should make sure that all efforts are made to acquire appropriate consent and assent from study participants. Further discussion of children and medical experimentation can be found in the ethical section of this chapter.

BOX 2-1

ELEMENTS OF INFORMED CONSENT FOR HUMAN SUBJECTS' RESEARCH

1. A statement that the study involves research.
2. An exploration of the purpose of the research, delineating the expected duration of the subject's participation.
3. A description of the procedures to be followed and identification of any procedures that are experimental.
4. A description of any reasonably foreseeable risks or discomforts to the subject.
5. A description of any benefits to the subject or to others that may reasonably be expected from the research.
6. A disclosure of appropriate alternative procedures or courses of treatment, if any, that might be advantageous to the subject.
7. A statement describing the extent to which anonymity and confidentiality of the records identifying the subjects will be maintained.
8. For research involving more than minimal risk, an explanation as to whether any medical treatments are available if injury occurs and, if so, what they consist of or where further information may be obtained.
9. An explanation about who to contact for answers to questions about the research and subject's rights, and who to contact in the event of a research-related injury to the subject.
10. A statement that participation is voluntary, that refusal to participate will not involve any penalty or loss of benefit to which the subject is otherwise entitled, and that the subject may discontinue participation at any time without penalty or loss of otherwise entitled benefits.

From: U.S. Department of Health and Human Services. (1994). Code of Federal Regulations, Title 45, Public Welfare. Part 46—Protection of Human Subjects (45 CFR 46). Washington, DC U.S. Government printing office.

CONFIDENTIALITY

The right to confidential health care is protected by the U.S. Constitution, federal and state laws, and the ethical codes of health care professionals. Confidentiality is an essential part of the relationship between client and health care provider. If clients do not feel secure about divulging their medical information to a provider, their care becomes restricted. Nurses play an important role in maintaining client confidentiality (Figure 2-2). They are legally and ethically responsible for keeping medical records and other types of client communications confidential. Most nurse practice acts define a nurse's duty of confidentiality. If a nurse breaches confidentiality, she or he can be held responsible for any damages that result. The nurse may also be disciplined by both the employer and the state board of nursing.

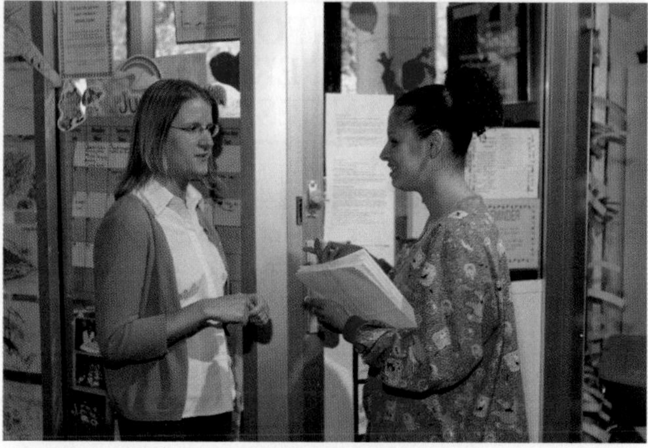

FIGURE 2-2 Nurses must respect client confidentiality and avoid discussing families and cases with co-workers not directly involved in care. DELMAR CENGAGE LEARNING.

WHEN A MINOR CAN RECEIVE CONFIDENTIAL CARE

As stated earlier, some states allow children to access confidential care for contraception, treatment of sexually transmitted infections, drug and alcohol treatment, and mental health care (Lerand, 2007). Some states also provide access to confidential human immunodeficiency virus (HIV) testing. It is important for nurses to be familiar with the laws and regulations concerning confidentiality in the state where they practice.

WHEN A HEALTH CARE PROVIDER CAN BREACH CONFIDENTIALITY

There are four recognized exceptions when a provider can breach client confidentiality. The first is mandatory reporting laws for child abuse. All 50 states have these laws (Gupta, 2007). Nurses need to know if their state defines child abuse to include witnessing domestic violence and at what age a child can consent to sexual relations if the reporting of statutory rape is mandated by their state (Sachs, Weinberg, & Wheeler, 2008). Statutory rape occurs when both partners consent to a sexual encounter but the law states that one or both partners were not old enough to give legal consent. Failure to report suspected abuse by a health care

RESEARCH Highlight

Informed Consent for Enrolling Minors in a Research Study

STUDY PURPOSE

To determine if preserving dignity was part of the delivery of health care to families with a child receiving care.

METHODS

In this qualitative study conducted at a Swedish university hospital pediatric unit, observations were used to collect data, focusing on care activity, place, point in time, professionals present, communication with health care providers and family members, emotional and physical expressions, and activities in the room. Field notes were kept describing observations of caring activities. Twenty families with a child with an acute or chronic illness participated in the study following receipt of parental consent and child assent. Ages of the children ranged from one week to 18 years.

FINDINGS

Major categories identified by the study included maintaining dignity, restoring dignity, and shattering dignity. Dignity was shattered when a focus on the individual and the family was not present. Dignity was restored when family perspectives were acknowledged. Dignity was maintained when there were collaborative relationships between providers and families.

IMPLICATIONS

The importance of family-centered care to the health and well-being of both parents and children was indicated. Ethical pediatric health care includes the preservation of dignity and demonstration of respect.

REFERENCE

Lundqvist, A., & Nilstun, T. (2007). Human dignity in pediatrics: The effects of health care. *Nursing Ethics*, *14*(2), 215–228.

provider may result in criminal charges. Most mandatory reporting laws carry the possibility of both fines and a term of imprisonment for failure to make a report. If a child receives additional injuries after the health care provider should have reported suspected abuse, the provider may be liable for malpractice for failing to appropriately diagnose and treat the abuse.

The second exception is mandatory injury reporting laws that apply to all clients who are injured by a weapon or criminal act. If a client is given care for a gunshot or stab wound, the provider may be required to breach confidentiality and report that information to law enforcement.

NURSING TIP

Mandatory Reporting Laws

When an adolescent is diagnosed with a sexually transmitted infection, it is important to explain to the client that you have an obligation to report the infection to the local health department. If the adolescent understands that the report is required by law and that the information will be handled in a sensitive and appropriate manner, there is a better chance of maintaining a relationship of trust between you and the adolescent.

A provider may also be required to follow public health laws for reporting infectious diseases to the local health department. Many states require providers to report cases of tuberculosis, HIV, hepatitis, and sexually transmitted diseases. Some states also require reporting of poisonings by pesticides or other agricultural products.

Providers may be required to breach confidentiality when there is a duty to warn third parties. In the case of *Tarasoff v. Regents of the University of California* (1976), a psychiatrist was held liable for the death of a woman who was murdered by her boyfriend. The boyfriend, a client of the psychiatrist, had disclosed during a therapy session his intent to kill his girlfriend. The family of the murdered woman sued the psychiatrist and won on the grounds that the physician had a duty to warn the woman about the threat to her life. In this case, the court decided that the risk of harm to a third party outweighed the client's right to confidential health care. The duty to breach confidentiality by warning a third party is required only when there is a specific threat to an identifiable person.

Finally, as the ability to detect risks for diseases through genetic testing increases, health care providers may have a duty to warn persons who have a genetically inherited disease risk. In the case of *Safer v. Estate of Pack* (1996), a physician failed to warn the child of a client that she could have a higher risk of colon cancer and should receive early and frequent screening. When colon cancer developed in the daughter, the physician was sued for failure to warn.

HIPAA AND PATIENT CONFIDENTIALITY

In 2003 the privacy regulations of the Health Insurance Portability and Accountability Act (HIPAA) became enforceable under federal law (42 U.S.C. § 201 et seq). With the computerization of health records and increased access of health information to entities other than health care providers and hospitals, the federal government saw a need to protect this

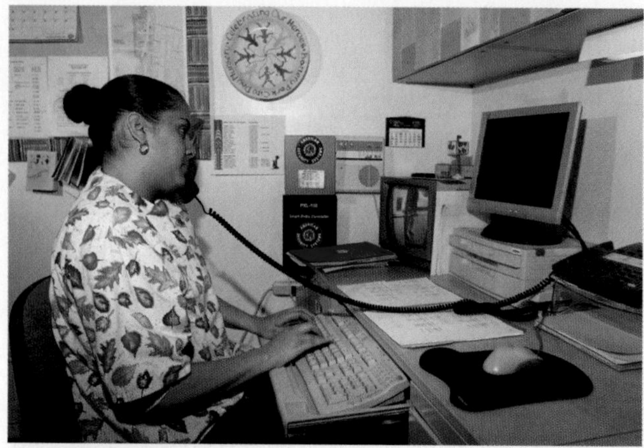

FIGURE 2-3 Under HIPAA regulations, nurses may not disclose client information over the phone without first confirming the identity of the caller and the caller's entitlement to that information. DELMAR CENGAGE LEARNING.

information from improper disclosure. HIPAA applies to all personal health information including electronic, written, or oral information.

To prevent unauthorized access or disclosure of electronic information, proper use of passwords and automatic screensavers should be used on all computers. Client information should not be released without proper consent or written authorization. Client information should not be given over the phone unless the nurse is able to verify that the person receiving the information is someone entitled to that information under the HIPAA regulations (Figure 2-3).

While this law creates many new obligations to maintain client privacy, HIPAA does not override mandatory reporting laws or state privacy laws that create a higher standard than the federal law. It is also important to understand that if a minor is entitled by state or federal law to confidential care, then the personal health information about that care cannot be released without the written authorization of the child. For example, if an adolescent can be seen at a clinic for confidential reproductive care, the parent cannot obtain the child's medical records unless written permission is given by the client.

Under HIPAA, health care providers including hospitals and clinics must appoint a privacy officer whose responsibility is to provide employees with training about privacy rules and procedures. It is important for nurses to be familiar with the privacy policies of their agency and to make sure proper procedures are followed when releasing the personal health information of a client.

MALPRACTICE IN THE PEDIATRIC SETTING

Anyone who works in the field of health care is constantly faced with the issue of negligence or malpractice. **Negligence** is defined as an occasion when a person owes a duty to another and, through failure to fulfill that duty, causes harm. **Malpractice** is professional negligence. It is important to understand that a bad outcome for a client in the hospital or clinic setting is not automatically malpractice. Even when a health care provider makes a mistake while providing care to a client, a malpractice lawsuit may not be a possibility. For a court to recognize a claim of malpractice or negligence, four legal elements must be present.

1. There must be a duty owed to the client by the nurse.
2. The nurse must breach that duty.
3. The breach of duty must be the cause of the damage.
4. There must be actual damage to the client.

When a claim of malpractice is made, the person making the claim (client) is the plaintiff. The nurse who is being accused of causing the injury is the defendant. Using the example of a medication error, let us look at the four elements required to prove a case of malpractice.

DUTY

Duty is the special relationship created when a person agrees to provide care to a client. The amount of time the duty is owed to the client will depend on the setting in which the care is given. When a nurse accepts an assignment of clients at the beginning of the day shift, under the laws of negligence, the nurse is considered to have a legal duty to provide care for those clients. After the shift is completed and the night shift nurse accepts the assignment of those clients, the first nurse is relieved of his or her duty to them. Thus, for example, if the night shift nurse gives a child gentamicin instead of the ampicillin that was ordered and the child suffers an anaphylactic reaction, the duty of the day nurse is not extended to the actions of the night nurse. The nurse from the day shift will not be held responsible for this medication error because that individual no longer owed a duty of providing the child with medication after the shift was completed.

BREACH OF DUTY

When a nurse fails to meet the standard of care, he or she has breached the duty to the client. In medication administration the standard of care is the right client, the right medication, the right dosage, the right time, by the right route. By giving the wrong medication in the previous example, the nurse breached the standard of care. Most malpractice cases require testimony from a nurse who is familiar with the particular area of nursing in question to determine whether the standard of care was breached. In other words, a labor and delivery nurse would not be able to testify about the standard of care for a pediatric client unless the individual could show prior experience in that area of nursing. Both the plaintiff and the defendant may each have a nurse testify about what is considered to be the standard of care.

CAUSATION

The injury to the child must be the result of the breach of the standard of care. If the child actually died because of respiratory failure that was unrelated to the medication error, malpractice did not occur. Causation is sometimes a difficult element to prove in a malpractice case. It may be impossible to determine whether the injury was the result of care given or if the child had a preexisting problem that caused the injury. Often medical expert testimony is required to establish causation.

DAMAGES

Unless there are damages when an error is made, there is no malpractice. If the nurse gave the antibiotic two hours late but the child had no adverse effects, there would be no claim for malpractice. Damages in a malpractice case may include lost wages, pain and suffering, and actual medical expenses. When a child is injured by malpractice, the actual cost of treating the injury is not the only money awarded. Costs will be awarded to pay for any care that will be required in the future because of the malpractice injury. An infant with severe brain damage will recover more money than an 80-year-old man because the cost of providing total care for the child will be multiplied by the child's life expectancy. A child with a 40-year life expectancy will be compensated more than an 80-year-old man with a 1-year life expectancy.

MALPRACTICE PREVENTION

Caring for pediatric clients can create situations that increase the risk for allegations of malpractice or negligence. Using the weight of a child to confirm a dosage can decrease medication errors, which are an area of special concern. Pediatric medications come in several forms, including elixir, pill, parenteral, and suspension; therefore, it is important to make sure any medication is given by the correct route. It is especially important to give accurate amounts of intravenous solutions, since an error in a small volume can create significant problems in a child or infant.

REFLECTIVE THINKING

Does the Threat of Malpractice Improve the Quality of Health Care?

A private health care provider can refuse to accept any client. In a small community, there was a law firm that had represented several clients in malpractice lawsuits against local health care providers. The lawyers and all of their employees were refused as clients by the local providers and forced to travel to another community for health care.

1. Would you refuse to provide care to these lawyers and their employees if you were a health care provider in this community? Why?
2. Does the ability to sue a health care provider improve the quality of care received by clients? Why?
3. What would happen to the quality of health care if physicians and nurses were immune to medical malpractice suits?

NURSING TIP

What Do You Do When a Client Is Injured?

It is very frightening when a client has a problem as the result of nursing care. Get immediate help for the client to prevent further injury. Document exactly the facts of the situation. Try not to discuss with other persons what happened. Notify appropriate personnel, including the client's physician, the nursing supervisor, and the hospital risk manager. Do not alter or falsify any medical records.

Child safety is another area of concern when caring for the pediatric client. It is important to keep side rails elevated to prevent small children from falling out of bed. Children are also more susceptible than adults to burns. Hot water bottles, heating pads, and heat lamps should be avoided or used only with extreme caution. Children are considered to be a vulnerable population; therefore, the nurse has a heightened duty of care with pediatric clients.

MEDICAL RECORDS

The client's chart is usually the most important document in a malpractice case. Charting is the nurse's opportunity to document the care given (Figure 2-4). This medical record will be the best evidence of both the chronology of events and what actually happened during a critical event. Always chart legibly and completely. When charting, avoid using judgmental terms—describe rather than label behavior. An example would be to chart that the caregiver has not performed the exercises that were prescribed by the physical therapist, rather than saying a caregiver is not cooperating with physical therapy. Never alter a medical record. In some states, altering a medical record is considered unprofessional conduct and can result in a formal complaint against a nurse's license. If you forget to chart an important detail, date and time a late entry.

LEGAL RESOURCES FOR PEDIATRIC NURSES

Every nurse should read and understand the Nurse Practice Act in the state where he or she is licensed to practice nursing. This act describes the scope of nursing practice and defines both illegal and unprofessional conduct for nurses. The state board of nursing is an excellent resource for assisting nurses with the resolution of legal issues. The

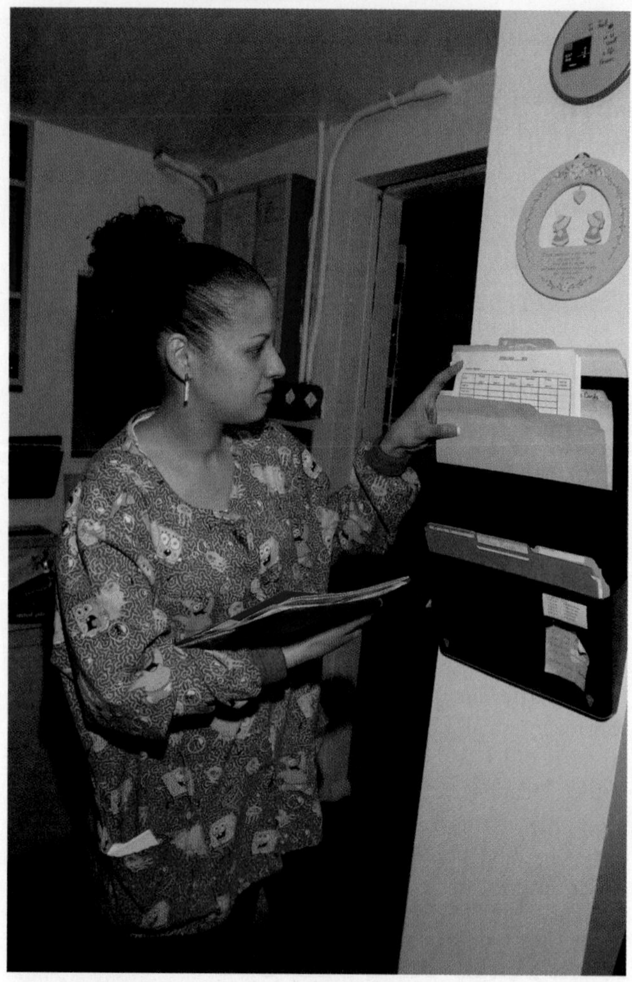

FIGURE 2-4 Proper and accurate charting is the nurse's first line of defense in a law suit. DELMAR CENGAGE LEARNING.

board of nursing can provide valuable guidance if there is a particular legal concern involving nursing practice in the state.

Nurses also need to be aware of other state laws that affect nursing practice. Does your state have a Good Samaritan Act that protects a nurse from liability when care is rendered voluntarily at the scene of the accident? Nurses also need to know their duty under the mandatory reporting laws of the state. All states require reporting child abuse. Your state may also require reporting of other types of abuse or injuries, including gunshot or stab wounds.

Find out if your hospital or health care facility employs a risk manager. In many health care facilities, the risk manager is a nurse with specialized training or a nurse who is also an attorney. The risk manager is responsible for making sure the facility conforms to state and federal laws. A risk manager should also review policies and procedures, which affect both client care and the legal rights of clients. Your facility should have policies and procedures dealing with informed consent, confidentiality, refusal of care, and other important legal issues (Figure 2-5).

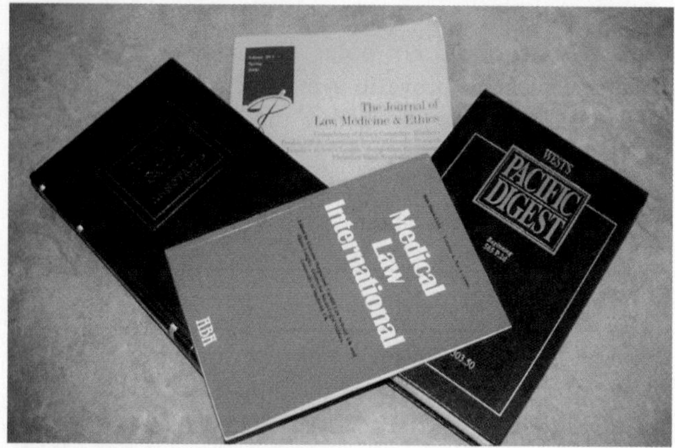

FIGURE 2-5 Legal Resources. DELMAR CENGAGE LEARNING.

If you work at a large health care institution, your hospital may have an ethics council. The role of this council is to provide a team of both professionals and laypersons to discuss and provide guidance when an ethical conflict arises. The ethics council may also facilitate communication between clients and health care providers when there is an ethical conflict. As with other aspects of health care, nurses should update their knowledge of legal issues on a regular basis. The law is constantly changing, and in order to provide appropriate care, a nurse must keep up with the changes that affect both nursing practice and the rights of clients.

CONCEPTS OF ETHICS

Pediatric nurses practice across health care settings and are referred to as "**boundary workers**" since they are required to negotiate their responsibilities to children, families, members of the health care delivery team, and the institution in which they work (Liaschenko & Peters, 2006). Nursing practice should be grounded in an ethical foundation (American Nurses Association, 2008). **Ethics** are principles that guide conduct. **Bioethics** refers to ethical conduct in health care providers, including those caring for children and families (Butts & Rich, 2008). Because bioethics is complex, ethical and moral decisions are not absolute black or white, but often involve shades of gray. There may not only be dilemmas that occur, but in some situations there may be more than three or more choices among competing and undesirable choices.

Moral behavior is often based on personal **values** or spiritual and religious beliefs and practices, including the right to die. Development of moral thinking in children occurs over time as discussed in Chapter 6. We make meaning out of the mortal experience through our values, which are influenced by how we are socialized. It is essential that nurses identify their personal values and recognize these may differ from those of others, and provide quality care regardless of those differences (Banks & Gallagher, 2009).

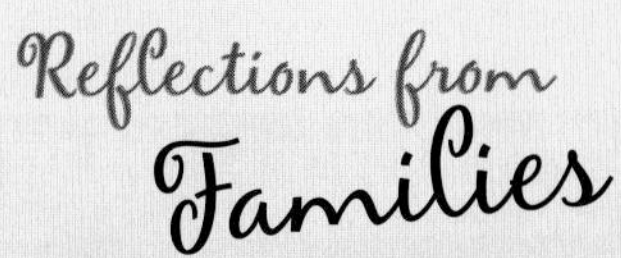

A 15-month-old who had been born at 23 weeks' gestation had only spent two weeks of his life outside the hospital. He had severe cognitive impairment and respiratory difficulties. The nurse felt his family was unrealistic and needed to face the magnitude of his condition, including the overwhelming emotional and economic costs. The child's grandmother came to spend the day with him and, while he didn't respond, the grandmother seemed happy just to hold his hand, stroke his head, and interact with him. Perhaps the joy of having him alive was greater than the sorrow of having a grandson with such significant impairments. The nurse then suspended judgment of this family, and this changed her approach in the provision of care.

All of us make small daily ethical decisions without even being aware we are doing so. These are very significant but often unseen compared to the dramatic ethical dilemmas highlighted in the media. But these daily decisions and actions shape our character and influence our moral and ethical character. Health care is becoming increasingly complex, with an increase in ethical dilemmas that are encountered by nurses. This is often very confusing when the nurse does not have past experiences on which to base ethical decision making. Conflicts may occur when members of the health care team have different perspectives and values. Ethical theories and principles can provide a framework for ethical nursing practice.

ETHICAL THEORIES

Ethical theories associated with health care include **deontologic theory** or Kantianism, **liberal individualism**, **communitarianism**, virtue theory, **care theory**, and **utilitarianism**. These theories frame ethical decision making (Butts & Rich, 2008).

In deontologic theory, right and wrong are clearly "black and white" to guide decision making regardless of the consequences. This theory is considered by many as appropriate to use in ethical decisions related to health care delivery. Liberal individualism focuses on protecting basic human rights and interests of individuals but may neglect the rights of the community. Communitarianism is considered the opposite of liberal individualism, focusing on communal values. Virtue theory focuses on the importance of character traits such as trustworthiness, integrity, and excellence to frame ethical decision making. Care theory is based on acting with empathy and caring to sensitively respond to individual concerns (Weaver, 2007).

ETHICAL PRINCIPLES

Ethical principles espoused by nurses include **autonomy**, **beneficence**, **nonmaleficence**, **justice**, **veracity**, and **fidelity**. Autonomy is the freedom for maturing children (adolescents) and families to make their own decisions about health care based on informed consent. Beneficence means "to do good," by taking positive actions to help another. Nonmaleficence is associated with the maxim "first, do no harm." This extends to not imposing a risk of harm.

Justice is the provision of fair and equitable care regardless of gender, culture or ethnicity, religious beliefs and practices, educational levels, or socioeconomic status. Unfortunately there are glaring health disparities in children who are vulnerable and underserved such as the uninsured, immigrants and refugees, those living in poverty, the homeless, or those living in dysfunctional families. Is it unjust to fail to provide health care to such children and their families?

Veracity is evident when there is clear and open communication between providers and parents and health care is transparent. Fidelity refers to keeping one's promise or word. For pediatric nurses, these ethical principles should be utilized in the provision of quality care for children and their families. See Table 2-2 for pediatric application.

PROFESSIONAL CODES OF ETHICS

Professional codes of ethics have been developed by the American Nurses Association (2008), the International Council of Nurses (2006), and the Canadian Nurses Association (2008). Nursing specialty organizations such as the American Association of Critical Care Nurses have also developed additional standards to guide nursing practice.

TABLE 2-2 Application of Ethical Principles in Pediatric Care

ETHICAL PRINCIPLE	APPLICATION
Autonomy	Giving children the opportunities to make age appropriate decisions (clothes, food) Engaging a family in a multi-disciplinary patient care conference about their child's case
Beneficence	Applying a topical analgesic to the site prior to inserting a peripheral IV in a toddler Using a child life specialist to provide appropriate play activities for a hospitalized child Facilitating a family's religious practices in a pediatric intensive care unit
Nonmaleficence	Using appropriate pain management strategies for a child in pain Notifying a health care provider that a child is allergic to a medication
Justice	Advocating for children without health care coverage to receive immunizations
Veracity	Telling parents the risks and benefits of a muscle biopsy to diagnose muscular dystrophy in their 6-year-old son Describing to a child what an injection will feel like
Fidelity	Suggesting to the orthopedic surgeon that a postoperative adolescent be provided with patient-controlled analgesia

THE ETHICAL DECISION-MAKING PROCESS

Ethical decision making involves thinking through what should be done based on ethical theories and principles. Many ethical decision-making models may be used in health care, but the decision-making process includes several basic steps.

The process starts with getting all of the information possible about the situation. The next step is defining what the dilemma actually is. The third step is determining who the stakeholders are and the values that are important to them. The fourth step is generating alternatives and weighing them, identifying all of the potential ways that the dilemma can be addressed or solved. This should include determining the advantages or disadvantages of each option. The fifth step is to decide on a course of action, including who should take action. Once that is accomplished, the choice of what to do is made and the action is completed. Having carried out the choice, the outcomes are assessed as the sixth and final step (Kurtz & Burr, 2009). Figure 2-6 summarizes this process.

ETHICAL DILEMMAS

Each health care encounter with children and their families has the potential to pose ethical concerns. Grappling with ethical dilemmas on a daily basis is part of nursing practice. Nurses with knowledge, skills, and a caring attitude can help children and families cope with these troubling situations. Pediatric nursing often presents heartrending circumstances with illnesses in young children. Some may represent sudden crises; others may be slow and insidious but nonetheless are challenging. Ethical dilemmas include conflicting rights and responsibilities, challenges of whether to disclose the truth and what informed consent truly entails, powerlessness versus authority, and autonomy versus vulnerability. The primary responsibility of the nurse is to act in the best interest of the pediatric patient and the family.

Moral distress occurs as the health care professional experiences conflict between one's own personal ethical beliefs and the inability for any number of reasons to not act in accordance at the workplace (Austin, Kelecevic, Goble, & Mekechuk, 2009). Moral distress is becoming increasingly acknowledged as an important concept in health ethics.

WITHHOLDING AND TERMINATION OF LIFE-SUSTAINING TREATMENT

Pediatric intensive care units and environments are fraught with multiple and complex ethical, moral, or religious dilemmas. Care of critically ill children presents ethical concerns for parents and the health care team, including the decision to implement "do not resuscitate" orders, limiting or withdrawing treatment, and determining when a child is brain dead. Moral and ethical decisions are often heart-wrenching, especially for parents.

Dramatic advances have been made in the care of infants born on the margin of viability who are not only extremely small (micro-premies) but also young (23 to 25 weeks gestational age). These newborns are at risk for poor long-term outcomes, which cannot be predicted in the first days of life. Often members of the health care team and parents may disagree about health care decisions and what the best interest of these vulnerable infants may be. Challenges to parents and providers are considerable (Chatfield, 2006; Obeidat, Bond, & Callister, 2009). Withholding and

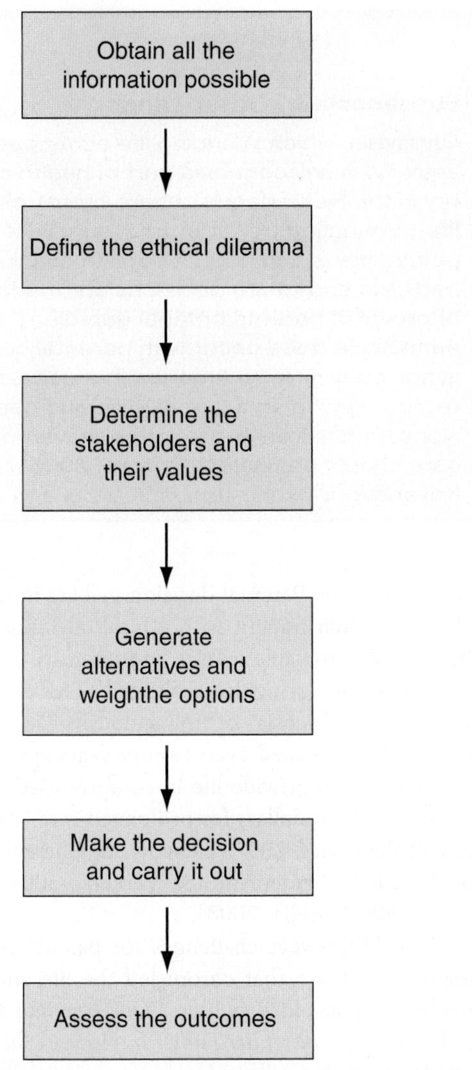

FIGURE 2-6 The Ethical Decision-Making Process. ADAPTED FROM KURTZ AND BURR 2009.

BOX 2-2

ATTRIBUTES OF AN EFFECTIVE ETHICAL DECISION MAKER

- Moral integrity
- Sensitivity, compassion, and caring
- Responsibility
- Empowerment
- Patience and willingness to deliberate

From Burkhardt, M. A., & Nathaniel, A. K. (2008). Ethics and issues in contemporary nursing (3rd ed.). Clifton Park, NY: Delmar Cengage Learning.

withdrawing treatment for critically ill newborns is fraught with ethical dilemmas, referred to as "playing God in the nursery" by Lyons in 1985 (Fleischman, 2008). Questions should be asked about long-term outcomes and future quality of life.

CRITICAL THINKING

Ethical Choices?

An adolescent mother unexpectedly gave birth at home at 26 weeks, claiming she was not aware that she was pregnant. The newborn was taken to the hospital, resuscitated, and put on a ventilator. Upon further examination, it was noted that there was incomplete brain development due to a carotid artery obstruction during pregnancy. The single, unemployed adolescent mother without a support system to rely on was informed about the severe impairment of her child. It was recommended that life support be removed. There are many ethical questions, such as: would it be in the best interest of a severely handicapped child to be raised by a young, inexperienced mother? Would it be in the best interest of the young mother to invest so much time and energy caring for this child? Would it be appropriate for the state to assume the immense costs of keeping the newborn alive with the provision of life-long specialized care?

The American Academy of Pediatrics has suggested that conferencing between the health care team and providers as well as the formation of infant bioethics committees are essential (American Academy of Pediatrics, 2008a). Applying the principle of beneficence when considering the best interest of critically ill infants is important, with the parents being the major decision makers as they attempt to make meaning out of a traumatic experience (Eden & Callister, 2009).

The support of caregivers is essential, especially when neonates are critically ill. Communicating clearly with the provision of complete information will help parents grasp the seriousness of the situation. Decisions need to be made whether aggressive intensive care interventions or palliative care will be provided. Situations where withholding or withdrawing life-sustaining treatment may be appropriate include when the child is brain dead, the child is in a permanent vegetative state, the "no chance" situation where there is great physical or mental impairment, and the "unbearable" situation where there is progressive and irreversible illness (Vince & Petros, 2007). Effective palliative pediatric pain control is essential (Peralta, 2007). Not only are such situations heart-wrenching for parents, they may also create moral distress in the pediatric health care team (Austin, Kelecevic, Goble, & Mekechuk, 2009).

Childbearing couples may also face decisions based on prenatal genetic testing. Prenatal genetic testing follows amniocentesis, fetal biopsy, or chorionic villus sampling, ultrasound scanning, and maternal serum screening. It includes over 500 tests and is offered routinely in many obstetric practices. In many instances, the legal, ethical, and social risks may outweigh the benefits (Ekberg, 2007; Lea, 2008).

REFLECTIVE THINKING

Survivability of Multiple Births

Because of dramatic advances in assisted reproductive technology, births of multiples are increasing. When high order multiples are expected, the chance increases that these infants will be born prematurely and compromised. A pressing ethical question is whether some of the multiples should be selectively aborted in order to provide increased opportunities for fewer fetuses to fully develop and be viable.

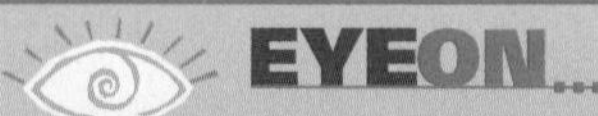

Euthanasia In Other Lands

Euthanasia, which is ending life either passively or actively, is a recognized part of health care delivery in the Netherlands, where clients may request life-terminating treatments. A survey of Dutch pediatricians and neonatologists concluded that pediatric end-of-life decisions are made with the approval of parents or legal guardians. Active euthanasia does occur with parental consent. This is not legal in North America, but debates continue regarding who should make life and death decisions for children and what palliative/end of life care should be (Gale & Brooks, 2006; Mooro, Kavanaugh, Okuno-Jones, & VanKleef, 2006).

Findings may include the presence of genetic disorders and congenital anomalies, including spina bifida, anencephaly, or trisomy disorders. Couples must decide whether they will abort the fetus, engage in prenatal fetal treatment if possible, decline treatment, or consent to aggressive critical care after the birth of the child.

Another ethical issue arises when the decision to treat a child is made by the health care team and/or the courts rather than the parents or legal guardians. Health care providers can be held liable for the "wrongful life" of a child with a disability. Parental decision making in newborn resuscitation is often fraught with ethical dilemmas, especially in the case of peri-viable infants and intensive care with "miracle babies" being highly publicized. The economic, social, and emotional costs of miraculously "saving" newborns that would have died even twenty years ago are significant. Expenditures to provide life in compromised newborns may exceed a million dollars for prolonged care (American Academy of Pediatrics, 2007; Eichenwald, Chervenak, & McCullough, 2008; Lindemann & Verkerk, 2008; Muraskas & Parsi, 2008; Vricella, 2008).

The bittersweet challenges for parents are voiced in a poignant obituary that chronicled the life and passing of a precious 3-year-old daughter: *"Our beautiful Grace returned to the waiting arms of her Father in Heaven. She was born with a perfect spirit but a flawed body due to partial trisomy 16 and partial monosomy 9. Our first wish was simply to meet and hold her before she returned home, but for three years she was our light, our joy, our daughter. Her beaming smile, her laugh, and the constant light in her eyes will forever be missed. She is survived by her heartbroken parents and the many whose lives and hearts she touched. Special thanks to the many people who cared for and loved our baby girl."*

EVIDENCE-BASED PRACTICE

Palliative Pediatric Care

CLINICAL PROBLEM

How do parents and the health care team determine what the most appropriate care is for a terminally ill child?

BEST CLINICAL PRACTICE

Venus, a 17-year-old African American girl died peacefully at home five years after having been diagnosed with a brainstem glioma. She had developed acute myelogenous leukemia as a side effect of chemotherapy. She and her parents were deeply religious and had to reconcile themselves with the inevitability of her death (Calabrese, 2007).

IMPLICATIONS FOR NURSING

- Nurses are involved in developing palliative protocols for children and adolescents based on the best possible evidence available and the preferences of the child and the family.
- Families should feel confident that they can trust the health care team to demonstrate beneficence, fidelity, and veracity regarding care of the dying child.
- Family-centered care should be provided by nurses.

Reference: Calabrese, C. L. (2007). ACT for pediatric palliative care. *Pediatric Nursing, 33*(6), 632–634.

NEWBORN SCREENING

Newborn screening for inherited and congenital conditions has been standard practice throughout the United States (approximately 98% of newborns are screened) since the 1960s but has been expanded considerably since that time based on the recommendations of the American College of Medical Genetics (Baily, 2008; Centers for Disease Control and Prevention's Division of Laboratory Sciences, http://www.cdc.gov/nceh/dls/newborn.htm; Retrieved February 1, 2009; Kenner, Lewis, Pressler, & Little, 2008). This now includes between 30–50 genetic disorders depending on the state (President's Council on Bioethics, 2008). Some of the conditions identified by screening are summarized in Table 2-3. Ethical dilemmas related to newborn

TABLE 2-3 Core Newborn Screening Conditions

CONDITION	EXAMPLES
Blood disorders	Sickle cell anemia, S-beta thalassemia, Sickle C anemia
Amino Acid disorders	Phenylketonuria, maple syrup urine disease, cystinuria, citrulinemia, argininosuccini academia, tyrosinemia type 1
Fatty Acid disorders	chain dehydrogenase deficiency, trifunctional protein deficiency, carnitine uptake defect
Other conditions	congenital hypothyroidism, biotinidase deficiency, congenital adrenal hyperplasia, hearing loss, cystic fibrosis, classical galactosemia

From Baily, M. A. (2008). Newborn screening. In Hastings Center (Ed.). From birth to death and bench to clinic, 125–128. Garrison, NY: Hastings Center.; Kaye, C. I., & the Committee on Genetics. (2006). Introduction to the newborn screening fact sheets. Pediatrics, *118*(3), 1304–1312.

screening are the constraint of scarce resources, the issue of screening being done without parental consent, the disposal of leftover blood spots for quality improvement, and predictive testing for adult-onset diseases which may create psychological harm (American Academy of Pediatrics, 2008b; Clayton, 2008; Fisher, 2006; Malpas, 2008; President's Council on Bioethics, 2008). The federal 2008 Newborn Screening Saves Lives Act was enacted to support state newborn screening programs. The recommendations of the President's Council on Bioethics are that "states mandate newborn screening only for diseases that meet traditional criteria, including the availability of an effective treatment." But the states are encouraged to implement pilot studies for newborn screening of conditions that do not meet the traditional criteria. Participants in these pilot studies should require the voluntary informed consent of the infant's parents (President's Council on Bioethics, 2008).

PERINATAL/NEONATAL AND PEDIATRIC POSTMORTEM EXAMINATION

Perinatal and pediatric postmortem examination poses many ethical challenges. Examination of the causes and contributing factors to the death of a child is essential in the case of homicide, suicide, puzzling circumstances, or an accident, yet some parents may feel that postmortem examinations are harmful to the grieving family. Alternatives include limited autopsies or radiography or magnetic resonance imaging (Putnam, 2007). Parental consent is required.

ORGAN DONATION AND TRANSPLANTATION

Organ transplantation is another ethical dilemma in pediatric nursing. Usually parents are desperate to find an organ match for their ill child, and yet may feel guilty about their desire since it generally means another child has to die for

Reflections from Families

A grief stricken mother spoke of her shock when her infant daughter unexpectedly died, with the assumed diagnosis of sudden infant death syndrome (SIDS): "I wanted an autopsy done to confirm what really happened. I felt comforted when the diagnosis was confirmed as SIDS and there was nothing that could have been done and it wasn't my fault."

REFLECTIVE THINKING

Palliative Care

Parents of infants born in the margin of viability (22-23 weeks gestation or "micro-premies", subject to a 34% death rate) (Eaton, 2006; MacDorman, Munson, & Kimeyer, 2007; Pignotti & Donzelli, 2008) or children with a terminal disease face the dilemma of instituting, continuing, or ending treatment and instead pursuing "compassionate" or palliative care (Eden & Callister, 2009; Wan & Ying, 2006). As a nurse, how would you respond to the query of a parent about changing the focus of care? What facts would you need in order to respond appropriately?

an organ to be procured. In some states it is required that in the case of a death or an impending death, family members are approached about organ donation. Solid organs including hearts and livers can be donated in infants greater than 35 days of life, kidneys greater than 6 months, lungs greater than 5 years, and pancreas greater than 8 years of age. Tissue donations including heart valves in infants greater than 34/40 weeks, corneas greater than 1 year, costal cartilage greater than 10 years and bone/skin greater than 16 years are considered ethical (Watts, 2006). Since the demand for human organs far exceeds the supply, value judgments are made as to who should receive the organ if there are several who have appropriate tissue matches for the same organ. Decisions about which child receives the organ should be made according to who will receive the most benefit (American Academy of Pediatrics, 2008c).

RELIGIOUS PREFERENCES AND IMMUNIZATIONS

Parents may decline to have their children immunized because of their religious beliefs. About 1% invoke non-medical exemptions to childhood immunization requirements. Some may believe in faith healing and others believe in complementary therapies. Parents may also have personal and philosophical objections to immunizations and invoke the "religious" exemption because of legal requirements in many states (Berlinger, 2006; Luthy, Beckstrand, & Callister, 2009). Suggestions have been made for nurses counseling parents who may decline to immunize their children.

Ethical dilemmas occur when a child is conceived to be a "donor child" for an older sibling who, for example, needs a bone marrow transplant. And what ethical dilemmas exist when a sibling is a perfect match for a brother or sister in need of a kidney, bone marrow, or portion of a liver (Ross, Thistlethwaite, & the Committee on Bioethics, 2008)? Is it appropriate to subject a child to the risks of an operative procedure, as well as the associated pain and potential suffering, in order to be a donor? For example, in the late 1980s the Ayala family had a daughter with chronic myelogenous leukemia who needed a bone marrow transplant. The parents purposely conceived a child to provide a bone marrow transplant for his sister, and that transplant saved their daughter's life. There is considerable debate over newborns with congenital anomalies that are incompatible with life being kept alive until their organs could be donated. In some states, transplantation from a child with anencephaly is legally prohibited.

Reflections from Families

A father described his experience when his 4-year-old son was fatally injured in a car accident: "When faced with the decision to donate his organs, our answer was 'yes'. We knew our baby would not recover; death was only a short time away. We knew our decision would allow another child a chance at a full life and would prevent another family from having to bury a child."

CRITICAL THINKING

Religious Beliefs and Immunizations

- Why would parents be uncomfortable for religious reasons with having their children immunized?
- How might you articulate your respect for the religious views of the parents while making clear that you believe immunization is best for their children's health?
- How can you educate parents about immunization recommendations and develop a compromise that is acceptable to the parents?

(Butts & Rich, 2008).

USING CHILDREN AS RESEARCH SUBJECTS

Research with children as subjects is conducted to document the effectiveness of health care interventions. Children are considered to be vulnerable subjects, and studies of children receive scrutiny regarding consent and assent. This is especially true when researchers give experimental drugs to children, including experimental therapies for childhood leukemia.

KIDS WANT TO KNOW

Where does my bone marrow transplant come from?

Since I'm getting a bone marrow transplant, did the other person give permission for me to get it or will the doctors just take it for me? The child should be told that the bone marrow is donated as a gift to help improve his health.

Following the development of the Nuremberg Code in 1949, which required the voluntary consent of individuals to be part of research studies, the National Commission for the Protection of Human Subjects of Biomedical and Behavioral Research (1979) issued the Belmont Report, in which guidelines were proposed for research involving human subjects. Informed consent and the voluntary agreement to be in a study were essential in these guidelines. Several groups of individuals were determined to be vulnerable subjects, including prisoners, mentally ill and mentally disabled individuals, pregnant women, and children. It was determined that, whenever possible, adults would be the subjects of research before children were used.

In 1994, the Code of Federal Regulations Title 45 stated that children who are developmentally able to decide for themselves must assent, or give their permission, to be in a research study. In addition, their parents or legal guardians must also voluntarily consent for their child to be in the study. Both assent and consent are required. If either the child or the parent declines, the child will not be in the study. The policy was expanded in 2000 to make sure that the benefits to children as participants are weighed along with the risks (Rice & Broome, 2004). Gaining access to children and adolescents to participate in research studies is sometimes challenging, with many gatekeepers including professionals and parents (Save & McCarron, 2009).

Ethical dilemmas in research arise when children are not asked for their assent to participate in a research study despite federal guidelines. In fact, it is possible for one parent to sign a consent for their child to be a human subject in an investigational study, while the other parent declines. In this case, the study can still proceed since only one signature is required. Furthermore, caregivers who are not the legal guardians sometimes refuse to allow a researcher to approach the parent or legal guardian about research when they have no legal right to prevent it.

Sometimes parents are willing and even anxious to enroll their child in a clinical study of an experimental treatment (Tomlinson, Bartels, Hendershot, Constantin, Wrathall, & Sung, 2007). The example is cited of a mother with her second child with stage IV brain cancer who desperately wanted her son enrolled in an NIH drug trial (Smith, 2006).

CRITICAL THINKING

Children in Research Studies

Jim S., a graduate nursing student, wishes to study children's perceptions of family-centered care utilized at the health care agency. The study would involve recruiting children ages 7 to 18 years receiving care in both inpatient and outpatient settings. How should Jim proceed to ensure the protection of the children in the sample as he plans his research methodology?

CHILDREN'S ASSENT TO TREATMENT

The rights of children to have access to health care have been established worldwide. An ethical dilemma develops when that child refuses health care. From a practical standpoint, it is obvious that health care workers would not refrain from giving care to a 4-year-old child who refuses an injection because it is painful. However, would that same nurse withhold care at the request of an intelligent, competent 16-year-old who is dying of leukemia? It is generally established that the parents or legal guardian make all consent decisions for their minor children. As assent to research participation is paramount, so is assent to treatment for children, or specifically, to refuse to receive care. The developmental and cognitive abilities of the child must be considered first. If the child is capable of abstract thinking and can understand the consequences of the refusal to receive what would be lifesaving care, then the wishes of the child may be granted. The maturity level of the child and his or her understanding of the situation must be taken into account along with the wishes of the parents so that a mutual decision is reached. In these instances, the values of the entire family, including the pediatric client, are the primary focus of the ethical decision-making process. The consent and assent of parents and children for treatment remain an area of concern based on the child's ethical and legal rights. Every situation will be resolved differently. Cultural preferences should be taken into consideration. For example, Chinese Confucian familism in decision making about life-saving medical care should be respected (Hui, 2008).

CULTURAL CONSIDERATION

Spotlight on Ethics

Increasingly, pediatric nurses are caring for culturally, ethnically, and linguistically diverse children and their families. Accordingly, this diversity is having a direct effect on how ethical principles need to be applied in pediatric health care. Ensuring effective communication with diverse pediatric populations is related to ethical principles such as autonomy, beneficence, and nonmaleficence. Translators should be available in compliance with TJC (The Joint Commission) standards of health care in all interactions with family members or legal guardians. Documents such as consent forms should be translated into the languages of populations commonly seen in health care facilities. Documents should be read aloud in those instances where the children and their families may be illiterate or sub-literate.

OTHER ETHICAL DILEMMAS

Greater numbers of newborn infants are testing positive for illegal drugs because of their mothers' substance abuse during pregnancy. Some governmental jurisdictions view this situation as child abuse and arrest the mother. This may result in the child, who is withdrawing from the drug, being placed in foster care away from his or her biological mother. The ethical dilemma comes from the paradox between the potential criminalization of the mother and the breakup of the family by the state. Nurses need to be aware of their legal obligations regarding notification of authorities in these instances. However, they also must be aware of their obligation to care for both the mother and the infant in the best possible way. The nurse must nonjudgmentally care for the mother and infant, knowing that willful actions of the mother have harmed the infant (Kenner & Altimier, 2008).

NEWBORN GENETIC SCREENING

Another pediatric ethical dilemma is newborn screening. The March of Dimes (http://www.marchofdimes.com/professionals; retrieved April 15, 2009) has endorsed newborn screening for 29 disorders which can be categorized as amino acid metabolism disorders, organic acid metabolism disorders, fatty acid oxidation disorders, hemoglobinopathies, and others. Congenital disorders can be detected by a single heel stick costing approximately $100 for all tests. This screening is done without parental consent. Some states test for additional disorders, and it has been suggested by the President's Council of Bioethics that routine screening be done, with informed consent obtained from parents for additional newborn screening (President's Council of Bioethics, 2008).

Community health nurses may encounter ethical dilemmas, such as "do not resuscitate orders" for children with disabilities, or adolescents asking for advice regarding contraception or abortion or treatment of sexually transmitted infections, and other challenging circumstances. The nurse must be prepared to make decisions effectively and with the rights of the child in mind.

EVIDENCE-BASED PRACTICE

Correctly Applying Research Protections to Children

CLINICAL PROBLEM

- Do research studies which represent minimal risks to children who are subjects have direct benefits to the children in the study?

BEST CLINICAL PRACTICE

- United States Federal Law requires that research involving children must have a potential benefit to the child.

IMPLICATIONS FOR NURSING

- Research involving children must involve risks to the clients that are comparable to the risks involved in living a regular life. Should there be a potential for harm in the children, the risk of having the children in the research is too high and the research should not be conducted.

Reference: Utah State Department of Health and Human Services. (2001). Protection for children in research. A report to Congress in accord with Section 1003 of P. L 106-310, Children's Health Act of 2000. Washington, DC: Author.

Shah, S., Whittle, A., Wilfond, B., Gensier, G., & Wendler, C. (2004). How do institutional review boards apply the federal risk and benefit standards for pediatric research? *Journal of the American Medical Association, 291*(4), 476–482.

EVIDENCE-BASED PRACTICE

Nurses, Knowledge of Do Not Resuscitate Orders

CLINICAL PROBLEM

- Are NICU nurses caring for terminally ill neonates knowledgeable about the legal definition and scope of do not resuscitate (DNR) orders?

BEST CLINICAL PRACTICE

- Complex issues surround DNR in terminally ill neonates

IMPLICATIONS FOR NURSING

- Nurses should be educated regarding the legal definition of DNR and be thoroughly oriented to NICU policies and procedures regarding DNR orders.

Reference: Bellini, S., & Damato, E. G. (2009). Nurses' knowledge, attitudes/beliefs, and care practices concerning do not resuscitate status for hospitalized neonates. *Journal of Obstetric, Gynecologic, and Neonatal Nursing, 38*(2), 195–205.

ETHICS COUNCILS

Ethics councils play key roles in resolving ethical dilemmas. The complexity and multitude of ethical situations confronting nursing and health care with the increase in technology and new treatments can be overwhelming. When a nurse and health care team are faced with difficult ethical decisions, these situations are now frequently being reviewed by ethics councils (Tabak & Zvi, 2008). Ethics councils can assist in promoting resolution in the ethical decision-making process. The roles of ethics councils are listed in Box 2-3.

BOX 2-3
ROLES OF ETHICS COUNCILS

1. Educate the health care team on utilization of the ethics council and issues involved in ethical decision making
2. Lead multidisciplinary discussion involving the health care team in conflict resolution and clarifying values
3. Allocate resources so outcomes represent quality care that is cost effective
4. Document and disseminate the health care facility's mission and vision
5. Formulate policies related to ethical standards
6. Consult and assist health care providers in difficult ethical decisions

Ethics councils include professional health care experts, community representatives, and those who bring a broad values perspective. Nursing staff representation usually includes nurse administrators and managers.

Ethics councils may be a sub-committee of the health care agency's governing board, a council appointed by the agency chief executive, or a sub-committee of the medical executive board (Figure 2-7).

Consultation provided by an ethics council varies from actual decision making to the provision of advice on specific ethical dilemmas. Input is provided by members of the health team, as well as the client and family and other stake holders in the ethical dilemma. The concerns of the ethics council are focused on the client. Such councils ensure quality care that is based on moral and ethical principles.

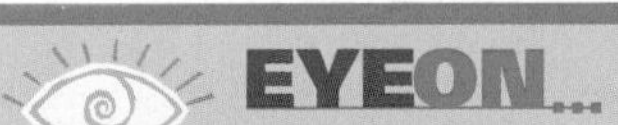

Educational Intervention for Ethical and Religious Dilemmas

A challenging ethical dilemma occurred in an NICU with a blind term infant with severe cortical damage and a painful decision about potentially withholding nutrition and fluids. When there was an impasse and a consultation was sought with the ethics committee, an educational intervention was designed to respond to moral distress experienced by the NICU nurses. This education increased the comfort levels of nurses caring for dying infants and reduced moral distress. The ethics council recommended multi-disciplinary debriefing sessions after each infant's death (Rogers, Babgi, & Gomez, 2008).

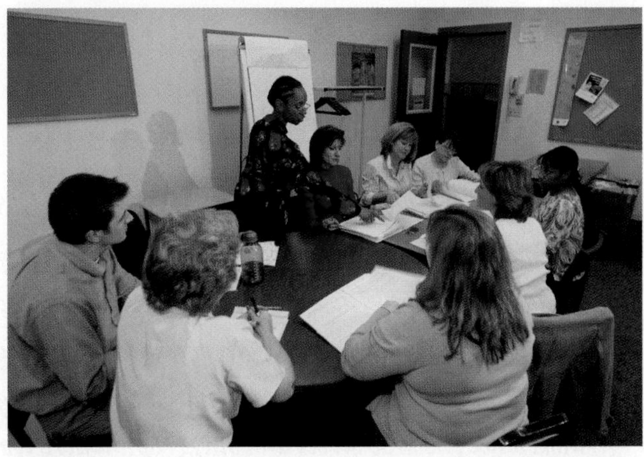

FIGURE 2-7 **A hospital ethics council may be engaged to provide input when decisions and judgments on moral or ethical implications are required.** DELMAR CENGAGE LEARNING.

REFLECTIVE THINKING

Maintaining Life

A family has a compromised newborn because of anoxia at birth in the NICU. The couple has two other children, 2 and 5 years old. Their daughter has been weaned from the ventilator but remains unconscious and is receiving parenteral nutrition. The parents request withdrawal of fluids and nutrition. The staff has mixed feelings about this request. Some of the nurses are feeling moral distress and the parents are also suffering and grieving the "loss" of the normal newborn they envisioned having (Butts & Rich, 2008). What are your feelings as a nurse caring for this neonate? When you meet with the neonatologists, the chaplain, and the social worker, how would you contribute to the discussion of this case? Would you suggest a consultation with the ethics committee? What role would the committee take in the decision making process?

FUTURE IMPLICATIONS FOR PEDIATRIC NURSING

Future ethical dilemmas in pediatric nursing are unpredictable, but may include such "hot topics" as stem cell research, with the potential for the development of new treatments using stem cells to help children with diseases such as leukemia or inherited immunological conditions (Nowlin, 2005). Nurses should focus on ways to promote moral and ethical care of children and families.

Reflections from Families

The father's plea was heartfelt and most unusual. "Stop the physical growth of my developmentally disabled little girl [with static encephalopathy]," he asked a panel of doctors, "so that we may be better able to care for her as years go by." The medical staff at Seattle's Children's Hospital agreed with the father's request. For doctors, stopping Ashley's growth presented two issues: Would the novel treatment improve her life? And would it cause harm? Ashley's parents shared the following statements on their website: "We call [Ashley] our Pillow Angel since she is so sweet and stays right where we place her—usually on a pillow."

Reference: Morehouse, M. (2007, January). Girl interrupted. *People*, 69–70.

IN THE REAL WORLD

This timeless and poignant question is frequently asked by families, "Nurse, if she were your child, what would you do?" When a family asked about continuing or discontinuing life support for a compromised newborn clinging to life, the nurse in the neonatal intensive care unit wanted to say, "Stop." Instead, the nurse told the parents it was their choice based on their knowledge of their daughter's tenuous condition and what they believed was appropriate for their daughter and their family. The nurse assured them that their decision would be honored and respected by the staff caring for their daughter.

Nurses play key roles in ethical issues in pediatrics, including:

- Obtaining informed consent and advocating for children and families.
- Communicating openly and honestly with children and parents and educating them appropriately about available options.
- Discussing curative versus palliative care for children as parents make end of life decisions.
- Respecting the dignity of the child and the family, reporting and refusing to participate in actions that are ethically objectionable (Butts & Rich, 2008).

CASE STUDY / CARE PLAN

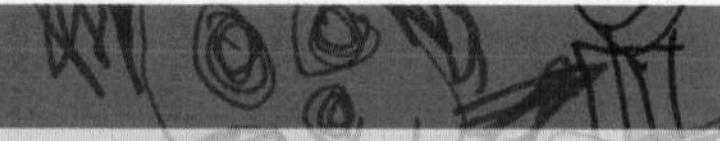

COMPARISON OF THE ETHICAL DECISION-MAKING PROCESS AND THE NURSING PROCESS

Sixteen-year-old Lindsay has end-stage renal disease and is receiving dialysis. Lindsay is on a waiting list for a kidney transplant. However, the health care team has told her that her overall health status has deteriorated such that should a kidney become available, she may not survive the stress of anesthesia and surgery. A meeting has been set up where Lindsay, her parents, the health care team, the medical center's ethics committee, organ donor services, and the transplant team can discuss whether she should be removed from the waiting list.

(Continues)

CASE STUDY / CARE PLAN (Continued)

Analyze the ways a decision can be reached by comparing ethical decision making and the nursing process.

ETHICAL DECISION-MAKING PROCESS	NURSING PROCESS
1. Obtain Information Lindsay's physiological status is deteriorating daily and she is exhausted and discouraged. Lindsay's parents have legal custody to give consent and Lindsay is capable of giving assent for health care.	1. Assessment
2. Identify the Ethical Dilemma Does Lindsay continue to be a viable candidate for a kidney transplant?	2. Nursing Diagnoses Impaired renal function Anticipatory grieving related to potential loss of Lindsay's life
3. List All Possible Ways to Solve the Dilemma How ill is Lindsay? What is her priority status on the transplant list? How soon may a compatible kidney become available?	3. Expected Outcomes Lindsay and her parents will verbalize understanding of the consequences of the decision to accept or to reject a kidney transplant.
4. Analyze Options Do Lindsay and her parents understand that she could die before organs become available? Does Lindsay want to stop treatment? Does everyone understand that Lindsay is a poor surgical risk? What are the chances that Lindsay's quality of life will improve after a kidney transplant?	4. Planning Same NOC: Acceptance: Health Status NIC: Decision-Making Support
5. Take Action	5. Intervention/Rationale Encourage continued active involvement by Lindsay in her health care. Maintains an understanding of her health status.
6. Evaluation Assess the situation in five months.	6. Evaluation Same

KEY CONCEPTS

- Laws that must be followed by nurses include state and federal statutes, agency regulations, and case law made by judges.
- Informed consent is used by health care providers to inform a client about the risks and benefits of health care treatments/procedures in order to get permission from the client to provide care. In most cases involving children, the caregiver or legal guardian provides informed consent for the child.

- Children may give their own informed consent when seeking care for pregnancy, sexually transmitted infections, HIV/AIDs, or substance abuse. Emancipated minors may also give informed consent.
- If a caregiver or legal guardian refuses needed health care for a child, the state may take custody of the child and obtain health care against the wishes of the child's caregivers or legal guardian.
- Genetic testing should not be performed on a child unless the results of the test will serve the best interests of the child.
- Federal law provides strict guidelines for using children as subjects of medical experiments.
- Nurses owe a duty of confidentiality to their clients to safeguard private health information from other persons unless the nurse has the consent of the client to divulge confidential information.
- Nurses may breach confidentiality when mandated by laws that require the disclosure of sexual, physical, or emotional abuse, infectious diseases, and situations in which one or more persons are at risk.
- Key ethical theories include deontology, liberal individualism, communitarianism, care theory, virtue theory, and utilitarianism.
- Use of an ethical decision-making process is of value in organizing thinking and clarifying issues in difficult moral situations.
- Children, based on their developmental level, must give assent to be a participant in research, and/or to assent to or refuse treatment.
- Ethics councils assist health care personnel in resolving difficult ethical situations since they offer a broad, community representation of viewpoints on the issue.

REVIEW ACTIVITIES

1. A nurse is volunteering at a community clinic. Where can she find out whether she is legally responsible if she does not provide appropriate treatment to a child at the clinic?
2. If a nurse is permitted to give intravenous narcotics in Idaho, should she assume that she can legally give intravenous narcotics in New Hampshire?
3. The Stone Drug Company wants to study a new antidepressant to see if it decreases sexual drive in adolescents. Would this study receive approval by an institutional review board?
4. You are taking care of a 3-year-old child who climbs out of the crib and breaks her arm. List the steps you would take to protect yourself from a possible malpractice suit
5. A 14-year-old with osteosarcoma (bone cancer) wants to receive an experimental chemotherapy treatment that the parents refuse. How would the nurse approach this situation?
6. The caregivers of a child who has been declared brain-dead following a car accident must be approached with information about donating the child's organs. Who would give permission for the organ donation?
7. A physician opts to treat a cognitively impaired adolescent seen in the clinic for a sexually transmitted infection (STI) without telling her or her parents of the diagnosis. How could the nurse use an ethics council in this situation? What factors must the ethics council consider?

STUDY QUESTIONS

1. Which statement below is correct about genetic testing of a 17-year-old child?
   a. A biological parent is the only person who can give consent for genetic testing.
   b. A court-appointed guardian is the only one who can give consent for genetic testing.
   c. Genetic testing should only be done if there is an immediate benefit to the child.
   d. Genetic testing should only be done if it is in the best interest of the child.
2. The Health Insurance Portability and Accountability Act (HIPAA) requires which of the following?

a. All adolescents must be given confidential health care.
b. Parents must have access to adolescent medical records.
c. Adolescents are entitled to confidential care and may control access to their medical records.
d. Abuse against adolescents cannot be reported without the adolescent's consent.

3. Which legal concept applies only to the pediatric patient?
a. informed consent
b. confidentiality
c. parens patrie
d. breach of duty

4. Under what circumstances would a living child be most likely NOT allowed to donate an organ or tissue?
a. significant risk of harm to the donor and the recipient is a sibling
b. minimal risk of harm to the donor and recipient is a stranger
c. significant risk of harm to the donor and recipient is a parent
d. minimal risk of harm to the donor and the recipient is a cousin

5. Malpractice requires which of the following?
a. duty, breach, causation, damages
b. duty, mistake, complications, causation
c. breach, causation, mistake, damages
d. breach, complications, damages, duty

6. A nurse overhears a fellow staff member talking about the mother of a child, telling her private information that the mother has shared. Which of the following responses by the nurse overhearing the conversation would be BEST?
a. Reporting this incident to the nurse manager.
b. Telling the mother what was being said about her.
c. Talking to the staff member privately about this.
d. Talking to the staff in general about confidentiality.

7. A 15-year-old female comes to the clinic with health concerns. What conditions can the nurse practitioner diagnose and treat (in most states) without parental consent?
a. pregnancy-related care
b. immunizations to meet school requirements
c. alopecia associated with an eating disorder
d. fracture of a humerus

8. What is informed consent referred to in children?
a. pediatric informed consent
b. child assent
c. joint parental/child consent
d. minor informed consent

9. Nurses are responsible for the direct care of their pediatric patients and:
a. limitations of health care organization policies.
b. acts of delegation of patient care activities to others, including other nurses.
c. practices of other health care professionals participating in patient care.
d. acts of delegation of patient care activities to others, except other nurses.

10. The American Nurses Association Code of Ethics relies partly on the ethical principle of justice. This means that nurses should:
a. avoid legislative activity, but engage in health care reform initiatives.
b. primarily focus their efforts on their area of expertise in their local communities.
c. be more concerned about economic disparities than providing care to culturally diverse children and their families.
d. be aware of health concerns such as poverty, human rights violations, and distribution of health care resources which have effects on children, their families, and communities.

REFERENCES

American Academy of Pediatrics. (2008a). *Communicating with children and families from everyday interaction to skills in conveying distressing information.* Retrieved February 21, 2009, from http://www.aap.org.

American Academy of Pediatrics. (2008b). *Ethical issues with genetic testing in pediatrics.* Retrieved February 22, 2009, from http://www.aap.org.

American Academy of Pediatrics. (2008c). *Pediatric organ donation and transplantation concerns.* Retrieved February 22, 2009, from http://www.aap.org.

American Academy of Pediatrics. (2007). Non-initiation of withdrawal of intensive care for high-risk newborns. *Pediatrics, 119*(2), 401–403.

American Nurses Association. (2008). *Code of ethics for nurses with interpretive statements.* Washington, DC: Author.

Americans with Disabilities Act of 1990, U.S.C.A. § 12101 et seq.

Austin, W., Kelecevic, J., Goble, E., & Mekechuk, J. (2009). An overview of moral distress and the pediatric intensive care team. *Nursing Ethics, 16*(1), 57–68.

Baily, M. A. (2008). Newborn screening. In Hastings Center (Ed.). From birth to death and bench to clinic, 125–128. Garrison, NY: Hastings Center.

Banks, S. & Gallagher, A. (2009). *Ethics in professional life: Virtues for health and social care.* London: Palgrave Macmillan.

Baren, J. M. (2006). Ethical dilemmas in the care of minors in the emergency department. *Emergency Medical Clinics of North America, 24,* 619–631.

Bellini, S., & Damato, E. G. (2009). Nurses' knowledge, attitudes/beliefs, and care practices concerning do not resuscitate status for hospitalized neonates. *Journal of Obstetric, Gynecologic, and Neonatal Nurses, 38*(2), 195–205.

Berlinger, N. (2006). Parental resistance to childhood immunizations: Clinical, ethical, and policy considerations. *American Medical Association Journal of Ethics, 8*(10), 681–684.

Bernard, D., Peters, M., & Makoroff, K. (2006). The evaluation of suspected pediatric sexual abuse. *Clinical Pediatric Emergency Medicine, 7,* 161–169.

Burkhardt, M. A., & Nathaniel, A. K. (2008). Ethics and issues in contemporary nursing (3rd ed.). Clifton Park, NY: Delmar Cengage Learning.

Butts, J. B., & Rich, K. L. (2008). *Nursing ethics* (2nd ed.). Sudbury, MA: Jones & Bartlett.

Calabrese, C. L. (2007). ACT for pediatric palliative care. *Pediatric Nursing, 33*(6), 632–634.

Caldwell v. Bechtol, 724 S.W.2d 739 (Tenn. 1987).

Canadian Nurses Association. (2008). *Code of ethics for registered nurses.* Ottawa, Canada: Author.

Centers for Disease Control and Prevention's Division of Laboratory Sciences, http://www.cdc.gov/nceh/dls/newborn.htm; Retrieved February 1, 2009.

Chatfield, A. (2006). How low shall we go? Is aggressive care always justifiable. *Journal of Neonatal Nursing, 12,* 216–221.

Chen, J. E. (2007). Family conflicts: The role of religion in refusing medical treatment for minors. *Hastings Law Journal, 58,* 643–669.

Curran v. Bosze, 566 N.E.2d 1319 (Ill. 1990).

Eaton, L. (2006). Ethics group rules on treating premature babies. *British Journal of Obstetrics and Gynecology, 333,* 1033.

Eden, L., & Callister, L. C. (2009). Parental involvement in end of life care and decision making in the newborn intensive care unit, in review.

E.G. v. E.G., 549 N.E.2d 322 (Ill. 1989).

Eichenwald, E. C., Chervenak, F. A., & McCullough, L. B. (2008). Physician and parental decision making in newborn resuscitation. *American Medical Association Journal of Ethics, 10*(10), 616–624.

Ekberg, M. (2007). Maximizing the benefits and minimizing the risks associated with prenatal genetic testing. *Health, Risk, and Society,* 9(1), 67–81.

Elrod, L. D. (2001). Reforming the system to protect children in high conflict custody cases. *William Mitchell Law Review, 28,* 495.

Fisher, C. B. (2006). Privacy and ethics in pediatric environmental health research. Part 1: Genetic and prenatal testing. *Environmental Health Perspectives, 114*(10), 1617–1621.

Fleischman, A. R. (2008). Neonatal care. In Hastings Center (Ed.). *From birth to death and bench to clinic,* 121–124. Garrison, New York: The Hastings Center.

Gale, G., & Brooks, A. (2006). Implementing a palliative care program in a newborn intensive care unit. *Advances in Neonatal Care, 6*(1), 37–53.

Gupta, M. (2007). Mandatory reporting laws and the emergency physician. *Annals of Emergency Medicine 49*(3), 369–376.

Health Insurance Portability and Accountability Act of 1996. 42 U.S.C. § 201 et seq.

Howell v. Michelin Tire Corp., 860 F. Supp. 1488 (M.D. Ala. 1994).

Hui, E. (2008). Parental refusal of life-saving treatments for adolescents: Chinese familism in medical decision-making. *Bioethics, 32*(5), 286–295.

International Council of Nurses. (2006). *ICN code of ethics for nurses.* Geneva, Switzerland: Author.

Kaye, C. I., & the Committee on Genetics. (2006). Introduction to the newborn screening fact sheets. *Pediatrics, 118*(3), 1304–1312.

Kenner, C., & Altimier, L. (2008). *Assessment of risk in the term newborn* (2nd ed.). White Plains, NY: March of Dimes.

Kenner, C., Lewis, J. A., Pressler, J. L., & Little, C. M. (2008). Neonatal genetic testing is more than screening. *Critical Care Nursing Clinics of North America, 20,* 233–237.

Kurtz, P., & Burr, R. L. (2009). Ethics and health. In K. S. Lundy & S. Jones (Eds.). *Community health nursing: Caring for the public's health* (2nd ed.), 248–269. Sudbury, MA: Jones & Bartlett.

Lea, D. H. (2008). Genetic and genomic healthcare: Ethical issues of importance to nurses. *Online Journal of Issues in Nursing, 13*(1), 1–4.

Lerand, S. J. (2007). Teach the teacher: Adolescent confidentiality and minor's consent. *Journal of Pediatric Gynecology 20,* 377–380.

Liaschenko, J., & Peters, E. (2006). Feminist ethics: A way of doing ethics. In A. Davis, V. Tschudin, & L. de Raeve (Eds.). (2006). *Essentials of teaching and learning in nursing ethics,* 181–190. Philadelphia, PA: Churchill Livingstone-Elsevier.

Lindemann, H., & Verkerk, M. (2008). Ending the life of a newborn. *Hastings Center Report,* January-February 2008, 47–51.

Lundqvist, A., & Nilstun, T. (2007). Human dignity in pediatrics: The effects of health care. Nursing Ethics, *14*(2), 216–228.

Luthy, K. E., Beckstrand, R., & Callister, L. C. (2009). Parents speak out: Parental hesitation in immunizing children. *Public Health Nursing,* in press.

MacDorman, M. F., Munson, M. L., & Kimeyer, S. (2007). Fetal and perinatal mortality, United States. *National Vital Statistics Report, 56*(3).

Malpas, P. J. (2008). Predictive genetic testing of children for adult-onset diseases and psychological harm. *Journal of Medical Ethics,* 34, 275–278.

March of Dimes. (2006) Recommended newborn screening tests: 29 disorders. Retrieved February 22, 2009, from http://www.marchofdimes.com/professionals.

Mooro, T., Kavanaugh, K., Okuno-Jones, & VanKleef, J. A. (2006). *Journal of Perinatal and Neonatal Nursing, 20*(3), 262–273.

Morehouse, M. (2007). Girl interrupted. *People*, Jan. 2007, 69–70.

Muraskas, J., & Parsi, K. (2008). Ethically responsible use of NICU capabilities. *American Medical Association Journal of Ethics, 10*(10), 613–615.

National Commission for the Protection of Human Subjects of Biomedical and Behavioral Research. (1979). Belmont report: Ethical principles and guidelines for research involving human subjects. Washington, DC: U.S. Government Printing Office.

Nowlin, A. (2005). The promise of stem cells. *RN, 68*(4), 48–52.

Obeidat, H., Bond, A. E., & Callister, L. C. (2009). The parental experiences of having an infant in the newborn intensive care unit. *Journal of Perinatal Education*, in press.

Peralta, A. (2007). Principles of palliative pediatric pain control. *International Journal of Pharmaceutical Compounding, 11*(1), 10–15.

Pignotti, M. S., & Donzelli, G. (2008). Perinatal care at the threshold of viability: An international comparison of practical guidelines for the treatment of extremely preterm births. *Pediatrics, 121*(1), e193–e198.

President's Council on Bioethics. (2008). The changing moral focus of newborn screening: An ethical analysis by the President's Council on Bioethics. Rockville, MD: Government Printing Office.

Putnam, M. A. (2007). Perinatal perimortem and postmortem examination. *Advances in Neonatal Care, 7*(6), 281–288.

Rice, M., & Broome, M. E. (2004). Incentives for children in research. *Journal of Nursing Scholarship, 36*(2), 167–172.

Roberson, A. J. (2007). Adolescent informed consent: Ethics, law and theory to guide policy and nursing research. *Journal of Nursing Law, 11*(4), 191–196.

Rogers, S., Babgi, A., & Gomez, C. (2008) Educational interventions in end of life care: Part 1. *Advances in Neonatal Care, 8*(1), 56–65.

Ross, L. F., Thistlethwaite, J. R., & the Committee on Bioethics. (2008). Minors as living solid-organ donors. *Pediatrics, 122*(2), 454–461.

Sachs, C. J., Weinberg, E., & Wheeler, M. W. (2008). Sexual assault nurse examiners' application of statutory rape laws. *Journal of Emergency Nursing 34*(5), 410–413.

Safer v. Estate of Pack, 677 A.2d 1188 (N.J. Super. Ct. App. Div. 1996).

Save, E., & McCarron, S. (2009). Research access to adolescents and young adults. *Applied Nursing Research, 22*, 63–67.

Schloendorff v. Society of N.Y. Hosp., 105 N.E. 93 (N.Y. 1914).

Schulter, J., Winch, S., Holzhauser, K., & Henderson, A. (2008). Nurses' moral sensitivity and hospital ethical climate. *Nursing Ethics, 15*(2), 305–321.

Shah, S., Whittle, A., Wilfond, B., Gensier, G., & Wendler, C. (2004). How do institutional review boards apply the federal risk and benefit standards for pediatric research? *Journal of the American Medical Association, 291*(4), 476–482.

Slonina, M. I. (2007). State v. physicians et al.: Legal standards guiding the mature minor doctrine and the bioethical judgment of pediatricians in life-sustaining medical treatment. *Health Matrix: Journal of Law and Medicine 17*, 181–214.

Smith, P. J. (2006). Clinical case: The desperate parent and the lures of experimental treatment. *American Medical Association Journal of Ethics, 8*(10), 649–653.

Stultiens, L., Nys, H., Cassiman, J. J., & Dierickx, K. (2006). Presymptomatic and predictive genetic testing in minors: A systematic review of guidelines and position papers. *Clinical Genetics 70*, 374–381.

Tabak, N., & Zvi, M. R (2008). When parents refuse a sick teenager the right to give informed consent: The nurse's role. *Australian Journal of Advanced Nursing, 25*(3), 106–111.

Tarasoff v. Regents of the University of California, 551 P.2d. 334 (Cal. 1976).

Tomlinson, D., Bartels, U., Hendershot, E., Constantin, J., Wrathall, G., & Sung, L. (2007). Challenges to participate in pediatric palliative care research: A review of the literature. *Palliative Medicine, 21*, 435–440.

Unguru, Y., Coppes, M. J., and Kamani, K. (2008). Rethinking pediatric assent: From requirement to ideal. *Pediatric Clinics of North America 55*, 211–222.

United States Department of Health and Human Services. (1994). Code of Federal Regulations, Title 45, Public Welfare. Department of Health and Human Services. Part 46—Protection of Human Subjects (45 CFR 46). Washington, DC: U.S. Government Printing Office.

United States Department of Justice Office of Violence Against Women. (2004). A National Protocol for Sexual Assault Medical Forensic Examinations: Adults/Adolescents. Retrieved February 22, 2009, from http://www.ncjrs.gov/pdffiles1/ovw/206554.pdf.

Utah Code Annotated 62A-4a-406.

Utah State Department of Health and Human Services. (2001). Protection for children in research. A report to Congress in accord with Section 1003 of P.L. 106-310. Children's Health Act of 2000. Washington DC: Author.

Vince, T., & Petros, A. (2007). Withdrawal of treatment in children. *British Journal of Hospital Medicine, 68*(12), 666–668.

Vricella, L. (2008). Ethically responsible use of NICU capabilities. *American Medical Association Journal of Ethics, 10*(10), 613–615.

Wan, S. Y., & Ying, S. (2006). Reflections of a critical care nurse regarding termination of life-sustaining support. *The World of Critical Care Nursing, 5*(2), 61–64.

Watts, C. E. (2006). Establishing the possibility of neonatal and pediatric organ/tissue donation. *Infant, 2*, 58–61.

Weaver, K. (2007). Ethical sensitivity: State of knowledge and needs for further research. *Nursing Ethics, 14*(2), 141–155.

SUGGESTED READINGS

Grace, P. J. (2009). *Nursing ethics and professional responsibility in advanced practice.* Sudbury, MA: Jones & Bartlett.

Judson, K., Harrison, C., & Hicks, S. (2009). Law and ethics for medical careers (5th ed.). New York: McGraw Hill.

Steinbock, B. (2008). A philosopher looks at assisted reproduction. In T. L. Beauchamp, L. Walters, J. P. Kahn, & A. C. Mastroianni (Eds.). *Contemporary issues in bioethics,* 316–323. Belmont, CA: Thomson Wadsworth.

RESOURCES

Refer to the online student StudyWARE for Potts & Mandleco at http://www.CengageBrain.com for additional content and study aids.

Organization: **American Association of Nurse Attorneys**
Description: The American Association of Nurse Attorneys (TAANA) members practice in private law practice, in academia, as litigators and defense attorneys, as legal counsel for health care entities, and in health care compliance among other settings. The website provides readers with information regarding attorney referrals, jobs, chapters and foundation purposes.
Website/Resource: http://www.taana.org

Organization: **American Academy of Pediatrics**
Description: The American Academy of Pediatrics is an organization of 60,000 pediatricians committed to the attainment of optimal physical, mental, and social health and well-being for all infants, children, adolescents, and young adults. This website offers general information related to child health as well as specific guidelines concerning many pediatric issues. In addition, the reader can access information regarding the Academy's many programs, activities, policies, guidelines, publications, and other child health resources.
Website/Resource: http://www.aap.org

Organization: **American Nurses Association**
Description: The American Nurses Association (ANA) is the only full-service professional organization representing the interests of the nation's 2.9 million registered nurses through its constituent member nurses associations, its organizational affiliates, and its workforce advocacy affiliate, the Center for American Nurses. This website offers the reader access to information regarding RN career updates, professional nursing practice guidelines, nursing ethnics, current health care policies, government affairs, and occupational environment information.
Website/Resource: http://www.nursingworld.org

Organization: **Find Law**
Description: Findlaw.com is a public resource that helps users access state and federal statutes as well as case law. The website offers information about finding lawyers, answering law questions, and common legal forms.
Website/Resource: http://www.findlaw.com

Organization: **Hastings Center Studies in Ethics**
Description: The Hastings Center is an independent, nonpartisan, and nonprofit bioethics research institute founded in 1969. The Center's mission is to address fundamental ethical issues in the areas of health, medicine, and the environment as they affect individuals, communities, and societies. The website offers users information regarding publications, research, and center news.
Website/Resource: http://www.thehastingscenter.org

Organization: Center for Democracy and Technology's **Health Privacy Project**
Description: This website provides information about health privacy statutes in each state.
Website/Resource: http://www.cdt.org

Organization: **International Association of Forensic Nurses**
Description: The International Association of Forensic Nurses (IAFN) is an international membership organization comprised of forensic nurses working around the world and other professionals who support and complement the work of forensic nursing. The mission of the IAFN is to provide leadership in forensic nursing practice by developing, promoting, and disseminating information internationally about forensic nursing science. The website offers users access to information regarding membership, certification, career options, and clinical programs.
Website/Resource: http://www.iafn.org

Organization: **HHS's Child Welfare Information Gateway**
Description: This website provides resources about child maltreatment, including definitions from federal and state laws, and resources that distinguish between discipline and abuse.
Website/Resource: http://www.childwelfare.gov

Organization: **National Council of State Boards of Nursing**
Description: The National Council of State Boards of Nursing (NCSBN) is a not-for-profit organization whose purpose is to provide an organization through which boards of nursing act and counsel together on matters of common interest and concern affecting public health, safety, and welfare, including the development of licensing examinations in nursing. The website offers users information regarding the NCLEX examination, nursing practice acts, and state board contact information.
Website/Resource: http://www.ncsbn.org

Organization: **National Institutes of Health**
Description: The National Institutes of Health (NIH), a part of the U.S. Department of Health and Human Services, is the primary federal agency for conducting and supporting medical research. NIH scientists investigate ways to prevent disease as well as the causes, treatments, and even cure for common and rare diseases. The NIH website offers readers information regarding countless health topics, clinical trials, grants, health related news, and current medical research.
Website/Resource: http://www.nih.gov

Organization: **National Newborn Screening and Genetics Research Center**

Description: The National Newborn Screening and Genetics Resource Center (NNSGRC) is a cooperative agreement between the Maternal and Child Health Bureau (MCHB). NNSGRC provides information and resources in the area of newborn screening and genetics to benefit health professionals, the public health community, consumers, and government officials. The website offers links to topics of special interest as well as information regarding events, professionals, and parent/family resources.

Website/Resource: http://genes-r-us.uthscsa.edu

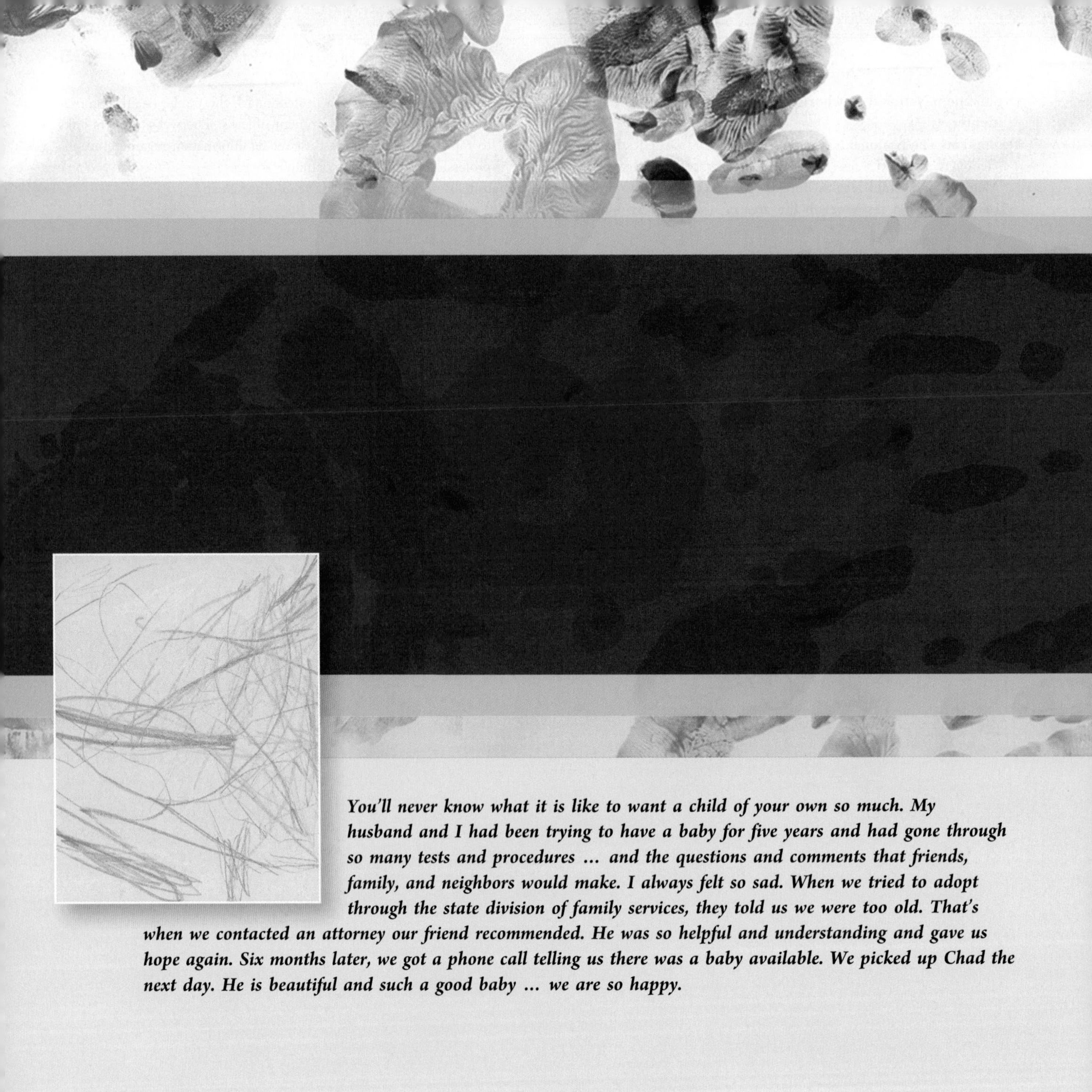

You'll never know what it is like to want a child of your own so much. My husband and I had been trying to have a baby for five years and had gone through so many tests and procedures … and the questions and comments that friends, family, and neighbors would make. I always felt so sad. When we tried to adopt through the state division of family services, they told us we were too old. That's when we contacted an attorney our friend recommended. He was so helpful and understanding and gave us hope again. Six months later, we got a phone call telling us there was a baby available. We picked up Chad the next day. He is beautiful and such a good baby … we are so happy.

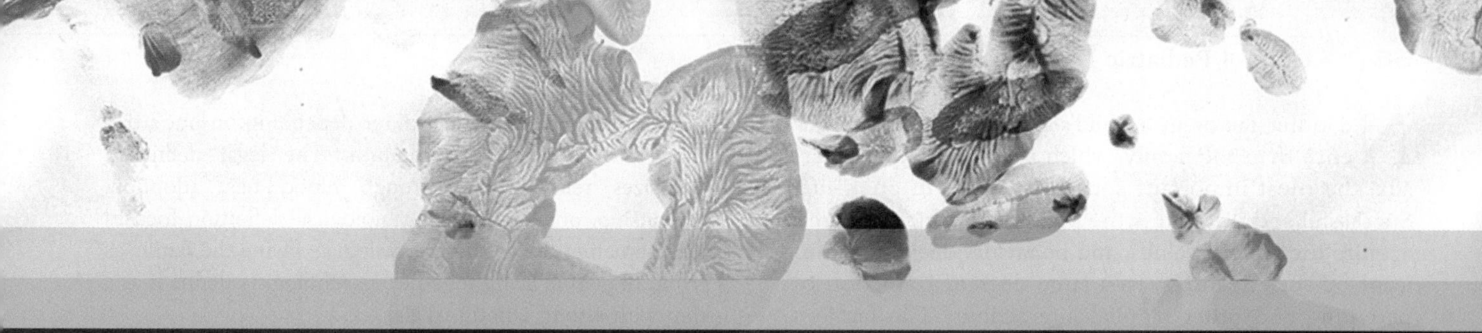

CHAPTER 3
The Child in Context of the Family

Barbara Mandleco, RN, PhD
Nicki L. Potts, RN, PhD

COMPETENCIES

Upon completion of this chapter, the reader will be able to:

- Discuss definitions of family, including one that encompasses the changing family structure.
- State some nursing theories that provide guidance for understanding families.
- Discuss social science theories that explain family dynamics, processes, and tasks.
- Identify family assessment measures that can be used in clinical practice, and state the advantages and disadvantages of each.
- Describe different types of family structures.
- Identify parenting tasks for the various stages of child development.
- Discuss the impact of various parenting styles on children and caregivers.
- Discuss the role of the nurse in supporting caregivers and their child rearing practices.
- Discuss cultural diversity and immigrant families and how that may impact nursing care delivered to these families.
- Successfully complete the games and activities in the online student StudyWARE.

No other factor in a child's life has a greater influence than the family, which is the first and, generally, the most important socializing agent in one's life. Successful socialization is the process by which children acquire the beliefs, values, and behaviors deemed significant by society and is, to a large degree, a function of parenting and other familial interactions. The family's organization, structure, and function have significant impacts on children during growth and development. Nurses caring for children must consider the entire family, rather than just the child, as the client.

Many stresses face today's families, but these stresses may seem worse than in the past because they are no longer ignored; we now have higher expectations of marriage and parenting. In fact, fathers in intact families today spend more time with their children than at any other time period in the past 100 years. This is good for children because hands-on fathers make better parents than those who leave all the nurturing and child care to mothers. Such fathers raise daughters who are likely to do well in school (math, science) and sons who are more expressive. Even though the amount of time the average mother spends at home with children has decreased since the early 1900s, there are fewer children per family and more attention is paid to each child. Mothers, including those who work outside the home, currently spend almost twice as much time with each child as mothers did in the 1920s (Coontz, 2006).

This chapter reviews several family theories relevant to pediatric nursing, discusses the various family structures in today's society, and concludes with a discussion of parenting.

DEFINITION OF THE FAMILY

The family, despite its changing and increasingly diverse nature, remains the basic social unit, and can be approached in one of four ways (Hanson, Gedaly-Duff, & Kaakinen, 2005). The first views the family as context; the second sees the family as a client. When families are treated as the context within which individuals are assessed, the emphasis is on the individual (**family as context**). Conversely, when the nurse treats the family as a set of interacting parts and emphasizes assessment of the dynamics among these parts rather than the individual parts themselves (family members), the family as a whole, rather than the individual members, becomes the client (**family as client**). The third approach sees the family as an interactional system, where the whole is greater than its parts. The interventions, therefore, focus on interactions between family members rather than on individual family members. The final approach sees the family as a social institution that is part of the larger society. The family in this view interacts as a whole with other institutions (educational, health, economic, religious) to give, receive, and exchange services and communication. In all cases, the nurse must grasp the interacting aspects of the family, understand the context within which the individual lives and to which she or he reacts, and work with the family as client.

Definitions of the family differ depending on one's discipline and theoretical orientation. The legal definition emphasizes relationships through blood ties, adoption, guardianship, or marriage. The biological definition focuses on perpetuating the species. Sociologists define the family as a group of people living together; psychologists define it as a group with strong emotional ties.

Traditional definitions usually include a legally married woman and man with their children. This narrow definition is reflected in the U.S. Bureau of the Census (2010) definition of family as a group of two or more persons related by birth, marriage, or adoption and residing together. The Census Bureau has used this same definition for years. However, this traditional definition fails to address the diversity of family structures present in U.S. society today. A broader definition of **family** is two or more persons joined by bonds of sharing and emotional closeness, and who identify themselves as members of the family (Friedman, Bowden, & Jones, 2003). Demo, Aquilino, and Fine (2005) see a family as a group of people who have long-term committed relationships, ongoing support, and responsibilities, rather than by biological ties, the law, or marriage. A final definition reflects contemporary society: Family is what the client says it is (Figure 3-1). Nurses working with families should first ask their clients who they consider to be in their family

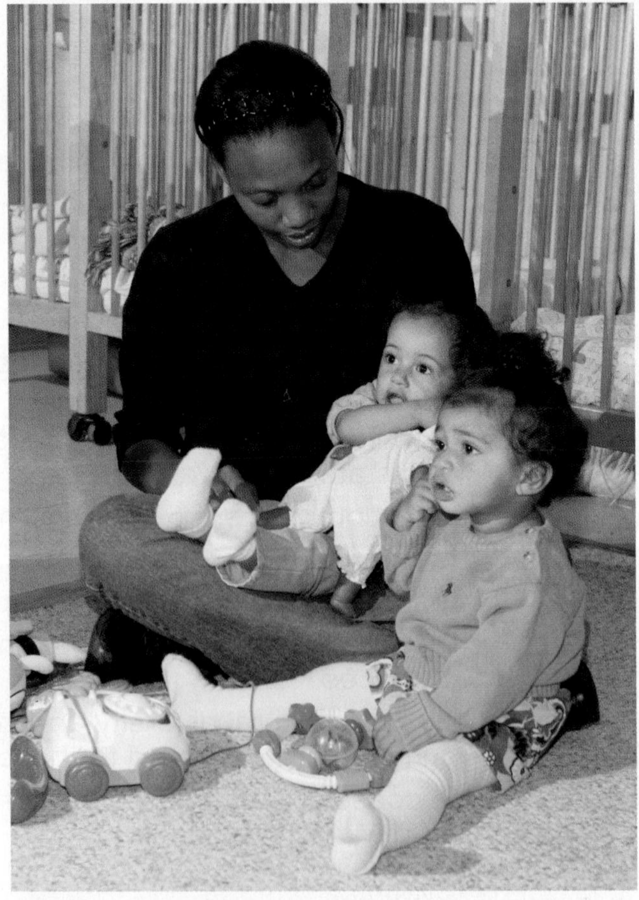

FIGURE 3-1 **Modern families come in all sizes, shapes, and configurations.** DELMAR CENGAGE LEARNING.

and then include those individuals in their health care planning.

THEORETICAL FOUNDATIONS OF FAMILY NURSING

Nursing has consistently had an interest in families and has acknowledged its importance in relation to health. A number of theories of families in nursing and social sciences give insight into understanding its dynamics and processes.

NURSING THEORIES

Early nursing theories focused on the individual and considered the family only as part of the client's context. However, some theorists have enlarged their perspectives to include the family as the client.

NEUMAN'S SYSTEM THEORY

Neuman's theory is consistent with a family systems approach (1972; 1983). Originally, her theory did not discuss the family as such, but it was later expanded to include the family as the recipient of nursing care (Neuman, 1995). The family is described as an appropriate target for both assessment and nursing interventions. The way each member expresses self influences the whole and creates the basic structure of the family. The major goal of the nurse is to help keep the structure stable within its environment.

KING'S OPEN SYSTEMS THEORY

King viewed the family as a social system that influences the growth and development of individuals (1981). The family is seen as both context (environment) and client. Her theory of goal attainment is useful for nurses when assisting families to set goals to maintain their health or cope with problems or illness. She believes nurses are partners with families. The role of nursing is to help members become healthy enough to function in their roles.

ROY'S ADAPTATION THEORY

In Roy's theory, the client is an individual, family, group, or community in constant interaction with a changing environment (1983). The family system is continually changing and attempting to adapt. When the family is confronted with unusual stresses and coping patterns are ineffective, problems in family functioning occur. The goal of nursing is to promote adaptation and minimize ineffective responses.

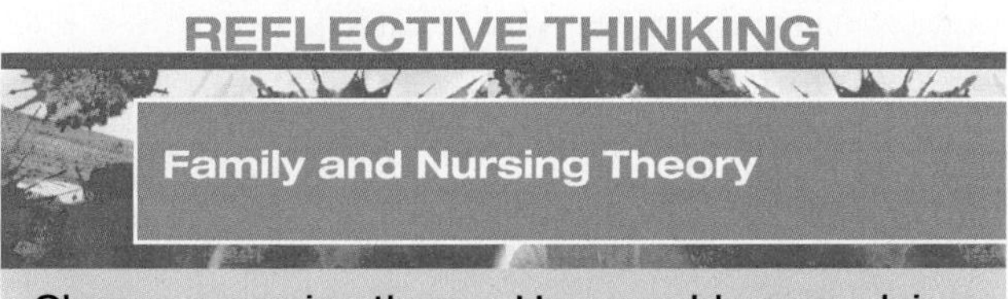

Choose a nursing theory. How would you explain family in terms of that theory? Do some theories fit your family life better than others? Or do they all seem to have relevance to your life experience?

SOCIAL SCIENCES THEORIES

A number of theories from the social sciences help to explain families; however, there is little consensus about which is the major one. Four will be examined: structural-functional, developmental, family systems, and family stress.

STRUCTURAL-FUNCTIONAL THEORY

The structural-functional theory emphasizes the organization or structure of the family and how this structure facilitates its functioning. It characterizes the family as a social system and examines the relationship between the members as they carry out family functions.

The theory, based on social philosophers such as Comte and Durkheim, suggests society (the family) is like the human body, which is made of various parts that need to function properly together so it can remain healthy (Smith, Hamon, Ingoldsby & Miller, 2008).

Basic assumptions of this theory are as follows:

- The family is viewed as part of the social system, with individuals being part of the family system.
- The family, as a social system, performs functions that serve both the individual and society.
- Individuals act in accordance with a set of internalized norms and values that are learned primarily in the family through socialization.

Family structure refers to the ordered set of relationships among the parts, and between the family and other social systems. Family structure or organization is evaluated based on how well it fulfills its functions, and the goals important to its members and society. The structure serves to facilitate the achievement of the functions. To determine family structure, the nurse must identify the individuals making up the family, their relationship to each other, and the relationship between the family and other social systems.

Family functions are the services provided by the family to society so the larger group survives. Five functions of the family have been identified that are important for nurses to understand (Friedman et al., 2003):

- affective
- socialization and social placement
- reproductive
- economic
- health care

The affective function is one of the most vital functions for the formation and continuation of the family unit. This function refers to the family meeting the need for love and belonging of each member. The family is a home base where the individuals can express their true feelings and thoughts without fear of rejection. It is the social milieu for the generation and maintenance of affection, where one is first loved and given to, and learns to love and give in return. Although the affective function is important for all families, those who must focus on providing the basic physical necessities of life have minimal energy remaining to meet the affective needs.

Socialization and social placement function refers to teaching children how to function and assume adult social roles in their culture. This function involves the acquisition of internal controls needed for self-discipline and values such as what is right and wrong according to society. Socialization occurs predominately in the family, and caregivers are the primary agent.

The continuity of both the family and society continues to be ensured through the reproductive function. In the past, marriage and the family were designed to control sexual behavior as well as reproduction. Individuals considered it their responsibility to marry, have many children, and rear those children within the bounds of marriage. The reproductive function is carried out very differently today. Many single people are having children, including adolescents, and many married couples are remaining childless. Reproduction has also been influenced by technological advances such as artificial insemination, *in vitro* fertilization, and surrogate mothers.

The economic function involves the family's provision of sufficient resources and their effective allocation. An assessment of the family's economic resources provides the nurse with information about their ability to appropriately allocate these resources to meet needs such as food, shelter, clothing, and health care. By gaining an understanding of how a family distributes its resources, the nurse can also obtain a perspective about their value system. One responsibility of the nurse is to assist families in obtaining appropriate community resources to meet their needs.

The health care function includes provision of physical necessities to keep the family healthy, such as food, clothing, and shelter, as well as health care (Friedman et al., 2003). The family keeps its members well by passing on attitudes, values, and behaviors that promote health and caring for them in times of illness.

The structural-functional approach is very useful for assessing family life because it enables the nurse to examine the family system holistically, in parts, and interactionally with other institutions and the wider society. A limitation of this theory is that it tends to present a static view of the family and minimizes the importance of growth and change (Friedman et al., 2003).

Even though the theory is helpful in examining families it has other limitations as well. First, structural-functionalism developed in a historically conservative time and reflects the values and traits of families that were popular at the time: unity, stability, and structure. As cultural values and political views have changed, support for the theory has declined. Second, even though families perform functions necessary to society, those functions are not reason enough for a family to exist. The theory, therefore, doesn't explain the historical processes of how different family types come to exist in a society. Finally, some functions traditionally assumed by women (or men), such as expressive tasks (maintaining morale and cooperation) may also be assumed by men (or women) (Smith et al., 2008).

Developmental Theory

Family developmental theory, which emerged in the late 1940s, was one of the first family-focused theories that was separate from sociology and psychology. The theory believes families are social groups influenced by developmental processes, much like those experienced by individuals. Family developmental theory suggests the family life cycle has two stages: expansion and contraction. Children are born and raised during expansion; children leave the family home during contraction (Smith et al., 2008).

The developmental or life-cycle theory is based on the premise that families evolve through predictable developmental stages, and experience growth and development in much the same way as individuals. Stages begin with marriage, followed by childbirth and child rearing. Each stage is characterized by specific issues and tasks. Developmental theories explain the changes that occur in human organisms or groups over time. This approach is based on the following assumptions (Duvall, 1977):

- Critical role transitions of individual members, such as birth, retirement, and death of a spouse, are viewed as resulting in a distinct change in the family life patterns.
- Families develop and change over time in predictable ways.
- Families and their members perform certain time-specific tasks that are decided upon by themselves, within their cultural and societal context.
- Family behavior is the sum of the previous experiences of its members as incorporated in the present and in their expectations for the future.

The best known formulation of the developmental stages comes from Duvall (1977; Duvall & Miller, 1985), who identified eight chronological stages the family passes through. Each stage includes predictable tasks that the family must master prior to proceeding to the next one. Table 3-1 delineates the stages of family development and tasks of each stage.

An advantage of the developmental approach is that it provides nurses with information about what to expect of families at different points in their life cycle and, thus, what teaching and counseling services may be needed.

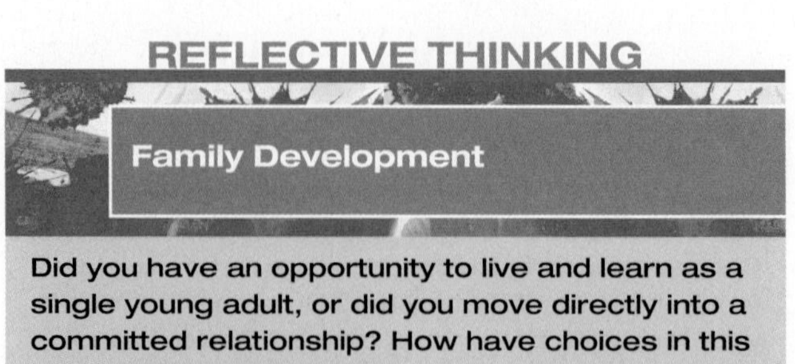

TABLE 3-1 Developmental Stages and Tasks of the Two-Parent Nuclear Family

STAGE	TASK
Beginning family	1. Establish couple identity and mutually satisfying marriage 2. Relate harmoniously to kin network 3. Make decisions about parenthood
Childbearing family	1. Integrate infant into family 2. Reconcile needs and conflicting developmental tasks of family members 3. Maintain a satisfying marital relationship 4. Expand relationships with extended family by adding parenting and grandparenting roles
Families with preschool children	1. Meet family members' needs for adequate space, privacy, safety, and housing 2. Socialize children 3. Integrate new children while still meeting needs of other children 4. Maintain healthy relationships within the family (marital and parent-child) and outside the family (extended family and community)
Families with school-age children	1. Promote school achievement; foster the healthy peer relations of children 2. Maintain a satisfying marital relationship 3. Meet the physical health needs of family members
Families with teenagers	1. Balance freedom with responsibility as teenagers mature and become more autonomous 2. Refocus on marital and career issues 3. Communicate openly between parent and children
Families launching young adults	1. Expand family circle to young adults, including new members acquired by the marriage of grown children 2. Assist aging and ill parents of husband and wife 3. Renew and renegotiate marital relationship
Middle-age parents	1. Provide health-promoting environment 2. Sustain satisfying relationships with aging parents and children 3. Strengthen marital relationship
Families in later years	1. Maintain satisfying living arrangement 2. Adjust to reduced income 3. Maintain marital relationship 4. Adjust to loss of spouse 5. Maintain intergenerational family ties 6. Continue to make sense of one's existence

Adapted from Duvall, E. M., & Miller, B. (1985). *Marriage and family development* (6th ed.). New York: Harper & Row; Friedman, M. M., Bowden, V., & Jones, E. (2003). *Family nursing: Research, theory and practice* (5th ed.). Stamford, CT: Appleton & Lange.

This theory also provides criteria for assessing a family's current stage and its ability to accomplish the tasks of this stage. The nurse is then able to support the family in order to progress smoothly from one stage to another.

There are several limitations of the developmental theory. It has a middle-class bias and assumes homogeneity (two caregivers, nuclear family) and that young adults marry in their early twenties before they develop a career. Additionally, this theory views the family from a traditional perspective. It does not take into consideration the diversity of family forms found in today's society, such as divorced, remarried, single-parent, and gay or lesbian families. The focus of the developmental approach is primarily child rearing; however, today this activity occupies less than half of a woman's adult life span. Thus, child rearing is no longer the central focus of the life cycle. The theory also does not provide much insight into what governs patterns of family behavior.

Family Systems Theory

The family systems approach is based on the general systems theory developed by Von Bertalanffy (1968), which describes principles that govern all living systems. One of the central propositions of the general systems theory is that the system is not the total sum of its parts but is characterized by wholeness and unity.

The family is therefore viewed as a system where all family members interact interdependently with one another. The theory emphasizes family elements and the processes that exist within and between families and their various environments; its principles and key concepts are:

1. Interdependency among family members holds the system together and defines the nature of family relationships.
2. Input and output reflects information the family receives that may impact family functioning and the way the family appears to those outside the family.
3. Boundaries determine how much information is allowed into or out of the family. Boundaries can be permeable or impermeable.
4. Hierarchy of subsystems reflects relationship patterns and power. Family subsystems are the parents and the children.
5. Rules prescribe members' roles, behaviors, communication patterns, authority, and emotional expression.
6. Goals change over time as the family grows and changes.
7. Feedback mechanisms monitor family status and functioning. Families strive to maintain equilibrium.
8. Nonsummativity means the family is greater than the sum of its parts.
9. Change occurs as families reorganize and adapt in response to information received from inside and outside the family.
10. Equifinality, the ability of a system to achieve a goal, occurs through various means or routes.

The family is defined as a system characterized by continual interaction between its members and with the environment. The interrelationships in a family system are closely tied together so that a change in one member results in a change in the other members. Therefore, one cannot understand the family as a whole by only knowing each of its members. The interrelationships of the members with each other and with the larger society must be analyzed.

There are three major criticisms of systems theory. The first is that the theory is too abstract and global, and therefore too general, to be useful. However, advocates of the theory would argue that since the world is diverse, systems help make connections between the social and natural world that more discipline-specific theories aren't capable of making. The second criticism is that some theorists view the theory as reality instead of using it as a model for understanding the family. The last criticism is that systems theory is not a true theory, but rather a model or flow chart. The major concepts to some are too vague for testing and cannot make predictions. Advocates, however, would suggest different models (such as this) could be used for different purposes (Smith et al., 2008).

Family Stress Theory

Families have always experienced stress. However, the scientific study of how families handle stress is relatively recent. Begun during the Great Depression of the 1930s, Angell (1936) and Cavan and Ranck (1938) were interested in learning how families were dealing with the stress and income loss accompanying unemployment. Angell found that the family's reaction to loss of income during the Depression depended on adaptability and integration: how flexible families were in talking about problems and making group decisions and how unified and economically interdependent they were. Those families who were adaptable and integrated were better able to deal with stress associated with the Depression. Cavan and Ranck (1938) found families who were cohesive and organized before the depression were better able to handle economic losses.

Koos (1946) and Hill (1949) followed Angell, Cavan, and Ranck in examining how families deal with economic loss (Koos) and stress (Hill). Hill's "profile of adjustment to crisis as a roller coaster" (p. 14) suggests families pass through four stages when faced with a crisis: crisis, disorganization, recovery, and reorganization. Disorganization follows the crisis as members cope with the situation, and then enter recovery, which can be either quick or long term. Families eventually achieve a new level of organization that will either be the same as before the crisis, better, or worse. This roller coaster model was followed by Hill's (1949) ABC-X model of family stress that described how families adjust to crisis caused by separation and reunion during wartime. Although some scholars have added to (McCubbin & Patterson, 1983), simplified (Burr & Klein, 1994), or built on (Lazarus & Folkman, 1984) the theory, the basics remain relatively the same (Smith et al., 2008). The assumptions are:

1. The stressor (A) can be either a positive (birth of a baby) or negative (death of a family member) event, and occur internal or external to the family. The stress can also be normative or nonnormative. Normative stress occurs in all families, is anticipated, and is short term rather than chronic. It is easier to handle normative stressors. Other criteria affecting the family's interpretation of the event are whether the stressor is

focused on one or all members of the family; how sudden, gradual, or severe is the stressor; how long families need to adjust to the situation; whether the stress is expected; whether it is natural or artificial (human made); and the family's perception of whether they can solve the crisis situation.

2. Resources (B) can be individual, family, or from the community. Individual resources include a family member's level of education, job and personal experiences, characteristics (perseverance), work ethic, skills, and abilities. Family resources include support and encouragement, and can be instrumental (help with household chores, writing a resume) or emotional. Community resources include churches, neighbors, friends, and community agencies that offer networking, help with problem-solving skills, and assistance in accessing valuable resources. Coping is another resource that considers what one does in attempting to handle the stressor. Coping, an interaction of resources and perceptions, may be intrapsychic, direct, or manifest by controlling emotions accompanying the situation. Intrapsychic coping refers to cognitively reframing the problem so it doesn't seem so overwhelming. Direct coping means actually doing something about the situation. Controlling emotions may involve talking about it, attending religious services, or possibly turning to drugs and alcohol. No matter how the family copes, returning the family to its previous state of functioning is the goal.
3. Definition of the situation (C) involves how a stressor is interpreted by the individual or family. This often determines how well resources are accessed. Cognitive appraisal and coping processes mediate psychological responses to stressors, and optimism helps one view a stressor as challenging rather than as threatening. If the family or individual is able to break the crisis or stressor into smaller, manageable parts, coping may be easier and results more positive. However, if the individual or family believes the stressor cannot be solved, failure is imminent.
4. Stress and Crisis (X). Whether or not the individual or family enters a state of stress or crisis is determined by the stressor itself, resources available to manage the stressor, and how the situation is defined. Crisis occurs when the individual or family can no longer maintain equilibrium. Family stress is an event experienced by the family that upsets the family's sense of normalcy or causes a change in the family. A crisis, however, is a state or period of disorganization rocking the family's foundation. The stress becomes a crisis when the family cannot maintain its status quo using existing resources, or is incapacitated because the stress is so overwhelming (Smith et al., 2008).

Even though the theory has been used widely since the 1930s, there are problems with it. The most common problem is that the ABC-X model is linear, and attempts to explain the complexity of family life, situations, and accumulation of normative and nonnormative events over time, which often causes families to be so stressed they are in crisis. The Double ABC-X model, developed by McCubbin and Patterson (1982), addresses this situation. The model (Figure 3-2) treats the traditional ABC-X model as the initial, precipitating event. The adjustment period (post-crisis) suggests families need to respond not only to the initial crisis, but also to the events preceding and following the event. The Double ABC-X model uses the ABC-X model as the base and then replicates the model with a different interpretation representing the post-crisis adjustment.

- The Double A Factor (aA): Stress and Change. The components include the initial stressor, changes in the family, and stressors resulting from coping with the initial

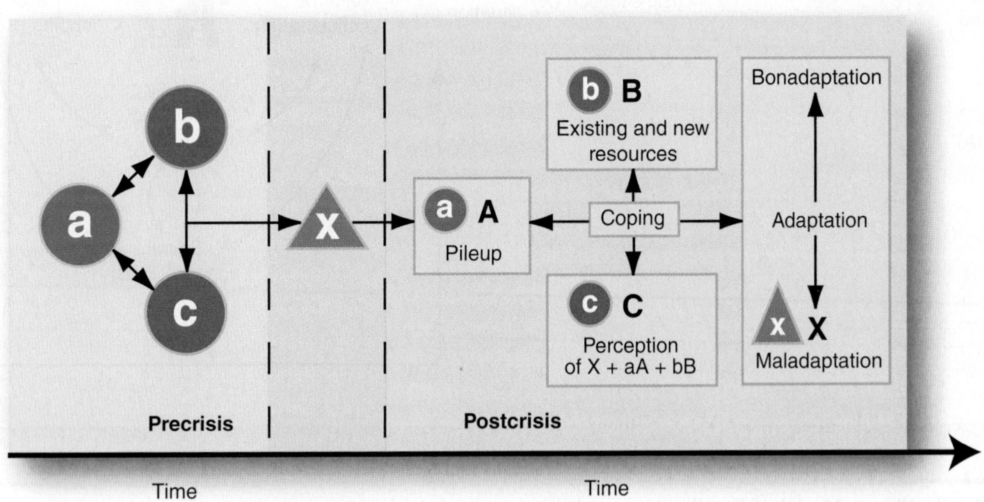

FIGURE 3-2 The Double ABC-X Model. USED WITH PERMISSION FROM MCCUBBIN, H. I., & PATTERSON, J. M. (EDS.). (1982). *FAMILY STRESS, COPING, AND SOCIAL SUPPORT (P. 46).* COURTESY OF CHARLES C. THOMAS PUBLISHER, LTD., SPRINGFIELD, ILLINOIS.

stressor. For example, if a husband loses his job, the family members may need to change roles (wife returns to work, husband does housework), which can be stressful. If resources need to be accessed to help with the situation (mother-in-law needed to help with child care), the resources themselves can be stressful. Multiple stressors occurring at the same time is termed stressor pileup.

- The Double B Factor (bB): Family Resources. These are new sources of support, and can include development of new skills, or strengthening of old skills because resources used to deal with the initial stressor did not avert a crisis state. This considers the fact that resources typically relied on cannot always help solve the problem. Therefore, new opportunities are sought.
- The Double C Factor (cC): Family Perception. This component of the model is concerned with the family's beliefs about or response to the initial stressor as well as how they interpret their responses to the crisis itself. The family's perception of its ability to respond to such situations determines coping.
- The Double X Factor (xX): Family Crisis and Adaptation. Post-crisis adaptation depends on how well the family has adapted not only to the new level of family functioning, but also to the initial crisis. That is, is the adaptation negative (maladaptation) or positive (bonadaptation)?

The Resiliency Model of Family Stress, Adjustment, and Adaptation

The **Resiliency Model of Family Stress, Adjustment, and Adaptation** (McCubbin & McCubbin, 1993; 1996) emphasizes adjustment and adaptation when families experience stressful life experiences (Figure 3-3). Built on Hill's ABC-X and other family stress models (McCubbin & McCubbin, 1989, 1993;

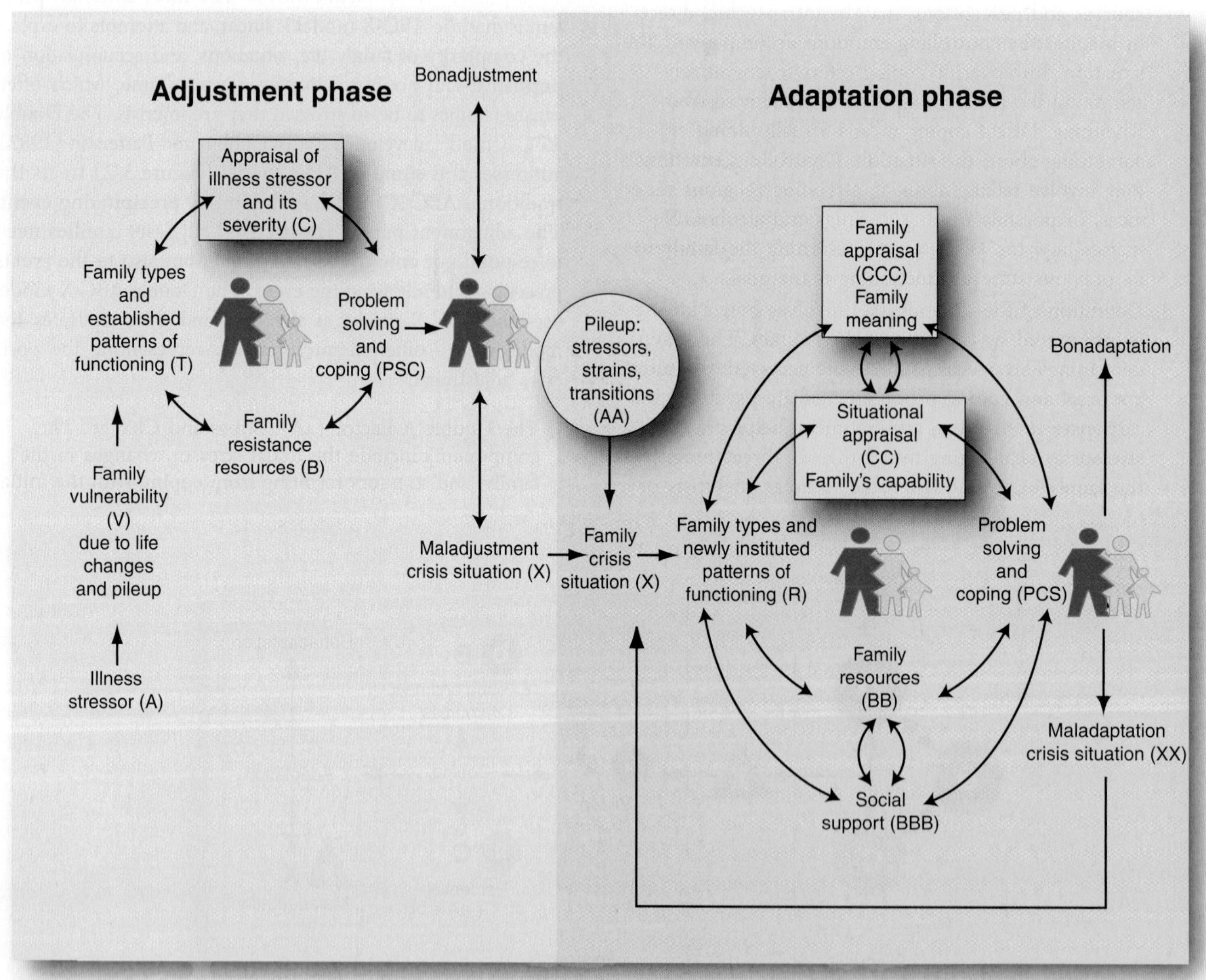

FIGURE 3-3 The Resiliency Model of Family Stress, Adjustment, and Adaptation. FROM MCCUBBIN, M., & MCCUBBIN H. (1993). *FAMILIES COPING WITH ILLNESS: THE RESILIENCY MODEL OF FAMILY STRESS, ADJUSTMENT, AND ADAPTATION.* IN C. DANIELSON, B. HAMEL-BISSEL, & P. WINSTEAD-FRY (EDS.), *FAMILIES, HEALTH, AND ILLNESS* (P. 391). ST. LOUIS, MO: MOSBY WITH PERMISSION FROM ELSEVIER.

McCubbin and Patterson, 1983), the model emphasizes family resilience (ability to recover from adverse life events), and considers family adjustment and family adaptation over time by highlighting family strengths and capabilities needed to overcome adversity. The Resiliency Model is based on the following four assumptions: (1) over time, families face natural and predictable changes and hardships; (2) individuals and the family as a unit develop strengths and capabilities that protect against major disruptions and foster growth and development when facing transitions and change; (3) the family is protected from unexpected and normative stressors by developing basic and unique strengths and capabilities; these same strengths and capabilities also help the family adapt after crises or major changes and transitions; (4) during times of family stress or crises, families contribute to and benefit from networks of relationships and resources within the community (McCubbin & McCubbin, 1991).

A family's response to transitions and stressful life events comes about in two phases: the adjustment phase and the adaptation phase. The **adjustment phase** reflects stress that is not a major hardship; the family maintains adaptation by making only minor adjustments or changes in its established patterns. For example, an acute illness with complete recovery in an otherwise healthy family member could be a situation requiring only minor adjustments. How the family defines the stressor of a minor illness (family appraisal), the existing resources, and problem-solving and coping abilities all determine how the family adjusts to the situation. Usually in such situations, families adjust by using their typical ways of functioning and make only minor changes (bonadjustment). However, the family moves into a crisis situation and the adaptation phase if these minor changes do not adequately manage the events (maladjustment).

During the **adaptation phase**, the family adjusts to the situation by making essential structural or systemic changes in functioning. Even though the crisis may not be detrimental or pathologic to the family, the family must make changes since old ways of doing things are no longer adequate; new solutions must be found. Adaptation can be required not only by developmental crises, but also by situational crises. During this phase, responses to the crisis situation are determined by the pileup of stressors, transitions, strains, and demands, as well as by the family unit's capabilities and strengths. Definitions of the major variables in the adaptation phase follow.

Pileup of Demands This variable refers to situations when families are dealing with more than one stress or strain at a time. The Resiliency Model identifies six categories of stresses or strains: (1) the stressor event and associated hardships (changes needed in the family or home when a member [child] suffers chronic asthma, such as making the home dust free, having no pets, asking family members not to smoke); (2) normative transitions (children entering school, or leaving home for college); (3) preexisting family strains (getting along with an ex-spouse, being a single parent); (4) situational demands (having hours one parent works increased or decreased); (5) consequences of the family's coping efforts (one parent has to take on a second job to help with medical expenses); and (6) intrafamily strains and social ambiguity (lack of guidelines regarding how to manage the situation).

Newly Instituted Patterns of Functioning The Resiliency Model emphasizes the importance of establishing new patterns of functioning when faced with a crisis. A regenerative family displays hardiness (feelings of being in control, committed to each other, seeing stresses as challenges to be overcome) and coherence. A rhythmic family focuses on family times and routines that help them cope with stress. A resilient family demonstrates flexibility and emotional closeness. Those families who are hardy, coherent, value time together, have set routines, and are flexible and emotionally close are better able to cope with stress.

Resources are family attributes and supports used in crisis situations. There are three different kinds of resources the family might use: individual (intelligence, knowledge, skills, personality traits, physical health, emotional health), family (decision-making abilities, conflict resolution skills), and community (friends, family, organizations).

Social support is important and includes emotional support (members believe they are loved and cared for), esteem support (members believe they are valued and respected), network support (members believe they belong to a network that provides understanding and mutual support), appraisal support (helps members look at how they are doing), and altruistic support (information received from others out of the goodness of their hearts).

Family appraisal includes not only the family's definition of the stressor as seen in the adjustment phase, but also the family's situational appraisal (shared assessment of the stressor, hardships related to the stressor, how well the family is managing) and its schema or worldview (shared values, expectations, goals developed over time). The worldview, which is quite stable unless the stress is very serious (premature death of a young mother), is influenced by adult member's family of origin, the family's cultural and religious background, and societal values and norms.

Problem Solving and Coping The Resiliency Model identifies four strategies used in coping. The first is actions to decrease demands (e.g., putting a grandparent with Alzheimer's disease in a care center). The second is obtaining additional resources (e.g., finding home care for a member with a chronic illness). The third is managing tensions or relieving stress (e.g., participating in an enjoyable activity). The last strategy is reappraising or reframing the situation (e.g., believing the family is doing all possible in the situation, being thankful for the good things in life).

Family adaptation describes outcomes of efforts to manage stressful situations. Family adaptation occurs with the individual in relation to the family and with the family in relation to the community. When families adapt well (bonadaptation) they are able to carry out their various functions

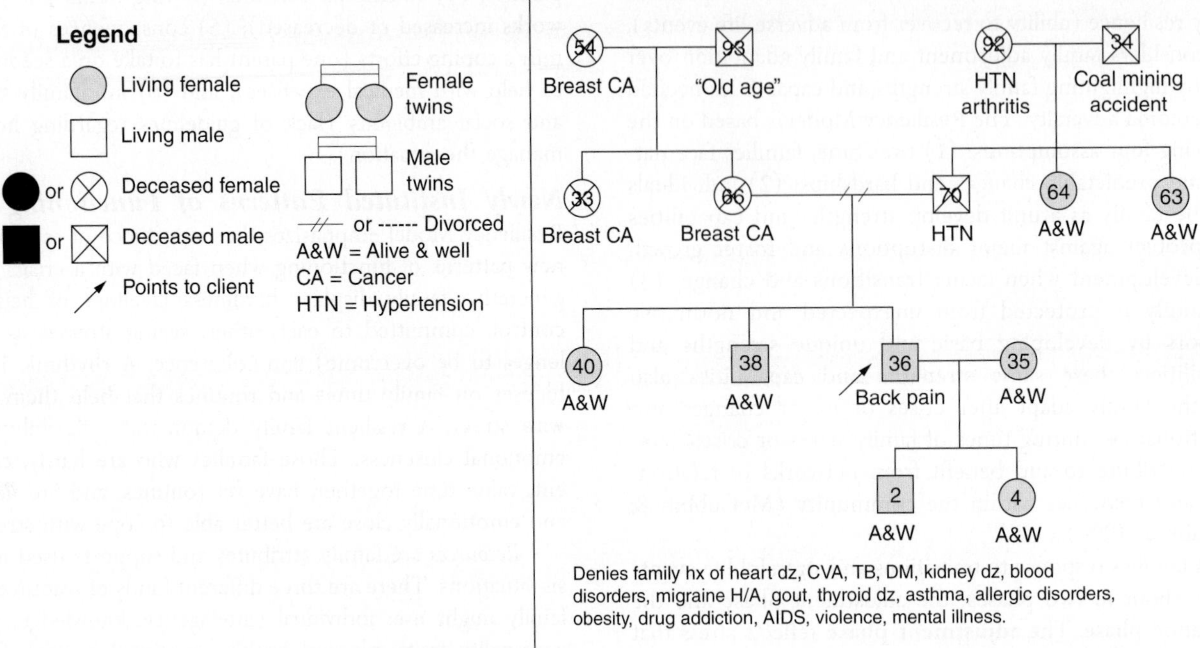

FIGURE 3-4 Family Genogram. DELMAR CENGAGE LEARNING.

(affective, health care, socialization) without compromising individual members and also at the same time to interact with the community appropriately. When they have difficulty adapting (maladaptation), they may move back into a crisis situation.

FAMILY ASSESSMENT

Family assessment is the process of collecting data about the family structure, and the relationships and interactions among individual members. A continuously evolving process, data about the family are systematically collected using predetermined guidelines or questions, and then classified and analyzed according to their meaning. Nursing diagnoses can then be generated, with goals and interventions for care created in collaboration with the child and caregivers.

ASSESSMENT INSTRUMENTS

Two of the most commonly used instruments for developing a family database are the genogram and the ecomap. Neither requires the purchase of a standardized assessment instrument, yet both have the advantage of providing a means for interacting with children and their family members in a nonthreatening way to obtain data about potentially complex and difficult issues.

A **genogram** is a format for drawing a family tree that records information about family members and their relationships over a period of time, usually three generations. It is a method of mapping the structure of the family and recording the health history of all members (morbidity, mortality, and onset of illnesses), thus revealing information about genetic and familial diseases. The genogram displays the family visually and graphically in a way that provides a quick overview of family complexities. It is also an efficient and nonjudgmental way to convey information about a family to other health care providers. Figure 3-4 is an example of a genogram.

An **ecomap** is a visual representation of a family in relation to the community. It demonstrates the nature and quality of family relationships and what kinds of resources or energies are going inside and outside of the family. Figure 3-5 shows a family ecomap. This assessment instrument is useful in identifying the strengths of family networks and what resources are available during stressful times or crises.

An in-depth family assessment requires a significant amount of time, and every family does not need a comprehensive assessment. However, when a nurse identifies a family at risk for dysfunction, such an assessment may be required. Referral to other health care professionals and community organizations is appropriate in these situations. Assessment information can be obtained through interviewing and questioning, observing interactions between members, and utilizing a family assessment instrument. Ideally, all family members are included in the interview, and it takes place in the home. At a minimum, the child and primary caregivers are assessed.

Many assessment instruments have been developed by family theorists, mostly nonnurses, and are used by the health care team to obtain information about family systems. Nurses have developed three assessment models: the Calgary Family Assessment Model (Wright & Leahey, 2009), the Friedman

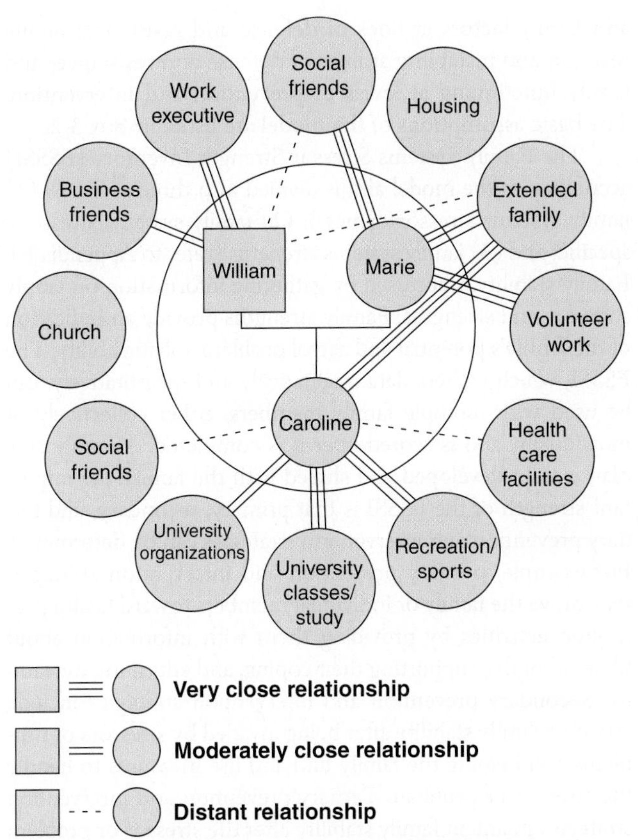

FIGURE 3-5 Family Ecomap. DELMAR CENGAGE LEARNING.

Family Assessment Model (Friedman et al., 2003), and the Family Assessment and Intervention Model and the Family Systems, Stressor-Strength Inventory (Hanson et al., 2005). Box 3-1 suggests criteria to use when selecting a family assessment instrument.

THE CALGARY FAMILY ASSESSMENT MODEL

The Calgary Family Assessment Model (CFAM) combines nursing and family therapy concepts and is based on systems theory, communication, and change theory, as well as cybernetics, and influenced by the biology of recognition and post-modernism (Wright & Leahy, 2009). The model consists of three major categories: structural, developmental, and functional, and assessment questions are organized into these groupings. The first major category is the family structure, which has internal, external, and contextual components (Figure 3-6). The internal family structure includes the family composition, gender of members, sexual orientation, rank order, subsystems, and boundaries. The external family structure includes the extended family and larger systems impacting the family. The family context involves the family ethnicity, race, social class, religion and/or spirituality, and environment. The genogram and ecomap are appropriate instruments to use in assessing the structure of the family.

BOX 3-1

CRITERIA TO USE WHEN SELECTING A FAMILY ASSESSMENT INSTRUMENT

1. Language should be at the sixth-grade level.
2. Measures should be completed within 10 to 15 minutes.
3. Measures should be sensitive to race, ethnic background, age, and gender.
4. Measures should be easy to score and provide information helpful in making decisions.

Adapted from Hanson, S., Gedaly-Duff, V., & Kaakinen, J. (2005). *Family health care nursing: Theory, practice, and research* (3rd ed.). Philadelphia: F. A. Davis.

Family development, the second major category, includes assessment of family stages, tasks, and attachments, and can be evaluated by examining developmental tasks that families go through as their children grow and develop. The third area for assessment is family functioning, which includes instrumental and expressive subcategories. Instrumental aspects of family functioning (how the family members behave in relation to each other) are activities of daily living such as sleeping, eating, meal preparation, and so forth. Expressive areas include emotional functioning, communication patterns, problem-solving methods, roles, influence and power, beliefs, and alliances. The CFAM is broad in perspective, though it focuses on internal relations within the family rather than on the family's relationship with the community. Assessment of every element is not always necessary. However, the nurse needs to decide which subcategories are relevant and should be assessed in order to develop an integrated picture of the many dimensions of family life.

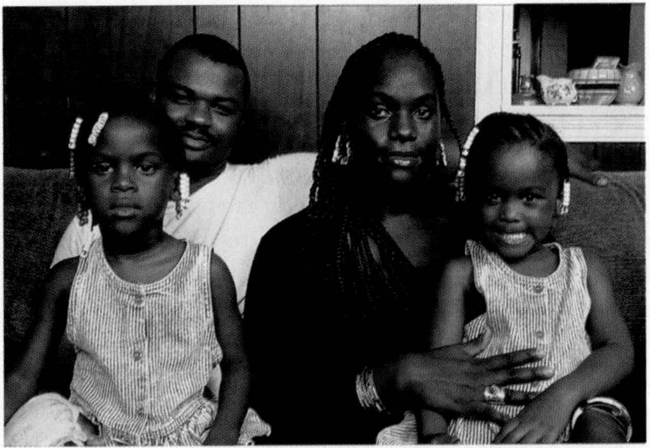

FIGURE 3-6 Family structure is different for every family; thus, the nurse needs to understand this structure to determine communication patterns and decision-making authority. DELMAR CENGAGE LEARNING.

Friedman Family Assessment Model

The Friedman Family Assessment Model is based on the structural-functional framework, as well as on developmental and systems theory. This model views the family as just one of the basic units of the wider society, along with institutions involving religion, education, and health. Its main focus is the family's structure and functions, and the family's relationships with other social systems. The Friedman Family Assessment Model consists of six broad categories of interview questions, each with numerous subcategories:

1. Identifying data (family last name, composition, ethnic background, religious identification, social class status)
2. Developmental stage and history of the family
3. Environmental data (characteristics of the home, neighborhood and larger community, geographic mobility, family's social support system)
4. Family structure (role structure, family values, communication patterns, and power structure)
5. Family functions (affective, socialization, reproductive, economic, health care)
6. Family coping (current stressors, coping strategies used, dysfunctional adaptive strategies used, problem areas in which family has achieved mastery)

This instrument exists in a short and a long form. The short form in Appendix A lists the six major categories and subcategories and questions. The long form is quite extensive, providing nine pages of questions to ask (Friedman et al., 2003). It may not be possible to collect all the data in one encounter. Additionally, all the categories of information listed may not be pertinent for every family. This instrument is broad and general, and is especially useful for viewing families in the context of their community. However, a disadvantage of this approach is that it provides large quantities of data with no clear direction about how to utilize it in developing nursing diagnoses, plans, and interventions (Hanson et al., 2005).

Family Assessment and Intervention Model

The Family Assessment and Intervention Model developed by Berkley-Mischke and Hanson (1991) extends Betty Neuman's (1995) Health Care Systems Model to focus on the family rather than the individual. According to the model (Figure 3-7), when stressors (i.e., problems) penetrate their defenses, families experience tensions. How well the family adapts and how deep the stressor penetrates the family unit impacts the family's reaction. The family's basic structure, including functions and energy resources, are protected at all costs by lines of resistance. Adaptation preserves or restores family stability after the lines of defense are penetrated and usual family functions are altered. Three areas are addressed in the model: health promotion, wellness activities, problem identification, and family factors at lines of defense and resistance; family reaction and instability at lines of defense and resistance; and family functioning at levels of prevention and intervention. The basic assumptions of the model are listed in Box 3-2.

The Family Systems Stressor-Strength Inventory (FSSSI) accompanies the model and is divided into three sections: (1) family systems stressors-general; (2) family systems stressors-specific; and (3) family systems strengths (refer to Appendix B). Family stability is accessed by gathering information on family stressors and strengths. Family strengths provide an indication of the family's potential and actual problem-solving ability. The FSSSI, which gathers data qualitatively and quantitatively, can be used with multiple family members, either collectively or individually, and is scored after it is completed. A family care plan is then developed and shared with the family. An important strength of the FSSSI is that primary, secondary, and tertiary prevention and intervention strategies can be determined. For example, primary prevention and intervention strategies may move the family or individual members toward health promotion activities by providing them with information about their strengths, supporting their coping, and educating the family. Secondary prevention and intervention strategies include attaining family stability after being invaded by stressors or problems and helping the family find and use measures to handle the stressor or problem. Tertiary prevention and intervention strategies maintain family stability after the stressor or problem has been handled (Hanson et al., 2005).

FAMILY STRUCTURE

The structure of the family refers to how it is organized (i.e., the manner in which members relate to one another, and the form it takes, such as nuclear or blended). During the past few decades, U.S. society has undergone vast economic and social changes that have transformed the structure of the family and the roles and responsibilities of women and men. Some of these societal changes are the increase in rates of divorce and remarriage, an increase in the number of mothers employed outside the home, the incidence of more adults waiting until they are older to marry or choosing to remain single, lower birth rates, and a longer life expectancy. Today, society is composed of a greater multiplicity of values, lifestyles, and family forms than ever before. The two-parent nuclear family consisting of a mother and father bonded by marriage with one or more children no longer reflects contemporary lifestyles. Knowledge of a child's family structure helps the nurse to determine the communication patterns and decision-making authority within the family unit. Such information is vital when the nurse asks the family for input regarding decisions related to health care.

NUCLEAR FAMILY

The nuclear family is defined as a husband, wife, and their children—biological, adopted, or both (Smith, et al., 2008)

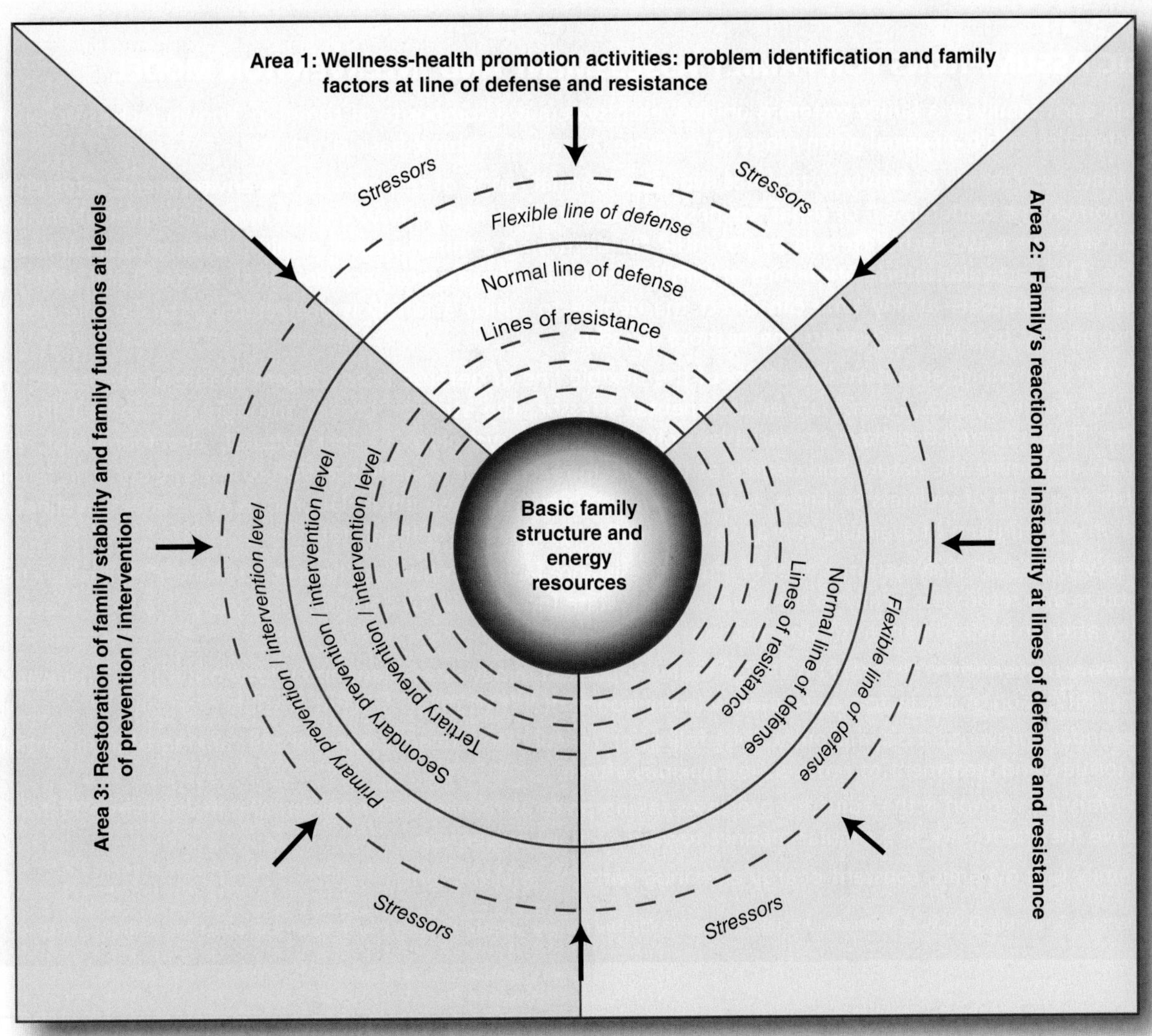

FIGURE 3-7 Family Assessment and Intervention Model. FROM HANSON, S., GEDALY-DUFF, V., & KAAKINEN, J (2005). *FAMILY HEALTH CARE NURSING: THEORY, PRACTICE AND RESEARCH* (3RD ED.). PHILADELPHIA, PA: F. A. DAVIS. USED WITH PERMISSION.

(Figure 3-8). No other individuals, relatives or nonrelatives, live in the household. The nuclear family form became common after World War II, and, until recently, it was considered the most common family form. However, with the increase in divorce rates, nonmarital childbearing, and cohabitation outside of marriage, family forms other than the nuclear family have proliferated. Currently, in the United States, families in the traditional pattern of a working father, homemaker mother, and one or more children are in the minority.

The nuclear family has been credited with providing stability for children. However, concern has been raised about the limited number of adult role models in this type of family structure. Additionally, in the nuclear family, the two adults have many expectations placed on them, such as working to meet financial needs, rearing the children, meeting the emotional needs of all members, and maintaining a home. In situations where both parents are employed, managing all of these responsibilities often results in significant stress in the family.

EXTENDED FAMILY

The extended family consists of those members of the nuclear family and other blood-related persons such as grandparents, aunts, uncles, and cousins (Figure 3-9). This family structure was prominent in the 1800s in the United States because the family was the main unit of economic production. Several generations of a family lived together, worked together, and shared resources and responsibilities. Children were reared by not only their parents but also by grandparents, aunts, and uncles and had a choice of adult role models. With the advent of the Industrial Revolution, families

BOX 3-2

BASIC ASSUMPTIONS FOR FAMILY ASSESSMENT AND INTERVENTION MODEL

Though each family as a family system is unique, each system is a composite of common, known factors or innate characteristics within a normal given range of response contained within a basic structure.

Over time, each family or family system has evolved a normal range of response to the environment, referred to as a "normal line of defense," or usual wellness or stability state. Many known, unknown, and universal environmental stressors exist. Each differs in its potential for disturbing a family's usual stability level, or normal line of defense. The particular interrelationships of family variables—physiological, psychological, sociocultural, developmental, and spiritual—at any time can affect the degree to which a family is protected by the flexible line of defense against possible reaction to one or more stressors.

When the cushioning, accordion-like effect of the flexible line of defense is no longer capable of protecting the family or family system against an environmental stressor, the stressor breaks through the normal line of defense. The interrelationships of variables—physiological, psychological, sociocultural, developmental, and spiritual—determine the nature and degree of the system reaction or possible reaction to the stressor. The family, whether in a state of wellness or illness, is a dynamic composite of these interrelationships of variables. Wellness is found on a continuum of available energy to support the system in its optimal state.

Implicit within each family system is a set of internal resistance factors, known as "lines of resistance," which function to stabilize and return the family to the usual wellness state (normal line of defense) or possibly to a higher level of stability after an environmental stressor reaction.

- *Primary prevention* is general knowledge that is applied in family assessment and intervention for identification and mitigation of risk factors associated with environmental stressors to prevent possible reaction.
- *Secondary prevention* is symptomatology following reaction to stressors, appropriate ranking of intervention priorities, and treatment to reduce their noxious effects.
- *Tertiary prevention* is the adjustive processes taking place as reconstitution begins and maintenance factors move the client back in a circular manner toward primary prevention.

The family is in dynamic, constant energy exchange with the environment.

From Hanson, S., Gedaly-Duff, V., & Kaakinen, J. (2005). *Family health care nursing: Theory, practice and research* (3rd ed.). Philadelphia: F. A. Davis.

were forced to move and seek employment in urban areas, and the nuclear family became more common. However, extended family situations are still seen. Situations include elderly parents moving in with adult children or an adult child and his or her spouse and children moving back into the home of the older parents for financial reasons.

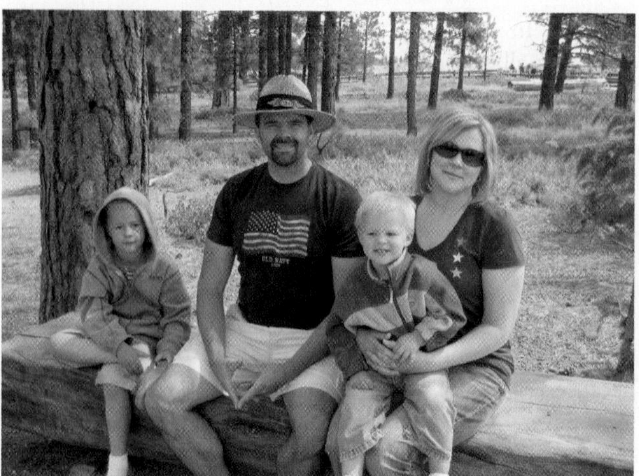

FIGURE 3-8 A nuclear family consists of a mother, a father, and children. DELMAR CENGAGE LEARNING.

BLENDED (OR STEP) FAMILY

A blended or stepfamily occurs when a divorced, widowed, or never-married single parent forms a household with a new partner; both or only one partner may have children. In fact, most divorced people eventually remarry and many

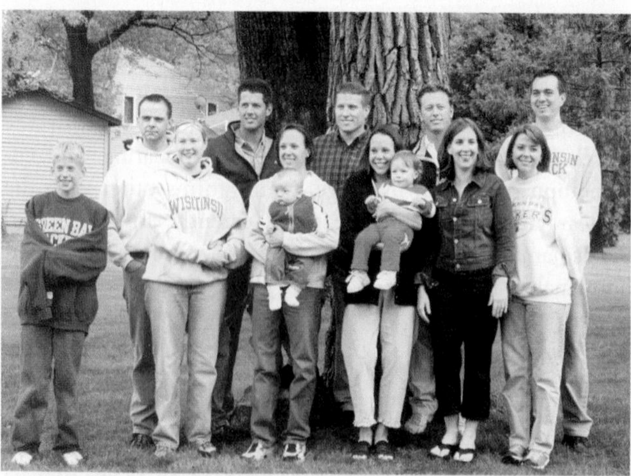

FIGURE 3-9 Members of an extended family benefit from sharing experiences and memories. DELMAR CENGAGE LEARNING.

of these remarriages involve children. Blended families can succeed by making a strong commitment, not only from the couple to each other, but also to the newly created family (Nance-Nash, 2009). The formation of a stepfamily can present many stresses for the parent, stepparent, and children. In the new stepfamily, there has been no time to blend family styles and traditions or to negotiate parenting. Additionally, there has not been time to establish or nurture the marriage. A remarried parent must deal with many strong emotions, and feeling a special loyalty to one's own biological children may create conflicts with the new spouse. The remarried couple may be unable to form a new spousal relationship because to do so would appear to be a betrayal of the intimacy between parent and child. This issue frequently conflicts with the needs of the new spouse, who may feel like an outsider in an established household. Stepfamilies where both adults have children from a previous marriage living with them have the greatest incidence of redivorce.

Stepparents and biological parents often believe the growth of the new family will be instantaneous, but the time required to create the stepfamily is usually longer than the adults expect. The stepparent should make clear to the children that she or he does not consider herself or himself to be a replacement for a dead or absent parent. Instead, the stepparent is another adult who can meet some of the child's needs for closeness and love since parental relationships need time to build. The transition to a stepfamily is also stressful for the children. Having suffered the loss of one of their parents and typically the loss of familiar surroundings, children may encounter a new series of losses and suffer loyalty conflicts and loss of control. The adults have chosen to make major changes in their lives; the children have had those changes imposed on them. Feelings of sibling rivalry are more intense in the stepfamily as the children may feel jealousy, insecurity, and a fear that a new sibling is more loved.

Children's responses to stepfamilies vary depending on their age. The stress of a remarriage often causes preschoolers to cling to parents and to regress behaviorally. With their magical thinking, preschoolers may believe their angry thoughts or behaviors led to the family disruption. They may also believe they can magically reunite the divorced parents. School-age children are often angry about their powerlessness to stop the dissolution of the family. Children at this stage are rarely able to express their feelings verbally and likely to act out their anger. They may have fights with siblings or classmates, develop psychosomatic symptoms, become accident prone, perform poorly in school, or even try to break up the new marriage. However, they may also act "angelic," thus hiding their inner turmoil. Adolescents are dealing with their own issues of identity and autonomy, making the new relationships even more difficult to accept. Additionally, they are dealing with their own sexuality at a time when the addition of a stepsibling or stepparent of the opposite sex can create sexual tensions, and divided loyalties may cause them to act out toward the stepparent.

RESEARCH Highlight

Does the Amount of Parental Conflict During Divorce Make a Difference in Child Outcomes?

STUDY PURPOSE

Because interparental conflict during divorce may have adverse effects on children, the purpose of this study was to discover the effects (immediate and short-term) of interparental conflict on children whose parents were divorcing. Specifically, the investigators wanted to know if there were differences in child outcomes depending on which level of divorce the parents were in: dissolution (agreement on all aspects of the divorce), divorce with little litigation (little disagreement), divorce with moderate litigation (referred for mediation), and divorce with high litigation (property hearing or custody investigation).

METHODS

Seventy-six parents (31 men and 45 women) between 22 and 53 years of age with children ranging in age from 2 to 17 years old completed The Divorce Adjustment Inventory–Revised immediately following the divorce hearing and again six months later.

FINDINGS

Children whose parents had a higher level of conflict exhibited poorer coping ability than those children whose parents displayed moderate and low levels of conflict. In addition, children from families going through dissolution were less vulnerable to maladjustment because of how the parents handled the separation and consequent divorce.

IMPLICATIONS

Practitioners need to understand that when a child's parents undergo divorce, the amount of conflict displayed by the parents may impact the child negatively. Therefore, appropriate interventions that help children whose parents are divorcing need to be provided, especially if the parents are experiencing a high level of conflict. In addition, parents undergoing divorce need to limit the amount of conflict they display towards each other in front of their children.

REFERENCE

Bing, N., Nelson, W., & Wesolowski, K., (2009). Comparing the effects of amount of conflict on children's adjustment following parental divorce. *Journal of Divorce & Remarriage, 50*, 159–171.

Finally, when comparing nuclear families to stepfamilies, at least six differences are apparent. First, there is little or no family loyalty and, initially, no family history. Second, the structure of stepfamilies is different from a nuclear family with a variety of coalitions, some preceding the remarriage. Third, there are a variety of family systems outside the stepfamily which affect functioning and coping. Fourth, many members may have experienced a loss and children may have more than two parenting figures. Fifth, family boundaries may be ambiguous, especially when biological parents not living with the family influence family decisions. Lastly, a solid couple relationship does not always mean stepchildren and stepparents will have a good relationship. In fact, in some stepfamilies, stepparents have little power and authority when compared to children (Visher & Visher, 1996).

SINGLE-PARENT FAMILY

While there have been a variety of shifts in family structures, none has been more dramatic than the shift toward families headed by a single parent. Single parenting occurs by means of divorce, separation, death of a spouse, or choice. A single-parent family can be created when a single person acquires a child through birth or adoption; however, most single-parent households have been created by divorce, and most are comprised of single mothers and their children. In fact, in 2006, 9% of households were headed by single parents; 10.4 million single mothers were raising children, and most single-parent families were Caucasian (Sugarman, 2007). However, not all single-family homes are headed by women: a number of single-parent homes are headed by men, most of whom are divorced. Some are widowed and a rare number are fathers of children born out of wedlock. When single men care for their children, they are often self supporting and tend to marry or remarry quickly (Sugarman, 2007).

Major concerns of single parents are limitations of available resources such as money, time, and physical and emotional energy. Increasingly, two incomes are needed to raise children at a decent standard of living. Single mothers are more likely to be poor when compared with other adults, and most poor children live in single-parent families. Single parents who are employed often feel overwhelmed in an attempt to provide adequate time for the family, the job, and the endless details of daily life. The single parent must also provide the majority of emotional support and sustenance for the children. Managing all of these responsibilities leaves little time for the parent's social or personal needs (Figure 3-10).

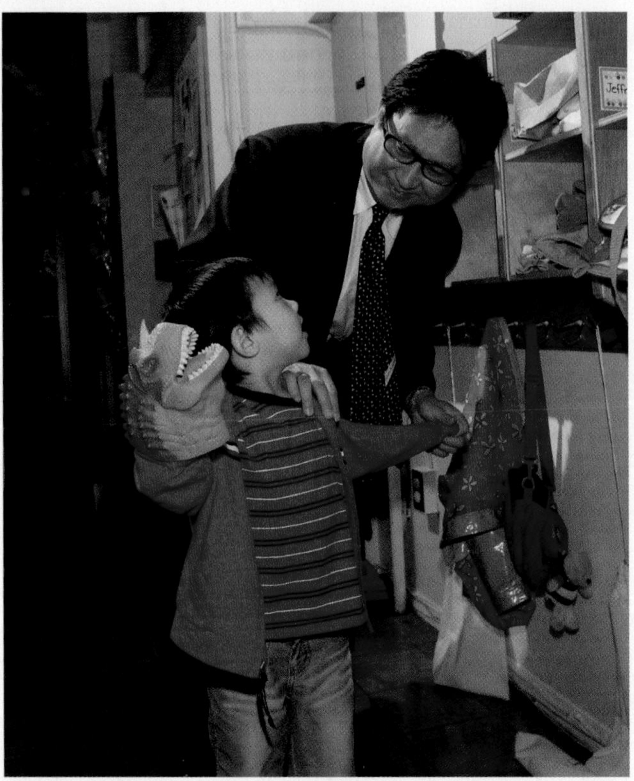

FIGURE 3-10 Major concerns of single parents are limitations of available resources such as money, time, and physical and emotional energy. DELMAR CENGAGE LEARNING.

Single-parent status is often born out of crisis such as separation or divorce. Such events have different meanings for the child than for the parent. For example, the parent may feel independence and relief due to the separation and divorce; however, the child may experience a sense of uncertainty, instability, and loss. There may be changes in the family home, the child's school, friends, and community. The subsequent transitional period is likely to be disorganized and tumultuous until a realignment of roles, schedules, and expectations can permit a new and stabilized family life.

Many children raised in single-parent families are at risk for adverse outcomes in three areas: academic performance, psychological functioning, and social functioning. On the other hand, some children benefit from being raised by single mothers because the mothers promote flexible attitudes toward gender roles and fewer gender role stereotypes. Single-parent families also tend to encourage independence, autonomy, responsibility, and maturity in their children. Successful single-parent families vary not only by parent gender and age, but also by race, ethnicity, employment status, educational level, living arrangements, and social factors (Hanson et al., 2005).

GAY AND LESBIAN FAMILIES

Gay and lesbian families are increasing in numbers. Such families are defined by the presence of two or more persons of the same sex or by the presence of at least one gay or lesbian adult rearing a child. The structure of these families is quite variable (Figure 3-11). Many lesbians, both single or in a relationship, are giving birth through artificial insemination. In addition, gay men are increasingly becoming parents through adoption or the use of a surrogate mother.

On the other hand, these families are faced with several legal barriers. Some of these include:

1. Same-sex relationships are often denied the legal benefits of marriage.
2. Gay and lesbian parents who were married are often denied custody or visitation with their children following divorce because of their sexual orientation.

RESEARCH Highlight

Do Grandparents Make a Difference in Single-Parent and Stepfamily Homes?

STUDY PURPOSE

Since an increased number of children/adolescents experience parental divorce, remarriage, or live in single-parent homes, the purpose of this study was to examine whether grandparent involvement varied in two-parent biological, single-parent, and stepparent families and then determine whether this involvement made a difference in the behavioral and emotional adjustment of adolescents according to their family structure.

METHODS

Children/adolescents (n = 1515) between the ages of 11 and 16 living with their two biological parents, in a single-parent home, or in a home with a stepparent completed the 25-item Strengths and Difficulties Questionnaire that measured adjustment difficulties (hyperactivity, emotional symptoms, conduct problems, and peer problems) and prosocial behavior. They also completed a grandparent-grandchild relationships scale that assessed the emotional closeness of the adolescents with their grandparents (the extent to which they could depend on their grandparents, were appreciated by their grandparents, experienced love or were cared for by their grandparents; believed their grandparents helped them in significant ways, and felt close to their grandparents compared to how other grandchildren felt to their grandparents).

FINDINGS

Results indicated that when grandparents were involved in the lives of their grandchildren, the grandchildren displayed fewer emotional problems ($p < .01$) and had more prosocial behavior ($p < .001$). In addition, if the grandchildren were from single-parent or stepparent homes, grandparent involvement was more strongly associated with reduced adjustment difficulties when compared to grandchildren from two-parent biological families.

IMPLICATIONS

Since grandparent involvement is important in the lives of grandchildren, it would be important to encourage grandparents to become part of and support their grandchildren, especially if they live in single-parent homes or with a stepparent.

REFERENCE

Attar-Schwartz, S., Tan, J., Buchanan, A., Flouri, E., & Griggs, J. (2009). Grandparenting and adolescent adjustment in two-parent biological, lone-parent, and step-families. *Journal of Family Psychology, 23*(1), 67–75.

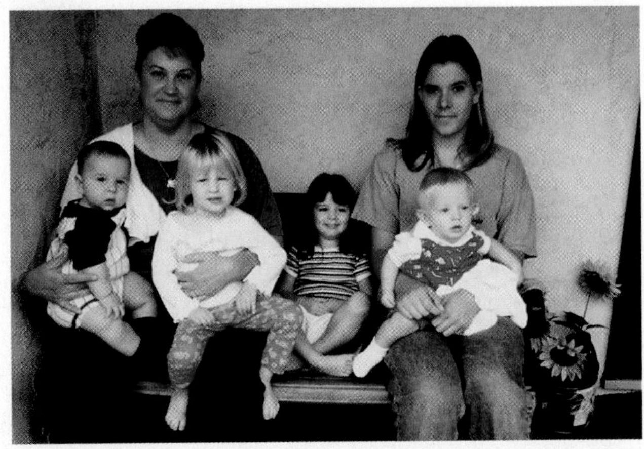

FIGURE 3-11 **The nurse must understand a family's system and structure to provide appropriate care and guidance.** DELMAR CENGAGE LEARNING.

3. In many states, regulations governing adoption and foster care make it difficult for lesbians and gays to adopt children or become foster parents.
4. Medical procedures often require approval of the biological parent, meaning that a durable power of attorney might be necessary for the nonbiological parent to legally authorize health services.

Contrary to common opinion, no significant differences have been found in gender identity and sex-role behaviors among children of gay and lesbian parents compared to children of heterosexual parents. Such children are no more likely to be lesbian or gay than are children with heterosexual parents. Another common misconception is that children raised by gay men and lesbians have psychological problems. However, such children do not differ from children with heterosexual parents in terms of psychological health. Finally, children of gay and lesbian parents are not different from children raised by heterosexual parents in their academic functioning (Dingfelder, 2008; Tellingator & Patterson, 2008).

NURSING ALERT

Working with Gay and Lesbian Families

When working with families, do not assume that all parents are heterosexual. In obtaining the family history, the following questions may be asked: (1) Who makes up your family? (2) Do you have a partner? (3) Do you share parenting responsibilities with anyone else? (4) Who else is responsible for the child's care if you are not available?

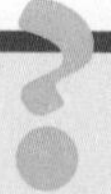

KIDS WANT TO KNOW

Will I grow up to identify as a lesbian since both of my parents are lesbians?

The nurse can answer this 10-year-old girl's question by stating that having lesbian parents does not mean she is more or less likely to be lesbian. This is a sensitive issue in U.S. society today because some conservative individuals maintain that homosexuals should not rear children because they will likely follow their parents' lifestyle. It is important to explain that gay or lesbian people do not make others gay or lesbian.

Children reared in a gay or lesbian family who discover they are homosexual often have fears of revealing this to their parents. Many feel they have failed their parents, who may believe their children's lives would be easier and less frustrating if they were straight.

CULTURAL INFLUENCES ON THE FAMILY

Because of growing proportions of ethnic minorities and immigrant families, the United States is becoming more culturally diverse. This diversity brings with it many challenges for health care providers. All families are shaped by their surrounding culture, which provides them with social norms. Some families are strongly influenced by their original culture, whereas others are more assimilated to the homogenous "American" culture. Many factors influence the extent to which families identify with a given culture and incorporate its customs and traditions into their daily lives: country of origin, language, level of education, religion, socioeconomic status, number of generations in this country, and urban versus rural lifestyle (Figure 3-12). Each culture has its own values, attitudes, and practices with regard to families and child rearing, yet there can be a wide range of beliefs and practices among families from the same cultural background.

For nurses working with families from cultures other than their own, the development of cultural sensitivity is paramount in order to respond accurately and sensitively

Reflections from Families

Because of my sexual orientation, people think of me as a lesbian, but I think mostly of myself as a woman and, now, a mother. I have been in a close and loving committed relationship with my partner for ten years. After living together for six years, we both realized that we very much wanted a child in our lives. We decided to try to have a baby through artificial insemination, but after many unsuccessful tries at getting pregnant, we found that we only wanted a child that much more. So we adopted our precious little son Jonah, who is now 6 years old and beginning public school.

When his classmates told him he was different because he had two mothers instead of a mother and a father, he was very confused. Yet the children and teachers all like him so much because of his happy nature and pleasant attitude towards school, and he rapidly adjusted to the school and socialization process much like all the other first graders. In fact, he has proven to be much better adjusted than some of them who do not come from such loving homes. We have gotten involved in school activities, and most of the other parents are now at ease with our parenting arrangement. Jonah has lots of friends, going often to visit at their homes or having them over here. In fact, some of the mothers we have gotten to know the best, after seeing how well two mothers can create a loving and nurturing home for a child, often ask us to care for their own children when they go out for an evening.

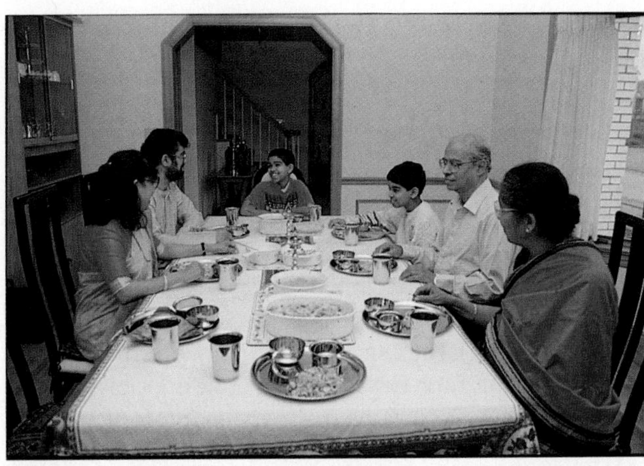

FIGURE 3-12 Respect for a family's cultural values and practices is important in providing culturally sensitive nursing care. DELMAR CENGAGE LEARNING.

to their needs and to provide care. **Cultural sensitivity** means having an awareness and appreciation of cultural influences in health care and being respectful of differences in cultural belief systems and values. Nurses can be most effective in their work if they adopt a multicultural perspective, which means using appropriate aspects of the family's cultural orientation to develop health care interventions. To provide culturally sensitive care to children and their families, nurses must first be aware of their own values and beliefs and recognize how they influence their attitudes and actions. Additionally, they should be knowledgeable about the different cultural groups they encounter in practice. Then they are able to determine whether a certain behavior is peculiar to the individual or characteristic of the culture.

CULTURAL CONSIDERATION

Jewish Families

The goal of Jewish parents is to raise a child to be a *mensch* (a person who cares and shares, loves and studies and acts righteously) and create a peaceful home (*shalom bayit*). Parental responsibilities are to teach children about religious and secular matters and to make their own decisions and respect their elders. The Sabbath, a building block of family peace, should be a day of rest. Hospitality is a sacred obligation, and many Jewish families will feed, clothe, and shelter others in need of basic necessities. Many homes contain ritual objects (*mezuzah, menorah, seder plates, kiddush*) and many families eat Kosher foods (meat and dairy cannot be mixed; meat must be from animals that chew a cud and have split hoofs and are slaughtered according to Jewish law). Jewish families read the Talmud (an encyclopedia of commentaries on Jewish law; written in Hebrew and Aaramaic), the Siddur (a daily book of prayer), and the Torah (the first five books of the Old Testament). Their spiritual leader is the Rabbi, who teaches, preaches, counsels, and represents the Jewish faith. Children may attend Day school, which is full time parochial education, or Religious (Hebrew) school, which is part time, after school/weekends. Members of the Jewish faith celebrate Rosh Hashanah (new year), Yom Kippur (day of atonement), Hannukah (the return of light in the heart of winter darkness), and Passover (the return of sunlight when the first spring fruits are on the table). Naming a child is important since it represents one's personal identity as well as familial and religious connections. Major celebrated life events include the bar and bat mitzvah. The breaking of glass at a Jewish wedding is a reminder that marriage is a transforming experience that leaves individuals forever changed.

Reference: Diamant, A., & Cooper, H. (1991). *Living a Jewish life.* Harper Collins.

IMMIGRANT FAMILIES

Over the past several years, the number of immigrant families has grown, and the ethnic background of these families has shifted from predominantly white Europeans to Latinos and Asians. In addition, immigrant families no longer are concentrated in states such as California, but rather are dispersed to new areas, leading to increases in immigrant populations in many small communities (Dinan, 2006).

To promote positive outcomes for children from immigrant families it is important to improve their education, health care, and economic security. This is because many of these children are not well represented in prekindergarten and early childhood education programs, even though by not participating they face problems in being ready for school. Immigrant families also have difficulty accessing needed health care and are more likely than native-born families to be living in poverty. Still, some immigrant families are economically secure and highly educated (Dinan, 2006; Shields & Behrman, 2004). In fact, immigrant families are noted to have a number of strengths including their healthy intact large extended families, strong work ethic and aspirations, and community cohesion (Shields & Behrman, 2004).

CULTURAL CONSIDERATION

Traditional Asian Families

The ideal Asian family is the extended family, involving at least three generations; parents, children, and grandchildren live in the same household or in the same neighborhood. Some marriages are arranged; the purpose of marriage is personal (emotional security) and social (socio-economic stability). The preference is for male children, especially the first child, to guarantee the family name will be carried into the future. The family is an important source for transmitting cultural traditions from one generation to the next, and interaction with grandparents strengthens children's sense of identity. Children are committed to care for their parents; parents are committed to care for children and grandchildren. Healthy seniors are actively engaged in family responsibilities; traditional gender roles are followed with domination of women by men (Quah, 2008).

CRITICAL THINKING

Culturally Sensitive Care

You are assigned to care for a Vietnamese boy who is in traction, hospitalized for a fractured femur. He speaks his native language as well as English. His caregivers, who also speak both languages, are present in the child's room when you enter to perform an initial nursing assessment. What considerations are important in order to provide culturally sensitive care?

PARENTING

Parenting is a dynamic process that evolves over time as parents acquire experience and mature as individuals. The social goal of parenting is to guide and nurture children so they become productive members of society. The personal goal of parenting is far more individualized, but, in general, reflects a desire to raise a child, see aspects of oneself continue to exist such as perpetuating the family line, upholding family traditions, or in some cases, fulfilling personal dreams through the child's accomplishments. Individuals approach the topic of parenting

CULTURAL CONSIDERATION

Muslim Families

Although Islam is the second largest and fastest growing religion in the world, there is diversity in how it is practiced. The two major groups have slightly different practices and beliefs: the Sunni (80%) and the Shia (15%). The Qur'an is read daily, and members of the Islamic faith believe in five basic principles or Pillars. The Pillars include the *shahada* (profession of faith that there is one God [Allah] and Muhammad is God's messenger); the *salat* (five daily prayers); *sawm* (fasting during the month of Ramadan); *zakat* (giving to the poor); and the *hajj* (pilgrimage to Mecca once in one's lifetime). Muslims believe that one will be resurrected and earn peace and companionship forever in paradise (*jannah*) if one behaves morally on earth. Consequently, members of the faith believe that life on earth is a test to see if they can obey God and follow his principles. Pride, arrogance, gossiping, slander, lying, theft, murder, adultery, greed, disrespect for parents, abuse of family members, and oppression of the poor as well as not following the five pillars are hurtful to others and sinful. However, Muslims believe sins can be forgiven in repentance. Shiekhs (religious scholars) issue *fatwas* (rulings) related to family matters including marriage, divorce, child custody, and inheritance. However, these fatwas can be subject to secular laws/civil courts. Since modesty is prescribed by the Qur'an many Muslim women wear head scarves, full-length dresses that cover the feet, and long-sleeved shirts. Adult children are required to care for their aged parents, and alcohol is forbidden.

Traditional Muslim societies are collectivist rather than individualistic. Therefore, all Muslims are brothers and sisters and should help one another as needed. In addition, Muslim families are part of the *ummah* (greater whole), which allows them to support each other in times of personal or family distress. Most Muslim families are patriarchal, and husbands are expected to be good examples of faith and right living and support their families. Even though women are usually encouraged to get an education or learn a useful skill, wives care for children, perform domestic chores, and protect/manage the household. However, some wives work outside the home with permission from their husbands. Marriages are often arranged, and unmarried women should not associate with marriageable men without being properly supervised. If they attend college, they do not live independently.

Reference: Springer, P., Abbott, D., & Reisbig, A. (2009). Therapy with Muslim couples and families: Basic guidelines for effective practice. *The Family Journal*, 17, 229–235.

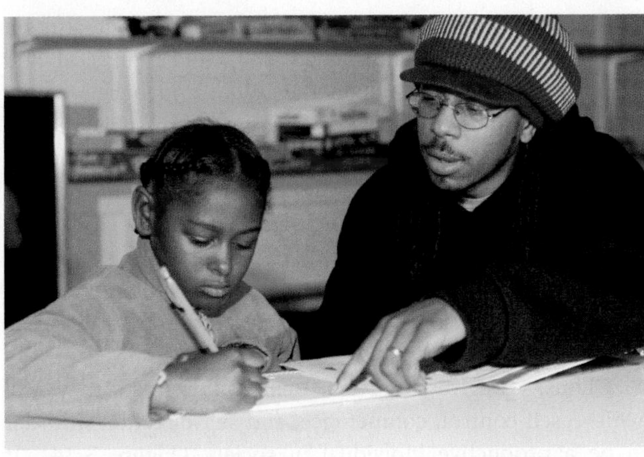

FIGURE 3-13 **This father displays a positive attitude toward school and learning by helping his daughter with her homework.** DELMAR CENGAGE LEARNING.

from a unique, experiential base: each has been parented. In the parenting role, women and men create models incorporating those elements they believe comprise "good" parenting. Whether this personal model is congruent with or antithetical to the parenting they received while growing up, it is nevertheless founded upon personal experiences, acquired knowledge, and beliefs about parents and children.

Social changes have influenced the timing of childbearing, so large numbers of young people are delaying the start of families to meet other social expectations. The need to complete one's education, initiate a career track, establish financial security, and build a committed relationship are fast becoming benchmarks to be achieved before one takes on the responsibility of raising a child. Parental roles are shaped by socially ascribed expectations for enacting the role; by family traditions, values, and cultural beliefs, which shape one's personal perceptions; and by legal and ethical role sanctions and expectations. Principal among these expectations is the responsibility of preparing the child to become a productive member of society. Children learn from their parents how to behave in a manner consistent with their role in the family and appropriate to their culture. While family traditions dictate much of the child rearing strategies used by parents, they do engage in a process of adapting their actions to fit their personal model of parenting. Such a reflective adaptation of child-rearing strategies may be stimulated when the traditional strategies are not effective, when the parent is confronted with new situations, or when the traditional strategy is incongruent with the parent's "good parent" model.

PARENTING BY DEVELOPMENTAL STAGE

Parenting is an evolving process that changes as parents and children grow and mature. Parents must actively adapt their parenting strategies to meet the needs of the growing child. The work of parenting is sustained by the attachment that develops between parents and their children—the strongest of all human relationships. Parents and children develop deep, personal attachments that enable them to care for and about each other, even when families experience great stress or the family system structure changes through divorce, death, or the addition of new family members. Such caring is essential for human survival. Indeed, small children cannot grow and thrive without care activities, including technical tasks like diapering and feeding, as well as those emotive, cognitive responses that support the growth of a centered, well-integrated person.

Nurturing and positive parenting practices help children develop secure attachments, positive self-esteem, and effective relationships with others. Positive parenting strategies show positive regard and attentiveness, respond to the child's need for individuality and autonomy, and utilize active listening (Figure 3-13). Specifically, that means parents should praise compliance and competency, apologize when appropriate, be consistent, communicate love and affection directly, label the child's behavior rather than the child, provide notice when requiring the child to change activities, and give directions firmly, specifically, and positively. In addition, positive parents allow children to make their own choices (if reasonable and appropriate); spend time with the child at a certain time every day with no interruptions, interrogations, or directions; frequently make positive comments about the child's behavior; respond with eye contact, physical contact, and smiles when a child seeks attention; and stay neutral and tell the child what behavior is preferred when a child misbehaves. Finally, it is important to use active listening. This means avoid using commands, editorializing, or judging; paraphrase what one thinks the child is saying; follow the child's lead in interacting and reflect what one thinks the child is feeling; and use the same affect the child is using in relation to tone of voice and posture.

PARENTING STYLES

Each child is unique in her or his own temperament and basic personality. Birth order, gender, and personality traits are a few of the characteristics a child brings to a family. The ways caregivers respond to these attributes and interact with the child are related to the individual's style of parenting. Four styles have been identified: (1) authoritarian or autocratic; (2) authoritative or democratic; (3) indulgent or permissive; and (4) indifferent or uninvolved (Macoby & Martin, 1983). Authoritarian caregivers value obedience over independence and favor punitive measures, harsh disapproval, and withdrawal of love when children question authority or disobey. They are likely to be less emotionally expressive and to use power to assert their will on their children. Deference and respect for authority are expected. They establish strict and rigid rules, which they don't discuss with their child. Children whose caregivers are authoritarian tend to be dependent, passive, and less intellectually curious. They usually lack social competence and spontaneity, and have low self-esteem.

Authoritative or democratic caregivers are warm but firm. They provide opportunities for their children to

REFLECTIVE THINKING

What Kind of Parent Are You or Do You Want to Be?

Consider the following questions as you clarify your personal view of parenting.

What are the sources of parenting that shape your ideal view of what it means to be a parent? Are there role models available who model the kind of parenting you give or want to give to your child? Which of your parents' strategies do you want to retain, and which do you want to avoid using?

develop a sense of autonomy and allow active involvement in decisions that affect them. They are consistent and clear about the expectations they have for their children and are firm when they are disobedient. They guide children's behavior by sharing reasons for their decisions, rules, and standards. Independence is valued, and they are receptive to the child's needs and desires. Children reared in this type of environment have self-control and high self-esteem and are socially competent and self-reliant.

Indulgent or permissive caregivers are interested and involved in their children's lives but place few demands on them and rarely attempt to control their behavior. With the indulgent style, there is an absence of restraints and maximum freedom for the child. Caregivers provide little input or direction and seldom punish their children because they are encouraged to develop their own standards of behavior (most of their behavior is considered acceptable by the caregivers). Although children are allowed freedom to set their own limits, most do not feel comfortable with this lack of direction. Additionally, the caregivers' permissiveness doesn't usually foster the development of internal control in these children, who tend to be disrespectful, defiant of authority, and irresponsible.

Indifferent or uninvolved caregivers attempt to minimize the amount of time and energy they must invest in their children's lives. They tend to be very self-centered and structure their home life primarily around their own needs and interests. They are rejecting of and unresponsive to their child's needs. The child receives little guidance, and discipline is inconsistent. Children from indifferent homes are often more impulsive, demonstrate disregard for other's rights, and are more likely to be involved in delinquent behavior (Macoby & Martin, 1983).

PARENTAL ROLE IN SOCIALIZATION OF CHILDREN

Socialization is a process of learning the rules and expected behaviors of a society. Expectations for a child's behavior depend not only on the society and culture, but also on the child's developmental stage, the child's physical and cognitive capabilities, and on the values and beliefs of the family and home. One goal of parenting is to socialize children, which includes teaching which behaviors are expected and appropriate, and fostering the development of self-control. Initially, during infancy and early childhood, caregivers provide external controls. Gradually and eventually, children guided by caregivers take responsibility for that control and integrate the adults' values, attitudes, and expectations into their behavior.

Thus, caregivers nurture their children so they will achieve self-control, competence, and self-direction in order to be a productive individual in society (Figure 3-14). It could be said this is also the goal of discipline, which comes from the root word *disciplinare*—to teach or instruct (American Academy of Pediatrics [AAP] Committee on Psychosocial Aspects of Child and Family Health, 1998). Discipline should be approached in the broadest sense of helping the child learn rules, regulations, and goals of living in a world with others—and not just as setting limits and punishing. In 1998 and again recently reaffirmed, the AAP suggests effective discipline should include three components: (1) a positive, supportive, nurturing caregiver-child relationship; (2) positive reinforcement techniques to increase desirable behaviors; and (3) removal of reinforcement or use of

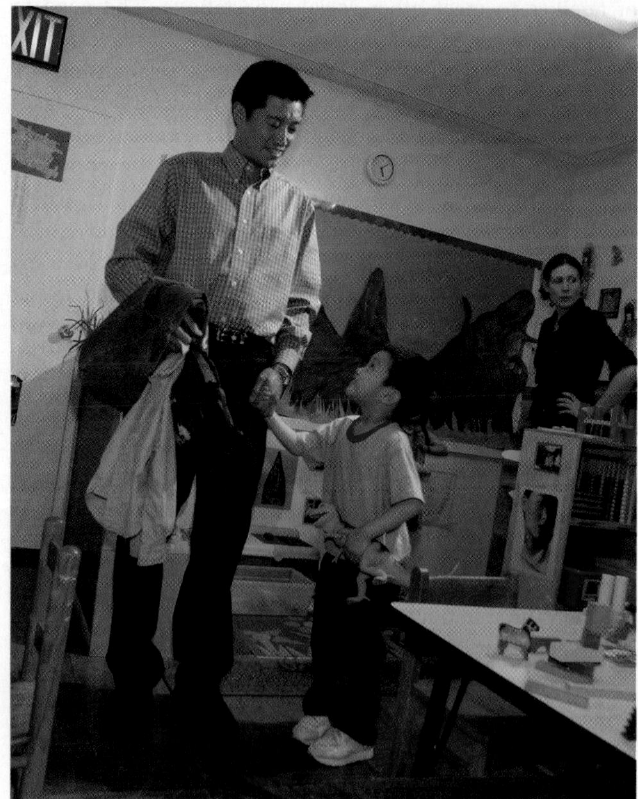

FIGURE 3-14 Modeling independence and self-direction are important parental responsibilities. DELMAR CENGAGE LEARNING.

BOX 3-3
EFFECTIVE DISCIPLINARY PRACTICES

- Use logical consequences
- Use natural consequences
- Withhold privileges
- Be aware of your child's abilities and limitations
- Think before you speak
- Remember children do what "works"
- Be consistent
- Pay attention to your child's feelings
- Learn to see mistakes

Adapted from the American Academy of Pediatrics (2007). *Parenting Corner Q & A: Discipline*. Retrieved June 28, 2009, from http://www.aap.org/pubed/ZZZLZ33YUSC.htm.

punishment to reduce or eliminate undesirable behaviors. Box 3-3 offers other suggestions for effective disciplinary practices.

Increasing Desirable Behavior

Many desirable behaviors occur as part of a child's normal development; however, others need to be taught, such as empathy, sharing, telling the truth (not lying), and good study habits. Family members can teach these behaviors by role modeling since children naturally learn through imitation. Other strategies that help children learn positive behaviors include: focusing on a child's improved behavior rather than on misbehavior; spending time with children doing what they like to do; asking children to share their happy and sad times during the day as tucking them in at night; talking with children about problems that need to be solved so they can provide solutions; giving children meaningful responsibilities congruent with their developmental level (setting the table, clearing the dinner table, picking up toys, etc.); giving children choices related to their responsibilities if appropriate; being sure children understand what is expected when assigning a responsibility; modeling and teaching respect for others; when disciplining children, being sure they know why they are being disciplined and what the discipline will entail; being sure consequences are respectful, reasonable, and related to the behavior expected; and involving children in deciding consequences for misbehavior. If children need to be disciplined, be sure they learn from their mistakes (Nelson, 2006). By implementing these strategies, the desired behavior is more likely to become internalized by the child, and the new behaviors will become a foundation for other desirable ones.

Reducing or Eliminating Undesirable Behaviors

When undesirable behaviors occur, discipline strategies are necessary to reduce or eliminate such behaviors. Undesirable behaviors are those that put the child or others in danger, do not comply with expectations of caregivers or other appropriate adults (e.g., teachers), and interfere with social interactions and self-discipline (AAP, 1998). However, effective discipline cannot occur if caregivers do not develop their abilities to be positive and rewarding. An important quality of discipline is that the consequences are effective, constructive, and not unduly harsh (Box 3-4).

Several disciplinary strategies are used by caregivers to deal with undesirable or unacceptable behaviors, including disapproval, verbal reprimands, time-out, and corporal punishment. Disapproval can be verbal or nonverbal and very effective. Tone of voice, facial expressions, and gestures often convey the caregiver's disapproval of a specific behavior. Even young children can learn when their caregiver is irritated by observing and responding to voice inflections, facial expressions, and gestures.

Many caregivers use disapproving verbal statements to alter undesired behavior. Such reprimands may be effective in immediately stopping or reducing the behavior when used infrequently and targeted toward specific behaviors. However, if caregivers use verbal reprimands frequently and indiscriminately, they may reinforce the undesired behavior because the child gets attention. It is important that reprimands refer to the child's behavior rather than him or her as a person, and not slander the child's character.

Time-out is an effective discipline strategy that involves removing positive reinforcement for unacceptable behavior. It is a defined period of time in which the child is removed

BOX 3-4
CHARACTERISTICS OF APPROPRIATE DISCIPLINE

- Set clear, reasonable, and developmentally appropriate rules.
- Explain the consequences that the child can expect when the problem behavior occurs.
- Develop consequences that are appropriate to the child's level of development and sufficient to be considered negative without being unduly harsh.
- Administer consequences as soon after the infraction occurs as possible.
- Administer consequences calmly without becoming angry.
- Praise the child when she or he behaves appropriately.

from activities and social interactions. The goal of time-out is to interrupt a pattern of negative behavior. The child should be placed in an area that is unstimulating and safe for a given amount of time (usually 1 minute per year of age). A timer can be used so the child knows when time is up. Verbal or physical interaction with the child tends to negate the effects of time-out because the child is given attention for unacceptable behavior. It is important to determine the behaviors that warrant a time-out and to provide the child with this information. The child should also be aware of the procedure to be followed and the "rules." Each time the child misbehaves, the time-out should take place. The use of time-out is advocated by many child care experts because it avoids the problems of other discipline methods such as corporal punishment. The advantage of time-out strategies is that they reduce direct confrontations between parent and child and allow for a "cooling off" period. Additionally, this technique has shown to increase compliance with caregiver expectations from 25% to 80% (AAP, 1998).

One cannot overlook the fact that many families believe **corporal punishment** is the only means for ensuring children behave as instructed. Corporal punishment involves the application of some form of physical pain in response to undesired behavior. Concerns have been raised about its negative effects, however. Still, one form of corporal punishment, spanking, remains a strategy commonly used to reduce undesirable behaviors (AAP, 1998; Kazdin & Benjet, 2009). Additionally, it continues to be sanctioned by many states in public schools in the United States (American Academy of Pediatrics Committee on School Health, 2000) and was recently reaffirmed by the AAP.

Corporal punishment may inhibit misbehavior, but at great cost. Its effectiveness decreases with subsequent use. The child becomes habituated to this strategy, and its intensity must be systematically increased each time it is used, which can quickly escalate into abuse. Further, corporal punishment increases the chance of physical injury, especially for infants and young children. It leads to altered caregiver-child relationships, making other forms of discipline more difficult when corporal punishment is no longer an option (e.g., with adolescents). Thus, because of the negative consequences of this type of punishment, caregivers should be encouraged and assisted to develop alternative methods in response to undesired behavior, such as using time-out and verbal reprimands. This is especially important for foster families, where caregivers may be prohibited from using corporal punishment but not know other strategies (Kazdin & Benjet, 2009).

SPECIAL PARENTING SITUATIONS

A variety of special family situations can increase the complexity of parenting and present different issues. These situations include parenting multiples, adolescent parents, adoption, grandparents as parents, and foster parents.

PARENTING MULTIPLES

Although parenting multiples may be similar to parenting singletons, there are still differences that are important to be aware of when working with these families. First, a pregnancy with twins or other multiples may be physically and emotionally difficult not only for the mother but also for the father. In addition, these families may be faced with health care issues if the mother needs to be on bed rest prior to the birth or if the twins are born early, as this is a common occurrence with multiples. Therefore, it would be important for the parents to be provided with written information about multiple births and local/national support organizations. Although some mothers may not feel it is possible to breastfeed multiples, it is possible, especially with support from fathers who tend to be more involved with multiples than singletons, and other family members or friends. Since the twins or other multiples may initially be eating and sleeping at different times, it would be important for parents to develop a plan/routine for eating and sleeping arrangements. It is also acceptable for the babies to sleep in the same crib at first since they have been together prior to birth (Leonard & Denton, 2006).

The literature suggests attachment is more complex with multiples since one may be favored over the other, or one may have an easier temperament than the other child. The parents may also be attached to the multiples as a unit rather than as separate children, so it would be important to help parents identify similarities/differences between each of the multiples, and seek ways to help them not show preference for one multiple over the other (Figure 3-15). If there are other children in the family they may feel more neglected and display behavior problems more commonly than if there was a singleton birth, because of the attention shown by parents or insensitive friends/family members. Consequently, parents may need advice on what to tell the siblings about the intended birth depending on sibling ages,

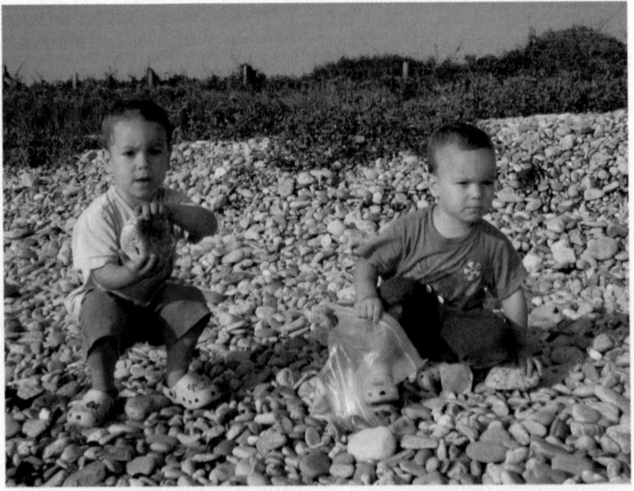

FIGURE 3-15 Parents of twin births often have challenges parents of singleton births do not have. DELMAR CENGAGE LEARNING.

and then involve them in simple caregiving activities, such as bringing items (diapers, toys, or clothes) as needed to care for the multiples (Leonard & Denton, 2006).

As the multiples grow older, competition between the children is not uncommon. Parents may have more disciplinary problems than they would have with singletons. Therefore, encouraging positive parent-child interactions and assisting them to reduce stress may be needed if the multiples' behaviors tax parental resources. Multiples may also not have the same opportunities as singletons due to the logistics of caring for more than one child of the same age, such as going to the store, interacting with other children of the same age, and feeding and dressing themselves. Therefore, it would be important to encourage parents to provide these experiences for the children and help them problem-solve how to provide these experiences (Leonard & Denton, 2006).

ADOLESCENT PARENTING

Adolescence is a time of considerable growth and development, with progression toward taking on adult roles and responsibilities. For some adolescents, this includes taking on the task of parenting at a time when they are still shaping their own identities (Klein, 2005) (Figure 3-16).

In America, the highest adolescent birth rates were before abortion was legal and contraceptives were developed (1950–1960). After 1973, when abortion was legalized, birth rates for United States females between 15 and 19 years of age decreased until 1986. Since then, however, the birth rates have continued to decrease including those for black, white, and Hispanic adolescents (Klein, 2005).

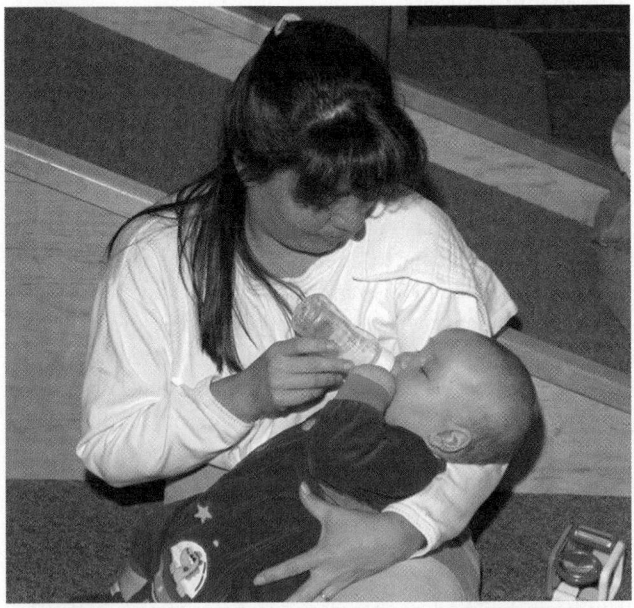

FIGURE 3-16 The adolescent parent and child face many challenges, yet many of these families have positive outcomes. DELMAR CENGAGE LEARNING.

Even though the adolescent birth rate has been decreasing in the United States, it is the highest when compared to comparable industrialized countries, even though sexual activity rates among Western European teens are similar to or higher than U.S. rates. Although unclear, reasons for the higher U.S. rate may be that welfare benefits are less generous in the United States than in Europe, some European countries have universal sexuality education in schools, and there may be more acceptance of and greater access to contraception in Europe than in the United States (Klein, 2005).

If the pregnancy was unintended, it affects not only the mother and child, but also the child's father and their respective families because adolescents are often not socially, emotionally, educationally, economically, or physically ready for pregnancy and parenthood. Several societal factors influencing the incidence of adolescent pregnancy include implied acceptance of intercourse outside marriage, a variety of adult behavioral values, media pressure, inadequate access to contraception, and the availability of public assistance or welfare for single young mothers. There are risks associated with adolescent pregnancies—medical and psychosocial. Medical risks include low birth weight (more than double the rate for adults) and neonatal death (almost three times as high as in adults). The mortality rate for the mother is twice as high as for adult pregnant women. Other problems include poor maternal weight gain, pregnancy-induced hypertension, sexually transmitted diseases, anemia, and premature births. Psychosocial problems include failure to complete school, persistent poverty, separation from the child's father, repeat pregnancy, limited vocational opportunities, and nonnurturing parenting strategies (Klein, 2005).

Children of adolescent mothers have an increased risk of developmental delay, academic difficulties, substance abuse, and behavioral problems. They are also at risk of dropping out of school and becoming adolescent parents themselves. It is hypothesized that these children do not fare as well as do children of adult mothers because teenagers do not possess the same level of parenting skills and maturity as do adults. Additionally, poverty and frequent changes of caregivers seem to play as much a role as the adolescent's parenting style. Two predictors of school and behavioral problems in these children are the mother's prolonged dependence on public assistance and an unstable relationship between the mother and father.

Despite these difficulties, some adolescents and their children have positive outcomes. Some studies have presented a more positive, hopeful view of adolescent mothers. Early parenthood enhances their personal strength and feelings of hope about the future, increases their motivation to improve their position in life, and improves their ability to bond to their family. Other mothers form a stronger identity and express more confidence in themselves and more engagement with their children (Herrman, 2008). Several factors have been associated with improved outcomes for adolescent mothers (Box 3-5).

When a pregnant adolescent is identified, comprehensive prenatal care is essential even if she decides to terminate the pregnancy. She should also receive information about available

BOX 3-5

FACTORS ASSOCIATED WITH IMPROVED OUTCOMES FOR ADOLESCENT MOTHERS

- Completion of high school before becoming pregnant
- Active participation in a program for pregnant teens
- Support from her family (financial assistance or child care) that allows her to finish school
- Little social isolation
- A sense of control over her life

options, including continuing the pregnancy, keeping and parenting the infant, creating an adoption plan, or terminating the pregnancy via abortion. The nurse can fulfill an important role in assisting the pregnant adolescent by promoting effective parenting skills through education, providing feedback for positive efforts, and providing referrals to community agencies, such as parenting classes, support groups, school-based programs, and infant stimulation programs.

Additionally, all health care professionals who work with teenage parents need to understand not only adolescent development and child development, but the factors that make teenage parenting particularly challenging. The primary source of support and advice for these parents is often their family of origin. In the event of a discrepancy or a difference of opinion about a child care issue between the professional and the family, the teenage parent will almost always adhere to the family's advice. To successfully support teenagers in the parenting role, it is necessary to clarify their knowledge and perceptions of child care issues. It is important to remember that it is the teenage parent who will make decisions for the child's care. The teenage parent needs information in order to arrive at an informed decision. In fact, the teenage parent may need more information than an older parent.

When caring for a child of a teenage parent who does not seem to adhere to professional advice, it is imperative that family health beliefs and strategies be explored. Although the teenage parent is the legal guardian and primary caretaker of the child, it may be necessary to encourage other family caregivers to participate in health visits so all persons who have a significant role to play in the care of the child are involved. In this way, issues can be openly discussed among all parties rather than having the teenage parent serve as the "go-between."

PARENTING THE ADOPTED CHILD

Adoption is a legal procedure where a relationship is established between a child and parents who are not related by birth. This process severs all legal ties between the adopted child and his or her biological parents, and establishes such ties between the adoptee and the adoptive parents. The adopted child has the same legal status with respect to his or her adoptive parents as do any biological children.

Several types of adoption exist: agency, independent or private, international, and transracial. Agency adoptions can be public or private, for profit or nonprofit. Costs of agency adoptions vary; however, public agency adoptions are usually less expensive or free. Independent adoptions (also known as private) are usually accomplished through individuals, such as physicians, attorneys, or social workers. Internationally adopted children may have incomplete information about health and medical histories. Because of their diverse origins, unknown backgrounds before adoption, and the inadequacy of health care in many developing countries, these children may be at risk for medical problems. Transracial adoptions of children from minority backgrounds continue to be challenging because of the limited availability of adoptive parents from the same race or ethnic group or caregivers from another race or ethnic group willing to adopt a transracial child.

Adoptions may also be open or closed. A **closed adoption** is when there is no contact between biological and adoptive parents. In **open adoption**, there is contact between the birth parents and adoptive parents and possibly between the child and his or her birth parents as well. Advocates of open adoption believe it will aid in lessening the identity struggles some teenage adoptees go through by having knowledge of their biological past. Additionally, the communication between both sets of parents provides better genetic, medical, and mental health background information for caring for the adopted child. Opponents argue, generally on privacy grounds for birth parents, that the effects on both adoptee and birth mother are not helpful, healthy, or positive, and can seriously threaten vital bonds of the adoptee with adoptive parents.

Arguments for both closed and open adoption reflect differences in philosophy rather than evidence obtained through research. Even though the value of open adoption has not been fully examined, openness has more positive than negative consequences. For example, adoptive mothers who experienced open adoption demonstrate favorable attitudes toward the birth mothers and adoptive child, and realized the birth mother was not going to attempt to reclaim the child. They also felt better able to answer questions the adopted child may ask. Birth mothers favor open adoption and felt lower levels of grief, regret about their decision, and worry about the baby. They were also able to come to terms with the loss of their baby, were able to play a more active role in the life of the child she gave up for adoption, and assured she would receive information about the child (Berge, Mendenhall, Weobel, Grotevant, & McRoy, 2007). Individuals who adopt a child in order to become parents are faced with the same tasks in child rearing as biological parents. However, the point at which they begin building an interdependent connection with their adoptive child presents distinctly unique challenges for these new parents. Unlike the biological parents, who begin developing connections with their child throughout pregnancy,

EVIDENCE-BASED PRACTICE

International Adoptions

CLINICAL PROBLEM

An increasing number of American families are adopting children born abroad, who have lived in conditions different than birth children. These experiences impact the child's adjustment and integration into the adoptive family.

BEST CLINICAL PRACTICE

Several issues and concerns need to be discussed with adoptive parents. These include:

1. Children available for international adoption often come from high-risk backgrounds (poverty, abuse, neglect, institutional environments, lack of consistent caregivers). They may also have medical or developmental concerns related to insufficient shelter, food, and clothing, and may have behavioral/attachment problems or conduct disorders.
2. The country of adoption may be an important consideration in the child's health and well-being because care received prior to adoption may vary according of the country of birth.
3. It will take time to integrate the child into the family.

IMPLICATIONS FOR NURSING

1. Educate adoptive parents about normal child development and how that may be altered when adopting a child from an at-risk environment.
2. Educate adoptive parents about issues that may surface.
3. Support adoptive parents in identifying, addressing, and ameliorating concerns.
4. Provide information about resources that can help adoptive parents integrate the adoptive child into their family and support the child's optimal development.

Reference: Hellerstedt, W., Madsen, N., Gunnar, M., Grotevant, H., Lee, R., & Johnson, D. (2008). The International adoption project: Population-based surveillance of Minnesota parents who adopted children internationally. *Maternal Child Health Journal, 12*: 162–171.

adoptive parents do not have this particular experience. They are presented with a stranger with whom they must build a loving, interdependent relationship. For a growing number of these families, the adoptive children are not infants; rather they are older children who have already experienced some form of parenting or caretaking, which will influence their responses to their new adoptive parents. However, since most adoptions frequently take a long time to execute, adoptive parents can go through their own transitional period of beginning the definition of "self-as-parents."

Unique to adoptive parents are the decisions of what and when to tell their child about the adoption. Parents now are advised to openly discuss adoption from the beginning, keeping in mind the child's developmental stage, cognitive abilities, and emotional needs. The child's understanding of the adoption will change with each stage. At the infant or toddler stage, when both the parents and child are adjusting to a changed environment and forming secure attachments, nurses can assist parents in the following ways: (1) allow them to discuss the actual adoption process with the provider; (2) encourage parents to discuss the process with relatives and close friends; (3) suggest or provide resources such as support groups, newsletters, or books; and (4) prepare them for the possibility of insensitive or unenlightened comments from other people (Lears, Guth, & Lewandowski, 1998).

The preschool years produce typical questions such as "Where do babies come from?" and "Where did I come from?" but also render adoption-specific questions such as "Why or how did you choose me?" "Why don't I look like you?" and "Can my birth parents or another family take me away?" Nurses can assist in the following ways: (1) remind parents that preschool children are preoperational and egocentric thinkers who can understand adoption only on a concrete level and not as an abstract concept (e.g., the adoptee may believe that if he or she was adopted, then all children must be adopted); (2) encourage parents to talk openly about the process of bringing the child into the family; (3) advise them to answer only the specific questions asked by the child and to answer questions truthfully; (4) emphasize similarities between the child and the family; and (5) reassure the child that the adoption is permanent (Lears et al., 1998).

In the middle childhood stage, questions posed by adoptees include such difficult topics as: "Why was I placed for adoption?" "If you're adopted, can you be unadopted?" and "Who do I look like?" Children at this age may begin searching for answers regarding their origins and reasons for relinquishment. Coping with the public stigma of adoption, peer reactions to adoption, and adoption-related losses and reactions (such as grief, sadness, or anger over the loss of biological parents) are key tasks for this age group. Nurses can help by (1) reminding parents to verbally acknowledge the loss adoptees may feel; (2) reassuring them that the child's feelings of grief, sadness, and anger typically dissipate with time; (3) supporting them in their own feelings that may arise as the child expresses thoughts and feelings about their origins; (4) encouraging them to continue to share factual information about the child's adoption; (5) proposing they work with the school to educate others about adoption; (6) advising them to refrain from making negative comments about the biological family since the child does integrate some of their identity into self; and (7) suggesting support groups and services for the parents and child (Lears et al., 1998).

In the adolescent stage, the prevailing question—"Who am I?"—assumes a different or additional meaning for adoptees. Adolescent adoptees have to deal with identity issues regarding both their adoptive parents as well as their biological parents. Since adolescents can now understand abstract processes, the implications and meaning of being adopted is a key area of exploration. Nurses can (1) remind parents that all adolescents deal with identity issues, but that adopted adolescents must deal with integration of both adopted and biological parent identities; (2) suggest they share the actual adoption papers with the adolescent; (3) prepare them for the possibility the child may search for the biological family; and (4) suggest both child and parent continue to use support groups (Lears et al., 1998).

PARENTING BY GRANDPARENTS

An increasing number of grandparents are raising their grandchildren. In 2006, there were 6.1 million children in the United States under 18 years living in the homes of their grandparents, and 2.5 million grandparents (most of them grandmothers) responsible for food, shelter, and clothing of one or more grandchildren who live with them. Many of these grandparents have an income below the poverty level (U.S. Bureau of the Census, 2008) (Figure 3-17). Grandparent-headed households are found in every socioeconomic, racial, and ethnic group and all geographic areas. However, more African-American grandmothers are raising their grandchildren than African-American males, European Americans, or Hispanic Americans (Goodman & Rao, 2007). On the other hand, families of ethnically diverse backgrounds are more likely to have grandparents with significant caretaking responsibilities because of societal or environmental factors, cultural beliefs and practices, or because of household arrangements.

Grandparents assume a parenting role for a variety of reasons, most of which revolve around problems related to the child's biological parent (Box 3-6). Grandparents cite four main reasons for rearing their grandchildren. They include: preserving family ties; reducing the trauma of separation for their grandchildren; providing community, ethnic, and cultural consistency; and the needs of the children (Linsk, Mason, Fendrich, Bass, Prubhughate, & Brown, 2009). Regardless of the reason, all result in a great deal of responsibility for those who take on the task.

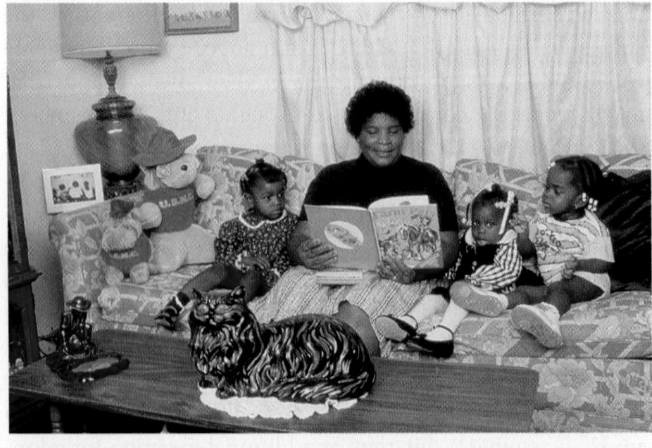

FIGURE 3-17 Grandparents may assume care of grandchildren in some families. DELMAR CENGAGE LEARNING.

BOX 3-6

ANTECEDENTS TO GRANDPARENTS RAISING GRANDCHILDREN

- Child abuse or neglect
- Divorce
- Substance abuse
- Death
- Adolescent pregnancy
- Unemployment
- Mental illness
- Incarceration
- Working in another location

Grandparent caregivers face a myriad of challenges and difficulties in almost all aspects of their lives when they assume the role of surrogate parent. For many their physical health is an issue. In fact, many seniors raising their grandchildren have health problems interfering with being able to hold a job, which makes it difficult to help with expenses. Closely related to health is the issue of stamina. Finally, many report feeling physically and emotionally drained and fatigued from caring for young children. They fear that, as a result of their tiredness and health problems, they may be unable to meet the demands of parenting (Casper & Bianchi, 2007).

Grandparents often experience emotional difficulties such as psychological distress, depression, disappointment, guilt, anger, and resentment. Social isolation and restrictions of the parenting role are related to psychological distress and depression. Disappointment, guilt, anger, and resentment are common feelings they have toward their own child. Many feel disappointed with the person their child has become as an adult and guilt about having raised a child that is incapable of being a competent parent. Anger and resentment are associated with having to assume the parent role because of their adult child's problems and incompetencies (Hayslip & Kaminski, 2005). The grandparents' lifestyle and relationships with family and friends are changed. They may become isolated from other members of their family who may resent the role they have taken on. It is not uncommon for grandparents' marriages to fall apart under the strain of once again parenting. This can be accompanied by family resentment and conflict because of little time and energy left for other grandchildren and children. Grandparents' circle of friends may also become smaller if grandparent friends do not want to be around the grandchildren.

Economic difficulties are common due to taking on the care of a child at a time in their lives when their income is dramatically decreased. Many grandparents are denied the financial benefits of foster parents because of their blood relation

CULTURAL CONSIDERATION

African-American Grandparents

African-American grandparents who care for their grandchildren:

1. View their role as critical to family survival
2. Exhibit no difference in quality of parenting between mothers and grandmothers
3. Have a favorable self-perception
4. Believe their strength lies in teaching grandchildren good manners, the need for lifelong learning, to care about the feelings of others, and a sense of right and wrong
5. Are satisfied with their role
6. Are not likely to complain even if experiencing physical, psychological, and economic challenges
7. Would like information about their role so they may feel prepared
8. Often downplay their own health problems

Adapted from Kataoka-Yahiro, Ceria, C, & Caulfield, R. (2004). Grandparent caregiving role in ethnically diverse families. *Journal of Pediatric Nursing, 19*(5), 315–328.

to the child, though some states have "kinship care" programs. Some financial assistance is available through the federal government (Medicaid, Social Security, Food Stamps, and Head Start programs).

Despite the negatives, there are also benefits to grandparents parenting a grandchild. Many experience a greater purpose for life and some feel young and alive (Hayslip & Kaminski, 2005). Raising a grandchild in a safe, nurturing environment and helping the child grow to be a productive person is rewarding. Grandparents are able to draw upon their own parenting experiences with the wisdom and knowledge they've accumulated over the years.

Grandparents and grandchildren need significant support from health care providers and social service agencies. Nurses can be instrumental in providing referrals to available services and supports (see Resources). Nurses who encounter grandparent-headed families in their practice should assess and intervene when issues such as physical and mental health problems are identified.

They can also act as consultants to settings where elderly are served, and help make intervention services easily accessible to grandparents. Improved policy and practice efforts that reach those grandparents especially at risk are needed so they can access social and health services for themselves and their families. Nurses can also initiate and facilitate support groups, parenting classes, and stress management programs to help grandparents who are ethnically diverse care for their grandchildren. These nurses can also act as consultants to community health agencies and schools in facilitating the development of services to grandparent caregivers that are culturally sensitive (Kataoka-Yahiro et al., 2004).

CULTURAL CONSIDERATION

Hispanic Grandparents

Research has shown that Hispanic-American grandparents who care for their grandchildren:

1. May show a need for information on grandparenting
2. May become frustrated when dealing with an adolescent if the adolescent does not speak Spanish
3. Often have grown up with a strong helping network within families where grandmothers take on the role of caregiver
4. Contribute to continual socialization of grandchildren
5. Are affected by societal changes that impact their health and well-being
6. Play important roles in the family network as a strong source of support
7. Prefer interdependent rather than dependent family situations
8. May act as babysitter, family historian, cook, celebrant of holidays and birthdays, gift exchanger, and surrogate parent
9. May care for grandchildren in times of need and crisis
10. May experience role strain due to constraining economic resources, erosion of social relationships, back migration, and life plan changes
11. Are generally positive about their own aging

Adapted from Kataoka-Yahiro, Ceria, C, & Caulfield, R. (2004). Grandparent caregiving role in ethnically diverse families. *Journal of Pediatric Nursing, 19*(5), 315–328.

FOSTER PARENTING

Foster care refers to all out-of-home placements for children unable to remain with their birth parents. Children in foster care are rapidly increasing in numbers, and meeting their psychosocial needs is a significant challenge. The majority of children placed in foster care as a result of neglect, physical abuse, parental substance abuse, or abandonment are infants and young children. In many cases, the caregiver is unable or unwilling to care for them because of substance

Adolescent Perceptions of Kinship and Nonkinship Foster Care

STUDY PURPOSE

African-American children are the second largest ethnic group needing foster care, and if placed with relatives, will remain more connected to people they know, compared to those placed with nonrelatives. Therefore, the purpose of this comparative, exploratory study was to explore relational context information according to whether the African-American adolescent was placed in kinship foster care or in nonkinship foster care. Specifically, the investigator was interested in discovering how family connections were maintained in each foster care family, and how the role dilemmas faced by adolescents in the two types of foster care differ.

METHODS

Eighteen African-American adolescents between 11 and 14 years of age who lived in nonrelative foster care ($n = 9$) or in relative foster care ($n = 9$) were asked whether or not their contact with members of their birth family had changed after being placed in foster care, and if living with their foster family changed the contact they had with their birth family compared to their living situation prior to being placed in foster care.

FINDINGS

Most (56%) adolescents living in kinship care were living with their grandparents, and had lived in fewer foster care homes than adolescents placed in nonrelative foster care. Those adolescents living in kinship care had stronger connections to people and places they knew prior to placement than those in nonkinship placements. However, they also experienced more role dilemmas, role conflicts, and role reversals in their relationships with their foster care parents and birth parents than those adolescents placed in nonfamily foster homes.

IMPLICATIONS

Since those placed in kinship foster homes experience fewer foster home placements and are able to maintain more contact with their biological parents and relatives than those placed in nonrelative foster care, it would be important to encourage kinship foster care whenever possible for African-American children/adolescents as well as children/adolescents of other ethnic groups. However, it would also be important if placing a child/adolescent in kinship foster care to apprise both the foster family and the child/adolescent of the issues that may arise related to role conflict, role reversal, and role dilemma so appropriate interventions can be provided and the impact of these role situations lessened.

REFERENCE

Schwartz, A. (2008). Connective complexity: African-American adolescents and the relational context of kinship foster care. *Child Welfare, 87*(2), 77–97.

abuse, mental illness, or major physical illness. The majority of children in out-of-home placements are living with relatives. These kinship caregivers, however, face more challenges as a foster parent than non-kin caregivers because they tend to be in poorer health, have lower incomes and less education, and are older. Kinship caregivers also may not have the support necessary to protect and nurture children in their care because they tend to receive fewer services and less supervision than nonkinship foster parents.

Children in foster care are at risk in many ways: having chronic health deficits, experiencing the trauma of abuse and neglect, and suffering from emotional challenges. They usually have experienced significant psychological stress during their early years and may not have had a nurturing, stable home environment, which is necessary for the development of optimal cognitive, language, and socialization skills. Additionally, multiple placements and interruptions in the continuity of caregivers are often detrimental to the child's well-being. Foster children are more likely to have unmet health needs and chronic health problems because they are often in and out of the health care system. Frequent changes in health care providers occur without the necessary transfer of medical information and records. Finally, many children in foster care also have attachment disorders, compromised brain functioning, and mental health difficulties. Former foster care children are also at risk for negative outcomes, including homelessness, substance abuse, and low educational attainment (Chamberlain, Price, Reid, & Landsverk, 2008; Fernandez, 2007). Reunifying children placed in foster care is the primary goal. However, reunification may not always work. Barriers to successful reunification variables are related to both birth parents and children's issues. Parental variables include ambivalence regarding the return of their children; a combination of mental illness, housing, and substance abuse problems; being a single parent; and the amount of contact with the child welfare system. Reunification may also be distressing to children if they have feelings of loss, grief, or fear at the prospect of leaving a foster home. Health care providers can be effective advocates for children in foster care in several ways. Those with expertise in child development and parenting can provide advice and support for foster and biological families. Caseworkers may need assistance in obtaining records from previous health care providers and interpreting the information. Individuals responsible for the child's care need an understanding of her or his physical and emotional problems. Providers can be proactive advisors for social services and the judicial system in determining what is in the best interest of the child and whether these interests can be met within the biological family or another family.

IMPLICATIONS FOR NURSING

Parenting is a highly valued activity both on a personal as well as a societal level. Good parenting is necessary for the healthy functioning of children and to produce successful members of society. It is learned through imitation, acquired knowledge, and practice. Nurses can play a vital role in supporting parenting as they work with families. This work must be done in collaboration with parents if positive results are to be achieved. Too often health care providers talk *to* parents rather than *with* them. Merely giving advice based on the providers' background and knowledge may fail to address the parents' personal and cultural beliefs. If the advice given is not congruent with the parents' valued beliefs, it will be ignored.

Assessment of parenting includes:

- the parent's views on parenting
- clarifying cultural and social expectations for parenting
- identifying issues or children's behaviors that are of concern to parents
- evaluating the interactions between children and their parents during health care encounters

Potential sources of problems can be identified from the assessment data. The identified problems should:

- be confirmed or clarified with parents
- be mutually agreed upon as the priority issues parents wish to address

When a problem is identified, then the parents and nurse can collaborate on creating a plan of care. Collaboration with parents can improve the success of the plan as parents will be involved with identifying:

- resources for implementing the plan
- strategies that are congruent with parental beliefs
- outcomes for determining effectiveness of the plan

The nurse will need to follow up with the parents at subsequent encounters to determine:

- how effective the plan of care was in achieving the stated outcomes
- any adaptations the family made in the plan of care
- the parent's satisfaction with this format for reducing or resolving the identified problem

It is crucial that nurses work with parents rather than against them if parenting is to be supported. Nurses should continually ask themselves whether they are imposing their personal beliefs about parenting when they evaluate others' parent-child relationships. Parenting issues or problems will not be resolved in a single encounter. The work of parenting is ongoing and dynamic. It will take weeks or months for a problem to be resolved. By establishing an open exchange of ideas, and respecting parents' personal and cultural values, nurses can support the work of parenting.

IN THE REAL WORLD

Heather, 12 years old, is my client at the mental health mental retardation (MHMR) clinic. When she was 8, her parents divorced, and she has been living with her mother since that time. Based on my conversation with her, I considered more deeply the profound effects that divorce and single parenting can have on a child and the family. I realized that some of my assumptions about them were not correct. As Heather talked, I realized that, more than anything else at the moment, she probably needed someone to just listen and empathize. She didn't need me to tell her what I thought. She just wanted me to listen. As she expressed feelings common to children whose parents divorced, my assumptions about her family changed. In other words, she allowed me to refine my perceptions of her family's experiences and thereby understand her situation and how she felt.

KEY CONCEPTS

- The definition of family varies widely. The most inclusive definition of family is when two or more persons are joined by bonds of sharing and emotional closeness and identify themselves as members of the family (Friedman et al., 2003).
- Four family theories from the social sciences that have major relevance to nursing are the structural-functional, the developmental, the systems theories, and stress theory.
- The process of family assessment includes data collected in a systematic fashion using a family

assessment measure where information is classified and analyzed as to its meaning.

- The traditional nuclear family structure no longer reflects contemporary U.S. lifestyles. Other forms such as the single parent, blended, and gay and lesbian families have emerged in recent years.
- Nurses have a responsibility to understand the influence of the cultural framework on a family's child rearing practices and attitudes about health and illness.
- As children grow and develop, parenting tasks change to both support their development and maintain family functioning.
- Parenting styles have an effect on the child's personality outcomes.
- A variety of special parenting situations can further increase the complexity of child rearing: parenting multiples, adolescent parents, adoption, grandparents as surrogate parents, and foster care.
- Nurses can play a vital role in supporting parents as they work with families. This work must be done in collaboration with parents if positive results are to be achieved.

REVIEW ACTIVITIES

1. How is the family conceptualized in various nursing theories?
2. How is the family conceptualized in the following frameworks: (a) structural-functional; (b) developmental; (c) systems theory; and (d) stress theory?
3. Identify the strengths and limitations of the four frameworks in question 2.
4. According to Duvall's developmental stages, what are the tasks for each of these families: (a) parents of an infant; (b) parents of an adolescent; and (c) a retired couple?
5. According to the structural-functional theory, what are four functions of the family?
6. Describe the family stress, double ABC-X, and Resiliency Model of Family Stress, Adjustment, and Adaptation.
7. Why is the view of the nuclear family not representative of contemporary families?
8. Discuss salient characteristics of the following types of family structure: (a) extended; (b) blended; (c) single parent; (d) gay or lesbian; (e) adoptive; and (f) foster; (g) immigrant families; and (h) families of multiples.
9. Discuss the importance of culture to nurses providing multicultural health care.
10. List some strengths of immigrant families.
11. What is the role of family time in successful parenting?
12. Discuss the impact of the following parenting situations on the child and parents: (a) parenting multiples; (b) adolescent parents; (c) adoption; (d) grandparents as surrogate parents; and (e) foster parents.

STUDY QUESTIONS

1. Nursing has consistently had an interest in families and has acknowledged its importance in relation to health. A number of theories of families in nursing and social sciences give insight into understanding its dynamics and processes. Which of the following theories views the family as both context (environment) and client, and believes the family influences the growth and development of individuals?
   a. Neuman's System Theory
   b. King's Open Systems Theory
   c. Roy's Adaptation Theory
   d. Family Stress Theory
2. In which theory is the family seen as having several primary responsibilities related to affection, socialization, reproduction, economics, and maintaining the health of its members?
   a. structural-functional theory
   b. developmental theory
   c. family systems theory
   d. the resiliency model of family stress, adjustment, and adaptation
3. Which of the family assessment models discusses primary, secondary, and tertiary prevention?
   a. The Calgary Family Assessment Model (Wright & Leahy)
   b. The Friedman Family Assessment Model (Friedman et al.)
   c. The Family Assessment and Intervention Model (Hanson et al.)

d. The Neuman Family Assessment Model (Neuman)

4. Which family structure was prominent in the 1800s in the United States because the family was the main unit of economic production?
   a. nuclear family
   b. extended family
   c. gay and lesbian family
   d. single-parent family
5. Which of these family structures may have a number of coalitions; little or no family loyalty and, initially, no family history; family boundaries that are ambiguous; and others outside the family that may affect its functioning and coping?
   a. adoptive family
   b. adolescent family
   c. immigrant family
   d. stepfamily
6. Which of the following statements about single-parent families is true?
   a. Children raised in single-parent families are at risk for adverse outcomes in academic performance, psychological functioning, and social functioning.
   b. Single mothers are rigid in their attitudes toward gender roles and gender stereotypes.
   c. Single-parent families encourage dependence and irresponsibility in their children.
   d. Single parents encourage immaturity in their children.
7. You are providing information to parents of young children on parent-child relationships. When giving advice it is important to:
   a. not give too much praise for compliance and competency.
   b. apologize when you have made an error.
   c. indirectly communicate love and affection.
   d. avoid letting children make their choices.
8. Parents who guide children's behavior by sharing reasons for their decisions, rules, and standards; value independence; and are receptive to the child's needs and desires are using what kind of parenting style?
   a. permissive
   b. authoritarian
   c. authoritative
   d. indulgent
9. Time-out is an effective discipline strategy that involves removing positive reinforcement for unacceptable behavior. However, when talking to parents about time-out it would be important to tell them:
   a. "Children need to be placed in an environment where there are a lot of things for them to do."
   b. "The amount of time spent in time-out is five minutes per year of age."
   c. "It is all right to talk to the children while in time-out."
   d. "Children need to know why they have been put in time-out."
10. Parents come to you asking about adoption. Which of the following statements is true?
   a. Children available for international adoption often come from high-risk backgrounds and may also have medical or developmental concerns.
   b. Most adoptions today are closed adoptions because it is less stressful for parents and the adopted child.
   c. "If a child is adopted, they should not be told they are adopted until they are adolescents."
   d. Birth parents are rarely interested in the life of the child they gave up for adoption.

REFERENCES

American Academy of Pediatrics. (2007). Parenting Corner Q & A: Discipline Retrieved June 28, 2009, from http://www.aap.org/pubed/ZZZLZ33YUSC.htm.

American Academy of Pediatrics Committee on Psychosocial Aspects of Child and Family Health. (1998). Guidance for effective discipline. *Pediatrics, 101*(4), 723–728.

American Academy of Pediatrics Committee on School Health. (2000). Corporal punishment in schools. *Pediatrics, 106*(2), 343. (Reaffirmed in May of 2006.)

Angell, R. C. (1936). *The family encounters the depression*. New York: Charles Scribner.

Attar-Schwartz, S., Tan, J., Buchanan, A., Flouri, E., & Griggs, J. (2009). Grandparenting and adolescent adjustment in two-parent biological, lone-parent, and step-families. *Journal of Family Psychology* 23(1), 67–75.

Berge, J., Mendenhall, T., Weobel, G., Grotevant, H., & McRoy, R. (2007). Adolescents' feelings about openness in adoption: Implications for adoption agencies. *Child Welfare, 85*(6), 1011–1039.

Berkley-Mischke, K. M., & Hanson, S. M. H. (1991). *Pocket guide to family assessment and intervention*. St. Louis: Mosby Year Book.

Bing, N., Nelson, W., & Wesolowski, K. (2009). Comparing the effects of amount of conflict on children's adjustment following parental divorce. *Journal of Divorce & Remarriage, 50*, 159–171.

Burr, W. R., & Klein, S. R. (1994). *Reexamining family stress: New theory and research*. Thousand Oaks, CA: Sage Publication, Inc.

Casper, L., & Bianchi, S. (2007). Grandparenting. In S. Ferguson, (Ed.). *Shifting the center: Understanding contemporary families* (3rd ed.). New York: McGraw Hill, pp. 473–486.

Cavan, R. S., & Ranck, K. H. (1938). *The family and the Depression*. Chicago: University of Chicago Press.

Chamberlain, P., Price, J., Reid, J., & Landsverk, J. (2008). Cascading implementation of a foster and kinship parent intervention. *Child Welfare, 87*(5), 27–48.

Coontz, S. (2006). The American family. In K. R. Gilbert (Ed.). *The family* (31st ed.). Dubuque, IA: McGraw-Hill/Dushkin, pp. 179–181.

Demo, D., Aquilino, W., & Fine, M. (2005). Family composition and family transitions. In V. Bengston, A. Acock, K. Allen, P. Dillworth-Anderson, & D. Klein, *Sourcebook of family theory and research.* Sage: Thousand Oaks, CA, pp. 119–142.

Diamant, A., & Cooper, H. (1991). *Living a Jewish life.* New York: Harper Collins.

Dingfelder, S. (2008). The kids are all right. In K. Gilbert (Ed.). *The family* (33rd ed.). Dubuque, IA: McGraw-Hill Contemporary Learning Series, pp. 112–114.

Dinan, K. (2006). Young children in immigrant families: The role of philanthropy, sharing knowledge, creating services, and building supportive policies. National center for children in poverty. Report of a Meeting, January 18–19, 2006. NY: NY.

Duvall, E. M. (1977). *Marriage and family development* (5th ed.). Philadelphia: J. B. Lippincott.

Duvall, E. M., & Miller, B. (1985). *Marriage and family development* (6th ed.). New York: Harper & Row.

Fernandez, E. (2007). How children experience fostering outcomes: Participatory research with children. *Child and Family Social Work, 12,* 349–359.

Friedman, M., Bowden, V., & Jones, E. (2003). *Family nursing: Research, theory, and practice* (5th ed.). Upper Saddle River, NJ: Prentice Hall.

Goodman, M., & Rao, S. (2007). Grandparents raising grandchildren in a U.S.-Mexico border community. *Qualitative Health Research, 17*(8), 1117–1136.

Hanson, S., Gedaly-Duff, V., & Kaakinen, J. (2005). *Family health care nursing: Theory, practice, and research* (3rd ed.). Philadelphia: F. A. Davis.

Hayslip, B., & Kaminski, P. (2005). Grandparents raising their grandchildren. *Marriage & Family Review, 37,* 147–169.

Hellerstedt, W., Madsen, N., Gunnar, M., Grotevant, H., Lee, R., & Johnson, D. (2008). The International adoption project: Population-based surveillance of Minnesota parents who adopted children internationally. *Maternal Child Health Journal, 12,* 162–171.

Herrman, J. (2008). Adolescent perceptions of teen births. *Journal of Obstetrics, Gynecological, and Neonatal Nursing, 37,* 42–50.

Hill, R. (1949). *Families under stress: Adjustment to the crisis of war separation and reunion.* New York: Harper and Brothers.

Kataoka-Yahiro, Ceria, C, & Caulfield, R. (2004). Grandparent caregiving role in ethnically diverse families. *Journal of Pediatric Nursing, 19*(5), 315–328.

Kazdin, A., & Benjet, C. (2009). Spanking children: Evidence and issues. In K. Gilbert (Ed.). *The family* (34th ed.). Dubuque, IA: McGraw-Hill Contemporary Learning Series, pp. 98–101.

King, I. (1981). A theory for nursing: Systems, concepts, process. New York: John Wiley.

Klein, J. D., American Academy of Pediatrics Committee on Adolescence. (2005, July). Adolescent pregnancy: Current trends and issues. *Pediatrics, 116*(1), 281–286.

Koos, E. L. (1946). *Families in trouble.* New York: Kings Crown Press.

Lazarus, R. S., & Folkman, S. (1984). *Stress, appraisal, and coping.* New York: Springer.

Lears, M., Guth, K., & Lewandowski, P. (1998). International adoption: A primer for pediatric nurses. *Pediatric Nursing, 24*(6), 578–586.

Leonard, L., & Denton, J. (2006). Preparation for parenting multiple birth children. *Early Human Development, 82,* 371–378.

Linsk, N., Mason, S., Fendrich, M., Bass, M., Prubhughate, P., & Brown, A. (2009). No matter what I do they still want their family: Stressors for African American grandparents and other relatives. *Journal of Family Social Work, 12,* 25–43.

Macoby, E. E., & Martin, J. A. (1983). Socialization in the context of the family: Parent-child interaction. In P. H. Mussen (Ed.). *Handbook of child psychology* (4th ed.)., *vol. 4.* New York: Wiley, pp. 37–56.

McCubbin, H. I., & Patterson, J. M. (1982). Family adaptation to crisis. In H. I. McCubbin, A. E. Cauble, & J. M. Patterson (Eds.). *Family stress, coping, and social support.* Springfield, IL: Charles C. Thomas, pp. 26–47.

McCubbin, H. I., & Patterson, J. M. (1983). The family stress process: The double ABC-X model of adjustment and adaptation. In H. I. McCubbin, M. B. Sussman, & J. Patterson (Eds.). Social stress and the family (Special issue). *Marriage and Family Review, 5*(1/2), 7–27.

McCubbin, M., & McCubbin, H. (1989). Theoretical orientations to family stress and coping. In C. R. Figley (Ed.). *Treating stress in families.* New York: Brunner/Mazel, pp. 3–44.

McCubbin, M., & McCubbin, H. (1991). Family stress theory and assessment: The resiliency model of family stress, adjustment, and adaptation. In H. McCubbin & A. Thompson (Eds.). *Family assessment inventories for research and practice.* Madison: University of Wisconsin, pp. 3–34.

McCubbin, M., & McCubbin, H. (1993). Families coping with illness: The resiliency model of family stress, adjustment, and adaptation. In C. Danielson, B. Hamel-Bissel, & P. Winstead-Fry (Eds.). *Families, health, and illness.* St. Louis, MO: Mosby, pp. 21–63.

McCubbin, M., & McCubbin, H. (1996). Resiliency in families: A conceptual model of family adjustment and adaptation in response to stress and crisis. In H. I. McCubbin, A. Thompson, & M. McCubbin (Eds.). *Family assessment: Resiliency, coping and adaptation—Inventories for research and practice.* Madison, WI: University of Wisconsin System, pp. 1–64.

Nance-Nash, S. (2009). Managing a blended family. In K. R. Gilbert (Ed.). *The family* (34th ed.). Dubuque, IA: McGraw-Hill/Dushkin, pp. 175–177.

Nelson, J. (2006). *Positive discipline.* New York: Ballantine Books.

Neuman, B. (1972). The Betty Neuman model: A total person approach to patient. *Nursing Research, 21*(3), 264–269.

Neuman, B. (1983). Family intervention using the Betty Neuman health care systems model. In J. Clements & F. Roberts (Eds.). *Family health: A theoretical approach to nursing care.* New York: John Wiley, pp. 161–175.

Neuman, B. (1995). The Neuman systems model. In *The Neuman systems model* (3rd ed.). Norwalk, CT: Appleton & Lange, pp. 3–44.

Quah, S. (2008). *Families in Asia: Home and kin.* Routledge: London.

Roy, Sr. C. (1983). Roy adaptation model. In I. Clements & F. Roberts (Eds.). *Family health: A theoretical approach to nursing care.* New York: John Wiley, pp. 161–175.

Shields, M., & Behrman, R. (2004). Children of immigrant families: Analysis and recommendations. *The future of children: Children of immigrant families, 14*(2), 4–16.

Smith, S., Hamon, R., Ingoldsby, B., & Miller, J. E. (2008). *Exploring family theories* (2nd ed.). Los Angeles: Roxbury.

Springer, P., Abbott, D., & Reisbig, A. (2009). Therapy with Muslim couples and families: Basic guidelines for effective practice. *The Family Journal, 17*, 229–235.

Sugarman, S. (2007). Single-parent families. In S. Ferguson (Ed.). *Shifting the center: Understanding contemporary families.* (3rd ed.). Boston, MA: McGraw Hill, pp. 287–299.

Schwartz, A. (2008). Connective complexity: African American adolescents and the relational context of kinship foster care. *Child Welfare, 87*(2), 77–97.

Telingator, C., & Patterson, C. (2008). Children and adolescents of lesbian and gay parents. *Journal of the American Academy of Child & Adolescent Psychiatry, 47*(12), 1364–1368.

U.S. Bureau of the Census. (2010). Current Population Survey (CPS)—Definitions and Explanations. Retrieved October 6, 2010, from http://www.census.gov/population/www/cps/cpsdef.html.

U.S. Bureau of the Census. (2008). Facts for features: Grandparents Day 2008. Retrieved June 27, 2009, from http://www.census.gov/Pressrelease/www/releases/archives/facts_for_features_special_editions/012095.html.

Visher, E. B., & Visher, J. S. (1996). *Therapy with stepfamilies.* New York: Brunner/Mazel.

Von Bertalanffy, L. (1968). *General systems theory.* London: Penguin Press.

Wright, L., & Leahey, M. (2009). *Nurses and families: A guide to family assessment and intervention* (5th ed.). Philadelphia: F. A. Davis.

SUGGESTED READINGS

Barber, J., & Delfabbro, P. (2004). *Children in foster care.* London: Routledge.

Bullock, K. (2005). Grandfathers and the impact of raising grandchildren. *Journal of Sociology & Social Welfare, 32*(1), 43–59.

Cosby, A., Greenberg, R., Southward, L., & Weitzman, M. (Eds.). (2005). *About children: An authoritative resource on the state of childhood today.* Elk Grove Village, IL: American Academy of Pediatrics.

Denham, S. (2003). *Family health.* Philadelphia: F.A. Davis Company.

Dolbin-MacNab, M. (2006). Just like raising our own? Grandmothers' perceptions of parenting a second time around. *Family Relations, 55*, 564–575.

Freeark, K., Rosenberg, E., Bornstein, J., Linkevich, M., Lohnes, K., & Jozefowicz-Simbeni, D. (2005). Gender differences and dynamics shaping the adoption life cycle: Review of the literature and recommendations. *American Journal of Orthopsychiatry, 75*(1), 86–101.

Fuller-Thomson, E., & Minklery, M. (2005). American Indian/Alaskan native grandparents raising grandchildren: Findings from the Census 2000 Supplementary survey. *Social Work, 50*(2), 131–139.

Green, R. (2004). The evolution of kinship care policy and practice. *Children in foster care.* London: Routledge, pp. 131–149.

Greenfeld, D. (2005). Reproduction in same sex couples: Quality of parenting and child development. *Current opinion in obstetrics and gynecology, 17*(3), 309–312.

Hansard, P., & McLean, C. (2006). The grandparent as parent. In K. R. Gilbert (Ed.). *The family* (31st ed.). Dubuque, IA: McGraw-Hill/Dushkin, pp. 129–133.

Henry, P., & McCue, J. (2009). The experience of nonresident stepmothers. *Journal of Divorce & Remarriage, 50*(3), 185–205.

Juffer, F., & van Jzendoorn, M. (2005). Behavior problems and mental health referrals of international adoptees: A meta-analysis. *Journal of the American Medical Association, 293*(20), 2501–2515.

Kim, S. (2005). Longitudinal pathways to psychological adjustment among black youth living in single-parent households. *Journal of Family Psychology, 19*(2), 305–313.

Leung, P. (2005). A comparison of family functioning in gay/lesbian, heterosexual and special needs adoptions. *Children & Youth Services Review, 27*(9), 1031–1044.

Lifton, B. (2002). The adoptee's journey. *Journal of Social Distress and the Homeless, 11*(2), 207–213.

Neff, D., Kinion, E., & Cardina, C. (2007). Nurse managed center: Access to primary health care for urban native Americans. *Journal of Community Health Nursing, 24*(1), 19–30.

Narad, C., & Mason, P. (2004). International adoptions: Myths and realities. *Pediatric Nursing, 30*(6), 483–487.

Robins, R., Scherman, A., Holeman, H., & Wilson, J. (2005). Roles of American Indian grandparents in times of cultural crisis. *Journal of Cultural Diversity, 12*(2), 62–68.

Twigg, R., & Swan, T. (2007). What research tells us about the experience of foster carers' children. *Adoption & Fostering Journal, 31*(4), 49–61.

Weber, S. (2008). Parenting, family life and well-being among sexual minorities: Nursing policy and practice implications. *Issues in Mental Health Nursing, 29*(6), 601–618.

Younes, M., & Harp, M. (2007). Addressing the impact of foster care on biological children and their families. *Child Welfare, 86*(4), 21–40.

Zarelli, D. (2009). Role-governed behaviors of stepfathers in families with a child with chronic illness. *Journal of Pediatric Nursing, 24*(2), 90–100.

RESOURCES

Refer to the online student StudyWARE for Potts & Mandleco at http://www.CengageBrain.com for additional content and study aids.

Organization: **About Twins & Multiples**
Description: Provides information for parents of twins and multiples related to issues that commonly arise.
Website/Resource: http://multiples.about.com

Organization: **AMA Archives of Pediatrics and Adolescent Medicine**
Description: Offers access to reliable medical resources including medical journals and information regarding careers in health care, advocacy, and medical news.
Website/Resource: http://www.ama-assn.org

Organization: **American Academy of Child and Adolescent Psychiatry (AACAP)**
Description: Provides information regarding mental illnesses, data concerning efforts to prevent mental illnesses, how to seek proper treatment, and access to services for children and adolescents.
Website/Resource: http://www.aacap.org

Organization: **American Academy of Family Physicians**
Description: Offers information regarding family physician careers, clinical research, advocacy, practice management, and recent news/publications.
Website/Resource: http://www.aafp.org

Organization: **American Academy of Pediatrics (AAP)**
Description: Offers general information related to child health, specific guidelines concerning many pediatric issues, information regarding AAP programs, activities, policies, guidelines, publications, and other child health resources.
Website/Resource: http://www.aap.org

Organization: **American Psychological Association (APA)**
Description: Offers readers information regarding psychology topics, publication, careers, news, and education, as well as the ability to access a psychology help center to address issues encountered in daily life.
Website/Resource: http://www.apa.org

Organization: **Centers for Disease Control and Prevention**
Description: Offers information regarding current disease conditions, emergency preparedness/response, life stages/populations, healthy living, workplace environment/health.
Website/Resource: http://www.cdc.gov

Organization: **Children's Defense Fund (CDF)**
Description: A nonprofit child advocacy organization; website offers information regarding CDF's policies and mission, child advocacy resources, and child research data.
Website/Resource: http://www.childrensdefense.org

Organization: **Families Like Mine**
Description: Website mission: decrease isolation for people who have parents who are lesbian/gay/bisexual/ transgender (LGBT); offers information about Abigail Garner and her literary works. (She wrote *Families Like Mine: Children of Gay Parents Tell It Like It Is*).
Website/Resource: http://www.familieslikemine.com

Organization: **Foster Care Alumni of America (FCAA)**
Description: Offers readers information regarding foster care resources, community involvement/support, and FCAA organizational chapters.
Website/Resource: http://www.fostercarealumni.org

Organization: **Grandparent Information Center: American Association of Retired Persons (AARP)**
Description: Offers information regarding grandparenting support/materials and grandparenting fact sheets.
Website/Resource: http://www.aarp.org

Organization: **Healthy People 2010**
Description: Offers information regarding the goals of *Healthy People 2010* as well as many helpful links to health related websites.
Website/Resource: http://health.gov

Organization: **Healthy People 2020**
Description: Reflects assessments of major risks to health and wellness, changing public health priorities, and emerging issues related to our nation's health preparedness and prevention
Website: http://www.healthypeople.gov/HP2020/

Organization: **Minority Health Network (MHNet)**
Description: Web based information source for individuals interested in minority health; offers information about different minority groups, diseases, publications, and upcoming events.
Website/Resource: http://www.mhnet.com

Organization: **Morbidity & Mortality Weekly Report**
Description: Provides information regarding current mortality findings/morbidity concerns as well as information regarding notifiable diseases and surveillance summaries.
Website/Resource: http://www.cdc.gov

Organization: **National Center for Biotechnology Information**
Description: Provides access to biomedical/genomic information; offers links to countless medical journals, including PubMed, PubChem, and GEO.
Website/Resource: http://www.ncbi.nlm.nih.gov

Organization: **National Center for Health Statistics (NCHS)**
Description: Compiles statistical information to guide actions/policies to improve health of Americans; website offers statistical reports concerning health employment, health data standards, and much more.
Website/Resource: http://www.cdc.gov

Organization: **National Council on Family Relations (NCFR)**
Description: Provides information regarding professional conferences, journals, and NCFR governance.
Website/Resource: http://www.ncfr.org

Organization: **National Foster Care Coalition (NFCC)**
Description: Offers information regarding foster care facts, policy issues, and newsrooms/resources.
Website/Resource: http://www.nationalfostercare.org

Organization: **National Foster Parent Association**
Description: Offers foster parents and others information regarding foster care, helpful tools/resources, and links to state organizations.
Website/Resource: http://www.nfpainc.org

Organization: **National Institute of Nursing Research (NINR)**
Description: Offers information regarding NINR supported research/funding, training, and basic NINR news/information.
Website/Resource: http://www.ninr.nih.gov

Organization: **National Institutes of Health**
Description: Offers information regarding countless health topics, clinical trials, grants, health related news, and current medical research.
Website/Resource: http://www.nih.gov

Organization: **National Network for Child Care (NNCC)**
Description: Offers information about child care, access to KIDCARE (email list allowing individuals to communicate with others concerned about child care), person-to-person contact with experts in child care, and access to newsletter.
Website/Resource: http://www.nncc.org

Organization: **National Safe Kids Campaign**
Description: Offers readers tips about child safety, news/information about Safe Kids, and support/funding information.
Website/Resource: http://www.safekids.org

Organization: **National Stepfamily Resource Center (NSRC)**
Description: Offers access to stepfamily programs/services and education resources, as well as facts, laws/policies, and research related to stepfamilies.
Website/Resource: http://www.stepfam.org

Organization: **Parents without Partners**
Description: Offers contact information, helpful resources, chapters, and news/updates related to single parents and their children.
Website/Resource: http://www.parentswithoutpartners.org

Organization: **Pediatrics (the journal)**
Description: Offers access to the current issue, past issues, topic collections, and journal supplements.
Website/Resource: http://www.pediatrics.org

Organization: **Stepfamily Association of America**
Description: Provides educational information/resources for anyone interested in stepfamilies; contains links to other sites specializing in family information, travel, fun, records, and origins.
Website/Resource: http://www.ssafamilies.org

Organization: **U.S. Census Bureau**
Description: Offers information on current censuses, jobs, data tools, and publications.
Website/Resource: http://www.census.gov

Organization: **U.S. Department of Health and Human Services (HHS)**
Description: Offers access to health information pertaining to family health, prevention, diseases, regulation, and preparedness.
Website/Resource: http://www.hhs.gov

Organization: **U.S. Department of Health and Human Services Children's Bureau**
Description: Offers information regarding services, policy/planning, and research/statistics offered by the US Department of HHS Children's Bureau.
Website/Resource: http://www.acf.hhs.gov/programs/cb/

Organization: **Youth Indicators 2007: Trends in the Well-Being of American Youth**
Description: Contains statistics that describe young people's lives both in school and beyond the schoolhouse; updated every two years.
Website/Resource: http://nces.ed.gov/pubs2005/2005050.pdf

Organization: **Youth Risk Behavior Surveillance**
Description: Offers access to fact sheets, results, publications and data files related to priority health-risk behaviors and the prevalence of obesity and asthma among youth and young adults. Updated every two years.
Website/Resource: http://www.cdc.gov

Organization: **Youth Info**
Description: A government Website helping create/maintain/strengthen effective youth programs. Includes facts, funding information, and tools to help assess community assets, generate maps of local/federal resources, search for evidence-based youth programs, and keep up-to-date on the latest, youth-related news.
Website/Resource: http://www.findyouthinfo.org

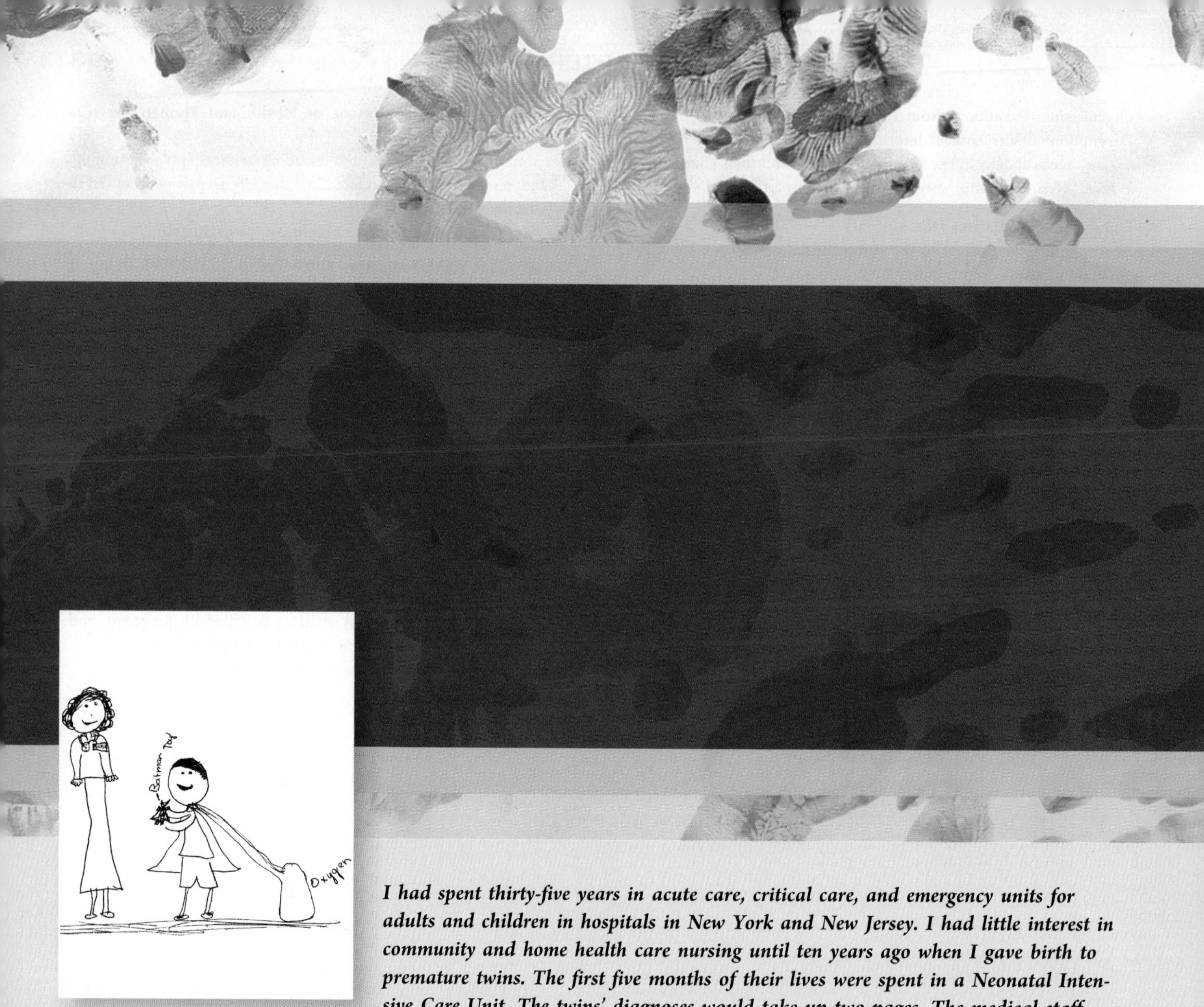

I had spent thirty-five years in acute care, critical care, and emergency units for adults and children in hospitals in New York and New Jersey. I had little interest in community and home health care nursing until ten years ago when I gave birth to premature twins. The first five months of their lives were spent in a Neonatal Intensive Care Unit. The twins' diagnoses would take up two pages. The medical staff gently yet constantly reminded us they would likely not survive. Six months after birth they were discharged home to mom, the nurse. I set up my battery of drugs, formulas, scales, apnea monitors, ostomy supplies and dressing kits much like I would have done in a hospital. One day I realized I could not be both mom and nurse. Near exhaustion I accepted home care nursing. The pediatric home care nurse was a wealth of knowledge and support. She coordinated the numerous early intervention therapists, scheduled the multitude of physician specialist appointments, ordered the Synagis injections, and explored ostomy supplies best suited for my sons. I will always remember her kindness when she told me, "Go take your shower, I will stay and watch the children." It is not only the knowledge home care nurses have in their practice but the caring they share with their clients that make the difference. I realized how lucky I was and decided to practice pediatric home care. Today I credit all the support I had during stressful times to all the professionals that helped me. The twins are in the fourth grade, and although we have our issues, they are thriving and happy. I believe in "giving back" to a community on a journey I was meant to travel. Pediatric home care nursing is the best it gets.

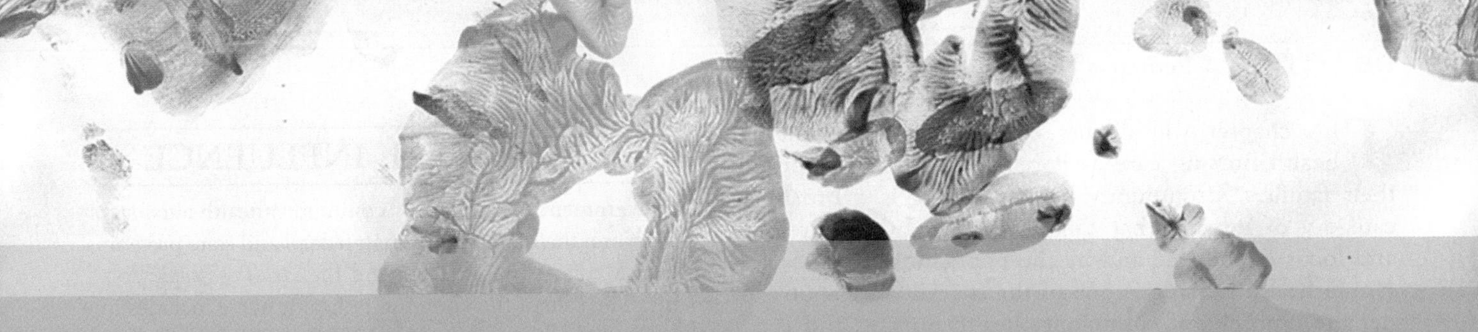

CHAPTER 4

Community and Home Health Nursing

KATHLEEN CERVASIO, RN, ACNS-BC, CCRN, PhD
MARY L. DOWELL, RN, BC, PhD

COMPETENCIES

Upon completion of this chapter, the reader will be able to:

- Review the history of community health nursing as it relates to children and their families, including the role government has played.
- Discuss how *Healthy People* objectives (health promotion, health protection, and disease prevention) relate to community health nursing care of children and their families.
- Describe the role of the community health nurse as it relates to assessment of the child, family, and community, and to environmental toxins.
- Compare types of home care agencies.
- Describe the role of the home health care nurse as it relates to skills, case management, and the home visit.
- Examine future trends in the area of community and home health care nursing for children and their families.
- Identify community resources that are available to help maintain the strength of the family and promote the child's health.
- Successfully complete the games and activities in the online student StudyWARE.

This chapter will discuss community and home health nursing care as it relates to children and their families. Community health nursing is a broad category of nursing that can be defined by the area and focus of practice and by the population it serves. Home health nursing is one of the specialty areas under the umbrella of community health nursing and is defined as a variety of services provided to people, in this instance a child, in their place of residence (Maurer & Smith, 2009).

Over the last several decades fewer nurses are working in community health settings. This trend may continue, although pending changes in access to health care may reverse it. Generally, about 15% of all registered nurses work in the community health setting. Approximately one in four community health nurses were employed by local and state health departments or community health centers. The largest percentage of community health nurses worked in home health. School health, occupational health, hospice, and other settings make up the remaining areas where community health nurses are employed. This chapter will focus on a broad discussion of community health nursing and home health nursing for children and their families.

COMMUNITY HEALTH NURSING

Community health nursing may be defined as "the synthesis of nursing practice and public health practice applied to promoting and preserving the health of populations" (Maurer & Smith, 2009, p. 3). The community health nurse has a focus on health promotion, disease prevention, and maintenance of health. While that focus may be on the individual or family, the well-being of the community as a whole is the final objective. The community health nurse can focus on health promotion at an individual (child) or family level while promoting the well-being of the community by conducting well-child assessments, giving immunizations, conducting screening tests, teaching, and making referrals for the child and family to other health care associates and resources. The community nurse also plays a pivotal role in immunization programs. Community health nursing, with its population-based focus and emphasis on health promotion and disease prevention, has a unique opportunity to be a leader in the national health objective of increasing the number of immunized children under age 3.

Community health nurses who care for children and their families practice in a variety of settings that teach health promotion and disease prevention, including the child's home, well-child clinics, migrant health clinics, neighborhood health centers, and centers that implement federally mandated or specific state-funded programs (Stanhope & Lancaster, 2008). The nurse may have a primary or team role during the delivery of services. Table 4-1 lists the various roles of community health nurses.

GOVERNMENTAL INFLUENCE

The government has influenced community health nursing for children and their families through federal and state programs such as Medicaid, public laws, and the *Healthy People* documents. The role of the community health nurse includes implementation of government-supported programs and referral of families who are eligible for these services. Children with disabilities and those with chronic conditions can receive assistance with health care services through the Title V Children with Special Health Care Needs (CSHCN) programs. Community health nurses can be instrumental in referring children and families for services under this program. Promotion of adequate nutrition for low-income families is important for growth and development and functioning in school (Maurer & Smith, 2009). Community and school nurses can assist families in obtaining services through the special supplemental nutrition program for Women, Infants, and Children (WIC) and the federally funded school breakfast and lunch programs.

In the mid-1980s, federal amendments to Medicaid expanded services to low-income pregnant women. As part of case management for these women, many states now reimburse for home visits by nurses employed by local health departments or health centers. In some states, New York being one, nursing visits are provided by third party payers and are considered case management. Nurses who make home visits focus on teaching caregivers to implement measures to promote growth, development, and safety; ensuring that the child is being provided with proper nutrition; and assessing the child's and family's health care for its adequacy and accessibility (Maurer & Smith, 2009). The Medicaid programs of the 1990s and beyond focused on managed care and cost-cutting initiatives but remained alarmed about the increase of unwanted pregnancies in young females.

Reflections from Families

I was a single mother with two small children. I felt embarrassed to go to the grocery store and use the coupons I had received from WIC. The nurse at WIC was always supportive and constantly focused on the importance of using the coupons, not because I wanted to get free food, but because I wanted to give my children nutritious meals. Thanks to her, I quit feeling so embarrassed when I went to the store.

TABLE 4-1 Various Roles of the Community Health Nurse

ROLES	FUNCTIONS	EXAMPLES
Clinician	Combines nursing, epidemiology, case management, resource coordination, expertise in working with families, into formulating health policy, assessing communities, and carrying out all phases of population-focused programs.	Provides information to a group of teenagers regarding safe sex practices. Plans, implements, and evaluates a program to decrease drug use by adolescents.
Advocate	Advocates for the child and his family by promoting their needs and desires.	Speaks for the needs of a soon-to-be-homeless family with a child who is dependent on technology.
Collaborator	Collaborates with other health care members, social service agencies, judicial systems, and schools to ensure holistic care.	Works with a caregiver, teacher, principal, physician, and social worker to develop a plan to facilitate the successful integration of a child with a disability into a public school setting.
Consultant	Serves as an expert (teacher, leader, resource person) who is able to propose solutions for identified problems.	Organizes a child and family health fair.
Counselor	Helps clients choose appropriate solutions to their problems.	Works with caregivers to decide if their child who is dependent on technology should attend school or be tutored at home.
Educator	Teaches health promotion and disease prevention activities as well as maintains optimal levels of health and wellness.	Teaches a prenatal class on nutrition and healthy habits.
Researcher	Partipates in research that will benefit the community. Should include identifying problem areas; collecting, analyzing, and interpreting data; applying findings; and evaluating, designing, and conducting research.	Identifies an area where environmental toxins near a popular playground are jeopardizing the health of children and develops solutions that will promote health and well-being.
Case manager	Develops and coordinates services for a selected client and family.	Coordinates all the services needed by a child recuperating from a hospital stay to ensure a healthy recovery; occupational therapy, physical therapy, tutoring, as well as financial resources for the caregivers.

Adapted from Hitchcock, J., Schubert, P., & Thomas, S. (2003). *Community Health Nursing: Caring in Action* (2nd ed.). Clifton Park, NY: Delmar Cengage Learning.

Recent years have seen the development of the Family Nurse Partnership, an evidence-based community health program focused on vulnerable first-time mothers. A community health nurse follows each family for two years to provide education, direction, and support. The results have been impressive: for example, there has been a 56% decrease in emergency room visits for routine health care. The beneficial outcomes of these types of programs have decreased family risk while containing costs.

The Early and Periodic Screening Diagnosis and Treatment Program (EPSDT) is funded through Medicaid (Title XIX of the Social Security Act). All states have an EPSDT program that offers early screening, diagnosis, treatment, and periodic follow-up services to children and youth who meet the financial eligibility requirements and who are under 21 years of age. Public Law 99-457, the Education of the Handicapped Act Amendments of 1986, directs states to develop and enact statewide coordinated, comprehensive, multidisciplinary interagency programs of early intervention (EI) services for infants and toddlers with disabilities, in addition to support services for these families in the home. In 1997, Public Law 105-17 reauthorized the Individuals with Disabilities Education Act (IDEA) mandating inclusion and appropriate services in the least restrictive environment for children with disabilities. Community nurses can provide

NURSING TIP

Lead Toxicity and Retained Bullet Fragments

Over the last three decades lead levels in North American children have been declining. However, lead toxicity remains a significant childhood environmental health hazard. Lead toxicity secondary to retained bullet fragments in children has been well-documented in the literature. Chelation therapy prior to surgical removal of bullets and their fragments is essential to prevent systemic lead toxicity.

many services for children covered under these government programs. They can assess and screen children in preschool settings, implement ongoing staff and client education, coordinate care with the health care team, become actively involved in community nursing networks, and develop health promotion programs for school personnel and family members (Scheffler, Vogel, Astern, & Burgess, 2007). Nurses can also play a role in early identification and referral of infants and toddlers who are eligible for early intervention (EI) services and serve as family advocates in coordination of care (Selekman, 2007).

HEALTHY PEOPLE 2010 OBJECTIVES

Changes and additions to the *Healthy People 2000* national health objectives, which were reflected in *Healthy People 2010* (U.S. DHHS, 2000b), will specifically affect community health care of children and their families. (At the time of publication, these goals for *Healthy People 2020* are not completed, but will be based upon the 2010 foundation). These include: (1) adding some new focus areas such as Medical Products Safety and Access to Quality Health Services and Programs; (2) combining violence and abusive behavior with unintentional injuries to become Injury/Violence Prevention; and (3) adding children to the maternal and infant priority area, becoming Maternal, Infant, and Child focus area. The relevant *Healthy People 2010* goals for children and their families are presented in Table 4-2. Some of the primary goals of community health nursing are also goals of *Healthy People 2010*

TABLE 4-2 *Healthy People 2010* Goals Relevant to Children and Their Families

	OBJECTIVE	BASE 2000	TARGET 2010
1-9a	Reduce pediatric hospitalizations for asthma (per 100,000 children)	23.0	17.3
6-9	Inclusion of children with disabilities in regular education programs	45%	60%
8-11	Eliminate elevated blood lead levels (BLLs) in children 1 to 5 years of age	4.4%	0%
14-22	Achieve and maintain effective vaccination in children 19 to 35 months of age for universally recommended vaccines	43–93%	90%
15-20	Increase use of child restraints	92%	100%
15-33	Reduce maltreatment and maltreatment fatalities of children (per 1,000 children)	13.9	11.1
16-1c	Reduce infant deaths (per 1,000 live births)	7.2	4.5
16-2	Reduce child death rates (per 100,000 children)		
	a. 1–4 years	34.2	25
	b. 5–9 years	17.6	14.3
16-10	Reduce		
	a. low birth weight	7.6%	5%
	b. very low birth weight	1.4%	0.9%
19-4	Reduce growth retardation in low-income children	8%	5%
21-2	Reduce untreated dental decay in young children	16%	9%
27-9	Reduce child tobacco exposure at home	27%	6%
28-4	Reduce blindness and visual impairment in children and adolescents (per 1,000 children)	25	20
28-12	Reduce otitis media in children and adolescents (visits per 1,000 children)	344.7	294

U.S. Department of Health and Human Services (2000b). *Healthy People 2010*. Washington, DC: Government Printing Office.

EYEON...

National Health Agenda

The Framework for *Healthy People 2010* has been established as a national health agenda that communicates a vision and a strategy for improving the health of the nation's population and achieving health equity. The preliminary goals that have been identified are:

- To eliminate preventable disease, disability, injury, and premature death.
- To achieve health equity, eliminate disparities, and improve the health of all groups.
- To create social and physical environments that promote good health for all.
- To promote healthy development and healthy behaviors across every stage of life.

Source: U.S. Department of Health and Human Services. *Healthy People Recommendations for 2020*. Washington, DC: Government Printing Office

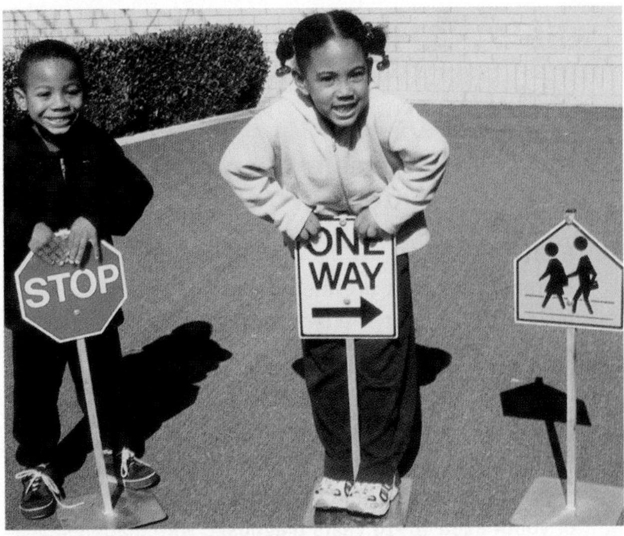

FIGURE 4-1 Health promotion can include learning safety signs and rules of the road. DELMAR CENGAGE LEARNING.

(USDHHS, 2000). These are health promotion, health protection, and disease prevention.

HEALTH PROMOTION

Health promotion is defined as "activities or interventions that identify risk factors related to disease; the lifestyle changes related to disease prevention; and the process of enabling individuals and communities to increase control over and improve their health. These activities or strategies are directed toward developing the resources of clients to maintain or enhance their physical, social, emotional, and spiritual well-being" (Hitchcock, Schubert, & Thomas, 2003, p. 891). Health promotion is a major goal of community health nursing practice. Community health nurses facilitate health in the population through direct nursing interventions for health promotion and disease prevention with individuals, families, groups, and populations. The community health nurse develops, implements, and evaluates health promotion programs in schools, work sites, hospitals, faith communities, prisons, and community settings (Maurer & Smith, 2009). These health promotion strategies are implemented by nurses through counseling, education, and anticipatory guidance. Some examples of health promotion activities conducted by community health nurses for children and their families are: well-child care clinics, safety programs (Figure 4-1), nutrition programs, environmental efforts (clean air programs), sanitation measures, and community parenting classes (Hockenberry & Wilson, 2011).

Reflections from Families

I went to a baby-care workshop after I had my first baby that was taught by a nurse from the local health department. I learned well-child care (e.g., bathing, feeding, holding, and diapering) as well as interpreting communication cues and average ages for achieving certain developmental milestones. My mother-in-law insisted that if a child was not rolling over by 2 months of age there was something wrong with him. Because of the workshop I could feel assured that my 3-month-old baby was not "slow" just because he was not rolling over yet. I offered to take my mother-in-law to the next class so she could learn about the average ages for achieving developmental milestones and she happily accepted.

RESEARCH Highlight

Diabetes in Hispanic American Youth

STUDY PURPOSE

To report the 2001 prevalence and 2002–2005 incidence of type 1 and type 2 diabetes in Hispanic youth in an effort to describe the clinical and behavioral characteristics of these youth.

METHODS

Data from the SEARCH for diabetes in youth study is a population-based multicenter observational study of youth aged 10–19 years diagnosed with diabetes. A large number of youth were used to estimate the prevalence and incidence of type 1 and type 2 diabetes. Information was obtained by a questionnaire, physical examination, blood, and urine samples.

FINDINGS

Among Hispanic youth type 1 diabetes was more prevalent than type 2 diabetes. There was no significant sex difference in type 1 or type 2 diabetes prevalence. The incidence of type 2 diabetes for females age 10–14 years was twice that of male subjects. Among youth age 15–19 years the incidence of type 2 diabetes exceeded that of type 1 diabetes for female subjects, but not for male subjects. Poor glycemic control as well as high LDL cholesterol and triglycerides were common among youth (male and female) 15 years of age with either type of diabetes. Forty-five percent of youth (male and female) with type 1 diabetes were overweight or obese.

IMPLICATIONS

Factors such as poor glycemic control, elevated lipids, and a high prevalence of overweight and obesity may put Hispanic youth with type 1 and type 2 diabetes at risk for future diabetes-related conditions.

REFERENCE

Lawrence, J., Mayer-Davis, E., Reynolds, K., Beyer, J., Pettitt, D., D'Agostino, R., Marcovina, S., Imperatore, G. & Hamman, R. (2009). Diabetes in Hispanic American youth: prevalence, incidence, demographics, and clinical characteristics: the SEARCH for Diabetes in Youth Study. *Diabetes Care, 32*(Suppl 2), S123–132.

Health Protection

Health protection is defined as "activities designed to maintain the current level of health, actively prevent disease, detect disease early, thwart disease processes, or maintain functioning within constraints of disease" (Hitchcock et al., 2003 p. 891). Screening programs for newborns, infants, children, and adolescents include blood lead levels, phenylketonuria (PKU), growth and development, serum cholesterol and glucose levels, blood pressure assessment, hearing and vision, dental health, scoliosis, behavior issues, and testicular and breast self-examination. Screening programs are conducted by nurses through health departments, home care agencies, clinics, schools, health fairs, community centers, and well-child clinics.

Firearm, playground safety, and car-seat loan programs are other examples of health protection programs. Community health nurses can assess these areas and provide guidance and educational resources for families who have needs in these areas. In 2004 drowning was the second leading cause of death in children 4–11 years old followed by motor vehicle accidents (National Center for Injury Prevention and Control, CDC, 2006). The implications for community health nurses in screening, educating, and evaluating recommendations to avoid injury or death are a vital part of each and every visit. Community nurses need to routinely inquire about potential safety hazards with children in the presence of their parents and use specific assessment tools to assure a safe environment.

Disease Prevention Services

"Disease prevention refers to those activities designed to protect persons from disease and its consequences" (Hitchcock et al., 2003 p.15). Programs included in the area of preventive services for children and their families include immunization programs, environmental screening programs, hearing and vision screening programs, and screening programs for children at risk for developmental delay. Community health nurses have a major role in administration of immunizations to children at well-child clinics, at immunization clinics, and during special immunization days at schools. They also assist in measuring serum lead levels, performing vision and hearing screenings, and administering assessments to screen for developmental delays. Once an area of risk is identified, the community health nurse follows through by making referrals as needed, following up with home visits, or arranging return visits to the clinic. These interventions may be initiated through community health centers, school-based clinics, home health programs, public health departments, or health maintenance organizations. The role of nurse as advocate and educator plays a vital role in the prevention of disease.

Standards

Standards of care and standards of professional performance have been developed by leaders of the Quad Council of Public Health Nursing Organizations (Quad Council of Public Health Nursing Organizations, 1999). The Quad Council represents nurses involved in population-focused and community-oriented nursing practice. The standards of care and standards of professional performance are widely available.

These standards reflect the steps of the nursing process and indicate that community health nurses are to apply this process to individuals, families, and groups to promote health and wellness throughout life. These standards provide guidelines for competent levels of practice and behavior for the community health nurse. They also help to define the scope and quality of community health nursing care (Maurer & Smith, 2009).

COMMUNITY ASSESSMENT

A community assessment is the process of compiling data regarding the health status and resources available for a community. This assessment is the foundation for nursing planning and advocacy. A needs assessment approach focuses on the health issues in a particular community (Clark, 2008). Some questions to include are:

- What are the child's neighborhood, school, and peer group like?
- Are there adequate community resources and agencies available?
- What is the availability and funding of health care resources, including managed care models?
- Is the community at large engaged to address the well-being of the population?
- What is the language spoken?
- What is the level of education of families?
- What are the unique cultural assessments?

The nurse's goal is to use knowledge gained during the community assessment to determine how the larger environment influences the health and development of the children and families.

Another community assessment the nurse can perform is a windshield survey. A **windshield survey** is a systematic assessment that is performed while the nurse travels through the community (Figure 4-2).

All of the senses should be used to look closely at the community and note housing, environment, common areas, and community development. The findings that have an impact on the health of children from the windshield survey could include safety hazards, loud sounds and noxious odors, unsafe air and water quality, lack of green space, homeless individuals or families, stray animals, limited public services, and inadequate public education systems. Attention should be paid to the environment in order to assess risk factors for safety and to prevent injury (Figure 4-3).

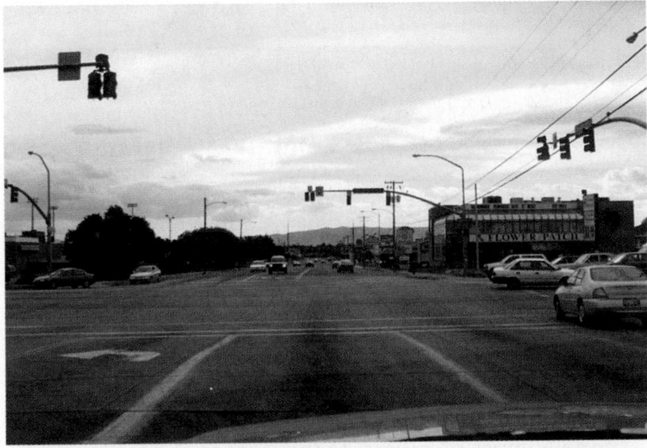

FIGURE 4-2 From the car, the nurse can directly observe a community and gain valuable assessment data. DELMAR CENGAGE LEARNING.

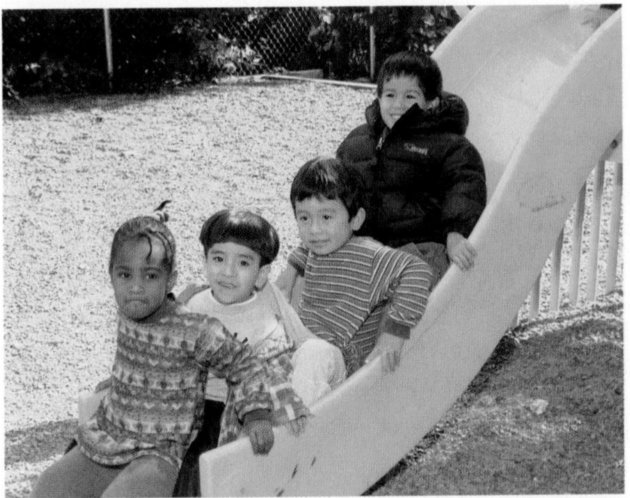

FIGURE 4-3 Safety of all the environments a child visits must be ensured. DELMAR CENGAGE LEARNING.

ENVIRONMENTAL TOXINS

The community health nurse can have an instrumental role in providing information and promoting safety and injury prevention. This role is especially important when assessing the child's environment. Community health nurses need to have a knowledge of how children, because of their unique physical, biologic, and social characteristics, are especially vulnerable to the adverse effects from interaction with polluted environments. Air pollution is a major threat to child health. Children are particularly vulnerable to the damaging effects of air pollution because their lungs are growing and their innate defenses against inhaled pollutants may be impaired. In addition, it is important to note that air pollution from the combustion of biomass fuels in or near homes is one of the most important global environmental threats to child health (Kulkarni & Grigg, 2008).

The illnesses caused by environmental hazards include asthma exacerbated by air pollution and secondhand cigarette smoke, developmental delays caused by lead in paint and contaminated drinking water, and increased respiratory symptoms from exposure to radon (a radioactive gas caused by the decaying of uranium that can enter homes through floors, cracks, and walls) (Maurer & Smith, 2009). Early recognition and prevention of exposure to environmental toxins is a goal of the community health nurse.

Assessment of the environment is the first step toward recognizing and preventing exposure to environmental toxins. Areas in the environment to be assessed include: radiation, lead and heavy metals, noise, infectious agents, insects and animals, plants, poisons, air pollution, lifestyle factors, occupations, and water pollution (Stanhope & Lancaster, 2008). Once assessment is completed the nurse can teach

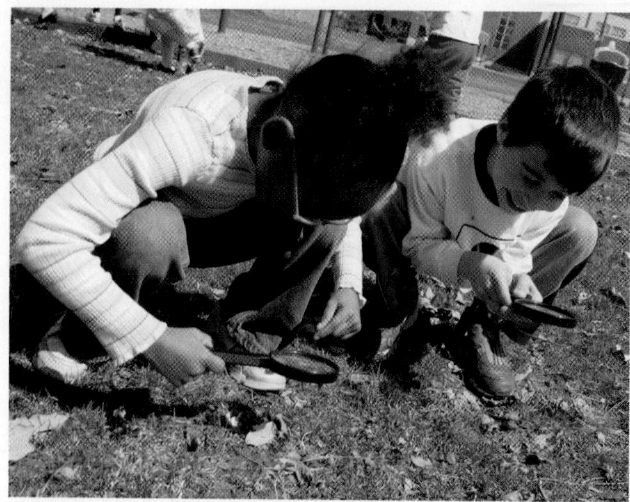

FIGURE 4-4 Children need play areas free of pollution and poisons. DELMAR CENGAGE LEARNING.

NURSING ALERT

Lead Poisoning

The effects of lead on the central nervous system are significant because they are believed not to be reversible. In the central nervous system, lead causes an increase in membrane permeability, causing a fluid shift into brain tissue, producing increased intracranial pressure, ischemia, and cellular destruction. Acute encephalopathy, manifested by hypertension, intellectual deficits, seizures, cerebral edema, coma, and even death may result. The nurse or family should seek immediate medical attention if the child has been exposed and lead levels are elevated, because lead can be removed from the body only by chelation therapy, which requires that the child be under the care of a health care provider.

the family ways to prevent exposure to environmental hazards (Figure 4-4). Teaching should include both primary and secondary preventive measures. Family teaching should include radiation, heavy metals, noise, infectious agents, insects and animals, plants, poisons, and air and water pollution. These secondary environmental hazards vary widely by community, city, and state. Hence, local health departments are excellent sources for local issues.

Families should be encouraged to minimize the use of household chemicals and pesticides, and to ensure safe (locked cabinet, out of reach) storage when they are not in use. Proper ventilation should be ensured when chemicals are used within the house. Families should be taught about the effects that secondhand smoke can have on children. Teaching about the prevalence of lead poisoning in children between the ages of 6 months and 6 years should also be conducted. Foods that contain high levels of pesticides should be properly washed to decrease contaminants. It is also vital to store and cook food and food products at the proper temperatures to assure safety.

The community health nurse is responsible to make appropriate referrals and provide needed resources on environmental health issues to families. Follow-up visits for evaluation is a critical component to the nursing process in the community setting.

FUTURE TRENDS

The care provided by community health nurses will continue to focus on promoting, restoring, and preserving the health of the total population or community. In the future, how this care is delivered and the role of the community nurse in delivering this care will change. Economic and technological trends will continue to influence the role of community health nurses. Improved medical advances will improve survival rates and quality of life issues for children with medical conditions. Community health nurses must continue to be involved in the implementation of programs that affect children's health. Medically fragile children will be cared for in community settings and schools with an emphasis on normalization of children with chronic conditions (Maurer & Smith, 2009).

The market-driven economic health policy has prompted a change in the health delivery system of community health for children and their families. Many of the services provided by the health department are being shifted to managed care systems or not-for-profit and proprietary home care agencies. Technology has introduced equipment in the home that has traditionally been in health care facilities. Some examples of technology include blood glucose monitoring, respiratory nebulizers, and ventilators. The growth of telemedicine programs empowers families to care for their child with support in care management utilizing computers. Advances in the availability of vaccinations for the prevention of numerous diseases continue to grow. The community health nurse role at the point of service will continue to evolve into an independent specialty practice utilizing alternative models of care (Clark, 2008).

CULTURAL CONSIDERATION

Food Spices and Lead

Most cases of elevated lead levels in children are caused by contaminated paint or dust in the environment. Spices bought in the Republic of Georgia and India for food preparation were found to have high levels of lead after families were diagnosed with lead poisoning. Families who travel internationally must be aware of this potential health risk (Woolf & Woolf, 2005).

HOME HEALTH NURSING

Home care can be defined as care provided to children in their home that is simple or complex for the purpose of health promotion, maintenance, or restoration. The health-related services provided for children and their families range from providing direct hourly nursing care to children who are dependent on technology, to intermittent visits from nurses, home health aids, physical therapists, occupational therapists, speech therapists, or social workers. Home care for children is growing in the area of referrals for home antibiotic therapy, pediatric hospice programs, nursing care for children who are dependent on technology, home phototherapy, private-duty nursing, and home visits to new mothers who are discharged with their babies after brief, routine hospital stays because of uncomplicated deliveries.

Home care services can be provided for either short-term or long-term needs. Referrals for home antibiotic therapy, home phototherapy, and home visits to new mothers are examples of children and families needing short-term home care services. The focus for short-term care is on primary and secondary prevention of disease. **Primary prevention** involves interventions for children that promote health and prevent disease processes from developing. Teaching new mothers how to perform infant care is one example of a home care service that is primary prevention. **Secondary prevention** aims to detect disease in the early stages before clinical signs and symptoms manifest in order to intervene with early diagnosis and treatment. The goal is to reverse or reduce the severity of the disease or provide a cure. Home phototherapy or short-term nursing visits to teach diabetes care would be examples of home care services that would provide secondary prevention. **Tertiary prevention** is directed toward children with clinically apparent disease. The aim is to improve the course of disease, reduce disability, or rehabilitate. Examples of tertiary prevention include services provided by home care agencies that are long term, such as provision of care for a child who is dependent on technology, or hospice care (Maurer & Smith, 2009).

Many different factors have an impact on home care for children and their families. The three factors this section will focus on include: (1) types of agencies and the impact of managed care on these agencies; (2) family needs (family and nurse interactions, respite care); and (3) the scope of nursing care (skills, case management, and the home visit).

HOME CARE AGENCIES AND MANAGED CARE

Home care agencies that provide care for children and their families fall into five categories: official, voluntary, combined, private, and hospital-based agencies. An explanation of these types of agencies is found in Table 4-3.

Managed care refers to cost-effective delivery of health care services. Home health care services are supported by managed care organizations in situations where they will result in shortened hospital stays. Caring for children at home with the assistance of home care services continues to be cost effective as compared with prolonged hospital stays. Early discharge programs are encouraged by managed care organizations because of their cost effectiveness. Children with acute and chronic illnesses are being affected by early discharge protocols.

Managed care, by supporting these early discharges, has created a need for comprehensive home care programs for children. Children are going home sicker, and families are required to assume more responsibility for their care. These children and families have special needs and require comprehensive nursing care and teaching.

TABLE 4-3 Types of Home Health Agencies

TYPE OF AGENCY	EXPLANATION
Official or public agencies	Receive power through statutes enacted by legislation, Early and Periodic Screening, Diagnosis, and Treatment (EPSDT) Program. Care includes well-child visits.
Voluntary agencies	Receive funds from contributions, fees for service, united community funds, contracts for services, and grants. Provide skilled nursing care in the home.
Combined governmental and voluntary agencies	Receive funds from official and nonofficial sources. Provide both health promotion and disease prevention services in addition to home health services.
Private agencies	Function as either for-profit or not-for-profit. Provide hourly nursing care for acutely or chronically ill children, as well as intermittent visits for short-term needs. Do not necessarily provide health promotion or disease prevention services.
Hospital-affiliated agencies	Receive majority of referrals from sponsoring hospital.
Specialty agencies	Specialize in particular population care (pediatric care or geriatric care).

FAMILY NEEDS

Children who are dependent on technology and those who need hospice care receive the majority of home care nursing hours. The other home care hours consist of teaching caregivers how to use apnea monitors, initiating short-term phototherapy, and administering medications through intravenous lines, performing dressing changes or teaching the caregiver how to administer tube feedings (Figure 4-5). The family who has a child dependent upon technology will often require private duty nursing for a number of hours a day at home and at school. These private duty nurses will require specialized training (Boroughs & Dougherty, 2009). This type of home care is long term in nature. Long-term home care programs continue to expand services to include nursing interventions for the management of burns, home traction for fractures, treatment of osteomyelitis, total parenteral nutrition (TPN), diabetes, ostomy, and long-term intravenous antibiotic therapy. Central line access devices are commonly seen in pediatric home care and require specialized nursing knowledge and intervention for appropriate and safe care.

Advantages and disadvantages of having an ill child at home, rather than in a hospital, have been identified by families. Advantages include a less-threatening environment, easier access to the child's loved ones, decreased need for travel to and from the hospital, strengthening of the family unit, and restoration of control of the child's care to the family (Boroughs & Dougherty, 2009). The disadvantages include intrusion of professionals on the family's privacy, financial pressures, and the impact on siblings of having the ill child at home. Another disadvantage reported by families is the stress of taking care of a child with special needs at home (Owens, 2008). Home health care nurses have an important role in alleviating the disadvantages families can experience with having the ill child at home. Healthy interpersonal relationships between the nurse and family can improve the family's adjustment to having home health care for their child. Nurses can provide referrals, within the boundaries of The Joint Commission confidentiality requirements, if the family is experiencing financial strain, and they can assist the siblings in adjusting to having an ill brother or sister at home. Numerous private and public resources exist to support the entire family unit when a child has a chronic illness.

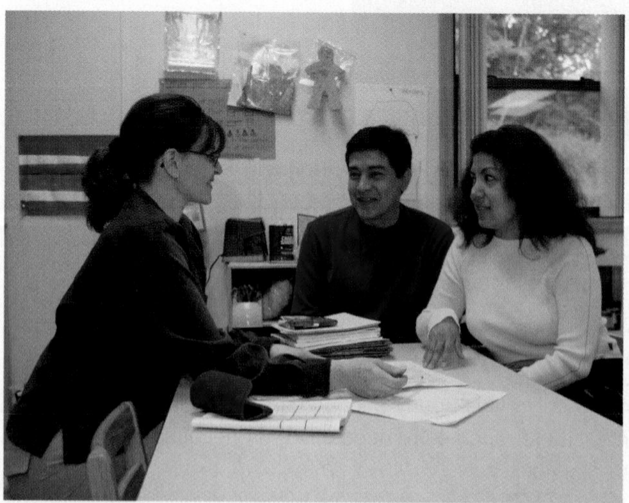

FIGURE 4-5 Nursing responsibilities include teaching families how to care for their children and manage the health equipment in the home. DELMAR CENGAGE LEARNING.

> **CRITICAL THINKING**
>
> **Managed Care Systems**
>
> **Managed care programs are concerned with cost containment. How will this concern with cost containment affect the quality of home care for children?**

INTERPERSONAL RELATIONSHIPS

Interpersonal relationships among the home care nurse, the child, and family can be described as collaborative—in other words, where mutual sharing and working together help to achieve common goals such that all persons or groups are recognized and growth is enhanced (Iglehart, 2008). During this collaborative relationship, the nurse should maintain professional boundaries. **Professional boundaries** are defined as the space between the nurse's power and the client's vulnerability. The power of the nurse comes from the professional position and the access to private knowledge about the client. Establishing boundaries allows the nurse to control this power differential and allows a safe connection to meet the client's needs (National Council of State Boards of Nursing, 1996). Williamson (2007) discusses how the child's caregivers need to have home care nurses listen to them and respect their knowledge and feelings because they are involved in care on a 24-hour, 7-day-a-week basis. Caregivers felt it was important when the home care nurse respected the family's wishes, was flexible, allowed them to participate in the child's care, communicated with the family, and talked to the caregivers directly and simply (Penz, 2008). Clarifying roles can assist the home care nurse to maintain professional boundaries. For instance, establishing house rules such as where to park and where to store belongings and defining issues such as routines, discipline, mealtime, and homework can help to clarify roles. Having professional support through nursing supervisors will also help the home care nurse to define appropriate family roles. Blurring of nurse-patient and family boundaries can be a significant problem. Caregivers may possess significant knowledge of their child's illness and needs from past experience, the library, and Internet re-

KIDS WANT TO KNOW

Why can't my home care nurse skip some of my treatments?

Sometimes I want my home care nurses to play games with me and skip some of my respiratory treatments. Why won't she do that?

Home care nurses are professionals who are there to help you maintain health. If the home care nurse can set up a schedule that ensures treatment protocols are being carried out, she may have time to play a game with you.

CRITICAL THINKING

Collaboration with the Family

You routinely perform home care for a child who has a tracheostomy and is dependent on oxygen. You prefer to do the bath and tracheostomy care in the early morning, but the child's caregivers prefer after lunch because this fits their afternoon and early evening schedule. How will you determine when the bath should be given? What factors will you consider?

sources. Including caregivers in the care plan and considering their judgment can facilitate or maintain a professional working relationship. Home health care nurses should recognize signs that they have crossed boundaries, including excessive self-disclosure, secretive behavior, "super nurse" behavior, selective communication, flirtations, and failure to protect the client (National Council of State Boards of Nursing, 1996).

The National Council of State Boards of Nursing (1996) states that every nurse-client relationship can be plotted on a continuum of professional behavior. This continuum ranges from under-involvement (distancing, disinterest, and neglect) to over-involvement (boundary crossings and boundary violations). The zone of helpfulness is in the center of the professional behavior continuum. This zone is where the majority of child and family interactions should occur to ensure effective nursing care. Home health care nurses are at risk of becoming over-involved with the family because of the informal home environment, casual, social conversations that occur with family members throughout the day, participation by family members in the care of the child, and attempts by some families to reduce the stress of having a stranger in the home by incorporating the nurse as a member of the family. Guidelines to determine professional boundaries and the continuum of professional behavior for the nurse are published by the National Council of State Boards of Nursing.

Guidelines important to the home health care nurse caring for children and their families are: delineation and maintenance of boundaries; examination of boundary crossings; variables of the care setting including actions that overstep established boundaries; and post-termination relationships. The nurse and family should be cognizant of feelings and behaviors and the nurse should always act in the best interests of the child and family.

By maintaining collaboration and professional boundaries, the home care nurse can begin to develop a trusting therapeutic relationship with the child and the family. Family caregivers report that nurses who come into the home offer them support for the physical and emotional challenges of caring for a child with a chronic illness at home. Without this support, caregivers are at risk for burnout and may need respite care.

Respite Care

Respite care is short-term, temporary care that is normally provided in the home for a child who requires specialized care; it provides relief for the caregivers, which may help to prevent burnout and increase the caregivers' ability to cope with stress. The home care nurse may provide this relief by referring the family to sources for respite care. The importance of respite care in assisting families to manage the extra stresses and problems of coping with children with complex health care needs is recognized as a vital aspect of care in chronically ill children maintained at home (Eaton, 2008). Families taking care of these children at home have complex and conflicting feelings about using respite care services if they are unfamiliar with the caretakers who will provide the respite care. Families want to be familiar with the person to whom they are entrusting the care of their child. When caretakers begin to think in terms of their need for a break, it is natural for them to turn to the home health care nurse to assist them in making arrangements.

Some agencies have successfully developed formal programs of respite care that are available to families taking care of children with a chronic illness at home. The agency ensures that if the child is to remain at home under the care of a nurse, and the caregiver is absent overnight, a designated substitute caretaker with power of attorney is appointed (Oresland, Määttä, Norberg, Lützén, 2009). When respite time is well planned, it can be therapeutic for the family and the child.

SCOPE OF NURSING PRACTICE

Nurses have many responsibilities when they care for the child and the family in the home. The scope of nursing practice will be discussed as it relates to these many responsibilities in the area of nursing skills, case management, and the home visit.

Home health care nurses provide direct care, assessments, instruction, support, screening, referrals, and case management (Maurer & Smith, 2009). The characteristics necessary for home care nurses to work effectively with children and families are flexibility, creativeness, sensitivity, and professionalism supported by nursing knowledge and skills. Although both hospital-based nurses and home health care nurses use acute care and high tech skills, the home visit requires nursing practice that is very different from the hospital setting. The home health care nurse must take into consideration the family's psychosocial resources, the neighborhood, and the presence or absence of community services (MacLeod, Misener, Banks, Morton, Vogt & Bentham, 2008).

Skills

The dimensions of home care for children are becoming more complex, requiring nurses to be competent in high tech care. The literature on medically fragile children living with their families is beginning to evolve with the introduction of the medical home concept (Volpintesta, 2009). The most frequently voiced positive aspect of having home care professionals in the home was that they were a support to the parent and family. Other positive aspects were genuine caring, respectful and collaborative interactions with the family, and competent and skillful delivery of care. Current practice techniques are essential for the home care nurse (see the evidence-based practice box for central venous catheter site care in children). Even nurses who are experienced in these technological skills in the hospital may encounter new challenges in the home setting. Competency-based curricula have been developed for home care nurses and caregivers to update or learn these skills and are now a part of the home care agency's orientation program for nurses. An example of such a curriculum has been developed for tracheostomy and ventilator care for caregivers, hospital-based nurses, home care nurses, nurse educators, school health nurses, educators, early intervention specialists, and training coordinators of home care agencies (Maurer & Smith, 2009).

Standards

Along with competency-based standards, the American Nurses Association (1999) has developed practice standards for home health care nurses that provide guidelines for competent levels of skills and practice behaviors. These guidelines are available as The Scope and Standards of Home Health Nursing Practice.

The standards of professional practice emphasize quality of care, performance appraisal, education, collegiality, ethics, collaboration, research, and resource utilization. These standards guide all facets of home health nurses' practice as they care for children and their families. The case management role of the home health care nurse is described in the scope of home health nursing practice as the promotion of continuity of care through discharge planning, case management, care management, and advocacy.

EVIDENCE-BASED PRACTICE

Central Venous Catheter Site Care

CLINICAL PROBLEM

Which solution is more effective for central venous catheter site care in children, chlorhexidine or povidone-iodine?

BEST CLINICAL PRACTICE

- Most studies found chlorhexidine to be superior to povidone-iodine for preventing microbial colonization of the central venous catheter site and the catheter tip, and for decreasing the risk of local site infection.
- However, conflicting evidence continues to exist regarding the efficacy of chlorhexidine versus povidone-iodine for preventing central venous catheter-related bacteremia.
- The safety of chlorhexidine in hospitalized infants and children has not been fully established.

IMPLICATIONS FOR NURSING

- Chlorhexidine gluconate appears to be a safe and effective solution for central venous catheter site care in older infants and children.
- Further study is necessary before practice changes can be made for low-birth-weight infants or infants born at less than 37 weeks' gestation.

Reference: Carson, S. (2004). Chlorhexidine versus povidone-iodine for central venous catheter site care in children. *Journal of Pediatric Nursing: Nursing Care of Children & Families, 19*(1), 74–80.

Case Management

Home health agencies may use nurses as case managers for children and their families. The home care nurse is concerned with providing continuous, comprehensive, cost-effective, quality care. Case management includes comprehensive nursing assessment of the child and family needs, coordination of the level of support needed for the care needs identified, and evaluation of the effectiveness of the coordination of care.

The case management approach includes a collaborative effort that takes place among the health care provider, family, home care providers, and case managers. The approach builds on the nursing process in order to assess, plan, implement, coordinate, monitor, and evaluate options and services specifically designed to meet children's and families' health needs to promote quality, cost-effective outcomes. As case manager, the nurse will be responsible for coordinating the care the child receives. As coordinator of care, the home care nurse must be knowledgeable about the availability of community resources not provided by the primary home care agency. Refer to the "Resources" section at the end of the chapter.

Case management nursing interventions frequently involve providing direct care, sharing community resource information with families, coordinating multidisciplinary care management and discharge planning efforts, and minimizing the family's anxiety about continuing care needs. These interventions are often implemented during the home visit. The kind of relationship that the nurse builds will often depend on how the nurse conducts the home visit.

The Home Visit

Hitchcock et al. (2003) describes how therapeutic relationships are developed between the nurse and caregivers when home visits are planned and implemented in phases. Following the initial phone call, the phases of the home visit are:

- Preinteraction: meeting the child and family and performing the assessments
- Engagement/active participation: outlining plans and initiating interventions
- Termination: evaluating the interventions and determining future rehabilitative needs

These phases can be generalized to most children who require home care nursing for either a short or long time.

Preinteraction Phase

The preinteraction phase includes activities performed prior to the first home visit. Before making the home visit the nurse will benefit from collaborating with the health care provider either through direct contact or through the health care providers, report sent to the agency. The provider's orders and the medical plan of care should be reviewed. Contact should be made with other interdisciplinary team members involved in the child's care.

The home health care nurse should review available family data, including referral information and previous records, and establish a plan for the visit. The family should be contacted by telephone and services briefly discussed. The nurse should prepare for a safe visit (e.g., identify exact location of home, consider safety issues in relation to the neighborhood being visited, and request escort or shared visit services if needed [Clark, 2008]). The neighborhood should also be assessed for environmental factors that may affect personal safety, including location of the home in relation to high crime areas and known drug and gang areas.

Engagement/Active Participation Phase

During this phase the home health care nurse begins to build the nurse-client relationship (Figure 4-6). The nurse carries out an initial client, family, and environmental assessment. Thorough assessments should be conducted. Collaboration with the child and caregivers and clarification of roles are done in the active participation phase.

Assessment of the adequacy and safety of the general living environment should be conducted. Some important areas to assess are (McEwen & Pullis, 2009):

- Adequacy of physical space, cooking facilities, and heating.
- Accessibility of the home environment for the child who may be wheelchair-bound.
- Presence and functioning of smoke and carbon dioxide detectors.

> **NURSING TIP**
>
> **Safety During the Home Visit**
>
> When traveling to make a home visit keep valuables, including any medical supplies, locked in the trunk of your car, out of sight. Carry a cellular phone in the car at all times and ensure that it is in working order and accessible. When using an elevator in a building always send it down then get on it on the way up. Never allow an elevator to control you, you control it. Avoid dimly lit areas, streets, or hallways; give travel route and arrival and departure times to your supervisor; and don't enter a situation you feel is unsafe (Anderson, 2008). Dress professionally, avoid wearing expensive jewelry, and park near the home. If you use public transportation know your route ahead of time. Always clarify the address and entry to any building with the family you are visiting.

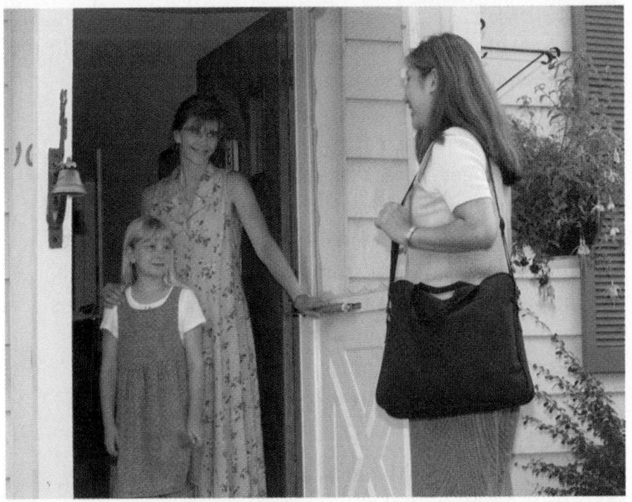

FIGURE 4-6 The nurse begins to build a relationship with the family on the first home visit. DELMAR CENGAGE LEARNING.

- Adequacy of electrical sources and back-up electrical source if the child has a respiratory ventilator that requires electricity.
- Condition of electrical cords and outlets. (Does the equipment require a three-pronged outlet but the outlets are two-pronged?)
- Functioning of telephones.
- Water sources.
- Presence of rodents, roaches, loose plaster, and paint chips.
- Proximity of neighbors.
- Education about age-specific safety measures followed in a child's home (i.e., gates on stairs for an active 15-month-old).
- Adequate heat or cooling systems.

Documentation of assessment findings is necessary through all phases of the visit. Home care equipment should be assessed during the initial visit and reassessed periodically

RESEARCH Highlight

Behavior Problems Among Inner-city Children with Asthma

STUDY PURPOSE

To determine the prevalence of behavior problems among urban children with asthma.

METHODS

Parents of kindergarten children completed a detailed survey regarding the child's background, medical history, and behavior with a focus on asthma. The study compared children with no asthma symptoms, and persistent asthma symptoms regarding positive peer social skills, negative peer social skills, task orientation, shy and anxious behavior utilizing validated scales and ranges. Multivariate regression was used to determine the independent association between symptom severity and behavioral outcomes.

FINDINGS

A total of 1619 children were included in the study with a response rate of 80% and mean age of 5.1 years. Asthma symptoms were reported in 15% of the participants (8% persistent, 7% intermittent). Average negative peer scores were worse for children with persistent asthma symptoms compared to children with intermittent or no asthma symptoms. Children with persistent symptoms scored worse than children with no symptoms on the task orientation and shy/anxious behavior. Children with persistent asthma symptoms scored lower on two or more scales, compared with children with intermittent or no asthma symptoms.

IMPLICATIONS

Urban children with persistent asthma symptoms demonstrate more behavior problems across several domains compared to children with no symptoms. These finding suggest a need for early biopsychosocial approach to care for vulnerable children with asthma.

REFERENCE

Halterman, J., Conn, K., Forbes-Jones, E., Fagnano, M., Hightower & Szilagyi, P. (2006). Behavior problems among inner-city children with asthma; Findings from a community-based sample, *Pediatrics 117*(2), 505–506.

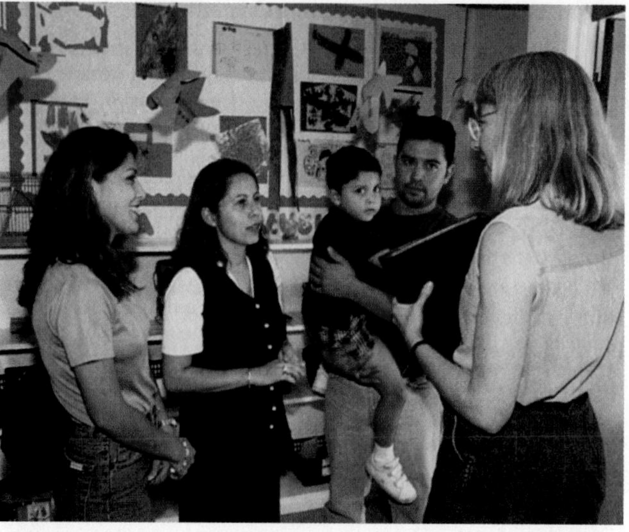

FIGURE 4-7 Cultural sensitivity and good communication skills will assist home care nurses in working with children and their families. DELMAR CENGAGE LEARNING.

BOX 4-1

PROVIDING CULTURALLY SENSITIVE NURSING CARE IN THE HOME

- Remember that the setting for care is controlled by the family and not by the health care provider.
- Engage in social conversation to facilitate rapport since the nurse is often viewed as a guest by the child and family.
- Be nonjudgmental about the condition of the home (e.g., presence of clutter or disarray).
- Show respect and consideration for the child and family. For example, wipe your feet or remove your shoes if it is a family custom before entering the home; ask permission before moving items in the child's room, and replace them after you have finished a task.
- Take advantage of the home environment to assess cultural values and norms. Cultural clues may include:
  Orderliness and decor of the home
  Assignment of family roles and tasks
  Types of family interactions
  Presence of religious objects in the home
  Value placed on privacy and possessions

for adequacy of routine and emergency maintenance and replacement, and the presence of explicit instructions about the care and operation of the equipment.

In the home, the family may initially view the nurse as a stranger or intruder since the nurse is basically a guest in the home. An awareness of and respect for the cultural and ethnic diversity of families is essential to gaining their trust. The family may have specific beliefs and practices about health and healing that the nurse should help them integrate into the treatment plan (Figure 4-7).

The nurse should inquire about social customs usually practiced, such as removing shoes before entering the house or avoiding eye contact when talking, which may be considered impolite behavior. If these customs are breached, it may prevent the nurse from being able to interact effectively with the child and family. Box 4-1 provides guidelines for providing culturally sensitive nursing care for children in the home.

Children who have complex medical conditions, are dependent on technology, and are being cared for in the home

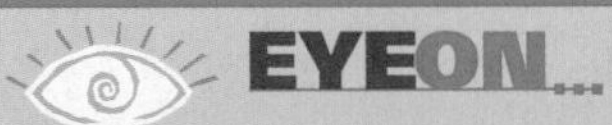

Cultural Assessment in the Home

Caring for a child with a cultural or ethnic background different from your own can be challenging, especially when you enter a family's home. For instance, it is important to know if a Jewish family observes kosher dietary laws. The kosher household will have different silverware for dairy and meat products. A Muslim or Asian household may require that you remove your shoes. The community health nurse needs to respect the cultural requirements in the home being visited.

may be at risk for developmental delays and problems. A developmental assessment should be performed by the home health care nurse initially and periodically. When the child is assessed at regular intervals, objective data can be obtained so small developmental changes can be noticed. When problems are detected, the nurse can provide interventions and refer the child for early intervention services or to the appropriate medical specialist. The nurse needs to provide feedback to families about their child's developmental level, strengths, and deficits; as well as instruction on maximizing the child's development through means such as therapeutic play. Caregivers need this information in order to meet the developmental needs of the child (Rubin & Crocker, 2006).

The home health care nurse should assess the appropriateness of third-party reimbursement systems and discuss with the caregivers the estimated length of service, including limits set by third-party payers. The home care nurse should become familiar with financial resources and therapeutic programs. Financial resources include private insurance; health maintenance organizations (HMOs); Medicaid; Supplemental Security Income (SSI); Women, Infants, and Children (WIC) programs; food stamps; and state programs for Children with Special Health Needs (CSHN). Therapeutic programs include infant stimulation, educational, occupational, physical, audiologic, and speech programs. Many of these therapeutic programs are mandated under the Early Intervention Service Program (Public Law 94-142 and its subsequent amendments 98-199, 99-457, and 101-476 [Individuals with Disabilities Education Act {IDEA}]).

Termination Phase The home health care nurse evaluates the child's status and the caretakers' ability to assume responsibility for the child's total care. Part of the termination process involves collaboration and coordination with other disciplines involved in the care of the child. Plans for terminating home care should begin during the engagement and active participation phase so that the continuity of care that was started can be maintained. During the termination phase, it may be necessary to continue with some rehabilitative services, such as speech, physical, or occupational therapies. Allowing for the family to evaluate the home care services is important at this time. The home care agency should have standard forms that are sent to families that allow them to routinely evaluate the home care service received. The home health care nurse will provide the physician and the agency with a summary discharge report so continuity of care is accomplished with the child.

FUTURE TRENDS

Home health care nursing for children and their families has grown significantly within the past decade, and it is

Reflections from Families

Our 6-month-old daughter Anna requires home health care for treatment of necrotizing enterocolitis. She is being treated by hyperalimentation, a process of feeding her nutrients through a central line to her heart. Anna's father and I find this treatment very frightening. It requires the presence of a home health nurse, as well as various technical personnel in our home at various times. Because Anna's condition is so delicate, we have moved her crib into our dining room so that we are able to watch her continually. It has been hard for our family to adjust to the loss of privacy and the disruption of routine. My two older daughters have begun to display behavioral problems because my husband and I have not been able to give them the time and attention they need. We have both become exhausted, which has been compounded by the fact that both of us are too anxious most of the time to get much sleep. We have tried getting out of the house for a little break, but respite care is very expensive, and it is hard to find anyone to care for a baby as sick as Anna, even for a little while.

REFLECTIVE THINKING

Third-Party Payment Systems

Third-party payments for home care services may run out before the child is rehabilitated fully or the family is ready to assume full responsibility for the child's care. What are your feelings on this discontinuation of services? What are the family's options?

IN THE REAL WORLD

I am a home health care nurse and have been caring for May, who is 4 years old and is dependent on a ventilator. For the past three months, I have visited May and her family four times a week. They have welcomed me into their home and are appreciative of everything I do for May. However, as time goes on, I have found it more and more difficult to maintain professional boundaries. I feel like they're beginning to see me as a family member. It's so easy for the boundaries to become blurred because of the informality of the home setting, the social conversation that occurs, and the involvement of the family in the child's care. But I know the signs of boundary crossing and will make changes if necessary.

predicted that this area of nursing will continue to grow. The cost of taking care of a child with chronic illness in the home is less than it would be in the hospital. However, in the future, cost containment for home care will become an issue, as insurance companies and the government try to manage the spiraling cost increase and need for medical care, whether inpatient or home care. The medical home concept is being implemented as chronicity increases in children's medical conditions. Competition in home health care for children and their families will increase as more home health care agencies offer pediatric care. The quality of service will continue to increase in response to this competition. As acuity in pediatric home care escalates, more specialized training and resources are required for the home care nurse to effectively serve this fragile population.

The home health care nurse will continue to care for the child who is dependent on technology. In addition to providing illness care, the nurse, increasingly, will provide health promotion and disease prevention care to children and their families. This is already beginning to happen as home health care nurses are providing home antibiotic therapy, home phototherapy, and home visits to children who are enrolled in early childhood intervention programs. It is vital that pediatric home care nurses be aware of the epidemiology of diseases and the infection control practices to be used both in the home and in the hospital. The increasing presence of organisms such as Methycillin Resistant *Staphlococcus Aureus* (MRSA) and other organisms continue to pose a threat to the health of children (Hinckley & Allen, 2008). The home health care nurse who cares for children and their families will need to have knowledge of acute care, community health, mental health, management, and pediatric acute and chronic illnesses as well as disaster preparedness protocols.

CASE STUDY / CARE PLAN

HOME CARE FOR A CHILD

Juan is a child who should receive eight hours of nursing home care each day. He is 4 years old and was born prematurely (week 29) with a ventricular septal defect (VSD) repaired at birth, and bronchopulmonary dysplasia (BPD) that developed after three months on a ventilator in the Neonatal Intensive Care Unit (NICU). Necrotizing enterocolitis (NEC) developed within the first five months of his life. It required surgery that removed a portion of his bowel and he has an ileostomy. Juan has a seizure disorder, eats poorly, requires oxygen as needed, and is developmentally delayed. Juan's family consists of his mother, father, and one older sister, Angelina, age 10. Juan's parents work and share the care of their son when the nurse is not available. Insurance coverage for Juan is through his father's work, and the plan has been changed so that some of the expenses of Juan's care, medical supplies, and medications are not covered. There are no family members in the neighborhood and friends typically work. Juan's parents express being overwhelmed with his care when help is not available. They do not have the time to spend with their daughter Angelina for homework and school functions. The parents have no social life and cannot afford vacations with the family.

(Continues)

CASE STUDY / CARE PLAN (Continued)

NURSING CARE PLAN

ASSESSMENT

You need to assess the family's knowledge of the child's medical condition and the necessary home treatment. Inquiring about their ability and willingness to assume the child's care is essential for home care to be effective. The physical resources of the family need to be evaluated, such as the appropriateness of the physical environment of the home. The adequacy of the caregivers' physical, intellectual, and mental energy for providing long-term care also needs to be carefully assessed and documented. Assessment of the family's financial resources for home care should include the cost to implement the treatment plan (e.g., equipment, supplies, and medications), insurance coverage, and changes in work situations outside the home.

NURSING DIAGNOSIS 1

Risk for powerlessness (family) related to financial stress.

EXPECTED OUTCOME

1. The family will verbalize feelings of having control over the financial situation.

NOC: Family Participation in Professional Care; Social Support

NIC: Family Involvement Promotion; Family Support

INTERVENTIONS/*RATIONALES*

1. Assess family's ability to understand financial changes associated with the insurance carrier. *Determines family's understanding of the current situation.*
2. Inform the family of additional avenues for financing care of the child's illness such as Aid to Families with Dependent Children (AFDC), Supplemental Security Income (SSI), or Medicaid waiver programs. *Information can increase family's feeling of being proactive in this situation.*
3. Explore ways to implement cost-containing measures, such as disinfecting equipment that can be reused instead of using disposable equipment. *Helps the family to take control of the situation.*
4. Encourage family to discuss feelings of powerlessness over benefit changes by their insurance company. *Allows the family to vent feelings of powerlessness and identify positive ways of coping.*

EVALUATION

The family verbalizes it is exploring avenues of additional financing to help with the costs of caring for the child at home, and members are planning to implement cost-containing measures.

NURSING DIAGNOSIS 2

Interrupted family processes related to the strain of caring at home for a child who is chronically ill.

EXPECTED OUTCOME

1. The family will regain ability to care for its chronically ill child and to meet the needs of all its members.

NOC: Family Coping; Family Functioning; Family Health Status

NIC: Family Integrity Promotion; Family Process Maintenance; Normalization Promotion

(Continues)

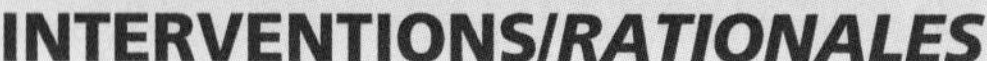

CASE STUDY / CARE PLAN (Continued)

INTERVENTIONS/*RATIONALES*

1. Assess the family dynamics (use a family assessment tool) and coping skills. *Assessment of these skills will allow the nurse to capitalize on the family's strength.*
2. Allow the family to verbalize feelings of guilt and inadequacy and stress the normalcy of these feelings. *Family will recognize the impact caring for a chronically ill child at home has on all family members.*
3. Discuss acceptable ways to modify the ill child's care to accommodate the usual family lifestyle. *Maintenance of a routine is important for family processes.*
4. Reinforce the importance of planning time for self, spouse, and the other children. *Allows family members to plan time away from the ill child without feeling guilty.*
5. Suggest that siblings be allowed to help in age-appropriate ways as family responsibilities are shifted to accommodate home care. *Sibling involvement can give them a feeling of worth and a sense of importance at a time when they might otherwise feel insecure.*

EVALUATION

The family is using appropriate coping skills, and they have worked out a schedule so that each family member can have some time away from caring for Juan. The sister Angelina has agreed to take on some responsibilities, for example helping Juan eat.

NURSING DIAGNOSIS 3

Risk for delayed development related to chronic illness and prolonged hospitalization.

EXPECTED OUTCOME

1. The child will display development that, as much as possible, meets age-appropriate norms.

NOC: Child Development: 12 Months, 2, 3, 4, and 5 years; Interaction Skills

NIC: Developmental Enhancement: Child

INTERVENTIONS/*RATIONALES*

1. Assess current developmental level. *To determine if there is a delay in development.*
2. Provide opportunities to enhance development (i.e., play that encourages motor development, contact with other children to encourage social development). *Providing opportunities allows the child chances to improve developmental level.*
3. Refer to the Early Childhood Intervention (ECI) program for assistance from the child development team and appropriate pre-school placement. *This community resource is skilled in improving the developmental level of a delayed child.*
4. Teach the caregivers strategies to foster improvement of developmental level. *Caregivers have the best opportunity for consistent interaction with the child.*
5. Collaborate with team members regarding developmental level and interventions. *Team approach ensures that concerns in all areas are addressed.*

EVALUATION

The child is making progress in meeting developmental norms.

(Continues)

CASE STUDY / CARE PLAN (Continued)

NURSING DIAGNOSIS 4

Caregiver role strain related to the requirements of caring for a child with a chronic illness.

EXPECTED OUTCOME

1. Caregiver will plan time away from the ill child.

NOC: Caregiver Emotional Health; Caregiver Lifestyle Disruption; Caregiver-Patient Relationship; Caregiver Performance: Direct Care; Caregiver Stressors

NIC: Caregiver Support; Respite Care; Role Enhancement; Health Education

INTERVENTION/*RATIONALES*

1. Identify support systems available, especially additional family members who can provide care for the child. *Provides respite care for the primary caregiver.*
2. Encourage the primary caregiver to express feelings and suggest joining a support group. *Helps the caregiver to vent and to recognize that feelings of strain are normal.*
3. Assist the primary caregiver to organize care, thereby reducing time spent on routine tasks. *Helps caregiver to manage time and to have more time for other activities.*

EVALUATION

The parents will occasionally plan to go out to dinner or to the movies during the time the home care nurse is with the child.

It is the responsibility of the home health care nurse to assess, teach, and evaluate the caregivers' capability and capacity to provide the necessary care for Juan that includes safety, ileostomy care, oxygen therapy, medications, physical assessment and recommendations in consultation with the physician and recognize signs and symptoms of decompensation for medical assistance. A chronically ill child needs many services including therapies, appropriate school placement, and accommodation.

KEY CONCEPTS

- Community health nursing is a broad category of nursing that can be defined by the focus of practice and by the population it serves; home health nursing is a specialty of community health nursing and is defined as a variety of services provided to children in their place of residence. The community health nurse collaborates with school nurses, physicians, and other professionals as needed.
- Activities that the community health nurse conducts to promote child and family wellness include well-child assessments, administering immunizations, screening, teaching, referring, and providing direct care.
- The government has influenced public health for children and their families through Medicaid, public laws, and outlining goals for health promotion, protection, and illness prevention through the publication of *Healthy People 2010* and the 2020 recommendations.
- The community health nurse assesses, intervenes, teaches, and refers families for health promotion, protection, and illness prevention services.
- The community health nurse who cares for children and their families has a variety of roles, including clinician, advocate, collaborator, consultant, counselor, educator, researcher, and case manager.
- Home health care nurses who care for children and their families provide direct care, assessments, instruction, support, screening, referrals, and case management.
- The types of home care agencies that provide services to children and their families are official, voluntary, combined, private, and hospital-based.
- Children who are dependent on technology and those who receive hospice care receive the majority of home health care nursing hours.
- The home health nurse must establish a therapeutic relationship with the child and family while at the same time respecting professional boundaries.
- The three phases of the home visit are preinteraction, engagement/active participation, and termination.
- Home health care for children and their families will continue to grow in the future.

REVIEW ACTIVITIES

1. How does the community health nurse promote health for children and their families?
2. What role does the government play in community health for children and their families?
3. Describe some of the resources that the community health nurse may use to promote and protect health and prevent illness for children and their families.
4. What role does the community health nurse have in promoting firearm safety, immunization programs, and environmental assessments?
5. What is the purpose of standards for community health nursing practice?
6. What is included in the assessment the community health nurse conducts for children and their families?
7. What is included in an environmental assessment?
8. What are some of the roles the home care nurse assumes when caring for children and their families?
9. Why has there been an increase in the need for home care for children and their families?
10. What are the types of home care agencies for children and their families?
11. How does the home care nurse relate therapeutically to children and their families?
12. What are some of the skills the home care nurse demonstrates?
13. How does a home care nurse conduct a home visit?
14. What are future trends for community health and home care nursing for children and their families?

STUDY QUESTIONS

1. The community health nurse is contracted to do a follow-up assessment on a 5-year-old child diagnosed with a ventricular septal defect (VSD). A postcardiac catheterization has been recommended this morning. The mother asks the nurse why her child requires further testing. The best response by the nurse is:
   a. "This test determines the exact location of the problem in the heart."
   b. "It is important to evaluate the strength of the heart muscle."
   c. "We need to assess the electrical function of the heart."
   d. "The presence of a murmur will be documented."
2. An 8-year-old boy bedridden at home needs a PPD test. The child refuses to allow the test. The community health nurse's most appropriate response is:
   a. "Your parents want you to have this test."
   b. "You are old enough to know that shots help you."
   c. "Your parents have consented to this so I must give it to you."
   d. "You seem to be really afraid of this injection so let's talk about it."
3. The community health nurse is teaching a class for mothers of toddlers at a local church. The nurse explains that household cleaning items, medications, and jewelry are kept out of reach because:
   a. toddlers have an increased appetite.
   b. toddlers have a heightened level of oral activity.
   c. toddlers will become rebellious teenagers if disciplined.
   d. toddlers consume many items that are not nutritious.
4. A child diagnosed with leukemia on chemotherapy is discharged home. The community health nurse assesses the parents' accurate knowledge of discharge instructions when the parents say:
   a. "I will allow my child to eat whatever and whenever she wants to eat."
   b. "My child cannot be around other children."
   c. "Every two hours I have a game for her to play."
   d. "We will go to the park daily."
5. The community health nurse is assessing a 3-year-old girl from a preschool with teacher concerns about development. The nurse refers the child to early intervention services based on which data?
   a. A ball is kicked twenty feet.
   b. Potty training is problematic.
   c. Stringing beads in art class is difficult.
   d. A twenty-word vocabulary.
6. A child on a ventilator with a tracheostomy is cared for at home by the parents with the assistance of a licensed practical nurse. The child has a pulse oximeter for daily oxygen saturation measurements. The community health nurse teaches the family to call 911 if:
   a. the pulse is above 100.
   b. the oxygen saturation is below 95%.
   c. the child has pink lips and nail beds.
   d. the child has a temperature of 99.4 degrees F.

7. A 12-year-old boy diagnosed with type 1 diabetes is referred to the community health nurse because of erratic blood glucose levels. The nurse suspects the child is not following the diet, based on behavioral cues during the visit. The child tells the nurse he is experiencing headaches. The most appropriate nursing action is to:
   a. test the urine for ketones.
   b. give the child a cup of milk.
   c. ask the child what and when was the last meal.
   d. obtain a blood glucose level via the accucheck.
8. An infant on home care services has a diagnosis of gastroesophageal reflux (GERD). The nurse teaches the caregivers best practice when feeding the child by stating:
   a. "Discontinue breastfeeding."
   b. "Keep the child in a prone position."
   c. "Thicken formula with rice cereal."
   d. "Obtain weights on a daily basis."
9. A mother of a 2-year-old girl with a seizure disorder is visited by the community health nurse. Seizure precautions are reviewed and the nurse prioritizes which action for the mother to follow during a seizure?
   a. Call 911.
   b. Hold the child during the seizure.
   c. Place the child on her side.
   d. Loosen the child's clothing.
10. Disaster preparedness is essential when chronically ill children are cared for in their home. The community health nurse is responsible to assist families in disaster preparation by identifying essential elements in a plan. Which of the following items are essential? Select all that apply.
   a. detailed list of medications
   b. flashlights and batteries
   c. canned foods and drinks
   d. equipment for blood pressure
   e. corded and cell phone
   f. emergency phone numbers

REFERENCES

American Nurses Association. (1999). *Scope and Standards of Home Health Nursing Practice.* Silver Spring, MD: Author.

Anderson, N. (2008). Safe in the city, *Home Healthcare Nurse, 26*(9), 534–540.

Boroughs, D. & Dougherty, J. (2009). Care of technology-dependent children in the home. *Home Healthcare Nurse, 27*(1), 37–42.

Carson, S. (2004). Chlorhexidine versus povidone-iodine for central venous catheter site care in children. *Journal of Pediatric Nursing: Nursing Care of Children & Families, 19*(1), 74–80.

Clark, M. (2008). *Community health nursing: Advocacy for population health* (5th ed.). Upper Saddle River, NJ: Prentice Hall.

Eaton, N. (2008). "I don't know how we coped before": A study of respite care for children in the home and hospice. *Journal of Clinical Nursing, 17*(23), 3196–3204.

Halterman, J., Conn, K., Forbes-Jones, E., Fagnano, M., Hightower, K., & Szilagyi, P. (2006). Behavior problems among inner-city children with asthma: Findings from a community-based sample. *Pediatrics, 117*(2), 505–506.

Hinckley, J. & Allen, P. (2008). Community-associated MRSA in the pediatric primary care setting. *Pediatric Nursing, 34*(1), 64–71.

Hitchcock, J., Schubert, P., & Thomas, S. (2003). *Community health nursing: Caring in action* (2nd ed.). Clifton Park, NY: Delmar Cengage Learning.

Hockenberry, M., & Wilson, D. (2011). *Wong's nursing care of infants and children* (9th ed.). St. Louis, MO: Elsevier.

Iglehart, J. (2008). No place like home: Testing a new model of care delivery. *The New England Journal of Medicine, 359*(12), 1200.

Kulkarni, N., & Grigg, J. (2008). Effect of air pollution on children. *Pediatrics and Child Health, 18*(5), 338–342.

Lawrence, J., Mayer-Davis, E., Reynolds, K., Beyer, J., Pettitt, D., D'Agostino, R., Marcovina, S., Imperatore, G., & Hamman, R. (2009). Diabetes in Hispanic American youth: prevalence, incidence, demographics, and clinical characteristics: the SEARCH for Diabetes in Youth Study. *Diabetes Care, 32*(2), 123–133.

MacLeod, M. L., Misener, R. M., Banks, K., Morton, A. M., Vogt, C., & Bentham, D. (2008). "I'm a different kind of nurse": Advice from nurses in rural and remote Canada. *Canadian Journal of Nursing Leadership, 21*(3), 40–53.

Maurer, F., & Smith, M. (2009). *Community/public health nursing* (4th ed.). Philadelphia: W. B. Saunders.

McEwen, M., & Pullis, B. (2009). *Community based nursing* (3rd ed.). St. Louis, MO: Mosby.

National Center for Injury Prevention and Control, Centers for Disease Control and Prevention. (2006). Retrieved March 20, 2009, from http://www.cdc.gov/injury/wisqars/dataandstats.html.

National Council of State Boards of Nursing. (1996). *Professional boundaries: A nurse's guide to the importance of appropriate professional boundaries. Updated pamphlets 2008.* Retrieved March 20, 2009, from https://www.ncsbn.org/247.htm. Chicago: National Council of State Boards of Nursing, Inc.

Oresland, S., Määttä, S., Norberg, A., & Lützén K. (2009). Patients as safeguard and nurses as substitute in home health care. *Nursing Ethics, 16*(2), 219–230.

Owens, J. (2008). *Working Mother, 31*(4), 61–66.

Penz, K. (2008). What are the potential factors that sustain registered nurses who provide home-based palliative and end-of-life? *Journal of Hospice & Palliative Nursing, 10*(5), 295–303.

Quad Council of Public Health Nursing Organizations. (1999). *Scope and standards of public health nurse practice.* Silver Spring, MD: Author.

Rubin, I., & Crocker, A. (2006). *Medical care for children and adults with developmental disabilities* (2nd ed.). Baltimore, MD: Brooks Publishing.

Scheffler, F., Vogel, D., Astern, R., & Burgess, J. (2007). Screening for communication and cognitive disorders in infants and toddlers. *Pediatric Nursing, 33*(6), 473–480.

Selekman, J. (2007). A review of the KySS guide. *Pediatric Nursing, 33*(6), 535–536.

Stanhope, M., & Lancaster, J. (2008). *Public health nursing: Population-Centered health Care in the Community* (7th ed.). St. Louis, MO: Mosby.

U.S. Department of Health and Human Services. (2000). *Healthy People 2010*. Washington, DC: Government Printing Office.

Volpintesta, E.J. (2009). The importance of healing skills in the medical home concept. *Annals of Internal Medicine, 150*(5), 360.

Williamson, K. M. (2007). Home health care nurses' perceptions of empowerment. *Journal of Community Health Nursing, 24*(3), 133–135.

Woolf, A., & Woolf, N. (2005). Childhood lead poisoning in 2 families associated with spices used in food preparation. *Pediatrics, 116*, 314–318.

SUGGESTED READINGS

Ackley, B., & Ladwig, G. (2008). *Nursing diagnosis handbook* (8th ed.). St. Louis, MO: Mosby.

Bagnato, S., Blair, K., Slater, J., & McNally, R. (2004). Developmental health care partnerships in early childhood intervention settings: The healthy child model. *Infants and Young Children, 17*(4), 301–318.

Berg, A. M., Snell, L., & Mahle, W. T. (2007). Home inotropic therapy in children. *The Journal of Heart and Lung Transplantation: The official publication of the International Society for Heart Transplantation. 26*(5), 453–457.

Brock Martin, A., Crawford, S., Probst, J., Smith, G., Saunders, R., Watkins, K., & Luchok, K. (2007). Medical homes for children with special health care needs. *Journal of Health Care for the Poor and Underserved, 18*(4), 916.

Broyles, B. (2006). *Clinical decision making: Case studies in pediatrics.* Clifton Park N.Y.: Delmar Cengage Learning.

Bulechek, G., Butcher, H., & Dochterman, J. (2008). *Nursing Interventions Classifications (NIC)* (5th ed.). St. Louis, MO: Mosby.

Chang, E., & Johnson, A. (2009). *Chronic illness and disability*, St. Louis, MO: Mosby.

Doolen, J., Alpert, P., Miller, S., & Doolen, J. (2009). Parental disconnect between perceived and actual weight status of children: A metasynthesis of the current research. *Journal of the American Academy of Nurse Practitioners, 21*(3), 160–166.

Lehoux, P., Richard, L., Pineault, R., & Saint-Arnaud, J. (2006). Delivery of high-tech homecare by hospital-based nursing units in Quebec: clinical and technical challenges. *Canadian Journal of Nursing Leadership, 19*(1), 44–55.

Moorhead, S., Johnson, M., Maas, M., & Swanson, E. (2008). *Nursing Outcomes Classification (NOC)* (4th ed.). St. Louis, MO: Mosby.

National Institutes of Health. (2008). *Diabetes and Youth.* Retrieved March 2, 2009, from http://www.ndep.nih.gov/diabetes/youth/youth_FS.html.

New York City Department of Health. (2008). *Children's health services.* Retrieved March 20, 2009, from http://www.nychealthplan.com/articles/medicaid-obstetrical-and-maternal-services-moms-program and http://www.nursefamilypartnership.org/resources/files/PDF/Fact_Sheets/NFP_Overview.pdf.

Occupational Safety and Health Administration (OSHA). (2007). *Workforce regulations.* Washington: DC. Retrieved March 20, 2009, from http://www.osha.gov/.

Overby, N., Margeirsdottir, H., Brunborg, C., Anderssen, S., Andersen, D., Jorgensen, K., & Overby, N. (2009). Physical activity and overweight children and adolescents using intensified insulin treatment. *Pediatric Diabetes, 10*(2), 135–141.

Patient- and Family-Centered Care and the Role of the Emergency Physician Providing Care to a Child in the Emergency Department. (2008). *Annals of Emergency Medicine, 48*(5), 643–645.

Yantzi, N., Rosenburg, M., & McKeever, P. (2006). Getting out of the house: the challenges mothers face when their children have long-term care needs. *Health and Social Care in the Community, 15*(1), 45–55.

RESOURCES

Refer to the online student StudyWARE for Potts & Mandleco at http://www.CengageBrain.com for additional content and study aids.

Organization: **Access to Respite Care Help (ARCH)**
Description: The mission of the ARCH National Respite Network is to assist and promote the development of quality respite and crisis care programs; to help families locate respite and crisis care services in their communities; and to serve as a strong voice for respite in all forums. The website offers readers access to fact sheets, products, memberships, and respite locators.
Website/Resource: http://chtop.org/ARCH.html

Organization: **Morbidity & Mortality Weekly Report**
Description: A subset of the Centers for Disease Control and Prevention (CDC), the Morbidity and Mortality Weekly Report provides information regarding current mortality findings and morbidity concerns. Besides the report itself, the website provides information regarding notifiable diseases and surveillance summaries.
Website/Resource: http://www.cdc.gov

Organization: **Division of Immunization, Centers for Disease Control and Prevention**
Description: This section of the CDC website offers readers information regarding immunization schedules, recommendations, and vaccine safety.
Website/Resource: http://www.cdc.gov

Organization: **March of Dimes**
Description: March of Dimes's mission is to improve the health of babies by preventing birth defects, premature birth, and infant mortality. The website provides information regarding March of Dimes professionals/researchers and pregnancy/newborn conditions.
Website/Resource: http://www.marchofdimes.com

Organization: **National Center for Environmental Health (CDC) Lead Poisoning Prevention**

Description: A program of the CDC, the Lead Poisoning Prevention program's mission is to develop programs to prevent childhood lead poisoning, provide funding to states to help with the prevention effort, educate the public and conduct research. The website offers users information regarding lead poisoning statistics/data, lead recalls, and prevention tips.
Phone: National Lead Information Center (800) LEAD-FYI
Website/Resource: http://www.cdc.gov

Organization: **National Center for Farmworker Health, Inc.**
Description: The National Center for Farmworker Health (NCFH) is a private nonprofit corporation, established in 1975, located in Buda, Texas. NCFH provides information services, technical assistance, and training to more than 500 private and federally funded migrant health centers as well as other organizations and individuals serving the farmworker population. The website offers information regarding farmworkers, migrant health centers, and health education.
Website/Resource: http://www.ncfh.org

Organization: **National Coalition of Hispanic Health & Human Services Organizations (COSSMHO)**
Description: The National Alliance for Hispanic Health is the premier science based organization focusing on Hispanic health. The website offers users access to information regarding action forums, community resources, and press/media news.
Website/Resource: http://www.hispanichealth.org

Organization: **National Council on Child Abuse and Family Violence**
Description: The National Council on Child Abuse and Family Violence (NCCAFV) provides intergenerational violence prevention services by bringing together community and national stakeholders, professionals, and volunteers to prevent family violence, child abuse and neglect, spouse/partner abuse, and elder abuse. The website offers users access to donation information and council news.
Website/Resource: http://www.nccafv.org

Organization: **National Hotlines for Child Abuse**
Phone: (800) 421-0353—Parents Anonymous
Phone: (800) 422-4453—National Abuse Hotline

Organization: **National Information Center for Children and Youth with Disabilities**
Description: The National Information Center on Children and Youth with Disabilities provides information to the nation on disabilities in children and youth, programs and services for infants, children, and youth with disabilities IDEA (the nation's special education law) No Child Left Behind (the nation's general education law) and research-based information on effective practices for children with disabilities. The website offers information about child disabilities for families/communities, early intervention providers, school/administration, and state agencies.
Website/Resource: http://www.nichcy.org

Organization: **National Rifle Association of America, The Eddie Eagle Gun Safety Program, NRA Safety and Education Division**
Description: The primary goal of the National Rifle Association of America (NRA) is to promote and encourage rifle shooting on a scientific basis. The Eddie Eagle GunSafe® Program (sponsored by NRA) teaches children in pre-K through third grade important steps to take if they find a gun. The website offers readers information regarding NRA programs and safety legislation.
Website/Resource: http://www.nra.org

Organization: **Nurse Family Partnership**
Description: When a young woman becomes pregnant before she's ready to take care of a child, the risk factors for the entire family escalates—often resulting in poverty, conflict and despair. Nurse-Family Partnership intervenes with a breakthrough solution: providing low-income first-time parents with a relationship they can count on. A trusted, respected and compassionate public health nurse visits the mom from pregnancy until the baby turns two years old. This evidence-based model of partnering nurses and first-time moms has more than 30 years of research and randomized, controlled trials that prove it works. The Nurse-Family Partnership National Service Office provides training and support services to ensure that the model is precisely replicated in communities.
Website/Resource: http://www.nursefamilypartnership.org

Organization: **Office on Smoking and Health, Centers for Disease Control and Prevention**
Description: The Centers for Disease Control and Prevention (CDC), through its Office on Smoking and Health (OSH), is the leading federal agency for comprehensive tobacco prevention and control. The website offers users access to information regarding smoking statistics, state/community resources, prevention/control programs, and publications.
Website/Resource: http://www.cdc.gov

Organization: **Sick Kids Need Involved People (SKIP)**
Description: SKIP of New York, Inc. is a 501 (c)(3) not-for profit agency. Too many medically fragile and developmentally disabled children remain in hospitals and institutions. SKIP helps these children live at home with their families. SKIP is an advocacy and case management agency. The website offers users information regarding helpful resources, family contacts, and donation information.
Website/Resource: http://www.skipofny.org

Organization: **U.S. Environmental Protection Agency**
Description: The mission of EPA is to protect human health and to safeguard the natural environment—air, water and land—upon which life depends. The website offers users access to information regarding current issues, science/technology, and laws/regulations.
Website/Resource: http://www.epa.gov

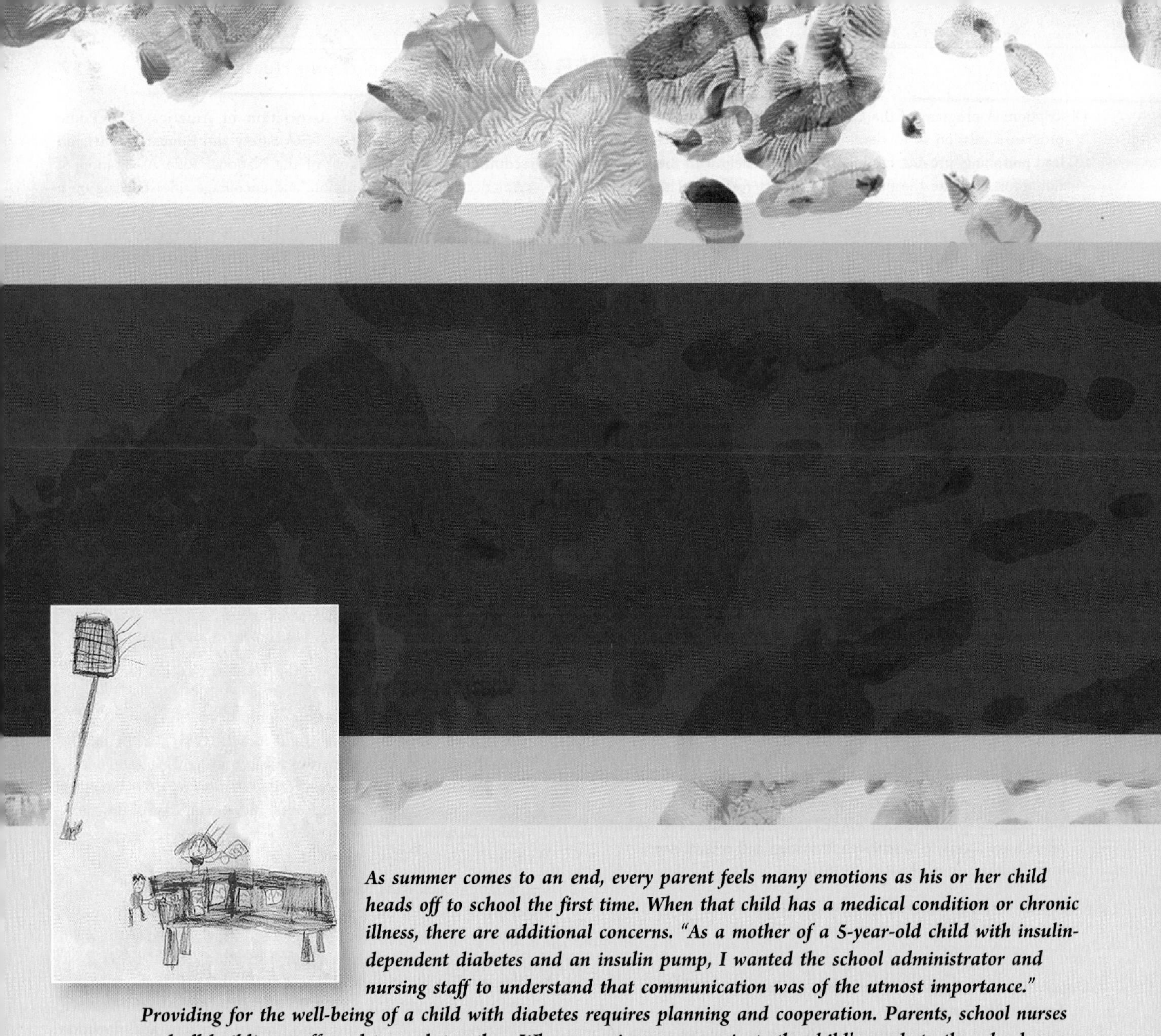

As summer comes to an end, every parent feels many emotions as his or her child heads off to school the first time. When that child has a medical condition or chronic illness, there are additional concerns. "As a mother of a 5-year-old child with insulin-dependent diabetes and an insulin pump, I wanted the school administrator and nursing staff to understand that communication was of the utmost importance." Providing for the well-being of a child with diabetes requires planning and cooperation. Parents, school nurses and all building staff need to work together. When caregivers communicate the child's needs to the school nurse, it is easier to provide a safe and healthy atmosphere, facilitating the child's ability to grow and learn in the school setting.

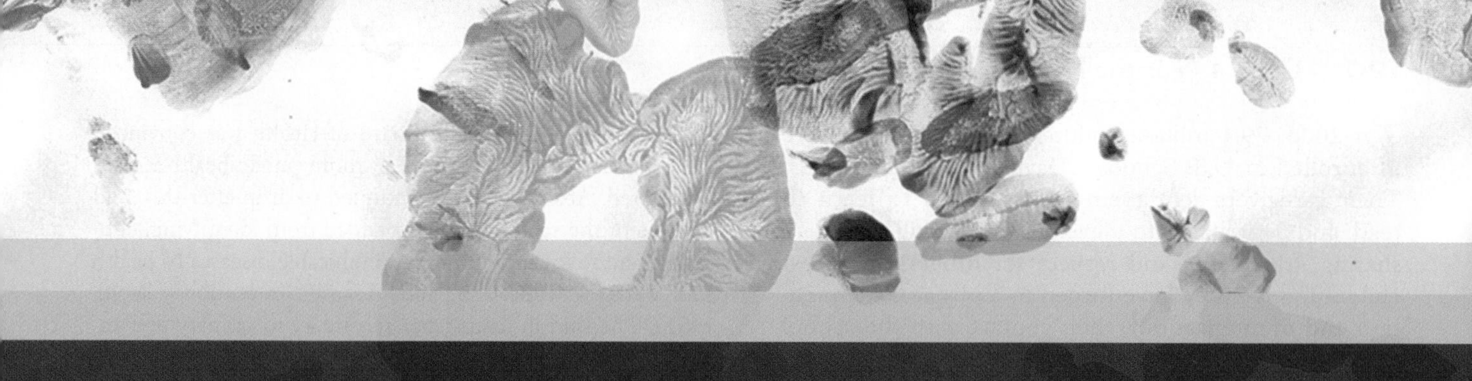

CHAPTER 5

School Nursing

MAUREEN L. LUE, RN, MS, CSN

COMPETENCIES

Upon completion of this chapter, the reader will be able to:

- Describe how political and social changes in history affected development of the school nurse's role.
- Describe three screenings often performed by nurses in the school setting.
- List common immunization requirements for children entering school, and explain strategies the school nurse employs for communicable disease control.
- Describe the school nurse's role in emergency care of children at school.
- Discuss the individual health plan and the role of the school nurse in its development.
- Identify and explain five content areas for health education the school nurse might teach.
- Explain how the school nurse works with other educators to enhance the child's learning experience.
- Discuss two current issues affecting school nurses.
- Successfully complete the games and activities in the online student StudyWARE.

In 2006, 79.1 million children ages 3 and up were enrolled in U.S. Schools (Davis & Bauman, 2008). Their caregivers sent them off to school to learn to read and write and to develop social skills such as sharing, friendship, and respect for others. For most children, once they have turned in a physical examination and immunizations, their contact with the school nurse is minimal. However, this is not the case for children who have a chronic illness or need medication during the day. To the caregivers of these children, the school nurse's role is as important as the teacher's. For students with a chronic condition or for those who need medication, the school nurse can make the transition from home to school smoother; and for other children, it would be impossible to attend school without a nurse.

What does the nurse do all day in the school? In a place where children are supposed to sit in class and learn all day, why would a nurse be needed? This chapter will provide a brief review of the history of school nursing; types of health services, including the various screenings performed by the nurse; health education programs taught; and psychological services offered in which the nurse may be involved. Ethical and legal issues such as Do Not Attempt to Resuscitate (DNAR) orders and delegation will be briefly discussed. Finally, the current roles of the school nurse will be described, as well as future issues facing her or him.

HISTORY OF SCHOOL NURSING

School nursing owes its beginnings in both the United States and Europe to the field of Community and Public Health Nursing (see Chapter 4). Public health nurses in England and France began extending their services to the schools in the mid-1800s. Social factors in the United States such as an increase in immigrants, overcrowded living conditions in urban areas, and activities of the reformists of the World War I era played a role in calling attention to the need for social services in schools (Passarelli, 1994; Wold, 1981). However, it was a public health nurse, investigating the number of children absent from school due to infectious diseases, who formulated the plan that led to school nursing in the United States.

Lillian Wald, a pioneer in community nursing and founder of the Henry Street Settlement, was astonished by the number of children who never returned to school after being excluded for a communicable disease. In 1893, she convinced the New York Board of Health to try an experiment: place a nurse in selected schools in New York City to screen for infectious diseases, provide education regarding their control, and follow-up by visiting the homes of children who had been excluded. The Board agreed, and in 1902 Lina Rogers became the first school nurse in the United States (Wold, 1981). Amazingly, exclusion rates dropped from 10,567 students in 1902 to just 1,101 in 1903 (Denehy, 2003). The Board of Health was convinced the program was helpful, and 25 more public health nurses were hired. Absentee rates continued to drop after this, and the role of the school nurse expanded from identifying, educating, and following-up on communicable diseases to health and wellness education and disease prevention (Wold, 1981). The shift in focus from secondary to primary prevention had begun.

During the 1920s, school nurses continued to identify children with communicable diseases and to provide home follow-up care to educate the students and their families about treatment. The role then expanded to identifying physical defects in children and providing referrals for their correction. By the 1930s, the school nurse worked as part of a team with physicians and school personnel to develop educational programs, including not only communicable disease prevention and treatment, but health-promotion topics such as hygiene, nutrition, and other basic needs of children. The growth and development of the student and their effects on the child's ability to learn became the focus of school nurses at this time. These changes in the duties of the school nurse also brought some role confusion. Cutbacks in funding due to World War II led nurses to delegate tasks to teachers and other school personnel. The school nurse was consequently caught between the roles of education and health professional.

After World War II, the focus in the United States changed and, again, so did the role of the school nurse. By 1945, teacher involvement in the health of the child was increased. Health education became a subject in and of itself in school curricula. Collaboration between the nurse, the student, the school, and the community was stressed, and the relationship between health behaviors at school and at home was explored. With these changes, the educational preparation of the school nurse also needed to change. Nurses now needed more technical knowledge, a wider background in education and family health, better-developed leadership skills, and the ability to work as part of an interdisciplinary team. At this time, sixteen states required special education courses and certification to become a school nurse (Wold, 1981).

The 1960s again brought about many changes in the United States. Social attitudes across the nation as well as financial changes in the schools affected the school nurse. Services not deemed essential were cut back, and the school nurse became a luxury, not a necessity. Changes in society brought about an increase in drug use and chemical dependence, sexual relations, and teen pregnancy. Students had new educational needs, and there was no one to address them.

Help came from professional nurses' organizations such as the American Nurses Association (ANA) and the American School Health Association (ASHA). The ANA formulated a broad definition of nursing in 1965, and in the 1970s it formulated minimum standards of practice for nurses. These guidelines helped better define the role of the nurse in various settings, including school nursing. In 1974, a philosophy of practice for school nurses was developed and endorsed by both the ANA and the ASHA, and guidelines for school nurses were developed. Professional nursing organizations became further involved in the educational preparation of the school nurse. Both the ANA and the ASHA recommended a minimum of a baccalaureate degree. By 1976, mandated certification requirements were in place in twenty-three states (Wold, 1981). The National Association of School Nurses (NASN), incorporated in 1979, further defined this specialized practice of nursing by providing a definition of school nursing which remains in place today. (Box 5-1).

During the 1970s, the federal government also played a part in the changing role of the school nurse. Although some federal laws addressing the educational needs of children with mental and physical handicaps were in place, it wasn't until 1975 that their education was guaranteed (Figure 5-1). The Education for All Handicapped Children Act (PL. 94-142), updated in 1990 to the Individuals with Disabilities Education Act (IDEA), and now named The Individuals with Disabilities Education Improvement Act of 2004, required all states to provide a free and appropriate education in the least restrictive environment to children with disabilities (Broussard, 2007; Special Education and Rehabilitative Services, 2006). Table 5-1 provides information on some laws affecting education and children with disabilities.

With special education now a right of students, schools found themselves responsible for educating children and adolescents with a multitude of physical, medical, and mental disabilities. In addition, IDEA included a mandate named Child-Find, a requirement that all school districts identify, locate, and evaluate all children with disabilities. This Child-Find mandate meant children began school at an earlier age. The numbers of children with chronic health conditions increased and school-based intervention programs were needed to provide adequate required care at school (Keehner, Guttu, Warren, & Swanson, 2008). School nurses needed additional expertise in caring for children with specialized needs as well as education on the laws impacting this selected group of children (Figure 5-2).

In 1992, there were approximately 26,000 registered professional nurses working in schools across the United States (Passarelli, 1994). In 2004 over 78,000 registered nurses were caring for over 52 million students in our schools (U.S. Dept. of Health and Human Services, 2004). Advances in medicine have improved the survival rates of premature infants and extremely sick children, which, in turn, have increased the prevalence of children with chronic health care conditions now seen in our nation's schools. The National Survey of Children with Special Health Care Needs estimates roughly 12.8% of children ages 0–17 years meet the Federal Maternal and Child Health Board's definition of having special needs (Tares & Brennan, 2008) (Figure 5-3). Because of the passage of federal laws such as the Individuals with Disabilities Education Act, children with disabilities now have the same right to an education as every other child in the United States, causing the role of the school nurse to continue to evolve and adapt. In fact, guidelines have been developed by ASHA, NASN, and *Healthy*

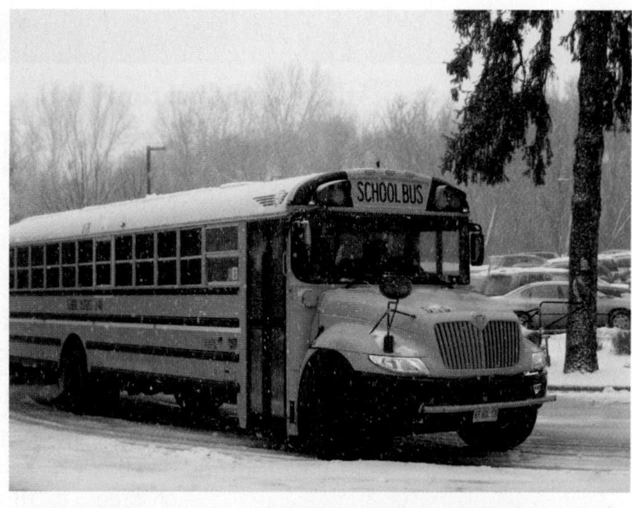

FIGURE 5-1 A number of children take the bus to school. Nurses and educators need to be aware of the challenges children with health alterations may face, both in the classroom and en route to school. DELMAR CENGAGE LEARNING.

BOX 5-1
DEFINITION OF SCHOOL NURSING

School nursing is the specialized practice of professional nursing that advances the well-being, academic success, and the life-long achievement of students. To that end, school nurses facilitate positive student responses to normal development; promote health and safety; intervene with actual and potential health problems; provide case management services; and actively collaborate with others to build student and family capacity for adaptation, self-management, self-advocacy, and learning.

Reprinted with permission of NASN. NASN (1999).

CRITICAL THINKING

Too Many Schools, Too Few Nurses

Recommended staff ratios are not possible in all areas, and some school nurses are responsible for several schools. You are the only school nurse in a district with seven elementary schools. Six of the seven buildings have children on medication, and two have children with complex medical needs and three have students with diabetes in need of blood glucose monitoring and insulin administration. How would you manage? What skills would you need? How would you prioritize your duties?

Table 5-1 Laws Affecting Education

YEAR	PUBLIC LAW	NAME AND SUMMARY
1965	89-10	Elementary and Secondary Education Act Addressed inequality of education for economically disadvantaged children.
1973	93-112	Rehabilitation Act of 1973 Provided for rehabilitation services to all individuals regardless of severity of disability. Civil rights enforced under Section 504.
1975	94-142	Education for All Handicapped Children Act Mandated free appropriate education for all children with disabilities. Mandated due process, least restrictive environment, and Individual Education Plans for children 3 to 18 years old.
1986	95-602	Education of the Handicapped Act Amendment Mandated services for preschoolers with disabilities ages 3 to 5 years and provided early intervention services from birth to 3 years.
1990	101-476	Individuals with Disabilities Education Act (IDEA)* Mandated transition services and assertive technology. Added autism and traumatic brain injury as disabilities. Extended services to 21 years.
1997	105-17	Reauthorization of IDEA Added modifications to IDEA regarding participation of students with disabilities in state or district testing, parental participation, evaluation requirements, transition teams for students at age 14 years, and disciplinary procedures for students with disabilities.
2001	107-110	No Child Left Behind Act of 2001 Amended the Elementary and Secondary Education Act of 1965 by making changes in federal efforts to support education from kindergarten to high school. Based on four concepts of accountability for results, education based on scientific research, expanded parent options, and local control.
2004	108-446	Individuals with Disability Education Improvement Act Preserves the basic structure and rights under IDEA but changes made to the definitions of "child with disability" and "related services." Age criteria for developmental disability now include children 3–9 years old. Tourette's syndrome is now included in Other Health Impaired, and "excessive costs" recalculated.

Adapted from Chauvin, V. (1994). *Students with special health care needs: A manual for school nurses.* Scarborough, ME: NASN (2003); and Office of Special Education and Rehabilitative Services.

People 2010 to address the changing needs of children in today's schools (Box 5-2). Unfortunately, this is only a recommendation and not a requirement of the school districts.

Staffing ratios and educational requirements for school nurses vary from state to state, and there is no national standard for school nurse certification requirements. Although NASN recommends and the American Academy of Pediatrics supports licensure as a registered nurse and a baccalaureate degree as the minimum standard, NASN does encourage national certification but only a few states actually require this level of practice. Educational preparation varies between states and some states employ LPNs as school nurses (Denehy, 2007a). Adding to the confusion, unless specified by a court decision, there is no federal mandate requiring schools to provide a nurse in the school.

The role of the school nurse continues to include identifying communicable diseases and enforcing immunization requirements. Preventive procedures such as vision and hearing screening; education in nutrition, healthy lifestyle, and safety practices; and a curriculum on drug-use and

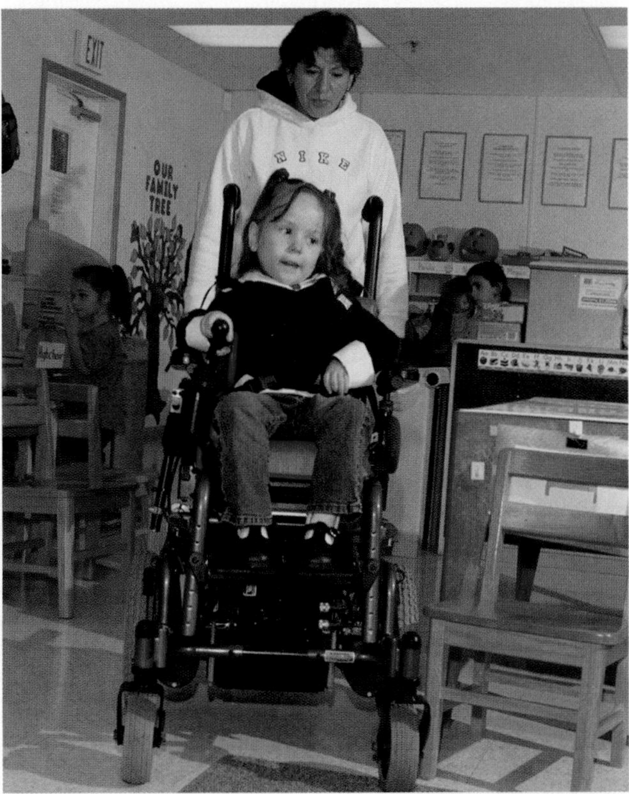

FIGURE 5-2 **Today's school nurse must be trained to care for children of all ability levels.** DELMAR CENGAGE LEARNING.

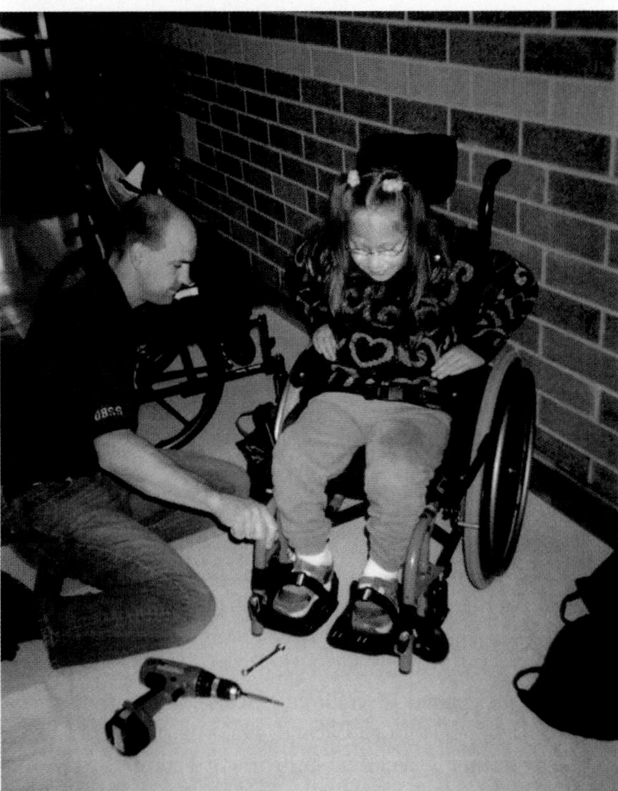

FIGURE 5-3 **Children with special health care needs often need a variety of support services. The school nurse works with therapists and other providers to help arrange services such as in-school wheelchair clinics, decreasing absences, and helping the child and family.** DELMAR CENGAGE LEARNING.

violence prevention have been added. But this role has changed dramatically and may now include more complex tasks such as ventilator care, gastrostomy feedings, and clean intermittent catheterization (Broussard, 2007). In addition, the increase of families living at or below the poverty level or those with no insurance has also changed the role of the school to first line access to health care. Sometimes, school nurses are the only health provider the child sees.

Financial constraints continue, and many school nurses must cover several schools even as their responsibilities have increased. In some states, the future of the school nurse as a certified professional is uncertain, although the need is greater than ever. Clarifying the importance of the nurse's role can assist in securing school nurses' positions now and in the future. Before others can see the need and value of nurses in the school, the individual must be confident about her or his worth in the health and education of today's children. It now rests with each individual nurse to document exactly how they influence and impact a child's ability to learn by contributing to and providing a safe health environment (Bonaiuto, 2007).

BOX 5-2
SCHOOL NURSE TO STUDENT RATIOS

It is the position of the National Association of School Nurses that the maximum ratio of nurse to student should be:

- One school health nurse to no more than 750 students in the general school population
- One school health nurse to no more than 225 students in the mainstreamed population
- One school health nurse to no more than 125 students in the severely chronically ill or developmentally disabled population
- In the medically fragile population, a ratio based on individual needs

Adapted from the NASN Position statement: Caseload assignments (2006b).

SCHOOL HEALTH SERVICES

The school nurse is involved in many school health services, including direct or indirect nursing care. **Direct services** include providing nursing procedures or care to individual students; **indirect services** include case management and consulting with staff on behalf of a child's health needs, providing community referrals and health education to children and their families. Health services also include screening programs, communicable disease control, emergency care, medication administration, and nursing care of children with specialized health care needs (Bonaiuto, 2007). Education and health promotion activities include presenting subjects such as personal care, nutrition, sex education, substance abuse, and violence prevention programs. **Healthy People 2010** guidelines have created a large shift towards health promotion and wellness programs. The school nurse may also collaborate with social workers and school psychologists to provide services to families after unusual events in a child's life.

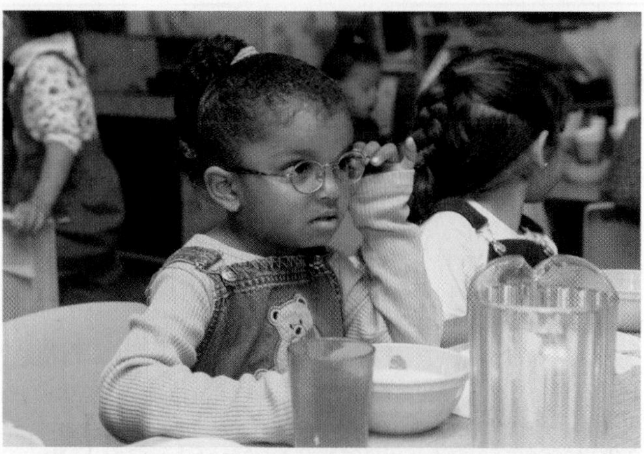

FIGURE 5-4 Early detection and treatment of vision problems improves children's learning success. DELMAR CENGAGE LEARNING.

SCREENINGS

One task of the school nurse is organizing and performing a variety of screening programs for school children. These screening programs assist in the early identification of possible problems related to children's health. When abnormalities are noted, the nurse plays a vital role in referring the child for further evaluation and/or correction. Traditional screening programs offered in the schools include vision and hearing testing; height and weight measurements; pediculosis screening; immunization monitoring; and, in some districts, orthopedic, dental, and tuberculosis screening (NASN, 2007a; American Academy of Pediatrics, 2008). The rapid increase in the incidence of obesity in children and number of cases of type 2 diabetes now seen in children has made body mass index (BMI) screening and research by the school nurse more prevalent.

VISION AND HEARING SCREENING

School nurses continue to play a large role in vision and hearing screening. Although it is recommended by the American Academy of Ophthalmology and the American Academy of Pediatrics as part of the routine school program, vision screening is not mandated in all states. Its purpose is to identify children with potential problems in visual acuity and muscle balance so treatment can begin early. School vision screenings have proven to be effective in identifying undiagnosed vision problems and coincide with the *Healthy People 2010* goal of improving vision through early detection, prevention, and treatment (NASN, 2006a). Preventing potential vision loss can positively influence a child's academic success (Clarke, Shacks, Kerr, Bottrell, Poulsen, & Yin, 2008).

Screening also includes inspecting the eye and evaluating visual acuity, muscle balance (**phoria**), excessive farsightedness (**hyperopia**), and color vision. Ideally, all students should be screened annually. A school-age child who does not have visual acuity of at least 20/30 should normally be referred for further evaluation; however, the school nurse must verify the state's referral criteria before referring children since all states do not follow the same criteria (Figure 5-4). Numerous instruments are available for assessing vision in children, and the school nurse needs to be familiar with these products. The traditional **Snellen chart**, which uses letters in various sizes, is also available in tumbling letters and pictures to match the age and ability level of the child being screened. Stereoscopic instruments, which use mirrors, lenses, and occluders to screen for vision problems and require special training, are also used in mass screening programs. Several populations are at a higher risk for vision problems including those with diabetes, cerebral palsy, born prematurely or with low APGAR scores (NASN, 2006a). The school nurse should be especially watchful of this subgroup of students.

Hearing screening is another responsibility of the school nurse (Figure 5-5). Hearing difficulties can have an impact on the child's ability to learn. If the child cannot hear

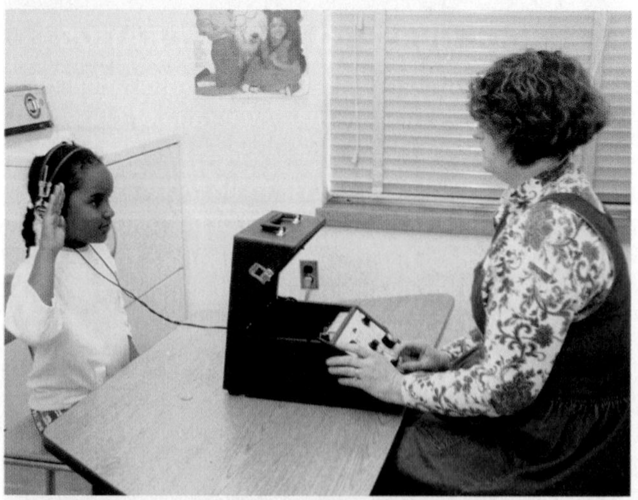

FIGURE 5-5 Performing annual hearing tests is one of the important screenings done by school nurses. DELMAR CENGAGE LEARNING.

adequately, directions and important information may be missed, speech development impaired, and reading affected. The nurse can help prevent or limit this problem by annually testing the child's hearing at 500, 1,000, 2,000, and 4,000 hertz in both ears at a fixed decibel (dB) level. Children with hearing loss between 70 and 90 dB are considered hard of hearing, and those with hearing loss greater than 90 dB are defined as having a severe or profound hearing loss (Bauman, 2008). Refer to Chapter 31 for more information on hearing.

As important as vision and hearing screenings are, without referral and follow-up practices in place there is little benefit. Ten million children have some form of vision disorder (AOA, 2008) and it is one of the most prevalent handicapping conditions seen in students. Because children with abnormal vision or hearing do not know their situation is not normal they often do not complain of any problems, and the deficit might be overlooked. Academic and behavioral difficulties can then result from missed learning opportunities (Box 5-3). Follow-up care after a failed vision or hearing screening may be extended due to lack of parent follow up, financial difficulties, or limited resources. The nurse can play a vital role in speeding up this process by individualizing follow up on students who failed screenings, and knowing about existing local resources to share with caregivers. The school nurse also needs to be aware of organizations that can assist families in obtaining vision and hearing services for their children. If a permanent vision or hearing loss is detected, the nurse can assist in obtaining specialized services or needed adaptations.

KIDS WANT TO KNOW

Getting Glasses

"My mom said I need to get glasses. It's been hard to see the chalkboard for awhile, but I was afraid to tell her. I don't want to get glasses. What if the kids laugh at me and call me names? I don't want to be different."

To help the child with this transition you can explain, in developmentally appropriate terms, why the child is getting glasses and how they will help him or her; point out other children and adults in the child's life who have glasses; encourage the parents to allow the child some choice in selecting the glasses, as appropriate; and supply developmentally appropriate books and videos to the student's family and teacher such as *Blueberry Eyes,* by M. Driscoll Beatty (1996); *Glasses for D.W.,* by M. Brown (1996); *Glasses, Glasses Oh What Do I See* by K. Smith Stair (2004), and *Magenta Gets Glasses* (Blues Clues #10) by Reber and Dujas (2008).

BOX 5-3
SIGNS OF A VISION PROBLEM: WHAT TO WATCH FOR IN CHILDREN

- Holds book close to face
- Looks with one eye or covers one eye
- Squints or rubs eyes
- Moves head while reading
- Omits words or letters; fails to recognize letters
- Complains of blurred or double vision
- Mistakes small words
- Blinks excessively
- Loses place when reading
- Complains of headache or blurry vision
- Writes slanting uphill or downhill along the paper
- Has difficulty copying from board to desk
- Demonstrates poor reading performance
- Has difficulty paying attention
- May have learning problems that need to be ruled out

Students with any of these symptoms warrant a request for a vision screening by a school nurse certified in visual screening procedures and referral for follow-up as needed.

Adapted from Clarke et al. (2008).

HEIGHT AND WEIGHT MEASUREMENT

Height and weight measurements are usually taken at the physician's office as part of a physical exam. However, some states require these measurements only on entry to kindergarten and ninth grade. Unless the child receives a yearly exam, height and weight can go unchecked for several years (Figure 5-6). The media constantly warns people of what health care professionals have discussed with parents for years: a significant population of children are overweight. In fact, the number of children considered overweight has tripled in the last 30 years (Murphy and Polivka, 2007; Harrington, 2008) with estimates of 16.3% of all children 2 to 19 years classified as obese or greater than 95th percentile BMI for age (Harrington, 2008). This weight increase in children comes with an increased incidence of type 2 diabetes, hypertension, and high cholesterol. Research has shown that 70% of obese teenagers become obese adults (Wilson, 2007; Story, 2009) often causing a financial burden on the health care system. A school nurse's annual measurements can provide valuable information for caregivers and health care professionals, alerting them to concerns before they become a dangerous health problem (Figure 5-7). School nurses also are in a key position to collaborate with administrators and legislators and influence local and federal decisions on policies regarding dietary choices and physical

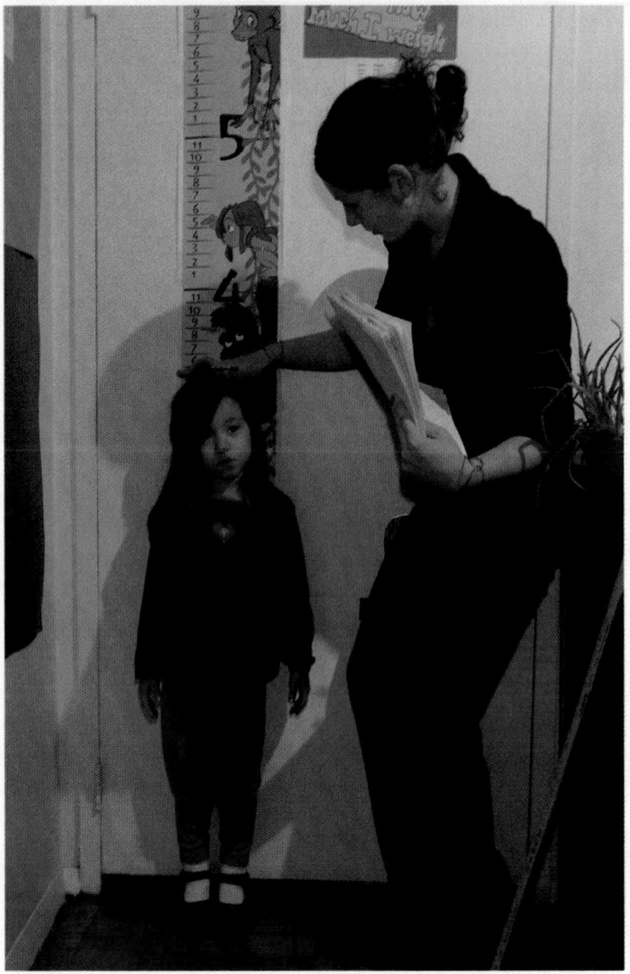

FIGURE 5-6 School nurses can monitor a child's growth and development through regular height measurements. DELMAR CENGAGE LEARNING.

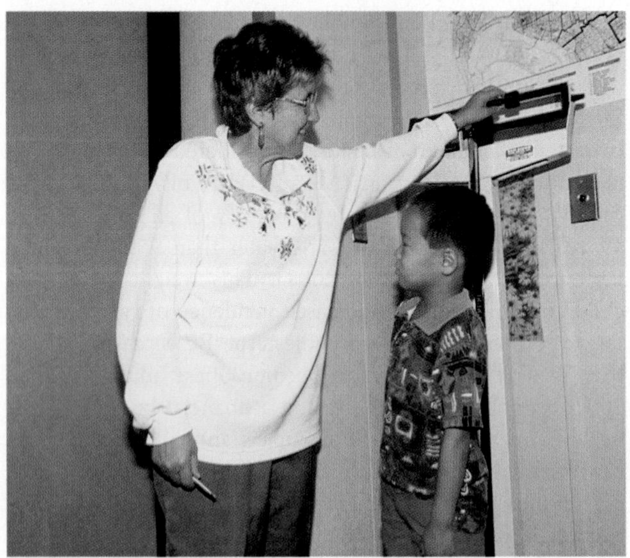

FIGURE 5-7 Weight screenings and calculating BMI can lead to early detection of obesity and help decrease health problems in later life. DELMAR CENGAGE LEARNING.

CULTURAL CONSIDERATION

Overweight and Obese Standards

What is considered normal weight to one culture may be considered too thin or a sign of illness in another. BMI standards for overweight or obese may be considered normal for families from other countries. Rice, beans, and tortilla are standard in many Hispanic's diets but are full of starches and carbohydrates. How do you approach a parent whose perception of a healthy weight or diet is different from American standards?

activity at school (Murphy and Polivka, 2007). For further information on normal height, weights, and body mass index measurements in children, see Chapter 14.

IMMUNIZATION MONITORING

Another important role of the school nurse is monitoring student immunization records. Since the introduction and use of vaccines, the occurrence of once devastating diseases such as diphtheria, tetanus, polio, and measles have decreased. New vaccines continue to be developed and researched, changing immunizations guidelines almost yearly. Families may have questions on these new vaccines, side effects, and scheduling. Keeping current with new vaccines and CDC guidelines allows the school nurse to better assist school families in obtaining correct information (Figure 5-8).

All states have written policies regarding immunization requirements at school entry (NASN, 2006d). Depending on individual state guidelines, a student could be denied entrance or excluded from school or required to obtain a physician-approved schedule for immunization when there

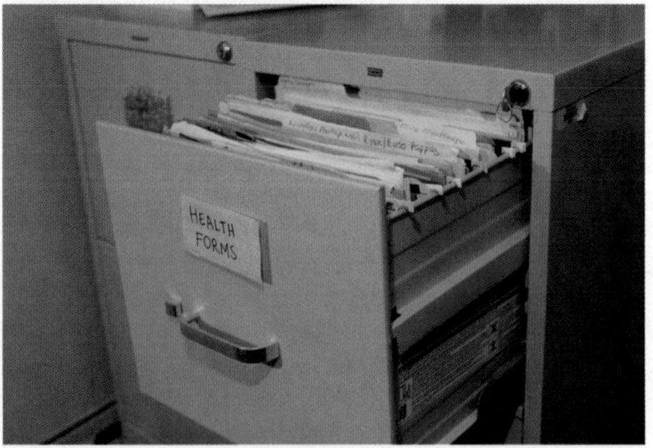

FIGURE 5-8 Most schools request an immunization history for every child. Keeping accurate records ensures all children are protected against major communicable diseases. DELMAR CENGAGE LEARNING.

> **NURSING TIP**
>
> **Communicable Disease Exclusion**
>
> Keeping a list of students enrolled in your school with medical or religious objections to immunizations or those with special health concerns that lessen their immunity makes exclusion of students easier in the event of an outbreak of a serious communicable disease such as measles.

is no verification of completed immunizations or a statement of religious or medical objection. However, not all states enforce their guidelines so close monitoring of records and communicable diseases remain an important responsibility of the school nurse.

COMMUNICABLE DISEASE CONTROL

Communicable disease control has been a major factor in developing school health services and the nurse's role in these services (Wold, 1981). NASN has determined the five roles the school nurse plays in disease control. These are to "prevent infections with vaccines, educate families on avoiding exposure, prevent transmission at school, provide the appropriate care to those ill and protect the confidentiality of the student" (NASN, 2007b). Monitoring immunization records has already been discussed. The school nurse can provide additional assistance by sponsoring clinics or immunization programs in schools as well as providing information to parents of local public health clinics. This will assist the families without a medical home or insurance in complying with school requirements (Figure 5-9).

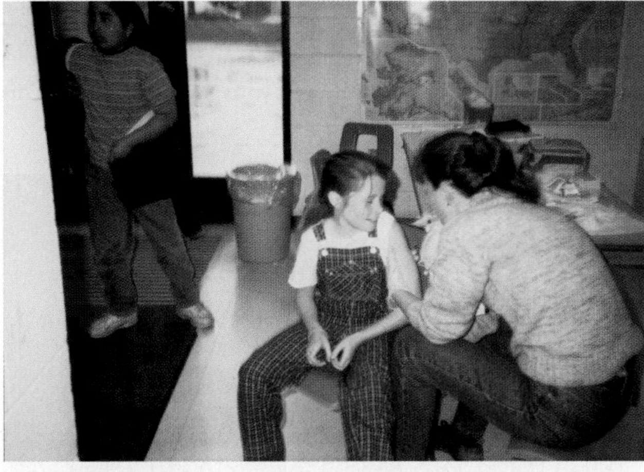

FIGURE 5-9 To assist parents in keeping their children up-to-date on immunizations, some school nurses administer immunizations in traveling clinics or work in partnership with government agencies in district sponsored immunization events. DELMAR CENGAGE LEARNING.

Education on how infectious diseases are spread can be provided in various media and across all grade levels. School nurse journals and state public health sites are full of creative ideas and kits to download to make learning about communicable disease more appealing to students. Hand washing has been especially targeted for the control of the spread of infectious diseases, and ties in with the school nurses' role of health prevention. In fact, research has shown that hand washing is the easiest, cheapest, and most effective way to control the spread of communicable diseases. Proper hand washing techniques can be shared with large groups through health education classes or any time a child visits the nurse's office. Working with the custodial staff to review specific cleaning methods during an outbreak is another way the nurse can be instrumental in preventing illness in a school. Of course, the school nurse continues the traditional role of providing care for a child who becomes ill at school. No matter what the communicable disease is that is currently being dealt with, confidentiality must be maintained to protect the rights of the child and in accordance with the federal and state HIPAA regulations. Almost all states have Health Department requirements requiring mandatory reporting and exclusion of certain communicable diseases; the school nurse needs to check with local or state health departments to determine which diseases are reportable. The nurses can also help decrease susceptibility to disease by providing education about health issues and promoting healthy living habits in students, especially in the early grades. Nutrition, exercise, adequate rest, and personal care can affect one's ability to fight off infectious diseases: these are possible topics for health promotion education.

Although the incidence of serious communicable diseases has decreased because of vaccination, other illnesses, such as strep throat, scabies, and lice still need to be monitored. Even though these diseases are less serious than measles, they can spread quickly through the classroom and lead to complications in some children. For children who are immunosuppressed, caregivers must be notified if these diseases occur in classmates because of the need for special monitoring or prophylactic treatment to prevent serious complications. Further information on communicable diseases can be found in Chapter 15.

EMERGENCY CARE

Emergency care of the child at school centers on two main concerns: (1) basic first aid care for a child with an illness or injury; and (2) emergencies requiring transport and more extensive treatment at a hospital. Because the school nurse is often the only health professional in the school, that individual must have excellent physical assessment skills and be able to make quick and accurate decisions regarding the extent of illnesses or injuries. Education in triage skills, including classification of illnesses or injuries as emergent, urgent, or nonurgent, will assist in making these decisions (University of New Mexico with New Mexico Department of Health, 2008).

Elementary School Nurse Interventions: Attendance and Health Outcomes

STUDY PURPOSE

To document the correlation of school nurse interventions and student attendance. To determine if students are referred to the school nurse for high absent rates.

METHODS

This was a retrospective descriptive study in three suburban elementary schools serving kindergarten to 5th grade. Two hundred and forty records were reviewed for nurse referrals, nursing interventions, nursing outcomes, student absent rate, and reasons for days missed. For the purpose of this study 11 days was considered a high absent rate. NIC codes were used to categorize nursing interventions and mean absent rates before and after nursing interventions were calculated.

FINDINGS

The school nurse was involved with 75% of the students with high absent rates and 66% with children who were absent 10 days or less. Seventeen percent of the children in the study had more then 11 days absent. There were no referrals to the school nurse specifically for absenteeism. More nursing interventions were documented with children with known health concerns on records. Records review found the standardized languages of NANDA, NIC, and NOC were inconsistent. When NIC codes were used they proved helpful for the sorting of health data.

IMPLICATIONS

A child's health can affect absent rates. Attendance can impact a child's learning. Funding for many schools is based on these attendance rates. High absenteeism rates can negatively impact the child's success and the school's budget. The school nurse is the ideal person to investigate and eliminate health barriers that may be causing missed school days. A referral system should be developed to alert the school nurse to a child with a high absent rate so that interventions can be planned and problems addressed. Without the referral process there is a missed opportunity for assistance. Using the standardized languages of NIC and NOC is an efficient way of documenting the nurse's interventions and outcomes and provides evidence of the direct effect the school nurse can have on the child's success in learning.

REFERENCE

Weismuller, P., Grasska, M., Alexander, M., White, C. & Kramer, P. (2007). Elementary school nurse interventions: Attendance and health outcomes. *Journal of School Nursing*, *23*(2), 111–118.

When a student comes into the nurse's office, an **across-the-room assessment** of the child is necessary in order to decide on the best course of action. The nurse must think:

How does the child look and act?

Are there visible signs of illness or injury?

Does the child say one thing, but body language or physical signs say another?

What brought this student to the nurse's office; what is his or her chief complaint?

Then the nurse should:

Assess the child from head to toe while the child talks about the reason for seeking out the nurse.

Check vital signs such as temperature, pulse, and respiration, as appropriate.

Look for signs of bruising or bleeding if an injury was the cause for the visit.

Allow the child to rest quietly, observe changes, or assist the child in washing a cut and applying a bandage or an ice pack, and always watch for signs of a more serious problem or complaint not relieved with these measures. This

NURSING TIP

Triage Off-Site

When the nurse is covering several buildings, providing a written checklist can assist in over-the-phone triaging. A printed list of questions to ask and symptoms that might be seen depending on the situation can be left with a secretary or other school staff and can be a valuable tool for those providing the information in an organized manner so the nurse can determine the best course of action.

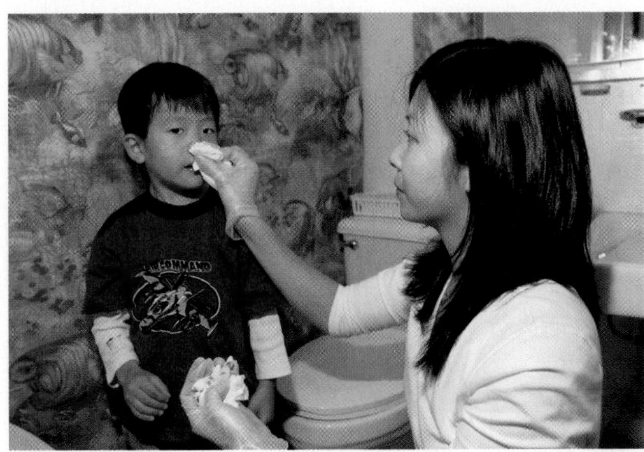

FIGURE 5-10 Caring for children with minor aches and sniffles is only one of the many responsibilities of the school nurse.
DELMAR CENGAGE LEARNING.

information can assist in deciding if the child's caregiver needs to be notified. Most school districts have developed a policy on specific instances when children need to be sent home. These policies may include a temperature over 100°F (37.8°C), an undiagnosed rash, and a constant productive cough (Figure 5-10). Sometimes physicians' standing orders allow the nurse to treat minor illnesses at school with medications such as acetaminophen or cough syrup. However, before dispensing any medications, the nurse must know the district medication policy. See Box 5-4 for a list of first aid supplies the school nurse should have readily available.

One would think school is the safest place for a child to be, but the potential for injuries in a school is nearly endless. Playground equipment, participation in gym and sports, and injuries in classes such as metal shop and chemistry can all lead to serious accidents. In the case of more serious injuries, such as a fall with a possible head injury or broken bone, additional assessment is essential. If the child has fallen in gym and is complaining of ankle pain and difficulty walking, the nurse should look for swelling, bruising, deformities, and decreased movement, circulation, and sensation in the extremity. If abnormalities are found, the extremity should be splinted as necessary. If there is a head injury, the child should never be left alone. Any bleeding should be controlled, and vital signs as well as vision disturbances, headaches, nausea, vomiting, and changes in level of consciousness or seizure activity should be noted. The caregiver should be notified and emergency services contacted as the assessment dictates. Knowing when to call for help when a child is injured is the most important aspect of caring for an injured child. Since extensive medical supplies and equipment are not always available in schools, help from paramedics who are often only minutes away can be essential.

Even though some days are filled with taking care of children with stomach aches and scraped knees, there is more to school nursing than just taking temperatures and supplying bandages. When the nurse assesses the child's illness or injury, she can also teach children to care for themselves, promote self-esteem, and encourage healthy habits.

BOX 5-4

FIRST AID SUPPLIES FOR SCHOOL HEALTH ROOM

- Soap and accessibility to running water
- Cool packs
- Thermometer
- Bandage scissors
- Tweezers
- Small flashlight
- Blanket
- Blood pressure cuff (adult and pediatric)
- Stethoscope
- Drug Book
- Dressing supplies
  —Bandages (various sizes)
  —Sterile gauze pads
  —Medical tape
  —Triangle bandage
  —Elastic bandages of various sizes
  —Splints (magazines can be used as splints if needed)
  —Eye pads or eye flush kit
- Sterile water and saline
- Peak flow meter
- Protective equipment
  —Gloves (non-latex)
  —Goggles
  —CPR shield
  —Sharps container
  —Biohazard container
- Plastic bags
- If allowed by school district (and standing orders are present)
  —Acetaminophen
  —Bee sting relief pads
  —Diphenhydramine
  —EpiPen
  —Oxygen
  —Glucose tabs
- AED machine (adult and child pads)
- First aid reference chart or book
- Poison control phone number (posted)
- Emergency rescue phone numbers (posted)

INJURIES AND ACCIDENTS

The National Health Interview Survey estimates 175,000 playground injuries occur each year, with swings and climbers

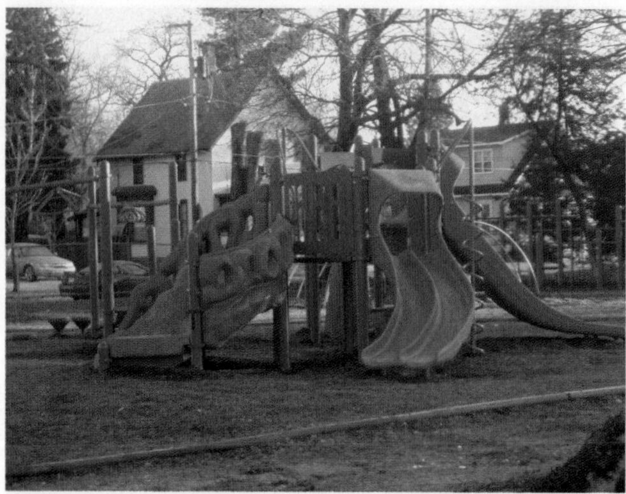

FIGURE 5-11 Playground equipment, although a favorite part of recess, can offer the highest potential for injury in the young school-age child. DELMAR CENGAGE LEARNING.

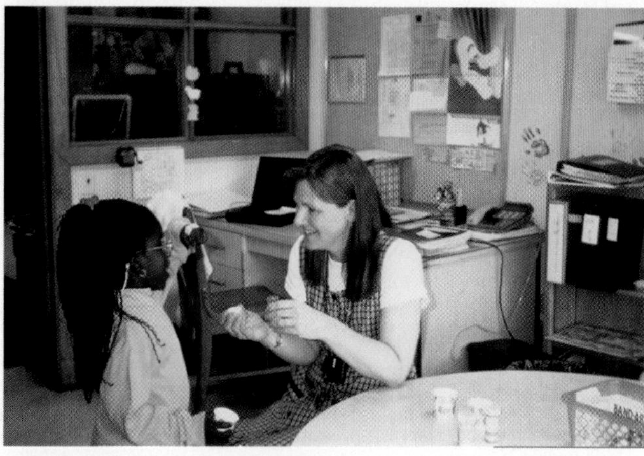

FIGURE 5-12 The school nurse often administers medications to children during the school day. Creative approaches allow medications to be organized and safely locked up. DELMAR CENGAGE LEARNING.

the top causes of injuries costing 1.2 million dollars a year (CDC, 2009). Eighty percent of all injuries at schools are on the playground (Olsen, Hudson & Thompson, 2008) (Figure 5-11). The school nurse can be instrumental in developing programs for students and staff related to injury prevention in the school. If a student or staff member needs to leave school because of an injury, it should be recorded on a standardized injury report form. These records can be important when examining data on injuries, looking for patterns, and developing plans to eliminate potential injuries. Curricula can include information on playground safety, the use of seat belts, school bus safety rules, bike helmet use, and injury prevention tips for sports activities. By becoming aware of legislation and policies on injury prevention within the school district and community, the nurse can help to decrease injuries and accidents.

MEDICATION ADMINISTRATION AND MONITORING

Another important service the school nurse provides is the monitoring and administration of medication children receive while at school (Figure 5-12). Although most children will not need to take medication during school hours, there are circumstances when it is necessary, as with chronic illnesses such as seizure disorder, diabetes, attention deficit hyperactivity disorder (ADHD), and asthma. Although the development of longer acting and extended release stimulants has decreased the number of children requiring medications at school there are still approximately 4–6% of students who will need this service (Clay, Farris, McCarthy, Kelly, & Howarth, 2008). Regulations for medication administration vary from state to state and even from district to district, but generally children who must receive medication at school have written orders from their physician as well as written permission from their caregivers. This is often recommended for over-the-counter medications as well. In some school districts a physician works with the school to provide standing orders for medications such as acetaminophen. For the safety of all students, medications must be stored in a locked cabinet and labeled by a pharmacy with the child's name, medication name, dose, and time to be administered. If the principal or other unlicensed personnel are to administer medications in the nurse's absence the nurse retains the responsibility for the medication and its administration. For this reason the school nurse must ensure adequate training on the medications, any adverse affects, and the six rights of medication administration (right client, right medication, right dose, right route, right time, and right documentation). Delegation of some nursing roles such as

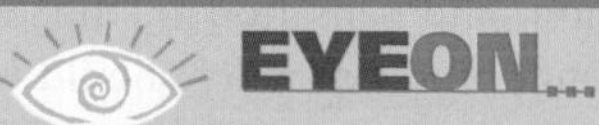

The Use of Herbal Therapies

In schools across the United States, children with a variety of diagnosed conditions are receiving prescription medications at school. Caregivers who worry about their child receiving Ritalin or psychotropic drugs are exploring the possibility of alternative treatments such as herbal therapies. Most school districts still require caregiver and physician permission for the use of herbal therapies at school even if they can be purchased over the counter. For the safety of students, you must remain current on popular herbal preparations and their side effects and contraindications.

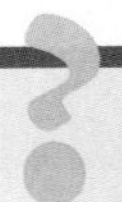

KIDS WANT TO KNOW

An Ambulance Ride

"What happens if I get hurt at school and have to go to the hospital? What's it like to ride in an ambulance? How will my parents find me?"

To help lessen the fears of students, the school nurse can:

- Arrange a visit from the local fire department so children can tour the ambulance
- Provide various pieces of equipment the children may see in the ambulance and emergency room for hands-on experiences
- Have a familiar staff person from the school ride in the ambulance with the child if possible and, if appropriate, reassure the child that caregivers will meet them at the hospital

medication administration is subject to state Nurse Practice Act and Board of Education rules so the nurse must investigate these sources before training others in medication administration.

Many children attending school are taking stimulant medications such as methylphenidate (Ritalin, Concerta, Focalin), amphetamine dextroamphetamine (Adderall), Lisdexam fetamine dimesylate (Vyvanse), or nonstimulants such as atomoxetine (Strattera) for attention deficit or attention deficit hyperactivity disorder (ADD/ADHD). In fact, ADHD is the most common neurobehavioral disorder seen in schools (Thorell & Rydell, 2008). The school nurse must be knowledgeable about the assessment procedures that acccompany the evaluation of ADD/ADHD and the various medications prescribed for children with these conditions. Many medications are controlled substances (Ritalin, Dexedrine) and must be treated as such. Children often have multiple diagnoses in addition to ADD/ADHD and may also be on antidepressants or other pychotropic medications. Research on ADD/ADHD continues and new medications and dosage options continue to become available so keeping up to date is imperative. Side effects of these medications still need to be monitored by the school nurse. Medication is not the only treatment these children receive. Other measures include behavior modification, psychological counseling, and classroom intervention. By being knowledgeable about all medications and interventions, the school nurse can assist students, families, and teachers in delivering appropriate care. For more information on ADD/ADHD and other mental health disorders, refer to Chapter 35.

NURSING TIP

Identifying Children Easily

Stapling a current photo of the child on his medication sheet can be helpful to nurses covering multiple buildings or substitute nurses, especially if the child has cognitive delays or is non-verbal.

INDIVIDUAL HEALTH PLANS

When a child enters or returns to school with a health concern that impacts his or her ability to learn, the school nurse must assess the child's health status; determine what, if any, specialized services are needed; and develop a plan for his or her care. In the hospital setting nurses write a nursing care plan, known in the school setting as the Individual Health Plan (IHP). An IHP is a document, based on the nurse's assessment of the child, which outlines the special health needs, goals, interventions, and outcomes necessary to improve or maintain the health of the child and allow him/her to remain in school. A health history, including a baseline of the child's vital signs and neurological status, medications at home or at school, dietary consideration or restrictions, and any specialized equipment is done before writing the IHP.

Using the diagnoses of the North American Nursing Diagnosis Association (NANDA) ensures continuity of care (NANDA, 2009). Standardized language also assists with data collection, funding by state and federal programs, and in the planning of health care services in the school district. Goals are written for each diagnosis in the form of nursing outcomes and guide what actions need to be taken by the nurse, student, or other staff. These outcomes and interventions also provide a basis for making appropriate decisions regarding the delegation of nursing tasks. Expected outcomes for each diagnosis are stated so the nurse can validate, by observing the student's behaviors, that goals have been met and the student has benefited from nursing care (Johnson, Bulechek, Butcher, McCloskey, Dochterman, Maas, Morehead, & Swanson, 2006). Professional nursing organizations are endorsing the use of the Nursing Intervention Classification (NIC) and the Nursing Outcome Classification (NOC). The use of standardized interventions and expected outcomes can benefit the school nurse as a professional. For further information on these systems please see Suggested Readings.

From the IHP the school nurse develops an Individual Emergency Plan (IEMP). This plan includes the basic steps to provide emergency care to the child for any potentially life-threatening event for which the child is at a high risk. It must be written in terms all staff can understand and be easily accessible to those who may need to provide emergency care in the absence of the nurse. By taking the time at the start of the school year to familiarize staff with the IEMPs, emergency care can be delivered to the student quickly and competently.

CASE STUDY / CARE PLAN

INDIVIDUAL HEALTH PLAN

Kevin is an 8-year-old Caucasian boy currently enrolled in second grade. He was diagnosed with asthma at age 4. Triggers for exacerbations include respiratory illnesses, sudden weather changes, and exposure to known allergens. He is also allergic to peanuts. His mother has noted an increase in asthma-related complaints and is wondering if they are related to stress. Kevin lives with his mother and younger sister. His parents are just recently separated and he sees his father infrequently. Kevin has just begun receiving Social Worker services.

ASSESSMENT

Baseline vital signs: HR 72, R 24, BP 84/58

Kevin is small for his age with a weight of 29 ¾ pounds (<5th percentile) and height of 41 inches (<5th percentile). His BMI is 12.6 (underweight). He presents as pale with dark circles under his eyes. His current diet is as tolerated with avoidance of peanuts or foods with peanut products in them. His mother tries to provide extra calories as snacks throughout the day. He pays for school lunch but on most days will eat very little of it.

Medications: Benadryl, Albuterol inhaler, Epipen Jr

Up to date on physical and immunizations.

Does not fully participate in gym due to complaints of being tired after a few minutes of activity.

NURSING DIAGNOSIS 1

Potential for ineffective airway clearance related to ingestion of allergen and environmental exposure.

EXPECTED OUTCOME

1. Kevin will maintain patent airway and avoid exposures to allergens.

NOC: Respiratory Status: Airway Patency

NIC: Airway Management; Anaphylaxis Management

INTERVENTIONS/*RATIONALES*

1. Establish baseline vital signs. *Baseline data provides for early recognition of alterations.*
2. Identify sources of allergens in school setting. *Sources of allergens need to be identified before they can be avoided.*
3. Administer Benadryl, Albuterol, and Epipen as ordered for allergic reaction. *Medications prescribed for reversal of allergic reaction and for bronchodilation.*
4. If exposure occurs monitor for signs of compromised airway (wheezing, decreased breath sounds, tight throat or hoarse voice). *Abnormality indicates respiratory compromise and increasing airway resistance.*
5. Establish and maintain patent airway. *Maintaining the airway is always the first priority.*
6. Call for EMS as appropriate. *To secure additional assistance and transport for higher level of care.*
7. Position client for maximum ventilation and comfort. *Promote better lung expansion and improved air exchange.*
8. Instruct in-service staff on signs of anaphylaxis and preventative measures. *Increased knowledge base provides for improved client care.*
9. Instruct client and alternate staff on Epipen usage as allowed by state regulations. *Provides for safety and continuity of care.*

(Continues)

CASE STUDY / CARE PLAN (Continued)

10. Develop IEMP and instruct in-service staff on appropriate emergency interventions. *Provides specific steps to take in an emergency situation.*

EVALUATION

Kevin's airway will remain patent and he will have no episodes of anaphylaxis.

NURSING DIAGNOSIS 2

Knowledge deficit related to disease process, diet, medications, and treatment regimen.

EXPECTED OUTCOME

1. Kevin will correctly state diagnoses, dietary restrictions, medication names, and what to do if he has difficulty breathing.

NOC: Knowledge: Asthma Management, Diet, Disease Process, Treatment Regimen, Medications
NIC: Teaching: Individual, Prescribed Diet, Disease Process, Prescribed Medications

INTERVENTIONS/*RATIONALES*

1. Assess current knowledge of asthma, allergies, dietary restrictions and medications. *Provides starting point and identifies gaps in knowledge for further teaching.*
2. Ensure teaching materials/instructions are at current developmental level. *Client education will vary depending on cognitive level.*
3. Determine cultural influences on health teaching. *Provides climate for acceptance allowing them to hold own beliefs as appropriate.*
4. Instruct on what asthma is, symptoms Kevin may notice, what he can do to prevent or help an attack. *Client education will vary depending on the acute or chronic disease state.*
5. Instruct client on dietary restrictions related to allergies and how to avoid these foods in home and school settings. *Knowledge should begin with simple information and build on this base.*
6. Review medications and what each medication does to improve breathing. *Knowing what medications do to assist in the breathing process can increase compliance.*
7. Assist Kevin in using information in his daily life. *Helping the client to incorporate learning into daily life may increase chance of behavior change.*
8. Include family and teacher in teaching. *Encourages ongoing support for client.*

EVALUATION

Kevin can correctly identify foods to avoid and what to do if he has difficulty breathing.

NURSING DIAGNOSIS 3

Fatigue/activity intolerance related to disease process and nutrition.

EXPECTED OUTCOME

1. Kevin's endurance with activity will increase as evidenced by participation in gym and recess.

NOC: Endurance; Activity Tolerance
NIC: Exercise Promotion; Energy Management; Nutrition Management; Asthma Management

(Continues)

CASE STUDY / CARE PLAN (Continued)

INTERVENTIONS/*RATIONALES*

1. Assess nutritional status. *Adequate energy reserves are required for activity.*
2. Assess the patient's usual level of exercise and physical activity. *Both increased physical exertion and limited levels of exercise can contribute to fatigue.*
3. Observe and document response to activity. *Close monitoring serves as a guide for optimal progression of activity.*
4. Establish guidelines and goals of activity with the client. *Motivation is enhanced if the patient participates in goal setting.*
5. Encourage adequate rest periods, especially before exercise sessions. *Rest between activities provides time for energy conservation.*
6. Progress activity and length of exercise gradually. *This prevents overexertion and promotes attainment of short-range goals.*

EVALUATION

Kevin will participate in gym and recess play to the best of his ability without fatigue.

NURSING DIAGNOSIS 4

Alterations in growth and development related to food allergies, nutritional status.

EXPECTED OUTCOME

1. Kevin will maintain or gain weight during the school year.

NOC: Growth

NIC: Health Screening; Health Education; Nutrition Management

INTERVENTIONS/*RATIONALES*

1. Establish baseline by measuring height and weight on school instrument. *Baseline data provides for early recognition of alterations.*
2. Provide for privacy and confidentiality during screening. *Patient confidentiality is mandated by HIPAA laws.*
3. Determine food preferences and allergies. *Finding foods the client likes or needs to avoid can assist in compliance to plan.*
4. Assess intake for nutritional adequacy. Ensures proper caloric requirements are being met for growth.
5. Encourage calorie intake appropriate to body weight and activities. To grow, adequate caloric needs must be met in relation to calories expended.
6. Allow time for mid-morning snack. *Small frequent meals can ensure adequate nutritional intake without discomfort of fullness.*
7. Weigh client at appropriate intervals and record on growth chart. *Shorter range goals may be more achievable and therefore reinforcing.*
8. Maintain communication between parent, nurse, and physician with permission of client. *To ensure continuity of care.*

EVALUATION

Kevin will maintain weight for height on CDC growth scale.

Additional diagnoses available: Family coping compromised; Risk for caregiver role Strain; Alteration in nutrition; Ineffective coping. (If social worker is not present in school the school nurse can expand on these diagnoses).

Individual Emergency Health Plan

Student: Kevin L. Student ID 13736 Birthdate: 9/5/2004
School: Holly Trails Grade/Room: 2nd Rm 105
Parent/Guardian: Thomas and Alvina L. Phone:
Primary Care Provider: Dr. Busse

PEANUT ALLERGY; ASTHMA

Medications:

Albuterol MDI. 2 puffs q4-6h prn;

Benadryl 2 tsp. q 4-6h as needed for allergic reaction;

Epipen JR. 1 injection IM as needed for anaphylaxis.

IF ANY OF THE FOLLOWING EMERGENCY SIGNS OCCUR CALL 911

Loss of consciousness
Struggling to breathe
Lips or nails gray or blue
Unable to talk

FOR PEANUT INGESTION:

- Call office for help
- If hives, itchy skin, give 2 teaspoons Benadryl by mouth
- If face puffy, tongue swelling, difficulty swallowing, administer Epipen JR
- Call 911, office notify parent

FOR ASTHMA ATTACK:

- Nurse or trained staff brings emergency kit and meds to location
- Coughing, wheezing, increased respirations, short of breath:
  - Give Albuterol inhaler 2 puffs
  - Position for comfort, rest
- Symptoms resolved—notify parent
- Continued or worsening symptoms call 911, office notify parent

HEALTH EDUCATION AND PROMOTION

Health education and health promotion principles have existed for many years, but their focus has changed over time. In the 1980s, health education dealt with learning experiences that changed one's behavior to be more health oriented. It then changed to individuals making informed decisions about matters affecting their personal health. The focus of health education now is prevention and wellness with appropriate curricula, continuity through the grade levels, cultural sensitivity, and a community focus. Health education can be planned or incidental and should help students see how the information given can be used in their own life (Streng, 2007).

One of the *Healthy People 2010* goals is planned health education for grades kindergarten through 12 (U.S. Department of Health and Human Services, 2000). In addition, the objectives new to *Healthy People 2020* related to early and middle childhood suggest the proportion of elementary, middle, and senior high schools requiring school health education be increased (U.S. Department of Health and Human Services, 2009). Teaching healthy living habits when children are young sets the stage for healthy habits as the child grows to adulthood. In addition, increased knowledge about health-related topics can influence attitudes and behaviors in health. The certified school nurse, with her background in health and additional preparation in education, can present this information to students or act as a resource for teachers who are planning lessons in health-related topics and act as a positive role model for students and staff.

Many health education curricula focus on strategic areas that may reduce injury or morbidity in children: (1) tobacco

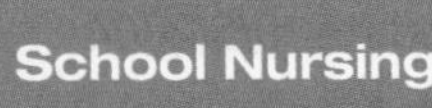

School Nursing

Many of today's schools are struggling with finances. New laws and changing policies force administrators to make important choices regarding which programs survive the budget cuts. Often, school nurses are called on to justify their positions. One way of doing this is by providing for an evidence-based practice. How many children with poor test scores have failed their vision screenings but have not received glasses? Will their scores go up after this is corrected? How can nutrition and exercise programs in schools help decrease the number of overweight children? Will this decrease in turn decrease the number of children diagnosed with type 2 diabetes? Can a hearing conservation program deter kids from playing their music into headphones so loudly? Can that decrease the incidence of hearing loss? How many children quit or never start smoking after completing an anti tobacco program? These are just a few ideas of the research projects open to school nurses that could make for healthier students who are more available for learning.

use; (2) alcohol and drug use; (3) sexual behaviors that lead to sexually transmitted diseases and pregnancy; (4) unhealthy diet; and (5) physical inactivity. Other important topics include personal and dental hygiene, safety, first aid, anger management, and conflict resolution. Since not all topics are appropriate for children of all ages, it is important to be sure the information presented is age-appropriate. The most common topics school nurses are involved in are personal and dental hygiene, sex education, antismoking campaigns, alcohol and drug prevention, and violence prevention instruction.

EVIDENCE-BASED PRACTICE

"I Feel Good!" A Weekly Wellness Radio Broadcast for Elementary School Children

CLINICAL PROBLEM:

Across the nation health education has been scaled back due to budgetary constraints. How can health education corresponding with learning standards be integrated into the school day within financial constraints?

BEST CLINICAL PRACTICE:

The teachable moment is providing health education to children in the school. The school nurse can teach about almost any subject when a child comes in to her office. But to reach a large group at one time has become trickier. Getting health education time in a classroom may now conflict with the extra curriculum that is provided for schools to meet the *No Child Left Behind* standards. A weekly broadcast over the school intercom set to imitate a radio program throughout the school year was developed. Topics ranged from health promotion, nutrition, dental care, drug awareness, cold weather advice, and what to do in an emergency, all aligning with educational standards. Evaluations by students were done by pre- and post-test on health topics.

IMPLICATIONS FOR NURSING:

- Similar programs can enhance students' knowledge on illness and health behaviors.
- Children with healthy behaviors may have decreased incidence of illness, decreasing absenteeism.
- The school nurse acts as an "agent of change" contributing to the nation's public health agenda.

Reference: Morton, J. (2008). "I Feel Good!" A weekly wellness radio broadcast for elementary school children. *Journal of School Nursing, 24*(2), 83–87.

PERSONAL AND DENTAL HYGIENE

Personal and dental hygiene information can be easily adapted for preschool through elementary levels and is a nice way for the school nurse to introduce herself to younger children. Many large companies offer free videos, supplies, and educational materials to schools, which can be useful in presenting information. If the budget allows, there are also numerous books, tapes, and instructional materials that can be purchased from medical supply catalogs, bookstores, and teacher centers. Many resources are available online under dental and health education sites.

One important personal hygiene topic to discuss is hand washing since it helps prevent the spread of infection and has been shown to decrease absentee rate 31–43% in school (Figure 5-13). Teaching hand washing when children are young can make it a more likely practice as they grow (Tousman et al., 2007). Instructions about hand washing can be presented by reading stories about cartoon germs, providing coloring books and activity sheets, viewing videotapes, using puppets, and making take-home charts. Presenting material in a variety of creative ways on how and when to wash one's hands and how germs are spread can hold young children's interest and make learning fun. For example, "Germs Are Not for Sharing" by Verdick & Heinlen (2006) or "Bill Nye the Science Guy's Big Book of Tiny Germs" (2005) are excellent stories about germs. Information on what germs are, how they get into one's body, how one can protect oneself from them, and the proper technique for washing hands should also be provided. The *Henry the Hand* program by

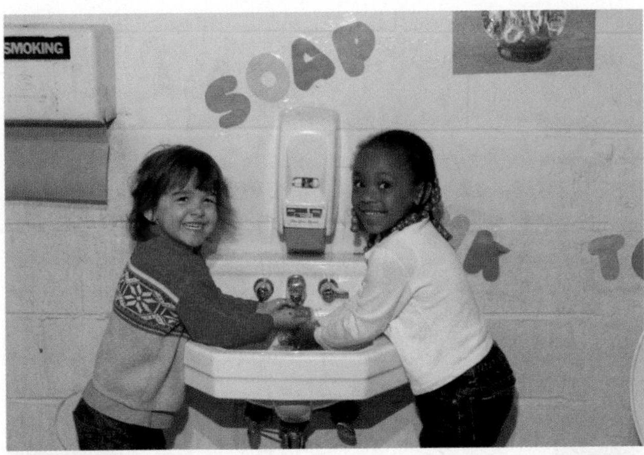
SMOKING
SOAP

FIGURE 5-13 Handwashing is a great way for the nurse to help control the spread of germs and teach children life long healthy habits. DELMAR CENGAGE LEARNING.

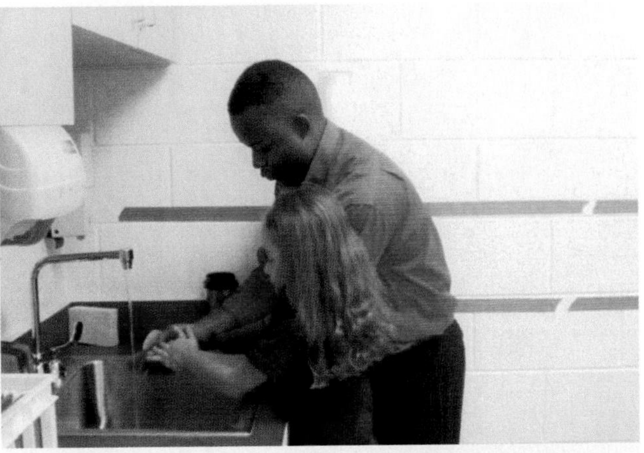

FIGURE 5-15 Education on handwashing can decrease the spread of communicable disease in the school and it doesn't have to be in a formal classroom setting. The school nurse can use the available moment, when the child comes to the health office for assistance, to teach a variety of subjects. DELMAR CENGAGE LEARNING.

William Sawyer (1999) is an example of a creative multimedia method of instruction (Figure 5-14). Videotapes, silly songs, and activity pages provide children information on hand washing.

A new program called *Glitterbug* by Breus Corporation uses a non-toxic fluorescent lotion with a UV lamp to see how well hands were washed and germs can travel. Whatever the child touches also lights up under the lamp. Children who have put their fingers in their mouth will have a glow around their lips, and table tops will show glowing fingerprints. New ideas and resources as well as facts, games, and coloring sheets that can be downloaded and used with students of various ages are available on the internet. However, whatever program is chosen, physically involving the child in the learning increases understanding (Figure 5-15).

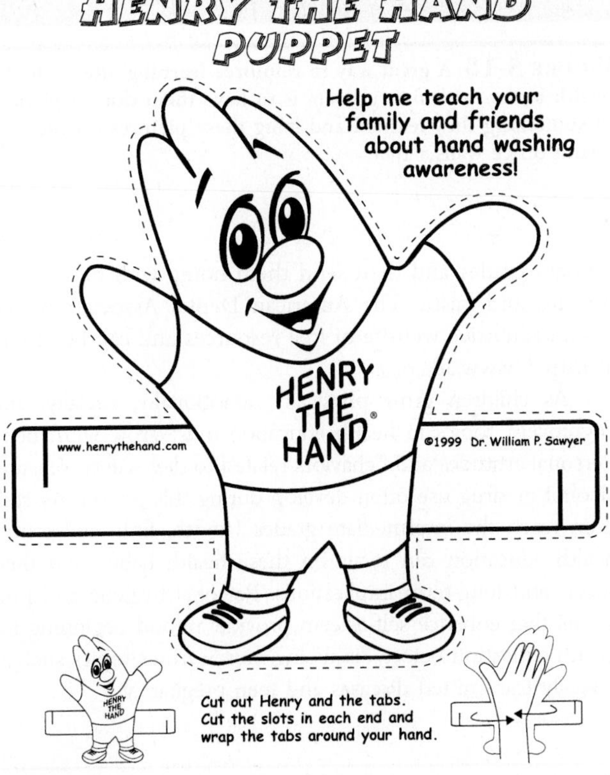
HENRY THE HAND®
PUPPET
Help me teach your family and friends about hand washing awareness!
HENRY THE HAND®
www.henrythehand.com
©1999 Dr. William P. Sawyer
Cut out Henry and the tabs.
Cut the slots in each end and wrap the tabs around your hand.

FIGURE 5-14 Pages and activity sheets to color can reinforce handwashing teaching. Here we see a hand puppet page for the primary school child to cut out and color. USED WITH PERMISSION OF DR. WILLIAM P. SAWYER ®.

Dental hygiene is another topic the school nurse can discuss with young children, since dental disease remains a major health problem for children (Figure 5-16). In fact, over half of children ages 5–9 years of age have had at least one cavity, and by age 17 years over 7% have lost a tooth to decay (CDC, 2004). Dental disease is responsible for millions of lost school days for students and workdays for their parents. Teaching preventive dental care could positively impact the dental health of children. Education on the correct way to brush teeth should begin in preschool, and as children get older, education can include when and why it is important to brush, how to floss, the importance of proper nutrition for dental health, and visiting a dentist. School nurses can request free dental education material from toothpaste companies and local dentists' offices. Children's books telling stories of favorite characters visiting the dentist are available in bookstores and libraries. A favorite method of teaching dental hygiene to young children is to use a giant set of teeth and a big toothbrush for demonstration or practice (Figure 5-17).

A take-home chart showing how often the child has brushed provides reinforcement and gets the family involved. Another method is to let the children show what they have learned by writing a story or drawing a picture (Figure 5-18). Hanging these pictures on the bulletin board

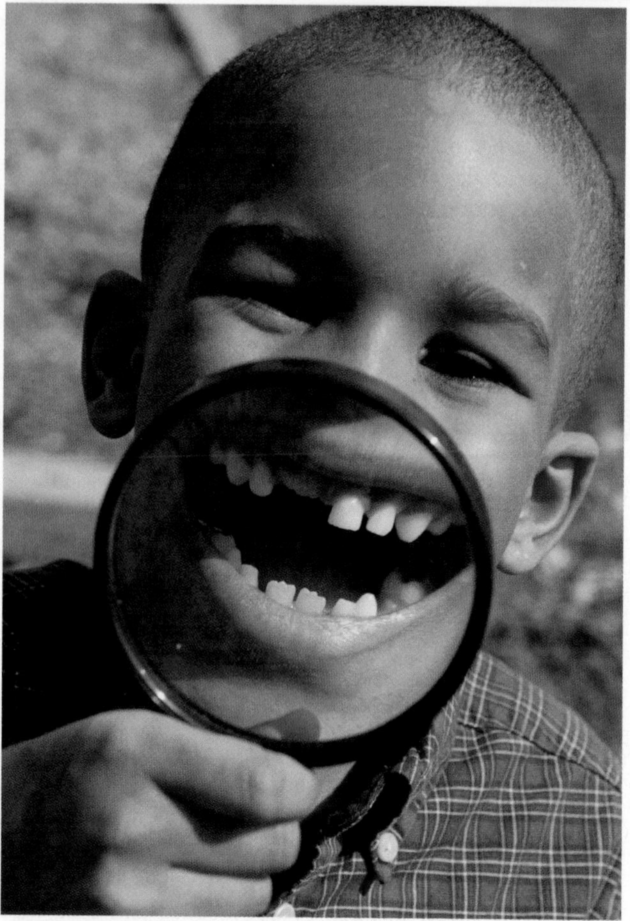

FIGURE 5-16 Proper dental health can be reinforced by the school nurse. DELMAR CENGAGE LEARNING.

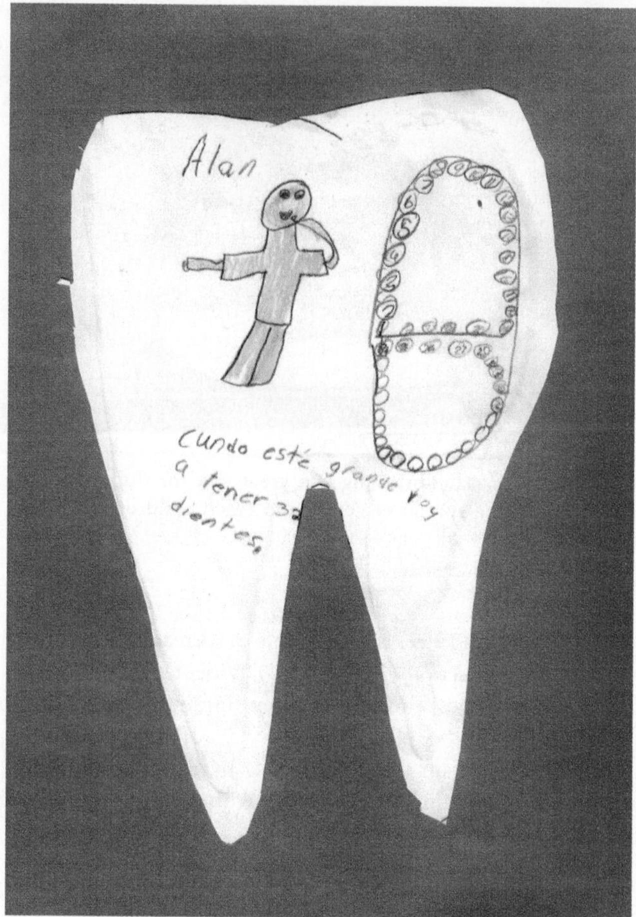

FIGURE 5-18 A great way to reinforce learning after a dental health lesson with first graders is to have them draw a picture of something they learned and hang these pictures on the health office walls. DELMAR CENGAGE LEARNING.

is a great way to celebrate Dental Health month during February. Some schools are teaming up with county agencies to provide materials and instruction on dental health. Some travel to schools and put on a fun assembly for the primary grades and then send them home with new toothbrushes and paste. The American Dental Association also has an extensive website of free resources and can be visited at http://www.ada.org.

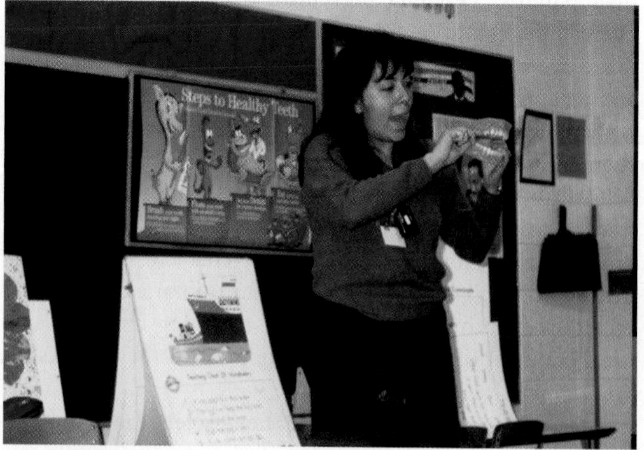

FIGURE 5-17 School nurses provide health education classes for students. Here, a nurse demonstrates how to properly brush your teeth. DELMAR CENGAGE LEARNING.

As children grow physically, emotionally, socially, and cognitively, topics in health education must grow with them. Personal attitudes and behaviors related to diet, safety, sex, and alcohol or drug use often develop during this period. As children reach the intermediate grades (fourth, fifth, and sixth), health education can focus on these health habits and their short- and long-term implications. Personal hygiene and programs that enhance self-esteem provide a good beginning for health education before discussing more serious topics such as sexually transmitted diseases and teen pregnancy.

SEX EDUCATION

As children reach the 5th and 6th grades, the school nurse is often asked by teachers or the parent-teacher organization to provide classroom materials or instruction on human growth

Reflections from Families

I have two children, Luke is in second grade and Sarah is in fourth. It's a daily battle to get them to brush their teeth before they leave for school. One day, Luke came home with a new toothbrush. Not only does he brush his teeth twice a day but he's been correcting Sarah's brushing techniques. He told me his school nurse came in the classroom with a set of really big teeth and showed him "the right way to brush his teeth." He even asked to bring his toothbrush to school.

and development and sex education (Figure 5-19). Finding materials and resources that are developmentally appropriate for this group of students is important. Over 22.2% of middle school students have already experienced sexual intercourse. This increases significantly to 46.8% for 9th through 12th graders (Kim-Godwin, Clements, Bullers, Maume & Demski, 2007). For that reason providing accurate information on this topic needs to be addressed at an early age. Since 37.2% of high school students fail to use condoms (Kim-Godwin et al., 2007), there are serious implications of teenage pregnancy, HIV/AIDS, and other sexually transmitted diseases to

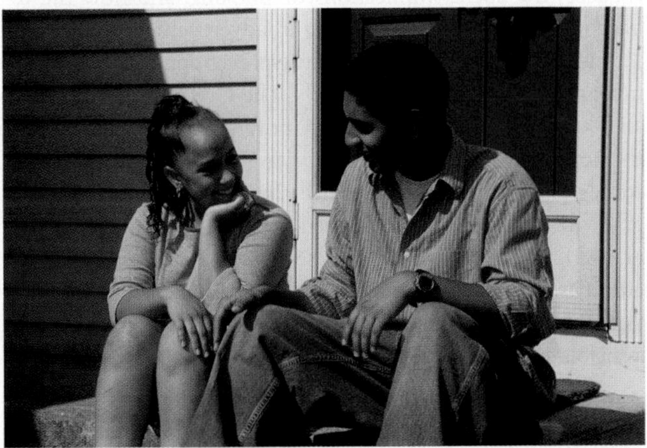

FIGURE 5-19 Nurses can be instrumental in relaying accurate information to teens on dating and sexual health. DELMAR CENGAGE LEARNING.

consider when planning a health education curriculum. The school nurse can be helpful in planning preventive programs and teaching these topics to students. In the past, having a sexually transmitted infection (STI) meant living with the physical complications and psychological stigma of diseases such as herpes or gonorrhea. Today, the outcome can be far more serious.

When preparing sex education curricula, the primary goal is to increase knowledge and encourage the student to make positive health choices. Programs designed to increase knowledge alone are not enough. Students also need instruction on values, decision making, and communication skills, presented in a nonjudgmental way. Gender and cultural differences as well as societal, physiologic, and psychological factors must be considered when planning a sex education program. Finding creative ways to reinforce material or opportunities for application of knowledge can foster healthy lifestyle choices. See Chapter 12 for more information on adolescent sexuality.

Sex education needs to focus on prevention. Four million new STIs are diagnosed in teens each year (Kim-Godwin et al., 2007). There are approximately 9.1 million people ages 15–24 with STIs and 33 million people living with HIV/AIDS (CDC, 2008b). Teens need information on how STIs are spread, precautions they can take, and treatments for the various diseases. Box 5-5 provides a quick HIV/AIDS fact sheet that can be used as an icebreaker for opening discussions with students.

Decision-making skills also need to be discussed and cultural and social values explored. Remembering the developmental level of the students is important. Adolescents are in various developmental stages. Many teens feel nothing bad can happen to them; bad things happen only to other people. Students need to know that if they are participating in unprotected sex, they may contract an STI; although abstinence can be encouraged, education aimed only at this option does not acknowledge that many teens are already sexually active. "Saying no" ignores this reality (Denehy, 2007b).

Sex education would not be complete without providing information on preventing pregnancy. However, there is controversy regarding teaching the use of contraception, so before developing or implementing an education program, the nurse must be familiar with the policies of the school district and the values of the community. Negative attitudes can be a barrier to sex education, so being aware of these attitudes and providing instruction with a nonjudgmental attitude are critical. Discussing sensitive information in an open, relaxed manner and letting students know the hours the school nurse is available is helpful. Helping students share personal information regarding sexual practices or possible pregnancies is challenging, and client confidentiality is of utmost importance. A student coming for help needs to know the school nurse is able and willing to help without notifying guardians. This presents a moral dilemma for some nurses. Answering questions and referring the student to appropriate resources is the key. For more information on confidentiality and ethics, see Chapter 2.

BOX 5-5
HIV/AIDS

Did you know?

1. Every state and most cities have reported cases of HIV. It's not just in low-income areas or big cities in the United States.
2. At the end of 2007, 468,578 people in the United States were living with AIDS.
3. There were 50,300 new cases of HIV in 2006, the last year complete data is available, and 14,561 people died of the disease.
4. You may not have AIDS if you are HIV infected, but you can still spread HIV to others.
5. In day-to-day contact, people with AIDS are more likely to pick up an infection from you than you are to get AIDS from them. However, sexual contact with a person with HIV/AIDS puts you at risk for contracting HIV/AIDS.
6. Advances in treatments have slowed the progress from HIV to AIDS but there is still no cure for AIDS.

Adapted from Centers for Disease Control and Prevention (2008b). HIV fact sheet. http://www.cdc.gov/hiv/topics/surveillance/basic.htm.

The nurse must also be prepared to assist a pregnant teen who remains in school until her baby is delivered. The nurse can provide instruction in prenatal care and referrals to appropriate community medical services. In fact, it is not uncommon for the school nurse to be the first contact the teen has with a health professional, and in some cases the only health care she receives. The nurse can develop and provide classes for a student so she can learn to care for herself during pregnancy as well as instruct her on infant care and parenting skills. The nurse can also be instrumental in helping the pregnant student stay in school and obtain community resources after giving birth. Finally, the nurse must be prepared if students go into labor at school. Any school where a pregnant student is enrolled should have an emergency delivery kit available. An IHP should also be developed for each pregnant student for school personnel to follow in case of emergency.

NURSING TIP

Teaching Preteens/Teens about Sex Education

When presenting sex education to groups of preteens/teens, having them write three questions on blank paper and dropping them in a box allows the nurse to answer specific questions without causing anxiety in the student.

ANTISMOKING EDUCATION

Despite media attention on lawsuits against tobacco companies, laws prohibiting smoking in many private and public places, and research showing the negative health risks of tobacco, the number of people who smoke cigarettes has not decreased significantly in recent years. In fact, approximately 23% of high school students reported regular cigarette use (Fritz, Crane-Wilder, Hardin, & Horrocks, 2008) and over 50% had reported trying tobacco (CDC, 2008a). Nicotine is a powerful drug, which causes physiologic dependence and adversely affects all ages. It has been linked to multiple medical problems, including cancer, heart disease, stroke, emphysema, chronic obstructive pulmonary disease, infertility, low-birth-weight infants, and drug interactions (Jannone & O'Connell, 2007). Diseases related to tobacco use cost the United States $157 billion a year and cause the premature deaths of 444,000 Americans a year (CDC, 2006). Tobacco, with its high addiction potential, is seen as a gateway drug and it is associated with experimentation and the use of alcohol and illegal substances. Experimentation at an early age increases the risk of regular smoking so much so that 74% of teen smokers still are smokers five years later (Jannone & O'Connell, 2007). Teen smokers are 3 times more likely to drink alcohol, 8 times more likely to use marijuana, and 22 times more likely to try cocaine (Fritz et al., 2008). Therefore, health education programs dealing with tobacco prevention and use need to be taught before middle school. Antismoking education must begin before the child tries the first cigarette and continue throughout all grade levels.

For teaching to be effective, it cannot be simply a lecture on the risks of smoking. It must be interactive, with teachers facilitating small peer discussion groups. Education regarding smoking should include both short- and long-term effects of tobacco, the social implications of smoking, and how the tobacco industry glorifies smoking in advertisements.

Multiple anti-tobacco and drug prevention programs exist, most at little or no cost to schools. The Quit 2 Win program is an 8-week school-based cessation program that helps students to stop smoking by teaching behavior changes and coping strategies (Jannone & O'Connell, 2007). TAR WARS, a program for fifth graders developed by Doctors Ought to Care (DOC), discourages tobacco use by increasing awareness of attitudes and effects of smoking. The American Lung Association also has valuable resources available. These programs are available online and can be requested by the school nurse.

Providing education is not enough. To see a significant decrease in the number of people who smoke, additional support is necessary. Ways to involve the family and the community need to be explored. Teachers need to be trained if they also provide anti-smoking instruction and follow-up to ongoing programs. The CDC recommends

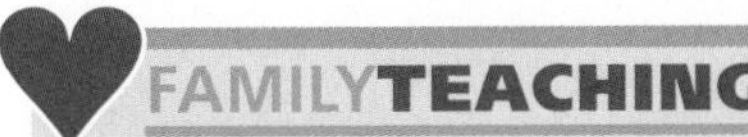

Parents Who Smoke

If parents smoke, they should be encouraged not to smoke in the house nor in front of their children.

that every school have a policy in place dealing with tobacco use as well as a smoking cessation program on site with staff trained on educating teens about tobacco. Making cigarettes less easy to obtain by enforcing these laws can help; despite laws prohibiting the sale of cigarettes to minors, adolescents have little difficulty purchasing them. Increasing anti-tobacco media, extending insurance coverage for treatment for smoking cessation, and increasing the federal excise tax need to be further explored. The school nurse can become involved with organizations such as the American Cancer Society or DOC and help promote anti tobacco education at the state and local level, while always evaluating existing programs and looking for ways to improve or expand antismoking education.

ALCOHOL AND DRUG ABUSE PREVENTION

Early experimentation with cigarette smoking has been linked to regular use of tobacco, alcohol, and marijuana. It continues to coexist with other unhealthy lifestyle behaviors including violence and unsafe sex practices (Dunn et al., 2008). It must be made clear that *use* and *abuse* are different terms, but both are a problem and can have serious long-term effects. Early use of illegal substances by adolescents leads to greater risk for later abuse and addiction. Alcohol use and drug use have been associated with truancy, poor academic performance, higher dropout rates, and low self-esteem. Forty-one percent of 8th graders have used alcohol with 19.5% self-reporting having been drunk (Dunn et al, 2008). Over one million adolescents reported trying inhalants (NIDA notes, 2007) and 4.4% of teens have experimented with methamphetamine (CDC, 2008a). An estimated 1.7 million teens reported using marijuana (NSDUH, 2009) (Figure 5-20).

Although risk-taking and experimentation are considered a normal part of the developmental stage adolescents go through on their way to independence, the long-term effects of experiences that lead to the regular use or abuse of alcohol and drugs can be serious. The best way to educate youths on the dangers of alcohol and drug use has been debated over the years. Curricula that present drug information, how to resist peer pressure, and social and communication skills have been incorporated into various programs. The goal of these programs is the prevention of drug and alcohol use. However, the reality of achieving that

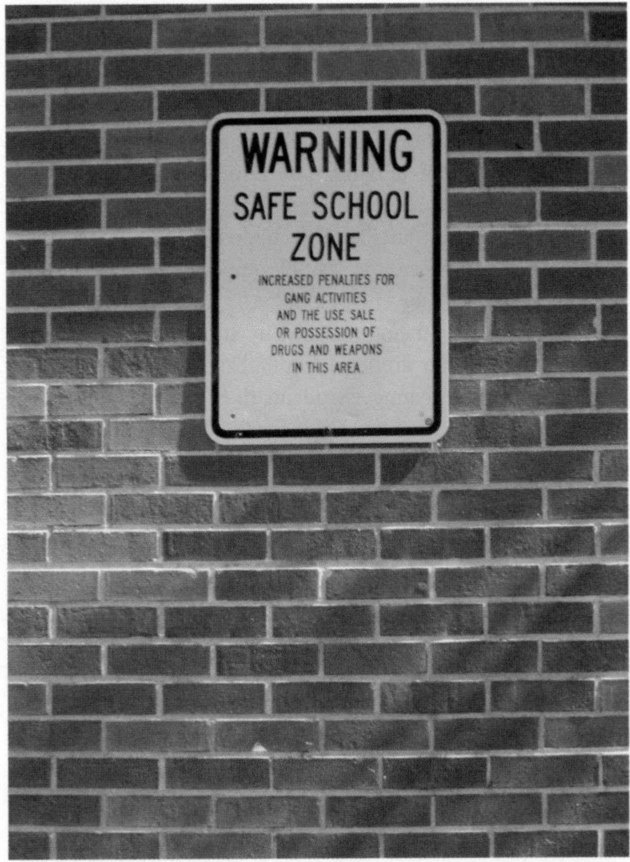
WARNING
SAFE SCHOOL ZONE
INCREASED PENALTIES FOR GANG ACTIVITIES AND THE USE SALE OR POSSESSION OF DRUGS AND WEAPONS IN THIS AREA

FIGURE 5-20 The school is a safety zone for all its students. Violence and anti-drug education is an important part of the school health curciculum. DELMAR CENGAGE LEARNING.

goal has been questioned, although harm reduction methods have been introduced with success in some countries.

Although research on how prevention programs influence adolescent behavior is becoming more available, studies showing specific program effects may not be valid across different ethnic and cultural groups of teens. When a teen makes the decision whether or not to try alcohol or drugs, multiple variables come into play: parental attitudes, support, and use; school policies and how they are enforced; geographic location; socioeconomic issues; and even friends or associates. The particular prevention program attended is also important. When planning or being part of a drug or alcohol prevention program the school nurse needs to consider the developmental level of the students being instructed, local district policy, and the community where the school is located. Knowledge of illegal drugs, how they are used, and their effects is important.

The U.S. Department of Education has developed grade-specific curricula for drug prevention education that provide a sound framework for the nurse to use or expand on when developing a more individualized program for particular students. It, along with a multitude of resources and information, is available free of charge from the National Clearinghouse for Drug and Alcohol Information. Many state and local governments have also developed educational programs and activities, and coordinating the school program with these community resources is ideal. No single program has proven superior in all groups of children. Like antismoking education, other skills that improve self-esteem and communication and increase knowledge are the focus and have been shown to be beneficial.

The use of inhalants among children and teens has been an increasing concern for school nurses. Aerosol products such as cleaners, solvents, adhesives, hair spray, or even whipped cream are being misused by students to get a high. In fact, because they are legal to purchase, they have become more popular with younger students than marijuana. Recently it has become the drug of choice for the "**tween**" population, 12–13 years olds (SAMHSA, 2008). This widespread problem has prompted some states to pass laws restricting the sale of spray paints and cold medicines.

Parents are often unaware of how these products are being misused, and children can be unaware of the dangers. "Sniffing" or "huffing" these products to get high is dangerous, as the chemicals dissolve the protective myelin around brain cells. This can result in mental impairment including disorientation, a drunken appearance, unconsciousness, slurred speech, bizarre behaviors, personality changes, and damage to the nervous, cardiovascular, and respiratory systems leading to sudden death (U.S. Department of Health and Human Services, 2008). School nurses need to be aware of the signs of inhalant use and be prepared to act in an emergency. When planning any drug prevention program, the dangers of inhalants must be included.

Statistics can be startling when the percentages of youths who use alcohol or take drugs are laid out in black and white. Alcohol and drug use in teens is not just a school problem but a problem that has an ongoing impact on society. Experimentation with these substances is starting at a younger age than any parent, educator, or health professional wants to believe. In addition, children are experimenting with prescription drugs of friends or family members.

TABLE 5-2 Signs of Inhalant Use

Inhalants are known as glue, kick, bang, sniff, huff, poppers, whippets, Texas shoeshine. Signs of use may include:

- Slurred speech
- Dazed, dizzy, or drunk-like appearance
- Unusual breath odor
- Chemical odor on clothing
- Frequent runny nose
- Red eyes

Adapted from Tips for Teens. (2008). U.S. Dept. of Health and Human Services.

FAMILY TEACHING

Helping Parents Be Aware of Drug/Alcohol Use in Their Children

It is important to teach parents the signs their children may be using drugs or alcohol including poor academic performance, higher dropout rates, low self-esteem, and withdrawal from family activities.

Providing children with the skills to make healthy choices and the ability to resist pressures must begin early. The school is the logical place for learning and practicing these skills. The nurse can be a resource, instructor, or coordinator for these programs and assist schools in meeting this important need. Chapter 35 provides further information on substance abuse in children.

VIOLENCE PREVENTION

The United States continues to have an alarming rate of violent crimes compared to other industrial nations. Homicide is in the top four in causes of death in 10- to 24-year-olds (CDC, 2008a). The scary truth is that violence occurs on school property. The Youth Risk Behavior Surveillance of 2007 (CDC, 2008a) reports 18% of students carried a weapon and admitted to bringing it to school. Five and a half percent of children reported being afraid to go to school because they felt unsafe at school or on the bus (CDC, 2008a). Violence is seen in inner city and suburban schools across the nation. Additional information on youth violence can be found in Chapter 12.

Newspaper headlines across the United States shock us with reports of school violence. Americans have read about children not only bringing guns to school but opening fire on classmates and staff. In 1998, we read about a student in Pennsylvania shooting a teacher; two Arkansas boys killing four girls and a teacher; a 15-year-old Oregon student opening fire in a cafeteria, killing 2 and wounding 22 students; and an Illinois student gunned down at an alternative school by a rival gang member. In 1999, we read about two Colorado students killing 15 and injuring many more in a shooting rampage that involved guns and explosives (National Education Association, 1999). In 2008, a student killed 6 and injured 18 in a campus lecture hall in DeKalb, Illinois (Twonney, Demirjian, & Gocca, 2008) and, as part of a gang initiation, a teen stabbed a high school teacher several times, blinding her for life in Elgin, Illinois (Fergus & Marrazzott, 2008). These are the extremes of violence in the school. But violence affects 55 million school children a year (CDC, 2008a), can include bullying and intimidation, and can be physical or emotional.

Long-term exposure to violence affects the cognitive, psychological, and moral development of children. Some researchers believe children who have experienced violence are prone to difficulties in school such as concentrating, mental impairment, uncaring behavior, powerlessness, aggressive play, and lasting symptoms of stress (CDC, 2008a). Media attention focuses on violence at school, but children experience violence at home and in the community as well.

The continued incidences of violence in schools have furthered the development of violence prevention programs. Some are grade level specific; others are more general and provide instruction for grades kindergarten through 12. Research is still evaluating the effectiveness of these programs. What they have discovered is that, for violence prevention programs to be effective, they must be matched to the developmental level of the child. Although violence prevention needs to begin in the early grades, teaching strategies and interventions that work in primary grades do not necessarily meet the needs of middle- or high-school students. Teaching needs to be interactive, allowing group work, role-playing, and practice time for skills across multiple environments. Education on nonviolent responses to situations, conflict management, self-esteem development, and crime prevention can build the base for further interventions. The use of metal detectors, locker searches, and dress codes reduces the possibility of violence. Providing adolescents with other outlets such as sports and after-school clubs reinforces school teachings and policies.

Training school staff is crucial to the success of any prevention program. Teachers and nurses may be uncomfortable with the topic, but they need to learn how to help students handle violence. The school must make violence prevention a priority. Education provided by a handful of teachers is less effective than education in a school system where the program starts early and builds through the grade levels. Having strategies available in class and during less structured times and having teachers and staff as role models is more effective. Developing a curriculum with culture and ethnic sensitivity is important but difficult to implement in schools with an interracial mix of students; it is better to stress that every child deserves courtesy and respect no matter their background. Parental and community support and involvement are needed for any program to be successful. Lastly, schools must develop set rules and policies on how violence will be dealt with on school grounds. Regulatory strategies, like those previously mentioned, lower the risk for violence with penalties and legal consequences.

An increasing concern in today's schools is bullying. Bullying can be violent or nonviolent harassment and can include threats or intimidations, verbal cursing, social isolation, and teasing. Many adults make light of this type of harassment but it remains a form of bullying. Bullying has been shown to leave long-term psychological effects on mental health and school performance. It has been correlated to increased absent rates, school drop out rates, anxiety, depression, and worsening grades (Meyer-Adams, 2008). The FBI has discovered that 71% of school shooters complained of experiencing bullying (Reuter-Rice, 2008). Fifteen to twenty percent of this nation's students reported verbal teasing and 90% of children 4–8 years of age reported being a victim of bullying (Reuter-Rice, 2008). Bullying may come to the school nurse's attention first because often the victim has frequent psychosomatic complaints or school avoidance. Other symptoms of being bullied are sleeplessness, depression, and attempted suicide. It is imperative the school nurse remains alert for signs of bullying or harassment. Being available and approachable to students and providing a caring presence and safe environment fosters confidence and a willingness to disclose sensitive information regarding a bullying incident. Like other acts of violence, school districts need to adopt a "zero tolerance" approach to bullying. The school nurse can be a strong advocate in the development and implementation of these policies.

> **NURSING TIP**
>
> **Bullying**
>
> Any one working in a school should read "Please Stop Laughing at Me" by Jodee Blanco (2003), a firsthand account from a young girl and an eye-opening view on the long term consequences of bullying.

PSYCHOLOGICAL SERVICES

School psychological services focus on issues such as child abuse, crisis intervention, suicide, and disaster preparedness. Child abuse includes physical, sexual, and emotional abuse, and emotional or physical neglect. All states have mandated reporting laws and the school nurse, being a health care professional, is included on that list. The school nurse's main focus in child abuse or neglect issues is awareness and recognition of the signs of abuse, and then reporting them to the appropriate authorities. Documenting assessment and history, if abuse is suspected, is extremely important since health records from the school can be admissible in court. However, before taking photographs of the child to document observable signs of abuse, it is important to check with local and state laws since digital photos may not be admissible in court because they can be altered, so use caution in obtaining the correct equipment. A report from a child indicating abuse must be documented in the child's exact words. Most states have official forms that are required to be completed and submitted to the caseworker assigned to the child. Because of the legal ramifications and the seriousness of this situation the school nurse must know the laws and procedures for his/her school district and state. The nurse can also be instrumental in prevention activities by either teaching or referring parents to local resources for improving parenting practices. For more information about child abuse and neglect see Chapter 36 and contact the National Committee to Prevent Child Abuse at 1-800-CHILDREN or the Child Welfare Information Gateway at http://www.childwelfare.gov.

DISASTER PREPAREDNESS IN THE SCHOOL/CRISIS INTERVENTIONS

As the only health professional on staff, the school nurse must be ready in case a crisis or traumatic event occurs. Traumatic events include natural disasters such as fires, tornadoes, hurricanes, and earthquakes, and acts of violence such as riots or random shootings similar to those reported in the media. Think back a few years to hurricane Katrina, which impacted and displaced families across multiple states. As far north as Illinois, schools were receiving children of families whose houses were gone. Bioterrorism and its effects on schoolchildren, unfortunately, have now also been added to this list. In any of these situations, the nurse's role involves planning, training, and identifying resources for referral. Every school should have an emergency plan for natural and human-made disasters that has been practiced so it can quickly and efficiently be put into action. The school nurse can be part of the team that develops, practices, and evaluates these plans and must also be prepared to handle all possible emergency situations. This requires training in emergency procedures, knowing triage and methods of handling mass trauma, and surveillance and precautions for biological agents and **bioterrorism protocols** since school personnel may expect the nurse to direct and lead them in such situations.

Finally, the school nurse can be an excellent resource for staff, parents, and students when handling the aftermath of disasters since children and adults may be affected after the actual crisis has passed. They may have seen a classmate severely injured or killed, have been injured themselves and unable to attend a friend's funeral, or simply not know what to do with the feelings they are experiencing when a friend commits suicide. Working closely with crisis counselors and social workers, the nurse can assist students and staff through this difficult period or provide referrals as appropriate.

However, psychological services do not have to be related to a crisis event that the whole school experiences. The school nurse may be needed to provide psychological services to students experiencing emotional stress due to a family situation such as separation, divorce, or death. Other students may be diagnosed with depression. The nurse may also learn about individual situations through a concerned teacher. In all these situations the nurse's focus should be on identifying signs of stress in the child and on

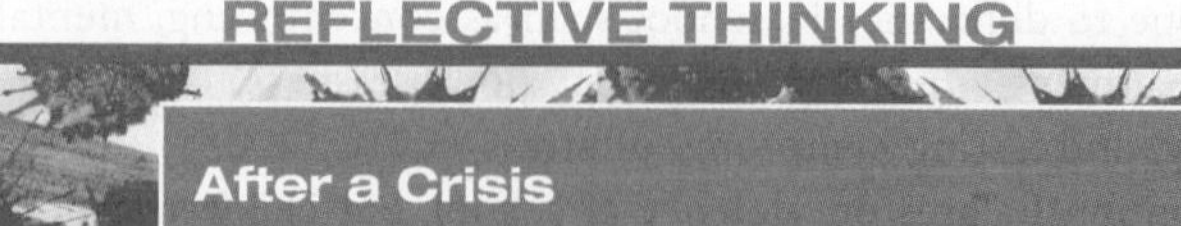

After a Crisis

A child from the school where you work was reported missing. Several weeks later, her body was found. During that period between when she went missing and when her body was found, the community was in fear of a stranger abducting their children. Sadly, it was a family member who took the life of the young girl. As the school nurse and a member of the community, how do you help deal with this loss in the school, the fear of parents and staff, and your own shock and fears? What plans might you make for providing an intervention or counseling for the student body?

Reflections from a Teacher

Jim is on multiple medications at home and at school. I know he has ADHD and sees a psychiatrist. Recently, I heard he has been diagnosed with depression. Sometimes around 10 A.M. he just gets too antsy sitting in the classroom. I know he has established a relationship with our school nurse. When his frustration level is about ready to top off, he asks to go to see her for an illness of some sort. I know he is not sick, but I allow him to go. The school nurse told me he comes in and just sits and talks about home, class, TV, whatever he wants, and she just sits and listens. Within 5 or 10 minutes, he's ready to come back to class. The simple act of walking to the nurse's office and expressing his frustrations or thoughts to someone he believes cares about him calms him down. He's more productive in his schoolwork when he returns.

working closely with the child, teacher, and social worker to provide support and to know when to refer for additional out-of-school support. If the child is under the care of a physician or psychiatrist, the nurse's role is to act as a liaison between the school and other health professionals and to monitor the administration and effects of prescribed medication. The goal, as always, is to assist the child and family through the crisis allowing the student to be available for learning.

MULTIDISCIPLINARY TEAMS

Besides giving first aid care, overseeing various screening services, and health promotion education, the school nurse plays an important role as part of a multidisciplinary team assessing and evaluating children for special education services. The **pupil personnel team**, or service team, is a team of professionals who work together with teachers to provide interventions for students having difficulties. The team may consist of the principal, social worker, school psychologist, speech therapist, regular education teacher, special education teacher, special education supervisor, and school nurse. Other specialists participate as appropriate. If a teacher feels a student is having trouble learning or concentrating or is displaying other difficulties, the situation may be informally discussed with colleagues in searching for different approaches. If these approaches do not work, the teacher asks the caregiver or guardian for permission to discuss the child with the team. The teacher and the caregiver then share with the team the concerns and what has been used in the past. The team brainstorms, offering additional information they may have about the student. Interventions are suggested and a date is set for the team to reconvene to determine if progress has been made. Before the team reconvenes, members may observe the child in various class situations, provide screenings, and gather more information. When the team meets again, they determine if the problem has been resolved. If the problem has been resolved, the teacher continues to monitor the child as needed. If difficulties are still present, special testing, often called a full case study, is needed. Permission from the child's guardian is necessary for this extensive evaluation, and specific Federal and State guidelines for testing must be followed.

Once permission is obtained, each team member has specific assessments or tests to perform, including IQ tests, processing tests, speech and language screenings or evaluations, adaptive skills and social developmental histories, and an in-depth health history. This health history can include information on prenatal complications, developmental milestones, past hospitalizations, past and current medical conditions, allergies, medications, and information on diet, sleep, fine and gross motor skills, and activities of daily living. A recent vision and hearing screening must be on file or be completed before other testing is begun. The idea is to determine if health-related issues are adversely affecting the child's ability to learn. In addition, screening tools for ADHD may be included if that is a concern. The school nurse can obtain written permission for the release of records from physicians' offices or medical testing if appropriate and can often provide additional information if the child has a diagnosed medical condition.

On completion of testing, the team sets up a meeting with the child's caregivers. All results are presented and explained, and eligibility for special education is determined using federal, state, and district guidelines (Table 5-3).

If the child needs special services, an **Individual Education Plan (IEP)**, a written plan spelling out the type and amount of services needed for that particular child, is developed. If health issues are adversely impacting the child's ability to learn, the school nurse will write goals to be included in the child's plan. All children do not qualify for special education services. Federal, state, and district eligibility criteria exist and must be followed. The team, including the nurse, strives to make sure accommodations are made so that the needs of all children are met so they can continue to learn and meet their potential. A child who does not qualify for special education services under state and federal laws, but has some type of disability may qualify for a **504 plan**. Please see Suggested Readings for further information on this law.

CHILDREN WITH UNIQUE HEALTH CONCERNS

For some school nurses, an increasing amount of the day is committed to the specialized care of students with unique health needs. Public schools are now providing education to children with complex medical diagnoses who a decade ago would not have lived or been able to attend their neighborhood school. In 1984, the U.S. Supreme Court ruled in favor of an 8-year-old girl, named Amber Tatro, who had spina bifida. The court ruling stated that the Irving Independent School District had to provide supportive services to Amber so she could attend school, including providing nursing services in the form of clean intermittent catheterization (CIC). Even though the school district argued that CIC was a medical service and too expensive to be provided at school (Vitello, 1989), Amber won the case. Other cases followed, but children who needed more extensive care were denied admission to school. In 1987, a Pennsylvania court ruled in favor of the school district in the case of a 7-year-old boy with multiple handicaps. The boy required extensive care, including oxygen, tracheotomy care, gastrostomy feedings, and chest physical therapy. Because a mucous plug could clog his breathing at any time, someone was needed at his side continuously. The court ruled that, in this case, services were medically extensive, expensive, and beyond the ordinary related services of a school nurse (Vitello, 1989). Admission to school was denied.

In 1999, however, things changed, because Garret Frey won his case against the Cedar Rapids, Iowa Community School District. Garret was a teen who was ventilator dependent, had a tracheotomy, and required gastrostomy feeding, tracheal suctioning, and catheterization. The U.S. Supreme

TABLE 5-3 Eligibility for Special Education

ELIGIBILTY	CRITERIA
Autism	Developmental disability significantly affecting verbal and nonverbal communication and social interaction, generally evident before age three.
Deaf-Blindness	Concomitant hearing and visual impairments, the combination of which causes such severe communication and other developmental and educational needs that they cannot be accommodated in special education programs solely for children with deafness or children with blindness.
Deafness	Hearing impairment so severe that the child is impaired in processing language through hearing.
Emotional Disturbance	Condition with one or more specified characteristics, time frames, or severities.
Hearing Impairment	Impairment in hearing, whether permanent or fluctuating, not included under the definition of deafness in this section.
Mental Retardation	Significantly subaverage general intellectual functioning along with adaptive behavior deficits.
Multiple Disablities	Concomitant impairments which, in combination, cause severe educational needs that cannot be accommodated in special education programs.
Orthopedic Impairment	Orthopedic impairment that adversely affects a child's educational performance. May include congenital anomaly, impairments caused by disease, and other causes (e.g., cerebral palsy, amputations).
Other Health Impairment	Limited strength, vitality, or alertness, including heightened alertness due to a chronic or acute health problem.
Specific Learning Disability	Disorder in one or more of the basic psychological processes involved in understanding or in using spoken or written language.
Speech and language Impairment	Communication disorder, such as stuttering, impaired articulation, a language impairment, or a voice impairment.
Traumatic Brain Injury	Acquired injury to the brain resulting in total or partial functional disability or psychosocial impairment; applies to open or closed head injuries resulting in impairments in one or more areas of brain functioning (congenital or degenerative or birth trauma do not apply).
Vision Impairment	An impairment in vision that, even with correction, adversely affects a child's educational performance. The term includes both partial sight and blindness.
Developmental Delay	A developmental delay in one or more of the following areas: physical development, cognitive development, communication development, social or emotional development, or adaptive development in children between 3 and 9 years of age.

Adapted from US Dept of Education. (2009) "Building the Legacy: IDEA 2004. Regulations: Part 300 Section 300.8. This list is not meant as full definitions of eligibilities. Please see website for exact criteria. http://www.idea.ed.gov.

Court ruled the school district had to provide nursing services to carry out Garret's extensive daily care. Without nursing care, he would have been unable to attend school (Gelfman & Schwab, 2000).

This case has an impact on children with disabilities across the nation, because ruling in Garret's favor could force school districts to expand their definition of related services and pay for nursing care for children with extensive health needs. With advances in technology and medical breakthroughs, premature babies are surviving at younger and younger gestational ages. Previously fatal childhood illnesses are controlled with extensive treatments and medications, and children who survive major traumas and head injuries are receiving rehabilitation services and recovering to their fullest potential. These children are entering or returning to school, and school nurses are extremely important in supporting their education. In fact, many would not be able to attend school without the services of a nurse. All of these children may not have health needs as complex as Garret's, but their cases are no less important.

The Individuals with Disabilities Education Act (IDEA) of 1990 required children with special needs to be educated in the least-restrictive environment. In 1992, parents in Chicago filed a suit against the Chicago Public School system, the Corey H. case, arguing children with complex medical and educational needs have the right to be educated in the regular classroom setting with nondisabled peers to the maximum extent appropriate (Asa, 1998). Most recently, lawsuits have been filed involving children with diabetes and their right to monitor their blood sugars and have appropriate personnel to assist them in administering insulin at school (Figure 5-21). As a result, children with disabilities, chronic illnesses, and high technology nursing needs are in their neighborhood schools. School nurses will need to organize their day so they are available to provide services like CIC or gastrostomy feedings. These additional responsibilities may mean traveling to several buildings in one day and keeping up to date with advances in direct services and community services.

Food allergies in children also create a potential problem in the school setting. Children with allergies to peanuts, milk, bee stings, latex, and other substances are scattered throughout schools throughout the country. Some of these allergies are mild and most problems can be prevented by the child simply avoiding eating certain foods. For other children exposure to an allergen can be life-threatening. The school nurse must be aware of each of these students and the severity of their allergies. Proper school personnel should be notified so that these children are not provided snacks or materials that may harm them. An Individualized Emergency Medical Plan must be written and available in the event of an allergic reaction. Proper medications and permissions must be in place and staff prepared to handle emergencies caused by allergic reactions. The child's school environment must be evaluated to ensure it is safe for him or her. This may mean establishing a "peanut-free lunchroom" or restricting certain snacks in the classroom. The school nurse is the coordinator of these services and liaison for the child, parent, doctor, and school to keep communication open and avoid, if at all possible, an exposure to known allergens. For further information about allergies and anaphylaxis please see Chapter 27.

With this increase in children with special needs and budget constraints, some school districts are also looking for new ways to provide for the health care needs of their students. Some districts are training assistance personnel or **unlincensed personnel (ULP)** to perform direct services, such as first aid, medication administration, glucose monitoring, tube feedings, and catheterizations. ULPs are individuals trained to work in an assistive role to the licensed registered

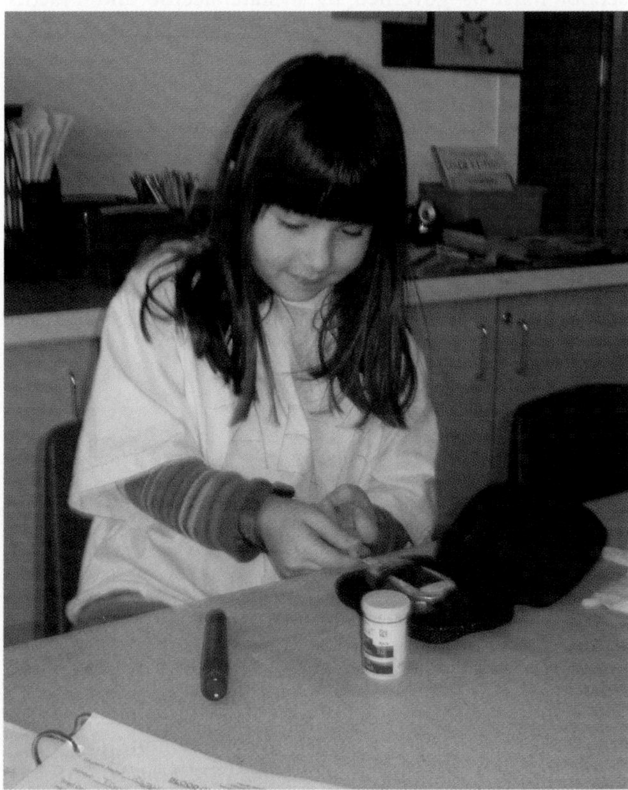

FIGURE 5-21 The growing number of children with diabetes in the school has forced the nurse to be creative in how to assist these children with blood glucose testing. DELMAR CENGAGE LEARNING.

IN THE REAL WORLD

I had been a pediatric nurse for 23 years. When I went back to school and became a school nurse, I admit I was looking forward to a slower pace. My nurse friends laughed at me and told me it would be a boring job. When I spent my first day in an elementary school building with 700 children, I realized this job was not what others believed. There was no sitting around giving out Band-Aids. In fact, there was no sitting around, period. There were tube feedings, asthma attacks, falls from playground equipment, hockey stick injuries, health classes to teach, medications to give, families in need of help getting their child glasses, blood sugars to check, multidisciplinary conferences to attend, and special education rules and regulations to learn. Yes, I gave out my share of Band-Aids, but with them came the opportunity to care for children, to teach them to care for themselves, to let them know someone cared about them. The best part of my job is when I'm out somewhere, maybe shopping, and hear a child call out, "Hey Mom, that's my nurse!"

REFLECTIVE THINKING

Special Services

You have been employed as a school nurse in a small school district for several years.

Your district has recently begun to return students with special needs to their home schools. Your new caseload will include daily tube feedings for a student in one building and catheterization assistance in another. How do you feel about providing such services? How do you balance taking care of these students and the needs of the rest of the students? Should the district be required to pay additional money for these services, or should insurance or the government provide assistance?

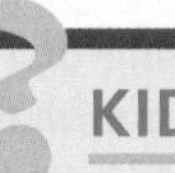

KIDS WANT TO KNOW

Why are some kids in my school in wheelchairs?

As the school nurse in a building with children with special needs, you can help by providing information appropriate to the developmental level of the children regarding disabilities and what they mean and why children use wheelchairs. It would also be helpful to allow time for questions, to read and have available books about children with disabilities, and to encourage teachers to include special education students in class time.

nurse to provide patient care as directed by and under the supervision of the nurse (NASN, 2006c). For a health care professional delegating means "granting legal authority for another person to perform a task which that person otherwise would not be permitted to do" (Texas Department of State Health Services, 2008). The controversy and ethical dilemma lies in the statement "would not otherwise be permitted to do." The nurse who delegates remains accountable for the task. Different states' Nurse Practice Acts have different regulations for delegation, and the school nurse must follow their state regulations and make sure the ULP function and delegation is within the scope of practice. Before delegating a task, the school nurse must ask if the procedure can be legally delegated in their state, who is available to perform the task, what the level of their training is, and whether the student's medical condition is stable. After deciding delegation is appropriate, the school nurse remains responsible for the initial assessment, care plan, training, and supervision of the ULP. NASN's position statement provides direction and recommendations for delegation stated in the "5 Rights of Delegation: right task, right person, right direction, right supervision and right circumstances" (NASN, 2006c).

School nurses remain apprehensive about the widespread use of ULPs for several reasons. First, there is the perceived threat that with budget cuts through school districts, the ULP will become the primary school health provider. School nurses may fear by opening the door a little for the additional help, ULPs will take over all nursing duties. Another reason may be because some school districts do not have clear policies regarding the use of ULPs, causing confusion for the school nurse and the ULPs. School administrators and other personnel may attempt to make decisions on the delegation of nursing tasks without knowing the school nurse retains the ultimate responsibility for the child's care. Third, some nurses may be concerned they are delegating duties to persons not qualified to perform them, but are feeling pressure from administration to delegate the duties against their better judgment or their Practice Act. This can be especially important, since procedures delegated to ULPs are still the responsibility of the nurse (NASN, 2006c). If ULPs are used in the school setting, the school nurse must be involved in developing their role and determining district policies regarding delegation and the ULP's role. Legal ramifications regarding delegation and supervision procedures need to be explored before policies are formalized. Administrators may not understand that the school nurse is governed by a state license and Practice Act which does not always meld with the Board of Education's policies.

Another ethical dilemma and potential legal controversy faced by school nurses today is a child with a "Do Not Attempt to Resuscitate" (DNAR) order at school. School Nurses are working with children with chronic and debilitating conditions and may encounter the situation in which a child's family has made the decision not to resuscitate their child in the event of a respiratory or cardiac failure. The school nurse has multiple roles in assisting this child and

NURSING ALERT

Delegation to Unlicensed Personnel

When unlicensed personnel (ULP) are assigned to provide services to children in the school, you remain accountable for the service. It is your responsibility to see that the ULP is properly trained and competent in the assigned skill before delegating the task. Written instructions, documentation of training, and ongoing supervision are important in delegation. Remember to always consult with your State Nurse Practice Act before delegating any task.

family. School staff is often frightened by a DNAR order at school and worry that "not doing anything" is legally or ethically wrong. The school nurse can advocate for the child and family and relieve the stress of the staff by providing information about how DNAR orders are managed at school. The nurse can notify appropriate local EMS providers and set up a plan so that if the child has an event at school, palliative care will be rendered and the family's wishes will be honored.

Guidelines vary from state to state and district to district but most are in agreement that for a DNAR order to be valid it must be signed by the child's parents and the doctor and dated within a one-year time frame. A DNAR order can be revoked verbally by a parent at any time. Again, check with your state and district policies. In some states, resuscitating a person with a written DNAR order present is considered assault and battery and punishable by law. The NASN recommends that each case should be considered individually and referred to the district's legal counsel. An Individual Health Plan and Individual Emergency Plan must be done in consultation with the caregivers and available to appropriate school staff (NASN, 2004).

SCHOOL NURSING TODAY

The school nurse's role has changed and grown since its experimental beginnings in New York. What started as a way to control communicable diseases in children has evolved into a complicated role that encompasses many different responsibilities and requires a variety of skills. This chapter has reviewed the technical components of the nurse's role and looked at the wide variety of topics included in health promotion education. Today's school nurse must have excellent skills in assessment and triage, communication, and diplomacy. In addition, school nurses must be able to educate children and provide them with a strong base for making healthy lifestyle choices. School nurses must be committed to continuing their education in the ever-changing world of children's health care, technical advances, and federal regulations. School nursing is a well-kept secret, where the responsibilities are endless but the opportunities for positively influencing children are tremendous, and the goal of enabling children to reach their full academic potential is rewarding.

KEY CONCEPTS

- The role of the school nurse, established to decrease the number of children out of school due to infectious diseases, is influenced by societal, political, economic, and educational changes. Starting as a health department position, the role evolved when absenteeism rates were noted to drop. Medical advances and economic changes in our country forced school districts to find ways to provide services to students and the nurse's role expanded.
- The school nurse provides vision/hearing screening, height/weight and BMI measurement, as well as immunization and communicable disease screening.
- Immunization requirements vary from state to state but most include proof of vaccination against DPT, polio, hepatitis B, measles, mumps, rubella, and varicella. Often states require a physical exam and diabetes screening. Some states are now mandating lead screenings for certain geographical areas.
- Emergency care of children in the school includes basic first aid, deciding when to transport to a hospital, and the development of emergency plans.
- An Individual Health Plan—including goals, how they will be met, expected outcomes, and types of services needed—is developed and updated annually and as needed for students with special medical conditions. Many nursing organizations are using the Nursing Interventions Classifications (NIC) and Nursing Outcomes Classifications (NOC) systems to help organize their care plans, provide consistency, and assist with Medicaid billing.
- The nurse's role in health education can include personal and dental hygiene, sex education, antismoking programs, alcohol and drug abuse prevention, and violence prevention information.
- Some school nurses work as part of a multidisciplinary team to provide direct care to children with complex medical needs in a school setting, offering the best environment available for the child's learning.
- Controversial issues now facing the school nurse are delegation and working with unlicensed personnel in the school and providing services to the child with a DNAR order at school.

REVIEW ACTIVITIES

1. Changes in society and government have influenced the role of the school nurse. Explain how the role has evolved over time.
2. Vision and hearing screenings are mandated in selected grade levels in many states. What other examples of secondary prevention are part of the school nurse's duties?
3. A first grader falls from the playground equipment; a group of children are around him with a teacher's assistant; he is crying loudly. Think of the order in

which you would proceed as you come upon the scene. What would you include in your initial assessment and interventions?

4. A 9-year-old child with diabetes has transferred into your school. Although he tests his own blood sugar, he has not yet learned to administer his own insulin. The personnel in the building are anxious because you are in the building only two days a week. How would you handle monitoring his blood sugar and the need for intermittent administration of insulin when you are not in the building? How would the use of ULPs fit in this scenario?

5. Health education is an important aspect of the school nurse's role. What information would you include when teaching second graders about dental health? What teaching strategies would be appropriate for this group's developmental level? What outside activities could you tie into the lesson? How would you evaluate the teaching?

6. You are the only school nurse covering four elementary schools. Your first priority is a student who needs a tube feeding, but several students in another building need medication at the same time. You have been asked to train the principal of the building to administer medications. What assessments are needed before delegating this task? What would you include in the training? How would you continue to supervise this procedure? What is your liability?

STUDY QUESTIONS

1. All of the following have affected the role development of the school nurse except:
   a. communicable disease rates.
   b. the development of charter schools.
   c. health education curriculum added to the school day.
   d. passage of laws such as the Education for All Handicapped Children Act.

2. This law's main focus was to address the inequality of education for economically disadvantaged children:
   a. IDEA
   b. No Child Left Behind
   c. Rehabilitative Act of 1973
   d. Elementary and Secondary School Act

3. The following rest within the scope of a school nurse's practice except:
   a. referring a 5th grader to the local clinic for his third hepatitis B immunization
   b. diagnosing an ear infection in a 4th grader
   c. presenting a growth and development class to a 6th grade class
   d. screening a 1st grader who is having a difficulty time reading the board

4. Routine vision screening of school-age children is mandated in certain grade levels. The school nurse, however, should be aware of special populations at risk. Which of the following is not a special population considered at risk?
   a. children with diabetes
   b. children who were born prematurely
   c. children whose BMI indicates obesity
   d. children with cerebral palsy

5. Which child would the school nurse not need to refer for further assessment?
   a. 2nd grader with weight of 85 lbs and a BMI of 25 with frequent trips to the bathroom
   b. 3-year-old preschool child with cognitive delays, living in a depressed economic area in an older home with no lead level on file
   c. 6th grade girl with lice
   d. 3rd grader with red conjunctiva, drainage from right eye, and complaint of itchy eyes

6. The most efficient way the school nurse can decrease the spread of infectious disease is to:
   a. provide immunizations at school.
   b. educate students on hand washing.
   c. provide sick day guidelines for parents.
   d. provide for a breakfast program.

7. To provide for the safety of a child with a severe peanut allergy at school the school nurse must first:
   a. develop a IEMP.
   b. post signs in the lunchroom.
   c. meet with caregivers and obtain a complete health history.
   d. notify staff.

8. Some health education topics of special importance for the nurse working with the adolescent population would include all but the following:
   a. sex education
   b. anti-tobacco education
   c. dental health
   d. anti-drug education

9. A 12-year-old boy is sent to the nurse's office with a drunk-like appearance, runny nose, red eyes, and an unusual odor to his breath. The nurse should suspect:
   a. marijuana use.
   b. alcohol use.
   c. inhalant use.
   d. cocaine use.

10. Two ethical and legal issues the nurse working in a school might face are:
    a. special education students and English language learners.
    b. unlicensed personnel (ULP) and special education students.
    c. DNAR orders and unlicensed personnel.
    d. English language learners and DNAR orders.

REFERENCES

American Academy of Pediatrics. (2008). Role of the school nurse in providing school health services. *Pediatrics, 21*(5), 1052–1056.

American Optometric Association. (2008). AOA, School nurses partner to link healthy vision and improved classroom learning. Press release December 10, 2008. http://www.aoa.org.

Asa, R. (1998). Special education entering new era. *Catalyst,* June. http://www.catalyst-chicago.org/arch/06-98/068main.htm; Retrieved October 9, 1010.

Bauman, N. (2008). Enter for hearing loss help. http://www.hearinglosshelp.com/articles/decibelsvspercent.htm. Retrieved February 9, 2009.

Bonaiuto, M. (2007). School nurse case management: Achieving health and educational outcomes. *Journal of School Nursing, 23*(4), 202–209.

Broussard, L. (2007). Empowerment in school nursing practice: A grounded theory approach. *Journal of School Nursing, 23*(6), 322–328.

Centers for Disease Control and Prevention. (2004). Children's Oral Health Fact Sheet, Division of Oral Health. http://www.cdc/gov/OralHealth/publications/factsheets.htm. Retrieved March 6, 2009.

Centers for Disease Control and Prevention. (2006). Cigarette use among high school students, United States, 1991–2005. *MMWR, 55*(26), 724–726.

Centers for Disease Control and Prevention. (2008a). YRBS 2007 Results. *MMWR, 57*(SS-4), June 6, 2008.

Centers for Disease Control and Prevention. (2008b). HIV in the United States. Factsheet. http://www.cdc.gov/hiv/resources/factsheet/us.htm. Retrieved February 13, 2009.

Centers of Disease Control and Prevention. (2009). Sports Injury Statistics Fact Sheet. http://www.cdc.gov/nalpc/factsheet/playgr.html. Retrieved February 23, 2009.

Chauvin, V. (1994). *Students with special health care needs: A manual for school nurses.* Scarborough, ME: NASN.

Clarke, N., Shacks, J., Kerr, A., Bottrell, C., Poulsen, M., & Yin, L. (2008). Use of noncycloplegic autorefractor to perform vision screening in preschools. *Journal of School Nursing, 24*(3). 158–163.

Clay, D., Farris, K., McCarthy, A., Kelly, M., & Howarth, R. (2008). Family perceptions of medication administration at school: Errors, risk factors and consequences. *Journal of School Nursing, 24*(2), 95–102.

Davis, J., & Bauman, K. (2008). School enrollment in United States: 2006 population characteristics.

Denehy, J. (2003). Documentation dilemma: What to record and why. *Journal of School Nursing, 19,* 187–90.

Denehy, J. (2007a). Educational preparation for school nurses. *Journal of School Nursing, 23*(4), 191–192.

Denehy, J. (2007b). Education about sexuality: Are we preparing our youth for today's realities? *Journal of School Nursing, 23*(5), 245–246.

Dunn, M., Ilapogui, V., Taylor, L., Nancy, C., Blackwell, R., Wilder, R., & Givens, C. (2008). Self-reported substance use and sexual behaviors among adolescents in a rural state. *Journal of School Health, 78*(11), 587–593.

Fergus, M., & Marrazzott. (2008). Teaching stabbing detailed. *Chicago Tribune,* Jan. 23, 2008.

Fritz, D., Crane-Wilder, L., Hardin, S., & Horrocks, M. (2008). Program strategies for adolescent smoking cessation. *Journal of School Nursing, 24*(1), 21–27.

Gelfman, M., & Schwab, N. (2000). School health services after Cedar Rapids Independent School District v. Garret F. *Journal of School Nursing, 16,* 54–59.

Harrington, S. (2008). The role of sugar-sweetened beverage consumption in adolescent obesity: A review of literature. *Journal of School Nursing, 24*(1), 3–12.

Jannone, L., & O'Connell, K. (2007). Coping strategies used by adolescents during smoking cessation. *Journal of School Nursing, 23*(3), 177–184.

Johnson, M., Bulechek G., McCloskey-Dochterman, J., Maas, M., Morehead, S., Swanson, E., & Butcher, H. (2006). *NANDA, NOC and NIC linkages: Nursing diagnosis, outcomes, and interventions.* St. Louis: Mosby Elsevier.

Keehner, M., Guttu, M., Warren, M., & Swanson, M. (2008). School nurse case management for children with chronic illness: Health, academic, and quality of life outcomes. *Journal of School Nursing, 24*(4), 205–214.

Kim-Godwin Y. S., Clements C., Bullers S., Maume M., & Demski E. (2007). Sexual behaviors and drinking patterns among middle school and high school students in southeastern North Carolina. *Journal of School Nursing, 23*(4), 214–221.

Meyer-Adams, N. (2008). School violence: Bullying behaviors and the psychosocial social environment in middle schools. *Children and Schools, 30*(4), 211–221.

Morton, J. (2008). "I Feel Good!" A weekly wellness radio broadcast for elementary school children. *Journal of School Nursing, 24*(2), 83–87.

Murphy, M., & Polivka, B. (2007). Parental perceptions of the school's role in addressing childhood obesity. *Journal of School Nursing, 23*(1), 40–46.

National Association of School Nurses. (1999). Definition of school nursing. Retrieved December 21, 2009, from http://www.nasn.org/Default.aspx?tabid=279.

National Association of School Nurses. (2003). *Annual State Affiliate Report Summary.* Scarbough, ME: NASN.

National Association of School Nurses. (2004). Position statement: DNR in the School. Retrieved January 23, 2010, from, http://www.nasn.org/Default.aspx?tabid=217.

National Association of School Nurses. (2006a). NASN Issue Brief: School nursing serves role in health care services: Vision screening. Retrieved January 23, 2010, from http://www.nasn.org/Default.aspx?tabid=284.

National Association of School Nurses. (2006b). Position statement: Caseload assignments. Retrieved January 23, 2010, from http://www.nasn.org/Default.aspx?tabid=209.

National Association of School Nurses. (2006c). Position statement: Delegation. Retrieved January 16, 2010, from http://www.nasn.org/Default.aspx?tabid=349.

National Association of School Nurses. (2006d). Position statement: Immunizations. Retrieved January 23, 2010, from http://www.nasn.org/Default.aspx?tabid=225.

National Association of School Nurses. (2007a). Healthy children learn better. School nurses make a difference. http://www.nasn.org. Retrieved January 3, 2009.

National Association of School Nurses. (2007b). Issue brief: School health nursing services role in health care. Role of the school nurse. Retrieved January 23, 2010, from http://www.nasn.org/Default.aspx?tabid=279.

National Education Association. (1999). Safe schools. *NEA Today, 17*, 4–6.

National Survey on Drug Use and Health (NSDUH). (2009). The NSDUH Report: Marijuana use and perceived risk of use among adolescents: 2002–2007. SAMSHA. Shortreports@samhsa.hhs.gov.

NIDA Notes. (2007). Adolescent inhalant use. *NIDA Notes, 21*(4), 17.

North American Nursing Diagnosis Association (NANDA, International). (2009). *Nursing diagnosis: Definitions and classification 2009–2011*. Wiley-Blackwell.

Olsen, H., Hudson, S., & Thompson, D. (2008). Developing a playground injury prevention plan. *Journal of School Nursing, 24*(3), 131–137.

Passarelli, C. (1994). School nursing: Trends for the future. *Journal of School Nursing, 64*, 141–150.

Reuter-Rice, K. (2008). Male adolescent bullying and the school shooter. *Journal of School Nursing, 24*(6), 350–359.

SAMHSA. (2008). SAMSHA Report. *Alcoholism and Drug Abuse Weekly, 20*(11), 5.

Sawyer, W. (1999). Henry the Hand Program. Retrieved January 23, 2010, from http://www.henrythehand.com.

Special Education and Rehabilitative Services. (2006). *Federal Register*. http://www.ed.gov/about/offices/list/osers/about.html.

Story, M. (2009). The third school nutrition dietary assessment study: Findings and policy implications for improving the health of US children. *Journal of the American Dietetic Association, 109*(2), S7–S13.

Streng, N. (2007). A follow-up study of former student health advocates. *Journal of School Nursing, 23*(6), 353–358.

Tares, H., & Brennan, J. (2008). Students with chronic disease: Nature of school physician support. *Journal of School Health, 78*(7), 389–396.

Texas Department of State Health Services. (2008). Delegation of health services in Texas public schools. http://www.dshs.state.tx.us/schoolhealth/delegate.shtm. Retrieved January 23, 2010.

Thorell, L., & Rydell, A. (2008) Behavior problems and social competence deficits associated with symptoms of attention deficit/hyperactivity disorder: Effects of age and gender. *Child Care, Health and Development, 34*(5), 584–595.

Tousman, S., Arnold, D., Helland, W., Roth, R., Heshelman, N., Casteneda, O., Fischer, E., O'Neil, K., & Bileto, S. (2007). Evaluation of a hand washing program for second graders. *Journal of School Nursing, 23*(6), 342–348.

Twonney, M., Demirjian, K., & Gocca, M. (2008). Elmhurst student identified as NIU shooting victim. *Chicago Tribune*. Feb. 15, 2008.

U.S. Department of Education. (2009). *Regulations, Part 300 Section 300.8: Building the Legacy: IDEA 2004*. Retrieved December 21, 2009, from http://www.idea.ed.gov.

U.S. Department of Health and Human Services. (2000). *Healthy People 2010*. Washington, DC: Government Printing Office.

U.S. Department of Health and Human Services. (2004). *The Registered Nurse Population: Findings from the 2004 National Sample Survey of Registered Nurses*.

U.S. Department of Health and Human Services. (2008). *Substance Abuse and Mental Health Services Administration*. "Tips for Teens." http://www.samhsa.gov.

U.S. Department of Health and Human Services. (2009). *Healthy People 2020*. Retrieved December 21, 2009, from http://www.healthypeople.gov/HP2020/Objectives/TopicArea.aspx?id=18&TopicArea=Early+and+Middle+Childhood.

University of New Mexico with New Mexico Department of Health. (2008). School nurse emergency preparedness program. http://www.unm.edu.

Vitello, S. (1989). The Detsel case: Limitations of school health services for special education students. *Journal of School Health, 59*, 37–38.

Weismuller, P., Grasska, M., Alexander, M., White, C., & Kramer, P. (2007). Elementary school nurse interventions: Attendance and health outcomes. *Journal of School Nursing, 23*(2), 111–118.

Wilson, L. (2007). Adolescents' attitudes about obesity and what they want in obesity prevention programs. *Journal of School Nursing, 23*(4), 229–238.

Wold, S. (1981). *School nursing: A framework for practice*. St. Louis, MO: Mosby.

SUGGESTED READINGS

Arnold, M., Silkworth, C., & Harrigan, J. (2005). *Individual health car Plans for School Nurses: Concepts, Frameworks and Applications for School Nursing Practice*. North Branch, MN: Sunrise River Press.

Blanco, J. (2003). *Please Stop Laughing At Me*. Avon, MA: Adams Media.

Bulechek, G., Butcher, H., & McCloskey-Dochterman, J. (2008). *Nursing Interventions Classifications (NIC)* (5th ed.). St. Louis, MO.: Mosby Elsevier.

Council of Administrators of Special Education. (2006). *Section 504 and ADA: Promoting student access* (3rd ed.). CASE.

Moorhead, S., Johnson, M., Maas, M., & Swanson, E. (2008) *Nursing Outcomes Classification (NOC)* (94th ed.). St. Louis, MO: Mosby.

National Association of School Nurses. (1994). *Students with special health care needs: A manual for school nurses*. Scarborough, ME: Author.

Nye, B. (2005). *Bill Nye the Science Guy's Great Big Book of Tiny Germs*.

Reber, D., & Dujas, T. (2008). *Magenta Gets Glasses (Blues Clues #10)*. Simon Spotlight: NY.

Smith Stair, K. (2004). *Glasses, Glasses Oh What Do I See*. Book Publishers Network: WA.

Verdick. E. (2006). *Germs Are Not for Sharing*. Free Spirit Publishing: Minneapolis, MN.

RESOURCES

Refer to the online student StudyWARE for Potts & Mandleco at http://www.CengageBrain.com for additional content and study aids.

Organization: **American Academy of Pediatrics**
Description: Offers general information related to child health, specific guidelines concerning many pediatric issues, information regarding AAP programs, activities, policies, guidelines, publications, and other child health resources.
Website/Resource: http://www.aap.org

Organization: **American School Health Association**
Description: Offers information regarding American School Health Association initiatives/projects, advocacy/resolutions, corporate support, continuing education, and conferences.
Website/Resource: http://www.ashaweb.org

Organization: **Child Abuse: Child Welfare Gateway**
Description: Provides access to print/electronic publications, websites, online databases covering a wide range of topics (child welfare, child abuse/neglect, adoption, search/reunion, etc.)
Website/Resource: http://www.childwelfare.gov

Organization: **Glitterbug Brevis Corporation**
Description: GlitterBug makes hand hygiene education interesting, fun, and memorable and offers products useful for teaching proper hand hygiene techniques; website offers product information, helpful downloads, shopping opportunities.
Website/Resource: http://www.glitterbug.com

Organization: **National Association of School Nurses (NASN)**
Description: Offers information regarding continuing education, helpful resources, education campaigns, policy/advocacy, and research, as well as professional information to active school nurses.
Website/Resource: http://www.nasn.org

Organization: **National Association of School Nurses** Position Statement: Medication Administration in the School Setting
Description: The article discusses current implementations of delegating medication administration to unlicensed assistive personnel.
Website/Resource: http://www.nasn.org/Default.aspx?tabid=230

Organization: **National Clearing House for Drug and Alcohol Information**
Description: Offers general information regarding many classes of drugs, drug/alcohol issues, and recent publications.
Website/Resource: http://www.ncadi.samhsa.gov

Organization: **Prevent Child Abuse America (PCA America)**
Description: Offers information about upcoming child abuse conferences, research, advocacy, and publications.
Website/Resource: http://www.preventchildabuse.org

Organization: **Tar Wars**
Description: Offers information about Tar Wars coordinators, national conferences, classroom presentations, and poster contests related to being tobacco free, making positive decisions regarding health, and promoting personal responsibility.
Website/Resource: http://www.tarwars.org

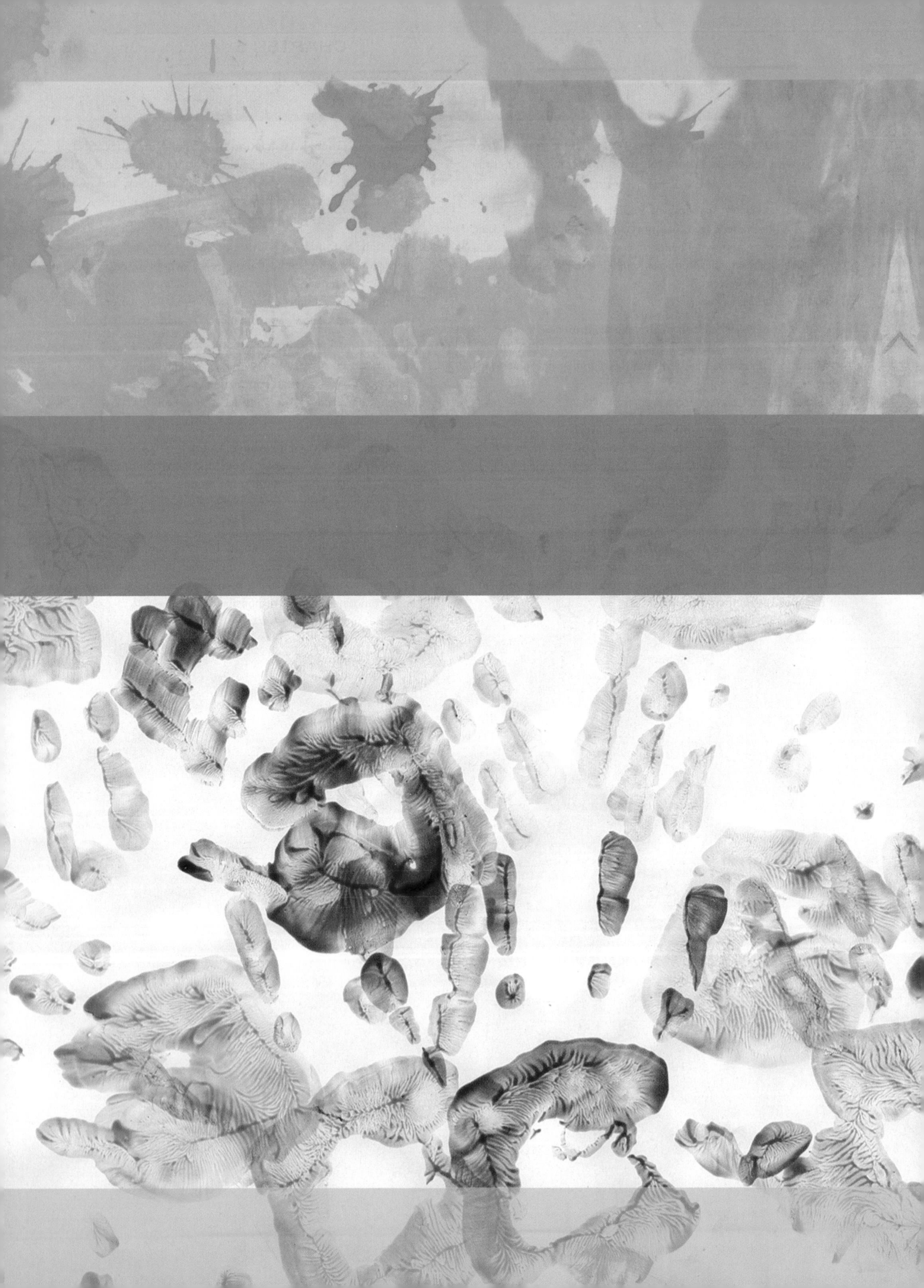

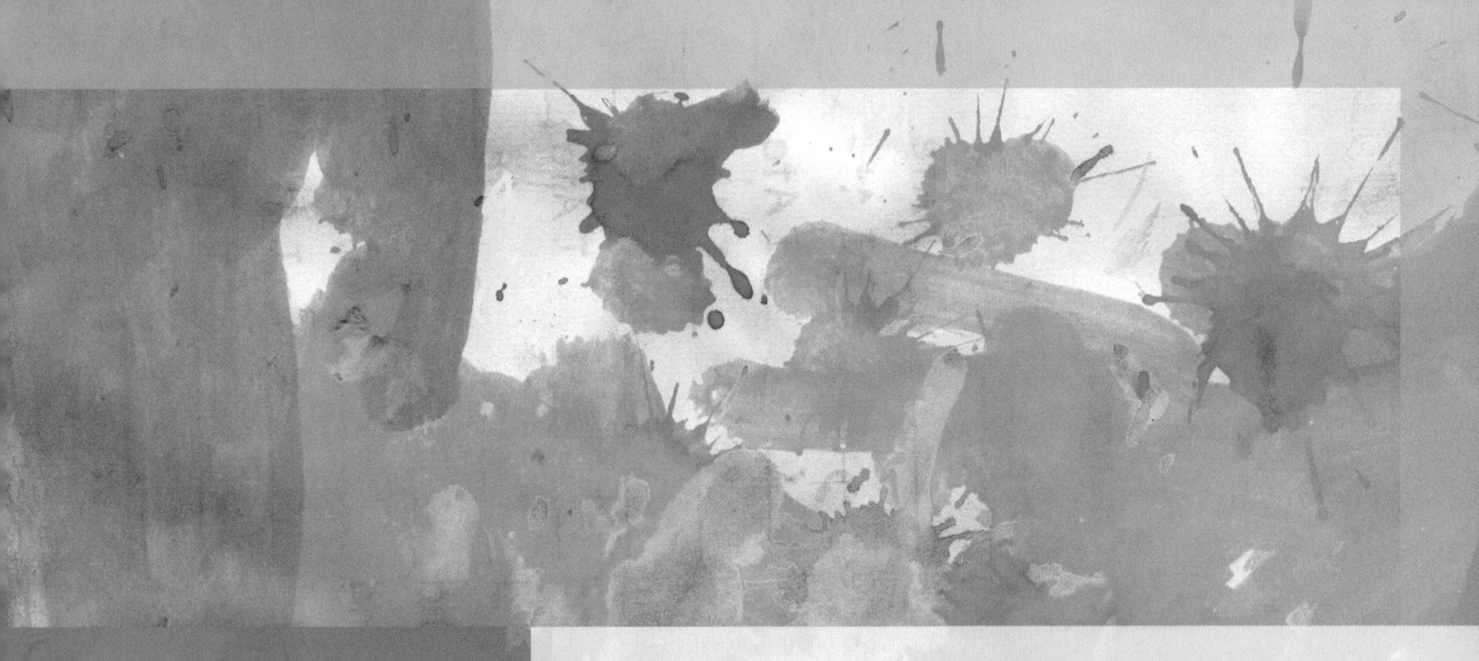

UNIT 2 Growth and Development of Children

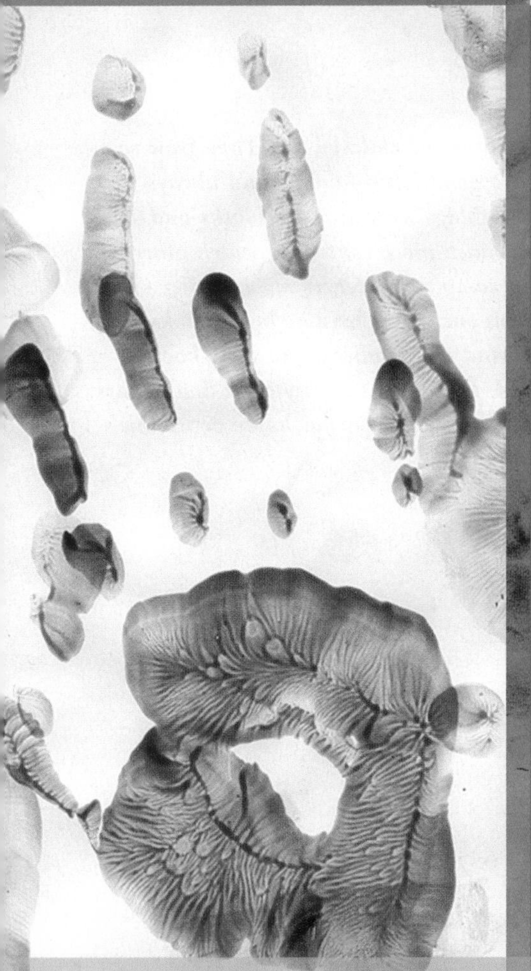

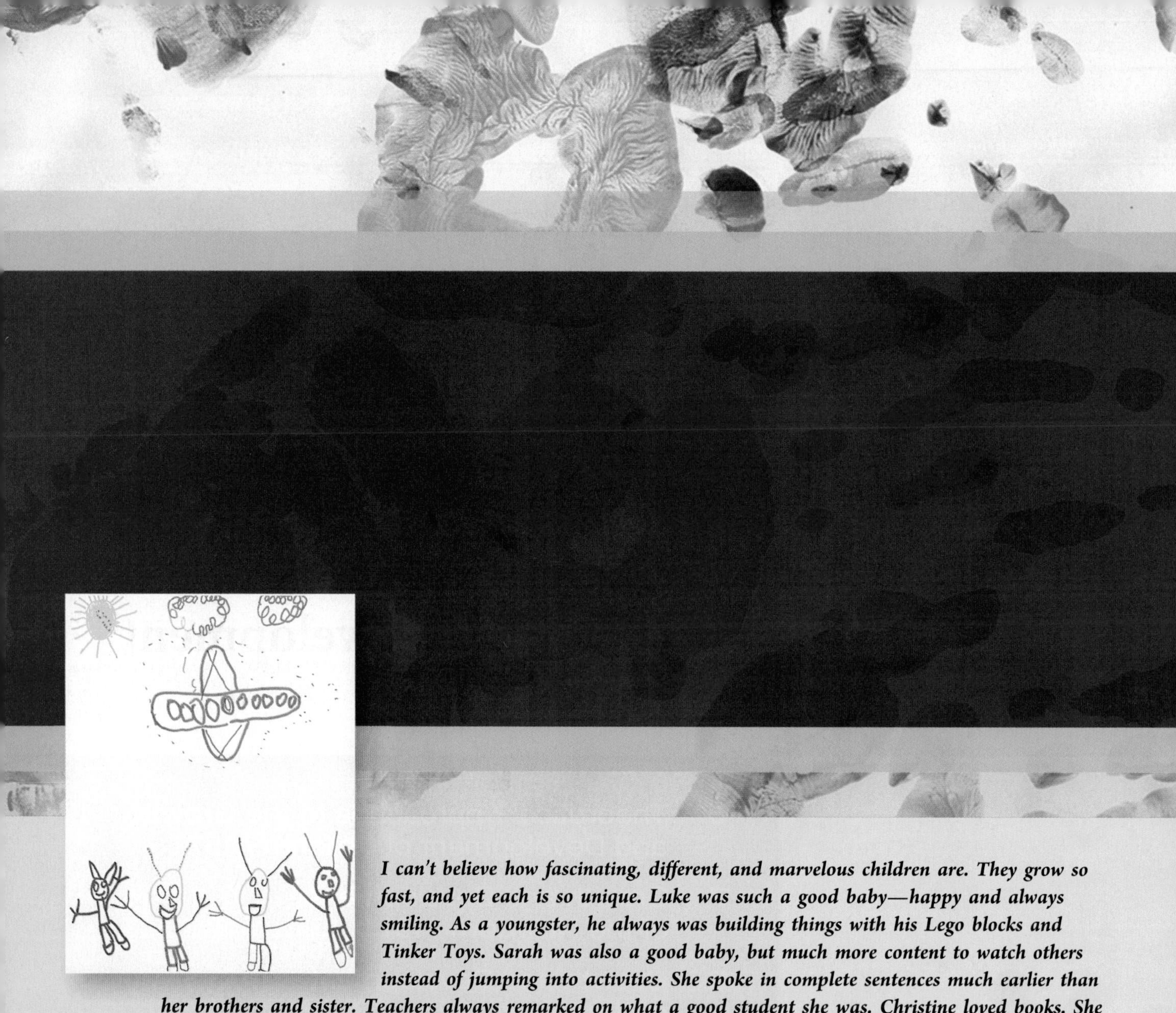

I can't believe how fascinating, different, and marvelous children are. They grow so fast, and yet each is so unique. Luke was such a good baby—happy and always smiling. As a youngster, he always was building things with his Lego blocks and Tinker Toys. Sarah was also a good baby, but much more content to watch others instead of jumping into activities. She spoke in complete sentences much earlier than her brothers and sister. Teachers always remarked on what a good student she was. Christine loved books. She would always climb on to her dad's lap with a book for him to read … and it was always the same book! I wondered why she never tired of hearing the story. Then there was Chad. He too was a busy child and always had friends over. When he was about 8, I think his friend Ronnie and he were either at our house or Ronnie's house for dinner every night during the summer months.

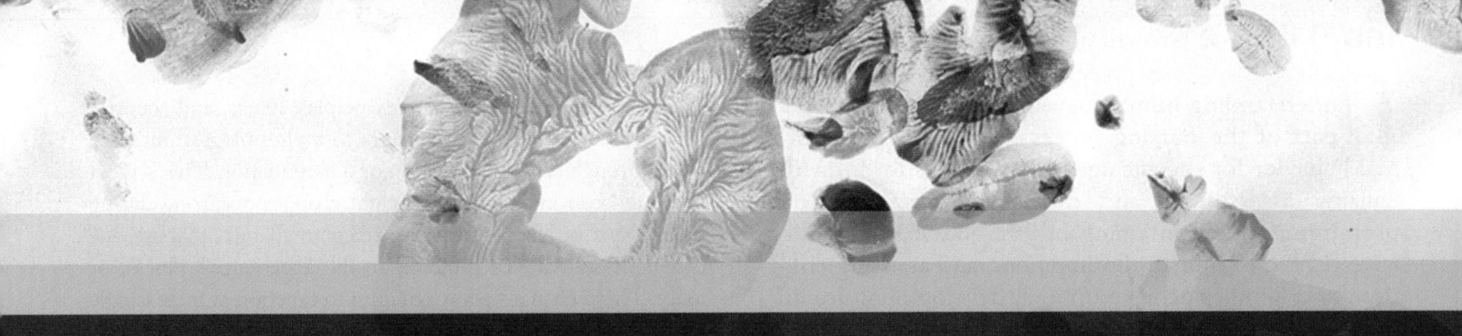

CHAPTER 6

Theoretical Approaches to the Growth and Development of Children

BARBARA L. MANDLECO, RN, PHD

COMPETENCIES

Upon completion of this chapter, the reader will be able to:

- Identify and describe eight principles of human development.
- Explain how these principles are applied to the various theories of human development.
- Compare and contrast the major theories of human development.
- Describe, compare, and contrast the major themes of human development.
- Explain how the major developmental themes can be applied to the theories of human development.
- Apply theories of human development to pediatric nursing practice.
- Successfully complete the games and activities in the online student StudyWARE

Understanding human development is an essential part of the nursing process. Knowledge of normal behavior for specific age groups allows for individualizing assessments and care plans. Emphasis on promoting and maintaining health, anticipatory guidance related to human development, and assisting children and families achieve optimal development are all important aspects of pediatric nursing. Knowledge of several principles, issues, and theories help nurses understand holistic optimal development and care. This chapter will describe the various principles and themes that are interwoven within the major developmental theories discussed. Each theory will be fully explained and analyzed. The discussion will also include ideas on how the nurse can apply the theories to practice.

GROWTH, MATURATION, AND DEVELOPMENT

Growth, maturation, and development are common terms used to describe human development. An explanation of these terms and of the age ranges associated with child development is needed before principles, issues, and theories can be understood. **Growth** refers to a physiological increase in size through cell multiplication or differentiation. This is most obviously seen in weight and height changes occurring during the first year of life. **Maturation** refers to changes that are due to genetic inheritance rather than life experiences, illness, or injury. These changes allow children to function at increasingly higher and more sophisticated levels as they get older. **Development** refers to the predictable physiological, psychosocial, and cognitive changes occurring over one's life span due to growth, maturation, and learning, and assumes that orderly and specific situations lead to new activities and behavior patterns (Shaffer & Kipp, 2010) (Figure 6-1).

The five stages and age ranges of human development relating specifically to pediatric nursing are found in Table 6-1.

PRINCIPLES OF GROWTH AND DEVELOPMENT

At least eight principles providing a framework for studying human development are embedded within the issues and theories discussed in the following pages. Although not all

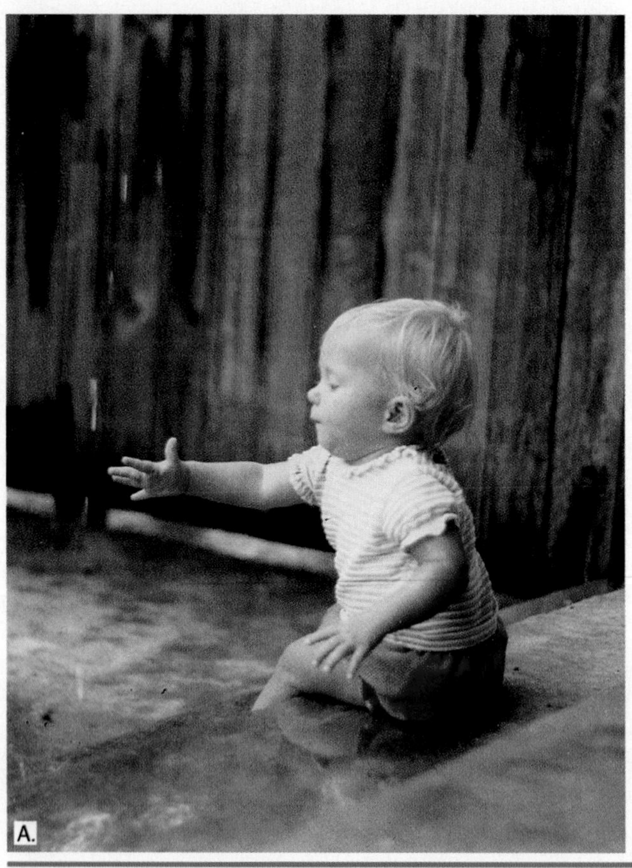

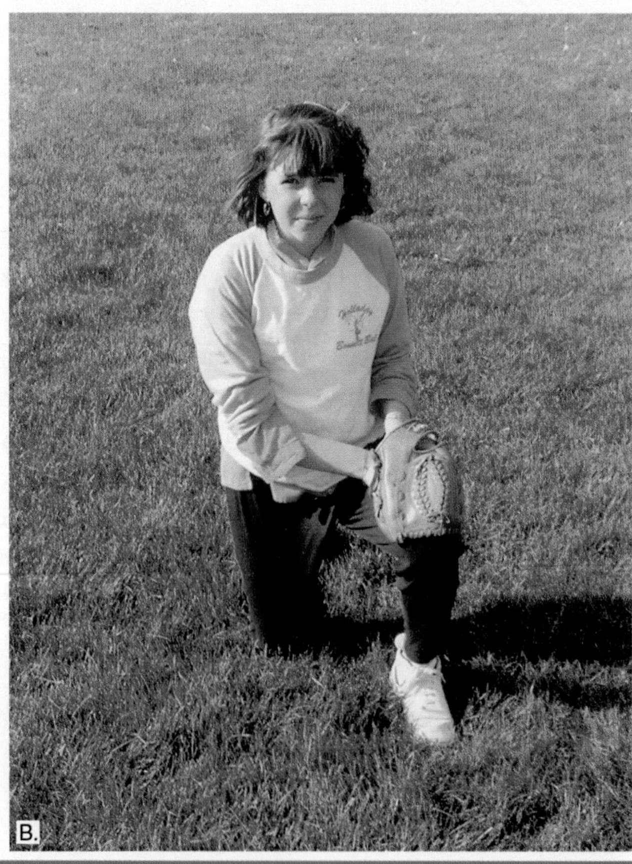

FIGURE 6-1 **(A) Toddlers are curious as they learn about the world around them. (B) School-age children often become involved in physical activities and team sports.** DELMAR CENGAGE LEARNING.

Table 6-1 Stages, Age Ranges, and Characteristics of Human Development Related to Pediatric Nursing

STAGE	AGE	CHARACTERISTICS
Infant	Birth to 1 year	Period of rapid growth and change; attachments to family members and other caregivers are formed; trust develops.
Toddler	1 to 3 years	Motor ability coordination, sensory skills developing; basic feelings, emotions, a sense of self, and being independent become important.
Preschooler	3 to 6 years	Continued physiological, psychological, and cognitive growth; better able to care for themselves, interested in playing with other children; beginning to develop a concept of who they are.
School age	6 to 12 years	Interested in achievement; ability to read, write, and complete academic work advances; understanding of the world broadens.
Adolescent	12 to 19 years, or later	Transition period between childhood and adulthood; physiological maturation occurs, formal operational thought begins; preparation for becoming an adult takes place.

of these principles are proven by research, they are often observed in children and generally assumed to be true (Shaffer & Kipp, 2010).

Development is orderly and sequential. This principle suggests that maturation follows a predictable and universal timetable. For example, children learn to crawl before they learn to walk, and they learn to walk before they learn to run. These changes occur rapidly during the first year of life and slowly during middle and late childhood. Even though the onset and length of each developmental change vary among children, the basic sequence is the same, allowing comparison to norms.

1. *Development is directional.* Skill development proceeds along two different pathways: cephalocaudal and proximodistal. **Cephalocaudal** development proceeds from the head downward. Therefore, areas closest to the brain or head develop first, followed by the trunk, then legs and feet. For example, head control is followed by sitting, then crawling, and then walking. **Proximodistal** development proceeds from the inside out. Controlled movements closest to the body's center (trunk, arms) develop before controlled movements distant to the body (fingers). For example, grasping changes from using the entire hand to just the fingers as infants get older (Figure 6-2).
2. *Development is unique for each child.* Every child has a unique timetable for physiological, psychosocial, cognitive, and moral development (Figure 6-3). For example, some children can name four colors by the time they are 3 years old, whereas others cannot name four colors until they are 4½ years old. Some children walk well at 11 months; others do not walk well until they are 14 months old.
3. *Development is interrelated.* Physiological, psychosocial, cognitive, and moral aspects of development affect and are affected by one another. For example, central nervous system maturation is necessary for cognitive development. Children cannot be independent in toileting if they are not aware of the urge to void and cannot independently remove clothing.
4. *Development becomes increasingly differentiated.* This means responses become more specific and skillful as the child grows. Young infants respond to stimuli in a generalized way involving the entire body, whereas older children respond to specific stimuli in a more

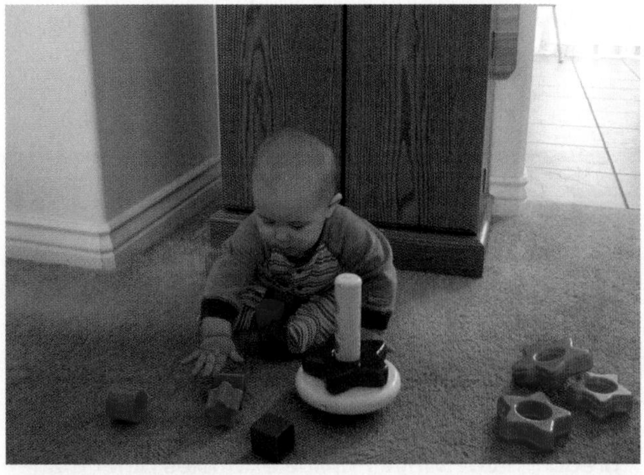

Figure 6-2 Infants' motor development improves with practice. DELMAR CENGAGE LEARNING.

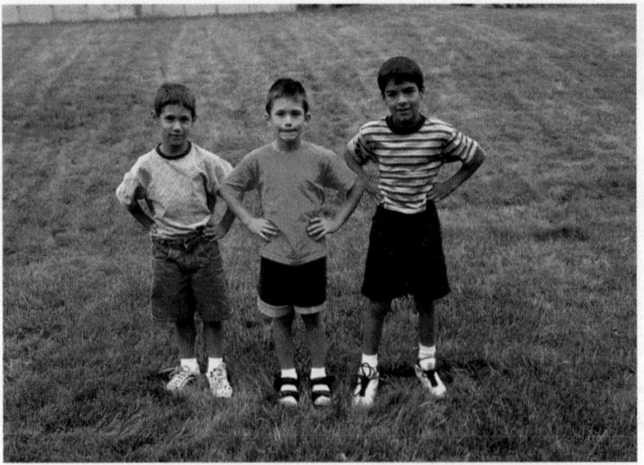

FIGURE 6-3 These children are the same age yet of different heights. DELMAR CENGAGE LEARNING.

FAMILY TEACHING

Principles of Development

- Teach caregivers that development, although orderly and sequential, may vary in individual children, so that some preschoolers may have advanced language skills and others may not.
- Remind caregivers of the importance of connections that exist among physiological, psychosocial, and cognitive development. Therefore, children need to know what it feels like to have a wet diaper and to be able to tell the caregiver that they are wet before they can be successfully toilet trained.

refined and specialized way. For example, infants will react with their entire body to pain by crying and withdrawing, whereas a child is able to localize the pain, can often identify its source, and may only withdraw the extremity experiencing the pain. An infant will use the entire hand to grab a toy before developing the fine motor ability necessary for the pincer grasp.

5. *Development becomes increasingly integrated and complex.* This means, as new skills are gained, more complex tasks are learned. For example, learning to drink from a cup initially requires eye-hand coordination, then grasping, and then hand-mouth coordination. Infants' cooing is followed by babbling, before these sounds are refined into the understandable speech of a child.
6. *Children are competent.* They possess qualities and abilities ensuring their survival and promoting their development. For example, newborns can cough, sneeze, suck, swallow, digest, breathe, and elicit caretaking responses from adults. Children make their needs known to caregivers in increasingly sophisticated ways so that others know if they are cold, hungry, or in pain.
7. *New skills predominate.* This occurs because of the strong drive to practice and perfect new abilities, especially early in life, when the child is not capable of coping well with several new skills simultaneously. For example, when children are learning to walk, talk, or feed themselves with utensils, their attention and effort is focused on developing that one skill; they do not usually learn to walk, talk, and feed themselves at the same time.

REFLECTIVE THINKING

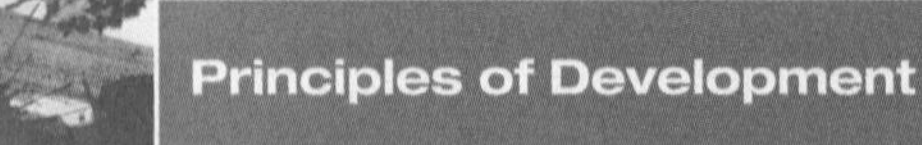

Principles of Development

Do you agree that development is orderly, sequential, directional, unique, and interrelated? Do you think development becomes increasingly differentiated, integrated, and complex as children get older? Are children competent? Do new skills predominate? Why? Provide examples other than those suggested in the text.

THEMES OF HUMAN DEVELOPMENT

Theories of growth and development are often considered from the perspective of seven themes. These themes help explain how development occurs and what humans are like, and can be applied to theories of human development. These themes answer questions related to the importance of biology or the environment on development; whether children are inherently good, bad, or actively involved in their own development; if development occurs gradually or abruptly; if children are more similar than different from one another; or if one's personality or way of interacting with others remains stable throughout life. The themes discussed include nature versus nurture, continuity versus discontinuity, passivity versus activity, critical versus sensitive periods, universality versus context specificity, assumptions about human nature, and behavioral consistency (Shaffer & Kipp, 2010).

NATURE VERSUS NURTURE

One of the more important and oldest themes discussed in human development is the nature versus nurture controversy. This debate concerns the influence that biology (nature) and the environment (nurture) have on an individual. **Nature** describes genetically inherited traits such as eye color or body type, or disease such as cystic fibrosis or hemophilia. This view sees development as predetermined by genetic factors and not altered by the environment. A person

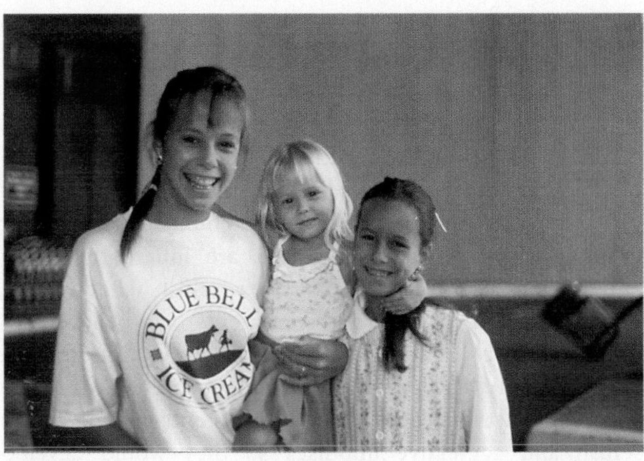

FIGURE 6-4 **Which of these children are sisters? Why do you think so?** DELMAR CENGAGE LEARNING.

believing in the principle of nature would suggest that all normal children achieve identical developmental milestones at a similar time due to maturational forces. If children differed in achieving these milestones, it would be because of differences in their genetic makeup. **Nurture** refers to the influences the environment has on development, and includes the influences child-rearing methods, culture, learning experiences, and societies have on development. A person believing in the principle of nurture would suggest development can take different paths depending on the experiences an individual has over a lifetime.

Today, most developmentalists believe both nature and nurture are important, and the relative contribution of each depends on the aspect of development studied. Developmentalists today are also more concerned about how biological and environmental factors interact to produce developmental differences and changes, rather than the importance of one over the other (Figure 6-4).

CONTINUITY VERSUS DISCONTINUITY

This theme addresses the nature of change across development. **Continuity** suggests change is orderly and built upon earlier experiences. Development is a gradual and smooth process without abrupt shifts; the course of development looks like a smooth growth curve. This theme also suggests early and late development are connected; aggressive toddlers become aggressive adults, curious infants become creative adolescents, and shy preschoolers become introverted adults. Finally, continuity proposes changes occur quantitatively, or in degrees. For example, when children grow older, they become taller, run faster, and learn more about the world around them.

Discontinuity suggests development is a series of discrete steps or stages that elevate the child to a more advanced or higher level of functioning with increased age. The course of development looks like a flight of stairs. There is no connection between early and later development; behavior seen later in life has replaced behavior seen earlier in life. For example, infants once comfortable around strangers may come to fear them as they get older; a shy and introverted preschooler may become an outgoing, extroverted adolescent. Discontinuity would also argue that adult behavior cannot be predicted by knowing what the person was like as a child. Finally, discontinuity implies qualitative change, or changes that make the individual different as growth occurs, as when a nonverbal infant becomes a toddler using language, or when a prepubertal child becomes a mature adolescent.

PASSIVITY VERSUS ACTIVITY

This theme views the child as either a passive recipient shaped by external environmental forces, or as internally driven and actively participating in development. The passive view suggests child-rearing beliefs, practices, and behaviors cause children to be either shy or assertive. Children become delinquent because of their association with an antisocial peer group. Talented and creative teachers deserve credit for a child's interest in mathematics or literature. Those disagreeing with this view believe children purposefully, creatively, and actively seek experiences to control, direct, and shape their development. Active children also modify caregiver, peer, and teacher behavior (Figure 6-5). For example, an inquisitive, friendly child may encourage that same behavior in an otherwise indifferent or unfriendly peer or adult.

CRITICAL VERSUS SENSITIVE PERIOD

This theme concerns the importance of different time periods in development and asks if some phases are more important than others in developing particular abilities, knowledge, or skills. The **critical period** refers to a limited time span when a child is biologically prepared to acquire

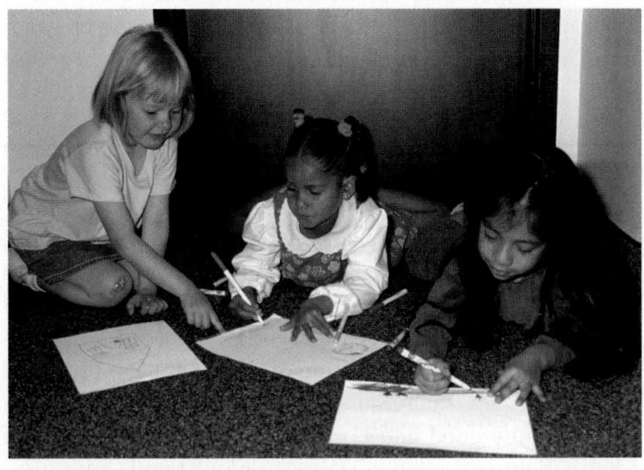

FIGURE 6-5 **Active children are interested in learning about other children's projects and art work.** DELMAR CENGAGE LEARNING.

certain behaviors, but needs the support of a suitably stimulating environment (Shaffer & Kipp, 2010). Indeed, there are some periods during development when children need to experience certain sensory and social input if their development is to proceed normally. The first three years of life are important for developing language, social, and emotional responsiveness. If there is little or no opportunity for these experiences during this time, children may have difficulty learning language, developing close friendships, or having an intimate emotional relationship later in life.

The **sensitive period**, however, is a time span that is optimal for certain capacities to emerge when the individual is especially receptive to environmental influences (Hutchinson, 2011; Shaffer & Kipp, 2010). Supporters of this view believe some behaviors can be modified during early development. For example, infants reared in an impoverished orphanage grew up without identifiable intellectual deficits if they were placed in a stimulating and nurturing adoptive home (Skeels, 1966). The fact early experiences can be modified suggests humans are malleable and adaptable and, for some areas of development, there are sensitive rather than critical periods.

UNIVERSALITY VERSUS CONTEXT SPECIFICITY

The importance of culture to development is embedded within this theme. Some theorists believe an individual's culture has a profound influence on development. Others suggest there are culture-free laws of development that apply to all children in all cultures. For example, **universality** would say humans follow similar developmental pathways regardless of their culture: language is acquired and used at 11–14 months of age, cognitive changes preparing children for school or higher learning occur during 5–7 years of age, and sexual maturity is reached during the preteen or teenage years. **Context specificity**, however, would suggest there are differences in children related to cultural values, beliefs, and experiences. For example, some societies encourage early walking by providing opportunities to exercise and practice these new skills, whereas in other societies carrying or swaddling infants is the norm, thereby reducing the chance of walking until older.

ASSUMPTIONS ABOUT HUMAN NATURE

The doctrine of **original sin**, used by Thomas Hobbes (1588–1679) to describe a child's nature, suggests children are inherently evil and selfish egotists who must be controlled by society. The doctrine of **innate purity**, proposed by Jean-Jacques Rousseau (1712–1778), suggests children are inherently good and born without an intuitive sense of what is right and wrong. The doctrine of **tabula rasa**, proposed by John Locke (1632–1704), suggests children are neither good nor evil, but rather enter the world as a blank slate without inborn tendencies, and are molded through life experiences. These assumptions are based on 17th- and 18th-century social philosophers and rarely addressed directly in theories of human development today. However, emphasis on positive or negative aspects of a child's character and a particular theorist's belief reflect an individual's orientation and assumptions about human nature. For example, if one believes children are inherently caring and helpful, or in contrast, innately selfish, child-rearing practices would vary. Permissive parents may believe children should be allowed to develop without interference (innate purity), whereas authoritarian parents may take an approach that would combat and control their child's selfish and aggressive impulses so they would develop positive behaviors (original sin).

BEHAVIORAL CONSISTENCY

This theme addresses whether or not a child's basic behavioral traits change according to the setting (school, neighborhood, family). Some theorists suggest individual personality characteristics and predispositions cause children to behave similarly no matter the setting (refer to Figure 6-6). Others suggest children's behavior changes from one setting to another. Those supporting the former view would say a particular child can always be described as honest, helpful, aggressive, or independent, no matter the situation. The latter view would argue children's behavior shifts according to the situation and who or what is present—friend in need, angry caregiver or teacher, competitive game, or a difficult test.

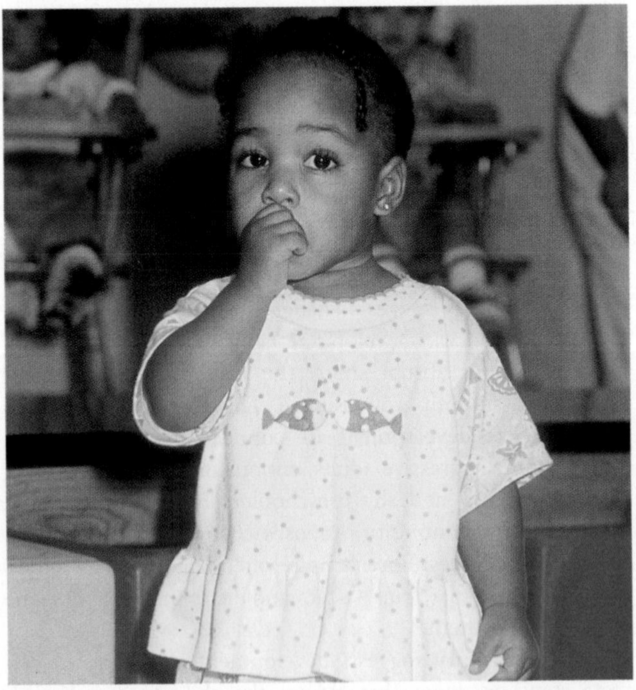

FIGURE 6-6 Some children are serious as toddlers and remain that way when older as well. DELMAR CENGAGE LEARNING.

REFLECTIVE THINKING

Experiences and the Child

What do you think the impact of providing young children with experiences formerly reserved for older children (academic preschool, computer technology) has on developing specific skills, habits, or relationships? What impact do political and social change have on a child's development in countries experiencing loss of traditional cultural values?

THEORIES OF HUMAN DEVELOPMENT

The following theoretical views present various ways of examining human development during childhood and adolescence. Although each theory may describe only one aspect of development, holistic pediatric care assumes all are important and need consideration when providing nursing interventions. Each theory focuses on particular areas of human development and has underlying assumptions, principles, strengths, and weaknesses that can help guide practice. Figure 6-7 provides a visualization of all theories discussed. Even though the figure is portrayed as a circle, consider it a sphere, with each part of the sphere a three-dimensional necessary part of the whole.

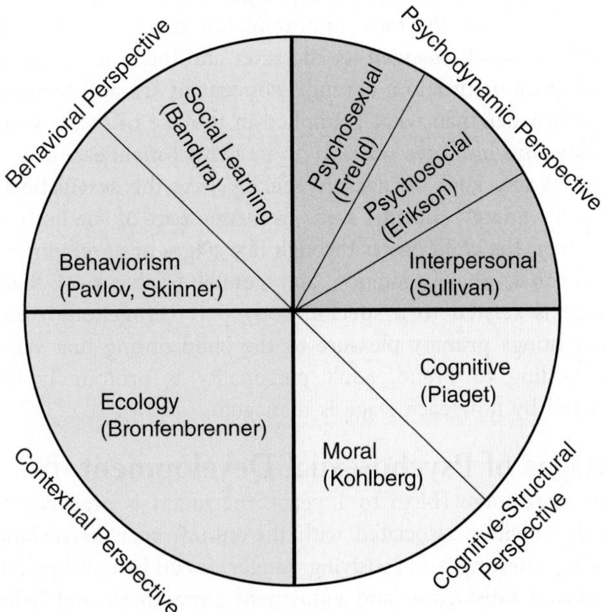

FIGURE 6-7 The Eclectic Nature of Human Development.

DELMAR CENGAGE LEARNING.

It is important to also evaluate the theories presented in relation to several criteria developed by Sidman (1960). These criteria relate to how useful the theory is and include inclusiveness, consistency, accuracy, relevance, fruitfulness, and simplicity. *Inclusiveness* refers to different phenomenon addressed in the theory, and asks the question, what kind of and how many events can the theory explain? For example, many theories of human development discuss a variety of aspects whereas theories of play would explain only small segments of a particular phenomenon. *Consistency* refers to how well the theory explains new information without having basic assumptions changed. When a theory is consistent, new discoveries are faithful to basic assumptions. For example, if a developmental psychologist discovers infant boys can recognize the sound of their mother's voices within the first six hours of life better than infant girls, and can easily explain that difference, the theory would be considered consistent. *Accuracy* refers to how well the theory explains past occurrences and predicts future outcomes. Accuracy is determined by how well a theory predicts relationships between variables. However, it is important to understand that some theories are more accurate than others, depending on the question asked. *Relevance* concerns how directly the theory relates to actual data collected. For example, prenatal nutrition is related to a child's intellectual development, and that theory has been proven by data collected during pregnancy and child outcome measures obtained during early childhood. How productive a theory is in generating new ideas and directions for research is defined as *fruitfulness.* This may be the most important criterion

CULTURAL CONSIDERATION

The Role of Culture and Gender

Understanding the influence culture and gender have on human development is crucial. An individual interacts with members of various cultures and different genders daily, and these interactions can affect school achievement and relationships with others. Although gender stereotyping is declining, it still occurs and can affect one's development, especially if children are treated according to rigid role characteristics. For example, if characteristics associated with a particular gender are limiting (girls can't do math and science), the effect can be negative. In addition, individuals from different cultures may value certain development or behavioral characteristics (attention to detail, quiet activities, deference to adults) that will affect a child's accomplishments and interactions, especially if those characteristics are not valued by the wider culture (Shaffer & Kipp, 2010).

when examining child development and behavior, since new questions always arise related to development or behavior that need to be answered. Finally, *simplicity* is concerned with the degree of detail needed to explain the theory. The most useful theories are parsimonious (simple, economical, and straightforward) rather than being so encumbered with many assumptions that their usefulness is doubtful. It is important, however, to keep in mind many theories of human development do not meet all Sidman's criteria, even though a theory that meets some criteria probably also meets others.

PSYCHODYNAMIC PERSPECTIVE

The psychodynamic perspective focuses on the emotional forces reflected in the individual's personality. These theories describe and define motivations and inner workings of the human mind during development, and answer questions related to the origin and development of personality and the outward expression of the inner self (mood, character traits, temperament, interaction patterns, and behaviors). Stages of development, unconscious motivation for behavior, and conflicts within the personality are emphasized (Shaffer & Kipp, 2010). The psychodynamic perspective is divided into the psychosexual (Freud), psychosocial or epigenetic (Erikson), and interpersonal (Sullivan) theories of development.

Freud and Psychosexual Development

Sigmund Freud (1856–1939), a Viennese physician, originated the **psychosexual** theory emphasizing the importance of unconscious motivation and early childhood experiences in influencing behavior, and describing concepts related to personality and stages of development (Freud, 1933). His ideas, considered radical when proposed early in the 20th century, became popular in the United States during the 1930s and continue to influence thinking about human development today.

Central to Freudian theory is the notion that two basic biological instincts (life and death) motivate behavior, must be satisfied, and compete for supremacy (Freud, 1933). The life instinct aims for survival and is responsible for such life-sustaining activities as eating, breathing, copulation, and behavior expressing self-preservation, love, and constructive conduct. The death instinct, however, is a destructive force expressed by self-centered and cruel behavior, hate, aggression, and destructive conduct. These instincts, the source of psychic energy that drives human behavior, have three components: id, ego, and superego. As the child matures, these components of personality become more rational and reality bound (Freud, 1933).

During infancy, all psychic energy resides in the **id**, the inborn element of personality that is driven by selfish urges. The id obeys the "pleasure principle," oriented toward maximizing pleasure and immediately satisfying needs, even when biologic needs cannot be appropriately or realistically met. The id is manifest as the irrational, selfish, impulsive part of personality (Freud, 1933).

As the infant develops, the **ego** or rational and controlling part of the personality emerges. The ego operates according to the "reality principle" as realistic ways of gratifying instinctual drives are discovered. Ego functions allow individuals to be successful and include memory, cognition, intelligence, problem solving, compromising, separating reality from fantasy, and incorporating experiences and learning into future behavior. Ego development continues during childhood and throughout the life span (Freud, 1933).

The third component of personality is the **superego** or conscience, which emerges when the child internalizes caregiver or societal values, roles, and morals. Superego development begins in infancy and becomes apparent in the preschool and school-age years when the child learns socially acceptable behavior. The superego strives for perfection rather than for pleasure or reality. After the superego emerges, children have a conscience that tells them the difference between right and wrong, and which behaviors are socially acceptable outlets for the id's undesirable impulses. The superego also serves as a disciplinarian by creating feelings of remorse and guilt for transgressing rules, and self-praise and pride for adhering to rules (Freud, 1933).

Conflict among the id, ego, and superego is inevitable throughout life. Mature, healthy personalities, however, are in a dynamic balance, with the id communicating its basic needs, the ego restraining the id until realistic ways are found to satisfy these needs, and the superego determining whether or not the ego's problem-solving strategies are morally acceptable. Freud believed defense mechanisms, such as regression, displacement, projection, and sublimation, were created as escape valves to repress painful experiences or threatening thoughts coming from the id's unsatisfied needs that were not managed by the ego or superego (Freud, 1933).

To Freud, the most important life instinct was the sex instinct, which changed its character and focus according to biological maturation. (Freud's concept of sex and sexuality was broader than what is implied in the use of these words today, and indicates sexuality in its genital manifestations as well as any kind of pleasure seeking.) As the sex instinct's psychic energy (**libido**) shifts from one part of the body to another, the child passes through five stages of development: oral, anal, phallic, latency, and genital (Table 6-2). Each stage is related to a specific body part (erogenous zone) that brings primary pleasure to the child during that stage. According to Freud, adult personality is profoundly impacted by how each stage is managed.

Stages of Psychosexual Development During the **oral stage** (birth to 1 year), the infant is preoccupied with activities associated with the mouth such as sucking, biting, chewing, and satisfying hunger. Freud believed infants received satisfaction and enjoyment from these oral behaviors and later development was affected by how well oral needs were met as well as how closely attached the infant was to the mother who usually met these needs. Children

TABLE 6-2 Stages of Freud's Psychosexual Development

STAGE	AGE	CHARACTERISTICS
Oral	Birth to 1 year	Receives satisfaction from oral needs being met; attachment to mother important because she usually meets infant's needs
Anal	1 to 3 years	Learns to control body functions, especially toileting
Phallic	3 to 6 years	Fascinated with gender differences, childbirth; Oedipal or Electra complex
Latency	6 to 11 years	Sexual drives submerged; appropriate gender roles adopted; learning about society
Genital	12 years and older	Sexual desires directed toward opposite gender; learns how to form loving relationships and manage sexual urges in socially appropriate ways

whose oral needs were not met appropriately could become thumb suckers, nail biters, or pencil chewers in childhood, and compulsive eaters or smokers later in life. They also could become overly dependent or have difficulty developing mature relations later if they were weaned too early or fed on a rigid schedule, thereby depriving them of oral gratification (Freud, 1933).

During the **anal stage** (1–3 years), sphincter muscles are maturing and children develop the ability to eliminate and retain fecal material. Sexual urges are gratified primarily by learning to voluntarily defecate. Freud suggested methods caregivers use to toilet train children during this period may have long-lasting effects on personality. For example, children who were products of rigid, severe toilet training could become obsessive about routines and schedules, or very meticulous and hypercritical. Children whose caregivers were overly attentive and concerned about success during this time could hoard possessions or use material objects to demonstrate love and affection when they are adults (Freud, 1933).

During the **phallic stage** (3–6 years), the child's psychic energy is redirected to the genitals. Children are curious about childbirth, fascinated with anatomic differences, and find pleasure in their own genitals. The phallus (penis) assumes a critical role in the development of both boys and girls. Girls wish they had a penis (penis envy) and occasionally believe they once had one that was removed by a jealous, hostile mother. Boys fear losing their penis due to an attack or injury by others (castration anxiety). During these years, children also develop a strong incestuous desire for the caregiver of the opposite gender. The **Oedipus complex** (attachment of a boy to his mother) and **Electra complex** (attachment of a girl to her father) produce anxiety that must be resolved and controlled. Resolution and control allow children to identify with the caregiver of the same gender and foster male and female identity (Freud, 1933).

At about age 6, children realize a sexual relationship with caregivers is impossible, and their energies and attention turn to the task of socialization. During this **latency stage** (6–11 years), sexual drives are submerged, appropriate gender roles are adopted, and the Oedipal or Electra conflicts are resolved. Since by now the superego has developed sufficiently to keep the id under control, children in this period rapidly learn about society and themselves while developing useful skills. They increasingly identify with the same-gender caregiver and become intensely involved with their same-gender peers. Energies are directed toward school, play, and increasing their problem-solving abilities (Freud, 1933) (Figure 6-8).

Freud's last period, the **genital stage**, begins at puberty (about age 12) and lasts throughout adulthood. Sexual desires reemerge due to physiological changes, fluctuating hormone levels, and changing social relationships (Figure 6-9). Before mature adult adjustment is possible, however, turmoil and adaptation are necessary. The adolescent vacillates between dependence and independence from parents, learns how to form loving relationships, and manages sexual urges

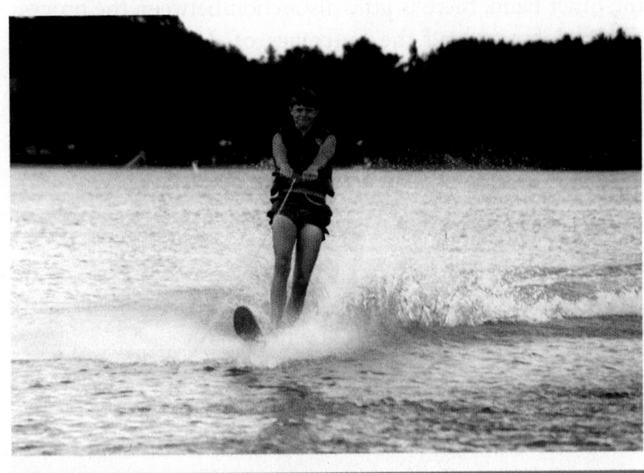

FIGURE 6-8 School-age children actively engage in a variety of activities. DELMAR CENGAGE LEARNING.

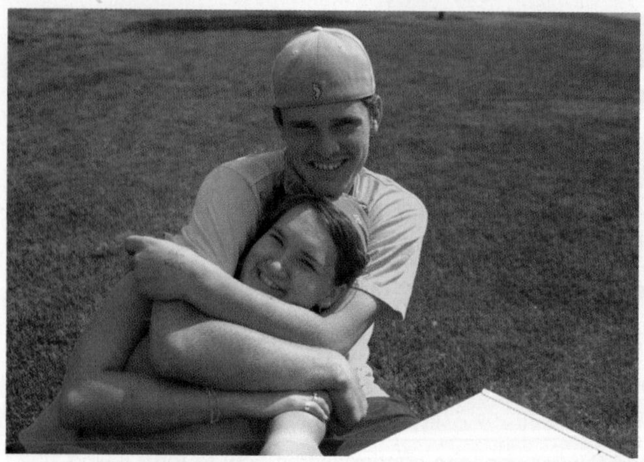

FIGURE 6-9 **Relationships with the opposite gender change during adolescence.** DELMAR CENGAGE LEARNING.

in societally appropriate ways. Some adolescents struggle with their sexuality, reexperience earlier conflicting feelings toward caregivers, and may consequently distance themselves from their caregivers as they defend against anxiety. These psychic conflicts are necessary for fully functioning and mature adult personality development (Freud, 1933).

Evaluation Freud has been criticized for developing a theory that is difficult to test, too narrow and simple, and based primarily on biological drives rather than sociocultural influences and learning. In addition, some of his theories are not always supported (Crain, 2005; Shaffer & Kipp, 2010); many preschoolers are ignorant of anatomical differences between genders. Freud's theory may also not be scientifically valid because it depends on instincts, defense mechanisms, and the unconscious; is based on retrospective memories of maladjusted adult clients, many of whom were women; and was not tested on children (Crain, 2005; Shaffer & Kipp, 2010; Sigelman & Rider, 2009).

In relation to Sidman's criteria, the psychosexual theory is quite content specific, and therefore not very inclusive. On the other hand, there is little distinction between the process of development and the outcomes of development. However, the theory is consistent, and can be easily and efficiently applied to behaviors different than those on which the theory originally was developed. The theory does not define any criterion for accuracy, and most predictions are done after the fact. In addition, there is minimal information on the exact factors responsible for changes in an individual's life. However, the theory produces a variety of new questions about human development.

However, Freud's theory did describe the concept of unconscious motivation for behavior and the importance of early family experiences on later development. Freud has also explored the emotional side of development (fear, anxieties, love), and has made us realize people are individuals who place meaning on different life experiences (Emde, 1992). His theory is also well developed and virtually unlimited in explaining a variety of behaviors from mate selection, habits, and art, to adversity and the meaning of dreams (Crain, 2005; Sigelman & Rider, 2009).

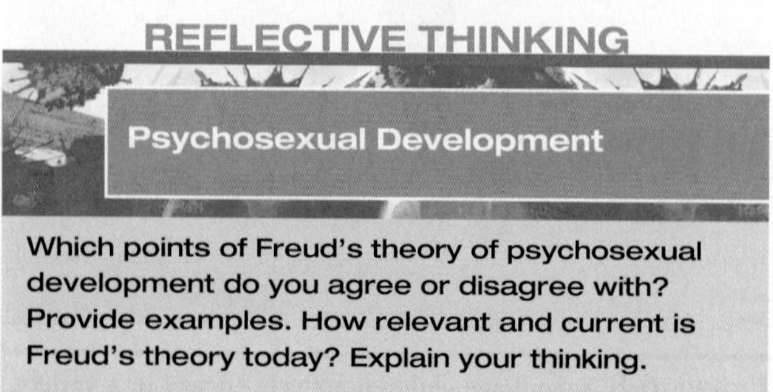

REFLECTIVE THINKING

Psychosexual Development

Which points of Freud's theory of psychosexual development do you agree or disagree with? Provide examples. How relevant and current is Freud's theory today? Explain your thinking.

Application Freud provides insight into human actions, and helps us understand others by realizing all behavior is meaningful and may hide inner needs or conflicts. Therefore, it is especially important to teach this information as well as normal behavior for the various stages to parents. Since during infancy comfort and pleasure are obtained through the mouth, it is important to offer babies a pacifier if they are NPO, or a bottle, pacifiers, or the breast after painful procedures. When hungry, they should be promptly fed (if not NPO). Providing plastic or rubber rings or other toys suitable for teething infants is also appropriate.

Toddlers are gratified by controlling body excretions. Therefore, when caring for children between 1 and 3 years of age, asking about the status of toileting and words and rituals used for elimination is important. It is wise to provide a child-sized potty chair and avoid starting toilet training during periods of illness or stress. In addition, toddlers should be reprimanded carefully if toilet training is difficult or if the child has accidents. Finally, parents need to be flexible and patient in toilet training and begin when the toddler indicates readiness.

Preschool children are concerned about sexuality and initially identify with the parent of the opposite gender. Nurses should teach parents that curiosity about gender differences and masturbation is normal. In addition, nurses should be aware of preschoolers who appear more comfortable with a particular nurse (no matter the gender), attempt to accommodate that situation, and encourage parents to participate in the care of their child. School-age children and adolescents should be encouraged to have contact with friends, and their questions answered honestly. Privacy for both school-age and adolescent clients should be ensured during physical examinations or when they are changing clothes or showering in gym class.

Erikson and Psychosocial Development

Erik Erikson (1902–1994) acknowledged the contribution of biologic factors to development, but felt the environment, culture, and society were also important. His **psychosocial** (epigenetic) **theory** of development stresses the complexity of interrelationships existing between emotional and physical variables during one's lifetime (Erikson, 1963). Erikson agreed with many of Freud's ideas regarding basic instincts and the three components of personality (id, ego, superego). In addition, he believed development was stage-like, and conflict resolution was necessary at each stage in order for the individual to successfully advance to the next stage. In fact, Erikson's first five stages of development and the approximate ages of each stage correspond closely with those outlined by Freud and others (Table 6-3). Erikson differs from Freud, however, in that he believes children actively adapt and explore their environment instead of being passively controlled and molded by caregivers and society. Erikson also assumes humans are rational creatures whose actions, feelings, and thoughts are controlled primarily by the ego instead of the id, superego, or conflicts between the three components of personality.

For Erikson, life-span development consisted of eight sequential stages. Five of these stages describe infants through adolescents (Table 6-4). Each stage is dominated by major

TABLE 6-3 Comparison of Stage Theories of Human Development

AGE PERIOD	FREUD	ERIKSON	SULLIVAN	PIAGET	KOHLBERG
Infancy (Birth to 1 year)	Oral (Birth to 1 year)	Trust/Mistrust (Birth to 1½ years)	Infant (Birth to 1½ years)	Sensorimotor (Birth to 2 years)	Preconventional (Birth to 7 years)
Toddler (1 to 3 years)	Anal (1 to 3 years)	Trust/Mistrust (continued)	Infant (continued)	Sensorimotor (continued)	Preconventional (continued)
		Autonomy/ Shame-Doubt (1½ to 3 years)	Early Childhood (1½ to 6 years)	Preoperational (2 to 7 years)	Preconventional (continued)
Preschool (3 to 6 years)	Phallic (3 to 6 years)	Initiative/Guilt (3 to 6 years)	Early Childhood (continued)	Preoperational (continued)	Preconventional (continued)
School age (6 to 12 years)	Latency (6 to 12 years)	Industry/Inferiority (6 to 12 years)	Late Childhood (6 to 9 years) Preadolescence (9 to 12 years)	Concrete Operations (7 to 11 years)	Conventional (7 to 12 years)
Adolescence (12 to 19 years)	Genital (12 years and older)	Identity/Role Confusion (12 to 18 years)	Early Adolescence (12 to 15 years) Late Adolescence (15 to 19 years)	Formal Operations (12 years and older)	Postconventional (12 years and older)

TABLE 6-4 Stages of Erikson's Psychosocial Theory of Development

STAGE	AGE	CHARACTERISTICS
Trust versus Mistrust	1 month to 1½ years	Learns world is good and can be trusted as basic needs are met
Autonomy versus Shame and Doubt	1½ to 3 years	Learns independent behaviors regarding toileting, bathing, feeding, dressing; exerts self; exercises choices
Initiative versus Guilt	3 to 6 years	Goal directed, competitive, demonstrates exploratory behavior; and imaginative play
Industry versus Inferiority	6 to 11 years	Learns self-worth as gains mastery of psychosocial, physiological, and cognitive skills; becomes society or peer focused
Identity versus Role Confusion	12 to 18 years	Develops sense of self; gains independence from parents; peers important

developmental conflicts or crises related to societal demands and expectations that must be addressed or resolved before the individual can progress to the next stage. The resolution of each conflict or crisis might be positive (favorable and growth enhancing) or negative (unfavorable, frustrating, and making later development difficult). Erikson believed major conflicts occurring during each stage are rarely completely resolved. Instead, they are of primary or dominant importance during a particular stage and then become less important or dominant as other conflicts arise in later stages. In addition, he suggests conflict is rarely completely resolved positively. Rather, the positive resolution predominates over the negative resolution during a particular stage. Failure to successfully master a crisis or developmental task does not destine the child to failure since delayed mastery is possible. It is true, however, that difficulty at one stage may affect progress through later stages (Erickson, 1963).

Stages of Psychosocial Development Erikson's first stage, **trust versus mistrust**, occurs during infancy (1 month to 1½ years) when the basic task is to establish trust rather than mistrust in relation to oneself and others. Infants whose needs for comfort, food, and warmth are effectively and consistently met by a nurturing caregiver learn that the world is not only predictable, but safe, reliable, and can be trusted (Figure 6-10). If caregivers are unpredictable,

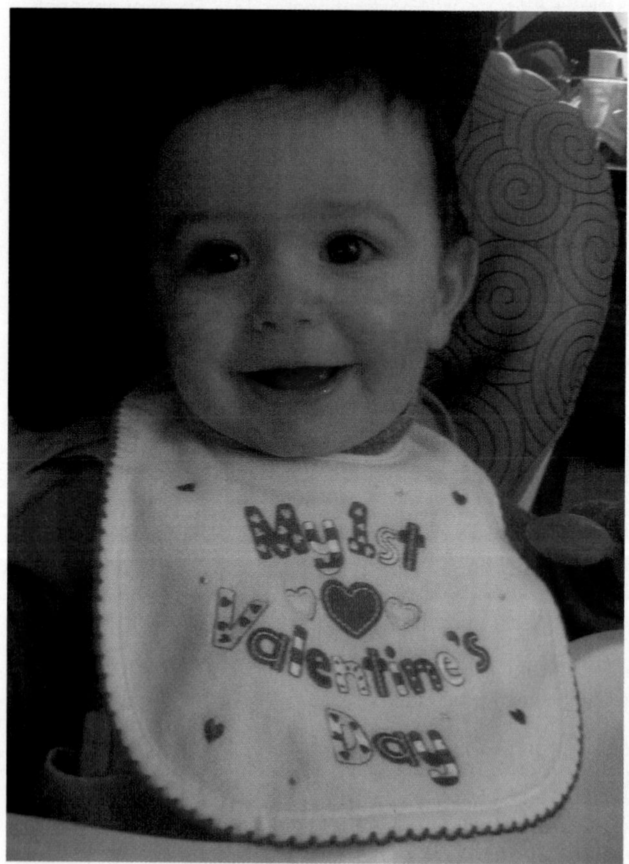

FIGURE 6-10 Infants whose needs for comfort, food, and warmth are consistently met will develop a sense of trust.

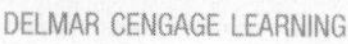
DELMAR CENGAGE LEARNING.

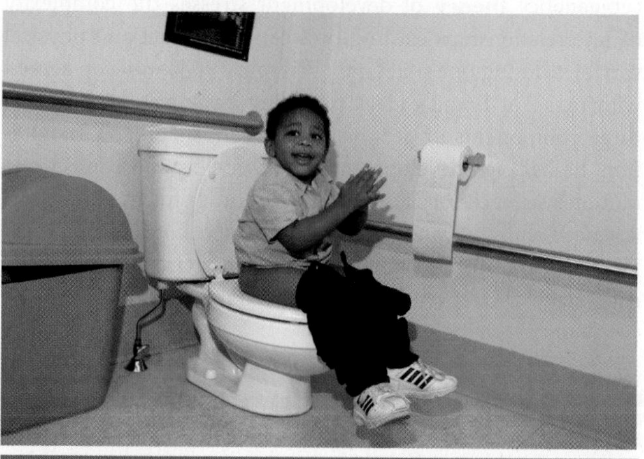

FIGURE 6-11 Toilet training is a significant milestone in the development of autonomy. DELMAR CENGAGE LEARNING.

inconsistent, inadequate, or convey a sense of confusion or chaos, the child learns to view the environment with mistrust or wariness, and may demonstrate restlessness, crying, whining, or physiological dysfunctions such as sleep disturbances, vomiting, or diarrhea (Erikson, 1963).

During the toddler years (1½ to 3 years), **autonomy versus shame and doubt** occurs. Autonomy develops as children discover their new mental and physical abilities while improving language and motor skills and learning competencies related to bathing, eating, toileting, and dressing (Figure 6-11). Shame occurs if assertiveness and independence are considered unacceptable or ineffective by caregivers. Doubt occurs if children learn to mistrust not only themselves but also others in the immediate environment. Children demonstrating dependency and constantly needing approval for their actions have not resolved this conflict (Erikson, 1963).

The third developmental stage (3–6 years) is **initiative versus guilt**. Initiative refers to a person's independently beginning an activity rather than merely responding to or imitating others. It occurs when a child tries out new ways of combining activities, invents creative ways to use skills and abilities, imagines what other people or things are like, and takes responsibility for one's own actions (Figure 6-12a, 6-12b). Guilt occurs when caregivers frequently reprimand behaviors reflecting initiative. Children experiencing severe restrictions and belittling feel guilty about their actions and thoughts, and may become passive, reluctant, or refuse to participate in activities (Erikson, 1963).

The major developmental task of the school-age years (6–11 years) is **industry versus inferiority**. Industry involves mastery of social, physical, and intellectual skills, and orientation toward and competition with peers. No longer interested in merely participating, school-age children in many western countries are interested in being the best, first, fastest, or smartest as they complete projects and compare their efforts to others. Attention and energy now are

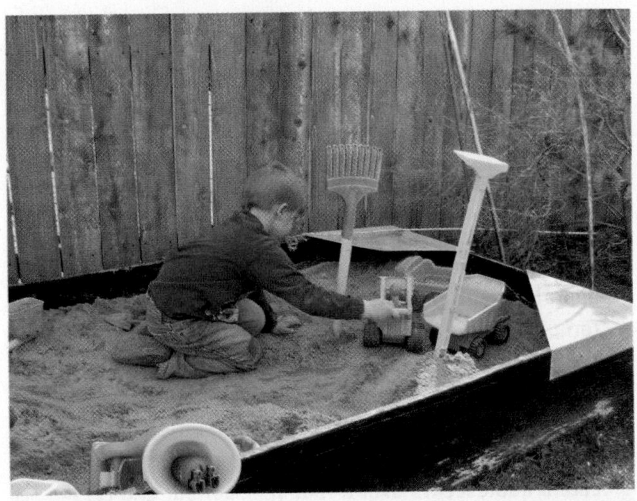

FIGURE 6-12A This preschooler is playing independently in his sandbox and inventing new ways to use his sand toys. DELMAR CENGAGE LEARNING.

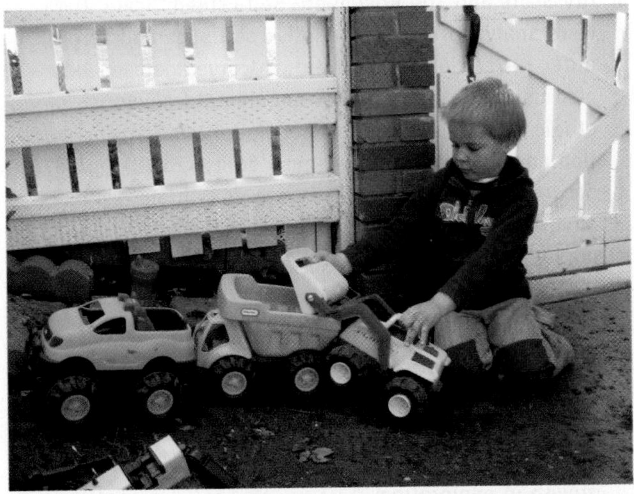

FIGURE 6-12B This preschooler demonstrates initiative as he lines up his trucks in the dirt. DELMAR CENGAGE LEARNING.

turned to learning academic skills and social roles, as the child becomes less family focused and more society and peer focused (Figure 6-13). Inferiority develops when school-age children are ridiculed by peers, don't measure up to adult or their own expectations, or lack certain skills so they are not always the best, first, fastest, or smartest (Erikson, 1963).

Adolescence (12–18 years) is characterized by **identity versus role confusion**. Identity involves achieving a sense of who one is intellectually, cognitively, behaviorally and emotionally, as emerging physical and sexual maturity is integrated with already existing skills and abilities. Erikson believed identity is attained as the young person's view of who one is becomes consistent with others' views. Identity achievement also requires resolution of subconflicts, including finding one's own political, social, economic, and religious ideology; adopting an appropriate gender identity; making an occupational or vocational choice; and adopting behaviors consistent with one's own self-concept. Considered a crucial stage in development, identity formation affects commitments and decisions made later in life. Role confusion occurs when the adolescent is unable to acquire a sense of direction, self, or place within the world (Erikson, 1963).

Erikson identified three other stages beyond identity versus role confusion that occur during adulthood. They are intimacy versus isolation, generativity versus stagnation, and integrity versus despair. In each of these stages, as with the earlier stages, conflict needs to be resolved before the next stage is reached.

Evaluation Erikson's theory is broader than Freud's and focuses on the importance of a variety of psychological motivations for behavior and the influence of both environmental and maturational factors on development. His theory also encompasses the entire life span and emphasizes the importance of assuming responsibility for self-development and methods of achieving healthy resolution of each stage.

Those criticizing Erikson believe he is biased against women and does not consider the differences between men and women in relation to social and cultural influences or experiences. In addition, he is criticized for being imprecise about the causes of psychosocial development, not able to articulate specifically how outcomes of one stage impact development at another stage, or specify the kinds of experiences needed to resolve or cope with conflicts. Instead, he describes development socially and emotionally, but does not explain well how or why development occurs. He also does not discuss observable behaviors indicating that trust, autonomy, initiative, industry, or identity has been achieved (Crain, 2005; Shaffer & Kipp, 2010; Sigelman & Rider, 2009).

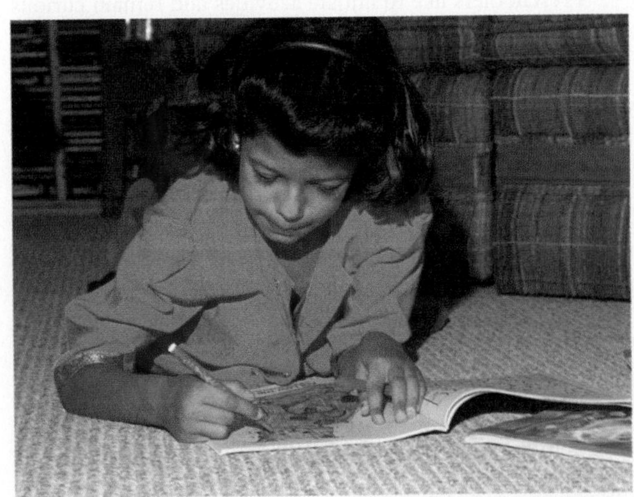

FIGURE 6-13 Industry is a task of school-age children. DELMAR CENGAGE LEARNING.

CRITICAL THINKING

Using Psychosocial Development in Practice

How would you identify children having difficulty developing trust, autonomy, initiative, industry, or identity? What suggestions would you give parents to help them help their children positively resolve each developmental crisis?

Application Erikson's theory provides us with a means of assessing and gaining insight into five developmental crises children and adolescents face, and allows us to use this knowledge to teach caregivers behaviors they can expect to see in their children. It also helps us realize the importance of societal influences on health and behavior, and that psychosocial development is a lifelong process.

Erikson's theory is easy to apply to practice. Health care provides a variety of situations and opportunities where a child's progression through stages can be facilitated, and caregivers taught how to encourage positive resolution of each developmental crisis. Since meeting basic needs (feeding, bathing, changing) in a timely and appropriate fashion during infancy results in the development of trust, it is critical that feeding and hygiene needs be met promptly. When an infant is ill, parents should be encouraged to spend as much time as possible with their infant.

For toddlers, independence is increasing and self-control gained by maintaining familiar daily routines. Allowing opportunities for the child to independently dress, feed, and do self-hygiene care is important (Figure 6-14). If restraint for procedures or treatments is necessary, explanations and comfort should be provided and caregivers encouraged to participate. Love, approval, and praise are important for toddlers and children in all stages.

Preschoolers like to initiate activities and remain curious and interested in the world around them. Opportunities to explore, ask questions, and create should be provided (Figure 6-15). Nurses should accept children's choices and negative expression of feelings, answer their questions, and allow them to play with medical equipment so their curiosity is satisfied and their knowledge about experiences broadened.

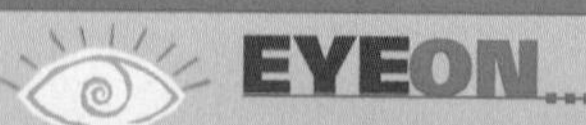

Psychosocial Development

The culture and beliefs that people grow up with will affect how they trust and express autonomy, initiative, industry, and identity. Examine how you demonstrate these elements, then compare your findings to someone else's who comes from a different cultural background.

RESEARCH Highlight

Adolescents' Ethnic Identity

STUDY PURPOSE

Since ethnic identity exploration and resolution for minority youth probably follows a developmental pattern, it would be important when working with adolescents to understand how they come to identify with their cultural heritage/background. Therefore, the purpose of this project was to discover: (1) if ethnic identity exploration, resolution, and affirmation grow in Latino adolescents over a four-year period; and (2) if self-esteem growth can be predicted by ethnic identity.

METHODS

Each year for four years, Latino adolescents from Midwestern high schools completed the Ethnic Identity Scale and The Rosenberg Self-Esteem Scale. Data were analyzed using descriptive statistics and zero-order correlations. Latent growth curve analyses were also used in examining developmental trajectories of ethnic identity exploration, resolution, and affirmation and determining if ethnic identity growth varied according to gender. Multivariate growth models examined the relationships between growth of the ethnic identity components and growth in self-esteem.

FINDINGS

For Latino girls, ethnic identity exploration, resolution, and affirmation increased significantly between middle and late adolescence. However, only affirmation increased significantly for Latino boys. Growth in boys' and girls' self-esteem was only predicted by growth in exploration.

IMPLICATIONS

When looking at growth in adolescent ethnic identity it is important to realize gender differences do exist. In addition, it would be important when working with adolescents of other cultures, to be aware of how patterns of growth in ethnic identity vary by gender and examine the contributions of identity exploration, resolution, and affirmation when determining an adolescent's ethnic identity.

REFERENCE

Umaña-Taylor, A., Gonzales-Backen, M., & Guimond, A. (2009). Latino adolescents' ethnic identity: Is there a developmental progression and does growth in ethnic identity predict growth in self-esteem? *Child Development*, *80*(2), 391–405.

For school-age children, involvement and success in a variety of activities provide a sense of self-worth and value. Nurses should provide the school-age child with

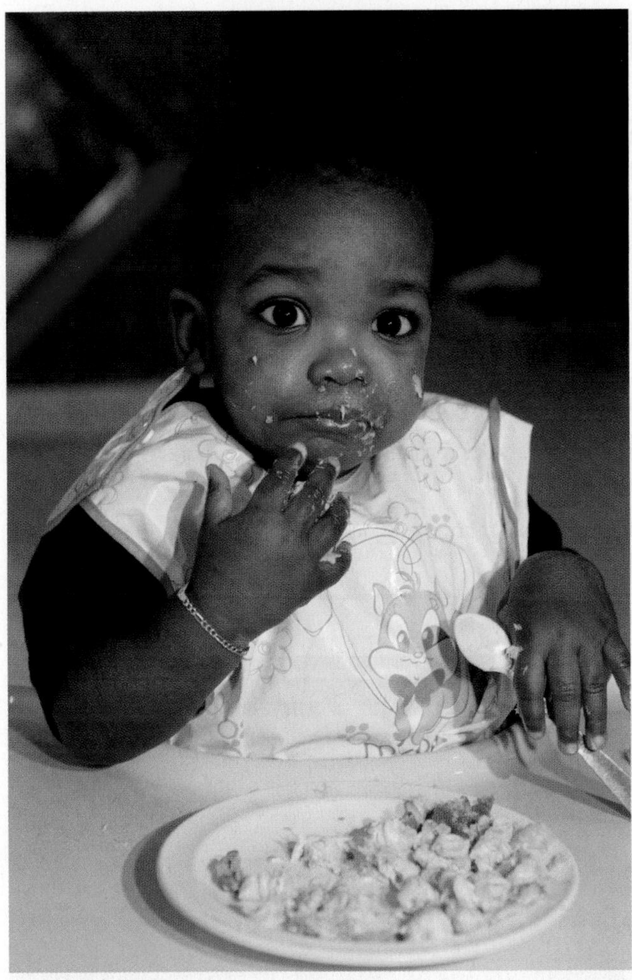

FIGURE 6-14 Letting toddlers feed themselves is important for the development of autonomy. DELMAR CENGAGE LEARNING.

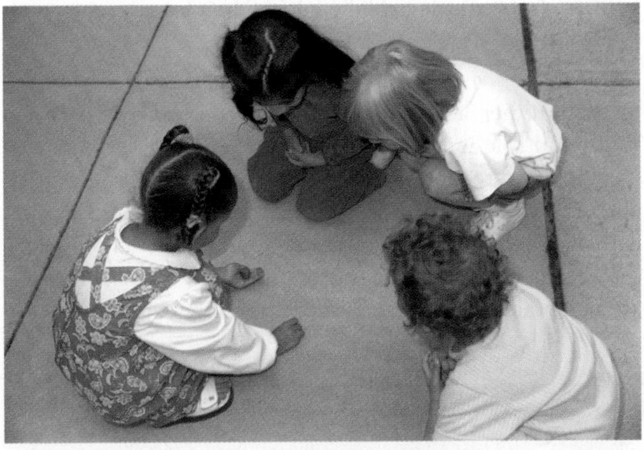

FIGURE 6-15 Children are curious about nature; these children are intrigued by a snail they discovered on the sidewalk. DELMAR CENGAGE LEARNING.

opportunities for continuing school work if hospitalized or ill, maintaining hobbies or activities, interacting with their peers, and adjusting to limitations imposed by illness or

FAMILY TEACHING

Erikson's Theory

- Teach parents to meet infant's basic needs in a timely and appropriate manner.
- Allow opportunities for toddlers to be independent.
- Provide preschoolers with a variety of experiences where they can explore, ask questions, and create.
- Encourage school-age children to interact with peers.
- Support adolescents' choices, be available to listen, and offer guidance.

hospitalization. Primary care nurses need to be in touch with school nurses when a child with a chronic condition is hospitalized and when this child is ready to return home and to school.

Adolescents are searching for who they will become independent from their parents. Nurses should allow adolescent clients to be as autonomous as possible, encourage them to take responsibility for their own actions, support their life choices, introduce them to other teens, and provide them with a separate recreation or activity area if in an acute care setting. Parental involvement in the care of adolescents is still important.

SULLIVAN AND INTERPERSONAL DEVELOPMENT

Harry Stack Sullivan (1892–1949) focused on interpersonal relations as important behavioral motivators and the source of psychological health. His **interpersonal theory** posits that self-concept is the key to personality development. He acknowledged the importance of the environment (especially the home), and also emphasized the role of social approval and disapproval in forming a child's self-concept. Sullivan believed personality development was largely the result of childhood experiences, interpersonal encounters, and the mother-child relationship. How well physiological needs were met in an interpersonal situation affected not only one's sense of satisfaction and security, but also allowed anxiety to be avoided. Poor environmental interactions caused anxiety and tension; a positive social relationship resulted in security, a major life goal (Sullivan, 1953).

Stages of Interpersonal Development Sullivan describes seven stages of interpersonal development (Sullivan, 1953); six relate specifically to infants through adolescents (Table 6-5). Sullivan believed each stage prepared the personality for the next stage and failure to successfully achieve stage activities limited personality development and opportunities

TABLE 6-5 Stages of Sullivan's Interpersonal Theory of Development

STAGE	AGE	CHARACTERISTICS
Infant	Birth to 18 months	Learns to rely on others, especially mother; "good me/bad me" emerges
Early childhood	18 months to 6 years	Learns to clarify communication; recognizes approval or disapproval; delays gratification
Late childhood	6 to 9 years	Increases intellectual abilities; learns to control behavior and own place in the world
Preadolescence	9 to 12 years	Is vulnerable to teasing; "chum" important
Early adolescence	12 to 15 years	Masters independence; develops relationships with persons of opposite gender
Late adolescence	15 to 19 years	Masters expression of sexual impulses; forms responsible and satisfying relationships with others

for a successful life. Refer to Table 6-3 for a comparison of Sullivan's first six stages with Freud's and Erikson's stages.

The first stage (infant) encompasses birth to when the child is able to use words that convey the same meaning to the child as they do to others (18 months). The primary task of this stage revolves around learning to rely on others, especially the primary caregiver, to gratify physiological needs and achieve satisfaction. When basic needs are met, infants are in a state of well-being. If these needs are not met, a fear-like state occurs, manifested by excessive crying or difficulties eating or sleeping. Infants are sensitive to other's negative and positive attitudes and emotions while these needs are being met. Sullivan felt one's self-image emerged according to how the infant interpreted the mother (primary caregiver)-infant relationship when these needs were met. "Good me" feelings occur when acceptance is sensed; "bad me" feelings occur when the infant experiences anxiety while interacting with caregivers. Excessive anxiety may cause children to believe they are bad, leading to feelings of inferiority or depression. "Good me" and "bad me" fuse around 18 months of age; but the dominant "me" can change with situational or maturational crises (Sullivan, 1953).

During the early childhood stage (18 months to 6 years), children are able to communicate better with others, thereby facilitating interpersonal relationships (Figure 6-16). As children learn to recognize signs indicating approval or disapproval of their behavior, they learn about controlling personal desires, delaying gratification, and accepting interference from others. Excess parental disapproval during this time may cause children to view themselves and the world as negative or hostile.

The third stage, late childhood (6–9 years), is characterized by increasing intellectual ability and developing internal control over behavior. Children learn to pay attention to others' wishes, form satisfying relations with peers of both genders, and sometimes oppose rules. They also learn to accept subordination from authority figures (parents, teachers, other adults) and develop a sense of their own status and role in society (Sullivan, 1953).

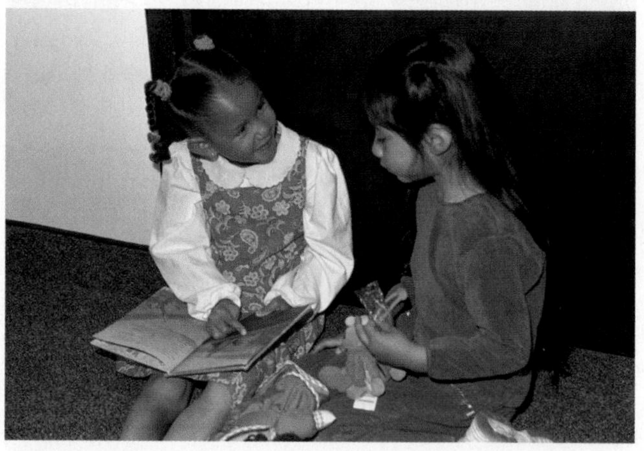

FIGURE 6-16 During childhood, children learn to communicate with others. DELMAR CENGAGE LEARNING.

During preadolescence (9–12 years), children participate in an expanding world that provides confrontation with rules and knowledge about themselves. They realize their status within the peer group is based on performance, are vulnerable to teasing, and become interested in relating

FAMILY TEACHING

Sullivan

- Teach caregivers their interactions with children should be positive, nurturing, and consistent.
- Remind caregivers children need special friends during the school-age years to share experiences, secrets, and dreams.

closely to a peer of the same gender, which Sullivan calls the "chum." This special friend allows the 9- to 12-year-old to participate in a genuine love relationship with another, furthers self-identity, and helps develop concern for others. "Chums" may share secrets, fantasies, dreams, and realities of life, and often collaborate, experiment, explore, and manipulate people and the environment. Preadolescents who do not have a chum may experience difficulty with relationships later (Sullivan, 1953).

During early adolescence (12–15 years), independence is mastered and satisfying relations with members of the opposite gender are established as attempts are made to integrate sexual urges with other aspects of personal relationships. Early adolescents may demonstrate a variety of behaviors including rebellion, dependence, cooperation, and collaboration as they become independent.

The sixth stage is termed late adolescence (15–19 years). Sullivan believes initial feelings of love for the opposite gender emerge here, as the individual learns to master expression of sexual impulses, form responsible and satisfying relationships, and use communication skills in interactions.

Evaluation There is little criticism of Sullivan's theory because most of his work (lectures, papers) was published after he died, was not systematic, and did not lead to replication. However, his view that social interactions are essential for personality development, and suggestions that personality can and does change, are meaningful contributions. Like Erikson, he emphasized the importance of caregivers, peers, other adults, and the wider social environment in shaping a child's self-concept.

Application Sullivan also has relevance to the nursing care of children. Perhaps the two most important points he made were to emphasize the significance of interpersonal relations with others on personality development, and meeting the child's basic needs in a timely and appropriate fashion. This does not mean, however, that caregivers protect children from all discomforts or meet needs before they are expressed. The key is to relieve unpleasant feelings associated with basic needs so feelings of security and attachment result in a "good me" rather than a "bad me." Sullivan also has helped us realize the important place chums have in a school-age child's life, and how this experience is critical for developing interpersonal relationships later in life.

Therefore, when children of any age are ill it is important to meet their basic needs and provide an opportunity for school-age children and adolescents to interact with others their same age. If children are hospitalized or have a chronic illness, caregivers should be involved in their child's care. Nurses also need to teach caregivers about Sullivan's theory so they may help their child develop a healthy personality, and realize the importance they have in a child's life.

> **REFLECTIVE THINKING**
>
> **Contributions of the Psychodynamic Perspective**
>
> Consider the contributions the psychodynamic perspective makes to the study of human development. Do you think that caregivers influence young children as much as Freud, Erikson, and Sullivan suggest? Why or why not? How would you explain children who grow up in dysfunctional environments but who overcome adversity and become well-adjusted and psychologically healthy adults?

BEHAVIORAL PERSPECTIVE

The **behavioral perspective** posits that human actions and interactions come from learned responses to environmental stimuli. Behavioral theorists study human behavior in a laboratory setting and then apply this information to the general population, and look for ways to alter or control the environment to change, modify, or teach desired behaviors. The past or unconscious motives are not the root of behavior and learning does not depend on maturation. These theorists believe children randomly respond to the environment consistent with developmental capabilities, and rewards or punishment influence behavior. Behavior resulting in punishment, pain, disappointment, or frustration often is discontinued, whereas behavior that is rewarded or viewed positively is retained and repeated in similar situations. The behavioral perspective is divided into behaviorism (classical and operant conditioning) and social learning (Crain, 2005; Shaffer & Kipp, 2010; Sigelman & Rider, 2009).

PAVLOV AND CLASSICAL CONDITIONING

Ivan Pavlov (1849–1936), a Russian physiologist, initially discovered linkages between a stimulus and a response while studying a dog's response to food. He learned a dog would respond (salivate) not only when he saw food (unconditioned stimulus), but also when he saw the person who fed him or heard a bell ring just before the food appeared (conditioned stimulus), because the dog had learned the bell or appearance of the man meant food would follow. This learning to respond to a new stimulus the same way a familiar stimulus was responded to is called **classical conditioning**, and suggests learning occurs when a response already part of the organism's normal activities (salivating) can be reproduced by an associated stimulus that previously would not have produced it—for example, the presence of a person or the sound of a bell (Crain, 2005; Shaffer & Kipp, 2010). Another example of classical conditioning would be when an infant, seeing the spoon used for feeding, becomes excited (waving hands and arms, kicking legs, making babbling sounds) because the spoon is associated with being fed and the infant knows feeding time is coming soon.

Skinner and Operant Conditioning

Operant conditioning, a term originated by B. F. Skinner (1904–1990), involves behavioral changes due to negative (punishment) or positive (reinforcers) consequences rather than just the occurrence of stimuli. If behavior is rewarded, the likelihood of it reoccurring increases; if behavior is punished, chances are it will not reoccur. Positive reinforcement includes friendly smiles, praise, or special treats and privileges; punishment includes criticism, a frown, or withdrawal of privileges. Skinner discovered behavioral change became more permanent when consequences were provided intermittently rather than continuously, and believed the essence of development involved constantly acquiring new behaviors or habits due to reinforcing or punishing stimuli. He emphasized why behaviors occur rather than simply describing the behavior seen (Skinner, 1953).

Bandura and Social Learning

A third kind of behaviorism is **social learning**, proposed by Albert Bandura (b. 1925). According to this view, children learn by imitating and observing others (a model), as well as by classical and operant conditioning. Social learning theorists also believe behavior is influenced by the environment and learned through various experiences. However, they do not believe behavioral change is a mindless response to stimuli. Rather, they suggest personality, past experiences, relationships with the model, the situation itself, and cognition also impact behavioral change (Bandura, 1977). Cognition plays a part because to successfully imitate behavior, a child must be capable of remembering, rehearsing, and organizing the behavior seen. Children often will think about connections between behavior and consequences and will likely be affected more by what they believe will be the consequences rather than what the consequences actually are. For example, learning to play a musical instrument is expensive for families and demanding and time-consuming for children. However, children and their parents continually tolerate the cost and inconvenience because they are anticipating rewards once the child learns to play the instrument.

Bandura also believes modeled behavior can be weakened or strengthened depending on whether it is punished or rewarded. Bandura suggests observational learning (learning that results from merely watching others), where children acquire a variety of new behaviors when "models" are merely pursuing their own interests and not attempting to teach, reward, or punish, is another important method of learning behaviors. For example, children who watch television violence frequently are more aggressive than those children who do not watch very much television violence. Finally, Bandura found children tend to model behavior of children and adults of their same gender more often than not, and males model behavior of others more often than females do (Crain, 2000; Shaffer & Kipp, 2010; Sigelman & Rider, 2009) (Figure 6-17).

Evaluation

Behavioral and learning theories are precise and testable since they can be replicated and observed; principles from these theories operate across the entire life span. They have practical applications, have been used to effectively treat developmental problems, and assist in optimizing development. They are also credited with introducing concepts of programmed instruction and computer learning, and emphasize the role of environmental influences in shaping behavior. They make adults aware of the example their behavior sets for children of all ages since it is not unusual for children to adopt behavior seen in their caregivers (smoking, crude language) even if these same caregivers talk to their children about not smoking, using crude language, or imitating their behavior.

However, critics say the behavioral perspective oversimplifies development by downplaying biological influences and places too much emphasis on environmental experiences. Children cannot achieve certain milestones until they are maturationally or developmentally ready. In addition, the perspective only examines one or two aspects of development instead of examining how all aspects fit together and misses spontaneity often seen in young children. Finally, the theory is viewed as too simplistic and unconnected; isolated aspects of behavior are described rather than examining how feelings, the unconscious, and psychodynamic factors fit into the holistic view of the child (Sigelman & Rider, 2009).

The behavioral theory is very inclusive since it addresses developmental processes with minimal concern for the behavior or content that characterizes the process. For example, the fact that many principles of operant conditioning apply to animals as well as humans illustrates decreased emphasis on behavioral content and increased emphasis on the process of behavioral development. This theory is also very consistent because it is content free and attempts to explain a variety of behaviors. In addition, the theory is accurate and,

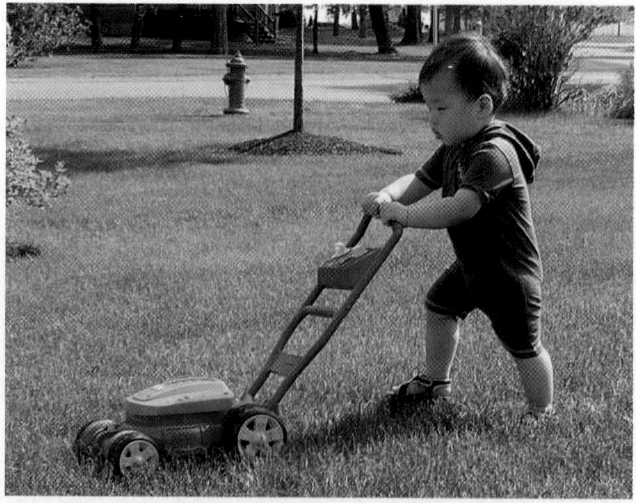

Figure 6-17 This preschooler is modeling behavior observed in others. DELMAR CENGAGE LEARNING.

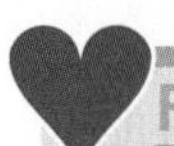

FAMILY **TEACHING**

Behavioral Perspective

- Reprimanding children for their unacceptable behavior should be consistent and appropriate.
- Children will model behavior they see in their parents even if parents talk to children about not modeling that same behavior.

under controlled conditions, behavioral outcomes can be predicted. The behavioral theory has a high degree of relevance since behaviors of interest are operationally defined. However, the theory is not very fruitful. Even though the theory has influenced parenting and child rearing, few new directions for future study have been identified. However, this is a very simple theory, and it explains behavior parsimoniously (Shaffer & Kipp, 2010).

Application Although behaviorism has been criticized for denying the inherent capabilities of persons to willfully respond to environmental situations and its relative elementary nature, it is useful in health care. Positive behaviors can be reinforced by encouragement, praise, and other rewards, and behaviors needing to be altered or removed from a child's repertoire can be extinguished by either ignoring or punishing. Parents commonly use these concepts when toilet training or teaching their children cooperation, compromise, helpfulness, and empathy. Some academic and preschool programs and parents use behavior modification and time-out activities to modify and change undesirable behavior in children. Operant conditioning can also help plan new or extinguish undesirable behavior by providing specific guidelines, determining available reinforcers, identifying responses acceptable for reinforcement, and planning how reinforcers will be scheduled so behavior is repeated.

Social learning theory is also readily applicable to health care. Children often will cooperate with procedures (blood draws, x-ray) if they see other children or adults they emulate cooperating for the same procedure. Nurses can help parents realize their appearance and behavior is often imitated by their children, and determines who might be significant role models. Finally, nurses can help by demonstrating nurturing approaches or discipline methods so parents learn effective parenting practices.

REFLECTIVE THINKING

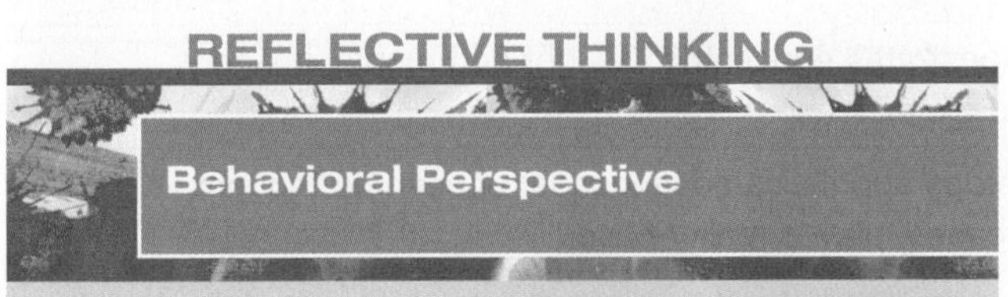

How would you use social learning and conditioning to change your child's behavior and attitudes toward responsibility and accountability?

Reflections from Families

I never realized the impact I have on my children until I heard 14-year-old Anna tell 5-year-old Harrison to "sit down and be quiet" when she was trying to study for a test she had the next day. She sounded just like me when I do not want to be bothered by one of the kids.

COGNITIVE-STRUCTURAL PERSPECTIVE

Cognitive-structural theorists are concerned with how children learn to reason, use language, and think, rather than what they learn. These theorists believe cognitive development is the result of the interaction between central nervous system maturation and active involvement with the environment. They also believe children constantly adapt to their world by integrating new knowledge with existing knowledge. The most significant cognitive-structural theorists are Jean Piaget and Lawrence Kohlberg.

Piaget and Cognitive Development

Jean Piaget (1896–1980) began studying children's intellectual development during the 1920s. He was fascinated by the process and steps children took as they discovered, reinvented, understood, and acquired knowledge of the world around them. He felt that from the moment of birth, children not only acted upon and transformed their environment, but also were shaped by the consequences of their actions. This constant interplay was responsible for intellectual growth.

Piaget believed intellectual growth followed an orderly progression based on the child's maturational level; experiences with physical objects; interactions with caregivers, other adults, and peers; and an internal self-regulating mechanism that responded to environmental stimuli. He used several terms (schema, assimilation, accommodation, and equilibrium) to describe cognitive development (Piaget, 1963).

To Piaget, interactions with the environment caused people to organize patterns of thought (**schema**), which

CRITICAL THINKING

Children and the Media

How would the behavioral perspective explain the effect the media (television, movies, videos, newspapers, the Internet) has on children and adolescents relative to violence, drug use, and promiscuity? What might you do to help caregivers concerned about this issue?

they used to interpret or make sense of their experiences. For example, young children who believe the sun is alive because it moves are operating on the schema that moving things are alive. As children develop, they may regard other moving objects they see (wind-up toy, animals) as alive as well, thereby demonstrating **assimilation**, or interpreting new information in terms of existing information. As they get older, children continually encounter animate and inanimate objects, and learn all objects are not alive. For example, trees do not move from one area of the yard to another even though they are alive. This more adequate understanding of differences between nonliving and living objects reflects **accommodation**, or revising, readjusting, or realigning existing schema to accept this new information. Assimilation and accommodation result in **equilibrium**, or harmonious relationships between thought processes and the environment (Piaget, 1963; Shaffer & Kipp, 2010; Wadsworth, 2003).

Stages of Cognitive Development According to Piaget, cognitive development occurs gradually, sequentially, and without regression. He postulated that development moves from simple to complex, begins with concrete situations and objects, and proceeds to abstraction. Piaget suggested cognitive development passes through four stages and several phases within some of these stages. Stages represented increased integration and organization, and although sequential, children could pass through them at different rates. Table 6-6 presents Piaget's stages of cognitive development. Refer back to Table 6-3 to compare Piaget's stages with Freud, Erikson, and Sullivan.

During the **sensorimotor stage** (birth to age 2), the foundation of future cognitive functioning is established and sensory and motor capabilities are used to gain a basic understanding of the world. Infants learn goal-directed

TABLE 6-6 Stages of Piaget's Theory of Cognitive Development

STAGE/PHASE	AGE	CHARACTERISTICS
Sensorimotor	Birth to 2 years	
Reflexive	Birth to 1 month	Demonstrates predictable, innate survival reflexes
Primary circular reactions	1 to 4 months	Responds purposefully to stimuli; initiates, respects satisfying behaviors
Secondary circular reactions	4 to 8 months	Learns from intentional behavior; motor skills/vision coordinated; recognizes familiar objects
Coordination of secondary schemes	8 to 12 months	Develops object permanence; anticipates others' actions; differentiates familiar/unfamiliar
Tertiary circular reactions	12 to 18 months	Interested in novelty, repetition; understands causality; solicits help from others
Mental combinations	18 to 24 months	Learns simple problem solving; imitates
Preoperational	2 to 7 years	
Preconceptual	2 to 4 years	Demonstrates egocentric thought and mental imagery; language increases
Intuitive	4 to 7 years	Develops sophisticated language; egocentric thought decreases; play is reality-based
Concrete operations	7 to 11 years	Understands relationships, classification, conservation, seriation, reversibility; logical reasoning limited; less egocentric thought
Formal operations	11 years and older	Is capable of systematic, abstract thought

behavior, alternate ways of achieving a goal, the connection between cause and effect, and that they can make things happen. Infants also acquire a primitive sense of who they are and their relation to others, and realize objects continue to exist even after they are out of sight (object permanence). For example, 6-month-old infants will continue to look for a rattle that has been dropped on the floor even though they cannot see it.

The sensorimotor stage is divided into six phases. The **reflexive phase** (birth to 1 month) is characterized by predictable, innate survival reflexes (sucking, grasping) becoming more efficient and generalized. During the **primary circular reaction phase** (1–4 months), the infant performs more complex, repetitive behaviors that appear to be responses to initial chance events centering on the infant's own body (following objects that disappear, expecting disappeared objects to reappear). They initiate and repeat satisfying behavior, and learn how their body feels. Infants during this phase commonly look and reach for objects in their environment. From 4 to 8 months (**secondary circular reaction phase**), the infant learns from intentional behavior (shaking rattle to hear sound), usually explores the world from a sitting position, and begins to show some understanding of objects (recognizes familiar objects, searches for objects at the point they disappear). Motor skills and vision become further coordinated and interest in the environment increases. The **coordination of secondary schemes phase** (8–12 months) occurs when the infant understands concepts of space and object permanence, learns to direct actions toward an intended goal (searches for hidden objects; drops, throws, examines objects), and anticipates actions of others (caregiver comes with crying). They can differentiate objects (caregiver and stranger; familiar toy and unfamiliar toy), and begin developing individual habits or ways of learning about the world. The **tertiary circular reaction phase** (12–18 months) is characterized by interest in novelty and repetition (continually hitting toy hammer on variety of surfaces or objects), awareness that objects which are out of sight continue to exist, understand causality (if I throw my toy out of the crib, I cannot reach it), and can solicit help (obtain an unreachable toy). Between 12 and 18 months, solutions to problems will be discovered, objects will be increasingly explored to learn how they work, and new behaviors developed (refer to Figure 6-18). During the **mental combinations phase** (18–24 months), young children are able to think before acting and use memory for simple trial and error problem solving. They can name and locate familiar objects, predict effects when observing causes, imitate behavior, and demonstrate symbolic and ritualistic play (Piaget, 1963).

During the **preoperational stage** (2–7 years), children use language and have a growing understanding of the past, present, and future. However, they have not yet developed the concept of irreversibility. That is, if one of two clay balls of the same size is flattened in front of the child, the child will not believe the two clay balls still contain the same amount of clay. They do not fully grasp the relationship between objects and events, and do not understand the process of transition (if A is less than B, and B is less than C, then A is less than C). They display egocentric thought (unable to take another's perspective), are easily fooled, respond to events and objects according to how they appear, are not able to understand the fundamental relationships among and between phenomena, and intermingle fantasy with reality. By the end of the stage they begin to realize others do not always perceive the world as they do (Piaget, 1963) (Figure 6-19).

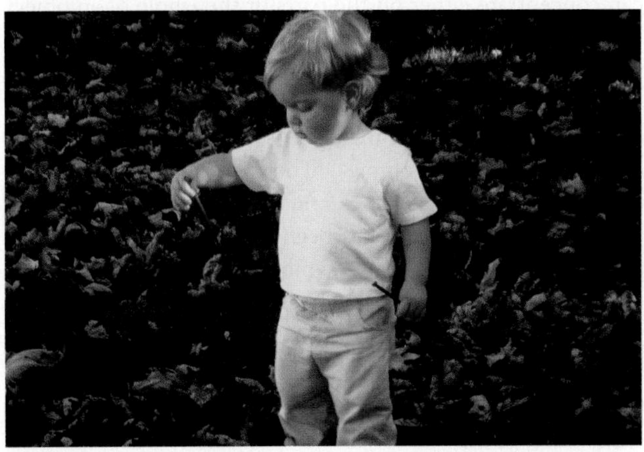

FIGURE 6-18 This 15-month-old is exploring sticks and leaves. DELMAR CENGAGE LEARNING.

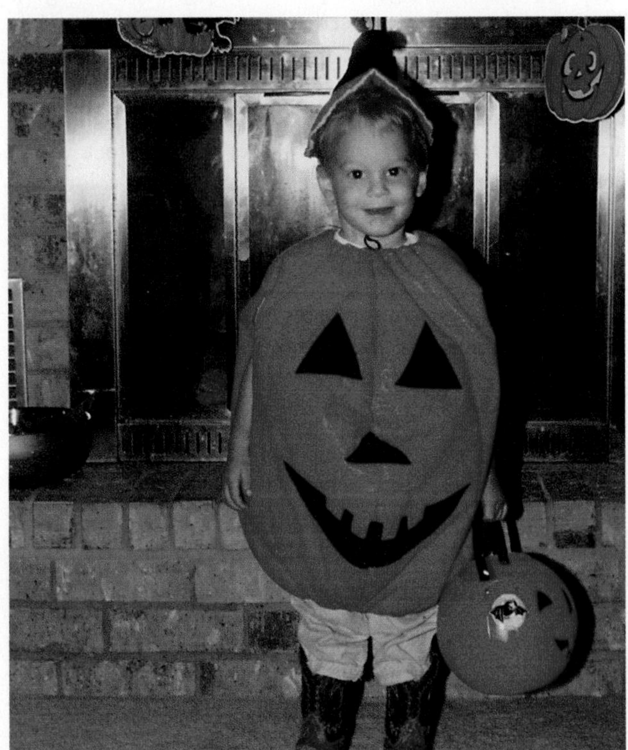

FIGURE 6-19 Toddlers often wear Halloween costumes throughout the year just to pretend and play dress-up. DELMAR CENGAGE LEARNING.

Piaget divides the preoperational stage into two phases, the preconceptual and intuitive phases. The **preconceptual phase** (2–4 years) is characterized by increasing use of language, egocentric thought, symbolic play, and mental imagery. During the **intuitive phase** (4–7 years), the child demonstrates more sophisticated language development, decreasing egocentrism, incessant questioning, and more reality-based play. Children during this phase are black and white in their thinking (cannot focus on more than one aspect of a situation at the same time, easily deluded by appearances, every question has a simple and direct answer), can concentrate either on the parts or the whole of an object but cannot relate to both at the same time, and cannot reverse actions, situations, or physical properties of objects (i.e., wide and tall containers do not contain the same amount of water even if the child is shown that the containers have the same volume). They also believe inanimate objects have human feelings and are capable of human actions, assume everything has been created either by humans or a supernatural force, use symbolic play (pieces of wood become boats, trucks, cars, animals), and play-act events experienced in their everyday life (Piaget, 1963).

Children acquire and use mental activities in the **concrete operations stage** (7–11 years) and begin understanding the basic properties of and relationships between objects and events (Figure 6-20). Their capability for logical reasoning is limited to their experiences. However, they are able to classify objects into several categories (size, shape, color), and understand the principle of conservation (things are the same even though shape or arrangement changes). They can also understand seriation according to a principle (arrange buttons according to size). Children in this stage tend to solve practical problems through trial and error, understand reversibility (a lump of clay contains the same volume when it is shaped into a ball or rolled into a rope), focus on several dimensions at the same time (color, size, shape), develop intricate rules, see others' viewpoints, and understand others' intentions (Piaget, 1963).

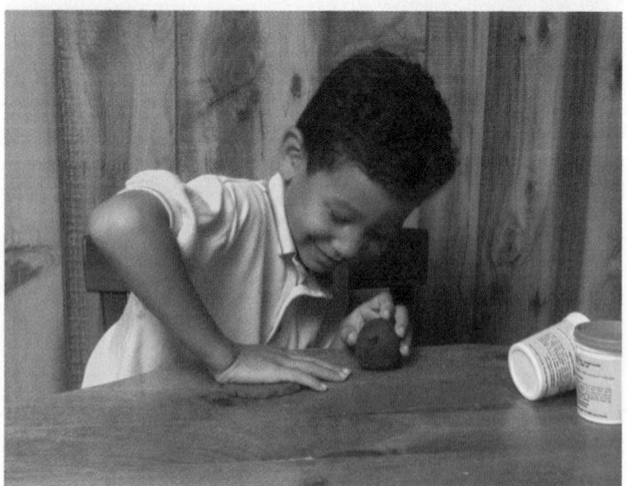

FIGURE 6-20 During concrete operations children begin to understand the principle of conservation. DELMAR CENGAGE LEARNING.

The **formal operations stage** (12 years and older) is characterized by systematic and abstract thought. Because they may enjoy thinking about hypothetical issues, children and adolescents in this stage may become idealistic. Their developing deductive reasoning abilities allow them to consider alternate solutions before choosing the correct answer. Their developing inductive reasoning ability allows them to organize and construct theories about their ideas. Children and adolescents in this stage move from what is real to what is possible, and can project themselves into and plan for the future. Finally, they have a better understanding of mathematics and scientific principles (proportion, variables) and are able to establish personal values and rules (Piaget, 1963).

Evaluation

Piaget has had a major influence on cognitive theory and caused developmental psychologists to focus on mental processes and their role in behavior. Today, most developmentalists accept Piaget's beliefs and have tested many of his propositions. They have demonstrated cognitive development is discontinuous and progresses through a series of different and increasingly complex stages. We now know children think differently than adults, and can only learn and do what they understand. Piaget's ideas influence child rearing and education by encouraging caregivers and teachers to be sure their efforts are understandable and children have firsthand experiences when learning about their world.

Those criticizing Piaget mention he defines his concepts rather loosely, pays little attention to the influences of emotions and motivation on learning, and underestimates the importance of adult interactions as a source of cognitive growth. They also suggest he does not fully explain how children progress from one stage to another and makes no allowance for cognitive growth continuing on through adulthood. In addition, he does not acknowledge people may advance to a certain cognitive level in one aspect of their lives but not in others, nor accept the idea that some people never reach the higher stages of abstract thought (Crain, 2005; Shaffer & Kipp, 2010; Sigelman & Rider, 2009).

The cognitive theories are inclusive since they are concerned with the process of learning rather than the content involved. However, the theory has limited consistency

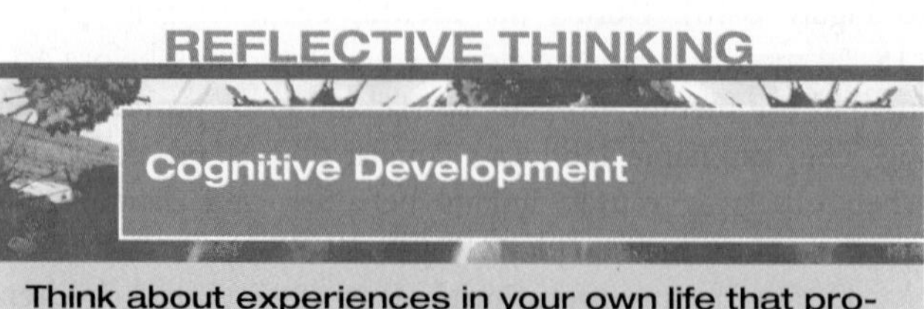

REFLECTIVE THINKING

Cognitive Development

Think about experiences in your own life that provide examples of Piaget's concepts of assimilation and accommodation. Describe them. Provide examples of formal and concrete operational thought. Do you use concrete operational thought more or less than formal operational thought? Explain your position.

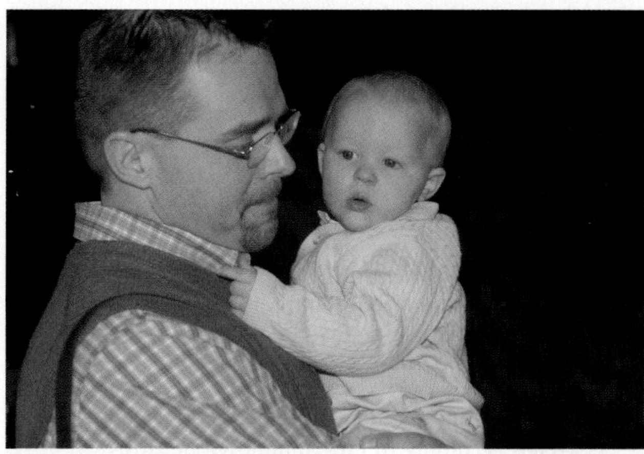

FIGURE 6-21 **Fathers are important in the lives of their children.** DELMAR CENGAGE LEARNING.

because the focus is exclusively on cognitive development, rather than on other areas of development. The cognitive theories are also not highly accurate. Even though the theory predicts the content and sequence of developmental stages, the lack of operational definitions is limiting. Relevance is also difficult to measure because definitions are vague and which variables are important is not always clear. However, this theory is fruitful because its application to the educational setting has raised a number of questions related to learning. Finally, somewhat simple, the theory requires more explanation than the behavioral theories but less explanation than the psychodynamic theory, because it includes few principles (organization, adaptation) but a detailed number of axioms and laws (Shaffer & Kipp, 2010).

Application Piaget's theory is especially important whenever communicating and interacting with children. This holds true not only when talking about health- and illness-related topics but also in any interactions at home, in the school, or in a community setting (Figure 6-21).

During the sensorimotor stage, infants use sight and motor skills to learn about the environment and become familiar with their abilities. Manipulative toys, mobiles, and bright pictures or photographs are helpful since young children in this stage receive comfort from these objects. The environment should be safe, and opportunities provided for exploring and manipulating objects. During the preoperational stage children become more verbal but are limited in thought processes. They may often believe they are the cause of illness in themselves or someone they love. Therefore, careful explanations of experiences in language the child will understand are important. Children also need to be reassured they are not responsible for illnesses in themselves or others.

School-age children are in the concrete operations stage. This means they are capable of mature thought, but need to manipulate or see objects to understand how they are related, change, or interact. Details are important when providing explanations, but care should be taken so the child understands the discussion. Allowing children to manipulate or at least see equipment used in treatments and procedures or items talked about in classes will help them understand their experiences better.

Adolescents are capable of abstract thought (formal operations). Therefore, providing complete and clearly understood information, both verbally and in writing, is important. If adolescents have a chronic, long-term illness such as diabetes or cystic fibrosis, reeducation or clarification may help them learn more about their disease and its care. However, since all adolescents may not have developed mature abstract thought, parents, nurses, and teachers should always be prepared to provide information at a more concrete or individualized level.

EVIDENCE-BASED PRACTICE

Does Culture Affect a Child's Cognitive Development?

CLINICAL PROBLEM

Children from different cultures develop different cognitive skills and abilities, because a number of factors specific to the culture play a role in a child's cognitive development. For example, childrearing practices and parental goals for children, resources, values, motivations, important developmental transitions that are culture specific, children's activities with other children or adults, and how one thinks and uses cultural tools and institutions will affect how children develop their cognitive skills.

BEST CLINICAL PRACTICE

When caring for children of different cultures it is important to be aware of cultural values that indicate why a particular cognitive skill is different for other children, why it is valued by parents and useful to the child, how the child learned the skills, how it is used in the culture, and how it may change over time or as the child grows older.

IMPLICATIONS FOR NURSING

- Be aware of specific values held by different cultures that may affect a child's cognitive development.
- Educate parents about the differences they may see in their child's cognitive development when compared to a child of a different culture.
- Encourage parents with strong cultural mores, values, and traditions to integrate these cultural mores, values, and traditions in to their child's cognitive development.

Reference: Maynard, A. (2008). What we thought we knew and how we came to know it: Four decades of cross-cultural research from a Piagetian point of view. *Human Development, 51*, 56–65.

KOHLBERG AND MORAL DEVELOPMENT

Lawrence Kohlberg (1927–1987), inspired by Piaget, formulated a theory of moral development that described changes in thinking about moral judgments and reflected societal

FAMILY TEACHING

Cognitive Development

- Remind caregivers their children may learn at different rates and in different ways. Even though adolescents are capable of formal operational thought, some still may use concrete operations.
- Encourage caregivers and family members to use simple language when talking with young children and help them understand directions may need to be repeated several times, or paired with a demonstration. Encourage family members to be patient with a child's questions as that is the way they learn about the world.

norms and values. In developing his theory, he asked children and adults to resolve a series of moral dilemmas, thereby challenging them to choose between obeying a rule, law, or authority figure and taking action to serve a human need that conflicts with these rules, laws, or authority figures. For example, should a mother who cannot afford an expensive drug that would save the life of her child steal the drug from a pharmacy? Kohlberg was interested in the underlying rationale for the moral decisions rather than the decision itself (Kohlberg, 1963).

He also believed the process of moral development was influenced by internal and external factors. Internal factors included empathy, intelligence, impulse control, and the ability to judge behavior. External factors included rewards, punishment, family structure, and parent and peer contacts (Lewis & Volkmar, 1990). Finally, he suggests moral growth progressed through universal and invariant sequences of three broad levels, each containing several stages. The stages cannot be skipped, and regression is not possible (Kohlberg, 1963). Table 6-7 presents Kohlberg's stages of moral development. Refer back to Table 6-3 for a comparison of Kohlberg's stages with Freud, Erikson, Sullivan, and Piaget.

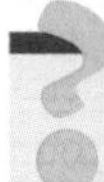

KIDS WANT TO KNOW

Helping with Homework

"How come Ryan doesn't understand the math problem? I've told him how to do it many times. It was easy for me" (question of a 13-year-old sibling when helping his 6-year-old brother with his homework).

Six-year-olds need lots of practice and explanations whenever you are helping them with homework. Some children catch on easily, but others need more time. Try to be patient and remember we all learn at our own pace.

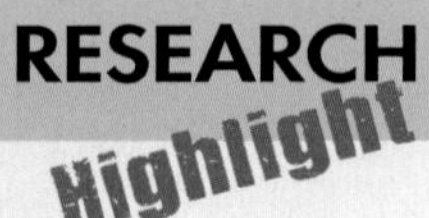

Fathers and Their Children's Cognitive Development

STUDY PURPOSE

To discover fathers' contribution to young children's cognitive development.

METHODS

Father–child and mother–child interactions were assessed according to how supportive or intrusive parenting was. Parent–child interactions were also videotaped in home visits when children were 2- and 3-years-old and right before entering kindergarten. Parent–child interactions were measured using scales adapted from the NICHD Study of Early Child Care's "Three Box" scales. Children's cognitive, language, and social and emotional development were assessed with the Bayley Scales of Infant Development, the Peabody-Picture Vocabulary Test-III, the Woodcock-Johnson Applied Problems and Letter-Word Identification, and the Leiter-Revised Examiner Rating Scale.

FINDINGS

Fathers were as sensitive as mothers and both parents showed low levels of intrusiveness. However, fathers with at least a high school education were less intrusive and more supportive than fathers with fewer resources. Fathers' supportiveness affected children's language and cognitive development at all ages as well as children's emotional and social behaviors, but less consistently. Father intrusiveness was related only to younger children's social and emotional behaviors.

IMPLICATIONS

It is important to educate parents on the impact of their supportiveness and intrusiveness on their children. It may be important to provide programs for fathers that promote/encourage positive parenting and further their education.

REFERENCE

Cabrera, N., Shannon, J., & Tamis-LeMonda, C. (2007). Fathers' influence on their children's cognitive and emotional development: From toddlers to pre-K. *Applied Development Science*, *11*(4), 208–213.

Stages of Moral Development The first level (**preconventional morality**), characterized by an egocentric focus, is divided into three stages. During stage 0 (**premoral stage**; birth to 2 years), impulses rule behavior. Infants and

TABLE 6-7 Stages of Kohlberg's Theory of Moral Development

STAGE/LEVEL	AGE	CHARACTERISTICS
Preconventional Level	Birth to 7 years	
Premoral stage	Birth to 2 years	Cannot differentiate right from wrong
Punishment and obedience orientation stage	2 to 3 years	Demonstrates conforming behavior based on fear of punishment
Instrumental realistic orientation stage	4 to 7 years	Displays conforming behavior based on rewards
Conventional Level	7 to 12 years	
Interpersonal concordance orientation stage	7 to 10 years	Evaluates behavior on intent and others' reactions
Authority and social order maintaining orientation stage	10 to 12 years	Obeys out of respect for laws, authority
Postconventional Level	12 years and older	
Social contract or legalistic orientation stage	12 years through adolescence	Believes laws should further human values and express majority views
Universal ethical principles orientation stage	Adolescence through adulthood	Defines right and wrong based on universal, comprehensive, and consistent, yet personal, ethical principles

young children are unable to differentiate right from wrong. What is good is pleasant or exciting; what is bad is painful or feared. Stage 1 (2–3 years) is the **punishment and obedience orientation stage**. During this stage, behaviors, decisions, and conformity to rules are based on fear of punishment rather than respect for authority ("I do it because you tell me to and I don't want to be punished"). A child's "goodness" and "badness" are defined by consequences; the more severe the punishment, the more "bad" the act. During stage 2, called the **instrumental realistic orientation stage** (4–7 years), rules are obeyed to gain rewards or satisfy personal objectives. Sometimes the child does something to please others, but other times, children will make decisions and behave out of self-satisfaction and self-concern; something is done to get something in return ("I do it because it makes me feel good"). There is no feeling of gratitude, loyalty, or justice (Kohlberg, 1963).

The second level (**conventional morality**) is seen in the school years. Here, the individual is concerned with maintaining and valuing the rules and expectations of the family, group, or society. Conformity and loyalty are reflected in good behavior and societal approval. Stage 3 is **interpersonal concordance orientation**, or the "good boy," "good girl" orientation (7–10 years). Here, behavior and decisions are evaluated on the basis of one's intent ("he means well") and concerns about others' reactions ("I'll do it because you expect it and will give me something"). Behavior may also be evaluated on the basis of how the other person feels ("I know what it's like to be cold, so I'll give you my sweater"). Stage 4 (10–12 years), **authority and social order maintaining orientation**, is characterized by believing laws should be obeyed because they are the laws and take precedence over any personal wishes, good intentions, or group beliefs. People conform to societal expectations because they want to preserve the social order, rather than because they are afraid of being punished (Kohlberg, 1963).

The third level is **postconventional morality** (12 years and older), with a universal focus where right, wrong, and moral values are defined autonomously and in terms of broad principles of justice that may conflict with authority figures or written laws. Stage 5 (**social contract or legalistic orientation**) reflects awareness that just laws should be followed because they further human values and express the majority will. However, laws compromising human rights or dignity are unjust and should be challenged. Social rules are not the only reason for behavior and decisions; there are higher moral principles (equality, justice, due process) which also need consideration. Stage 6 (**universal ethical principles orientation**) is attained by few. Considered the highest moral state, right and wrong are defined on universal, comprehensive, and consistent, yet personal, ethical principles. These ethical principles are abstract moral guidelines that include respect for individual rights and that transcend any law or social contract. People at this stage are able to see the perspective of anyone affected by a moral decision and can make a decision considered fair for everyone. They believe there is a higher order than the social order, and accept pain, death, and injustice as an integral part of existence (Kohlberg, 1963).

Evaluation Kohlberg's theory is important, and offers a detailed stage sequence for moral thinking (Crain, 2005). However, Kohlberg's stages seem more helpful in describing the moral reasoning of adolescents and adults rather than young children. The stages are also clearly related to a person's level of cognitive development. In addition, proficiency at role-taking may be necessary for conventional morality since reasoning here requires the ability to recognize another's point of view before being able to evaluate intentions capable of winning approval. Kohlberg also suggests intellectual growth does not guarantee moral development since those able to achieve the highest level of intellect may continue to reason about moral issues at the preconventional or conventional level. Two ingredients necessary for moral development have also been left out: perspective taking (the ability to see a situation from another's point of view) and empathy (the ability to understand another's emotional condition) (Hutchinson, 2011).

Another criticism of Kohlberg's theory is its bias against women because his subjects were all male (Gilligan, 1977). Gilligan argues women develop a different moral orientation than men because of how they are raised. Men are raised to consider moral dilemmas as inevitable conflicts between individuals that laws and other social conventions are designed to resolve (**morality of justice**). Women, however, are taught to be empathetic, nurturant, and concerned about others, and often define their sense of "goodness" in terms of their interpersonal relations (**morality of care**). However, there is little evidence women emphasize morality of care more than men do and they travel different moral paths. Both men and women are concerned with issues of

Moral Motivation, Sympathy, and Prosocial Behavior

STUDY PURPOSE

To examine the effects of moral motivation and sympathy on prosocial behavior in a representative longitudinal sample of Swiss kindergarten children. Initially, the moderating role of moral motivation on the relationship between sympathy and prosocial behavior was investigated to discover if sympathy predicted prosocial behavior; children with high moral motivation were expected to compensate for a relative lack of sympathy by displaying high levels of prosocial behavior. Then, the connection between moral motivation and prosocial behavior was examined. High levels of moral motivation were expected to be positively associated with prosocial behavior.

METHODS

In both arms of the study, sympathy was assessed by; (a) children's self-reports; (b) mothers' ratings; and (c) kindergarten teachers' ratings. Children's prosocial behavior was assessed in both arms of the study by; (a) mothers' and kindergarten teachers' ratings; and (b) spontaneous sharing behavior. Moral motivation was measured in the first study by having children respond to two hypothetical rule violations: not sharing a pencil; and stealing another child's chocolate. In the second study moral motivation was measured using two hypothetical situations: (a) neglecting prosocial moral duties (i.e., not supporting a needy child, not sharing a pencil and (b) violating a strict moral duty by committing psychological /physical harm (i.e., stealing another child's chocolate, pushing a child off a swing).

FINDINGS

Mothers and teachers rated girls more prosocial than boys. Girls were also rated more sympathetic than boys by mothers and teachers early in the study. Sympathy and prosocial behavior were related. Children with high moral motivation scored high on teacher-rated prosocial behavior, regardless of their level of sympathy. If children had low moral motivation, they showed increased prosocial behavior with increasing levels of sympathy. Girls shared more than boys and revealed more moral motivation in the context of harm than boys, and also showed more prosocial behavior and sympathy than boys.

IMPLICATIONS

Because children's moral motivation and sympathy are related to prosocial behaviors, it would be important to promote children's moral growth.

REFERENCE

Malti, T., Keller, M., Gummerum, M., & Buchmann, M. (2009). Children's moral motivation, sympathy, and prosocial behavior. *Child Development*, *80*(2), 442–460.

FAMILY TEACHING

Moral Development

- Explain to caregivers and other family members how moral development changes during childhood and why children of certain ages respond the way they do.
- Teach caregivers appropriate ways to help children learn ethical behavior.
- Provide examples of appropriate disciplinary practices caregivers can use for children of various ages based on their level of moral development.

individual rights, justice, and the law, and raise issues of compassion and interpersonal responsibility when reasoning about real-life moral dilemmas

Application Although Kohlberg offered age guidelines for his stages, they are approximate but many people do not reach the highest stage (Crain, 2005; Sigelman & Rider, 2009). Therefore, adults, including nurses, teachers, and parents, need to understand the stage a particular child is in relative to moral development. Parents need to be educated about normal behavior at each stage so behavioral expectations are appropriate and discipline is fair. For example, young children may stop hitting each other because of fear of being punished rather than because it is morally wrong, and show no remorse for their behavior. Parents also need to know that only when young children show interest in another's well-being will they truly understand why it is wrong to hit others. In addition, children may participate in an activity for the wrong reason (to please others, to avoid punishment), and not fully understand the decisions they are making. In addition, whether or not rules are internalized may affect how well a new regime of care is accepted. Therefore, it is important to give clear and specific reasons for requests or treatment regimes and be patient if there are questions or more information is needed. When moral dilemmas arise (should I do it if it is against my parent's wishes? Will the new treatment really help or just prolong a painful condition?), clarifying, explaining, and validating concerns may help contribute to moral development.

REFLECTIVE THINKING

Moral Standards

Think about a moral dilemma that has affected you. Why do some people have higher moral standards than others? Apply your answer to Kohlberg's theory. How can you assist children and adolescents to develop high moral standards?

CONTEXTUAL PERSPECTIVE

The contextual perspective adopts a broader focus by viewing human development as a lifelong process affected by other individuals or groups of individuals, and the historical, cultural, political, and economic context one lives in. Ecological theory is an example of the contextual perspective.

Ecological theory stresses the importance of understanding how relationships between the individual and a variety of environmental systems affect human development. The theory proposes changes in the environment produce changes in the individual, and changes in the individual produce changes in the environment. These interchanges occur simultaneously and continuously. Children are seen as active participants in creating their environments, and although biology is important, the main emphasis is on environmental systems. Development is viewed as continuous; experiences throughout the life span are important. However, situational influences have more impact on development than individual characteristics, and there are culture-bound principles explaining differences between individuals raised in different cultures (Asian, Italian, Swedish) and at different historical time periods (1920s, 1950s, 1980s).

BRONFENBRENNER AND ECOLOGICAL THEORY

Urie Bronfenbrenner (1917–2005) offers an organizational framework for examining the environmental systems' influences on human development (Bronfenbrenner, 1979). For him, the child's world is like a set of nested Russian dolls, with these systems (microsystem, exosystem, macrosystem) ranging from the most immediate setting or context (family, peer group) to the more remote setting or context (the government). The developing individual, embedded within the center of these systems, has a unique heritage (physical appearance, maturation rate, emotionality, innate intelligence, physical health, gender), which is different from any other person. As individuals mature, they impact and are impacted by these changing systems and relationships differently.

The broadest context or system affecting development is the **macrosystem**. This system is large, enduring, and contains cultural and subcultural ideologies and beliefs, hazards, resources, or lifestyles. Although macrosystem effects may not be obviously apparent in the life of any one individual, the macrosystem profoundly affects development (Bronfenbrenner, 1979). For example, children living in poverty or an inner city ghetto (the macrosystem) are exposed to beliefs and values that are different than those of children living in an affluent suburb.

The **exosystem**, or middle system, indirectly affects development and is the linkage between microsystems and larger institutions affecting the system. It includes social settings the individual never directly experiences even though these experiences provide an important influence (Bronfenbrenner, 1979). Examples of the exosystem are caregiver work settings, social networks, or educational level; one's neighborhood (including environmental noise or pollution); and community decision-making bodies. For example, when a caregiver travels a great deal or works different shifts, the child's family life may change. Children can be affected by whether or not a caregiver's work is satisfying or stressful, or if the caregiver has supportive social relationships. If a planning and zoning commission decides to build a highway through a neighborhood playground, the child's recreational life changes.

The **microsystem** is the child's immediate environment and includes daily face to face interactions with others (family, peers, teachers, neighbors, religious leaders) or community resources (school, church) (Bronfenbrenner, 1979). The importance of the microsystem changes across development; during infancy, the family and home are of primary importance, whereas in middle childhood and adolescence, the peer group and school become more important (Figure 6-22).

The **mesosystem** is the interrelationship among two or more microsystems and includes the networks of microsystems of a given person. For example, the interrelationship among the home, school, and peer group make up a child's mesosystem. For an adult, the mesosystem typically consists of family, employment situations, and friends. If the mesosystem has positive interrelationships, development will progress normally and optimally. If the mesosystem has negative interrelationships, development may not progress normally or optimally.

Bronfenbrenner has also refined his original theory (Bronfenbrenner & Morris, 2000) to include bioecological factors that influence development according to the contributions individuals themselves make to their environment

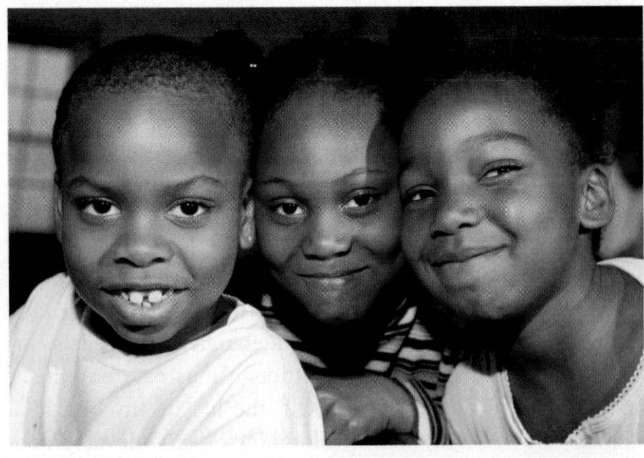

FIGURE 6-22 Family is important and the connections made in childhood last throughout a lifetime. DELMAR CENGAGE LEARNING.

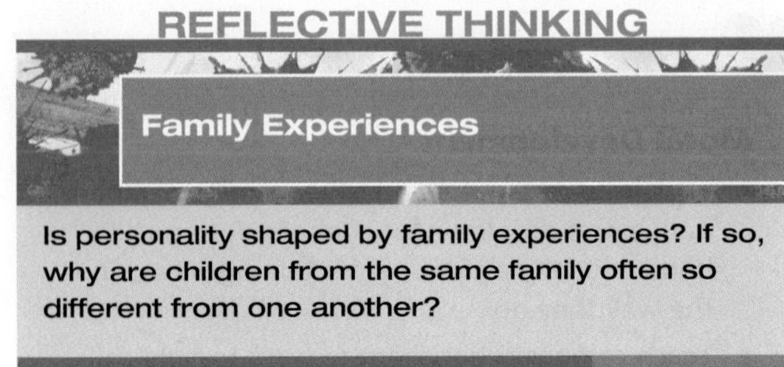

REFLECTIVE THINKING

Family Experiences

Is personality shaped by family experiences? If so, why are children from the same family often so different from one another?

(proximal processes). He proposes, therefore, that: (1) individuals need to actively contribute to their environment in order for development to occur; (2) these contributions need to occur regularly and over time; (3) the contributions need to become more complex over time; (4) reciprocity occurs as individuals and groups influence each other; (5) although interactions with individuals are important, interactions with objects in the environment are also important; and (6) the role and importance of these processes change over time as the individual and the environment also change.

Evaluation Bronfenbrenner brings a unique and essential perspective to the study of human development: the importance of analyzing relationships between the child and environmental systems. He also has emphasized the importance of examining connections between systems, and reminds us children and their environments are always changing and influencing one another. It also encourages us to examine development naturally where it occurs rather than in laboratory settings. One weakness of ecological theory is it does not discuss the influence of biology or cognitive processes on development, and does not describe how these processes influence and are influenced by environmental systems. The theory also provides a limited view of development since it does not give a clear picture of the course of human development over the life span and may not represent what the real world is actually about. Initially, it is difficult to generate principles about development true for most people (Shaffer & Kipp, 2010; Sigelman & Rider, 2009).

Application Bronfenbrenner provides a view of the child impacted by his environment in a way that is different from the behavioral perspective. In the ecological theory, the child is viewed holistically, as a member of a unique family, neighborhood, and cultural belief system, that impact development. The behavioral perspective, however, proposes behavior is impacted by the environment consisting of models, rewards, or punishment only. Ecological theory also suggests the important influence parents have on their children, it reminds us home and cultural environments are not the same, and why those

CRITICAL THINKING

Developmental Theories

How do the issues discussed in the early part of the chapter relate to the theories described in the later part of the chapter? That is, how does Freud or Erikson or Bandura or Piaget view the child: active or passive; innately pure or of original sin? How would Bronfenbrenner view the impact culture has on a child?

home resources and facilities must be assessed before discharge or prescribing home treatment or procedures.

The model is responsible for helping us recognize the impact social and economic status (SES) has on children, since, in addition to income, SES is related to parental employment, education, and social networks. Therefore, the better the parents' education, the more likely they are to work, have a work ethic, and possess organizational skills. Working parents are also more likely to provide activities for children that build academic, physical, and social skills, consequently connecting them to other members of the community. Finally, children living in families with higher SES status have better access to health care than families with lower SES status.

Finally, ecological theory helps us understand human development can proceed along several different pathways depending on the interplay of internal and external forces within the individual. All children in the same family really may come from different families, since a first child's experiences with parents may be different than a second or third child's experiences in the same family. Bronfenbrenner also reminds us the influence children have on parents and other family members is as important as the effect family members and parents have on children. It also teaches us to realize stress or illness in one family member will affect the entire family system. Parents with a hospitalized or ill child cannot always be at home with siblings or spouses; siblings may worry about, miss, or feel responsible for the ill child or, in contrast, resent the attention the ill child receives.

Therefore, nurses implementing Bronfenbrenner's perspective in acute care and in the community will need to understand children in their environmental context, teach this information to parents, and allow for family differences. Other nursing considerations include educating parents and other family members (especially siblings), and appropriately conveying understanding and support of parents struggling with setting priorities relative to family and work commitments. Finally, nurses need to encourage sibling visits and contact with peers and extended family members.

CONCLUSION

There is no single principle, issue, or theory capable of holistically explaining human development. Therefore, it is important for nurses to be aware of the contribution each makes to understanding development and apply each in context. For example, behaviorists and social learning theorists help us understand how various stimuli, reinforcers, and models influence behavior. Psychoanalytic theory helps us understand the unconscious mind, reasons for abnormal behaviors, and the importance of the past in influencing present behavior. Erikson helps us realize the best solution to a stage crisis is not always positive; exposure to the negative conflict is sometimes inevitable and helpful. The cognitive theories, oriented toward explaining how we acquire and process information and become

REFLECTIVE THINKING

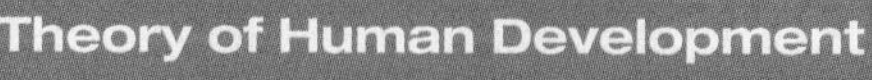

Theory of Human Development

If you could develop a theory of human development, what would you propose? Upon which theoretical orientation do you lean most heavily in constructing your theory? What personal experiences have you had that might influence the developmental theory you would construct?

IN THE REAL WORLD

I never realized how important understanding the theories of human development was when I was in school. They all were so confusing and abstract. They didn't make any sense. I didn't understand why I needed to learn them. But now I know I cannot effectively care for children unless I use that knowledge. It is important to know that a 3-year-old needs to be encouraged to learn about the world, a 7-year-old needs friends to visit, an infant needs a primary nurse who meets needs promptly, and an adolescent may have many questions about his care and treatment regime. Now I know why we learn about the important influence parents have on their children and why siblings need to be included in care. I use those theories every day. I always did, I just didn't know it.

knowledgeable about the world, help us learn not only what to expect cognitively from children of all ages, but also help us understand how to challenge and stimulate learning at any age. Ecological theories remind us of the importance of the family, culture, and society in development. Therefore, it is essential nurses develop an eclectic approach to human development, borrowing and using whatever is appropriate with individual children and their families as they practice holistic care.

KEY CONCEPTS

- Principles providing a framework for studying humans suggest development is orderly, sequential, directional, and interrelated; becomes increasingly differentiated, integrated, and complex as the child grows; and is unique for each child. Also, children are competent and possess qualities and abilities ensuring their survival and promoting their development, and they tend to learn one new skill at a time.
- Seven themes related to human development include nature versus nurture, continuity versus discontinuity, passivity versus activity, cultural versus sensitive periods, assumptions of human nature, universality versus context specificity, and behavioral consistency.
- The psychodynamic perspective of human development is divided into the psychosexual, psychosocial, and interpersonal theories. Major theorists are Freud, Erikson, and Sullivan.
- Behaviorism (classical and operant conditioning) and social learning emphasize the importance of the environment on human development. Major theorists include Pavlov, Skinner, and Bandura.
- Cognitive-structural theorists (Piaget, Kohlberg) are concerned about how children learn to think, use language, and develop moral reasoning.
- The contextual perspective suggests a variety of systems (microsystem, exosystem, macrosystem, mesosystem) and historical, cultural, political, and economic environments interact to impact human development. One major theorist is Bronfenbrenner.
- Each theory of human development contributes to our understanding of human behavior. Whenever caring for an individual child, the eclectic approach to human development will help provide holistic care.

REVIEW ACTIVITIES

1. List the eight principles characteristic of human development and explain what each means.
2. List the seven themes characteristic of human development and explain each.
3. Summarize the main points of each theory. Which theorists describe life-span development?
4. Suppose a caregiver comes to you with questions regarding sibling rivalry. Using Piaget's theory, what advice would you offer?
5. Using the stages of moral development, provide examples of children's actions or behaviors indicative of each stage.
6. Compare and contrast the theories discussed in the chapter.

STUDY QUESTIONS

1. The predictable physiological, psychosocial, and cognitive changes occurring over one's life is termed:
   a. growth.
   b. maturation.
   c. development.
   d. behavioral consistency.
2. Which of the following statements refers to the continuity/discontinuity theme?
   a. Development is predestined.
   b. Environment influences development.
   c. Development is smooth and gradual.
   d. Children are born as blank slates.

3. Which of the following statements refers to the cultural universal/cultural relativism theme?
   a. Behavior is shaped by external forces.
   b. Each period of development is important.
   c. Children actively interact with their environment.
   d. Humans follow similar pathways, no matter where they live.

4. According to psychoanalytic theory, human development is influenced by:
   a. a past history of reinforcement and punishment.
   b. unconscious drives and motives.
   c. the pleasure principle.
   d. active involvement with the environment.

5. According to Erikson's theory, we should expect toddlers to:
   a. want to feed and dress themselves without interference.
   b. be reluctant to give up sucking on a pacifier.
   c. maintain a very close proximity to their mothers.
   d. readily agree with most parental suggestions.

6. Which of the following theorists suggests social interactions are essential for personality development, personality can and does change, and chums are important for school-age children?
   a. Watson
   b. Sullivan
   c. Gilligan
   d. Bandura

7. A child constantly hits other children. According to operant conditioning this behavior occurs because:
   a. of innate tendencies.
   b. similar behavior has been observed in others.
   c. frustration leads to aggression.
   d. it has been reinforced.

8. Which of the following is an example of Piaget's concrete operations?
   a. A 4-year-old child insists that a ball of clay "has more" once it is shaped into a snake.
   b. A 5-year-old child demonstrates the ability to read a paragraph to decode the words.
   c. A 7-year-old child maintains that a ball of clay weighs the same amount after it has been shaped into a snake.
   d. An 8-year-old child must recalculate basic mathematic facts each time he attempts to solve a word problem.

9. During which stage of moral development is the individual concerned with maintaining and valuing the rules and expectations of the family, group, or society?
   a. conventional morality stage
   b. preconventional morality stage
   c. postconventional morality stage
   d. universal ethical principles stage

10. Brofenbrenner suggested which of the following statements?
   a. The interrelationships between changing organisms and their world affect human development over a lifetime.
   b. Species-specific behavior is preselected to increase chances of survival.
   c. It is important to answer four questions: What causes behavior? How did it develop? What are its biologic consequences? How did it evolve?
   d. It is important to understand the relationship between environmental systems when examining human development.

REFERENCES

Bandura, A. (1977). *Social learning theory.* Upper Saddle River, NJ: Prentice Hall.

Bronfenbrenner, U. (1979). *The ecology of human development.* Cambridge, MA: Harvard University Press.

Bronfenbrenner, U., & Morris, P. A. (2000). The ecology of developmental processes. In W. Damon (Series Ed.) & R. M. Lerner (Vol. Ed.), *Handbook of child psychology: Vol. 1. Theoretical models of human development* (5th ed., pp. 993–1028). New York: John Wiley.

Cabrera, N., Shannon, J., & Tamis-LeMonda, C. (2007). Fathers' influence on their children's cognitive and emotional development: From toddlers to pre-K. *Applied Development Science, 11*(4), 208–213.

Crain, W. (2005). *Theories of development: Concepts and applications* (5th ed.). Upper Saddle River, NJ: Prentice Hall.

Emde, R. N. (1992). Individual meaning and increasing complexity: Contributions of Sigmund Freud and Rene Spitz to developmental psychology. *Developmental Psychology, 28,* 347–359.

Erikson, E. (1963). *Childhood and society* (2nd ed.). New York: Norton.

Freud, S. (1933). *New introductory lectures in psychoanalysis.* New York: Norton.

Gilligan, C. (1977). In a different voice: Women's conceptions of self and of morality. *Harvard Educational Review, 47*(4), 481–517.

Hutchinson, E. D. (2011). *Dimensions of human behavior: The changing life course* (4th ed.). Thousand Oaks, CA: Sage Publications Inc.

Kohlberg, L. (1963). The development of children's orientation toward a moral order: Sequence in the development of moral thought. *Vita Humana, 6,* 11–33.

Lewis, M., & Volkmar, F. (1990). *Clinical aspects of child and adolescent development* (3rd ed.). Philadelphia: Lea and Febiger.

Maynard, A. (2008). What we thought we knew and how we came to know it: Four decades of cross-cultural research from a Piagetian point of view. *Human Development, 51,* 56–65.

Malti, T., Keller, M., Gummerum, M., & Buchmann, M. (2009). Children's moral motivation, sympathy, and prosocial behavior. *Child Development, 80*(2), 442–460.

Piaget, J. (1963). *The origins of intelligence in children.* New York: Norton.

Shaffer, D., & Kipp, K. (2010). Developmental psychology: Childhood and adolescence (8th ed.). Belmont, CA: Wadsworth Cengage Learning.

Sidman, M. (1960). *Tactics of scientific research.* New York: Basic Books.

Sigelman, C., & Rider, E. (2009). *Life-span human development* (6th ed.). Belmont, CA: Wadsworth Cengage Learning.

Skeels, H. (1966). Adult status of children with contrasting early life experiences. *Monographs of the Society for Research in Child Development, 31*(9).

Skinner, B. F. (1953). *Science and human behavior.* New York: Macmillan.

Sullivan, H. S. (1953). *The interpersonal theory of psychiatry.* New York: Norton.

Umaña-Taylor, A., Gonzales-Backen, M., & Guimond, A. (2009). Latino adolescents' ethnic identity: Is there a developmental progression and does growth in ethnic identity predict growth in self-esteem? *Child Development, 80*(2), 391–405.

Wadsworth, B. (2003). *Piaget's theory of cognitive and affective development* (5th ed.). New York: Longman.

SUGGESTED READINGS

Angoff, W. (1988). The nature-nurture debate, aptitudes, and group differences. *American Psychologist, 43,* 713–720.

Bandura, A. (1986). *Social foundations of thought and action.* Englewood Cliffs, NJ: Prentice Hall.

Bornstein, M. H. (1989). Sensitive periods in development: Structural characteristics and causal interpretations. *Psychological Bulletin, 105,* 179–197.

Bronfenbrenner, U. (1986). Ecology of the family as a context for human development: Research perspectives. *Developmental Psychology, 22,* 723–742.

Buckley, K. W. (1989). *Mechanical man: John Broadus Watson and the beginnings of behaviorism.* New York: Guilford Press.

Child Development and Developmental Psychology. These journals are two leading research journals in the field of child development and discuss the research interests of developmentalists over the years.

Colby, A., & Kohlberg, L. (1987). *The measurement of moral judgment. Vol. 1: Theoretical foundations and research validation.* Cambridge, U.K.: Cambridge University Press.

Forman, D., Aksan, N., & Kochanska, G. (2004). Toddlers' responsive imitation predicts preschool-age conscience. *Journal of Psychological Science, 15*(10), 699–704.

Gedo, J. E. (2001). The enduring scientific contributions of Sigmund Freud. In J. A. Winer & J. W. Anderson (Eds.), *The annual of psychoanalysis: Vol. 29. Sigmund Freud and his impact on the modern world* (pp. 105–115). Hillsdale, NJ: Analytic Press.

Gewirtz, J. L., & Pelaez-Nogueras, M. (1992). Skinner, B. F.: Legacy to human infant behavior and development. *American Psychologist, 47,* 1411–1422.

Horowitz, F. D. (1992). John B. Watson's legacy: Learning and environment. *Developmental Psychology, 28,* 360–367.

Kohlberg, L. (Ed.). (1973). *Collected papers on moral development and moral education.* Cambridge, MA: Moral Educational Research Foundation.

Mullahy, P. (1970). *Psychoanalysis and interpersonal psychiatry: The contributions of Harry Stack Sullivan.* New York: Science House.

O'Donohue, W., & Ferguson, K. E. (2001). *The psychology of B. F. Skinner.* Thousand Oaks, CA: Sage Publications Inc.

Smetana, J., Campione-Barr, N., & Yell, N. (2003). Children's moral and affective judgments regarding provocation and retaliation. *Merrill-Palmer Quarterly, 49*(2), 209–236.

RESOURCES

Refer to the online student StudyWARE for Potts & Mandleco at http://www.CengageBrain.com for additional content and study aids.

Organization: **American Academy of Child and Adolescent Psychiatry (AACAP)**
Description: Provides information regarding mental illnesses, data concerning efforts to prevent mental illnesses, how to seek proper treatment, and access to services for children and adolescents.
Website/Resource: http://www.aacap.org

Organization: **American Academy of Family Physicians**
Description: Offers information regarding family physician careers, clinical research, advocacy, practice management, and recent news/publications.
Website/Resource: http://www.aafp.org

Organization: **American Academy of Pediatrics**
Description: Offers general information related to child health, specific guidelines concerning many pediatric issues, information regarding AAP programs, activities, policies, guidelines, publications, and other child health resources.
Website/Resource: http://www.aap.org

Organization: **American Pediatric Society**
Description: Offers information regarding the American Pediatric Society, including abstracts, research, publications, and scientific meetings.
Website/Resource: http://www.aps-spr.org

Organization: **American Psychological Association**
Description: Offers readers information regarding psychology topics, publication, careers, news, and education, as well as the ability to access a psychology help center to address issues encountered in daily life.
Website/Resource: http://www.apa.org

Organization: **Children's Defense Fund (CDF)**
Description: A nonprofit child advocacy organization; website offers information regarding CDF's policies and mission, child advocacy resources, and child research data.
Website/Resource: http://www.childrensdefense.org

Organization: **Pediatrics (the journal)**
Description: Offers access to the current issue, past issues, topic collections, and journal supplements.
Website/Resource: http://www.pediatrics.org

Organization: **Society for Research in Child Development (SRCD)**
Description: Offers information regarding SRCD membership, publications, and policies.
Website/Resource: http://www.srcd.org

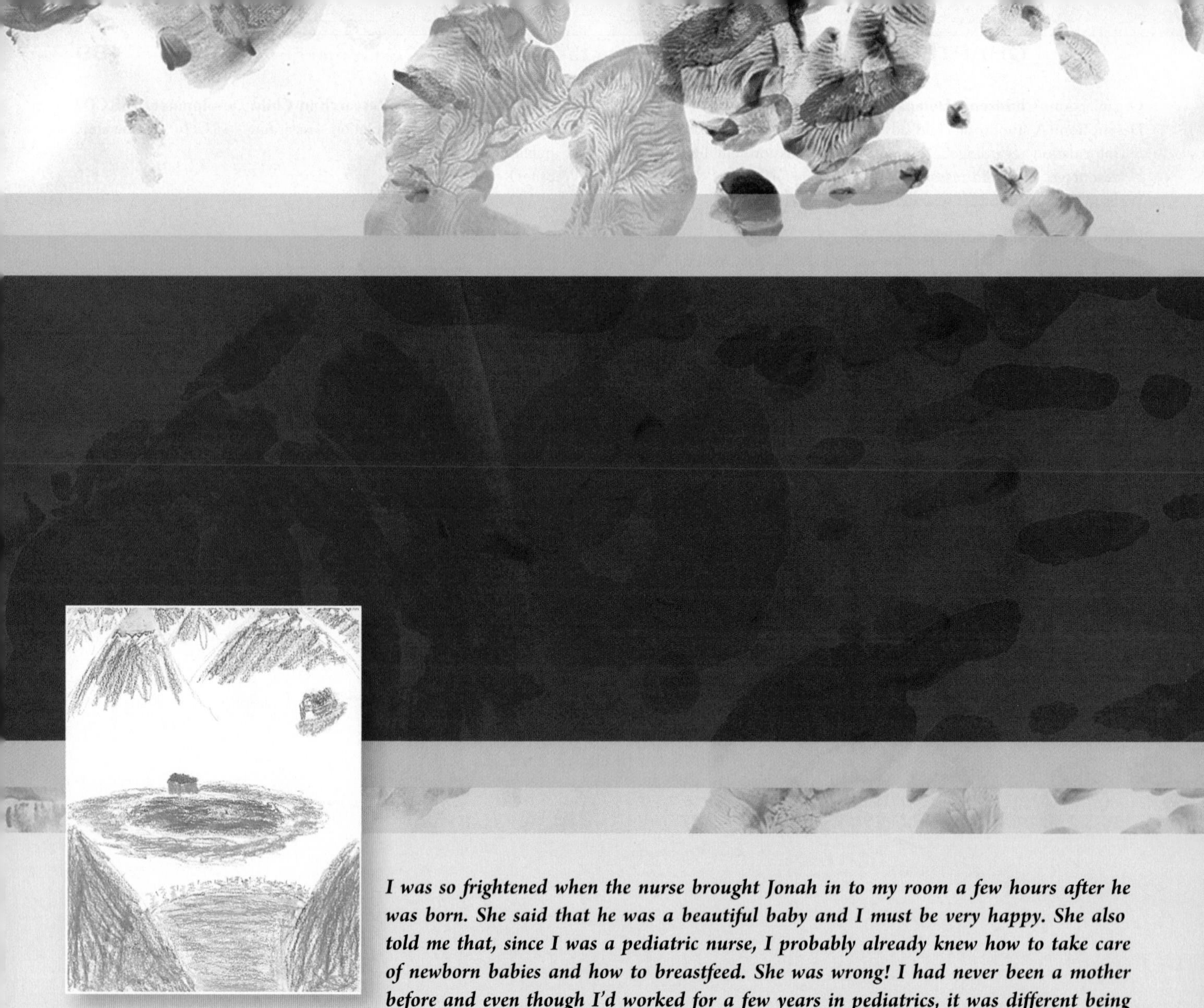

I was so frightened when the nurse brought Jonah in to my room a few hours after he was born. She said that he was a beautiful baby and I must be very happy. She also told me that, since I was a pediatric nurse, I probably already knew how to take care of newborn babies and how to breastfeed. She was wrong! I had never been a mother before and even though I'd worked for a few years in pediatrics, it was different being the mother, not the nurse. I wanted her to teach me everything new mothers are taught and to treat me like I was just like any other new mother.

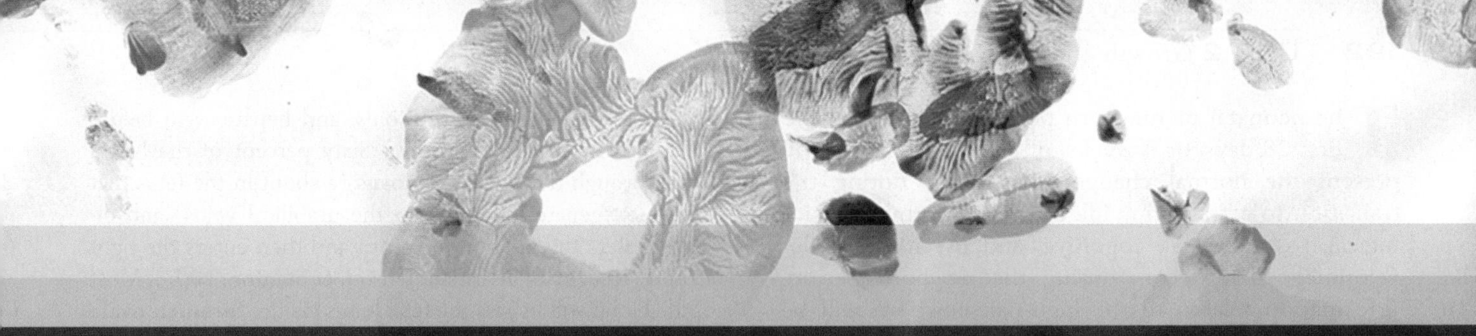

CHAPTER 7

Growth and Development of the Newborn

Patricia King, RN, FNP, MS; Natalie Annen, RN, BS
Barbara L. Mandleco, RN, PhD

COMPETENCIES

Upon completion of this chapter, the reader will be able to:

- Identify the adaptive changes that occur during the transition to extrauterine life.
- Describe the typical physiological development of the newborn.
- Discuss the psychosexual, cognitive, and psychosocial development of the newborn.
- Identify and explain aspects of health promotion and maintenance pertinent to the newborn.
- Explain the nutritional needs of the typical newborn. Describe family educational needs regarding health promotion of the newborn.
- Discuss potential cultural and ethnic aspects that may affect newborn care.
- Explain the etiology and treatment of the high-risk newborn.
- Discuss the nurse's role in caring for healthy and high-risk newborns.
- Successfully complete the games and activities in the online student StudyWARE.

The neonatal or newborn period is defined as the first 28 days, or 4 weeks, of life. This chapter will present the normal changes that occur during the transition to extrauterine life as well as normal physiological, psychosexual, cognitive, and psychosocial development that occurs during the newborn period. Information related to the high-risk newborn will be presented also. Nursing care related to the normal and high-risk newborn will be discussed.

EXTRAUTERINE TRANSITION

Fetal circulation is different from neonatal circulation due to structural differences that include the: (1) placenta; (2) umbilical arteries and vein; (3) ductus venosus; (4) foramen ovale; and (5) ductus arteriosus. The placenta provides oxygen and nutrients for the fetus and removes carbon dioxide and other waste products. The umbilical cord connects the fetus to the placenta, and contains two arteries and one vein. The blood from the placenta flows through the umbilical vein to the abdominal wall of the fetus where it then divides into two branches. A small portion of the blood flows through one branch and to the liver, sinusoids, and hepatic vein before entering the inferior vena cava. Sixty percent of the blood flows through the **ductus venosus** (a shunt in the fetus that carries oxygenated blood from the umbilical veins) and directly enters the inferior vena cava and then enters the right atrium (Kliegman, Behrman, Jenson, & Stanton, 2007). Most of the blood will bypass the fetal lungs via the **foramen ovale** (an opening between the right and left atria) and enter the left atrium. From the left atrium, the blood enters the left ventricle and is pumped into the aorta to the hypogastric arteries. The small amount of blood that does pass from the right atrium to the right ventricle will pass into the pulmonary artery. From the pulmonary artery, a small amount will go to the nonfunctional lungs into the pulmonary vein, left atrium, left ventricle, and to the aorta. The remainder of the blood will pass through the **ductus arteriosus** (channel between the main pulmonary artery and the aorta) to the aorta. The hypogastric arteries lead to the iliac arteries and give rise to the umbilical arteries, and then return the blood to the placenta. Figure 7-1 represents fetal blood flow.

The transition to extrauterine life begins with the cutting of the umbilical cord and the initiation of respirations. With the initiation of respirations, the PaO_2 levels are

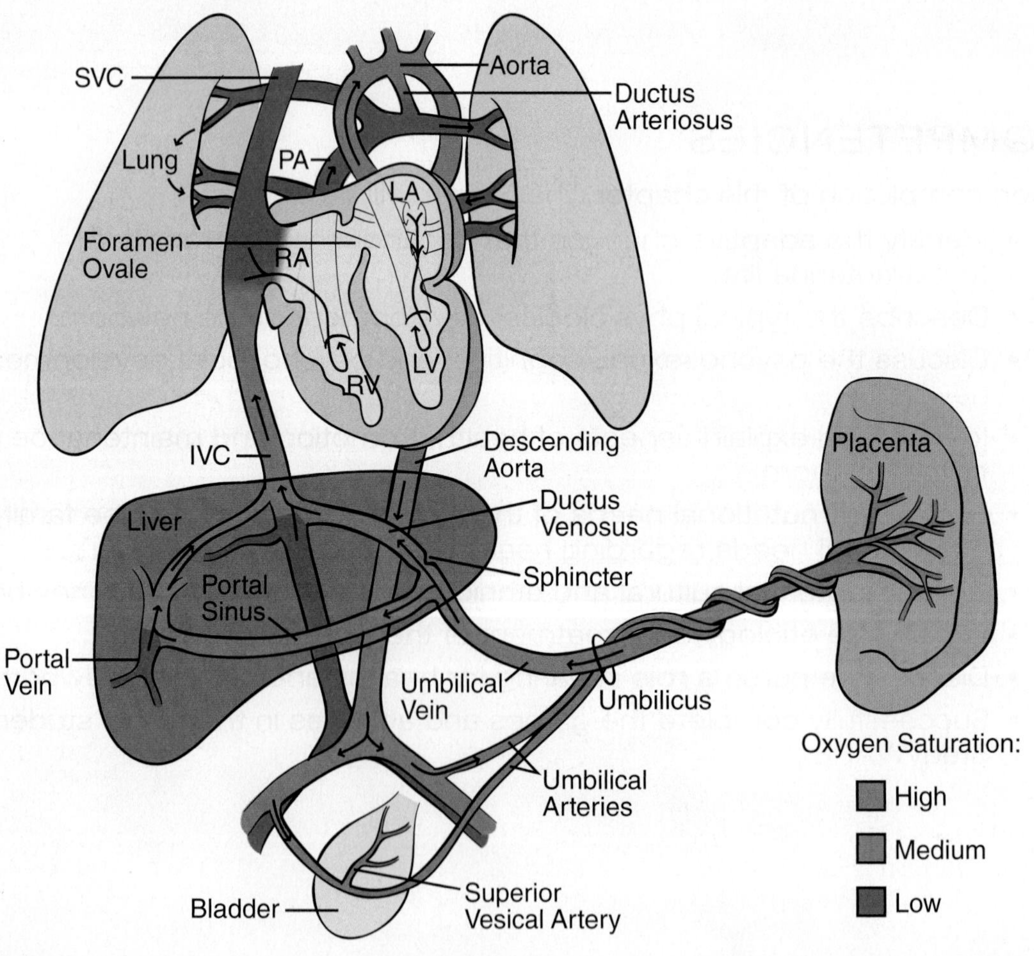

FIGURE 7-1 Fetal Circulation. DELMAR CENGAGE LEARNING.

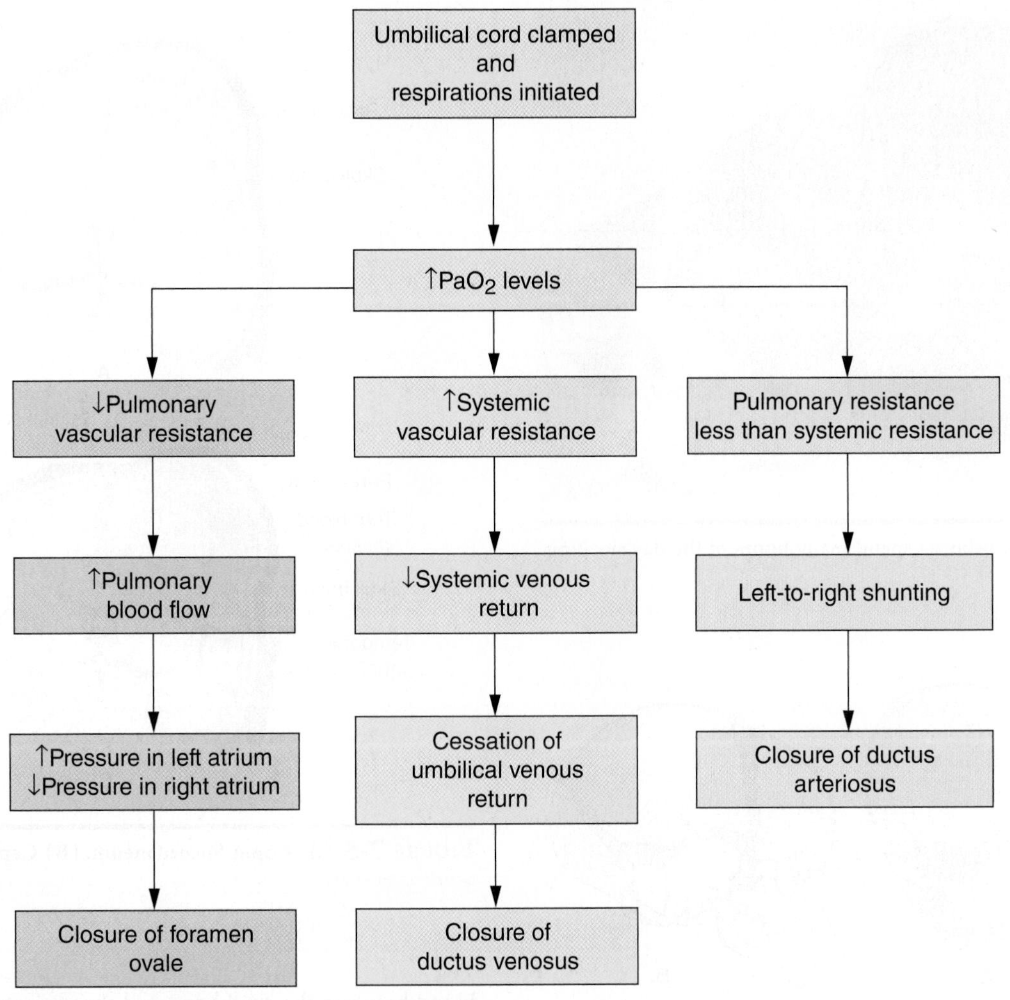

FIGURE 7-2 Transition to Extrauterine Life. DELMAR CENGAGE LEARNING.

increased and several changes occur. The decreased pulmonary vascular resistance results in increased pulmonary blood flow, causing an increase in the pressure of the left atrium, a decrease in pressure of the right atrium, and closure of the foramen ovale. The foramen ovale closes shortly after birth and then undergoes fusion of the tissue margins during early childhood. The increased PaO_2 levels also lead to an increase in systemic vascular resistance, a decrease in systemic venous return, cessation of umbilical venous return, and closure of the ductus venosus. The closure of the ductus venosus occurs gradually over a period of about 2 weeks. Since systemic resistance is greater than pulmonary resistance, a left-to-right shunt occurs within the heart, resulting in closure of the ductus arteriosus (usually within 24 hours of birth) and gradual obliteration over the next month (Kliegman et al., 2007). Figure 7-2 represents transition to extrauterine life.

The average period of transition is 6 to 12 hours, but may be shorter or longer depending on the newborn's ability to adjust to the stresses of labor, delivery, and a new environment (Kliegman et al., 2007). Therefore, during this transition period, the newborn needs to be closely observed for any difficulties so appropriate interventions may be initiated.

PHYSIOLOGICAL DEVELOPMENT

GENERAL APPEARANCE

Most people visualize a newborn as the baby seen in advertisements (Figure 7-3); however, the actual appearance may be a surprise to the caregivers. The newborn's head, which is one-quarter of the total body size, may appear out of proportion to the body and be misshapen due to the labor and delivery process (**molding**; Figure 7-4). After a long labor a **caput succedaneum** may be present. A caput is the swelling of the soft tissues of the scalp and may extend across the suture lines. A caput is evident within 24 hours after birth and usually resolves within a few days. The collection of

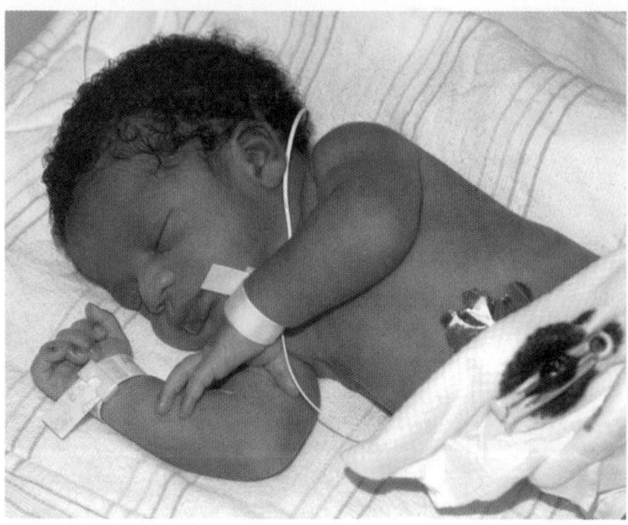

FIGURE 7-3 Newborns spend many hours of the day sleeping. DELMAR CENGAGE LEARNING.

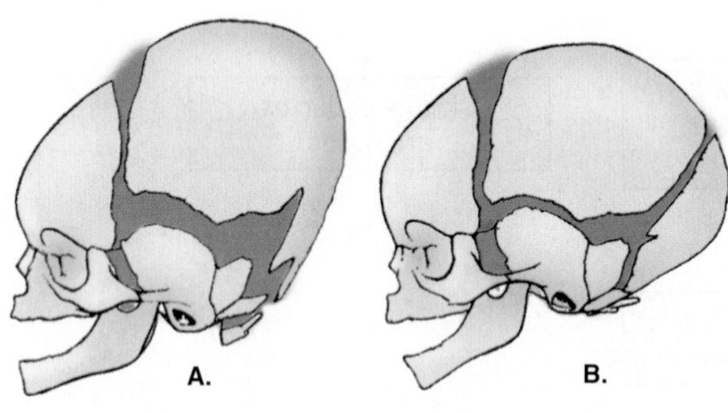

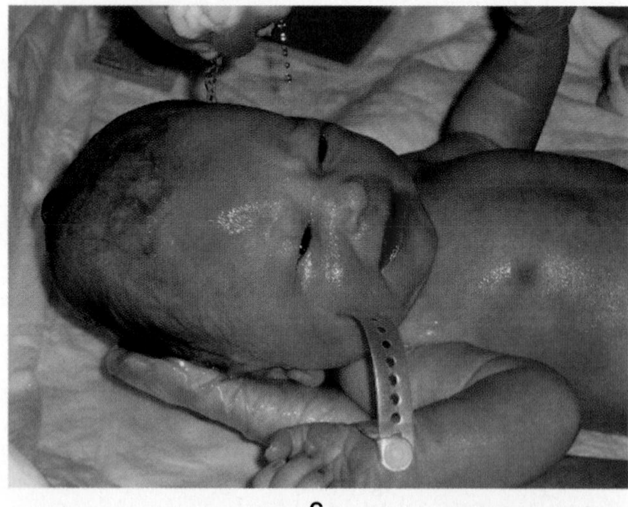

FIGURE 7-4 Molding. (A) Movement of Cranial Bones During Labor. (B) Cranial bones return to their proper placement in 2 to 3 days. (C) Newborn Exhibiting Molding. DELMAR CENGAGE LEARNING.

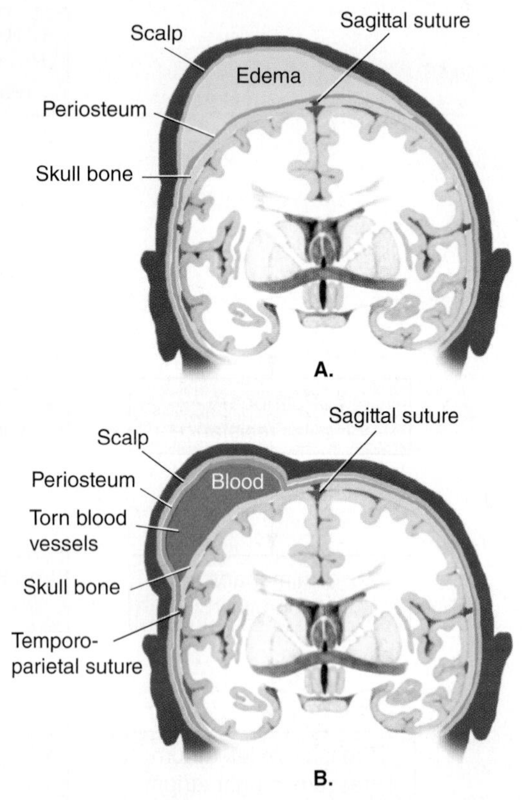

FIGURE 7-5 (A) Caput Succedaneum. (B) Cephalohematoma. DELMAR CENGAGE LEARNING.

blood between the skull bone and the periosteum as a result of the rupture of blood vessels secondary to head trauma from the birth process may result in a **cephalohematoma**. A cephalohematoma develops 24–48 hours after birth and will not cross suture lines (Figure 7-5). A cephalohematoma may take 2 to 3 weeks to resolve. Providing reassurance to the caregivers is needed with the explanation that many of these characteristics will change over the next several weeks. The newborn will soon begin to take on the appearance of a "normal" baby.

The newborn's eyelids may be puffy and the eye color may be indistinguishable. In addition, the newborn has a large, round abdomen with an umbilical area that may protrude for several weeks until the cord stump falls off. The caregiver needs to be instructed on appropriate umbilical cord care.

The extremities may appear short in comparison to the body, but hands should be able to touch the upper thighs when extended. The legs may appear to be bowed and the newborn typically remains in a position with the extremities flexed. The skin is delicate, often mottled and **acrocyanosis** may be present. Acrocyanosis is the bluish discoloration of the hands and feet caused by the instability of the peripheral circulation system (Figure 7-6).

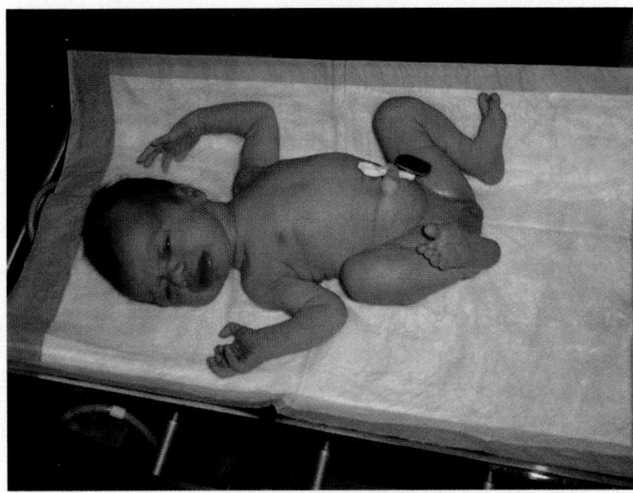

FIGURE 7-6 This newborn has acrocyanosis and also demonstrates flexion of the arms and legs. DELMAR CENGAGE LEARNING.

> **FAMILY TEACHING**
>
> **Cord Care**
>
> - The diaper needs to be folded or diapers with a notch may be used to provide air circulation to the cord.
> - Cord care with 70% isopropyl alcohol or hydrogen peroxide should be performed during diaper changes. It is important to make sure the substance is applied to the base of the cord, next to the skin. It is normal for a small amount of blood to appear on the diaper when the cord falls off.
> - Continue to provide cord care after the cord falls off until the skin appears normal.
> - Never pull the cord off or attempt to loosen it.

Many caregivers are afraid to touch the baby's head or "soft spot" due to the fear of causing damage. The soft spots, or **fontanels**, occur at the junctions or suture lines of the skull bones, allowing for the adaptation to the pelvis shape during delivery and growth of the brain over the coming year (Figure 7-7). The posterior fontanel typically closes by 3 months of age, while the anterior fontanel closes around 8 to 18 months of age. Caregivers need reassurance that many of the newborn's characteristics will change during these first few weeks and months and the newborn will then begin to take on the appearance of a "typical" baby.

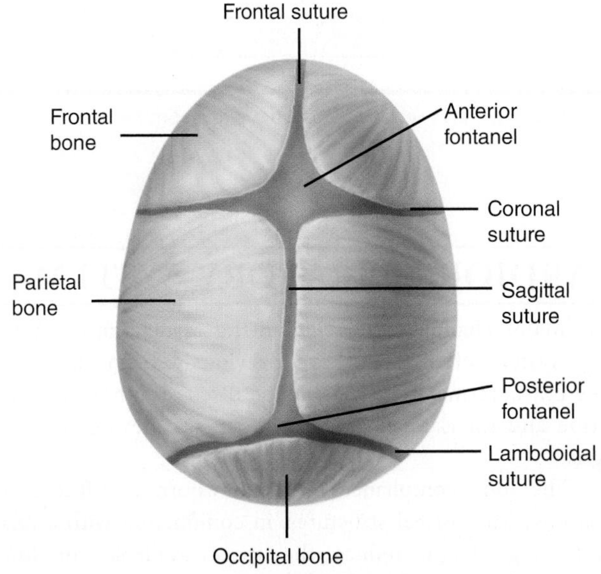

FIGURE 7-7 Placement of Sutures and Fontanels. DELMAR CENGAGE LEARNING.

NEUROLOGICAL SYSTEM

The initial neurological examination includes the observation of the newborn's position and response to handling and stimulation. The use of the Ballard Assessment Scale assists in determining the gestational age of the newborn. For accuracy and validity the examination should be completed within the first 12 hours of life (Ballard, Khoury, Wedig, Wang, Eilers-Walsman, & Lipp, 1991) (refer to Figure 7-8 for the Ballard Assessment Scale of Gestational Age). After the determination of gestational age, the newborn is classified as (1) **large for gestational age (LGA)**, (2) **appropriate for gestational age (AGA)**, or (3) **small for gestational age (SGA)**. Newborns that fall above the 90th percentile are classified as LGA. The AGA newborn is one who falls between the 10th and 90th percentile. The SGA newborn will be below the 10th percentile. Determination of gestational age assists in developing appropriate care and may influence the newborn's optimal neurological development and functioning. Refer to the high-risk section of this chapter for more information on LGA and SGA newborns.

Most of the time the newborn is in a sleep state with short periods of wakefulness between those states. These periods of wakefulness provide for caregiver interaction. As the newborn advances to the infant stage, the length of time of these periods will increase, allowing for more interactions. The newborn responds to the environment and stimulation by changing expression (smiling, grimacing, and crying). The caregivers will learn how to decipher these signals into a specific meaning for their baby.

Reflexes are primitive, innate behaviors seen in the newborn. Deep tendon reflexes can be elicited in the newborn but have limited value. The reflexes the newborn exhibits serve a variety of purposes and can be categorized into

NEWBORN MATURITY RATING & CLASSIFICATION

ESTIMATION OF GESTATIONAL AGE BY MATURITY RATING

SYMBOLS: X - 1ST EXAM O - 2ND EXAM

Gestation by Dates ________________wks

Birth Date ____________ Hour ____________ am/pm

APGAR ____________ 1 min ____________ 5 min

NEUROMUSCULAR MATURITY

	-1	0	1	2	3	4	5
Posture							
Square Window (wrist)	>90	90	60	45	30	0	
Arm Recoil		180	140-180	110-140	90-110	<90	
Popliteal Angle	180	160	140	120	100	90	<90
Scarf Sign							
Heel to Ear							

PHYSICAL MATURITY

Skin	sticky friable transparent	gelatinous red, translucent	smooth pink,visible veins	superficial peeling and or rash few veins	cracking pale areas rare veins	parchment deep cracking no vessels	feathery cracked wrinkled
Lanugo	none	sparse	abundant	thinning	bald areas	mostly bald	
Planiar Surface	heel-toe 40 - 50min: -1 <40 min: -2	>50mm no crease	faint red marks	anterior transverse crease only	creases ant. 2/3	creases over entire sole	
Breast	imperceptible	barely perceptible	flat areola no bud	stippled areola 1-2mm bud	raised areola 3-4mm bud	full areola 5-10mm bud	
Eye/Ear	lids fused loosely: -1 tightly: -2	lids open pinna flat stays folded	sl. curved pinna; soft slow recoil	well curved pinna; soft but ready recoil	formed and firm instant recoil	thick cartilage ear stiff	
Genitals Male	scrotum flat, smooth	scrotum empty faint rugae	testes in upper canal rare rugae	testes descending few rugae	testes down good rugae	testes pendulous deep rugae	
Genitals Female	clitoris prominant labia flat	prominant clitoris small labia minora	prominant clitoris enlarging minora	majora & minora equally prominant	majora large minora small	majora cover clitoris and minors	

MATURITY RATING

score	weeks
-10	20
-5	22
0	24
5	26
10	28
15	30
20	32
25	34
30	36
35	38
40	40
45	42
50	44

SCORING SECTION

	1st Exam=X	2nd Exam=O
Estimating Gest Age by Maturity Rating	______Weeks	______Weeks
Time of Exam	Date ______ Hour______ am/pm	Date ______ Hour______ am/pm
Age at Exam	______Hours	______Hours
Signature of Examiner	______M.D.	______M.D.

FIGURE 7-8 Ballard Assessment Scale. REPRINTED FROM *JOURNAL OF PEDIATRICS, 119*(3), BY J. L. BALLARD ET AL., "NEW BALLARD SCORE," P. 418, COPYRIGHT 1991 MOSBY, WITH PERMISSION FROM ELSEVIER.

localized or generalized. They are further separated into those that are of a primitive or survival nature. Refer to Table 7-1 for newborn reflexes.

> **KIDS WANT TO KNOW**
>
> **How come Maggie always has such funny positions and always grabs my finger?**
>
> They are normal reflexes that all newborns have. They will go away within the next few months.

CARDIORESPIRATORY SYSTEM

The major changes that occur in the cardiac and respiratory system after birth have previously been discussed (see Extrauterine Transition). The discussion here will describe and focus on characteristics of the newborn's vital signs.

The lung compliance of the newborn is affected by anatomy. Mediastinal structures, in conjunction with a relatively large heart, reduce the space available for lung expansion. The newborn's large abdomen also affects lung space by increasing upward pressure on the diaphragm. The structures of the thorax, including weak intercostal muscles, horizontally positioned ribs, and high diaphragm restrict lung expansion space. Finally, airway resistance is affected

Table 7-1 Neonatal Reflexes

REFLEX	STIMULI	RESPONSE	DISAPPEARS	PATHOLOGY IF ABNORMAL
LOCALIZED REFLEXES				
Eyes				
Blinking or corneal reflex*	Sudden appearance of a bright light or approach of an object toward cornea	Infant blinks	Persists throughout life	Neurological damage
Doll's eye	Head moved slowly to right or left	Eyes lag behind and do not immediately adjust to new position of head	As ability to fixate develops	Neurological damage
Pupillary*	Bright light shines toward pupil	Pupil constricts	Persists throughout life	Neurological damage
Nose				
Sneeze*	Irritation or obstruction in nasal passages	Sneezing	Persists throughout life	Neurological damage
Mouth and Throat				
Cough	Irritation of laryngeal or tracheobronchial tree mucous membranes	Coughing	Persists throughout life	Neurological damage
Extrusion	Depressing or touching the tongue	Tongue is forced outward	4 months	
Gag*	Food, suction, or passing a tube stimulating the posterior pharynx	Gagging	Persists throughout life	Neurological damage
Rooting*	Stroke or touch cheek	Head turns toward stimuli	Approximately 4 months	Central neurological system disease (frontal lobe lesion)
Sucking*	Object touching lips or placed in mouth	Sucking	7 months	Prematurity; CNS depression in full-term breastfed newborn whose mother has ingested barbiturates
Yawn	Decreased oxygen	Baby yawns	Persists throughout life	

* Survival reflex

(Continues)

Table 7-1 Neonatal Reflexes (*Continued*)

REFLEX	STIMULI	RESPONSE	DISAPPEARS	PATHOLOGY IF ABNORMAL
Extremities				
Babinski†	Lateral aspect of the sole is stroked from heel upward and across ball of foot	Hypertension of the toes	1 year	Cerebral palsy
Grasp†	Palms of hands or soles of feet are touched near base of digits	Flexion of hands and toes	8 months	Frontal lobe lesions
Palmar grasp†	Stimulate the palm	Object is grasped	4 months	
Plantar grasp†	Place the finger at the base of the newborn's toes	Toes will curl downward	8 months	Cerebral palsy; obstructive CNS lesion (abscess, tumor)
MASS REFLEXES				
Crawl	Infant placed on abdomen	Makes crawling movements with arms and legs	6 weeks	Neurological damage
Dance or step†	Newborn is held upright, one foot is allowed to touch a flat surface	Alternate stepping movements	4 months	Cerebral palsy
Moro†	Sudden changes in position or jarring	Arms extend, head moves back, fingers spread apart with thumb and forefinger forming a "c" followed by arms being brought back to center with hands clenched, spine and lower extremities extended	3–4 months	Neurological damage

† *Primitive reflex*

(*Continues*)

Table 7-1 Neonatal Reflexes (*Continued*)

REFLEX	STIMULI	RESPONSE	DISAPPEARS	PATHOLOGY IF ABNORMAL
Placing	Held upright; dorsal surface of the feet touch the edge of the table	Flexion of the knees and hips and movement of the legs up the table surface	4 months	Breech paralysis; cerebral cortex abnormalities
Tonic neck	Head turned to one side when supine	Arm and leg extend on the side head is turned toward; arm and leg flexed on opposite side	3–4 months	Neurological damage
Trunk incurvation (Galant)	Firmly stroke the back in a downward motion for about 5 cm (2 in.) when in prone position	Body curves to the side of the stimulus; important to check both sides	2–3 months	Spinal cord lesion

by the length, radius, and number of airways. Since the newborn has smaller airways and is an obligatory nose breather; any obstruction will cause respiratory distress.

The respiratory rate is typically 30 to 60 breaths per minute. The respirations are primarily abdominal and shallow, with irregular depth and rhythm. Short periods of apnea may be seen. The newborn's state of consciousness will affect the respiratory pattern. When the newborn is in a deep sleep, the respiratory pattern is quite regular. Irregular breathing is more noticeable when the newborn is in a light sleep or active state.

The newborn's heart rate will initially accelerate up to 180 beats per minute following the first breath (Davidson, London, & Ladewig, 2008). The heart rate will range from 100 beats per minute while asleep to 150 beats per minute while awake. The blood pressure is affected by the changes in blood volume that occur during transition, as well as the newborn's birth weight and activity state.

GASTROINTESTINAL SYSTEM

Gastrointestinal system motility gradually matures during the first few years of life and is significantly slower in the newborn period than in the adult period. The stomach's capacity is approximately 60 mL and gradually increases during infancy. The typical emptying time of the stomach is 2½ to 3 hours, and increases to 3 to 6 hours during infancy. Gastroesophageal reflux is common as a result of diminished lower esophageal sphincter function or inappropriate relaxation in conjunction with delayed gastric emptying. Refer to Chapter 23 for more information about gastroesophageal reflux. See Figure 7-9 for a description of stools produced by the infant.

The liver, from a gastrointestinal standpoint, is an exocrine gland that produces bile to digest fats. Because the liver has reduced bile salt secretion and the pancreas works less efficiently in the newborn, the newborn is less capable of

A. Meconium—First bowel movement; black and tarry; usually occurs within 24–48 hours of birth
B. Breastfed—Yellow to golden, pasty, sour-milk odor
C. Formula-fed—Pale to light yellow, firmer, strong odor

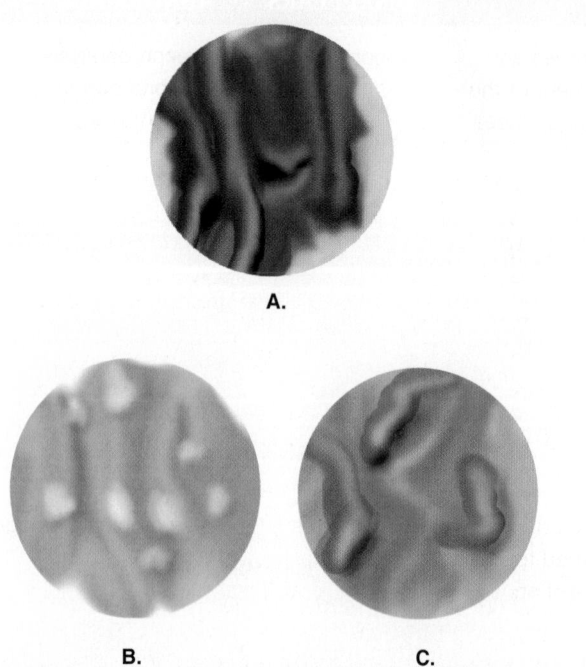

FIGURE 7-9 Stool Patterns of Newborn (A) Meconium. (B) Stool of Breastfed Newborn. (C) Stool of Formula-fed Newborn. DELMAR CENGAGE LEARNING.

absorbing fat. A discussion of the nutritional needs of the newborn will follow later in this chapter.

During uterine life, more hemoglobin is required to carry oxygen as the oxygen tension available to the fetus is decreased. After delivery, the newborn no longer requires this extra hemoglobin and the excess cells are destroyed by the reticuloendothelial system and are not replaced. As the erythrocytes are broken down, the end products of metabolism are formed, and the hemoglobin becomes a protein consisting of globin and heme. Unconjugated (indirect) bilirubin is formed in the liver and plasma concentrations may become elevated (Davidson et al., 2008).

The liver contains specialized cells that remove unconjugated bilirubin from the bloodstream and convert it to conjugated bilirubin. Since conjugated bilirubin is water soluble, it can then be excreted through the stool as bile. However, the newborn's immature liver is not always able to adequately alter and remove the excess bilirubin, and as the amounts accumulate, visible **jaundice**, the yellowish discoloration of the skin and eyes caused by excess bilirubin, occurs (Figure 7-10).

The American Academy of Pediatrics (2004) recommends that all newborns be assessed no less than every 8–12 hours for the development of jaundice. Assessing levels

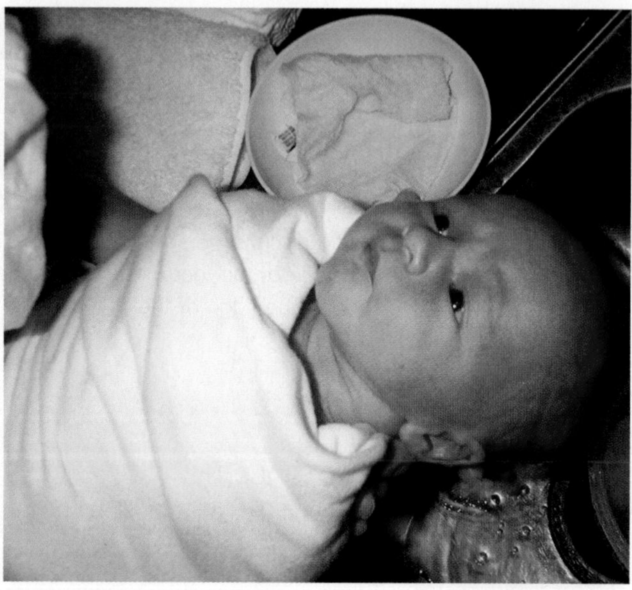

FIGURE 7-10 Notice the sclera on this newborn appears yellowish. DELMAR CENGAGE LEARNING.

may include obtaining a transcutaneous bilirubin (TcB) measure or total serum bilirubin (TSB) (Beachy & Nash, 2007; Maisels, 2005a; 2005b; Stokowski, 2007). The use of visual estimation, such as blanching the skin, may lead to errors in estimation of the jaundice's severity and therefore should not be utilized.

Over the past decade, with the initiation of early discharge, the incidence of severe hyperbilirubinemia has increased (AAP, 2004; Maisels, 2005a; 2005b). The American Academy of Pediatrics (2004) therefore recommends assessing each newborn for risk factors for developing severe hyperbilirubinemia before discharge. If indicated, measurement of the transcutaneous or total serum bilirubin is obtained and plotted on a nomogram based on the newborn's age in hours. This nomogram places the newborn in a risk zone ranging from low risk to high-risk of developing severe hyperbilirubinemia (AAP, 2004; Maisels, 2005a; 2005b). Each hospital nursery should develop protocols for the identification and evaluation indicating jaundice. This protocol should include a standing order indicating when nursing staff should obtain a transcutaneous or total serum bilirubin measurement.

Bilirubin encephalopathy is the clinical central nervous system finding resulting from toxicity to the basal ganglia and brainstem nuclei. **Kernicterus** is the chronic and permanent sequelae of bilirubin toxicity (AAP, 2004; Beachy & Nash, 2007; Maisels, 2005a; 2005b). This condition may lead to cerebral palsy, auditory neuropathy, gaze and vision abnormalities, and dental enamel hypoplasia.

In the mid-1950s, a nurse in England would take the infants outside to be exposed to the healing forces of the fresh air and sun (Stokowski, 2007). This was the beginning of phototherapy. **Phototherapy**, or the use of special high-intensity fluorescent lights, is generally an effective method of reducing serum bilirubin levels and preventing kernicterus. The phototherapy light oxidizes the unconjugated bilirubin

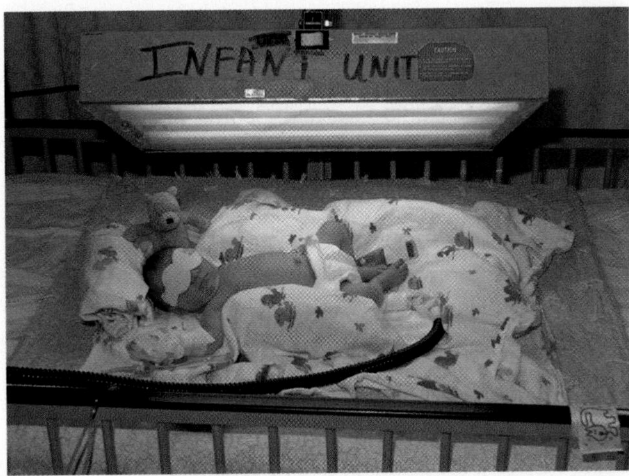

FIGURE 7-11 Newborn with Jaundice Receiving Phototherapy. DELMAR CENGAGE LEARNING.

in the skin, which then becomes soluble in water and is excreted in the stool and urine. The use of phototherapy, ordered by the primary care provider, may be administered in the newborn nursery or at home (Figure 7-11). The newborn's eyes should be shielded with special patches to prevent possible retinal damage when undergoing phototherapy, and the genital area covered with a surgical mask to provide protection to the gonads, since maximum exposure is accomplished when the newborn is unclothed.

Serial serum bilirubin levels, obtained every 8–12 hours while under phototherapy, may be used to assess treatment effectiveness. When the level returns to the normal range, phototherapy may be discontinued. Sometimes a rebound elevation of bilirubin occurs initially after phototherapy has been discontinued, but it should soon return to an acceptable level.

The options for providing phototherapy have advanced from the first unit that was developed in 1958 (Stokowski, 2007). The decision as to which system to use will depend on the size of the newborn, the degree of hyperbilirubinemia, and the location where the therapy will be provided (Stokowski, 2007). In some cases, a combination of systems may be warranted.

The use of blue-green high irradiance light that has low heat generation is one choice. With this unit one has the option to switch between single or double phototherapy. A second choice is the use of a single quartz halogen bulb. A disadvantage with this system is the heat that is generated. The use of fluorescent tubes was one of the original phototherapy systems. There are a variety of tubes available with a special blue being noted to be the most effective (Stokowski, 2007).

The introduction of fiber optics afforded the opportunity for the development of more convenient phototherapy units such as the bili blanket, which contains fiber optic fibers and can be placed under and around the newborn. This facilitates caregiver contact as the newborn may be held (Stokowski, 2007).

NURSING ALERT

Care of the Newborn during Phototherapy

The newborn's eyes need to be protected while under phototherapy (Beachy & Nash, 2007; Stokowski, 2007). The eye protectors need to be opaque to protect the retina from potential damage (Stokowski, 2007). Periodic examination and care of the eyes and skin should be performed. In addition, the newborn should be repositioned every 2 hours. Many newborns experience loose stools and increased urine output that may lead to dehydration and excoriation of the skin in the perianal area (Beachy & Nash, 2007; Stokowski, 2007).

GENITOURINARY SYSTEM

The kidneys are responsible for the regulation of fluid and electrolyte balance, arterial blood pressure, and removal of several toxins. The fetus does not begin urine production with glomerular filtration until 9–12 weeks' gestation, with renal development continuing until 36 weeks' gestation (Kliegman et al., 2007). The term newborn's kidneys have a full complement of glomeruli and even though the glomeruli are small, the surface area for filtration, in respect to body weight, is higher than the adult's. The newborn's renal tubules are short, narrow, and less able to concentrate urine due to the inability to reabsorb water, sodium, glucose, and other solutes back into the blood; the ability to concentrate urine completely will not be achieved until 3 months of age.

Urine output depends on the glomerular filtration rate and tubular reabsorption of water. Normal urinary output for a newborn is 15 mL/kg/day (Davidson et al., 2008). This is equivalent to approximately 2 to 6 voidings per day. The urine output is typically low during the first day of life and increases as daily intake increases. Renal function should be evaluated in a newborn that does not void in the first 24 hours of life. Normal newborn urine values are identified in Table 7-2.

TABLE 7-2 Normal Values for Newborn Urine

Color	Pale yellow
Glucose	Negative
pH	4.5–8
Protein	<5–10 mg/dL
RBC	Negative
Specific gravity	1.001–1.020
WBC	Negative

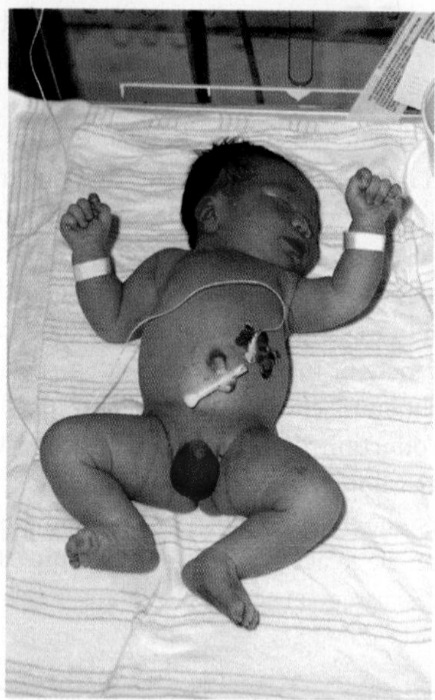

FIGURE 7-12 **Notice the pendulous scrotum on this full-term newborn.** DELMAR CENGAGE LEARNING.

Male genitals are evaluated for the presence of testes and the appearance of the rugae on the scrotal sac. Prior to 36 weeks' gestation, the scrotum is small with few rugae (folds), the testes have not descended to the scrotum, and they remain in the inguinal canal. The term newborn, however, will demonstrate a pendulous scrotum covered with rugae, with testes palpable in the lower portion of the scrotal sac (Figure 7-12). If the scrotum is distended, the use of a transilluminator may reveal a **hydrocele** or a collection of fluid between the parietal and visceral layers of the tunica vaginalis, the outermost covering of the testes. No treatment is usually necessary unless the hydrocele persists beyond the first year of life. Caregivers may need reassurance that this is normal and will soon disappear.

Circumcision, which originated over 15,000 years ago (the oldest documented evidence is found in ancient Egypt), is the surgical removal of the foreskin, which is the skin that covers the glans, or head, of the penis. This is considered an elective procedure when performed on the newborn. Initially, circumcisions were based on a ritual from religious practices or "rites of passage" to manhood. This ritual continues in some religions and societies today.

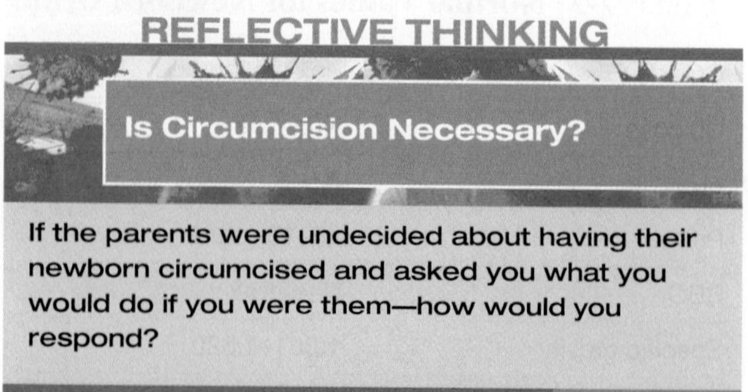

REFLECTIVE THINKING

Is Circumcision Necessary?

If the parents were undecided about having their newborn circumcised and asked you what you would do if you were them—how would you respond?

The World Health Organization (2007) estimates 30% of males worldwide are circumcised. It is very common in Africa, North America, New Zealand, and Australia, almost universal in the Middle East and Central Asia, and uncommon in Asia (except in the Philippines and South Korea), Central America, South America, the United Kingdom, Europe, and Russia.

The decision to have the newborn male circumcised is left up to the parents. Factors that may affect their decision include cleanliness, tradition, possible prevention of cancer, and personal preference. As with any surgery there are risks involved when a circumcision is performed. Although rare, they may include hemorrhage; infection; injury to the penis, urethra, and scrotum; deformity; and scarring. Refer to Table 7-3 for a list of the pros and cons related to circumcision that parents may use in making their decision whether or not to circumcise their male infants. Newborns that warrant a circumcision not being performed or having it delayed include those who are premature, ill, distressed at birth, or have hemophilia or any genitourinary abnormality. If circumcision is done, procedural anesthesia should be used (AAP, 1999).

The appearance of female genitalia depends on subcutaneous fat deposition and gestational age. In the newborn less than 36 weeks' gestation the clitoris is prominent with the labia majora small and widely separated. The term newborn will have the clitoris and labia minora covered by the labia majora. Vernix caseosa may be present between the labia. Occasionally, the hymenal tag may protrude from the floor of the vagina. Withdrawal of the maternal hormones at the time of delivery may result in blood being observed on the diaper. This is called **pseudomenstruation** and caregivers may need reassurance that this is normal and will soon disappear (Figure 7-13).

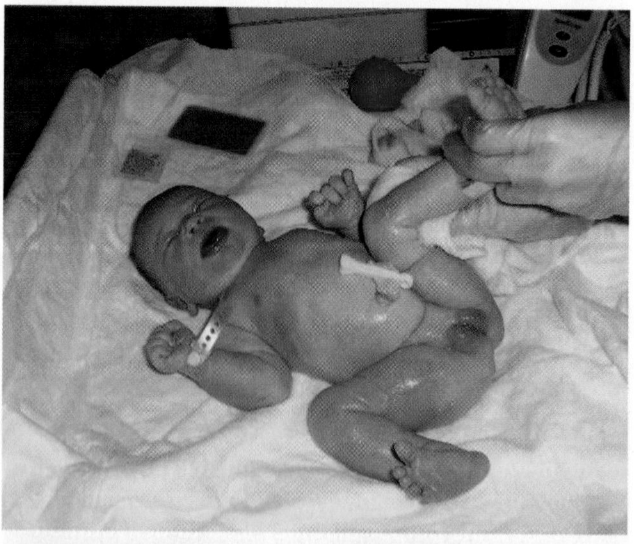

FIGURE 7-13 **Female newborn. Note labia majora as well as cyanotic color to the hands and feet.** DELMAR CENGAGE LEARNING.

TABLE 7-3 Pros and Cons related to Circumcision

POINTS OF DISCUSSION	FOR CIRCUMCISION	AGAINST CIRCUMCISION
Mutilation	Disfigurement/aesthetics is in the eye of the beholder; if the majority of males are circumcised, a young male may be embarrassed if he is not circumcised and to him it would be a disfigurement if he was not circumcised.	Removing the foreskin is mutilation.
Pain	Dorsal penile nerve block is very effective and should be used during the procedure.	Circumcision has been practiced without any or inadequate analgesia and it is a painful procedure.
Complications	The incidence of clinically significant complications is around 0.19% to 1.5%.	The procedure carries a risk of bleeding and sepsis. Major complications have included denuded penile shaft, laceration or necrosis of the glans, urethral fistula, and death.
Penile cancer	The evidence suggests that neonatal circumcision is associated with a lower incidence of the more severe forms of penile cancer.	None of the studies are ideal or definitive—retrospective, small sample sizes, and use of self-report, so this argument seems weak.
Urinary tract infections	The consensus in medical literature is that circumcision is associated with a lower incidence of urinary tract infections.	The absolute incidence of urinary tract infections is low: 0.15% of circumcised and 1.5% of uncircumcised male infants. That means urinary tract infections do not occur in 99.85% of circumcised males and 98.5% of uncircumcised males.
Sexually transmitted disease (not HIV)	Circumcised males may be less at risk for syphilis.	Studies have conflicting results. The only consistent trend is an increased susceptibility to genital ulcer disease.
HIV	Increased risk of genital ulcer disease increases risk of HIV. The foreskin mucosa contains accessible HIV-1 target cells close to the epithelial surface. The cells are directly exposed to vaginal secretions during intercourse.	Association between circumcision and susceptibility to HIV infection is strongest in high-risk populations. (all studies done in Africa).

Adapted from Benatar, M., and Benatar, D. (2003). Between prophylaxis and child abuse: The ethics of neonatal male circumcision. *American Journal of Bioethics*, 3(2), 35–48; World Health Organization. (2007). *Male circumcision: Global trends and determinants of prevalence, safety and acceptability.* Retrieved January 23, 2010 from http://whqlibdoc.who.int/publications/2007/9789241596169_eng.pdf

MUSCULOSKELETAL SYSTEM

The term newborn exhibits hypertonic flexion of all extremities. Flexion development occurs in the lower extremities first; therefore, during examination, the legs should be assessed first. To begin, place the newborn on a flat surface with the legs in flexion while manipulating the hip joint and placing a hand on the newborn's knees. After flexing the legs, extend them onto the flat surface and release. The term newborn's legs should recoil and quickly return to a flexed position. When examining the elbows, flex them by holding them for 5 seconds and then extending them. The term newborn's elbows form an angle of less than 90°

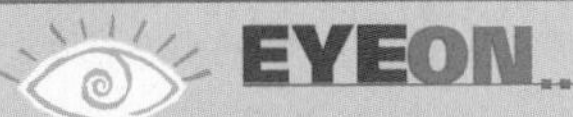

Circumcision

Male Jewish newborns may be circumcised on the eighth day of life at a religious ceremony. The circumcision is performed by a mohel, a person trained in performing circumcisions. Parents should be taught circumcision care prior to leaving the hospital even though the circumcision is done in the home. Anesthesia is not used. The infant is often given a bit of wine as part of the ceremony.

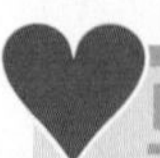

FAMILY**TEACHING**

Circumcision Care

The immediate care of the circumcised newborn is dependent on the procedure performed. If the *Plastibell* is utilized, it is left on the penis. Instruct the caregiver to gently lift the ring and squeeze warm water from a cotton ball on to the tip of the penis when changing the diaper. The ring of the *Plastibell* will fall off in 7–10 days when the circumcision has healed—do *not* pull it off. *If the ring was not used,* there may be gauze on the penis. This may or may not be replaced depending on the person who performed the circumcision. Diapers should be changed often so urine and stool do not irritate the site. A thin layer of petrolatum jelly may be applied to prevent the diaper from adhering to the circumcision site. Yellow exudate may be seen on the second day after the circumcision. This is granulation tissue and is normal and should not be removed.

NURSING TIP

Care of the Uncircumcised Newborn

The caregiver should be instructed to wash the outside of the penis to decrease the chance of odor and infection. **Smegma,** a collection of cells that shed from the outer layer of skin, gathers under the foreskin. Odor and infection may develop if the smegma is not removed. In the uncircumcised male the foreskin remains intact. The foreskin may not be retractable until the child is around 3 years of age. Caregivers must be cognizant of this so that they do not attempt to retract the foreskin and cause damage.

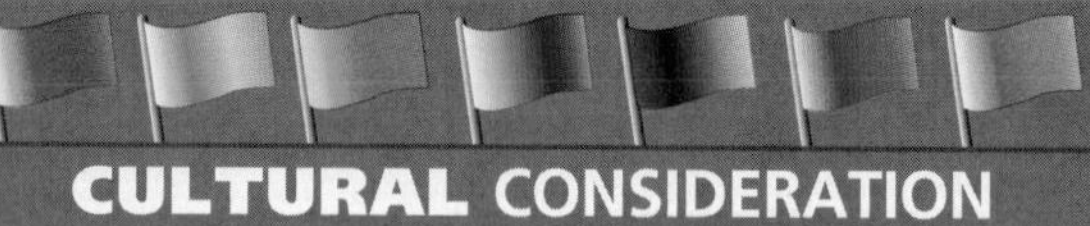

CULTURAL CONSIDERATION

Circumcision

For members of the Jewish faith, male circumcision is an outward sign of the Abrahamic covenant and a positive commandment obligatory for Jewish males. It is only postponed/abrogated if the child's health is threatened. Muslims are the largest religious group to practice male circumcision, and it is part of their Abrahamic faith. However, unlike those of the Jewish faith, there is no clearly prescribed age for circumcision. Circumcision is not specifically prescribed or prohibited by any Christian denomination.

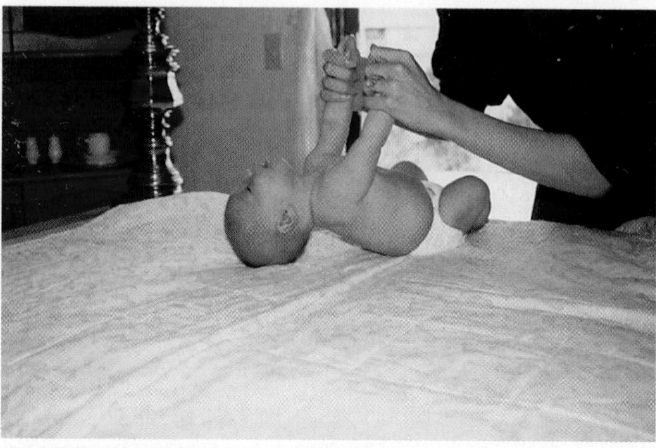

FIGURE 7-14 **Head lag is seen when the newborn is supine and the body lifted.** DELMAR CENGAGE LEARNING.

and rapidly recoil back to a flexed position. Because a healthy but fatigued newborn may elicit a slower response, this test should be delayed until after the first hour after birth.

Muscles in the extremities are not well defined, and muscle tone is not fully developed. Therefore, the newborn cannot support the full weight of the head, and head lag is seen if the newborn is pulled from a supine to a sitting position (Figure 7-14). However, in the prone position, the newborn is able to slightly raise the head (Figure 7-15). In addition, the hands should reach to the upper thighs when the upper extremities are extended. The legs should be of equal length with symmetrical gluteal skin folds.

Intrauterine positioning of the newborn's feet may result in a unilateral or bilateral talipes deformity or clubfoot. Usually, no treatment is needed if the foot can easily be manipulated to midline. When the foot cannot be aligned readily, an orthopedic consult should be considered. The spine, examined with the newborn in a prone position, should be straight and flat. The lumbar and sacral curves do not develop until the infant begins to sit (refer to Chapter 34 for more information on these conditions). The

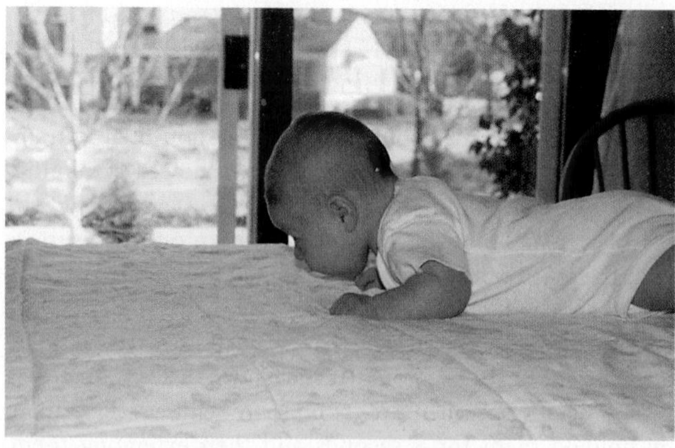

FIGURE 7-15 **Newborns can hold their heads up when placed in a prone position.** DELMAR CENGAGE LEARNING.

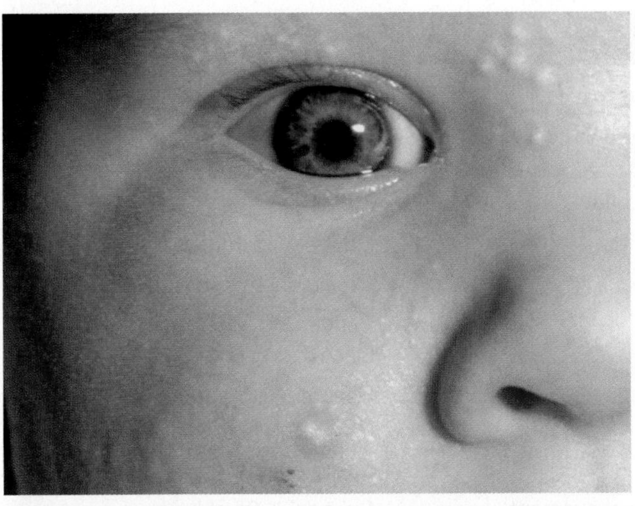

FIGURE 7-16 **Milia on the Face of a Newborn.** © LOGICAL IMAGES, INC.

base of the spine should be closely observed for any deformities such as **spina bifida** (a congenital defect in the walls of the spinal cord caused by a lack of union between the laminae of the vertebrae). Refer to Chapter 32 for more information on this condition.

INTEGUMENTARY SYSTEM

The newborn's skin is delicate and often mottled, and acrocyanosis may be present. The skin should be observed for other characteristics such as color and color change that may occur during activity, racial features, rashes, milia, birthmarks, and petechiae. **Milia** are small white papules on the nose, face, forehead, and upper torso caused by the plugging of the sebaceous gland (Figure 7-16). **Petechiae** are small, pinpoint, nonraised, perfectly round, purplish red spots, which are a result of an intradermal or submucosal hemorrhage. Petechiae may be a normal finding if located in the area of the presenting part. However, if petechiae are found elsewhere on the body, an investigation of possible causes such as sepsis should be pursued. A **mongolian spot** is an irregularly dark pigmented area on the posterior lumbar region. It has no clinical significance but may be noted in newborns of various racial backgrounds such as African American, Asian, and Native American (Figure 7-17). **Desquamation**, or peeling of the skin, may also be present. The degree of peeling depends on the maturity of the newborn with preterm newborns experiencing less and post term newborns experiencing more. **Telangiectatic nevi** are capillary hemangiomas commonly called "stork bites," which are usually found on the nape of the neck and the bridge of the nose. These typically disappear with time. **Nevus flammeus**, or **port wine stain**, is a hemangioma or vascular tumor that will not disappear with time. Some newborns may experience a transient newborn rash that is characterized by a red macular base with a white vesicular center, referred to as **erythema toxicum**.

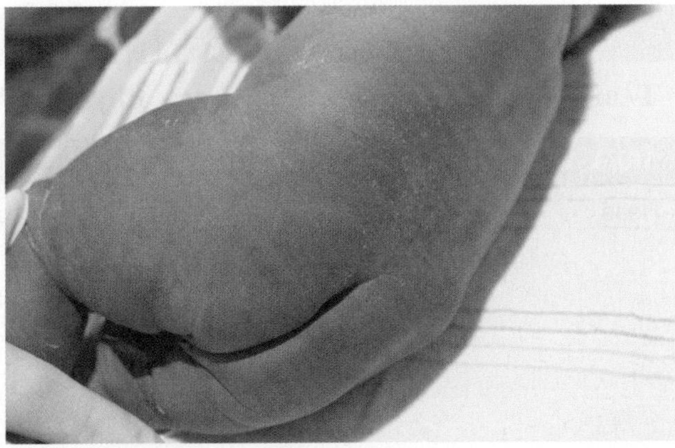

FIGURE 7-17 **Mongolian spot on the buttocks of a newborn.** DELMAR CENGAGE LEARNING.

Table 7-4 provides a summary of the normal and acceptable variations found when performing a newborn assessment.

PSYCHOSEXUAL DEVELOPMENT

At the time of conception, the gender of the fetus is biologically determined. However, the primitive gonads that develop by the fifth or sixth week of gestation are bipotential, containing both ovarian and testicular components (Kliegman, 2007). This genetic information directs development of either ovaries or testes, and in the presence of a Y chromosome, the bipotential primitive gonads develop into testes by 6–7 weeks of gestation. In the presence of two X chromosomes and the absence of a Y chromosome, the primitive gonads will develop into ovaries by 10 weeks of gestation. Psychosexual development continues after birth as the newborn finds satisfaction from oral stimuli, from physical contact with the caregiver, and from being held and cuddled (Figure 7-19).

COGNITIVE DEVELOPMENT

Cognitive development refers to the development of thinking and the gaining and use of knowledge. T. Berry Brazelton (1994) has shown that the newborn has the ability to interact with the environment as well as signal needs and gratitude when those needs are met. Learning, which is a function of the cerebral cortex, occurs through imitation and habituation. The newborn as young as 12 days of age is able to imitate facial and manual gestures of adults and prefers sharply contrasting colors, large squares, medium-bright objects, and ovoid objects with eyes and a mouth.

The newborn also has the ability to respond to auditory stimuli by turning the head and "looking" with the eyes to find the source. The frequency and intensity of the auditory stimulus, however, affects the response. High-frequency signals are

TABLE 7-4 Summary of Newborn Physical Assessment

AREA ASSESSED	NORMAL FINDINGS	ACCEPTABLE VARIANCES
Head	Anterior fontanel diamond-shaped, soft and flat Posterior fontanel triangle-shaped Head circumference 33–35 cm (13–14 in.) Refer to Figure 7-18	Molding Caput succedaneum Cephalohematoma Puncture mark from internal scalp electrode Head circumference 32.5–37.5 cm (12.5–14.5 in.)
Face and eyes	Symmetrical facial features and movement Eyes symmetrical in shape, placement, and movement	Eyelid edema Subconjunctival hemorrhage
Thorax	Symmetrical movement Circumference equal to or less than head circumference Nipples symmetrical Breath sounds clear and equal bilaterally Heart with regular rate and rhythm S2 split	Breast engorgement Supernumerary nipples Noticeable ribs on deep inspiration Functional heart murmur
Abdomen	Soft, nondistended Umbilical cord with two arteries and one vein Bowel sounds present	Irregular bowel sounds Reducible umbilical hernia
Genitalia	**Male** • Meatal opening in center of glans • Strong, arching urinary stream • Penile erection when voiding or with stimulation • Scrotum with rugae and pink or dark brown in color (depends on ethnic background) • Both testes descended	Hydrocele (accumulation of fluid in the scrotal sac) Testes at external inguinal ring
	Female • White or pink vaginal discharge • Edematous clitoris and labia majora • Increased pigmentation	Vaginal or hymenal tag Fusion of labia minora
Anus and rectum	Patent anus Meconium passage by 24 hours	Meconium within 48 hours
Extremities	Flexed position Symmetrical and equal movement Full range of motion Hands reach upper thighs when upper extremities are extended	Extended knees if breech
Spine	Straight Moves head from side to side when prone Can lift head when prone	

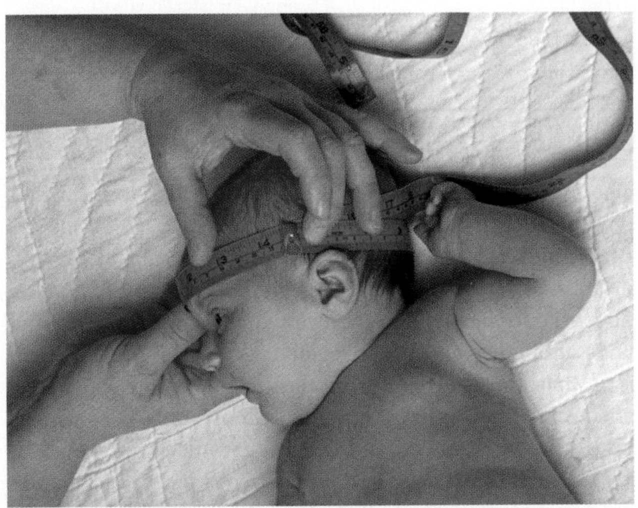

FIGURE 7-18 **Measuring Head Circumference.** DELMAR CENGAGE LEARNING.

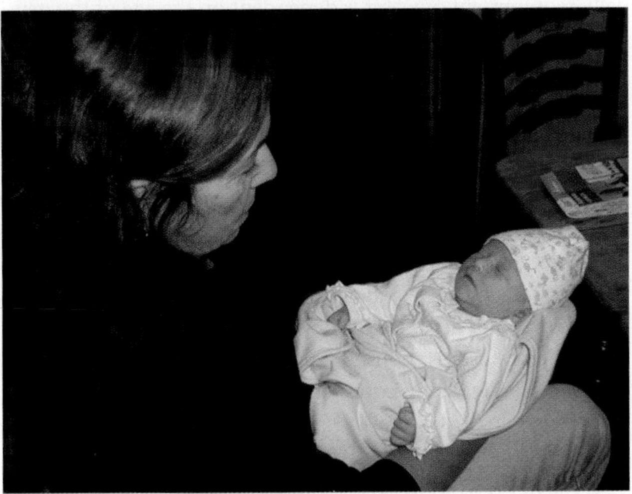

FIGURE 7-19 **All family members including grandmothers are important to newborns.** DELMAR CENGAGE LEARNING.

more likely to produce a response, but it may be a distress response whereas lower-intensity signals inhibit distress.

In addition, the newborn is sensitive to touch and handling. If a newborn is quiet, a rapid, intrusive touch will elicit an alert state. When the newborn is upset and crying, a slow soft touch will be calming. If some form of central nervous system irritation exists, there is increasing irritability with stimuli (especially tactile stimulation) and further evaluation is required (Figure 7-20).

The newborn's response to various stimuli affects the caregiver–newborn bond. Since nonverbal communications between caregiver and newborn are the initial stages of attachment, caregivers should provide the newborn with stimuli that evoke a response, thus enhancing attachment. Caregivers should also be taught to look for cues that the infant may be over-stimulated or becoming habituated.

Habituation, the ability to decrease responses to disturbing stimuli, is a defensive state that the newborn may

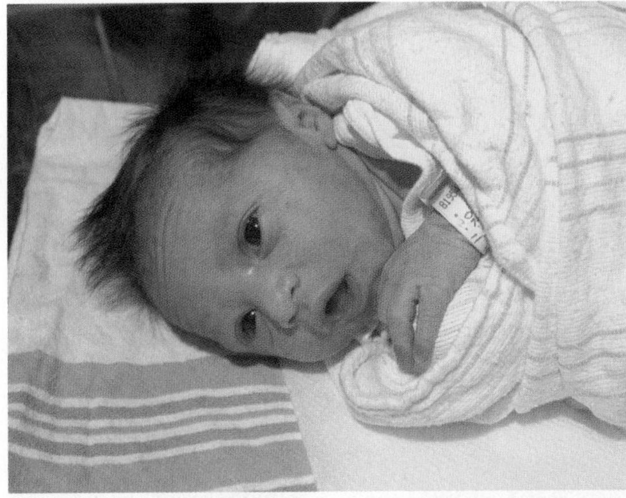

FIGURE 7-20 **Notice how awake and alert this newborn appears.** DELMAR CENGAGE LEARNING.

enter in response to noxious stimuli. Habituation protects the newborn from overstimulation and frees energy to meet physiologic demands. A newborn who cannot habituate will continue to react vigorously to repeated stimuli.

PSYCHOSOCIAL DEVELOPMENT

Child psychoanalyst Erik Erikson has divided the human life span into eight stages. In each of these stages, a human is faced with social and emotional conflicts. The first stage, infancy, which includes the newborn, is trust versus mistrust. Here, the newborn relies on others to fulfill needs, and develops basic trust when the caregivers meet these needs (Figure 7-21). Through a supportive, nurturing, and loving environment, the newborn will form an attachment to the caregiver and develop positive relationships (refer to Chapter 6 for more information).

HEALTH PROMOTION AND MAINTENANCE

Shortly after birth, all newborns receive antibiotic ophthalmic drops or ointment. Even though the incidence of mothers infected with gonorrhea and chlamydia at the time of delivery is less than 3%, the importance of preventing blindness makes this procedure mandatory for all newborns (Davidson et al., 2008).

Hemorrhagic disease of the newborn due to vitamin K deficiency may be prevented by administering phytonadione within one hour of birth. The dosage is usually 1 mg intramuscularly for the full-term newborn or 0.5 mg for preterm infants (Davidson et al., 2008). Prior to discharge from the hospital, the newborn should have a screening blood test to rule out the presence of various disorders including phenylketonuria (PKU), hypothyroidism, and sickle cell disorders.

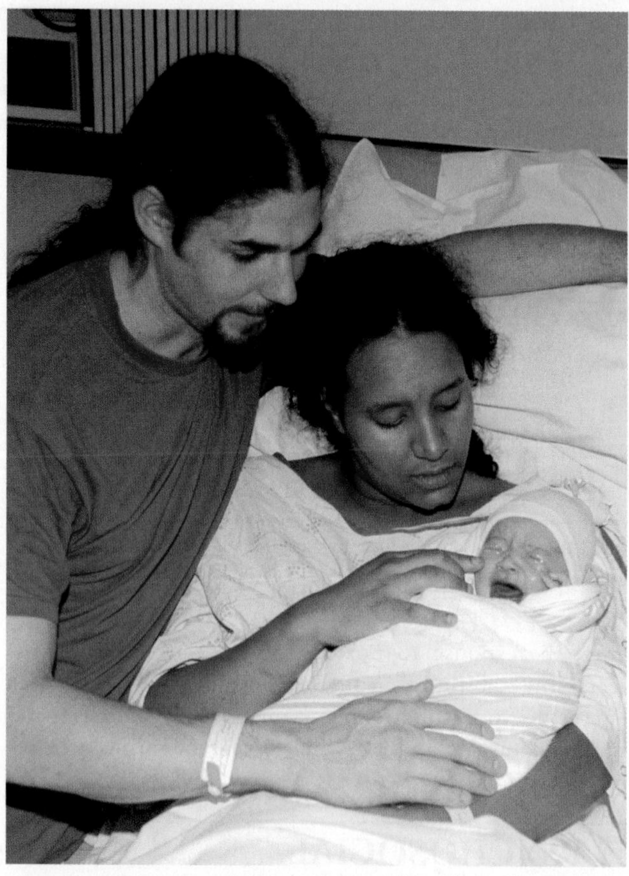

FIGURE 7-21 Newborns are often given to their mothers to hold soon after birth so attachment can begin early. DELMAR CENGAGE LEARNING.

Immunizations to promote disease resistance and prevention are essential for all newborns and infants. Caregivers should be informed of the importance of obtaining recommended immunizations and receive a written immunization schedule (see Appendix C for immunization schedule). Recommendations for routine well-baby checkups vary among practitioners. Some primary care providers will see breastfed newborns two to three days after discharge to check their weight, while others will have all newborns return to the office at 2 weeks of age. Finally, caregivers should receive a recommended schedule for follow-up care.

NEWBORN SCREENING

Required screening for newborns differs from state to state. The most common requirements involve phenylketonuria, congenital hypothyroidism, galactosemia, and sickle cell disease (Kaye and the Committee on Genetics, American Academy of Pediatrics, 2006; Kliegman et al., 2007). Check with your institution regarding screenings mandated in your state.

The AAP suggests that all newborns go through a hearing screen to identify possible hearing loss. The AAP Joint Committee on Infant Hearing (1995) suggests the goal of universal detection of hearing loss before 3 months of age and appropriate intervention at no more than 6 months of age (AAP, 2007).

ANTICIPATORY GUIDANCE

NUTRITION

The American Academy of Pediatrics (AAP) recommends breastfeeding for the first 6–12 months of life (AAP, 2005). Breast milk has many advantages over formula: (1) requires no mixing; (2) always at the correct temperature; (3) requires no sterilization; (4) is easily digested and absorbed; (5) contains antibodies and immunoglobulins to many microorganisms that are passed from mother to baby; and (6) is cost effective. Many women, however, choose not to breastfeed for a variety of reasons and the mother's decision should be respected. If breastfeeding is not selected, a variety of commercial formulas is available that attempt to mimic human milk (Gregory, 2005). The nutritional needs of the newborn are dependent on the clinical condition and the gestational age. Water comprises up to 75% of a term newborn's weight. The daily requirement of water is dependent on the age of the newborn and varies from 80 mL/kg/day up to 150 mL/kg/day (Gregory, 2005). The variations in fluid requirements compensate for changes in urinary output, stool output, and insensible water loss that occur with thermoregulation, respiration, and the development of new tissues (Gregory, 2005).

Caloric intake must meet the needs of a growing newborn to ensure appropriate growth and development. The term newborn requires 100 to 115 kcal/kg/day for the first month (Gregory, 2005). The balance of nutrients is necessary to promote health and decrease the development of disease. The only carbohydrate that is found in human milk is lactose which has also been replicated in commercial formulas (Gregory, 2005). Since carbohydrates are the primary source of energy they should represent at least 40–50% of the total daily calories.

When the body's reserve supply of carbohydrates has been exhausted, the body will turn to fat for energy (Gregory, 2005). Fat also serves the newborn to protect from temperature changes and cushions body organs from damage. For the first six months of life the fat requirement is 31 grams per day with a decrease to 30 grams per day thereafter (Gregory, 2005).

Protein is composed of essential and nonessential amino acids. The production of body proteins, hormones, and enzymes relies on the intake of adequate protein. A term newborn requires 1.5 grams/kg/day starting on the first or second day of life (Gregory, 2005).

NURSING TIP

Infant Immunity

The newborn immune system is very immature with a small amount of immunity being passed across the placenta (Davidson et al., 2008). As early as 1934, studies have reported that immunity is associated with breastfeeding (Newburg, 2005).

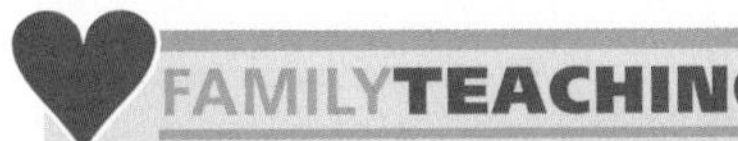

FAMILY TEACHING

Newborn Feeding

The most ideal form of nutrition for the newborn is breastfeeding (Gregory, 2005; Newburg, 2005). In addition to the nutritional advantages there are multiple potential protective mechanisms, including reduction of sudden infant death syndrome, childhood obesity, Crohn's disease, otitis media, and asthma (Gregory, 2005). A successful start with breastfeeding may be the determining factor as to whether the mother continues to breastfeed (Figure 7-22).

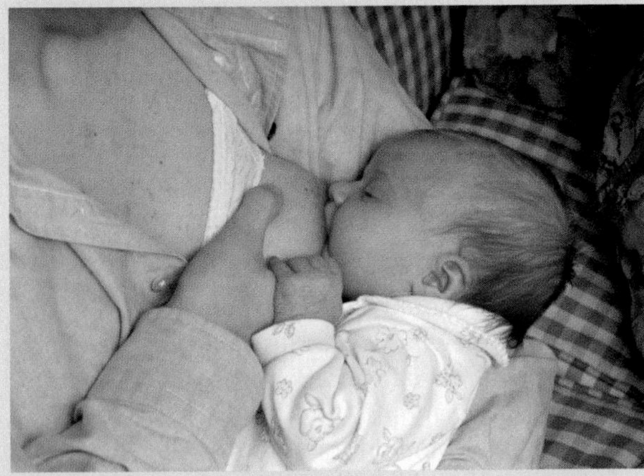

FIGURE 7-22 Breastfeeding is an important method of feeding a newborn. DELMAR CENGAGE LEARNING.

Recent research studies have reviewed the role of docosahexaenoic acid (DHA), an omega-3 fatty acid, in the photoreceptor portion of the retina and arachidonic acid (ARA), an omega-6 fatty acid found in other neural tissue (Gregory, 2005). Their function in growth, cognitive development, and visual acuity came under scrutiny when several studies revealed that breastfed infants had scored higher on neurocognitive developmental testing (Gregory, 2005).

Education of the caregiver on the importance of how to properly mix the formula is a crucial nursing responsibility. Formula is available in a variety of styles including ready-to-feed, concentrate, and powder. It is important that the water used in reconstituting the powder or concentrate be appropriate. Water sources can be from the tap, a well, distilled, or bottled. However, soft water should be avoided. Improper mixing may lead to dehydration due to the formula being too concentrated. On the other hand, water intoxication may occur when formula is diluted in an attempt to stretch it.

Cow's milk should not be used to feed infants until recommended by the primary care provider. The composition of cow's milk is designed for a rapidly growing animal and differs significantly from human milk or commercial formula. It contains more protein, fat, sugar, calcium, sodium, potassium, magnesium, sulfur, and phosphorous than human milk or commercial formulas. The caregivers should be instructed on these differences and the importance of maintaining the newborn and infant on breast milk or commercial formula.

Soy protein may be substituted for milk protein for those newborns with a milk (lactose) intolerance, symptoms of which include abdominal pain, diarrhea, distention, and flatus after ingesting milk products. Special formulas have also been developed to meet the needs of babies with PKU, fat malabsorption problems, or those requiring increased calories (e.g., preterm infants). The choice of formula is often decided by the provider and hospital staff unless the caregiver requests a specific formula.

CRITICAL THINKING

Baby Friendly Hospital Initiative

Although recognized as the most beneficial method of feeding, the percentage of mothers who begin and continue breastfeeding continues to remain low (Philipp & Radford, 2006). In 1991 the World Health Organization (WHO) and the United Nations Children's Fund (UNICEF) introduced the *Baby-Friendly Hospital Initiative* (BFHI) in an effort to enhance maternity care and facilitate breastfeeding (Baby Friendly USA, 2009; Philipp & Radford, 2006; World Health Organization, 2009). Criteria have been established that, with the cooperation of the BFHI, provides breastfeeding mothers with the information and support to be successful (Friendly USA, 2009; Philipp & Radford, 2006; World Health Organization, 2009). A birthing center or hospital is recognized with *Baby-Friendly* status when they have met the ten steps outlined by the BFHI, WHO, and UNICEF (2004).

A key component of the BFHI is the education of the nursing staff. The implementation of this program requires major practice change including: (1) initiation of breastfeeding within the first hour of delivery; (2) no supplementation of breastfed newborns; (3) on-demand/unrestricted breast-feeding; (4) elimination of pacifiers; (5) rooming in care for the mother and newborn to stay together at all times; and (6) information on community support available to the breastfeeding mother (Baby Friendly USA, 2009; Philipp & Radford, 2006). As of March 2009 the United States had 79 *Baby Friendly* birth centers and hospitals (Baby Friendly USA, 2009).

However, if mothers choose not to breastfeed, they should not be made to feel guilty as the most important outcome is a healthy newborn rather than the method of feeding or the staff's feelings about bottle feeding.

What are some practical, hands-on suggestions you could offer your facility to help achieve BFHI status?

The method of feeding is important, but the procedure for feeding also has a significant impact on the newborn. It is also important that if a mother chooses to bottle feed her newborn, she be given encouragement and information on how to mix the formula, how to hold the infant, and how often to feed the infant. Feeding time is crucial to the development of the caregiver-newborn attachment since it is a time for the newborn and caregiver to interact and learn about each other, whether the mother chooses to bottle feed or breastfeed the infant. If the newborn remains in the crib or in an infant seat with the bottle propped, the attachment process can be delayed. If the newborn is held and cuddled during feeding, both caregiver and newborn experience a feeling of closeness as well as close proximity eye contact.

In past years, newborns were placed on a specific feeding schedule. However, current practice is for **on-demand feeds**. This involves feeding when the newborn is hungry instead of by a prearranged time schedule. Because formula is digested more slowly, formula-fed newborns may go longer between feedings and usually establish a pattern of feeding every 3 to 4 hours, whereas a breastfed newborn may nurse every 1 1/2 to 3 hours. For the first few feedings, the newborn may only consume one half to one ounce, and progress to 6 to 8 feedings of 2 to 3 ounces per feeding after the first week of life. By 1 month of age, the newborn is eating 5 to 6 feedings per day and taking 3 to 4 ounces per feeding (Figure 7-23). The newborn will gain approximately 5 to 7 ounces per week. Head circumference and length will increase approximately 1 inch per month.

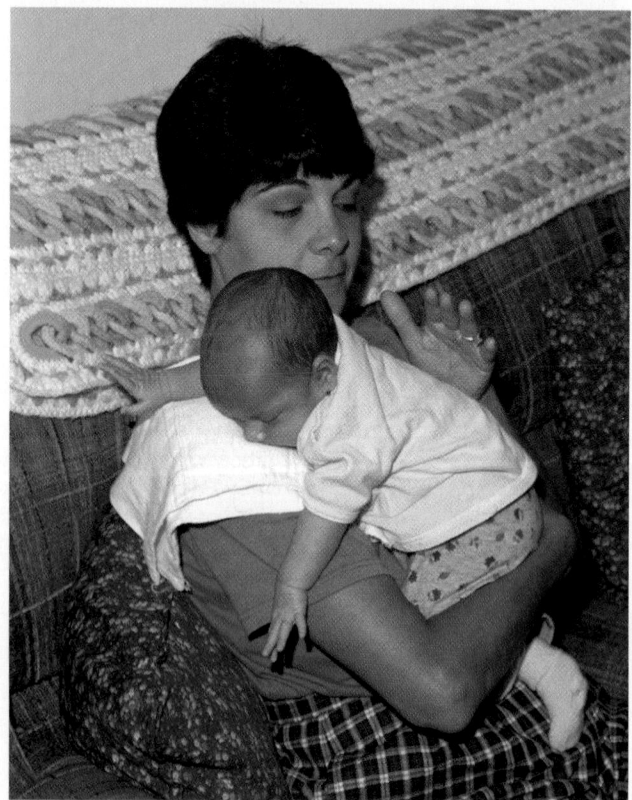

FIGURE 7-23 Burping after feeding is important. DELMAR CENGAGE LEARNING.

FAMILY TEACHING

Breastfeeding

1. Breasts may be firm but feel softer after nursing.
2. Nurse at least 10–15 minutes on each side.
3. To prevent nipple tenderness, hold infant correctly: cradle hold, football hold, or side lying down.
4. Make sure the newborn's lips are behind the nipple, encircling the areola.
5. Release the suction before the newborn is removed from the breast by placing a finger in the side of the mouth and between the jaws.
6. After nursing, express a little breast milk, massage into the nipples and areola, and allow to air dry.
7. Do not use soap or alcohol on breasts or nipples. Clean with water during showering or bathing.
8. Baby's urine should be light yellow with soft yellow stools.
9. Burp baby between breasts and at the end of feeding.

Bottle Feeding

1. Formula should be iron-fortified.
2. All the newborn's nutritional needs are met by formula. Cereal, juice, or other baby foods are not necessary.
3. Formula comes in three forms: ready to feed, concentrated liquid, and powdered.
4. Be sure formula is diluted correctly if in concentrated or powder form. Never add more or less water to the formula than is recommended by the manufacturer.
5. Once opened or mixed, a can of formula or prepared bottle should be refrigerated and used within 48 hours.
6. If the newborn drinks part of a bottle, it can be left at room temperature, but it must be used within 1 hour.
7. Do not add fresh formula to a partially used bottle or reuse a bottle that has been out for longer than 1 hour.
8. Do not heat bottles in a microwave. This leads to uneven heating and can cause severe burns to the newborn's mouth and throat.
9. Most babies are satisfied in about 20 minutes. Feedings should not last longer than 30 minutes.
10. Burp after half of the feeding and again at the end of the feeding.
11. Never prop the bottle or leave the newborn unattended.
12. Do not allow the newborn to drink from a bottle for long periods, especially when sleeping. This practice can cause "nursing bottle syndrome" or the development of dental caries and has also been linked to an increased incidence of otitis media.

THERMOREGULATION

Temperature regulation, or thermoregulation, is controlled by the hypothalamus. Body temperature is altered by changes in metabolism, motor tone and activity, vasomotor activity, and sweating. The adult human is capable of maintaining a constant body temperature over a wide range. The newborn is also capable of maintaining body temperature but not as effectively as a more mature person. Therefore, the newborn is more vulnerable to underheating and overheating because of a relatively large body surface area, poor thermal insulation, limited shivering response, and increased metabolic rate.

Heat exchange occurs through convection, conduction, radiation, evaporation, and over a heat gradient, or from a higher to lower temperature. The transfer of heat between a solid surface and air or liquid is convection. This type of heat exchange would occur between the newborn and liquid during a bath. Conduction of heat occurs between two solid objects that come in contact with each other. For example, when the infant's body comes in contact with a cold scale or counter, heat is lost. The transfer of heat between solid objects that are not in contact is radiation. Placing the newborn next to a cold window, despite the room being warm, will cause heat loss through radiation. Evaporative heat loss occurs when water on or in the body changes from a liquid to a gas. If an infant is not dried thoroughly after birth or a bath, the body temperature will drop secondary to evaporation.

If the newborn is exposed to temperature variations, multiple physiological responses occur. An increase in environmental temperature may cause vasodilation of the skin arterioles, resulting in increased blood flow from the body core to the periphery in an attempt to dissipate the heat and produce a cooling effect. A decrease in environmental temperature will result in vasoconstriction of the skin arterioles and reduction of heat from the body core. Shivering, a specialized muscular response that increases oxygen consumption and muscle metabolic rate, is limited in the newborn.

The primary form of heat production in the newborn is through brown adipose tissue metabolism. This **brown fat** is found primarily in the subscapular, axillary, adrenal, and mediastinal regions, and increases cellular metabolic rates and oxygen consumption, resulting in heat. Brown fat cells differ from other adipose tissue because of the fat vacuoles, number of mitochondria, and glycogen stores, and enhance the responsiveness of brown fat to thermal stimuli.

FAMILY TEACHING

Keeping the Newborn Warm

1. Explain how the newborn loses heat:
   a. Convection
   b. Conduction
   c. Radiation
   d. Evaporation
2. Provide information on how to reduce heat exchange:
   a. Reduce the area exposed during a bath.
   b. Limit exposure to drafts created by doors, ventilation systems, and traffic flow around the newborn's bed.
   c. Warm solid surfaces between the newborn by placing a blanket on the scale or counter.
   d. Place the newborn's crib on an inside wall in the room, away from the window.
   e. Block sunlight on the newborn in the car to prevent overheating.

REFLECTIVE THINKING

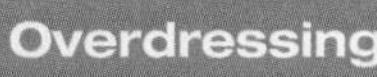

Overdressing

You enter a room to find the thermostat set at 80°F (36.3°C). The newborn is dressed in a T-shirt, sleeper, socks, and bundled in a quilt. How do you approach the mother to explain how overdressing and over bundling can affect the newborn's temperature? What if the mom states she's doing this because of her cultural background?

SLEEP

Term newborns have two sleep states: deep and light. During deep sleep, the eyes are firmly closed and still, no rapid eye movements occur, and little or no motor activity is present, except for occasional startles. During light sleep, rapid eye movements occur during 10-second intervals, and activity ranges from stretching to minor twitches. The newborn will sleep between 16 and 19 hours a day, with sleep cycles averaging 45–50 minutes (Kliegman et al., 2007).

Circadian rhythm, the cyclic variations in bodily functions that occur in a 24-hour period, is controlled by the central nervous system. Often the newborn's "clock" does not coincide with the family's and can result in conflict and disruption. This discrepancy may lead the family to perceive the newborn as "difficult." However, through alterations in care giving and patience, the newborn's schedule can become synchronous with the family's schedule.

In 1992, the AAP recommended the supine or side lying position (2000). In recent studies from various countries, the back sleeping position has shown a large and sustained decrease in the incidence of sudden infant death syndrome (SIDS). The type of bedding the newborn is

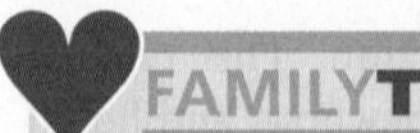

FAMILY TEACHING

Sleeping

1. Explain the American Academy of Pediatrics Recommendation for "back to sleep":
   a. Do not position newborn prone.
   b. Position newborn supine.
2. Provide information on the type of bedding to avoid:
   a. Soft bedding
   b. Pillows
   c. Comforters
   d. Sheepskin
   e. Water beds
3. Explain that over-swaddling or increased room temperature, in combination with the prone position, may increase the likelihood of SIDS threefold.

placed on has also been implicated in SIDS, with a higher incidence occurring on soft bedding such as pillows, comforters, blankets, or sheepskin (AAP, 2000). Refer to Chapter 8 for more information about SIDS.

DIAPER CARE

When changing the diaper of a female, instruct caregivers to wipe from front to back. This will control feces contamination of the vaginal area. Keeping the diaper clean and dry is the best prevention against diaper rash. The AAP recommends using plain water and absorbent cotton or a fresh washcloth. There is no need to use commercial wipes. However, if they are used, the wipes should be designed for babies, not adults. The adult wipes contain alcohol that can dry babies' skin.

The causes of diaper rash include:

- Too much moisture next to skin
- Chafing or rubbing
- Prolonged skin contact with urine, feces, or both
- Use of antibiotics (yeast infection)
- Allergic reaction to diaper material

Symptoms of diaper rash can be mild to severe and include red skin; painful open sores; and rash around the abdomen, genital area, or inside the skin folds of thighs and buttocks. Treatment includes changing the diaper often, using clear water to clean the diaper area, and applying a layer of protective ointment or cream (zinc oxide or petrolatum). Caregivers should contact a health care practitioner if the rash doesn't go away within 48–72 hours or gets worse, including open sores and blisters.

RESEARCH Highlight

Sleep Patterns in Parents when the Newborn is Breastfed

STUDY PURPOSE

To compare sleep patterns of first-time parents when the mother either exclusively breastfeeds the newborn or uses supplementation during the night or evening.

METHODS

A randomized clinical trial using feeding and sleep data from 133 new mothers and fathers.

FINDINGS

Parents of infants who received supplemental feedings in the evening and night reported more sleep disturbances and slept an average of 40–45 minutes less than parents whose infants were exclusively breastfed.

IMPLICATIONS

If parents choose to use supplemental feedings during the evening or night they may benefit from learning this may result in loss of sleep which can affect their daytime functioning.

REFERENCE

Doan, T., Gardiner, A., Gay, C., & Lee, K. (2007). Breast-feeding increases sleep duration of new parents. *Journal of Perinatal & Neonatal Nursing*, *21*(3), 200–206.

SAFETY PROMOTION AND INJURY PREVENTION

Contrary to popular belief, a newborn is not immobile. Newborns can wiggle themselves into a variety of positions that may become a safety hazard. The caregivers should be cognizant of this. Therefore, the only place to leave a newborn unattended is in the crib with side rails up. The caregiver should always keep one hand on the newborn when the newborn is on top of any object, since the newborn can quickly roll off.

NURSING ALERT

Safety for Newborns

When a pacifier is used, it should be of solid, one-piece construction. It should not be tied to a string or rope and placed around the newborn's neck as this poses a strangulation hazard.

Bathing can be a fun time for caregiver and the newborn, but the newborn should never be left unattended for any reason. Therefore, the caregiver should be taught to not answer the phone or door bell when bathing the newborn, unless the newborn is bundled up and taken with the caregiver.

Motor vehicle crashes can plague every age group, and all children need to be properly restrained. Recent information has shown that the front passenger seat is a dangerous place; so the newborn should be secured in an appropriate sized car seat in the rear, facing backward. The caregiver should know how the car seat should be installed and how it works prior to use. If the family is involved in an accident the car seat needs to be replaced even if there is no visible damage. Placing the crib away from heat sources, covering unused electrical outlets, and not holding the newborn while drinking hot coffee or other hot liquids help prevent injury or accidents.

Since the incidence of recurrent otitis media and respiratory infections has been linked to secondhand smoke, smoking around the newborn should be avoided. If family members need to smoke, they should go outside, and also avoid smoking in the car.

NURSE'S ROLE IN FOSTERING HEALTHY NEWBORNS

Although the time allowed for mothers and newborns to remain in the hospital following delivery has decreased in recent years, nurses can still have an impact on their care, as they are in an excellent position to teach parents about their newborn and what to expect in the upcoming months. Education should begin early in the hospital stay and not wait until the day of discharge. Frequent reinforcement with a variety of formats will accommodate various learning styles. One-on-one or classroom instruction, videotapes, written handouts, or demonstration are appropriate methods. Information needs to be individualized for each newborn and caregiver with consideration given for cultural, ethnic, religious beliefs, and educational levels.

The nurse is in an excellent position to ensure a caregiver feels comfortable before the newborn is sent home. The caregiver should be provided with information about community resources that may be helpful. The nurse should also instruct the caregiver on the importance of follow-up care, including well-baby checkups and routine immunizations, as well as helping siblings to get to know the newborn (Figure 7-24).

NURSING ALERT

Water Temperature for Bathing

Water heaters should be set no higher than 120°F (56.6°C). Exposure to hot water for even a brief time may result in second or third degree burns. At a water temperature of 155°F (73.1°C), a burn may occur in one second. At a temperature of 120°F (56.6°C), a burn occurs in 5 minutes. After filling the bath tub, turn off the hot water first and then the cold. The water temperature should always be checked before the newborn is placed in the tub.

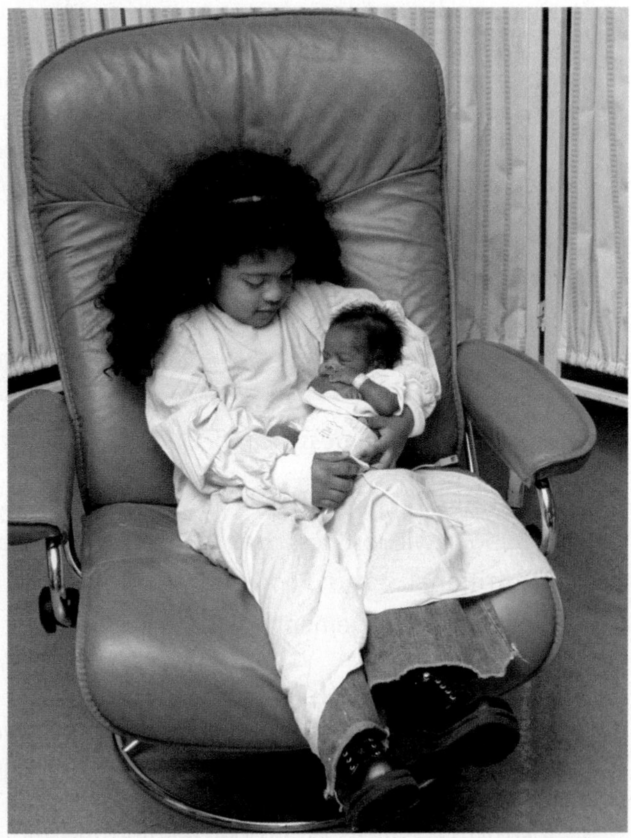

FIGURE 7-24 Young children love to hold newborn siblings.

DELMAR CENGAGE LEARNING.

CASE STUDY / CARE PLAN

NEWBORN

Joshua is a 2-hour-old Caucasian male who was delivered vaginally after an uneventful term pregnancy. Joshua's mother is a 23-year-old first-time mother. This is a study of his first hours and days.

NURSING DIAGNOSIS 1

Ineffective peripheral tissue perfusion related to decreased thermoregulation.

EXPECTED OUTCOMES

1. Newborn's temperature remains between 36.5° to 37°C (97.7° to 98.6°F).
2. Skin will be pink in room air.

NOC: Thermoregulation: Neonate.

NIC: Temperature Regulation

INTERVENTIONS/*RATIONALES*

1. Place under radiant warmer on servo control until temperature is stable (97.7°F). *The new born's ability to regulate temperature is immature. Exposing the newborn may result in hypothermia.*
2. Place newborn in T-shirt, diaper, and bundle in a blanket when temperature is stable. *Prevents heat loss through radiation or conduction.*
3. Keep ambient temperature of room at approximately 70°F (28.2°C). *So infant does not get chilled.*
4. Keep newborn out of drafts. *Prevents loss of heat through convection.*

EVALUATION

Child's temperature is maintained between 36.5° to 37°C (97.7° to 98.6°F).

NURSING DIAGNOSIS 2

Imbalanced nutrition: less than body requirements related to limited nutritional/fluid intake.

EXPECTED OUTCOME

1. Newborn will lose less than 10% of birth weight by 4 days of age.

NOC: Nutritional Status: Food and Fluid Intake

NIC: Nutrition Management

INTERVENTIONS/*RATIONALES*

1. Obtain weight on admission to nursery. *Obtains a baseline measurement.*
2. Begin feedings as soon as newborn is stable and able to eat. *Limits weight loss and establishes feeding pattern.*
3. Instruct caregivers on proper feeding techniques and cues that the newborn is feeding appropriate amounts. *Teaching assists caregivers on appropriately caring for their newborn.*
4. Weigh newborn prior to discharge. *Determines amount of weight loss.*
5. If weight gain is questionable, have caregivers return to primary care provider's office within 1 week for a weight check. *Determines if weight loss is transient and whether or not infant regained amount lost earlier.*

(Continues)

CASE STUDY / CARE PLAN (Continued)

EVALUATION

Child's weight loss is minimal and remains less than 10%.

NURSING DIAGNOSIS 3

Ineffective airway clearance related to secretion obstruction.

EXPECTED OUTCOMES

1. Newborn will maintain a patent airway.
2. Newborn will remain pink or appropriate color to race in room air.
3. Newborn will not demonstrate signs and symptoms of airway obstruction.

NOC: Aspiration Prevention

NIC: Airway Management

INTERVENTIONS/*RATIONALES*

1. Position newborn on back. *Prevents or treats aspiration.*
2. Have bulb syringe readily available in crib. *Clears airway of secretions.*
3. Teach caregivers on the proper use of bulb syringe and newborn positioning. *Educating caregivers assists them to provide appropriate care to their newborn.*
4. Assess for sign or symptoms of airway obstruction. *Assesses maintenance of patent airway.*

EVALUATION

Child is pink, airway remains open, and there is no sign of respiratory obstruction.

NURSING DIAGNOSIS 4

Deficient caregiver knowledge related to lack of experience with a newborn

EXPECTED OUTCOMES

1. Caregiver will verbalize or demonstrate appropriate newborn care.
2. Caregiver will verbalize when to contact the newborn's primary care provider.

NOC: Knowledge: Infant Care; Knowledge: Parenting

NIC: Family Integrity Promotion: Childbearing Family; Newborn Care; Parent Education: Infant; Teaching: Infant Nutrition, Safety

INTERVENTIONS/*RATIONALES*

1. Assess caregiver's educational needs. *Determines what needs to be taught.*
2. Adjust teaching technique to caregiver needs. *Caregiver is able to learn.*
3. Discuss major aspects of newborn care (safety measures, feeding techniques, bathing, general care, when to call primary care provider). *Education on care of newborn will help caregivers become more confident and knowledgeable so they are able to provide effective and appropriate care.*

EVALUATION

Caregiver is successfully able to care for newborn and knows when to contact pediatrician.

THE HIGH-RISK NEWBORN

Transition to extrauterine life is more difficult for some newborns than for others. Specifically, large for gestational age (LGA), small for gestational age (SGA), preterm (<37 weeks' gestation), and post term (>42 weeks' gestation) infants have special challenges that they must overcome to survive and thrive in their new environment. Unfortunately, these and other risk factors are not always determined before birth. It is important to assess and discover these conditions as soon as possible so appropriate care can be provided. Each condition requires special consideration in care and assessment abilities.

LARGE FOR GESTATIONAL AGE (LGA)

The LGA or macrosomic infant can be defined as being above the 90th percentile or two standard deviations above the mean for weight. A variety of obstetrical situations can result in an LGA infant: a high maternal weight or gestational weight gain, multiparity, a history of large infants, or maternal disease such as diabetes (Lawrence, 2007; Derbyshire, 2008). The infant can also have a genetic predisposition for largeness, or genetic aberrations such as Beckwith Wiedemann Syndrome (refer to Figure 7-8, the Ballard Assessment Scale). As compared with an appropriate for gestational age (AGA) infant, an LGA infant has an increased potential for neonatal morbidity since a frequent complication is birth trauma, especially caput succedaneum or cephalohematoma (refer to Figure 7-5). You may also see bruising or laceration secondary to a forceps delivery. Facial nerve palsy may also be evident. Other injuries the LGA newborn is at risk for developing include a broken clavicle and a fractured humerus. A broken clavicle is suspected if there is swelling, pain, or tenderness in the affected area, or a reluctance to use the affected extremity. Care should be taken to not manipulate the extremity, though splinting or complete immobilization is rarely needed. A humeral fracture will present similarly, with pain, tenderness, edema, and decreased movement. However, the humerus will need to be immobilized upon diagnosis. These diagnoses can be verified through radiological imaging. A brachial plexus injury can also accompany upper extremity trauma. In extreme cases of birth trauma, you may see subgaleal hemorrhage, asphyxia, spinal cord injury, and even death.

If there is a concern the LGA infant has suffered birth trauma, a neonatal neurological examination is important to determine to what extent the neurological system is affected. Physical, occupational, and speech therapies may be indicated (Lawrence, 2007).

Hypoglycemia is also commonly seen in the LGA infant. Oftentimes, insulin-dependent or gestationally diabetic mothers will give birth to LGA infants. These infants can develop a transient hyperinsulinemia in response to maternal hyperglycemia. After birth, this infant will continue to overproduce insulin and can be at risk for hypoglycemia. To prevent neonatal hypoglycemia, it is important to monitor serum glucose, initiate early enteral feedings, and supplement as necessary with an IV glucose solution. LGA infants born of normoglycemic mothers also have a higher incidence of hypoglycemia and need close monitoring (Lawrence, 2007).

SMALL FOR GESTATIONAL AGE (SGA)

An SGA infant is defined as an infant who has a weight to gestational age ratio that is below the 10th percentile or two standard deviations below the mean for weight (Lawrence, 2006). A moderately low-birth-weight (LBW) infant can be defined as a child weighing 2,500 to 1,501 grams. An infant less than 1,500 grams is considered very low birth weight (VLBW), while less than 1,000 grams is extremely low birth weight (ELBW). Maternal situations which may result in an SGA infant include low socioeconomic status, hypertension, cardiac disease, renal disease, medications or other drugs, cigarette smoking, placental insufficiencies, uterine anomalies, multiple gestation, small maternal stature, and a history of late spontaneous abortion or previous SGA infant. Fetal conditions which contribute to intrauterine growth restriction (IUGR) are congenital malformations such as Potter's syndrome or anencephaly, osteogenesis imperfecta, inborn errors of metabolism, and congenital infection.

Upon examination of an SGA infant, you may see a baby who is lacking subcutaneous fat, has a scaphoid abdomen, a general appearance of malnutrition, and a head that is disproportionally large for the body. This infant's head, although of normal size or slightly small for gestational age, is perceived as large because of the relative small size of the body. These infants have been fortunate to a point: though their nutrition is suboptimal, their body has attempted to optimize the nutrition going to vital areas, most notably the brain. This is representative of asymmetric intrauterine growth-restriction (Lawrence, 2006). An infant that has experienced symmetric intrauterine growth restriction has generally had a longer standing nutritional deficit or a chromosomal abnormality. These infants are proportionally small, with both body size and occipital-frontal circumference (OFC) below the 10th percentile on the neonatal growth charts.

Postnatal complications for the SGA infant include increased susceptibility to infection, respiratory compromise, neurological challenges, or death. Hypoglycemia can also be present. It is therefore important to monitor serum glucose until adequate enteral feedings are tolerated. This may be a bit of a challenge, as SGA infants are at higher risk for gastrointestinal complications including intestinal perforation. Temperature instability which may also occur is secondary to the lack of stored fat, which serves as both an

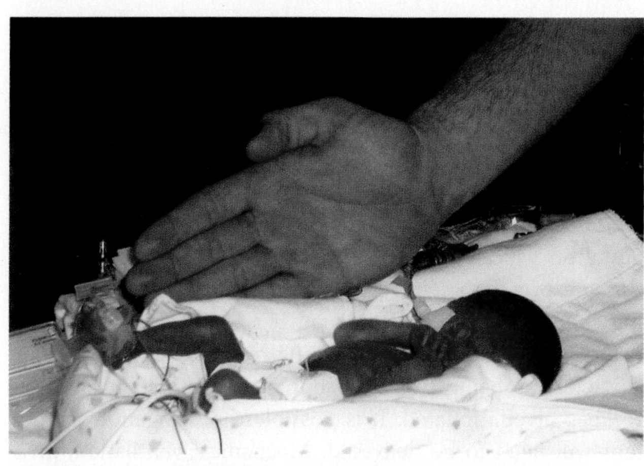

FIGURE 7-25 **Premature infant. Note how small she is compared to the nurse's hand.** DELMAR CENGAGE LEARNING.

insulator and a heat producer. Therefore, the SGA newborn should be monitored closely for hypothermia, dressed warmly, and placed in an artificial heat source such as an isolette, radiant warmer, or hybrid bed as necessary. Supplemental oxygen or assisted ventilation may also be needed. Long term sequelae of IUGR include developmental and neurological deficits. These deficits will be more significant in the symmetrically growth-restricted infants (Lawrence, 2006).

Figure 7-25 illustrates the size of a premature infant in comparison to an adult hand.

THE PRETERM INFANT

The preterm infant is born earlier than 37 weeks' gestation. Preterm infants can be classified by weight as well as gestational age. You will see preterm infants falling in the LBW, VLBW, or ELBW categories or gestational age categories. The extremely preterm infant is <27 weeks' gestation (Stoelhorst, Rijken et al., 2005), a very preterm infant is <32 weeks, and a moderately preterm, 32–36 weeks' gestation (Cloherty, 2008). This latter group is divided further into the subgroup *late preterm.*

The number of preterm deliveries, about 12% of live births in the United States, has actually been increasing (Gibson, 2007). Factors precipitating a preterm birth can include maternal hypertension, preeclampsia, multiple gestation, renal disease, cardiac disease, and a history of preterm pregnancies or labor. Also, late initiation of prenatal care, a lower socioeconomic level, and substance use and abuse can contribute to a preterm delivery. Common complications for the preterm infant are similar to those of the SGA infant, and include hypoglycemia, hypothermia respiratory instability, neurological problems, necrotizing enterocolitis, and visual compromise (Cloherty et al., 2008). Please refer to figure 7-26 for problems commonly associated with prematurity.

Respiratory distress syndrome (RDS) is defined as an inadequate production of surfactant, a mixture of phospholipids and apoproteins that adhere to the internal surfaces of the alveoli, reduce the surface tension of these surfaces, and improve the lung's ability to remain inflated during exhalation. Without adequate production of this substance, respiratory difficulty increases. Though primarily seen in the preterm infant, RDS is also seen in more mature infants. Precipitating factors include prematurity, cesarean delivery without labor, maternal diabetes, and multiple gestations. Symptoms of RDS include tachypnea (60 breaths or more per minute); intercostal, subcostal, and sternal retractions; nasal flaring; and audible grunting. Poor aeration of the lung fields despite great respiratory effort will be heard upon auscultation. Symptoms can worsen to the point where supplemental oxygen or mechanical ventilation may be required. In these situations, surfactant replacement can be administered, but the infant will need to receive ventilatory support until able to adequately assume respiratory and other functions independently (Cloherty et al., 2008). Prolonged ventilatory support can lead to bronchopulmonary dysplasia (BPD). This is a chronic lung disease characterized by cellular hyperplasia, muscular hypertrophy, increased reactivity, decreased compliance, and decreased surface area for gas exchange (Cloherty et al., 2008).

Preterm infants are at increased risk for neurological complications. Rarely seen in more mature infants, intraventricular hemorrhage (IVH) is seen in 15–20% of infants born at <32 weeks' gestation. The increased incidence of this complication is multifactorial. These immature infants are at a higher risk of hypoxia and ischemia. They may require fluid resuscitation or correction of acid-base imbalances. They may have hypotension followed by a reperfusion that this fragile compromised vascular system cannot handle. These hemorrhages are graded by severity. A Grade I hemorrhage is usually defined as bleeding that is isolated in the germinal matrix. Grades II–IV first moves into the ventricles, then causes ventricular dilation, and finally extends into the parenchymal tissue. You may suspect an IVH if you see hypotonia, bulging fontanels, or abnormal eye movements. Definitive diagnosis is made by cranial ultrasound (Cloherty et al., 2008). Premature and SGA infants who have experienced an IVH are at greater risk for cerebral palsy and other significant developmental issues (Kelly, 2006a; 2006b).

The increased incidence of necrotizing enterocolitis or NEC in the preterm infant is, like IVH, due to a combination of several factors. An immature gastrointestinal tract, mucosal injury secondary to hypoxia, ischemia, or infection, and enteral feedings have all been associated with an increased incidence of NEC. Indications of NEC can include symptoms of sepsis, poor feeding, emesis, increased girth, discolored abdomen, and bloody stool. Radiologic studies may show thickening of the bowel wall secondary to edema, pneumatosis intestinalis (visible air within the bowel wall), portal air, or pnuemoperitoneum (free air in the abdominal cavity). Mortality for NEC may be as high as 28%. Morbidity includes intestinal strictures, adhesions, malabsorption, short gut, and dumping syndrome (Cloherty et al., 2008).

Retinopathy of prematurity (ROP) can be seen in as many as 65% of infants born under 1,250 grams. ROP can be described as an aberrant vascularization of the retina. This process begins with an insult such as hypotension, hypoxia, or hyperoxia which disrupts the normal vascularization process of the retina. When vascularization resumes, especially in a hyperoxic environment, the vessels can be tortuous, and permeable. This can lead to retinal hemorrhage and detachment. These infants are also at higher risk of refractory errors, myopia, strabismus, and glaucoma (Cloherty et al., 2008). With many of the complications of prematurity, probability and severity increase as the gestational age and size of the infant decreases (Cloherty et al., 2008) (Figure 7-26).

The late preterm infant is one born at 34–36 6/7 weeks' gestation. This gestational age infant is gaining recognition for several different reasons. The incidence of late preterm birth has increased significantly over the past decade. Over 70% of all preterm births will fall into this category. Unlike the stereotypical preterm infant these neonates can look and act a bit like full term infants. However, these infants are not term as the name indicates. These infants are at greater risk for a number of complications related to the general immaturity of all of their body systems (Figure 7-27). You will see infants of this gestational age with hypoglycemia, hyperbilirubinemia, temperature instability, respiratory distress, and feeding difficulties (Shaw, 2008). Late preterm infants are more likely to require hospital readmission, and have a mortality rate three times higher than the term infant (Engle, Tomashek et al., 2007).

The very preterm infant born at less than 32 weeks gestation will also experience those complications listed for the late preterm infant. These infants are significantly lacking subcutaneous and brown fat. It is likely that an artificial heat source will be needed. During respiratory development, surfactant is being produced but not in sufficient amounts to keep alveoli inflated. It is possible that exogenous surfactant will need to be delivered. Mechanical ventilation, invasive or non-invasive, may need to be utilized until the infant can independently maintain oxygenation and ventilation. If supplemental oxygen is required, use caution. To decrease the severity of ROP, maintaining tight saturation parameters would be prudent (Cloherty et al., 2008). During fetal development, the coordination of sucking and swallowing does not start to develop until the 34th week of gestation

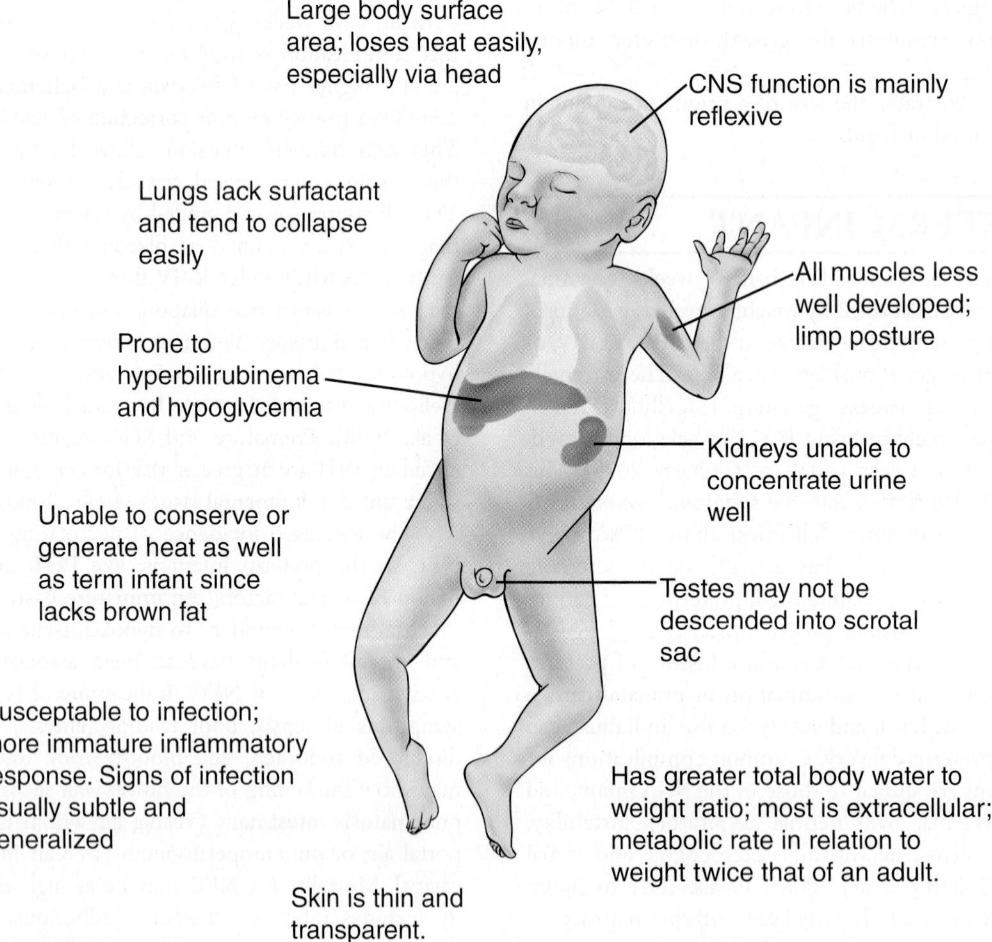

FIGURE 7-26 Premature Infant and Associated Problems. DELMAR CENGAGE LEARNING.

(Bakewell-Sachs, 2007). The infant born at 32 weeks' is at a disadvantage in regards to oral feedings. The coordination will develop, but the infant will likely require gavage feedings for a couple of weeks or longer. Of course, this neonate is at greater risk for developing NEC. It is important to assess girth and residuals with each feed. This will indicate how well the infant is tolerating the feedings.

The infant born at less than 27 weeks' gestation will see these difficulties to a greater degree. A heat and humidity source will be necessary. Surfactant therapy, supplemental oxygen, and invasive mechanical ventilation are likely to be needed. The invasive mechanical ventilation and supplemental oxygen may be prolonged, which can lead to chronic lung changes. Again, when utilizing respiratory support, utilize an eye-protective strategy. Any enteral feeding will need to be provided via a gavage tube until suck-swallow coordination and adequate strength can be obtained by the infant. Again, it is very important to determine if the infant is tolerating the feedings. Early intervention in an episode of NEC is important in limiting its damaging effects (Gibson, 2007).

Infants born at 22–25 weeks' gestation are at the threshold of viability (Kelly 2006a; 2006b). Though statistics have improved over the last twenty years, these infants continue to have a very high morbidity and mortality rate. It is suggested that heroic measures should not be taken, especially with the infant less than 23 weeks' gestation. This difficult decision continues to challenge both health care professionals and families. The ultimate decision lies with the parents. They should be aware of their options, and what the future may hold for them and their child. Once the decision is made, it should be respected, as long as it is medically feasible (Hurst, 2005).

EVIDENCE-BASED PRACTICE

Kangaroo Care for Preterm Infants

CLINICAL PROBLEM

Although premature infants (born at <37 weeks) are only a minority of the population of total births, they present a significant clinical challenge. Due to their immature organs and underdeveloped extra-utero adaptation abilities, premature babies experience significantly more complications, including unstable respiratory status, temperature regulation, breastfeeding ability, etc. Research has been conducted to determine better and more cost-effective forms of care to help decrease these complications. Kangaroo care (KC) or skin-to-skin contact, first implemented in 1983, by Edgar Rey and Hector Martinez, in Bogota, Colombia, has been identified as one method that not only is inexpensive, but also can decrease complications in premature infants. KC consists of placing the unclothed newborn on a parent's (usually the mother's) bare chest, tummy to tummy. The original form of KC also required the baby be exclusively breastfed and involved early discharge from the hospital. In developed countries such as the United States, the main feature of KC, skin-to-skin contact between a mother and her baby, has received increasing attention over the years. Many positive outcomes with no negative consequences have been documented. However, in spite of emerging evidence in favor of KC, it has not been widely adopted in the clinical setting.

BEST CLINICAL PRACTICE

Premature infants receiving kangaroo care:

- Can maintain their body temperature (36.5–37.5°C) for up to 3 hours.
- Have a higher average body temperature as opposed to those receiving traditional incubator care.
- Had significantly ($p<0.017$) greater weight gain, and increases in overall growth and development.
- Showed more effective behavioral organization and emotional regulation, including more organized sleep-wake cycles and more engagement and bonding with the mother.
- Are more likely to breastfeed successfully.
- Are clinically more stable.

IMPLICATIONS FOR NURSING

- Kangaroo care should be taught to and practiced by mothers of preterm infants daily. Encourage three 2–3 hr sessions per day.
- Intubated preterm infants can and should participate in KC. It has been determined safe by several studies and shown to benefit the infant and have better outcomes.

  Specific infant transferring guidelines are outlined in the Ludington-Hoe et al., 2008 article.
- Provide a supportive environment for KC.
- Provide education for staff and facility on: safety of KC, simplicity of KC, and benefits of KC.

References: Johnson, A. N. (2007a). Factors influencing implementation of kangaroo holding in a special care nursery. *American Journal of Maternal Child Nursing, 32*(1), 25–29; Johnson, A. N. (2007b). The maternal experience of kangaroo holding; *Journal of Obstetric, Gynecologic, & Neonatal Nursing, 36*(6), 568–573; Leonard, A. (2008). Parents' lived experience of providing care to their preterm infants. *Health, 13*(4), 16–28; Ludington-Hoe, S. M., Morgan, K., & Abouelfettoh, A. (2008). A clinical guideline for implementation of kangaroo care with premature infants of 30 or more weeks' postmenstrual age. *Advances in Neonatal Care, 8*(3S), S3–23; Moore E. R., Anderson, G. C., & Bergman, N. (2007). Early skin to skin contact for mothers and their healthy newborn infants. *Cochrane Database of Systematic Reviews*, (3) (journal article - research, systematic review) ISSN: 1469-493X CINAHL AN: 2009823774; Chiu, S. H., Anderson, C., & Burkhammer, M. (2005). Newborn temperature during skin-to-skin breastfeeding in couples having breastfeeding difficulties. *Birth, 32*(2); and van Zanten, H. A., Havenaar, A. J., Stigt, H. J. H., Ligthart, P. A. H., & Walther, F. J. (2007). The kangaroo method is safe for premature infants under 30 weeks of gestation during ventilatory support. *Journal of Neonatal Nursing, 13*(5), 186–189.

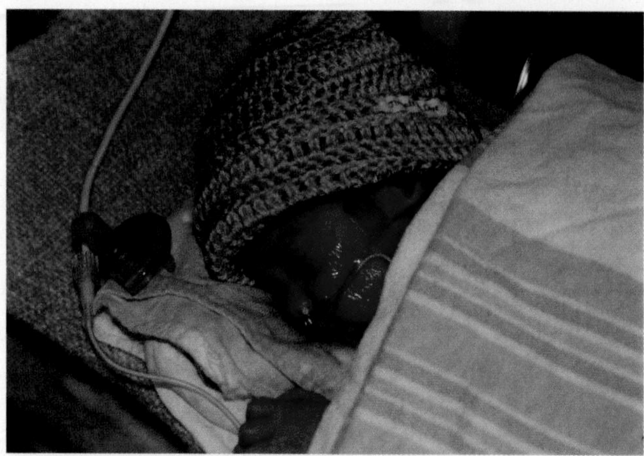

FIGURE 7-27 **This sleeping premature infant is wearing a hat to prevent heat loss from his head and is receiving an NG feeding.** DELMAR CENGAGE LEARNING.

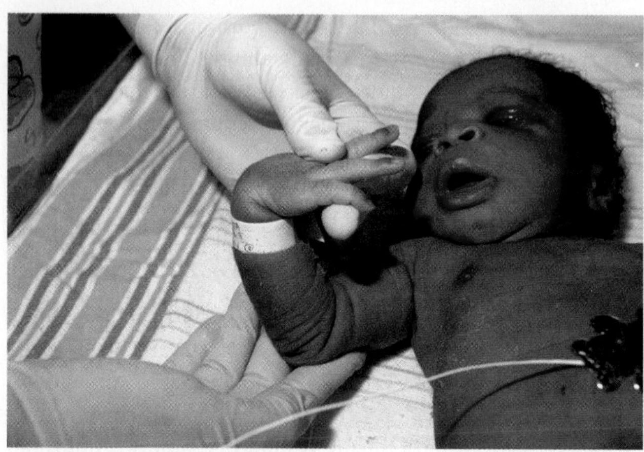

FIGURE 7-28 **Postmature Infant with Peeling Skin.** DELMAR CENGAGE LEARNING.

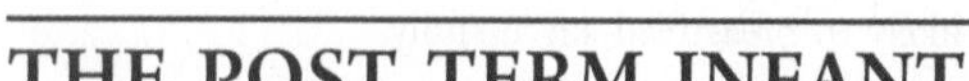

THE POST TERM INFANT

About 5–10% of pregnancies will fall in this category. By 42 weeks gestation, the mortality rate has doubled over the term infant (Briscoe et al., 2005). Around the 36th week of pregnancy, the placenta begins to lose its ability to transport nutrients, oxygen, and waste products. The placenta becomes increasingly insufficient the farther a pregnancy goes past term. The increase in neonatal morbidity and mortality in the post term infant may be secondary to this placental insufficiency. Problems of post term infants include meconium aspiration, malnutrition, asphyxia, and death. Physical exam will show a child with dry, cracking skin, the absence of vernix and lanugo, and long and thin extremities; the skin may appear green if meconium was passed *in utero* (Kliegman et al., 2007). (Figure 7-28.)

CARE OF THE HIGH-RISK NEWBORN

Early intervention in any high-risk situation is essential. This begins by first recognizing the high-risk pregnancy. If an extremely preterm baby is anticipated, maternal transport or immediate neonatal transport to a tertiary center should be attempted. This will not always be possible. If this is not possible, the labor and delivery and newborn unit nurses should ask for additional medical staff to attend this or any high-risk delivery. After delivery, nurses should be prepared to perform or initiate assisted ventilation, cardiopulmonary resuscitation, and

RESEARCH Highlight

Music and the Preterm Infants

STUDY PURPOSE

To discover whether live music or recorded music will improve physiological and behavioral parameters of stable preterm infants in the NICU.

METHODS

Over 3 days in a row, 31 stable preterm infants randomly received live music, recorded music, or no music. Music lasted 30 minutes.

FINDINGS

Although preterm infants who received live music for 30 minutes did not show any significant effect on behavioral or physiological parameters during the therapy, they did show a significantly reduced heart rate and a deeper sleep state 30 minutes after the therapy. Staff preferred either live or recorded music to no music but parents believed live music was more effective than recorded music or no music.

IMPLICATIONS

Using live music (female voice, frame drum, harp) in the neonatal intensive care unit may be helpful for improving preterm infants' cardiac rate and sleep states, and should be provided if feasible for stable preterm infants.

REFERENCE

Amon, S., Shapsa, A., Forman, L., Regev, R., Bauer, S., Litmanovitz, I., & Dolfin, T. (2006). *Live music is beneficial to preterm infants in the neonatal intensive care unit environment. Birth, 33*(2), 131–136.

establish vascular access, while not forgetting to dry and keep the baby warm. The baby will then need to be transported from the delivery room to the nursery. The high-risk infant may be cared for in the birth hospital. A detailed exam will determine cardiovascular stability, neurological appropriateness, respiratory status, and temperature. If physiological homeostasis cannot be maintained at the birth hospital, it will become necessary to transfer the infant to a tertiary center (Figure 7-29).

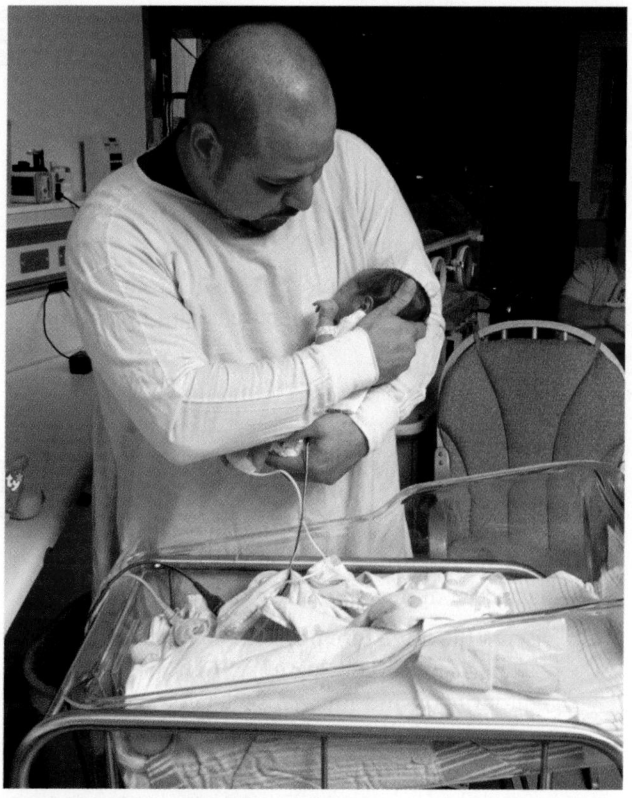

FIGURE 7-29 **All high-risk infants need contact with, and to be held by, their parents.** DELMAR CENGAGE LEARNING.

IN THE REAL WORLD

Those babies are so small and fragile; one wonders how they could possibly survive. when I first began to work in the newborn intensive care unit, I was very anxious and afraid that I would hurt them whenever I cared for them. I learned, however, that although small, and indeed fragile, they are also resilient and many are really strong. I know that the care I give makes a difference, and I really love what I do. I would not want to work on another unit.

Reflections from Families

I was in labor with my second child. I was very excited because my first child was born cesarean, but this time I was having a vaginal delivery. As my daughter Heather was delivered she aspirated fluid. Needless to say she spent the first few days of her life hooked up to a respirator and on antibiotics. This was a very difficult time. I was discharged from the hospital within 2 days. But every day I would go to the hospital and feed her and hold her. Heather was discharged, and is none the worse for wear. Now she is a healthy 4-year-old who has had no repercussions from her first week of life.

KEY CONCEPTS

- The transition to extrauterine life involves changes in the cardiovascular and respiratory systems.
- A variety of reflexes are present during the newborn period that can be separated into primitive, survival, localized, or generalized.
- The newborn's musculoskeletal, gastrointestinal, integumentary, and renal systems are immature at birth.
- The newborn can interact with the environment and, within two weeks of birth, is able to imitate facial and manual gestures of adults.
- Education on the care of the newborn should begin at birth and include positioning, nutrition, safety, bathing, immunizations, normal growth and development, and schedules for well-baby examinations.
- High-risk newborns (LGA, SGA, preterm, post-term) need careful monitoring and interventions.

REVIEW ACTIVITIES

1. Describe the principal cardiorespiratory changes that occur during the transition to extrauterine life.
2. Discuss the immature physiologic functioning of the neurological, cardiorespiratory, gastrointestinal, genitourinary, and musculoskeletal system in the newborn, and their relationship to the nursing care of the neonate.
3. Describe the expected normal findings of a newborn physical assessment.
4. Discuss the prominent anticipatory guidance concerns for caregivers during the neonatal period.
5. Describe areas addressed in teaching caregivers about safety promotion and injury prevention for the neonate.
6. Describe the etiology and care of the high-risk newborn.

STUDY QUESTIONS

1. The mother of full-term newborn Henry is concerned because her baby is now 10 hours old and he seems sleepy and does not breastfeed as well as her other children. The best response to this mother is:
   a. "It is not unusual for the newborn transition to last between six and ten hours after birth. Let's wait a few more hours and see how he feeds."
   b. "Don't worry; I am sure he'll be fine."
   c. "I'd be worried too. Let me call the doctor."
   d. "I'm new to the unit even though I have worked in a newborn nursery for several years. I'll ask the charge nurse what she thinks."
2. Which of the following reflexes is a survival reflex?
   a. Babinski
   b. Rooting
   c. Palmar Grasp
   d. Moro
3. The first-time mother of Madison asks you about the small white papules on the nose, face, forehead, and upper torso of her daughter. You tell her they are caused by the plugging of the sebaceous gland and called:
   a. Mongolian spots.
   b. Petechiae.
   c. Milia.
   d. Telangiectatic nevi.
4. The mother of newborn Jonah is wondering about whether to breastfeed or bottle feed her son. When giving her advice it would be important to tell her:
   a. "Commercial formula only comes in powder form."
   b. "Since cow's milk is designed for a rapidly growing animal it is all right for her to use that during the first month of Jonah's life."
   c. "Breast milk has many advantages over formula."
   d. "Soy formula should not be used if the newborn has a lactose intolerance."
5. The mother of newborn Noah asks about his head and notices there are two soft spots. Which of the following responses would be most appropriate for the nurse?

a. "Those soft spots are fontanels. The small one usually closes by 3 months of age; the large one closes between 8 and 18 months."
b. "Those soft spots are seen when the newborn tries to grasp objects placed in his hand."
c. "Those soft spots are unusual and are an early sign of mental retardation."
d. "Those soft spots indicate the baby has iron deficiency anemia; if you feed him iron-fortified formula they will disappear in a few weeks."

6. The mother of newborn Anna is concerned about her daughter's sleeping habits when she leaves the hospital. The best response by the nurse would be:
   a. "Anna should be placed on her side or stomach when you put her in her crib to sleep."
   b. "Often the newborn's sleep "clock" coincides with the family's sleep schedule."
   c. "Anna will sleep between 16 and 19 hours a day, with sleep cycles averaging 45-50 minutes."
   d. "Be sure Anna has soft bedding such as pillows, comforters, blankets, or sheepskin when you put her to bed in her crib."
7. Baby girl Jones was born at 31 weeks' gestation. She has been in the hospital for two months and has had a reasonably uncomplicated course. She is on full enteral feedings and doesn't require supplemental oxygen. She had a cranial ultrasound a week before discharge and it was read as normal. She has an appointment in the clinic in a week. Her family should:
   a. Keep her appointment as ordered.
   b. Disregard her appointment for neonatal developmental follow-up and treat her the same as they treated her older sister who was born at term.
   c. Keep the appointment for follow-up, only if they see problems.
   d. Start developmental follow-up once they start to teach her letters and numbers.
8. Which of the following statements about high-risk newborns is not true?
   a. They should be cared for as any normal newborn at delivery.
   b. They should be monitored for hypoglycemia.
   c. They should be observed for signs of respiratory compromise.
   d. They should be observed for temperature instability.
9. Baby Boy Pugh has a birth weight of 5.2 kg. When giving him his first bath, you notice that he is not moving his right arm. He becomes irritable whenever you touch the extremity. Your next action should be:
   a. Dress the infant and take him out to his mother. It is probably just a soft tissue injury that will heal on its own.
   b. Notify his pediatrician and mention that you suspect injury to the right arm. Keep the limb immobilized and assist the radiology technologist with an x-ray, as ordered.
   c. Continue to manipulate the arm to assure that the arm is indeed tender, before you bother the pediatrician.
   d. Immobilize the arm, take the infant out to his mother and tell her to be careful with her son, because you think he has a clavicular fracture.
10. Baby girl Andreas was born at 42 2/7 weeks gestation. She is not at risk for:
   a. Meconium staining and aspiration.
   b. Hypoglycemia.
   c. Retinopathy of prematurity.
   d. Dry, cracking and peeling skin.

REFERENCES

American Academy of Pediatrics. (1999). Circumcision policy statement. *Pediatrics, 103*(3), 686–693.

American Academy of Pediatrics. (2004). Management of hyperbilirubinemia in the newborn infant 35 or more weeks of gestation: Clinical practice guideline. *Pediatrics, 114*(4), 297–316.

American Academy of Pediatrics Task Force on Infant Sleep Position and Sudden Infant Death Syndrome. (2000). Changing concepts of sudden infant death syndrome: Implications for infant sleeping environment and sleep position (RE9946). *Pediatrics, 105*, 650–656.

American Academy of Pediatrics Joint Committee on Infant Hearing. (2007). Year 2007 position statement: Principles and guidelines for early hearing detection and intervention programs. *Pediatrics, 120*(4), 898–921.

Amon, S., Shapsa, A., Forman, L., Regev, R., Bauer, S., Litmanovitz, I., & Dolfin, T. (2006). Live music is beneficial to preterm infants in the neonatal intensive care unit environment. *Birth, 33*(2), 131–136.

Baby Friendly USA. (2009). What is the Baby-Friendly Hospital Initiative and why do we need it? Retrieved January 23, 2010, from http://www.babyfriendlyusa.org/eng/01.html.

Bakewell-Sachs, S. (2007). Near-term/late preterm infants. *Newborn & Infant Nursing Reviews* 7(2), 67.

Ballard, J. L., Khoury, J. C., Wedig, K., Wang, L., Eilers-Walsman, B. L., & Lipp, R. (1991). New Ballard Score, expanded to include extremely premature infants. *Journal of Pediatrics. 119*(3), 417–423.

Beachy, J., & Nash, P. (2007). Investigating jaundice in the newborn. *Neonatal Network, 26*(5), 327–333.

Benatar, M., & Benatar, D. (2003). Between prophylaxis and child abuse: The ethics of neonatal male circumcision. *American Journal of Bioethics*, 3(2), 35–48.

Brazelton, T. B. (1994). Behavioral competence. In G. B. Avery, M. A. Fletcher, & M. G. MacDonald (Eds.), *Neonatology: Pathophysiology and management of the newborn* (4th ed.). Philadelphia: Lippincott, 289–300.

Briscoe, D., Nguyen, H., Mencer, M. et al., 2005. Management of pregnancy beyond 40 weeks' gestation. American Family Physician, *71*(10), 1935–1941.

Cloherty, J. P. E., Eric, C., & Stark, A. R. (2008). *Manual of neonatal care*. Philadelphia, PA: Lippincott, Williams & Wilkins.

Chiu, S. H., Anderson, C., & Burkhammer, M. (2005). Newborn temperature during skin-to-skin breastfeeding in couples having breastfeeding difficulties. *Birth*, *32*(2), 115–21.

Davidson, M., London, M., & Laedwig, P. (2008). *Old's maternal-newborn nursing & women's health across the lifespan* (8th ed.). Upper Saddle River, NJ: Pearson Education.

Derbyshire, E. (2008). Implications of high maternal weight during pregnancy. *Nursing Standards, 22*(49), 42–46.

Doan, T., Gardiner, A., Gay, C., & Lee, K. (2007). Breast-feeding increases sleep duration of new parents. *Journal of Perinatal & Neonatal Nursing, 21*(3), 200–206.

Engle, W. A., Tomashek, K. M., Wallman C., & Committee on Fetus and Newborn, American Academy of Pediatrics. (2007). Late-preterm infants: A population at risk. *Pediatrics, 120*(6), 1390–1401.

Gibson, A. T. (2007). Outcome following preterm birth. *Best Practice & Research Clinical Obstetrics & Gynaecology, 21*(5), 869–882.

Gregory, K. (2005). Update on nutrition for preterm and full-term infants. *Journal of Obstetric, Gynecologic, and Neonatal Nursing, 34*(1), 98–108.

Hurst, I. (2005). The legal landscape at the threshold of viability for extremely premature infants: A nursing perspective, part II. *Journal of Perinatal & Neonatal Nursing, 19*(3), 253–264.

Johnson, A. N. (2007a). Factors influencing implementation of kangaroo holding in a special care nursery. *American Journal of Maternal Child Nursing, 32*(1), 25–29.

Johnson, A. N. (2007b). The maternal experience of kangaroo holding. *Journal of Obstetric, Gynecologic, & Neonatal Nursing, 36*(6), 568–573.

Kaye, C., & the Committee on Genetics, American Academy of Pediatrics. (2006). *Newborn Screening Fact Sheets.* Retrieved May 5, 2009, from http://www.pediatrics.org/cgi/doi/10.1542/peds.2006-1783.

Kelly, M. M. (2006a). The basics of prematurity. *Journal of Pediatric Health Care 20*(4), 238–244.

Kelly, M. M. (2006b). The medically complex premature infant in primary care. *Journal of Pediatric Health Care 20*(6), 367–373.

Kliegman, R., Behrman, R., Jenson, H., & Stanton, B. (2007). *Nelson's textbook of pediatrics*, (18th ed.). Philadelphia, PA: Saunders/Elsevier.

Lawrence, E. J. (2006). A matter of size: Part 1. Evaluating the growth-restricted neonate. *Advanced Neonatal Care 6*(6), 313–322.

Lawrence, E. J. (2007). A matter of size: Part 2. Evaluating the large-for-gestational-age neonate. *Advanced Neonatal Care 7*(4), 187–199.

Leonard, A. (2008). Parents' lived experience of providing care to their preterm infants. *Health, 13*(4), 16–28.

Ludington-Hoe, S. M., Morgan, K., & Abouelfettoh, A. (2008). A clinical guideline for implementation of kangaroo care with premature infants of 30 or more weeks' postmenstrual age. *Advances in Neonatal Care,* 8(3S), S3–S23.

Maisels, J. (2005a). Jaundice in a newborn: Answers to questions about a common clinical problem. First of two parts. *Contemporary Pediatrics, 5*, 34–40.

Maisels, J. (2005b). Jaundice in a newborn: How to head off an urgent situation. Second of two parts. *Contemporary Pediatrics, 5*, 41–42, 45–46, 48–49.

Moore, E. R., Anderson, G. C., & Bergman, N. (2007). Early skin to skin contact for mothers and their healthy newborn infants. *Cochrane Database of Systematic Reviews,* (3) (journal article – research, systematic review) ISSN: 1469-493X CINAHL AN: 2009823774.

Newburg, D. (2005). Innate immunity and human milk. *Journal of Nutrition, 135*, 1308–1312.

Philipp, B., & Radford, A. (2006). Baby-Friendly: Snappy slogan or standard of care? *Archives of Disease in Childhood—Fetal and Neonatal Edition, 91*, F145–F149.

Shaw, R. R. (2008). Late preterm birth: A new nursing issue. *American Journal of Maternal Child Nursing, 33*(5), 287.

Stoelhorst, G. M., Rijken, M. et al. (2005). Changes in neonatology: comparison of two cohorts of very preterm infants (gestational age <32 weeks): The project on preterm and small for gestational age infants 1983 and the Leiden follow-up project on prematurity 1996–1997. *Pediatrics 115*(2), 396–405.

Stokowski, L. (2007). Fundamentals of phototherapy for neonatal jaundice. *Advances in Neonatal Care, 6*(6), 303–312.

van Zanten, H. A., Havenaar, A. J., Stigt, H. J. H., Ligthart, P. A. H., & Walther, F. J. (2007). The kangaroo method is safe for premature infants under 30 weeks of gestation during ventilatory support. *Journal of Neonatal Nursing, 13*(5), 186–189.

World Health Organization. (2007). *Male circumcision: Global trends and determinants of prevalence, safety and acceptability.* Retrieved January 23, 2010, from http://whqlibdoc.who.int/publications/2007/9789241596169_eng.pdf.

World Health Organization (2009). Baby-friendly Hospital Initiative. Retrieved May 7, 2009, from http://www.who.int/nutrition/topics/bfhi/en/print.html.

SUGGESTED READINGS

Blackman, J. A. (2007). NICU Micropreemies; how do they fare? *Contemporary Pediatrics, 24*(2), 64.

Chow, J. M., & Douglas, D. (2008). Fluid and electrolyte management in the premature infant. *Neonatal Network, 27*(6), 379–386.

Engle, W. A. (2006). A recommendation for the definition of "late preterm" (near-term) and the birth weight-gestational age classification system. *Semin Perinatol, 30*(1), 2–7.

Hashim, M. J., & Guillet, R. (2002). Common issues in the care of sick neonates. *American Family Physician, 66*(9), 1685.

Hurst, I. (2005). The legal landscape at the threshold of viability for extremely premature infants: a nursing perspective, part I. *Journal of Perinatal & Neonatal Nursing, 19*(2), 155–168.

Jain, A., Aggarwal, R., Jeevasanker, M., Deorari, A. K., & Paul, V. K. (2008). Hypoglycemia in the newborn. *Indian Journal of Pediatrics, 75*(1), 63–67.

Kelly, M. M. (2006). Primary care issues for the healthy premature infant. *Journal of Pediatric Health Care, 20*(5), 293–299.

Lucey, J. F., Rowan, C. A. et al. (2004). Fetal infants: The fate of 4172 infants with birth weights of 401 to 500 grams—the Vermont Oxford Network experience (1996–2000). *Pediatrics, 113*(6), 1559–1566.

Mandruzzato, G., Antsaklis, A. et al. (2008). Intrauterine restriction (IUGR). *Journal of Perinatal & Neonatal Nursing, 36*(4), 277–281.

McFarlin, B. L. (2009). Solving the puzzle of prematurity. *American Journal of Nursing, 109*(1), 60–63.

Moos, M. K. (2004). Understanding prematurity. Sorting fact from fiction. *AWHONN Lifelines, 8*(1), 32–37.

Rosenberg, A. (2008). The IUGR newborn. *Semin Perinatol, 32*(3), 219–224.

Sasidharan, C. K., Gokul, E., Anoop, P., & Vijaykumar, M. (2005). Benefits of maternal participation in newborn nurseries. *Indian Journal of Pediatrics, 72*(10), 829–833.

Shapiro-Mendoza, C. K., Tomashek, K. M., Kotelchuck, M., Barfield, W., Weiss, J., & Evans, S. (2006). Risk factors for neonatal morbidity and mortality among "healthy," late preterm newborns. *Semin Perinatol, 30*(2), 54–60.

Tomashek, K. M., Shapiro-Mendoza, C. K. et al. (2006). Early discharge among late preterm and term newborns and risk of neonatal morbidity. *Semin Perinatol, 30*(2), 61–68.

Tyson, J. E., Parikh, N. A., Langer, J., Green, C., Higgins, R.D., & National Institute of Child Health and Human Development Neonatal Research Network. (2008). Intensive care for extreme prematurity—moving beyond gestational age. *New England Journal of Medicine 358*(16), 1672–1681.

Tyson, J. E., & Saigal, S. (2005). "Outcomes for extremely low-birth-weight infants: Disappointing news." *Journal of the American Medical Association, 294*(3), 371–373.

RESOURCES

Refer to the online student StudyWARE for Potts & Mandleco at http://www.CengageBrain.com for additional content and study aids.

Organization: **American Academy of Pediatrics**
Description: Offers general information related to child health, specific guidelines concerning many pediatric issues, information regarding AAP programs, activities, policies, guidelines, publications, and other child health resources.
Website/Resource: http://www.aap.org

Organization: **La Leche League International**
Description: Offers information regarding forums and helpful resources for breastfeeding mothers in several languages; access to an online marketplace/store.
Website/Resource: http://www.llli.org

Organization: **National Association of Neonatal Nurses (NANN)**
Description: Offers information regarding education/jobs, meetings, publications, and membership as well as access to an online store.
Website/Resource: http://www.nann.org

Organization: **National Association of Pediatric Nurse Associates and Practitioners (NAPNAP)**
Description: Offers information regarding NAPNAP's mission/efforts, upcoming events, associated programs, and access to NAPNAP's online store.
Website/Resource: http://www.napnap.org

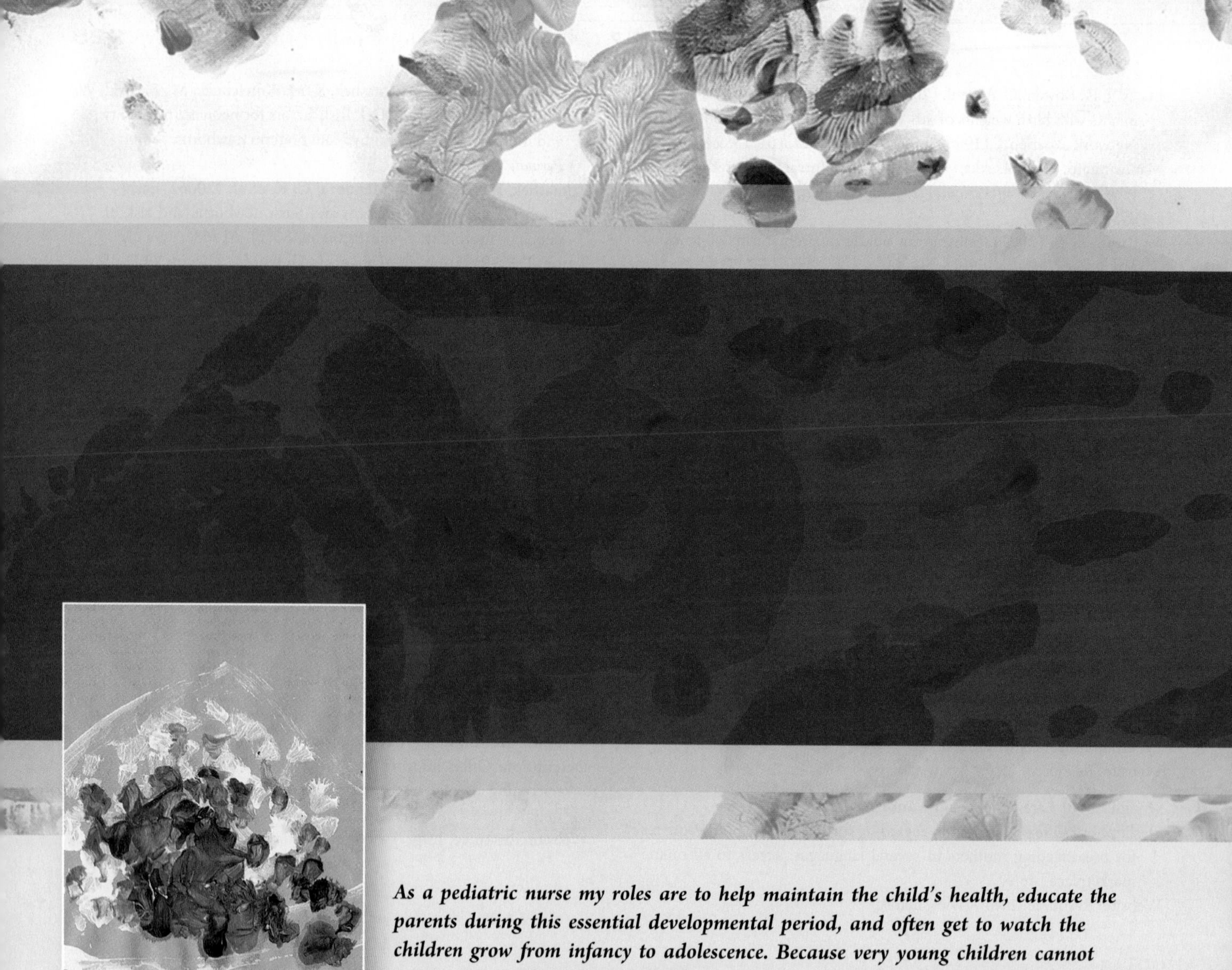

As a pediatric nurse my roles are to help maintain the child's health, educate the parents during this essential developmental period, and often get to watch the children grow from infancy to adolescence. Because very young children cannot communicate what they are feeling or thinking, my basic tools to assess them are my eyes, ears, and hands. These require an extensive knowledge of growth and development, basic cognitive development, and appropriate equipment to use for different ages and sizes. Open-mindedness is crucial when relating to them and more importantly, acknowledgment of the expertise of the family when caring for their child.

But there is something distinctive about me being a pediatric nurse, and that is being a mother as well. I can relate more to the children and their families because I am mother of two young children (Harrison and Jonah). Those sick children could be my own and I feel so much empathy for them. This feeling makes me a more caring and understanding nurse, which makes my job special.

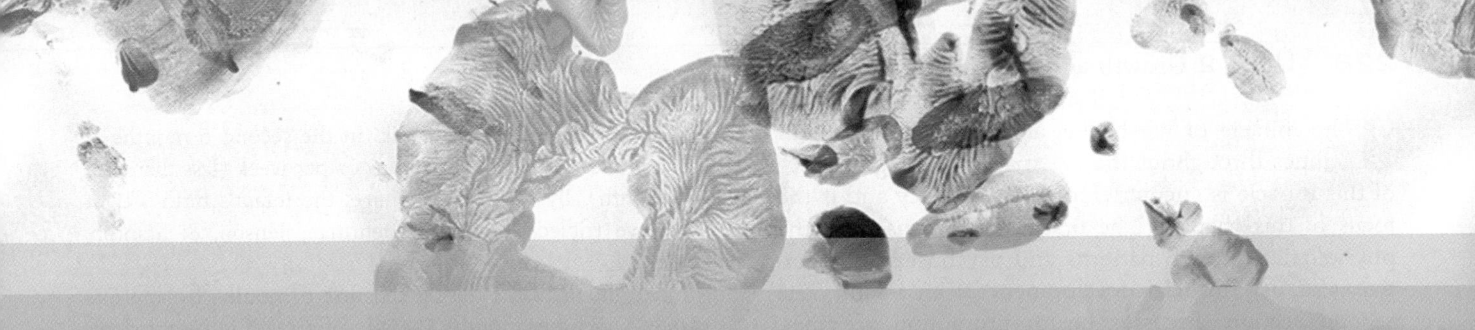

CHAPTER 8
Growth and Development of the Infant

Maria G. Rosario-Sim, RNC, EdD, PNP, BC; Barbara L. Mandleco, RN, PhD; and Janice Vincent, CRNP, DSN

COMPETENCIES

Upon completion of this chapter, the reader will be able to:

- Assess physiological growth and developmental milestones of infants.
- Apply the process and principles of infant fine and gross motor development to nursing care.
- Describe infant psychosexual, cognitive, and psychosocial development.
- Discuss health promotion and maintenance activities for infants.
- Discuss caloric and fluid requirements for infants.
- Design play activities for infants.
- Discuss educational strategies for infant caregivers related to nutritional needs, growth and developmental patterns, stranger and separation anxiety, and safety.
- Describe the millennium development goals in relation to poverty and nutrition.
- Successfully complete the games and activities in the online student StudyWARE.

The miracle of life begins at conception and continues throughout the life span. The magnificence of this miracle is encountered during infancy and is the focus of this chapter. The first section focuses on the physiological growth patterns and psychosexual, cognitive, and psychosocial development of an infant. The second section discusses health promotion activities, including health screening, dental care, and nutrition. Educational strategies parents can use to promote an infant's optimal development will then be presented.

Infancy is the period between 1 month and 1 year of age. Rapid growth and development enables maturation to unfold in a relatively short time. Health status is based on the infant's ability to adapt to these rapid changes. As health care providers, nurses must have an understanding of these changes to ensure the infant and his or her family maintains an optimal level of health.

The nurse can help the family integrate the infant into the existing family unit. The nurse also has the opportunity to educate the family, assist in problem identification, and facilitate decision making. By asking questions, interpreting feelings, and providing information to the family, the nurse is able to reinforce the self-confidence of each family member in caring for the infant.

PHYSIOLOGICAL DEVELOPMENT

The rapid changes seen during infancy will never be encountered again throughout the life span. As the body matures, skill development progresses in an orderly fashion to enable the infant to respond to and cope with the world. Gross and fine motor skills develop in a cephalocaudal (head-to-toe) and proximal-distal (central-to-peripheral) fashion; gross motor abilities develop before fine motor abilities.

The infant's physical growth is influenced by genetics, the environment, ethnic background, and biology. Physical growth patterns include weight, height, and head circumference changes. The infant's growth measurements should be plotted on a growth chart and, over time, compared to the infant's own growth curve (see Appendix B for growth charts).

WEIGHT AND HEIGHT

During the first 6 months of life, the infant's birth weight typically doubles. The approximate weight gain is 1.5 lb per month, or 5–7 oz per week. In the second 6 months of life, the infant will gain about 3–5 oz per week (less than 1 lb per month). By 12 months of age, the infant's birth weight will have tripled (Kliegman, Behrman, Jenson, & Stanton, 2007).

Height increases during the first 6 months by approximately 1 inch per month. The rate of growth in height slows to approximately 0.5 inch (1.27 cm) per month by 12 months of age, resulting in almost a 50% increase in height from the birth length (Kliegman et al., 2007).

HEAD GROWTH

The size of the head changes rapidly during infancy, reflecting rapid brain growth. By the age of 12 months, the infant's brain will be two-thirds the size of an adult's. During the first 6 months of life, head circumference will increase by approximately 0.5 inch (1.27 cm) per month. During the second 6 months of life, head circumference will slow to approximately 0.25 inch (0.635 cm) per month. As the head grows, the fontanels gradually close; the posterior fontanel closing by 2 months of age and the anterior fontanel closing by 12–18 months of age (Kliegman et al., 2007).

CHEST GROWTH

The chest circumference averages from 12 to 14 inches (30 to 35 cm); approximately 2.54 cm, or 1 inch less than the head circumference at birth (Davidson, London, & Ladewig, 2008; Ricci, Kyle, & Kyle, 2008). By 1 to 2 years of age, the head circumference and the chest circumference are approximately equal. During childhood, the chest circumference should outgrow the head circumference by 5.0–7.62 cm (2–3 inches). The chest circumference is measured by placing the tape at the lower edge of the scapulas and brought around anteriorly over the nipple line (Kliegman et al., 2007).

MOTOR DEVELOPMENT

Motor development is strongly related to physical, cognitive, and social development. Motor growth includes gross and fine motor development, which provides the infant with the means and freedom to explore the environment. Chapter 6

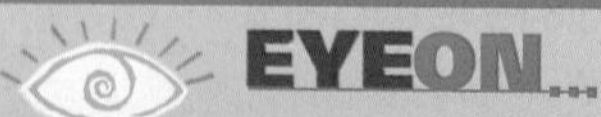

Cultural Weight Differences

Birth weights differ among ethnic groups. For instance, Native American infants are often heavier at birth than European American infants. Infants of Asian descent are typically shorter and lighter than European American infants.

CRITICAL THINKING

Posterior Fontanel

During 4-month-old Peyton's assessment, the nurse notes that his anterior fontanel is closed. How should the nurse interpret the findings? What action should the nurse take at this time? Why?

discusses growth and development in detail. General principles associated with motor development include:

- Voluntary behaviors follow the disappearance of primitive reflexes. To be able to willingly grasp an object, the infant must first lose the involuntary grasp reflex.
- Pronation occurs before supination. The infant must be able to pick up an object (pronation) before being able to put the object in the mouth (supination).
- The ability to grasp an object precedes the ability to release it (Dixon & Stein, 2006).

Gross Motor

Gross motor development is the ability to use large muscle groups to maintain balance and postural control or locomotion. A major task for the infant in obtaining postural control is head control, which is mastered in the prone as well as the upright positions (e.g., standing and sitting). These developmental milestones are not exact, but do occur in a predictable order and usually within 1–2 months of the expected target age. By the age of 1 month, the infant can turn the head to the side while prone and, at 4 months of age, can hold the head up and use the forearms for support (Figure 8-1). At 5 to 6 months of age, the infant has the ability to hold the head, chest, and abdomen up by bearing weight with the hands (Figure 8-2). Once weight bearing with the hands has occurred, the infant will have the ability to turn readily from a prone to a supine position and, one month later will be able to turn from a supine position to a prone position.

Infant head control is judged by the presence or absence of head lag. The amount of head lag can be determined when the infant is pulled by the arms from a supine to a sitting position. At 1 month of age, the infant's back is completely rounded while in a sitting position, with the head falling forward. By 2 months, partial head lag is evident, and the infant can hold the head erect with minimal head bobbing while sitting. At 4 months, the infant has no head lag and good head control while sitting (Figure 8-3).

Once head control is established, the infant begins to sit without support. At 4 months of age, the infant can sit only

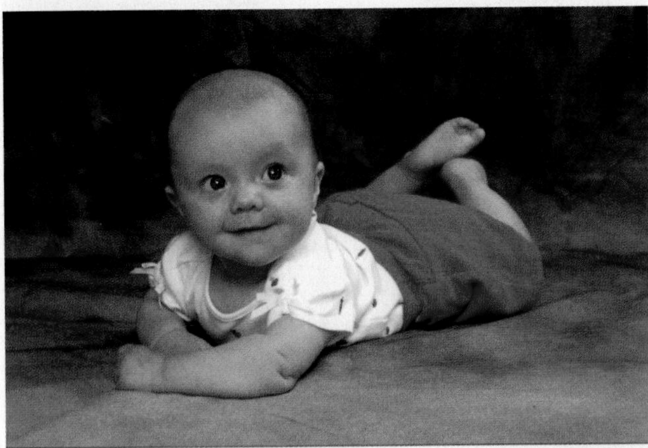

Figure 8-1 This 4-month-old infant can lift her head and support herself on her forearms. DELMAR CENGAGE LEARNING.

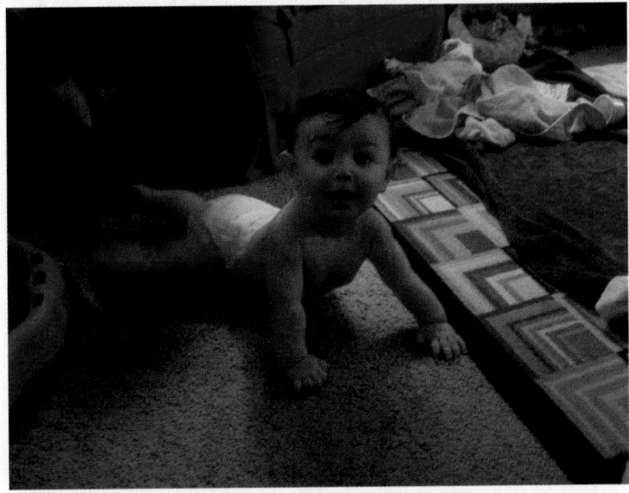

Figure 8-2 At 5 to 6 months, the infant can bear weight on his arms and lift his head, chest, and abdomen. DELMAR CENGAGE LEARNING.

with support. By 6 months of age, the infant can sit alone while using the hands for support. Between 7 and 8 months, the infant is able to sit alone steadily without any support and, by 12 months, sits alone well (Figure 8-4). When the infant is able to sit alone without support, then he or she can explore the environment by scooting or moving on the floor while sitting.

Locomotion, the ability to move from place to place without assistance, is dependent on head control and sitting without support. A variety of skills such as rolling over, bearing weight, moving forward on all extremities, and standing upright without assistance are also necessary for locomotion (Figure 8-5). Once these skills are developed, the infant will be able to move forward (walk), first with assistance, then alone.

By 6 months, the infant can bear most of the body's weight on legs when held in a standing position, and by 8 months can bear weight. From 8 to 10 months of age, the infant demonstrates increasing mobility first by **crawling** (pulling self forward with abdomen touching the floor) and then by **creeping** (moving on hands and knees with abdomen off the floor). By the time infants are creeping, they are able to pull themselves to a standing position. However, there are variations as not all infants creep or crawl before standing and walking.

CRITICAL THINKING

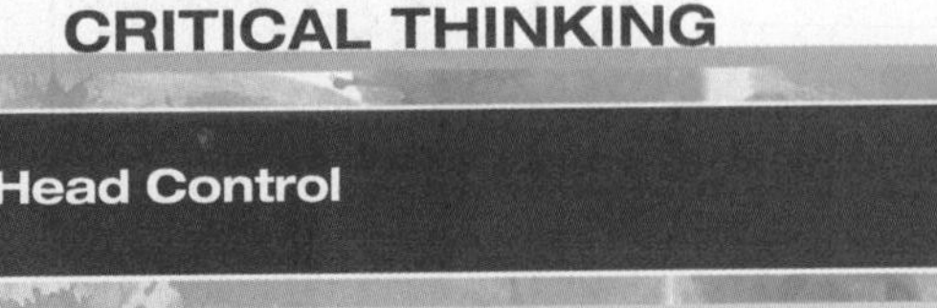

During physical assessment, a nurse finds a 6-month-old infant with a head lag. What priority action should the nurse take?

What is the best way to promote the development of head and neck muscles during infancy?

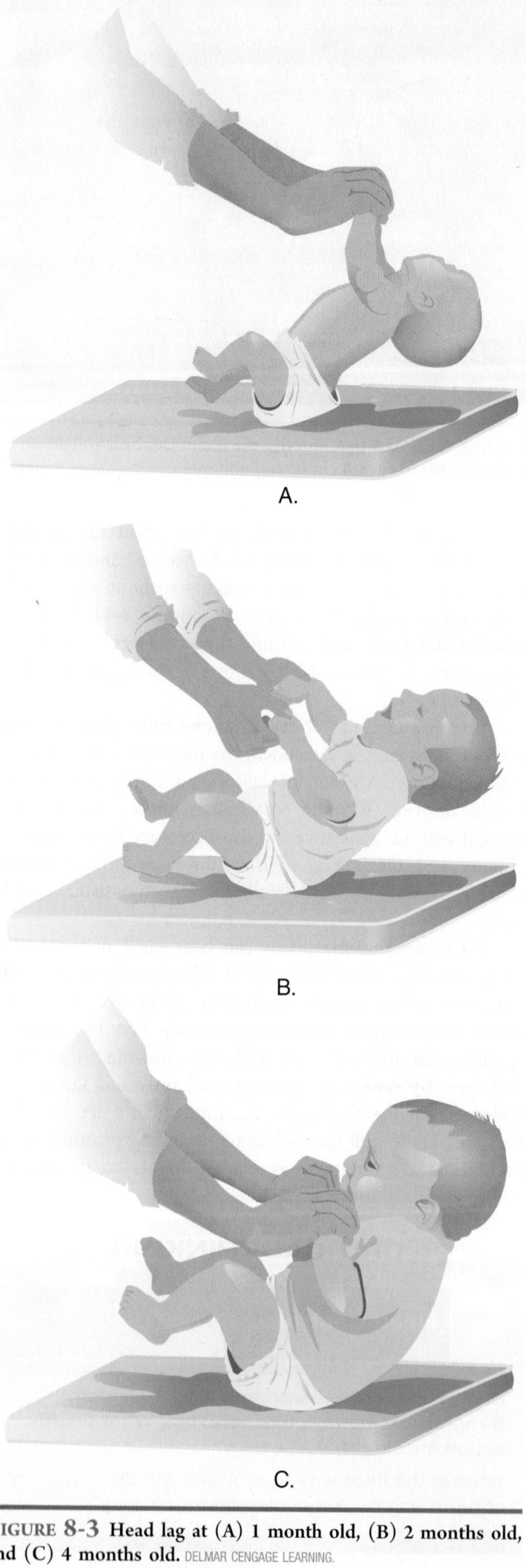

A.

B.

C.

FIGURE 8-3 Head lag at (A) 1 month old, (B) 2 months old, and (C) 4 months old. DELMAR CENGAGE LEARNING.

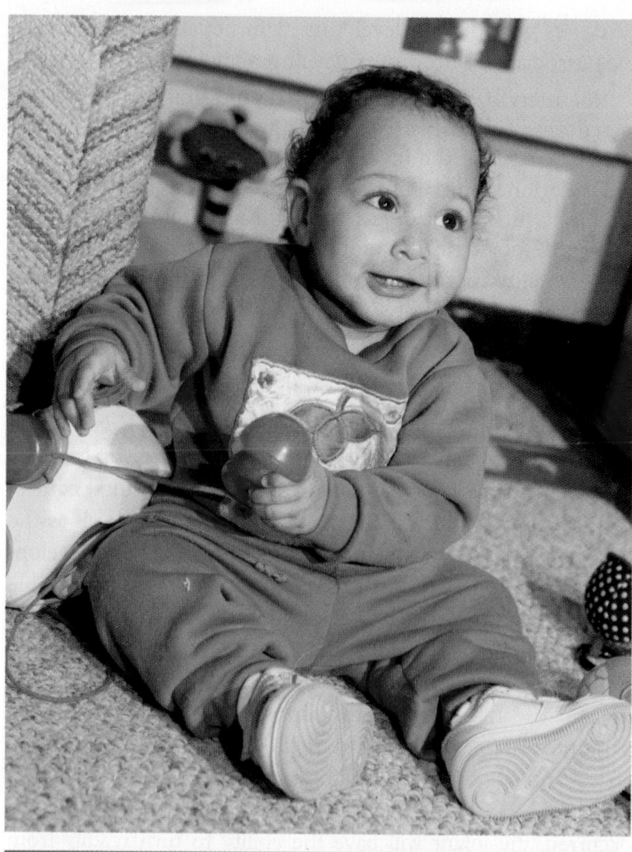

FIGURE 8-4 This 8-month-old infant can sit alone well without support. DELMAR CENGAGE LEARNING.

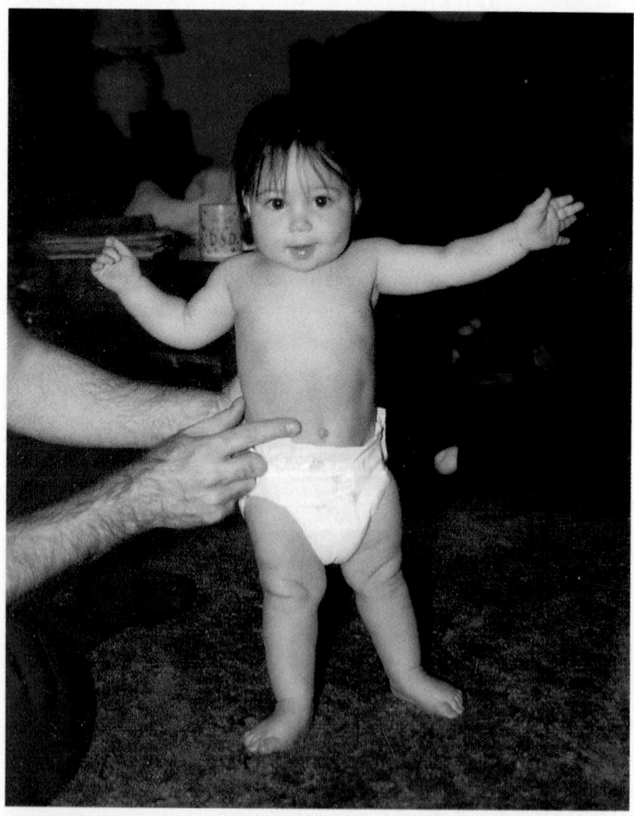

FIGURE 8-5 At 8-10 months of age, the infant can bear weight with support. DELMAR CENGAGE LEARNING.

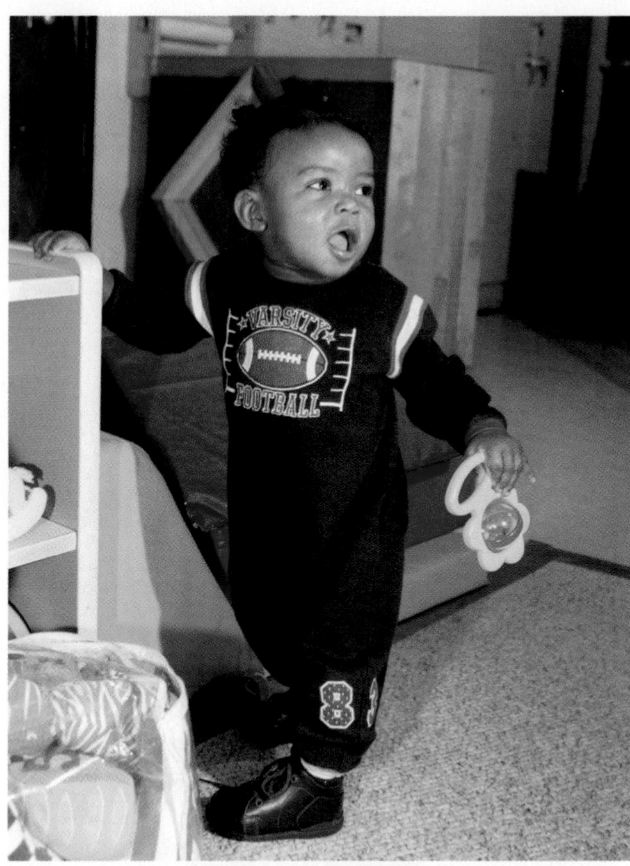

FIGURE 8-6 **This 12-month-old infant is able to cruise by holding on to furniture.** DELMAR CENGAGE LEARNING.

From 10 to 12 months, infant locomotion progresses rapidly. During this time, deliberate steps will be taken while holding onto something (**cruising**). The infant will start to walk sideways while holding onto furniture, before walking or standing alone (Figure 8-6). Once infants can stand alone, they will attempt to take a few steps alone. A summary of gross motor skills can be found in Table 8-1.

TABLE 8-1 Summary of Gross Motor Development

AGE IN MONTHS	GROSS MOTOR SKILLS
2–3 months	Some head lag when pulled to sitting position
	Holds head up and supports weight on forearms when prone
	Some head bobbing while supported in sitting position
	Rolls from abdomen to back
	Tonic neck and Moro reflexes disappearing
4–6 months	Good head control with no head lag
	Holds chest and abdomen up with weight supported by hands while prone
	Sits with support
	Rolls from back to abdomen
	Bears weight in standing position with support
7–8 months	Sits alone without support
	Bears weight in standing position with less support than when 4–6 months of age
9–12 months	Moves from prone to supine to sitting to standing positions without assistance
	Stands alone without support
	Goes from crawling to creeping to cruising
	Attempts to walk alone

FINE MOTOR

As development progresses, the infant begins to utilize the hands and eyes to explore and manipulate the environment. Fine motor development is the ability to coordinate hand-eye movement in an orderly and progressive manner.

During the first month of life, a primitive grasp reflex enables the infant to hold objects with a tightly clenched fist. By the end of 2 months, this primitive reflex fades and the infant begins to actively grasp and momentarily hold an object before dropping it.

At 3 months of age, the infant has the ability to hold the hand open, look at the fingers, and place them in the mouth, and by 4 months, the infant can look from hand to hand. By 5 months of age, the infant can voluntarily grasp an object with the whole hand (palmar grasp), can actively manipulate all grasped objects, and can place them in the mouth. Between 6 and 7 months of age, the infant can hold a bottle securely, and readily grasp the feet and pull them to the mouth. In addition, the infant can willingly drop any grasped object.

As the infant's fine motor development progresses, the palmar grasp is replaced with a thumb and finger pincer grasp at approximately 8 months of age (Figure 8-7). At first, the infant can only crudely grasp objects in a pincer fashion with the thumb and index finger. As the infant practices the grasp, a dominant hand begins to emerge. During this developmental time, the infant continues to test new abilities by reaching for objects, banging them together, and transferring them from hand to hand.

By 10 months of age, the infant's pincer grasp is more refined and reflected in the ability to grasp small finger foods such as small cereals shaped like boxes or the letter O. Between 10 and 12 months of age, infants' hand movements become very deliberate, as they purposefully drop or place small objects into a container and remove them. The infant can even hold and mark paper with a crayon. By 12 months of age, the infant will be able to turn multiple pages in a book. A summary of fine motor development can be found in Table 8-2.

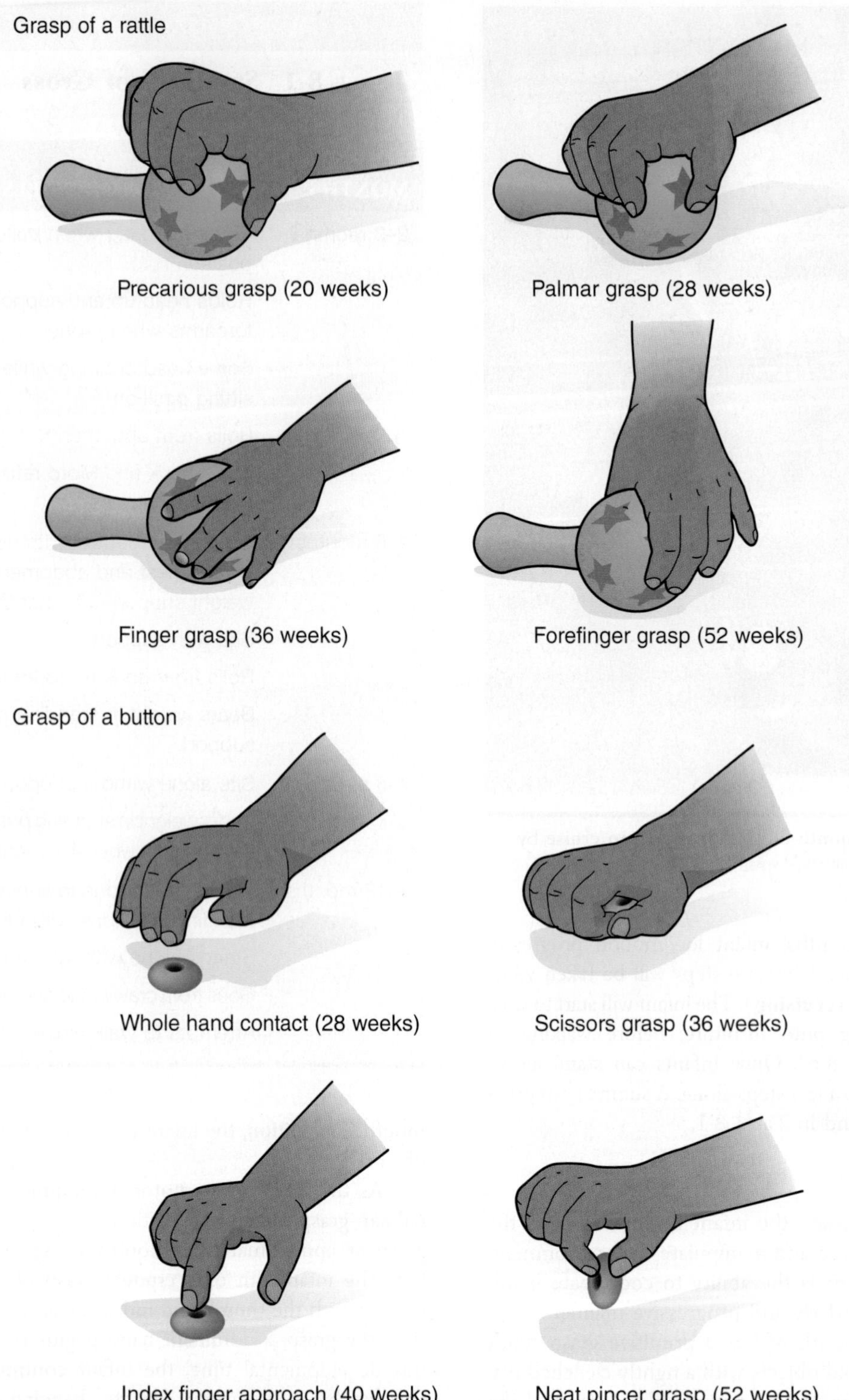

FIGURE 8-7 Development of Prehension. DELMAR CENGAGE LEARNING.

PSYCHOSEXUAL DEVELOPMENT

Psychosexual development is based on the individual's need to seek pleasure. The individual must be able to balance pleasure seeking with societal expectations. According to Freud's theory (1933), the infant is in the oral stage of development (birth to 1 year), during which the need for pleasure dominates life. Oral stimulation or sucking is the central focus of this stage (Dixon & Stein, 2006), and according to Freud (1933), feeding or nutritive sucking becomes the most important source of pleasure and satisfaction. See Chapter 6 for more information on Freud's theory.

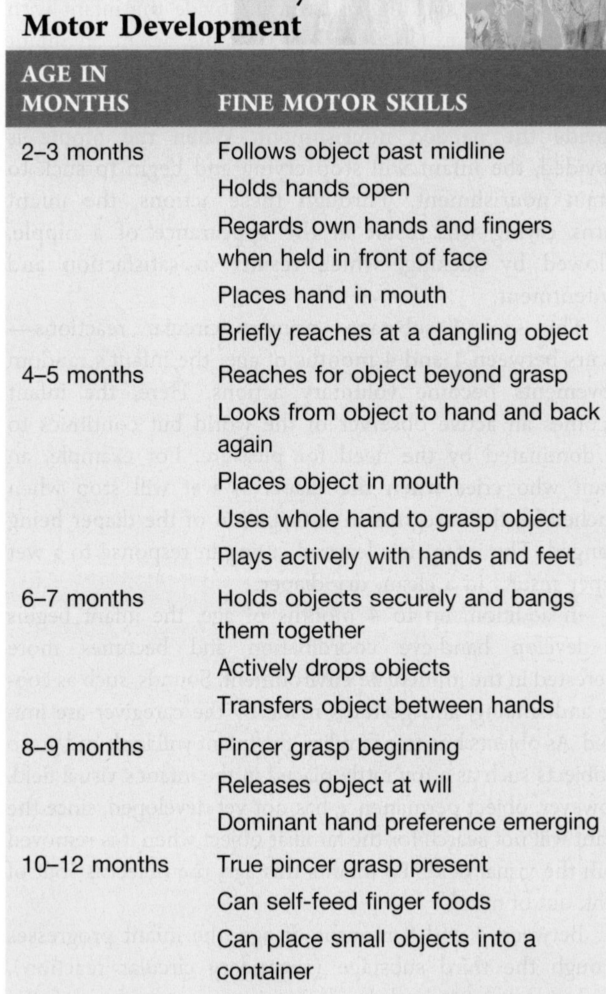

Table 8-2 Summary of Fine Motor Development

AGE IN MONTHS	FINE MOTOR SKILLS
2–3 months	Follows object past midline
	Holds hands open
	Regards own hands and fingers when held in front of face
	Places hand in mouth
	Briefly reaches at a dangling object
4–5 months	Reaches for object beyond grasp
	Looks from object to hand and back again
	Places object in mouth
	Uses whole hand to grasp object
	Plays actively with hands and feet
6–7 months	Holds objects securely and bangs them together
	Actively drops objects
	Transfers object between hands
8–9 months	Pincer grasp beginning
	Releases object at will
	Dominant hand preference emerging
10–12 months	True pincer grasp present
	Can self-feed finger foods
	Can place small objects into a container
	Can remove small objects from a container
	Can hold and mark with a crayon
	Can turn multiple pages in a book

As development progresses, the infant learns to connect actions with end results. For example, the infant learns that cries of hunger result in being fed; eventually the caregiver's touch will be associated with feeding needs being met as infants learn to delay the need for immediate gratification in anticipation of being fed. If the infant is not fed within a few minutes of being held, the infant will start to cry as a signal that the need for the pleasure or comfort from the feeding has not been met.

In addition to feeding, another source of pleasure and satisfaction for the infant is obtained through nonnutritive sucking (Figure 8-8). With the infant's natural tendency to suck, non-nutritive sucking occurs first by accident through the reflex of rooting and then purposefully by actively placing objects, such as toys, fingers, or a pacifier in the mouth.

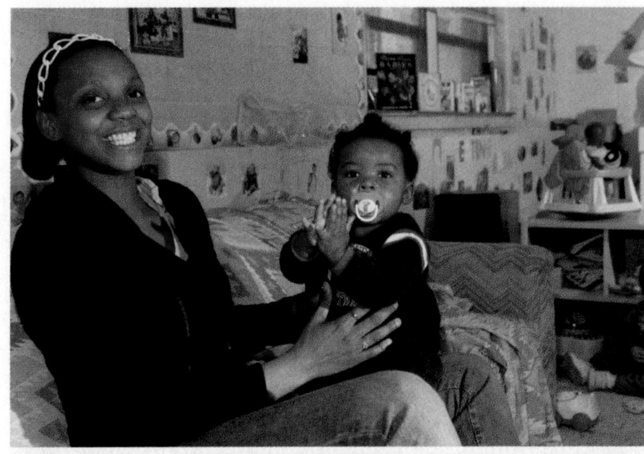

Figure 8-8 Nonnutritive sucking is a source of pleasure and satisfaction for infants. DELMAR CENGAGE LEARNING.

PSYCHOSOCIAL DEVELOPMENT

The psychosocial development of an infant, as defined by Erikson (1963), is centered on the concept of trust versus mistrust. According to Erikson, trust is developed when the basic needs of feeding, clothing, and comforting are met by caretakers. If these needs are not met, the infant will develop a mistrust of others.

However, trust development involves more than just meeting basic needs. The quality of the caregiver-infant interaction while providing care also plays a major role. If the caregiver consistently demonstrates nurturing behaviors such as talking, playing, smiling, dressing, and comforting, the infant will develop a strong sense of trust. If these behaviors are absent, trust development may be delayed. Furthermore, the caregiver and infant must learn together ways to achieve satisfaction and decrease frustration during daily routines (Figure 8-9).

Should the infant be in an alternative child care situation (child care setting, baby sitters, child care workers), the trust

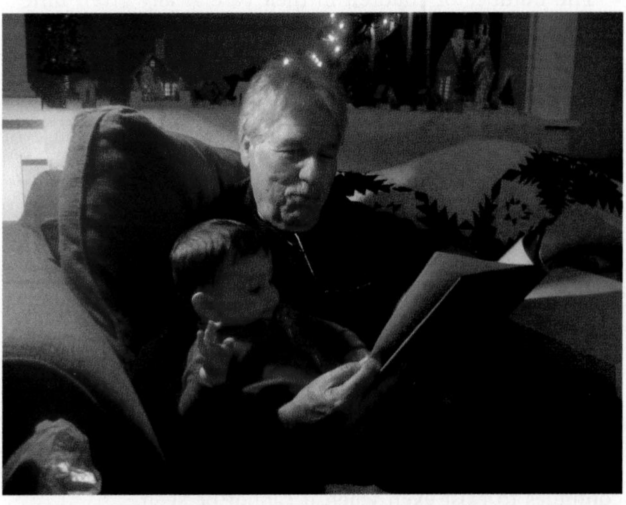

Figure 8-9 Grandparents are important caregivers for infants. DELMAR CENGAGE LEARNING.

> **NURSING TIP**
>
> **Understanding Psychosocial Development**
>
> To improve your understanding of the infant's psychosocial development and the caregiver's knowledge of psychosocial development, ask yourself:
>
> - Does the infant demonstrate trust in the environment?
> - What does the caregiver know about developing the infant's sense of trust?
> - Does the caregiver have other situations (e.g., divorce, financial problems, and health problems) that might interfere with the infant developing a sense of trust?
> - Are there any environmental and/or cultural biases that might impede the caregiver's ability to assist the infant in developing a trusting relationship?

development is continued by the child care provider. Therefore it is critical to inform the child care provider of the following:

- Usual home routines
- Sleep patterns
- Eating habits
- Cues given when frustrated
- Response to comforting methods
- Favorite toys, games, songs, music

Confidence in the child care provider's ability to provide a trusting environment is very important. The caregiver should inquire about:

- The child care provider's experience with infants
- How the child care provider comforts a fussy infant
- Whether there are other children in their care
- The number of children in their care at any given time

If the infant's needs are met in a consistent manner by the caregiver or alternative child care provider, trust in self as well as trust in others and the surrounding environment will develop. If not, the infant will eventually develop a sense of mistrust.

COGNITIVE DEVELOPMENT

According to Piaget (1952), an infant is in the sensorimotor stage (birth to 24 months) of cognitive development when knowledge is acquired about an object through interaction with that object and use of the senses. The major task for the infant, according to Piaget, is **object permanence**, where the infant learns an object is not an extension of the self and continues to exist even when it cannot be seen.

Piaget's sensorimotor stage consists of six substages. During the first year of life, the infant will pass through the first four of these substages. In the first substage, the newborn (birth to 1 month) learns about the world through repetitive use of involuntary reflexes. These repetitive acts, such as rooting, sucking, or crying, provide the infant with cause-and-effect experiences. For example, when an infant is hungry, crying will signal the infant has a need. The caregiver understands this cry is due to hunger and will provide the needed nourishment. When the nipple is provided, the infant will stop crying and begin to suck to obtain nourishment. Through these actions, the infant learns crying will result in the appearance of a nipple, followed by sucking, which results in satisfaction and contentment.

The second substage—primary circular reactions—occurs between 1 and 4 months of age; the infant's random movements become voluntary actions. Here, the infant becomes an active observer of the world but continues to be dominated by the need for pleasure. For example, an infant who cries when the diaper is wet will stop when touched by the caregiver in anticipation of the diaper being changed. The infant has learned crying in response to a wet diaper results in a clean, dry diaper.

In addition, up to 4 months of age, the infant begins to develop hand-eye coordination and becomes more interested in the immediate environment. Sounds, such as cooing and smiling, and gestures made by the caregiver are imitated. As objects become familiar, the infant will look and grasp at objects such as a toy rattle placed in the infant's visual field. However, object permanence has not yet developed, since the infant will not search for the familiar object when it is removed from the visual field. To infants this age, the object is "out of sight, out of mind."

Between 4 and 8 months of age, the infant progresses through the third substage (secondary circular reaction), which is characterized by becoming more aware of the surrounding environment and mastering voluntary actions. The concept of play becomes evident during this period as

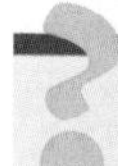

> **KIDS WANT TO KNOW**
>
> **Sibling rivalry: I want my mommy all to myself**
>
> It would be important in this situation for the mother to assure the sibling that he/she is loved, but explain to the sibling that she needs to also spend time with the infant. The sibling can be allowed and encouraged to help with the infant's care, but it would also be important for the parent to spend time with the older sibling in an activity which is normally off limits when the infant is around, such as painting, reading a book, or going for a walk.

BOX 8-1

THE MILLENNIUM DEVELOPMENT GOALS (MDGS)

The United Nations Millennium Development Goals (MDGs) are time-bound and quantified targets for addressing extreme poverty across the world in its many dimensions: income poverty, hunger, disease, lack of adequate shelter, and exclusion-while promoting gender equality, education, and environmental sustainability (UN MDGs Report, 2008).

The number one goal of the MDGs is to eradicate extreme poverty and hunger with a target to reduce by half the proportion of people who suffer from hunger by 2015. According to the Millennium Project Task Force on Hunger, it is now more than halfway towards the target date—2015—by which the MDGs are to be achieved (UN MDGs Report, 2008). Halving Hunger calls for the implementation of seven recommendations in the areas of political action, national policy reforms, increased agricultural productivity for insecure farmers, improved nutrition for the chronically hungry, productive safety nets for the acutely hungry, improved rural incomes and markets, and restoration and conservation of natural resources essential for food security (UN MDGs Report, 2008).

Another MDG goal is to reduce under-5 mortality rate by two-thirds by 2015. In low-income countries, 1 out of every 10 children dies before the age of 5. In wealthier nations, this number is only 1 out of 143. Eleven million children under the age of 5 die in the world every year from easily preventable or treatable causes. The leading causes of deaths are pneumonia, diarrhea, malaria, and measles (UN MDGs Report, 2008). Malnutrition is estimated to be an underlying cause in more than one third of all deaths in children under 5. Of the under-5 deaths, 37% occur in the first month of life. Improved neonatal and maternal care could save these newborns.

Measures to achieve the necessary reductions in child mortality:

- Ensure full coverage of immunization programs.
- Scale up vitamin A supplementation.
- Pursue exclusive breastfeeding for children under 6 months of age and breastfeeding plus appropriate complementary feeding for children aged 6 months to 2 years.
- Provide adequate nourishment for children of poor families.
- Promote hand-washing and treatment of home drinking water.
- Target the underlying socioeconomic causes of child mortality such as access to reproductive health, education, and employment.
- Prevent and provide effective treatment of pneumonia, diarrhea, malaria, and other infectious diseases.
- Promote comprehensive and universal coverage of primary health-care systems.

Achieving the Goals

With the help of donor aid and UN organizations, the world governments started an aggressive approach to reducing child mortality and increasing the number of children vaccinated from 9.6% in 1991 to 76% in 2002. This was done using the Integrated Management of Childhood Illnesses (IMCI) method, a holistic way of looking at the life of infants and young children. Health workers were trained in IMCI methods in prevention and cure of diseases, focusing on the well-being of the entire child including launching an aggressive vaccination campaign (UN MDGs Report, 2008).

Source: United Nations Millennium Development Goals Report 2008. *Goal 4: Reduce child mortality fact sheet.* Retrieved May 22, 2010, from http://www.un.org/millenniumgoals/2008highlevel/pdf/newsroom/Goal%204%20FINAL.pdf.

well (Figure 8–10). Here, the infant's actions are more intentional and not solely directed by pleasure, as the infant learns through repetitive actions to create interesting sights and sounds and begins to focus on the effects of the actions. For instance, the infant may repeatedly bang a toy just to produce a sound.

The beginning of object permanence is evident during this substage, as an object is no longer seen as an extension of the infant but rather as a separate entity. While interacting with a familiar object, the infant will now search for the object if it is removed from the visual field. Although infants will look for the object, they quickly lose interest if it is not readily found. Another example of object permanence is the infant's development of stranger anxiety when left with a new babysitter. Here, the infant actively searches for the caregiver after the caregiver has left and may begin crying when the caregiver is not found.

The infant applies newly mastered skills to new experiences in the fourth substage (8 to 12 months), called coordination of secondary schema, and is able to put several events together to accomplish an end result. For example, the infant is able to put blocks into a container with various shaped holes and understand simple words and commands (e.g., no-no, bye-bye, cracker).

Object permanence is apparent and demonstrated when the infant actively seeks a hidden object. The beginning of

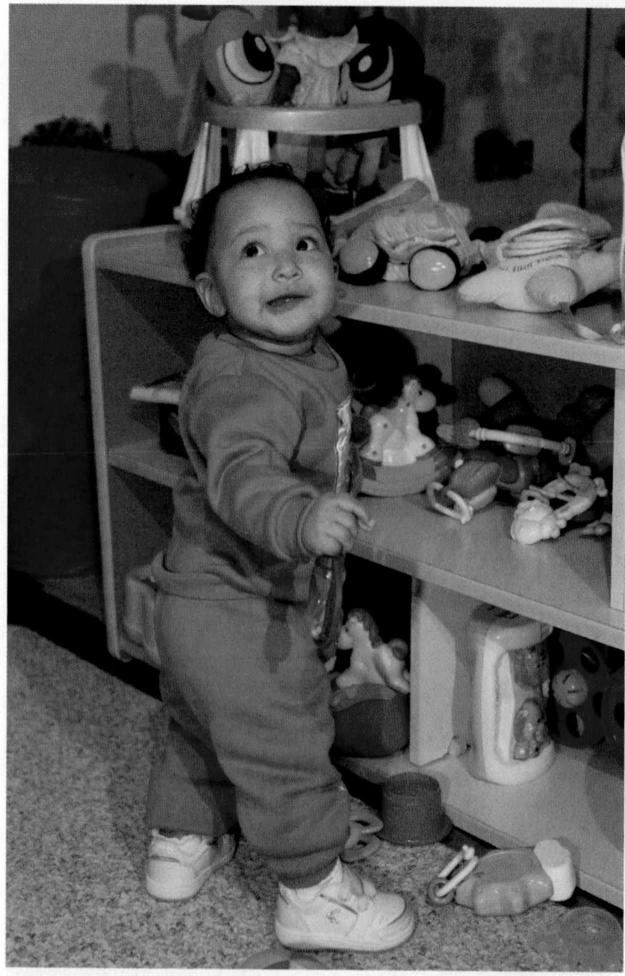

FIGURE 8-10 **This older infant is able to remember and find toys that he has played with in the past.** DELMAR CENGAGE LEARNING.

reasoning is evident when the infant moves any obstacle to uncover a hidden object.

BOX 8-2

THE BABY-FRIENDLY HOSPITAL INITIATIVE

The Baby-Friendly Hospital Initiative (BFHI) is an effort by World Health Organization (WHO) and the United Nations Children's Fund (UNICEF) designed to help hospitals maximize their ability to help mothers breastfeed. A maternity facility can be designated 'baby-friendly' when it does not accept free or low-cost breast milk substitutes, feeding bottles or teats, and has implemented 10 specific steps to support successful breastfeeding. The following are the ten steps to become designated a baby friendly hospital:

1. Maintain a written breastfeeding policy that is routinely communicated to all health care staff.
2. Train all health care staff in skills necessary to implement this policy.
3. Inform all pregnant women about the benefits and management of breastfeeding.
4. Help mothers initiate breastfeeding within one hour of birth.
5. Show mothers how to breastfeed and how to maintain lactation, even if they are separated from their infants.
6. Give infants no food or drink other than breast milk, unless medically indicated.
7. Practice "rooming in"—allow mothers and infants to remain together 24 hours a day.
8. Encourage unrestricted breastfeeding.
9. Give no pacifiers or artificial nipples to breastfeeding infants.
10. Foster the establishment of breastfeeding support groups and refer mothers to them on discharge from the hospital or clinic.

Source: *The Baby-Friendly Hospital Initiative. (2010).* Retrieved May 22, 2010, from http://www.unicef.org/programme/breastfeeding/baby.htm#10 and www.babyfriendlyusa.org.

HEALTH PROMOTION

The health status of the infant, a major concern for caregivers, is based on the ability to adapt to rapid changes. Therefore, the caregiver needs to know the expected physical, emotional, and developmental growth patterns of the infant. As health care providers, nurses are able to assist the caregiver in understanding these patterns. Through education, counseling, anticipatory guidance, and understanding the family's cultural needs, the nurse can assist the caregiver and family and ensure that the infant maintains an optimal level of health and development (Box 8-1).

HEALTH SCREENING

Health promotion and maintenance are important since health status is a good indicator of the infant's ability to adapt to the rapid changes of growth and development. Optimal health enables the infant to adjust to these changes without placing undue stress on the body.

Health screening provides the opportunity to assess for and detect any problems the infant may have and includes tests to detect phenylketonuria (PKU), iron deficiency anemia, lead poisoning, and hypothyroidism. The infant's health screening actually begins immediately after birth with the first Apgar scoring and physical examination. Once discharged home, the infant's health promotion and maintenance becomes the responsibility of the caregiver, who should be encouraged to contact the health care provider for any health concerns.

In the first year, well-child visits are usually scheduled when the infant is 2 weeks, and 2, 4, 6, 9, and 12 months old. The visit typically includes health assessment, physical

RESEARCH Highlight

Are U.S. Mothers Meeting the *Healthy People 2010* Breastfeeding Targets for Initiation, Duration, and Exclusivity?

STUDY PURPOSE

To determine the characteristics of groups meeting the *Healthy People 2010* breastfeeding targets for initiation, duration, and exclusivity.

METHODS

Using data from the National Immunization Surveys (2003 and 2004), the authors model the influence of child, maternal, and state- or metropolitan-level factors on the initiation, duration, and exclusivity of breastfeeding.

FINDINGS

Analyses indicate that only children of college graduates meet the targets for breastfeeding at initiation, 6 months, and 12 months; no groups meet the target for exclusive breastfeeding. Results also found a low prevalence of breastfeeding among children of single mothers, less educated mothers, participants in the Women, Children, and Infants program, and those living in nonwestern states and in areas of high newborn risk. Hispanic children, children of college graduates, and children living in the West consistently have higher odds of breastfeeding.

IMPLICATIONS

U.S. mothers are not meeting the *Healthy People 2010* breastfeeding targets for initiation, duration, and exclusivity. Only the prevalence of breastfeeding early postpartum is near the *Healthy People 2010* target of 75%; the percentages for 6 or 12 months and exclusive breastfeeding are well below.

REFERENCE

Forste, R., & Hoffmann, J. P. (2008). Are U.S. mothers meeting the *Healthy People 2010* breastfeeding targets for initiation, duration, and exclusivity? The 2003 and 2004 national immunization surveys. *Journal of Human Lactation, 24*(3), 278–288.

NURSING TIP

Family Database

To be more effective in the promotion of optimal health and development, it is important to be familiar with family circumstances, including the following:

- Composition of the household
- Language spoken in the household
- Identity of the primary caregiver
- Caregivers' health status
- Caregivers' employment status
- Caregivers' educational level
- Caregivers' financial status
- Caregivers' use of alcohol, tobacco, and other substances
- Adequacy of house size to accommodate family
- Cultural influences
- Religious affiliation
- Social support or conflict
- Environmental/community factors impacting family

examination, growth indicators (weight, height, head circumference), anticipatory guidance, assessment of parental concerns, and administration of scheduled immunizations. Table 8-3 provides an outline of the specific kinds of assessments that are performed during well-child visits during the first year of life.

During the visit, the caregiver will probably have questions and concerns regarding the infant's ongoing needs and care. The nurse can be instrumental in providing information related to physical development, nutrition, safety, immunizations, and play. With guidance, the caregiver will be better able to understand the infant's needs and the care required to meet those needs.

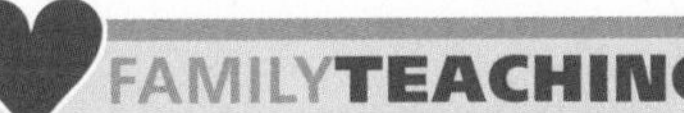

When to Call Your Health Care Provider

The following signs and symptoms may indicate the need to contact the health care provider:

- Fever: under 2 months, 38°C (100.4°F); 3 to 6 months, 38.3°C (101°F); over 6 months, 39.4°C (103°F)
- Feeding poorly: lack of interest, poor sucking effort, failure to awaken for feeding
- Vomiting
- Decreased activity or alertness: appears listless
- Inconsolable crying
- Abnormal movement: unusual jerking of body
- Unusual skin color: pale or mottled skin color, bluish around the lips
- Increased frequency of wet diapers
- Signs of dehydration: absence of tears, fewer wet diapers than normal, dry mouth

TABLE 8-3 Health Screening Visits

EMPHASIS OF VISIT	1 MONTH	2 MONTHS	4 MONTHS	6 MONTHS	9 MONTHS	12 MONTHS
Assessments: Developmental milestones, hearing and vision, nutritional	✓	✓	✓	✓	✓	✓
Physical examination	✓	✓	✓	✓	✓	✓
Growth measurements: Height, weight, head circumference	✓	✓	✓	✓	✓	✓
Immunizations*						
Anticipatory guidance: Infant care, expected growth, developmental milestones, safety, dental health	✓	✓	✓	✓	✓	✓
Screenings:						
PKU	✓ (if not done as newborn)					
Thyroid	✓ (if not done as newborn)					
Hematocrit, hemoglobin	✓ (if not done as newborn)				✓	
Lead				✓ (if at high risk)	✓	or ✓
Parental concerns	✓	✓	✓	✓	✓	✓

*Refer to Appendix C for latest immunization schedule.

Adapted from American Academy of Pediatrics. (2009a). Recommendations for Preventative Pediatric Health Care (RE9535). Committee on Practice and Ambulatory Health Care. Retrieved January 23, 2010, from http://aappolicy.aappublications.org/cgi/reprint/pediatrics;105/3/645.pdf.

IMMUNIZATIONS

The recommended childhood immunization schedule can be found in Appendix C.

Prior to administering any immunization, the nurse assesses for contraindications to administration. Immunizations are usually not contraindicated when a mild illness such as allergic rhinitis, mild diarrhea, or mild respiratory infection is present (see Chapter 15 for an extensive discussion on contraindication to immunizations). The nurse also provides the caregiver with information about the benefits and risks of the immunizations and answers questions about them. In addition, the caregiver should receive information about possible reactions the infant might experience after receiving the immunizations (Centers for Disease Control, and Prevention 2009; 2010).

VISION

The visual system is not fully developed at birth. Research however, has shown that even newborns have full visual array with acuity of 20/100 to 20/200 (Kliegman et al., 2007). Therefore, it is important that problems with vision be detected early to prevent significant delays in motor development since visual and auditory abilities have an impact on perception and understanding of the surrounding environment. To enhance visual development, a variety of stimuli should be introduced into the infant's life.

Why Do Parents Hesitate to Have their Infants/Children Immunized?

STUDY PURPOSE

To determine why parents do not immunize their infants/children according to the published schedule.

METHODS

Eighty-six parents completed a questionnaire during a well-child visit seeking reasons why they did not or were hesitant to immunize their infants/children.

FINDINGS

Reasons parents delayed getting their infants/children immunized were that the schedule was confusing, they were concerned about vaccination safety, they had difficulty finding time to schedule the immunization, they were waiting until the infant/child was older, and they did not have a current immunization record so did not know what the infant/child had had or needed. Parents also voiced concerns related to childhood immunizations that included the child's panic/anxiety before, during and after the immunization, the short-term adverse effects of the immunization (fever, pain), the overall safety of the vaccines, the possibility of overloading the infant/child's immune system, and the number of vaccines that were combined into one administration. Finally, the study discovered the most common sources parents used to obtain information about immunizations were health care providers, family members, the local health department, and an Internet Website.

IMPLICATIONS

When interacting with parents during well-child visits, discuss and provide a copy of the immunization schedule along with expected side effects and reasons for obtaining the immunizations. In addition it would be important to always check on the infant/child's immunization status during these visits and answer any questions or respond to any concerns voiced by parents related to immunizations. Finally, it would be critical to talk with parents on ways to help infants/children cope with the immunization experience.

REFERENCE

Luthy, K. E., Beckstrand, R. L., & Peterson, N. E. (2008). Parental hesitation as a factor in delayed childhood immunization. *Journal of Pediatric Health Care, 23*(6), 388–393.

FAMILY TEACHING

Home Care with Immunizations

Most common reactions usually last 1–2 days:

- Irritability
- Mild loss of appetite
- Low-grade fever (101°F) (38.3°C)
- Redness, swelling, and tenderness at the injection site

General treatment of reaction:

- Administer acetaminophen every 4–6 hours for a total of three doses

Immunization-specific reaction:

- Diphtheria, tetanus, pertussis (DTaP)—low-grade fever with redness, swelling, and tenderness at injection site
- Inactivated polio vaccine (IPV)—tenderness at injection site
- Hepatitis B (hep B)—irritability and redness, swelling, and tenderness at injection site
- Measles, mumps, rubella (MMR)—mild rash, low-grade fever, and drowsiness beginning 7–10 days after immunization

Contact the health care provider immediately if the infant develops any symptoms other than the common reactions or if the mild reactions persist longer than 2 days (CDC, 2010).

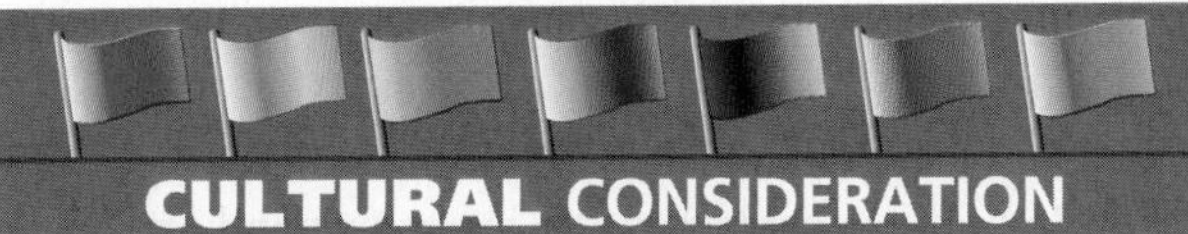

CULTURAL CONSIDERATION

Barriers to Immunizations for African American Children

African American children are less likely to receive immunizations when compared to children of other ethnic groups, even when socioeconomic status is controlled. Reasons for not being up to date on immunizations included family composition (single parent/blended families), lack of trust of medical care system in general even though parents might trust their child's pediatrician, low priority (only needed for entrance to school or preschool/day care), mild illness in the child, parental perception that immunization against some diseases is not necessary, and desire for parental control over child's health care.

Reference: Darden, P., Blue, A., Brooks, D., Taylor, J., Hendricks, J., & Bocian, A. (2006). Staff and parent perceptions of barriers to immunization for African-American children: A study from PROS and NMAPEDSNET. Accessed January 23, 2010, from http://www.aap.org/research/abstracts/05abstract18.htm.

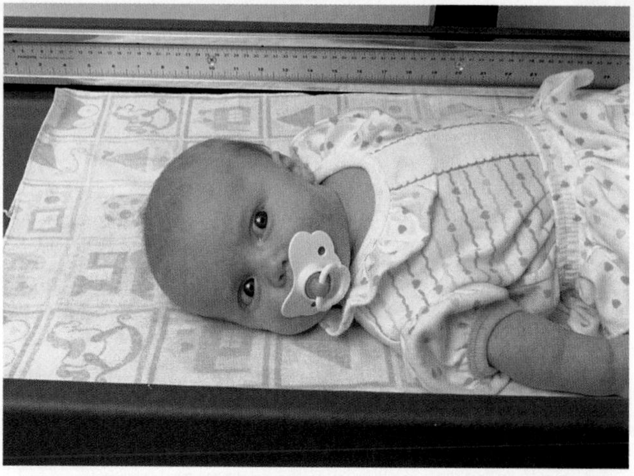

FIGURE 8-11 At 2 months of age, infants can track objects in their visual field. DELMAR CENGAGE LEARNING.

Visual development is demonstrated by the infant's ability to follow a light or object placed within the visual field and the cessation of body movements after fixating on the object (Figure 8-11). Infants prefer the human face, demonstrated by visual attentiveness when interacting with the caregiver. By 6 months, the infant can recognize familiar faces and may experience stranger anxiety. As visual acuity improves and motor skills develop, the infant begins to respond to the variety of colors and shapes in the environment. There is a preference for contrast such as black and white designs, especially checkerboards and designs with angles. By 1 year, both near and distant acuities are good (in the 20/50 range); there is ability to focus and the child has depth perception; he/she can discriminate between simple geometric forms, scribbles with a crayon, and is visually interested in pictures (Monitoring Visual Development, 2007). Any caregiver concern regarding visual responsiveness or lack of eye contact in the infant may indicate visual or other problems that should receive a follow-up evaluation.

Once the skills of reaching and picking up objects have developed, play behavior can be observed to evaluate vision, since the ability to easily find and pick up small toys is a good indicator of vision in children under 3 years of age. If milestones in visual development are not consistently demonstrated, the infant should be referred for further evaluation (Kliegman et al., 2007).

HEARING

The intensity of the infant's response to auditory stimuli may vary depending on the state of alertness. The human voice is an important and readily available sound stimulus, and infants prefer the sound of a human voice to other sounds in their environment. The infant also responds well to musical toys and those making different sounds (Figure 8-12).

Hearing problems should be detected early in life to prevent significant delays in speech development. An infant's development can be profoundly affected by the inability to see or hear. Children with hearing loss who had universal newborn hearing screening have better language outcomes at school age than those who were not screened. Infants identified with hearing loss through universal screening have significantly earlier referral, diagnosis, and treatment than those identified in other ways (Nelson, Bougatsos, & Nygren, 2008). Therefore, it is important that the infant's vision and hearing be assessed regularly.

NURSING ALERT

Infant Behaviors Related to Vision Problems

- Absence of blink
- Absence of doll's eye reflex (movement of head to the right or left, in which eyes lag behind and do not immediately adjust to the new position; disappears as infant is able to focus)
- Does not follow objects by 1 month of age
- Does not fixate on objects by 3 to 4 months of age
- Does not watch own hands and feet by 4 months of age
- Does not reach for objects by 5 months of age
- Absent or poor hand-eye coordination by 7 months of age
- Does not watch objects fall when dropped

DENTAL CARE

Tooth development and eruption are affected by genetics, gender, race, and growth patterns. **Deciduous teeth**, also

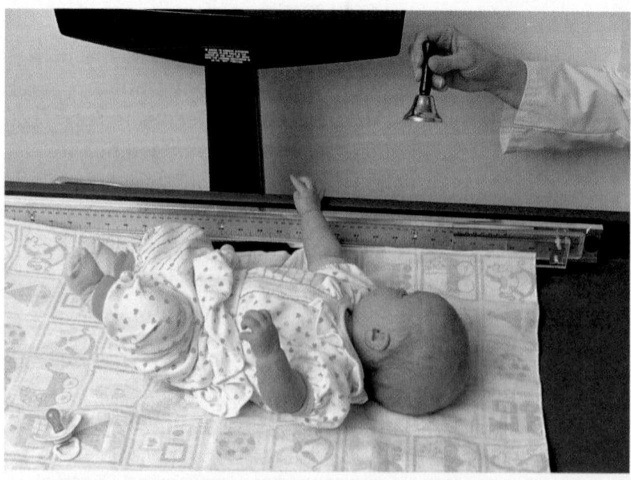

FIGURE 8-12 At 2 months of age, infants can localize sounds. DELMAR CENGAGE LEARNING.

NURSING TIP

Parental Concerns about Infant Hearing and Vision

Caregivers are in constant interaction with their infant and are usually the first to notice something is wrong with vision or hearing. Be alert to any concerns expressed by the caregiver regarding the infant's lack of response or inability to achieve milestones associated with vision or hearing.

NURSING ALERT

Infant Behaviors Related to Hearing Problems

- Lack of startle reflex or blink with a loud sound
- Failure to be awakened by loud noises in the environment
- Lack of cooing or babbling by 3 months
- Failure to turn head toward a sound by 6 months of age
- General indifference to sound
- Lack of response to the spoken word

Reflections from Families

How could he be deaf? We could not believe what was being said about our baby. But in reality, we had known for some time that something was wrong. By the time Aiden was 2 months old, we became increasingly concerned that he might have a hearing problem. We decided to get him checked since Aiden did not seem to respond to loud noises or to turn his head to the sound of our voices. Now, we have been told that he is deaf. What will happen now?

referred to as primary or baby teeth, are the first teeth to develop and erupt. The eruption of teeth varies among children, but the teething process typically begins around 3–4 months of age. The first teeth to erupt are usually the lower central incisors, followed by the upper central incisors after approximately 4–8 weeks (Kliegman et al., 2007) (Figure 8-13).

Good dental hygiene and care begins prior to pregnancy. Maternal nutrition before and during pregnancy as well as breastfeeding are essential to good dental health during infancy and childhood. The American Academy of Pediatrics (AAP) Section on Pediatric Dentistry and Oral Health (2008a) developed a policy using scientific evidence designed to improve oral health outcomes for all children and especially children at significant risk of dental decay. The policy statements emphasize the importance of promoting healthy eating behaviors. To decrease the risk of dental caries and ensure the best possible health and developmental outcomes, it is recommended that parents do the following: breastfeed infants during the first year of life and beyond as is mutually desired, remove the nipple from a sleeping infant's mouth and cleanse the gums and teeth after feedings and before bedtime, limit sugary foods and drinks at mealtimes, and avoid carbonated beverages and juice drinks (AAP Section on Pediatric Dentistry and Oral Health, 2008a).

Fluoride is a naturally occurring element that has been instrumental in the widespread decrease in dental caries. Fluoride reduces enamel dissolution while it encourages remineralization (AAP Section on Pediatric Dentistry and Oral Health, 2008a). For infants who get most of their nutrition from formula during their first 12 months, ready-to-feed formula is preferred to help ensure that their fluoride intake does not exceed the optimal amount. If liquid concentrate or powdered infant formula is the primary source of nutrition, it can be mixed with water that is fluoride-free or contains low levels of fluoride to reduce the risk of fluorosis (American Academy of Pediatric Dentistry [AAPD], 2006). Because of the risk for dental fluorosis, and the lack of demonstrable benefit from ingesting fluoride before teeth erupt, the AAPD recommends that children under 12 months of age should not consume fluoridated water while babies under 6 months of age should not receive any fluoride drops. The latest recommendation is to give children 6 months to 3 years of age 0.25 mg of fluoride daily if water content is less than 0.3 ppm (parts per million) (AAPD, 2006); refer to Table 8-4. Parents can ask the local health department or their infant's health care provider about the fluoride content of their water source if they do not know what the fluoride content of their water is.

Dental caries can also occur in infants who have frequent or prolonged exposure to sugars found in milk, formula, or juice. The longer the sugar stays on the tooth enamel, the more opportunity there is for bacteria in the mouth to combine with sugar to form dental caries (AAP, 2006). This type of dental caries, known as **nursing** or **bottle-mouth caries** or early childhood caries, is commonly

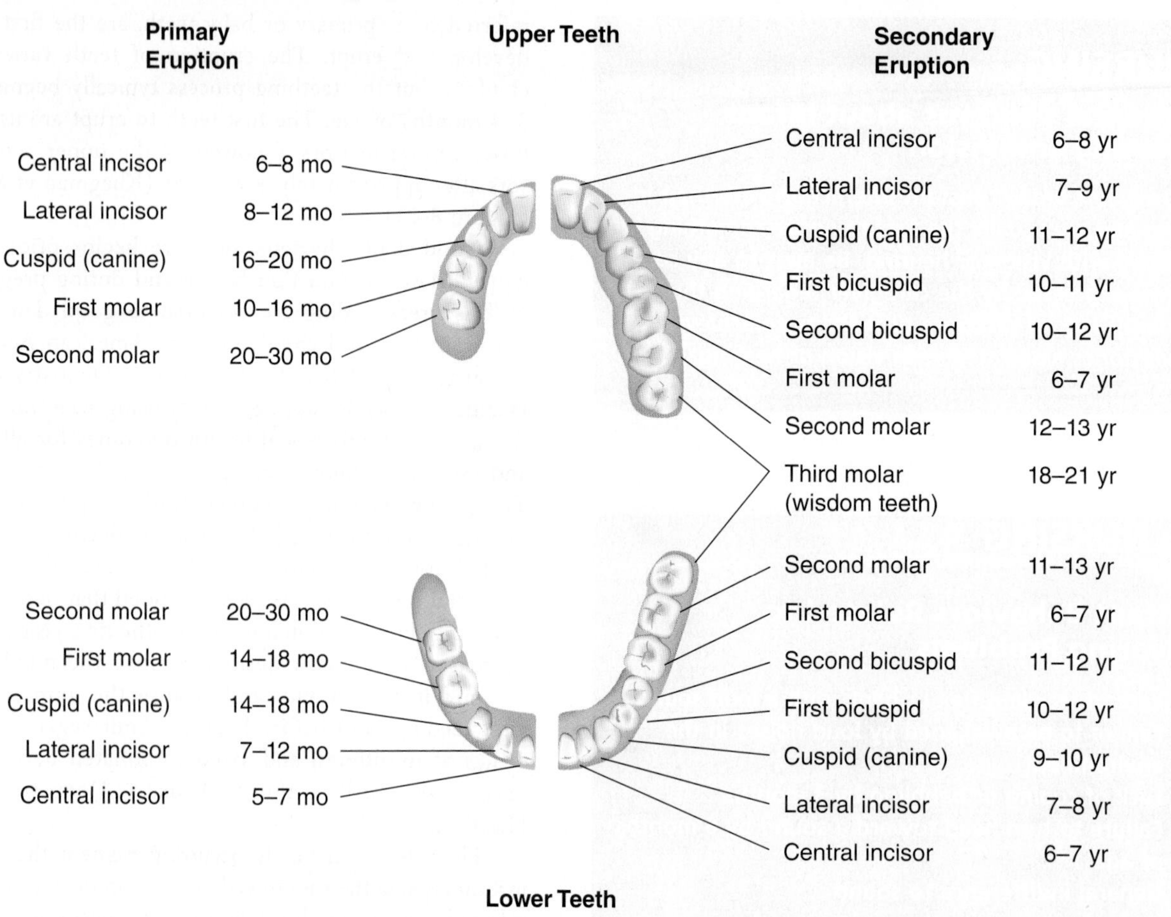

FIGURE 8-13 **Sequence of Tooth Eruption.** DELMAR CENGAGE LEARNING.

seen in infants who receive a bottle filled with formula or juice at nap or bedtime. The problem also occurs when a young child is allowed to breastfeed for long periods, especially when sleeping, or if the parent gives the infant a bottle of formula/milk at bedtime or naptime (Figure 8-14).

TABLE 8-4 Daily Fluoride Supplementation*

	FLUORIDE CONTENT OF WATER		
CHILD'S AGE	< 0.3 PPM	0.3–0.6 PPM	> 0.6 PPM
Birth–6 months	0	0	0
6 months–3 years	0.25	0	0
3–6 years	0.50	0.25	0
6–12 years	1.00	0.50	0

**Fluoride dose given in milligrams.*

Adapted from the recommendations of the American Academy of Pediatrics (2006) and the American Academy of Pediatric Dentistry (2006).

Dental hygiene also includes routine visits to the dentist. Most dentists suggest this first visit occur between the eruption of the first tooth and the first birthday (AAP, 2006). The initial dental visit should include discussion with parents regarding how to care for an infant's or toddler's mouth, appropriate use of fluoride for the child, oral

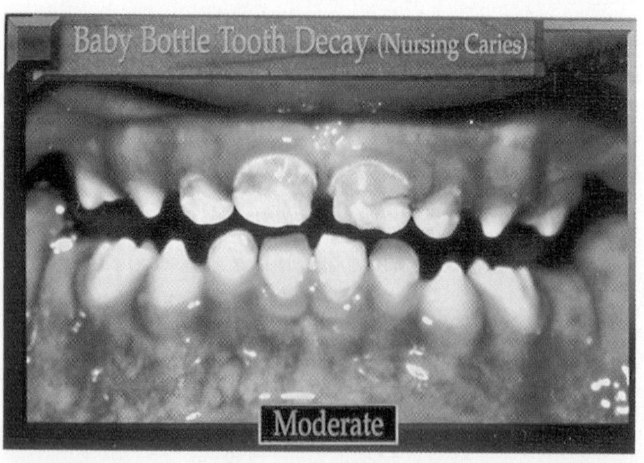

FIGURE 8-14 **Moderate Baby-Bottle Tooth Decay.** REPRINTED WITH THE PERMISSION OF THE AMERICAN ACADEMY OF PEDIATRIC DENTISTRY.

EVIDENCE-BASED PRACTICE

Oral Infant Health

CLINICAL PROBLEM

The most common chronic disease in young children is dental caries, which can develop soon after the teeth erupt. Dental caries, an infectious bacterial disease of teeth, is most often caused by *streptococci mutans*, which metabolize sugars (monosaccharides, disaccharides) to produce acids that demineralize teeth and cause cavities.

BEST CLINICAL PRACTICE

- "Baby-bottle tooth decay" or "nursing caries" is a multifactorial disease rather than being caused only by inappropriate and prolonged use of the bottle. Caries result when frequent sugar consumption occurs in the presence of *streptococci mutans*.
- Dental caries (which are five times more common than asthma) can be prevented.
- Many children do not receive dental care until 3 years of age.
- Addressing oral health during well-child visits within the first year of life can easily be integrated into parent teaching and is not time consuming.

IMPLICATIONS FOR NURSING

- Educate parents about the importance of good oral hygiene.
- Teach parents the importance of not propping an infant's bottle.
- Teach parents that when finger foods are introduced, foods containing sugar should be limited to meal times, and "grazing" should be avoided by establishing regular patterns of meal time and snack time.
- Encourage parents to limit a child's intake of sweetened liquids including fruit juices and snacks.
- Teach parents to introduce a Sippy cup at 6 months of age. Juice, limited to 4–6 ounces, should be consumed in cups and at meal time.
- Diluting fruit juices by using half water and half juice can help prevent dental caries.
- Encourage parents to give child systemic fluoride if the drinking water does not contain fluoride (0.6 ppm).
- Encourage parents to brush their child's teeth (after 6 months of age) with a small soft brush and toothpaste (size of rice grain) that does not contain fluoride, focusing on the junction between the teeth and gums.
- All children should visit a dentist by the time they are 12 months of age (or earlier if there are concerns) especially those at risk for developing dental caries (a mother with a number of cavities, enamel defects, high sugar intake, premature birth, low socioeconomic status, special health care needs, inadequate dental care, and poor oral hygiene).

Reference: Gussy, M. G., Waters, E. G., Walsh, O., & Kilpatrick, N. M. (2006). Early childhood caries: Current evidence for aetiology and prevention. *Journal of Paediatrics & Child Health, 42*(1/2), 37–43.

habits, including finger and thumb sucking, ways to prevent oral and facial accidents and trauma, teething and developmental milestones, and the relationship between diet and oral health.

TEETHING

During infancy, the period of eruption of deciduous teeth is called **teething** and occurs over several months. During eruption, the periodontal membrane becomes slightly swollen, red, and tender. The infant may have increased drooling and fussiness, mild anorexia, and an increased desire to bite. A low-grade fever has also been attributed to teething (Kliegman et al., 2007). The accompanying Family Teaching box contains several measures to soothe the infant during the teething process.

NUTRITION

Since the infant experiences rapid changes in growth and development over a relatively short time, a good nutritional foundation is necessary. The responsibility for meeting the

NURSING TIP

Estimation of Deciduous Teeth Related to Child's Age

Caregivers are usually concerned about the number of teeth their child should have at a certain age. While each child gets teeth at a different rate, the following formula is used by many clinicians as a guide to determine the expected number of teeth a child should have at a certain age: Subtract 6 from the child's age in months to equal the total number of teeth expected. For example by 12 months the infant should have 6 teeth.

FAMILY TEACHING

Soothing Swollen, Tender Gums

To soothe swollen, red gums, try:

- Frozen teething ring
- Ice cube in a washcloth
- Zwieback, toast, or teething biscuits
- Hard rubber toy
- Topical application of an oral anesthetic such as Orajel or Anbesol
- For irritability or a low-grade temperature, give acetaminophen according to recommended dosage

infant's nutritional needs falls on the caregiver; needs are normally evaluated during a routine assessment or when the caregiver expresses a concern over the infant's pattern of growth and development. During the assessment, the nurse should also take the opportunity to discuss the infant's developmental skills and feeding milestones.

For the first few months of the child's life, the infant will be either breastfed, formula-fed, or a combination of the two. Both breast and formula feedings are nutritionally sound, easy to digest, and provide the infant with the needed nutrients to grow. They also provide approximately 20 kcal/oz. (See Chapter 7 for a discussion of formulas). The infant's nutritional requirements are based on the physical activity and rate of growth needed to support life. At one month, energy requirements are 110–115 kcal/kg/day. They gradually decrease to 85–95 kcal/kg/day from 6–12 months of age (Gregory, 2005), because of the gradual decline in metabolic needs as the infant's growth slows. In addition to energy requirements, the infant must have adequate fluid intake, which is based on daily energy expenditure. Infant fluid requirements range from 80–150 mL/kg/day during the newborn period to 120–135 mL/kg/day by 1 year (Gregory, 2005) (Figure 8-15).

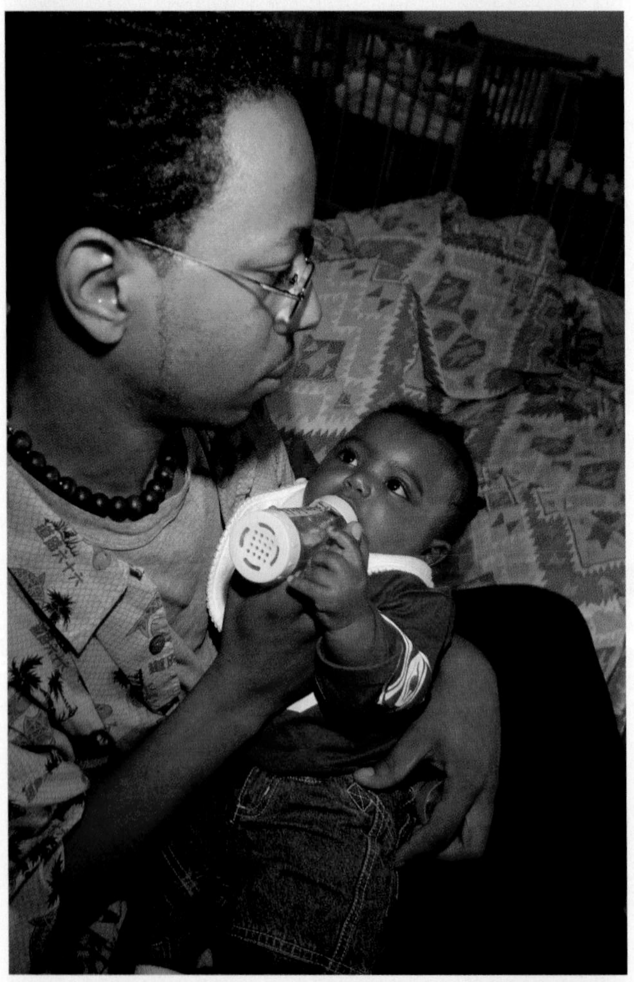

FIGURE 8-15 Infant being bottle fed; one method of providing appropriate nutritional requirements. DELMAR CENGAGE LEARNING.

SOLID FOODS

The American Academy of Pediatrics (2009b) recommends introducing semi-solid foods (e.g., single-grain infant cereal and applesauce) when the infant can sit well with support, tongue thrusting (extrusion reflex) has decreased, and the infant's hunger seems unsatisfied after nursing or bottle feeding; this usually occurs between 4 and 6 months of age. Introduction of solids before this time can contribute to food allergies; increased calorie intake, resulting in an overweight infant; and the danger of choking. The decision to introduce solid foods should be individualized after consulting with the child's health care provider (Figure 8-16). Developmental behaviors related to feeding can be found in Table 8-5.

The caregiver may express concern about the sequence of adding solid foods to the diet. Usually, the first food introduced is iron-fortified rice cereal, since it is the easiest to digest and the least likely to cause allergies. The cereal can be mixed with formula or expressed breast milk and, later, fruit or juice. Because of the infant's need for iron, the nurse should stress the benefit of feeding iron-fortified cereal during infancy. Fruits or vegetables are usually the next foods introduced; one food at a time. Encourage the caregiver to introduce vegetables before fruits since some infants become accustomed to the sweet taste of fruits. By 8–10 months of age, most fruits and vegetables should have been introduced and strained meats can be added to the infant's diet. Fruit juices, a good source of vitamin C, which enhances absorption of iron in the cereal, are usually offered the same time as fruits. Because of cultural variations, it is important for the nurse to ask what the infant is eating and support good nutritional habits that are culturally appropriate.

Due to the potential for an allergic reaction during the infant's first year, the Family Teaching box identifies foods that need to be avoided until the second half of the first year.

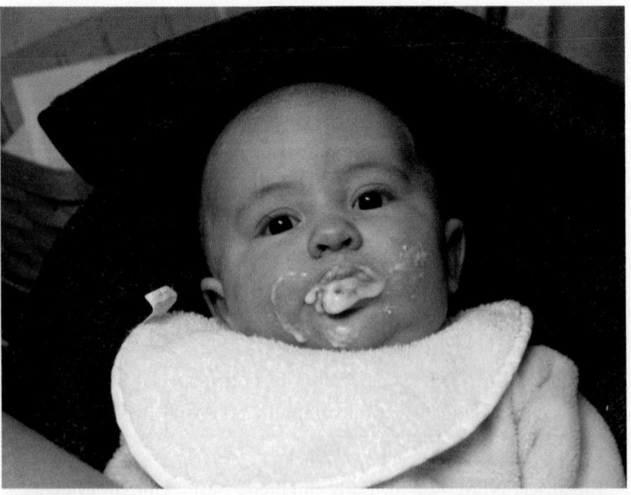

FIGURE 8-16 Feeding solid foods to infants can sometimes be messy. DELMAR CENGAGE LEARNING.

TABLE 8-5 Developmental Behaviors Related to Feeding

AGE	SKILL
Newborn–2 months	Primitive reflexes facilitate feeding Hunger cry initiates feeding interaction
2–4 months	More alert and interactive during feeding Beginning ability to wait for food Associates caregiver's smell, voice, and cradling with feeding Hand-to-mouth behavior quiets infant
4–6 months	Readiness for solids Excellent head and trunk control Reaching for objects Loss of extrusion reflex of tongue
6–8 months	Sits alone with steady head during feedings Chewing mechanism developed Holds bottle Vocal eagerness during meal preparation Much more motor activity during feeding
8–10 months	Readiness for finger foods Grasps spoon but cannot use it effectively Enjoys new textures, tastes Emerging independence
10–12 months	Increasing determination to feed self Neat pincer grasp Holds cup but frequently spills contents More verbal and motor behavior during feeding

When infants can sit steadily, they are usually allowed to drink from a cup with help. Finger foods are introduced during the second half of the first year as the finger grasp develops, teeth begin to erupt, and hand-eye coordination improves. Table 8-6 is a guide for introducing solid foods.

When discussing the infant's developmental readiness for solid foods, the nurse should stress to the caregiver the importance of self-feeding. To encourage autonomy, the infant needs to be given the opportunity to explore the texture, smell, color, and taste of food. The caregiver should expect that self-feeding will be messy. Anticipatory guidance can help this experience become a valuable lesson for the infant.

NURSING TIP

Calculation of Infant's Caloric and Fluid Needs

Infant's weight = 4.5 kg; formula = 20 kcal/oz (30 mL). (However, this may vary depending on the infant's age, gender, and individual needs/circumstances.)

1. Caloric need: 115 kcal/kg/day
   115 kcal × 4.5 kg = 495 kcal/day
   Amount of formula needed per day:
   495 kcal ÷ 20 kcal/oz = 25 oz of formula
2. Fluid need: 1 to 1.5 mL/kcal/day
   495 kcal × 1 mL = 495 mL/day
   495 kcal × 1.5 mL = 745 mL/day
   Amount of formula needed per day (in ounces):
   495 mL ÷ 30 mL/oz = 17 oz of formula
   745 mL ÷ 30 mL/oz = 25 oz of formula

NURSING TIP

Salt and Sugar Content of Commercially Prepared Strained Foods

The caregiver should be cautioned about the salt and sugar content of commercially preprared strained foods. Extra sugar intake can contribute to excessive calorie intake. Salt contributes to an increase in extracellular fluid and a slight rise in blood pressure. Consequently, excessive use of sweet and salty foods should be avoided in the infant's diet (Haydu & Sundquist, 2006).

TABLE 8-6 Guide for Introduction of Solid Foods

AGE	FOOD	FREQUENCY
4–6 months	Cereal	Twice a day
6–8 months	Vegetables	Twice a day
	Fruits	Once a day
	Juices	Once a day (small amounts)
8–10 months	Meats	Once a day
9–12 months	Finger foods	At least daily
10–12 months	Egg yolks	Once a day
10–12 months	Plain water	As needed

FAMILY**TEACHING**

Feeding Infant Solid Foods

Stress the importance of the infant's need to practice the new skill of eating solids (chewing and swallowing) instead of sucking.

- Introducing one new food at a time at 4-day intervals allows for identifying food intolerances and gives the infant the chance to become accustomed to the new food.
- Feed solids with a spoon. Put a small amount of food on an infant-sized spoon and place toward the middle to back of the infant's mouth. This enables the infant to overcome the diminishing extrusion reflex and facilitates the newly acquired skills of chewing and swallowing.
- Give solid foods when the infant is hungry, and then follow with formula or breast milk. This encourages the infant to eat the solids instead of becoming satiated with fluids.
- Gradually increase solid foods to approximately 4 oz per feeding. As solid food intake advances, the infant's daily intake of breast milk or formula will decrease to approximately 24 oz at 12 months of age.

FAMILY**TEACHING**

Food Allergy

Food allergy is defined as an adverse immune response to food proteins and affects as many as 6% of young children. Cow's milk allergy is the most common food allergy in the first year of life, affecting 2.2% to 2.8% of infants (Sicherer & Sampson, 2009). Therefore, exclusive breastfeeding remains the preferred method for providing infant nutrition, particularly during the first 4 to 6 months of life. Maternal avoidance of some proteins during lactation is an appropriate first-line measure against manifestations of food allergy in exclusively breastfed infants (AAP, 2005). The role of specialized formulas, even in infants at risk for developing atopic disease, remains uncertain (Bauchner, 2008).

FAMILY**TEACHING**

Helpful Hints for Infant Self-Feeding

- Place high chair in an area that can be easily cleaned.
- Place infant in a high chair and fasten safety belt.
- Use a large plastic bib.
- Dress in easily removable and washable clothes.

Weaning

Weaning is a process of giving up one method of feeding for another, such as the transition from breast to cup or bottle, and from bottle to cup. There is no right way or time to wean an infant. Weaning can be accomplished with the infant's needs as a guide (Lawrence & Lawrence, 2005). Behaviors consistent with weaning include eating from a spoon, holding the bottle, feeding self with fingers or a spoon, eating foods that require chewing, and the decreasing desire to be held during feeding. The American Academy of Pediatrics (AAP) (2005) recommends feeding babies only breast milk for the first 6 months of life. After that, the AAP recommends that a combination of solid foods and breast milk be given until a baby is at least 1 year old. Some experts say that after the first birthday is the best time to begin weaning because kids are more adaptable to change at that age. (A 2-year-old toddler, for example, is likely to be much more attached to breastfeeding and less flexible about giving it up). A 1-year-old baby is also eating more solid foods and so may naturally lose interest in nursing.

If the infant is weaned too soon from breast milk or formula, iron deficiency anemia may occur (Gregory, 2005). Weaning from the breast to a bottle is often associated with the mother's confidence in her breastfeeding ability, and her perception of the impact of breastfeeding on the comfort and well-being of both herself and her infant (O'Brien, Fallon, Brodribb, & Hegney, 2007). Weaning should be a process in which breastfeeding sessions are gradually replaced by a bottle, or the bottle-feeding sessions are gradually replaced by increased amounts of solid foods and drinking from a cup.

Pacifiers

Oral stimulation or sucking is one of the most important sources of pleasure and satisfaction for the infant, and one of the first coordinated muscular activities. There are two forms of sucking, nutritive and nonnutritive. Nutritive sucking enables the infant to obtain nutrients necessary for life through either bottle- or breastfeeding. Nonnutritive sucking, such as that with a pacifier, is used as a source of pleasure and satisfaction. It also calms the infant, especially when undergoing painful procedures (Miller, 2007; South, Strauss, South, Boggess, & Thorp, 2005). However, pacifiers should rarely be used after 9–12 months of age.

Since sucking provides the infant with pleasure and satisfaction, caregivers need to understand the difference

FAMILY TEACHING

Finger Foods

Many finger foods should not be provided until the infant is around 6 months or has good eye-hand coordination. However when introducing finger foods, the rule of thumb is that pieces of food should be the size of the infant's thumb. In addition, food items that are hard, round, smooth, and small should be avoided since they can slip easily into the infant's throat and may cause choking.

Foods to avoid:

- Nuts, popcorn, whole kernel corn, chunks of meat (e.g., hot dogs), chips, pretzels, berries, grapes, cherries, raw fruit and vegetables (e.g., apples, carrots, celery)
- Sticky, stringy, and chewy foods (e.g., peanut butter, caramel, honey)
- Small, hard, or round candy (e.g., jelly beans, peppermints, butterscotch, m & ms)

between nutritive and nonnutritive sucking. If the infant is fussy and crying, the caregiver may offer a pacifier as a soothing method without understanding the infant's true need. If the infant is hungry, however, offering a pacifier will not calm the infant for long.

In an attempt to understand infant needs, caregivers are encouraged to note the time and circumstances around their infant's distress. Distress may be due to a need for sleep or food, to be held, or simply to suck if the infant simply wants to suck. The caregiver may select a pacifier to meet this need, or infants may start sucking on their fingers. As time goes on the infant will decide which method of nonnutritive sucking is the favorite.

NURSING ALERT

Being Safe with Pacifiers

- Look for one-piece construction.
- The mouth guard should be wider than the infant's mouth.
- Ventilation holes should be present on the mouth guard.
- Keep the pacifier clean.
- Never put a pacifier on a string.
- Do not leave a pacifier in a sleeping infant's mouth.
- Mothers should not use their mouths to clean the pacifer.

If a pacifier is selected, it is important that the caregiver receive appropriate information about pacifier use and safety considerations (see Nursing Alert Box). It should be stressed that the pacifier should not be used as a substitute for general caregiving, nor as an attempt to meet needs other than for nonnutritive sucking. When the caregiver selects a pacifier, the shape should correspond with the shape of the nipple used for infant feeding. Many lactation consultants stress caution in introducing a pacifier if the infant is being breastfed. In fact, nipple confusion and even refusal to breastfeed can occur if a pacifier is introduced before the nursing relationship has been established (Huang & Huang, 2006; Marter & Agruss, 2007; Nelson, Yu, Williams, & International Child Care Practices Study Group Members, 2005).

COMMUNICATION

Communication enables the infant to express needs and emotions, and involves central nervous system maturation, cognitive abilities, and social interaction. The infant's initial means of communication—crying and smiling—elicit different responses from the caregiver. When the infant cries, the caregiver responds with soothing behaviors such as speaking softly, holding, and establishing eye contact. Caregiver's reactions to an infant's smile include talking, cooing, smiling, and playing. Even though the infant begins smiling as a reflex, by 2 months the infant has a "social" smile used to gain attention and amazement from the caregiver.

The infant's ability to communicate through language follows a predictable course. As maturation progresses so do language abilities. During infancy, **receptive language** (the ability to understand words) is greater than **expressive language** (the ability to speak words). By the end of the first year, the infant can say several words such as "dada" and "mama" as well as understand simple commands such as "bye-bye," "point to your belly," and "no-no." A summary of language development during infancy can be found in Table 8-7.

The nurse's awareness of the expected pattern of language development is important during the infant's routine health screening visits. The American Academy of Pediatrics (2008b) recommends administration of standardized developmental screening instruments during well-child visits to facilitate timely identification of developmental delay. Assessing the infant's language development by using the Denver II screening tool enables the health care provider to detect any potential problems (Frankenburg, Dodds, Archer, Shapiro, & Bresnick, 1992). Language patterns can provide anticipatory guidance to the caregiver to enhance language development as well. Therefore, the caregiver should be encouraged to talk to the infant, make eye contact, and smile during feeding and diaper changes, as well as read to the baby. Once the infant starts to vocalize, the caregiver should repeat these sounds in response to the infant's vocalizations. The names of objects or people should be emphasized when talking to the infant and the caregiver should always be observant of the infant's response to adult vocalization.

TABLE 8-7 Summary of Language Development in Infancy

AGE	EXPRESSIVE SKILLS	RECEPTIVE SKILLS
Birth–2 months	Crying Comfort sound with feeding Coos Vocalizes to familiar voice	Sounds elicit startle reflex Turns and looks for sounds Prefers human voice
3–6 months	Vocalizes during play and pleasure Squeals Laughs aloud Cries less Uses vowels and consonant sounds that resemble syllables (ma, mu, ba, ga, ah, da)	Watches speaking mouth Shifts gaze between sounds Understands own name Uses sound to get attention
7–9 months	Increases vowel and consonant sounds Uses two-syllable sounds (baba, dada) Talks along with others	Associates words with activity Responds to simple commands ("no-no") Understands familiar words
10–12 months	Says "mama" and "dada" to identify caregivers Repeats sounds made by others Makes intentional gestures Learns three to five words	Recognizes family members' names Recognizes objects by name Understands simple commands (say "bye-bye")

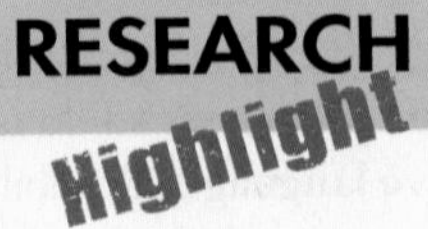

Pacifiers and Breastfeeding: A Systematic Review

STUDY PURPOSE

To summarize current evidence on the association between infant pacifier use and breastfeeding.

METHODS

A literature search for English-language records (from January 1950 through August 2006) containing the Medical Subject Heading terms *pacifiers* and *breastfeeding* was conducted, from MEDLINE, CINAHL, the Cochrane Library, EMBASE, POPLINE, and bibliographies of identified articles resulting in 1098 reports. Duplicate and irrelevant studies were excluded, yielding 29 studies that fit inclusion criteria for the review (4 randomized controlled trials, 20 cohort studies, and 5 cross-sectional studies). Outcome measures were breastfeeding duration or exclusivity.

FINDINGS

Results from 4 randomized controlled trials revealed no difference in breastfeeding outcomes with different pacifier interventions such as when the infant is fed though a nasogastric tube or when a pacifier is used at any time after delivery. Most observational studies reported an association between pacifier use and shortened duration of breastfeeding.

IMPLICATIONS

The findings do not support an adverse relationship between pacifier use and breastfeeding duration or exclusivity. The association between shortened duration of breastfeeding and pacifier use in observational studies likely reflects a number of other complex factors, such as breastfeeding difficulties or intent to wean. Additional quantitative and qualitative research is needed to better understand the relationship between pacifier use and breastfeeding.

REFERENCE

O'Connor, N. R., Tanabe, K. O., Siadaty, M. S., & Hauck, F. R. (2009). Pacifiers and breastfeeding: A systematic review. *Archives of Pediatric and Adolescent Medicine, 163*(4), 378–382.

TEMPERAMENT

Temperament is the way a child interacts with the surrounding environment. Children are thought to be genetically endowed with specific temperamental characteristics. When these characteristics are combined with the caregiver's personality, a characteristic pattern of social interaction between the child and the environment occurs (Figure 8-17).

Temperamental characteristics are behavioral tendencies, not implications of a good or bad child, and can be categorized into nine attributes (Thomas, Chess, & Birch, 1968; 1970):

1. *Activity*—intensity and frequency of physical activity
2. *Rhythmicity*—regularity of repetitive physiological functions (e.g., sleep cycle, eating patterns, elimination patterns)
3. *Approach-withdrawal*—initial reaction to a given stimulus (e.g., people, situations)
4. *Adaptability*—ease or difficulty with which the child reacts or adapts to a given stimulus
5. *Intensity of response*—degree of energy used by the child to react to the stimulus
6. *Threshold of responsiveness*—amount of stimulation needed to evoke a child's response
7. *Mood*—amount of happiness versus unhappiness or pleasant and friendly behavior versus unpleasant and unfriendly behavior exhibited in various situations
8. *Distractibility*—effectiveness of the stimulus to alter the direction of the ongoing behavior
9. *Attention span and persistence*—length of time the child pursues an activity and the continuation of an activity despite the obstacles

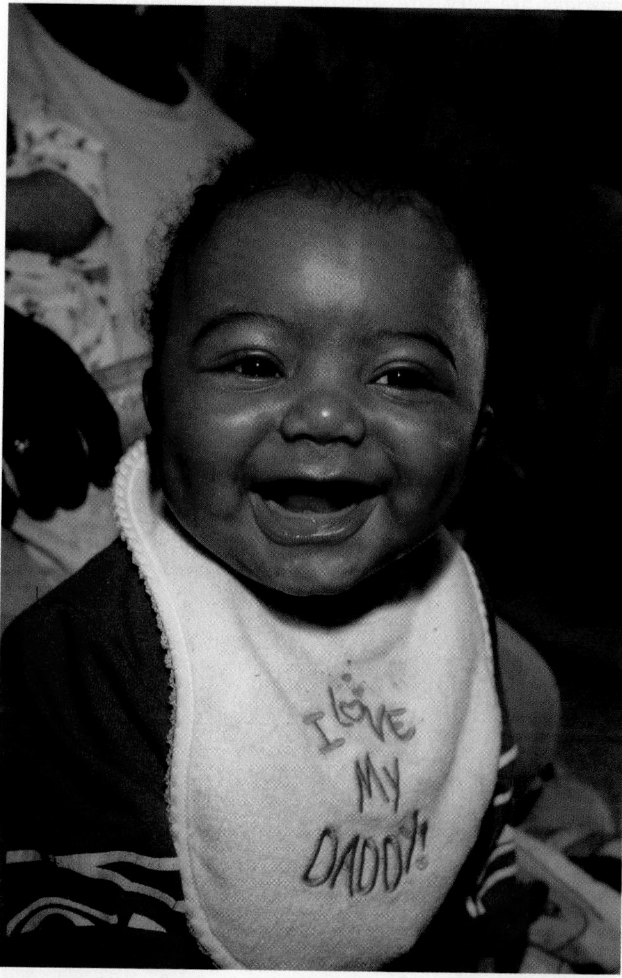

FIGURE 8-17 A child's temperament is considered to be a combination of genetics and caregivers' personalities. DELMAR CENGAGE LEARNING.

The attributes provide a framework for three distinct personality types, as described in Table 8-8. Not all children can be placed into these categories easily; children often exhibit a variety of personality types.

The knowledge of temperament can be very useful in understanding the caregiver-infant relationship (Hane, Fox, Polak-Toste, Ghera, & Guner, 2006). The nurse can be instrumental in helping the caregiver understand the uniqueness of the child's personality and provide a guide in child-rearing

TABLE 8-8 Summary of Personality Types

PERSONALITY TYPE	CHARACTERISTICS
Easy	Easygoing and adapts rapidly to stimuli
	Has an overall positive mood
	Likes to be around people
	Sleeps and eats well
	Has regular and predictable behaviors
Difficult	Adapts slowly to stimuli
	Has an overall negative mood
	Requires a structured environment
	Likes people but can do well alone
	Seems to be in constant motion
	Has irregular patterns of behavior
Slow-to-warm-up	Adapts slowly to stimuli but is watchful
	Quietly withdraws and usually moody
	Primarily a loner and socially shy
	Oversensitive and slow to mature
	Primarily inactive
	Reacts passively to changes in routine

Adapted from Thomas, A., Chess, S., and Birch, H. (1970). The origin of personality. *Scientific American, 223*(2), 106–117.

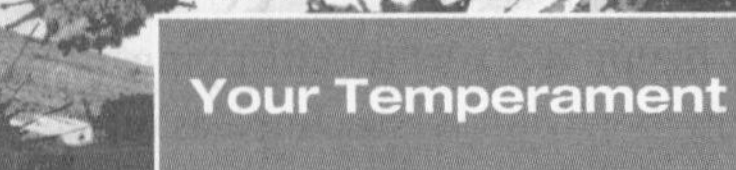

REFLECTIVE THINKING

Your Temperament

Recall when you were a child. How would you classify your temperament? Is it similar to how you would classify yourself today? Do others see you the same way?

NURSING TIP

Goodness of Fit

The nurse can assist the caregiver by:

- Being aware of the cultural norms of the caregiver
- Taking time to ask about the infant's general behavior characteristics
- Asking how the caregiver interprets the infant's behavior
- Asking questions about areas that may be problematic
- Encouraging the expression of feelings about infant-caregiver interactions

techniques. For example, a consistent routine is important for the child who is easily overwhelmed by changes. If the child has problems falling asleep, it may be helpful to provide a calm and quiet environment during the bedtime ritual. For the child who is easily distracted while eating, the caregiver should minimize all distractions by providing a quiet setting during the meal.

By increasing caregiver's understanding of the child's personality, a more effective plan of care can be developed to meet infant needs. Thus, when needs are met, a trusting relationship develops, and the caregiver's frustrations associated with child rearing may be diminished.

COLIC (INFANT IRRITABILITY)

Colic, now often termed infant irritability, is one of the most common health problems seen in infants younger than 3 months of age, and describes recurrent episodes of unexplained crying and the inability to be consoled. The onset varies, but it usually occurs around 1–2 weeks of age and subsides spontaneously by approximately 16 weeks of age.

The colicky episode is characterized by loud, persistent crying and flexing of the hips toward the abdomen. These physical characteristics are thought to be a result of paroxysmal abdominal cramping. The "rule of 3" used to define colic (Cohen-Silver & Ratnapalan, 2009) states that colic is present if crying occurs during the first 3 months of life, lasts longer than 3 hours per day, occurs more than 3 days in any 1 week, and continues for at least 3 weeks.

Even though colic usually resolves spontaneously, the episodes are very stressful. The family is usually fatigued, frustrated, and expresses feelings of helplessness; caregivers often blame themselves for not being able to console the infant.

Colic management begins by recognizing a problem exists. First and foremost, it is important for the health care provider to eliminate an infectious or organic cause for the infant's discomfort. Once a medical condition has been ruled out, colic should be approached in terms of managing the infant's episodes as well as the emotional turmoil experienced by the family. In managing the infant's episodes, the nurse should assess the infant's daily routine and discuss the infant's normal patterns. Refer to Figure 8-18 for some

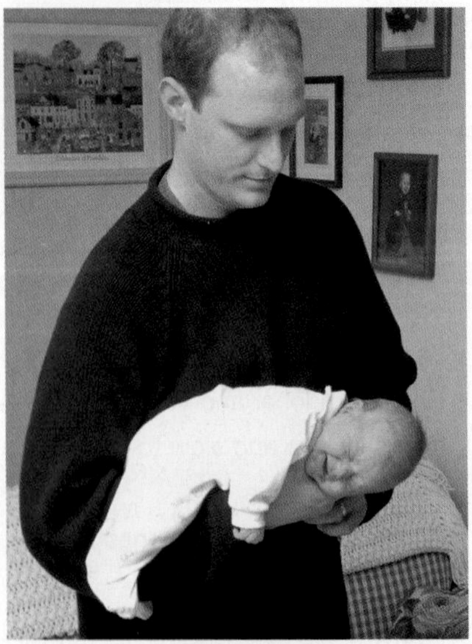

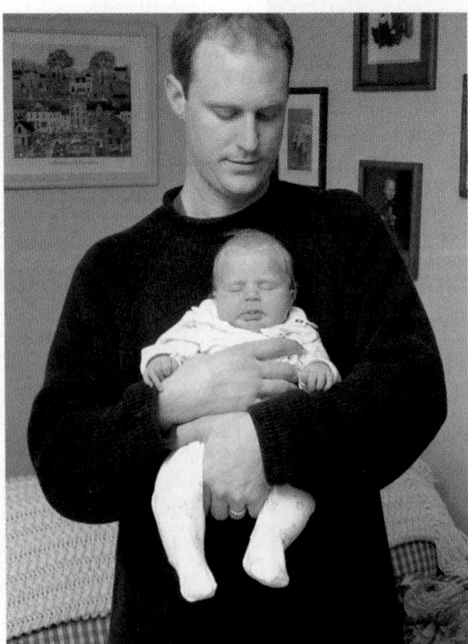

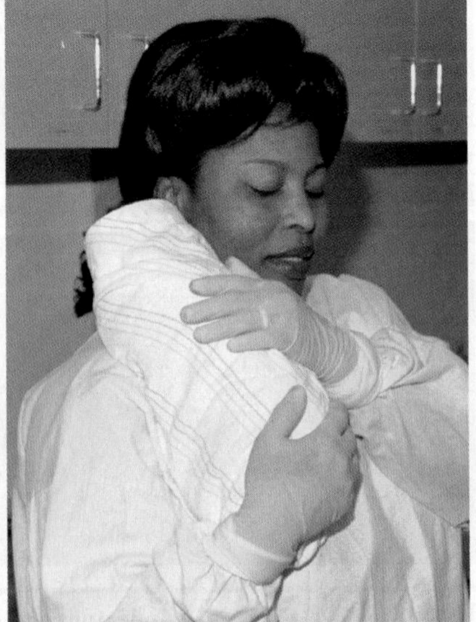

FIGURE 8-18 **Different types of infant carries that may alleviate colic (infant irritability).** DELMAR CENGAGE LEARNING.

carrying techniques that may soothe a colicky infant. Some suggestions for easing the discomfort of colic include:

1. Feed the infant slowly, burp frequently, and keep in upright position during feeding to decrease the amount of air swallowed. Do not over-feed the infant, which can be determined by calculating the infant's required caloric needs by body weight.
2. When breastfeeding, avoid eating foods that may contribute to gas formation. Typically these include foods such as onions, cabbage, collards, and dry beans, which cause gas in the caregiver. This is a trial-and-error approach and may take a week before results are seen.
3. Swaddle the infant to decrease self-stimulation by jerky or sudden movements. A front carrier for body contact, swaddling, or gentle movement may be useful.
4. Take the infant for a car ride. Almost all colicky children respond favorably to vibration and movement.
5. Use a swing for at least 20 minutes. This provides movement and allows the family time for a rest period between interactions with the infant.
6. Walk or rock the infant while applying gentle pressure to the infant's abdomen.
7. Gently massage the infant's back while the infant is lying down.
8. Supply background or "white" noise (hair dryer, vacuum cleaner, fan) or play a mothers' heart beat or some soft music.
9. Place the infant in a quiet, darkened room to reduce environmental stimuli.
10. Let the infant cry it out in the crib when other measures do not work. Sometimes only fatigue will make the infant fall asleep.
11. Place warm towel or washcloth on infant's abdomen.
12. Do not shake the infant if frustrated with the crying and irritability.

NURSING TIP

Care of the Infant with Colic/Irritability

To help the caregiver manage colic:

- Stress that no one is to blame!
- Explain the possible reasons for colic.
- Give suggestions for relieving colicky episodes.
- Explain that colic usually disappears by 16 weeks of age.
- Be supportive, and encourage expression of concerns.
- Encourage talking with others who have experienced a colicky infant.
- Encourage brief periods away from the crying infant.

REFLECTIVE THINKING

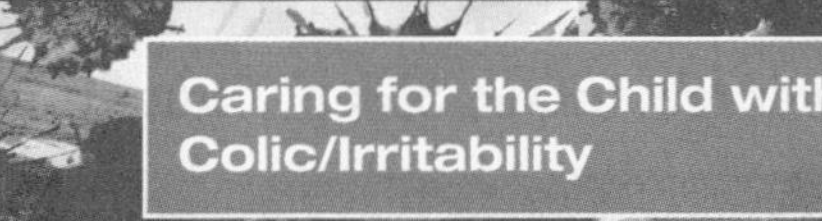

To improve your understanding of colic and the caregiver's situation, ask yourself:

1. **How would you personally feel if your infant cried constantly while you provided the care? Would you feel that people thought you were not a good caregiver?**
2. **What coping techniques would you use?**
3. **Who would you call when reaching the point of exasperation?**

The nurse should encourage the caregiver to avoid the tendency to take the episode personally, to keep a positive attitude, and to remain calm. The caregiver may be encouraged to try breathing techniques to relax, taking some time away from the care of the infant, doing something special when away from the ongoing care of the infant, or asking a relative to help in the infant's care.

SLEEP

Infants have variable sleep patterns that are influenced by temperament, satisfaction with feedings, caregivers' responses to periodic awakenings, and environmental conditions (Porter, 2007). There is a transition from neonatal sleeping, which is shorter with multiple sleep periods, to the more organized central nervous system maturation after the third month (Table 8-9). As the child matures, the sleep-wake cycle evolves into a pattern of being awake during the day and asleep at night (Dixon & Stein, 2006; Porter, 2007).

During the first months of life, infants sleep approximately 16 hours a day and experience more rapid eye movement (REM) sleep than at any other time in life (Porter, 2007). Sleep provides the time needed to rebuild reserves necessary for rapid physical growth and development. In addition, the central nervous system and neurons undergo a great deal of development during REM sleep (Porter, 2007).

As the infant matures, the amount of REM sleep diminishes, the required hours for sleep gradually decrease, and sleep-wake periods develop into a day and night cycle. This occurs over time and by the time the infant is 3 to 4 months of age, sleep patterns are well established. This developmental milestone of "sleeping through the night" or "settling-in" is a time the caregiver has been anxiously awaiting. Napping also occurs during this time. The number of naps per day varies with each infant, but generally the infant will take one or two naps by the age of 1 year (Sadeh, Mindell, Luedtke, & Wiegand, 2009).

Table 8-9 Average Infant Sleep Time

AGE IN MONTHS	AWAKE	DAY SLEEP	NIGHT SLEEP
0–2	7.5 hours	8 hours	8.5 hours
3–5	10.75 hours	4 hours	9.25 hours
6–8	10.85 hours	3.75 hours	9 hours
9–11	11.25 hours	3.25 hours	9.5 hours

Adapted from Sadeh, A. Mindell, J. Luedtke, K., & Wiegand, B. (2009). Sleep and sleep ecology in the first 3 years: A web-based study. *Journal of Sleep Research*, *18*(1), 60–73.

After regular sleep patterns develop, the infant may begin to experience periods of awakening during the night, referred to as night wakings. These night wakings seem to coincide with the development of separation anxiety. Even though this is a transient phase, night waking can result in a strained caregiver-infant relationship. During this time, it is not uncommon for the infant to have difficulty falling asleep at night and nap times as well as falling back to sleep if awakened. Methods such as rocking and providing a pacifier and a dim light (night light) may assist the infant in returning to sleep. Usually, the infant can settle back to sleep if left alone during the awakenings that occur every 2–4 hours during the sleep times.

The infant's sleep state can also be influenced by sleeping arrangements. Sleeping arrangements for an infant vary widely from family to family. For the first few months of the child's life or when the infant is ill, the sleeping arrangement known as co-sleeping is a relatively common practice used by many cultures (Blair, 2008).

Part of the nurse's developmental assessment of the infant is the evaluation of sleep patterns. The nurse should also keep in mind that the infant's sleep pattern is a common concern for the caregiver (Figures 8-19). When concern is expressed, the nurse should elicit information related to the history of the problem, daily sleep routine, sleeping position, sleeping arrangements, changes in feeding, environmental problems, and occurrence of stressors in the family unit.

The best way to prevent sleep problems is to assist the caregiver in understanding the infant's individual needs. The caregiver should be given information relevant to healthy sleep patterns and signs of maturation in the infant. When providing this information, the nurse should take the caregiver's cultural practices and personal preferences into consideration. In addition, the nurse should suggest measures that will foster healthy sleep patterns including:

- Establish a bedtime routine for the infant such as giving a bath, reading a book, telling a story, singing, holding, or rocking.
- Provide a quiet, relaxed environment in a cozy, safe crib.
- Use warm sleep garments.

FAMILY TEACHING

Family Bed Concerns

Once you share the bed you will always share the family bed.
No, but you should be prepared for it to take several months or more to ease the infant out of your bed if you prefer the infant not sleep your bed.

Sharing the family bed will encourage your infant to be overly dependent on you.
No, there is no evidence to support this idea.

Sleeping with your infant increases the risk of suffocation.
Yes, if the family bed is chosen, then risk of suffocation may be minimized by:

- Not placing pillows, blankets, or comforters under infant
- Not sleeping on a waterbed, sheepskin, or featherbed
- Not overdressing or overbundling infant for sleep
- Not indulging in drugs, alcohol, or prescription medication that results in unusual grogginess or sleepiness

Sharing the family bed will increase the risk for sudden infant death syndrome
Yes, bed sharing is associated with an increased risk of SIDS for infants younger than 11 weeks of age (risk to be greatest among infants younger than 3 to 4 months). Sharing a couch for sleep should be strongly discouraged at any age. Researchers have identified elevated risk for SIDS among bed-sharing infants in case-control studies. The risk appeared to be greatest among infants younger than 3-4 months.

Ruys, J. H., De Jonge, G. A., Brand, R., Engelberts, A. C., & Semmekrot, B. A. (2007). Bed-sharing in the first four months of life: A risk factor for sudden infant death. *Acta Paediatrica*, 96(10), 1399–1403; Tappin, D., Ecob, R., & Brooke, H. (2005). Bedsharing, roomsharing, and sudden infant death syndrome in Scotland: A case-control study. *Journal of Pediatrics*, 147(1), 32–37.

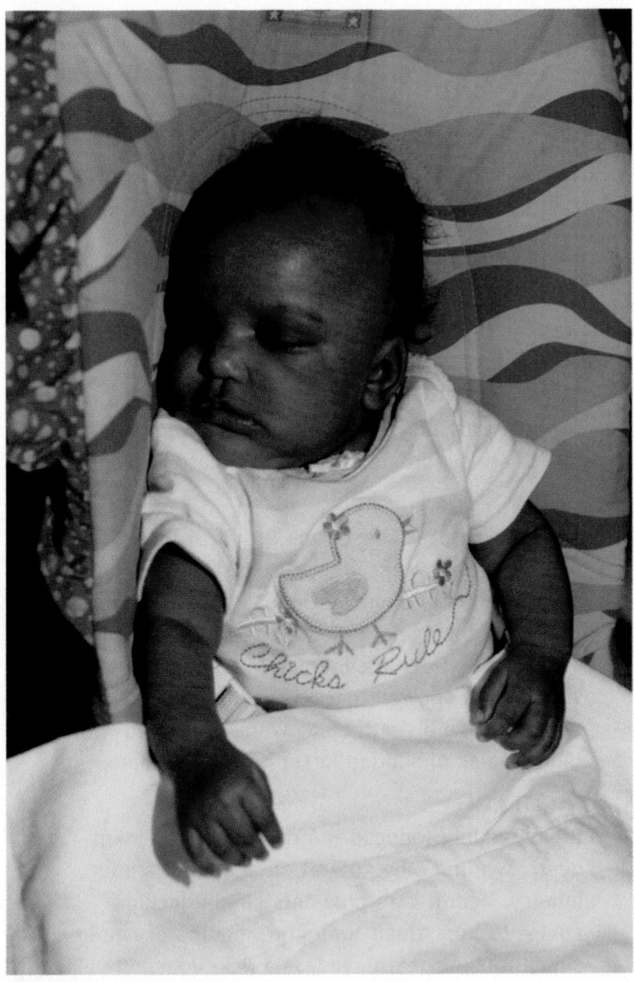

FIGURE 8-19 **Infants typically take one to two naps during the day, and will establish their own sleep pattern.** DELMAR CENGAGE LEARNING.

- Do not use the crib as a playpen.
- Place infant in the crib when drowsy but not asleep.
- Place infant supine for sleep.
- Do not feed infant during the night if infant generally sleeps through the night; if feeding is necessary, make it brief.
- Do not awaken infant to feed or change a diaper.

The sleeping position of the infant is also important. Even though some infants may seem to sleep better or more soundly on their stomachs (prone), sudden infant death syndrome has been associated with this sleeping position, and the American Academy of Pediatrics recommends infants be placed on their back (supine) while sleeping (Dewar, 2008).

SUDDEN INFANT DEATH SYNDROME

Sudden infant death syndrome (SIDS) is the sudden, unexplained death of an infant between 1 month and 1 year of age after all known causes have been ruled out through autopsy, death scene investigation, and review of medical history (Hunt & Hauck, 2007). Most SIDS deaths happen when babies are between two and four months of age (NICHD, 2006). After the initiation of the Back to Sleep campaign in 1994, the incidence of SIDS progressively declined and leveled off by 2002. The decline in the number of SIDS deaths in the United States and other countries around the world has been attributed to the increasing use of the supine position for sleep. Several other countries have decreased prone sleeping prevalence to less than 2%, but in the United States, 13% were still placed in prone position in 2004 (Hunt & Hauck, 2007). Other risk factors associated with SIDS can be found in the Nursing Tip box. Generally, it is not known what causes SIDS, but the AAP (2000) proposes the following mechanisms:

- A delayed development of arousal or cardiorespiratory control
- Maldevelopment or malnutrition in the brain region involved with hypercapnic ventilatory response, chemosensitivity, and blood pressure
- Rebreathing, with associated hypoxia and hypercarbia providing noxious stimuli
- Arousal responses to laryngeal chemoreflex diminished, leading to apnea and bradycardia

The incidence of SIDS in the United States is highest in American Indians and African Americans, with a rate of two to three times that of the national average. Due to these factors and incidence, it is important caregivers are given information about SIDS and strategies to reduce the risk of SIDS. Strategies to reduce the risk can be found in the Family Teaching box.

BATHING

Infants do not need much bathing during the first year of life. During the bath, caregivers should never leave the infant unattended to answer the telephone or doorbell. Even though sponge baths are used until the umbilical cord stump falls off, it is always important to keep the diaper area clean to avoid diaper rash. Before bathing, caregivers should gather all supplies, including a basin of lukewarm water, a washcloth, towels, baby shampoo, mild soap, and cotton balls. While giving a sponge bath, the caregiver should expose only those areas on the infant being washed to avoid chilling the infant. A cotton ball can be used to clean the eyes first, moving from the inner to outer areas, before using a washcloth for the remainder of the face. The perineal area is always washed last. It is important to clean all body creases thoroughly, especially the neck folds and perineal area, and wash and dry each body part before moving on to the next area. To prevent **cradle cap** (seborrhea), a dry, scaly scalp condition, hair should be washed every other day using a mild baby shampoo. If cradle cap does develop, a soft-bristle toothbrush can be used to remove the crusts and

NURSING TIP

Risk Factors Associated with SIDS

INFANT

- Prematurity
- Low birth weight
- Male gender
- Multiple birth
- Age under 6 months

ENVIRONMENTAL

- Exposure to cigarette smoke
- Co sleeping or bed-sharing under 4 months (Ruys et al., 2007)
- Maternal smoking (Anderson, Johnson, & Batal, 2005)
- Prone sleeping position
- Bottle-feeding in the crib
- Overbundling for sleep
- Overheating
- Soft sleep surfaces
- Loose bedding or excessive bedding or items in crib
- Inadequate room ventilation (Coleman-Phox, Odouli, & Li, 2008)

mineral oil or petroleum jelly can be used to soften the patches. After the cord stump falls off, the infant can be bathed in a sink or plastic tub in about 2 inches of warm water. A towel can be placed on the bottom to prevent the infant from slipping. While bathing infants, caregivers should always hold or use a tub ring to stabilize the infant even though the child may be able to sit upright without much support. Since bathing can be an important time for bonding and play, it should be unhurried and not stressful.

FAMILY TEACHING

Use of a Fan during Sleep

Although placing infants on their backs has decreased the SIDS rate, another potential modifiable risk factor is room ventilation. For example, inadequate ventilation in the infant's room may result in carbon dioxide pooling around the infant's nose and mouth and consequently increasing re-breathing of that gas. However, use of a fan or open window to improve ventilation in the room where the infant is sleeping has been shown to decrease SIDS risks in infants.

Coleman-Phox, K., Odouli, R., & Li, D. O. (2008). Uses of a fan during sleep and the risk of sudden infant death syndrome. *Archives of Pediatric and Adolescent Medicine, 162*(10), 963–968.

RESEARCH

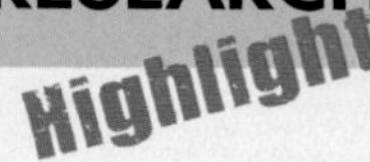

Does Breastfeeding Reduce the Risk of Sudden Infant Death Syndrome?

STUDY PURPOSE

To examine the association between type of infant feeding and sudden infant death syndrome.

METHODS

The German Study of Sudden Infant Death is a case-control study of 333 infants who died of sudden infant death syndrome and 998 age-matched controls.

FINDINGS

A total of 49.6% of cases and 82.9% of controls were breastfed at 2 weeks of age. Exclusive breastfeeding at 1 month of age halved the risk, partial breastfeeding at the age of 1 month also reduced the risk of sudden infant death syndrome. Breastfeeding survival curves showed that both partial breastfeeding and exclusive breastfeeding were associated with a reduced risk of sudden infant death syndrome.

IMPLICATIONS

Breastfeeding reduced the risk of sudden infant death syndrome by 50% at all ages throughout infancy. Health care providers should include advice to breastfeed through 6 months of age in sudden infant death syndrome risk-reduction messages.

REFERENCE

Vennemann, M., Bajanowski, T., Brinkmann, B., Jorch, G., Yücesan, K., Mitchell, E. A.; GeSID Study Group. (2009). Does breastfeeding reduce the risk of sudden infant death syndrome? *Pediatrics, 123*(3), e406–e410.

SKIN AND NAIL CARE

Generally, infants do not need lotions or baby powder. If lotions are used, they should be hypoallergenic and initially placed on the hands of the adult for warming before being rubbed on the infant's skin. Baby powder, typically a mixture of hydrous magnesium silicate (talc) and other silicates, can cause severe aspiration pneumonia, which can often be fatal. Therefore, parents should be told of its danger and discouraged from using it or encouraged to use a corn starch preparation in its place. A nail clipper can be used to keep fingernails and toenails short to prevent infants from scratching themselves. The best time to clip the nails is right after the bath because nails are softer. Finally, frequently changing and then cleaning the infant after a wet or soiled diaper is critically important to maintaining skin integrity.

STRANGER AND SEPARATION ANXIETY

Stranger and separation anxiety emerge at approximately 8–12 months of age, when the infant develops a sense of object permanence. Stranger and separation anxiety usually peak at 15–18 months and disappear by 2 years of age. **Separation anxiety** behaviors are demonstrated when an infant is separated from the caregiver. **Stranger anxiety** behaviors are demonstrated by an infant when a stranger appears.

When these anxieties emerge, developmentally, the infant can produce a mental image of the caregiver and recall that image even after a separation. Separation anxiety occurs because the infant does not understand the caregiver will return. However, as time goes on and with repeated episodes of separation, the infant will no longer demonstrate the behaviors (Dixon & Stein, 2006).

The infant's ability to produce a mental image of the caregiver enables the infant to also detect a difference in the appearance of an unfamiliar person. For the 8-month-old infant, the ability to recognize a discrepancy occurs rapidly when the stranger and familiar caregiver are seen together. As the child becomes older, the caregiver will not need to be present for the infant to identify a stranger (Figure 8-20).

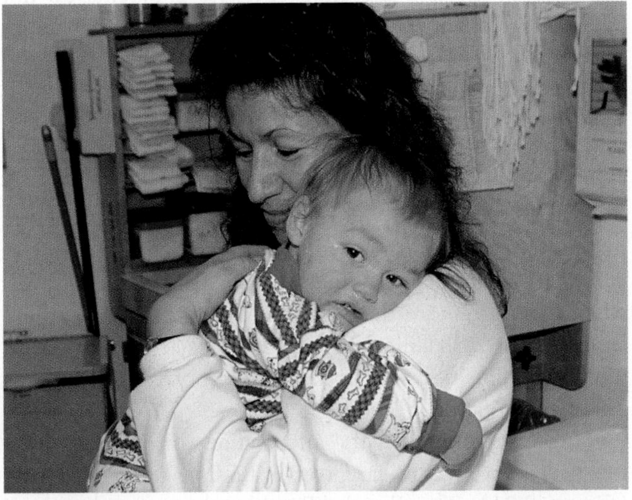

FIGURE 8-20 With ample time, an infant will warm up to a stranger. DELMAR CENGAGE LEARNING.

Typically, the infant who is experiencing stranger and/or separation anxiety will demonstrate overt distress by withdrawing, frowning, whimpering, crying, and clinging. Separation anxiety is more likely to occur if the infant is left in an unfamiliar place or with an unfamiliar person. With stranger anxiety, the stranger's approach influences the infant's reaction to the stranger. The infant will usually become anxious if the stranger immediately tries to reach out and touch or pick the child up. When time is provided for adjustment or adaptation to the unknown person, the infant usually reacts with less distress. The caregiver's reaction to the infant's behavior can also either reassure the infant or increase the infant's anxiety (Bowlby, 2007).

Stranger and separation anxieties can be disturbing for the caregiver, especially the caregiver who works away from the home. Therefore, it is important to help the caregiver understand these anxieties are a normal part of infant development. In addition, information related to the time of occurrence, the rationale for the occurrence, the characteristic behaviors expected, and when these anxieties usually disappear should be provided. The nurse should also give suggestions to ease the infant's discomfort.

FAMILY**TEACHING**

Relieving Stranger and Separation Anxiety

STRANGER ANXIETY

- Encourage friends and relatives to visit often.
- Let the infant see the caregiver's expression when a stranger approaches.
- Have the caregiver talk to the stranger first.
- Encourage the stranger to avoid intrusive movements or expressions.
- Have the caregiver maintain a safe distance from the stranger.
- Allow the infant to warm up to the stranger.
- Encourage the stranger to approach on the infant's level and use a soothing tone of voice.

SEPARATION ANXIETY

- Leave the infant in a familiar place or with a familiar person.
- Encourage the caregiver to talk to the infant before leaving.
- Do not leave the infant without saying good-bye.
- Leave a security object with the infant (e.g., a familiar toy or an object belonging to the caregiver).
- Encourage the infant to explore at his or her own pace.

Reflections from Families

Separation anxiety is a perfectly normal part of childhood development, but it can be unsettling. I remember the times I left my son, Carl, at the child care center when he was 9 months old. Teary-eyes and tantrum-filled good-byes were a common part of those times. I probably felt more separation anxiety than he did. I felt guilty leaving him to go to work and felt overwhelmed by the thought of the amount of attention he seemed to need from me.

I realized that my initial unwillingness to leave him was a good sign of healthy attachments between us. I was reassured by the caregivers that he always calmed down and happily interacted with other infants shortly after those teary episodes, and eventually remembered that I returned and that was enough comfort for us both. This experience, although distressing, was important in developing his independence and coping skills.

Some helpful hints for the relief of stranger and separation anxiety can be found in the accompanying Family Teaching box.

ALTERNATIVE CHILD CARE

When faced with having to leave their infant with another person, caregivers are challenged to find quality child care (care that is responsive and developmentally appropriate and provides an environment where the infant is safe, nurtured, and challenged to learn). The caregiver must become an informed consumer when searching for quality child care and learn the ages of infants/children served at the facility. The nurse should keep caregivers informed on alternative child care issues such as availability, affordability, and quality. Prior to any investigation into alternative child care, the nurse should stress it is important for the caregiver to:

- Be realistic about challenges inherent in using child care such as hours of operation, policies when the child is ill, and who is able to pick up the infant if the parent is not able to do so.
- Think carefully about whether or not alternative child care is appropriate.
- Learn to adapt.
- Set priorities based on family values.
- Keep communications open.
- Identify any financial concerns.

Table 8-10 provides information on the various types of child care providers available, with advantages and disadvantages of each, and Table 8-11 provides guidelines for choosing quality child care.

While searching for quality child care, the caregiver may inquire about the long-term effects of child care on infant development. Even though this area needs further study, research shows those who are in child care for many hours starting in infancy may be at increased risk for stress-related behavioral problems. In addition, behavioral problems occur more frequently and the child struggles if parents do not provide high quality child care and if the child has difficulties interacting with peers. On the other hand, child care arrangements may be advantageous for poor children in relation to their language development and achievement, especially if the care is of high quality. In fact, children in child care arrangements meeting the American Academy of Pediatrics standards are more likely to have better developmental outcomes and receive better care than those not in child care situations that meet those standards. However, when there are more than six children in the setting, there is an increased likelihood of being exposed to more communicable illnesses and upper respiratory tract infections (Bradley & Vandell, 2007).

Once equipped with information on quality care, the next step for the caregiver is finding good child care (Figure 8-21). The Family Teaching box provides some suggestions for locating such a setting.

TABLE 8-10 Types of Alternative Child Care

TYPES	ADVANTAGES	DISADVANTAGES
Center-based care	• Group care for two or more children • Located usually in a home, school, church, or building designed for group care • Include nursery school, preschool, parent cooperative • Licensed by local or state agencies • Staff usually trained in child care and development • Structured program of activities for children usually available • Has specific hours of operation	• Regulations vary from area to area • May be placed on a waiting list for admission • Fewer adults per child • Care may not be individualized
Family child care	• Small group care • Good adult/child ratio • Located in provider's home • Special arrangements are easier to make	• May include provider's children • May not be licensed by local or state agencies that expect certain adult/child ratios or other standards • Provider(s) may not be trained in child care and development • Hours of operation may not be reliable

Adapted from: American Academy of Pediatrics (2009c). Parent's guide to choosing safe and healthy child care. Retrieved May 12, 2009, from www.aap.org/sections/scan/practicingsafety/Toolkit_Resources/Module3/ParentsGuide.pdf - 2010-03-12; Quality child care: Recognizing and choosing the best for your children. *The Daily Parent,* 49. Retrieved January 23, 2010, from http://www.childcareaware.org/en/subscriptions/dailyparent/volume.php?id=39.

Lastly, only the caregiver can make the final decision regarding child care. As an informed consumer, it is most important for the caregiver to be sure to:

- Interview the child care provider by calling first and then visiting.
- Check references.
- Make the decision on what is heard and seen.
- Always stay involved.
- Ask child care provider if he/she has made contingency plans (arrange for an alternate child care provider, call parent) if for any reason the child care provider is not able to adequately care for or tolerate the child during a particular day.

PLAY

Play enhances the infant's maturation and provides an opportunity to practice newly acquired motor skills as well as learn about the environment and the people around them. Play enhances bodily gracefulness; promotes social skills; sharpens cognitive and language skills; and extends attention span, persistence, and sense of mastery (Honig, 2006).

Play for the infant moves rapidly from accidental pleasure-producing activities to purposeful, repetitive activities with an increasing awareness of the surrounding environment. By 6 months to 1 year, the infant engages in repetitive activities involving voices, sounds, music, and a variety of toys, which enhance the development of language and sensorimotor skills (Figure 8-22).

The caregiver's involvement and responsiveness influence the quality of play; interpersonal contact is essential. The infant needs to be played with, not just allowed to play, because the richest play occurs when the caregiver takes an active role. Caregiver play nurtures the relationship through shared activities, accomplishments, and joys. If the caregiver is uncomfortable playing with the infant, the nurse can be instrumental in insisting the caregiver become involved. Suggestions from *Bright Futures* (2009) and Dixon and Stein (2006) to aid the caregiver in being involved in infant play include:

- Be sure toys are developmentally appropriate and safe.
- Provide toys to stimulate all five senses.

TABLE 8-11 Choosing Child Care

Does Child Care Provider	
Appear warm and friendly?	Accept and respect your family's cultural values?
Seem calm and gentle?	Seem to enjoy cuddling infants?
Seem easy to talk with?	Meet infant physical needs?
Seem to like themselves and the job?	Provide infant stimulation?
Treat each child as special?	Provide dependable and consistent care?
Understand children's stages of development?	Provide consistency between home and child care?
Encourage good health habits?	Seem to have time for all infants?
Have previous experience and trained staff?	Have first aid or CPR certification?
Does the Child Care Setting Have	
Up-to-date license or registration certificate?	Smoke detectors?
A clean and comfortable look?	Covered radiators and protected heaters?
Enough room to allow children to move freely and safely?	Strong screens or bars on windows above first floor?
Appropriate staff/child ratio?	Nutritious meals and snacks?
Late pick-up policy?	A separate place to care for sick children?
Child-proofed environment?	A first-aid kit?
Enough heat, light?	Safe gates at top and bottom of stairs?
Enough furnishings for all children?	A clean, safe place to change diapers, sanitized after each use?
Furnishings that are safe and in good repair?	Cribs with firm mattresses?
Adequate number of clean bathrooms?	Separate linen for each crib?
Fire safety plan and adequate exits?	Safe play areas?
Fire extinguishers?	Safety issues related to toys or the environment?
	Measures to prevent/reduce infection transmission?
Are There Opportunities for the Child to	
Play quietly and actively?	Learn to get along, share, and respect themselves and others?
Play alone?	Learn about their own and others' cultures?
Follow a schedule that meets young children's needs?	Crawl and explore safely?
Learn new developmental skills?	Play outside in a safe, contained environment?

Adapted from: Is This the Right Place for My Child? Checklist Helps Parents Identify High-Quality Child Care. (2010). Retrieved January 23, 2010, from http://www.naccrra.org/publications/naccrra-publications/is-this-the-right-place-for-my-child; Recognizing and choosing the best for your children. *The Daily Parent, 49*. Retrieved April 4, 2009, from http://www.childcareaware.org/en/subscriptions/dailyparent/volume.php?id=39.

- Place the infant in a variety of positions throughout the day (e.g., stomach, side, back [if the infant can turn from supine to prone position or if the caregiver is present]).
- Encourage the use of hands and feet in play.
- Offer a few new experiences each day.
- Encourage banging toys together.
- Praise often.
- Read to the infant often (before nap time; before bed time).

During routine infant assessment, the nurse should ask the caregiver about the nature of the infant's play. With the emergence of voluntary reach and grasp, it is important to investigate the infant's motor competency, visual-motor

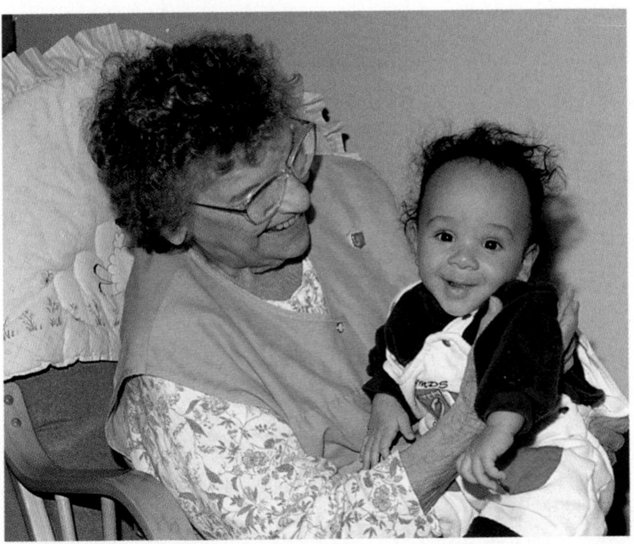

FIGURE 8-21 Finding quality child care takes effort, time and patience. DELMAR CENGAGE LEARNING.

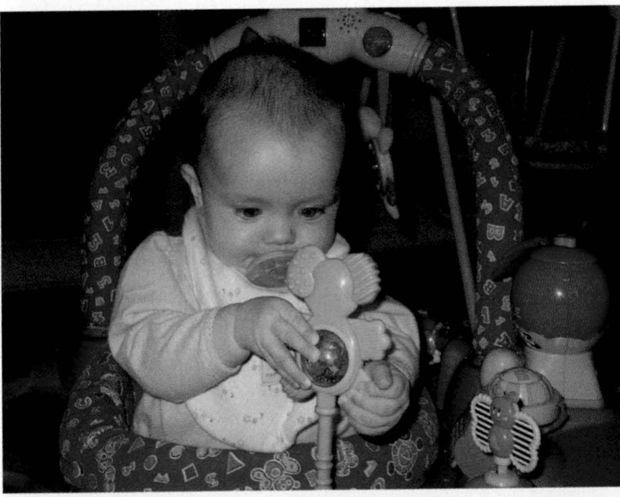

FIGURE 8-22 This infant is intent on learning about her toys. DELMAR CENGAGE LEARNING.

REFLECTIVE THINKING

Alternative Child Care

What are your feelings about alternative child care? Provide statements for and against both parents working outside the home and requiring alternative child care.

FAMILY TEACHING

Ways to Find Quality Child Care

- Ask friends and neighbors how they found child care.
- Look in the Yellow Pages of the telephone directory under "Child Care Centers."
- Check classified ads in the local newspaper.
- Talk with family child care associations or provider support groups.
- Ask the local affiliate of the National Association for the Education of Young Children.
- Contact the local Human Development Extension agent (usually a person with a college degree in human development or child psychology who works for the county or state).

coordination, and the appropriateness of the environment in exploring the object world. To facilitate the infant's continued development, the caregiver should be given information relevant to the toys and activities appropriate for the infant (Dixon & Stein, 2006). Table 8-12 provides a list of developmentally appropriate toys and activities for the infant.

When inquiring about the nature of the infant's play, the nurse should also listen for details about the quality and complexity of play to determine if it is age-appropriate. The caregiver's description of play behavior can be beneficial in screening for problems such as developmental delays, neurologic problems, delayed social skills, autism, learning disabilities, and emotional disturbances (Dixon & Stein, 2006).

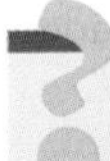

KIDS WANT TO KNOW

Disappointed sibling

I waited for so long for this baby to come, and she is not fun. She doesn't play or laugh. What is wrong with her?

- First of all assure the child that there is nothing wrong with the baby—this is what babies do. Explain that very young babies eat and sleep a lot so that they can get enough energy to grow and be able to play.
- Encourage the child to keep talking and singing to the infant, so that the baby loves the sibling's voice.
- Explain that in a month or two the baby will watch the older child run around, dance, and sing and before you know it the baby will be old enough to join in.

NURSING TIP

Motor Skills and Coordination

To have a clearer understanding of the infant's motor competency and visual-motor coordination, ask yourself the following questions when caring for an infant:

- What motor skills does the infant demonstrate?
- Are these motor skills appropriate for the age of the infant?
- How does the infant use hand and mouth in exploration?
- What toy does the infant choose?
- Does the infant use both hands and arms equally?
- Are the infant's movements smooth?
- How does the caregiver facilitate the infant's play?

SAFETY PROMOTION AND INJURY PREVENTION

Infants are in a state of perpetual development and refinement of motor skills. In addition, infants have an insatiable curiosity about the environment. When this perpetual change and curiosity are combined, the infant is at risk for accidental injury, the leading cause of infant deaths, especially between 6 and 12 months of age. To ensure a safe environment for the infant, the caregiver must be aware of the safety concerns most associated with each stage of motor development. The nurse and caregiver should discuss the environmental hazards associated with specific motor development. Anticipatory guidance (preparing caregivers for the normal growth and development of their child), provided prior to the skill development, should include:

- The reason why infants are prone to injury
- The importance of injury prevention
- The importance of setting age-appropriate limits
- The importance of always anticipating danger and removing the child from the danger

One way to prevent accidental injury is to childproof the home. A general safety checklist can be found in Box 8-3.

Of all the places in the home, the infant's bedroom should be monitored most closely because it harbors many hazards. First and foremost, the bedroom furniture should meet Consumer Product Safety Commission standards. The crib should be located away from windows and electrical outlets. The head or footboard should have no cutouts where the infant's head could be trapped, and the spaces between the bed rail slats should be no more than 2 3⁄8 inches. The side rails should be locked in the highest position when the infant is in the crib to prevent falling. The

TABLE 8-12 Toys and Activities Appropriate for the Infant

AGE	TOYS/ACTIVITY
Birth–3 months	Black-and-white pattern cards
	Soft, cuddle toys
	Nonbreakable mirror
	Rattles
	Mobiles
	Music boxes
	Talking and singing
	Rocking and holding
	Gentle massage
	Interaction with other people
3–6 months	Hand-held infant toys
	Squeaky toys
	Teething rings
	Different textured toys
	Noise-making toys
	Talking and singing
	Playing pat-a-cake and peek-a-boo
	Interacting with other people
	Reading/looking at picture books
6–9 months	Safe place to creep and crawl
	Bath tub toys
	Jack-in-the-box
	Nested toys
	Large soft blocks
	Toys to bang together
	Talking and singing
	Playing peek-a-boo
	Interacting with other people
9–12 months	Continue with toys for 6–9 months
	Safe place for exploration
	Push-pull and motion toys
	Colorful cloth books
	Paper for tearing
	Building blocks
	Plastic bowls and containers
	Toys that have different shapes and colors
	Interacting with other people

BOX 8-3
GENERAL SAFETY CHECKLIST

House

- All cleaning supplies, medicines, and cosmetics locked up or out of reach
- All knives or sharp edged objects out of reach
- Poisonous plants removed
- All firearms removed/locked in a cabinet
- Ammunition stored separately from firearms
- Fans and heaters out of reach
- Smoke and carbon monoxide detectors working (replace batteries every six months)
- All small objects picked up and out of sight
- No small parts on toys
- Plastic bags and all balloons stored out of reach
- Unused large appliances kept locked
- Pool area gated and fenced
- Water hazards (buckets) removed or out of reach
- Locks on refrigerators
- Bathroom doors kept closed to prevent infant's access to the toilet and/or bath tub
- All unused electrical outlets covered with safety caps
- Electrical cords out of sight and access to a crawling infant
- Cords for blinds or curtains out of reach

Falls

- Gates in front of stairs/steps
- All electrical wires out of reach or hidden
- Furniture sturdy and in good repair
- Edge protectors used on end and coffee tables
- Inspect cribs for loose bolts and/or screws
- Remove breakable items, glass topped tables, heavy objects
- Walkways clear of any obstacles
- Stairway gated
- Sturdy handrails on all stairs or steps
- Window screens in good repair
- Use of window guards
- Use of non-skid rugs
- Use of door knob covers
- Adequate lighting
- Infant/child safety seats in automobiles
- No infant walkers; instead use jumper seats/saucers

Burns

- No smoking around infant; all cigarettes and matches out of reach
- Guards on front of heating appliances, furnace, fireplace
- Hot water heater thermostat set at 120°F (45.2°C)
- Clothes dryer set at low heat
- Clothes dryer/washer doors closed
- Infant removed from kitchen during meal preparation unless in infant seat or high chair
- All cooking utensil handles to the back of stove
- Electric cords for kitchen appliances out of reach
- No drinking or handling hot liquids around infant
- Smoke detectors working correctly (replace batteries every six months)
- Fire extinguishers easily accessible for adults

Emergency Needs

- Post all emergency numbers by telephones including poison control
- Post house address and phone number by each telephone
- First-aid kit up to date
- Have and practice an emergency exit plan in case of a fire
- Caregivers know CPR

Adapted from: Baby: Protecting your family. Preventing accidental injury. Accessed January 23, 2010, from http://www.usa.safekids.org/tier3_cd.cfm?content_item_id=288&folder_id=167; Dixon, S., & Stein, M. (2006). *Encounters with children: Pediatric behaviors and development* (4th ed.). St. Louis: Elsevier.

mattress should fit snugly against the frame so the infant cannot slip between the mattress and frame. Bumper pads or pillows should not be used, nor should any object be hung on the crib (Keeping your Child Safe in Today's World, 2009). When the infant begins to stand, the mattress should be placed in the lowest setting.

As the infant's ability to explore the environment increases daily, so do the hazards encountered. The caregiver needs to be reminded that the ability to roll and turn makes the infant susceptible to falling if left unattended on the bed, changing table, or counter top. When the infant can reach for and grasp items and bring them to the mouth, the caregiver must be cautious in leaving objects within the infant's reach (Figure 8-23). With the ability to creep and crawl, the infant can move farther and faster than the caregiver might expect, so the floor should be kept free of small objects and child-proof latches used in cupboards (Figure 8-24). As locomotion improves, the infant is soon able to stand and walk (cruise) around objects. Once this occurs, the caregiver must constantly be vigilant since the infant is now susceptible to falling, suffocating, and drowning (Figure 8-25). Table 8-13 provides information related to the appropriate infant safety measures associated with specific developmental achievements and type of injury.

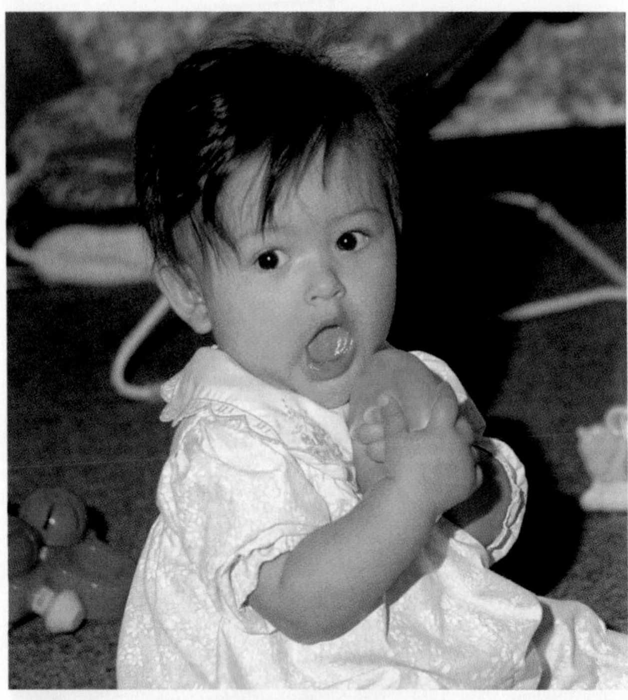

FIGURE 8-23 For safety reasons make sure all toys in reach of an infant are age appropriate. DELMAR CENGAGE LEARNING.

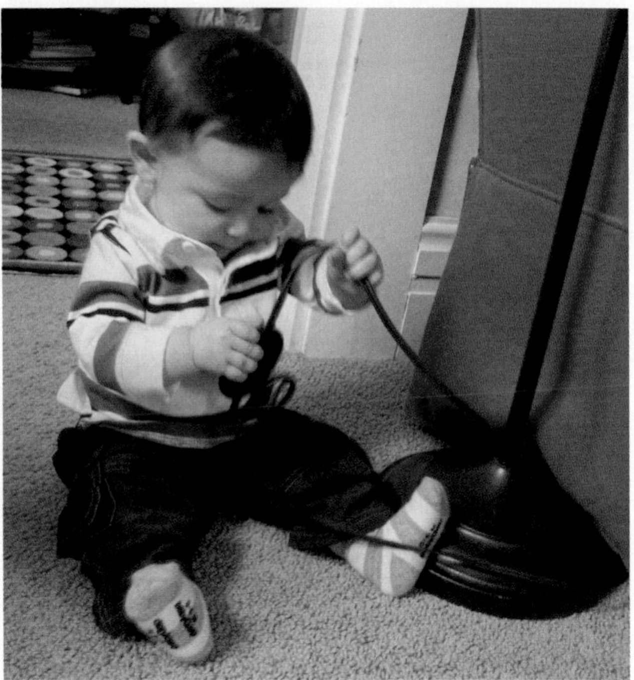

FIGURE 8-24 Electrical cords must be kept out of reach and out of sight of curious infants. DELMAR CENGAGE LEARNING.

FAMILY TEACHING

Check for Hidden Dangers

To ensure the infant's safety, the caregiver is encouraged to crouch down at what is the child's eye level, close to the floor, to survey the environment for hazards the infant might encounter. It may even be necessary to crawl around to find any hidden dangers. Infants should also be placed in appropriate child safety restraints in the middle of the back seat whenever riding in automobiles. See Chapter 7 for further information about child-restraint seats.

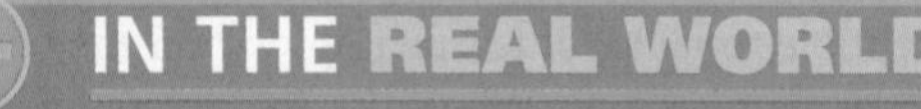

IN THE REAL WORLD

A number of developmental changes occur during infancy. The infant begins life as a completely dependent being and ends as an independent individual in perpetual motion. As a nurse, I watch this period of life with such awe and fascination and count myself lucky to be called a caregiver. Infants deserve only the best from caregivers, who will influence their outlook on this wonderful thing called life. As a child health nurse, my responsibility is to provide necessary information and guidance and to answer any question asked by caregivers so the infant will have the potential to achieve optimal growth and development.

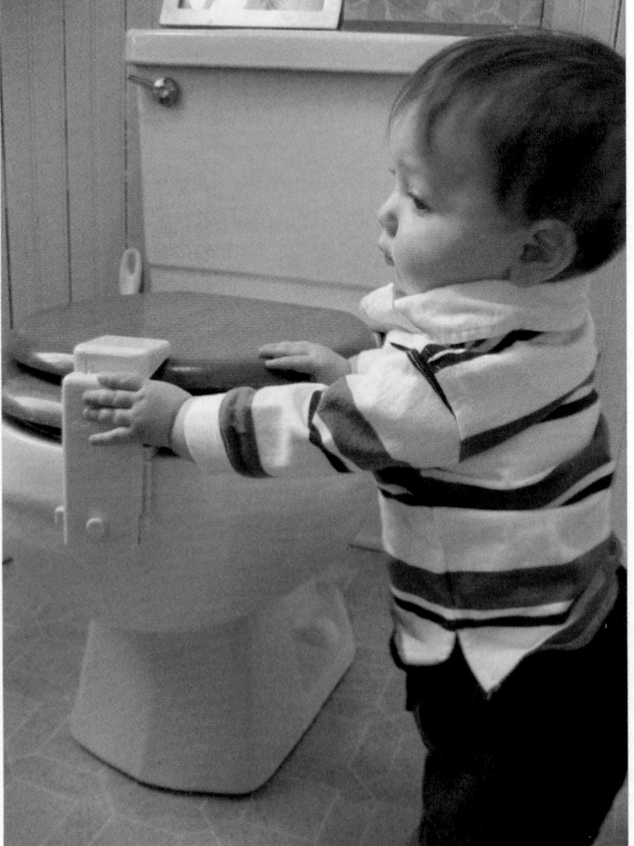

FIGURE 8-25 Toilet lids should be kept latched, and bathroom doors closed, to prevent accidental drowning and injury. DELMAR CENGAGE LEARNING.

Table 8-13 Infant Safety

AGE AND DEVELOPMENT ACHIEVEMENTS	TYPE OF INJURY	SAFETY CHECKLIST
Birth to 4 Months		
Rolls from side to back	Falls	Keep crib rails up.
Reaches for objects		Never leave infant unattended on a high surface.
Places objects in mouth		
	Drowning	Never leave infant unattended in bathtub.
	Burns	Keep hot water heater temperature <45.2°C (120°F).
		Always check bath water temperature.
		Do not hold or drink hot liquids when holding infant.
		Install smoke and carbon monoxide detectors in home.
		Avoid sun over exposure.
		Use sunscreen.
		Do not use microwave oven for warming formula or food.
		Always check temperature of formula and food prior to feeding (should be room temperature).
	Suffocation	Do not use pillows in the infant's bed.
		No co-sleeping.
		Keep plastic bags or wrap, and balloons out of reach.
	Strangulation	Be sure crib slats are <2⅜ inches apart.
		Be sure mattress fits tightly against slats.
		Do not tie anything to crib.
		Keep infant's crib away from curtain or blind cords.
		Never tie any string around infant's neck.
	Motor vehicle accident	Use only an approved infant-restraint system in the car.
		Do not leave infant unsecured in car seat.
		Always put car seat in the back seat facing rear.
		Never place car seat in front seat unless there is no other alternative and air bag is turned off.
	Choking	Keep small objects out of reach.
		Never leave infant unattended on the floor.
	Ingestion	Have poison control number available.
4 to 7 Months		(In addition to those listed for birth to 4 months)
Sits with support	Choking and strangulation	Keep floor free of small objects.
Rolls from back to side		Keep infant's crib away from curtain or blind cords.

(Continues)

Table 8-13 Infant Safety (*Continued*)

AGE AND DEVELOPMENT ACHIEVEMENTS	TYPE OF INJURY	SAFETY CHECKLIST
4 to 7 Months (Continued)		
Bears weight in standing position with support		
Reaches for object beyond grasp		
Actively drops objects		
	Burns	Cover all unused electrical outlets with safety caps.
		Put manufacturer-approved protective covering over heaters, furnaces.
	Falls	Restrain infant in high chair.
		Do not use walkers.
		Gate all stairways.
	Ingestion	Use child-proof latches on cupboards and drawers.
		Never leave infant unattended on the floor.
		Keep toxic substances (and plants) out of reach in locked cabinet.
		Post poison control number by telephone.
		Do not smoke around infant.
8 to 12 Months		(In addition to those listed for 1–7 months)
Drops object at will	Burns	Turn cooking handles toward back of stove.
Uses pincer grasp		Do not use a dangling tablecloth.
Can self-feed finger foods		Never leave unattended in bathroom.
Places and removes small objects in a container		Keep electrical wires or cords out of reach.
Sits alone without support	Drowning	Never leave unattended in bathroom.
Can move from prone to sitting to standing		Never leave unattended in the yard, pool, or playground.
Stands alone without support	Falls	Fence all stairways.
Progresses from crawling to creeping to cruising		Be sure furniture is sturdy.
Attempts to walk alone		Never leave unattended in the yard or playground.
		Put infant's bed in lowest position.
	Ingestion	Keep medicines, cosmetics, and toxic substances or plants out of reach.
		Never leave unattended in the yard or playground.

(Continues)

TABLE 8-13 Infant Safety (*Continued*)

AGE AND DEVELOPMENT ACHIEVEMENTS	TYPE OF INJURY	SAFETY CHECKLIST
8 to 12 Months (Continued)	Choking	Use caution with finger foods (e.g., berries, grapes, cherries, carrots, popcorn, hot dogs) and coins. Never leave unattended in the yard or playground.
	Motor vehicle	Leave infant in the back seat and switch to forward-facing car seat at 20 lb and at least 1 year.

Adapted from: American Academy of Pediatrics. (2002). Selecting and using the most appropriate car safety seats for growing children: Guidelines for counseling parents. *Pediatrics, 109*(3), 550–553; and CDC (1995) Air-bag associated fatal injuries to infants and children riding in front passenger seats—United States. *Morbidity and Mortality Weekly Report, 44*(45), 845–847. Retrieved January 23, 2010, from http://www.cdc.gov/mmwr/preview/mmwrhtml/00039562.htm.

KEY CONCEPTS

- It is essential for the nurse to have an understanding of infant growth and development to ensure the infant and family maintain an optimal level of health.
- Motor skill development progresses in an orderly fashion. Gross motor development occurs before fine motor development, and the infant must be able to reach before being able to grasp an object.
- An infant is in the sensorimotor stage of cognitive development. Knowledge is acquired about an object through interaction with that object. The major task for the infant is object permanence.
- Trust can be developed by promptly meeting the infant's basic needs of feeding, clothing, and comforting.
- Health screening includes health assessment, physical examination, and administration of scheduled immunizations and provides the health care provider with the opportunity to detect and evaluate any problems.
- Nutritional requirements are based on physical activity and rate of growth. Energy requirements range from 110–115 kcal/kg/day at birth to 100 kcal/kg/day by 1 year of age. Fluid requirement is 1–1.5 mL/kcal expended per day.
- Anticipatory guidance provides information on expected milestones and methods to encourage optimal development.
- During infancy, receptive language is greater than expressive language.
- Temperamental characteristics and the caregiver's personality produce a characteristic pattern of social interaction between the child and the environment.
- Infants have variable sleep patterns that are influenced by temperament, satisfaction with feedings, caregiver's response to periodic awakenings, and environmental conditions.
- Play provides the infant the opportunity to practice newly acquired motor skills and to learn about the environment and the people around them.
- The infant's inherent curiosity coupled with limited cognitive ability places them at risk for accidental injuries.

REVIEW ACTIVITIES

1. What are the physiological growth and developmental milestones of infants, and why are they important?
2. What are the fine and gross motor developmental milestones of infancy? Why are the principles associated with them important?

3. Why are an infant's psychosexual, cognitive, and psychosocial development important, and how do they interrelate?
4. What health promotion and maintenance activities for infants do nurses need to know about and why?
5. What is the recommended immunization schedule during the first year? What are the contraindications for administering immunizations in infants? What information should parents receive regarding immunizations?
6. What information should a nurse provide for a parent of an infant related to calorie and fluid requirements?
7. How does infant play change during the first year of life? What activities would a nurse suggest parents provide for their infant to facilitate growth and development?
8. What are the important anticipatory guidance interventions caregivers of infants need to know related to nutritional needs, growth and development patterns, and stranger and separation anxiety?
9. How do infant nutritional needs vary from birth to 3 months, from 4 to 6 months, and from 6 to 12 months?
10. What are the safety concerns for families with infants? How can families prevent injury to the infants?

STUDY QUESTIONS

1. A nurse takes the weight of a 12-month-old child who is brought by the mother for checkup. If the child weighed 6 lbs, 3 oz. at birth, which of these weights should the nurse expect to find during the 12-month-old well-child checkup?
   a. 12 lbs, 6 oz.
   b. 18 lbs, 9 oz.
   c. 22 lbs, 12 oz.
   d. 28 lbs, 15 oz.
2. Which of these behaviors, if observed on a 10-month-old infant, would suggest to a nurse that the infant is developing the concept of object permanence?
   a. The infant babbles to the mirror image when placed in front of the mirror.
   b. After seeing the mother put the toy in a container, the infant takes a toy from the container.
   c. The infant cries and holds on to the mother when the nurse greets the infant.
   d. The infant waves bye-bye to the nurses when the infant leaves the health clinic.
3. A nurse in the well-baby clinic is conducting an assessment on a 6-month-old infant. Which of these observations would warrant further investigation?
   a. Crying when the rattle is removed
   b. Crying when the nurse approaches
   c. Only rolls from abdomen to back
   d. Absence of moro reflex
4. A nurse is obtaining growth measurements on a 1-year-old child. The nurse should recognize which of these measurements as a normal finding for this age?
   a. The head is one inch larger than the chest.
   b. The head and chest are approximately equal.
   c. The chest is one inch larger than the head.
   d. The chest is two inches larger than the head.
5. The father brings his 4-month-old son for well-baby checkup. Which of the following instructions is most appropriate?
   a. "Do not allow your son to chew paint from the window ledges because he might absorb too much lead."
   b. "Lock the crib sides securely because your son may stand and lean against them and fall out of bed."
   c. "You must supervise your son whenever on a high surface because he might fall when he learns to roll over."
   d. "You do not need to cover electric outlets and lock cabinets around the area where your son crawls or creeps."
6. When a mother of a 6-month-old infant asks a nurse how to reduce the likelihood of sudden infant death syndrome (SIDS) happening to her child, which of these responses by the nurse would be appropriate?
   a. "Limit your child's exposure to public places."
   b. "Follow the recommended schedule for well-child checkups."
   c. "Avoid overfeeding your child."
   d. "It is advisable to put your child on her back to sleep."
7. You are caring for a 2-month-old infant whose mother says he has colic. Which of the following is incorrect as you respond to the mother?

a. "It is important to feed the infant slowly, burp frequently, and keep him in an upright position during feeding to decrease the amount of air swallowed."
b. "When breastfeeding, avoid eating foods that may contribute to gas formation (onions, cabbage, collards, and dry beans)."
c. "Swaddling the infant is helpful to decrease self-stimulation by jerky or sudden movements."
d. "It is not helpful to use an infant swing, rock the infant in a rocking chair or massage the infant's back."

8. A mother brings her 8-month-old daughter to the clinic for well-child care. The mother says to a nurse, "My daughter loves to suck her thumb, and I'm worried this habit will cause permanent damage to her teeth." Which of these responses should the nurse give to the mother?
   a. "You should wrap your daughter's thumb with adhesive tape."
   b. "Offer her favorite toy to distract her from sucking her thumb."
   c. "Infants need sucking; it's okay to let your daughter suck her thumb."
   d. "Remove her thumb from her mouth when you see her thumbsucking."
9. A mother asks a nurse when solid foods should be introduced into the infant's diet. Which of these responses should the nurse give the mother?
   a. "Introduce solid foods at 2 to 3 months of age."
   b. "Start introducing solid foods at 5 to 6 months of age."
   c. "Give solid foods when the birth weight has tripled."
   d. "Offer solid foods when tooth eruption has started."
10. A mother tells a nurse that she plans to discontinue breastfeeding her 5-month-old infant. The nurse instructs the mother on the type of feedings the mother should give when she weans the child from breastfeeding. Which of these feedings, if chosen by the mother, would indicate that the mother understood the teaching?
   a. Skim milk
   b. Whole cow's milk
   c. Iron-fortified formula
   d. Formula without iron

REFERENCES

American Academy of Pediatric Dentistry. (2006). Guideline on infant oral health care. In *AAPD Reference Manual 2005–2006*.

American Academy of Pediatrics. (2000). Changing concepts of sudden infant death syndrome: Implications for infant sleeping environment and sleep position. *Pediatrics, 105*, 650–656.

American Academy of Pediatrics. (2002). Selecting and using the most appropriate car safety seats for growing children: Guidelines for counseling parents. *Pediatrics, 109*(3), 550–553.

American Academy of Pediatrics. (2005). Breastfeeding and the use of human milk. Policy statement. *Pediatrics, 115*(2), 496–506.

American Academy of Pediatrics. (2006). Baby bottle tooth decay. Retrieved January 16, 2006, from http://www.aap.org/pubed/ZZZKBW52R7C.htm?&sub_cat511.

American Academy of Pediatrics. (2008a). Section on Pediatric Dentistry and Oral Health. Preventive oral health intervention for pediatricians. *Pediatrics, 122*(6), 1387–1394.

American Academy of Pediatrics. (2008b). Screening Initiatives: Developmental/Behavioral. Retrieved May 13, 2009, from http://www.medicalhomeinfo.org/screening/cdc_rev1.html.

American Academy of Pediatrics. (2009a). Recommendations for Preventative Pediatric Health Care (RE9535). Committee on Practice and Ambulatory Health Care. Retrieved January 23, 2010, from http://aappolicy.aappublications.org/cgi/reprint/pediatrics;105/3/645.pdf.

American Academy of Pediatrics. (2009b). Parenting corner: Starting Solid foods. Retrieved May 12, 2009, from http://www.aap.org/publiced/BR_Solids.htm.

American Academy of Pediatrics. (2009c). Parent's Guide to choosing Safe and Healthy Child Care, available from http://www.aap.org/sections/scan/practicingsafety/Toolkit_Resources/Module3/ParentsGuide.pdf - 2010-03-12.

Anderson, M. E., Johnson, C. D., & Batal, H. A. (2005). Sudden infant death syndrome and prenatal maternal smoking: Rising attributed risk in the *Back to Sleep* era. *BioMed Central Medicine, 3*(4). Retrieved January 23, 2010, from http://www.pubmedcentral.nih.gov/articlerender.fcgi?artid=545061.

Baby: Protecting your family. Preventing accidental injury. (2010). Accessed January 23, 2010, from http://www.usa.safekids.org/tier3_cd.cfm?content_item_id=288&folder_id=167.

Baby Friendly USA. (2009). What is the Baby-Friendly Hospital Initiative and why do we need it? Retrieved January 8, 2010, from http://www.babyfriendlyusa.org/eng/01.html.

Bauchner, H. (2008). Early nutrition and development of atopic disease. *Journal Watch Pediatrics and Adolescent Medicine*. Retrieved April 1, 2009, from http://pediatrics.jwatch.org/cgi/content/full/2008/220/.

Blair, S. (2008). Putting co-sleeping into perspective. *Jornal de Pediatra, 8*(2). n. p. Retrieved January 23, 2010, from http://www.scielo.br/scielo.php?pid=S0021-75572008000200001&script=sci_arttext&tlng=en.

Bowlby, J. (2007). Babies and toddlers in non-parental day care can avoid stress and anxiety if they develop a lasting secondary attachment bond with one caregiver who is consistently available to them. *Attachment & Human Development, 9*(4), 307–314.

Bradley R. H., & Vandell, D. L. (2007). Child care and the well-being of children. *Archives of Pediatric & Adolescent Medicine, 161*(7), 669–676.

Bright Futures: Guidelines for Health Supervision of Infants, Children, and Adolescents. Promoting Physical Activity. (2009). Accessed January 23, 2010, from http://brightfutures.aap.org/pdfs/Guidelines_PDF/7-Promoting_Physical_Activity.pdf.

Centers for Disease Control and Prevention. (1995). Air-Bag Associated Fatal Injuries to Infants and Children Riding in Front Passenger Seats—United States. *Morbidity and Mortality Weekly Report, 44*(45), 845–847. Retrieved January 23, 2010, from http://www.cdc.gov/mmwr/preview/mmwrhtml/00039562.htm.

Centers for Disease Control and Prevention. (2009). Immunization Schedules. Accessed January 23, 2010, from http://www.cdc.gov/vaccines/recs/schedules/default.htm.

Centers for Disease Control and Prevention. (2010). Vaccine Information Statements. Retrieved January 23, 2010, from http://www.cdc.gov/vaccines/pubs/vis/default.htm.

Coleman-Phox, K., Odouli, R., & Li, D. O. (2008). Uses of a fan during sleep and the risk of sudden infant death syndrome. *Archives of Pediatric and Adolescent Medicine, 162*(10), 963–968.

Cohen-Silver, J., & Ratnapalan, S. (2009). Management of infantile colic: A review. *Clinical Pediatrics, 48*(1), 14–17.

Darden, P., Blue, A., Brooks, D., Taylor, J., Hendricks, J., & Bocian, A. (2006). Staff and parent perceptions of barriers to immunization for African-American children: A study from PROS and NMA-PEDSNET. Accessed January 23, 2010, from http://www.aap.org/research/abstracts/05abstract18.htm.

Davidson, M., London, M., & Laedwig, P. (2008). *Old's maternal-newborn nursing & women's health across the lifespan* (8th ed.). Upper Saddle River, NJ: Pearson Education.

Dewar, G. (2008). Baby sleep patterns: A guide for the science-minded parent. *Parenting Science*. Accessed January 23, 2010, from http://www.parentingscience.com/baby-sleep-patterns.html.

Dixon, S., & Stein, M. (2006). *Encounters with children: Pediatric behaviors and development* (4th ed.). St. Louis, MO: Elsevier.

Erikson, E. E. (1963). *Childhood and society* (2nd ed.). New York: Norton.

Forste, R., & Hoffmann, J. P. (2008). Are US mothers meeting the *Healthy People 2010* breastfeeding targets for initiation, duration, and exclusivity? The 2003 and 2004 national immunization surveys. *Journal of Human Lactation, 24*(3), 278–288.

Frankenburg, W. K., Dodds, J., Archer, P., Shapiro, H., & Bresnick, B. (1992). The Denver II: A major revision and restandardization of the Denver developmental screening test. *Pediatrics, 89*, 91–97.

Freud, S. (1933). *New introductory lectures in psychoanalysis*. New York: Norton.

Gregory, K. (2005). Update on nutrition for preterm and full-term infants. *Journal of Obstetric, Gynecologic, and Neonatal Nursing, 34*(1), 98–108.

Gussy, M. G., Waters, E. G., Walsh, O., & Kilpatrick, N. M. (2006). Early childhood caries: Current evidence for aetiology and prevention. *Journal of Pediatrics & Child Health, 42*(1/2), 37–43.

Hane, A., Fox, N., Polak-Toste, C., Ghera, M., & Guner, B. (2006). Contextual basis of maternal perceptions of infant temperament. *Developmental Psychology, 42*(6), 1077–1088.

Haydu, S., & Sundquist, J. (2006). Normal infant feeding (0–12 months). Accessed January 23, 2010, from http://www.cdph.ca.gov/HealthInfo/healthyliving/childfamily/Documents/MO-InfantFeeding0-12mo.pdf.

Honig, A. S. (2006). What infants, toddlers, and preschoolers learn from play: 12 ideas. Montessori Life. FindArticles.com. Accessed January 23, 2010, from http://findarticles.com/p/articles/mi_qa4097/is_200601/ai_n17188806/.

Huang, Y., & Huang, C. (2006). Nipple confusion and breastfeeding: A literature review. *Journal of Nursing, 53*(2), 73–79.

Hunt, C. E., & Hauck, F. R. (2007). In R. M. Kliegman, R. Behrman, H. B. Jenson, & B. F. Stanton (Eds.), *Nelson textbook of pediatrics* (18th ed.). Philadelphia, PA: Saunders, 1736–1742.

Keeping your child safe in today's world. (2009). *The Daily Parent 22*. Retrieved April 28, 2009, from http://www.childcareaware.org/en/subscriptions/dailyparent/volume.php?id=22.

Kliegman, R. M., Behrman, R. Jenson, H. B., & Stanton, B. F. (Eds.). (2007). *Nelson textbook of pediatrics* (18th ed.). Philadelphia, PA: Saunders.

Lawrence, R. A., & Lawrence, R. M. (2005). *Breastfeeding: A guide for the medical profession* (6th ed.). St. Louis, MO: Mosby.

Luthy, K. E., Beckstrand, R. L., & Peterson, N. E. (2008). Parental hesitation as a factor in delayed childhood immunization. *Journal of Pediatric Health Care, 23*(6), 388–393.

Marter, A., & Agruss, J. C. (2007). Pacifiers: an update on use and misuse. *Journal for Specialists in Pediatric Nursing, 12*(4), 278–285.

Miller, J. L. (2007). Preliminary ultrasound observation of lingual movement patterns during nutritive versus non-nutritive sucking in a premature infant. *Dysphasia, 22*(2), 150–160.

Monitoring Visual Development. (2007). Accessed January 23, 2010, from http://www.tsbvi.edu/Education/infant/page7.htm.

Nelson, E., Yu, L., Williams, S., & International Child Care Practices Study Group Members. (2005). International Child Care Practices Study: Breastfeeding and Pacifier Use. *Journal of Human Lactation, 21*, 289–295.

Nelson, H. D., Bougatsos, C., & Nygren, P. (2008). Universal newborn screening systematic review to update the 2001 US Preventive Services Task Force Recommendation. *Pediatrics, 122*(1), e266–e276.

National Association of Child Care Resource & Referral Agencies. *Is This the Right Place for My Child? Checklist Helps Parents Identify High-Quality Child Care.* (2010) Accessed January 23, 2010, from http://www.naccrra.org/publications/naccrra-publications/is-this-the-right-place-for-my-child.

National Institute of Child Health Development and Human Services. NICHD alerts parents to winter SIDS risk and updated AAP recommendations. (2006). National Institute of Child Health Development and Human Services.

O'Brien, M., Fallon A., Brodribb, W., & Hegney, D. (2007). Reasons for stopping breastfeeding: What are they, what characteristics relate to them, and are there underlying factors? *Birth Issues, 15*(3–4), 105–113.

O'Connor, N. R., Tanabe, K. O., Siadaty, M. S., & Hauck, F. R. (2009). Pacifiers and breastfeeding: A systematic review. *Archives of Pediatric and Adolescent Medicine, 163*(4), 378–382.

Piaget, J. (1952). *The origins of intelligence in children*. New York: International Universities Press.

Porter, L. (2007). All night long: understanding the world of infant sleep. *Breastfeeding Review, 15*(3), 11–15.

Recognizing and choosing the best for your children. (2010). *The Daily Parent, 49*. Retrieved January 23, 2010, from http://www.childcareaware.org/en/subscriptions/dailyparent/volume.php?id=39.

Ricci, S. S., Kyle, T., & Kyle, T. (2008). *Maternity and pediatric nursing.* Philadelphia, PA: Lippincott Williams & Wilkins.

Ruys, J. H., De Jonge, G. A., Brand, R., Engelberts, A. C., & Semmekrot, B. A. (2007). Bed-sharing in the first four months of life: A risk factor for sudden infant death. *Acta Paediatrica, 96*(10), 1399–1403.

Sadeh, A., Mindell, J., Luedtke, K., & Wiegand, B. (2009). Sleep and sleep ecology in the first 3 years: A web-based study. *Journal of Sleep Research, 18*(1), 60–73.

Sicherer, S. H., & Sampson, H. A. (2009). Food allergy: Recent advances in pathophysiology and treatment. *Annual Review of Medicine,* [Epub ahead of print]. Accessed January 23, 2010, from http://www.ncbi.nlm.nih.gov/pubmed/18729729.

South, M. T., Strauss, R. A., South, A. P., Boggess, J. F., & Thorp, J. M. (2005). The use of non-nutritive sucking to decrease the physiologic pain response during neonatal circumcision: A randomized controlled trial. *American Journal of Obstetrics and Gynecology, 193*(2), 537–543.

Tappin, D., Ecob, R., & Brooke, H. (2005). Bedsharing, roomsharing, and sudden infant death syndrome in Scotland: A case-control study. *Journal of Pediatrics, 147*(1), 32–37.

The Baby-Friendly Hospital Initiative. (2010). Accessed May 22, 2010, from http://www.unicef.org/programme/breastfeeding/baby.htm#10 and 65www.babyfriendlyusa.org.

Thomas, A., Chess, S., & Birch, H. (1968). *Temperament and behavior disorders in children.* New York: New York University Press.

Thomas, A., Chess, S., & Birch, H. (1970). The origin of personality. *Scientific American, 223*(2), 106–117.

United Nations Millennium Development Goals Report. (2008). Goal 4: Reduce child mortality fact sheet. Accessed May 22, 2010, from http://www.un.org/millenniumgoals/2008highlevel/pdf/newsroom/Goal%204%20FINAL.pdf.

Vennemann, M., Bajanowski, T., Brinkmann, B., Jorch, G., Yücesan, K., Mitchell, E.A.; GeSID Study Group. (2009). Does breastfeeding reduce the risk of sudden infant death syndrome? *Pediatrics, 123*(3), e406–e410.

SUGGESTED READINGS

A Science-Based Framework for Early Childhood Policy: Using Evidence to Improve Outcomes in Learning, Behavior, and Health for Vulnerable Children. National Scientific Council on the Developing Child. Harvard University. (2009). Retrieved May 11, 2009, from http://www.developingchild.harvard.edu/content/downloads/Policy_Framework.pdf.

American Academy of Pediatrics. (2009). Car safety seats check up. Retrieved May 13, 2009, from http://www.aap.org/publiced/br_carseatcheckup.htm.

American Academy of Pediatrics. (2009). Car safety seats: A guide for families 2009. Retrieved May 4, 2009, from http://www.aap.org/family/Carseatguide.htm.

American Academy of Pediatrics. (2009). Tips for a Healthier New Year. Retrieved May 13, 2009, from http://www.aap.org/advocacy/releases/jantips.cfm.

Bailey, G. (2004). Your infant's visual development. Retrieved May 13, 2009, from www.allaboutvision.com/parents/infants.htm.

Barrett, S. (2009). Dietary Guidelines for infants. Retrieved April 2, 2009, from http://www.quackwatch.org/03HealthPromotion/dgi.html.

Blood-Siegfried, J., Rambaud, C., Nyska, A., & Germolec, D. R. (2008). Evidence for infection, inflammation and shock in sudden infant death: Parallels between a neonatal rat model of sudden death and infants who died of sudden infant death syndrome. *Innate Immunity, 14*(3), 145–152.

Bolton, T. A., Chow, T., Benton, P. A., & Olson, B. H. (2009). Characteristics associated with longer breastfeeding duration: An analysis of a peer counseling support program. *Journal of Human Lactation, 25*(1), 18–27.

Chase, J. D. (2009). Baby talk: Infant language development starts in the womb. *About.com.* Retrieved May 10, 2009, from http://babyparenting.about.com/od/childdevelopment/a/babytalk.htm.

Children's nutrition: 20 tips for picky eaters. Is your child a picky eater? Use these practical tips to avoid mealtime battles. (2009). *MayoClinic.com.* Retrieved May 10, 2009, from http://www.mayoclinic.com/print/childrens-health/HQ01107/.

Consumer Reports. (2009). *Pacifiers: The good and bad news.* Retrieved May 13, 2009, from http://blogs.consumerreports.org/baby/2009/04/pacifiers-and-teeth-breastfeeding-breastfed-babies.html.

Courage, M., & Cowan, N. (Eds.). (2008). *The development of memory in infancy and childhood.* London: Psychology Press.

Dental Health Center 101. (2009). All about fluoride. Retrieved May 13, 2009, from http://www.everydayhealth.com/dental-health/101/all-about-fluoride.aspx.

Dewey, K. G. (2009). Infant feeding and growth. *Advances in Experimental Medicine and Biology, 639,* 57–66.

First connections with families. (2009). Birth to 18 months. Retrieved May 13, 2009, from http://www.nde.state.ne.us/ech/fcwf/Birthto18months.pdf.

McKenna, K. M., & Shankar, R. T. (2009). The practice of prelacteal feeding to newborns among Hindu and Muslim families. *Journal of Midwifery and Women's Health, 54*(1), 78–81.

Ozanne, S.E. (2009). The long term effects of early postnatal diet on adult health. *Advances in Experimental Medicine and Biology, 639,* 135–144.

Perez-Escamilla, R. (2007). Evidence based breast-feeding promotion: The baby-friendly hospital initiative. *Journal of Nutrition, 137,* 484–487.

Porter, P., & Collins, G. M. (Eds.). (2008). Ciba Foundation Symposium 89: Temperamental differences in infants and young children. *Novartis Foundation Symposia.*

Rovee-Collier, R. (2007). Infant learning and memory. In G. Bremner & A. Fogel, *Blackwell handbook of infant development.* Boston: Blackwell Publishing.

Shealy, K. R., Scanlon, K. S., Labiner-Wolfe, J., Fein, S. B., & Grummer-Strawn, L. M. (2008). Characteristics of breastfeeding practices among U.S. mothers. *Pediatrics, 122,* S50–S55.

Sices, L., Drotar, D., Keilman, A., Kirchner, H. L., Roberts, D., & Stancin, T. (2008). Communication about child development during well-child visits: Impact of parents' evaluation of developmental status screener with or without an informational video. *Pediatrics, 122*(5), e1091–e1099.

Spruyt, K., Aitken, R. J., So, K., Charlton, M., Adamson, T. M., & Horne, R. S. (2008). Relationship between sleep/wake patterns, temperament and overall development in term infants over the first year of life. *Early Human Development, 84*(5), 289–296.

Stark, R. E. (2006). Infant vocalization: A comprehensive view. *Infant Mental Health Journal,* 2(2), 118–128.

Szucs, K. A., Axline, S. E., & Rosenman, M. B. (2009). Quintuplets and a mother's determination to provide human milk: It takes a village to raise a baby—how about five? *Journal of Human Lactation,* 25(1), 79–84.

Ward Platt, M. P. (2009). Demand weaning: Infants' answer to professionals' dilemmas. *Archives of Disease in Childhood, 94*(2), 79–80.

Wojcik, K. Y., Rechtman, D. J., Lee, M. L., Montoya, A., & Medo, E. T. (2009). Macronutrient analysis of a nationwide sample of donor breast milk. *Journal of the American Dietetic Association, 109*(1), 137–140.

World Health Organization. (2009). Model chapter for textbooks for medical students and allied professionals. In *Infant and young child feeding.* Retrieved May 10, 2009, from http://whqlibdoc.who.int/publications/2009/9789241597494_eng.pdf.

Yew, K. S., Webber, B., Hodges, J., & Carter, N. J. (2009). Clinical inquiries: Are there any known health risks to early introduction of solids to an infant's diet? *Journal of Family Practice, 58*(4), 219–220.

Zeisel, S. H. (2009). Is maternal diet supplementation beneficial? Optimal development of infant depends on mother's diet. *American Journal of Clinical Nutrition, 89*(2), 685S–687S.

RESOURCES

Refer to the online student StudyWARE for Potts & Mandleco at http://www.CengageBrain.com for additional content and study aids.

Organization: **American Academy of Pediatrics**
Description: Offers general information related to child health, specific guidelines concerning many pediatric issues, information regarding AAP programs, activities, policies, guidelines, publications, and other child health resources.
Website/Resource: http://www.aap.org

Organization: **Consumer Product Safety Commission**
Description: Charged with protecting public from unreasonable risks of serious injury/death from consumer products; offers information about consumer safely/business regulations; access to library.
Website/Resource: http://www.cpsc.gov

Organization: **Guide to Teething Parenting.com**
Description: Articles published in Parenting Magazine discusses the basics of teething in young children and provides a developmental timetable.
Website/Resource: http://www.parenting.com/article/Baby/Health/Teething

Organization: **Healthy Living Newsletter**
Description: The Health Living Newsletter is distributed by Health Net Federal Services.
Website/Resource: https://www.hnfs.net

Organization: **I Am Your Child**
Description: Raises awareness about the importance the prenatal period through the first early years plays in a child's healthy brain development; offers access to product information and an online store.
Website/Resource: http://www.iamyourchild.org

Organization: **National Association of Neonatal Nurses (NANN)**
Description: Offers information regarding education/jobs, meetings, publications, and membership as well as access to an online store.
Website/Resource: http://www.nann.org

Organization: **National Association of Pediatric Nurse Associates and Practitioners (NAPNAP)**
Description: Offers information regarding NAPNAP's mission/efforts, upcoming events, associated programs, and access to NAPNAP's online store.
Website/Resource: http://www.napnap.org

Organization: **National Network for Child Care (NNCC)**
Description: Offers information about child care, access to KIDCARE (email list allowing individuals to communicate with others concerned about child care), person-to-person contact with experts in child care, and access to newsletter.
Website/Resource: http://www.nncc.org

Organization: **National Sudden Infant Death Syndrome Resource Center**
Description: Offers information regarding helpful topics, contacts, FAQs, links and publications related to sudden infant death syndrome.
Website/Resource: http://www.sidscenter.org

Organization: **The Shaken Baby Alliance**
Description: Offers information regarding family/professional support, prevention/awareness, and products related to shaken baby syndrome.
Website/Resource: http://www.shakenbaby.com

Organization: **Vaccine Information Statements**
Description: Provides instructions for statement use as well as CDC information sheets explaining to vaccine recipients/parents/legal representatives the benefits and risks of a vaccine.
Website/Resource: http://www.cdc.gov/vaccines/pubs/vis/default.htm

Organization: **Vision Development: Milestone in Vision Development**
Description: This article was written by Troy Bedinghaus O.D. It discusses normal child visiondevelopment and five important milestones.
Website/Resource: http://vision.about.com/od/childrensvision/tp/vision_develop.htm

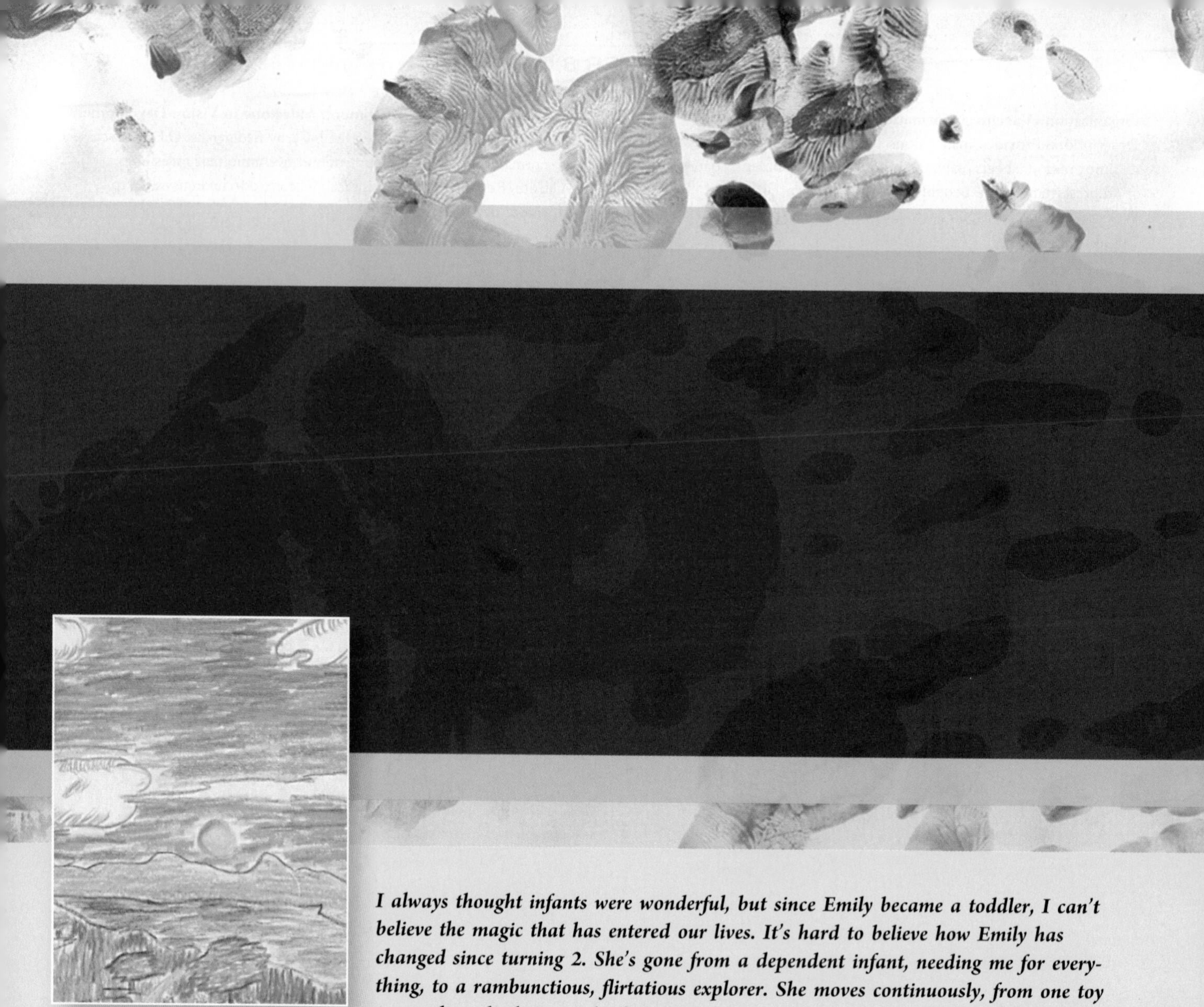

I always thought infants were wonderful, but since Emily became a toddler, I can't believe the magic that has entered our lives. It's hard to believe how Emily has changed since turning 2. She's gone from a dependent infant, needing me for everything, to a rambunctious, flirtatious explorer. She moves continuously, from one toy to another, climbing on the furniture, trying to do and be everything. I can hardly keep up with her! She's independent and wanting to do things her way one minute, clinging to me the next.

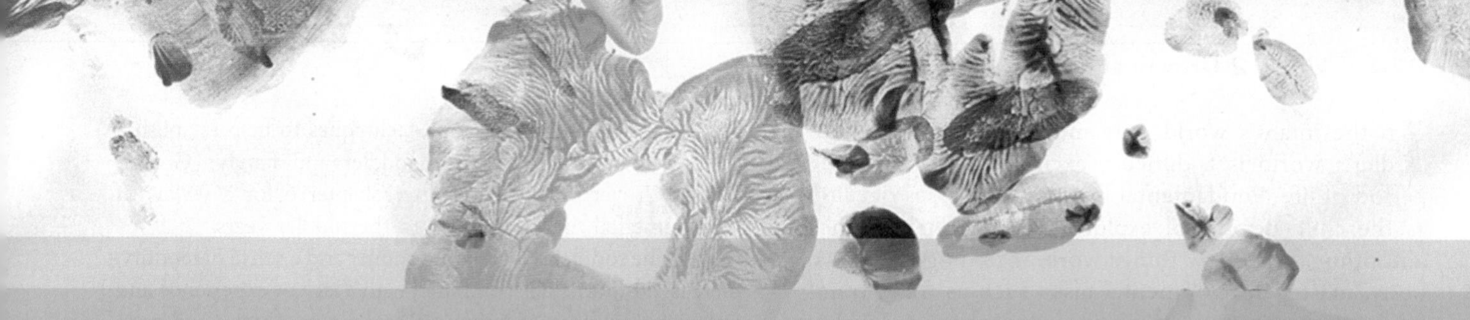

CHAPTER 9
Growth and Development of the Toddler

DEBRA ANN MILLS, RN, MS
BARBARA C. WOODRING, RN, EdD

COMPETENCIES

Upon completion of this chapter, the reader will be able to:

- Discuss the developmental changes of the toddler: physiological, psychosexual, psychosocial, cognitive, and moral.
- Apply the various aspects of a toddler's development to nursing interventions.
- Apply interventions for temper tantrums, negativism, regression, and ritualism to practice.
- Promote strategies caregivers can use when developing a disciplinary plan.
- Discuss sibling rivalry and apply appropriate interventions to practice.
- Assess physiological and psychosocial signs of readiness for toilet training and apply that information to practice.
- Develop strategies for health promotion, including play, nutrition, sleep, safety, development, and dental hygiene.
- Evaluate the impact of social, economic, and cultural factors that impact health promotion and developmental perspectives of the toddler.
- Successfully complete the games and activities in the online student StudyWARE.

In the infant's world only months before, the toddler's world is a difficult, exciting, and interesting period of life. Fundamental learning processes develop as the child begins to: explore the world, experience autonomy, learn how things work, including their own body, master developmental tasks such as toilet training, tolerate limitations, express desires, and develop relationships. The toddler's excitement and frustration make this a period of incredible challenge for caregivers and health care providers alike.

Toddlerhood is the magical time of childhood encompassing the tumultuous twos and the terrific threes. This 24-month-span (12–36 months of age) reflects periods of rapid, unprecedented maturation, and change in the life of the child and family. The toddler evolves from a dependent infant, with limited mobility and communication skills, into a more independent, very mobile, verbal, and inquisitive member of the family (Figure 9-1).

Promoting toddler health and maintaining wellness involve knowledge of normal growth and developmental processes. These include the impact of genetic and cultural factors, an understanding of common significant milestones, the ability to anticipate deviations that may occur within the individual child, and awareness of health surveillance and screening. Knowledge of concepts and theories that support toddler development is very important. It is also important to use therapeutic communication techniques to help establish a trusting relationship with the toddler and family (Grover, 2008a; Grover, 2008b). Refer to Chapter 6 for a review of developmental theories related to the toddler years.

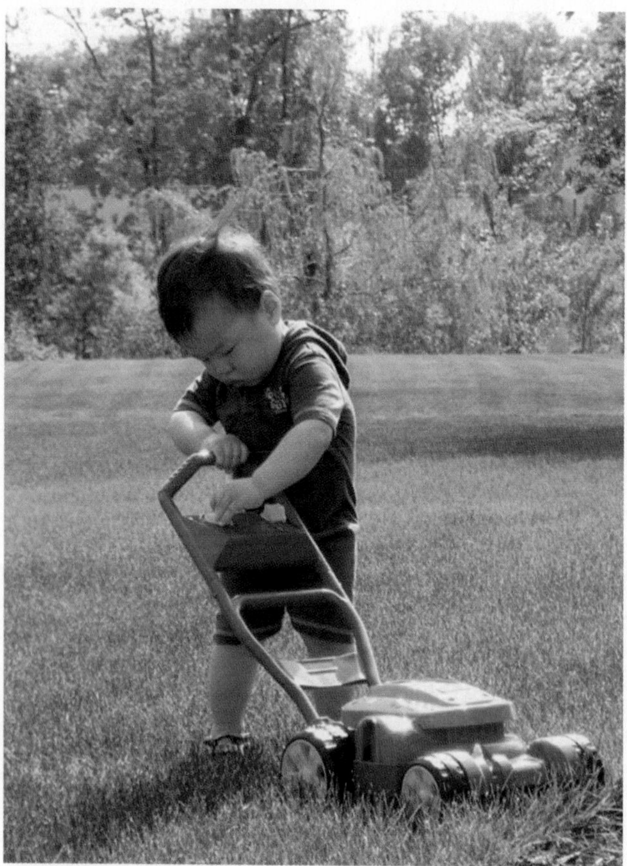

FIGURE 9-1 **This toddler is learning about cutting the grass with his lawnmower.** DELMAR CENGAGE LEARNING.

As the toddler develops autonomy and a sense of identity, increased motor skills combined with a lack of experience and judgment can present innumerable dangers. Nurses and caregivers, therefore, need to utilize strategies to promote and assist the toddler's mastery of major developmental skills. They must also protect the child from environmental dangers, provide structured guidelines and loving discipline, and promote a sense of independence and inquisitiveness.

Toddler physiological, psychosexual, psychosocial, cognitive, and moral development will be discussed in the following pages. It is always important to remember, however, that development in each area significantly impacts overall growth, development, and maturation, and no area of development can be viewed in isolation. Information about issues commonly arising during the toddler stage will also be presented.

PHYSIOLOGICAL DEVELOPMENT

The physical changes of toddlerhood occur in a fairly predictable manner; however, no child can be held to a rigid time frame as to when those milestones will be reached. While some children initially direct their energy toward accomplishing motor activities first, others initially concentrate on verbal mastery. Generally, this does not mean one toddler is advanced and another delayed, but rather it means both will accomplish desired developmental tasks within a normal range of time, but at their own pace. It is important to provide caregivers with information to help them understand and anticipate developmental sequences. It is also essential, however, that they realize the information provides flexible guidelines rather than hard and fast rules.

Physical growth, so rapid in infancy, slows during toddlerhood; on the other hand, the toddler should show a steady increase in growth, with an average weight gain of about 5 pounds per year and an increase in height averaging 3 inches per year. This slowed growth rate is evidenced by the toddler's decline in appetite and erratic eating habits.

EYE ON...

Health care providers also need to be sensitive to cultural and ethnic variations when comparing children to pre-established norms. For instance, attention should be given to the height and weight assessment of Asian children. A single evaluation of a child of Asian ancestry, compared to standard U.S. Caucasian norms, may lead to an inaccurate judgment that the child is short in stature or malnourished for age, when actually this should be attributed to genetic makeup.

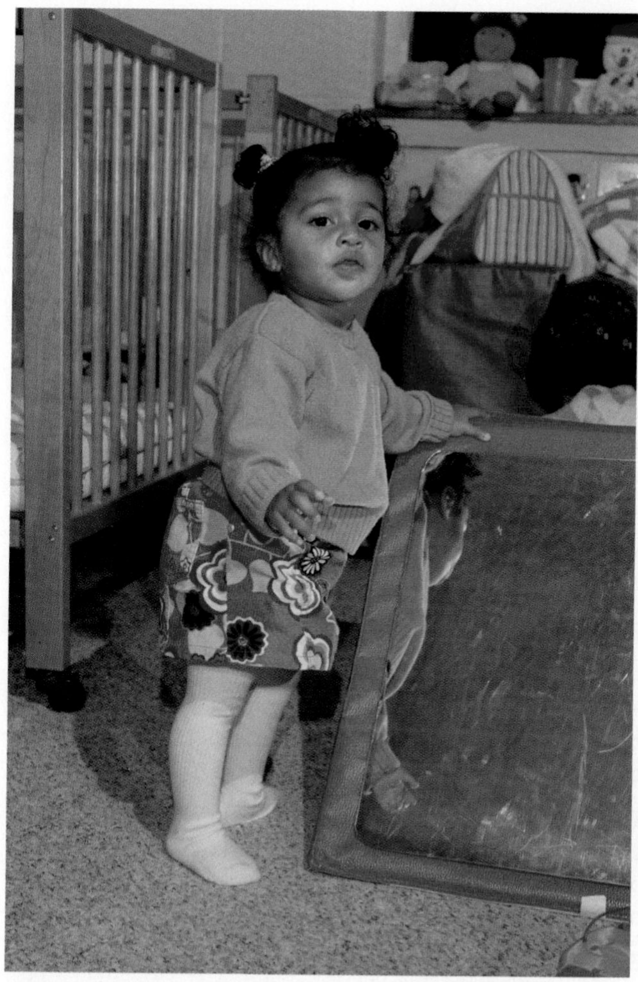

FIGURE 9-2 Balance and coordination develop as the toddler's neurological and musculoskeletal systems mature. DELMAR CENGAGE LEARNING.

Physical appearance also changes markedly. The head gains a more proportional dimension to the rest of the body, reflecting slower brain growth, as the extremities lengthen (refer to Figure 9-2). Chest circumference increases and soon exceeds the abdominal girth; the top-heavy, wide base (feet spread) pot-bellied stance and toddling gait of young toddlers eventually gives way to a well-balanced appearance and gait as bones lengthen and strengthen and abdominal muscle replaces adipose tissue. Children learn to walk at various ages, with some beginning as early as 9–12 months; however, most toddlers are walking by 15 months and climbing stairs by 18 months—and spending a great deal of time perfecting their efforts, compelled to repeat the process over and over again until the skill is mastered.

NEUROLOGICAL SYSTEM

The toddler engages in many behaviors reflecting central and peripheral nervous system maturation. Brain growth continues slowly, corresponding to advancing intellectual skills and fine motor development by 2 years. Improved coordination and

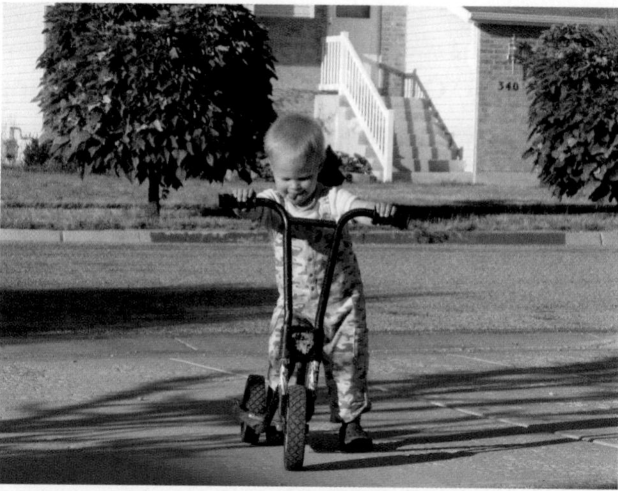

FIGURE 9-3 This toddler is learning to ride a scooter. However, because his balance and coordination are not yet mature, he will need close adult supervision as well as safety devices, such as a helmet and knee pads. DELMAR CENGAGE LEARNING.

equilibrium parallels the almost complete myelinization of the spinal cord as evidenced by the toddler's refined skill in walking, jumping, and climbing (Figure 9-3).

Increasing eye-hand coordination, manual dexterity, and walking and running skills contribute significantly to the toddler's locomotion and socialization. These skills promote throwing and retrieving a variety of objects, opening and closing containers with lids, and building objects with blocks before knocking them down (Figure 9-4). The neurophysiological

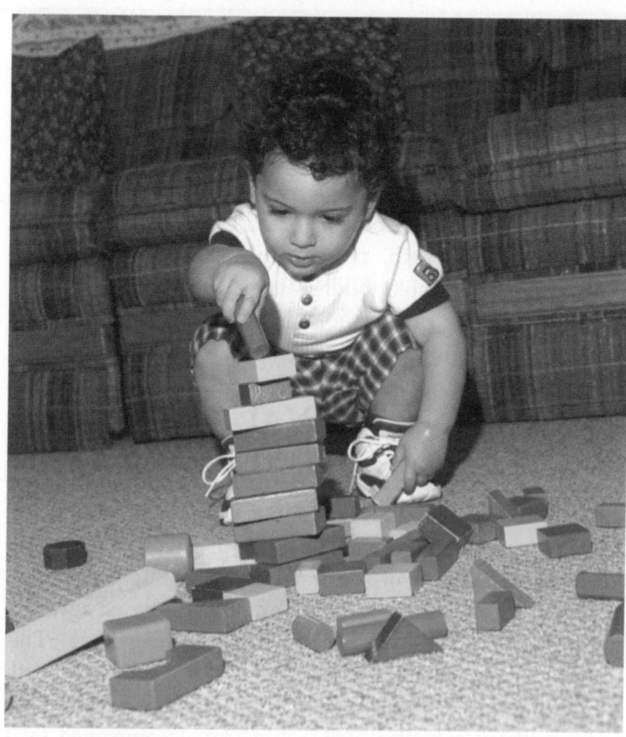

FIGURE 9-4 Increased eye-hand coordination and fine motor development allow the toddler to arrange and stack blocks. DELMAR CENGAGE LEARNING.

TABLE 9-1 Overview of Neurological Changes of Toddlerhood

SIGNIFICANT CHANGES	NURSING OR CAREGIVER IMPLICATIONS
Anterior cranial fontanel closes at approximately the time of cord myelinization (12–18 months).	Be alert for premature closure as it can impinge on brain growth and function. Prior to closure, a bulging fontanel indicates increased intracranial pressure; sunken fontanel indicates dehydration.
Brain growth continues, reaching 80%–90% of adult size by 3 years.	Increasing head circumference is stimulated by brain growth; small circumference may suggest growth abnormalities, which place child at risk for developmental delay; enlarged circumference may indicate genetic syndromes, hydrocephalus, or familial characteristics.
Cognitive development is demonstrated by rapidly expanding vocabulary.	The child begins toddlerhood with a vocabulary of a few words and, by 3 years, uses 300–900 words and two-or three-word phrases.
Control gained over most reflex activity.	Persistence of primitive reflexes may suggest defective cortical development.
Head circumference should approximate chest circumference, with chest enlarging more rapidly after 24 months.	Head circumference should increase 1 inch (2.5 cm) or less per year until school age. Always measure head using a paper tape measure placed 1 inch above top of the ears.
Myelinization completed around 24 months of age.	The child is not able to walk well until myelinization has been completed. Walking well is an indication that myelinization has occurred and the child is physiologically capable of bladder and bowel control.
Spinal cord and vertebral column grow at variable rates.	Be alert for positioning the toddler for lumbar punctures.

changes that have the greatest impact upon family and child education and suggested nursing interventions are listed in Table 9-1.

MUSCULOSKELETAL SYSTEM

Increased bone length, muscle maturation, and increased muscle strength enable toddlers to develop autonomy. Major advances occurring in the musculoskeletal system during toddlerhood are reflected in Table 9-2.

GASTROINTESTINAL AND GENITOURINARY SYSTEMS

The gastrointestinal and genitourinary systems continue to mature during these years. The stomach enlarges in size, allowing consumption of the traditional 3 meals per day, all deciduous teeth generally erupt by 30 months of age, and improved eye-hand coordination enables self-feeding. This would seem to set the perfect scenario for a toddler growth spurt; however, this does not generally occur. Instead, the toddler enjoys a gradual increase in size, accompanied by a decreased appetite and a ritualistic interest in limited types of food. Toddlers also vary in their energy requirements, eating large amounts of food one day and very little food the next. Food likes and dislikes also differ from day to day. This period of decreased appetite as a result of decreased caloric need is often referred to as a time of **physiologic anorexia**. Parents may need reassurance that this is normal.

Even though caloric needs diminish during this time, protein requirements, though less, remain higher than for other age groups. Vitamin and mineral requirements—particularly calcium, phosphorous, and iron (essential for bone and muscle growth)—increase slightly. This can create concern since the eating patterns and behaviors often consist of food fads and decreased food intake. Measures should be taken to help reduce the amount of fat in the toddler's diet by providing low-fat meats and limiting foods that are high in salt and other additives. It is also important to advise parents to offer nutritious foods during mealtimes as well as for snacks. This issue is especially important with the explosion of data related to childhood obesity and the link to health concerns such as diabetes and hypertension (see Research Highlight). Toddlerhood is an opportune time to develop healthy eating habits as well as including daily physical activities (Refer to Figure 9-5).

Bladder and bowel control is typically achieved during this time period, and children are able to retain urine up to 4 hours before needing to void. Specific gastrointestinal and genitourinary changes that can be expected and accompanying nursing interventions are found in Table 9-3.

TABLE 9-2 Overview of Musculoskeletal Changes of Toddlerhood

SPECIFIC CHANGES	NURSING OR CAREGIVER IMPLICATIONS
Bone length increases due to ossification and long bone growth.	Gains 4–6 inches (10–12 cm) in height per year until school-age.
• By 36 months, children at the 50th percentile for height should be 38 inches (97 cm) tall	• Deviations may indicate endocrine or hormonal abnormalities
Pot-belly appearance is generally due to weak abdominal musculature.	Poor nutritional intake or constipation can also create pot-bellied appearance; assess carefully to ascertain cause.
Between 12–18 Months	
• Increases ability and steadiness of gait from taking a few steps with support to navigating stairs	• Consider safety issues with increased mobility (falls on stairs or onto furniture with sharp edges)
• Finger dexterity and coordination improve to enable: turning of pages, removing shoes and socks, pulling of toys, zipping zippers, stacking up to four blocks	• Select toys and activities that encourage fine and gross motor development (finger foods, activity books, blocks), but remain alert for choking risks from toys and household items
Between 19–30 Months	
• Climbs stairs alone (places both feet on one step before going to next)	• Encourage use of handrail for safety
• Kicks ball forward without losing balance	• Begin teaching basic safety rules (stop and look both ways before crossing street)
• Rides tricycle	• Encourage to wear helmet
• Holds crayons with fingers, not fist; turns door knobs, brushes teeth	• Encourage interest in pictures and drawing (is able to copy horizontal and vertical lines)
• Binocular vision developed	
• Dresses self with supervision (manages buttons and snaps, but not shoes)	
By 36 months, large and small muscle groups enlarge and physically observable actions are refined.	

CARDIORESPIRATORY SYSTEM

During toddlerhood, the cardiorespiratory system continues to mature; vital signs become less variable and move closer to adult norms. Respiratory and cardiac rates slow, while blood pressure rises. Other significant factors related to cardiopulmonary assessment can be found in Table 9-4.

SENSORY SYSTEM

In addition to the physiologic changes noted in Tables 9-1 to 9-4, the senses of hearing, smell, taste, touch, and vision develop and begin to connect, as toddlers utilize all five senses to explore the world and exert autonomy and independence. Caregivers and health care providers need to be aware of behaviors reflecting hearing and vision difficulties such as failure to develop language, unusual responses to loud sounds, or increased falls. Baseline hearing and vision screening should be performed during toddlerhood and appropriate strategies begun immediately, if necessary (Grover, 2008c). Refer to Chapter 31 for more information.

Toddler vision should range from 20/20 to 20/40, with full binocular capabilities reached shortly after 12 months of age. Depth perception continues to develop throughout the toddler years. Developing depth perception, combined with inquisitiveness, poor judgment, and occasional lack of coordination, puts the toddler at risk for frequent falls when learning to walk, run, and climb.

PSYCHOSEXUAL DEVELOPMENT

Attitudes related to gender identity, sex roles, and sexuality are mostly determined by the values and morals of the caregiver and the environment. Toddlers are generally able to recognize gender differences by 2 years of age and begin to explore and recognize body parts, most often during toilet training.

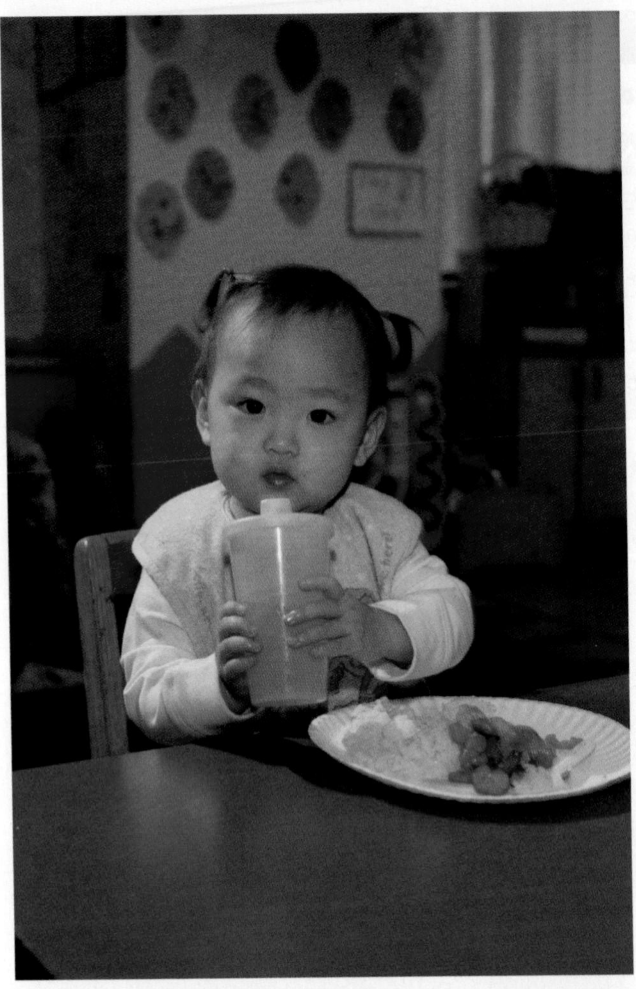

FIGURE 9-5 **This toddler's improved motor development and coordination make it possible for her to hold her own cup and feed herself.** DELMAR CENGAGE LEARNING.

According to Freud (1957), toddlers are in the anal stage of development (refer to Chapter 6 for more information on Freud). Freud also first pointed out the tension revolving around toddler bowel and bladder training, and viewed toilet training as a possible way of resolving conflict and handling stress. He believed improperly managed toilet training could lead to lifelong psychological trauma with accompanying physical bowel and bladder responses (Freud, 1957).

Many thoughts and activities of both the caregiver and the toddler tend to be focused on toilet training and, because of the close proximity of the genitalia to the urinary and anal orifices, toddlers tend to manually manipulate and inspect these areas. Masturbation is common and should be handled in a matter-of-fact-manner, thereby lessening the child's anxiety and feelings of shame. The inquisitive nature of toddlers, combined with their need to explore, the concept of object permanence, and the desire to know about their bodies influences toddler behaviors related to toileting (AAP, 2010c).

Domestic mimicry, or imitation of domestic or role activity, is one way toddlers express their understanding of gender roles. For example, in imaginative play, the child takes the role of "mommy," "daddy," or "baby." Caregiver responses to boys playing with dolls or cooking in the play kitchen, and girls taking a truck apart or building houses in the mud, can influence later role-related thinking patterns and experiences (Figure 9-6).

In a similar fashion, the caregiver's response to the toddler's sexually related actions and questions can influence future sexual attitudes. Therefore, the caregiver needs to clarify what the child really wants to know before beginning detailed explanations. For example, when the 2½-year-old asks, "Where does baby come from?" the child may really want to know that the baby *doll* was a gift from Aunt Barb, not the physiological process of reproduction.

TABLE 9-3 Overview of Gastrointestinal and Genitourinary Changes of Toddlerhood

SPECIFIC CHANGES	NURSING OR CAREGIVER IMPLICATIONS
Increased eye coordination: grasps spoon (15 months), drinks from cup without spilling (18 months).	Encourage self-feeding. Finger foods and appropriately shaped cups and utensils are important to foster independence and dexterity.
Gains 4–6 lbs (1.8-2.5 kg) per year, average weight by 3 years = 30–32 lbs (14–15 kg)	Need for protein and calorie intake remains high; toddler needs 1,000–1,500 kcal per day to support growth and 115 mL per kg of liquids per day to maintain fluid balance; weight should reveal a consistent incline on growth chart.
Slowed growth needs produce physiologic anorexia at 18 months; stomach capacity increases to allow for less frequent, larger meals.	Toddlers become "picky" eaters. Do not use food as a disciplinary tool or cookies and sweets as behavioral rewards. Do not dissolve medications in essential food or fluids (e.g., milk).
Poor eating habits and prolonged use of a bottle can create nutritional anemia and tooth decay.	Obtain an accurate food history; teach caregivers alternatives to bottle feeding, especially at bedtime (e.g., sipper cups, finger foods); expand food options; encourage child to make healthy selections as appropriate; add one new food at a time to avoid overlooking food allergies.
Primary dentition (20 deciduous teeth) is completed by 30 months.	Encourage tooth brushing after meals. Assess need for adding dietary fluoride to assure dental health if the fluoride level in the water is low.

(Continues)

TABLE 9-3 Overview of Gastrointestinal and Genitourinary Changes of Toddlerhood (*Continued*)

SPECIFIC CHANGES	NURSING OR CAREGIVER IMPLICATIONS
Sphincter control enables bladder and bowel training.	Encourage caregivers to develop realistic expectations related to potty training based on child's developmental abilities and physiologic capabilities; encourage food with high-fiber content (such as whole grain cereals, fruits, and vegetables) and adequate fruit juices and water to prevent constipation; large quantities of fruit juices, especially apple juice, can produce diarrhea.
Bladder capacity increases, to allow the retention of urine for 2–4 hours; bladder and kidneys reach near-adult functional levels at about 16–24 months, which normally coincides with the ability to walk.	Urinary output should equal or exceed 1 mL/kg/hr.
Urinary bladder is positioned higher in the abdominal cavity than in adults.	Palpate bladder between umbilicus and symphysis pubis.
Urethral structures are short (1–3 inches, versus 4 inches in adult female and 8 inches in adult male). Female toddlers are susceptible to urinary tract infections because of their short, straight urethra.	Keep perineal area clean, especially during toilet training. Begin teaching child to cleanse self from front to back; encourage child to take breaks while playing to empty bladder, which prevents incontinence and infections from urinary retention. Use plain water only to bathe toddler females.

TABLE 9-4 Overview of Cardiorespiratory Changes of Toddlerhood

SPECIFIC CHANGES	NURSING OR CAREGIVER IMPLICATIONS
Vessels are easily compressed, obliterating the pulse.	Take pulse apically for 1 full minute. Awake = 70–110; asleep = 60–100 beats/min.; respirations = 25–30 breaths/min.; blood pressure = 90/50 mm Hg.
Circulating blood volume is less than in adult.	Small blood loss, including multiple blood tests, can compromise circulating volume; hypotension is a late sign of circulatory compromise; child may remain normotensive until 25% of blood volume is lost; assess capillary refill as indicator of peripheral circulation status (should refill in 2 seconds).
Lengthening body and decreasing adipose tissues produce thinner chest wall.	Breath sounds are easily heard.
Airway is small and easily compromised.	Asthma, reactive airway, acute allergic reactions, and infectious processes may rapidly escalate into respiratory distress; observe for nasal flaring, retractions, and dyspnea.
Cough reflex remains.	Avoid suppressing cough through the use of antitussive medications.
Tracheal diameter approximates size of adult's small finger.	Toddler rapidly reacts with signs of respiratory distress with even small amounts of mucus or obstruction.
Tongue is large in proportion to the size of the mouth.	Airway may become obstructed by tongue if child seizes or loses consciousness.
Laryngeal cartilage is softer than in adults and is positioned more anteriorly.	Hyperextension of neck may occlude airway, increasing the risk of aspiration or obstruction.
Alveoli are not fully functional.	Watch for rapid onset of respiratory distress due to the tendency for bronchioles to collapse.
Ear and throat internal structures remain relatively short and straight; tonsils and adenoids are large.	Otitis media, tonsilitis, and upper respiratory infections are common.

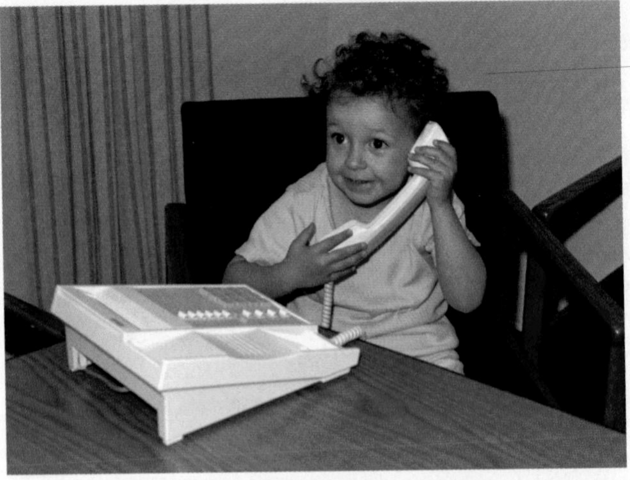

FIGURE 9-6 It is not uncommon for toddlers to mimic the behavior they observe in others. DELMAR CENGAGE LEARNING.

Since the child's gender identity is formulated during toddlerhood, continual rewards for responding in a manner consistent with a specific gender internalize that identity. Gender identity is reinforced by observing same and opposite sex caregivers enact their gender roles, attitudes, and values, and by experiencing the way adults treat children of different genders differently. Refer to the Family Teaching display for guidelines to use in assisting caregivers to encourage appropriate psychological development.

PSYCHOSOCIAL DEVELOPMENT

The major psychosocial tasks of toddlerhood are gaining self-control, developing autonomy, and increasing independence.

FAMILY TEACHING

Accomplishing Positive Psychosexual Outcomes with Toddlers

- Avoid using slang, baby talk, or confusing terms. Teach the child correct anatomical names.
- Provide positive reinforcement as the toddler experiments with various gender-related behaviors. Do not confuse the child with statements such as "big boys don't cry" or "only boys play with trucks."
- Accept manipulation of genitalia and masturbation as a natural, private behavior of toddlerhood.
- Respond to questions with age-appropriate language.
- Do not make toilet training a major confrontational issue; try to tie in educational aspects when possible (e.g., always wash hands, wipe front-to-back).

Progress toward autonomy can be judged through observing specific behaviors such as:

- Tolerating separation from caregiver (stays with sitter or in child care without prolonged crying or distress)
- Withstanding delayed gratification (waits, without a temper tantrum, until toy is removed from box to play)
- Increasing control over bowel or bladder function (maintains dryness for more than 2 hours)
- Learning to use socially acceptable behavior and language (fewer temper tantrums and biting behaviors as child progresses through toddlerhood)
- Walking well and seeking new experiences in the environment
- Interacting with others in a less id-centric or egocentric manner (shares toys more willingly as progresses through toddlerhood)

In the process of mastering self-control, autonomy, and independence, the toddler must also grapple with new, confusing, and frightening situations. The way the child responds to these situations culminates in what Erikson refers to as autonomy versus shame and doubt (Erikson, 1963). Either the child masters the situation and autonomy and self-concept are strengthened, or he is unsuccessful and doubts his abilities to succeed in such situations in the future. Several common psychosocial issues of toddlerhood are identified in Table 9-5. For more information on Erikson's theory, refer to Chapter 6.

TABLE 9-5 Psychosocial Issues

AGE	DESCRIPTION
15 months	Fears being alone, being abandoned, strangers, objects, and places. Expresses independence by trying to feed and undress self; may display temper tantrums.
18 months	Negativism predominates; sometimes fears water. Temper tantrums and awareness of own gender begins.
24 months	May resist bedtime and naps, fears the dark and animals; temper tantrums, negativism, and dawdling continue. Bedtime rituals important. Explores genitalia. Shows readiness for bowel or bladder control.
36 months	Temper tantrums, negativism, and dawdling behaviors subside; self-esteem increases due to increased independence in eating, elimination, and dressing. Explores many emotions in pretend play. Separation fears generally subside; may develop a fear of monsters.

COGNITIVE DEVELOPMENT

The social smile and babbling language of infancy give way to meaningful hand and arm gestures punctuated with rapidly increasing development of speech skills during the toddler years (Figure 9-7). Language ability develops rapidly. However, it is dependent upon physical maturity as well as environmental influences (parental encouragement and participation). In most toddlers, their comprehension of words is greater than their ability to verbalize. By 36 months of age children are able to converse and begin to acknowledge different points of view. Vocabulary expands from a few words to over 900 words in 2 short years. Speaking in short sentences, using pronouns, and understanding directional commands (Table 9-6) also occur during this time. These advancements suggest toddlers' language is more mature than their thinking processes since the meanings of all verbalizations are not always understood. Reasoning skills also remain undeveloped during this time, although an understanding of causal relationships is emerging. Guidelines to enhance communication are found in Nursing Tip: Talking with Toddlers. Refer to Chapter 31 for more information on language development.

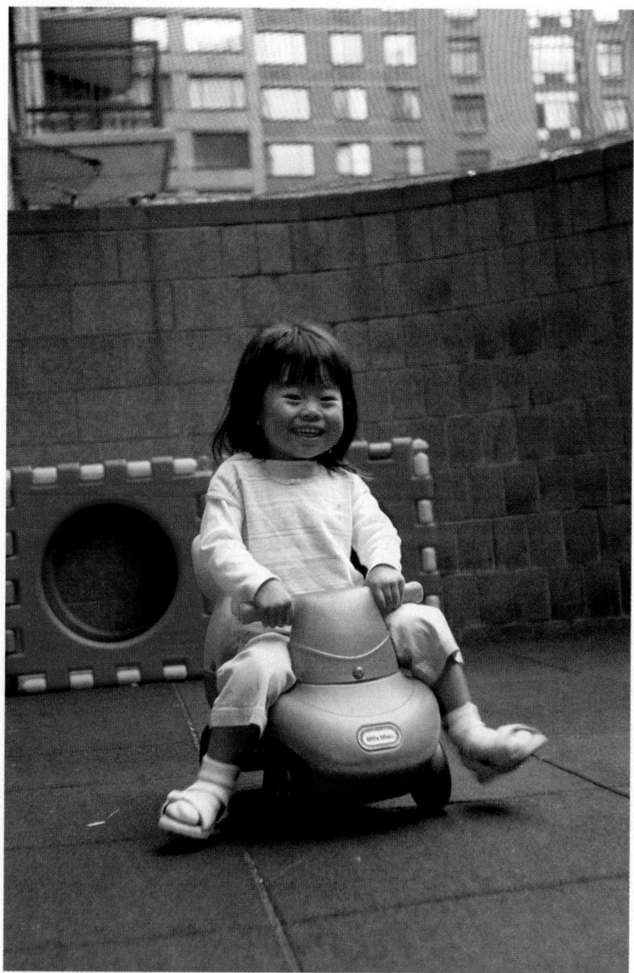

FIGURE 9-7 An engaging social smile is a hallmark of toddlerhood. DELMAR CENGAGE LEARNING.

NURSING TIP

Talking with Toddlers

- Ask family or caregiver about culturally specific terms, actions, or rituals that, if incorporated into care, would make the toddler more comfortable.
- Relate time and scheduled events to familiar occurrences (e.g., after lunch); child's attention span is not as long as older children.
- Position self at the child's eye-level before speaking; use short, specific terms the child understands; use the child's nickname or familiar name.
- Avoid use of literal terms (e.g., "cough your head off").
- Use play to gain insight and information (e.g., "if you had a wish ...").
- Set limits firmly, but gently; reward acceptable behavior (avoid using food as a reward).

TABLE 9-6 Toddler Cognitive-Communication Milestones

AGE	COGNITIVE ADVANCEMENT	COMMUNICATION PATTERNS
12–15 months	Expresses self in refined hand and arm gestures Learns by repetitive experiences and trial and error	Develops own language; speaks three to four words understood by others
18 months	Develops concept of object permanence	Speaks 10 or more words; frequently uses jargon used in home (e.g., nicknames or cultural terms)
24 months	Engages in symbolic play and domestic mimicry; egocentric thinking evident in speech and play	Uses pronouns; refers to self by name; speaks in two- to three-word sentences
36 months	States full name; names body parts	Speaks in three- to five-word sentences; uses approximately 900 different words—most understandable to others

Cognitively, toddlers are able to recognize and distinguish between shapes of objects, but they are only beginning to classify objects into categories of use. In the mind of a toddler, all objects that look alike have the same function and are therefore treated equally. For example, a pail is used to collect sand from the sandbox, hold water to scrub the floor, and hold paint. So, in the child's mind, if the toddler is allowed to overturn the pail of sand, then he or she is also allowed to overturn the water pail and the paint pail (Figure 9-8).

Piaget (1952) was concerned primarily with how knowledge is acquired and learning takes place; he systematically explained how children processed experiences and situations that touched their lives (culture, neighbors, other children, etc.). According to Piaget (1952), toddler cognitive development is broken into age-based behavioral and cognitive changes as described in Table 9-7.

MORAL DEVELOPMENT

Toddlers have little concept of right and wrong even though Kohlberg's (1976) theory of moral development could be applied to toddlers because of their willful desire to make independent decisions and their increasing cognitive capacities (refer to Chapter 6 for more information on Kohlberg). However, a child's ability to actually make moral decisions is based upon multiple cognitive and social interactions that exceed the abilities of a toddler. On the other hand, Fowler (1974) made a strong case for the consideration of early stages of faith development in this age group. Fowler defined faith as a relational phenomenon, an active relationship with another, a commitment, belief, love, and hope, which may be directed toward family, religion, God, or friends. As such, undifferentiated faith, as a foundation for other faith development, may occur as early as 2 years of age. Although religious rituals and symbols may not be understood at this time, the child does enjoy interacting with adults and children around simple religious stories.

HEALTH PROMOTION

Pediatric nurses are integral in the promotion of health and well-being of children and their families, regardless of the location of practice. Their role includes advocating for children's rights, such as access to adequate nutrition, health care, and safe living environments. The pediatric nurse's best practice for promoting health must include an awareness of the implications of culture, ethnicity, social structures, illiteracy, socio-economic factors (such as poverty

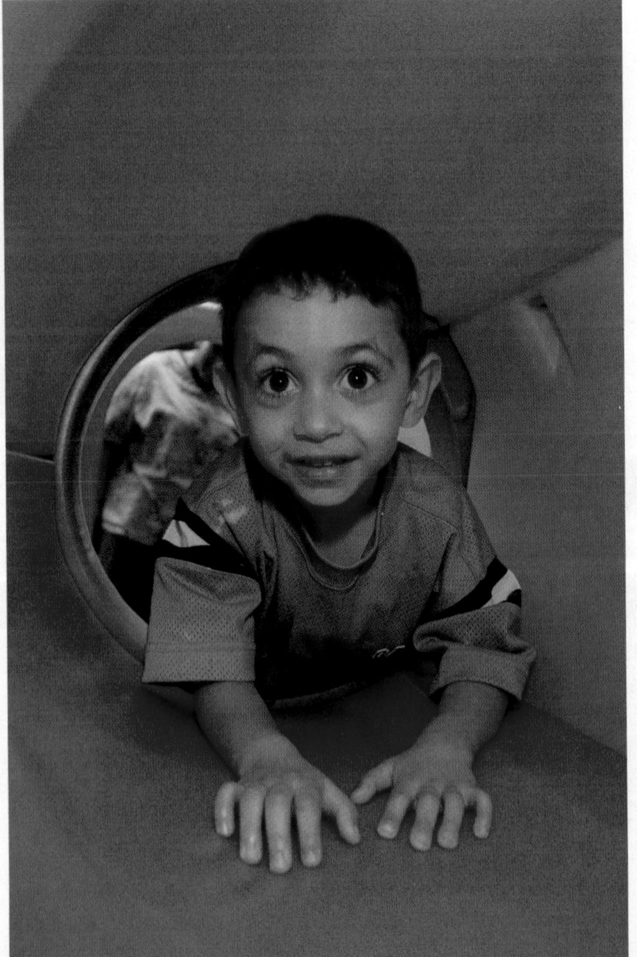

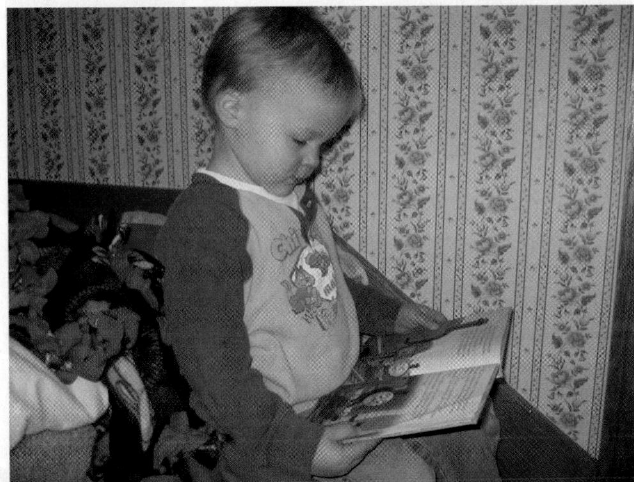

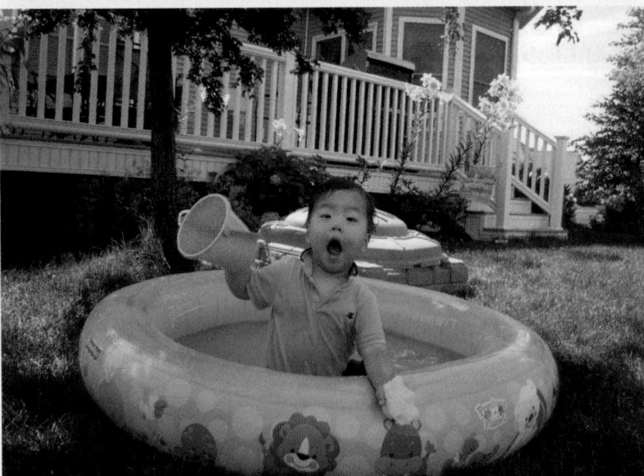

FIGURE 9-8 Toddlers need a variety of experiences to develop their cognitive and motor abilities. DELMAR CENGAGE LEARNING.

TABLE 9-7 Sensorimotor and Preconceptual Phases of Toddler Development (Piaget)

STAGE OR AGE	COGNITIVE CHANGES	BEHAVIORAL CHANGES
Sensorimotor		
Tertiary circular reactions, 15–18 months	Experiences as many new situations as possible to achieve new skills and abilities. Combines new and old knowledge to experiment and begin early reasoning. Understanding of object permanence is enhanced. Learns to differentiate self from objects. Develops awareness of spatial and causal concepts.	Inquisitive and curious about "world." Uses all senses to explore and test environment. Increases use of physical skills to increase abilities (e.g., transitions from walking to climbing to reach a higher shelf). Places items in and out of containers; recognizes items out of sight exist (box of crackers in cupboard). Is comforted by parents' voices, even if they are unseen. Extends separation time from caretakers.
Mental combinations, 18–24 months	Can infer a cause even if only experiencing the effect (threw a toy, child disciplined, and toy put out of reach). Beginning to think before acting. Imitation becomes more symbolic. Beginning sense of memory in early problem solving. Better sense of time relationships. Egocentric in actions and thinking.	Follows directions and understands requests (don't run, you will fall; put your toy here). Imitates role model's speaking (words and animal sounds). Demonstrates domestic mimicry. Uses simple words with meaning (sit, go, up, down). Engages in parallel play and senses ownership (my truck). Refers to self by name. Comfort level requires routine schedule and rituals.
Preconceptual, 2–4 years	Thoughts, play, and actions continue to be egocentric. Sense of time, space, and causality improve. Use of language as mental representation increases. Develops cognitive connection between new experience and things that occurred in the past (refuses to eat food because something before didn't taste good, "icky"). Uses trial and error learning.	Increased vocabulary with phrases of two to three words. Has difficulty sharing and is possessive of toys, family members, and other items (mine or my). Uses future oriented vocabulary terms (tomorrow). Can follow more complex directions (put this toy in the box behind you). Can put shoes on even if on wrong foot, repeats procedure again and again.

and homelessness), mass media, genetics and genomics, and health disparity. As nurses who focus their efforts on meeting the needs of children and their families, we must be aware of these factors as we provide informational and educational supports to equip caregivers so they can be as well prepared as possible to meet the mounting challenges presented by growing children. When caregivers are informed of expected growth patterns and developmental changes, they can anticipate what should come next, plan for the changes, and note quickly when the expected changes do not occur. The nurse's knowledge of health beliefs and practices, constraints, and resources may greatly impact health promotion for families that are faced with disparity concerns and should be considered when planning and implementing a nursing plan of care.

A recent patient survey found that minority patients have worse health care experiences than Caucasian patients. These racial and ethnic disparities suggest pediatric nurses in community and acute care settings should provide patient centered culturally competent nursing care that focuses on

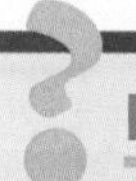

KIDS WANT TO KNOW

Cognitive Development

I babysit two little boys every Saturday. Charlie is 2 years old and his cousin Jackson is 2½ years old. Most of the time, they are pretty good, but they can't seem to play together very well. I give them each a toy and say, "Have fun"! The next thing I know, Jackson has Charlie's toy. Charlie is crying and sometimes has a red mark from being hit by Jackson. I try to make them share, but it just doesn't work. If Jackson isn't taking Charlie's toys, Charlie's taking Jackson's. I feel frustrated when this happens, and I don't know what to do!

Your feelings of frustration are not uncommon, but it might help if you know why they act this way. Toddlers live in a world of their own. They only see their side of things and don't see another person's perspective, such as sharing. Each toddler is concerned only with playing with the toy. Charlie doesn't realize that taking it away from Jackson will make him unhappy, and vice versa.

health promotion and disease prevention. These interventions need to reflect knowledge about patient beliefs and traditions related to health behaviors, particularly in regards to dietary preferences, e.g., vegetarian, vegan, and routines and preferences in accessing health care (Beller, 2005).

Parenting is a journey one is often not prepared to begin. Therefore, parents or caregivers of toddlers need preparation and patience to deal with the emotional periods their child will experience during these volatile 24 months of excitement and frustration. Gemelli (1996) has identified three essential roles for parents of toddlers:

- Protecting the toddler from experiencing too many episodes of distressing, over- or under-stimulation such as violent television shows or long periods without interaction
- Teaching the toddler how to gratify innate needs while keeping within the limits and rules set by the family and society, such as eating off of their own plate at mealtimes
- Providing empathy, encouragement, support, and love, while teaching their toddler that autonomy has limits and restrictions, such as praising the child for trying a new food item or disciplining when a disliked food item is thrown

Nurses need to provide assistance and guidance to caretakers for common issues such as nutrition, sleep, dental hygiene, safety and injury prevention, health screening, negativism, ritualism, regression, discipline, sibling rivalry, temper tantrums, toilet training, child care, and play. Each of these topics will be addressed briefly. It is important for the nurse to remember that encounters with toddlers and their families of many different racial and ethnic origins occur in all types of settings. Although some of these families may have adopted health promotion practices consistent with those of the United States, others may continue to follow ethnic and cultural traditions. Nurses can be most effective in working to promote health and maintain wellness by practicing with a multicultural perspective and considering a cultural orientation when providing support and education for the toddler and family regarding common health promotion issues.

REFLECTIVE THINKING

Access to Health Care

Children who do not have access to health care coverage often are from families where at least one parent is working. How is health promotion and disease prevention impacted? What health care risks will you anticipate for the toddler that lacks access to health care?

ROUTINE HEALTH SCREENINGS

Routine health visits to a primary health care provider begun in infancy should continue through toddlerhood. Caregivers should be encouraged to schedule well-child visits at 15, 18, 24, 30, and 36 months of age; additional visits should be made if illness occurs. The routine visits are needed for health monitoring and updating or beginning immunizations if not initiated during infancy. The American Academy of Pediatrics (2010a) has published a revised immunization schedule, which indicates toddlers need boosters of diphtheria, tetanus, and pertussis (DTaP), H. influenza (HIB), polio, and hepatitis B (if not received at 6 months of age) by 18 months of age. They also need initial doses of measles, mumps, rubella (MMR), varicella or chicken pox (Var), and hepatitis A vaccines. See Appendix C for the schedule of recommendations for all childhood immunizations. Caregivers should be encouraged to complete the initial immunization series in a timely manner to protect their child and to prevent delayed school entry.

Health screening should always include a complete physical examination (including blood pressure, height, and weight), evaluation of hemoglobin (for iron-deficiency anemia), dental evaluation, and vision and hearing assessment. The head circumference should be measured at all visits until 36 months of age. In addition, serum lead levels should be obtained in children exhibiting poor growth patterns or neurological irritability, or in those living in high-risk areas.

NUTRITION

Today nutrition is an important aspect of promoting health. Nutritional habits are influenced by ethnic and cultural traditions and backgrounds as well as economic sustainability

Reflections from Families

I am a single mother and know that I should be feeding my 2-year-old fruits and vegetables more often, but they are so expensive and I don't like very many of them myself. I decided that I needed to do a better job and have tried to buy more fresh fruits. I cut up some carrots and bananas for Sam, but he refused to eat the carrots and only a few bites of the banana. Instead he just cried and asked for "chips." I don't know what to do, should we do without something in order to buy fresh produce or should I just let him eat the snacks that he loves because they are so much cheaper? It's really hard to be healthy!

that allow access to and preparation of good foods. Statistics from national sources show an alarming increase in childhood obesity, including children from 2–5 years of age. There also continues to be significant difference in obesity according to race/ethnicity. In response *Healthy People 2010* has identified obesity as a leading health indicator (Ogden, Carroll, Curtin, McDowell, Tabak, & Flegal, 2006; U.S. Department of Health and Human Services, 2000). As nurses provide nutritional counseling it is important to teach that introduction of good eating habits and good foods, such as fresh fruits and vegetables, low-fat protein sources, and complex carbohydrates during the toddler years fosters growth and development and is instrumental in helping reduce future health risks such as anemia, nonorganic failure to thrive, dental decay, as well as obesity related health risks.

As families begin the process of transitioning infants/toddlers from high density liquids to solid food, it is important to remember that food habits and attitudes developed during toddlerhood have long lasting effects. Parents can help make mealtimes enjoyable rather than stressful by setting meal times where everyone eats together. Mealtimes continue to be messy during this age. Toddlers are still in the process of becoming proficient with a spoon and often spill. Caregivers should be encouraged to provide praise and positive reinforcement since scolding causes tension and stress. Eating habits are established in the first 2–3 years, and forcing food or creating periods of extended tension at mealtime are not healthy (Hui & Grover, 2008; Toddler Nutrition, 2009a; Toddler Nutrition 2009b).

Caregivers may need reminding that toddlers are able to chew and swallow well; their ability to use utensils improves, and they begin to develop personal preferences in food choices. Other considerations for caretakers include limiting eating fast food to less than once or twice a week, offering healthy snacks, and considering portion size and toddler preferences. Most adult food can be provided with some modifications; however, toddlers may not like a new food the first time it is introduced. Juice should be limited to 4 ounces per day, because it is a nutrient-dense food that often replaces calories that should come from more nutritious foods. Caretakers who understand these ideas will be better able to introduce new foods reflecting the child's abilities (Hui & Grover, 2008).

Caregivers tend to become concerned about the child's decreased food intake or the fact that, for weeks, the toddler may eat only cereal (or go on other food jags). Caregivers need to be assured the child will not starve and generally will eat when hungry. A general rule of thumb to use in determining adequacy in the meal is to offer 1 tablespoon of each

REFLECTIVE THINKING

Effect of Poverty on Toddler Nutrition and Development

Many children in poverty stricken families experience hunger and nutritional deficiencies. This may include Hispanic, African-American, or Caucasian toddlers who consume snacks and other foods high in carbohydrates because they can be purchased at lower cost. However the calories consumed rarely support an appropriate level of dietary energy and these children may be either overweight or underweight. What are other implications of poverty or low income on toddlers' physical, social, and psychological development? What nursing actions can be taken to help families experiencing poverty or low income to access resources that can help to provide adequate and appropriate nutrition for their toddlers and their families?

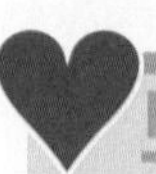

FAMILY**TEACHING**

The Picky Eater

1. Provide healthy snacks every 1–2 hours; place them where the toddler can independently reach them.
2. Plan snacks for the day; regulate their timing with meals.
3. Provide small amounts of food which can be increased upon demand.
4. Carry crackers or fruit snacks while traveling in the car.
5. Be patient, food jags will pass; the child may eat only grilled cheese sandwiches for a month, but will move on to another favorite food in time.
6. Keep distractions to a minimum; turn off the television during mealtimes.
7. Respect the child's speed of eating.
8. Encourage the child to participate in meal preparation.

If the child . . .	Offer . . .
Is not a big milk drinker and needs calcium	Yogurt, frozen yogurt, hot cocoa, pudding
Does not eat meat and needs iron	Fortified breakfast cereal (not presweetened), raisins, fortified breakfast bars, leafy green vegetables, eggs
Eats only white bread and needs more fiber	Fresh fruit and vegetables, bran muffins, bean or pea soup
Does not eat vegetables and needs vitamin A	Vegetable juice, apricots

food group for each year of age. For example, a 3-year-old would need 3 tablespoons of meat, 3 tablespoons of carbohydrate (rice or potato), 3 tablespoons of vegetable, and 3 tablespoons of fruit.

Different strategies may also be used. Offering smaller amounts of food may encourage the toddler to ask for more. For others, frequent nutritious snacks throughout the day may be more enjoyable. Nurses should also remind caretakers to acknowledge the toddler's ritualistic needs (e.g., same plate, same cup). Encouraging the toddler to explore the world of food should be accompanied by clear limits. The Family Teaching box on picky eaters provides some helpful guidelines in coping with these stressors. Many experts believe mealtime experiences and picky eating are part of the toddler's developmental process, and as such can be trying for both parents and child. Safety is another consideration for nurses and caregivers. It is important to avoid foods that may be major choking hazards (e.g., pieces of hot dogs, popcorn, nuts, hard candy) (AAP, 2009; 2010b Proper Foods and Amounts for Toddlers, 2008). Caregivers should consider the toddler's abilities by cutting food into small bits, offering dipping sauces, and serving small portions.

Although obesity is generally not noted in the average toddler, the prevalence of pediatric obesity is increasing and can originate during early childhood. The most important factor in preventing obesity is parental influences in developing food attitudes and practices as well as including physical activity in the family life. Parental strategies that set positive food consumption and activity patterns may prevent the onset of childhood obesity and the risk of both short-term and long-term health implications. Pediatric nurses

CRITICAL THINKING

To Test or Not to Test

You are the nurse working in a small Native American health clinic. Mrs. Tso and her mother Mrs. Small Bear have come to the clinic with Mrs. Tso's 18-month-old son BJ. You observe that BJ is a very round and "rolly polly" child who smiles and says several words. You know from previous visits that BJ is well above the 98th percentile for his weight on the standardized growth chart. Today you notice that his weight is even higher than before. You are aware of the national trend of increasing numbers of obese children, the significant risk for health concerns such as diabetes and hypertension, and the new cholesterol screening recommendations from the American Academy of Pediatrics (2010b).

1. **Would you consider recommending to Mrs. Tso that BJ have the cholesterol screening so medication therapy can be started?**
2. **What cultural and traditional factors influence the nutrition of Native American children and their families?**
3. **What will be your plan of care to help Mrs. Tso understand the importance of feeding her family foods lower in non-essential calories and high in nutritive value? What resources would you consider if Mrs. Tso was considered impoverished?**

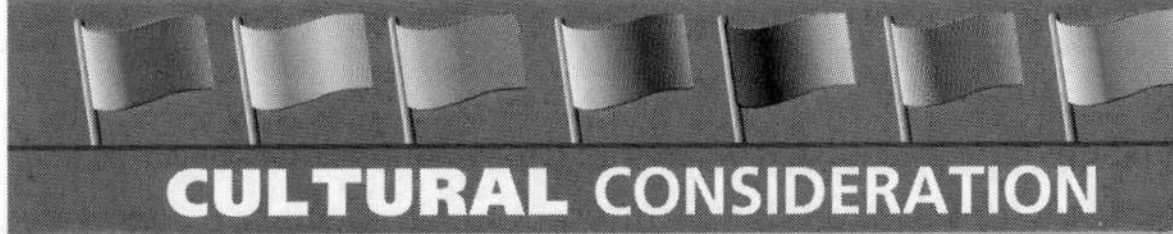

CULTURAL CONSIDERATION

Snack and Mealtime Habits of Hispanic Toddlers

Hispanic toddlers are fed on average 7 times a day, and 90% consume an afternoon snack. These afternoon snacks often contain more fiber than the snacks of non-Hispanic toddlers. Hispanic toddlers also receive lower percentages of energy from saturated fat and unsaturated fat, and consume a higher percentage of carbohydrates at lunch when compared with non-Hispanic toddlers. Compared to non-Hispanic toddlers, these children also consume less fat and saturated fat at dinnertime. Most foods consumed at snack and meal times lack whole grains, fruits, and vegetables.

Reference: Ziegler, P., Hanson, C., Ponza, M., Novak, T., & Hendricks, K. (2006). Feeding infants and toddlers study: Meal and snack intake of Hispanic and non-Hispanic infants and toddlers. *Journal of the American Dietetic Association*, *106*, S107–S123 Suppl. 1 January.

RESEARCH

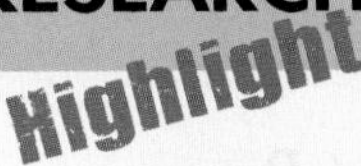

Low-Income, African-American Adolescent Mothers and Their Toddlers Exhibit Similar Dietary Variety Patterns

STUDY PURPOSE

To examine the relationship between maternal and toddler dietary choices.

METHODS

Data from this longitudinal study were collected in the homes of 100 primiparous, low-income, African-American adolescent mothers (mean age 17.5 years) and their toddlers. Data were collected when the toddler was 13 and 24 months old.

FINDINGS

Analysis indicated maternal and toddler consumption of fruits, vegetables, meats, dairy, snacks, and sodas were significantly correlated. No association was found between adolescent maternal and toddler diet choices and obesity at 24 months of age. However, adolescent mothers who purchased their own food consumed more fruits and vegetables compared to adolescent mothers who did not purchase their own food, but relied on others to purchase their food.

IMPLICATIONS

Pediatric nurses should help adolescent mothers develop the ability to shop for, select, and prepare healthy food choices for themselves and their toddlers. This is particularly important to help prevent nutritional issues such as obesity or malnutrition, which both have adverse effects on their child's growth and development.

REFERENCE

Papas, M. A., Hurley, K. M., Quigg, A. M., Oberlander, S. E., & Black, M. M. (2009). Low-Income, African American Adolescent Mothers and Their Toddlers Exhibit Similar Dietary Variety Patterns. *Journal of Nutrition Education and Behavior*, *41*, 87–94.

should recognize their role in identifying at-risk toddlers, educate parents about appropriate nutrition, and support family strategies to create an environment for food selection, quality, and quantity. It is also important for the nurse to understand what high risk factors can be modified and what cannot. For example, children of African-American and Native American descent are at higher risk for developing obesity. However, other risk factors such as low family income and maternal obesity are factors that can be addressed (Fuller, Keller, Olson, & Plymale, 2005; Ogden et al., 2006; Vaughn & Valdrop, 2007; Wofford, 2008).

Despite obesity being a major concern in children, pediatric nurses should be mindful of other considerations which may require intervention. These considerations may include: lack of access to good food due to socio-economic barriers, cultural or traditional food preferences that may lack essential nutrients or that may be related to unhealthy practices, and genetic disease-related factors such as phenylketonuria (PKU). The nurse should complete a nutritional assessment for the whole family and determine what resources or education may be needed to help establish or maintain health of the child and family.

SLEEP

Most 2-year-olds require 10-12 hours of sleep each day with a nap generally in the late morning and afternoon. Self-elimination of a second nap is a normal part of development for 2-year-olds. The toddler may also resist going into the crib at nap time or spend nap time playing in the crib. Sleep is important to re-energize the toddler and promote growth and development. Lack of sleep makes the toddler feel tired, cranky, and irritable. To help the toddler obtain adequate sleep and rest, caretakers can develop naptime and bedtime routines (Figure 9-9). Bedtime protests can be reduced by beginning a winding down period when toddlers are bathed, cuddled, and/or read to prior to being put to bed for the night. Firm consistent limits are needed when the child resists going to bed and dawdles or stalls (asking for water) (Murray, Zentner, & Yakimo, 2009).

Approximately 20%–25% of toddlers wake in the middle of the night and may have trouble returning to sleep. It is

EVIDENCE-BASED PRACTICE

Group Based Treatment Programs

CLINICAL PROBLEM

Pediatric obesity is a serious global health issue that is impacting more children 2- to 5-years old than in the past. These children are at risk for metabolic abnormalities, hypertension, type 2 diabetes, and other metabolic and cardiovascular issues if obesity persists into adulthood.

BEST CLINICAL PRACTICE

Early interventions that focus on increasing physical activity, education on nutrition, and strategies to help reduce stress and increase coping benefit children and families.

IMPLICATIONS FOR NURSING

Pediatric nurses need to track toddlers' height and weight during regular childhood health care visits. Using this data, nurses should identify those children who are obese or at risk for developing obesity. Pediatric nurses can also offer effective interventions in small group settings that can help families establish a healthy lifestyle. Topics to be considered should include physical activity, nutrition education, and strategies for coping with stress and other potential issues.

Reference: Weigel, C., Kokocinski, K., Lederer, P., Dorsch, J., Rascher, W., & Knerr, I. (2008). Childhood obesity: Concept, feasibility, and interim results of a local group-based, long-term treatment program. *Journal of Nutrition and Behavior, 40,* 369–373.

FAMILY TEACHING

Positive Mealtime Interaction

Childhood obesity has increased for children of all ethnic and cultural backgrounds, especially in low income children, and has been linked to mealtime practices. Having the TV on during toddler mealtime is associated with lower mealtime interaction. It is also noted that parents are less likely to be sitting and eating with their toddler and that the family consumes less fruits and vegetables and more snack foods such as chips and popcorn. The American Academy of Pediatrics recommends children under 2 years of age not watch TV. It is important for nurses and parents to promote positive mealtime interactions thereby also encouraging healthy food consumption.

Source: American Academy of Pediatrics—Committee of Public Education. (2001). Children, adolescents and television. *Pediatrics, 107*(2), 423–426; DiNardo, K. (2005, January 7). 15 things you must do for your baby. *USA Weekend*, p. 7, Horodynski, M. A., Strommel, M., Weatherspoon, L., & Brophy-Herb, H. (2009). Association between toddler mealtime televsion viewing, mealtime interaction, and dietary consumption in low-income Aftrican American and white families. *Journal of Nutrition Education and Behavior, 40,* S27.

NURSING TIP

Nursing Interventions to Assist in the Prevention of Obesity in Children

The following are excerpts of interventions recommended by the Society of Pediatric Nurses to address the rising national crisis of obesity, especially as seen in overweight children and adolescents:

- Identify overweight children and adolescents by screening for height, weight, skin fold, and BMI measurements while encouraging individual diversity and a positive self-image.
- Promote primary prevention through education on proper nutrition, identification of high- and low-fat and carbohydrate foods, reading food labels, appropriate portions size, and suggestions of low-fat food planning and preparation while remaining conscious of resources available to vulnerable populations.
- Encourage children and adolescents to eat only when hungry and to eat together as a family whenever possible.
- Advocate for daily physical exercise for grades K–12 with a focus on culturally appropriate and appealing activities that reflect diversity, abilities, and interests.
- Promote the reduction of sedentary time children spend in front of television, computer, or video games.
- Promote research into attitudes, beliefs, and perceptions related to exercise, eating, and excess weight in a wide range of cultural groups in order to design culturally and developmentally appropriate interventions.

Society of Pediatric Nurses. (2004a). *Position statement: Overweight children and adolescents.* Retrieved January 15, 2010, from https://www.pedsnurses.org/component/option,com_docman/task,cat_view/gid,49/.

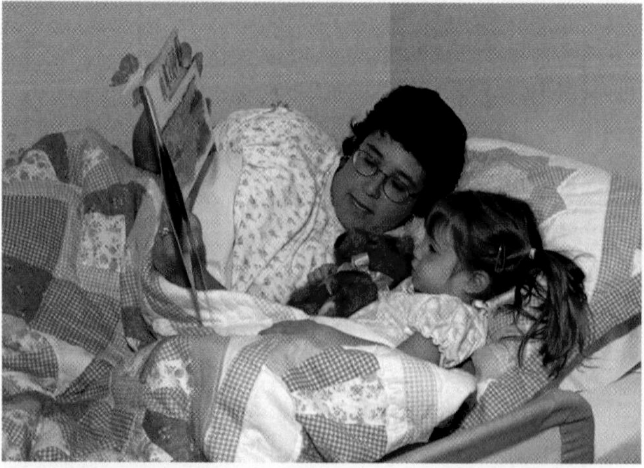

FIGURE 9-9 Nighttime rituals are especially important to toddlers. DELMAR CENGAGE LEARNING.

important to let the child cry for a short time since this assists the child to learn self-calming and comforting measures. If crying continues, caregivers can offer a hug, backrub, or drink before leaving the room again. A favorite blanket or toy coupled with a calm reassurance can also help facilitate the child's return to sleep. Nightmares are common in toddlerhood since their dreams seem very real (Grover, 2008d). The toddler will generally respond to gentle reassurances and most often return to sleep and not remember the dream the next day.

DENTAL HEALTH

In addition to routine health care visits, toddlers should also see a dentist for dental care. The presence of dental caries is a common infectious disease in children and can result in harmful consequences, including gingivitis, tooth loss, and systematic infections. Failing to seek dental health care is a common unmet health care need, often due to lack of ability to pay for the services needed and lack of trained dental personnel. Important aspects of the visit are assessment of oral health, education of caretakers regarding correct methods of dental hygiene, and counseling on strategies to prevent caries (Donahue, Waddell, Plough, del Aguila, & Garland, 2005; Lewis, 2008; Nainar & Mohummed, 2004).

Young children are unable to brush all areas of the mouth, and, as a result, caretakers will need to assume some responsibility for effective teeth cleaning (Figure 9-10). Toddlers may use only water, disliking the taste and foam of toothpaste. There is, however, some danger if fluoridated toothpaste is swallowed, so caregivers should be cautioned that, if toothpaste is used, it be used sparingly or wiped from the teeth/mouth with a clean cloth. Caregivers should select small toothbrushes that are soft with short, rounded bristles. After cleansing the teeth, flossing is recommended to remove debris below the gum line and prevent gingivitis (Lewis, 2008).

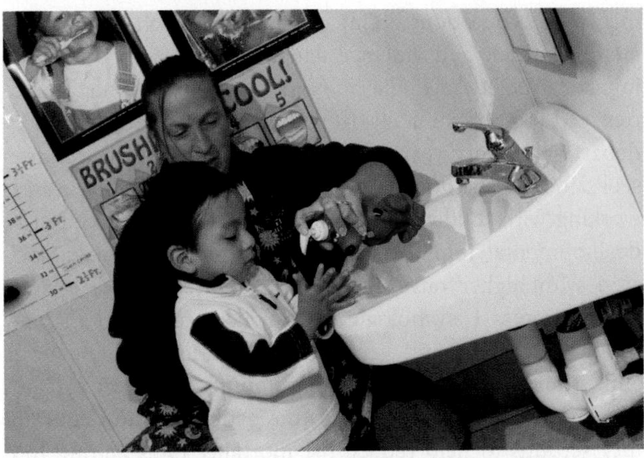

FIGURE 9-10 Toddlers need to be supervised when learning to brush their teeth and wash their hands. DELMAR CENGAGE LEARNING.

The use of fluoride is an effective method to lessen the extent of tooth decay and promote tooth health (American Academy of Pediatrics Committee on Nutrition, 1986). Tooth enamel resists developing caries when adequate amounts of fluoride are consumed before the teeth erupt. The nurse should educate caregivers regarding correct administration of fluoride supplements if fluoridation of water does not exist in the community.

Another consideration for the pediatric nurse is that children who are at low income socioeconomic levels may not have access to dental services on an ongoing annual basis. Only one in five Medicaid-eligible children has access to dental health care. These toddlers may also fail to brush their teeth daily and are more likely to consume foods high in fructose/sucrose such as sodas. This places them at greater risk for dental caries and other possible dental issues. For a nurse advocate it will be important to identify and link these families to resources that may offer no-cost or low-cost dental care as well as provide teaching about dental care. In addition, many pediatric health care providers provide dental assessments and fluoride for those having dental access care difficulties.

CULTURAL CONSIDERATION

Sleeping Traditions

For most families in Western countries an anticipated goal for parents is to have their toddler sleep in his/her own bed. However, there are many cultures that share a "family bed" with infants and small children. This can be a health concern as there is evidence that accidental asphyxia or overheating may occur. Nurses need to be aware of "sleeping traditions" and if appropriate provide education to families about the safety risk for their toddler and offer guidance if parents desire to make changes in their sleeping behaviors.

SAFETY PROMOTION AND INJURY PREVENTION

The coupling of an inquisitive mind and a tottering, but mobile body places toddlers at increased risk for injury through accidents. The types of accidents and injuries experienced are directly related to the child's developmental progression. Most injuries and deaths to toddlers are due to airway obstruction, poisonings, drowning, falls, burns, and automobiles (*Online Safety Project,* 2001). Drowning is the second most common cause of death due to unintentional injury for children ages 1–4 years (CDC, 2010). An increasing concern for nurses and families is the presence of firearms in the home. Nurses have the opportunity to incorporate questions about guns and to teach parents and children about gun violence and the prevention of firearm injuries (Society of Pediatric Nurses, 2004b). Nonfatal injuries lead to approximately 10 million visits to the emergency department every year. Each year 1 out of every 5 children seeks medical help for an injury. It is important that nurses working with toddlers and families know that in addition to developmental implications, there are other factors associated with higher rates of pediatric injuries. These include gender, stress (psychological, financial, presence of a new sibling), environment, geographical location, income level, and ethnicity. This is key in developing a plan of care for the toddler and family in both the acute care and community settings to help reduce the mortality rates among toddlers due to unintentional injuries.

Auto Safety

Motor vehicle accidents are the leading cause of death during infancy and childhood. State and federal laws related to child safety seats and seat belt use have produced a marked decrease in injuries and deaths among children; however, the laws are of little value unless caregivers follow them. Toddlers should *always* be strapped into a child-safety seat, appropriate for weight and size. The safety seat should be placed in the *back seat* of the vehicle in the middle seat if possible (Figure 9-11). Toddlers should *not* ride in the front seat of a vehicle that has an airbag. A booster seat (one without side arms) is not appropriate until a child weighs at least 30 pounds. Transition of a child from a booster seat to lap-shoulder belts should not occur until the child reaches at least 4 years of age, 85 pounds, or 4 feet tall. Toddlers should ride rear-facing for as long as possible, generally until they reach the highest weight or height allowed by the car seat's manufacturer. Nurses should review child passenger safety information with caregivers at every opportunity and remind them to be a good role model and never leave their child unattended in or around vehicles (AAP, 2010d).

Keeping toddlers from darting into streets in front of vehicles requires constant attention and repeated teaching. By 3 years of age, the child should begin to understand the concept of stopping and looking both ways before moving into a street. Even if toddlers do not understand the concept of oncoming danger, repetition of the stop–look sequence helps build the concept of safety.

Home and Environmental Safety

Homes and surrounding play areas need to be childproofed to prevent drowning, falls, and accidental poisonings. Even when caregivers make a conscious effort to protect toddlers, toddlers need to learn which things they may and may not play with in a home (Figures 9-12 and 9-13). All medications and toxic substances (e.g., gasoline, pesticides, and household cleaning products) must be kept out of the child's

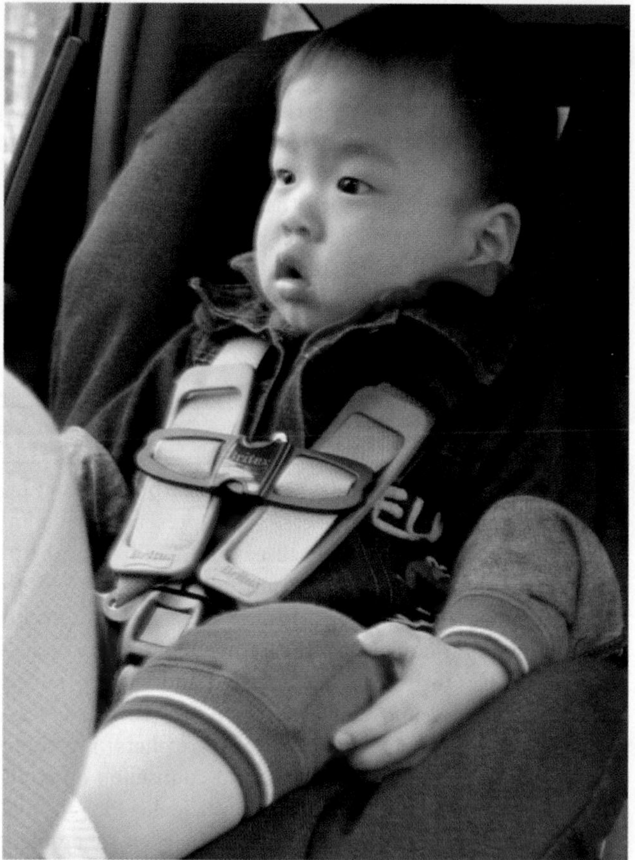

Figure 9-11 Toddlers should always be buckled into a child safety seat which is placed in the back seat of a vehicle. DELMAR CENGAGE LEARNING.

reach and preferably locked away. These items should *never* be stored in familiar containers (such as soft drink bottles) and should have a "Mr. Yuck" or similar poison alert symbol affixed. Never tell a child medication is candy to encourage taking it and never leave medications (including vitamins) sitting on tables or in the diaper bag or purse.

Water Safety

Alertness to water safety issues continues from infancy. The toddler's anatomical configuration (larger head and shorter

> **NURSING ALERT**
>
> **Common Car Seat Mistakes**
>
> - A harness is not used with car seat or harness is too loose.
> - Infant car seat is facing forward.
> - Putting a baby in a car seat that is meant for larger child.

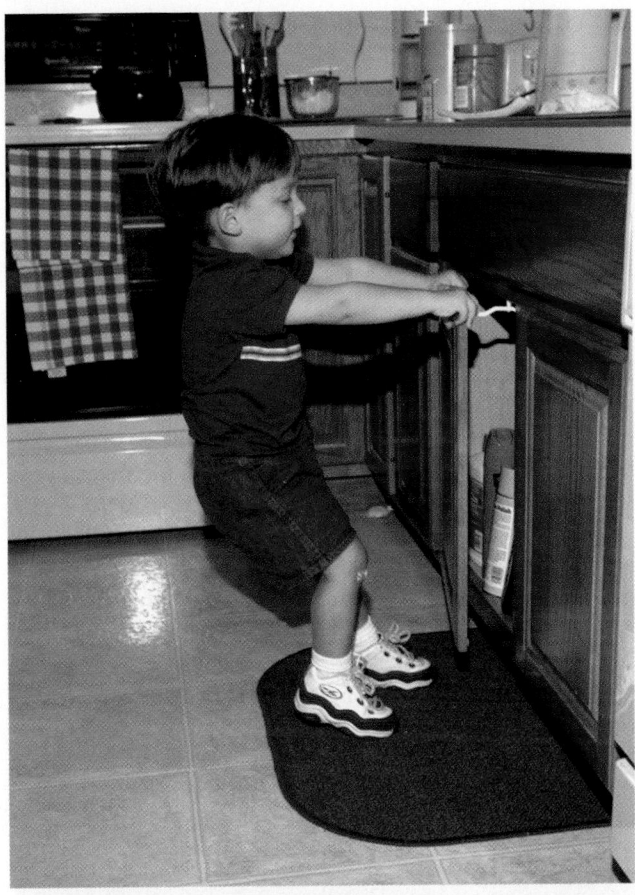

FIGURE 9-12 A toddler's curiosity may require caregivers to be sure low cabinets have a child safety lock. DELMAR CENGAGE LEARNING.

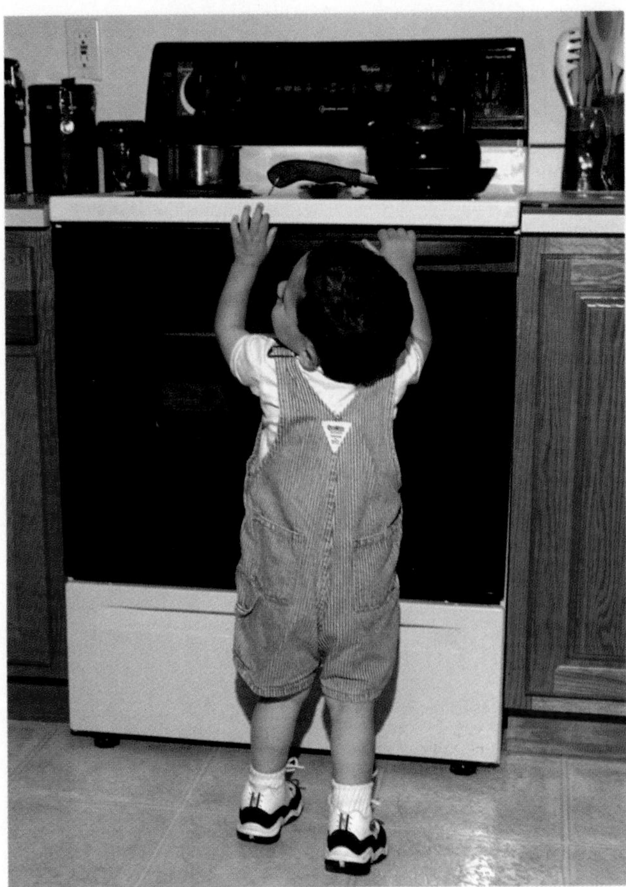

FIGURE 9-13 All homes where toddlers live or visit need to be childproofed. Be sure all pot handles are always turned away from the front of the store. DELMAR CENGAGE LEARNING.

lower extremities) creates a higher center of gravity and, when combined with an unsteady gait and insatiable curiosity, increases the risk of injury near bodies of water. The fact that a child may drown in one inch of water makes every bathtub and mud puddle a potential hazard. Therefore, a toddler should *never* be left alone in a bathtub or pool since the child's attempts to stand may result in a fall. The fall could injure bones, fracture skulls, cause unconsciousness, or precipitate drowning. Being alone in the tub may also encourage the inquisitive toddler to turn on the hot water faucet, producing scalding water burns. Therefore, the water temperature on a water heater should be turned down to 120° F. Standing water should never be left in uncovered children's pools, and a locked fence should surround larger outdoor pools and ponds. Toddlers should not be allowed to go near any standing water without adult supervision; life jackets are recommended at poolside and required whenever the toddler is on any boat.

Toy Injuries and Gun Safety

Injuries related to the toys children play with are central to toddler safety (Figure 9-14). Toys must be strong, safe, and large enough to prevent swallowing. Popped balloons are a major culprit, and for this reason, the use of latex balloons should be discouraged. Mylar, foil-type balloons are the only ones recommended as safe for young children, but should be out of reach or the child supervised if around balloons.

Another category of concern to toddler safety is gun safety. It is impossible to teach toddlers the differences between toy guns and real guns since their cognitive abilities are not well enough developed to comprehend gun safety. Therefore, if guns are in the house, they must always be kept locked away from the inquisitive toddler (Society of Pediatric Nurses, 2004b). The absence of guns from children's homes is the most reliable and effective strategy for preventing firearm incidents.

NEGATIVISM

Negativism is an expression of the toddler's constant search for autonomy. The toddler may not like being given directions and not allowed to explore what is desired in an expanding environment. Characteristically, the toddler seems to delight in doing the opposite of what is asked

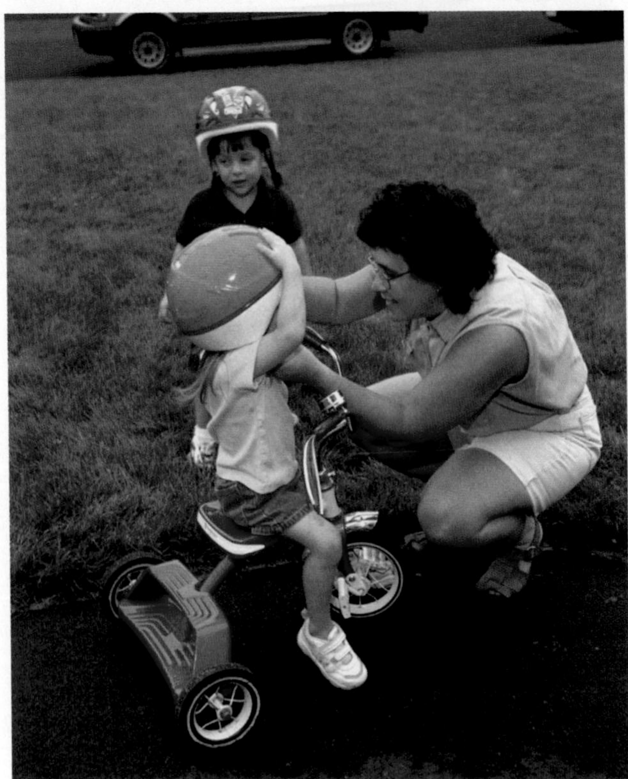

FIGURE 9-14 Even children as young as toddlers need to learn to wear helmets when riding their bicycles. DELMAR CENGAGE LEARNING.

and responding "no" to all requests, even if the child does not really mean "no." Caregivers are frequently frustrated when trying to deal with toddler negativism and delighted to learn this period typically passes by about 30 months of age.

Caregivers, however, will have to select their own method of dealing with their child's negativism. As with any attention-seeking behavior, it is best to ignore the action as much as future behavior-related issues.

RITUALISM AND REGRESSION

As disrupting as negativism can be, another characteristic developing simultaneously is **ritualism**, or the need to maintain sameness (same cup, same spoon). The toddler needs stability within the expanding environment and to know, when in a new play area, familiar people and places will still be available (Figure 9-15). Rituals, such as mealtime and bedtime routines, provide repetition where the child may gain comfort and security. If rituals are disrupted, as when a child is ill or hospitalized, the child experiences stress, responds by exerting autonomy, and frequently **regresses** (returns to an earlier, safer, more familiar behavior) to dependence and negativism (Erikson's concept of autonomy versus shame and doubt) to cope with the situation.

FAMILY TEACHING

Handling "No!"

- Reduce the opportunity to say "no." Do not give the child an option if one doesn't really exist. **Do not ask:** "Do you want lunch now?" **Ask:** "Do you want a peanut butter or a cheese sandwich for lunch?"
- Avoid complex requests or over stimulating situations (such as trips to the grocery store) when the toddler is tired or hungry.
- Do not draw attention to negative behaviors, but if you are going to deal with them, do it immediately; otherwise, the child will have forgotten why reprimanding occurred.
- Do not threaten the child, especially as a reaction of frustration or anger. State disciplinary guidelines briefly, in simple terms. Be sure the child understands the consequence. The toddler may not remember both the terms and the consequence with a lengthy explanation. Example: "You need to brush your teeth so we can read your bedtime story," ***not*** "If you don't hurry up and brush your teeth there will be no story tonight."

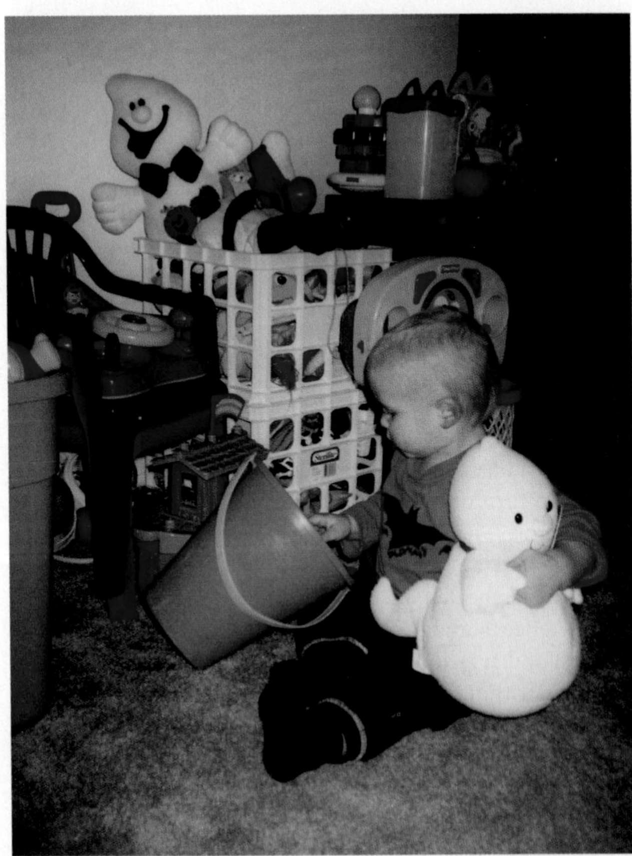

FIGURE 9-15 Toddlers often have a special object of affection such as a blanket, special toy, doll, or stuffed animal that provides them with comfort. DELMAR CENGAGE LEARNING.

FAMILY**TEACHING**

Routines That Work

1. Set a schedule fitting both the caregiver's lifestyle and the child's personality whenever possible. For example, if the caregiver works the night shift and the child is an early riser, plan enjoyable activities early in the day (e.g., playing outside, going shopping, doing the bath time routine), so both can rest in the early afternoon.
2. Stick to a schedule, since routines provide security for toddlers. Establish a routine and time for sleep (e.g., change clothes, brush teeth, read story). Adhere to these unless exceptional circumstances arise.
3. Use a consistent alternate caregiver. It is much easier to develop trust and separate from the primary caregiver if the same person cares for the toddler in the caregiver's absence.

Many caregivers feel they become slaves to the schedules of their 2-year-old. When a toddler demands things be done in the same way at the same time, the child is not acting out of stubbornness, but asking for needs to be met. Routines provide a sense of security and give a framework to master new skills while providing a sense of control over the environment.

The best initial approach is to ignore regression while complimenting the child on positive attributes and behaviors. When caregivers assess the toddler's behavior, they often assume regression is an act of defiance or willful disobedience. Since the loss of a newly acquired skill is frightening to the toddler, regression should be disciplined cautiously.

It is not uncommon for toddlers to demonstrate a variety of behaviors when stressed. These behaviors include aggression, avoidance, distraction, isolation, seeking information, self-consoling activities, and emotional expressions (Figure 9-16). That is why toddlers may use a security blanket, have a favorite teddy bear, ask many questions, argue, cry, or have temper tantrums.

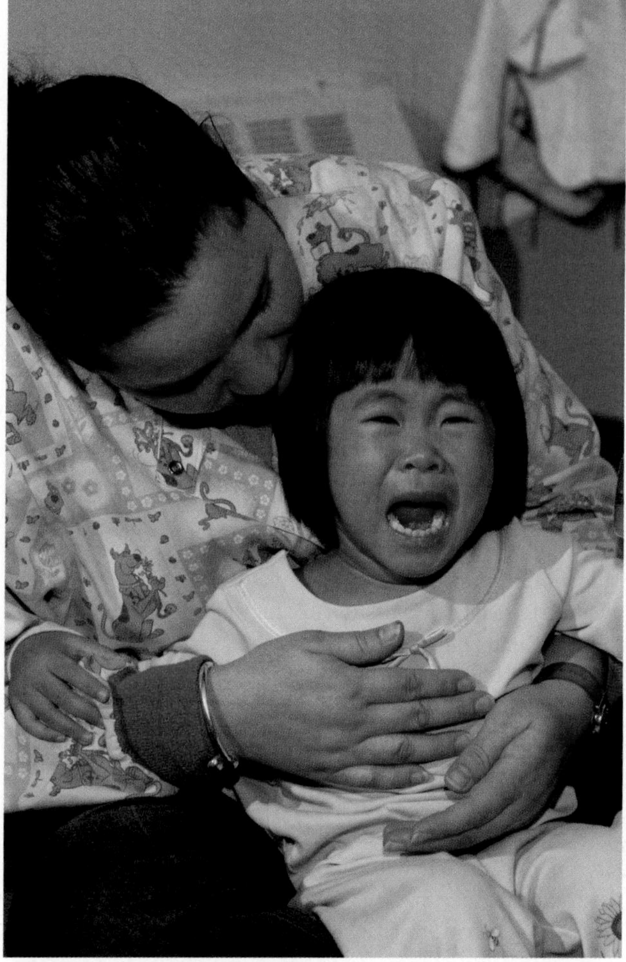

FIGURE 9-16 Toddlers need assurance they are loved even when certain behaviors are inappropriate. DELMAR CENGAGE LEARNING.

DISCIPLINE

In light of their evolving concept of ritualism and the need for familiar routines, toddlers are assisted in developing self-control by consistently applied discipline. Regardless of the methods used, teaching children the reasons for the discipline is essential to help them learn how to behave in a socially accepted manner (American Academy of Pediatrics, 1998; Berkowitz, 2008a).

Limit setting (letting the child know what he or she is able to do and not do in a situation) is an important part of toddler discipline since we all tend to function better when both the expectations and limits defining actions are known. These limits may be established by the child, adult caregivers, or the external environment. Caregivers who provide the toddler with clear and concise limits facilitate autonomy development and help the child gain a sense of order, control, and security (Berkowitz, 2008a).

FAMILY**TEACHING**

Avoiding or Managing Regression

- Attempt to identify overwhelming stressors, and consider various options to help the toddler manage the situation.
- Alternate activities and provide more caregiver attention and interaction to help the child develop behavioral stability.
- Remember, regression is a normal expression and generally does not have long-lasting effects. However, it may be related to autism or similar developmental conditions so needs to be monitored over time.

Caregivers should agree upon both the limits not to be exceeded and the type of discipline used when established boundaries are pushed. The American Academy of Pediatrics (1998) identifies three essential components of successful and effective discipline: (1) a supportive and loving relationship between parent(s) and child; (2) use of positive reinforcement to promote desired behaviors; and (3) removing reinforcement to reduce and eliminate undesired behaviors.

To support and facilitate consistency, all caregivers, including grandparents and babysitters, should be told about established limits and disciplinary actions. Providing *consistent* discipline is critical for understanding, gaining responsibility, and experiencing positive behavioral outcomes. Refer to the Family Teaching box for more information.

The type of discipline utilized will vary from family to family and culture to culture; however, approximately 90% of parents in the United States use corporal punishment (physical punishment) in disciplining their children (AAP, 1998). Corporal punishment may bring about an immediate change in behavior, but the long-term effect is questionable for toddlers. Use of caregiver role modeling (Bandura, 1986) has been successful in disciplining toddlers, but requires the child to: (1) see the correct behavior enacted; (2) remember what the role model did; (3) be physically able to repeat the role model's action; and (4) be motivated to engage in the modeled behavior. This works especially well where a strong trust relationship exists with the role model (Figure 9-17). Role modeling, use of the teaching process, scolding, ignoring, or time-out (placing the child in a nonstimulating environment) seem to be among the most widely used methods of achieving behavioral change with toddlers (Berkowitz, 2008a).

NURSING ALERT

Toddler Discipline

1. Nurses should never physically discipline a child. Physical punishment may legally be administered only by a parent or legal guardian and the type and degrees of such punishment are currently under scrutiny. The American Academy of Pediatrics' (1998) statements related to spanking, discipline, and punishment are accepted as the professional standard and can be found on their website.
2. If the child is hospitalized, discuss with caregivers how you may support their methods of discipline. Explain hospitalized children frequently display regressive behavioral patterns, and carefully think before implementing any disciplinary measures related to regressive behavior.
3. If you observe inappropriate verbal or physical discipline, as a professional you are mandated to report it. The reporting mechanism will differ from state to state, but your responsibility does not change.

TEMPER TANTRUMS

Temper tantrums are outward explosive reactions to inward stressful or frustrating situations that are a normal part of toddler life. Between 2 and 3 years of age, the child is faced with new environments, new rules, and new fears. Toddlers need to express their feelings, wishes, and frustrations, but lack the language skills to do this. All of these new experiences, coupled with the child's

FAMILY TEACHING

Appropriate Toddler Discipline

- Predetermine and communicate limits to the child.
- Allow limit testing.
- Assist in achieving mastery of socially acceptable behaviors.
- Provide ways for channeling undesirable feelings into constructive activities.
- Avoid disciplining in the wrong place, with the wrong motive, or the wrong timing.
- Avoid threats to discipline; always follow through.
- Follow discipline with love and positive encouragement.

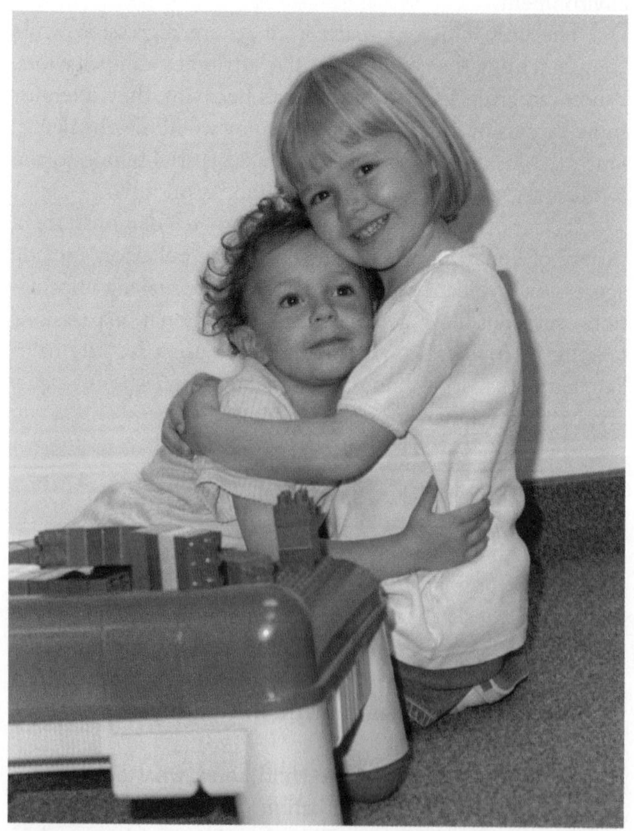

FIGURE 9-17 Toddlers often receive comfort from an older sibling. DELMAR CENGAGE LEARNING.

quest for autonomy, may create tension and erupt into a tantrum. Tantrums are ways toddlers say, "I have needs, I am important, I need to have some control." A typical temper tantrum—occurring when the toddler cannot control his or her emotions, feels overwhelmed, or does not get what is wanted when it is wanted—may involve crying, screaming, falling onto the floor, kicking the feet, flailing the arms, banging the head, and breath holding (Grover, 2008e). Head banging requires intervention if it is continuous or unsafe; to prevent injury, the caregiver should hold the child's head, make few comments (to prevent reinforcement of the negative behavior), or provide a protective mat or pillow. Beyond this, as with any attention-seeking behavior, the tantrum should be ignored. Speaking softly and calmly, recognizing the child's feelings, and holding can help.

When breath holding occurs and the child appears to faint or stop breathing, caregivers frequently become frightened and rush into frenzied action, which only reinforces the tantrum behavior. Therefore, caregivers must be taught that breath holding is usually harmless. The child may "faint," but will automatically begin breathing again as soon as carbon dioxide builds up and stimulates the respiratory center. Although caregivers are not encouraged to intervene during a tantrum, they should remain close by to prevent traumatic injuries. It is also helpful to remove the child from public attention.

At the conclusion of the tantrum, the caregiver should offer a toy or option not related to the incident-producing difficulty. ("Why don't we play with your new tea set?") This will redirect the toddler's attention. Disciplining a child after a tantrum usually is of little value. However, if the caregivers have told the child there would be a consequence to this behavior, they should follow through as promised.

Tantrums cannot always be controlled, but caretakers can take measures to lessen their frequency or intensity, including developing a regular schedule for the toddler, reducing the need to say "no," allowing choices, rewarding good behavior, and staying calm. Tantrums can sometimes be avoided by using time-outs or by placing a child in a bedroom before the behavior escalates. Temper tantrums are considered a normal developmental response of toddlerhood but should disappear by 4 years of age.

SIBLING RIVALRY

Sibling rivalry, defined as intense feelings of jealousy between siblings, often is seen when an infant is born into a family with a toddler. The arrival of this new baby can be devastating to toddlers since now they must compete for a caregiver's attention and fear loss of love or abandonment (Berkowitz, 2008b) (Figure 9-18a). See the Family Teaching box for some suggestions for handling this common problem.

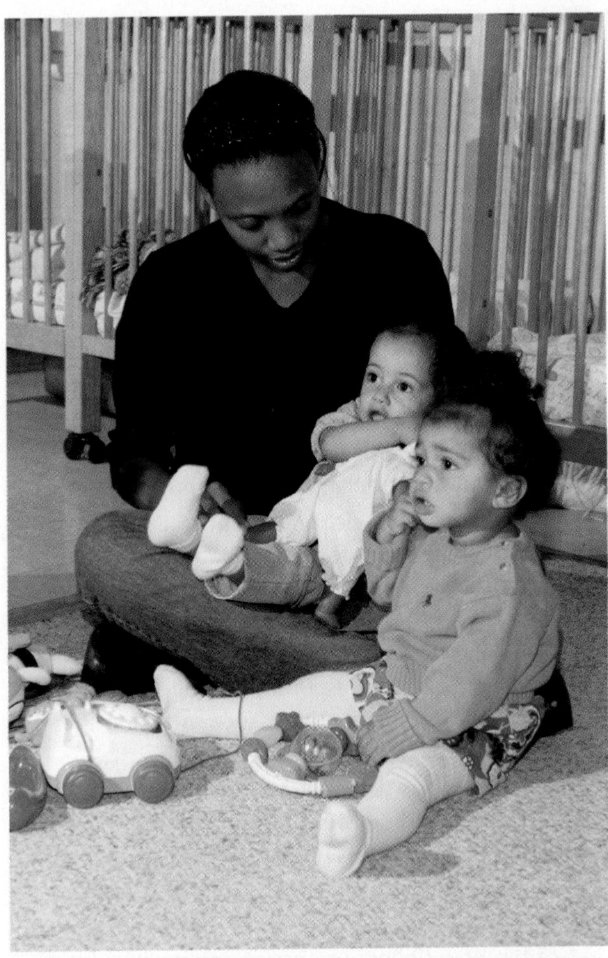

FIGURE 9-18A The arrival of a new sibling can be less traumatic for the toddler who is involved in the baby's care and made to feel an important member of the family. DELMAR CENGAGE LEARNING.

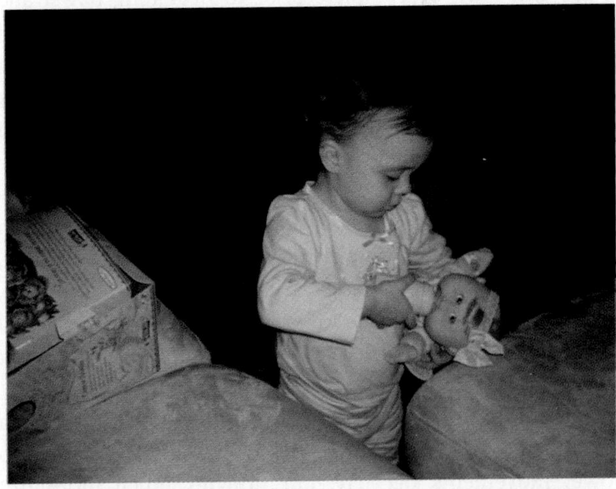

FIGURE 9-18B This toddler feeds her doll baby similar to how she sees her mother feeding her new brother. DELMAR CENGAGE LEARNING.

TOILET TRAINING

A major factor contributing to the toddler's goals of independence and autonomy is accomplishing bowel and bladder control. Success, however, depends on the readiness of both the child and the caregiver. Caregivers who understand normal child growth and development will have more realistic expectations and less frustration during toilet training.

Myelinization of the spinal cord and development of sphincter muscle control occur at approximately 12–18 months

FAMILY TEACHING

Tips for Dealing with Sibling Rivalry

- Establish a time frame when attention is focused exclusively on the toddler.
- Maintain the toddler's rituals as long as needed.
- Do not introduce new developmental tasks (e.g., toilet training or weaning from nighttime bottle) near the time when a new baby is expected.
- Have the toddler "sleep over" in the home of the grandparent or individual who will be caring for him or her when the mother is in the hospital several times before the birth occurs. Reassure the child that his or her mother will return.
- If the toddler will be moved out of a nursery or crib to make room for a new baby, make the move several months in advance, and do not announce the real purpose of the move. Emphasize positive aspects: "You're getting to be so big."
- Be alert for subtle responses (not all sibling rivalry is overt) of sibling jealousy, such as taking the baby's bottle, pacifier, or toys.
- When toddlers demonstrate rivalry, set limits and consistently administer discipline with love.
- Plan joint time with children, equalizing attention as much as possible.
- Encourage participation in the play-time and care of the new sibling; use praise and positive interactions (Figure 9-18b).

NURSING TIP

Atraumatic Toilet Training

- The child needs to achieve this level of independence at her or his own speed.
- Caregivers must reach agreement as to how the toilet training will be handled and determine acceptable words used to describe the activities; a consistent approach and vocabulary must be maintained.
- The child must be physiologically (able to walk well, can pull pants up and down, usually 24–30 months of age) and psychologically (dislikes feeling of wet diapers, wants to go to preschool but cannot in a diaper) ready to be potty trained.
- Caretakers should ignore helpful advice from grandparents, aunts, neighbors, and day care workers: focus on the unique characteristics of this child.
- Avoid scolding, punishing, or overreacting to accidental soiling.
- Have a child-sized potty available.
- Praise the child for each attempt, either verbally or with favorite stickers, whether successful or not.

of age and must be complete prior to beginning bowel and bladder training since the average toddler is ready to begin toilet training at approximately 18–24 months. The time to begin toilet training, however, varies from culture to culture and family to family. Nurses should educate parents about the signs of readiness for toilet training, which include the ability to demonstrate cognitive awareness of elimination (diaper is wet), follow directions and communicate understanding of elimination needs to the caregiver (pulls on diaper, asks for diaper change), remain dry for longer periods of time (more than 2 hours), independently dress and undress, and sit, squat, and walk well (AAP, 2010c; Blum, Taubman, & Nemeth, 2003; Choby & George, 2008; Smith, 2008).

Bladder control is often more difficult to attain than bowel control. The toddler usually has only one to two bowel movements per day, but urinates much more frequently. Often, accidental urinary incontinence occurs because the toddler becomes so involved in play activities the urge to urinate is ignored until it is too late to reach the bathroom. When the toddler is attempting to remain dry and learn bowel control, an emotional tug-of-war often develops between the child and the caregivers, leaving both frustrated and angry. Punishment and coercion can lead to shame and feelings of inferiority. A helpful strategy is giving the child control over the process. Telling the child how the body makes "pee" and "poop" daily and helping the toddler succeed can encourage participation and responsibility. A relaxed approach, with positive reinforcement and praise, will aid in toilet training, as will avoiding constant reminders and providing incentives for using the toilet correctly. Recording the child's progress and not punishing accidents are also important. For some children completion of toilet training is occurring at an older age. This may be related to initiating the training at an older age, stool toileting refusal, and issues with constipation. Parents should be given encouragement and reassurance. Consistent day and night dryness should be achieved by 5 years of age, or further evaluation for physical or psychological problems is warranted (AAP, 2010c; Smith, 2008).

REFLECTIVE THINKING

Toilet Training

Sarah, the mother of a 20-month-old daughter (Rylin), is returning to work in a week and is concerned about placing her daughter in child care. Sarah feels that Rylin should be potty trained prior to entering child care, and she wants to know if this can be accomplished during the next week. Considering your understanding of growth and development and the signs of toilet training readiness, what is your response?

EVIDENCE-BASED PRACTICE

Children Who Are Difficult to Toilet Train

CLINICAL PROBLEM

Most children are toilet trained by the time they are 3 years of age. On the other hand, there is a group of children who have difficulty being toilet trained, and this is a concern for parents and health care practitioners. Information is needed on what differentiates those children who are easy to toilet train from those children who are difficult to toilet train.

BEST CLINICAL PRACTICE

Children found to be difficult to toilet train had a temperament that was less persistent and adaptable, more negative in mood, and lower in approach than children who were easier to train. They were also more likely to be constipated than other children. However, children who were difficult to toilet train have appropriate developmental skills necessary for toilet training, even though some hide when stooling. Parenting practices were not correlated with toilet training difficulties.

IMPLICATIONS FOR NURSING

- When children are difficult to toilet train, encourage parents to consider constipation as a cause and provide referrals to health care providers who can investigate and suggest treatment for constipation.
- Assist parents in developing strategies for helping their child toilet train that avoid conflict and consider the child's temperament.
- Teach parents that their style of parenting is not the cause of toilet training difficulties.

Reference: Schonwald, A., Stadtler, A., & Bridgemohan, C. (2004). Factors associated with difficult toilet training. *Pediatrics, 113*(6), 1753–1757.

Stress may either interfere with toilet training or precipitate regressive bowel or bladder continence. Caregivers need to be informed that such regressions are usually temporary, and understanding, gentle support, reinforcement, and encouragement will assist the toddler to regain a sense of independence and success.

ALTERNATIVE CHILD CARE

Placing the toddler in a child care setting if both parents are employed outside the home may be necessary in some situations. However, the child care setting may pose additional threats to the toddler's health and well-being. Caregivers might need assurance from professionals that use of such facilities is perfectly acceptable in today's society. Refer to Chapter 7 for more information on the use of alternative child care.

PLAY

Play has been described as "the work of childhood." Certainly, this is an appropriate description since it is through active play and manipulation that toddlers learn about the environment (Figure 9-19). Object exploration also enhances fine and

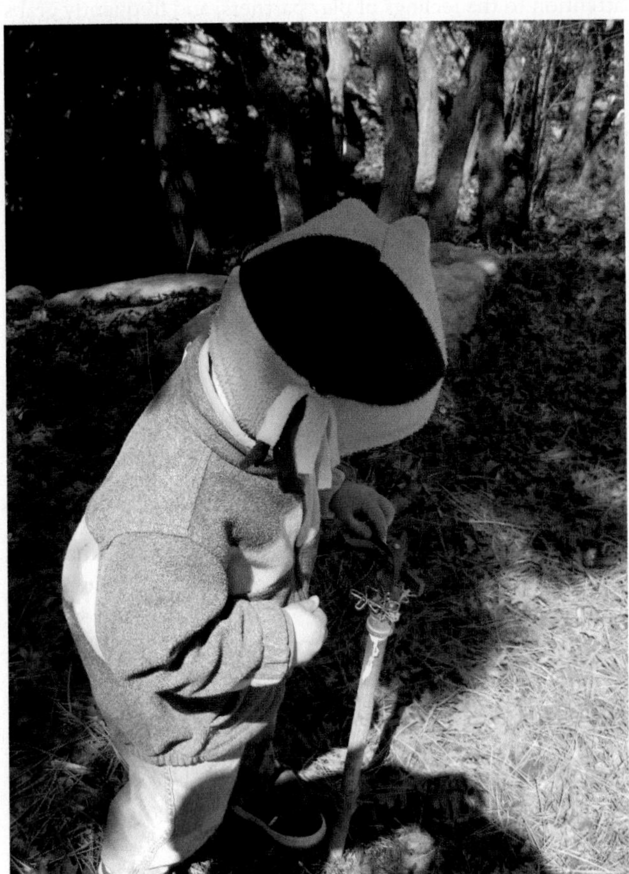

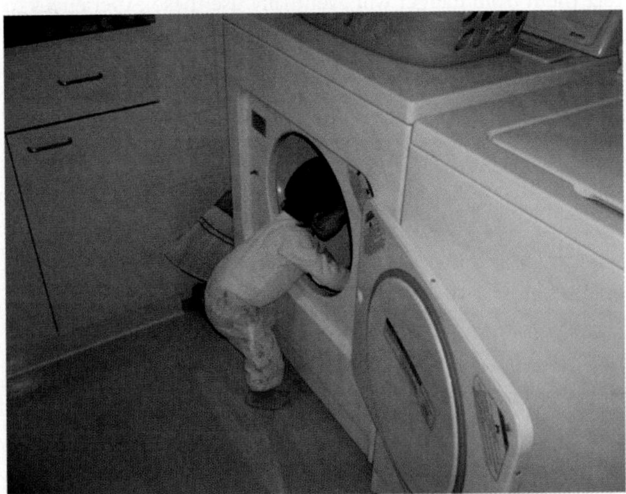

FIGURE 9-19 Toddlers often explore items in their environment so they can learn more about what they do and how they work. Caregivers must be diligent about ensuring the safety of all environments to which toddlers have access. DELMAR CENGAGE LEARNING.

gross muscle development and coordination. According to Gemelli (1996), play is the primary way toddlers teach themselves; they do not necessarily view their play as play, but a natural aspect of life. As one 2½-year-old replied when asked why he liked to play, "I don't play. This is what I do!" Toddlers most often play alongside, rather than with other children (**parallel play**) (Figure 9-20). The toddler demonstrates little attention to the feelings of play partners, and frequently grabs desired toys or hits others to keep a favorite toy.

Play fulfills three functions for toddlers, including facilitating cognitive development by permitting exploration of the environment, learning about objects, and solving problems. It also advances social development particularly through fantasy play when acting out roles. Finally, it permits problem solving, vents frustrations, uses excess energy, and assists in coping with inner conflicts and anxieties in nonthreatening ways.

Each time a new toy is introduced into the toddler's world, the teaching–learning process should occur: introduce the toy, instruct the child how to use the toy, allow the child to play or practice with the item, and provide feedback and reinforcement on how well the child has done. Caregivers may need some instruction about this process, but once established, it provides the basis for a life-long educational process. The initiation of "why?" and "why not?" questions, which accompany play, especially with a new toy or game, enhances the child's ability to gather data and make decisions (Figure 9-21).

Age-appropriate play does not require expensive, shiny, developmentally approved toys. It does, however, require a patient and innovative caregiver who views play activities as major educational and socializing events in the child's life.

A portion of the play experience involves make-believe, pretending, or fantasy. Fantasy and make-believe help conceptualize what and how a child wishes the world to be. Fantasy helps the toddler cope with parental expectations and aids in denying aspects of reality they prefer to ignore (Figures 9-22 and 9-23). Toddlers who trust their caregiver's ability to protect them from danger will eventually use these experiences to reconstruct their fantasies into reality-based beliefs (Gemelli, 1996).

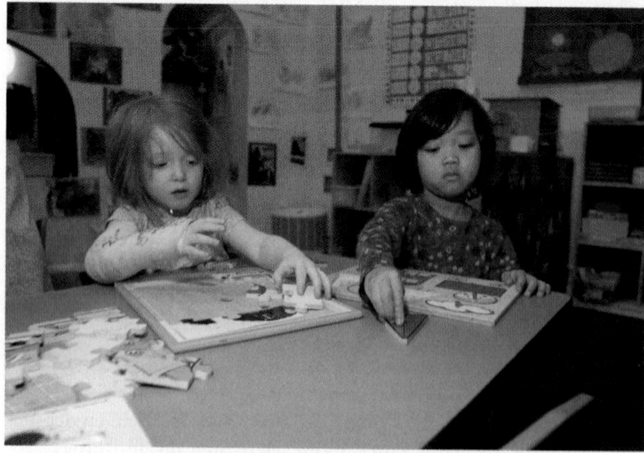

FIGURE 9-20 Parallel play: toddlers involved in similar activities but not playing with one another. DELMAR CENGAGE LEARNING.

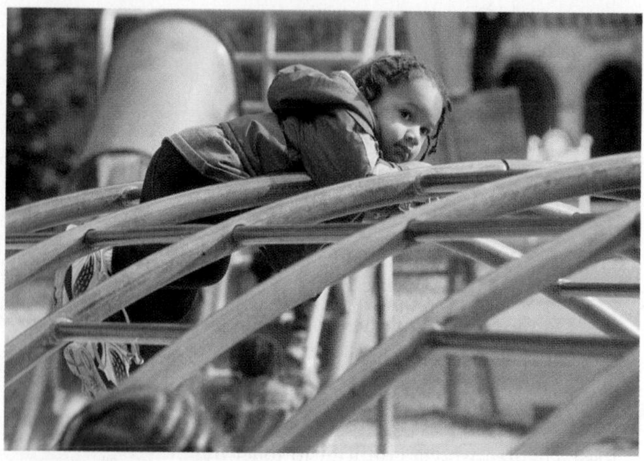

FIGURE 9-21 This toddler is exploring her world and demonstrating mastery of both the physiological and cognitive dimensions of development in her play. DELMAR CENGAGE LEARNING.

PHYSICAL ACTIVITY

It is important that physical activity become a part of family life that can provide toddlers and children with a strong foundation for good health, encourage future motor development, and help to prevent childhood obesity. Parents play a key role in helping their toddler develop a positive attitude and health habits, including exercise. Some possible suggestions include choosing fun activities that involve all family members, selecting activities that the child enjoys such as throwing or rolling balls, jumping up and down, and using toys such as cars in an active fashion. It is recommended that children and adults spend about 60 minutes a day in physical activity. A key factor is making the time for the activity; often children are overscheduled with various nonphysical activities. Turn off the TV; use the free time for physical activity. It is important that parents be role models (Gunner, Atkinson, Nichols, & Eissa, 2005).

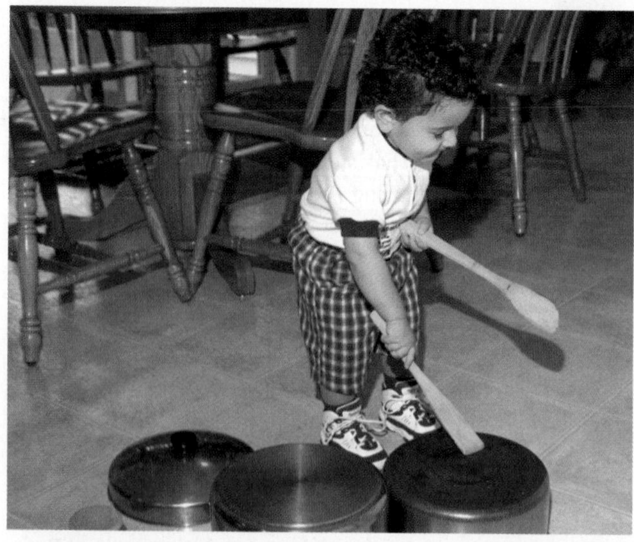

FIGURE 9-22 Toddlers have very active imaginations and can make toys out of just about anything. DELMAR CENGAGE LEARNING.

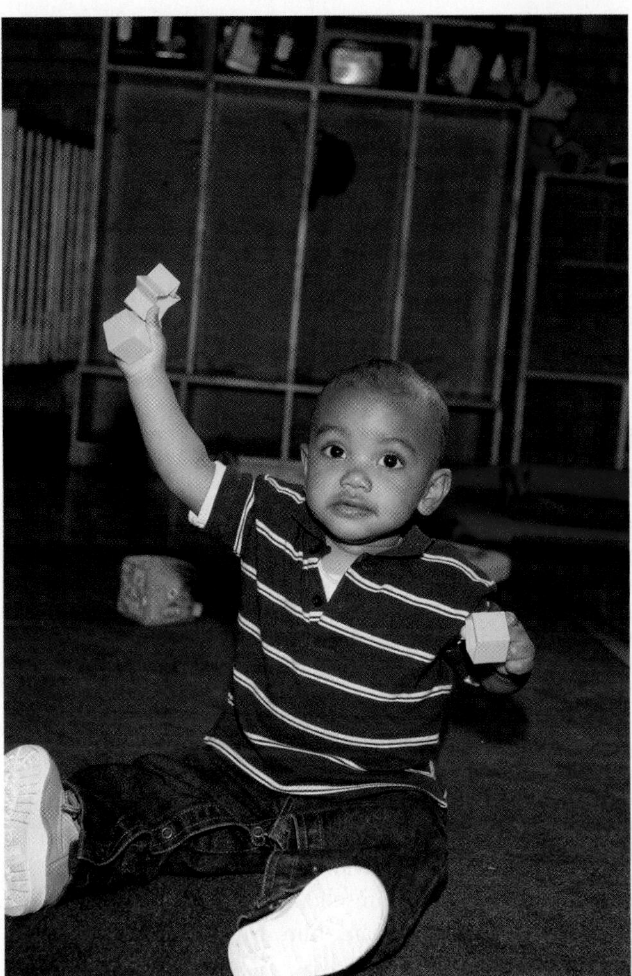

FIGURE 9-23 **Caregivers need to be sensitive to a toddler's abilities and provide play and learning opportunities in line with the child's developmental level.** DELMAR CENGAGE LEARNING.

NURSING MANAGEMENT

The nurse's role in toddler health promotion is critical. Education should provide ideas, suggestions, and concepts surrounding growth, development, and parenting skills. This knowledge will allow caregivers to become independent in promoting health with respect to nutrition, sleep, dental needs, safety, elimination, and growth and development. Nurses can be advocates for toddlers and families and identify those children at risk due to environmental, economical, sociological, and physiological factors. Nurses should also be involved as a leader and help establish laws and policies that will promote children's health and well-being (e.g., funding for safety education, developing programs for accessing low- or no-cost health promotion services, education regarding nutrition and physical activities).

IN THE REAL WORLD

I hadn't cared for a toddler before and when I did, boy did I learn a lot! Teddy, age 21/2 years, was admitted for pneumonia because of his cystic fibrosis. I needed to draw blood, start oxygen, begin medications, and call respiratory therapy. The first thing I did was try to explain about the blood collection: "Teddy, it won't hurt for very long." The screaming began: "I don't want a stick in my arm, the leaves will look funny!" I'd forgotten about toddler's thinking. I began again using simple terms and getting help from one of the nurses. Although it was a challenge to take care of him, I loved his energy, his sweetness, and his durability.

KEY CONCEPTS

- Toddlerhood is a period characterized by Erikson's task of autonomy versus shame and doubt. The toddler struggles to separate from caretakers and develop a sense of self.
- Major developmental tasks surround the toddler's developing locomotion, language, and cognitive development.
- Socio-economic, cultural, and ethnic factors play key roles in the toddler's growth and development, ability to participate in health promotion and disease prevention activities, and may be health risk indicators which the pediatric nurse may need to identify.
- Toddler physical growth slows, resulting in decreased appetite and relatively less demand for calories (physiologic anorexia). Nutritional needs continue, particularly for protein, calcium, magnesium, and iron, to support growth. Caregivers should be educated to facilitate this period of growth, but discourage foods contributing to obesity.
- The combination of increased motor skills (fine and gross), desire to explore, lack of experience (judgment), and immaturity places the toddler at risk for accidental injury. Caretakers should be provided with education and guidance in creating a safe home environment.

- The provision of structure, guidance, and limit setting is critical for the toddler's development of autonomy, self-control, and mastery of skills. Effective disciplinary techniques are consistent and firm, and may include time-outs, diversion, and positive reinforcement.
- Sibling rivalry reflects the toddler's fear, anxiety, and lack of understanding when a new infant enters the family. It can be minimized with methods such as including the toddler in preparations for the baby, affirming the toddler is loved and very special, and setting appropriate limits.
- Nurses can assist caretakers to understand their toddler's readiness for toilet training (recognizing physical and psychological signs) and provide guidance for strategies for success.
- Nurses need to educate caretakers on health promotion such as nutrition, sleep, immunizations, hygiene, and safety.

REVIEW ACTIVITIES

1. Jamie is wearing mom's sweater and her eyeglasses while pouring make-believe tea for her playmate. Which of the following best describes this toddler's behavior?
   a. Role anxiety
   b. Separation anxiety
   c. Parallel play
   d. Domestic mimicry
2. Of the physiologic changes that occur during toddlerhood, which of these is *essential* before a child is capable of walking?
   a. Calcification of long bones
   b. Myelinization of spinal cord
   c. Readiness for separation (from caregiver)
   d. Stabilization of muscles of the legs
3. There are several major developmental milestones of toddlerhood. Which of these should *not* be included in the list?
   a. Seeks independence
   b. Walks well
   c. Plays well with friends
   d. Uses over 300 words
4. When a toddler is not able to accomplish a task (such as tying his shoe), he may go quietly into a corner and pout. This behavior demonstrates which of the following theories?
   a. Erickson's industry versus inferiority
   b. Piaget's sensory-motor stage
   c. Erickson's autonomy versus shame
   d. Piaget's preconceptual stage
5. A 2-year-old child has been crying ever since his mother left his hospital room. The nurse begins playing an audiotape of his mother's voice, and he quiets immediately. This response is evidence of:
   a. An increased concept of object permanence
   b. Differentiation of self from others
   c. Symbolic imitation
   d. Egocentrism
6. A 2 ½ -year-old boy is having a temper tantrum in the middle of a large family gathering. Which response would you recommend to the caregiver as being *most appropriate* in this situation?
   a. Immediately pick him up and carry him from the middle of activities.
   b. Toss water in his face when he begins holding his breath.
   c. Ignore his behavior completely as long as he is not injuring himself.
   d. Threaten to spank him if he doesn't stop his kicking immediately.
7. In assessing a toddler's physical growth, which of these factors would suggest intervention was needed?
   a. His weight at 3 years is 15 pounds.
   b. She has all of her deciduous teeth by 27 months.
   c. His anterior fontanel has not closed by 13 months.
   d. She is 28 months old and still not potty trained.
8. The *primary* reason for discontinuing a bedtime bottle of milk is to:
   a. Prevent tooth decay
   b. Assist in maintaining nighttime dryness
   c. Encourage more mature eating habits
   d. Prevent dental deformity
9. When planning to meet a toddler's nutritional needs, one should include which of the following?
   a. 500 kcal/kg, high fiber
   b. 1,000 kcal/day, high protein
   c. 2,000 kcal/day, low fat
   d. 150 kcal/kg, wide variety of components

10. From the factors listed below, select the primary purpose for disciplining a child:
    a. To identify who is in control
    b. To display evidence of good parenting skills
    c. To teach punishment and reward system
    d. To protect child and others
11. In general, potty training a child can best be accomplished by which of these means?
    a. Same-sex parental role modeling
    b. Setting specific behavioral limits and adhering to them
    c. Describing socially acceptable behaviors to toddler
    d. Threatening to withhold items of pleasure (e.g., favorite toy, dessert)

STUDY QUESTIONS

1. Mrs. Valdez has brought two-year-old Mario to the Family Clinic because he has been ill with a "bad cold" for the past two weeks. Collecting data from Mrs. Valdez you learn that Mario received immunizations at his two-month checkup, but that she has not brought him to the clinic since then. What is your next action?
    a. Educate Mrs. Valdez about the possible consequences of not having Mario immunized according to the schedule recommended by the Centers for Disease Control.
    b. Educate Mrs. Valdez about the immunizations Mario needs and arrange for him to receive the first catch-up series.
    c. Suggest that Mrs. Valdez bring Mario back to the clinic when he is no longer experiencing upper respiratory symptoms for his catch-up immunizations.
    d. Arrange for Mrs. Valdez to take Mario to a free immunization clinic in a week to ten days once his upper respiratory symptoms have gone.
2. Mrs. Jenkins has brought Jessica, her 2-year-old, to the primary care provider because she is concerned about her lack of appetite and her refusal to try eating new foods. As you prepare to provide education to Mrs. Jenkins about her daughter's eating habits you understand that appetite lags occur for all of the following reasons except:
    a. Jessica is rebelling in response to her parents' new restrictions.
    b. Jessica is experiencing physiological anorexia.
    c. Jessica has a preference for one type of food.
    d. Jessica has a high level of activity and exploration.
3. Toddlers often regress during periods of stress primarily because they:
    a. Forget the skills that have been learned.
    b. May be responding to parents' preferences for less mature behavior.
    c. Return to behaviors that increase a sense of security during stressful situations.
    d. Experience growth progression best following regression which allows growth spurts.
4. Mara and Cassie are both 2 ½ years old. They both want to play with the same toy and are fighting, grabbing the toy back and forth. Mara's mother is very upset and asks the nurse why they just can't get along. You would most likely suggest that she do which of the following based on your understanding of development?
    a. Suggest to the mothers that they reprimand the children and tell them to share the toy.
    b. Suggest to the mothers that they give each child a toy to play with. Have two toys on hand.
    c. Suggest that when the children begin to fight over a toy that they have the toy removed and then place the children in separate parts of the room.
    d. Suggest that they tell the children it is not necessary to fight, there are "plenty of toys," and provide another toy for one of the children.
5. Parents often need reassurance about disciplining their toddler. You assure them that setting limits is important because limits:
    a. Provide parents control over their toddler's actions and behaviors.
    b. Provide clearly defined rules that toddlers can understand and consistently follow.
    c. Provide parents with the feeling that they are "right."
    d. Provide toddlers with a sense of security and comfort.
6. Temperament is a key part of the development of toddlers and can influence the choice of discipline strategies. Which of the following would be

effective strategies when working with the "difficult toddler"?
a. Using a stern voice and sustained eye contact when the child is exhibiting the challenging behavior
b. Using a quick, nonviolent spanking with an explanation to the toddler why the spanking occurred
c. Providing time to gradually introduce the child into new situations
d. Providing a "friendly" warning to stop the activity, followed by a set time-out if the behavior continues

7. Sam, age 3 years, is seeing a dentist for the first time. This is important because:
a. Dental caries is a common infectious disease.
b. Toddlers may have several misaligned teeth that need bracing.
c. Toddlers may have speech issues secondary to dental concerns.
d. The first dental visit should always occur by the age of three years.

8. An important goal of Healthy People 2010 is to reduce mortality rates in toddlers. A primary risk for toddlers is:
a. Falls.
b. Burns.
c. Drowning.
d. Poisonings.

9. Pediatric nurses need to be aware of and sensitive to cultural and ethnic variations when assessing and comparing children to preestablished norms. Particular attention should be paid to:
a. Head circumference and height.
b. Fine motor skills.
c. Height and weight.
d. Weight and muscle build.

10. Mr. Harold has come with Helene, his 2-year-old, for her checkup. He verbalizes his concern that Helene is very challenging to care for and help sometimes because she wants things done the same way all the time and cries and becomes distraught if her routine is changed. You understand that she is currently experiencing "ritualism." You explain that this is a normal part of her development and recommend which of the following approaches?
a. Follow Helene's clues and set a daily schedule which she seems most comfortable with, knowing that she will soon outgrow this stage.
b. Ignore Helene's regression behaviors while complimenting her on positive attributes and behaviors.
c. Ignore Helene's regression behaviors, providing stern verbal warnings that she "can't always have her own way."
d. Slowly begin to introduce Helene to new routines while helping her to understand that she can't have her own way all the time.

REFERENCES

American Academy of Pediatrics Committee on Nutrition. (1986). Fluoride supplements. *Pediatrics, 77*, 58–761.

American Academy of Pediatrics Committee on Psychosocial Aspects of Child and Family Health. (1998). Guidance for effective discipline. *Pediatrics, 101*, 723–728.

American Academy of Pediatrics Committee of Public Education, (2001). Children, adolescents and television. *Pediatrics, 1078*(2), 423–426.

American Academy of Pediatrics Committee on Nutrition. (2009). Retrieved February 2, 2009, from http://www.aap.org/visit/cmte25.htm.

American Academy of Pediatrics Committee on Infectious Disease. (2010a). 2010 Childhood immunization schedule and catch-up schedule. Retrieved May 24, 2010, from http://aapredbook.aappublications.org/resources/IZScheduleCatchup.pdf.

American Academy of Pediatrics. (2010b). Parenting Corner Q&A: Nutrition. Retrieved May 24, 2010, from http://www.healthychildren.org/english/healthy-living/nutrition/pages/Hassle-Free-Meal-Time.aspx?nfstatus=401&nftoken=00000000-0000-0000-0000-000000000000&nfstatusdescription=ERROR%3a+No+local+token.

American Academy of Pediatrics. (2010c). Parenting Corner Q&A: Toilet Training. Retrieved January 23, 2010, from http://www.aap.org/publiced/BR_ToiletTrain.htm.

American Academy of Pediatrics, Car Safety Seats: Information for families. (2010d). Retrieved May 24, 2010, from http://www.healthychildren.org/English/safety-prevention/on-the-go/pages/Car-Safety-Seats-Information-for-Families-2010.aspx.

Bandura, A. (1986). *Social foundation of thought and actions: A social cognitive theory*. Englewood Cliffs, NJ: Prentice Hall.

Beller, G. (2005). Disparities in health care in racial and ethnic minorities. *Journal of Nuclear Cardiology, 12*, 617–619.

Berkowitz, C. (2008a). Discipline. In *Berkowitz's Pediatrics: A primary care approach* (3rd ed.). American Academy of Pediatrics: Elk Grove Village, IL, 193–198.

Berkowitz, C. (2008b). Sibling rivalry. In *Berkowitz's Pediatrics: A primary care approach* (3rd ed.). American Academy of Pediatrics: Elk Grove Village, IL, 179–182.

Blum, N. J., Taubman, B., & Nemeth, N. (2003). Relationship between age at initiation of toilet training and duration of training: A prospective study. *Pediatrics, 111,* 810–814.

Centers for Disease Control and Prevention (CDC). (2010). Water Related Injuries: Fact Sheet. Retrieved January 23, 2010, from http://www.cdc.gov/HomeandRecreationalSafety/Water-Safety/waterinjuries-factsheet.htm.

Choby, B. A., & George, S. (2008). Toilet training. *American Family Physician, 78,* 1059–1064.

DiNardo, K. (2005, Jan. 7). 15 things you must do for your baby. *USA Weekend,* p. 7.

Donahue, G. J., Waddell, N., Plough, A. L., del Aguila, M. A., & Garland, T. E. (2005). The ABCDs of treating the most prevalent childhood disease. *American Journal of Public Health, 95,* 1322–1329.

Erikson, E. (1963). *Childhood and society.* New York: Norton.

Fowler, J. (1974). Toward a developmental perspective of faith. *Religious Education, 69,* 207–219.

Freud, S. (1957). In J. Strachey (Ed.), *The standard edition of the complete psychological works of Sigmund Freud* (Vol. 18). London: Hogarth.

Fuller, C., Keller, L., Olson, J., & Plymale, A. (2005). Helping preschoolers become healthy eaters. *Journal of Pediatric Health Care, 19,* 178–182.

Gemelli, R. (1996). *Normal child and adolescent development.* Washington, D.C: American Psychiatric Press.

Grover, G. (2008a). Talking with children. In *Berkowitz's Pediatrics: A primary care approach* (3rd ed.). American Academy of Pediatrics: Elk Grove Village, IL, 11–14.

Grover, G. (2008b). Normal development and developmental surveillance, screening, and evaluation. In *Berkowitz's Pediatrics: A primary care approach* (3rd ed.). American Academy of Pediatrics: Elk Grove Village, IL, 87–94.

Grover, G. (2008c). Language development: Speech and hearing assessment. In *Berkowitz's Pediatrics: A primary care approach* (3rd ed.). American Academy of Pediatrics: Elk Grove Village, IL, 95–99.

Grover, G. (2008d). Sleep: Normal patterns and common disorders. In *Berkowitz's Pediatrics: A primary care approach* (3rd ed.). American Academy of Pediatrics: Elk Grove Village, IL, 75–80.

Grover, G. (2008e). Temper tantrums. In *Berkowitz's Pediatrics: A primary care approach* (3rd ed.). American Academy of Pediatrics: Elk Grove Village, IL, 199–202.

Gunner, K. B., Atkinson, P. M., Nichols, J., & Eissa, M.A. (2005). Health promotion strategies to encourage physical activity in infants, toddlers, and preschoolers. *Journal of Pediatric Health Care, 19,* 253–258.

Horodynski, M. A., Stommel, M., Weatherspoon, L., & Brophy-Herb, H. (2009). Association between toddler mealtime television viewing, mealtime interaction, and dietary consumption in low-income African-American and white families. *Journal of Nutrition Education and Behavior, 40,* S27.

Hui, W. T., & Grover, G. (2008). Nutritional needs. In *Berkowitz's Pediatrics: A primary care approach* (3rd ed.). American Academy of Pediatrics: Elk Grove Village, IL, 63–70.

Kohlberg, L. (1976). Moral stages and moralization: The cognitive-developmental approach. In T. Likona (Ed.), *Moral development and behavior.* New York: Holt, Rinehart, & Winston.

Lewis, C. W. (2008). Oral health and dental disorders. In *Berkowitz's Pediatrics: A primary care approach* (3rd ed.). American Academy of Pediatrics: Elk Grove Village, IL, 81–86.

Murray, R., Zentner, J., & Yakimo, R. (2009). *Health promotion strategies through the life span* (8th ed.). Prentice Hall: Upper Saddle River, NJ.

Nainar, S. M. H., & Mohummed, S. (2004). Role of infant feeding practices on the dental health of children. *Clinical Pediatrics, 43,* 129–133.

Ogden, C. L., Carroll, M. D., Curtin, L. R., McDowell, M. A., Tabak, C. J., & Flegal, K. M. (2006). Prevalence of overweight and obesity in the United States, 1999–2004. *Journal of the American Medical Association, 295,* 1549–1555.

Online Safety Project. (2001). Available: http://www.safekids.com.

Papas, M. A., Hurley, K. M., Quigg, A. M., Oberlander, S. E., & Black, M. M. (2009). Low-income, African American adolescent mothers and their toddlers exhibit similar dietary variety patterns. *Journal of Nutrition Education and Behavior, 41,* 87–94.

Piaget, J. (1952). *The origin of intelligence in children.* New York: International University Press.

Proper Foods and Amounts for Toddlers. (2008). Retrieved January 15, 2010, from http://www.uri.edu/ce/efnep/toddler/toddler_amt.html.

Schonwald, A., Stadtler, A., & Bridgemohan, C. (2004). Factors associated with difficult toilet training. *Pediatrics, 113*(6), 1753–1757.

Smith, L.M. (2008). Toilet training. In *Berkowitz's Pediatrics: A primary care approach* (3rd ed.). American Academy of Pediatrics: Elk Grove Village, IL, 11–14.

Society of Pediatric Nurses. (2004a). *Position statement: Overweight children and adolescents.* Retrieved January 15, 2010, from https://www.pedsnurses.org/component/option,com_docman/task,cat_view/gid,49/.

Society of Pediatric Nurses. (2004b). Policy statement for prevention of pediatric firearm injuries. In *SPN policy manual:* Author.

Toddler Nutrition (Part 1). (2009a). Nutrient intakes of toddlers vs recommendations. *Pediatric Perspectives,* Mead Johnson & Co.

Toddler Nutrition (Part 2). (2009b). Metabolic programming and overweight status and risk. *Pediatric Perspectives,* Mead Johnson & Co.

U.S. Department of Health and Human Services. (2000). What are the leading health indicators? Washington, D.C.: Government Printing Office. Retrieved January 15, 2010, from http://www.healthypeople.gov/LHI/lhiwhat.htm.

Vaughn, K., & Valdrop, J. (2007). Parent education key to beating early childhood obesity. *The Nurse Practitioner, 32,* 37–41.

Weigel, C., Kokocinski, K., Lederer, P., Dorsch, J., Rascher, W., & Knerr, I. (2008). Childhood obesity: Concept, feasibility, and interim results of a local group-based, long-term treatment program. *Journal of Nutrition and Behavior, 40*, 369–373.

Wofford, L. G. (2008). Systematic review of childhood obesity prevention. *Journal of Pediatric Nursing, 23*, 5–19.

Ziegler, P., Hanson, C., Ponza, M., Novak, T., & Hendricks, K. (2006, January 1). Feeding infants and toddlers study: Meal and snack intake of Hispanic and non-Hispanic infants and toddlers. *Journal of the American Dietetic Association, 106*(1), S107–S123.

SUGGESTED READINGS

American Academy of Pediatric Dentistry recommendations for 2008. (2008). Retrieved January 15, 2010, from http://www.aapd.org/media/Policies_Guidelines/P_ECCClassifications.pdf.

American Academy of Pediatrics Committee on Injury and Poison Prevention. (1996). Selecting and using the most appropriate car safety seats for growing children: Guidelines for counseling parents. *Pediatrics, 97*(5), 761–763.

American Academy of Pediatrics Committee on Sports Medicine and Fitness and Council on School Health. (2006). *Active healthy living: Prevention of childhood obesity through increased physical activity.* Retrieved February 9, 2010, from http://www.aaplorg/advocacy/release/may06_physicalactivity.htm.

Biagioli, F. (2002). Proper use of child safety seats. *American Family Physician, 65*, 2085–2090.

Car safety seats: A guide for families. (2002). Elk Grove Village, IL: American Academy of Pediatrics. Retrieved February 9, 2010, from www.aap.org/family/carseatguide.htm.

Cathy, M., & Gaylord, N. (2004). *Picky eating: A toddler's continuing approach to mealtime. Pediatrics, 30*, 101–107.

Guzman-Armstrong, S. (2005). Rampant caries. *Journal of School Nursing, 21*, 272–278.

Horn, I. B., Brenner, R., Rao, M., & Cheng, T. L. (2006). Beliefs about the appropriate age for iniating toilet training: Are there racial and socioeconomic differences? *Journal of Pediatrics, 149*, 165–168.

Horodynski, M. A. O., Hoerr, S., & Coleman, G. (2004). Nutrition education aimed at toddlers: A pilot program for rural, low-income families. *Family & Community Health, 27*, 103–113.

Kenney, G. M., McFeeters, J. R., & Yee, J. Y. (2005). Preventative dental care and unmet dental needs among low-income children. *American Journal of Public Health, 95*, 1360–1366.

McConahy, K. L., Smiciklas-Wright, H., Mitchell, D. C., & Picciano, M. F. (2004). Portion size of common foods predicts energy intake among preschool-aged children. *Journal of the American Dietetic Association, 104*, 975–979.

National Highway Traffic Safety Administration. (n.d.). Proper child safety seat use chart. Washington, DC: Author. Retrieved February 9, 2010, from http://www.nhstsa.dot.gov/people/injury/childps.

Passehl, B., McCarroll, C., Buechner, J., Gearring, C., Smith, A. E., & Trowbridge, F. (2004). Preventing childhood obesity: Establishing healthy lifestyle habits in the preschool years. *Journal of Pediatric Health Care, 18*, 315–319.

Rugolotto, S., Min, S., Blum, N. J., & Taubman, B. (2004). Toilet training. *Pediatrics, 113*, 1802.

Summerbell, C. D., Waters, E., Edmunds, L. D., Kelly, S., Brown, T., & Campbell, K. J. (2006). Interventions for preventing obesity in children. *The Cochrane Database of Systematic Reviews*, 1. doi: 10.100214651858, CD001871.pub2.

RESOURCES

Refer to the online student StudyWARE for Potts & Mandleco at http://www.CengageBrain.com for additional content and study aids.

Organization: **American Academy of Family Physicians**
Description: Offers information regarding family physician careers, clinical research, advocacy, practice management, and recent news/publications.
Website/Resource: http://www.aafp.org

Organization: **American Academy of Pediatrics**
Description: Offers general information related to child health, specific guidelines concerning many pediatric issues, information regarding AAP programs, activities, policies, guidelines, publications, and other child health resources.
Website/Resource: http://www.aap.org

Organization: **Centers for Disease Control and Prevention**
Description: Offers information regarding current disease conditions, emergency preparedness/response, life stages/populations, healthy living, workplace environment/health.
Website/Resource: http://www.cdc.gov

Organization: **Family Doctor: "Toddlers: When yours doesn't want to eat"**
Description: Provides health information for families; toddler section is about how much children should eat, what to do if child is a picky eater, when to offer snack, how to make mealtimes easier.
Website/Resource: http://www.familydoctor.org

Organization: **Kid Source Online**
Description: Online community allowing parents to share values/goals in raising, educating and providing for children; access to parenting/education/recreation/organizations/product information.
Website/Resource: http://www.kidsource.com

Organization: **National Center for Infants, Toddlers and Families; Zero to Three**
Description: Offers access to an online store as well as information about key topics, leadership, authors, and training.
Website/Resource: http://www.zerotothree.org

Organization: **National Institute of Child Health & Human Development (NICHD)**
Description: Offers information regarding general health information, research, funding, and recent news/media related to child health and development.
Website/Resource: http://www.nichd.nih.gov

Organization: **National Network for Child Care (NNCC)**
Description: Offers information about child care, access to KIDCARE (email list allowing individuals to communicate with others concerned about child care), person-to-person contact with experts in child care, and access to newsletter.
Website/Resource: http://www.nncc.org

Organization: **The Online Safety Project**
Description: Provides information concerning many aspects about child safety as well as links to other informative sites.
Website/Resource: http://www.safekids.com

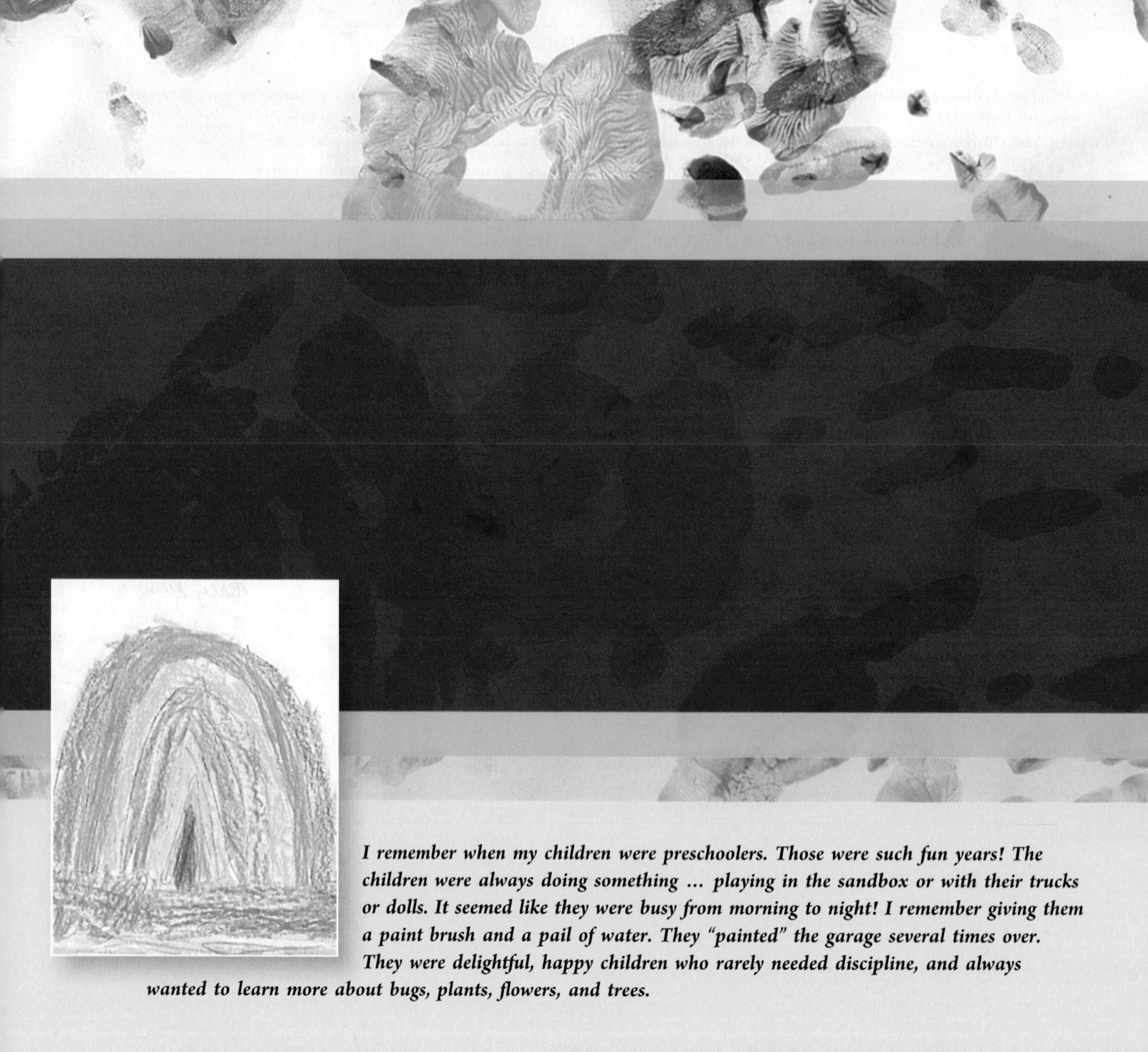

I remember when my children were preschoolers. Those were such fun years! The children were always doing something … playing in the sandbox or with their trucks or dolls. It seemed like they were busy from morning to night! I remember giving them a paint brush and a pail of water. They "painted" the garage several times over. They were delightful, happy children who rarely needed discipline, and always wanted to learn more about bugs, plants, flowers, and trees.

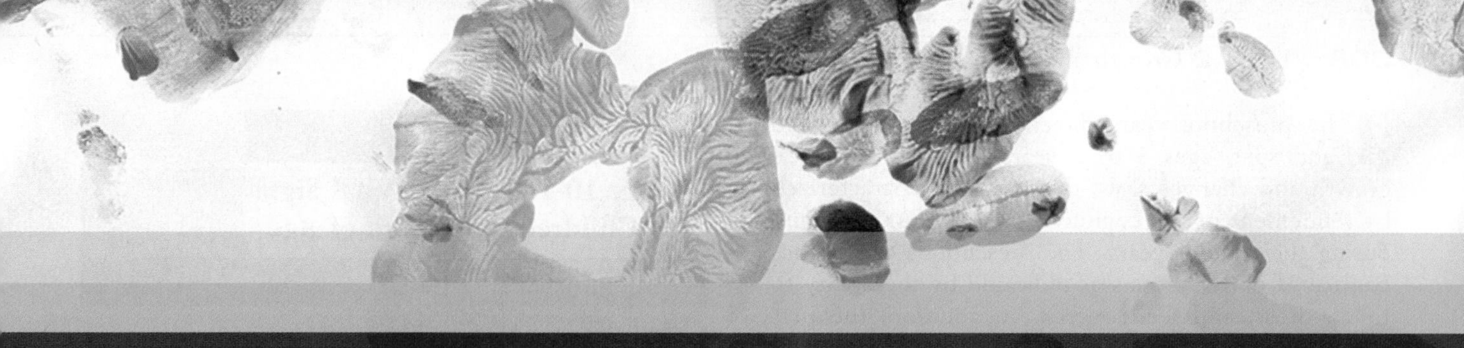

CHAPTER 10

Growth and Development of the Preschooler

CAROLYN C. REYNOLDS, APRN, MS

COMPETENCIES

Upon completion of this chapter, the reader will be able to:

- Discuss normal physiological changes that occur during the preschool years.
- Discuss changes in gross and fine motor movement, and identify appropriate activities to help develop these skills.
- Formulate examples of Piaget's preoperational phase of cognitive development.
- Apply the skills obtained during Erikson's phase of developing a sense of initiative versus guilt.
- Discuss activities of daily living (ADLs) the preschool child is capable of independently performing.
- Describe how a preschooler determines right from wrong.
- Promote ways to maintain optimal health through nutrition, activity, and sleep and rest.
- Classify activities and toys a preschooler would enjoy.
- Develop plans for injury prevention when a family is raising a preschool-age child.
- Describe ways to evaluate readiness and preparation for school.
- Discuss appropriate methods of discipline and limit-setting.
- Successfully complete the games and activities in the online student StudyWARE.

The preschool years directly follow toddlerhood and span ages 3 to 6 years. Although physical growth and changes slow, this is a time characterized by refinement of the cognitive and social skills begun during the toddler years. The preschooler establishes control of body systems as indicated by the ability to toilet, dress, and feed oneself. In addition, the preschooler is able to tolerate longer periods of separation from caregivers, and interact cooperatively with adults and other children. The preschooler can use language in a sophisticated manner and has an increased attention span and memory. The refinement of these skills prepares the child for entrance into school (Figure 10-1).

The changes typically occurring in the physiological, psychosexual, cognitive, psychosocial, and moral realms of development during the preschool years are described in the following pages. Health promotion, safety, and common concerns related to normal growth and development during the preschool years are also presented.

PHYSIOLOGICAL DEVELOPMENT

PHYSICAL GROWTH

During the preschool years, the rate of physical growth and change slows as compared to the rate experienced during the infant and toddler years. Generally, children will gain an average of 2.3 kg or 5 pounds per year in weight and 7.5 cm or 3 inches per year in height (Feigelman, 2007).

The preschooler's body contour also changes. The prominent abdomen, **lordosis**, and wide-legged gait characteristic of the toddler years gives way to a slimmer, taller, more posturally-erect contour.

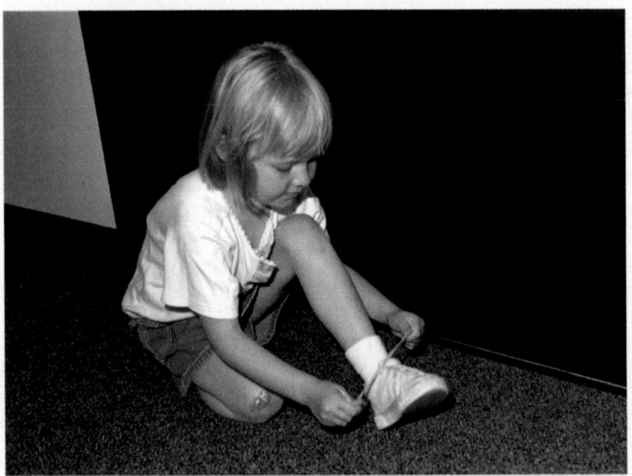

FIGURE 10-1 During the preschool years, as fine motor skills refine, the child learns how to tie her own shoelaces.
DELMAR CENGAGE LEARNING.

TABLE 10-1 Normal Vital Signs for Children 3–6 Years of Age

VITAL SIGN	VALUE
Heart rate	65–110 beats per minute
Respiratory rate	20–25 breaths per minute
Blood Pressure	Systolic rate: 95–110 Diastolic rate: 60–75

Adapted from Agrawal, S. (2008). Normal vital signs in children: Heart rate, respirations, temperature, and blood pressure. *Complex Child E-Magazine*. Retrieved January 5, 2010, from http://www.articles.complexchild.com/march2009/00114.pdf.

Body systems also continue to mature and stabilize. All the senses mature, and visual acuity reaches 20/20 with intact color vision (Green & Palfrey, 2008). Tonsils may grow and levels of antibodies may increase to assist the preschooler in better fighting infection. Children generally have all 20 of their deciduous teeth by 3 years of age. By the end of the preschool years, the eruption of permanent teeth may begin (Cleveland Clinic, 2009b). Their vital signs have also changed a bit from the toddler years. Refer to Table 10-1 for normal vital signs for children between 3 and 6 years of age.

Hand preference is established by the end of the preschool years. Muscle and bone growth continues, but maturity is not reached yet. Excessive activity and overexertion can damage growing tissue. Care should be taken to ensure the preschooler receives adequate rest, nutrition, and exercise to promote optimum development of the musculoskeletal system.

Bowel and bladder control, including nighttime control, is generally achieved during this period of development as well. However, accidents may still occur if the child becomes absorbed in an activity. Sleep patterns also become more organized with longer periods of night time sleep and daytime wakefulness.

GROSS AND FINE MOTOR SKILLS

The preschool period is a time of refinement of eye-hand coordination and muscle coordination. Walking, running, and jumping are well established by the preschool years, and by 3 years of age the child is able to ride a tricycle, balance on one foot for a few seconds, jump off the bottom step, and use alternate feet when going up the stairs. At age 4, the child can skip and hop on one foot, walk forward heel-to-toe, catch a ball with both arms, and use alternate feet when going down the stairs. Then, by 5 years of age , the child is able to skip on alternate feet, jump from a height of 12 inches and land on toes, throw and catch a ball well, walk backward heel-to-toe,

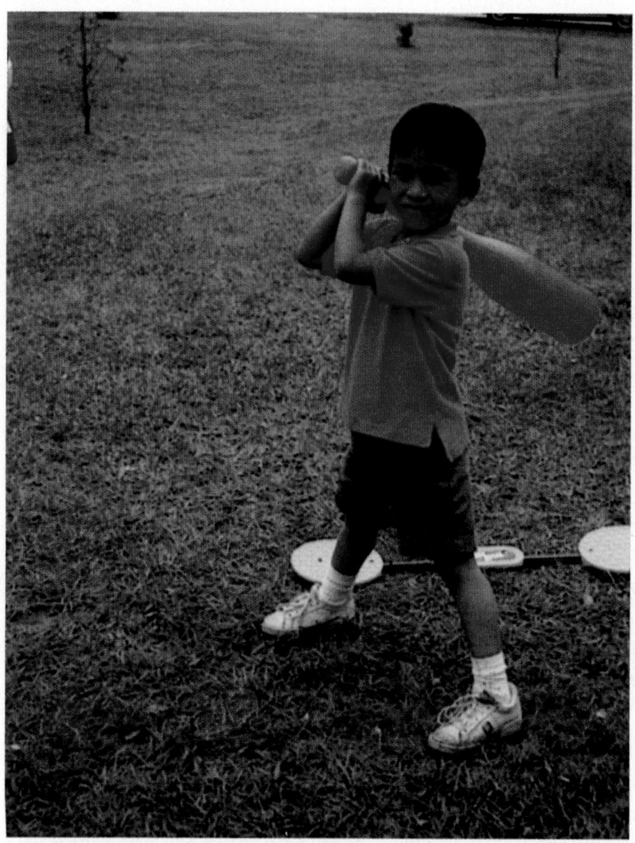

FIGURE 10-2A As the child progresses through the preschool years, gross and fine motor coordination improves and he becomes more proficient in hitting a ball. DELMAR CENGAGE LEARNING.

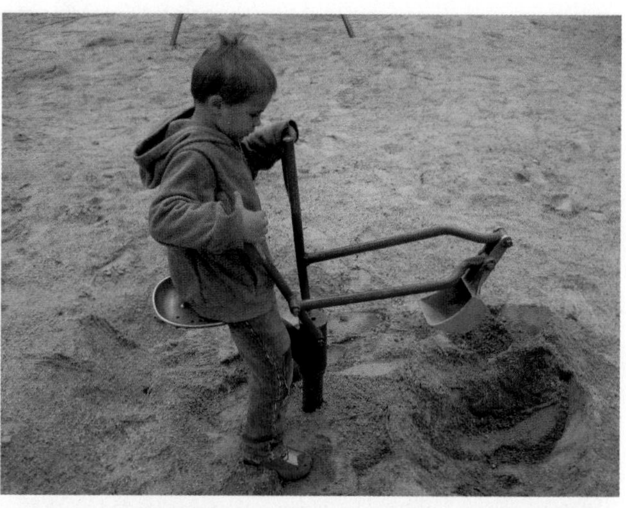

FIGURE 10-2B This preschooler is improving his eye-hand coordination by learning to use a sand shovel. DELMAR CENGAGE LEARNING.

and begin to learn many other motor skills, including skating, swimming, dancing, tumbling, and hitting a ball (Dixon & Stein, 2006) (Figure 10-2a; Figure 10-2b).

Fine motor skills also develop at an advanced rate. These skills can be tested through the use of the Denver Developmental Screening Test (Denver II), a standardized development test in wide use throughout the United States. The child who is 3 years old can build a tower of nine to ten cubes, build a bridge with blocks, copy a circle and may add facial features, and dress and undress oneself. The 4-year-old child can use scissors successfully, draw a stick figure with three parts, lace shoes, do up simple buttons, copy a square or trace a cross or diamond, and show hand preference. The 5-year-old child can begin to tie shoelaces, copy a square and triangle, and draw a person with at least six parts. The 5-year-old also becomes increasingly skilled with the use of a pencil and scissors.

The refinement and mastery of gross and fine motor skills encourage expression and independence, which leads to a greater sense of self-achievement and success as the child gets ready to enter school (Figure 10-3). Table 10-2 summarizes the preschooler's physiological development.

TABLE 10-2 Preschool Developmental Milestones

	3RD YEAR	4TH YEAR	5TH YEAR
Physiological Development			
Growth	**Weight** increases 4–6 lb (1.8-2.7 kg) per year. Average weight is 32 lb (14.6 kg).	**Weight** increases at a rate similar to the prior year. Average weight is 37 lb (16.7 kg).	**Weight** increases at a similar rate. Average weight is 41½ lb (18.7 kg).
	Height increases 3 in (7.5 cm) per year. Average height is 37½ inches (95 cm).	**Height** increase at same rate. Average height is 40½ inches (103 cm). Birth length is doubled.	**Height** increases at same rate.
			Handedness is established.
	Visual acuity is 20/20. Color vision is fully intact. May have achieved nighttime control of bowel and bladder.	Maximum potential for development of amblyopia. Cooperates with Snellen test.	Eruption of permanent teeth may begin. Pulse and respiration rates decrease slightly.

(Continues)

Table 10-2 Preschool Developmental Milestones (*Continued*)

	3RD YEAR	4TH YEAR	5TH YEAR
Gross Motor	Walking, running, and jumping are well established. Rides tricycle. Jumps off bottom step. Balances on one foot for a few seconds. Alternates feet going up stairs.	Skips and hops on one foot. Alternates feet going up and down stairs. Able to walk forward heel-to-toe, climbs jungle gym, and catches ball with both arms.	Skips on alternate feet and jumps rope. Jumps from height of 12 inches and lands on toes. Begins to skate and swim. Throws and catches ball well. Rides bike with training wheels. Able to walk backwards heel-to-toe and run on toes. Arms are coordinated with legs when running. Proficient climber.
Fine Motor	Builds towers of 9–10 cubes. Cannot draw a stick figure but may make a circle with facial features. Copies circle and can build a bridge. Dresses and undresses self.	Uses scissors successfully. Draws stick figures with 3 parts. Can lace shoes but may not be able to tie shoes. Copies a square and traces a cross or diamond. Shows hand preference.	Begins to tie shoelaces. Improved cutting with scissors. Uses a pencil very well. Copies square and triangle. Draws person with at least 6 parts.
Psychosexual Development			
Sexuality	Knows own and others' gender. Begins to adopt culturally prescribed behavior and roles.	Masturbation may increase. Displays sexual curiosity and interest in bodily differences between girls and boys. May explore differences in gender through play ("doctor" and "nurse"). May have own ideas to explain sexual differences and reproduction.	Displays gender stereotypic roles. Curiosity and sexual exploration continues. Able to understand potential for sexual abuse.
Cognitive Development			
Cognition	Preoperational thinking characterized by egocentrisim, concrete or tangible thinking, transductive reasoning, magical thinking, and the inability to distiguish between one's own perception and that of someone else. This is a period of magical thinking and the inability to reason logically. Concepts of time, space, and causality are primitive.		
	Attention span is still short but is increasing. Learns through observing and imitating. Continues to be very self-centered. Believes objects have human qualities (animism). Begins to learn concepts of time. Asks questions about environment. Fears are more specific, including fear of bodily harm. Active imagination! Color and number recognition begins.	Less self-centered and developing social awareness. Comprehends some simple analogies such as "if fire is hot, ice is cold". Better understanding of time. Understands concepts of long and short, light and heavy, and so on. Can sort objects into like categories. Usually separates from family easily. Starts, but may not complete projects.	Questions parents' thinking and principles by comparing to peers and other adults. Learns the "rules" of the culture (values and acceptable behavior). Beginning to see other perspectives but tolerates differences rather than understanding them. Very curious about factual information about the world. Shows more realistic sense of causality. Classifies objects according to similarities. Personality qualities are noticeable (see Figure 10-4).
Language	Knows name and age. Forms sentences of three to four words. Asks many questions. Uses	Use of longer sentences (four to five words). Tells exaggerated stories. Questioning is at peak.	Use of longer sentences (six to eight words) and uses prepositions, past verb tenses,

(Continues)

Table 10-2 Preschool Developmental Milestones (*Continued*)

	3RD YEAR	4TH YEAR	5TH YEAR
	mainly "telegraphic" speech. Correct use of plurals and pronouns. May use personal, made-up words and may carry on conversation with self. Vocabulary of about 900 words.	Correct use of some prepositions. Names one or more colors. Vocabulary of about 1,500 words.	adjectives, and so on correctly. Vocabulary of about 2,100 words by the end of the 5th year of age. Names four or more colors. Knows names of days of week, months, and other time-associated words. Follows three commands in succession.
Psychosocial Development			
Psycho-Social	Developing a sense of initiative vs. guilt (Erikson) This is a period of very energetic play and the child can develop a sense of accomplishment and satisfaction in his or her activities. As the child oversteps his or her limits, he or she experiences a feeling of guilt for not having behaved appropriately. This is the beginning of the development of a conscience (**superego**). The child has mostly overcome stranger anxiety and separation anxiety. More sociable and willing to please. Likes being a helper.		
Family Relations	Likes to please parents and conform with their wishes. Is less jealous of younger siblings (may be an opportune time for birth of additional sibling). Is aware of family relationships and sex-role functions.	Takes aggression and frustrations out on parents or siblings. "Do's" and "Don'ts" become important. Rivalry with older and younger siblings increases. May "run away" from home. Is able to run simple errands outside the home.	Gets along well with parents. May seek out parent for reassurance and security, especially when starting school. Begins to question parent's thinking and principles. Enjoys activities such as sports, cooking, shopping, or working.
Social	Feeds self completely and dresses with minimal help. Has increased attention span. Can help to set the table and do the dishes.	Very independent in dressing and feeding. Tends to be selfish, impatient, and physically aggressive. Has mood swings. Shows off dramatically to entertain others. Tells family stories to others without restraint.	Less rebellious and quarrelsome. More settled and eager to please. Tries to live by the rules. Trustworthy and can take on responsibilities. Has fewer fears. Has better manners.
Coping	Temper tantrums, negativism, and ritualism begin to decrease. Coping behaviors may include regression, denial, projection, displacement, attack, rationalization, and sublimation. Active imagination (may have an imaginary friend).	Begins to verbalize fears about body integrity, animals, or the dark. Uses play and fantasy.	Verbalizes feelings in later preschool years, may temporarily regress. May display independence through non-compliance or express confusion over inconsistent limits.
Play	Learns through play and imitation of adult behaviors. Will play cooperatively with other children and share toys. Plays group games with simple rules. Also likes dramatic play and is very imaginative and creative.		

(Continues)

Table 10-2 Preschool Developmental Milestones (*Continued*)

	3RD YEAR	4TH YEAR	5TH YEAR
Moral Development			
Moral	Kohlberg Stage 3 (Conventional Level): Child desires to please others or seek approval through behaviors. Shows concern for others.		
Spiritual	Learns to imitate the religious affect and behavior of parents. Mimics religious gestures although does not comprehend the meaning. Cannot separate feeling from thoughts. Formulates imagined descriptions of God, in other words, God is a friend the child can communicate with.		

Every child is unique and has an individual personality. While these descriptors are generally applicable, each child must be assessed as an individual.

Compiled with information from Charlesworth, R. (2011). *Understanding child development* (8th ed.). Clifton Park, NY: Delmar Cengage Learning: Dixon, S. D., & Stein, M. T. (2006). *Encounters with children: Pediatric behavior and development* (4th ed.). St. Louis: Mosby; Erikson, E. H. (1963). *Childhood and society*. New York: Norton; Freud, S. (1959). *Collected papers*. New York: Basic Books; Green, M., & Palfrey, J. S. (Eds.). (2008). *Bright futures: Guidelines for health supervision of infants, children, and adolescents* (3rd ed.). Arlington, VA: *National Center for Education in Maternal and Child Health*; Kohlberg, L. (1981). *The philosophy of moral development, moral states, and the idea of justice*. New York: Harper & Row; and Piaget, J. (1969). *The theory of stages in cognitive development*. New York: McGraw-Hill.

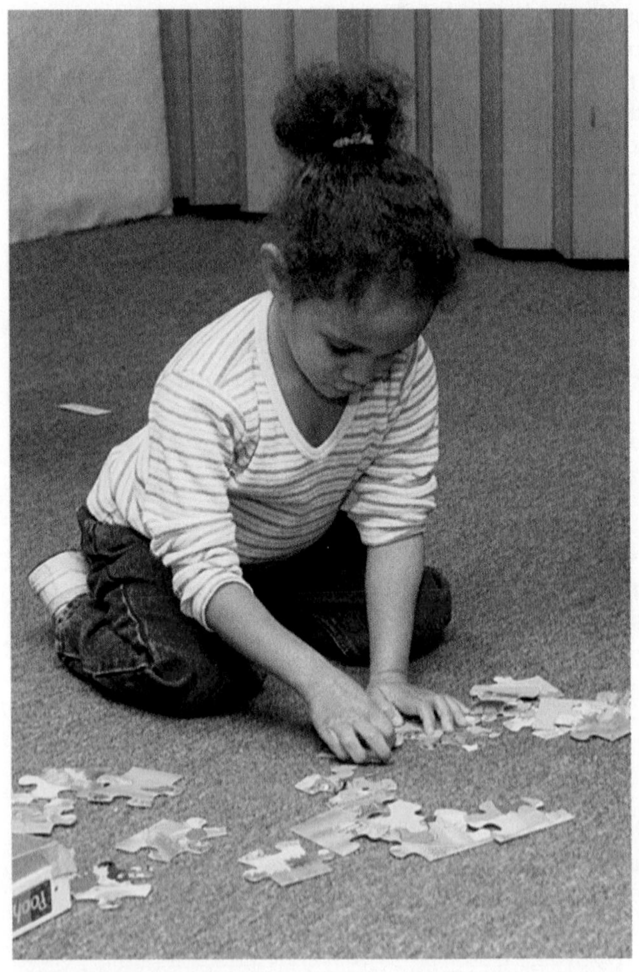

Figure 10-3 Preschoolers are increasingly able to complete puzzles and enjoy doing the same puzzle over and over. DELMAR CENGAGE LEARNING.

PSYCHOSEXUAL DEVELOPMENT

During the preschool years, the child is curious about his or her body, and learns about the physical differences between boys and girls. Freud described this period of time as the Oedipal, or phallic, stage of psychosexual development (Freud, 1959). During this stage the child experiences subconscious conflicts and an intense attraction and love for the parent of the opposite sex. In turn, the child feels competition with the parent of the same sex for the attraction and affection of the other parent. This is termed the **Oedipus** (preschool boy to his mother) or **Electra** (preschool girl to her father) **complex**. Caregivers can be reassured this phenomenon of competition and romance is normal, but may need help handling feelings of anger and jealousy that may arise. The resolution of the Oedipus or Electra complex comes as the child identifies with the parent of the same sex (Freud, 1959). (See Chapter 6 for more information.)

During this stage, the child becomes aware of himself or herself as a male or female, and begins to take on the behavior of the same-sex caregiver (Charlesworth, 2011). For example, a young girl sees her mother putting make-up on and wants to do the same. Or a young boy sees his father vacuuming and wants to help.

Children will display sexual curiosity and interest in bodily differences according to gender. They may explore these differences through play such as "doctor" and "nurse," or ask many questions. If these questions are not answered by an adult, the children might come up with their own answers, which often are inaccurate (Brazelton & Sparrow, 2006). Therefore, caregivers

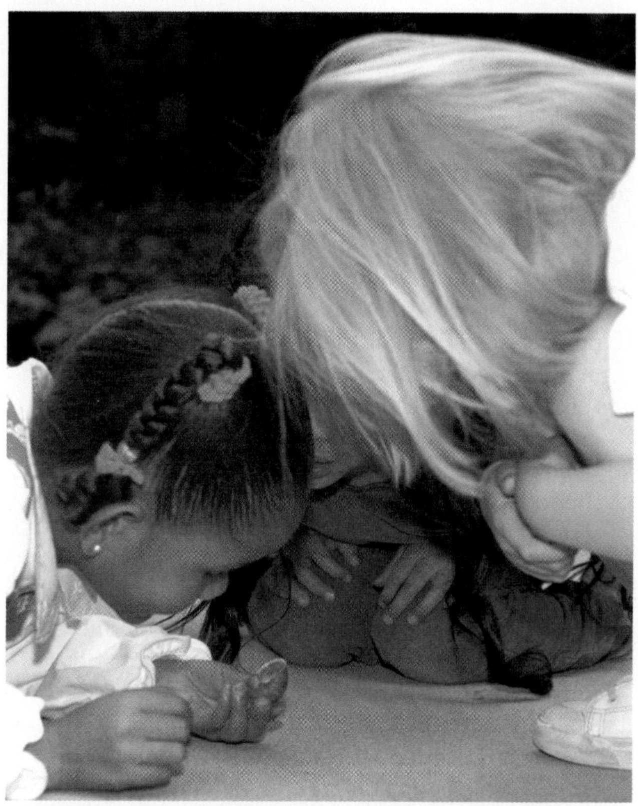

FIGURE 10-4 As they look at an empty snail shell, these preschoolers wonder where the snail is. DELMAR CENGAGE LEARNING.

REFLECTIVE THINKING

Differences between Boys and Girls

A mother comes to you with concerns about her preschool son Peter's inquisitiveness related to physiological differences between boys and girls. How would you respond? Would you feel awkward in responding? Why? Why not?

should answer questions simply, by using correct terms for all body parts, including genitalia. Caregivers should be cautioned to only answer questions asked, since often the child is curious only about one aspect of sexuality and not interested in hearing a complete description. This is also an optimum time to teach children that certain body parts are private and should not be touched by any other person. Table 10-2 summarizes the preschooler's psychosexual development.

PSYCHOSOCIAL DEVELOPMENT

The development of a sense of initiative versus guilt is the chief psychosocial task described by Erikson (1963). (See Chapter 6 for more information.) This is a time of very energetic learning, as the child participates in play and works with energy and enthusiasm, and develops a sense of accomplishment and satisfaction in activities. This increases the child's ability to use initiative, but as established limits are overstepped, feelings of guilt for not behaving appropriately may appear. A feeling of conflict may also arise as the child realizes actions were not appropriate. Feelings of guilt may come from thoughts the child has that are different from expected behaviors.

As the child learns to distinguish between the feelings of initiative and guilt, the child also begins to develop a conscience (superego). Learning right from wrong and good from bad is the beginning of moral development (Figure 10-5). However, preschoolers generally do not understand the reasons that something is acceptable or unacceptable; rather, preschoolers become aware of appropriate behavior through punishments and rewards handed out by caregivers or other adults. Reliance on caregivers and adults assists preschoolers in developing moral judgment.

In this age group, verbal reminders of established limits are effective, and the preschooler will understand the danger of running out into the road without looking. A reminder of what to do when crossing the street will be sufficient. The preschooler may disagree and question limits, which allows

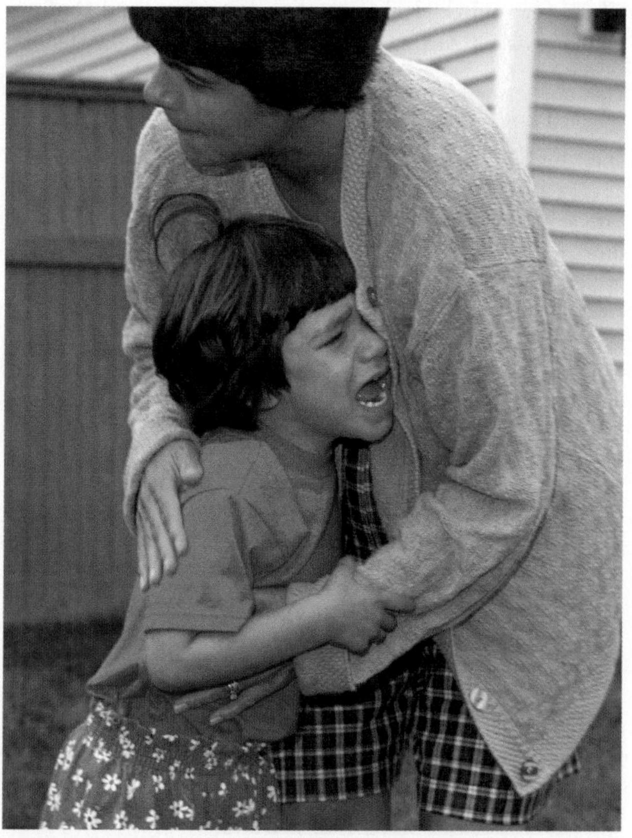

FIGURE 10-5 Distinguishing right from wrong is a concept learned in the preschool years. DELMAR CENGAGE LEARNING.

development of independence in thought and action as well as socially acceptable behaviors.

SOCIALIZATION

The preschool years are also critical years for the development of social skills—both the skills to care for self (dressing, bathing, eating, acting appropriately in social settings and manners) and the skills to get along with others. The preschool-age child is less egocentric, more capable of sharing, and able to enjoy play groups, since playing with other children helps teach relating to others and encourages imitation of adults. Preschool play is also dramatic, imaginative, and creative (Figure 10-6).

As the preschool-age child matures, arguing with others appears and may progress to the point where the child uses physical aggression to make a point. Although this may appear to be regressive behavior, this is actually normal behavior needed to identify and test roles in the social group and family. The child will gradually become less rebellious and quarrelsome and, by the end of the preschool years, will be more eager to please and take on additional responsibilities. The child will also try to live by established rules and enjoys playing group games with simple rules (Brazelton & Sparrow, 2006).

FAMILY RELATIONS

The 3-year-old child likes to please caregivers and conform to their wishes. At this age, the child is also less jealous of a younger sibling, so this may be an opportune time for the birth of an additional sibling. The 3-year-old is also aware of his or her place in the family and understands sex-role functions well.

As the child turns 4 years old, there is a dramatic increase in aggressive behavior, and frustrations may be shown through physical aggression. Rivalry with older and younger siblings increases. The 4-year-old may act out if she doesn't

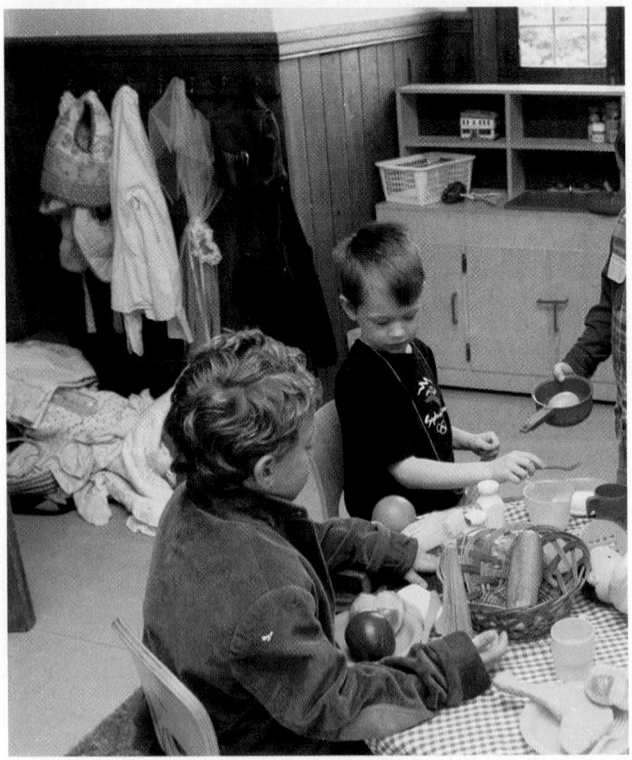

FIGURE 10-6 Preschoolers often engage in imaginative play.
DELMAR CENGAGE LEARNING.

CULTURAL CONSIDERATION

Collectivism and Familism

Collectivism and familism, two cultural dimensions describing the relationship of individuals to their social groups, are found in Latino families. Collectivism is characterized by a willingness to make personal sacrifices for the welfare of the group and high levels of empathy (Brewer & Chen, 2007). Familism is characterized by high family contact and unity, positive interpersonal relationships within the family, interdependence in role function, and social support (Schwartz, 2007). Familism is a very important and constant cultural characteristic Latino subgroups share, and is related to a family members' psychological functioning, help-seeking behaviors, and academic outcomes. It also provides emotional support for a child as she or he develops close bonds to the immediate and extended family network (Gamble & Modry-Mandell, 2008). According to the 2007 census, Latino families are usually larger and younger than African-American and European-American families (U.S. Bureau of the Census, 2007). Often childrearing is a shared responsibility for older siblings, parents, and extended family members (Maynard, 2002). Extended family members commonly reside in the same household or neighborhood. A strong positive significance is placed on Latino sibling relationships; siblings, lives are intertwined daily and companionship and shared caretaking are typical.

Reference: Brewer, M. B., & Chen, Y. R. (2007). Where (who) are collectives in collectivism? Toward conceptual clarification of individualism and collectivism. *Psychological Review*, *114*, 133–151; Gamble, W., & Modry-Mandell, K. (2008). Family relations and the adjustment of young children of Mexican descent: Do family cultural values moderate these associations? *Social Development*, *17*(2), 358–379; Maynard, A. (2002). Cultural teaching: The development of teaching skills in Maya sibling interactions. *Child Development*, *73*, 969–982; Schwartz, S. (2007). The applicability of familism to diverse ethnic groups: A preliminary study. *Journal of Social Psychology*, *147*(2), 101–118; and U.S. Bureau of the Census. (2007). *Mapping census 2007: The geography of U.S. diversity.* Retrieved March 13, 2009, from http://www.census.gov/population.

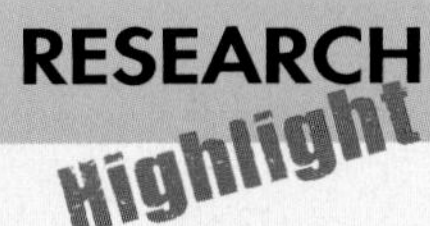

Do Family Relationships and Cultural Values make a Difference in Preschooler's Behavior and Relations with Others?

STUDY PURPOSE

To discover (1) if preschoolers of Mexican descent who had close and warm relations with siblings and mothers and would have fewer behavior problems and better, more positive peer and emotional adjustment in their Head Start classrooms; and (2) if familism and simpaticia would moderate these associations.

METHODS

Fifty-five mothers of Mexican descent with preschoolers (mean age 57.5 months; 51% male) completed instruments measuring familism, simpatía, mother–child relationship quality, child behavioral problems, and sibling relationships. Six months later, the preschool child's teachers completed instruments describing the child's social functioning with peers and emotional adjustment.

FINDINGS

Those children who had a close relationship with their mothers had fewer internalizing problems. Preschoolers with warm sibling relationships had positive social and emotional functioning: fewer behavior problems and positive relationships with peers. Finally, close and warm relationships with family members along with familism encouraged positive outcomes for preschool children.

IMPLICATIONS

A family's cultural beliefs and values as well as the quality of their relationships need to be considered when encouraging optimal development of preschool children. For those families of Mexican ethnicity, familism should be encouraged since it promotes young children's adjustment not only within the family but also with peers.

REFERENCE

Gamble. W., & Modry-Mandell, K. (2008). Family relations and the adjustment of young children of Mexican descent: Do family cultural values moderate these associations? *Social Development*, *17*(2), 358–379.

get her way. However, the 4-year-old child is also becoming increasingly able to run simple errands, such as getting a diaper for an infant the parent is changing or a book from another room, and to complete assigned tasks.

As the child turns 5, behavior within the family stabilizes and the child gets along well with family members. Parents are looked to for reassurance and a sense of security as the time for attending school nears. The 5-year-old also enjoys helping with cooking, shopping, chores, or other family activities.

COGNITIVE DEVELOPMENT

During the preschool years, many changes in the child's cognitive abilities are also occurring. **Cognitive ability**, or the capacity to understand and use phenomena in the world around us, is best explained by Piaget (Piaget, 1969). Piaget saw the child as an active participant in life, constantly assimilating and incorporating experiences into mental and physical structures of action (**schema**). These schema change over time as the child confronts new experiences and seeks to modify behavior and mental structures to handle the change. This change is called accommodation. (See Chapter 6 for more information.)

PREOPERATIONAL PHASE

Piaget's **preoperational stage** occurs between the ages of 2 and 6 years (Piaget, 1969). During this period, the child develops the ability to perform mental operations governed by personal perceptions and linkage to events previously experienced. The preschool child can understand experiences only from his or her own point of view, and cannot imagine that another person would have a different perspective (**egocentrism**). There is no separation of internal and external reality. The preschooler uses a personal system for organizing objects and events in his or her mind (**idiosyncratic**) and reasons from one particular to another, often by unrelated events (**transductive reasoning**), when in reality the particulars are not linked at all. **Animism** (belief that objects have human qualities) is also a part of the preschooler's thinking (Dixon & Stein, 2006). See Table 10-3 for examples.

The 3-year-old child's attention span is increasing, but it lasts for only a short time. Learning occurs through observation and imitation, as the 3-year-old asks many questions about the surrounding world, has a beginning concept of time, and begins to recognize colors and numbers (Figure 10-6). Due to the 3-year-old's active imagination, fears, including fears of bodily harm, may be experienced at this time (Charlesworth, 2011).

The 4-year-old child is less self-centered and has an increasing awareness of others and can comprehend simple analogies, for example, "if fire is hot, ice is cold." The child can also understand time better as well as the concept of opposites, for example, heavy and light and long and short. Finally, the 4-year-old can sort objects into like piles (Charlesworth, 2011).

The 5-year-old is busy learning the values and acceptable behavior of the culture, will question parent's thinking

TABLE 10-3 Preoperational Thinking

	QUESTION	CONCLUSION
Egocentrism	Why do cars go?	Cars go to take me to the park.
	Why does the sun shine?	The sun shines to see me when I play outside.
	Why did I get sick?	I hit my sister.
Animism	How did you get hurt?	The bike threw me off.
	Why did you hit the door?	The door hit me in the head.
Transductive reasoning	Daddy is home.	It must be time for dinner.
	The doctor put that thing in my ear.	I have an earache.
	I ate cookies right before dinner.	The cookies made me get sick.

by comparing with peers and other adults, and has a fairly good estimate of time. In addition, the 5-year-old begins to see other perspectives but only *tolerates* differences, rather than understanding them. The 5-year-old also demonstrates a more realistic understanding of cause and effect (Charlesworth, 2011).

FEAR

Preschoolers can become fearful of real or imagined things (bugs, the dark, animals). It is best to counsel the caregiver to tackle the problem directly. Instruct caregivers to find realistic ways to overcome or deal with the fear. For instance, keep a night light on at night. In some cases, continuous exposure to the fear stimulus may diminish the fear. However, it is important to not force a child. For example, if a child has a fear of swimming, the caregiver should encourage the child to put on a swimsuit and lifesaving gear, and sit by the edge of the pool. As the child witnesses the safe fun that other children and caregivers are experiencing, they may realize that there is nothing to be afraid of.

LANGUAGE

Another method of assessing cognition is through the child's use of language. The 3-year-old child has a vocabulary of about 500 words, forms sentences that are three to four words in length (**telegraphic speech**), uses plurals and pronouns correctly, and may make up words or carry on a conversation with himself or herself (Dixon & Stein, 2006).

The 4-year-old has a vocabulary of about 1,500 words, and uses longer sentences (about four to five words long) and some prepositions correctly. This is the age when questioning is at a peak; the child may tell exaggerated stories at this time too (Dixon & Stein, 2006).

The 5-year-old has a vocabulary of about 2,100 words, speaks in longer sentences (six to eight words long), and uses prepositions, adjectives, and past verb tenses correctly. In addition, the 5-year-old can name four or more colors and recognize time-associated words, such as the days of the week and the months of the year (Dixon & Stein, 2006).

Promote language development by talking with the child. Ask "how" and "why" questions to learn what the preschooler thinks. Answer questions with simple, short answers. Conversation helps the child build vocabulary and boost self-esteem.

MORAL AND SPIRITUAL DEVELOPMENT

Children of preschool age are in the **preconventional** or **premoral** stage of moral development as described by Kohlberg (Kohlberg, 1981). (See Chapter 6 for more information.) The child's moral judgment is at the most basic level, and right and wrong are determined from rules parents have established. Additionally, right and wrong are determined through rewards or punishments the child receives in response to an action. However, the preschool child has little understanding of why something is right or wrong, and if questioned will often say "because my mother says so." Young preschoolers may have difficulty applying known rules to a different situation. For example, if a parent says "there is no jumping on the couch in our house," the preschooler may jump on the couch in a friend's house. Later, the child is able to direct actions toward satisfying personal needs rather than the needs of others, and develops a concrete sense of justice and fairness.

The preschoolers' knowledge of faith or religion is learned from parents and other important adults in their lives. The preschooler may have a concrete concept of a Supreme Being with physical characteristics often like an imaginary friend. The child understands simple religious stories and memorizes short prayers. However, understanding the meaning of these rituals is limited, and participation in religious rituals occurs out of self-interest rather than out of a strong spiritual motivation.

HEALTH PROMOTION

As with any age group, it is important to look at the ways normal growth and development impact daily activities and the health of the child. In the preschool period, families play a major role in ensuring health and preventing injury and illness. The following sections explore the unique issues a preschooler may encounter related to health promotion and injury prevention as well as offer a discussion of important health screenings that need to occur during the preschool period.

HEALTH SCREENINGS

Health supervision and screenings are important in ensuring the ongoing health of the preschool-age child. Healthy habits are built through regular screenings, helping avert issues that may turn into problems later. A preschooler should see a health care provider yearly, including a physical examination with care taken to assess growth parameters, and vision, hearing, and blood pressure screening. If the young child is uncooperative with the vision screening, another appointment should be scheduled 6 months later.

The preschooler will also need to be kept current on immunizations, especially prior to starting school. If the child has received all the recommended vaccine doses as an infant and toddler, then only booster doses of diphtheria, tetanus, and acellular pertussis (DTaP), varicella vaccine, inactivated polio vaccine (IPV), and measles, mumps, and rubella (MMR) will be needed. Refer to Appendix C for the current schedule of immunizations.

The health screening should also include an assessment for the risk for hyperlipidemia, high-dose exposure to lead, and a tuberculin (TB) test. The TB test is required only once prior to school entrance unless there are risk factors present; then the test can be done annually with the health screening (Dixon & Stein, 2006).

One of the most common and preventable health problems in the United States is lead poisoning. Common sites of exposure include older homes and apartments that may have peeling lead-based paint, older lead water pipes, or lead dust from renovation of older homes. Extremely high blood lead levels can cause mental retardation, coma, or seizures. However, chronic low-level lead exposure is more common and leads to learning disabilities, impaired growth, anemia, and hearing loss. During the health screening, it is important to determine whether or not the child is at risk for exposure to lead. If there is a risk, a venous blood lead level should be drawn as well as a complete blood cell count. If the blood lead level is 10 mcg/dL, medical treatment is necessary (AAP, 2005).

The common health problems of the preschool years include mostly minor illnesses such as otitis media, colds, or gastrointestinal disturbances. In fact, during the preschool years, minor illnesses are more common than at any other age. This is probably because children start playing together more frequently, attend child care, or start preschool or school activities, resulting in more exposure to illness. Therefore, teaching children hand washing principles (after using the bathroom and before eating) may decrease the incidence of illnesses.

> **NURSING ALERT**
>
> **Antibiotic Resistance**
>
> Not every minor illness should be treated with antibiotics. Evidence is showing that resistance to antibiotics is increasing due to the indiscriminate use of antibiotics during childhood. Antibiotics should only be used for confirmed cases of bacterial infection, such as a positive streptococcal throat culture.

NUTRITION

Nutritional health is important in the preschool years as in other ages because of the impact good nutrition has on growth and also for the value of establishing good health habits for the rest of one's life. By 3 years of age, a child should be eating table foods. The diet of a preschool child should revolve around the principles of the U.S. Department of Agriculture's MyPyramid, which suggests a diet that contains whole grains, vegetables, fruits, milk, small amounts of meat, and beans. Fats and sweets should be taken sparingly. In addition, this is a good time to switch the preschooler to low-fat or skim milk, to decrease the amount of fat intake, since total fat intake should be no more than 30% of total caloric intake per day (NICHD Information Resource Center, 2005; U.S. Department of Agriculture, 2005). Tips for families from MyPyramid include: make half the grains whole; vary vegetables provided; focus on fruits; eat calcium rich foods; go lean with protein; change the type of oil used; and don't sugarcoat it (U.S. Department of Agriculture, 2005).

Planning meals and snacks around MyPyramid will give the child a well-balanced diet providing all the nutrients necessary to maintain health. If the child is eating a well-balanced diet, it shouldn't be necessary to supplement the diet with vitamins or minerals. If the child does not get a balanced diet, it may be necessary to start vitamins.

> **NURSING TIP**
>
> **Vitamins**
>
> Children's vitamins look fun and taste good, so children may be tempted to take more than the one per day. Be sure all vitamins are stored with other medications in a locked cupboard so the preschooler cannot "get into" the vitamins and take too many.

It is overwhelming to a preschooler to be served too much of any one food. Because of the decreased rate of growth during the preschool years, the appetite will also be decreased and the child may not be able to eat a large serving at one time. A helpful rule to follow is to serve 1 tablespoon of every kind of food per every year of age per meal. It is also a good idea to vary the types of foods offered (Brazelton & Sparrow, 2006). Some children may be labeled "picky eaters," but this is an age of exploration, and something the child refuses one day may be eaten another day. Experimenting with various ways of preparing foods, as well as letting the child help prepare the foods, may also increase intake (Green & Palfrey, 2008).

Some preschoolers will go on a "feeding strike" where they will refuse to eat much for a few days. This is normal, since children will often self-regulate their needs and eat when hungry. Other children may have "food jags" or go through a period of time when they will only eat one food or only foods of one color. Once again it is all right for children to make these choices. Caregivers should not fall into the trap of making eating and mealtimes a power struggle. Instead, mealtimes should be happy and enjoyable times for the family.

Preschoolers learn principles of good nutrition at home. Parents may struggle with knowing how to help the child learn good nutrition, especially with the many negative influences found in the media and society in general. Parents can assist preschoolers' learning by encouraging children to try new foods, not forcing any foods to avoid any negative associations, providing small meals with planned, nutritious snacks in-between meals (NICHD Information Resource Center, 2005), and allowing them to help in food preparation (Figure 10-7). In addition, make mealtimes a time when the whole family enjoys being together.

CHILDHOOD OBESITY

Today, there is an increasing incidence of childhood obesity. In fact, obesity prevalence among low-income, preschool-aged children has increased from 12.4% in 1998 to 14.6% in 2008. This might relate to the growing number of obese adults since studies have shown, prior to three years of age, parental obesity is the biggest predictor of a child's risk of developing obesity in adulthood (CDC, 2009a; Daniels et al., 2005; Ogden, Carroll, Curtin, McDowell, Tabak, & Flegal, 2006). Childhood obesity has both immediate and long-term physical and psychosocial effects. The physical effects may be hyperlipidemia, obstructive apnea, pancreatitis, gallbladder disease, noninsulin-dependent diabetes, and hypertension, which often lead to long-term cardiovasular diseases (CDC, 2009b). The obese child also often has lower self-esteem and may find it hard to "fit in" with a group of peers in those cultures that do not consider obesity attractive (Starr, 2009).

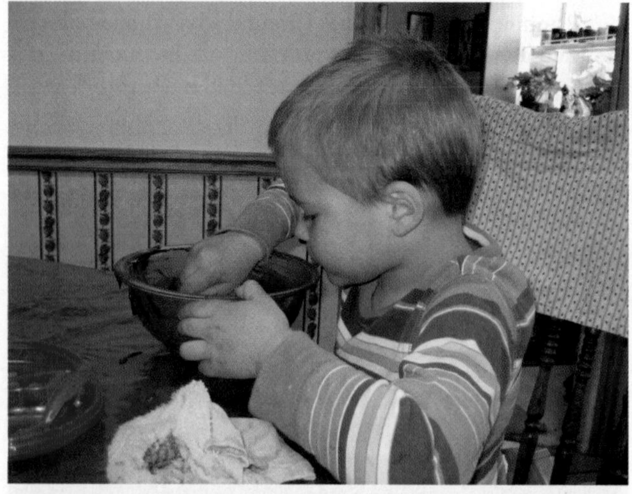

FIGURE 10-7 This preschooler is helping prepare the dessert for dinner. DELMAR CENGAGE LEARNING.

The prevention of childhood obesity starts by establishing healthy lifestyle habits during the child's early years. Healthy lifestyles are learned within the context of the family and should include: (1) developing practical ways to become physically active every day; (2) establishing the roles of parent and child in regards to food and eating: (3) determining the do's and don'ts for mealtime management; (4) promoting increased water intake, decreased sweetened beverage consumption, and prevention of overeating; and (5) reducing time spent in sedentary activities (American Dietetic Association, 2009; Hassink, 2007; Skelton & Rudolph, 2007).

SLEEP AND REST

Sleep patterns begin to change during the preschool years, and may vary from child to child. Generally, the preschooler will sleep a total of 12 hours every day. Some children sleep 10.5 hours a night and another 1.5 hours during an afternoon nap. Others will sleep for 12 hours every night. If children participate in preschool or day care centers, they will generally have a nap time. Even though many preschoolers will not sleep during nap time, it is important to have the children at least rest (Brazelton & Sparrow, 2003b; Cleveland Clinic, 2009a).

It is also critical to establish a bedtime routine for the child, and hopefully, those rituals started during the infant and toddler years can be continued. If bedtime rituals have not been started earlier, this is the time to establish routines that prepare the child for sleep. By participating in the routine consistently, the child will enjoy bedtime and the household will not be disturbed as much (Brazelton & Sparrow, 2003b; Cleveland Clinic, 2009a).

It is also important to help the child relax and prepare for sleep. Some children like to take a bath, play a quiet game, read a bedtime story, have a chat, say "goodnight moon," listen to soothing music, or have a light left on. All of these can help the child relax, learn how to be calm, and fall asleep (Figure 10-8).

SLEEP DISTURBANCES

An increase in the number and kind of sleep problems is common and normal during the preschool years. They should resolve and diminish, however, as the child gets

RESEARCH Highlight

Prevention and Early Treatment of Overweight and Obesity in Young Children

STUDY PURPOSE

To identify effective early treatment or prevention interventions that could be used in pediatric primary care practices with young children who are overweight, obese, or at high risk for later life obesity to decrease the trajectory of child weight gain, promote healthy weight attainment, and decrease the incidence of chronic comorbidities that are associated with overweight and obesity.

METHODS

Reviewed and critically appraised evidence from 12 randomized controlled trials conducted to determine the effectiveness of treatment or prevention intervention programs that included young children (4 to 7 years).

FINDINGS

Based on this evidence review, there are very few published rigorous studies to guide primary care providers in the prevention or early treatment of childhood obesity. Despite the lack of generalizable research, there is some evidence to guide health care providers who care for obese and overweight young children. These intervention strategies include: a) a combination of nutritional and activity information, b) a cognitive-behavioral aspect to the intervention, c) parent-directed activities, d) limiting sedentary child behaviors, and e) positive approaches with children by parents and practitioners.

IMPLICATIONS

Nurses should incorporate these practices, i.e. calculation and assessment of child's BMI at every visit, inclusion of a BMI percentile of 85 or greater on the problem list, and regular evaluation of history and physical information that suggest a child is at increased risk for overweight or obesity. In addition, adherence to current clinical practice guidelines that include the above interventions to prevent or treat childhood overweight or obesity is critical in addressing this growing public health problem.

REFERENCE

Small, L., Anderson, D., & Melnyk, B. M. (2007) Prevention and early treatment of overweight and obesity in young children: A critical review and appraisal of the evidence. *Pediatric Nursing, 33*(2), 149–161.

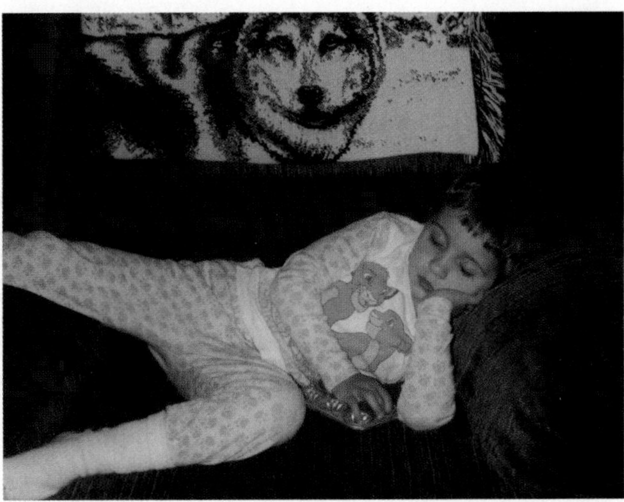

FIGURE 10-8 This preschool child, although ready for bed, fell asleep in a living room chair. DELMAR CENGAGE LEARNING.

older, since many are related to irregular sleep habits or anxiety about going to bed and falling asleep. By following a bedtime routine and teaching the child ways to become calm and relaxed before bed, the caregiver can minimize the incidence of these problems. Other children suffer from bedtime fears, which may be helped by using a night light and by having an open discussion to resolve those fears (Cleveland Clinic, 2009a).

Nightmares, which are also fairly common, often involve a major threat to the child who wakes up crying because of being scared. If nightmares awaken a child, the parent should comfort and reassure the child that the nightmares are not real, and help the child remain in bed and fall back to sleep. In addition, the parent should not talk about the nightmare a lot during the day as this may cause the child to feel bad about oneself. It will also help reduce the stresses on the child during the day as nightmares are often

FAMILY TEACHING

Establishing a Bedtime Routine

The bedtime routine should include:

- Establishing a go-to-bed time and sticking to it
- Establishing a wake-up time and sticking to it
- Avoiding stimulants such as sugar or caffeine, or roughhousing near bedtime
- Making the bedroom cozy and inviting
- Avoiding non-sleep activities in bed, for example, watching television
- Maintaining quiet in and near the bedroom
- Making bedtime a fun time to be with the child
- Providing a quiet activity (reading a story) prior to going to bed

Reflections from Families

It was always hard to get Joshua and Anna to bed when they were preschoolers, especially in the late spring and summer when it was daylight savings time and they could hear their friends playing outside. While this time of year brought the bellyaching of wanting to play with friends, I had established a routine when they were toddlers. I would give them a bath, have them brush their teeth, read them a favorite story, have them say their prayers, and then tuck them in. I also made sure their room was dark by pulling the blinds. While not every day was easy, sticking with a routine was definitely a plus.

associated with times of increased stress in the child's life (Brazelton & Sparrow, 2003b; Cleveland Clinic, 2009a).

Night terrors, talking in the sleep, and sleepwalking are other sleep disturbances occurring during the preschool years. In these situations, the child may appear to be awake but in actuality is confused and can't communicate clearly. Most often, children will just experience a single or an occasional episode of sleep disturbance. If the episodes occur several times a night or nightly, the child should be seen by a health care provider. Fortunately, as children mature, these sleep problems should diminish (Brazelton & Sparrow, 2003b; Cleveland Clinic, 2009a).

DENTAL HEALTH

By the beginning of the preschool period, the eruption of the deciduous (primary) teeth is complete. It is essential to preserve these primary and temporary teeth so the permanent teeth will have room to form correctly and the dental arch will not be narrowed. Since the preschooler is also very willing to be involved in brushing his or her teeth, this is an appropriate time to establish good dental habits that will last a lifetime.

The number one dental problem in the preschool years is dental caries or tooth decay, which may cause the premature loss of teeth and a consequent alteration of the dental arch, compromising development of the permanent teeth. Prevention of dental caries is accomplished through daily brushing and flossing of teeth; in addition, preschoolers enjoy imitating parents and older siblings brushing their own teeth. Parents or other adults should assist the child to ensure even the back teeth are brushed thoroughly (Figure 10-9). If toothpaste containing fluoride is used, only a pea-sized amount of toothpaste should be used (AAP, 2007b). The preschool-age child will also need assistance flossing because motor skills are lacking.

The preschool child should visit a dentist at least every 6 months. The first time the child visits the dentist, the child should not be told there will be no pain because, if pain is felt, trust will be lost and the child will become frightened (AAP, 2008). Most dentists prepare children according to their developmental level before any work begins. The dentist will determine if the child needs to take fluoride

CRITICAL THINKING

Nighttime Fears

The parents of 3-year-old Noah tell you he keeps the whole family awake at night because he is afraid of the dark. How would you help this family?

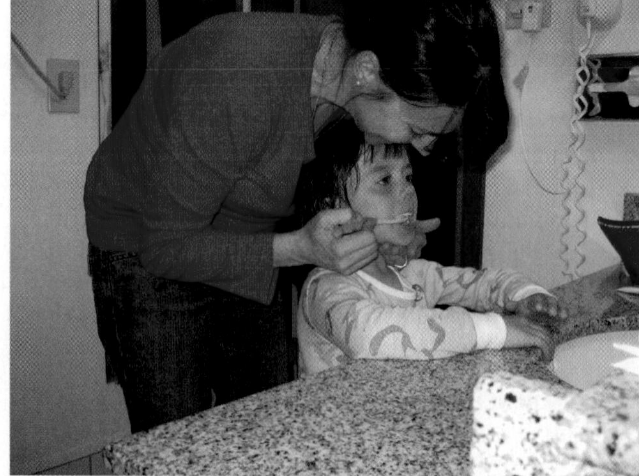

FIGURE 10-9 Sometimes preschoolers need help brushing their teeth, especially the back teeth. DELMAR CENGAGE LEARNING.

supplements depending on the amount of fluoride in the drinking water.

Lastly, children should avoid sugary snacks that may predispose them to dental caries. Instead, parents should provide healthy snacks such as fruit, vegetables, or cheese. When the child is ready to chew gum, it should be sugar-free. When the child does have a sugary treat, the child should brush or at least rinse the mouth out with plain water (Green & Palfrey, 2008).

NIGHT GRINDING

Some children grind their teeth at night. This is common during the preschool years and may be a way to release tension and calm oneself in order to fall asleep. Generally, tooth grinding lasts for a short time as the child slips into sleep. Tooth grinding may worsen during periods of stress in the child's life or prior to another developmental change. If tooth grinding is excessive, the child should be referred to a dentist who may prescribe a protective soft mouthpiece to wear during sleep (Brazelton & Sparrow, 2003b). Children with cerebral palsy, however, grind their teeth due to jaw muscle spasticity.

ACTIVITY

As detailed previously, the preschool child is refining both gross and fine motor coordination and skill. This allows the child to participate in more physical games and sports where motor activity is used (Figure 10-10). An emphasis on physical fitness has emerged in the last few years, and regular physical activity can benefit a child in many ways—for example, improved ability to perform motor skills; enhanced self-confidence and body image; development of lifetime habits; and prevention of disease processes associated with inactivity (Council on Sports Medicine and Fitness, Council on School Health, 2006). Physical activity can also help get rid of tension and excess energy.

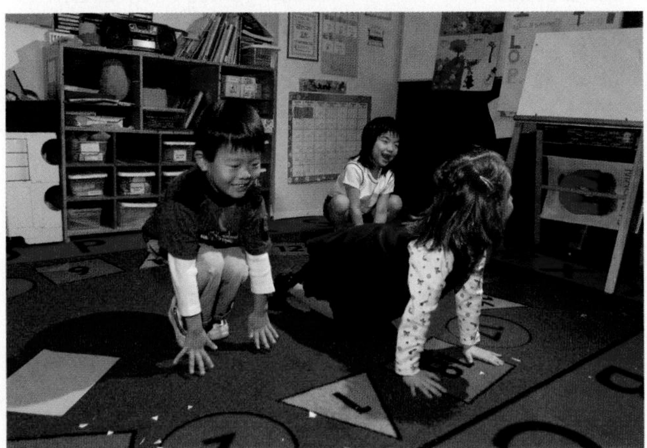

FIGURE 10-10 These preschoolers are enjoying hopping, dancing, and playing. DELMAR CENGAGE LEARNING.

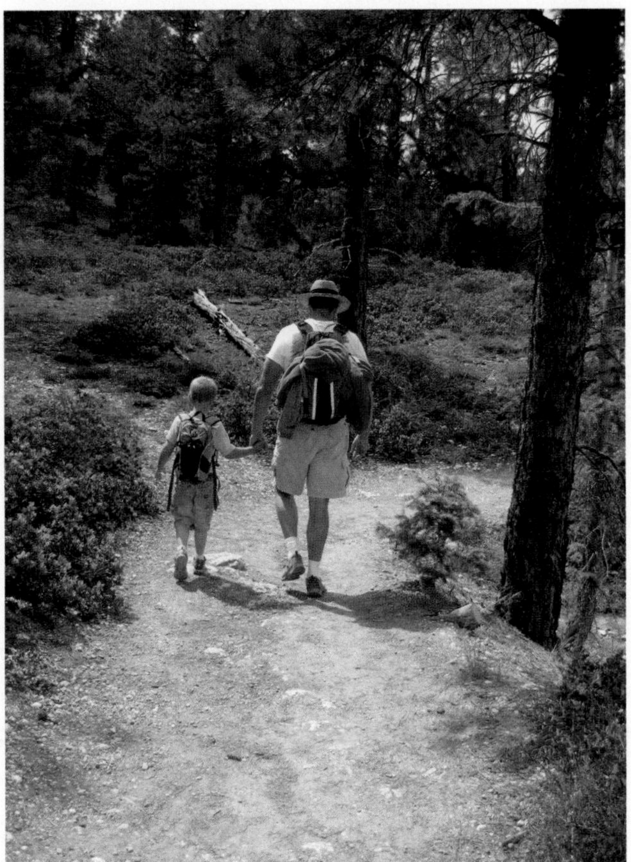

FIGURE 10-11 Hiking with parents provides physical activity which is important and can be enjoyable for preschoolers if the path is not too strenuous. DELMAR CENGAGE LEARNING.

By introducing the preschooler to sports activities and exercise, physical fitness can improve. Therefore, the main goal of sports for this age is to have fun, get exercise, and learn to enjoy the activity. However, since not all children will enjoy every sport or activity, it is important to find the right one for each child in order to make it a positive experience. The American Academy of Pediatrics (2006) suggests caregivers encourage a variety of physical activities in a non-competitive environment, with an emphasis on fun and safety. Some sports meeting these criteria are T-ball, karate, gymnastics, bicycling, or dance. However, not all activities have to be organized. Kids get great benefit from participating in physical activities like walking, bicycling, jumping rope, dancing, playing street games, and so on (Figure 10-11).

PLAY

Preschoolers enjoy group play, and also engage in imitative, dramatic, and imaginative play.

A 3-year-old still plays in an egocentric manner but is developing more tolerance of playmates. Play at this age is associative where there starts to be some interaction with other children and some toy sharing. Appropriate toys and activities for this age may include a tricycle, pounding bench, big blocks, musical or rhythm toys, show and tell, guessing games, and puzzles (Figure 10-12).

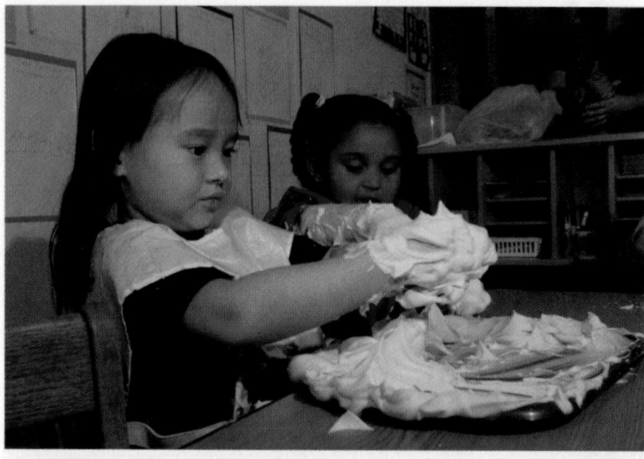

FIGURE 10-12 These preschoolers are enjoying the tactile nature of their art creation. DELMAR CENGAGE LEARNING.

A 4-year-old's play is interactive. The child cooperates with another child and actively shares toys. The child can also obey limits and often has an imaginary friend. This imaginary friend is often given up by the time the child enters school. Toys and activities may include construction toys, puzzles, memory games, fantasy play, books, and music.

A 5-year-old has achieved impulse control and plays well in groups, so this is an optimal time to introduce the child to group sports and games. The 5-year-old child enjoys dramatic or pretend play, puppets, dress-up, books, and art activities (Dixon & Stein, 2006) (Table 10-4).

TABLE 10-4 Toys and Activities that Stimulate Development

SKILL	TOY/ACTIVITY
Hand-eye coordination	Bubbles Coloring books Scissors Video games Large beads to string Stickers Markers or paint Large building set
Small motor	Crayons Sewing cards Art projects Play dough
Gross motor	Playing catch Kicking a ball Riding a tricycle Building blocks
Dramatic play	Play tools Kitchenette with dishes Dolls Magic wand Dress-up supplies Action figures Cars, trucks, trains Play people and animals
Cognitive	Books Puzzles Educational videos
Problem-solving	Puzzles Shape sorter Board games
Socialization	Group games such as London Bridge and Red Rover Board games Pretend play

LITERACY

The child's love of reading and interest in obtaining the skill is established during this time period when caregivers spend time reading to young children. The child will show early literacy skills by reciting the name of the books he or she wants to read; retelling the stories in the book; asking questions about the story; pretending to read a favorite book; correcting the reader if a page is skipped; and paying attention through the entire story (AAP, 2009).

Preschoolers will also enjoy books with more words that tell stories, especially if the book has lots of pictures. Books about children with similar experiences, including going to the doctor, going to the park, and going to school, or books about friends and families are also appropriate for children this age. Lastly, books with a predictable story line and repeated phrases help keep the child's attention (Figure 10-13).

TELEVISION AND MEDIA

The influence of television and other media on children has become controversial even though it can be constructive and positive. Television, however, is not a substitute for education and play. Some programs can reinforce learning, promote creativity, and encourage cognitive growth by teaching colors, numbers, the alphabet, and social skills in a creative and stimulating manner. However, some programs are inappropriate for young children. Since preschoolers often believe what they see is real; they cannot differentiate between reality and fantasy in television programs. Inappropriate programs give children a distorted view of how to deal with problems, such as violence (AAP, 2007a).

While the television should not be used as a babysitter, it is virtually impossible to "ban" television viewing. Instead, caregivers should closely monitor and control what a child

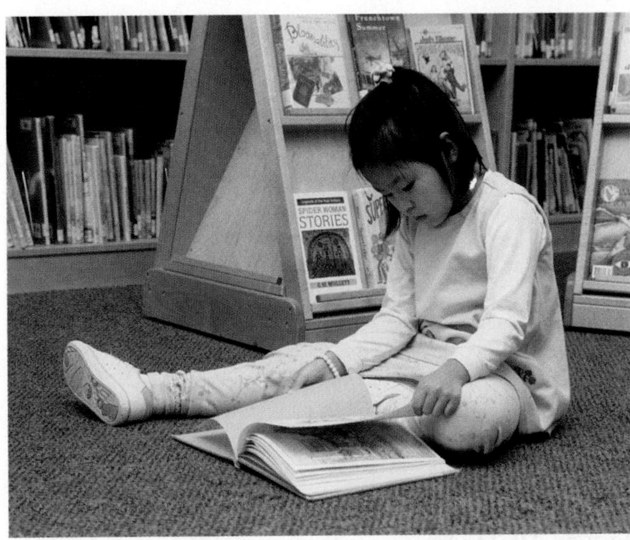

FIGURE 10-13 **Regular visits to the library for story hour and borrowing books encourage a love of reading.** DELMAR CENGAGE LEARNING.

EVIDENCE-BASED PRACTICE

The Effect of Home Literacy Practices on Preschoolers

CLINICAL PROBLEM

Children who have difficulty learning to read most likely will have reading problems throughout much of their school years. Literacy skills (attitude, knowledge, skills) necessary for developing reading and writing are linked to later reading success.

BEST CLINICAL PRACTICE

Specific literacy practices (frequently reading books, the child's interest in books, book reading strategies [asking open-ended questions, adding information], parental sensitivity and responsiveness) are important in helping children's language and emergent literacy skills. However, the home environment (responsive, sensitive, and accepting of child's behavior; positive emotional climate; stimulating toys and interactions; structure and organization) was the most consistent predictor of children's literacy skills and language.

IMPLICATIONS FOR NURSING

- Educate parents on the importance of reading to their young children; encourage them to read frequently, ask open-ended questions about the story being read, and be sensitive and responsive to their children while reading.
- Encourage parents to provide a home environment that is sensitive, responsive, accepting, positive, structured, organized, and provides stimulating toys and interactions.

Reference: Roberts, J., Jurgens, J., & Burchinal, M. (2005, April). The role of home literacy practices in preschool children's language and emergent literacy skills. *Journal of Speech, Language, and Hearing Research, 48*, 345–359.

BOX 10-1
GUIDELINES FOR TELEVISION AND VIDEO VIEWING

- Set limits
- Plan your child's viewing
- Watch TV with your child
- Find the right message
- Help your child resist the commercials
- Look for quality children's videos
- Give other options
- Set a good example
- Express your views

Adapted from AAP. (2007a). *Television and the Family*. Retrieved March 13, 2009, from http://www.aap.org/publiced/BR_TV.htm.

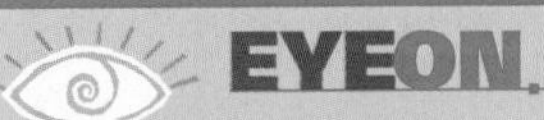

Toys that Teach

Through advertisements, some toys are promoted as "toys that teach," meaning they teach, for example, "cause and effect" and "manual dexterity." While these toys are safe and attractive, the nurse must caution caregivers to be cognizant of deceptive advertising. For instance, an advertisement may imply that, if children do not have this toy, they will be developmentally delayed or that this toy is an adequate substitute for caregiver-child interaction. These claims are not true.

watches. The AAP recommends a preschooler only watch 1–2 hours of television per day. See Box 10-1.

SAFETY AND INJURY PREVENTION

With the increase in motor skills and coordination, the preschool-age child is less prone to falls common during the toddler years. However, due to their increased mobility and skills, there are now other dangers. One of the greatest areas of concern is playing near the street or driveway since preschool children still need close, constant supervision by adults to remain safe (Figures 10-14 and 10-15).

It is also important to remember that the preschool-age child is less reckless, but will listen more to rules, and is aware of potential dangers such as hot objects, sharp instruments, or dangerous heights. This makes it easier for adults who are supervising preschoolers to set limits and expect obedience. However, as this is a time when the child likes to imitate whatever adults do, it is critical adults also abide by the same rules, for example, putting on a seat belt before the car moves (Green & Palfrey, 2008).

Box 10-2 gives guidelines for injury prevention.

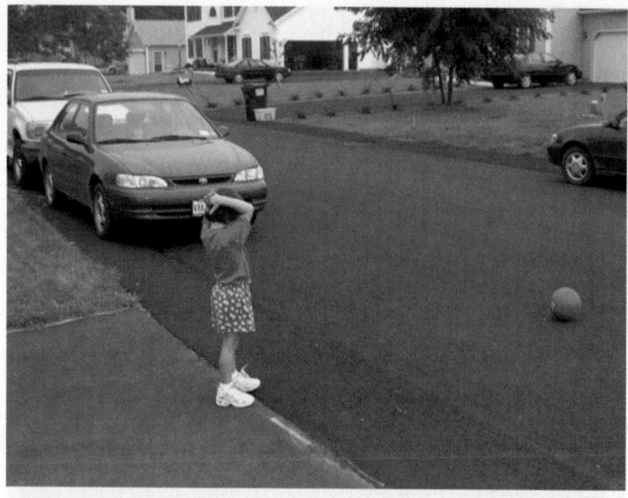

FIGURE 10-14 Injury prevention includes teaching the preschooler how to cross the street and not to run after a ball that has rolled into the street. DELMAR CENGAGE LEARNING.

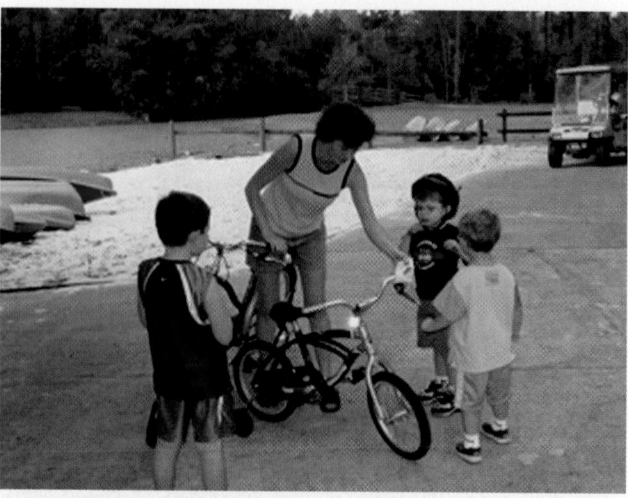

FIGURE 10-15 These preschoolers are being reminded to wear their helmets when learning to ride a bicycle. DELMAR CENGAGE LEARNING.

BOX 10-2
INJURY PREVENTION GUIDELINES

Home Safety

- Establish and enforce consistent, explicit, and firm rules for safe behavior.
- Never leave the child alone in the house.
- Test smoke detectors to ensure that they work properly. Change batteries yearly.
- Keep all poisonous substances, cleaning agents, health and beauty supplies, medicines, and home improvement materials in a locked, safe place. Have safety caps on all medications.
- Keep cigarettes, lighters, matches, and alcohol out of the child's sight and reach.
- Ensure guns, if in the home, are locked up and the ammunition is stored separately.

Play Safety

- Ensure playgrounds are safe. Check for impact- or energy-absorbing surfaces under playground equipment.
- Teach the child about playground safety.
- Teach the child about sports safety, including the need to wear protective sports gear.

Water Safety

- Ensure home and neighborhood swimming pools are enclosed by a four-sided fence with a self-closing, self-latching gate. Children should be supervised by an adult whenever they are in or around water.
- Ensure the child wears a life vest if boating.
- Teach the child how to swim.
- Teach the child safety rules for swimming pools.

Car Safety

- Continue to use a car seat or a properly secured booster seat until the child's head is higher than the back of the seat or the child weighs 85 pounds or is four feet tall. When the child moves out of a booster seat, ensure the seat belt is always fastened when the car is moving.
- The child should always ride in the back seat.
- Never leave the child alone in the car.

(Continues)

BOX 10-2
INJURY PREVENTION GUIDELINES *(Continued)*

Safety with Others

- Keep the child away from cigarette smoke. Do not allow smoking in the home or in the car.
- Choose sitters carefully. Discuss with them their attitudes about behavior in relation to discipline.
- Teach the child safety rules regarding interacting with people he or she does not know.
- Ensure the child is supervised before and after school in a safe environment.
- Teach the child his or her phone number and address in case he or she becomes lost.

Outdoor Safety

- Put sunscreen on before going outside to play.
- Supervise all play near streets or driveways.
- Teach the child pedestrian and neighborhood safety skills.
- Teach the child about safety rules for getting to and from school.
- Teach the child about safety rules for bicycles. Teach the correct signals for traffic safety.
- Ensure the child wears a bicycle helmet when riding a bicycle, tricycle, scooter, or skates.

Emergency Preparedness

- Keep your address and phone number posted near the phone.
- Keep your list of emergency numbers (doctor, hospital, nearest neighbor, poison control center, etc.) near the phone.

Adapted from Green, M., & Palfrey, J. S. (Eds.). (2008). *Bright futures: Guidelines for health supervision of infants, children, and adolescents* (3rd ed.). Arlington, VA: National Center for Education in Maternal and Child Health.

KIDS WANT TO KNOW

Why do I have to wear my helmet?

It is safer to wear your helmet when riding your bike because it will protect your head from getting hurt if you fall. Everyone should wear a helmet when riding a bike.

DISCIPLINE AND LIMIT SETTING

Poor behavior is normal for all children. As a toddler, the child has learned to throw temper tantrums to get what is wanted. As the child becomes a preschooler, the same kind of tactics may be used. Limits are needed to help the child learn acceptable behavior. Initially, the child will test limits, but in the end, the child will welcome the limits because they define expected behaviors. If the child crosses over these boundaries, disciplinary action must be taken, and the child's behavior redirected in as positive a manner as possible (Brazelton & Sparrow, 2003a; Green & Palfrey, 2008).

Time-outs can also be an effective method of discipline. No longer than 1 minute per each year of age, time-outs teach the child how to calm down and will give the child enough time to calm down but not too much time to become resentful (Brazelton & Sparrow, 2003a).

One of the challenges of working with preschoolers is diverting aggressive behavior. Preschoolers tend to engage in instrumental aggression, that is, aggression designed to unblock a blocked goal such as getting back an object, territory, or privilege. The caregiver needs to encourage sharing and nonaggressive ways of resolving conflict. Preschoolers engage in modeling, which is imitating behavior they witness. It is important for caregivers to not only model positive behavior but also reward positive behavior (Charlesworth, 2011).

An effective tool for teaching appropriate behavior is **reverse attention**. Our society tends to give attention to bad behavior and ignores good behavior. The news is filled with reports of robberies, murders, and other bad behavior. Rarely does the news highlight a person who never causes any trouble, pays bills on time, and takes good care of his or her family. This trend toward focusing on negative behavior is also seen within the family. The child who is quietly coloring is left alone, but when the child colors on the walls, parents discipline the behavior. Caregivers need to be taught to reward good behavior in addition to disciplining negative behavior (Brazelton & Sparrow, 2003a).

PREPARATION FOR SCHOOL

During the preschool years, many children attend some type of early childhood program, either child care or preschool, which provides an excellent opportunity to encourage development. The experience can bring increased time for

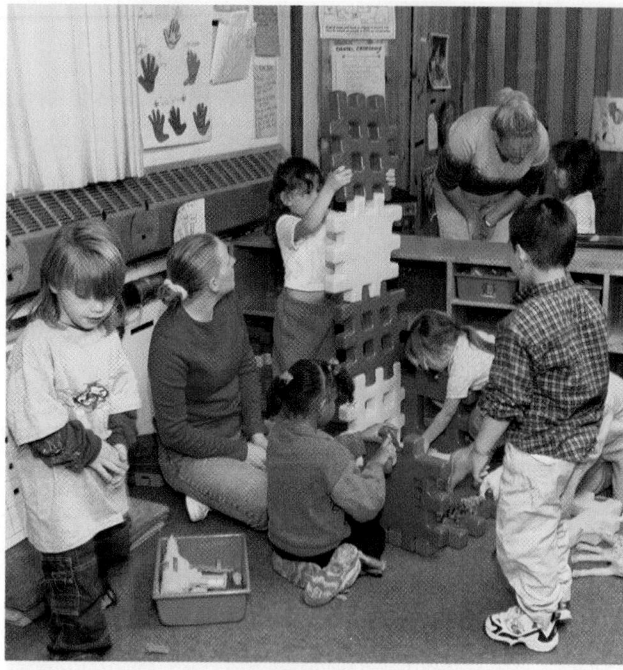

FIGURE 10-16 Preschoolers learn to cooperate in their play.
DELMAR CENGAGE LEARNING.

interaction with other children of the same age; teach group cooperation skills; stimulate language, physical, and social development; and help them cope with frustration and dissatisfaction (Brazelton & Sparrow, 2006; Dixon & Stein, 2006) (Figure 10-16).

Most early childhood programs include quiet play; active, outdoor activities; group activities and games; art projects; creative or free play; snack time; and rest time. All activities are tailored to provide mastery of skills and to give the child an increased sense of achievement, confidence, and success.

Caregivers often ask health care providers for advice on knowing when the child is ready to attend preschool or school. Even though there are no absolute indicators of school success, the child's social maturity (age, physical abilities, and ability to play with other children) and potential to participate in learning (can follow instructions and has an attention span that is long enough to be able to participate in activities) can provide an indication of readiness (Dixon & Stein, 2006).

Preparation for attending preschool or school can help the transition. Since there will be separation issues when the child initially starts school, this can be lessened by helping the child understand what will happen at school if the experience is presented as fun and exciting. If the child thinks school is an adventure and learning can be fun, the change may be embraced quicker.

FAMILY TEACHING

Preparation for the First Day of School

- Send detailed information about the child to the school, including familiar routines, favorite activities, food preferences, and names of siblings and parents.
- Put the child on a "school" schedule a few weeks before school actually starts. This will assist the child to feel comfortable with the routine before school actually begins.
- Practice school-type activities: ride the bus, have school lunch at home (play cafeteria), sit in chair at table to color, practice printing name, tie shoes, and have a rest period or quiet time.
- Introduce child to the school, surroundings, and the teacher.
- Stay with the child on the first day if possible. Be available but not conspicuous.

IN THE REAL WORLD

I never thought I would get used to the questions my preschool clients asked. But now, preschool age is my favorite age to take care of. They are so honest, inquisitive, interested in learning all they can about what is going on around them, and willing to help. I love reading them stories. Many times they know the story by heart and will tell me if I forget to read a paragraph or talk about one of the pictures. Isn't it too bad that, as children get older, they lose the openness they had as preschoolers?

KEY CONCEPTS

- The preschool years are characterized by the refinement of physical, motor, cognitive, and social skills.
- The preschooler is in the preoperational stage of cognitive development where he learns to perform mental operations that are governed by his own perception and understanding of events.
- During the preschool years, the child develops a sense of initiative versus guilt.
- The preschooler learns activities of daily living including how to dress oneself, tie shoes, and brush teeth.
- The preschool child learns to cooperate with other children, and enjoys associative and cooperative play.

- The beginning of moral judgment is seen as the child learns what is right and wrong based on the punishments and rewards established by caregivers.
- Health promotion is directed toward proper nutrition, sleep or rest, activity, and dental health.
- Preschoolers need close supervision in the home, by water, outdoors, and on the playground in order to prevent injury.
- The preschool child should visit a health care provider on a yearly basis for a routine assessment of health and development.
- A child's readiness for participation in school is determined by the child's social maturity and readiness to learn.
- Give attention for good behavior, and ignore negative behavior.

REVIEW ACTIVITIES

1. Describe physical growth during the preschool years.
2. List several tests of motor function for a 3-year-old that are included on the Denver II.
3. Give an example of animism and transductive reasoning.
4. Explain the language development skills of the preschooler.
5. Describe how a child who has achieved a sense of initiative may react to a new situation.
6. Is it normal for the preschooler to have an imaginary friend? When would you be concerned about this imaginary friend?
7. What is a rule to follow when serving food to a preschooler?
8. List some common sleep disturbances that may occur during the preschool years.
9. Why would a preschooler grind his or her teeth at night?
10. When can a preschooler stop riding in a car safety seat?

STUDY QUESTIONS

(Questions 1 through 5) A 4-year-and-4-month-old girl presents for her prekindergarten check-up. The family is expecting a new baby in two months. The child's history is significant for recurrent otitis media with effusion, with resulting tympanostomy tubes at 3 years of age, and a urinary tract infection at 4 years of age. She is starting kindergarten in the fall and her mother has concerns about her adjustment to a new baby in the family. Additionally, she has been awakening with nightmares over the past two months. Her history and physical exam is normal for her age.

1. Among the following options, what is the best response to the family regarding the child's sleep problems?
   a. "It is abnormal for healthy preschool children to have nightmares."
   b. "Preschool children have night terrors more often than nightmares."
   c. "Nightmares are common during preschool years and during times of stress."
   d. "Don't use a night light as the shadows cast by the light may make her more frightened."
2. Which of the following skills would be beyond the developmental level of the 4-year-old girl?
   a. Copies a circle
   b. Recites her full name
   c. Rides a tricycle
   d. Can count ten objects
3. This child's visual acuity using the Allen Picture Cards was 20/50 in the right eye. The best course of action would be:
   a. Refer to an ophthalmologist for evaluation
   b. Retest in 3 months
   c. Nothing; results are normal for this age
   d. Retest in 1 year
4. Which of the following would be normal for a 4-year-old?
   a. Skips on alternate feet and jumps rope
   b. Throws and catches ball well
   c. Able to walk forward heel-to-toe
   d. Begins to tie shoelaces
5. Recommendations regarding preventive pediatric dental care include which of the following?
   a. Fluoride supplementation to children who are drinking water with fluoride
   b. Weaning bottle-fed infants by 24 months of age
   c. Fluoride supplementation to exclusively breast-fed infants
   d. First dental visits during the preschool years

(Questions 6 through 10) Five-year-old Adam is admitted for an asthma exacerbation. His history is significant for attention deficit/hyperactivity disorder. He has been on Ritalin for the past six months. His weight percentile is 90th and his height is 40th. His parent states that he has been difficult to discipline at home. She has tried spanking, but he seems to keep repeating the same behaviors.

6. Effective discipline requires:
   a. Harsh punishment.
   b. Ignoring inappropriate behaviors.
   c. Instilling fear.
   d. Using physical force.
7. In addressing the child's current growth, his weight and height percentile indicate that:
   a. He is overweight for his height.
   b. His height is greater than his weight percentiles.
   c. He has appropriate height for his weight.
   d. He is shorter than he should be for his age.
8. What healthy lifestyle habits could this family institute to assist their child in growing into his weight?
   a. Participate in physical activities at least once a month
   b. Increase intake of sweetened beverages
   c. Avoid having meals together as a family
   d. Promote increased water intake
9. An average preschooler is recommended to watch no more than how many hours of TV per week?
   a. 25-30
   b. 15-20
   c. 10-15
   d. 20-25
10. When taking a history regarding a behavioral problem, it is best to get information from:
    a. The mother and father alone.
    b. The child by himself/herself.
    c. Each parent individually.
    d. All household members.

REFERENCES

Agrawal, S. (2008). Normal vital signs in children: Heart rate, respirations, temperature, and blood pressure. *Complex Child E-Magazine.* Retrieved January 5, 2010, from http://www.articles.complexchild.com/march2009/00114.pdf.

American Academy of Pediatrics. (2005). Lead exposure in children: Prevention, detection, and management. *Pediatrics 116*(4), 1036–1046.

American Academy of Pediatrics. (2007a). Television and the family. Retrieved March 13, 2009, from http://www.aap.org/publiced/BR_TV.htm.

American Academy of Pediatrics. (2007b). How to prevent tooth decay in your baby's teeth. Retrieved March 13, 2009, from http://www.aap.org/publiced/BR_ToothDecay.htm.

American Academy of Pediatrics. (2008). Preventive oral health intervention for pediatricians. *Pediatrics, 122*(6), 1387–1394.

American Academy of Pediatrics. (2009). Read me a story: Reading checkup guide. Retrieved January 24, 2010, from http://www.aap.org/family/readmeastory.htm.

American Dietetic Association. (2009). *Guidance for parents on preventing childhood weight gain and obesity.* Retrieved July 13, 2009, from http://www.eatright.org/cps/rde/xchg/ada/hs.xsl/media_5482_ENU_HTML.htm.

Brazelton, T. B., & Sparrow, J. D. (2003a). *Discipline: The Brazelton way.* Cambridge, MA: DaCapo Press.

Brazelton, T. B., & Sparrow, J. D. (2003b). *Sleep: The Brazelton way.* Cambridge, MA: Perseus Publishing.

Brazelton, T. B., & Sparrow, J. D. (2006). *Touchpoints: Three to six* (2nd ed.). Cambridge, MA: DeCapo Press.

Brewer, M. B., & Chen, Y. R. (2007). Where (who) are collectives in collectivism? Toward conceptual clarification of individualism and collectivism. *Psychological Review, 114,* 133–151.

Centers for Disease Control and Prevention, and National Center for Chronic Disease Prevention and Health Promotion. Improving Health and Quality of Life for all People. (2009a). Obesity at a glance: Halting the epidemic by making health easier.

Centers for Disease Control and Prevention. (2009b). Obesity prevalence among low-income, preschool-aged children—United States, 1998–2008. *Morbidity and Mortality Weekly Report* 58(No. 28), 769–73.

Charlesworth, R. (2011). *Understanding child development* (8th ed.). Clifton Park, NY: Delmar Cengage Learning.

Cleveland Clinic. (2009a). Sleep in toddlers and preschoolers and sleep disorders. Retrieved March 13, 2009, from http://my.clevelandclinic.org/disorders/sleep_disorders.htm.

Cleveland Clinic. (2009b). Teeth eruption timetable—children. Retrieved March 13, 2009, from http://my.clevelandclini.org/services/dental_care.htm.

Council on Sports Medicine and Fitness, Council on School Health. (2006). Active healthy living: Prevention of childhood obesity through increased physical activity. *Pediatrics, 117*(5), 1834–1842.

Daniels, S. R., Arnett, D. K., Eckel, R. H., Gidding, S. S., Hayman, L. L., Kumanyika, S., Robinson, T. N., Scott, B. J., St. Jeor, S., & Williams, C. L. (2005). Overweight in children and adolescents: Pathophysiology, consequences, prevention, and treatment. *Circulation, 111,* 1999–2012.

Dixon, S. D., & Stein, M. T. (2006). *Encounters with children: Pediatric behavior and development* (4th ed.). St. Louis: Mosby.

Erikson, E. H. (1963). *Childhood and society.* New York: Norton.

Feigelman, S. (2007). The preschool years. In R. Kleigman, R. Behrman, H. Jenson, & B. Stanton. (Eds.), *Nelson's textbook of pediatrics* (18th ed.). Philadelphia, PA: Saunders/Elsevier, 54–57.

Freud, S. (1959). *Collected papers.* New York: Basic Books.

Gamble, W., & Modry-Mandell, K. (2008). Family relations and the adjustment of young children of Mexican descent: Do family cultural values moderate these associations? *Social Development, 17*(2), 358–379.

Green, M., & Palfrey, J. S. (Eds.). (2008). *Bright futures: Guidelines for health supervision of infants, children, and adolescents* (3rd ed.). Arlington, VA: National Center for Education in Maternal and Child Health.

Hassink, S. (2007). *Pediatric obesity: Prevention, intervention, and treatment strategies for primary care.* Elk Grove Village, IL: American Academy of Pediatrics.

Kohlberg, L. (1981). *The philosophy of moral development, moral states, and the idea of justice.* New York: Harper & Row.

Maynard, A. (2002). Cultural teaching: The development of teaching skills in Maya sibling interactions. *Child Development, 73*, 969–982.

NICHD Information Resource Center. (2005). *Milk matters for your child's health*. NIH Publication no. 05-4521.

Ogden, C. L., Carroll, M. D., Curtin, L. R., McDowell, M. A., Tabak, C. J., & Flegal, K. M. (2006). Prevalence of overweight and obesity in the United States, 1999–2004. *Journal of the American Medical Association, 295*, 1549–1555.

Piaget, J. (1969). *The theory of stages in cognitive development*. New York: McGraw-Hill.

Roberts, J., Jurgens, J., & Burchinal, M. (2005, April). The role of home literacy practices in preschool children's language and emergent literacy skills. *Journal of Speech, Language, and Hearing Research, 48*, 345–359.

Schwartz, S. (2007). The applicability of familism to diverse ethnic groups: A preliminary study. *Journal of Social Psychology, 147*(2), 101–118.

Skelton, J., & Rudolph, C. (2007). Overweight and obesity. In R. Kleigman, R. Behrman, H. Jenson, & B. Stanton. (Eds.), *Nelson's textbook of pediatrics* (18th ed.). Philadelphia, PA: Saunders/Elsevier, 232–242

Small, L., Anderson, D., & Melnyk, B. M. (2007). Prevention and early treatment of overweight and obesity in young children: A critical review and appraisal of the evidence. *Pediatric Nursing, 33*(2), 149–161.

Starr, N. (2009). Self perception issues. In C. Burns, A. Dunn, M. Brady, N. Starr, & C. Blosser (Eds.), *Pediatric primary care* (4th ed.). St. Louis, MO: Saunders Elsevier, 347–365.

U.S. Bureau of the Census. (2007). *Mapping census 2007: The geography of U.S. diversity*. Retrieved March 13, 2009, from http://www.census.gov/population.

U.S. Department of Agriculture. (2005). *My Pyramid*. Retrieved March 13, 2009, from http://www.myPyramid.gov.

SUGGESTED READINGS

American Dental Association. (2009). Water fluoridation: Nature's way to prevent tooth decay. Retrieved March 13, 2009, from http://www.ada.org/goto/fluoride.

DeOnis, M., Garza, C., Victoria, C. G., Bhan, M. K., Novum, K. R., guest editors. (2004). The WHO multicentre growth reference study (MGRS): Rationale, planning, & implementation. *Food & Nutrition Bulletin, 25*(1), supp 1.

Henry, L. L. (2005). Childhood obesity: What can be done to help today's youth? *Pediatric Nursing, 31*(1), 13–16.

Lewis, C., Lynch, H., & Richardson, L. (2005). Fluoride varnish use in primary care: What do providers think? *Pediatrics, 115*(1), e69–e76.

NICHD Information Resource Center. (2005). *Autism overview: What we know*. NIH Publication no. 05-5592.

Society for Nutrition Education, Weight Realities Division. (2003). Guidelines for childhood obesity prevention programs: Promoting healthy weight in children. *Journal of Nutrition Education and Behavior, 35*(1), 1–4.

Vismara, L. A., & Rogers, S. J. (2008). The early start Denver model: A case study of an innovative practice. *Journal of Early Intervention, 31*(1), 91–108.

Welsh, J. A., Cogswell, M. E., Rogers, S., Rockett, H., Mei, Z., & Grummer-Strawn, L. M. (2005). Overweight among low-income preschool children associated with the consumption of sweet drinks: Missouri, 1999–2002. *Pediatrics, 115*, 223–229.

RESOURCES

Refer to the online student StudyWARE for Potts & Mandleco at http://www.CengageBrain.com for additional content and study aids.

Organization: **American Academy of Family Physicians**
Description: Offers information regarding family physician careers, clinical research, advocacy, practice management, and recent news/publications.
Website/Resource: http://www.aafp.org

Organization: **American Academy of Pediatrics**
Description: Offers general information related to child health, specific guidelines concerning many pediatric issues, information regarding AAP programs, activities, policies, guidelines, publications, and other child health resources.
Website/Resource: http://www.aap.org

Organization: **Centers for Disease Control and Prevention**
Description: Offers information regarding current disease conditions, emergency preparedness/response, life stages/populations, healthy living, workplace environment/health.
Website/Resource: http://www.cdc.gov

Organization: **Kid Source Online**
Description: Online community allowing parents to share values/goals in raising, educating, and providing for children; access to parenting/education/recreation/organizations/product information.
Website/Resource: http://www.kidsource.com

Organization: **MedlinePlus: Trusted Health Information for You**
Description: Access to the National Library of Medicine for directories, medical encyclopedia/dictionary, tutorials on common conditions/tests/treatments, information on prescription/nonprescription drugs, health information/links to clinical trials.
Website/Resource: http://medlineplus.nlm.nih.gov/

Organization: **National Institute of Child Health & Human Development (NICHD)**
Description: Offers information regarding general health information, research, funding, and recent news/media related to child health and development.
Website/Resource: http://www.nichd.nih.gov

Organization: **National Safe Kids Campaign**
Description: Offers readers tips about child safety, news/information about Safe Kids, and support/funding information.
Website/Resource: http://www.safekids.org

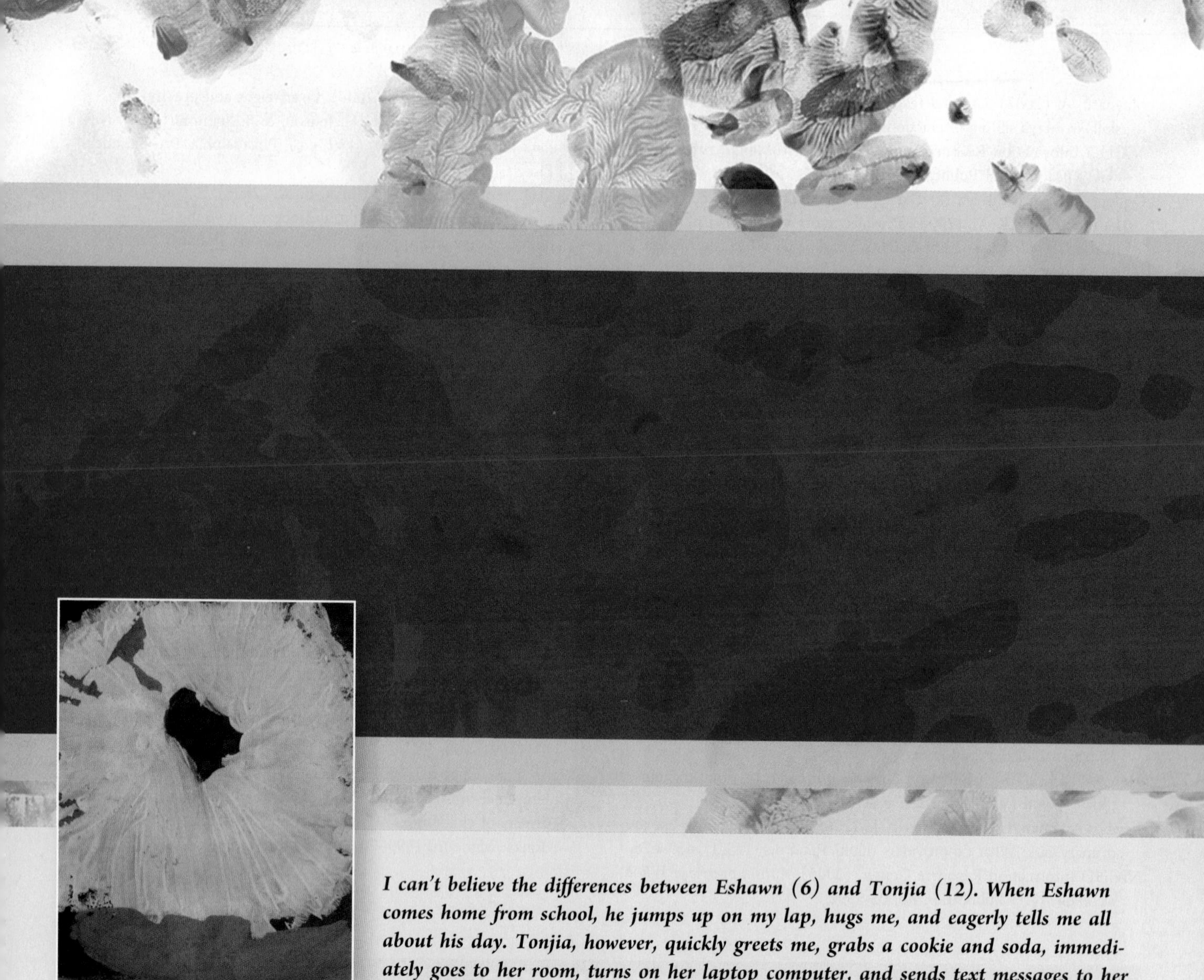

I can't believe the differences between Eshawn (6) and Tonjia (12). When Eshawn comes home from school, he jumps up on my lap, hugs me, and eagerly tells me all about his day. Tonjia, however, quickly greets me, grabs a cookie and soda, immediately goes to her room, turns on her laptop computer, and sends text messages to her girlfriends. They also are "into" different things. Eshawn enjoys puttering around the house on Saturdays with his dad, but Tonjia would rather spend the day at the mall with her friends. What a difference six years make in children!

CHAPTER 11

Growth and Development of the School-Age Child

Susan O'Conner-Von, RN, PhD

COMPETENCIES

Upon completion of this chapter, the reader will be able to:

- Describe the normal physical growth pattern for the school-age child.
- Discuss Freud's latency phase of psychosexual development.
- Offer examples of concrete operations of the school-age child.
- Explain Erikson's major task of school-age psychosocial development.
- Describe the characteristics of moral development during school-age years.
- Explain the nurse's role in caring for school-age children.
- Discuss the significance of school and peers for the school-age child.
- Identify common stressors of the school-age child and coping strategies to help them manage.
- Discuss health promotion activities for the school-age child.
- Successfully complete the games and activities in the online student StudyWARE.

The phase of development from 6 to 12 years, the **school-age years**, is crucial to establishing positive self-esteem, a sense of belonging, and feelings of competence. During this time, the child moves from egocentric thought to experiencing the world through peers, online social networks, and the school environment. Today's child entering school also experiences the world beyond the classroom with the help of the Internet, electronic mail, and satellite television.

This chapter begins with a description of the normal growth and development parameters of the school-age child, including physiological, psychosexual, cognitive, psychosocial, and moral development, and concludes with health promotion and the nurses' role in health promotion activities.

PHYSIOLOGICAL DEVELOPMENT

The school-age years are marked by a steady rate of physical growth. However, caregivers and nurses need to keep in mind that each child is unique and growth is affected by genetic background, gender, the presence of acute or chronic illness, and environmental factors (Deloian & Berry, 2009). A vital mechanism influencing physical development during the school-age years is growth hormones, which stimulate cells throughout the body. The pituitary gland and hypothalamus, located at the base of the brain, are believed to play key roles in stimulating physical growth. The brain and skull growth slows down during the school-age years and will increase little from that point. The brain is adult size by about 12 years of age (Gance-Cleveland & Yousey, 2009).

MUSCULOSKELETAL

During the school-age years, the child's weight increases by 7 pounds per year and height increases by 2.5 inches per year (Feigelman, 2007). At 6 years, the average boy weighs 45 pounds and is 46 inches tall; the average girl weighs 43 pounds and is 45 inches tall. At 12 years, the average male weighs 88 pounds and is 59 inches tall; the average female weighs 91 pounds and is 60 inches tall. Skeletal growth is particularly noticeable in the long bones of the extremities.

KIDS WANT TO KNOW

Why do I wake up at night with cramps in my legs?

Growing pains are temporary and caused by bones growing faster than muscles. The discomfort is usually located in the knees, heels, calves, and thighs. Comfort measures that can be used at home include analgesics, gentle massage, and a warm bath. Shoes that are sturdy and supportive are also helpful.

CRITICAL THINKING

Physiological Development

Ryan and Wally have come to the office for a physical. Ryan, an eight-year-old, weighs 43 pounds and is 45 inches tall. Wally, a ten-year-old, weighs 68 pounds and is 50 inches tall. The boys are accompanied by their mother, who is worried about their weight and height. Why is she showing concern? What does the nurse need to consider when answering the mother?

Growing pains, affecting 25–40% of school-age children (American Academy of Pediatrics, 2007a), commonly occur between the ages of 8 to 12 years; girls are affected up to two times as often as males (American Academy of Pediatrics, 2007a).

Muscle strength and size also increase at a gradual rate during school-age years (Figure 11-1), and six basic gross motor skills (balancing, catching, throwing, running, jumping, climbing) continue to be refined. At the same time, improved balance and coordination enable the school-age child to explore new physical activities, such as bike riding and rollerblading. These newly found activities are often met with enthusiasm. However, muscles can be easily injured so physical activities should be selected according to the child's development.

Boys have a greater number of muscle cells than girls, so it is common to find they do well with gross motor activities, such as throwing and running. In contrast, girls tend to have better dexterity of fingers and hands, so they are more adept at fine motor (small muscle) skills during the school-age years. As eye-hand coordination and motor skills improve, the school-age child is able to write, tie shoes, and become autonomous in dressing. Motor development progresses in a cephalocaudal and proximal to distal direction, with refinement of both gross motor and fine motor skills occurring as the central nervous system matures (Deloian & Berry, 2009).

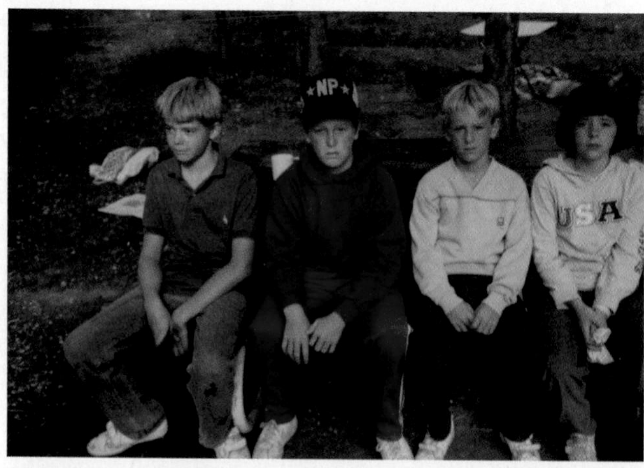

FIGURE 11-1 School-age children mature at different rates.
DELMAR CENGAGE LEARNING.

KIDS WANT TO KNOW

Will I have to undress during my check-up? What is happening to my body?

By the time a child reaches 9 years of age, honest discussion by caregivers is warranted about upcoming physical examinations and changes. Caregivers are encouraged to use correct terms when discussing these changes, be aware of the importance of modesty, and stay with their child during an exam to offer support.

Reflections from Families

My father never told me about sex; instead, I learned about it from the other guys on my Little League baseball team. At that point in my life, the thought of sex was repulsive and I thought there is no way I could even think about it. Now that I am a father, I plan to be honest with my son and talk to him about sex.

To meet the increased activity levels during the school-age years, the cardiovascular and respiratory systems develop in size and capacity. Heart growth slows, the heart assumes a more vertical position in the chest, and the diaphragm descends to allow for lung expansion. As the cardiac and respiratory systems become more efficient, the pulse and respiratory rates slow down. The average apical pulse rate for the school-age child is 90 to 95 beats per minute while at rest. The average respiratory rate for the school-age child is 20 breaths per minute while at rest.

NURSING ALERT

Innocent Heart Murmur

As many as 50% of all school-age children between 6 and 10 years of age have an "innocent" heart murmur. These murmurs are not clinically significant, but may be a concern to the caregiver if found during a routine physical exam.

FAMILY TEACHING

Innocent Heart Murmur

- Explain to caregivers that an "innocent" murmur is created from the sound of the blood flowing through the heart and can be heard because of the child's thin chest wall.
- Reassure the child and caregiver the murmur is not associated with heart disease and will no longer be heard when the child reaches adolescence.
- Provide the school nurse with medical documentation confirming the presence of an innocent heart murmur.
- Provide athletic coaches with medical documentation confirming the presence of an innocent heart murmur.

During the preschool years, children are exposed to and develop immunity to a variety of microorganisms. Therefore, the school-age years are often among the healthiest phases of life (Santrock, 2009). Antibodies are produced by the lymphatic system and reach their peak by age 7 years. For example, IgA, which protects the respiratory and gastrointestinal tracts from pathogens, and IgG, which activates destruction of bacteria, are found at adult levels during this time. Because of the increase in body size and maturity of the immune system, school-age children are able to respond to illnesses in a similar manner to adults.

PSYCHOSEXUAL DEVELOPMENT

Freud (1923) believed the first five years of life were the most critical to psychosexual development. Starting at age 6 years and throughout school-age, the child enters a calm period in the development of sexuality, called latency. Freud theorized the school-age child identifies with the same-sex parent by modeling the behaviors and emotions of this parent (see Chapter 6 for more information on Freud's theory). The child also learns about sex-role behavior and identity by observing caregiver interactions, the media, and friendships with children of the same gender.

SEXUAL DEVELOPMENT

The last years of the school-age period are called prepubescence, meaning the two years before **puberty** (Figure 11-2). Puberty comes from the Latin word *pubertas,* meaning adult, and is considered the stage of human maturation when secondary sex characteristics begin to develop and females have their first period (**menarche**) (see Chapter 12). The first

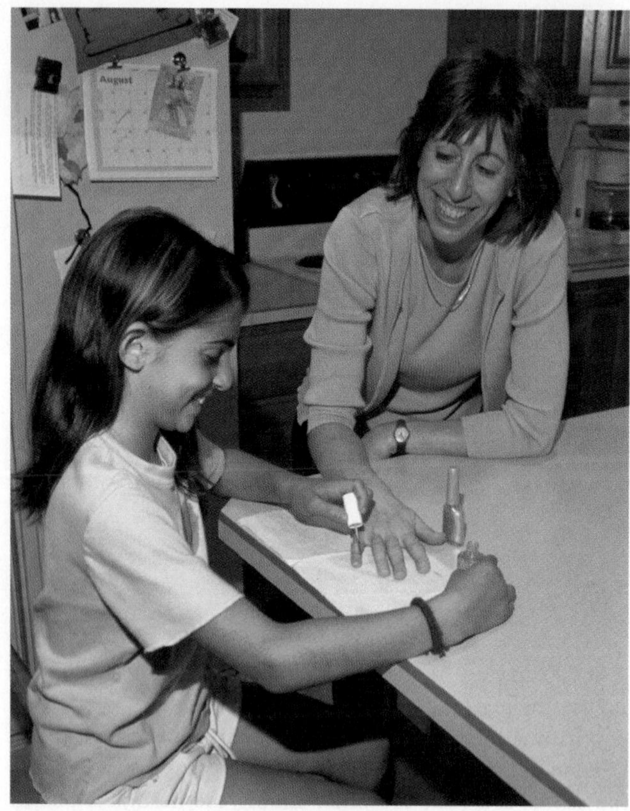

FIGURE 11-2 Prebuscence starts between 8 and 13 years of age in females. DELMAR CENGAGE LEARNING.

physiological signs of prepubescence, such as breast tissue development, appear between 8 to 13 years of age in females and from 10 to 14 years in males (American Academy of Pediatrics, 2007b).

PSYCHOSOCIAL DEVELOPMENT

The school-age years introduce the child to the world of peers and school. As each child interacts within this new context, a more realistic sense of self and place in this world evolves. A newfound independence from caregivers is discovered and peers become a major socializing agent. Because they are the major socializing agents at this time, children behave according to what they deem is acceptable to their friends. Although school-age children need the love and support provided by caregivers, peers provide the support needed to gain independence from family, and are central to development as increased amounts of time are spent with peers of the same gender (Huston & Ripke, 2006). At age 2 years, children interact with peers 10% of their day; between the ages of 7 and 11 years, children interact with peers more than 30% of their day (Damon & Lerner, 2006).

The developmental theory of Erik Erikson (1963) identified the major task of the school-age period as industry (the ability to be useful or productive) versus inferiority. (See Chapter 6 for more information on Erikson's theory.)

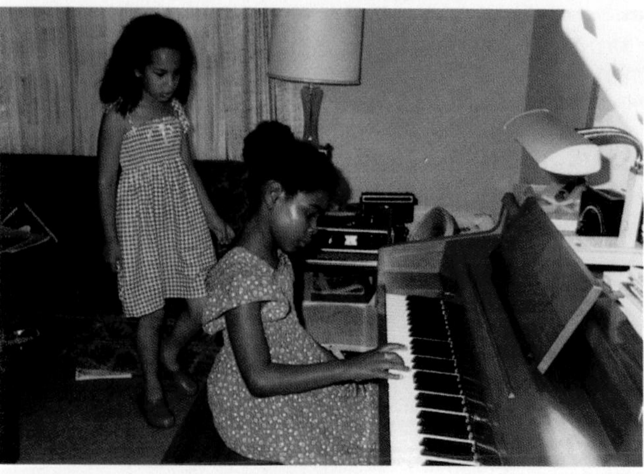

FIGURE 11-3 Playing the piano provides a sense of accomplishment to this school-age child. DELMAR CENGAGE LEARNING.

During this time, energy is channeled into activities such as school projects, sports, and hobbies. These concrete endeavors become the child's work and bring a sense of accomplishment and worth (Figure 11-3). During this stage, the school-age child also develops the ability to work with others on school projects and athletic teams in preparation for becoming a citizen of the world.

Erikson (1963) believed development is a continual process based on prior success, and if children are not able to realize a sense of industry, feelings of inferiority may develop. This occurs when children believe they cannot live up to the expectations of caregivers or teachers, or when they feel different from peers. In order for school-age children to feel a sense of competence, it is imperative they have a positive relationship with an affirming adult (Figure 11-4). If unable to receive the support needed from caregivers or teachers, a school nurse, club leader, or coach may be instrumental in instilling this positive sense of competence.

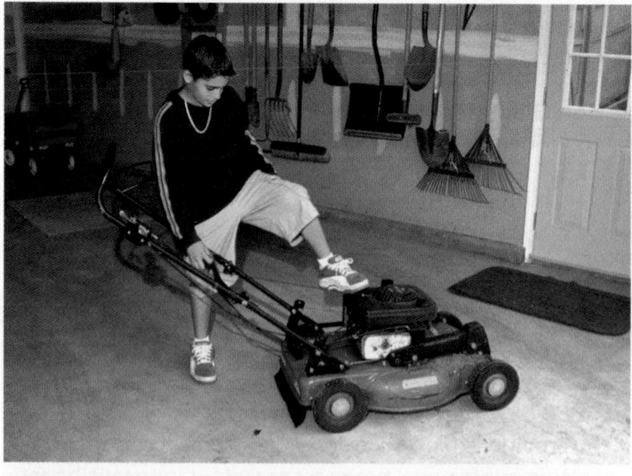

FIGURE 11-4 School-age boys can learn role behavior by watching caregivers as they work around the house. DELMAR CENGAGE LEARNING.

SELF-CONCEPT

The development of a positive self-concept and self-esteem are critical at this time. Self-concept is influenced by physical appearance, athletic ability, academic achievement, approval from caregivers, and shaped by comparisons with peers (Santrock, 2009). Caregivers and peers also play a role in determining self-esteem, a global evaluation of self also known as self-image or self-worth. The closer the perceived self is to the ideal self (how the child would like to be) the higher the child's self-esteem. Acceptance by peers also influences a child's sense of self-worth and healthy body image. Examples of positive self-esteem include the ability to express an opinion, work cooperatively with others, and initiate a conversation. A child with low self-esteem may be self-critical, feel shame and inadequacy, show signs of regression, and have an increased risk of depression, anxiety, resentment, and eating disorders (American Academy of Pediatrics, 2007c).

> **NURSING TIP**
>
> **Understanding the Concepts of Time, Height, Weight, and Volume**
>
> Because of the child's skill in concrete operations, more detail can be included when preparing the child for new health care experiences. For example, in preparing a child for an upper gastrointestinal series, the nurse can explain the scheduled date and time of the procedure, demonstrate how the procedure will be performed, and show the child the amount of barium to be used. The need for detailed explanation, as well as the school-age child's increased interest and desire to participate in self-care and treatment, are important to consider when caring for children in this developmental stage (Vessey & Sullivan, 2010).

COGNITIVE DEVELOPMENT

Piaget (1962) suggested that children around 6 years of age start to move from the egocentric view of the preschool age to the more open and flexible thought of the school-age child. Piaget described this stage of cognitive development as concrete operations. As children learn about the ideas of their peers and adults, they are able to see things from another's point of view.

Expanded cognitive abilities enable the child to imagine the world without having to experience it. However, because abstract thought has not been developed, the child is limited to thinking concretely and in the present time frame. During these **concrete operations**, the child gains the skills of **classification** (the ability to group items according to common characteristics), **conservation** (the ability to acknowledge that a change in shape does not mean a change in amount), and **reversibility** (the ability to recognize that actions can move in reverse order). For example, the child who has mastered classification can group animals according to the dog, cat, or horse family, and often collects baseball cards, coins, and rocks. Conservation emerges as the child's egocentric thinking is replaced by cognitive reasoning, develops over time, and begins with the conservation of numbers, followed by mass, weight, and volume. Reversibility is important when learning addition and subtraction and is seen when a child can reassemble a toy or play a game in reverse order (Figure 11-5 and Figure 11-6).

Original	Physical Change	Question	Nonconserving Response	Conserving Response
Child agrees that the same amount of drink is contained in each glass. 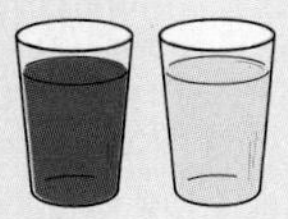	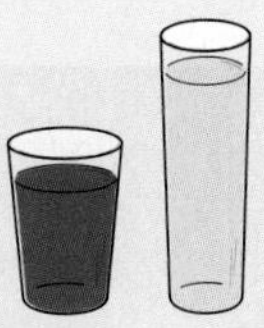	Is there still the same amount of drink in each glass, or does one glass have more?	No, they are not the same; there is more in the tall glass.	Yes, they have the same amount; you just put the drink in a different size glass. It is taller, but it is also thinner.
Child agrees each ball contains the same amount of clay. 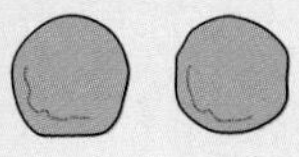	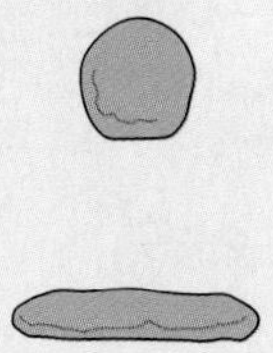	Is there still the same amount of clay in the ball and the snake, or does one have more?	No, there is more clay in the snake because it is longer (or more in the ball because it is fatter).	Yes, they have the same amount. You just rolled one ball out in a different shape.

FIGURE 11-5 Physical Changes in Conservation Tasks. DELMAR CENGAGE LEARNING.

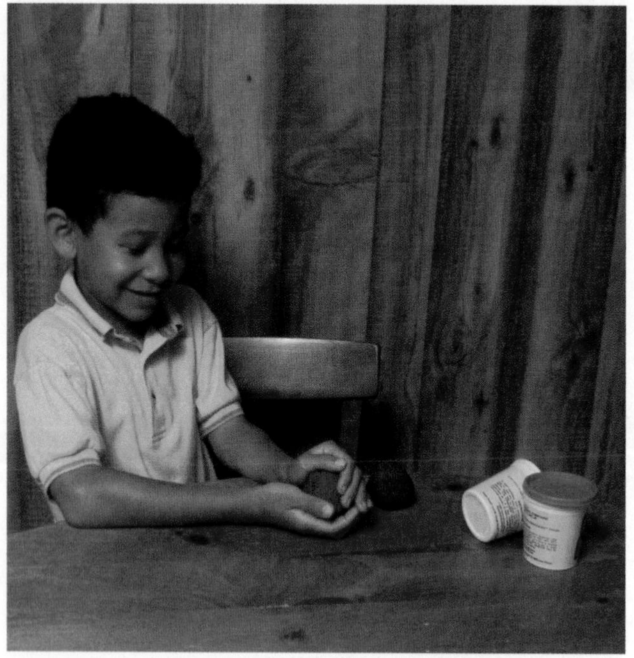

FIGURE 11-6 **This young school-age child will master the concepts of conservation, reversibility, and classification before moving on to adolescence.** DELMAR CENGAGE LEARNING.

LANGUAGE AND READING

During the school-age years, the child's ability to use language is enhanced and vocabulary increases fourfold (Berk, 2008). By age 6 years, the school-age child has begun to master the grammatical rules of language, and has a vocabulary of 10,000 words. By the end of the school-age years, the child's vocabulary exceeds 40,000 words (Berk, 2008). In addition, by 6, the school-age child uses six-word sentences and can follow a story without the use of pictures. By 7, the school-age child understands time and the difference between right and left; by 8, the child can use language as a tool for reasoning (Santrock, 2009). School-age children also can learn the literal meaning of words and are beginning to understand a word's nonliteral meaning. By 11 years of age, metaphors are understood and used in conversation, such as when describing a headache as "drums pounding in my head." However, temperament, social and cultural factors, and verbal and language environment affect language acquisition. This is especially true of expressive verbal skills, which entail the ability to recall required words effortlessly and to construct paragraphs and stories (Santrock, 2009).

Besides a tool for communication, language becomes a tool for socialization as the school-age child's language becomes less egocentric. However, because their mental capacity and control of language is not fully developed, nurses need to use words school-age children can understand and carefully assess their comprehension.

During the school-age years children begin to acquire the ability to read through letter identification, telling a story from looking at the pictures, and being read to. Reading should be encouraged by choosing books the child enjoys, being read to by an adult, and reading alone.

NURSING TIP

Explain Medical Terms

Language unites groups and cultures. Medicine has a distinct language from mainstream society. Therefore, when caring for school-age children, it is important to use correct terminology they will understand. Since children of this age may interpret each word literally, avoid using terms such as "taking a CAT scan" or "being put to sleep." Instead, explain the sequence of events the child will experience and exactly what will happen, such as "the machine will take a picture" or "you will fall asleep."

MORAL DEVELOPMENT

Kohlberg (1969) proposed eight stages of moral development (see Chapter 6 for more information on Kohlberg's theory). The school-age child is at the **conventional level** (Stages 3 and 4) of moral development, when the conscience develops an internal set of "rules" that must be followed in order to "be good." During Stage 3 (ages 6–10 years), the child's morality is based on avoiding the disapproval of others, and maintaining a positive relationship with friends, family, and teachers (Figure 11-7). Accidents can be viewed as punishment for disobeying. For instance, a toy breaking may be punishment for spilling milk in the family room where drinking is prohibited. During Stage 4 (ages 11 and 12 years), the child is concerned with doing the "right" thing and showing respect for authority figures. Children at this level can also demonstrate rigid behavior in an effort to obey the law. These children can take into account circumstances surrounding an incident rather than just looking at the result. Older school-age children understand the need to treat others as they would like to be treated.

Table 11-1 describes key milestones for school-age children.

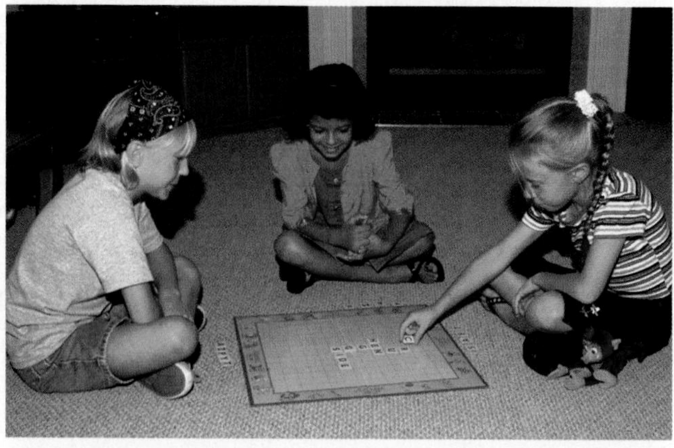

FIGURE 11-7 **School-age children learn how to abide by rules, making board games a popular choice for leisure time.** DELMAR CENGAGE LEARNING.

TABLE 11-1 School-Age Milestones

GROSS AND FINE MOTOR SKILLS	COGNITIVE DEVELOPMENT	SOCIAL DEVELOPMENT
6 to 7 Years		
Legibly prints letters. Uses knife, fork, and spoon. Rides 2-wheel bike. Masters all skills on the DDST. Improved dexterity. Cuts, pastes, folds paper. Ties shoe laces. Throws overhand. Copies a diamond. Walks a straight line.	Learning to tell time. Learning to read. Can read from memory. Understands right and left. Knows value of currency. Interested in magic and fantasy. Defines common objects according to their use. Understands concept of numbers. Attention span increasing. Enjoys word and spelling games. Obeys three commands. Likes to help. Knows right and left hand. Concrete, animistic thinking. Attends first and second grades. Reflective.	Able to bathe and dress self. Able to fix own hair. Enjoys games with peers of same gender. Shares and cooperates. May be jealous of younger siblings. Needs praise and recognition. Fewer mood swings. Enjoys helping around the house. Participates in school and community activities. Attentive listener. Demonstrates independence. Spends time in quiet play.
8 to 9 Years		
Developing eye-hand coordination. More fluid movement. Plays team sports. Body becomes flexible. Able to use household tools. Writes using cursive. Dresses self completely. Jumps, skips, draws three-dimensional figures.	Understands concept of time. Knows the date and month. Collects and classifies objects. Increased ability to read. Learning fractions. Understands space, cause, effect, conservation. Knows similarities and differences of objects. Counts backward from 20. Shows interest in music lessons. Can make change (small currency). Helps around the house. Can be critical of accomplishment and failure. Learns from experiences. Punctual. Improvises simple activities. Less animistic in thinking. Attends third and fourth grades.	Likes competitive games and sports. Runs errands. Social, well behaved. Modest. Demanding and critical of others. Compares self with others. Looks up to adults. Dependable, responsible. Rules are important. Able to do household chores. Best friends are important. Tolerant and accepting of others.

(Continues)

Table 11-1 School-Age Milestones (*Continued*)

GROSS AND FINE MOTOR SKILLS	COGNITIVE DEVELOPMENT	SOCIAL DEVELOPMENT
10 to 12 Years		
Eye-hand coordination well developed. Fine motor skills well developed. Gross motor skills may become awkward with growth spurt. Balances on one foot for 15 seconds. Catches a fly ball. Cooks and sews.	Developing ability for abstract thought. Able to write stories. Drawings are detailed. Easily distracted. Knows death is irreversible. More realistic than idealistic. Truthful. Reads for enjoyment; reads well. Knows limits. Interested in the future. Likes to memorize and identify facts. Likes to discuss and debate. Unaware of effect on others. Beginning formal operations.	Rules are important. Interest in opposite sex. Quarrelsome with siblings. Developing social competence. Self-disciplined. Easy to please. Obedient. May have best friend. Becoming diplomatic. Affectionate, sensitive. Respects parents. Self-directed and independent. Can stay at home alone for short periods of time. Increased interest in family.

NURSING TIP

Modeling Moral Behavior

It is imperative nurses model moral behavior and use sound moral judgment in caring for school-age children and families (Click & Parker, 2009). They also need to assist these youngsters to make decisions regarding their health care, keeping in mind that children may agree with suggestions in order to do the "right thing." Nurses also need to present good health care options and encourage school-agers to choose the option that works best for them.

HEALTH PROMOTION AND MAINTENANCE

NUTRITION

During the school-age years, the child becomes aware of how the body works and can more fully understand physical development and how to remain healthy, because a steady rate of physical development is also occurring at this time. The nutritional needs of the school-age child should remain relatively steady and children should be encouraged to make independent food choices. Eating a healthy breakfast before school is encouraged as a means to provide the essential nutrients needed for academic and physical performance. While at school, nutrition education must be a part of the curriculum so the school-age child will have the knowledge to select the most nutritious and appropriate quantities of food (Figure 11-8).

Although school-age children are more independent in making food choices, the influences of culture and caregivers cannot be ignored as eating habits established during childhood

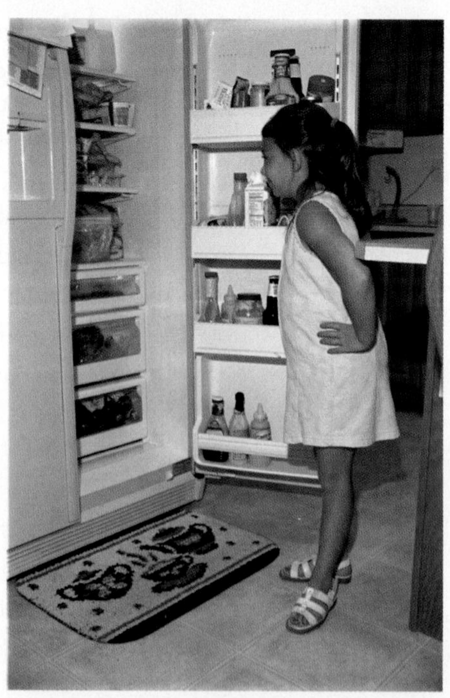

Figure 11-8 School-age children are able to choose nutritious foods when they are available and should be encouraged to do so. DELMAR CENGAGE LEARNING.

may be difficult to alter later in life. Leading a fast-paced life is common for many families today, so nutritious foods like fruits and vegetables must be readily available in order to avoid the temptation to live on fast-foods, which are often high in calories, fat, and sodium and low in vitamins and minerals. If consumed on a regular basis, fast-foods can lead to obesity, a fact that probably contributes to the increase in obesity in children during the past three decades. In 1970, 4% of children in the United States, ages 6–12 years, were considered overweight; currently, 17% of children suffer from obesity (Berk, 2008) and 32% are obese or overweight (Ogden, Carroll, & Flegal, 2008). Thus, the obesity rate for school-age children has quadrupled during the last four decades (National Association of State Boards of Education, 2009).

Obesity is considered the most serious health risk facing children in the United States (Katzmarzyk et al., 2008), yet most parents of overweight children tend to underestimate their child's weight problem (Towns & D'Auria, 2009). Although obesity occurs in all populations, ethnic minority children in the United States are at higher risk for obesity (Gottesman, Brady, Gance-Cleveland & Duderstadt, 2010). For example, 38% of Mexican-American children are obese or overweight and 34% of African-American children are obese or overweight (Ogden et al., 2008).

Childhood obesity presents a variety of physical health problems with a long-range proclivity for hypertension, heart disease, diabetes, cancer, and sleep disorders (Berk, 2008). Obesity also poses a potential for psychological harm. A survey of obese children ranked their quality of life at the same low level as children undergoing chemotherapy for cancer treatment (Walker, 2005). See the Family Teaching Box for steps in preventing childhood obesity.

Caregivers may be hesitant to limit the dietary intake of their school-age child because of their concern regarding the nutrients needed for physical growth. However, the early school-age period, ages 5–7 years, is a critical time when the onset of obesity is likely to persist into the adult years. In fact, research shows that children who are overweight by age 8 are more likely to be obese adults (National Association of State Boards of Education, 2009). Careful meal planning, setting a schedule for snacks and meals, and physical activity are crucial for the physical and emotional health of the school-age child. Table 11-2 includes the nutritional needs of the school-age child (Figure 11-9).

TABLE 11-2 Nutritional Needs of the School-Age Child

FOOD	DAILY SERVINGS
Milk (milk, cheese, yogurt)	2–3
Meat (lean meat, chicken, fish, beans, eggs, peanut butter)	3 or more
Bread (bread, cereal, rice, pasta)	6–9
Vegetables	3–5

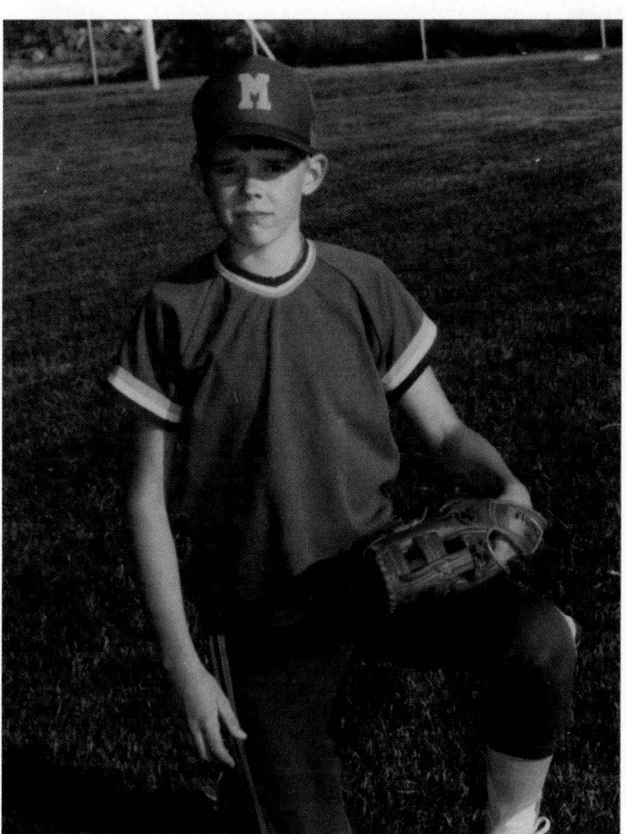

FIGURE 11-9 Outside activities help prevent obesity in childhood and promote self-esteem. DELMAR CENGAGE LEARNING.

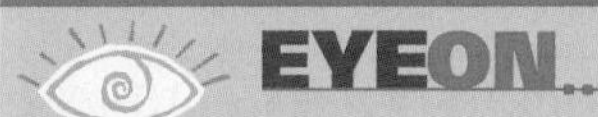

Dietary Differences

The diet of children raised in a traditional Native-American household can be high (35–50%) in fat and carbohydrates. The diet of children raised in traditional Hispanic American households usually consists of beans, salsa, tortillas, and rice with hot spices, and there is a tendency for these children to be heavier than their counterparts. Nurses need to be cognizant of family and ethnic traditions when counseling on nutrition and try to work these traditions into dietary planning.

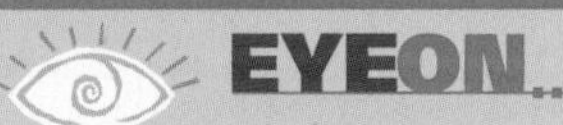

Vegetarian Diets

In the United States, vegetarian diets are common among some immigrant populations. School-age children who prefer a pure vegetarian (vegan) diet may not be receiving enough protein or calcium needed for growth. Since most school lunch programs serve a menu of meat and dairy, these children will need to bring a packed lunch from home with foods high in protein or calcium such as green leafy vegetables, nuts, legumes, and enriched bread or cereal. They may also need supplements of vitamin B12 and vitamin D.

FAMILY TEACHING

Steps in Preventing Childhood Obesity

1. Offer a variety of healthy foods, especially fruits and vegetables.
2. Encourage school-age children to help with meal preparation.
3. Avoid eating snacks and meals in front of the television or computer.
4. Limit the consumption of high calorie fast food or drinks.
5. Teach children how to handle stress instead of eating.
6. Encourage eating only when hungry.
7. Eat together as a family and make it a positive experience.
8. Limit computer, video game, and television time to less than 2 hours per day.
9. Encourage physical activity for at least 60 minutes per day.
10. Serve as a role model by adopting an active lifestyle.
11. Consult a pediatrician if concerned about a child's weight

Source: Society of Pediatric Nurses, 2010a & 2010b.

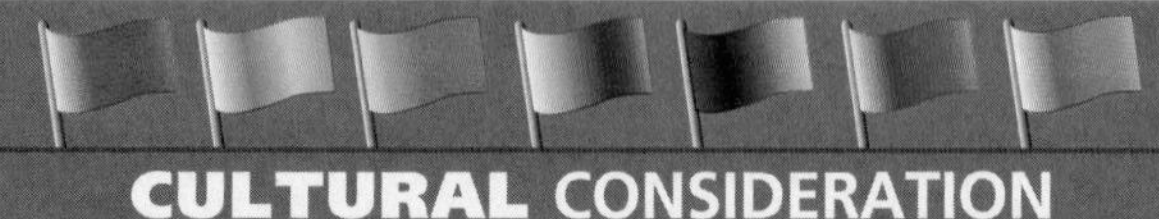

CULTURAL CONSIDERATION

Sleep Behavior in School-Age Children

Many school-aged children sleep less than 9 hours a night, which is the recommended amount of sleep this age group needs. However ethnic minority children have a delayed bed time (11 pm or later) when compared to nonminority children. In addition, ethnic minority males slept less (significantly) than minority females and nonminority males and females. An understanding of environmental and social influences related to children's bedtime behavior is needed when interacting with ethnic minorities.

SLEEP AND REST

Sleep is essential to optimal growth and development; however, by the time children reach school-age, most do not need to nap. Although nighttime sleep habits may vary, at 6 years children require at least 10 hours of sleep, and at 12 years children require 8 to 9 hours of sleep. Sleep is essential during the school-age years to foster physical growth and academic performance, and failure to receive adequate rest can lead to irritability and lack of attention span at school, which may lead to falling asleep and the potential of failing grades.

Parasomnias such as nightmares, night terrors, and sleepwalking usually begin between age 3 and 8 years (Ward, Rankin, & Lee, 2007). Nightmares and night terrors are less common during the school-age years and rarely result in daytime sleepiness. However, it is estimated **somnambulism**, or sleepwalking, occurs in 15% of all school-age children and is common between 4 and 8 years of age. The sleepwalking event is usually not remembered in the morning, occurs more frequently in boys, and can be associated with nocturnal enuresis. Most children outgrow sleepwalking by adolescence. Safety is a priority and should include locking outside doors and placing a bell on the child's bedroom door to alert caregivers (Ward, Rankin, & Lee, 2007). **Somniloquy**, or sleep talking, can occur at any age across the life span and does not indicate a health concern or need for intervention.

DENTAL HEALTH

During the school-age years, the 20 deciduous or baby teeth are shed and the permanent teeth appear. This process usually starts at age 5 years and is complete before adolescence, except for the third molars (wisdom teeth). The first permanent teeth appear by age 6 years and are called the central incisors and first molars. Over the next five years, deciduous teeth are replaced at a rate of four teeth per year (Feigelman, 2007). When children start to lose their teeth, the rate of loss is determined by genetics and gender. It is common for girls to lose their teeth earlier than boys. However, for children of both genders, by the end of the school-age years, the 20 deciduous teeth are replaced by 28 of the 32 permanent teeth (Stedman's Medical Dictionary, 2008). That is why the permanent front teeth seem too large for the face, giving the child an odd look (Figure 11-10).

During the school-age period, **malocclusion** or an abnormality of the coming together of the teeth can occur when the permanent upper and lower teeth do not approximate, leaving them crowded or uneven. Malocclusion occurs in 30% of school-age children and requires a referral to an orthodontist (Berk, 2008). If braces are needed, frequent brushing and flossing are critical in preventing dental caries. An **evulsed tooth** (tooth that is knocked out) should be picked up, rinsed gently under water, and placed back in its socket. The child should hold the tooth in place and a dentist should be contacted immediately. If the tooth cannot be held in place, it should be put in cold milk or held in the mouth, under child's or caregiver's tongue, until seen by a dentist.

SAFETY AND INJURY PREVENTION

The leading cause of death in this age group is accidents, so health education should be focused on accident prevention (Martin et al., 2008). The estimated medical costs and lost

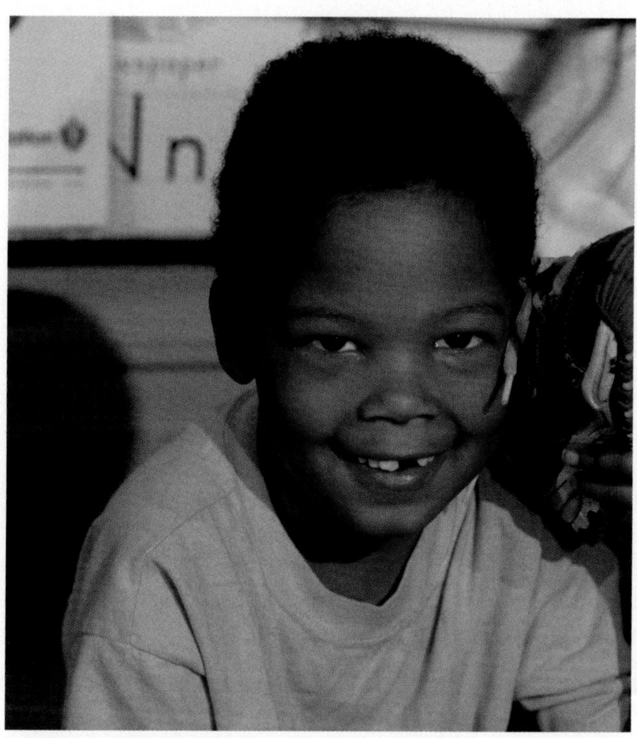

FIGURE 11-10 **During ages 6–11 a child loses his or her deciduous teeth.** DELMAR CENGAGE LEARNING.

FAMILY**TEACHING**

Dental Health

To maintain proper dental health, regular brushing and flossing are important during the school-age years. It is important for the nurse to assess the school-age child for correct brushing and flossing technique because of the child's relative lack of manual dexterity, and to advise caregivers to monitor the school-age child at home, including encouraging brushing at least twice a day with fluoride tooth paste and scheduling yearly visits to the dentist. Since the child's first visits to the dentist can greatly influence future visits, seek a pediatric dentist (American Academy of Pediatrics, 2009a). In addition, nurses should suggest caregivers purchase a toothbrush with a small brush head and soft bristles for their school-age child and replace it every 2 to 3 months.

productivity related to unintentional injuries for school-age children is more than 50 billion dollars (Finkelstein, Corso, & Miller, 2006). Factors contributing to the high incidence of accidents for this group are the child's increased independence, desire to have peer approval, and increased involvement in physically challenging activities. Most childhood accidents are related to motor vehicles either as a passenger or a pedestrian (Santrock, 2009). Each year 900 child pedestrians are killed and 51,000 are injured (American Academy of Pediatrics, 2009b). During the 1980s, firearm injuries for children ages 10 to 14 continued to increase steadily and by 1990, 1 of 8 deaths among children ages 10 to 14 years was caused by a firearm (Fingerhut, 1993). However, over the past two decades, unintentional firearm fatalities have dropped by 74% (Safe Kids Worldwide, 2007), probably because of education regarding firearm dangers.

Because school-age children may understand but resist rules established by adults in an effort to gain independence and peer approval, safety rules must be clearly defined through education and enforced with discipline. Rules related to motor vehicle, bike, skateboard, and swimming safety, and avoidance of firearms and strangers, are critical. School-age children's behavior can be influenced by parental example; the safety behaviors they plan to use as adults are best predicted by current parental practices (Morrongiello, Corbett, & Bellissimo, 2008). The Family Teaching box offers examples of important rules that need to be established and enforced by caregivers, nurses, and teachers.

HEALTH SCREENING

When compared to traditional standards, school-age children enjoy excellent health (Feigelman, 2007); when school-age children are sick, it is typically for a minor illness. School-age children average two health care visits each year. The American Academy of Pediatrics (AAP) recommends routine medical exams for the school-age child at least every two years, and suggests they occur at ages 5, 6, 8, 10, 11, and 12 years. These exams should include height, weight, vital signs, physical exam, vision and hearing screening, and assessment of dietary intake and use of tobacco, alcohol, and drugs. In addition, use of the HEADSS mnemonic (*h*ome, *e*ducation and employment, peer *a*ctivities, *d*rugs, *s*exuality, and *s*uicide or depression) will aid in completing a holistic assessment of the school-age child (Behrman, Kliegman, Jenson, & Stanton, 2007). Scoliosis screening is also recommended (see Chapter 34 for more information). In addition, annual tuberculosis testing is recommended for any high-risk children.

IMMUNIZATIONS

By the time they enter kindergarten, most children have received all the recommended immunizations. For the school-age child, booster shots of diphtheria, tetanus, and pertussis (DTaP), and measles, mumps, and rubella vaccine (MMR) are recommended between the ages of 4 and 6 years. If the MMR booster is not given at this time, it is given at ages 11 to 12 years, as is the Td (tetanus and diphtheria) booster, which is then repeated every ten years as well. Refer to Appendix C for the current immunization schedule. The 2010 Recommended Immunization Schedule for Persons Aged 7–18 Years is available on the CDC website and in the Appendix.

FAMILY TEACHING

Safety Rules for School-Age Children

Motor vehicle	Always wear a seat belt, sit in backseat, especially in car with airbags.
Bicycle/skateboard/inline skates	Wear helmet, elbow, and knee pads.
Pedestrian	Use caution when crossing streets, and obey traffic lights.
Trampolines	Use should be discouraged.
Swimming	Learn how to swim, never swim alone. Wear a life jacket while in a boat. Do not dive in shallow water.
Firearms	Avoid guns; do not assume a gun is not loaded.
Strangers	Do not talk to strangers or accept rides from strangers. Learn home address and telephone number. Use 911 if needed and know how to call a safe neighbor. Medicines should be kept out of reach; explain consequences of taking the drugs.
Drug use and smoking	Teach about illicit drugs; counsel on why and how to avoid their use.
Fire/burns	Teach escape route; cook and bake under supervision of adult.

NURSING ALERT

Children, Pickup Trucks, and Automobiles

- Children riding in the cargo area of pickup trucks are at risk for death or injury if the vehicle is involved in an accident. Caregivers should be reminded not to allow their children to ride in that area.
- Children seated in the front seats of vehicles are at increased risk of death and injury in crashes. This holds especially true in vehicles with passenger-side airbags. Almost all children killed by airbags were either unrestrained or improperly restrained at the time of the crash. Children under 12 years of age should sit in the back seat.
- Seat belts fit correctly when the lap portion of the belt rides low over the hips. The well-fit shoulder belt crosses the sternum and shoulder. Correct seat belt fit is usually not achieved until the child is 9 years old.

SCHOOL

School is an exciting new world because it provides the arena for physical, intellectual, and social development. Schools affect the evolving character of the school-age child, and every school has the potential to actively encourage prosocial behavior. School-age children who feel their school is a caring environment and have caring relationships are less likely to miss school or drop out (Santrock, 2009). The teacher can guide and provide a structured environment where learning can take place, and regulate what is being learned, how it is being learned, with whom it is being learned, and in what context the learning occurs.

Teachers serve as role models: they strive to stimulate intellectual development; are in a position to influence the child's attitudes and values; and can be an important factor in determining school success. The child facing extreme difficulties of poverty, abuse, and violence may find a safe haven at school and learn to cope with life stressors because of a teacher's positive influence (Click & Parker, 2009). Dedicated teachers must be credited with keeping students' performance at a steady pace when considering the conditions many children and families have faced over the past decades.

As social interaction and communication develop between school-age children, so does their role in facilitating the transmission of knowledge. Vygotsky (1962) suggested when a child of one stage of development helps another child of the same level of development, both benefit. Nurses can also use cooperative learning as an effective method of teaching the school-age child in the health care setting.

HOMEWORK

School-age children may occasionally have homework assignments, although many teachers try to allow time within the school day to complete assignments. If children do have school work that needs to be completed at home, caregivers should:

1. Provide a positive atmosphere where children can work without being distracted. This means a quiet area with no television that is well-lit and free of clutter.

2. Show interest in the child's work. Check to see the homework is complete and be prepared to explain the assignment if the child does not understand what the teacher has asked the child to do.
3. Be prepared to help the child in a particular subject that is difficult by providing guidance, not answers. You may need to consider using a tutor.
4. Re-evaluate the after-school activities the child is involved in, especially if these activities leave little time to complete their homework assignments.
5. Be positive about homework so your child will acquire your attitude.
6. Watch for signs of frustration, and encourage your child to take short breaks as needed.
7. Reward progress in homework and reinforce the positive effort.

(Keep Kids Healthy, 2010a)

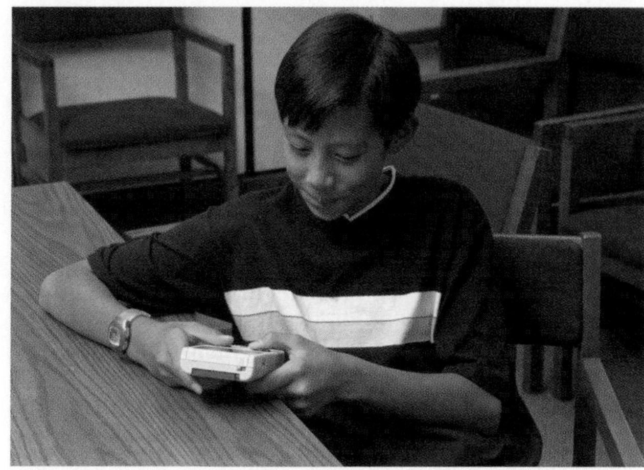

FIGURE 11-11 **Handheld computer games are popular with school-age children. Their use should be limited as this is a sedentary activity.** DELMAR CENGAGE LEARNING.

PLAY

Piaget (1962) described play during the school-age years as games with rules as the child is able to think more objectively, thus making group activities a possibility. Socially, school-age children are beginning to understand the concept of cooperation and reflect this in their play as they work together for the good of their team. Strict adherence to rules provides the framework for playing the game and creating a sense of security. Children of this age enjoy video games and watching television. In fact, recent studies indicate that boys ages 8 to 13 years spend on average 7.5 hours per week playing computer video games (Strasburger, Wilson, & Jordan, 2009). These activities should be limited as they are sedentary activities (Figure 11-11).

Play also provides the opportunity to learn what the body is physically capable of as gross and fine motor development are stimulated. By the time the school-age child is 6 years old, the physical strength and stamina for team sports have developed, contributing to physical health and release of frustrations. Children enjoy playing board games; starting collections; participating in, listening to, or playing music; and water activities (Figure 11-12). Lastly, since school-age children use play as an outlet to express their emotions, caregivers should participate in play with their children as a means of developing a stronger emotional connection (Click & Parker, 2009).

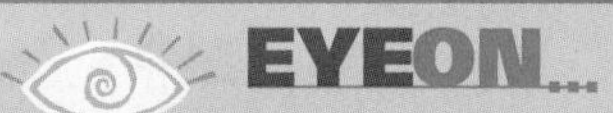

United Nations Millennium Development Goal 2: Achieve Universal Primary Education

Target: Ensure that by 2015, boys and girls alike will be able to complete a full course of primary schooling

According to the United Nations *The Millennium Development Goals Report (2009),* 72 million children worldwide were denied the right to education in 2007. Almost 50% of these children live in sub-Saharan Africa, followed by southern Asia, with 18 million children out of school. Evidence reveals an association between mothers with a primary or secondary education and a decrease in child mortality and malnourishment. Unfortunately, these families face barriers to attending primary school and receiving an adequate education as they lack the basic needs of food, clean water, and clothing; live far from school and do not have transportation; or may be fearful of leaving home because crime and violence is commonplace in their neighborhood.

PHYSICAL ACTIVITY

Although physical activity is essential for overall health, in 1999 only 35% of middle school children participated in

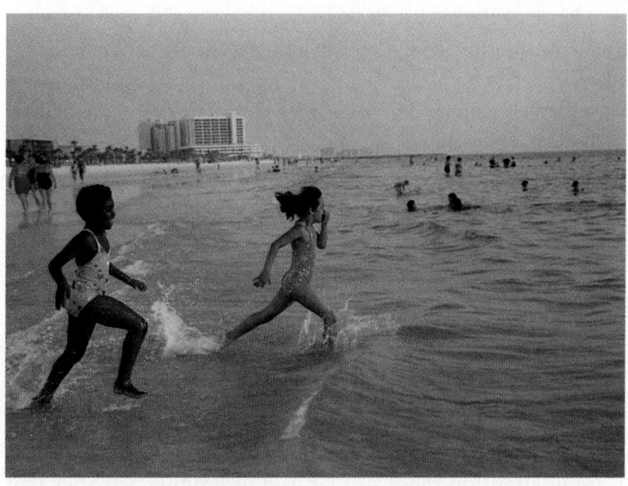

FIGURE 11-12 **These school-age children are enjoying water activities.** DELMAR CENGAGE LEARNING.

NURSING TIP

Encouraging Play

During play children enact what they cannot verbalize or physically demonstrate. Therefore nurses can incorporate play into health care experiences as a way of helping children express needs and actively cope with experiences. Scribbling, finger painting, coloring, and drawing are useful tension-reducing methods, which are inexpensive and can foster a child's creativity (Ryan-Wenger, 1998).

daily physical education classes, compared to 57% of middle school children in 1991 (Dalton, 2004). More recently, of U.S. private and public schools, only 8% of elementary and 6.4% of middle schools provide daily physical education classes (American Academy of Pediatrics, 2006). Specifically, the average American school-age child receives only one hour and 20 minutes of physical education at school every week (Berk, 2008). Although most school-age children are physically active, a concern remains related to their decreased physical activity and increased sedentary activities, such as watching television or playing computer games. The average child in the United States spends 15,000 hours watching television every year (Society of Pediatric Nurses, 2010a). For the overweight child, physical activity can help with weight reduction; for the child with type 2 diabetes, it can improve insulin sensitivity. Physical activity is also associated with psychological benefits such as a more positive self-concept and self-esteem, along with a decreased incidence of depression and anxiety (American Academy of Pediatrics, 2006). Physical activity for school-age children can take many forms and includes walking, hiking, dancing, spontaneous sports activities, or being a member of an organized community team (soccer, baseball). It is important for each child to find something enjoyable, as the health benefits of physical activity will be felt for life (American Academy of Pediatrics, 2006).

Considering the physical and psychological benefits of physical activity, children with physical or emotional limitations should be encouraged to participate in an activity that uses their abilities. Nurses should also promote growth and development for children with special health care needs (Allen, 2010).

Sports

As the child's skeleton and muscle size continue to grow at a gradual rate, the gross motor skills of jumping, running, throwing, and catching continue to be refined. However, the child's muscles and bones are easily injured because of immaturity, so athletic activities must be carefully selected according to the child's physical development and not the caregiver's wishes. Careful attention must also be paid to limiting activities that stress the child's physical development and endurance, such as contact sports and long distance running. The sports most likely associated with injury for the school-age child are baseball, football, and soccer (Rappley & Kallman, 2009).

As the child seeks cooperative play with rules, team sports become interesting. Team play can contribute to physical and social development as the youngsters learn to play as team members and work for common goals. Sports should encourage everyone to participate and recognize all team members for their contributions, not just a select few. However, during the school-age years, the child is also exposed to the high value placed on winning and competing, and should learn a healthy balance between playing for the sake of playing and always winning or competing (Figure 11-13).

PEERS

During the school-age years, children transition from the central focus of their home and caregivers to a world of school and peers. As school-age children become older, gain more independence, and spend more time with peers of the same gender, friendships develop that may influence them for the rest of their life. Peers help each other learn about the world and all its possibilities, influence self-esteem and self-confidence, and are important sounding boards for issues needing to be discussed. Child-child interactions provide opportunities to learn a wide variety of social behaviors and how to negotiate in situations involving

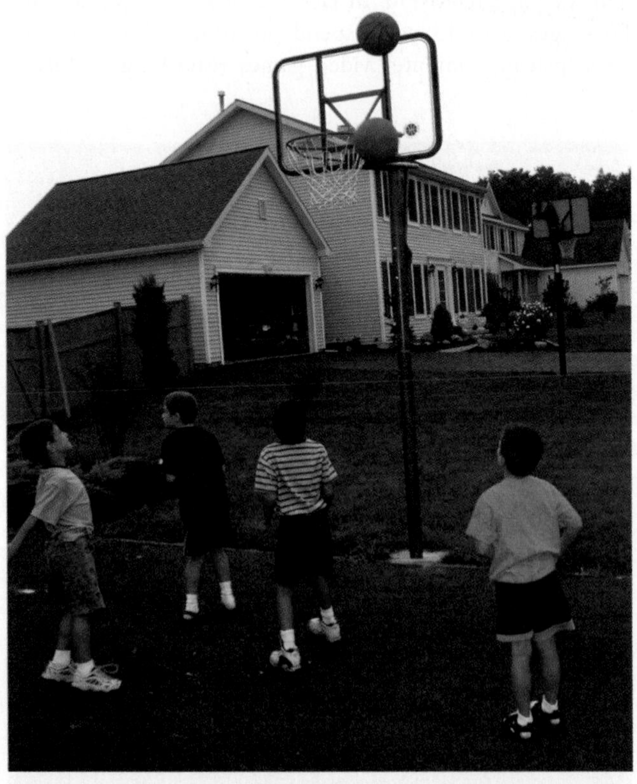

FIGURE 11-13 These children are enjoying a game of pickup basketball. DELMAR CENGAGE LEARNING.

competition, aggression, disagreement, and rejection (Youngblade, Storch, & Nackashi, 2009).

BODY IMAGE

School-age children are knowledgeable about their bodies and often will compare how they look to how their peers or adults look. Children also are acutely aware of physical differences related to height or weight and know if they are not as coordinated as their friends. School-age children who are especially sensitive about these differences may be uncomfortable in a swimming suit or shorts and not participate in activities where their "differences" may become apparent. If the child has a physical disability, it is not uncommon for other children to call attention to the disability, exclude them from activities and, at the same time, worry that they themselves have a similar disability. Caregivers and nurses need to be sure children know each child is different in a special way, yet at the same time, identical to their friends in many other ways. Children who call attention to physical disabilities in others need to realize such comments may have lasting effects; they should be discouraged from making hurtful comments.

BULLYING

Developing social skills is one of the primary tasks of the school-age years (Click & Parker, 2009). For children who lack such skills, one of the ways to express their anger is the act of bullying, inflicting verbal or physical harm on another. Studies indicate that almost 50% of all children are bullied at some time during their school-age years (American Academy of Child & Adolescent Psychiatry, 2008). Recent studies indicate that 20% of students ages 11–18 years have been bullied online, known as cyberbullying (Click & Parker, 2009).

Boys are more likely to engage in bullying than girls, and to use physical intimidation. Children who bully try to control or dominate others and have often been bullied themselves. Bullying behavior is more intense in middle school, and declines in high school. Children with emotional or physical disabilities are bullied more often (Wells & Stein, 2006) than those children who do not have disabilities. Signs of bullying can include physical scratches and bruises, requests for extra money for school, and resistance to attend school. The effects of bullying may negatively impact school performance, decrease self esteem, and increase anxiety (Click & Parker, 2009). If bullying continues, the victim can become depressed, withdrawn, and even suicidal (American Academy of Child & Adolescent Psychiatry, 2008). Victims of bullying tend to feel that they do not belong at their school (Glew, Fan, Katon, & Rivara, 2008). School nurses can play a vital role in identifying both the victims and perpetrators of bullying behavior and must take action for the safety and well-being of all involved as some of the recent incidences of school violence and shootings were carried out by students who were bullied by peers. Taking action includes notification of the school principal, teaching staff, and caregivers of the involved children, plus taking the lead in the development and delivery of an antiviolence program.

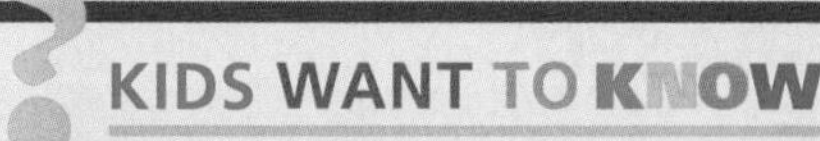

Hey Mom, can I join Facebook?

Many school-age children have accounts at social networking websites such as Facebook. Parents should have a discussion with their children and be mindful of their child's level of maturity and understanding before granting access to such sites. School-age children do not necessarily have the maturity or experience to embrace how some of these sites work, or understand that by posting comments and photos, the user surrenders all rights and control over where those comments and photos can be sent or shared by other users. There also have been instances of "cyber-bullying", where kids post mean and hurtful comments onto these social networking sites, in some cases with dire consequences for the target of the abuse. Parents who grant their children access to social networking sites may want to consider signing up themselves, so they can monitor their children's activity.

CRITICAL THINKING

Dealing with Bullying Behavior

Consider the following situation: You are a school nurse in a large urban school. Over the past month, 11-year-old Spencer, who is new to your school, has been stopping in your office on a weekly basis with complaints of headache and stomachache. You noticed at this visit that he has a number of bruises on his face. Spencer reluctantly responds to your question about the bruises and admits that a group of bullies have been "beating him up" because he would not steal for them. He tells you he is scared to tell his mother, as she cannot afford to send him to another school.

1. **Determine the approach you should use with Spencer.**
2. **Discuss ways you could intervene to prevent future harm.**
3. **Describe how you would address Spencer's concern about notifying his mother.**
4. **Would you notify school administrators? If so, how would you do this?**
5. **Identify school and community resources that could help this family.**

EVIDENCE-BASED PRACTICE

Bullying in School-Age Children

CLINICAL PROBLEM

Bullying, a common form of youth violence, can escalate into other forms of antisocial behavior and is a major problem in schools. It affects almost one in three children. Those children who are bullied may, in turn, bully others.

BEST CLINICAL PRACTICE

Several strategies used to help decrease bullying include creating a warm and involved school environment with firm limits placed on unacceptable behavior, using adults as role models, and applying non-hostile consequences when rules are violated. Another strategy is to teach students how to get adult help, stand up to bullies, and reach out to those students who may be involved in bullying situations. The bully needs to be counseled on restitution, empathy development, or acknowledging behaviors. Victims need to be provided with support groups made up of other victims, physical protection, or individual therapy. Children who have high-quality friendships rarely are bullies or victims of bullying.

IMPLICATIONS FOR NURSING

- Educate caregivers and teachers about bullying.
- Provide support and help to children who are victims of bullying, including making and maintaining friendships with peers.
- Provide children who bully with alternative means of interacting with peers, including social skills training.

References: American Academy of Child & Adolescent Psychiatry. (2008). Facts for families: Bullying; Click, P., & Parker, J. (2009). *Caring for school-age children.* Clifton Park, NY: Delmar Cengage Learning; Keep Kids Healthy. (2010b). How do you deal with bullies? www.keepkidshealthy.com/schoolage.

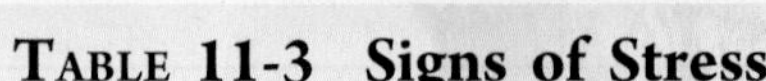

TABLE 11-3 Signs of Stress

Fatigue
Irritability
Anxiety
Low self-esteem
Change in sleep pattern
Emotional eating
Complaints of headache, stomachache, backache, or neck pain
Substance abuse
Drop in academic performance
Social withdrawal

Adapted from Washington, T. (2009). Psychological stress and anxiety in middle to late childhood and early adolescence: Manifestations and management. *Journal of Pediatric Nursing, 24*(4), 302–313.

STRESS

Consider the following situations:

1. Twelve-year-old Karl is admitted to the emergency room with an exacerbation of his asthma.
2. Ten-year-old Mary brings home a report card with all A's and one B.
3. Six-year-old Chad is admitted to the hospital for same-day surgery.
4. Eight-year-old Christine's father is diagnosed with cancer and is scheduled for a bone marrow transplant.

Without knowing the children in these situations we cannot know if they experienced stress. We do know, however, that stress is a part of life for everyone, including school-age children. The school-age child in today's world is constantly exposed to stress. Like never before, children are subjected to the effects of a high divorce rate, peer pressure, and use of illicit drugs and alcohol. A situation is considered stressful for a child when there is a discrepancy between demands placed on the child and the child's perceived ability to meet these demands (Menke, 1981). In addition, what is stressful for one school-age child may not be stressful for another; if the child feels resources and supports are available it may be viewed as a positive challenge instead of a negative threat. If stress is viewed as a negative threat and beyond their ability to handle, children may exhibit some of the signs listed in Table 11-3 and need assistance in working through the experience.

Health care experiences can be potential stressors for children as they deal with separation from friends and family, interruption of school, and the threat of injury or pain. Surgery is an example of a health care stressor that results from the potential loss of control, fear of pain, concern for modesty, and separation from caregivers and friends. Therefore, school-age children need to be prepared at least a week in advance of a stressful event such as surgery, so they can have their questions answered and formulate coping strategies. Caregivers also need to be prepared because, if prepared, they will be less anxious and better able to provide positive support for their child.

LATCHKEY CHILDREN

Today, in both single- and two-caregiver families, more caregivers are working outside the home. It is estimated that parents of more than 28 million school-age children work outside the home (Afterschool Alliance, 2008). As a result, many children come home after school to an empty house and are home alone for a period of time without adult

RESEARCH Highlight

Stress and Coping Related to School Testing

STUDY PURPOSE

To assess the change in school-age childrens' appraisal of proficiency tests, concurrent stressors, stress symptoms, and coping strategies during the course of one academic year.

METHODS

The convenience sample consisted of 53 Caucasian children (24 boys, 29 girls) in fourth grade at one Midwestern elementary school. Using a repeated measures design, each child was asked to complete the following instruments during the months of October, February, March, and April: Proficiency Test Stress Visual Analog Scale (VAS), Children's Source of Stress Scale, Children's Stress Symptom Scale, and the School-Ager's Coping Strategies Inventory.

FINDINGS

Results indicated that the children were the most stressed about proficiency testing at the beginning of the school year. Reasons for what makes these tests stressful were: fear of failure, uncertainty, and pressure from others to succeed. Identified sources of stress before the proficiency tests included: fighting with siblings, missing family members, playing sports, tests, and feeling left out. Reported symptoms of stress were: hunger, headache, nervousness, fatigue, and confusion. The following coping strategies–drawing, eating, and watching television–were included in the top five at each time point. Of interest, prayer was one of the top five coping strategies only during test week.

IMPLICATIONS

The "No Child Left Behind" Act has led to an increased focus on proficiency testing as a means of evaluating teacher and school performance. As a result, school-age children may feel increased pressure for academic excellence. This study underscores the importance of assessing each child's stress level related to school performance. School nurses need to work with teachers, counselors, and parents to identify children with school related stress. By taking a direct approach, the child's stressors can be identified and addressed in order to foster healthy coping strategies and ensure academic success.

REFERENCE

Skybo, T., & Buck, J. (2007). Stress and coping responses to proficiency testing in school-age children. *Pediatric Nursing, 33*(5), 410–418.

NURSING TIP

Stress Reduction Strategies

Nurses have a responsibility to recognize common manifestations of stress and must work in partnership with the child and family to determine effective methods of stress reduction (Washington, 2009). Since school-age children often enjoy writing, they can be encouraged to write about their experiences in order to cope. Additional stress reducing techniques such as relaxation, guided imagery, or distraction may also help some children.

supervision (**latchkey children**) (Figure 11-14). The current number of latchkey children in this country is difficult to estimate, but may be as high as 14 million school-age children (National Institute on Out-of-School Time, 2006). An even greater number of children whose caregivers work are cared for by an older sibling. Because of this lack of adult supervision, latchkey children are at risk for developing physical and social problems and anxiety. The hours between 3 p.m. and 6 p.m. are peak times for juvenile crime and experimentation with sex, smoking, and drinking alcohol. Unfortunately, there is a chronic shortage of after-school programs in the United States, although 76% of Americans agree that Congress, state, and local officials should increase funding for such programs (Afterschool Alliance, 2008).

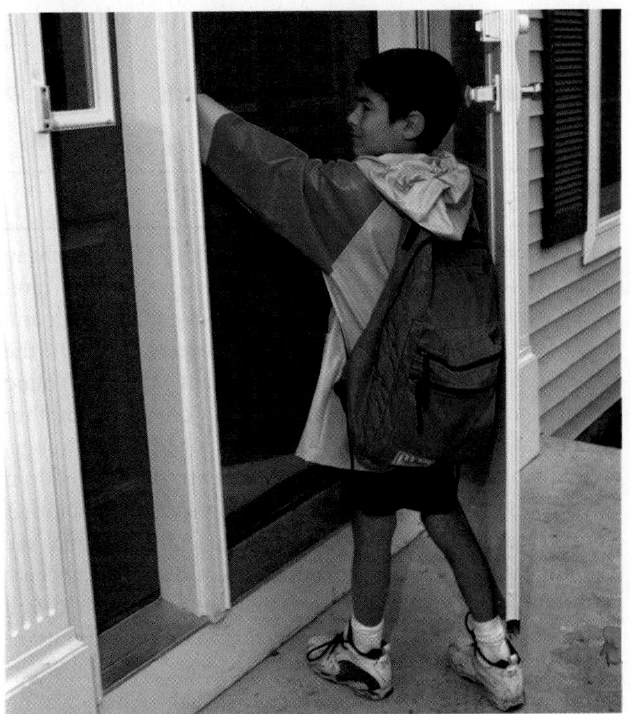

FIGURE 11-14 Latchkey children usually spend a few hours home alone after school before their adult caregivers come home from work. DELMAR CENGAGE LEARNING.

KIDS WANT TO KNOW

My friends tell me that surgery is gross and will hurt a lot. Can I put it off?

Ronnie, age 10 years, is scheduled for outpatient surgery next week. This is his first surgery. Ronnie has not verbalized any concerns about the surgery until today. Upon arriving home from school, Ronnie says his friends warned him about the horrible pain he would have and told him he would be naked during surgery. Ronnie asked that the surgery be postponed.

Without knowing the accuracy of his friends' statements, his caregivers decided to seek the answers. They contacted his surgeon and found their hospital offered a presurgery preparation program for children and caregivers. At the program they were told about the surgery and assured their child's safety and welfare was the primary goal. Ronnie and his caregivers were also told pain management was an important intervention and medication would be available throughout the stay. Finally, the caregivers received information about postoperative pain management at home. Ronnie was relieved to know he would be covered during surgery and his caregivers could visit before surgery, attend the anesthesia induction, and stay with him after the surgery. Attending the presurgery preparation program greatly reduced the stress and allowed Ronnie and his caregivers to be more fully informed about the surgical experience.

HONESTY

It is not uncommon for school-age children to steal, cheat, or lie. Although these behaviors may be upsetting for caregivers, they are often just a phase the child goes through and may be related to immature cognitive development. On the other hand, it may indicate a more serious problem. Young children may steal because they want something another person has, feel they were treated unfairly and want revenge, or want to be able to bribe other children. Other children may observe family members take things from one another (money out of a purse, clothes from a drawer) and see nothing wrong in doing the same thing. Children may cheat because they want to win a game they are playing or do well on an examination. If winning or being the best is important to their caregivers, or if they see caregivers cheat, children are more likely to model that same behavior. Finally, young school-age children may lie to cover up misbehavior or avoid being punished, whereas older children lie because they may not meet expectations of teachers or caregivers.

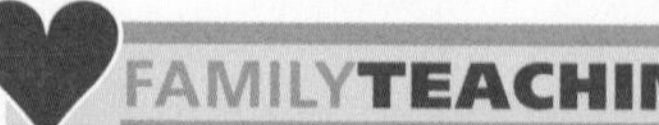

FAMILY TEACHING

Tips for Latchkey Children

Nurses should take a proactive role in promoting quality after-school programs in communities by encouraging students who go home to an empty house to discuss safe rules to abide by while they are alone. The following tips can be communicated to caregivers as well.

1. Do not open the door to anyone you do not know.
2. Do not tell a telephone caller you are home without a caregiver.
3. Make a list of emergency phone numbers and the phone number for a neighbor who can be trusted. Keep this list in a safe place near the phone. Review use of 911.
4. Create an after-school routine such as homework, household chores, or caring for pets.
5. Make sure firearms are locked and unloaded, or removed from the home.
6. No access allowed to adult cable TV or Internet sites.

FAMILY TEACHING

Tips about Honesty

1. Role model the behavior you want to see in your child by being honest and respectful of others
2. Try to understand the motive behind your child's lying.
3. Discuss the consequences of lying without being angry.
4. Reinforce the benefits of being honest.

Reference: Stott, F. (2009). The truth about lying. Retrieved May 22, 2009, from http://www2.scholastic.com/browse/article.jsp?id=702&print=2.

While lying is a normal aspect of development, it should not be dismissed. The above tips will help children understand the importance of being honest.

LIMIT SETTING AND DISCIPLINE

Nurturant caregivers include discipline in a warm, supportive, and empathetic relationship with their school-age child. By providing clear limits of behavior and positive reinforcement for good behavior, the caregiver is better able to help the child develop self-confidence. In effect, caregivers who model responsible behavior can easily be examples of effective values.

Implicit in discipline approaches is a fundamental attitude toward the child. Taking the child seriously and treating the child as a person whose feelings and questions

Hospitalized Children's Perceptions of Nurses

STUDY PURPOSE

To describe children's perceptions of nurses and nurse behaviors and to identify any differences in children's perceptions of nurses when examined by demographic variables (age, gender, ethnicity, chronicity, length of stay, parental presence).

METHODS

This qualitative study was conducted at a children's hospital in the Midwest. Sixty-five children (34 boys, 31 girls) participated in the study. Participant age groups were:
5–7 years (n = 12), 8–10 years (n = 15), 11–13 years (n = 12) and 14–18 years (n = 26).
A questionnaire, developed by the first author, was used with all participants and consisted of 8 demographic questions that were completed by a staff nurse researcher, followed by 8 participant questions. Younger participants were interviewed by one of the 8 staff nurse researchers and older participants completed the questionnaire on their own.

FINDINGS

Participants in this study had been hospitalized for at least 2 nights, functioned at an age-appropriate level and spoke English. Eighty-eight percent (n = 57) had a parent with them at the hospital. The following seven themes of nurse behaviors were identified: (1) positive attitude; (2) physical comfort; (3) humor; (4) advocacy; (5) basic needs; (6) acknowledgment; and (7) reassurance. All of the children had positive feelings about nurses and used such terms as helper, protector, caring, honest, concerned, and gentle to describe them. Some of the advice from children included "Just listen more and be more sensitive to patients and families" and "Say it's alright if we are scared."

IMPLICATIONS

Nurses caring for school-age children in the hospital should remember that they are children first by providing age-appropriate activities that will foster growth and development. At the same time, nurses should be cognizant of the sources of stress for hospitalized children, (separation from family and friends, loss of control, pain, procedures, fear of the unknown) and provide holistic interventions to decrease these stressors. Children in this study described admission as frightening, so careful attention should be paid at this particular time by explaining your role and reassuring them of your care.

REFERENCE

Schmidt, C., Bernaix, L., Koski, A., Weese, J., Chiappetta, M., & Sandrik, K. (2007). Hospitalized children's perceptions of nurses and nurse behaviors. *MCN: The American Journal of Maternal/Child Nursing, 32*(6), 336–342.

matter is critical. The child's preference, however, cannot always be accommodated but should be considered and never dismissed. The school-age child is someone with a distinctive point of view and a unique set of needs. The caregiver needs to be not only warm and empathetic but also needs to model for the school-age child the values of honesty and prosocial behavior (helping, sharing, and caring). Reasoning capabilities of the school-age child are being developed, so talking about and explaining a negative behavior and clear understanding of consequences should be encouraged. Withdrawing privileges is often a satisfying method of discipline (Feigelman, 2007).

REFLECTIVE THINKING

Caring for a Latchkey Child

1. How would you feel if a 7-year-old boy you are caring for in a health care setting told you he was left alone for many hours every day without adult supervision?
2. How would you feel about his caregivers and what actions would be appropriate?

SEXUALITY

School-age children may engage in some form of sex play during the late school-age years. This is normal behavior. Caregivers should avoid drawing attention to it or laying on guilt. At a very early age, children are exposed to sexually explicit information through the media. Unless caregivers are honest and open about sexual issues, children will seek answers to their questions from peers. All too often the information from peers is inaccurate; therefore, it is imperative nurses be available to provide education regarding sexuality to children and caregivers. In providing education, it is important to use the appropriate anatomical terms and encourage open discussion between children and caregivers. Caregivers should use truthful information and not shy away from the discussion.

NURSE'S ROLE IN FOSTERING HEALTHY SCHOOL-AGE CHILDREN

The school-age years are an exciting time, because during this time the child learns how to master skills and relate to others. How successful the child feels during this period can shape his or her future success in work and relationships. Although their world revolves around school and relationships with peers, childrens' caregivers still play a critical role in their lives. The nurse caring for a school-age child is in an ideal position to serve as a positive role model and teacher for both child and caregiver. Nurses should encourage caregivers to foster independence within their child by promoting acceptable limit-setting and allowing choices. Education about nutrition, exercise, rest, sexuality, and safety can foster healthy habits for life. The rewards are many when a school-age child is able to realize his or her full potential as a healthy, self-assured individual.

IN THE REAL WORLD

I love caring for school-age children! They are always so inquisitive and want to learn everything they can about their disease or illness. Most recuperate quite quickly from surgery unless there are complications, and, once their pain is under control, are out in the halls talking to nurses, caregivers, and other clients. They are also so willing to help the nurses in any way they can. It is not unusual to see a school-age child sitting at the desk talking to the nurses, especially during the evening hours when things are beginning to wind down on the units. Of course, there are those children who are not like this, but I have not seen too many and when I do, all it takes on my part is a little extra time and attention as they are usually just scared.

KEY CONCEPTS

- During school-age, the child's weight increases by 7 pounds per year, height increases by 2.5 inches per year, 20 deciduous teeth are shed, and 28 of the 32 permanent teeth appear.
- During latency, the child ignores his or her own sexuality and instead identifies with the same-sex caregiver.
- According to Erikson's theory of psychosocial development, the major task of the school-age period is industry versus inferiority where the child's work brings a sense of accomplishment and worth.
- Concrete operations, where thoughts are less egocentric and become more open and flexible, allow the child to gain the skills of classification, conservation, and reversibility.
- Kohlberg proposed the school-age child is at the conventional level of moral development when the conscience develops an internal set of "rules" that must be followed in order to be "good."
- Schools, teachers, and peers play important roles in the school-age child's development.
- Play for school-age children includes quiet time, board games, and sports.
- Bullying has become an increasing problem in school-age children and can result in long term consequences.
- Latchkey children are at risk for problems associated with poor or lack of adult supervision.
- Factors contributing to the high incidence of accidents involving school-age children are increased independence from caregiver supervision, desire to meet the approval of peers, and increased involvement in physically challenging activities.
- Nursing care of school-age children involves teaching caregivers and children about nutrition, immunizations, health and safety issues, activity, rest and sleep, and expected developmental changes.

REVIEW ACTIVITIES

1. Describe the physiological changes occurring during the school-age period.
2. What developmental milestones occur during school-age?
3. Define the cognitive skills of classification, conservation, and reversibility. Offer examples of each. Explain the importance of gaining these skills in terms of the nurse's plan of care in a health care setting.

4. What are the major influences on moral development of the school-age child?
5. Why are peers, teachers, and schools so important for the school-age child?
6. Explain the risks associated with latchkey children.
7. Describe why bullying is a problem and offer suggestions to decrease its increase.
8. List several safety promotion and injury prevention techniques for school-age children and their caregivers.
9. Put together a response for a child who asks "how a baby gets in his mother's tummy?."

STUDY QUESTIONS

1. Which of the following statements accurately describes a physiological change during the school-age period?
   a. The child will grow in height an average of 2.5 inches per year.
   b. The child's weight will triple during the school-age period.
   c. The child's hair color and texture will change.
   d. The child's vision will improve every year.
2. Freud described the school-age years as which period of psychosexual development?
   a. Anal
   b. Latency
   c. Oedipal
   d. Oral
3. What is the psychosocial developmental goal for the school-age child according to Erikson?
   a. Trust
   b. Initiative
   c. Guilt
   d. Industry
4. According to Piaget, the expanded cognitive abilities of the school-age child include which of the following?
   a. Animism
   b. Rationalization
   c. Inferiority
   d. Reversibility
5. According to Kohlberg, the school-age child is at the conventional level of moral development. Which of the following statements accurately represents this level?
   a. Children do not seek the approval of others.
   b. Children show no respect for authority figures.
   c. The child's morality is based on the approval of younger siblings.
   d. The child's conscience develops an internal set of rules.
6. Children who come home alone after school and are without adult supervision are called:
   a. Latchkey children.
   b. Juvenile delinquents.
   c. Foster children.
   d. Truants.
7. Javan is a 10-year-old boy who has seen the school nurse multiple times for vague complaints. He tells the nurse he is being bullied by some of the older boys in the school. Which of the following signs or symptoms are often reported by children in response to fear of being bullied?
   a. Sleep problems
   b. Fever
   c. Ear infection
   d. Sprained ankle
8. When providing a talk to caregivers of school-age children concerning motor vehicle safety, the nurse includes which of the following statements?
   a. Children age 8 years and older should sit in the front seat of the vehicle.
   b. Children can sit in the cargo area of pickup trucks.
   c. Correct seat belt fit is usually not achieved until the child is 9 years old.
   d. Seat belts fit correctly when the lap portion of the belt rides across the stomach.
9. The leading cause of death for school-age children in the United States is:
   a. Cancer.
   b. Malnutrition.
   c. Accidents.
   d. AIDS.
10. Tymm, age 8 years, is scheduled to have a tonsillectomy. The best time for Tymm to receive preoperative preparation is:
    a. Two hours before surgery.
    b. Two days before surgery.
    c. One week before surgery.
    d. One month before surgery.

REFERENCES

Afterschool Alliance. (2008). Afterschool programs: Making a difference in America's communities by improving academic achievement, keeping kids safe and helping working families. Retrieved July 1, 2009, from http://www.afterschoolalliance.org.

Allen, P. (2010). The primary care provider and children with chronic conditions. In P. Allen, J. Vessey, & N. Schapiro (Eds.). *Primary care of the child with a chronic condition*. St. Louis, MO: Mosby Elsevier, pp. 3–21.

American Academy of Child & Adolescent Psychiatry. (2008). Facts for families: Bullying. Retrieved April 9, 2010, from http://www.aacap.org/cs/root/facts_for_families/bullying.

American Academy of Pediatrics. (2006). Policy Statement–Active healthy living: Prevention of childhood obesity through increased physical activity. *Pediatrics, 117*(5), 1834–1842.

American Academy of Pediatrics. (2007a). Healthy children. Retrieved June 1, 2009, from http://www.aap.org/healthychildren.

American Academy of Pediatrics. (2007b). What is puberty? Retrieved July 3, 2009, from http://www.aap.org/publiced/BR_Teen_Puberty.htm.

American Academy of Pediatrics. (2007c). What are the signs of low self-esteem? Retrieved April 9, 2010, from http://www.aap.org/publiced/BK5_SelfEsteem_Low.htm.

American Academy of Pediatrics. (2009a). *Plain language pediatrics*. Elk Grove Village, IL: Author.

American Academy of Pediatrics. (2009b). Policy Statement–Pedestrian safety. *Pediatrics, 124*(2), 802–812.

Berk, L. (2008). *Infants and children*. New York: Pearson Education.

Click, P., & Parker, J. (2009). *Caring for school-age children*. Clifton Park, NY: Delmar Cengage Learning.

Dalton, S. (2004). Schools and the rising rate of overweight children: Prevention and intervention strategies. *Topics in Clinical Nutrition, 19*(1), 34–40.

Damon, W., & Lerner, R. (2006). *Handbook of child psychology*. Hoboken, NJ: John Wiley & Sons.

Deloian, B., & Berry, A. (2009). Developmental management in pediatric primary care. In C. Burns, A. Dunn, M. Brady, N. Starr, & C. Blosser (Eds.). *Pediatric primary care*. St. Louis, MO: Saunders, pp. 53–70.

Erikson, E. (1963). *Childhood and society*. New York: Norton.

Feigelman, S. (2007). Middle childhood. In R. Kliegman, R. Behrman, H. Jenson, & B. Stanton (Eds.). *Nelson textbook of pediatrics* (18th ed.). Philadelphia, PA: Saunders, pp. 57–60.

Fingerhut, L. (1993). Firearm mortality among children, youth, and young adults 1–34 years of age: Trends and current status. United States Department of Health and Human Services. CDC, No. 231.

Finkelstein, E., Corso, P., & Miller, T. (2006). *Incidence and economic burden of injuries in the United States*. New York: Oxford University Press.

Freud, S. (1923). *The ego and the id*. London: Hogarth Press.

Gance-Cleveland, B., & Yousey, Y. (2009). Developmental management of school-age children. In C. Burns, A. Dunn, M. Brady, N. Starr, & C. Blosser (Eds.), *Pediatric primary care*. St. Louis, MO: Saunders, pp. 109–131.

Glew, G., Fan, M., Katon, W., & Rivara, F. (2008). Bullying and school safety. *Journal of Pediatrics, 152*, 123–128.

Gottesman, M., Brady, M., Gance-Cleveland, B., & Duderstadt, K. (2010). Obesity. In P. Jackson-Allen, J. Vessey, & N. Schapiro (Eds.). *Primary care of the child with a chronic condition*. St. Louis, MO: Mosby Elsevier, pp. 686–714.

Huston, A., & Ripke, M. (2006). *Developmental contexts in middle childhood*. New York: Cambridge University Press.

Katzmarzyk, P., Baur, L., Blair, S., Lambert, E., Oppert, J., & Riddoch, C. (2008). International conference on physical activity and obesity in children: Summary statement and recommendations. *International Journal of Pediatric Obesity, 3*, 3–21.

Keep Kids Healthy. (2010a). Homework tips for parents. Retrieved April 9, 2010, from http://keepkidshealthy.com/schoolage/homework_tips.html.

Keep Kids Healthy. (2010b). How do you deal with bullies? Retrieved April 9, 2010, from http://keepkidshealthy.com/schoolage/schoolagequicktips/bullys.html.

Kliegman, R., Behrman, R., Jenson, H., & Stanton, B. (2007). *Nelson textbook of pediatrics* (18th ed.). Philadelphia, PA: Saunders.

Kohlberg, L. (1969). *Stages in development of moral thought and action*. New York: Holt, Rinehart, & Winston.

Martin, J., Kung, H., & Mathews, T. Hoyert, D. L., Strobino, D. M., Guyer, B., & Sutton, S. R. (2008). Annual summary of vital statistics: 2006. *Pediatrics, 121*(4), 788–801.

Menke, E. (1981). School-aged children's perception of stress in the hospital. *Journal of the Association for the Care of Children's Health, 9*(30), 80–86.

Morrongiello, B., Corbett, M., & Bellissimo, A. (2008). "Do as I say, not as I do": Family influences on children's safety and risk behaviors. *Health Psychology, 27*(4), 498–503.

National Association of State Boards of Education. (2009). Preventing childhood obesity: A school health policy guide. Arlington, VA: Author.

National Institute on Out-of-School Time. (2006). Making the case: A fact sheet on children and youth in out-of-school time. Retrieved April 9, 2010 from http://www.niost.org/pdf/factsheet2009.pdf.

Ogden, C., Carroll, M., & Flegal, K. (2008). High body mass index for age among U.S. children and adolescents, 2003–2006. *Journal of the American Medical Association, 299*(20), 2401–2405.

Piaget, J. (1962). *Play, dreams and imitation in childhood*. New York: Norton.

Rappley, M., & Kallman, J. (2009). Middle childhood. In W. Carey, W. Coleman, A. Crocker, E. Elias, & H. Feldman (Eds.). *Developmental-behavioral pediatrics*. Philadelphia, PA: Saunders.

Ryan-Wegner, N. (1998). Children's drawings: An invaluable source of information for nurses. *Journal of Pediatric Health Care, 12*(3), 109–110.

Safe Kids Worldwide. (2007). Childhood Injury Trends Fact Sheet. Retrieved July 11, 2009, from http://www.usa.safekids.org.

Santrock, J. (2009). *Child development*. Boston: McGraw-Hill.

Schmidt, C., Bernaix, L., Koski, A., Weese, J., Chiappetta, M., & Sandrik, K. (2007). Hospitalized children's perceptions of nurses and nurse behaviors. *MCN: The American Journal of Maternal/Child Nursing, 32*(6), 336–342.

Skybo, T., & Buck, J. (2007). Stress and coping responses to proficiency testing in school-age children. *Pediatric Nursing, 33*(5), 410–418.

Society of Pediatric Nurses. (2010a). Position statement on exercise and physical activity. Retrieved April 9, 2010, from https://www.pedsnurses.org/component/option,com_docman/Itemid,0/task,doc_view/gid,63/.

Society of Pediatric Nurses. (2010b). Position statement on overweight children and adolescents. Retrieved April 9, 2010, from https://www.pedsnurses.org/component/option,com_docman/Itemid,117/task,doc_view/gid,66/.

Stedman, T. (2008). *Stedman's medical dictionary* (6th ed.). Philadelphia: Wolters Kluwer Health/Lippincott, Williams & Wilkins.

Stott, F. (2009). The truth about lying. Retrieved May 22, 2009, from http://www2.scholastic.com/browse/article.jsp?id=702&print=2.

Strasburger, V., Wilson, B., & Jordan, A. (2009). *Children, adolescents, and the media.* Los Angeles, CA: Sage.

Towns, N., & D'Auria, J. (2009). Parental perceptions of their child's overweight: An integrative review of the literature. *Journal of Pediatric Nursing, 24*(2), 115–130.

United Nations. (2009). *The Millennium Development Goals Report 2009.* New York, NY: author.

Vessey, J., & Sullivan, B. (2010). Chronic conditions and child development. In P. Allen, J. Vessey, & N. Schapiro (Eds.). *Primary care of the child with a chronic condition.* St. Louis, MO: Mosby Elsevier, pp. 22–41.

Vygotsky, L. (1962). *Thought and language.* New York: Wiley.

Walker, W. (2005). *The Harvard Medical School guide to healthy eating for kids: Eat, play, and be healthy.* New York: McGraw Hill.

Ward, T., Rankin, S., & Lee, K. (2007). Caring for children with sleep problems. *Journal of Pediatric Nursing, 22*(4), 283–296.

Washington, T. (2009). Psychological stress and anxiety in middle to late childhood and early adolescence: Manifestations and management. *Journal of Pediatric Nursing, 24*(4), 302–313.

Wells, R., & Stein, M. (2006). Seven to ten years: World of middle childhood. In S. Dixon & M. Stein (Eds.). *Encounters with children: Pediatric behavior and development.* Philadelphia, PA: Mosby Elsevier, pp. 505–533.

Youngblade, L., Storch, E., & Nackashi, J. (2009). Peers. In W. Carey, W. Crocker, A. Crocker, E. Elias, & H. Feldman (Eds.). *Developmental-behavioral pediatrics.* Philadephia, PA: Saunders, pp. 152–158.

SUGGESTED READINGS

American Academy of Pediatrics. (2006). Menstruation in girls and adolescents: Using the menstrual cycle as a vital sign. *Pediatrics, 118*(5), 2245–2250.

American Academy of Pediatrics. (2007). Policy Statement – Professionalism in pediatrics: Statement of principles. *Pediatrics, 120*(4), 895–897.

American Academy of Pediatrics. (2008). Policy Statement–Role of the school nurse in providing school health services. *Pediatrics, 121*(5), 1052–1056.

Annie E. Casey Foundation. (2009). The 2009 kids count data book. Retrieved April 9, 2010, from http://datacenter.kidscount.org/databook/2009/Default.aspx.

Atkins, R. (2007). The association of personality type in childhood with violence in adolescence. *Research in Nursing and Health, 30*, 308–319.

Bagdi, A., & Pfister, I. (2006). Childhood stressors and coping actions: A comparison of children and parents' perspectives. *Child & Youth Care Forum, 35*(1), 21–40.

Bingham, M., Harrell, J., Takada, H., Washino, K., Bradley, C., Berry, D., Park, H., & Charles, M. (2009). Obesity and cholesterol in Japanese, French, and U.S. children. *Journal of Pediatric Nursing, 24*(4), 314–322.

Brendgen, M., Vitaro, F., Boivin, M., Girard, A., Bukowski, W., Dionne, G., Tremblay, R., & Perusse, D. (2009). Gene-environment interplay between peer rejection and depressive behavior in children. *Journal of Child Psychology and Psychiatry, 50*(8), 1009–1017.

Cave, K. (2009). Influences of disordered eating in prepubescent children. *Journal of Psychosocial Nursing, 47*(2), 21–24.

Children's Defense Fund. (2008). *The state of America's children.* Washington, DC.: Author.

Christensen, P., & Mikkelsen, M. (2008). Jumping off and being careful: Children's strategies of risk management in everyday life. *Sociology of Health & Illness, 30*(1), 112–130.

Coll, C., & Marks, A. (2009). *Immigrant stories: Ethnicity and academics in middle childhood.* New York: Oxford University Press.

Crosnoe, R. (2006). Health and the education of children from racial/ethnic minority and immigrant families. *Journal of Health and Behavior, 47*, 77–93.

Ewing, B. (2008). Children's wishes: Holistic revelations in art. *Journal of Holistic Nursing, 26*(2), 147–154.

Greenman, P., Schneider, B., & Tomada, G. (2009). Stability and change in patterns of peer rejection: Implications for children's academic performance over time. *School Psychology International, 30*(2), 163–183.

Kennedy, C., & Chen, J. (2009). Changes in childhood risk taking and safety behavior after a peer group media intervention. *Nursing Research, 58*(4), 264–273.

Kennedy, C., & Floriani, V. (2008). Translating research on healthy lifestyles for children: Meeting the needs of diverse populations. *Nursing Clinics of North America, 43*(3), 397–417.

Krause-Parello, C. (2008). Loneliness in the school setting. *Journal of School Nursing, 24*(2), 66–70.

Ladd, G., Herald-Brown, S., & Reiser, M. (2008). Does chronic classroom peer rejection predict the development of children's classroom participation during the grade school years? *Child Development, 79*(4), 1001–1015.

Li, Y., Jackson, J., & Zhang, J. (2008). Overweight is associated with decreased cognitive functioning among school-age children and adolescents. *Obesity, 16*(8), 1809–1815.

Meizi, H., Harris, S., Piche, L., & Beynon, C. (2009). Understanding screen-related sedentary behavior and its contributing factors among school-aged children: A social-ecologic exploration. *American Journal of Health Promotion, 23*(5), 299–308.

Moore, J., Pawloski, L., Goldberg, P., Kyeung, M., Stoehr, A., & Baghi, H. (2009). Childhood obesity study: A pilot study of the effect of the nutrition education program Color My Pyramid. *Journal of School Nursing, 25*(3), 230–239.

Morrongiello, B., & Lasenby, J. (2007). Psychological determinants of risk taking by children: An integrative model and implications for interventions. *Injury Prevention, 13*, 20–25.

National Agricultural Library USDA, Food and Nutrition Information Center. (2009). Childhood obesity: A resource list for educators and researchers. Retrieved April 9, 2010, from http://www.nal.usda.gov/fnic/pubs/bibs/topics/weight/childhoodobesity.pdf.

Nixon, G., Thompson, J., Becroft, D., Clark, P., Robinson, E., Wild, C., & Black, P. (2008). Short sleep duration in middle childhood: Risk factors and consequences. *Sleep, 31*(1), 71–78.

Pelander, T., Lehtonen, K., & Leino-Kilpi, H. (2007). Children in the hospital: Elements of quality in drawings. *Journal of Pediatric Nursing, 22*(4), 333–341.

Pong, S., & Hao, L. (2007). Neighborhood and school factors in the school performance of immigrants' children. *International Migration Review, 41*(1), 206–241.

Randall, D., Brook, G., & Stammers, P. (2008). How to make good children's nurses: Children's views. *Paediatric Nursing, 20*(5), 22–25.

Reijntjes, A., Stegge, H., & Terwogt, M. (2006). Children's coping with peer rejection: The role of depressive symptoms, social competence, and gender. *Infant and Child Development, 15*, 89–107.

Shaya, F., Flores, D., Gbarayor, C., & Wang, J. (2008). School-based obesity interventions: A literature review. *Journal of School Health, 78*(4), 189–196.

Shoup, J., Gattshall, M., Dandamudi, P., & Estabrooks, P. (2008). Physical activity, quality of life, and weight status in overweight children. *Quality of Life Research, 17*, 407–412.

Skybo, T., Ryan-Wenger, N., & Su, Y. (2007). Human figure drawings as a measure of children's emotional status: Critical review for practice. *Journal of Pediatric Nursing, 22*(1), 15–28.

Society of Pediatric Nurses. (2009). Position statement on child welfare. *Journal of Pediatric Nursing, 24*(1), 75–76.

UNICEF. (2009). The *state of the world's children 2009*. Retrieved April 9, 2010, from http://www.unicef.org/publications.

Wilson, B. (2008). Media and children's aggression, fear, and altruism. *Future of Children, 18*(1), 87–118.

Wittmeier, K., Mollard, R., & Kriellaars, D. (2008). Physical activity intensity and risk of overweight and adiposity in children. *Obesity, 16*(2), 415–420.

RESOURCES

Refer to the online student StudyWARE for Potts & Mandleco at http://www.CengageBrain.com for additional content and study aids.

Organization: **About Our Kids**
Description: Offers access to information about NYU Child Study Center research, education, news, and impacts as well as links to local doctor offices and specific information for families.
Website/Resource: http://www.aboutourkids.org

Organization: **After School Alliance**
Description: Works to ensure all children have access to affordable, quality afterschool programs; contains information about current programs, facts, research, publications, newsletters, and helpful links.
Website/Resource: http://www.afterschoolalliance.org

Organization: **American Academy of Child and Adolescent Psychiatry (AACAP)**
Description: Provides information regarding mental illnesses, data concerning efforts to prevent mental illnesses, how to seek proper treatment, and access to services for children and adolescents.
Website/Resource: http://www.aacap.org

Organization: **American Academy of Family Physicians**
Description: Offers information regarding family physician careers, clinical research, advocacy, practice management, and recent news/publications.
Website/Resource: http://www.aafp.org

Organization: **American Academy of Pediatrics**
Description: Offers general information related to child health, specific guidelines concerning many pediatric issues, information regarding AAP programs, activities, policies, guidelines, publications, and other child health resources.
Website/Resource: http://www.aap.org

Organization: **American School Health Association**
Description Offers information regarding American School Health Association initiatives/projects, advocacy/resolutions, corporate support, continuing education, and conferences.
Website/Resource: http://www.ashaweb.org

Organization: **American School Health Association**
Description Offers information regarding American School Health Association initiatives/projects, advocacy/resolutions, corporate support, continuing education, and conferences.
Website/Resource: http://www.ashaweb.org

Organization: **Bright Futures**
Description: Offers access to helpful multimedia/materials, family resources, and information about clinical practice related to children's health promotion and disease prevention.
Website/Resource: http://www.brightfutures.aap.org

Organization: **Child Advocate**
Description: Serves needs of children/families/professionals; addresses mental health/medical/educational/legal/legislative issues; offers information about mental health, education, psychiatric assistance, and legislative/governmental involvement.
Website/Resource: http://www.childadvocate.net

Organization: **Child Development Institute**
Description: Provides current, relevant, and easy to attain parent education including readers' development, parenting, psychology, learning, and health/safety.
Website/Resource: http://www.childdevelopmentinfo.com

Organization: **Children's Defense Fund (CDF)**
Description: A non-profit child advocacy organization; website offers information regarding CDF's policies and mission, child advocacy resources, and child research data.
Website/Resource: http://www.childrensdefense.org

Organization: **Connect for Kids—Guidance for Grownups**
Description: Offers information/tools needed to learn about issues affecting children, families, and communities and to take action to improve policies and programs.
Website/Resource: http://www.connectforkids.org

Organization: **Consumer Product Safety Commission**
Description: Charged with protecting public from unreasonable risks of serious injury/death from consumer products; offers information about consumer safely/business regulations; access to library.
Website/Resource: http://www.cpsc.gov

Organization: **Keep Kids Healthy**
Description: Free parenting advice, news updates, immunization schedule, growth charts, asthma/breastfeeding centers, BMI calculator, height predictor, lead poisoning screening quiz, nutrition, growth, development, common problems/diseases/conditions/ infections in children.
Website/Resource: http://www.keepkidshealthy.com

Organization: **Kidlink**
Description: Offers information about free educational programs that motivate learning by helping teachers relate local curriculum guidelines to students' personal interests and goals.
Website/Resource: http://www.kidlink.org

Organization: **Kids Health Organization**
Description: Provides advice about a wide range of physical, emotional, and behavioral issues that affect children and teens.
Website/Resource: http://www.kidshealth.org

Organization: **Kid Source Online**
Description: Online community allowing parents to share values/goals in raising, educating, and providing for children; access to parenting/education/recreation/organizations/product information.
Website/Resource: http://www.kidsource.com

Organization: **Maternal and Child Health Bureau (MCHB)**
Description: Offers information regarding current MCHB programs, funding opportunities, reports and resources/publications.
Website/Resource: http://mchb.hrsa.gov

Organization: **National Association of School Nurses (NASN)**
Description: Offers information regarding continuing education, helpful resources, education campaigns, policy/advocacy, and research, as well as professional information to active school nurses.
Website/Resource: http://www.nasn.org

Organization: **National Center for Children Exposed to Violence (NCCEV)**
Description: Offers information concerning childhood violence, resource centers, and NCCEV initiatives.
Website/Resource: http://www.nccev.org

Organization: **National Federation of Families for Children's Mental Health**
Description: Offers information regarding program contacts/ resources/events related to families and children/youth with emotional, behavioral and mental health challenges.
Website/Resource: http://www.ffcm.org

Organization: **National Institute of Child Health & Human Development (NICHD)**
Description: Offers information regarding general health information, research, funding, and recent news/media related to child health and development.
Website/Resource: http://www.nichd.nih.gov

Organization: **National Institute on Out-of-School Time (NIOST)**
Description: Offers information regarding the institute's work, publications, news/events, and resources related to programs, activities, and opportunities for children during non-school hours.
Website/Resource: http://www.niost.org

Organization: **National Runaway Switchboard**
Description: Offers access to information regarding runaway prevention curriculum, helpful links, research and education/promotional materials.
Website/Resource: http://www.nrscrisisline.org

Organization: **Safer Child**
Description: Allows blogging opportunities as well as access to headlines/news, advocacy, and statistics related to child safety.
Website/Resource: http://www.saferchild.org

Organization: **Stand for Children**
Description: Offers access to state affiliates, events, and membership opportunities to help children get excellent public education/ strong support needed to thrive.
Website/Resource: http://www.stand.org

Organization: **United Nations Children's Fund (UNICEF)**
Description: Provides information regarding UNICEF programs, country situations, and the state of the world's children.
Website/Resource: http://www.unicef.org

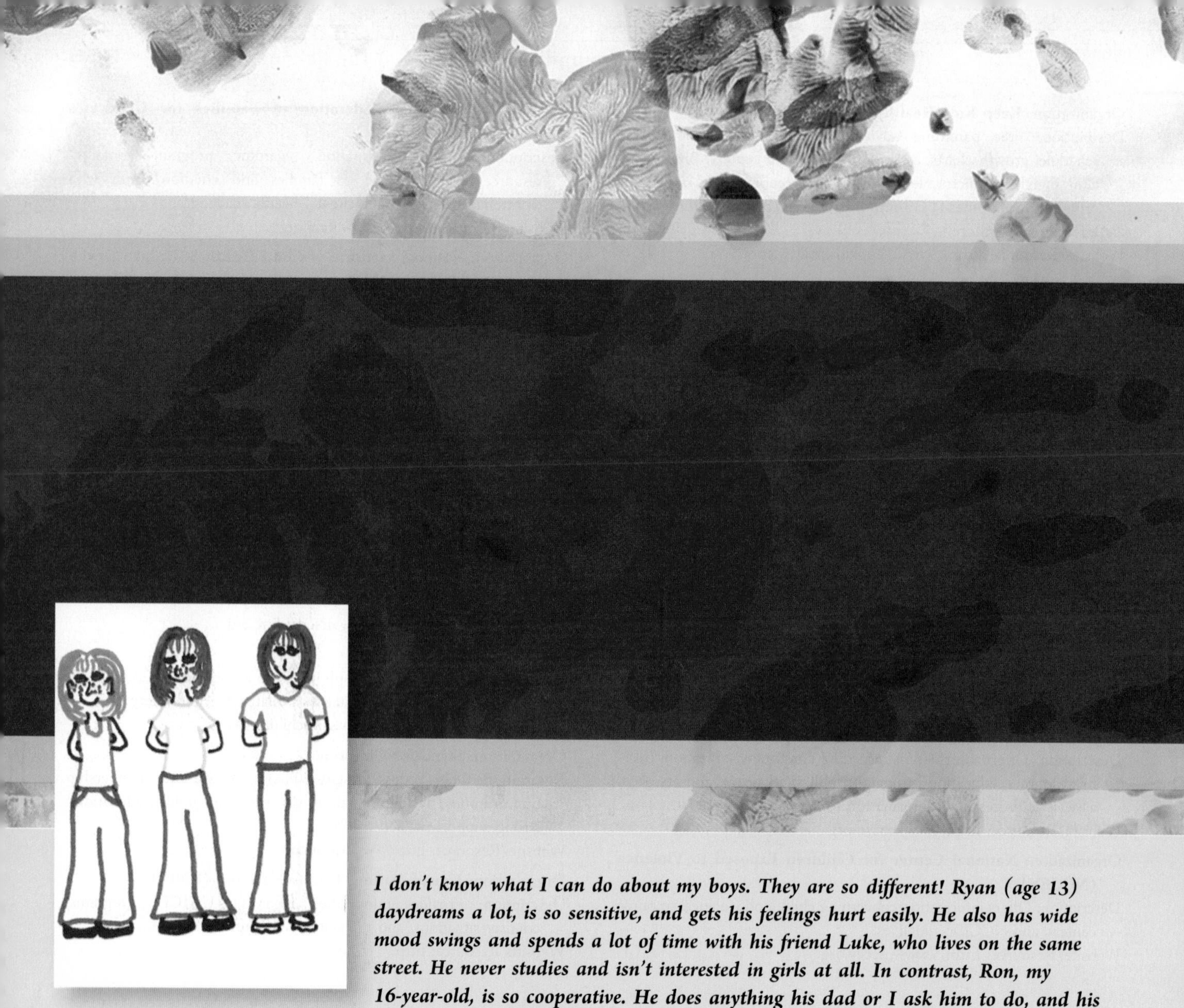

I don't know what I can do about my boys. They are so different! Ryan (age 13) daydreams a lot, is so sensitive, and gets his feelings hurt easily. He also has wide mood swings and spends a lot of time with his friend Luke, who lives on the same street. He never studies and isn't interested in girls at all. In contrast, Ron, my 16-year-old, is so cooperative. He does anything his dad or I ask him to do, and his room is so neat! He has started to date Penelope, a girl in his Spanish class at school; works part time at his dad's office; and plans to major in accounting when he attends college.

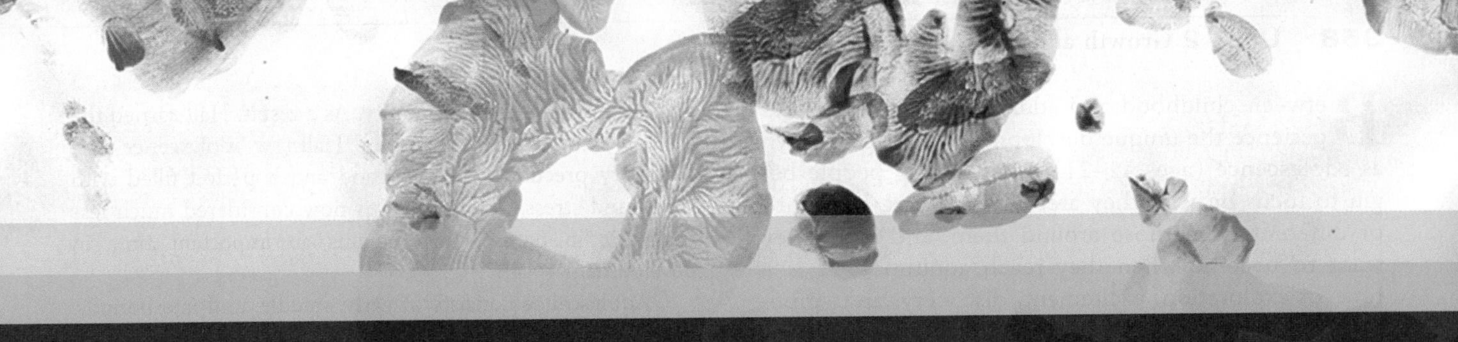

CHAPTER 12

Growth and Development of the Adolescent

BARBARA L. MANDLECO, RN, PhD
J. KELLY MCCOY, PhD

COMPETENCIES

Upon completion of this chapter, the reader will be able to:

- Explain the importance and timing of physiological development in adolescence.
- Discuss the importance of psychosexual, psychosocial, cognitive, and moral development in adolescence.
- Discuss the impact school, peers, work, and leisure time have on adolescent development.
- Describe the major developmental tasks of adolescence, and discuss why they are important for the transition to adulthood.
- Discuss several nursing interventions for effectively working with adolescents.
- Discuss several health promotion and screening activities related to adolescence and the appropriate nursing interventions.
- Discuss several issues or problems facing adolescents today and the appropriate nursing interventions.
- Successfully complete the games and activities in the online student StudyWARE.

Between childhood and adulthood, individuals experience the unique developmental period known as adolescence (ages 12–21), when young people begin to focus on who they are, how they are similar to or different from those around them, and what they want to become when they reach adulthood. It is a time of exploration, excitement, discovery, and sometimes confusion and despair (Figure 12-1).

Adolescence is second only to infancy in the amount of change individuals encounter physiologically and psychosocially. In order to effectively identify issues and problems commonly seen in adolescence, and consequently deliver appropriate and individualized nursing care, it is important to consider the physiological, psychosexual, psychosocial, cognitive, and moral transformations occurring during this time, as well as changes in adolescents' rapidly expanding social context, including the family, school, and peers.

The concept of an adolescent stage of development is actually a relatively recent phenomenon. Not until the beginning of the 20th century did society begin to recognize adolescence as a unique period of development, different from both childhood and adulthood. As the early industrialization of the 19th century shifted work opportunities from agriculture toward urban factories, the cheap, unskilled labor produced by an adolescent workforce was viewed as an economic asset. However, as industry began to utilize other sources of power and the machinery used became increasingly complex and dangerous, the labor provided by children and adolescents shifted toward being more of a liability. The increasing need to protect children and adolescents in an increasingly sophisticated workplace resulted in child labor laws being enacted. As automation made unskilled jobs more dangerous and scarcer, and therefore necessitated a more educated workforce, a compulsory secondary education system was developed to better prepare and supervise the growing number of unemployable adolescents. At the same time, the 1904 publication of G. Stanley Hall's two-volume set of books titled *Adolescence* resulted in many changes regarding how the second decade of life was conceptualized among the scientific community. As a result, Hall earned the title of "Father of Adolescence." Hall saw adolescence as a necessary precursor to adulthood and a period filled with storm and stress. Adolescence is now considered much less traumatic in nature, but remains an important time in development.

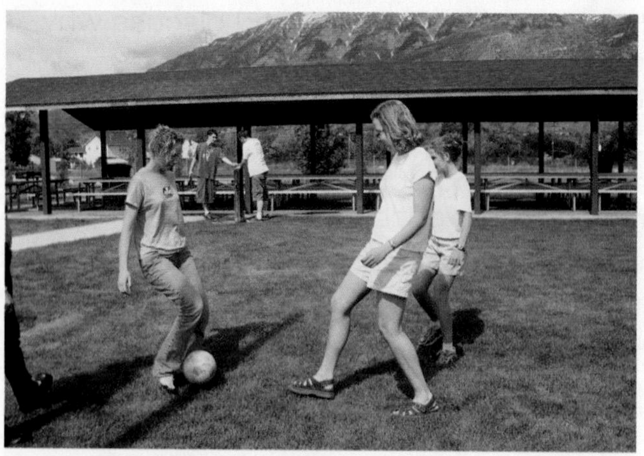

FIGURE 12-1 Adolescence can be a time of excitement, discovery, and despair. DELMAR CENGAGE LEARNING.

Adolescence consists of early, middle, and late periods. Each is distinguished by several different aspects of adolescents' lives and constitutes the ages of 12–14, 15–17, and 18–21 years. Another way to differentiate these periods relates to physiological development: **prepubertal** (early), **pubertal** (middle), and **postpubertal** (late adolescence). A third way relates to the level of education—early, middle, and late adolescence are associated with middle school, high school, and post-high school.

PHYSIOLOGICAL DEVELOPMENT

The physiological changes occurring during adolescence are extensive, do not occur in isolation, and have an impact on the adolescent's psychosexual, psychosocial, and cognitive development. These changes also affect the experiences adolescents have with family members, peers, and others in their social world, as well as their own body image and self-esteem.

Clarification of two terms commonly associated with this period is needed, however, before discussing the actual physiological changes occurring. **Puberty** is the state of physical development (between ages 12 and 16 for males and ages 10 and 14 for females) when secondary sex characteristics begin to appear: increased body hair, growth of the breasts in females, increased muscle mass, voice changes (in males), widening of the hips (female), and changes in body fat distribution. Sexual organs mature, reproduction first becomes possible, and the adolescent growth spurt starts (Dunn, 2009a; Steinberg, 2008).

Adolescence begins with puberty and ends when the individual is physically and psychologically mature and able to assume adult responsibilities. The age when puberty begins and how long adolescence lasts varies individually and cross-culturally (Marcell, 2007).

Before puberty, the primary hormone regulating growth is somatotropin, also called growth hormone. However, during puberty the gonadal hormones are responsible for many of the significant physiological changes seen in various body systems (Katchadourian, 1977).

MUSCULOSKELETAL SYSTEM

During the **adolescent growth spurt (AGS)**, which lasts about 4.5 years, the body assumes an adult appearance. Girls may begin their spurt as early as 7.5 or as late as 12 years of age, whereas boys typically begin their growth spurt by age 13. During the AGS, there is rapid acceleration in weight and height; boys gain 12–14 lb and grow 3–6 inches; girls gain 8–10 lb and grow 2.5–5 inches.

The AGS is not uniform; weight begins to increase first, followed in 4–6 months by a rapid increase in height. The age of onset, intensity, and duration of the AGS vary from individual to individual, and differs for boys and girls (Figure 12-2). In females, the AGS accompanies the first signs of puberty (pubic hair, breast development), and peaks when breast development is between Tanner stages 2 and 3. However, the AGS for males occurs during Tanner Stages 3 and 4 (mid-puberty) as testosterone levels rise rapidly (Abbassi, 1998; Marcell, 2007).

Typically, height begins increasing in early adolescence for females and in midadolescence for males. Females achieve **peak height velocity (PHV)**, the maximum annual rate of growth in height during the AGS, at about 11 years of age, or 6–12 months before menarche. Very few females grow more than 2 inches after menarche (Marcell, 2007). Males reach PHV at about age 13, after axillary and mature pubic hair appears, and growth of the penis and testes begins. Most males do not grow in height after 18 or 20 years of age. See Figures 12-3 and 12-4 for linear growth curves during childhood and adolescence.

Weight increases for adolescents tend to follow the same growth curve as height. **Peak weight velocity (PWV)**, the period when weight gain is the most rapid, is greater for males than females, and occurs simultaneously with PHV. PWV for females occurs about 6 months after PHV. Females frequently are heavier than their male counterparts during the AGS and tend to weigh more than males until about age 14, when their weight gain begins to level off. Weight gain in adolescent males is due primarily to increases in muscle mass and height, whereas in females, it is due primarily to increases in fat and height. Males continue gaining weight until about 22 years of age (Marcell, 2007). Diet, gastric motility, exercise, socioeconomic status, lifestyle, and hereditary factors affect adolescent weight gain.

Significant changes also occur in skeletal size, muscle mass, skin, and adipose tissue. Full bone length is first reached in the extremities and moves inward. Trunk growth begins with lengthening and widening of the hips, especially

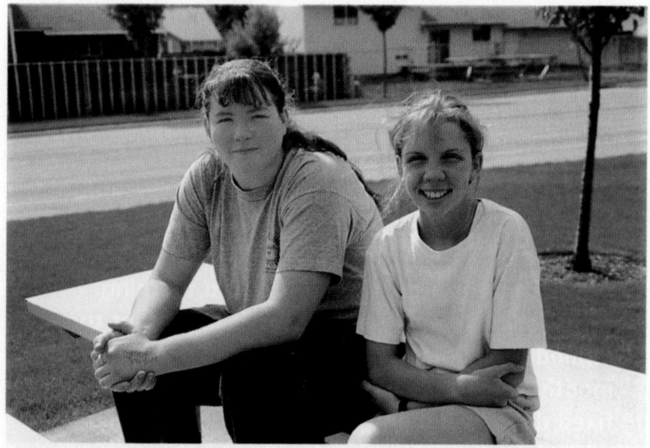

FIGURE 12-2 Adolescents develop at very different rates. What is considered normal varies greatly. DELMAR CENGAGE LEARNING.

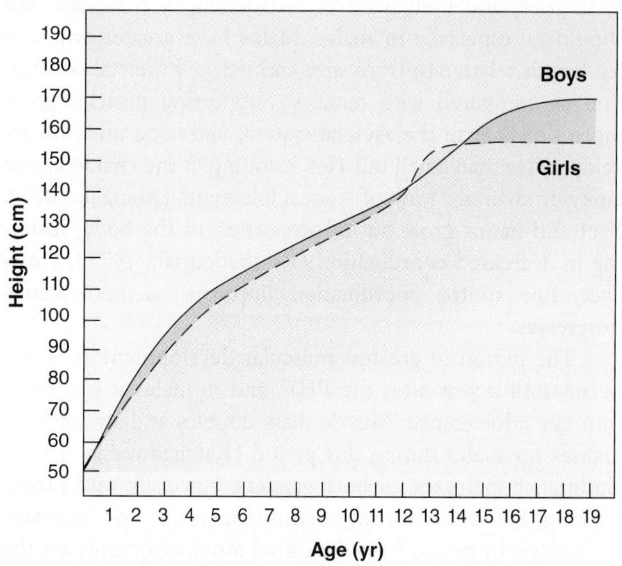

FIGURE 12-3 Linear Growth Throughout Childhood. FROM TANNER, J., WHITEHOUSE, R. H., & TAKAISHI, M. (1966). STANDARDS FROM BIRTH TO MATURITY FOR HEIGHT, WEIGHT, HEIGHT VELOCITY, AND WEIGHT VELOCITY: BRITISH CHILDREN, 1965. *ARCHIVES OF DISEASES OF CHILDREN*, 41, 454-471. REPRODUCED WITH PERMISSION FROM THE BMJ PUBLISHING GROUP.

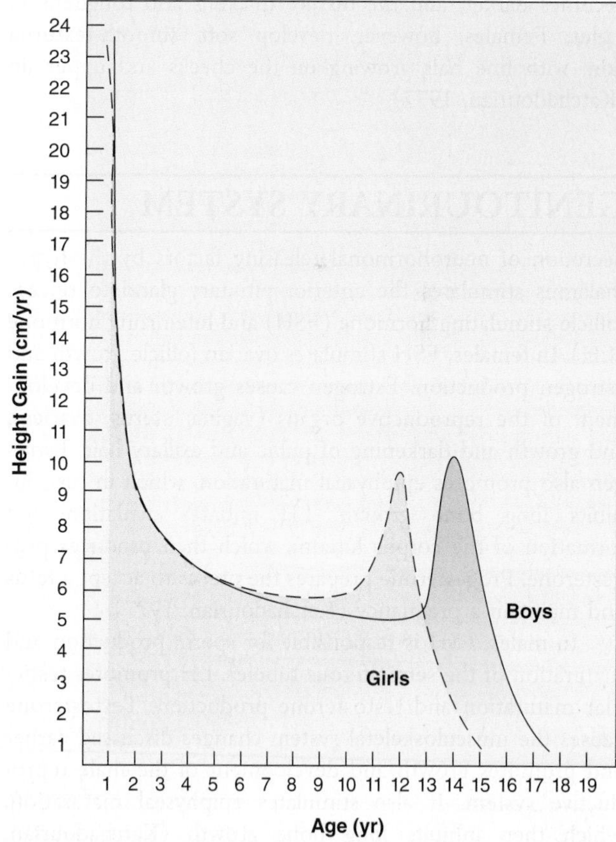

FIGURE 12-4 Linear Growth in Centimeters per Year. FROM TANNER, J., WHITEHOUSE, R. H., & TAKAISHI, M. (1966). STANDARDS FROM BIRTH TO MATURITY FOR HEIGHT, WEIGHT, HEIGHT VELOCITY, AND WEIGHT VELOCITY: BRITISH CHILDREN, 1965. *ARCHIVES OF DISEASES OF CHILDREN*, 41, 454-471. REPRODUCED WITH PERMISSION FROM THE BMJ PUBLISHING GROUP.

in females, and then involves broadening of the chest and shoulders, especially in males. Males have greater arm and leg length relative to trunk size and delayed skeletal ossification as compared with females. Supporting muscles grow more slowly than the skeletal system, and large muscles develop faster than small muscles, resulting in the characteristic lanky or awkward look of some adolescents (Marcell, 2007). Feet and hands grow out of proportion to the body, resulting in decreased coordination (Katchadourian, 1977). However, fine motor coordination improves as adolescence progresses.

The period of greatest muscular development does not occur until a year after the PHV, and in males it continues into late adolescence. Muscle mass doubles and strength increases for males during this period (Katchadourian, 1977). Endurance increases for both genders, especially with fitness training. Subcutaneous fat decreases in males and increases in females. In males, fat is deposited more commonly on the trunk, whereas in females, it is deposited over the thighs, buttocks, and breasts.

Sebaceous glands increase in size as they become active for both genders (Steinberg, 2008). Eccrine and apocrine glands mature as well, leading to increased amounts of, and a distinct odor to, perspiration. Perspiration is also now secreted in response to emotional stimuli. The skin becomes darker, and the texture thickens and toughens in males. Females, however, develop soft, smooth-textured skin, with fine hair growing on the cheeks and upper lip (Katchadourian, 1977).

GENITOURINARY SYSTEM

Secretion of neurohormonal releasing factors by the hypothalamus stimulates the anterior pituitary gland to release follicle-stimulating hormone (FSH) and luteinizing hormone (LH). In females, FSH stimulates ovarian follicle growth and estrogen production. Estrogen causes growth and development of the reproductive organs (vagina, uterus, ovaries), and growth and darkening of pubic and axillary hair. Estrogen also promotes epiphyseal maturation, which in turn inhibits long bone growth. LH initiates ovulation and formation of the corpus luteum, which then produces progesterone. Progesterone prepares the uterus to accept a fetus and maintain a pregnancy (Katchadourian, 1977).

In males, FSH is responsible for sperm production and maturation of the seminiferous tubules. LH promotes testicular maturation and testosterone production. Testosterone causes the musculoskeletal system changes discussed earlier and promotes growth and development of the male reproductive system. It also stimulates epiphyseal maturation, which then inhibits long bone growth (Katchadourian, 1977).

These reproductive hormones are also responsible for the predictable sequence of the appearance of secondary sexual characteristics that occurs during puberty. The age when the changes occur and the rate of progression vary.

KIDS WANT TO KNOW

Asymmetrical Breast Size

Why is one of my breasts larger than the other one? Will they ever be the same size? Is something wrong with me? Reassure the adolescent that it is not uncommon and in fact normal for female breasts to be different sizes. Often the only one who is aware of the size discrepancy is the teen herself.

In fact, cross-cultural studies show the onset of these secondary sexual changes varies with environmental conditions, race and ethnicity, geographical location, and nutrition (Eveleth & Tanner, 1990; Garibaldi, 2007a; Marcell, 2007).

This sequence of secondary sexual characteristics has been divided into five stages, called the **Tanner stages**. For females, the stages describe breast and pubic hair growth. For males, the stages describe growth of the testes, penis, scrotum, and pubic hair.

The first visible sign of female sexual maturation is breast development, which may not be symmetrical. This is followed by growth of pubic hair, which begins on average between 11 and 12 years of age, and is complete by about age 14 (Katchadourian, 1977; Marshall & Tanner, 1969). Breast development and pubic hair growth for females is described in Appendix D. Figure 12-5 illustrates the approximate timing of developmental changes in females.

In females, **menarche** (first menstrual period) indicates puberty and sexual maturity. Most adolescent females are ambivalent about menarche; they are happy for the proof they are women, yet view it as a burden since they are unable to control their bodies. Often, the response reflects feelings about growing up and femininity, and can be influenced by messages and attitudes of peers and parents.

Even though regular menstrual cycles and ovulation typically begin 6–14 months after menarche, adolescent females can become pregnant after their first menstrual period. Menarche occurs about two years after breast development starts

NURSING TIP

Breast Self-Examination

Adolescence is a good time to begin teaching breast self-examination (BSE). It is important to remind the adolescent to perform BSE once per month, eight days following menses or on a given fixed date each month. BSE should be avoided when breasts are tender due to menstruation or ovulation.

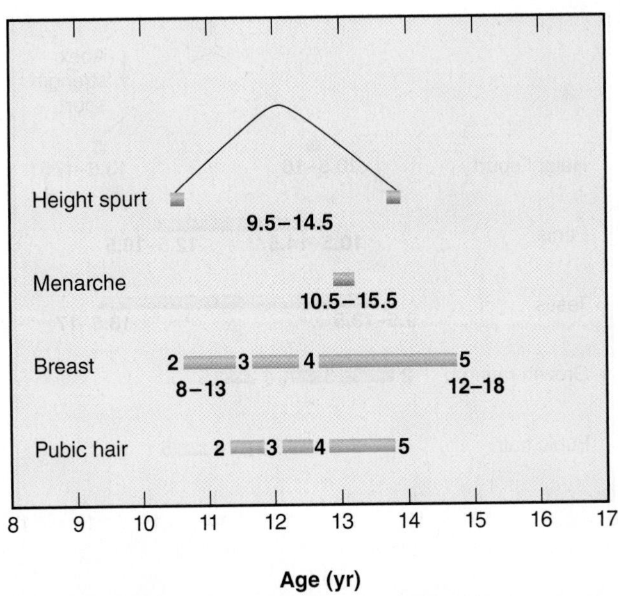

FIGURE 12-5 Approximate timing of developmental changes in females. Numbers appearing in the pubic hair and breast category indicate the Tanner stage of development. Ranges of ages during which the height spurt, menarche, and breast development may begin or end are indicated by inclusive numbers below the categories. The PHV is illustrated by the apex of the line indicating the timing when the height spurt occurs. FROM MARSHALL, W. A., & TANNER, J. M. (1969). VARIATIONS IN THE PATTERN OF PUBERTAL CHANGES IN GIRLS. *ARCHIVES OF DISEASES IN CHILDREN*, 45, 22. REPRODUCED WITH PERMISSION FROM THE BMJ PUBLISHING GROUP.

and after the AGS peaks. The exact time menarche begins, however, varies among populations and is influenced by nutrition, exercise, weight, breast development, health, metabolism, heredity, stress, depressive affect, family relations, and other environmental influences (Dunn, 2009a; Garibaldi, 2007a; Jenkins, 2007a; Marcell, 2007). For example, total calories, amount of dietary fat, and the type of protein consumed are related to the onset of puberty. Therefore, heavier children of both genders begin puberty earlier whereas those adolescents who exercise excessively or are underweight may have delayed or arrested pubertal development (Garibaldi, 2007b). Usually, 17% of body fat is needed for menarche and around 22% is needed to initiate and maintain regular ovulation (Jenkins, 2007a). Typically, females enter puberty with 80% lean body weight and 20% body fat, but by the time puberty ends, lean body mass has dropped 5% (Dunn, 2009a).

The average age of menarche has declined an average of 2.3 months from 1988 to 2002, and in 2002 was 12.52 years for non-Hispanic whites, and 12.09 years for Blacks and Mexican Americans (Jenkins, 2007a). Puberty is considered delayed (in the United States) if sexual maturation has not occurred by age 13, if the menarche has not started by age 16, or if menarche does not occur within 5 years of the onset of puberty (Jenkins, 2007a).

For males, puberty and sexual maturity are initially indicated by growth of the penis and testes, spermatogenesis, and seminal emissions. The first ejaculate, however, usually does not contain mature sperm, and occurs about one year after the penis begins its adolescent growth. Testicular enlargement begins between 10 and 13 years of age and is usually complete by age 18 (Katchadourian, 1977; Marshall & Tanner, 1970). Sexual maturity for males varies according to race. Non-Hispanic black males had earlier mean and median ages for sexual maturity stages when compared to Mexican-American and non-Hispanic white boys (Sun, Schubert, Chumlea, Roche, Kulen, Lee, Himes, & Ryan, 2002). The onset of sperm emission ranges from 11.7–15.3 years with a mean age of 13.4 years (Neinstein & Kaufman, 2002). For males, puberty is considered delayed

Reflections from Families

First of all, I think one of the biggest ways that I felt I was growing up and becoming a woman was when I got my first period. I thought this was a huge deal. My friends and I would talk about it and saw it as a sign that we were growing up. I also thought that getting my first bra was such a big deal. I wanted to wear a bra because it meant I was growing up and becoming an adult. There were many other things I looked forward to too, like shaving my legs, wearing nylons and high heels. I have a sister who is 4 years older than me and she was doing all those things. I wanted to be like her. I felt these were signs that I was an adult.

KIDS WANT TO KNOW

Gynecomastia and Nocturnal Emissions in Males

Why does it look like I'm growing breasts? Will it ever go away? How long will it last? Why are my pajamas damp in the morning when I get up? What causes it? Is it normal? Reassure boys that many adolescents experience temporary breast enlargement and nocturnal emissions. These situations are normal and will disappear as they progress through puberty.

KIDS WANT TO KNOW

Why do I seem to be developing more slowly than my friends?

Sexual maturation and physical development vary considerably from adolescent to adolescent. Assure the adolescent that if development of his secondary sexual characteristics has begun, maturity will soon follow.

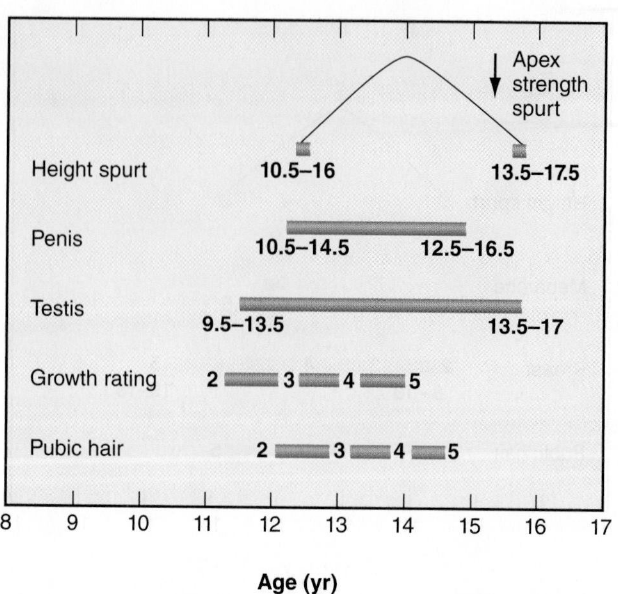

FIGURE 12-6 Approximate timing of developmental changes in males. Numbers appearing in the pubic hair and growth rating indicate the Tanner stage of development. Ranges of ages during which the height spurt and penis and testis development may begin or end are indicated by inclusive numbers below the categories. The PHV is illustrated by the apex of the line indicating the timing when the height spurt occurs. FROM MARSHALL, W. A., & TANNER, J. M. (1970). VARIATIONS IN THE PATTERN OF PUBERTAL CHANGES IN BOYS. *ARCHIVES OF DISEASES IN CHILDREN*, 45, 22. REPRODUCED WITH PERMISSION FROM THE BMJ PUBLISHING GROUP.

if it does not become apparent by 14 years of age (Burchett, Hanna, & Steiner, 2009; Pinyerd & Zipf, 2005). A description of male external genitalia development and pubic hair growth is found in Appendix D. Figure 12-6 illustrates the approximate time developmental changes occur for males according to Tanner staging and age ranges.

During this time, it is not uncommon for one side of the scrotum to grow faster than the other; 60% of males experience transient breast enlargement (gynecomastia), and many after the age of 14 experience nocturnal emissions (loss of seminal fluid during sleep). These situations can be disturbing, and adolescent males may have uncomfortable and embarrassing feelings related to the changes their body undergoes during this period. They are sensitive to suspected deviance and constantly compare their body and appearance to their peers. Teens can also be reassured that as they get older, their body will slim down and fat will be redistributed.

CARDIORESPIRATORY SYSTEM

The heart almost doubles in weight and increases in size by about one half during adolescence (Malina & Bouchard, 1991). Although the heart continues to enlarge until age 17 or 18, the rate of growth is slower in comparison with other body systems and the pumping mechanism is somewhat inefficient. This may be one cause of fatigue and symptoms of inadequate oxygenation some adolescents complain about. Systolic blood pressure accelerates during puberty, before achieving adult values by the end of adolescence. Average blood pressure is 100–120/50–70 mm Hg. The pulse drops from childhood rates to average 60–70 beats per minute. Females have a slightly lower systolic blood pressure and a slightly higher pulse and body temperature than males (Katchadourian, 1977). Red blood cell mass and hemoglobin concentrations increase and the white blood cell count is decreased in both genders during adolescence. Platelet count and sedimentation rates are increased in females, whereas hematocrit levels and blood volume are increased in males (Katchadourian, 1977).

The lungs increase in length and diameter during adolescence, and the respiratory rate averages 16–20 breaths per minute. Males have greater vital capacity, volume, and rate because of their greater shoulder width and chest size. Their lung capacity, however, matures later than in females, probably due to their general later maturation. The slowness of respiratory system growth relative to the growth of other body systems may be another cause of the

CRITICAL THINKING

Physiological Development

How can you help adolescents struggling with the physiological changes their body undergoes when they have not received correct information from their parents or peers or when they are developing slower than their age-mates? How can you help parents explain correct physiological development to their teenagers?

FAMILY TEACHING

Physiological Development

Physiological development can be worrisome and embarrassing to adolescents, especially if they are maturing earlier or later than their peers. You need to discuss the importance of frequent showering, and using deodorant and body powders.

HOME

Teach caregivers and teens that physiological development may vary among individuals, and even though development may be early or late, these are "normal" and temporary situations. However, if females do not begin breast development by age 13 and males do not demonstrate testicular enlargement of 2.5 cm by age 14, referral may be warranted.

Avoid ridiculing and blaming adolescents about their hygiene; they are trying to gain acceptance from peers and control over their changing body at a time in life when self-esteem is fragile.

SCHOOL

Teachers need to be aware of different maturity levels of their students and realize late maturers may not feel comfortable showering in front of early maturing peers. Allow ample opportunity for showering after physical education classes.

COMMUNITY

Coaches need to be aware of physiological development of their athletes, especially if the adolescents are late maturers. This is important because late maturers may not be physiologically mature enough to engage in sports, especially contact sports like football.

inadequate oxygenation and fatigue sometimes experienced by adolescents.

NEUROLOGICAL SYSTEM

One of the most exciting areas of research about adolescents during the past decade has been the work identifying changes in adolescents' brains. Until recently, it was generally believed brain development was largely complete before adolescence, with children's brains reaching 90% of adult weight at 5 years, and 95% at 10 years (Katchadourian, 1977). However, using innovative technology like magnetic resonance imaging (MRI), a whole new understanding of the adolescent brain has occurred. Although fully developed in size, the brain actually continues to change in numerous ways during adolescence. For example, the corpus callosum, the cable of nerve fibers that connect the right and left hemispheres of the brain, continues to thicken and process information more efficiently during adolescence (Giedd, 2008). The prefrontal cortex, which is responsible for such "executive" functions as self-control, judgment, emotional regulation, organization, and planning, undergoes significant change between puberty and young adulthood (Giedd, 2008). The presence of cortical gray matter begins to decrease at about 11 years in girls and 12 years in boys as a result of a "pruning" process that occurs for many of the neuron connections present during childhood. This pruning phase is based on the "use it or lose it" principle, in which unused connections will wither and die (Giedd, 2008). Simultaneous to this pruning of cortical gray matter, there is an increase in the white matter or myelination in the brain. Myelination is a result of the neuronal axons being wrapped in a fatty sheath that speeds up the transmission between neurons as much as 100 times that of unmyelinated neurons (Giedd, 2008). Finally, there is some evidence that during the pruning process in the prefrontal cortex there appear to be higher levels of activity in the amygdala during cognitive processing—which is involved in emotion—compared to that of adults who are more likely to process the same information using the prefrontal cortex. This has been interpreted to mean adolescents may respond with "gut" reactions to emotional stimuli while adults are more likely to respond in a more logical manner.

GASTROINTESTINAL SYSTEM

Rapid maturation of the gastrointestinal system occurs during adolescence, and by the 21st birthday, all 32 teeth have erupted. Gastric acidity and capacity increase (up to 1,500 mL) to accommodate and facilitate digestion of the increased food intake that occurs in response to rapid growth. Adult size, function, and location of the liver is attained, as are adult elimination patterns (Katchadourian, 1977).

A summary of physiological milestones appears in Table 12-1.

TABLE 12-1 Physiological Milestones in Adolescence

STAGE	BOYS	GIRLS	BOTH
Early (11–14)	Testes, scrotum, penis growing Pubic hair curly, abundant Facial hair fine, downy Axillary hair present PHV 9.4 cm/yr Gynecomastia	Breast development occurs Menarche Ovulation Pubic hair curly, thick, triangular distribution PHV 8.3 cm/yr Heavier than males	Appetite increases PWV achieved Immature cardiovascular pumping mechanism Muscle mass increases Gangly, awkward Fine motor coordination increases Permanent teeth present
Middle (15–17)	Adult genitalia Mature sperm production Facial and body hair present Muscle mass and strength greater than females Increased appetite Gynecomastia decreases Voice changes	Skeletal growth ends Sexual maturation achieved Percent of body fat decreases Appetite decreases Height gain 6–10.4 cm/yr	Increased fine motor coordination Physical endurance increases Sweat glands function Increased capacity of cardiovascular system Acne
Late (18–21)	Skeletal growth ends		Cardiovascular, respiratory, gastrointestinal, hematopoietic, and sexual maturity achieved Stable appetite Motor activity increases Endurance increases Dentition complete

SELF UNDERSTANDING

Two major tasks for adolescents are figuring out who they are and what their unique place is in the world. In reality, these two characteristics cannot be separated; adolescents, like all of us, cannot understand who they are without understanding how they fit into their home, community, or broader society. Adolescents' motivation to make sense of their lives has been explained in different ways by different theorists. Some have argued the need to define oneself is a function of heredity, others contend it is a function of the hormonal changes that emerge during adolescence, while others believe it is a response to changes in adolescents' interactions with those in their social contexts. For example, G. Stanley Hall (Arnett, 1999) argued the struggles of adolescents as they approached adulthood reflect the challenges faced by our prehistoric ancestors as they advanced toward a civilized state. In contrast, Freud, in his psychosexual theory of development, contended it was psychological struggles resulting from physiological changes (i.e., blaming teens' behavior on their raging hormones) that brought about a need to define oneself. By contrast, Erik Erikson's theory of identity development (1968) provides one of the most enduring explanations regarding the establishment of selfhood. His psychosocial theory of development provided an explanation of identity formation that focused on adolescents' changing interactions with those in their most immediate social contexts, particularly their interactions with family, peers, and school. In the sections that follow we will examine in greater detail a few of the explanations for adolescents' eventual establishment of an adult sense of self-understanding.

PSYCHOSEXUAL DEVELOPMENT

The basic assertion of Freud's psychosexual theory (Cloninger, 2008, also see Chapter 6) is that we are motivated by two competing forces; one compels us to appease our inherent biological drives while the other fosters the desire to live in a social community. Freud contended that virtually all psychological development is an adaptive response to the upsurge in our physiologically based "drives" and our attempts to satisfy these drives while coexisting with others. While these instinctive drives are motivated by several biologic needs (hunger, fatigue, etc.), the sexual instinct, or id, is the most important in establishing individuals' psychological makeup or personality. For Freud, the physical changes of puberty reawaken the sexual and aggressive energies felt toward parents during early childhood, but repressed during latency or late childhood. To effectively cope, adolescents need to redirect these newly reemerging energies from parental relationships to nonfamilial relationships (friendships, love interests) and career endeavors. For this to occur, a separation or detachment from parents is necessary, sometimes resulting in conflict between adolescents and their parents. As adolescents struggle with the inner tension brought on by pubertal change, Freud believed anxiety, heightened distress over how to act out their inner conflict, and a likely demonstration of psychologically regressive or immature behavior occurred (Cloninger, 2008).

Thus, Freud argued, many psychological issues adolescents face are attributable to physiological changes. Most researchers now contend the implications of these physiological changes are much more complex than Freud or the psychosexual perspective originally indicated and, in fact, are more a result of how individual adolescents and others around them respond to the adolescents' physiological changes than of the changes themselves.

BODY IMAGE

A primary example of interaction between the psychological and physiological attributes of adolescents is evident in their evolving sense of body image or mental conception of their physical appearance. **Body image** encompasses positive or negative feelings, and the self-perception of physical attractiveness. Implicit in the definition is the assumption that one's body image varies with maturation, and changes across time, situations, and experiences one has with others (Figure 12-7). Constant changes in appearance—including increases in weight and height, appearance of body hair, oversized hands and feet, developing sex organs, and facial blemishes—present the adolescent with new challenges, both real and imagined, that affect his or her body image.

This is particularly significant during adolescence because the adjustment required by rapid physiological changes affect self-esteem; few adolescents are satisfied with their physical appearance (Pinyerd & Zipf, 2005). Adolescent females tend to be more dissatisfied with their appearance and more likely to be concerned about particular parts of their bodies than their male counterparts (Rosenblum & Lewis, 1999). Often, they perceive themselves as weighing more than they actually do. In fact, in a 2009 survey of American high school students, almost 28% of students nationwide believed they were overweight, and 44.4% reported they were trying to lose weight. Of these findings,

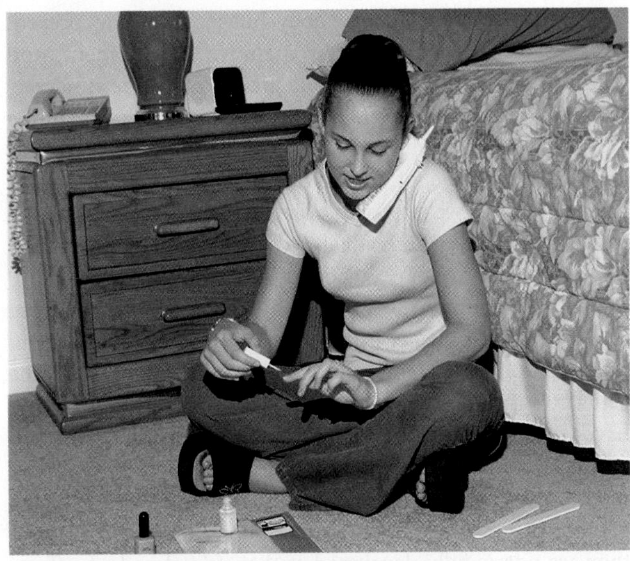

FIGURE 12-7 As adolescents begin to take on adult features during puberty, their interests and activities begin to change.
DELMAR CENGAGE LEARNING.

female students were 50% more likely than male students to report being overweight (33.1% of the female students reported being overweight compared to 22.7% of the male students) and almost twice as likely to report trying to lose weight (59.3% of the female students reported trying to lose weight compared to 30.5% of the male students) (Eaton, Kann, Kinchen, Shanklin et al., 2010). This distortion of body image is not only a potentially significant emotional problem for adolescents, but also may motivate the adolescent female to engage in potentially dangerous and life-threatening weight-reducing behaviors such as binge eating and purging vigorous aerobic exercise, or special diets (Weinshenker, 2002). In fact, 5.1% of high school students report trying to lose weight by taking diet pills (6.3% of the female students compared to 3.8% of the male students), and 4% of high school students had vomited or taken laxatives to lose or avoid gaining weight (5.4% of the female students compared to 2.1% of the male students) (Eaton et al., 2010).

While developing a sense of body image, most adolescents look to the cultural ideal valued by their society. In Western culture, this traditionally has been the shapely, thin woman and the muscular, tall man. However, few adolescents, or any individual for that matter, can successfully measure up to these standards (McCabe & Ricciardelli, 2005). More than vanity, the adolescent's preoccupation with appearance is recognition of the role physical attractiveness plays in gaining the attention and admiration of the opposite sex. The fact physique is valued by both genders is understandable. There is a strong relationship between how adolescents feel about themselves and how they feel about their bodies. Looking "awful" or believing others view them as looking "awful" is the same as being "awful." These feelings may be reinforced by the fact that physically unattractive teens tend to have fewer friends than attractive teens (Sprinthall & Collins, 1995).

Many factors influence body image, including present and past experiences, level of cognitive development, and identity formation. Other factors are one's degree of attractiveness, size and physique appropriate to gender (including weight and body type), name or nickname, cultural ideals and values, degree of identification with same-sex parent, peer and sibling relationships, level of aspiration, and ability to reach societal or individual ideals as portrayed in the media (Wiseman, Sunday, & Becker, 2005). The rate and timing of maturation can also be an important factor in an adolescent's self-image. In fact, pubertal timing has a greater influence on behavioral and emotional problems than the actual transition to puberty itself. The young people who have the most difficult time adjusting to their physical development and body image are those whose body is on a different schedule from their peers. For example, late maturing adolescents may feel a sense of failure about their body if they are not as fully developed as their friends, which affects self-esteem and causes them to feel uncomfortable and insecure. Since, on average, early maturing males and females are shorter than their later maturing counterparts, they too may have difficulties with body image as their later maturing peers catch up and overtake them in height.

Social experiences are different for early and late maturing males and females. For boys, early maturation is associated with more favorable social status, greater popularity, and greater self perceptions of positive affect, attention, feeling strong, and being in love. These reported experiences are likely due to early maturing boys, earlier increased muscle mass and appearance of secondary sexual characteristics. Since for boys physical ability is most valued, it appears that those who develop early have the edge in almost all realms; at least initially. One cautionary note, although early maturation is largely advantageous for males, some studies have suggested that they may become involved sooner in delinquency and alcohol use and abuse.

In contrast, early pubertal development among adolescent girls is not nearly so positive. Although some findings suggest early maturation for girls is associated with high social status and prestige in the peer group, most findings indicate early maturation is associated with greater vulnerability to social pressures leading to problems in social adjustment, which often persist into adulthood (Graber, Brooks-Gunn, & Warren, 2006). Early maturing females may be socially disadvantaged because they are out of step with their peer group. They may become lonely and experience pressure to become involved in sexual relationships beyond the level of their maturity and coping ability. This can result in damaged self-esteem. Often, those who are taller and more developed early on relative to their classmates discover there are few peers who share common interests or problems. As a result, they often attract the attention of older boys, resulting in their heightened risk for engaging in delinquent behavior and greater vulnerability to eating disorders, depression, and deviant peer pressures as compared with their late maturing or on-time peers (Graber et al., 2006).

REFLECTIVE THINKING

Your Own Adolescence

Were you an early or late maturer? How did puberty affect you as a young adolescent? Has puberty had any long-term effects on you? What advice would you give an adolescent about the rate and timing of maturation?

While early maturation appears to be difficult for females, late maturation appears to be most problematic for males, but to a lesser degree. Later maturing males tend to be less relaxed, poised, and popular with peers; and feel more restless, talkative, socially inadequate, and inferior. As adults they tend to hold fewer leadership positions in their jobs or organizations, and are less responsible, dominant, and controlling.

PSYCHOSOCIAL DEVELOPMENT

PSYCHOSOCIAL IDENTITY

According to Erikson (1968), the major task of adolescence is establishing a personal sense of **identity**. Adolescents define themselves according to several distinct physiological,

NURSING TIP

Concerns about Body Image

You need to be aware of the importance physical appearance has to adolescents, and offer reassurance and encouragement to late maturing adolescents that they will catch up with their counterparts. Suggestions for becoming involved in activities they may enjoy or do well in can help maintain self-esteem and perhaps make up for slower physiologic development or unhappiness with body type, height, or weight. Early maturing adolescents can be directed to activities where they will succeed and encouraged to be understanding of their later maturing peers. Parents need to understand the importance of body image to adolescents and refrain from commenting negatively about weight and general appearance. If comments are necessary, they should be couched with tact, understanding, and nurturance.

psychological, and social events and experiences, including: (1) adolescents' own pubertal development and the biological changes of their agemates; (2) their shift to abstract reasoning, the resulting changes in behavior, and the moral explanations that come to justify that behavior; (3) the individual (parents, peers, teachers, folk heroes) and group ("my gang," "our generation," other blacks, other Americans) identifications they established during childhood; (4) the increasing level of responsibility they assume at home, at school, and in the workplace; (5) the need to begin thinking about their careers; and, to a lesser extent, (6) the need to begin considering their religious beliefs and political ideology. Based on these events, adolescents establish a unique sense of individual identity.

Marcia (1980) explains that *identity* is adolescents' definition of who they are based on their cumulative understanding of their inherent motivations, personal belief systems, and previous experiences. When adolescents have a strong sense of identity, their actions will be more self-determined and they will have a more secure sense of who they are, and how they are similar to, and different from, those around them (Figure 12-8).

Adolescents' sense of identity is based on three primary factors: (1) individual identifications (parents, peers, teachers, folk heroes) as well as group ones ("my group of friends," "our generation," other blacks, other Americans) established during childhood; (2) their ability to master each developmental task (i.e., trust versus mistrust, autonomy versus shame and doubt) presented to them by society; and (3) the establishment of their own ideology, based on the social, political, and religious attitudes and values they adopt.

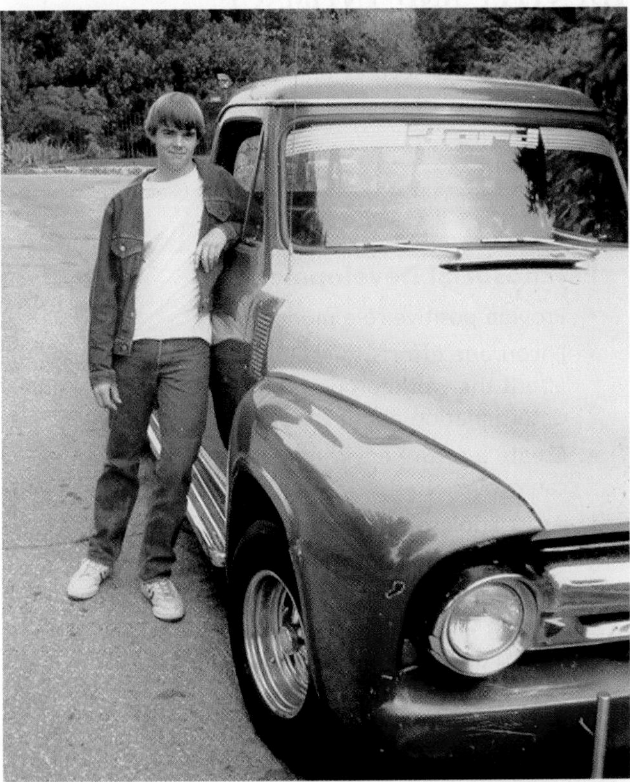

FIGURE 12-8 There are many aspects of adolescents' lives that contribute to their sense of identity, including relationships, talents, beliefs, and material possessions.

DELMAR CENGAGE LEARNING.

IDENTITY STATUSES

Not all individuals arrive at a definitive answer about who they are during adolescence. Many will spend much of their lives either avoiding or failing to see a need for establishing a sense of identity. Although many young people won't establish their identity until young adulthood, the process generally begins during adolescence.

Marcia (1980) recognized there are different paths young people take in establishing a sense of identity, and identified two dimensions critical to the identity process: exploration and commitment. Based on Erikson's work, Marcia recognized adolescents, en route to establishing a personal identity, needed to experience a period of active questioning which should result in a personal commitment to a set of beliefs and corresponding actions that define for themselves who they are. Using different combinations of the exploration and commitment dimensions, Marcia defined four different identity statuses: identity achievement, foreclosure, identity diffusion, and moratorium. While the eventual goal is identity achievement, young people will not necessarily pass through each of the other three statuses en route to achieving an identity. **Identity achievement** indicates individuals have experienced a process of exploration and established a relatively firm set of commitments. These individuals are generally well-adjusted, stable, and mature. **Foreclosed** individuals demonstrate a strong sense of commitment, but have not explored the principles upon which their commitments are based. These individuals may appear to have very strong belief systems, but on closer inspection have difficulty explaining their commitments, typically having "borrowed" or been given their ideologies or career aspirations by their parents or other authority figures. **Identity diffusion** refers to individuals who have not experienced any active exploration nor made a commitment to any ideological or occupational direction. These individuals are less mature and are more likely to follow popular fads or trends. Finally, **moratorium** status indicates individuals are currently exploring or questioning different occupational or ideological choices, but have yet to establish a firm set of commitments.

Psychosocial moratorium, Erikson's term referring to the period of exploration many young people engage in as they attempt to determine their life's course, is particularly evident among young people who attend college, an experience that allows them time to further explore career options before making a final decision. Adolescents entering the workforce directly after high school are more likely to be identity achieved when compared to their college-bound peers.

An important determinant of adolescents' identity status appears to be the parenting to which they are exposed. Of particular importance is the extent to which parents promote a strong sense of connectedness among family members while providing their adolescents appropriate opportunities for developing a sense of individuality. Individuality includes the ability to present one's own point of view and verbally define who one is. Identity achieved adolescents are more likely to come from homes that promote a strong sense of connectedness and individuality (Grotevant & Cooper, 1998). In contrast, adolescents whose homes were high in connectedness, but weak in individuality, are more likely to promote a foreclosed identity style, while homes that were weak in connectedness, regardless of individuality, are likely to promote a diffused identity status.

Cognitive Reasoning and Personal Identity

An important part of adolescents' ability to develop a personal identity is their capacity to think in more complex and abstract ways, allowing them to consider the more psychological characteristics that define them. For example, when asked to describe themselves, early adolescents are likely to identify themselves using physical attributes, preferred activities, and the roles that define them, such as being a boy or girl, a football player, a dancer, a student, or someone who enjoys working on computers. The same question to older adolescents is likely to evoke descriptions of the more abstract characteristics, beliefs, and ideologies that make up their personalities, such as being a happy person, a religious person, or a caring person.

As adolescents initially begin to think in increasingly complex ways, they begin to demonstrate increased levels of differentiation in how they define themselves (Harter, 2001). For example, they may begin to recognize that they behave one way when at school, another way with their families, and still another way when they are with their best friends. The contradictions in these situationally defined self-definitions can initially go unnoticed by young people, but as they pass through middle adolescence, they are likely to begin recognizing the contradictions in their self-definitions that arise from their different ways of responding in different settings. During this stage adolescents question which of their situational responses define their true self ("If I behave so differently in different settings, in which setting am I really me?"). Eventually, adolescents come to recognize there is a core sense of who they are that transcends or incorporates the diverse self-definitions that now represent them (Harter, 2001).

Gender Identity

Gender identity refers to the way we think about ourselves as either male or female, and is a culmination of biological makeup, personal and social expectations, and recommendations about how males and females should think and behave. From the moment children are born, the world will respond to them differently depending on whether they are male or female. As young children first come to understand the differences between boys and girls they are likely to demonstrate very strong preferences toward gender-appropriate behavior. During late childhood, children continue to recognize the need to engage in gender-appropriate behavior, but become more accepting of themselves and others engaging in behaviors normally identified with the opposite sex. However, as young people approach adolescence there is a reorientation regarding what is considered acceptable behavior for those of each gender. Adolescents are much more traditional in their gender attitudes and behavior compared to older children or adults. This shift during adolescence is referred to as the gender intensification hypothesis (Hill & Lynch, 1983; Lobel, Nov-Krispin, Schiller, Lobel, & Feldman, 2004). The greater attitudinal and behavioral differences that emerge between early adolescent boys and girls are likely due to the adolescents' and others' (i.e., caregivers, teachers, peers) responses to the pubertal changes experienced by the adolescents that cause them to look increasingly different as they take on adult male and female physiological characteristics. Erikson (1968) considered gender to be an important part of establishing young people's individual identity. In fact, one explanation for adolescents' more intolerant attitudes about certain cross-sex behaviors is that this more rigid perspective may help adolescents as they attempt to make sense of who they are.

Identity and Intimacy

Following Erikson's stage of identity formation, Erikson's (1968) sixth stage focuses on the task of intimacy versus isolation. During this stage individuals face the task of

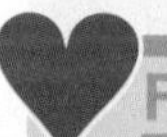

FAMILY**TEACHING**

Psychosocial Development

- Provide positive role models.
- Encourage efforts to establish a sense of hope about the world around them and a purpose and determination about themselves.
- Create a secure environment where adolescents can grow.
- Assist adolescents in finding and developing unique strengths.
- Allow adolescents to participate in family decision making while providing guidance and structure regarding the decisions they make about themselves.
- Create a learning and social environment where young people are encouraged to think and solve problems for themselves.
- Provide opportunities to begin exploring various career options.

Reflections from Families

I felt a great responsibility to not openly trouble my parents or cause them to worry. I felt that I needed to prove to them and to everyone else that they were still good parents despite my brother's problems. Inwardly there was a constant struggle going on between who I thought people wanted me to be and who I really was. I constantly thought about it—struggling between my feelings of responsibility and the pressure to just once quit being me and be the irresponsible, bad child. It became vital to me that I do things for the right reason. Was I doing it because it was right or because my parents wanted me to? Was I pushing myself to succeed because that was what I wanted or because that would help my parents believe that they hadn't failed?

forming intimate relationships with others. Erikson contends once young people have achieved a sense of who they are, they are better able to commit themselves intimately to another person (Figure 12-9). Marcia (1980) states the paradox of intimacy is that "it is a strength that can be acquired only through vulnerability; and vulnerability is possible only with the internal assurance of a firm identity" (p. 160). According to Erikson (1968), the youth who is not sure of his identity "shies away from interpersonal intimacy or throws himself into acts of intimacy which are 'promiscuous'" (p. 135). Such an individual may be involved in intimate relationships, but is likely to settle for highly stereotyped interpersonal relations resulting in a lack of fulfillment and "a deep sense of isolation." It is interesting that while we often think of elderly people as the loneliest individuals, adolescents and young adults may also feel a great sense of loneliness or isolation.

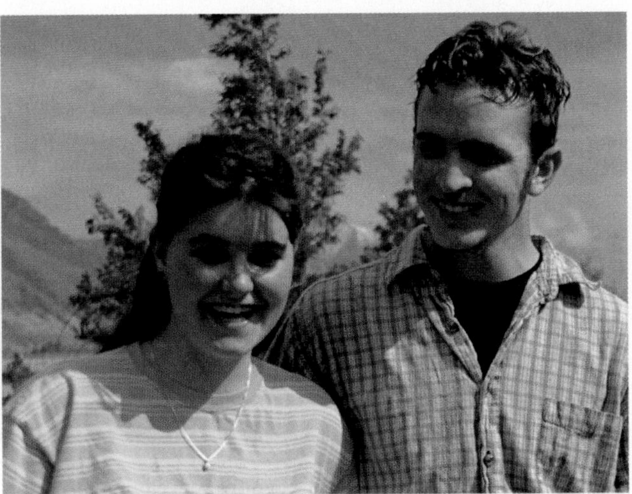

FIGURE 12-9 Learning about intimacy becomes a significant part of many late adolescents' lives. DELMAR CENGAGE LEARNING.

COGNITIVE DEVELOPMENT

Although physiological changes associated with puberty are the most apparent indicators of development, equally important to young people's movement toward adulthood are the cognitive changes that occur during this time. As young people's thought processes become more sophisticated, their ability to think about themselves and the world around them changes radically. Piaget, Vygotsky, Selman, and Elkind describe the cognitive changes occurring during adolescence from a variety of perspectives. Most research about the changes in young people's thought processes is the result of Jean Piaget's (1972) theoretical ideas (see Chapter 6). During adolescence (Piaget's stage of formal operations), the most distinct feature of young people's thinking is that they can now consider what is possible rather than just what is real. Thinking is no longer constrained by the concrete, physical world of their existence; rather, they are now capable of considering abstract possibilities. No longer are potential solutions based only on previous experiences; young people are able to consider all possible solutions to a problem, both real and abstract, and they can assess options and determine the best solution. Young people can now consider their own thoughts as real objects which can be studied and analyzed—they are now able to think about their own thoughts in a way not previously possible.

One outcome of adolescents' ability to consider abstract possibilities is that they begin to recognize the distinction between how things are and how things could be (the difference between the "real" and the "ideal"). During earlier stages of development, the "real" and the "ideal" are largely the same. However, as adolescents' thinking ability moves beyond the limitations of reality, they begin to conceive of the possible. Out of this ability comes a new sense of idealism and a new set of standards by which they begin evaluating themselves and the world around them. Adolescents' new ability to critically assess their world is often seen in their more discordant interactions with their parents, and in the emergence of their social, political, and religious identities.

Another significant cognitive change is language development. Compared to children, adolescents are generally more sophisticated in their ability to understand words and their related abstract concepts (Figure 12-10). Because of this increased sophistication, adolescents develop a new understanding and appreciation of words and their meanings, including the use of metaphors and satire. Regarding metaphors, children can generally identify the obvious story that exists in a book or movie, but it is often not until adolescence that they begin to understand the more abstract metaphorical meaning. During adolescence, young people also begin to find great joy in the double meaning of puns, satire, and parodies. An example of this new-found appreciation can be seen in adolescents' increased enjoyment of such movies as *Shrek,* and Disney's *Aladdin* and *Hercules,* which poke fun at all aspects of our culture. Whereas a child is only likely to understand the basic meaning of the dialogue in these movies, an adolescent can now enjoy the satire simultaneously communicated by the same dialogue. In addition, adolescents can now appreciate and engage in the use of irony, where they begin to understand that subtle changes in voice inflections can change words or statements to represent something opposite of the literal meaning.

The shift to formal operational thought occurs gradually and varies individually. Formal operational thought consists of two sub-periods: early and late. When adolescents first acquire the abilities associated with formal operational thought, their new-found skill to think in hypothetical ways produces unconstrained thoughts with unlimited possibilities. This early stage of thinking results in an inordinate attempt to fit newly available abstract information into their existing immature understanding of how the world works, resulting in a subjective and idealist perception of the world (Lapsley, 1990), which can be observed in the almost zealous, simplistic way they frequently embrace political or social causes. As adolescents become more cognitively mature, they are better able to adjust their thinking strategies to fit new information now available to them. Finally, there is a question related to whether a link exists between physiological maturation and cognitive development; however, no substantial association between these two areas of growth has been found (Keating, 2009). As mentioned in the neurological systems portion of this chapter, there are many recent advances in our understanding of brain development that may provide a better understanding of how cognitive abilities and the other changes occurring during adolescence may be linked (Giedd, 2008). What is being discovered would indicate that no simple explanation of cognitive development will adequately explain the changes evident in adolescents' thinking; rather, a model based on an interdependence of multiple mechanisms will be required (Keating, 2009).

COGNITIVE SOCIALIZATION

Lev Vygotsky, a Soviet cognitive theorist who was a contemporary of—but whose work was not influenced by—Piaget, considered the differences in adolescents' cognitive abilities to be more a function of identifiable features of their cognitive environment (Wertsch & Tulviste, 1999), and emphasized the way society promotes cognitive growth (Figure 12-11). One of Vygotsky's most important concepts is the **zone of proximal development (ZPD)**, which consists of tasks too difficult for individuals to master alone, but which can be

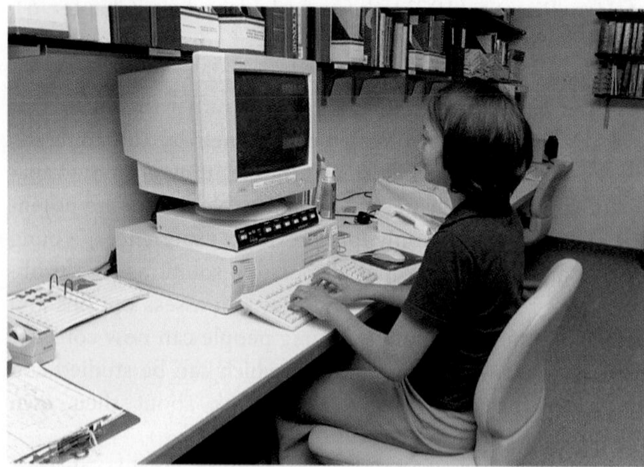

FIGURE 12-10 As adolescents' ability to think abstractly begins to emerge, their understanding and use of language becomes more sophisticated. DELMAR CENGAGE LEARNING.

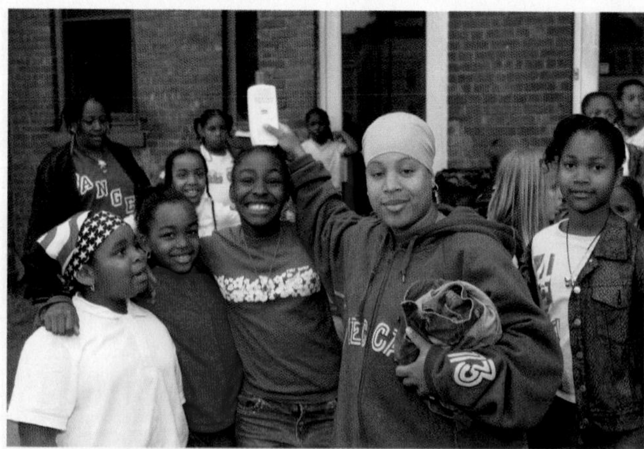

FIGURE 12-11 One aspect of cognitive development important to adolescents' acceptance among peers is their ability to recognize and correctly interpret the thoughts and emotions of those around them. DELMAR CENGAGE LEARNING.

mastered with the guidance and assistance of adults or more skilled peers (Santrock, 2010). The lower limit of this "zone" is the level of problem solving reached by the adolescent working independently; the upper limit is the level of additional understanding the adolescent can achieve with assistance. Above the upper limit of this "zone" an adolescent is unlikely to be able to master a skill or understand a concept even with the assistance of an experienced other. According to Vygotsky, the greatest growth occurs when adolescents are stretched to perform at the upper limit of their ZPD. For Vygotsky, cognitive development is a function of the social relationships adolescents experience and the extent to which they are challenged within these relationships to think at a level beyond their independent capability. For example, most seventh-grade students would be overwhelmed if they were placed in a college-level calculus course. However, these same students are capable of understanding far more complex ideas (e.g., math operations) if they are coached by an adult or peer who is sensitive to their potential upper limit of understanding and can push them to think at that higher level. According to Vygotsky's theory, learning can most effectively occur when the person giving guidance initially provides much support and structure, but correspondingly decreases the support as the learned concepts or skills are mastered. This process is often likened to the use of scaffolding to support a building that is being constructed; as the building becomes able to support itself, the scaffolding is progressively removed. Once introduced to new skills, young people can increasingly internalize and make use of them on their own (Kozulin, 1990).

ADOLESCENT EGOCENTRISM

Formal operational thought enables adolescents to think about their own thoughts, and also permits them to realize that other people's thoughts are separate and distinct from their own. According to Elkind (1967), this capacity to consider other people's thoughts is the crux of adolescent **egocentrism**, when one is unable to appropriately differentiate between oneself and the objects of one's attention. Although some egocentrism is present at each developmental stage, it is most commonly associated with adolescents' thinking. With the onset of formal operational thought, adolescents are now able to consider the thoughts of others. However, their cognitive immaturity presents difficulties in differentiating their own thoughts and others' thoughts. Although adolescents realize others' thoughts are not the same as their own, they have the mistaken notion that others know what they are thinking, and assume others are as obsessed with the adolescents' behavior and appearance as they are themselves, resulting in an even greater sense of self-consciousness (Figure 12-12).

As a function of this egocentrism, Elkind identified two types of social thinking particularly evident during early adolescence—imaginary audience and personal fable. **Imaginary audience** refers to the adolescents' beliefs of always being on stage. Because adolescents often impose their own thoughts and concerns in their attempts to understand what others are thinking, they are likely to believe others are as concerned about their appearance and behavior as they are. For example, numerous adolescents have experienced dreading going to school on a particular day because they

Reflections from Families

I can remember how my thinking changed. I was able to solve problems more easily. I felt like all of a sudden, I had problem-solving skills. I was not only able to work out some of my own problems, but I was able to help out my peers with their problems. I also remember spending a lot of time thinking about things. It always seemed as if there was something to think about or something to wonder about. I even sometimes would ask myself why I was thinking about what I was thinking. I found myself looking at other people's perspectives. I also thought about hypothetical situations, wondering what I'd do and planning what to do ahead of time before those situations could come up. I remember comparing myself to others, wanting to acquire others' ideal characteristics. I remember asking myself really thought-provoking questions and pondering deep subjects such as "What am I? Why am I here? Who do I want to become? What is important in life?"

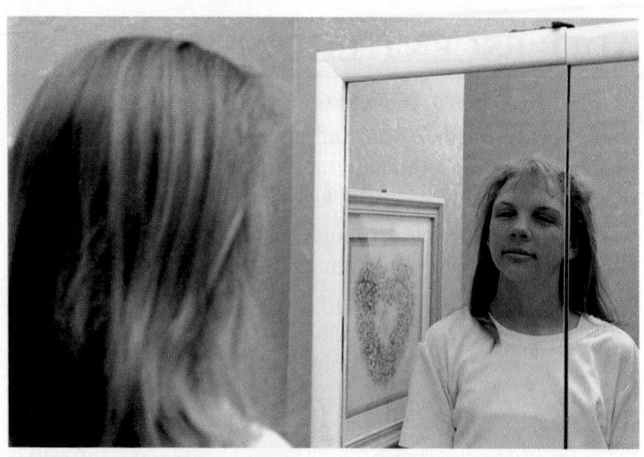

FIGURE 12-12 **Appearance is important for adolescents, and illustrates their egocentrism.** DELMAR CENGAGE LEARNING.

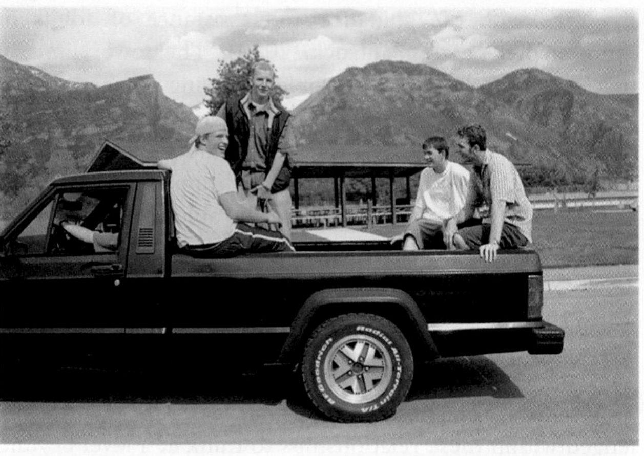

FIGURE 12-13 **The sense of immortality that accompanies adolescents' formation of a personal fable is evidenced by their increased likelihood of engaging in risky behavior.** DELMAR CENGAGE LEARNING.

FAMILY**TEACHING**

Cognitive Development

- Adolescents are likely to begin questioning many things previously learned and are capable of reasoning problems out for themselves.
- Adolescents will often begin reexamining many parental rules, values, and explanations.
- Adolescents need opportunities to explore the reasons for different religious and political values, attitudes about sexuality and social responsibility, or explanations about injustices they see.
- Adolescents need clear explanations of values and the reasoning behind them.
- Adolescents need others to demonstrate greater willingness to listen to and understand adolescents' evolving opinions.

were sure everyone else at school would be as conscious as they are of the unusually large pimple on their nose. These experiences often result in adolescents responding to the anticipated behaviors of an imaginary audience, rather than the actual behaviors of those around them (Elkind, 1985).

Connected to the adolescents' imaginary audience is their belief in what Elkind calls their own **personal fable**, in which adolescents have an exaggerated notion of their own uniqueness. Because adolescents frequently believe they are important to so many people (i.e., the imaginary audience), they regard themselves, and particularly their feelings, as special and unique. This personal uniqueness is expressed in two ways—an extreme sense of isolation, believing no one has ever had to endure the feelings or difficult situations they are experiencing (thus the phrase, "You just don't understand"), or the belief that they are immortal and thus immune to the bad things that happen to others, including death (Figure 12-13). This sense of immortality is frequently evidenced in adolescents' behaviors relating to driving, substance abuse, and sexuality.

SOCIAL PERSPECTIVE TAKING

Another important aspect of adolescents' cognitive development is their broadening ability to assume another person's perspective. Based on Piaget's work and the symbolic interaction theory of George Herbert Mead, Selman (1980) proposed that an individual's interactions are in large part due to their **social perspective taking ability**. For Selman, an adolescent interacts or communicates with others according to the social-cognitive understanding they have about who they are in relation to those around them. Maturation and social experience changes this over time. Selman argues that between early and late childhood the distinction between self and others moves from one that is behaviorally based to one that is capable of distinguishing between the actions and motives of others or the reasoning behind others' behavior. Young children have difficulty understanding that others' intentions are not always consistent with their resulting behavior; for example, a caregiver's attempt to remove a sliver from the child's hand is meant to be helpful, but it hurts. During adolescence, cognitive reasoning continues to become more complex, where simultaneous, mutual (third-person) perspective taking becomes possible. This allows young people to think not about what is best for each individual in an interaction, but rather what would be best for the relationship between them. Early adolescents' initial attempts to focus on the relationship between self and others is particularly evident in their best friendships, where there is a high expectation regarding uniformity in dress, interests, and activities, and individual differences are considered threats to friendship. According to Selman, as this mutual perspective taking ability matures, young people come to recognize that relationship needs can be fulfilled through more than one or two relationships, and individual differences can be an asset rather than a threat.

MORAL DEVELOPMENT

An important aspect of young people's cognitive maturation is their ever-increasing ability to consider the complexity of their own and others' moral and ethical reasoning. As a result of their gradual movement away from the solitary influence of the home and toward the diverse influence of society and the adult world, and because of their increasing need for self-definition, the concern for moral values and standards is likely to never be more relevant than during adolescence. Several theorists have attempted to explain adolescents' increased interest in and ability to establish moral reasoning during adolescence.

From a psychoanalytic perspective, moral development arises out of the individual's fear of rejection as a result of his or her inability to control unconscious impulses. Thus, young people adopt as their own the rules and prohibitions defined by society generally, and their parents specifically. Freud referred to this internal set of rules or moral values as the superego.

From a social learning perspective, moral development is a result of early experiences and the reinforcement children and adolescents receive for their different behaviors. In addition, parental discipline, and more specifically the discipline techniques applied, is also crucial in determining whether a response to a moral situation will be internalized. For example, children whose parents give explanations or reasons for desired behavioral changes, rather than demanding change based on their authority, are much more likely to internalize the reasoning behind the behavior rather than merely conforming temporarily to the desired changes in behavior.

While these perspectives are insightful, the major contributor to our current thinking regarding moral development is Kohlberg (1976). His theory is based largely on the work of Piaget. Kohlberg's conventional level of moral reasoning, which emerges during adolescence and persists as the predominate stage of moral functioning throughout adulthood, focuses on the acceptance by individuals of those norms and rules defined either by their close social network or by the more formal governmental systems of their culture and society (i.e., local, state, or federal laws). This level of moral thinking is occupied by two stages or primary orientations, stage 3, or the relationship-maintenance stage of decision making; and stage 4, or the authority-maintaining stage of decision making, where upholding the laws and order of society becomes central. Some researchers have argued that there is a difference in moral reasoning based on gender—Gilligan argued that adolescent males are more likely to reflect the authority-maintaining-based reasoning of the fourth stage of moral thinking, whereas female adolescents are more likely to reflect the relationship-based reasoning of the third stage (Gilligan, 1982; Gilligan, Lyons, & Hanmer, 1990)—however, others have failed to find similar gender differences in moral reasoning (Walker, 1989). The ability to consider the moral implications of their own and others' thoughts and actions is crucial to adolescents' developing a personal belief system, which largely defines their social, political, and religious identities.

REFLECTIVE THINKING

Personal Fable

Do you remember any friends you had as a teenager who clearly demonstrated a personal fable, thinking they could engage in risky behavior (e.g., drinking and driving, unprotected sexual intercourse, daredevil stunts) without any concern that the existing dangers might happen to them? Did you ever experience a personal fable, where you thought your circumstances were particularly unique or you were immune from the typical dangers of a particular behavior? What was it?

RELIGIOSITY

For many adolescents, an important part of their moral development is the formation of their own religious beliefs and personal patterns of religiosity. Religion appears to have positive implications for adolescents with greater religiosity demonstrating an inverse association with risk-taking behavior and a positive one with greater social competency. However, to assess the significance of religiosity for adolescents, it is necessary to differentiate between the different types of religious observance adolescents are likely to engage in.

Too often religiosity is defined solely by attendance at organized activities. While this is important, outward activity may have little to do with adolescents' inner commitments to their religious beliefs. As a result, many researchers now consider both the "public" and "private" levels of adolescents' religious observance (Nonnemaker, McNeely, & Blum, 2003). Public observance is generally represented by participation in different religious activities. In contrast to the high number who reported a belief in a god, only 48% of adolescents surveyed in the Gallup poll reported attending church in the last seven days, with lower percentage scores for older adolescents. To understand the importance of private religious observance, such activities as personal prayer, meditation, and reading of sacred scripture are generally examined. In these areas of worship, teens' commitment appears to vary greatly.

Adolescents' religious involvement is both predicted by their social context and predictive of how much they contribute to their social context. Adolescents' church attendance continues to primarily be influenced by their parents, but is also predicted by the attendance patterns of their friends and, to a lesser extent, schoolmates (Regnerus, Smith, & Smith, 2004).

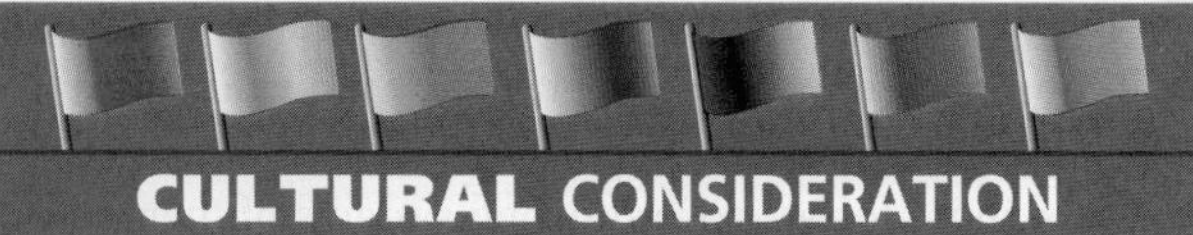

CULTURAL CONSIDERATION

Differences in Constructs about Death

People who have no religious beliefs and those who practice folk religions (Taoist, Buddhist) tend to have more emotional states surrounding death than do those of other religious beliefs, including Western religions. Various religious groups also express grief differently. For example, Buddhist or Taoist ceremonies show more expressions of sadness relative to death and expect mourners to express sorrow openly and demonstrate reluctance at having a family member die. Their belief in the importance of suffering accompanying transmigration or inferno after death is also painful. Those with no religious beliefs think the world after death is strange and abstract. They have no idea what to expect and display a low understanding of others' beliefs about death.

Reference: Yang, S. C., & Chen, S. (2006). Content analysis of free-response narratives to personal meanings of death among Chinese children and adolescents. *Death Studies*, *30*, 217–241.

ADOLESCENTS IN CONTEXT

FAMILIES

The family is the first and, in general, the most important socializing agent in one's life. Successful socialization is the process by which children acquire the beliefs, values, and behavior deemed significant by older members of their society (Shaffer, 2009), and is, to a large degree, a function of the parenting and other familial interactions experienced while growing up. But do familial experiences change as young people pass through the adolescent period? In particular, do caregiver–child relationships differ as youths move through the second decade of life?

Several changes are likely to have an impact on the type of interactions and quality of relationships adolescents and their caregivers have with one another. First, adolescents experience physiological changes associated with puberty that cause both they and their caregivers to think and respond differently to one another; caregivers begin to expect adolescents to act more like adults. And while they may not always act more mature, adolescents begin to believe they should be treated more like adults. These changes in adolescents' interpersonal interactions with caregivers may be linked to the onset of puberty and the hormonal changes that occur during this period, resulting in greater conflict particularly when adolescents experience precocious, or early, pubertal development.

The cognitive shift to formal operational thinking has an impact on young people's relationships with caregivers as well. Abstract thinking allows adolescents to better distinguish their real and ideal worlds, resulting in caregivers' observed behavior no longer defining adolescents' ideal standard, which is now measured according to what ideal caregivers should be like. In addition, as adolescents are better able to articulate their own concerns when caregivers make requests they disagree with, they are less likely to comply. If caregivers are not sensitive to adolescents' desires to test their newly found cognitive skills, adolescents are likely to be incorrectly perceived as defiant.

In seeking their own identity, adolescents begin to explore the attitudes and values they have been taught in order to establish what best defines who they are. This exploration process often increases the level of tension between adolescents and parents, particularly when this exploration causes parents to reexamine their own rationale for who they are and what they are doing in their lives. This process may be threatening to parents as they confront their own mortality and the notion they are approaching a new stage in their own lives.

Parent Socialization

Parents' significance to children and adolescents has been identified to primarily be a function of their behavior within two domains: responsiveness and demandingness (Maccoby & Martin, 1983). **Parental responsiveness** refers to the degree to which parents are responsive to their children's needs in an accepting, supportive manner. **Parental demandingness** is the extent to which parents expect and demand mature, responsible behavior from their children (Steinberg, 2008). The optimal situation for positive adolescent outcomes is when parents use a high amount of both responsiveness and demandingness. Adolescents are likely to face various struggles when either one, or both, of these elements is missing from the parenting they experience. For example, adolescents reared in authoritarian homes (where parents are less responsive and more demanding) are more dependent and passive, and less intellectually curious; those from indulgent homes (where parents are very responsive, but not at all demanding) are more irresponsible and less able to assume positions of leadership. Adolescents from indifferent homes (where parents are low in both responsiveness and demandingness) are often more impulsive and more likely to be involved in delinquent behavior. In contrast, adolescents from authoritative homes (where parents are responsive and demanding) tend to be more responsible, self-assured, and creative.

Demandingness has been described as constituting both positive and negative forms of control (Barber, 2002). Adolescents whose parents engaged in more **behavioral control**, or regulation of their adolescents' behavior, are less likely to be involved in antisocial behaviors. However, when parents exhibit greater **psychological control**, or inappropriate intrusion into or manipulation of adolescents' decision-making abilities, adolescents have more difficulty establishing their own sense of individuation or identity, and are less confident in facing the world (Barber & Harmon, 2002). Thus, while parental demandingness has been positively linked to adolescents' well-being, it is increasingly evident that some forms of demandingness can diminish adolescents' well-being.

Attachment and Autonomy

As young people approach adulthood, they want more autonomy and need to have a sense of self-direction and independence. Caregivers, however, are often unsure of how to provide opportunities for establishing autonomy. They may even feel threatened by their child's desire for more independence, therefore responding by exerting ever greater control.

The interesting dilemma for adolescents is that although they are attempting to establish a sense of autonomy and, as a result, often act as if they would rather die than be seen with their parents, the unsureness of this period makes the safety found in the caregiver–child relationship no less important (Figure 12-14). The task for caregivers is to recognize the normalcy of their adolescents' need to push away to begin exploring the world around them, while at the same time recognizing their need to know there is still a secure base to return to if their world becomes too unfamiliar or frightening. Indeed, adolescents' attachment to caregivers (both mothers and fathers) is important to characteristics such as self-esteem, emotional adjustment, and autonomy formation (Becker-Stoll, Fremmer-Bombik, Wartner, Zimmermann, & Grossmann, 2008), as well as the quality of the adolescents' peer relationships, their level of depressive symptoms, and their involvement in negative behaviors towards others (Allen, Porter, McFarland, McElhaney, & Marsh, 2007).

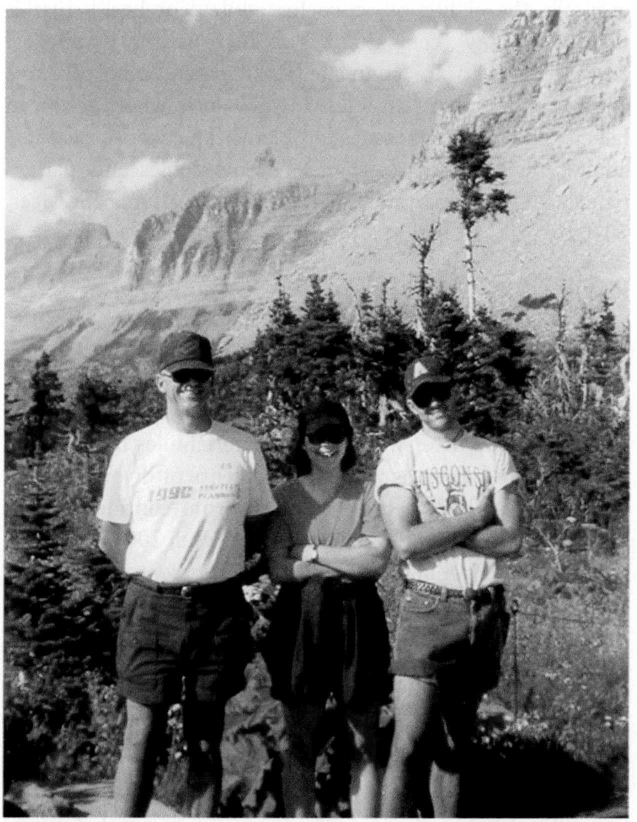

FIGURE 12-14 Contrary to what many caregivers would guess, they generally continue to be an important part of adolescents' lives. DELMAR CENGAGE LEARNING.

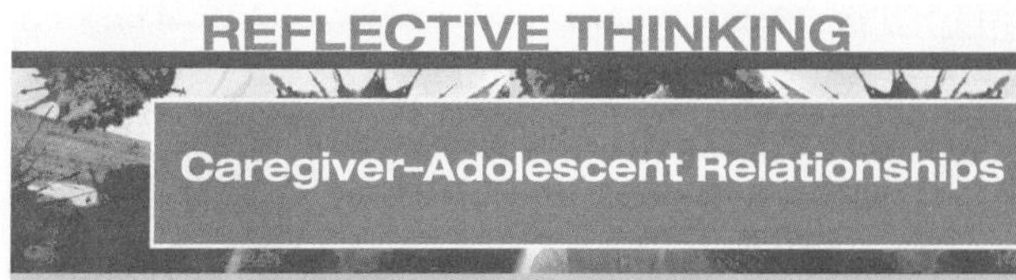

Caregiver-Adolescent Relationships

Think back to your adolescence. Do you recall ever feeling embarrassed that your parents were with you when you were at the mall or at a dance, even though you may have enjoyed doing things with them when you were around the house? Why do you think you felt uncomfortable? What suggestions would you give an adolescent who is embarrassed to be seen with his or her parents?

Caregiver–Adolescent Conflict

Conflicts between parents and adolescents occur because either parents want adolescents to follow directions or they want the adolescent to avoid making the same mistakes the parents did when they were adolescents. In addition, Smetana (1989) found parents felt conflict with their adolescent children was primarily about issues related to maintaining authority, upholding conventional standards, or regulating the household. Adolescents, in contrast, felt the conflicts were primarily issues related to personal control. The conflict may be related to generational differences in attitudes, beliefs, and values during a time of major transitions that is in and of itself stressful. In addition, many parents and adolescents do not possess adequate communication and coping skills to handle the stress associated with the transitions (Figure 12-15).

In 2000, Riesch, Bush, Nelson, Ohm, Portz, Abell, Wightman, and Jenkins discovered adolescents viewed their conflicts with fathers revolved around fighting with siblings, helping around the house, determining time for going to bed, getting low grades, using the television, and doing homework; whereas conflicts with mothers revolved around cleaning up their room, fighting with siblings, doing homework, helping around the house, and putting their clothes away. These topics of adolescent–parent conflict are interesting because most conflict occurs over apparently typical, everyday topics (fighting with siblings, cleaning room), whereas sensitive topics such as dating, sex, alcohol,

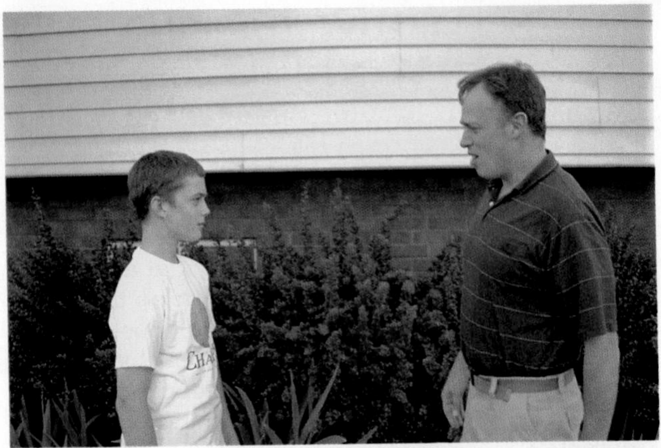

FIGURE 12-15 **Changes in both teens and their caregivers during the adolescent period often result in more conflict between them.** DELMAR CENGAGE LEARNING.

> **NURSING TIP**
>
> **Caregiver-Adolescent Conflict**
>
> Adolescents' attempts for greater autonomy can often result in an escalation in the amount of conflict they have with their caregivers. Discuss with caregivers why adolescents may disagree with rules and expectations. Suggest that caregivers "choose their battles" with adolescents. That is, keeping a bedroom neat and clean may not need to be as important as who their adolescent chooses as peers or what time they need to be home at night. Sometimes allowing adolescents to "win" may be all it takes for them to realize they are "in control" over some parts of their life.

smoking, and drugs are rarely discussed, and perhaps purposely avoided.

Conflict between adolescents and their parents is higher during early and middle adolescence. In fact, Barber, Hall, and Armistead (2003) discovered mid-range adolescents had a poorer relationship with their mothers than older adolescents. In addition, Riesch, Jackson, and Chanchong (2003) found most young (between 11 and 14) adolescent–parent conflict tended to be negative, confrontational or avoidant, and reactive, whereas ten years later the conflict tended to be more direct, healthy, and less negative.

Coughlin and Malis (2004) examined the type of conflict occurring between parents and adolescents. They discovered that when demand or withdraw conflict (one person nags or criticizes while the other person avoids the topic) was high when discussing issues important to parents, issues important to adolescents, and drug and alcohol use among teens, both parents and teens had low self-esteem and high use of drugs and alcohol. A parent's use of psychological control (controlling a person's behavior by use of such psychological mechanisms as guilt induction, which is psychologically intrusive in manipulating and constraining), when interacting with adolescents can also be related to parent and adolescent conflictual relations (Barber & Harmon, 2002; Stone, Buehler, & Barber, 2002). In fact, Kerr and Stattin (2000) discovered adolescents exhibited expectations of failure, low self-esteem, and high levels of depressed mood if they felt controlled by their parents.

Conflict between parents also affects adolescents. For example, Grych, Raynor, and Fosco (2004) discovered if adolescents were exposed to intense, frequent, and poorly resolved interparental conflict, they were more likely to feel triangulated, or torn between the warring parties. However, this feeling was moderated by the alliances created with each parent. If the adolescent had stronger alliances with one parent over the other, they were likely to feel more triangulated. However, supportive parent–child relationships lowered an adolescent's appraisal of self-blame and threat for interparental conflict. In another study examining the effect of interparental conflict on adolescents, Clark and Phares (2004) discovered interparental conflict was negatively related to parental availability and perceptions of the parent–adolescent relationship.

Relationships adolescents have with their parents or other significant adult caregivers is also acknowledged as important today because one of the *Healthy People 2020* goals for adolescents specifically discusses these adults. For example, the eighth objective for adolescent health that is new to *Healthy People 2020* is to increase the number of adolescents who are connected to a parent/other positive adult caregiver, have an adult in their lives whom they can talk to about serious issues/problems, and whose parents/adult caregivers attend activities/events adolescents participate in (U.S. Department of Health and Human Services, 2010).

DIVORCE AND REMARRIAGE

During the past several decades divorce has become a significant part of almost all adolescents' lives. Even if their own parents do not divorce, virtually all adolescents will have friends or classmates whose immediate families have experienced divorce. Even as adults, adolescents of divorce exhibit lower levels of well-being than those from continuously intact families of origin (Amato & Sobolewski, 2001; Amato & Cheadle, 2005). Children with divorced parents score lower than children of continuously married parents on measures of academic success, conduct (substance use), psychological adjustment, self concept, and social competence (Amato, 2000). Young people who experience divorce as adolescents are more likely to have drug problems than adolescents whose parents divorced when they were children or those who grew up living with both biological parents. Sons living in mother-headed, single-parent homes had more behavioral and interpersonal problems both at home and at school that persisted or accelerated as they moved from childhood through adolescence than girls in single-mothered homes and children in non-divorced homes (Hetherington, Anderson, & Hagan, 1991). Daughters of divorce fare better during childhood, but have more difficulties during adolescence with maternal conflict, lower self-esteem, and difficulties in heterosexual relationships. When divorce occurs before adolescence, girls appear to particularly struggle as they approach adolescent dating experiences; they seek more attention and contact from male adults and peers, and become sexually active earlier than girls whose fathers had either been present during childhood or whose fathers' absence was due to death. Hetherington, Stanley-Hagan, and Anderson (1989) found adolescent girls from single-mother divorced homes are more likely to marry early, be pregnant at the time of their marriage, and marry unstable or immature men. Some findings also suggest that adolescent girls may struggle more as their parents' marriage approaches divorce, while adolescent boys struggle more after the divorce has occurred (Doherty & Needle, 1991).

Although numerous studies have demonstrated that adolescents of divorced parents tend to be more at-risk for socio-emotional, behavioral, and cognitive disturbances (Amato, 2000; Amato & Sobolewski, 2001; Hetherington et al., 1991), the level of conflict in parental relationships, in either intact or divorced homes, may actually be a stronger indicator of adolescents' overall well-being than whether or not the adolescents' parents are divorced (Amato & Booth, 2002; Amato & Sobolewski, 2001).

Since a number of divorced individuals will remarry, many adolescents must not only adjust to their parents' divorce, but also attempt to reintegrate into a new family structure that often includes other children. When children become part of a stepfamily as a function of their custodial parent remarrying, it appears that girls and older children are the ones most likely to have difficulty adjusting to the new family structure. Many children will eventually develop a positive relationship with their stepparent, which has been related to fewer adolescent problems particularly for adolescent boys. Some children have more adjustment problems in more complex stepfamily structures (i.e., whether both the husband and the wife have children from previous marriages, and whether those children reside in the same household or not).

Sibling Relationships

Siblings provide a unique relationship for adolescents because they are generally close in age and are likely to spend a great deal of time with one another. Interestingly, their relationship is one in which there is no choice about membership. Thus, while conflict in friendships may be avoided in order to preserve the relationship, sibling relationships have more warmth and conflict since they do not operate under the same threat of termination (McCoy, Brody, & Stoneman, 2002).

Siblings can have an impact on one another for both good and ill. For example, older adolescents' involvement

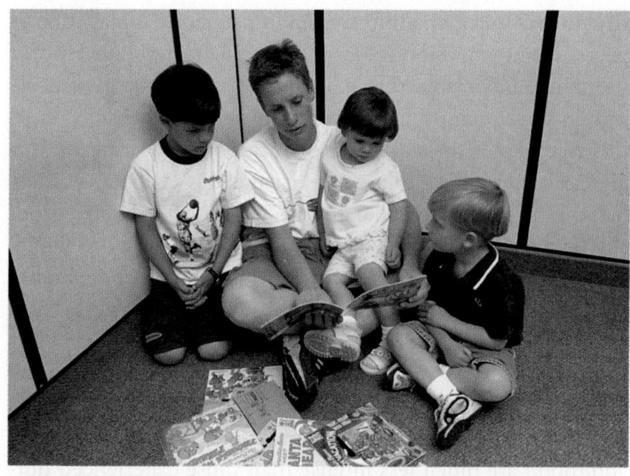

FIGURE 12-16 Sibling relationships can provide adolescents with significant opportunities for learning how to teach, help, and care about others. DELMAR CENGAGE LEARNING.

in illicit drugs and alcohol, as well as deviant and sexual behavior are predictive of their younger siblings' involvement in similar behavior. In contrast, siblings also provide a buffering effect against challenging experiences such as parental divorce or poor peer relationships.

As youths approach adolescence, several changes occur in relationships with siblings. Often, progression through adolescence was associated with a reduction in perceived sibling support and a corresponding increase in perceived sibling conflict, which apexes between the ages of 12 and 13 years old, followed by an increase in support and a decrease in conflict when youths reached the age of 15 or 16. In addition, siblings are important socializing agents for adolescents as they transition into the world outside their family since they may provide young people with an environment where they can learn appropriate interpersonal skills in preparation for their nonfamilial interactions, particularly with peers (Figure 12-16).

For adolescents who are "only" children, there appears to be little research indicating they are at a loss because of the absence of a brother or sister. However, only children tend to have a fairly high sense of self-esteem and achievement motivation as compared with those with siblings. This may be a result of their increased level of interaction with parents and other adults.

PEERS

Friends have long been considered to be of central importance to adolescents. Erikson (1968) believed the peer group provides a sanctuary of group identity while a young person is passing between the dependency of childhood and the independence of adulthood. Piaget considered peer relationships crucial to youths' understanding of rules and moral behavior and argued while young children's interactions with adults and siblings tended to emphasize the divine structure of rules, the informal and unsupervised play among peers during childhood and adolescence fosters the kind of spontaneous, flexible rule making and rule enforcing necessary in developing a mature moral orientation.

Because of the developmental importance of peers during early to middle adolescence, friendships experienced during this period are unlike those encountered at any other stage of life (Brown & Klute, 2006; Elkind, 1984; Selman, 1980). Friendships during this period demonstrate higher levels of mutuality, interaction, and interdependency. Thus, during childhood, peers are more appropriately characterized as playmates rather than as friends, and their coming together is based more on proximity and common activities than on relationship issues. Conversely, the friendships of adulthood are much less intense than those experienced during adolescence as a result of adults' greater sense of individuality and the consequent reduction in their need to "share thoughts with others."

Peer relationships generally exist at one of four levels: the friendship dyad, the clique, the crowd, and the age cohort. The **friendship dyad** is the most fundamental peer relation and the one most likely to be based on similar interests and emotional support. **Cliques** comprise a small group of peers who regularly interact with one another and who generally exhibit a strong sense of shared closeness (Brown, 2004; Dunphy, 1963). Adolescents' cliques have been described as constituting an alternative family structure for its members as they acclimate to the world outside of the home (Dunphy, 1963). Same-sex cliques define the majority of early adolescents' peer experiences. As youths approach middle adolescence the **crowd** becomes an increasingly important part of their peer experiences (Figure 12-17). Dunphy originally defined crowds as an association of two to four cliques in which relations are less intimate than in the smaller groups (1963), while others believe peer groups at this level are more symbolic than interactional. Formation of the crowd is usually based on shared distinguishing characteristics, evidenced by the labels often associated with different adolescent crowds (e.g., "preppies," "brains," "jocks," "normals," "druggies") (Brown & Klute, 2006). Finally, the **age cohort** is often regarded as constituting adolescents' classmates or same-age schoolmates. Although friendship is typically not a part of this level of peer interaction, these peer dynamics are a very important part of the adolescent experience. This level of peer association is important to adolescents' identity formation and to their opportunities for heterosexual interactions (Dunphy, 1963). It is also at this level that adolescents come to understand general notions of social competence and their level of peer status or popularity. The importance of the peer group at each level varies across adolescence as a function of individual development (Selman, 1980) and the developmental stage of the individual's peer interactions (Dunphy, 1963).

The structure of youths' peer relationships changes as they pass through five stages of peer development (Figure 12-18) (Dunphy, 1963). Beginning with the solitary, unisexual

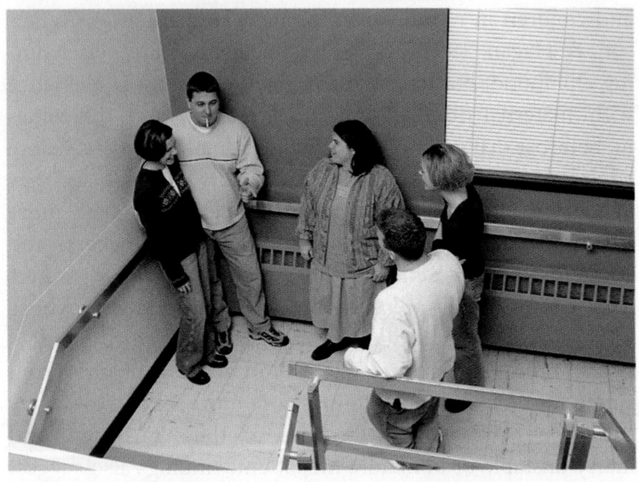

FIGURE 12-17 Male and female friend groups are often found among adolescents. DELMAR CENGAGE LEARNING.

cliques established during childhood, early adolescents begin to explore, within the safety of their unisexual cliques, interactions with cliques of the opposite sex. During this early period, interaction with the opposite sex is most likely to occur among the higher status members of the different cliques. Unisexual cliques eventually begin to merge to form heterosexual crowds, which provide adolescents with a temporary sense of identity and with introduction into dating behavior. In late adolescence, crowds no longer serve a purpose and are replaced by loosely associated groups of heterosexual couples.

Same-sex identity formation of adolescents in peers is either similar to or different from heterosexual peer group development based on the timing of their transition toward a homosexual identity; a shift to the gay community as a source of close relationships is the pivotal step.

Adolescents' peer status and the quality of their friendships affect their general well-being. Children who are less popular or more rejected by their peers are more likely to subsequently drop out of school and become involved in later juvenile and adult criminal activity (Coie, 2004).

Another important aspect of adolescents' peer relationships is the *quality* of the friendships. Quality friendships are characterized by high levels of mutual caring, respect, and trust, in a context of balanced give and take. Adolescents who experience these types of close friendships generally report more intimate self-disclosure, more prosocial behavior, and more emotional support or encouragement from their friends, while also reporting less conflictual, domineering, or rivalrous behavior. Although present in childhood friendships, these characteristics probably become much more pronounced during preadolescence and adolescence.

For most adolescents, ethnicity or culture appear to be very important in determining who they select as friends. The importance of ethnicity to affiliation is particularly evident among tight-knit cliques, as compared to loose-knit peer groups. For example, in integrated schools, many

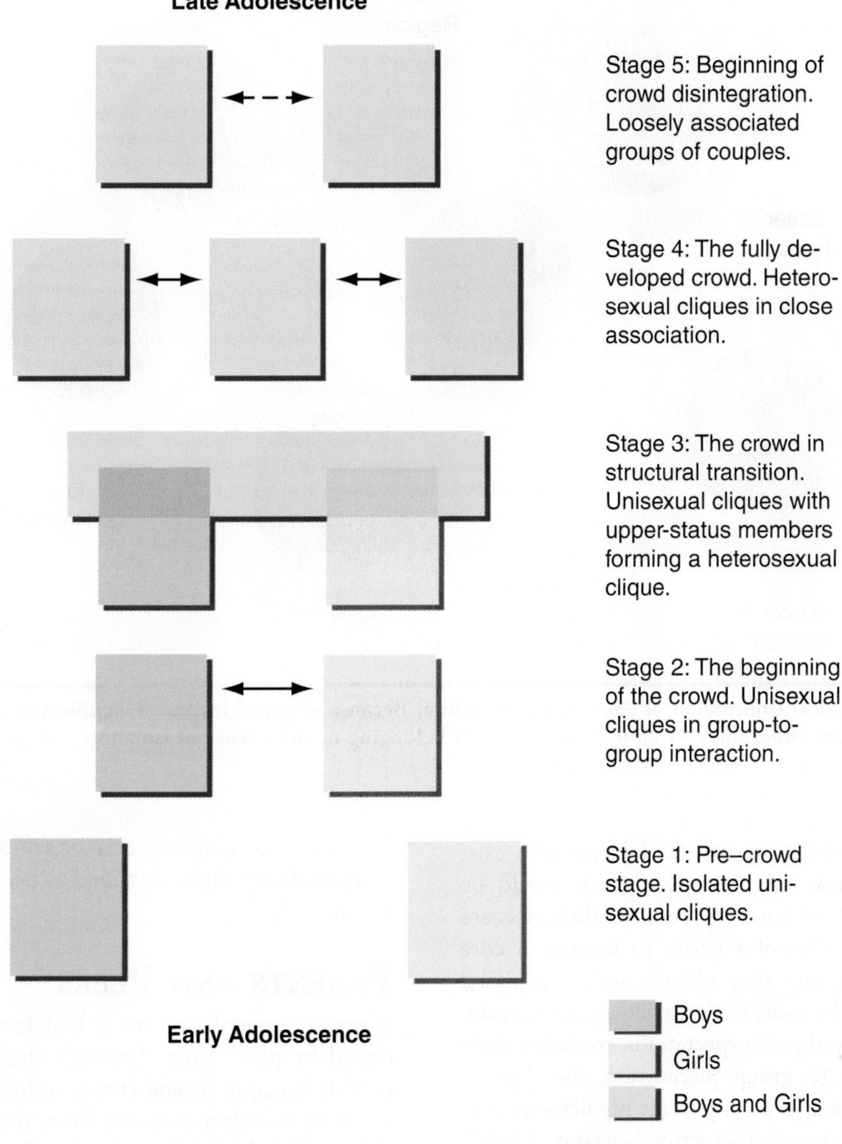

FIGURE 12-18 Stages of Group Development in Adolescence. PUBLISHED BY THE AMERICAN SOCIOLOGICAL ASSOCIATION.

students have an other ethnic school friend; few have contact with these friends outside of school. For many ethnic minority youths, especially immigrants, peer relations formed from their own ethnic group can provide an adaptive support against the sense of isolation that can often exist among their peers of the majority population (Santrock, 2010).

PEER INFLUENCE

A major concern for many parents is whether their adolescents are being adversely influenced by their friends. The extent to which adolescents influence friends or are influenced by them varies according to their ability to establish and maintain supportive peer relationships as well as the type of group they belong to. Teevan (1972) contends compliance with peers is often based on the expectation that "such conformity will be rewarded with eventual acceptance into the group" (p. 283). Whether responding to actual peer pressure or merely to perceived expectations, young people who are less secure in their relations with friends are more likely to engage in behavior they would otherwise avoid. The importance of peer influence may be evaluated according to how closely associated the individual is to their friendship group or clique (Figure 12-19). Most adolescents would be expected to fit into the *core* of a particular peer circle, where there is a strong sense of commitment and collegiality. However, many adolescents instead fit into the *peripheral* region of one or more groups, where there is frequently a sense of tentative belonging and a desire to become a part of the core group. These individuals are sometimes termed "wannabes" (Figure 12-20). Finally, others float unattached, *outside* any particular peer group. This lack of peer group connectedness

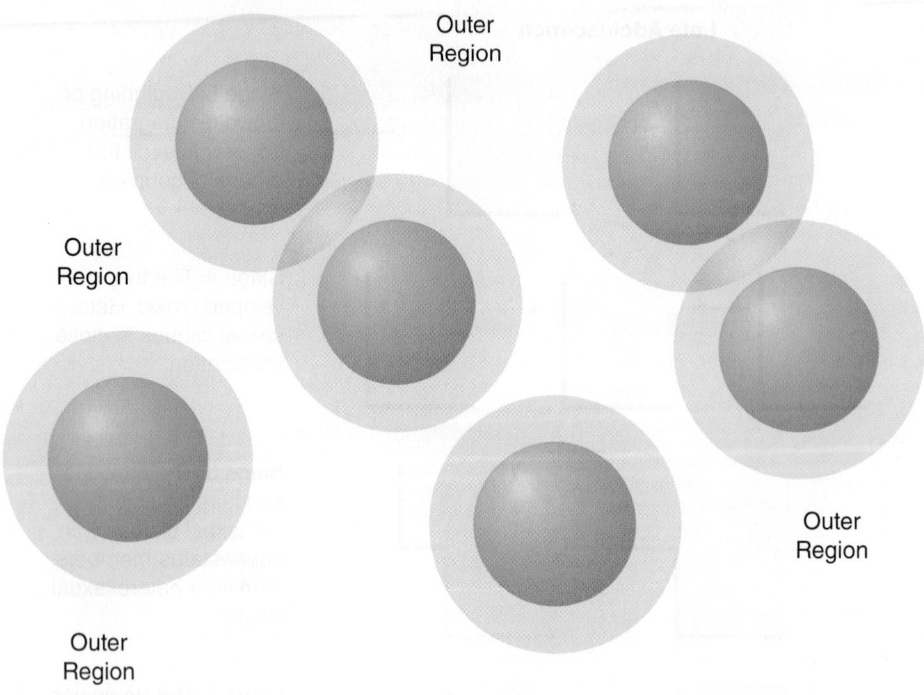

FIGURE 12-19 Theoretical Conception of Peer Group Structure. Because of peers' increased significance during adolescence, experiences with peers can either increase adolescents' sense of belonging or their sense of isolation. REPRINTED WITH PERMISSION OF J. KELLY MCCOY.

can be either self- or other-imposed. Adolescents who exist at the periphery of their identified peer group would be most vulnerable to peer influence as a result of their insecure position in the group. Out of a desire to become a core member of the peer group they identify with, peripheral group members would be most likely to allow peer expectations, or at least perceived peer expectations, to dictate their behaviors. In addition to group placements, the type of group one belongs to is also an important predictor of participation in antisocial or self-destructive behavior. Adolescents identified as being in the "druggies" or "toughs" peer groups are much more likely to report participating in groups encouraging antisocial or self-destructive behaviors as compared with those identified as being "populars," "brains," or "normals."

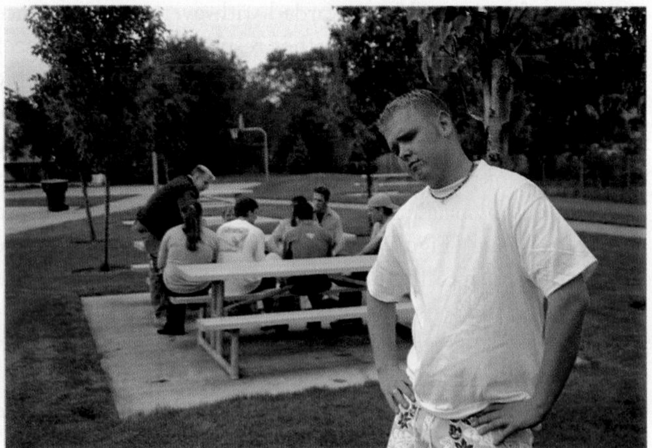

FIGURE 12-20 Adolescents typically want to be a member of the group. DELMAR CENGAGE LEARNING.

PARENTS AND PEERS

A major parental concern is that family values will be displaced by peer values. Although there is some justification for this concern, several factors influence whom adolescents are likely to select as peers. First, there is usually considerable overlap between parental and peer values because of common backgrounds; many adolescents select friends whose values are congruent with their parents'. Second, parents often are unsure of appropriate expectations for certain areas of adolescents' lives, and are thus willing to defer to the expectations of their adolescents' friends. This is especially apparent in current fashions, music, and leisure activities. Third, parents and peers have an impact on different aspects of adolescents' lives; peers are more likely to be influential in matters of current importance (i.e., tastes in music and entertainment, fashions in clothing and language, dating and friendship behavior), whereas parents are more likely to be influential in matters of greater and longer-term permanence (i.e., moral and social values, educational aspirations, and occupational choice). Fourth, when adolescents do turn to peers for support, frequently it is not a displacement of parental influence but rather an attempt to fill a void left by parents' lack of support and involvement. Finally, adolescents' orientations toward parents as compared with peers vary as a function of individual differences within

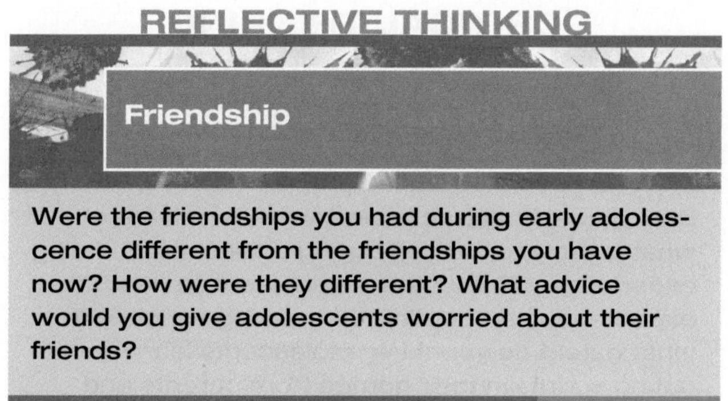

Were the friendships you had during early adolescence different from the friendships you have now? How were they different? What advice would you give adolescents worried about their friends?

adolescents and their social contexts. As a result, the degree of conflict between parental and peer influence is less than generally assumed.

Adolescents' behavior is strongly predicted by peers' behavior. Much of this similarity may actually result from young people seeking out friends with attitudes and behavior similar to their own. For example, a girl who becomes sexually active may cease to feel comfortable around her friends who are not sexually active, thus, she is likely to seek out new friends who have a similar sexual status. Because the similarity among friends is just as likely to be a result of selection as influence, the resemblance found in the attitudes and behavior of adolescent friendships is just as likely to be a function of characteristics developed in the home and in other non-peer contexts as it is in the friendships themselves.

Caregivers have both direct and indirect effects on children's and adolescents' peer relationships. Caregivers' indirect influence on children's and adolescents' peer relationships is thought to generally be a result of the caregivers' interactions with their own children or by the parenting behaviors they use in rearing their children. In fact, the quality of adolescents' relationships with caregivers is reflected in the quality of their best friendships or closest group of friends, and parenting received by adolescents is likely to be important to the quality of their friendships or broader peer experiences.

Caregivers can also have a more direct effect on children's and adolescents' peer experiences. This more direct influence is a result of caregivers' interactions with or about their children's friendships. Caregivers can directly influence young children's peer relationships in four ways: designing, mediating, supervising, and consulting. Caregivers *design* children's peer experiences by controlling or influencing the settings in which children are likely to meet and interact with peers. Caregivers *mediate* by actively assisting children to successfully meet and interact with peers. Caregivers *supervise* by providing oversight or regulation of children's peer experiences. Caregivers *advise* children about peer interactions by sharing advice or "coaching" children about how to maintain more positive friendships. All of these direct peer involvement processes have been associated with young children having more positive peer experiences.

Most research about caregivers' direct influence on adolescent peer relationships has generally focused on caregivers' managing adolescents' peer interactions. This is because caregivers' involvement in children's peer relationships must become qualitatively different as the children become adolescents. Whereas optimal parental involvement in younger children's peer relationships consists of more direct management of their peer relations, caregivers' direct management of adolescents' peer relations must become less overt. Although less evident in the adolescent literature, caregivers' direct facilitating behaviors have similarly been found to be significant to early adolescents' formation of positive peer relationships. In fact, caregivers' efforts to encourage more positive friendship experiences are significantly related to the quality of adolescents' friendships, and although caregivers spent a relatively small amount of time with adolescents' friends, adolescents' reports of parent involvement behavior were still predictive of greater intimacy and less negativity in best friendships, particularly for boys.

DATING

As previously mentioned, youths' passage through adolescence is marked by the increased significance of peer relationships. This process begins with same-sex friendships. However, during middle and late adolescence, young people begin to explore opposite-sex relationships—frequently through dating. Up until the early part of the past century, dating was a courtship experience overseen by parents used largely to identify an appropriate mate. Since World War II, we have seen a dramatic shift in the purpose and events that define adolescent dating. Although some adolescents still view early dating experiences as a means of sorting and selecting an appropriate mate, for most, dating has taken on much more of a recreational role. In addition, dating is seen as providing other functions, including a source of status and achievement; a unique socializing experience in which to learn about intimacy, sexuality, and a sense of identity; and an opportunity to develop new and deeper forms of companionship (Bouchey & Furman, 2006).

A major shift in the dating experience has been the age when it is likely to begin. Dating now typically begins around age 12 and 13 for most girls, and between ages 13 and 14 for boys. Although the onset of dating would seem most likely to be triggered by adolescents' individual pubertal development, socially defined factors are much better predictors of dating onset than an individual adolescents' pubertal status.

As dating becomes more important to adolescents, their motivation for dating and their selection of a potential partner changes. Adolescents' focus on a dating partner shifts with age; early adolescents tend to be more egocentric, focusing on issues of immediate gratification (e.g., recreation and status) regarding who and why they date, whereas older adolescents focus more on long-term aspects of the dating experience (i.e., companionship and mate selection issues). There are also several gender differences regarding dating choices. Males more frequently listed "sexual activity" as a reason for dating while females were more likely to list "intimacy." Similarly, when 15-year-old males and females were asked what they liked about their girlfriend or boyfriend, boys were more likely to mention physical attractiveness, whereas girls were more likely to mention support and intimacy.

Another important part of the dating process involves the **dating scripts** adolescents learn and internalize regarding what is expected of them and what they should expect from their dating partners. Dating scripts will vary based on regional location, community size, socioeconomic status, religious affiliation, and peer group, but they are most differentiated by gender. Dating scripts for males and females differ, with males being responsible for initiating, planning, and paying for the date and for initiating the level of sexual interaction; females are generally responsible for appropriately responding to males' attempts to initiate and carry out the date as well as their initiation of sexual gestures. Although these gender-defined scripts have changed somewhat over the past decade—giving males and females more flexibility in what is considered appropriate—they appear to have remained largely unchanged.

The extent to which adolescents' dating experiences have an impact on individual development remains largely unknown. Although this area has received limited exploration, there are some ways dating has been found to be important. First, because boys are not encouraged to develop the capacity to be emotionally expressive in their same-sex peer relationships, opposite-sex relationships may provide boys with an opportunity to explore intimacy development in a context that is much more socially acceptable (Steinberg, 2008). Second, becoming seriously involved in a steady dating relationship before age 15 may have a somewhat stunting effect on adolescents' psychosocial development, particularly for girls. Girls who begin early to date seriously have been found to be less mature, less imaginative, less oriented toward achievement, less happy with who they are, and more superficial. In contrast, adolescent girls who have not dated at all by the time they reach late adolescence may have a more retarded social development, excessive dependency on their parents, and greater feelings of insecurity.

If adolescents postpone dating, and dating behavior remains light to moderate, it can provide a positive opportunity for social development. What has been difficult to determine is whether adolescents' dating experiences are themselves an important positive factor for social development or whether more socially advanced adolescents are simply more likely to date.

Adolescents' dating experiences are likely to be impacted by, and have an impact on, both their family and peer relationships. Regarding adolescents' family relationships, a primary source of difficulty may be the changing amounts of time adolescents spend with their family; those adolescents involved in romantic relationships spend less time with family members. Dating can also often be an increased source of tension and conflict between adolescents and their caregivers; parents often struggle with their own changing relationship with their adolescents as the adolescents increasingly turn to a romantic partner for support. Similarly, although adolescents' same-sex friendships often provide initial access to romantic relationships with those of the opposite sex, friends are also likely to experience competition for adolescents' time as they become involved in romantic relationships.

Finally, as Bouchey and Furman (2006) have pointed out, little theoretical and empirical work has focused on gay and lesbian youths' romantic experiences. Indeed, few sexual-minority youth enter into romantic relationships with same-sex peers during adolescence due largely to the limited opportunities available to them. Those who have researched the development of sexual-minority youths' romantic experiences have concluded that there is no singular "sexual-minority developmental trajectory" (Diamond & Savin-Williams, 2006). In particular, gender appears to be a significant discriminating factor. While male sexual-minority youths often pursue sexual contact during their early teen years, the majority of sexual-minority women do not have same-sex contact until late adolescence or young adulthood.

CRITICAL THINKING

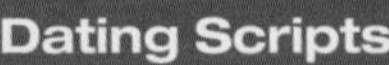

Dating Scripts

Dating scripts are an important determinant of what is likely to happen during adolescents' dating experiences. But where do adolescents learn the expectations that define their dating scripts? To what extent do you think adolescents learn about dating scripts in their homes from parents and siblings? To what extent are these scripts learned from the media? How important are peers in determining the dating scripts adolescents establish?

SCHOOLS

Schools and academic achievement are important in shaping the developing adolescents' sense of autonomy and identity. This is because almost 90% of adolescents attend public secondary school (grades 9 to 12), and they spend an average of 180 days per year in school. In fact, during most of the year, typical adolescents spend more than one-third of their waking hours every week in school or school-related activities. In addition, adolescents remain in school for more years now than they did in the past (Steinberg, 2008). This is due to not having to drop out to support their families. Academic achievement during adolescence is important because it often reflects not only how well the individual accomplishes long- and short-term goals, but also the feelings of success one has in one's own as well as society's eyes. To

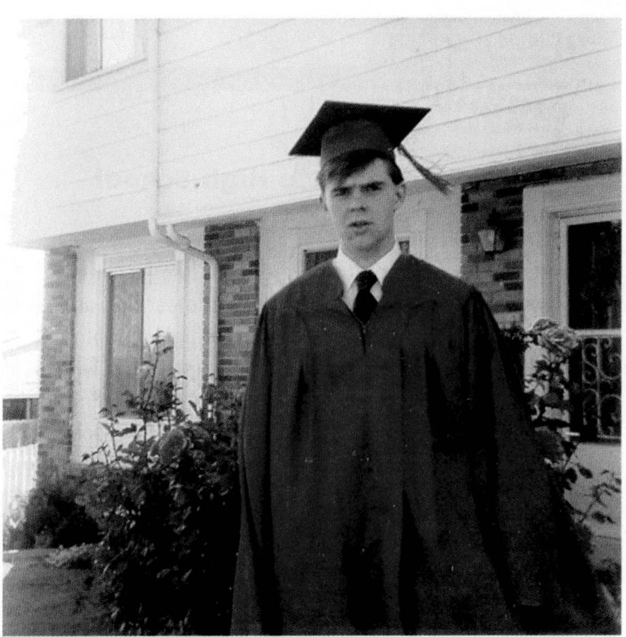

FIGURE 12-21 High school graduation is an important milestone and accomplishment for teens. DELMAR CENGAGE LEARNING.

be effective, schools and curricula for adolescents should be based on principles of learning and development and provide a climate that encourages exploring future directions and goals (Figure 12-21).

School is also important because it is a critical setting for adolescent development. In fact, most developmental milestones related to competence (academic achievement, involvement in athletic activities, peer relationships, prosocial behavior) are related to behavior or defined in the school context). In addition, adolescents' psychological functioning is strongly related to their school experiences. Those who feel connected to school reported higher levels of well-being than those who do not feel connected, and those who feel connected to school during seventh and eighth grade had fewer psychological problems than students who did not feel as connected (Faircloth, 2009; Ozer, 2005).

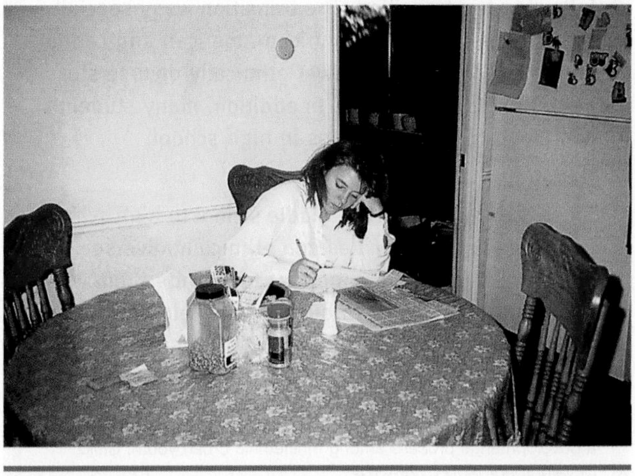

FIGURE 12-22 Studying and keeping up with homework assignments help adolescents succeed in school. DELMAR CENGAGE LEARNING.

Schools can have a positive or negative effect on adolescents. Often, a student's experience varies according to parent and family context, peer group, size of the school, extracurricular activities, and academic track. An adolescent's adjustment to school is also influenced not only by the behavior of his or her friends, but also by the characteristics of the friendship and by teachers. Students whose friends described them as disruptive in the fall of the academic year described themselves as increasing their disruptive behavior during the year. Students whose friendships had positive features increased their involvement in activities during the year; students whose friendships had more negative features were less involved in activities and became more disruptive as the year progressed (Figure 12-22).

For some adolescents, school is a stabilizing, friendly force in their lives. It can encourage cognitive development, establish a climate for social interaction, and provide an environment that encourages task completion. School also allows adolescents to have contact with peers and teachers, test new ideas, and validate their thoughts (Figure 12-23). In fact, across different cultures and ethnicities, positive and supportive student–teacher relationships can decrease an adolescent's risk for school failure, externalizing behaviors, emotional distress, suicide ideations, violence, and substance abuse as well as improve academic functioning and enhance peer relations (Suldo, Friedrich, White, Farmer, Minch, & Michalowski, 2009). Activities and opportunities at school can provide safe, acceptable outlets for their energy and foster development. Groups such as the honor society, musical and dance groups, student council, athletic teams, school yearbook and newspaper staff, debate teams, special interest clubs, pep squads, cheerleading, and ethnic-identity groups give adolescents a chance to participate in activities with young people who have similar interests, provide experiences in organizations working toward common goals, and allow development of cohesiveness and group loyalty.

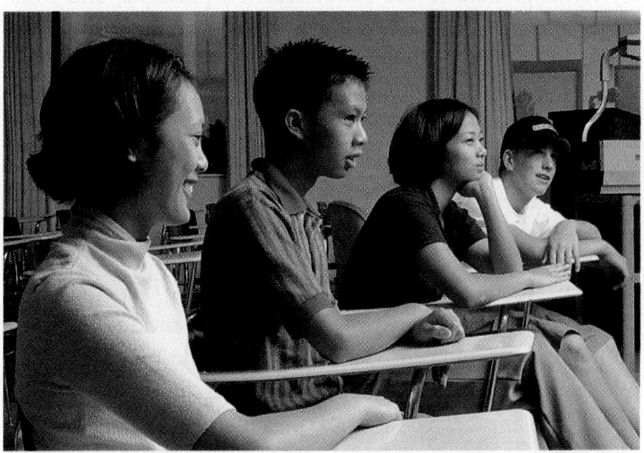

FIGURE 12-23 Classroom interactions allow for varying points of view and new experiences with teens of different cultures. DELMAR CENGAGE LEARNING.

Schools also can help break barriers related to ethnicity, social class, race, and gender.

School is more likely to have a positive effect on adolescents if they have close friends before, during, and after the transition to secondary school. Academically talented and economically advantaged students also tend to have a more positive experience as compared with their less-affluent or less capable counterparts. These adolescents are more likely to hold positions of leadership, experience classes that are challenging and enjoyable, and have teachers who pay more attention to them (Steinberg, 2008). In fact, an important prediction for adolescent healthy behaviors and well-being is successful school performance.

For other adolescents, however, school can be a source of stress, where threats to safety and self-esteem and constant change occur. Some adolescents may experience depression, decreases in perceptions of their athletic and academic abilities or actual academic and athletic performances, dissatisfaction with school, or discrimination based on race and consequently drop out or skip classes. In fact, class skipping, chronic absenteeism, and other kinds of school avoidance need in-depth assessment because they may indicate an underlying mental health problem (Dunn 2009a). Moving from an elementary school, where they were the oldest and tallest, to a middle school or high school where they are now the youngest and shortest may also cause stress. This "top-dog" phenomenon, where students move from the top position in elementary school to the lowest position in middle school, can be difficult and may result in less commitment and satisfaction with school as well as liking their teachers less than they did in earlier years. There are also shifts from the personal to the impersonal; from smaller to larger classes and buildings; from the same class with the same peers and teachers to different classes, different peers, and different teachers; from simple to complex classroom organization; and from slower-paced to faster-paced curricula. The transition from middle school to high school can also provide negative experiences. For example, it is not uncommon when moving to high school for ninth graders to see lower teacher, principal, and assistant principal support, less teacher monitoring, less involvement in school activities, higher depression, lower self-esteem, lower level of liking school, and a perceived need for more school organization.

In addition, adolescents are dealing with physiological, psychosocial, and cognitive changes that affect their adjustment; junior and senior high schools often have a more open, frightening, combative, and academically taxing environment than elementary school. Learning activities may often emphasize individual achievement and competition rather than learning for learning's sake. As a result, students may be alienated from the subject matter since these experiences and approaches are not well matched to their developmental needs of greater autonomy and independence. Perhaps that is why levels of unexcused absenteeism, dropout rates, grade failure, and suspensions are higher during

The Transition to High School

STUDY PURPOSE

Adolescents of color face different challenges when compared to non-ethnically diverse adolescents as they transition from middle school to high school. Therefore, guided by the life course perspective, which suggests that social ties both influence and are influenced by life transitions, this study sought to discover the high school transition experiences of adolescents from different racial/ethnic groups. Specifically, the investigators were interested in learning how participants' perceptions of the school climate and their psychological functioning and academic behaviors changed across the transition from middle school to high school, and how those perceptions affected the adolescents' first two years of high school.

METHODS

During this quantitative descriptive longitudinal study, an urban sample of 1,979 adolescents were followed from seventh to tenth grade (mean age = 14.6, SD = .37 in seventh grade). Data were gathered two times each year. School climate was measured by asking the students how much they liked school and how much they felt like they belonged. Psychological functioning was assessed by using a shortened version of the Social Anxiety Scale for Adolescents, and the Loneliness Scale. Academic behavior was measured by Grade point average (GPA) and attendance.

FINDINGS

Most adolescents were doing well before moving from middle school to high school but experienced disruptions in grades, attendance, and psychological functioning (lonelier and more anxious) immediately following the transition. The transition was especially challenging for girls and African-American and Latino students (if there were fewer ethnically diverse students in the new school). In addition, many students continued to have struggles in high school.

IMPLICATIONS

Since the transition from middle school to high school is challenging for females and ethnically diverse students, it would be important to provide them with support as they move through this developmental period of life.

REFERENCE

Benner, A. & Graham, S. (2009). The transition to high school as a developmental process among multiethnic urban youth. *Child Development*, *80*(2), 356–376.

Reflections from Families

Even though my folks spend a lot of time helping me with my homework, sometimes I just don't get it. I am the biggest kid in my class because I was sick a lot when I was younger, missed a year of school, and never did catch up. The teacher is nice, but lots of the kids are weird. They make noise and are always jumping around. It is hard to concentrate on my work.

this time. Indeed, it is no wonder adolescents with more psychological and academic problems before the transition to secondary school cope less well with the transition to this new environment (Steinberg, 2008).

It is difficult to generalize about the role school plays in adolescent development, however, since different adolescents have different experiences within the same school. Many schools do not promote psychosocial development and have higher dropout rates because of their focus on obedience and conformity and their lack of encouragement for self-reliance, creativity, and independence. However, there are also many good schools that emphasize these qualities and intellectual activities, have classrooms where students actively participate in their own learning, employ committed and autonomous teachers who continually evaluate their programs, and invite parent involvement. They also encourage adolescents to learn about themselves, their relationships with others, the academic material, and society so the students are better able to experience the challenges of adulthood.

Finally, school is such an important part of an adolescent's life that three of the *Healthy People 2020* goals for adolescents relate to school achievement and school experiences. One of the goals involves the educational achievement of adolescents as indicated by increasing the number of students who graduate from high school four years after starting ninth grade, the number of students with reading and mathematic skills at or above their grade level, and the number of adolescents who are active and involved in school, as well as decreasing the number of school days missed due to injury or illness (U.S. Department of Health and Human Services, 2010). Other goals of *Healthy People 2020* related to adolescents and school are to increase the number of middle and high schools prohibiting sexual orientation or gender identity harassment, and decrease the number of adolescents who choose not to attend school at least one time a month because they feared for their safety, and who, on school property, have been offered, sold, or given an illegal drug (U.S. Department of Health and Human Services, 2010).

REFLECTIVE THINKING

School Experiences

What do you remember about the high school you attended? Was the experience primarily negative or positive? Why? What suggestions would you give an adolescent concerned about school experiences?

Nurses can work closely with parents and school officials to provide accurate, objective information related to health promotion activities and issues adolescents are concerned about and see as important. School-based health centers (SBHCs) afford unique opportunities for nurses to provide accurate information and nonjudgmental counseling about adolescent issues. Located in or adjacent to schools, these centers provide physical examinations; health education programs; screenings; counseling related to substance abuse, mental health, and sexuality; dental care; and treatment of minor injuries. Often set up to serve poor young people, who are less likely to receive health care than more affluent students, these local centers are in a position to address important adolescent health issues, such as confidentiality, underused services, and preventable diseases (Steinberg, 2008). Adolescents who use SBHCs are more likely to use them for mental health, medical, and substance abuse counseling. See Chapter 5 for a more thorough discussion on school-based health clinics.

WORK AND CAREER DEVELOPMENT

Part-Time Employment

One important way adolescents become aware of the adult world is through their increasing exploration of potential career opportunities and part-time employment experiences. Adolescents' part-time employment has received a great deal of attention in the past, particularly regarding employment while attending school. In some of the earliest research on this topic, Greenberger and Steinberg (1986) identified three areas needing further consideration: the number of adolescents working and the amount of time they worked; the type of work adolescents were now involved in compared to the past; and the implications of the work experience on adolescents' lives.

They found nearly two-thirds of all 16-year-olds in the United States had some kind of part-time work while attending school (Greenberger & Steinberg, 1986). Although there is a general conception that adolescents today are lazy, adolescents often have some kind of part-time employment as compared with adolescents in 1960, when only one-third of all adolescents worked part-time while attending school. In addition, older students are more likely to work than younger ones, males are more likely to work than females, white students are more likely to work than nonwhite students, and students from middle-economic status families are more likely to work compared to youths from upper- and lower-economic status families.

Secondly, over half of all adolescent work opportunities fall into one of two areas: fast food and retail sales. In the past young people were likely to receive training to prepare them for the jobs they would take on as adults; however, most of the work available to adolescents today is dull and repetitious. Because adolescents were found to spend only about 5 minutes per hour using skills they were likely to have learned in school, there was little opportunity for gaining skills with long-term benefits. However, a possible benefit of adolescents' part-time work experience is their potential exposure to the adult workplace and the opportunity to better prepare for full-time entry into the adult world. Again, most adolescents worked in agesegregated workplaces, where teens are generally supervised by other teens, and have little opportunity for adult contact or to learn how to interact more effectively in the adult world.

Finally, a critical aspect of adolescents' part-time employment has to do with the number of hours worked while attending school. The average number of hours worked during a week is between 19 and 20 hours for employed senior males and between 17 and 19 hours for employed senior females. With this in mind, we can more accurately identify the final point identified by Greenberger and Steinberg regarding the implications or risks and benefits to adolescents that may result from part-time work experience. While a number of benefits do appear to be related to adolescents working (e.g., learning about the business world, learning how to manage money, a greater sense of control over one's own life, and the opportunity to develop a sense of pride in one's abilities and accomplishments), these benefits are most evident among adolescents who work a limited number of hours per week and when adolescents see their work experiences as stimulating and good preparation for later life. However, when adolescents work more hours per week or are employed in jobs that seem to provide little personal growth, there appear to be a number of potentially negative outcomes. For example, those adolescents who work probably have a lower investment in schooling, higher rates of school tardiness and absences, a greater likelihood of lying about incomplete homework, more propensity to engage in deviant acts—including higher rates of alcohol and marijuana use—greater cynicism and tolerance for cheating, less investment in schoolwork, and fewer extracurricular activities than those students who do not work while in high school.

Career Development

Another important aspect of adolescents' interactions with the workplace is their exploration of a career or occupation. But, how do adolescents go about choosing a career, since they often do not stay in their choice of careers much longer than three years?

Several researchers have developed theories about the process adolescents go through in their selection of a career (refer to Santrock, 2010, and Vondracek & Porfeli, 2006, for a more thorough review). Of particular interest is the developmental theory of career selection proposed by Ginzberg (1972), who believed there are three stages of career exploration young people are likely to experience as they move toward a final career choice: fantasy, tentative, and realistic. During the **fantasy stage** (until about age 11), career opportunities are likely to be limited only by children's imagination. When asked what they would like to be when they grow up, children in this stage will likely select careers they are currently the most impassioned about, without considering possible constraints. Between the ages of 11 and 16 years, young people move into the **tentative stage** during which they begin to consider how they might fit in with the various career options they are interested in. They first evaluate what they are really interested in (11 to 12 years), then evaluate how careers of interest match their own capabilities (13 to 14 years), and then finally determine what types of work are most congruent with the principles they most value (15 to 16 years). Ginzberg identified late adolescence through young adulthood as the **realistic stage**, or the stage when young people begin to more extensively explore available careers and the steps required to enter their chosen career and specific job within that career.

Factors that appear to be important to adolescents' career selection include their own personalities, the attitudes and expectations of their parents and peers, and their broader social context (Steinberg, 2008). First, career selection is a reflection of adolescents' basic personality style; once individuals have found a career that fits their personality, they are more likely to enjoy their work and stay with it. Adolescents are also very much influenced by the attitudes and values of their parents and peers. Although peer educational and occupational plans are important predictors of adolescents' career aspirations, it is parents who appear to have a greater influence on the types of career paths adolescents are likely to choose, since adolescents raised in homes with values more characteristic of middle-class jobs (i.e., autonomy, self-direction, and independence) are more likely to seek those types of jobs regardless of whether their family situations are more middle class or working class in nature. Also, while gender is an important factor in adolescents' decisions about the type of career they will select, parents' modeling gender-related career choices is

REFLECTIVE THINKING

Career Selection

Do you recall when you first began thinking about what you wanted to do for a living once you had grown up? What did you first want to be? Do you recall the process of selection that you went through to get to the point of career preparation that you are at currently?

also important to adolescents' sex-stereotyped attitudes about work.

HEALTH PROMOTION

GENERAL NURSING INTERACTIONS

Any adolescent health promotion effort needs to incorporate the adolescents' perspective of what health means and consider their priorities and concerns relative to health and health care services, as well as the level of their cognitive development. Often, developmental tasks and crises in the physiological, psychosexual, psychosocial, or cognitive domains have an impact on adolescent concerns related to health since the concerns usually have something to do with their own point of view or context. Many adolescents are reluctant to seek health care even though the fourth objective of *Healthy People 2020* is to increase the number of adolescents who have a yearly wellness checkup (U.S. Department of Health and Human Services, 2010) because of financial concerns, geographical access, characteristics of the health care provider, or the perceived notion of unavailability of confidential services. Therefore, it is critical providers be respectful; demonstrate openness, competence, honesty, warmth, compassion, and understanding; and have the ability to communicate effectively with adolescents and their families (Figure 12-24). It is also important for nurses working with adolescents to know that for adolescents, mental and emotional well-being tend to be related to one another. Therefore, interventions aimed at improving one aspect of well-being may also have positive effects on others. In addition, emotional and mental well-being is related to a teen's environments, which can include school, neighborhood, and community characteristics, as well as parents and families. Consequently, positive experiences in one area (school, peers, and family) can lessen negative effects in other areas.

Several guidelines are also important for nurses to remember when interacting with adolescents. First, the environment should be caring—positive relationships are encouraged, individual differences are valued, and strengths and weaknesses are acknowledged. Second, nurses need to treat adolescents with dignity and make it a priority to know them as individuals. Third, assessment with the purpose of improving health, describing health promoting behaviors, and understanding is crucial. Fourth, relationships with families are important to develop and maintain. This means frequent communication between nurses, adolescents, and families and encouraging family participation in many health and other issues.

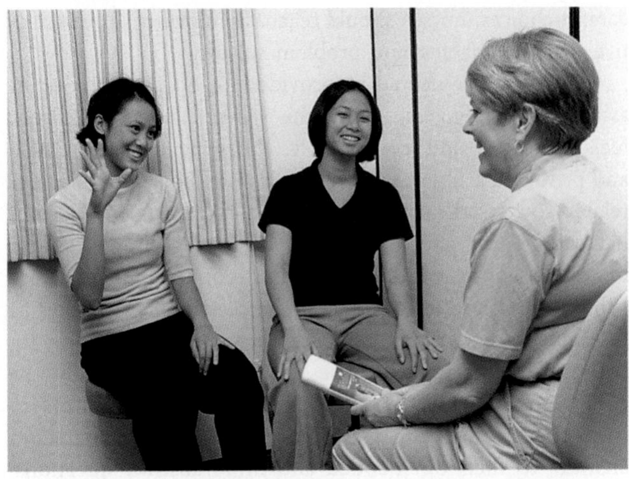

FIGURE 12-24 Nurse–adolescent interactions need to be relaxed, warm, and accepting. DELMAR CENGAGE LEARNING.

Effective nurses also need to know and understand that age, maturational level, and physiological changes have an impact on development, and also understand the specific psychosocial needs and developmental changes expected during adolescence. Interactions should always be individualized, and communications need to convey honesty, general concern, and acceptance. Confidentiality and trust can be important issues for adolescents, which nurses must acknowledge. The physiological, psychosexual, psychosocial, and cognitive changes that normally occur during this period and the many issues and concerns adolescents face today need discussion and explanation. Any program developed for adolescents or their caregivers should present information objectively and accurately, and adolescents themselves should be allowed and encouraged to identify and discuss issues and problems they consider important and provide input into planning.

To work effectively with adolescents, nurses should demonstrate poise, tolerance, warmth, and empathy. They should encourage independence and be aware of hidden adolescent fears or concerns that may be subtly expressed. Nurses also need to be aware of their own biases, which may have an impact on interactions or care delivered. Adolescents should be allowed and encouraged to be responsible for as much of their own personal health care as possible, and helped as needed. Finally, adolescents should be assisted in making appropriate decisions that have an impact on their lives. If they do not know how to make wise decisions and careful choices, nurses should teach them principles of effective decision making and problem solving.

Nursing care should be provided in settings, sometimes away from caregivers, where the self-conscious adolescent feels welcome and comfortable. Allowing sufficient time and privacy for all interactions is essential, so sensitive topics related to physiological growth, sexuality, personal goals, and behaviors (drug abuse, gang membership, promiscuity) can be discussed in an unhurried and nonjudgmental atmosphere. It is not uncommon for successful interactions to resemble conversations between persons with common interests. The interviewer applies developmental principles, so concrete-thinking early adolescents understand answers to their specific questions and older adolescents understand answers to their open-ended and more abstract questions. Confidentiality issues should be discussed early in interactions, since adolescents may confide information to nurses they prefer their caregivers not know about. It is important to make clear early on, however, some issues may need to be shared with caregivers, especially when they are younger adolescents still living at home.

Even though adolescence is generally a time of wellness, these young people will seek health care for skin conditions, minor illnesses, school and sports physicals, management of chronic illness, high-risk behaviors, and conditions related to sexuality. Therefore, all adolescents should have not only vital signs, height, weight, and BMI measured at all visits, but also an assessment of the growth trajectory to determine deviations from normal. In addition, at each visit the Tanner stages should be recorded so progression of pubertal changes can be evaluated. Assessment should also be done annually that checks for scoliosis and goiter. Finally, adolescents should be questioned about their attitudes related to their own physical growth and development, since dissatisfaction may warrant additional probing to elicit unhealthy behaviors such as steroid use, purging, or binging (Dunn, 2009a).

The *Healthy People 2010* (U.S. Department of Health and Human Services, 2000) goals for adolescent health promotion included immunizations, nutrition, oral health, fitness, physical activity, unintentional injury, risky behaviors, violence, substance abuse, sexual behavior, and mental health. These areas are relevant to adolescents because they are the major sources of morbidity and mortality for the adolescent age group. The twelve *Healthy People 2020* (U.S. Department of Health and Human Services, 2010) goals for adolescent health promotion relate to educational achievement, involvement in extracurricular and out-of-school activities, being tested for HIV, having yearly wellness checkups, prohibiting harassment, decreasing the number of adolescents who do not go to school, decreasing violence, encouraging adolescents to be connected to a parent or other positive adult caregiver, decreasing illegal drug activities on school property, helping those with special health care needs transition into an independent and self sufficient adulthood, decreasing criminal activity, and increasing the number of school breakfast programs for adolescents. The *Healthy People 2020* goals for adolescents are particularly relevant to this age group because they reflect advances in scientific knowledge, changing public health priorities, issues related to the country's health preparedness, and major risks to adolescent health/wellness (U.S. Department of Health and Human Services, 2010). A discussion of the 2010 and some of the 2020 goals as well as appropriate nursing interventions follows.

IMMUNIZATIONS

Until recently, immunization or vaccination programs have not focused on improving coverage for adolescents. Since adolescents continue to be adversely affected by preventable diseases such as measles, rubella, hepatitis B, pertussis and varicella, it is important to improve the delivery of immunization services to this age group by implementing the recommended childhood immunization schedule (see Appendix C).

NUTRITION

Adolescence is a time of rapid growth in muscle mass, weight, and height. These physical changes mean increased nutritional needs, especially calories, proteins, and minerals (calcium, riboflavin, niacin, folate, zinc, and iron) (Dunn, 2009a). Calcium is needed to meet skeletal growth requirements, prevent fractures, and help prevent osteoporosis later in life. Zinc is necessary for final body growth and sexual maturation. Iron intake should be increased to meet normally expanding blood volume needs, the increase in lean body mass, and to replace iron lost through menstruation. Males will need more calories than females, especially if they are involved in athletics. Typically, female requirements are around 2,000 calories per day; males will need from 2,500 to 3,000 calories per day (Dietary Guidelines for Americans, 2005). Protein needs also increase. The recommended allowance for females is 46 grams per day and for males is 52 grams per day (Food and Nutrition Board, 2003).

Adolescents always seem hungry but often do not eat appropriate, well-balanced meals. Instead, they prefer snack foods that are easy to prepare, popular with their peers, and often full of empty calories. Perhaps that is why one of the new *Healthy People 2020* goals for adolescents is to increase the percentage of schools with a school breakfast program (U.S. Department of Health and Human Services, 2010). Adolescent food habits are influenced by concerns of their body image, peer pressure, emotional problems, their busy schedules, or unsupervised meal preparation and purchase. It is also not unusual for teenagers to skip meals (breakfast most commonly), eat fast foods, or snack frequently. Therefore, nurses can help caregivers and adolescents improve their nutrition by explaining the importance of a good diet and encouraging adolescents to be involved in meal planning. Caregivers also need to realize that the adolescents' need for freedom, independence, and peer acceptance may be reflected in their eating habits. If nutritious foods and snacks are available (milk, cheese, yogurt, fruits, vegetables, juices), adolescents are regularly allowed to be responsible for preparing family meals, and food preferences (hamburgers, pizza, burritos) are integrated into meal plans, conflicts about nutritional concerns may decrease. Adolescents and their caregivers also need to be aware of the recommended dietary allowances, and know which foods are high in calcium (milk and milk products), iron (green vegetables, meats), and zinc (milk, meat, fish, eggs). Adolescents should also receive information about nutritious snacks and fast foods available in restaurants (salads, pasta, grilled meats, vegetables, fruits).

All health screening visits for adolescents need to include height and weight measurements as well as BP, BMI, and questions about eating habits, including dieting, changes in weight, meal patterns, and consumption of empty-calorie, high-fat, high-salt foods. Nutritional evaluations should also include information about family cultural preferences related to food, whether psychological or psychosocial problems affect eating, and whether nutritional requirements are understood or being met.

At least three issues related to nutrition may surface during the nutritional assessment: obesity, anorexia nervosa, and bulimia nervosa. Obesity is one of the most serious health problems facing today's children and adolescents, and, even though there has been a decrease in dietary fat intake since 1990, obesity rates for childhood and adulthood have dramatically increased (Dunn, 2009a). Obesity in adolescents is the result of environmental, genetic, and physiologic factors that are complexly related (Dunn, 2009b). Children today are more sedentary as compared with a generation ago. The Youth Risk Behavior Surveillance Survey for the United States in 2009 indicated 67.7% of students exercised or participated in physical activities that made them breathe hard and sweat for more than 20 minutes a day between 3 and 7 days preceding the survey (Eaton et al., 2008). One reason for this decline in physical activity may be that mandatory physical education classes are decreasing in schools as children get older, and television, computer games, and video games are popular with young people (Dunn, 2009b). Second, today's children's diets (high in fat, low in fruits and vegetables and complex carbohydrates) promote obesity. High-fat foods tend to be palatable, less satiating, and higher in total energy, and of smaller volume, leading to overconsumption. In addition, fruits, vegetables, and complex carbohydrates may not be popular with children and adolescents. In fact, the Youth Risk Behavior Surveillance Survey of 2009 found only 22.3% of adolescents had eaten fruits and vegetables more than five times a day and only 18% had drunk more than three glasses of milk a day during the week preceding the survey (Eaton et al., 2008).

Finally, factors related to the home environment—parental obesity (more often maternal than paternal), low family income, lower levels of cognitive stimulation in the home, parental occupation, and parenting practices—promote obesity in children and adolescents. Parental obesity is an important risk factor because of child–parent modeling and genetics (Skelton & Rudolph, 2007). Low family income may be related to obesity because of less healthy eating patterns, decreased activity, and an environment that provides high-fat foods and few fruits and vegetables. Lower levels of cognitive development may be related to obesity in children and adolescents because children raised in stimulating and interactive home environments may engage in fewer sedentary activities (television, video games) and more regular physical activity. Parental occupation is a factor if a parent's education is not used in the occupation or if the occupation is nonprofessional. Parenting practices, especially if dysfunctional, have also been linked to obesity. Those suffering from abuse or neglect or having over controlling parents may turn to food for solace and comfort, resulting in obesity (Dunn, 2009b). All these factors are important independent of other socioeconomic factors, including race and caregiver marital status or education.

Obesity in adolescence may also be connected to not being able or wanting to master the psychosocial and psychosexual tasks of adolescence. Overeating compensates as a regression tactic for self-satisfaction or as a coping mechanism for stress. The resulting obesity becomes yet another obstacle to overcome in achieving developmental milestones. Obesity can ward off the pressures associated with puberty and societal expectations and, as long as an adolescent is obese, can repress emotional maturation. For some, obesity can be the reason for their disappointments and eating a method of coping that keeps them connected to their family. This dependence on food and family also interferes with the developmental tasks of separation and individuation. In addition, obesity can interfere with sexuality issues; excess weight protects the adolescent from unwanted sexual advances or attention. Obesity may also represent a way to bring embarrassment and shame to others (caregiver, family), a way of becoming larger than a person not liked (peer), or aggression directed at the self. It is not unusual for obese adolescents to dislike their own physical appearance, express admiration for thin people, and judge others in terms of their own weight. Psychological counseling as well as nutritional and activity counseling may help adolescents develop more mature methods of coping if their obesity is connected to psychosocial or psychosexual issues.

The obese adolescent's sense of identity can also be affected by derogatory comments made by others, leading to guilt, shame, and consequent overeating, which results in more weight gain, more derogatory comments, and even more poor self-esteem. Box 12-1 provides suggestions on ways to help overweight or obese adolescents lose weight.

Mechanical methods of weight loss frequently advertised in popular magazines are another option that can be used alone or in combination with diet and exercise programs. These methods include steam baths, sauna suits, spot reducers, and special exercise outfits. However, they offer only short-term weight loss. Use of appetite-suppressant drugs is typically reserved for adolescents who are severely obese. This option should be managed by a

> **BOX 12-1**
> **HELPING ADOLESCENTS WITH THEIR WEIGHT**
>
> Instruct obese adolescents to:
>
> 1. Avoid purchasing empty-calorie foods; remove empty-calorie snack foods from home.
> 2. Ask self before eating, "Am I hungry?"
> 3. Make dining pleasurable.
> 4. Eat only at mealtimes and at the table; avoid empty-calorie snacks, reduce dietary intake by at least 500 calories daily to lose 1 lb a week.
> 5. Serve individual portions on smaller plates; avoid second helpings.
> 6. Eat slowly by cutting food into small mouthfuls and putting eating utensils down between bites.
> 7. Keep a food diary; examine for empty calories and to see if you are eating traditional food groups.
> 8. Participate in regular exercise (walking, bicycle riding, swimming, etc.).
> 9. Maintain attractive appearance and proper posture.
> 10. Avoid using food as a reward.
> 11. Praise and feel proud of small weight losses.

physician or nurse practitioner. On a final note, it is uncommon for weight-reduction plans to be successful with adolescents, even though many are used. A more realistic alternative goal for those who have difficulty losing weight and keeping it off may be just to not gain any additional weight.

Two other issues related to nutrition in adolescence are anorexia nervosa and bulimia nervosa. Although related, they may have different causes and long-term complications. Both, more commonly seen in females (Dunn, 2009b), are characterized by having a distorted self-image and are psychological illnesses with accompanying physical symptoms. People with anorexia nervosa severely limit their food intake; those with bulimia nervosa have repeated episodes of binge eating followed by the use of laxatives or vomiting. The diagnosis of either should be considered when the adolescent appears underweight, has not achieved normal reproductive milestones for gender, follows a poor diet, or has not achieved anticipated height (Dunn, 2009b). It is important to refer these clients to professionals who specialize in treating clients with eating disorders. See Chapter 35 for a more detailed discussion of adolescent eating disorders.

ORAL HEALTH

During adolescence dental visits occur twice a year, good oral hygiene habits have been established, the majority of orthodontic work has begun, and most permanent teeth have erupted. Third molars (wisdom teeth), however, may erupt in later adolescence (Milgrom, Tut, Chi, Draye, & Acker, 2009) or may become impacted, requiring surgical removal. Although the incidence of dental caries decreases during this time, fluoride supplements (or the need for fluoridated water) should continue until age 16 (Milgrom et al., 2009).

During adolescence, malocclusion, gingivitis, and dental trauma may occur. Malocclusion occurs due to dental crowding or mandibular and facial bone growth changes. Usually, braces are needed to redirect facial and mandibular growth and correct tooth positioning (Figure 12-25). Gingivitis, the inflammation and consequent breakdown of the gingival epithelium, may be seen during adolescence because of ineffective cleaning, high sugar and simple carbohydrate diets, or increased hormonal activity. The gums may bleed easily and appear swollen and pale. Treatment involves brushing the teeth at least twice a day using a soft-bristled brush and fluoride toothpaste, flossing daily, eating a well-balanced diet, and regular dental visits (American Dental Association, 2009a).

Dental trauma, more common in males, often accompanies sports injuries and involves fractured or avulsed teeth, lacerations of the oral mucosa or gums, or jaw fracture. If tooth avulsion (tooth knocked out of socket) occurs, it is important to rinse off the root of the tooth in water if it is dirty by holding the tooth by the crown and then gently insert and hold the tooth back in its socket. If the tooth

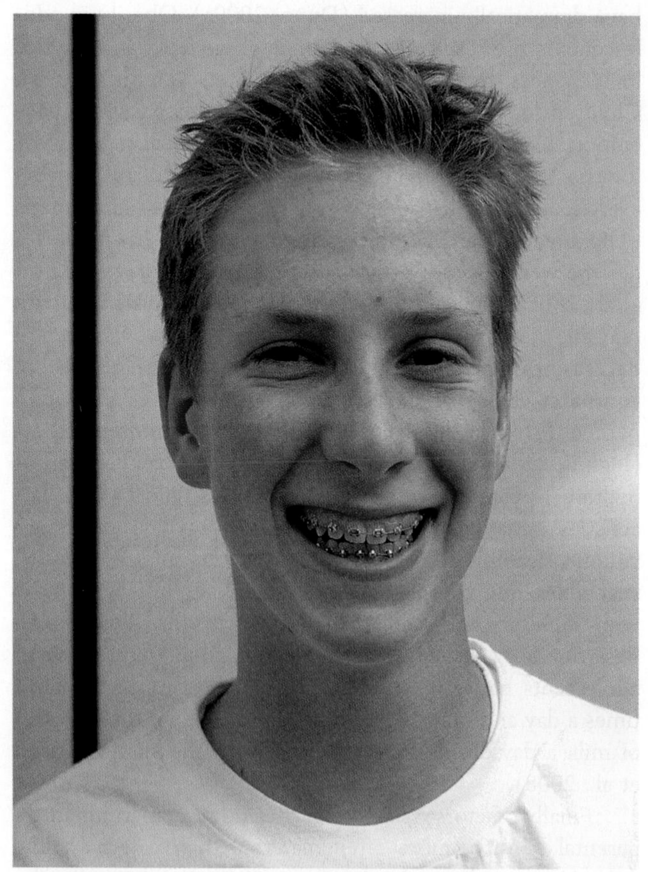

FIGURE 12-25 It is not uncommon to see adolescents wearing braces to treat malocclusions. DELMAR CENGAGE LEARNING.

cannot be repositioned in the socket, it should be placed in a container of milk, and the adolescent taken immediately to the dentist (American Dental Association, 2009b). All cases of dental trauma should be treated as an emergency and a dentist seen as soon as possible.

SLEEP, REST, AND ACTIVITY

Adolescents need approximately 8 hours of sleep per night. Because of their busy schedules (social activities, obligations at school, employment commitments) and rapid physical growth, adolescents often do not receive enough sleep. Many appear fatigued, their schoolwork may suffer, and parents may complain their teens rarely have time to help around the house. Nurses need to educate both parents and adolescents on the importance of adequate rest and sleep and encourage teens to have realistic activity schedules that do not overextend them. An adolescent's excessive anxiety and fatigue may also result in sleep disturbances, which can continue into adulthood since adult sleep cycles and habits are formed during adolescence.

Many adolescents are not as physically active as they should be, even though they are very busy (see previous discussion of nutrition). Perhaps that is why one of the goals for adolescents considered for *Healthy People 2020* is to increase the number of adolescents who participate in extracurricular and out-of-school activities (U.S. Department of Health and Human Services, 2010). There are several health benefits of regular physical activity during childhood and adolescence. Benefits of higher activity levels include increased bone mineral mass, lower levels of alcohol and tobacco use, and lower levels of body fat (American Academy of Pediatrics and the Committee on Sports Medicine and Fitness, 2008). However, only 33% of students enroll in a daily physical education class, and older adolescents were less likely to be enrolled in P.E. classes when compared to younger adolescents (Eaton et al., 2008). Others exercise regularly and develop physically fit bodies. Often, fitness behaviors adopted during adolescence are predictors of fitness habits later in life (Hagan, Shaw, & Duncan, 2008). Adolescents need daily exercise to provide an outlet for tension and anxiety and to maintain muscle tone and development. Regular exercise will also promote healthy sleep patterns and enhance emotional development. Physical activity and fitness may also reduce cardiovascular disease risk factors such as hyperlipidemia, hypertension, and obesity.

The Physical Guidelines for Americans (2008) suggest adolescents should be involved in moderate to vigorous physical activity three or more times a week for at least 30 minutes per session, and be active daily, or nearly every day. *Healthy People 2010* (U.S. Department of Health and Human Services, 2000) goals for adolescents validate these recommendations by encouraging adolescents to increase vigorous activity to at least 20 minutes or more a day for 3 days a week in at least 75% of children and adolescents. However, strength training (known as resistance training) in adolescence can occasionally lead to significant musculoskeletal injury, such as ruptured intervertebral disks, and injuries in the wrist and apophyseal injuries in the spine from weight lifting in skeletally immature individuals (American Academy of Pediatrics and the Council on Sports Medicine and Fitness, 2008). Injuries can be lessened or prevented if the program followed is based on the physical maturity of the individual. Adolescents should be encouraged to participate in sports according to their size rather than according to their chronologic age. Weight-lifting is especially dangerous if the body is not physiologically ready. Sports injuries to late maturing boys are more likely to occur if they participate in contact sports with early maturing, muscular age-mates. It is better to direct adolescents into activities where they will succeed rather than those where they will experience physical and psychological failure. Tennis, swimming, and horsemanship may be some suggestions for alternative, more appropriate activities for adolescents who develop more slowly.

Even though being involved in sports is advantageous for adolescents and participation is increasing, injuries do occur. Most injuries involve falls or being struck by or against objects. Injury rates are higher for males than females, and even noncontact sports (soccer, basketball, baseball, bicycling) may result in head injuries and collisions with other persons.

Nurses can help adolescents increase their physical activity as appropriate to meet the physical activity guidelines for adolescents and avoid injury by considering the adolescent's physical development and capabilities. Therefore, nurses need to inquire about an adolescent's activity program, including frequency, vigor, and preferences, before making any recommendations, as well as determine Tanner staging. Adolescents can also be encouraged to develop interests in sports, recreation, active play, or exercise at home, school, or in the community (Figure 12-26). Any prescribed programs, however, should allow for warm-up and cool-down periods and develop fitness gradually instead of overnight. Adolescents involved in sports need to wear appropriate protective gear, including helmets, pads, and guards, and be aware of safety rules and regulations.

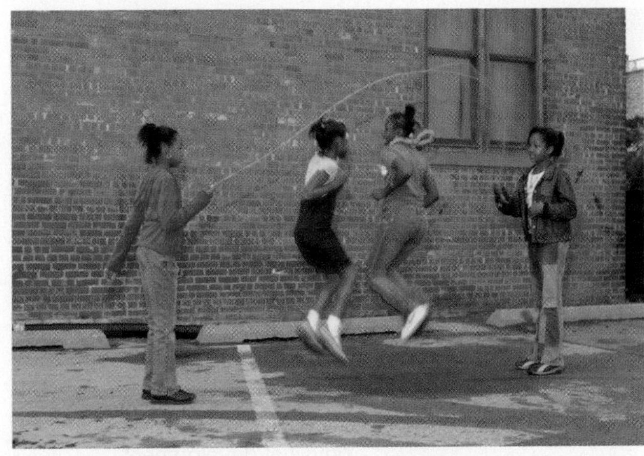

FIGURE 12-26 Physical activity is a popular activity for adolescents, either alone or with others. DELMAR CENGAGE LEARNING.

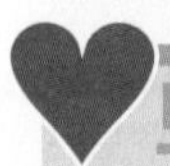

FAMILY TEACHING

Activity

- Initiate exercise programs that are enjoyable, realistic, and consider physical limitations and capabilities. 30 to 60 minutes per day three to four times per week will enhance fitness and set the stage for a lifetime of health. However, sports involving physical contact are not recommended until after PHV.
- Seek out physical education courses at times and places conducive to adolescent participation.
- Evaluate physical development regarding PHV before allowing participation in contact sports.

SAFETY AND INJURY PREVENTION

According to the 2009 Youth Risk Behavioral Surveillance Survey (YRBSS), almost one third of deaths occurring to individuals between ages 16 and 19 are caused by motor vehicle accidents, and drivers in this age group are four times more likely to crash per mile than older drivers (Eaton et al., 2010). Automobiles, motorcycles, motor scooters, mopeds, snowmobiles, minibikes, and all-terrain vehicles cause many adolescent skeletal, head, and spinal cord injuries and abrasions and burns. Approximately 9.7% of teens report they rarely or never wear seat belts. The prevalence of rarely or never worn seat belts was higher in males than in females. In addition, within the last 7 days of the survey, 28.3% of students had ridden in a vehicle of some kind driven by a driver who had been drinking alcohol. In addition, 84.7% rarely or never wear helmets when riding their bicycles (Eaton et al., 2010). Adolescents are also more at risk for sports-related injuries and accidents. Therefore, accident prevention and safety promotion programs are extremely important for the adolescent. Nurses can initiate such programs or become involved in them through clinics, schools, or community agencies serving adolescents. In addition, nurses need to educate adolescents and their caregivers about safety issues and accident prevention (seat belts, helmets while riding bicycles, motorcycles, skateboards, and the use of protective equipment while participating in baseball, football, and soccer), and remind them they are not immortal or immune from being injured (personal fable) if they take unnecessary chances. Table 12-2 presents various hazards and developmental characteristics of adolescents as well as appropriate intervention strategies.

TABLE 12-2 Injury Prevention in Adolescents

HAZARD	DEVELOPMENTAL CHARACTERISTICS	NURSING IMPLICATIONS
Firearms	Independent, believe they are invulnerable	Do not carry or use a weapon to deal with conflict resolution Follow firearm safety rules
Motor vehicles	Take unnecessary risks Like to impress friends	Enroll in drivers' education courses Wear seat belts (driver and passengers) Follow traffic rules and speed limit Do not drink and drive
Poisoning sports	Need peer approval	Be aware of dangers of drug and alcohol use
Contact sports	Physically active	Encourage to stay active and conditioned Wear protective gear, including padding, helmets, and clothing when participating in contact sports or riding bicycles, all-terrain vehicles, motorcycles, skateboards Proper use of sports equipment
Exercise programs	Responsible for self and others	Assess exercise and fitness programs for safety and ability
Outdoor activities	Curious	Integrate safety information about outdoor activities (hiking, camping, fishing, backpacking, etc.) into behavior
Water craft, swimming	Overestimate abilities, stamina, physical development	Avoid drinking alcohol when boating or swimming Learn how to swim Follow rules regarding water safety

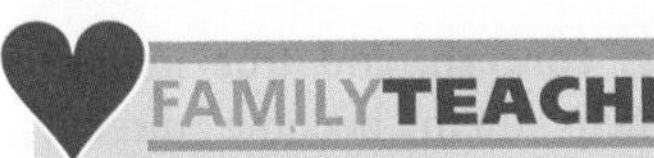

Health Promotion

- Adopt a flexible approach to meals.
- Provide healthy snacks.
- Set realistic sleeping schedules that provide an average of 8 hours of sleep per night.
- Participate in sports according to size rather than according to chronological age.
- Encourage schools to offer nutritious options that appeal to adolescents.
- Search for a variety of activities (tennis, basketball, baseball, softball, hockey, skateboarding, etc.).

RISKY BEHAVIORS

Adolescents also engage in risky behaviors affecting their health and well-being. Two behaviors discussed in the following paragraphs are substance abuse and smoking.

Substance abuse is a maladaptive pattern of alcohol or drug use resulting in significant distress or impairment. Onset often occurs in adolescence and is related to several factors, including positive family history, negative life events, ineffective coping, dysfunctional family relationships, and psychiatric conditions (ADHD, depression, conduct disorders) (Gottesman & Houck, 2009). In fact, according to the 2009 Youth Risk Behavioral Surveillance Survey, 72.5% of students had drunk alcohol, 41.8% of students had consumed one or more drinks of alcohol 30 days before the survey, and 24.2% had consumed more than five drinks in a row and within a couple of hours. Almost 38% had used marijuana and almost 21% had used marijuana one or more times within 30 days of the survey (Eaton et al., 2010). When an adolescent is suspected of substance abuse, it is important to complete a careful assessment that includes an accepting, nonthreatening, nonjudgmental attitude. Behavioral changes indicative of substance abuse include loss of appetite, less attention to hygiene than usual, angry or violent outbursts, withdrawal from family and usual friends, decline in academic performance, deviant or risk-taking behavior, and loss of interest in previously enjoyed activities (Gottesman & Houck, 2009). Refer to Chapter 35 for additional information on substance abuse.

Smoking is another risky behavior seen during adolescence. Smoking is considered a risk-taking behavior because adolescent smokers are more likely than their nonsmoking peers to sell drugs, drop out of school, use marijuana and hard drugs, experience early pregnancy and parenthood, and have multiple drug problems. Those adolescents are also at risk for using predatory and relational violence, low academic performance, behavioral problems at school, and stealing and other delinquent behaviors (Dunn, 2009c). Smoking is positively related to advertising, parent smoking, and portrayal of smoking in films, as well as access to tobacco products in the home and whether a close friend or sibling smokes (Dunn, 2009c).

Nationwide data from the 2009 Youth Risk Behavioral Surveillance Survey showed 46.3% of students tried cigarette smoking and almost 20% of students surveyed smoked more than once during the 30 days preceding the survey. Over 10% of students smoked a cigarette before they were 13 years old. Current cigarette use was highest for males, (19.5%) white (22.5%) and 12th-grade students (25.2%) (Eaton et al., 2010). Adolescent tobacco use can be managed two ways. The first is to prevent use; the second is cessation for those adolescents who do smoke. Prevention strategies include antismoking campaigns directed at teens, increasing the cost of tobacco products, implementing school-based programs, and supporting parenting practices discouraging smoking. Strategies helpful for smoking cessation include informing the adolescent about the health risks of tobacco and how one becomes addicted to nicotine, emphasizing it is easier to stop earlier than later, helping the adolescent identify barriers to stopping, and then implementing strategies to overcome those barriers, determining a realistic stop date, providing information about self help and support groups, and if parents smoke, encouraging them to stop smoking and support them in their efforts (Dunn, 2009c).

VIOLENCE

Older adolescents are more likely to be violent than younger teens; males are more likely to be violent than females. However, since violence is a concern related to all adolescents, the *Healthy People 2020* goals for adolescents include two for this age group related to violence and criminal activity. One involves decreasing the number of public middle and high schools who participate in a violent incident. The other relates to decreasing the number of adolescents involved in criminal activity by decreasing the number of youth involved in violent crimes, the rate of minors' and serious property crimes committed by this age group, and the number of adolescents who are victims of violent crimes (U.S. Department of Health and Human Services, 2010).

A number of variables are related to violent behavior including family factors, individual factors, economic factors, and societal and environmental factors (Brady & Dunn, 2009). Family factors include authoritarian parenting, low parental education, inconsistent disciplinary practices, and poor family functioning. Individual factors include low IQ, poor behavioral control, emotional problems, hyperactivity, substance abuse, and learning disabilities. The economic factor includes living in poverty. Finally, societal and environmental factors include exposure to violence in the media and at school, easy access to drugs, alcohol or weapons, as well as low levels of community participation, coming from a socially disorganized neighborhood, and diminished economic opportunities (Brady & Dunn, 2009).

Violence is a great threat to the lives of adolescents, and those exposed to violence when young are likely to develop depression or PTSD which hinders development (Ozer, 2005). Those factors identified as protective when exposed to violence include social support from peers and adults and connection to school.

The 2009 Youth Risk Behavioral Surveillance Survey suggests the third leading cause of death (16%) for youths and young adults is homicide (Eaton et al., 2010). In addition, 5.9% of students reported they had carried a gun during the past 30 days; 17.5% reported they had carried some form of weapon at least once during the past year. Furthermore, 31.5% of students participated in a physical fight at least once over the past year, and it was higher for males (39.3%) than females (22.9%), and 3.8% of adolescents needed to be treated by a doctor or nurse because of injuries caused by fighting. In addition, 11.1% of the students participated in a physical fight on school property over the last year (Eaton et al., 2010).

During 2009, there was an increasing likelihood of violence having an impact on adolescents. Almost 6% of students felt too unsafe to go to school and said they had carried a gun, knife, or club onto school property at least once in the month preceding the survey. Almost 8% claimed they had been injured or threatened with a weapon on school property during the year before being surveyed (Eaton et al., 2010).

Prevention programs targeted to stem the tide of teen violence are essential and need to involve health care providers, including nurses, caregivers, schools, and other community agencies. Adolescents need connectedness (feelings of warmth, love, caring) with caregivers and schools so they feel a sense of belonging, concern, and true interest in their welfare. This will help them become directly involved and begin to feel some ownership in programs beneficial to their health and well-being. Intervention efforts directed toward creating prosocial environments in the home and school may help prevent and reduce aggressive and violent behavior as well. Affection, involvement, cohesiveness, effective supervision, and acceptance can assist in preventing delinquency and subsequent violent behavior.

CRITICAL THINKING

Violence in the Home

How do you help children who live in a home that puts them at risk for violence?

NURSING TIP

Violence

When working with youths who are victims of violence, ask about the victim's relationship to the perpetrator, circumstances surrounding the event, use of alcohol or drugs, predisposing risk factors (violence in the family, unemployment, truancy), and intentions regarding seeking revenge (Brady & Dunn, 2009).

SEXUAL ACTIVITY

Sexual decision making and behaviors are traditionally controlled by family and societal values. In the past, these values were rather conservative and congruent. Today, however, teenagers have more options than in the past, and are faced with family and societal values that are more liberal and may not be as congruous as they once were. Today, 46% of high school students have engaged in sexual intercourse, 8.9% experience intercourse before they turn 13 years of age, and almost 14% have had sexual intercourse with four or more persons (Eaton et al., 2010). Sexual activity is also related to self-esteem issues; those adolescents most vulnerable and more likely to engage in risk-taking activities associated with sexuality are those adolescents with low self-esteem.

The 2009 YRBSS found the prevalence of sexual activity is higher among black (47.7%) than white (32%) and Hispanic (34.6 %) students (Eaton et al., 2010). Over one-third (34.2%) of adolescents participated in sexual intercourse within three months of being surveyed, and participation was higher among white female (35.4%) and black male (50.3%) than white male (28.9%) and black female (45%) youth. However, 61.1% of sexually active adolescents or their partners used a condom during the last sexual encounter, and 19.8% reported either they or their partner used birth control pills (Eaton et al., 2008).

Adolescents' reasons for becoming sexually active include but are not limited to feeling grown-up; to enhance self-esteem; to experiment; to be accepted by friends; to have someone to care about, love, and be close to; for pleasure; to gain control over one's life; to seek revenge; and to prove they are "normal" (American Academy of Pediatrics Committee on Adolescence, 2000; Herrman, 2008). Since few adolescents have the ego strength or decision-making skills to counter peer pressure from sexually active friends, they may become sexually active against the wishes of their families and some health care providers.

Predictors of early sexual activity include lack of attentive or nurturing parents, early pubertal development, poverty, history of sexual abuse, cultural and family patterns of early sexual experience, poor school performance, lack of school or career goals, and dropping out of school. (Jenkins, 2007b; Klein and the Committee on Adolescence, 2005).

Costs and Rewards of being Pregnant as a Teen

STUDY PURPOSE

To discover adolescents' perceptions of: (1) the personal and social rewards and costs of being pregnant; (2) who in their lives was supportive during their pregnancy; and (3) what would be the most effective intervention strategies to help these teens.

METHODS

During this qualitative descriptive study, 120 adolescents (72 females, 48 males, and mean age 16.1 years) were asked about their lives and stresses, and the costs and rewards related to teen births during seventeen focus groups. Five of the participants were pregnant, 19 of the participants had children, and all but 6 of the students were in school at the time of the study; 68% were African American, 19% were White, 11% were Hispanic.

FINDINGS

The costs and rewards of teen births were organized into three domains. The first domain was the impact on their relationships with friends, their intimate partner, their family, and the public. The second domain was the impact on their vocation, including their education, their future career and ability to work, and finances associated with the pregnancy. The third domain was the impact on the self, including their perception of themselves and parenting. The teens also mentioned several people in their lives who were helpful and supportive including their parents, siblings, other relatives, adult advocates, and some of their friends. Finally, the participants thought adolescents should be educated and given the tools to make responsible decisions; birth control should be more accessible; teen parents should share their personal stories and the realities of teen pregnancy with their non-parenting peers; and the importance of having someone to communicate with about sexuality and pregnancy should be emphasized.

IMPLICATIONS

It would be important for nurses to provide programs for teens based on these data including the costs and rewards of teen pregnancy, participants' ideas on how to prevent pregnancies, and the importance of supportive adults, especially parents, in the lives of teens, whether they are pregnant or not.

REFERENCE

Herrman, J. (2008). Adolescent perceptions of teen births. *JOGNN*, 37, 42–50.

Sexually active young people participate in behaviors that put them at risk for sexually transmitted diseases and pregnancy because they frequently have multiple partners or do not use condoms or other forms of contraception. Sexually transmitted infections (STIs), defined as any disease spread from person to person during sexual contact, are highly communicable, currently considered a public health epidemic, and affect an increasing number of persons. Perhaps that is why one of the *Healthy People 2020* projected goals for adolescents is to increase the number of adolescents who have been tested for HIV (U.S. Department of Health and Human Services, 2010). Reasons for the increased incidence of sexually transmitted diseases include lack of understanding about transmission; breakdown of the family unit; decreased use of contraceptives; changing sexual patterns, attitudes, and mores; the feeling "it can't happen

EVIDENCE-BASED PRACTICE

Parent–Adolescent Relations and Sexual Activity

CLINICAL PROBLEM

Parental caring is associated with less chance their teens will initiate sex, less frequent disagreements about dating, more communications about sex, how much parents monitor teens' behaviors related to dating, and the amount of independence teens are given. This suggests parental caring is important and that parents understand their adolescents need support as they strive for autonomy. However, as teens pass through adolescence, they are less likely to be affected by their parents, especially related to dating decisions and initiating sexual activity.

BEST CLINICAL PRACTICE

Helping parents and adolescents maintain nurturing relationships during adolescence is important. However, as youths get older parents need to encourage independent decisions in a number of areas, including dating.

IMPLICATIONS FOR NURSING

Developing interventions to delay teens' sexual activity must consider the importance of parents. Therefore, nurses should encourage the development and maintenance of warm relationships between parents and their children/adolescents. In addition, parents have to learn that respecting autonomy and allowing growth in teens may help decrease the need to adopt risky behaviors. Such relationships may also help parents maintain credibility when it comes to talking to their adolescents about risky behaviors.

Reference: Longmore, M., Eng, A., Giordano, P., & Manning, W. (2009). Parenting and adolescents' sexual initiation. *Journal of Marriage & the Family, 71*(4), 969–982.

to me"; and increased societal mobility. Common STIs include chlamydia papilloma infections, genital herpes, gonorrhea, trichomonas, and acquired immunodeficiency syndrome (AIDS).

Although birth rates to women under 20 have declined since the 1990s, the United States continues to have one of the highest teenage pregnancy rates among developed countries (Elfenbein, Felice, & Jenkins, 2007; Klein and the Committee on Adolescence, 2005). Many teenage mothers are unmarried, and the resulting unplanned pregnancy affects not only the mother and child, but also the child's father and the respective families because adolescents are often not socially, emotionally, educationally, economically, or physically ready for pregnancy and parenthood.

Several factors related to individual, family and friend, and society influence the incidence of adolescent pregnancy. Individual factors include self-destructive or self-hate feelings and behaviors, egocentrism, low self-esteem, loneliness, recent loss, early maturation, independence from family, lack of responsibility, plea for attention, personal fable, self-punishment, and need to prove one's womanhood. Family and friend factors include having a close relative who has experienced an adolescent pregnancy, conflictual mother-daughter or father–daughter relationships, sexually permissive peer group, inadequate communication, history of sexual abuse or incest, few girlfriends, an older boyfriend, lack of religious affiliation, substance abuse by family and friends, and fulfilling caregiver prophecy when parents suggest their daughter will become pregnant if she does not change her behavior. Societal factors include implied acceptance of intercourse outside marriage, a variety of adult behavioral values, media pressure, inadequate access to contraception, and the availability of public assistance and welfare for single young mothers (Klein and the Committee on Adolescence, 2005).

There are risks associated with adolescent pregnancies—medical and psychological. Medical risks include low birth weight (more than double the rate for adults) and neonatal death (almost three times as high as in adults). The mortality rate for the teenaged pregnant woman is twice as high as for adult pregnant women. Other problems include poor maternal weight gain, pregnancy-induced hypertension, STIs, anemia, and prematurity. Psychological complications include persistent poverty, separation from the child's father, repeat pregnancy, divorce, school interruption, and limited vocational opportunities (Klein and the Committee on Adolescence, 2005).

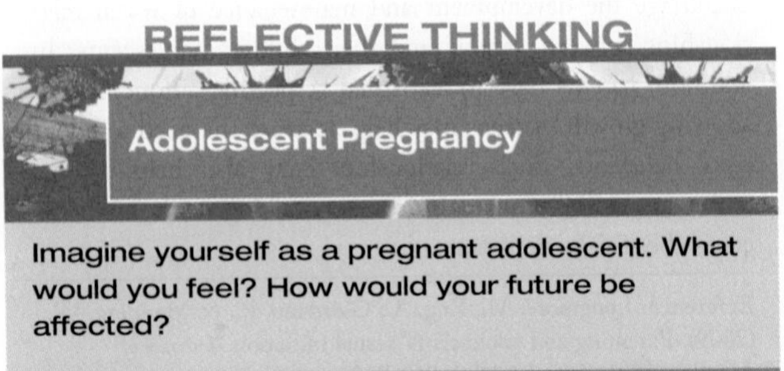

Imagine yourself as a pregnant adolescent. What would you feel? How would your future be affected?

> **NURSING TIP**
>
> **Sexual Activity**
>
> **Assess adolescents' knowledge, feelings, and concerns about sexual preference and activity. Provide accurate information using correct terminology. Refer to appropriate agencies, resources, or caregivers. Ensure adolescents understand that what they are experiencing is a normal part of moving into adulthood.**

Improved methods of contraception and the increased number of sex education courses in the schools reach only a small percentage of adolescents. Not all those students who are sexually active attend such courses or have them readily available, and those adolescents who do participate in the courses may not integrate this information into their behavior because they do not see pregnancy as a concern for themselves or their partners. Therefore, during routine interactions or health assessments, nurses should determine how much an adolescent understands about intercourse, contraception, and reproduction before screening or providing necessary information and support. This includes assessing their understanding and accurate interpretation of risks of being sexually active and then discussing sexual responsibility, including abstinence, how STIs are transmitted, and possible consequences of infection and pregnancy. Adolescents who are sexually active should also receive information about the potential outcomes of their behavior, including ways to reduce their risk of becoming pregnant or infected with STIs or AIDS by limiting the number of sexual partners, using appropriate birth control methods, and consistently using condoms. When adolescents with STIs are identified, they should receive appropriate counseling and medical care. When pregnant adolescents are identified, comprehensive prenatal care is essential to reduce maternal and neonatal complications. Pregnant adolescents should also receive information about available options. Teens who keep their infants need help becoming effective, secure, and comfortable parents. Information about normal infant growth, development, and care should be provided in an accepting, nurturing environment.

HOMOSEXUALITY

Adolescence is an important time for developing one's sexual orientation. During adolescence, individuals typically experience a variety of behaviors and attractions: some reflect experimentation and curiosity; some reflect one's sexual orientation; and some reflect social pressure. Sexual orientation is an early developing, essential, stable predisposition to be sexually attracted to persons of the same sex, the other sex, or both sexes, and includes sexual imagery (attraction), self identity (as bisexual, heterosexual, or homosexual), and sexual behavior (Gerit, Blosser, & Dunn, 2009; Remafedi, 2007). Development of one's sexual orientation is related to genetic, environmental, and hormonal factors (Gerit et al, 2009; Remafedi, 2007), and those with same-sex orientation have most likely experienced the onset of their same-sex sexuality at an early age and more exclusively than those who do not truly have same-sex orientation. In addition, they have childhood indicators of homosexuality (gender atypical behaviors) and have presumed their sexuality.

On average, gay teens come out just before or after high school graduation, and have their first sexual encounter at age 14. However, those who come out earlier tend to have a harder time with their friends, parents, and at school. Acknowledgement of one's attraction to the same sex has changed over time. In the 1960s the age of first same-sex attraction for males was 14 years, whereas in the 1990s males had their first same-sex attraction at around 10 years of age (Savin-Williams, 2005). Most gay adolescents felt different from other boys as children. Many say they initially try to deny their identity as a gay person and many were confused when they first became aware of their preference.

In contrast, development of a same-sex orientation for females is likely to occur later and more abruptly (Diamond, 1998). The age of first sexual contact for lesbians is 16, and in the 1990s females had their first same-sex attraction at age 12. This is earlier than in the 1970s when the average age of same-sex attraction was 17 (Savin-Williams, 2005). Although development of a same-sex identity for many adolescent females will be similar to the developmental trajectory of adolescent males, most females' progression toward a same-sex orientation is likely to be more subject to nonsexual influences (emotions, personal experience, ideological or political beliefs), less associated with childhood indicators (early and pervasive sense of feeling different and gender-atypical behavior or ideation during childhood), and less stable as compared with adolescent males' development of a same-sex orientation (Diamond, 1998). Savin-Williams and Ream (2002) found gay adolescents of both genders were more likely to disclose their sexual orientation to their mothers rather than to their fathers, and to do it in face-to-face encounters. Mothers were told first because the gay adolescent wanted to share his or her life with the mother or because the mother asked. Fathers were told by a person other than the adolescent or by the adolescent because the time was right. If gay adolescents did not tell their fathers, it was because they weren't close, and they did not tell their mothers because it wasn't the right time. Although sons feared their parents' negative reactions more than daughters, parents were slightly negative and supportive for both genders. Parental relationships either improved or didn't change after disclosure. When acknowledging their sexual orientation, adolescent reactions ranged from being happy and relieved to depressed, anxious, and having suicidal thoughts (Santrock, 2010).

Nurses need to recognize that even though many young people explore their own sexual orientation or homosexual attractions, few who engage in homosexual behavior during adolescence continue the practice into adulthood (Santrock, 2010). Thus, nurses and caregivers need to help young people recognize that homosexual experimentation is not the same as establishing a homosexual orientation, and phrase questions about sexuality and sexual activity carefully and respectfully.

EFFECT OF TELEVISION AND OTHER MEDIA ON ADOLESCENTS

Media in America contribute to more adverse health outcomes than to prosocial or positive outcomes. This is especially true with regard to violence, guns, sex, and drugs. For example, cross-sectional, naturalistic, and longitudinal studies as well as several meta-analyses suggest there is a relationship between media violence, real-life aggression, and acceptance of aggressive attitudes. Those exposed to violence on television and the media tend to be more likely to commit violent acts. Research also suggests adolescents exposed to greater amounts of alcohol or tobacco advertising are more likely to use or intend to use those products as compared with those adolescents who are not exposed to those products. One-third of teens who smoke could link their smoking to tobacco promotional activities. Research also shows adolescent drinkers are more likely to have been exposed to alcohol via the media than non-adolescent drinkers (American Academy of Pediatrics and the Committee on Communications, 2006).

Box 12-2 lists the effects of television and other media on adolescents. The dominant youth media today are TV and music. In fact 15- to 18-year-olds spend about 2 1/2 hours a day watching TV and 1 1/2 hours a day listening to music. In addition, they spend just over 1 hour a day on computers outside of school or work and just less than 1/2 hour a day playing video games (Rideout, Roberts, & Foehr, 2005). Most homes where 8- to 18-year-olds live have an average of 3.6 CD or tape players, 3.5 TVs, 3.3 radios, 2.9 DVD players, 2.1 video game consoles, and 1.5 computers. It is also not uncommon for adolescents to spend additional time during a day using the Internet, computers, and video games while not reducing the time spent with television, music, and print media. In fact, two-thirds of 8- to 18-year-olds have a television in their bedrooms, 54% have a VCR or DVD, 49% have a video game player, 37% have satellite or cable TV, 31% have a computer, and 20% have Internet access in their bedroom. Most adolescents eat, talk on the phone, or do homework while watching TV (Rideout et al., 2005).

Even though those young people who watch more than 5 hours of TV a day reported spending more time with their

BOX 12-2

EFFECT OF TELEVISION AND OTHER MEDIA ON ADOLESCENTS

1. 2–3 hours/day means less physical activity, reading, and interaction with friends.
2. 10,000 acts of violence viewed/year; 26% involved use of guns.
3. 15,000 sexual references, innuendoes, jokes per year; 170 deal with abstinence, birth control, pregnancy, STIs.
4. 70% of content from prime-time dramatic programs contains references to alcohol, tobacco, illicit drugs; over 50% of movies contain references to tobacco or smoking; for every "just say no" public service announcement, 25–50 beer and wine advertisements will be viewed.

parents than other groups, it is unclear exactly the type of interaction is occurring between parent and children. When examining how content 8- to 18-year-olds are, those who are less content spend more time using media than those 8- to 18-year-olds who are "most content." In addition, those youth with the lowest grades spend less time reading and more time playing video games than those with the best grades (Rideout et al., 2005).

Caregivers need to control or monitor the media programming their teens watch, and remove television sets from teens' bedrooms. Specifically, this means to limit all media use to no more than 1 to 2 hours per day, view television with their adolescents, and monitor their child or adolescent's use of the media.

IN THE REAL WORLD

This past week I cared for 16-year-old Noah, who had had a ureteral resection. Madison (the other nurse) and I spoke with him frankly about procedures, care plans, and equipment. At one point I explained how a pulse oximeter worked to measure oxygen-carrying productivity. This 6-foot, 90-kg young man did not need to be babied, but he did need to be respected and supported in his recovery. Recognizing adolescents' general desire for privacy and sensitivity about anatomy, I tried to keep him well-covered and work as professionally as possible. Noah was appreciative, polite, and cooperative.

KEY CONCEPTS

- In order to effectively identify issues and problems commonly seen in adolescence and consequently deliver appropriate and individualized nursing care, the physiological, psychosexual, psychosocial, cognitive, and moral transformations occurring during this time, as well as changes in adolescents' rapidly expanding social context, including the family, school, and peers should be considered.
- The physiological changes that occur during adolescence are extensive, do not occur in isolation, and have an impact on the adolescent's psychosexual, psychosocial, and cognitive development. These changes also affect the experiences adolescents have with family members, peers, and others in their social world, as well as their own body image and self-esteem.
- Young people are able to consider all possible solutions to a problem, both real and abstract, and can assess options and determine the best solution.
- Elkind identified two types of social thinking particularly evident during adolescence—imaginary audience and personal fable.
- Adolescents' psychosocial orientation is affected by their family, peers, and school experiences.
- Adolescents' identity is based on individual and group identifications established during childhood; their ability to master each developmental task presented to them by society; and establishing their own ideology, based on social, political, and religious attitudes and values.
- Nurses working with adolescents need to be respectful and demonstrate openness, competence, honesty, warmth, compassion, and understanding and have the ability to communicate effectively with adolescents and their families.
- Adolescents' health promotion topics include immunizations, nutrition, oral health, fitness, physical activity, unintentional injury, risky behaviors, violence, substance abuse, sexual behavior, and mental health.

REVIEW ACTIVITIES

1. Why is adolescence such an important period of life?
2. What are the Tanner stages and why are they important?
3. How do thinking processes change during adolescence? How are adolescents helped to learn?
4. What factors are important in adolescent identity development?
5. What identity statuses do adolescents experience as they attempt to answer the question, "Who am I?"
6. How do parents, siblings, and peers influence adolescent development?
7. Why does school have such a profound influence on adolescents? What are the positive and negative effects of schools on adolescents?
8. How do work experiences influence adolescents?
9. What are at least five issues adolescents face that have an impact on their health and well-being?
10. How might a nurse interact effectively with adolescents?
11. What are the health promotion or screening activities nurses need to be concerned about with adolescents?

STUDY QUESTIONS

1. Which of the following statements about physiological development of adolescents is true?
   a. The physiological changes that occur during adolescence occur in isolation and therefore are not related to psychosexual, cognitive, or psychological development.
   b. The age of onset, intensity, and duration of the adolescent growth spurt does not vary across gender or individually.
   c. Although fully developed in size, the right and left hemispheres of the brain continue to thicken and process information more efficiently during adolescence.
   d. For females the first sign of sexual maturation is growth of pubic hair; for males, the first sign of sexual maturation is darkening of the scrotum.
2. Which of the following statements is true about psychosexual or psychosocial development?
   a. An adolescent's body image is often influenced by present/past experiences, level of cognitive development, identity formation, as well as one's degree of attractiveness, size, and physique appropriate to gender.
   b. Two major tasks of adolescence (figuring out who they are and what their unique place is in the world) occur in isolation.
   c. An adolescent with a foreclosed identity has not experienced any active exploration of what the possibilities are, nor made any commitment toward an occupation.
   d. In order to facilitate adolescent psychosocial development it would be important to allow adolescents to take little part in family decision making and discourage exploration of career options.
3. The following statements relate to adolescent cognitive development. Which statement is true?
   a. Piaget suggests adolescent cognitive development involves being aware of what is real rather than the possibilities of what may be real.
   b. The zone of proximal development suggests students are capable of understanding difficult concepts if they are coached by a teacher who pushes them to think at a higher level and is sensitive to their potential.
   c. The imaginary audience and personal fable rarely affect adolescent behaviors because they are aware of their own uniqueness and are proud of their skills and abilities.
   d. Social perspective-taking allows an adolescent to ignore relationships with others and therefore think and dress as one wants rather than as peers may think and dress.
4. The statements below discuss parent–adolescent conflict. If parents come to you for advice about conflicts they are having with their adolescent, which of the following statements can you use in discussing the issue?
   a. "Conflict between adolescents and their parents is highest during late adolescence."
   b. "Topics of conflicts adolescents have with their mothers are different than topics of conflicts they have with their fathers."
   c. "If parents use psychological control (controlling a person's behavior by guilt induction), the adolescent is at risk for failing, having low self-esteem, and becoming depressed."
   d. "Conflict between parents and adolescents is rare and should not be a concern to parents."

5. The following statements relate to adolescent–peer relationships. Which is correct?
   a. Peer relationships are not important to adolescents, especially if they have positive self-esteem.
   b. Adolescent crowds provide an alternate family structure for adolescents and are usually made up of both gender adolescents.
   c. Adolescents who are secure in their relationships with others are more likely to engage in behavior they would otherwise avoid.
   d. Adolescents who are on the periphery of their peer group are most vulnerable to peer influences because of their position within the group.
6. School is important for adolescents. Which of the following statements is true?
   a. Those adolescents who do not feel connected to school report lower levels of well-being and have more psychological problems than those who feel connected to their school.
   b. An adolescent's feelings of connection to school depend mainly on parents' views of the school.
   c. Skipping school is common during adolescence and is an issue that should be ignored by parents.
   d. The transition from middle school to high school rarely affects adolescents because relationships with teachers are similar to those of middle school.
7. Adolescents are faced with several issues and nurses need to be aware of not only how to interact with adolescents but also how best to help them through these issues. Consequently which of the following statements is not true?
   a. To work effectively with adolescents, nurses should demonstrate poise, tolerance, warmth, and empathy.
   b. Nurses do not need to be aware of their own biases, since they rarely have an impact on interactions or care delivered.
   c. Nursing care should be provided in settings, sometimes away from caregivers, where the self-conscious adolescent feels welcome and comfortable.
   d. Allowing sufficient time and privacy for all interactions is essential, so sensitive topics can be discussed in an unhurried and nonjudgmental atmosphere.
8. Below are several statements related to adolescents; only one is correct.
   a. Caregivers need to realize that adolescents' need for freedom, independence, and peer acceptance is rarely reflected in their eating habits.
   b. Obesity in adolescence may also be connected to not wanting or being able to master the psychosocial and psychosexual tasks of adolescence.
   c. It is difficult to provide helpful suggestions to adolescents struggling with their weight because suggestions rarely work.
   d. Adolescents should not be concerned about their activity levels since they often are more active than they need to be.
9. The statements below relate to suggestions to help adolescents remain healthy. Which one is incorrect?
   a. Nurses need to inquire about an adolescent's activity program, including frequency, vigor, and preferences, before making any recommendations.
   b. Nurses need to educate adolescents and their caregivers about safety issues and accident prevention, and remind them they are not immortal or immune from being injured (personal fable) if they take unnecessary chances.
   c. When working with youths who are victims of violence, ask about the victim's relationship to the perpetrator, circumstances surrounding the event, use of alcohol or drugs, and predisposing risk factors.
   d. Since smoking is not common in adolescents, nurses do not need to talk to them about prevention strategies or risks to their health if they choose to smoke.
10. Adolescent pregnancy is a concern to parents and teens. Which of the following statements would be the best response to parents who ask you to talk to them about adolescent pregnancy?
    a. "Adolescents' reasons for becoming sexually active include feeling grown-up; to enhance self-esteem; to experiment; to be accepted by friends; to have someone to care about, love, and be close to; for pleasure; to gain control over one's life; to seek revenge; and to prove they are 'normal.'"
    b. "Sexually active young people rarely are exposed to sexually transmitted disease because they usually have one partner and use condoms or other forms of contraception."
    c. "There are few risks associated with adolescent pregnancies since those teens that become pregnant are usually healthy and the rate of neonatal death is low for these mothers."
    d. "Improved methods of contraception and the increased number of sex education courses in the schools reach most adolescents who then integrate this information into their behavior."

REFERENCES

Abbassi, V. (1998). Growth and normal puberty. *Pediatrics, 102,* 507–511.

Allen, J. P., Porter, M., McFarland, C., McElhaney, K. B., & Marsh, P. (2007). The relation of attachment security to adolescents' paternal and peer relationships, depression, and externalizing behavior. *Child Development, 78*(4), 1222–1239.

Amato, P. R. (2000). The consequences of divorce for adults and children. *Journal of Marriage & Family, 62*(4), 1269–1287.

Amato, P. R., & Cheadle, J. (2005). The long reach of divorce: Divorce and child well-being across three generations. *Journal of Marriage & Family, 67*(1), 191–206.

Amato, P. R., & Sobolewski, J. M. (2001). The effects of divorce and marital discord on adult children's psychological well-being. *American Sociological Review, 66*(6), 900–921.

Amato Booth, 379.

American Academy of Pediatrics and the Council on Sports Medicine and Fitness. (2008). Policy statement: Strength Training by Children and Adolescents. *Pediatrics, 121*(4), 835–840.

American Academy of Pediatrics and the Committee on Communications. (2006). Children, adolescents, and advertising. *Pediatrics, 11,* 2563–2569.

American Academy of Pediatrics Committee on Adolescence. (2000). Adolescent pregnancy—Current trends and issues: 1998. *Pediatrics, 103*(2), 516–520.

American Dental Association. (2009a). Oral health topics: Periodontal (gum) diseases. Retrieved August 20, 2009, from http://www.ada.org/public/topics/periodontal_diseases_faq.asp.

American Dental Association. (2009b). Dental emergencies and injuries. Retrieved August 20, 2009, from http://www.ada.org/public/manage/emergencies.asp#broken.

Arnett, J. (1999). Adolescent storm and stress, reconsidered. *American Psychologist, 54*(5), 317–326.

Barber, B. K. (2002). Reintroducing parental psychological control. In B. K. Barber (Ed.). *Intrusive parenting: How psychological control affects children and adolescents.* Washington, DC: American Psychological Association: 3–13.

Barber, B. K., & Harmon, E. L. (2002). Violating the self: Parental psychological control of children and adolescents. In B. K. Barber (Ed.). *Intrusive parenting: How psychological control affects children and adolescents.* Washington, DC: American Psychological Association: 15–52.

Barber, C. N., Hall, J., & Armistead, L. (2003). Parent–adolescent relationship and adolescent psychological functioning among African-American female adolescents. *Journal of Child & Family Studies, 12*(3), 361–374.

Becker-Stoll, F., Fremmer-Bombik, E., Wartner, U., Zimmermann, P., & Grossmann, K. E. (2008). Is attachment at ages 1, 6 and 16 related to autonomy and relatedness behavior of adolescents in interaction towards their mothers? *International Journal of Behavioral Development, 32*(5), 372–380.

Benner, A., & Graham, S. (2009). The transition to high school as a developmental process among multiethnic urban youth. *Child Development, 80*(2), 356–376.

Bouchey, H. A., & Furman, W. (2006) Dating and romantic experiences in adolescence. In G. R. Adams & M. D. Berzonsky (Eds.). *Blackwell handbook of adolescence.* Malden, MA: Blackwell.

Brady, M., & Dunn, A. (2009). Role relationships. In C. E. Burns, A. M. Dunn, M. A. Brady, N. B. Starr, & C. G. Blosser (Eds.), *Pediatric primary care* (4th ed.). St. Louis: Saunders, 366–394.

Brown, B. B. (2004). Adolescents' relationships with peers. In R. M. Lerner & L. Steinberg (Eds.). *Handbook of adolescent psychology* (2nd ed.). Hoboken, NJ: John Wiley & Sons: 363–394.

Brown, B. B., & Klute, C. (2006). Friendships, cliques, and crowds. In G. R. Adams & M. D. Berzonsky (Eds.). *Blackwell handbook of adolescence.* Malden, MA: Blackwell.

Burchett, M., Hanna, C., & Steiner, R. (2009). Endocrine and metabolic disorders, In Burns CE, Dunn AM, Brady MA et al., (Eds.). *Pediatric Primary Care* (4th ed.), 2009; 584–590.

Chandra, A., Martino, S., Collins, R., Elliott, M., Berry, S., Kanouse, D., & Miu, A., (2008). Does watching sex on television predict teen pregnancy? Findings from a national longitudinal survey of youth. *Pediatrics, 122,* 1047–1054. DOI: 10.1542/peds.2007-3066.

Clark, T. R., & Phares, V. (2004). Feelings in the family: Interparental conflict, anger, and expressiveness in families with older adolescents. *Family Journal, 12*(2), 129–138.

Cloninger, S. C. (2008). *Theories of personality: Understanding persons* (5th ed.). Upper Saddle River, NJ: Prentice Hall.

Coie, J. D. (2004). The impact of negative social experiences on the development of antisocial behavior. In J. B. Kupersmidt & K. A. Dodge (Eds.). *Children's peer relations: From development to intervention.* Washington, DC: American Psychological Association.

Coughlin, J. P., & Malis, R. S. (2004). Demand/withdraw communication between parents and adolescents: Connections with self-esteem and substance use. *Journal of Social and Personal Relationships, 21*(1), 125–148.

Diamond, L. M. (1998). Development of sexual orientation among adolescent and young adult women. *Developmental Psychology, 34,* 1085–1095.

Diamond, L. M., & Savin-Williams, R. C. (2006). The intimate relationships of sexual-minority youths. In G. R. Adams & M. D. Berzonsky (Eds.). *Blackwell handbook of adolescence.* Malden, MA: Blackwell.

Dietary Guidelines for Americans. (2005). Retrieved April 9, 2010, from http://www.health.gov/dietaryguidelines/dga2005/document/html/chapter2.htm.

Doherty, W. J., & Needle, R. H. (1991). Psychological adjustment and substance use among adolescents before and after a parental divorce. *Child Development, 62*(2), 328.

Dunn, A. (2009a). Developmental management of adolescents. In C. E. Burns, A. M. Dunn, M. A. Brady, N. B. Starr, & C. G. Blosser (Eds.). *Pediatric primary care* (4th ed.). St. Louis: Saunders, 132–150.

Dunn, A. (2009b). Nutrition. In C. E. Burns, A. M. Dunn, M. A. Brady, N. B. Starr, & C. G. Blosser (Eds.). *Pediatric primary care* (4th ed.). St. Louis: Saunders, 191–234.

Dunn, A. (2009c). Health perception and health management patterns. In C. E. Burns, A. M. Dunn, M. A. Brady, N. B. Starr, & C. G. Blosser (Eds.). *Pediatric primary care* (4th ed.). St. Louis: Saunders, 168–190.

Dunphy, D. C. (1963). The social structure of urban adolescent peer groups. *Sociometry, 26,* 230–246.

Eaton, D., Kann, L., Kinchen, S., Shanklin, S., Ross, J., Hawkins, J. et al. (2010). *Youth Risk Behavior Surveillance—United States, 2009. Morbidity and Mortality Weekly Report*, June 4, 2010/Vol. 59/ No. SS-5.

Elfenbein, D., Felice, M., & Jenkins, F. (2007). Adolescent pregnancy. In R. Kliegman, R. Behrman, H. Jenson, & B. Stanton. *Nelson's textbook of pediatrics* (18th ed.). Philadelphia, PA: Saunders/ Elsevier, 850–853.

Elkind, D. (1967). Egocentrism in adolescence. *Child Development, 38*, 1025–1034.

Elkind, D. (1984). *All grown up and no place to go: Teenagers in crisis.* Reading, MA: Addison-Wesley.

Elkind, D. (1985). Egocentrism redux. *Developmental Review, 5*(3), 218–226.

Erikson, E. H. (1968). *Identity: Youth and crisis.* New York: Norton.

Eveleth, P. B., & Tanner, J. M. (1990). *Worldwide variation in human growth* (2nd ed.). Cambridge, UK: Cambridge University Press.

Faircloth, B. (2009). Making the most of adolescence: Harnessing the search for identity to understand classroom belonging. *Journal of Adolescent Research, 24*, 321–348.

Food and Nutrition Board. (2003). *Dietary reference intakes for energy, carbohydrate, fiber, fat, fatty acids, cholesterol, protein, and amino acids.* Washington DC: Institute of Medicine.

Garibaldi, L. (2007a). Physiology of puberty. In R. Kliegman, R. Behrman, H. Jenson, & B. Stanton. *Nelson's textbook of pediatrics* (18th ed.). Philadelphia, PA: Saunders/Elsevier, 2308.

Garibaldi, L. (2007b). Disorders of pubertal development, In R. Kliegman, R. Behrman, H. Jenson, & B. Stanton. *Nelson's textbook of pediatrics* (18th ed.). Philadelphia, PA: Saunders/Elsevier, 2309–2316.

Gerit, T., Blosser, C., & Dunn, A. (2009). Sexuality. In C. E. Burns, A. M. Dunn, M. A. Brady, N. B. Starr, & C. G. Blosser (Eds.). *Pediatric primary care* (4th ed.). St. Louis: Saunders, 395–410.

Giedd, J. (2008). The teen brain: Insights from neuroimaging. *Journal of Adolescent Health, 42*(4), 335–343.

Gilligan, C. (1982). *In a different voice.* Cambridge, MA: Harvard University Press.

Gilligan, C., Lyons, N., & Hanmer, T. (Eds.). (1990). *Making connections: The relational worlds of adolescent girls at Emma Willard School.* Cambridge, MA: Harvard University Press.

Ginzberg, E. (1972). Toward a theory of occupational choice: A restatement. *Vocational Guidance Quarterly, 20*, 169–176.

Gottesman, M., & Houck, G. (2009). Coping and stress tolerance: Mental health problems of children and adolescents. In C. E. Burns, A. M. Dunn, M. A. Brady, N. B. Starr, & C. G. Blosser (Eds.). *Pediatric primary care* (4th ed.). St. Louis: Saunders, 411–440.

Graber, J. A., Brooks-Gunn, J., & Warren, M. P. (2006). Pubertal effects on adjustment in girls: Moving from demonstrating effects to identifying pathways. *Journal of Youth and Adolescence, 35*(3), 413–423.

Greenberger, E., & Steinberg, L. (1986) *When teenagers work.* New York: Basic Books.

Grotevant, H. D., & Cooper, C. R. (1998). Individuality and connectedness in adolescent development: Review and prospects for research on identity, relationships, and context. In E. E. A. Skoe & A. L. von der Lippe (Eds.). *Personality development in adolescence: A cross national and life span perspective.* Florence, KY: Taylor & Frances/Routledge, 3–37.

Grych, J. H., Raynor, S. R., & Fosco, G. M. (2004). Family processes that shape the impact of interparental conflict on adolescents. *Development & Psychopathology, 16*(3), 649–665.

Hagan, J., Shaw, J., & Duncan, P. (2008). *Bright futures: Guidelines for health supervision of infants, children, and adolescents.* Elk Grove Village, IL: American Academy of Pediatrics.

Harter, S., (2001). *The construction of the self: A developmental perspective.* Guilford Press. NY.

Herrman, J. (2008). Adolescent perceptions of teen births. *JOGGN, 37*, 42–50.

Hetherington, E. M., Stanley-Hagan, M., & Anderson, E. R. (1989). Marital transitions: A child's perspective. *American Psychologist, 44*(2), 303–312.

Hetherington, E. M., Anderson, E. R., & Hagan, M. S. (1991). Divorce: Effects on adolescents. In R. M. Lerner, A. D. Petersen, & J. Brooks-Gunn (Eds.). *Encyclopedia of adolescence (Vol. 1).* New York: Garland.

Hill, J. P., & Lynch, M. E. (1983). *The intensification of gender-related role expectations during early adolescence.* New York: Plenum.

Jenkins, R. (2007a). Menstrual problems. In R. Kliegman, R. Behrman, H. Jenson, & B. Stanton. *Nelson's textbook of pediatrics* (18th ed.). Philadelphia, PA: Saunders/Elsevier, 836–844.

Jenkins, R. (2007b). Contraception. In R. Kliegman, R. Behrman, H. Jenson, & B. Stanton. *Nelson's textbook of pediatrics* (18th ed.). Philadelphia, PA: Saunders/Elsevier, 844–850.

Katchadourian, H. (1977). *The biology of adolescence.* San Francisco: Freeman.

Keating, D. (2009). Cognitive and brain development. In R. M. Lerner & L. Steinberg (Eds.). *Handbook of adolescent psychology* (3rd ed.). Hoboken, NJ: John Wiley & Sons, 45–84.

Kerr, M., & Stattin, H. (2000). What parents know, how they know it, and several forms of adolescent adjustment: Further support for a reinterpretation of monitoring. *Developmental Psychology, 36*, 366–380.

Klein, J. D., & the Committee on Adolescence. (2005). Adolescent pregnancy: Current trends and issues. *Pediatrics, 116*(1), 281–286.

Kohlberg, L. (1976). Moral stages and moralization: The cognitive-development approach. In T. Lickona (Ed.). *Moral development and behavior.* New York: Holt, Rinehart and Winston.

Kozulin, A. (1990). *Vygotsky's psychology: A biography of ideas.* Cambridge, MA: Harvard University Press.

Lapsley, D. K. (1990). Continuity and discontinuity in adolescent social cognitive development. In R. Montemayor, G. Adams, & T. Gullotta (Eds.). *From childhood to adolescence: A transitional period?* Newbury Park, CA: Sage.

Lobel, T. E., Nov-Krispin, N., Schiller, D., Lobel, O., & Feldman, A. (2004). Gender discriminatory behavior during adolescence and young adulthood: A developmental analysis. *Journal of Youth & Adolescence, 33*(6), 535–546.

Longmore, M., Eng, A., Giordano, P., & Manning, W. (2009). Parenting and adolescents' sexual initiation. *Journal of Marriage & the Family, 71*(4), 969–982.

Maccoby, E. E., & Martin, J. A. (1983). Socialization in the context of the family: Parent–child interaction. In P. H. Mussen & E. M. Hetherington (Eds.). *Handbook of child psychology: Vol. 4. Socialization, personality, and social development* (4th ed.). New York: Wiley, 1–101.

Malina, R., & Bouchard, C. (1991). *Growth maturation and physical activity*. Champaign, IL: Human Kinetics.

Marcell, A. (2007). Adolescence. In R. Kliegman, R. Behrman, H. Jenson, & B. Stanton. *Nelson's textbook of pediatrics* (18th ed.). Philadelphia, PA: Saunders/Elsevier, 60–65.

Marcia, J. E. (1980). Identity in adolescence. In *Handbook of adolescent psychology*. New York: John Wiley & Sons, 159–187.

Marshall, W. A., & Tanner, J. M. (1969). Variations in the pattern of pubertal changes in girls. *Archives of Disease in Childhood, 44*, 291–303.

Marshall, W. A., & Tanner, J. M. (1970). Variations in the pattern of pubertal changes in boys. *Archives of Disease in Childhood, 45*, 13–23.

McCabe, M. P., & Ricciardelli, L. A. (2005). A prospective study of pressures from parents, peers, and the media on extreme weight change behaviors among adolescent boys and girls. *Behaviour Research and Therapy, 43*(5), 653–668.

McCoy, J. K., Brody, G. H., & Stoneman, Z. (2002). Temperament and the quality of best friendships: Effect of same-sex sibling relationships. *Family Relations, 51*(3), 248.

Milgrom, P., Tut, O., Chi, D., Draye, M., & Acker, M. (2009). Dental and oral disorders. In C. E. Burns, A. M. Dunn, M. A. Brady, N. B. Starr, & C. G. Blosser (Eds.). *Pediatric primary care* (4th ed.). St. Louis: Saunders, 845–865.

Neinstein, L. S., & Kaufman, F. R. (2002). Normal physical growth and development. In L. S. Neinstein (Ed.). *Adolescent health care: A practical guide* (3rd ed.). Baltimore: Williams & Wilkins, 3–58.

Nonnemaker, J. M., McNeely, C. A., & Blum, R. W. (2003). Public and private domains of religiosity and adolescent health risk behaviors: Evidence from the national longitudinal study of adolescent health. *Social Science & Medicine, 57*(11), 2049.

Ozer, E. J. (2005). The impact of violence on urban adolescents: Longitudinal effects of perceived school connection and family support. *Journal of Adolescent Research, 20*(2), 167–192.

Physical Guidelines for Americans. (2008). Chapter 3: Active Children and Adolescents. Retrieved April 9, 2010, from http://www.health.gov/paguidelines/guidelines/chapter3.aspx.

Piaget, J. (1972). Intellectual evolution from adolescence to adulthood. *Human Development, 15*, 1–12.

Pinyerd, B., & Zipf, W. B. (2005). Puberty—timing is everything! *Journal of Pediatric Nursing, 20*(2), 75–82.

Regnerus, p. 375.

Remafedi, G. (2007). Adolescent homosexuality. In R. Kliegman, R. Behrman, H. Jenson, & B. Stanton. *Nelson's textbook of pediatrics* (18th ed.). Philadelphia, PA: Saunders/Elsevier, 68–70.

Rideout, V., Roberts, D. F., & Foehr, U. G. (2005). *Generation M: Media in the lives of 8–18 year olds*. Menlo Park, CA: The Henry J. Kaiser Family Foundation.

Riesch, S. K., Bush, L., Nelson, C. J., Ohm, B. J., Portz, P. A., Abell, B., Wightman, M. R., and Jenkins, P. (2000). Topics of conflict between parents and young adolescents. *Journal of the Society for Pediatric Nurses, 5*(1), 27–39.

Riesch, S. K., Jackson, N. M., and Chanchong, W. (2003). Communication approaches to parent-child conflict: Young adolescence to young adult. *Journal of Pediatric Nursing, 18*(4), 244-256.

Rosenblum, G. D., & Lewis, M. (1999). The relations among body image, physical attractiveness and body mass in adolescence. *Child Development, 70*, 50–64.

Santrock, J. W. (2010). *Adolescence* (13th ed.). Boston: McGraw-Hill.

Savin-Williams, R. C. (2005). *The new gay teenager (adolescent lives)*. Cambridge, MA: Harvard University Press.

Savin-Williams, R. C., & Ream, G. L. (2002). Sex variations in the disclosure to parents of same-sex attractions. *Journal of Family Psychology, 17*(3), 429–438.

Selman, R. L. (1980). *The growth of interpersonal understanding*. New York: Academic.

Shaffer, D. R. (2009). *Social and personality development* (6th ed.). Belmont, CA: Wadsworth Publishing.

Skelton, J., & Rudolph, C. (2007). Overweight and Obesity. In R. Kliegman, R. Behrman, H. Jenson, & B. Stanton. *Nelson's textbook of pediatrics* (18th ed.). Philadelphia, PA: Saunders/Elsevier, 232–242.

Smetana, J. G. (1989). Adolescents' and parents' reasoning about actual family conflict. *Child Development, 60*, 1052–1067.

Sprinthall, N. A., & Collins, W. A. (1995). *Adolescent psychology: A developmental view*. New York: McGraw-Hill.

Steinberg, L. (1990). Autonomy, conflict, and harmony in the family relationship. In S. S. Feldman & G. R. Elliott (Eds.). *At the threshold: The developing adolescent*. Cambridge, MA: Harvard University Press, 255–276.

Steinberg, L. (2008). *Adolescence* (8th ed.). Boston: McGraw-Hill.

Steinburg, 388.

Stone, G., Buehler, C., & Barber, B. K. (2002). Interparental conflict, parental psychological control, and youth problem behavior. In B. K. Barber (Ed.). *Intrusive parenting: How psychological control affects children and adolescents*. Washington, DC: American Psychological Association, 53–95.

Suldo, S., Friedrich, A., White, T., Farmer, J., Minch, D., & Michalowski, J. (2009). Teacher support and adolescents' subjective well-being: A mixed-methods investigation. *School Psychology Review, 38*(1), 67–85.

Sun, S. S., Schubert, C. M., Chumlea, W. C., Roche, A. F., Kulen, H. E., Lee, P. A., Himes, J. C., & Ryan, A. (2002). National estimates of the timing of sexual maturation and racial differences among U.S. children. *Pediatrics, 110*(5), 911–919.

Tanner, J., Whitehouse, R. H., & Takaishi, M. (1966). Standards from birth to maturity for height, weight, height velocity, and weight velocity: British Children, 1965. *Archives of Diseases of Children, 41*, 454–471. Reproduced with permission from the BMJ Publishing Group.

Teevan, J. J., Jr. (1972). Reference groups and premarital sexual behavior. *Journal of Marriage and the Family, 34*, 283–291.

U.S. Department of Health and Human Services. (2000). *Healthy People 2010*: National health promotion and disease prevention objectives. Washington DC: Author.

U.S. Department of Health and Human Services. (2010). *Healthy People 2020*: Retrieved May 25, 2010, from http://www.healthypeople.gov/hp2020/Objectives/TopicArea.aspx?id=11&TopicArea=Adolescent+Health.

Vondracek, F. W., & Porfeli, E. J. (2006). The world of work and careers. In G. R. Adams & M. D. Berzonsky (Eds.). *Handbook of adolescence*. Malden, MA: Blackwell, 109–128.

Walker, M. (1989). What does the different voice say? Gilligan's women and moral philosophy. *The Journal of Value Inquiry, 23*(7), 123–134.

Weinshenker, N. (2002). Adolescence and body image. *School Nurse News, 19*, 12–16.

Wertsch, J. V., & Tulviste, P. (1999). L. S. Vygotsky and contemporary developmental psychology. In P. Lloyd & C. Fernyhough

(Eds.). *Lev Vygotsky: Critical assessments: Vygotsky's theory* (vol. I). Florence, KY: Taylor & Frances/Routledge, 109–128.

Wiseman, C. V., Sunday, S. R., & Becker, A. E. (2005). Impact of the media on adolescent body image. *Child & Adolescent Psychiatric Clinics of North America, 14*(3), 453–471.

Yang, S. C., & Chen, S. (2006). Content analysis of free-response narratives to personal meanings of death among Chinese children and adolescents. *Death Studies, 30,* 217–241.

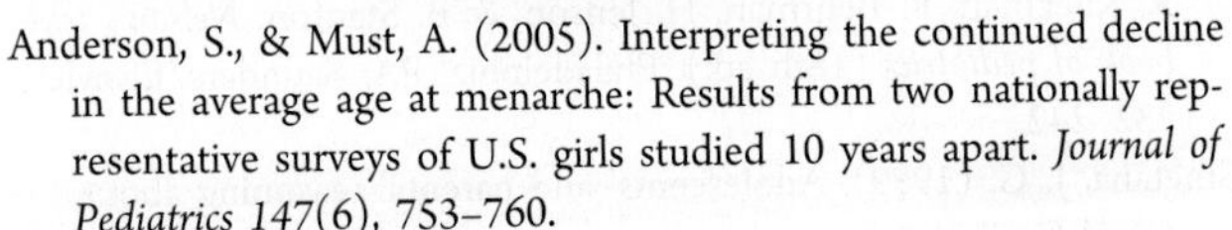

SUGGESTED READINGS

Anderson, S., & Must, A. (2005). Interpreting the continued decline in the average age at menarche: Results from two nationally representative surveys of U.S. girls studied 10 years apart. *Journal of Pediatrics 147*(6), 753–760.

Barber, J. G., & Delfabbro, P. (2000). Predictors of adolescent adjustment: Parent–peer relationships and parent–child conflict. *Child and Adolescent Social Work Journal, 17*(4), 275–288.

Carroll, J., Padilla-Walker, L., Nelson, L., Olson, C., McNamara, C., & Madsen, S. (2008). Generation XXX: Pornography acceptance and use among emerging adults. *Journal of Adolescent Research, 23,* 6–30.

Feldman, A., & Matjasko, J. (2007). Profiles and portfolios of adolescent school-based extra-curricular activity participation. *Journal of Adolescence, 30:* 313–332.

Guilamo-Ramos, V., Jaccard, J., Dittus, P., & Bouris, A. (2006). Parental expertise, trustworthiness, and accessibility: Parent–adolescent communication and adolescent risk behavior. *Journal of Marriage and Family, 68*(5), 1229–1246.

Hill, N., Bromell, L., Tyson, D., & Flint, R. (2007). Developmental commentary: Ecological perspectives on parental influences during adolescence. *Journal of Clinical Child and Adolescent Psychology, 36*(3), 367–377.

Renk, K., Liljequist, L., Simpson, J. E., & Phares, V. (2005). Gender and age differences in the topics of parent–adolescent conflict. *The Family Journal: Counseling and Therapy for Couples and Families, 13*(2), 139–149.

Sinha, J., Cnaan, R., & Gelles, R. (2007). Adolescent risk behaviors and religion: Findings from a national study. *Journal of Adolescence, 30,* 231–249.

Sullivan, H. S. (1953). *The interpersonal theory of psychiatry.* New York: Norton.

Wickman, M., Anderson, N., & Greenberg, C. (2008). The adolescent perception of invincibility and its influence on teen acceptance of health promotion strategies. *Journal of Pediatric Nursing, 23*(6), 460–468.

RESOURCES

Refer to the online student StudyWARE for Potts & Mandleco at http://www.CengageBrain.com for additional content and study aids.

Organization: **Adolescence Directory On-Line (ADOL)**
Description: Associated with the Center for Adolescent and Family Studies at Indiana University; offers information concerning current adolescence issues as well as a teens only section offering help links.
Website/Resource: http://www.education.indiana.edu

Organization: **AMA Archives of Pediatrics and Adolescent Medicine**
Description: Offers access to reliable medical resources including medical journals and information regarding careers in health care, advocacy, and medical news.
Website/Resource: http://www.ama-assn.org

Organization: **American Academy of Child and Adolescent Psychiatry (AACAP)**
Description: Provides information regarding mental illnesses, data concerning efforts to prevent mental illnesses, how to seek proper treatment, and access to services for children and adolescents.
Website/Resource: http://www.aacap.org

Organization: **American Academy of Family Physicians**
Description: Offers information regarding family physician careers, clinical research, advocacy, practice management, and recent news/publications.
Website/Resource: http://www.aafp.org

Organization: **American Academy of Pediatrics**
Description: Offers general information related to child health, specific guidelines concerning many pediatric issues, information regarding AAP programs, activities, policies, guidelines, publications, and other child health resources.
Website/Resource: http://www.aap.org

Organization: **Youth Indicators 2007: Trends in the Well-Being of American Youth**
Description: Contains statistics that describe young people's lives both in school and beyond the schoolhouse. Updated every two years.
Website/Resource: http://www.nces.ed.gov

Organization: **Youth Risk Behavior Surveillance**

Description: Offers access to fact sheets, results, publications and data files related to priority health-risk behaviors and the prevalence of obesity and asthma among youth and young adults. Updated every two years.

Website/Resource: http://www.cdc.gov

Organization: **Youth Info**

Description: A government Website helping create/maintain/strengthen effective youth programs. Includes facts, funding information, tools to help assess community assets, generate maps of local/federal resources, search for evidence-based youth programs, and keep up-to-date on the latest, youth-related news.

Website/Resource: http://www.findyouthinfo.org

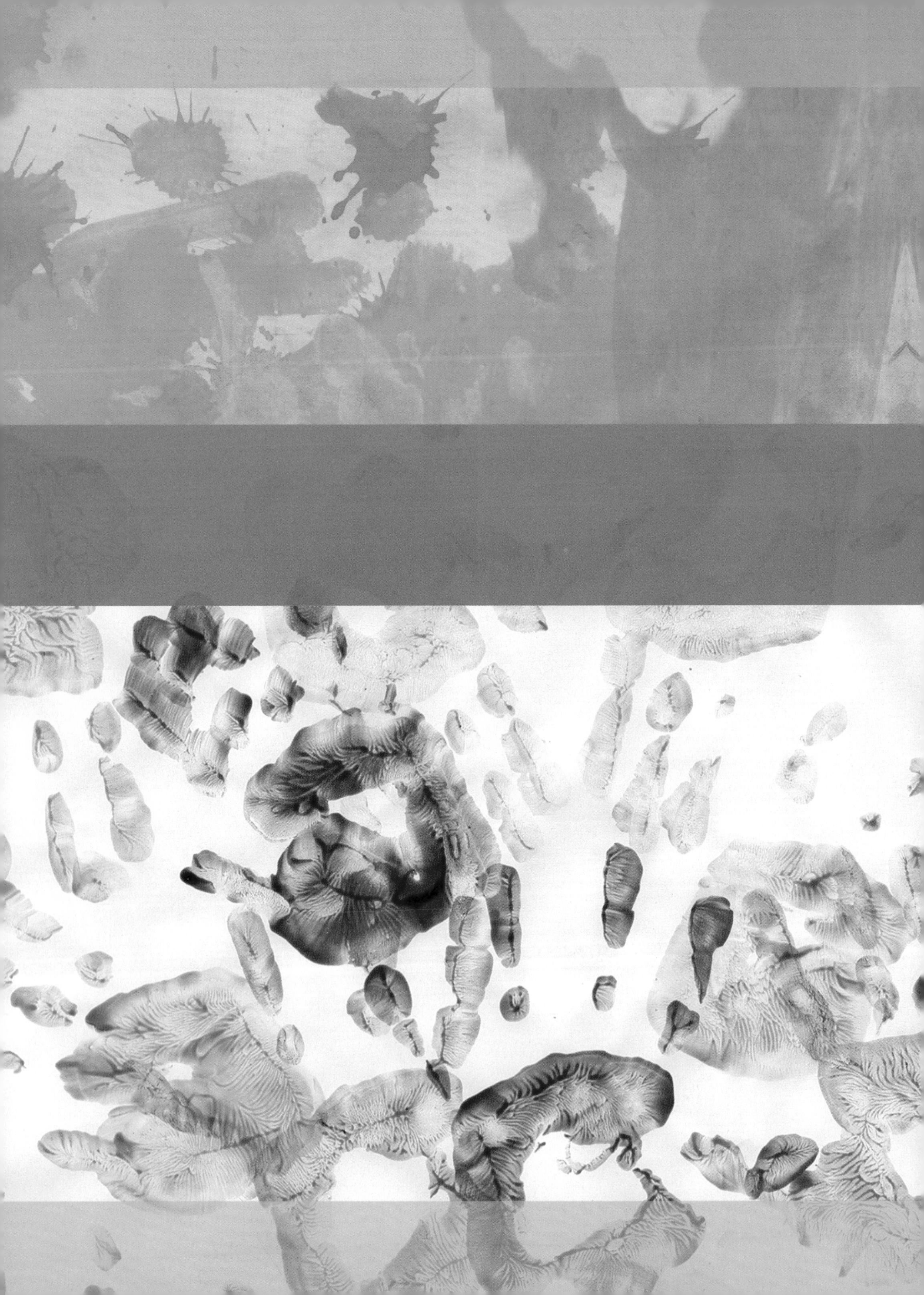

UNIT 3 Unique Considerations in Children

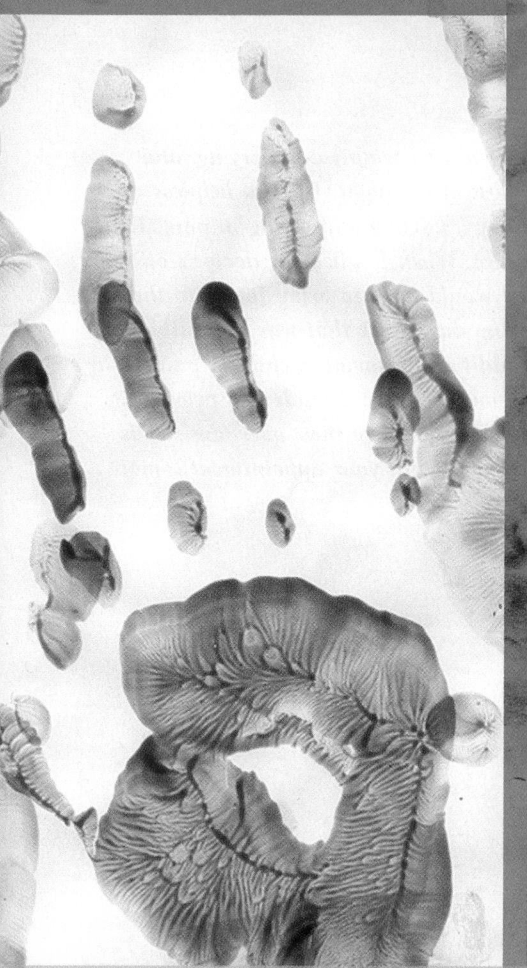

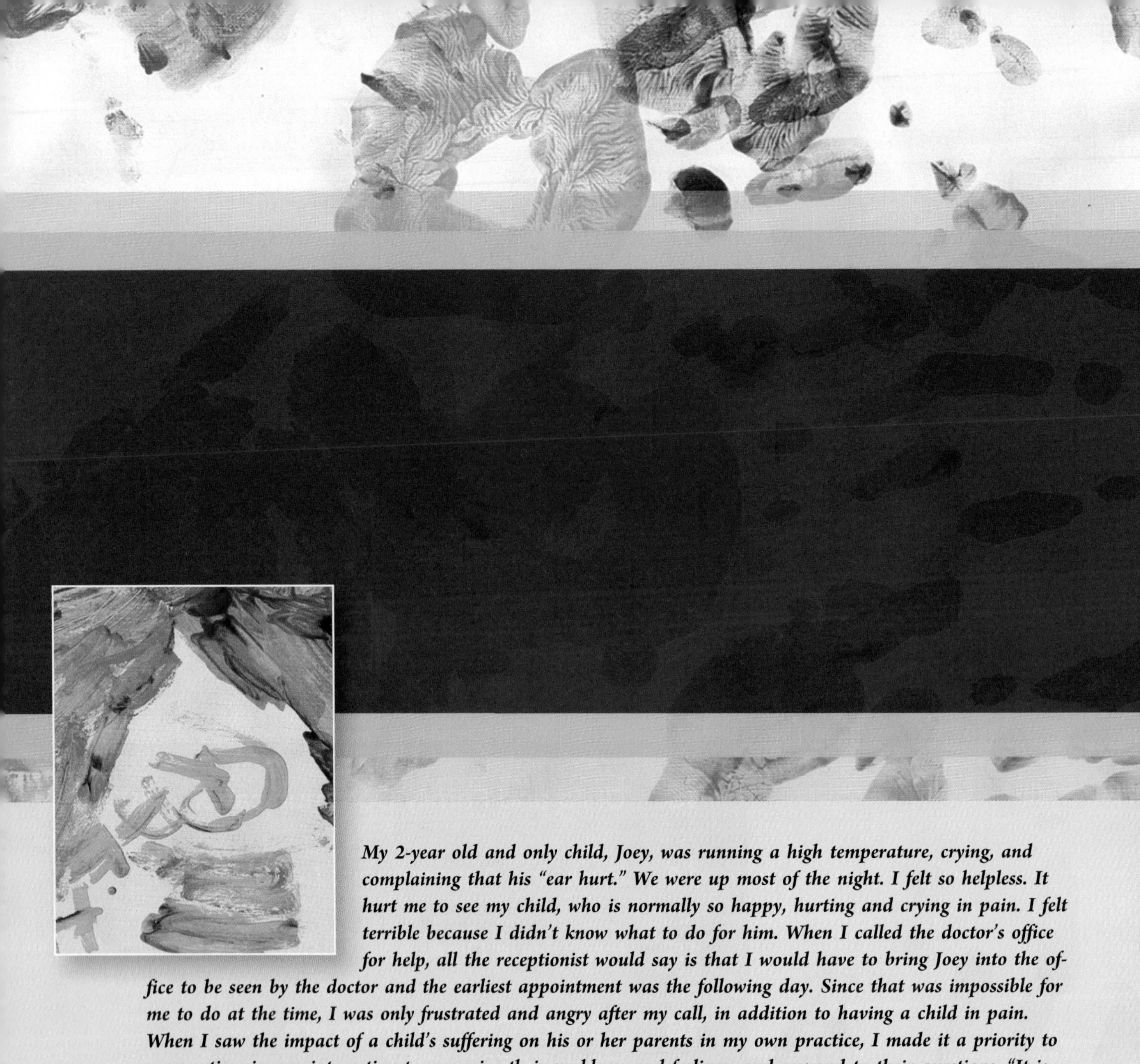

My 2-year old and only child, Joey, was running a high temperature, crying, and complaining that his "ear hurt." We were up most of the night. I felt so helpless. It hurt me to see my child, who is normally so happy, hurting and crying in pain. I felt terrible because I didn't know what to do for him. When I called the doctor's office for help, all the receptionist would say is that I would have to bring Joey into the office to be seen by the doctor and the earliest appointment was the following day. Since that was impossible for me to do at the time, I was only frustrated and angry after my call, in addition to having a child in pain. When I saw the impact of a child's suffering on his or her parents in my own practice, I made it a priority to reserve time in any interaction to recognize their problems and feelings, and respond to their questions. "It is very difficult to deal with a child in pain particularly when they are our own. Until your appointment tomorrow, are there questions I can help you with?"

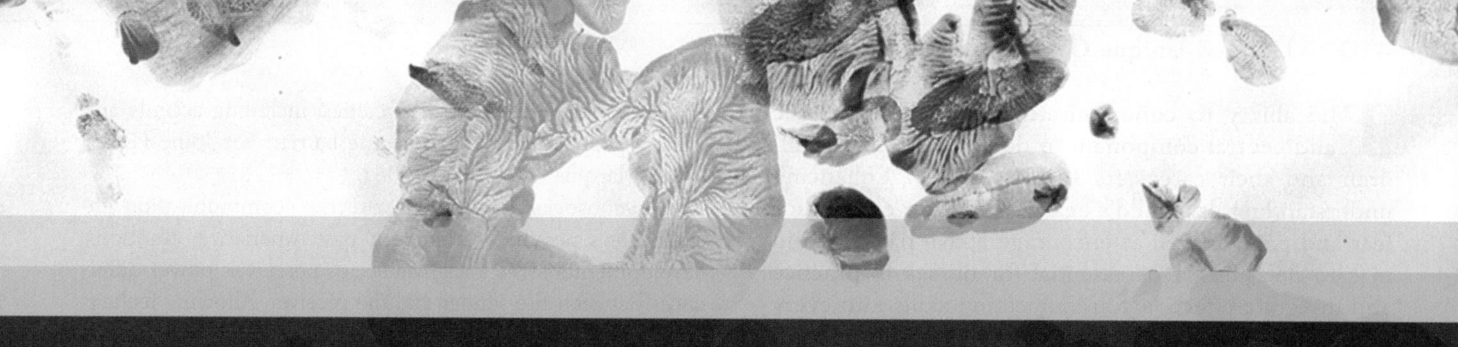

CHAPTER 13

Child and Family Communication

FRANCES J. DOTTON, RN, PhD
BARBARA L. MANDLECO, RN, PhD

COMPETENCIES

Upon completion of this chapter, the reader will be able to:

- Explain what communication is and its importance in developing positive relationships with children and their families.
- Discuss barriers encountered in communication.
- Describe verbal and nonverbal communication.
- Discuss the elements of communication, including rapport and trust, respect, empathy, listening, providing feedback, and conflict management.
- Describe the impact and challenges a child's developmental level has on communication.
- Describe effective communication strategies that assist nurses' work with infants, children, and adolescents.
- Discuss the impact a person's cultural background may have on his or her communication patterns.
- Explain the concept of communicating with children who have special needs.
- Successfully complete the games and activities in the online student StudyWARE.

The ability to communicate effectively is a basic and central component in delivering care to children and their caregivers (Stuart, 2009). Enhancing understanding of a child's health condition can reduce fear and pain, as well as encourage active participation in care decisions. It is essential for nurses to practice and integrate effective communication skills into every facet of interaction. An authentic, nonjudgmental, empathetic manner improves not only the quality of care but also determines the success of relationships established in delivering care. Communication skills can be compared to aseptic skills: once one understands the principles behind effective communication, one can integrate these principles into practice.

THE COMMUNICATION PROCESS

Communication is defined as the exchange of meanings between and among individuals through a shared system of symbols. The sender, message, channel, receiver, and feedback are major components of the communication process. The **sender** generates a message in response to a need to relate to others, to create meaning, and to understand various situations. The **message** is a verbal or nonverbal stimulus produced by a sender and responded to by a receiver. The **channel** is the medium through which a message is transmitted. It may be visual, auditory, or kinesthetic. Visual channels include sight, observation, and perception. Auditory channels include the spoken word and cues. Kinesthetic channels include sensations experienced, as in touch. The **receiver** is the person interpreting the sender's message. **Feedback** provides the sender with information from the receiver about the message. The sender can then adjust the message so it is understood more effectively by the receiver the next time it is sent (Estes, 2010).

Communication is both talking and listening. Nurses must be able to not only use words to explain information to caregivers and children, but also listen to what caregivers and children say. The ability to prepare and present ideas, feelings, and thoughts accurately (by talking) and respond to messages accurately (by listening) reduces distortion and results in effective communication.

BARRIERS TO COMMUNICATION

Barriers to communication may be physical factors or psychological factors. Physical or environmental factors include the physical space or distance between the receiver and sender, the temperature or ventilation in the environment, distracting noises such as the radio or television, or the patient's health status, especially if the child (or family) is disoriented or has a hearing or visual handicap. Effective communication will not occur when children and families do not understand the medical terminology used, so explanations should include common words and simple terms. Finally, hearing or speech difficulties, including accents and speech impediments, may become barriers for some (Estes, 2010; Marquis & Huston, 2008).

Psychosocial barriers to effective communication include one's personal judgments, past experience, emotions, developmental level, social values, or perceived power differences between the sender and the receiver. Allowing feelings or preconceptions to influence behavior, opinions, or beliefs may also be problematic. Personal opinions need to be carefully shared with children and their caregivers because nurses represent authority figures. Even facial expressions that convey disapproval may become a psychosocial barrier if the child or family suspects disapproval (Estes, 2010; Marquis & Huston, 2008).

MODES OF COMMUNICATION

Formal communication refers to communication that occurs in an organized way, with a particular agenda, such as when teaching a child's care to the caregiver upon discharge. Formal communication must be clear and understandable. **Informal communication** occurs when individuals talk using no particular agenda or protocol. Often, informal communication occurs sporadically when caring for children and their caregivers in day-to-day interactions (Figure 13-1).

VERBAL COMMUNICATION

Verbal communication refers to messages that are communicated through words and language (Estes, 2010). Verbal communication is most effective if it is brief, clear, effectively toned, paced appropriately, relevant, and well timed. The receiver will be confused if more words than necessary are used or if the speaker does not speak slowly and clearly. Important points should be repeated and medical jargon avoided, especially when talking to children and their caregivers and families. Messages also need appropriate pacing; they should not be too slow or fast, and there should be few pauses and periods of silence. Only important and relevant

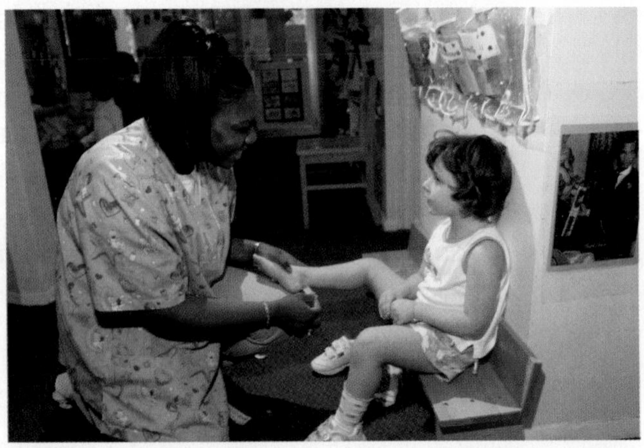

FIGURE 13-1 While tending to a minor scrape, a school nurse can get a sense for a child's overall sense of health and well-being. DELMAR CENGAGE LEARNING.

information should be conveyed, and the tone should be pleasant.

Messages should also be sent at the appropriate time. For example, teaching will not be effective if delivered when children are in pain or have visitors, or when caregivers are preoccupied with personal thoughts. When interacting with families, it is also essential to convey interest and warmth; to avoid distractions, yes or no questions, and personal bias; and not monopolize the conversation. **Paraverbal cues**, also part of verbal communication, include the tone and pitch of the voice; volume, inflection, and speed; and grunts or other vocalizations not considered language (Burnard & Gill, 2008; Munoz & Luckman, 2005). These cues add meaning to the words spoken and can and often do

RESEARCH Highlight

Kangaroo Mother Care (KMC) Diminishes Pain from Heel Lance in Very Preterm Neonates: A Crossover Trial

STUDY PURPOSE

The purpose of this study was to determine if KMC (skin-to-skin contact) would also be efficacious in very preterm neonates. (Figure 13-2).

METHODS

The sample consisted of preterm neonates (n = 61) between 28 0/7 and 31 6/7 weeks gestational age in three Level III NICUs in Canada. A single-blind randomized crossover design was employed. In the experimental condition, the infant was held in KMC for 15 minutes prior to and throughout heel lance procedure. In the control condition the infant was swaddled in a blanket in the prone position in the incubator. The primary outcome used was the Premature Infant Pain Profile (PIPP), which is comprised of three facial actions, maximum heart rate, and minimum oxygen saturation levels from baseline in 30-second blocks from heel lance. The secondary outcome was time to recover, defined as heart rate return to baseline. Continuous video, heart rate, and oxygen saturation monitoring were recorded with event markers during the procedure and were subsequently analyzed. Repeated measures analysis-of-variance was employed.

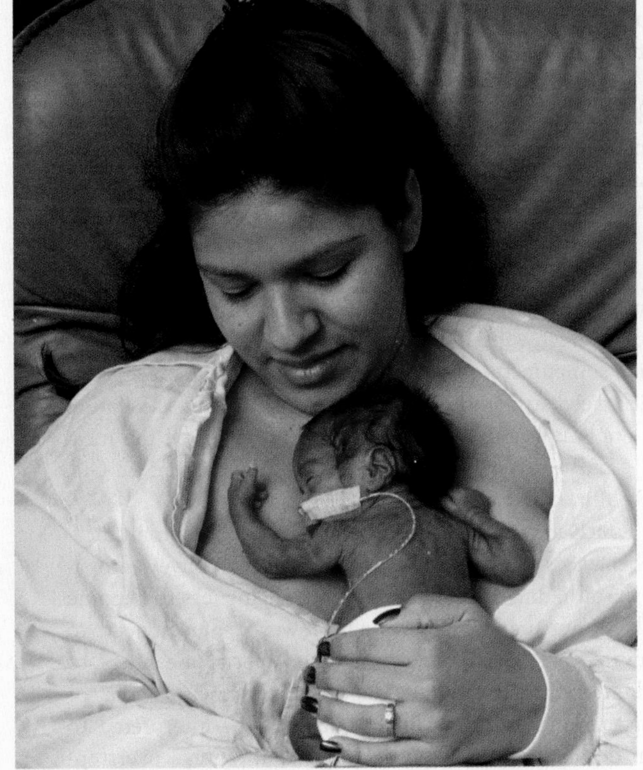

FIGURE 13-2 Kangaroo care, or skin-to-skin holding, has many benefits for the parent and infant. DELMAR CENGAGE LEARNING.

FINDINGS

PIPP scores at 90 seconds post lance were significantly lower in the KMC condition (8.871 (95%C1 7.852–9.889 (10.677: 95%C1 9.563–11.792) p ‹.001). Non-significant mean differences ranging from 1.2 to 1.8. Time to recovery was significantly shorter, by a minute (123 seconds (95%C1 103–142 versus 193 seconds (95%C1 158–227).

IMPLICATIONS

Very preterm neonates appear to have internal mechanisms elicited through skin-to-skin maternal contact that decrease pain response, but are not as powerful as in older preterm neonates. The shorter recovery time in KMC is clinically important in helping maintain homeostasis and should be encouraged if possible.

REFERENCE

Johnston, C. C., Fillon, F., Campbell-Yeo, M., Goulet, C., Bell, L., McNaughton, K., Byron, J., Aita, M., Findlay, G. A., & Walker, C. D. (2008). Kangaroo mother care diminishes pain from heel lance in very preterm neonates: A crossover trial. *BMC Pediatrics*, 8, 13.

influence the listener more than the actual words themselves (Estes, 2010). Confusion results when verbal messages are inaccurate or unreliable, or contradict paraverbal cues.

Nonverbal Communication

Nonverbal communication conveys feelings, attitudes, and intentions (Burnard & Gill, 2008; Munoz & Luckman, 2005). It enables one to interpret verbal communication and transcend the literal content of the message. Nonverbal communication is especially apparent when emotions cause observable body changes, and comes through more powerfully and effectively when there is incongruence between the verbal and the nonverbal message. In fact, most communication is nonverbal, and most verbal communication contradicts nonverbal messages. Listeners will believe the nonverbal message rather than the verbal message if they contradict each other. Therefore, it is critical to always consider nonverbal communication in any interaction since it contributes to what others "hear." The nurse should use language consistent with the child's developmental level and deliver the message so the language is consistent with the nonverbal cues. For example, never smile or laugh when giving care that may be frightening or painful. Avoid words that have violent or scary connotations, such as *stick, shot,* and *sting.*

Nonverbal communication includes: spatial relationships (the distance between participants); appearance (clothing, grooming, hair style); eye contact; body posture (slouching, standing erect with the head leaning to receiver); gestures (which sometimes add emphasis to words); facial expressions (which need to agree with the message); timing (hesitation may imply untruthfulness or diminish the effect of the message); and, with children especially, touch (Burnard & Gill, 2008; Munoz & Luckman, 2005) (Figure 13-3).

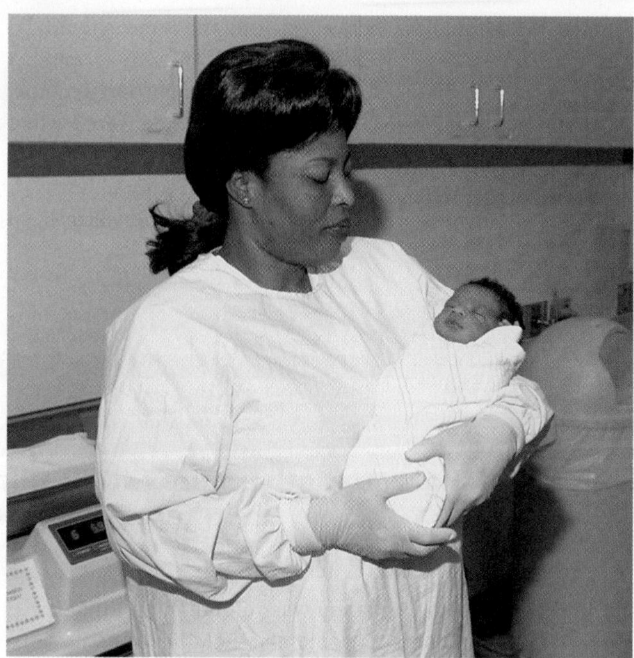

FIGURE 13-3 Nurses should recognize that their general appearance and demeanor, including clothing and accessories worn on their uniforms, body posture and movement, and nonverbal behaviors such as facial expressions, eye contact, and expressions of affect such as smiling, impact their interactions with children and their families as much as their language. DELMAR CENGAGE LEARNING.

Touch may be one of the most important communicative behaviors nurses use, because to many it conveys empathy, warmth, understanding, affection, willingness to become involved, nurturance, and caring. However, nurses need to be aware that touch may have other special meanings to children and their families, depending on their gender or ethnic background. For some, touch may be interpreted to mean dominance, or taken as a sign of the nurse overstepping his or her bounds. For others, touch may signify an inappropriate desire for intimacy and lead to discomfort.

NURSE, CHILD, AND FAMILY COMMUNICATION

Effective communication requires sensitivity to the child and family's needs and a well-developed and carefully thought-out plan. In fact, the nurse's ability to establish a therapeutic relationship with children and their caregivers is strongly tied to communication abilities and must be a high priority for all nurses as they interact with clients and families. Nurses always need to be aware of client and family needs for education and use communicative interactions as an entree into providing new or reinforcing old information. Increasing knowledge and providing information regarding a child's illness, symptoms, care needed, or developmental level can empower families and ultimately increase well-being. Before communication can be effective, several key elements must be addressed, including establishing rapport, building trust, showing respect, conveying empathy, listening actively, providing appropriate feedback, managing conflict, and establishing professional boundaries (Figure 13-4).

RAPPORT AND TRUST

Nurses must develop trust and rapport with clients and clients must be willing to talk, listen, and provide honest answers. Nurses may also need to be available and open to questions caregivers and children may have. To build rapport with the child and caregivers, the nurse must be accepted by them and willing to discuss non-health-related issues to convey warmth and friendliness. To establish trust, a nurse must follow through on promises, keep appointments, respect client confidentiality, and carefully explain procedures in a way that is acceptable to the family (Burnard & Gill, 2008; Munoz & Luckman, 2005).

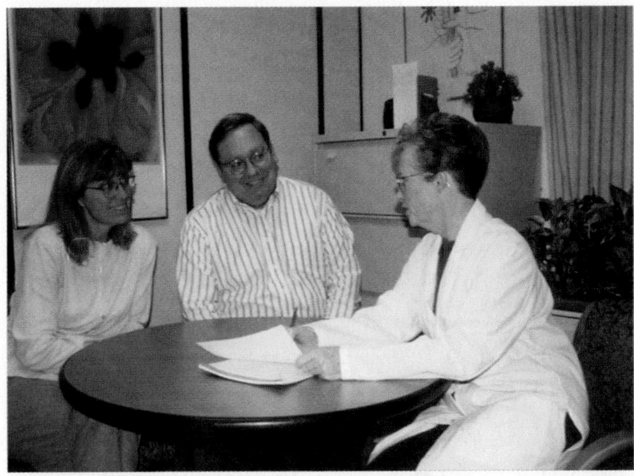

FIGURE 13-4 Nurses should make the environment conducive to effective communication when interacting with family members. The environment most effective for teaching or learning, discussions, and meetings should be comfortable, quiet, and private. DELMAR CENGAGE LEARNING.

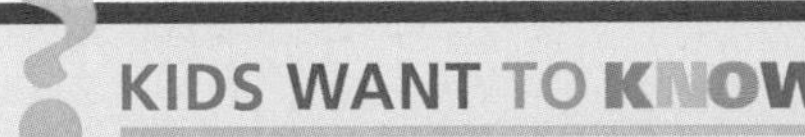

KIDS WANT TO KNOW

Taking Medication

Child: "I don't want to take that. It tastes yucky."
Nurse: "I feel so proud of you when you take your medicine. I understand it doesn't taste good and you don't like to do it. I am pleased you want to help yourself feel better by taking your medicine." Feelings are emphasized, and the "I" statements express ownership of the feelings. Empathy is illustrated when the child understands what the nurse is thinking.

RESPECT

To establish respect, the nurse should address the child by first name (the formal name unless given permission to use a nickname) and the caregivers by Mr., Ms., or Mrs. and then the last name. Before addressing the caregivers by first name, it is imperative caregivers give their consent. Respect is also conveyed by considering the family's feelings, cultural views, and values. Nurses need to convey they have time to spend with the child and the family. This will allow the family to share thoughts and concerns and ask questions. If nurses nonverbally communicate they do not have time, for example, by standing near the doorway, frequently looking at the clock while talking, or confiding to the child and family how busy they are, caregivers and children will soon believe the nurse is too busy or doesn't really care. These messages interfere with establishing trust and respect and should be avoided. Interference in establishing respect also occurs when a child is in isolation and nurses are required to wear gloves and masks. Indeed, children in these situations may feel isolated since they are not visited frequently and verbal communication is muffled or difficult to understand. Therefore, the nurse should make a concerted effort to speak more clearly without appearing as if yelling. Smiling is also important; although the child may not see a smile from the nurse's mouth, if it will be covered by a mask, the child will see it in the nurse's eyes.

EMPATHY

Empathy forms the basis of a helping relationship and is an important element in communication. **Empathy** refers to the ability to put one's self in the other person's shoes—to feel as well as to intellectually know what the other person is experiencing (Burnard & Gill, 2008; Munoz & Luckman, 2005). Empathetic nurses are able to appreciate and understand children and caregivers as unique individuals and allow them to feel cared about and accepted. For this to happen, the nurse's empathy needs to be integrated with verbal and nonverbal behavior.

Empathy, however, is not to be confused with sympathy. The empathetic nurse maintains a sense of objectivity and is supportive, understanding, and able to plan and implement helpful behaviors by teaching and giving examples that facilitate the ability of the child and the caregivers to function in difficult and sad situations. The sympathetic nurse, however, offers condolence and pity and is not able to develop or carry out behaviors that engage the child or parent in activities that help them maintain their relationship and ability to function in difficult situations. For example, Shawn, an 11-year-old boy with an inoperable brain tumor, is being cared for at home by his parents. The nurse sympathizer feels sorry for Shawn and is often near tears when she looks at him and tries to talk to his parents. She assumes all of Shawn's care. The nurse empathizer would teach the parents how to participate in Shawn's care, make suggestions on how to conserve Shawn's energy, and outline diversional activities that all might enjoy together given Shawn's condition. The nurse empathizer would direct energy toward finding ways to enable the parents to have quality time and experiences with Shawn and might even "share tears with" the parents as they talk about what to expect in the end. The nurse empathizer is able to establish an accurate understanding of the child and the caregivers from their perspective, build rapport, and relate to the child and caregivers in such a way as to allow them to express their feelings and concerns.

LISTENING

Listening consists of providing verbal and nonverbal cues that communicate interest. It is an activity that requires

BOX 13-1
FOUR BS OF EFFECTIVE LISTENING

- Be attentive; eliminate distractions.
- Be clear about the message; clarify if necessary.
- Be empathetic; convey concern and caring.
- Be open minded; avoid prejudices.

attention and effort: one not only listens to the words of the child and caregivers, but also to how words are used and decides whether what is said is what is meant. Accurate listening does not happen without effort. It requires actively attending to what is verbalized, observed, and created by the entire communication context. It is important not to allow one's mind to wander, to daydream, to prejudge what is being said, or to think about what will be said as a response; one must listen attentively and wait for others to finish what they are saying. Attentive listening goes beyond hearing and includes what is not said or what is conveyed through gestures. Active listening also includes maintaining eye contact, taking an open and relaxed posture, and facing the child or caregivers (Burnard & Gill, 2008; Munoz & Luckman, 2005). See Box 13-1 for more information on effective listening. However, remember, giving and receiving eye contact is a culturally determined behavior.

When working with children and caregivers, the nurse should encourage and allow each to give input, discuss concerns, express feelings, and acknowledge problems. Respecting other's feelings and views, and appreciating each other's understandings and fears even though different than one's own, are also important. While listening to children, the nurse must consider their developmental level, cognition, and emotional behavior. Children who are social and verbal may seem to be more in control and able to understand, and think more logically and rationally than children who engage in shy, clinging, and dependent behaviors. Nurses should use developmentally appropriate language and behavior with children and attend to their behavioral cues for clues as to their concerns and fears (Figure 13-5). For example, a child may continue talking and asking questions in order to avoid beginning a treatment.

PROVIDING FEEDBACK

Providing feedback can include nodding of the head, reflecting back to the client what was said, asking questions to clarify, seeking validation from the client to ensure one is talking about the same thing, and focusing on a single idea and exploring it further. Focusing means to direct the conversation based on a statement made by the client. For instance, during a conversation with a child regarding her broken leg, the child mentions another child on the playground has been pushing her around. The nurse may want to direct the conversation and delve more deeply into the fear the child may be experiencing due to the playground incident, other violent interactions the child may have had in the past, and what may occur during interactions in the future.

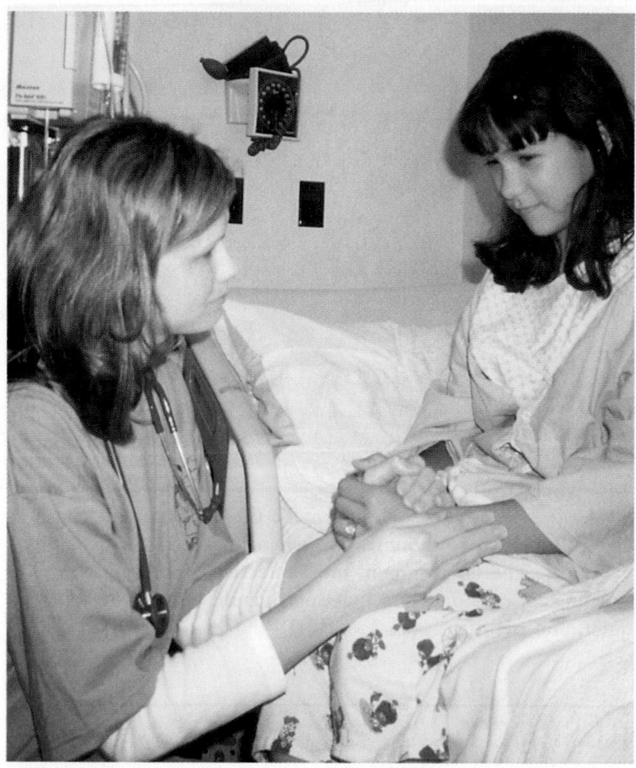

FIGURE 13-5 Adolescents often need reassurance when they are to undergo treatments or procedures. The nurse reassuring them should take the time to listen to their concerns, give explanations, and share how and what can be done to help the adolescent's experience be a positive one. USED WITH PERMISSION OF BAYSTATE MEDICAL CENTER CHILDREN'S HOSPITAL.

CONFLICT MANAGEMENT

There are four ways to approach conflict resolution: win-win, lose-win, win-lose, and lose-lose. The win-win approach

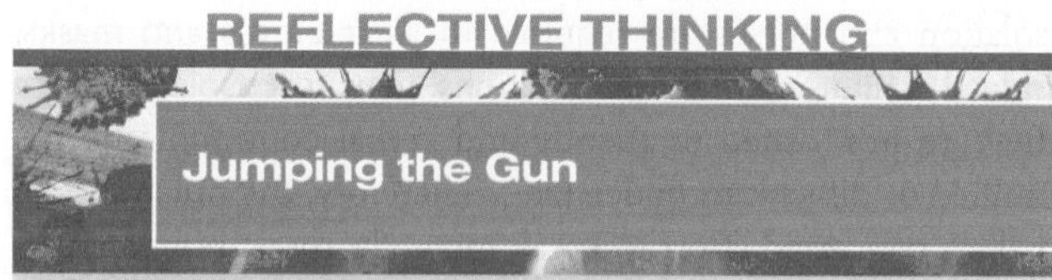

Active listening takes conscious effort, time, and practice. When you listen, you are able to convey in your own words what children and their caregivers have said and the feelings expressed. If you construct responses before children or caregivers finish speaking, or answer questions while they are being asked, listening isn't occurring. Can you in your own words express the thoughts and feelings of children and caregivers? If you cannot, you are not listening. Evaluate yourself. How well do you listen?

NURSING TIP

Healing Chitchats

Provide a quiet, private time to talk without interruption about troubles a child or the caregivers may be experiencing. No feedback should be offered or judgments made. An opportunity to verbalize hurt feelings and discuss problems without reproach is a step toward healing.

occurs when both parties are committed to solving the conflict. They work together toward a resolution, searching for a variety of ways to resolve the problem so they are able to finally arrive at a solution acceptable to all parties. The lose-win situation occurs when one person allows a resolution at his or her own expense; the win-lose approach occurs when one person resolves the conflict by having his or her needs and wants satisfied, but forces others to agree with the solution. Lose-lose occurs when neither party is happy with the outcome of the conflict. It is important for the nurse to strive for the win-win approach. This allows the child and caregivers to feel in control, and there is more likelihood of adherence to whatever decisions are made.

PROFESSIONAL BOUNDARIES

The nurse should create and maintain professional boundaries in relationships with children and their caregivers. Therapeutic relationships should be caring and empathetic, but should avoid emotional over-involvement and overprotectiveness. It is always helpful to explain to children and families the type of care to be provided, when the care will be provided, and how both parents and children can assist in the care. Identifying needs and establishing expectations will enhance and facilitate interactions. The nurse should never interfere with the relationship between the child and the caregivers. Rather, the nurse best serves the child by assisting the caregivers in caring for and nurturing the child, and by recognizing the need of the caregivers to feel accepted by the professionals and to be recognized as important to the child's well-being. Finally, nurses should avoid personal behaviors that signal over-involvement such as socializing with the child or their family, sharing personal information such as home addresses or telephone numbers, and giving or accepting gifts. See Box 13-2 for more information about how to avoid becoming over-involved.

FAMILY TEACHING

Resolution through Communication

The way conflict is handled within the family unit will determine how children learn to manage disagreement (Figure 13-6). The nurse should assist parents to learn the skills of conflict resolution by teaching and helping them practice in clinical encounters to:

- Actively listen to their child
- Clarify points of their differences
- Take each other's feelings seriously
- Generate alternative solutions together and
- Negotiate the solution

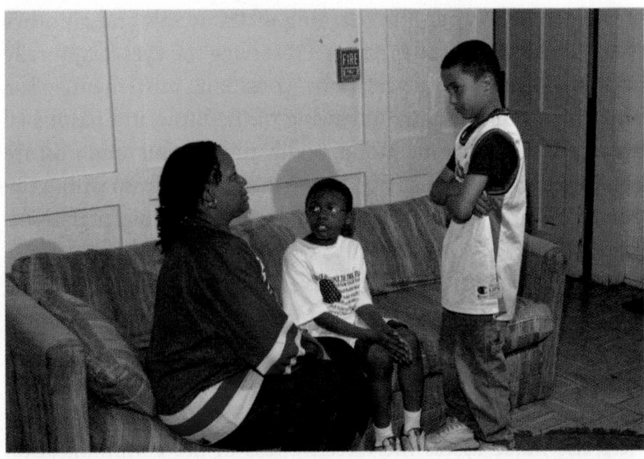

FIGURE 13-6 Understanding how families manage conflict will give the nurse insight into the family's coping skills and behaviors. DELMAR CENGAGE LEARNING.

ADDITIONAL SKILLS USEFUL IN COMMUNICATING

Several additional skills are useful when communicating with children and their caregivers. These include observation, silence, being aware of the environment, humor, play, writing, drawing, using third parties, and storytelling.

OBSERVATION

Observational skills enable the nurse to validate and interpret what children and caregivers do not say. Nonverbal behavior provides meaningful information about what the child and caregivers are communicating to each other and to the nurse. How words are delivered is as important as what words are used.

BOX 13-2
TO AVOID OVER-INVOLVEMENT

- Do not have contact with children and families after discharge.
- Do not purchase gifts for children and families.
- Do not share personal information with children and families.
- Request assignment change if you feel boundaries are getting blurred.

Congruence between the meaning of the words and all other behaviors validates the message. Observing the eyes if culturally acceptable during conversations (position, movement, gaze, and expression), mouth, furrowing of the brow and nasolabial area, general emotional mood, bodily movements, and posture are important. Cues also need to be interpreted from within the child's cultural perspective to avoid erroneous interpretations. For example, in some cultures, eye contact and directness are signs of paying attention. However, in other cultures, looking someone directly in the eye is considered rude. The nurse should also observe the ways children and caregivers respond to each other's request for attention, and behave and interact in disciplinary or nurturing situations. These observations can help the nurse assess the effectiveness of the communication patterns between children and caregivers and allow development of health-related strategies respectful of the relationship.

SILENCE

Silence may be another method used to communicate. Silence should be interpreted in relation to the environment where communication occurs and the normal behavior of those interacting. A child who is shy and hesitant with strangers may be silent when the nurse approaches for care. A caregiver who is silent after being told of a child's terminal diagnosis is likely to be experiencing shock and disbelief and trying to come to grips with the reality of what was just heard. Children may be silent out of separation anxiety and fear, as in the case of a 4-year-old child who is hospitalized and must spend time in a strange environment without caregivers nearby. Silence also may demonstrate comfort, respect, and concern as when a nurse sits with parents after upsetting news is heard or when the child is falling asleep after an upsetting procedure.

ENVIRONMENT

The environment can affect communication events among the nurse, the child, and the caregivers even more than the spoken words. The way nurses exist in the environment and use space to make people more or less comfortable as they seek care is important. Nurses who are effective in nurse-client communication develop and demonstrate a respect for the client's sense of physical and personal space. For example, when sensitive issues or feelings of anxiety need to be discussed and the environment is a four-bed unit where roommates can overhear the conversation, sharing fears and anxieties and asking questions may be difficult. A quiet, private environment should be provided before discussion begins (Figure 13-7). Nursing behaviors such as knocking before entering a child's room, asking permission to enter if the curtain is closed around the child's bed, calling the child and caregivers by name, addressing each directly, and asking permission to examine demonstrate respect and engender a sense of ownership over physical and personal space. Clients in care-giving settings such as hospitals and clinics will experience less stress, irritability, and fatigue when they remain in relative control of their physical and personal space. Environments that facilitate therapeutic communication reduce psychological distress so children can attend to their health care situation. When children are relaxed or not experiencing fear, they are able to cope with people and the environment and to converse more willingly. However, children may vary in their communication levels based on their personality, temperament, experiences, and developmental abilities. The nurse should use concern, care, and knowledge of child development, and be willing to use a variety of communication approaches with the same child during different interactions or with different children in similar interactions.

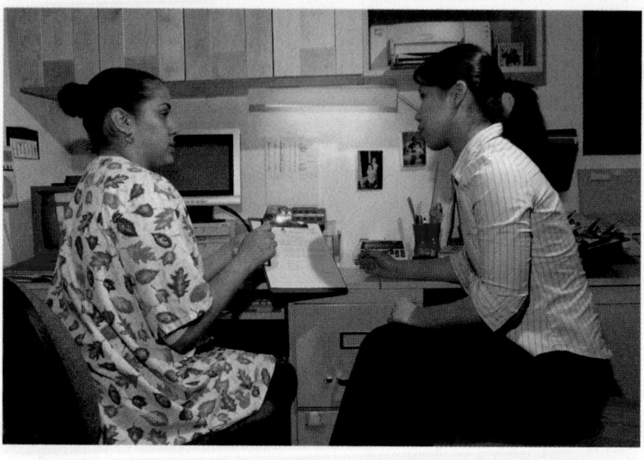

FIGURE 13-7 Nurses should discuss health information with families in a private environment and be prepared to answer questions and explain procedures. DELMAR CENGAGE LEARNING.

> **NURSING TIP**
>
> **Managing Aggressive Family members**
>
> When dealing with a client or family member who is verbally aggressive (using profanity, threats or sarcastic comments):
> - Remain calm and ask them to remain calm.
> - Speak in low, slow, assertive manner.
> - Try to identify the cause of the anger.
> - Encourage cooperation to find the solution.
> - State that you want to understand the problem.
> - Provide privacy to avoid involvement of non-essential persons and/or onlookers.

HUMOR

Humor is healing and can bridge communicative gaps even when the direct communication is feared or offensive (Andrews & Boyle, 2007; Martin, 2007). It is recognized as an effective method of helping children and adolescents cope with illness, pain, and hospitalization (May, 1999). For example, nurses who are able to laugh at themselves may be forgiven, and nurses who can make others laugh can't be all bad (or frightening). The nurse should use tasteful humor in dealing with pediatric clients and their caregivers to promote therapeutic interactions. However, if using humor, it is important to know if humor is appropriate for the child's cultural or ethnic background. It is also important to be sure the child understands the terms used.

Play

Play, a natural childhood behavior, should be encouraged in health care environments and employed as a method of communicating (May, 1999). Using puppets, dolls, or stuffed animals, drawing pictures with crayons and paints, or employing a storytelling approach to give information engages the child (Figure 13-8). Because play is familiar and a daily form of natural behavior, children do not associate it with stress, anxiety, or fear. Play helps the child relax and shed inhibitions brought about by health care environments. The nurse who engages in play is likely to be legitimized as someone who can be trusted in communication. For more information about children's play, see Chapter 16.

Writing and Drawing

An especially effective method of communicating with older school-age children and adolescents, writing can include keeping a journal or diary, or writing a letter that is not delivered. Other examples include encouraging the child or adolescent to write down thoughts or feelings not easy to express verbally, keep track in written form of experiences related to a health care situation, or write a story or essay about an experience (Hamama & Ronen, 2009; Lester, Masten, & McEwen, 2006). Sometimes just being able to articulate thoughts and feelings in writing can serve as a springboard for later discussions or concerns.

Drawing can be helpful for younger children since it provides clues to a child's emotional state and feelings (Hamama & Ronen, 2009; Lester et al., 2006). Evaluating the drawings or having a child tell a story about the drawing allows the nurse a window into the child's inner self. One needs to be cautious, however, since the evaluation of drawings should take place in conjunction with the evaluation of other

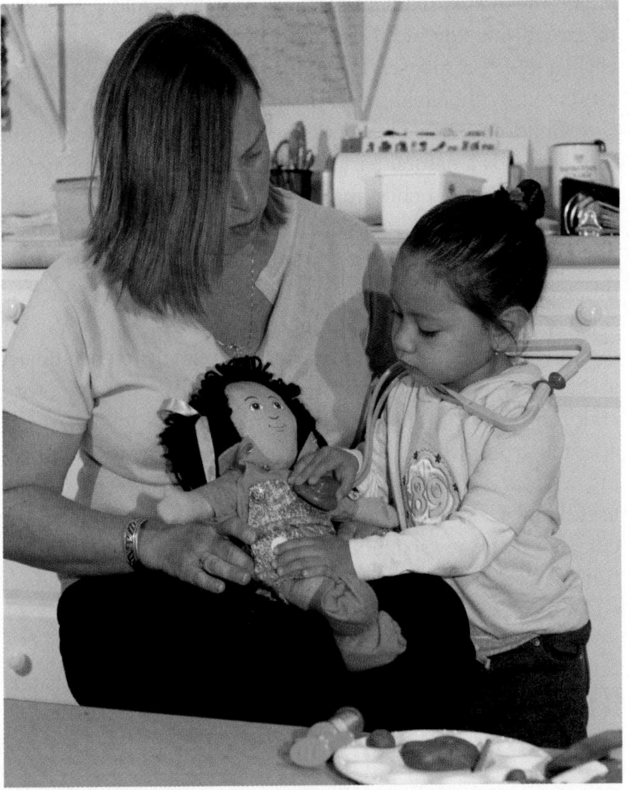

Figure 13-8 Nurses can help allay a child's fears by encouraging play with a doll and toy stethoscope. DELMAR CENGAGE LEARNING.

EVIDENCE-BASED PRACTICE

Using Music as Therapy with Children

CLINICAL PROBLEM

Children do not often have the cognitive ability or language development to convey and process their experiences through words. Therefore, art, play, and other auditory, visual, and kinesthetic imageries need to be used to help them communicate.

BEST CLINICAL PRACTICE

Nurses need to use symbolic modes of engagement and communication in addition to verbal modes when working with children. Use of alternative modes of communication can increase trust and allow the nurse to better understand the child's needs so appropriate interventions can be offered. One of these alternative modes is music. Music has been linked to religion, spiritual practices, and healing. It can reduce tension, distract, create dream-like states, and help one remember experiences and past events. It also can be used to express emotion and communicate thoughts and feelings. Parents often sing to infants and young children, and these songs can become transitional objects when the parent leaves. Music therapy is often used with individuals who have speech or communication difficulties, autism, mental illness, or were sexually abused. Music has a range of therapeutic benefits including enhancing personal growth, communication, and self expression.

IMPLICATIONS FOR NURSING

Consider using music as another way of communicating with children. An electronic keyboard or piano allows the caregiver and child to experiment with different ways of playing the same tune. Harmonic (cymbals, castanets, maracas, bells, tambourines, drums) as well as pre-recorded rhythmic accompaniments may also be useful. A child's sense of self can be supported if music created is recorded and then played back. Writing and then singing songs not only encourage creativity but also can be self affirming. Using pre-recorded music may provide opportunities for a child's deep seated feelings and thoughts to surface or provoke imagery. Whenever selecting music for children, be sure to ask the child what kind of music he/she prefers or would like to hear. If "real instruments" are not available, the nurse and patient can make them (drums from plates or bowls, a guitar from a tissue box and rubber bands).

Reference: Ockelford, A. (2008). *Music for children and young people with complex needs.* Oxford Music Education Series. Oxford, England: Oxford University Press; Baby Einstein Music Box Orchestra & Weisbach, B. (2008). *Sing & Play.* Burbank, CA: Walt Disney Records; Lefevre, M. (2004). Playing with sound: The therapeutic use of music in direct work with children. *Child and Family Social Work, 9,* 333–345.

information such as observation of behavior and communication with the child directly. Examination of drawings should include the evaluation of the gender of figures, the order in which the figures are drawn, the position of each in relation to other figures in the drawing, the exclusion of certain individuals, the accentuation or absence of particular body parts, the placement and size of the drawing on the page, whether or not the drawing is made with bold or light strokes, and the colors used (Hamama & Ronen, 2009).

Third-Party Communication (Toys and Dolls)

The nurse can promote dialogue with children by using indirect methods such as employing a third party. Here, the nurse directs her attention to the child through a trusted friend (e.g., a stuffed toy). By doing this, the nurse is taking an interest in the child's normal activity, is employing a stress-reducing communication method to create a therapeutic environment, and is helping the child focus on the content of the message rather than on anxieties and fears. See Box 13-3.

Another third-party approach used with older children and adolescents is to attribute feelings or thoughts to other children. This method can be a safe form of interaction that uses the thoughts and feeling of the group rather than of the child or adolescent directly. Using group feelings helps a child or adolescent feel comfortable talking to an adult because someone else is talking; the adult is told what the third person thinks without the child or adolescent being held responsible for the statement since the statement is made by the third person. For example, when explaining how one learns how to give oneself insulin injections, monitor blood glucose, or manage the diet during daytime hours while at school, the nurse could state that Christine, one of her 16-year-old clients, often will excuse herself from her friends, go to the restroom to check her sugar levels, and give herself insulin if needed. The nurse could also mention that Christine has told her friends she is diabetic, wears a med alert bracelet, and always carries hard candy in her purse.

BOX 13-3
USING A TOY TO COMMUNICATE

A 4-year-old boy is sitting in bed holding a stuffed bear. Instead of directly addressing the child, the nurse approaches and uses the toy as a medium for introduction.

Nurse: Hi Mr. Teddy Bear! How are you? My name is ___. What is your name? (Wait for an answer). Oh, I guess I'll have to call you Mr. "No name" bear. Mr. "No Name" bear, who is your friend?

Child: His name is Billy Bear! (In clinical practice, it has been found that even shy children will not let their friend be called Mr. "No Name" and will quickly provide their teddy bear friend's name.)

Nurse: Billy Bear! What a nice name. I bet he is fun to play with.

CRITICAL THINKING

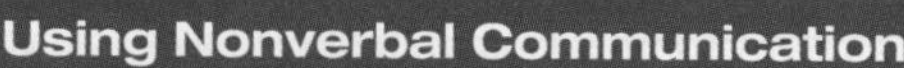

Using Nonverbal Communication

You are taking care of a school-age child who refuses to talk to you about how he feels. What might you do to encourage him to express his feelings?

Storytelling

Storytelling is an effective communication strategy nurses may use to promote therapeutic environments with children. Storytelling techniques can be used to establish rapport, assess and help resolve children's anxieties and fears, explain treatments and procedures, teach health, and prepare for painful or emotional events. The nurse can devise or use stories so the child can adopt either of the two story-telling roles: teller and listener. For example, a child can be read to or told a story about a boy who had surgery, or be asked to tell a story about a boy who has had surgery. The former might be used to explain what will happen when going to surgery. The latter might be used to elicit information about the child's experience when the nurse devises a story and takes turns with the child to fill in the content. Called "mutual story-telling" (Gardner, 1986), the nurse might say, "I'll start the story, and when I nod, you fill in the next part of the story." The nurse begins with, "Once upon a time a boy broke his leg and had to have surgery. He ..." The nurse nods to the child to fill in the blank. The nurse then uses the child's response to extend the story a bit, followed by nodding to the child to elicit another response. The nurse then analyzes the themes presented by the child, which may reveal important feelings.

Children begin to experience storytelling as infants and toddlers. It is a natural part of their early lives, and the use of story plots helps a child make the transition from preoperational to concrete operational thinking (Arnold & Boggs, 2007). For nurses, however, storytelling is a skill, and confidence and competence are gained through use and practice. Storytelling may be carried out in a variety of ways, for example, by telling stories from books related to the subject at hand, telling stories based on previous experiences with children or told to you by other children, and telling stories adapted from articles printed in nursing journals. Composing a story specific to the child and content area can be useful as well. Using drawings, dances, mime, poetry, or cut-outs from newspapers, comics, or magazines for illustration may also encourage communication between children and nurses. Refer to Box 13-4 for further information.

Developmental Factors Affecting Communication

Effective communication will enhance the preparation of a child and caregivers for their experiences related to health and illness (McDonald & Rushforth, 2006). However, the nurse must

BOX 13-4
PRINCIPLES OF EFFECTIVE COMMUNICATION IN PEDIATRIC SETTINGS

1. Talk to caregivers initially if child is shy or appears hesitant, but always look at child during conversations with caregivers.
2. Use objects (toys, dolls, stuffed animals) instead of questioning child directly.
3. Provide opportunities for older children and adolescents to talk privately with the nurse or other care provider.
4. Use clear, specific, simple phrases in confident, quiet, unhurried speech.
5. Position yourself so communication is at eye level.
6. Allow expression of thoughts and feelings.
7. Provide honest answers.
8. Offer choices only if they exist; for example, would you like to take your pills with apple juice or water? Do you want the injection in your right or left arm?
9. Use a variety of age-appropriate methods and techniques.

incorporate knowledge of human growth and development when communicating with children. Children should be encouraged to become active contributors to their health as soon as they are developmentally able to understand and carry out health-promoting behaviors. Until then, the nurse works directly with caregivers and reinforces their self-confidence in caring for and teaching the child. Refer to Chapter 31 for additional information on language development, which is critical when communicating with children, and to Table 13-1 for general principles of communicating with children of various ages.

TABLE 13-1 Communication Principles Based on Developmental Level

DEVELOPMENTAL LEVEL	COMMUNICATION PRINCIPLES
Infants	Allow the infant time to warm up to strangers.
	Respond to the infant's cries in a timely manner.
	Use motherese*, and a soothing and calm voice.
	Talk to the infant directly.
	Approach at eye level if possible.
Toddlers	Approach the toddler carefully; the child may be fearful.
	Integrate the toddler's words for familiar objects or activities into care.
	Prepare for procedures right before they are to be carried out.
	Integrate dolls, storytelling, and picture books into conversations.
	Stand at eye level.
Preschoolers	Allow choices as appropriate.
	Use play, storytelling, puppets, and third parties.
	Speak honestly, use simple language, and be concise.
	Prepare for procedures 1 hour or less before they are to be experienced.
School-age children	Use books, diagrams, and videos in preparing for procedures.
	Prepare for procedures several days in advance.
	Allow for honest expression of feelings and adequate time for questions to be answered.
Adolescents	Prepare for up to 1 week prior to experiences.
	Respect the adolescent's need for privacy.
	Use appropriate medical terminology.
	Use creative methods to explain experiences and procedures.
	Respect the adolescent's right to refuse treatment.

*Motherese is child-directed speech that adults use when talking to young children. It uses simple, short sentences, spoken slowly in a high-pitched voice. There is also repetition and exaggerated emphasis on key words, which are usually words for activities and objects.

Reflections from Families

When Helen was first born, I was so frightened. You see, I was a single mother in my early thirties with little to no experience taking care of children. While I am an outgoing, personable person who is verbally adept and observant, this whole experience of becoming a mother threw me for a loop. Even with supportive people around me, the highs and lows of raising a child alone were staggering.

Helen is 5 years old now. I am much more relaxed, even though I sometimes find myself at wit's end with the constant chatter and questions and relentless energy of my soon to be kindergarten student. As I think back on some of the nurses I have interacted with these last several years, only a few stand out "softly and brightly" in my mind. There are the few who asked me how I was getting along and actually waited for an answer. There are the few who were not too busy to listen, and then suggested alternatives as to how I might want to handle Helen's health problems. I wish all nurses, and doctors for that matter, could learn to empower a parent as I know these few nurses did for me. After all, it is the parent who raises a child; nurses and doctors only help.

INFANTS

Infancy is a time when communication is achieved through nonverbal means. Even though the adult may use language to relate to an infant, the tone, pitch, and speed of words as well as touch and the bodily movements accompanying the words generate meaning to the infant rather than the words used. However, loud, sudden noises may cause startle reactions and crying, while soft, song-like tones delivered in an upbeat tempo may soothe and comfort. Gentle rubbing or patting while securely holding an infant is also a method to communicate pleasure and security. Infant responses are nonverbal, such as vocal cues, including crying, cooing, and whining. Body language, such as stiffness or relaxation, arm or leg movement, pushing away with hands and feet against the adult, opening or closing the mouth, and gripping or pushing objects such as rattles and blankets are other nonverbal methods infants use. Infant expressions of comfort and discomfort become more direct and overtly explicit with age. That is, a 2-week-old infant will cry and flail arms and legs when hungry, while a 6-month-old infant may kick the legs and arm-wave, or suck on toys, fingers, or blankets when hungry. Caregivers soon learn to distinguish their infant's cries and will differentiate the cry of hunger from the cry of pain or anger. As the caregiver understands the meaning of infant behavior, satisfaction and attachment increase. As the caregiver learns how to turn the infant's tears into satiation, contented sleep, or cooing wakefulness, interactions and communication are positively reinforced.

FAMILY TEACHING

Communicating with Caregivers

1. Explain equipment and procedures thoroughly.
2. Address the questions and concerns of caregivers honestly.
3. Teach caregivers what to expect the child will look like and feel like during treatment.
4. Help caregivers understand the bigger picture—that is, the long-range as well as the short-range effect of treatment.
5. Teach and allow the caregiver to carry out as many aspects of the child's care as feasible.
6. Make reassurance a part of family interactions; ask caregivers how they are doing as time passes.
7. Respect caregivers' concerns even if they seem trivial.

Prior to developing stranger anxiety, infants will respond positively to the nurse and other strangers who provide comforting behaviors through feeding, diapering, rocking, and other forms of nonverbal communication. After the onset of stranger anxiety, incorporating the caregiver into the health care procedures reduces the infant's discomfort. Whenever the nurse needs to hold or give an infant care, caregivers should be involved. If this is not possible, the nurse should

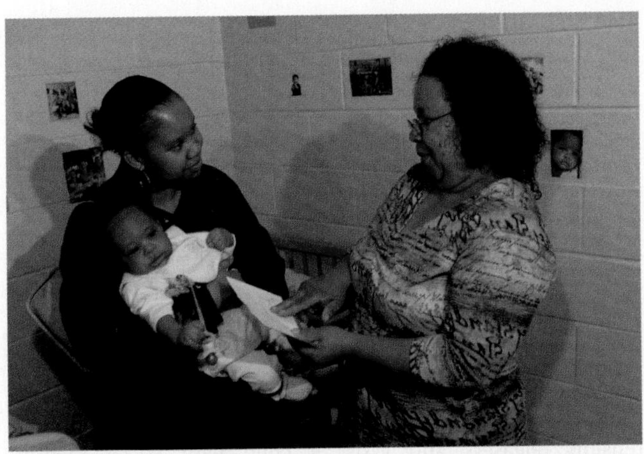

FIGURE 13-9 Nurses interacting with infants should move slowly and incorporate the parent in their examination of the infant; for example, by allowing the mother to hold and manipulate the infant's position when listening to breath sounds.

DELMAR CENGAGE LEARNING.

CRITICAL THINKING

Communicating with Infants

Ronnie, a 6-month-old infant diagnosed with meningitis, is fussy whenever you enter his room. How could you communicate with him when providing care?

hold the infant so the caregiver is in view. The nurse's movement should be firm and gentle, allowing time for the infant to get to know the nurse; abrupt movements will only increase the infant's distress. Using calm, soft, and soothing vocalizations and purposeful, slow movements enhances therapeutic communication with infants (Figure 13-9). For more information, refer to Chapter 8.

TODDLERS

The toddler continues to experience the world through hearing, seeing, smelling, tasting, and touching, and remains dependent on caregivers. Independence emerges, and satisfaction is derived from repetition and routine as the environment is explored. Language in the form of two-word combinations emerges as well as the ability to participate in turn-taking rules of social communication, such as the fact that an answer follows a question and someone listens when someone speaks. Gestures and simple language are used to convey wants and needs. One-word sentences that are part babble with "bye-bye" may be used to express whole ideas, aided by accompanying gestures that provide clues to the meaning. "Bye-bye" with hat in hand may mean "I want to go out and play," while "bye-bye" after being kissed by dad prior to walking out the door may mean "I want to go bye-bye with Dad." Two-word utterances become common at about 2 years of age. The two-word sentence consists of a noun and verb such as "me do." By the age of 3 years, complete sentences are constructed using all parts of speech, and the child's vocabulary has progressed to approximately 900–1,000 words. Toddlers also engage in monologues as a way of practicing speech, and as they mature, egocentric thought and monologue speech become more socialized. Increasingly, they engage in more conversation with others (Albertson, 2007; Grover, 2008; Puckett, Black, & Moriarity, 2007).

Nurses interacting with toddlers should be observant of the situation surrounding one-word utterances and gestures. They should also learn the words toddlers use for common items or behaviors, and use them in conversation. For instance, instead of saying it is "time for bed," the nurse may want to use an expression that for the child means bedtime, such as "it is time to hear the night-night angel sing." Using the expression that indicates bed- or naptime, while following the child's ritual of falling asleep while a music box plays, is a comforting, familiar way of interacting that brings safe and familiar experiences to the child's mind. Using play or books to demonstrate or describe activities or procedures immediately before they are to occur is a good way to prepare toddlers for experiences. Refraining from wordy explanations and having all necessary supplies and equipment ready to accomplish procedures expeditiously is also toddler friendly. Being aware of the child's response and approaching the child calmly and positively are important, since toddlers may withdraw and reject people and/or objects when they are fearful or distressed. For more information, see Chapter 9.

PRESCHOOLERS

During the preschool years, a child's articulation becomes clearer, there are improvements in correct grammatical usage, and an expansion of word combining occurs. The child's vocabulary rapidly expands, and the child is able to use words appropriately even when the meaning is not fully appreciated. Since the preschooler is striving for independence, but still needs adult encouragement and support, it is important to allow the child to initiate activities and make choices if possible. For example, let the child decide whether to have "water or a mouthful of Jell-O after your medicine." Nurses may need to remind children how to cooperate in an activity or to wait for their turn. Asking the child's cooperation by giving them something to do or hold may engage them cooperatively and allow the procedure to be performed. Using picture books, stuffed toys, and puppets to prepare a child for a procedure will allow the child to experience the procedure in a nonthreatening way (Figure 13-10). A child may also answer the nurse's question through a teddy bear: "Hi, Mr. Teddy bear, do you think your friend Johnny would like some Jell-O after his medicine or would a mouthful of chocolate pudding be better?"

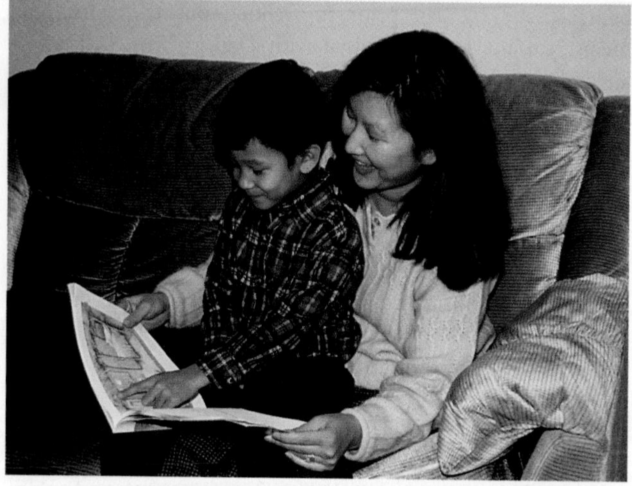

FIGURE 13-10 **Storytelling, particularly with the use of storybooks, helps a nurse develop rapport with preschoolers. Hand puppets and dolls are also engaging methods used to decrease a child's anxiety in first-time encounters.** DELMAR CENGAGE LEARNING.

Preschoolers are egocentric, and magical thinking predominates; these children see things only from their perspective. When they lack information or do not understand something, they fill in the gaps with their imagination. Since an avid imagination can be far worse than any reality, it is better to communicate with honesty, in simple sentences using concrete language. The nurse should never smile or laugh when giving an injection, say something won't hurt when it will, or use words with double or literal meanings such as a "shot" or a "stick in the arm." It is also not helpful to tell the child about others or what "good boys or girls" do. Allowing preschoolers to touch and manipulate equipment they will see and experience is essential. Telling preschoolers how it will feel when they come in contact with the equipment (cold, warm, pressure, tickles, etc.) and how they can behave is also important. For example, tell them that it is okay to squeeze the teddy bear, cry, yell, or bang on the bed with their hand, and so on. It is also important to use positive statements such as "while you are getting the injection, this other nurse is going to help you hold still," instead of saying "the nurse is going to hold you still." For more information, see Chapter 10.

KIDS WANT TO KNOW

Why do they have to do that test? Will it hurt?

Whenever talking to preschoolers, use simple words that answer the questions asked; avoid detailed answers. "You will go to the X-ray department so they can take a picture of your tummy. They want to find out why you have a tummy ache. The bed you lie on will be cool, but they will put a blanket on you to keep you warm. The test will not hurt." It may also be appropriate to say something like, "be sure you smile or make a funny face when your picture is taken."

SCHOOL-AGE CHILDREN

A school-age child's relational experiences expand to include people and environments outside the family and home. They are taught rhymes, chants, and rituals by other children, which can serve as a means of emotional-social control in frightening and confusing contexts. We all remember examples, such as "cross your heart and hope to die," "star light, star bright, first star I see tonight," and "knock on wood," which we used to minimize the bad that could befall us. Humor and riddles are tension releasers and assist a child with social identity (i.e., "knock, knock, who's there?"). During early school years, interaction with other children increases and close friendships are developed. Children of this age group may be verbally aggressive, bossy, opinionated, and argumentative.

School-age children learn to accept responsibility for their actions, they understand rules, and they become oriented to rules and sanctions. They are interested in learning and have increased attention spans. They learn to master classification, serialization, and spatial, temporal, and numerical concepts. Concrete thinking emerges and predominates. They learn to focus on more than one aspect of an experience and to explore and consider many alternatives to a problem. They are increasingly able to understand their body and their environment and to use language as a means of control and appreciate it as a method used by others to control them. School-age children also have expanding vocabularies that enable them to describe feelings, thoughts, and concepts. They are able to carry on conversations with others and to appreciate their viewpoints. However, words with multiple meanings and words that describe things they have not experienced are still not thoroughly understood.

When working with the school-age child, the nurse should spend time with the child to explain treatments and procedures well in advance of the scheduled time (Figure 13-11). Photographs, books, drawings, and videos may be used to aid understanding and assist in answering questions. Immediate and subsequent opportunities should be allowed for questions, and repetition of explanations and enhanced details of what will happen to them should be provided. Fears and concerns about body integrity should be assessed and truthfully answered. Conversation that encourages critical thinking should be promoted. For more information, see Chapter 11.

ADOLESCENTS

Adolescents are able to think logically and abstractly, and are able to verbalize and comprehend most adult concepts. They are able to create hypothetical situations and generate explanations for and about situations they encounter. Privacy and independence are sought in activities and relationships. Adolescents make personal discoveries about their relationships and events, and will discuss these discoveries with peers and trusted adults in an effort to construct ideals.

Table 13-2 Traditional Communication Patterns of Various Cultures (*Continued*)

CULTURAL GROUP	COMMUNICATION STYLES
Hispanic American (Mexican)	• Sensitive to incongruence between verbal and nonverbal messages • Tend to test those in the majority before submitting to their suggestions and care • Use direct eye contact • Use gestures and voice tone changes in speech • Unassertive if others appear busy or rushed • Offended by a hurried attitude • Value politeness and respond to being called by title or complete name • May smile and nod even if they do not understand • Perceive touch as reassuring, comforting, and sympathetic • Although many are bilingual, may use nonstandard English • View small talk as important before serious discussion • Appreciate open-ended questions and a nondirective approach
Puerto Rican	• Value personal and family privacy; questions regarding family are considered presumptuous and disrespectful • Possess a relaxed concept of time • May not use standard English • Many are bilingual • New immigrants and older individuals may speak Spanish
Cuban	• Most new immigrants are bilingual • Consider small talk important before serious discussion
Native American	• Value nonverbal communication • Consider silence essential to understanding and respecting another • Consider direct eye contact insulting • May be reticent in forming opinions of health care providers • Pauses after being questioned are common; pauses signify thoughtful consideration • Hesitant to discuss personal affairs unless trust has developed and prefer these discussions occur with a person of the same gender • Sensitive about having their behaviors and words written down • Believe it is ethically wrong to speak for another
Middle Eastern	• Use silence to show respect • Men and women do not touch each other unless they are in the immediate family or are married • Touching or embracing is common among those of the same gender • Devout Muslims may not want to talk to female nurses or physicians
European American	• Tolerate hugs or embraces among intimates and close friends only • Note understanding or agreement by nods • Use neutral facial expressions in public • Individuals separate into gender-specific groups at social events, unless the activity is for couples • Prefer personal space • Speak warmly and pleasantly and smile to put others at ease • A firm handshake symbolizes goodwill; a pat on shoulder or back denotes camaraderie

Adapted from Estes, M. E. Z. (2010). *Health assessment & physical examination* (4th ed.). Clifton Park, NY: Delmar Cengage Learning; Martin, J. N. (2009). *Intercultural communication in contexts.* New York: McGraw-Hill; and Pullen, R. (2007). Tips for communicating with a patient from another culture. *Nursing 2007, 37,* 48–49.

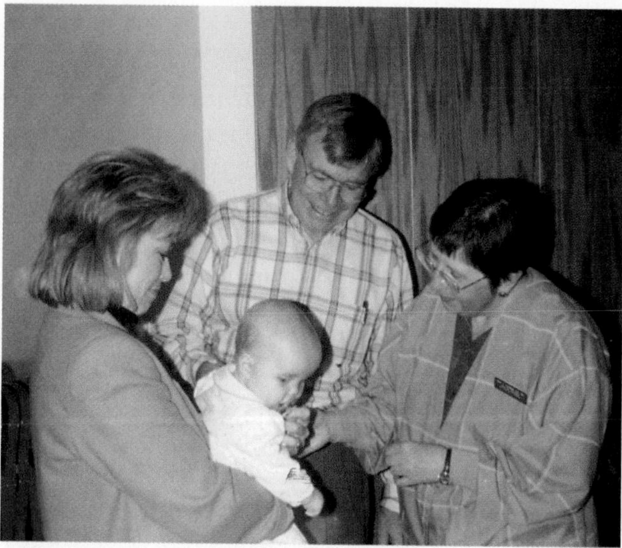

FIGURE 13-13 Nurses understand the importance of interacting with family members when caring for infants, children, and adolescents. When the family is informed and involved in the health and well-being of their children, they are likely to thrive. DELMAR CENGAGE LEARNING.

Consideration box for information about using an interpreter. Chapter 3 also has additional information about families from other cultures. Remember, what is most important is to treat and understand each person as an individual who may or may not incorporate the communication patterns of their ethnic group into their value system.

The care planned and implemented with a child or caregiver should be congruent with their values and consistent with their understanding of health care. During contact, the nurse needs to incorporate questions and make observations that elicit information about family practices that may impact care (Figure 13-13). These include questions about their communication and decision-making strategies, child rearing, and health and illness practices. Once this information is obtained, it can be used to determine priorities and develop an individualized treatment plan culturally consistent with the family's values and beliefs and that will engender their commitment and compliance See Box 13-5 for more information.

For caregivers who would normally depend on their extended family for support and find themselves without them in their present environment, extra time or assistance may be necessary to help them make critical health care decisions. Anticipating the arrival of members who must travel to reach a child and family, or providing a quiet place for the family to telephone distant extended family members are also appropriate nursing interventions.

BOX 13-5

QUESTIONS TO ELICIT PERTINENT INFORMATION ABOUT HEALTH CARE PRACTICES AND BELIEFS

When caring for children and their families, bear in mind that health care practices and beliefs can be influenced by many different sources. Consider incorporating questions such as these into your client interactions:

- Who do you discuss your child's health or illness problems with?
- Who assists you in making decisions about your child's health or illness problems?
- Who assists you or your family when you need help related to health care?
- Which other family members (such as grandparents) would you like to have involved in this discussion of your health care needs?
- Is there a religious or spiritual leader you would like us to contact to assist you in making some of your health care decisions?
- Would you like to refer to a certain book, credo, or teaching (such as the Bible or Koran) when considering your health care options?

CRITICAL THINKING

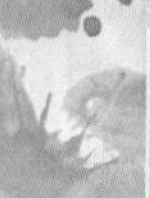

Communicating with Children from Another Culture

You are caring for a child who does not speak English. What nursing interventions can you use when an interpreter is not available?

COMMUNICATING WITH CHILDREN WITH SPECIAL NEEDS

Communicating with children who have special needs can be particularly challenging and may require adopting alternative methods of interacting. Whenever communicating with children with special needs, it is imperative to involve families and to carefully assess the child's skills and abilities. Principles of communicating with children with special needs and their families are the same as those discussed in this chapter. However, refer to Chapter 31 for specific information on communicating with children who have a visual or hearing impairment and to Chapter 33 for specific information on communicating with children who have a significant cognitive impairment.

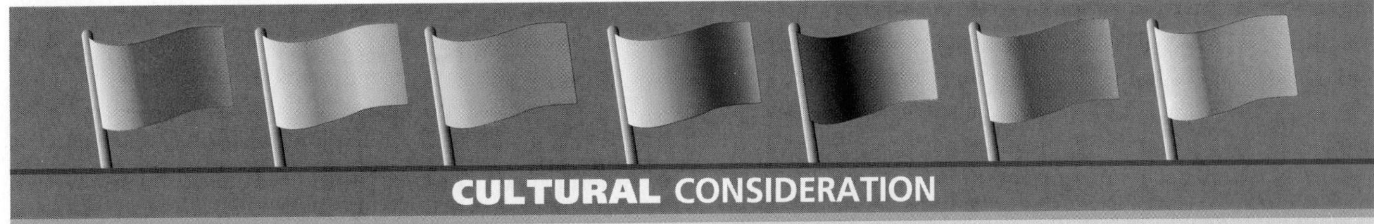

CULTURAL CONSIDERATION

Surmounting Language Barriers between Health Care Providers and Children or Families

A. With an interpreter

1. Determine language(s) and dialect (if relevant) a client is familiar with and speaks at home; the language may not be identical to the one commonly used in their country of origin. Some clients may be multilingual, and a language other than their mother tongue can be used.
2. Be sensitive to and make allowances for differences with regard to age, culture, gender, and socioeconomic status between the client and interpreter.
3. Request as verbatim a translation as possible.
4. Assure confidentiality.
5. Preferably request an interpreter that is the same sex as the patient.
6. Have the interpreter remain as unnoticed as possible within the nurse-patient relationship.
7. The nurse should control the conversation.
8. The interpreter should be fluent in both the nurse's and the patient's language.
9. Ideally, the interpreter should understand medical terminology and medical and nursing procedures.
10. Be mindful of HIPAA laws when using an interpreter

B. Without an interpreter

1. Always be polite, formal, patient, and attentive to the client's (or client's family's) attempts to communicate.
2. When greeting the client, smile, use the client's complete or last name, indicate your name by saying it while gesturing to oneself, and offer a handshake or nod.
3. Speak in a low and moderate tone; avoid raising your voice.
4. Assure the patient that your communication is confidential.
5. If possible, use words from the client's language.
6. Use simple words—no idiom, no jargon (medical or otherwise), no slang. Avoid the use of contractions and pronouns, which may be unclear to the client.
7. Give instructions clearly, in simple language (with a minimum of words), and in the correct order.
8. Talk about one topic at a time.
9. Use hand signs freely and act out actions while talking.
10. Check client's understanding by requesting he/she describe or illustrate the procedure, pantomime the meaning, or repeat the instructions.
11. Try using Latin phrases or phrases from other languages that have become universal.
12. Write simple sentences in English or another language, since some people understand the written, but not spoken languages, and some accents may be confusing.
13. Use phrase books and flash cards.
14. Use Internet options such as Google to help with translation.

Adapted from Burnard, P., & Gill, P. (2008). *Culture, communication, and nursing.* Harlow, England: Pearson Education; Munoz C., & Luckman, J. (2005). *Transcultural communication in nursing* (2nd ed.). Clifton Park, NY: Delmar Cengage Learning; Smith, L. S. (2007). Speaking up for medical language interpreters. *Nursing 2007, 37*, 49.

NURSING TIP

Be Proactive for Children or Caregivers Who Speak English as a Second Language

- Enunciate clearly, and speak slowly.
- Avoid situations that prevent the listener from seeing lip movements, facial expressions, or gestures.
- Speak in the active voice.
- Avoid using contractions, slang, and idioms.

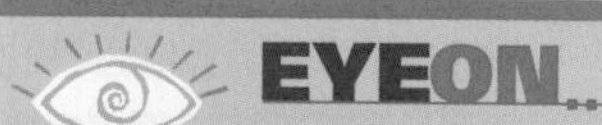

EYE ON...

Touch

Avoid touching a Cambodian, Vietnamese, Thai, or Hmong child on the head during an initial assessment or conversation, since the head has traditionally been considered the site of the soul for these cultures. However, Hispanics view touch as a gesture of sincerity and are used to gentle embraces. Therefore, when caring for Hispanic children and families, shaking hands and sitting or standing closer are important, as is gentle touch on the hand or head.

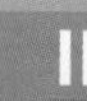

IN THE REAL WORLD

Because of his age (12), I tried to allow Luke (admitted for incision and drainage of an abscess on his leg) to be as modest and independent as possible. As I helped him with his bed bath, he began to open up about his interests, friends, and hospital stay. Although I only spent 20–30 minutes performing these simple activities, the time allowed for trust to develop and communication lasted throughout the day. Furthermore, he was more relaxed and cheerful. When I changed him from a PCA to oral pain meds, I explained the importance of staying on top of the pain and he indicated he understood. Later on that day, when his IV line was heplocked, I let him help me. By letting Luke become more involved in the procedure, I think it became less scary for him and I communicated my trust.

The definition of communication includes transferring knowledge and information. Besides discussing pain control and heplocks with Luke, I do not feel I did a lot of client teaching. However, I did transfer knowledge about feelings and trust, and I believe this is especially important since often pediatric clients may not understand why procedures need to be done. Communicating information has an empowering effect on clients and allows them to assume more control of their environment and care. With empowerment comes an increased effort to improve and a better attitude about treatment. Communication is that aspect of therapeutic nursing interventions which helps standards of practice be effective.

KEY CONCEPTS

- The ability to communicate effectively is recognized as a basic and central component in delivering care to children and their caregivers.
- The sender, message, channel, receiver, and feedback are major components of the communication process.
- Barriers to successful communication will impede the message, and include physical factors and psychological factors.
- Communication can be formal or informal and verbal or nonverbal.
- Empathy, listening effectively, observing accurately, using silence appropriately, being aware of the environment, humor, play, writing, drawing, and using third parties are effective methods of communicating with children and adolescents.
- Effective communication requires sensitivity to and an understanding of the child's developmental level and the needs of the child and family, and a well-developed and carefully thought-out plan.
- Cultural background can play a role in the determination of an individual's communication pattern.
- Communication with children with special needs requires knowledge of their skill and ability level, and may require adopting alternative methods of interacting.

REVIEW ACTIVITIES

1. Describe a developmentally appropriate communication approach for each of the following age groups: infant (0–12 months), toddler (1–2 years), preschooler (3–5 years), school-age child (6–11 years), and adolescent (12 years plus).
2. Describe two behaviors that negatively affect communication between nurse and child, or nurse and caregiver, and discuss each.
3. Describe two behaviors that positively affect the relationship between nurse and child, or nurse and caregiver, and discuss each.
4. Describe three nonverbal behaviors that, if engaged in, would contradict the nurse's spoken words.
5. Give an example of a professional yet empathetic phone greeting when calling clients.
6. Describe how play can be used to develop rapport and trust, or give information to an infant, a 5-year-old, and a 10-year-old.

STUDY QUESTIONS

1. When the nurse talks to the client during procedures, the type of discourse is best described as which of the following types of communication?
   a. Spontaneous
   b. Informal
   c. Sporadic
   d. Formal
2. When caring for a client the nurse expresses attitudes and feelings through which of the following behaviors?
   a. Compliments
   b. Smiles
   c. Praise
   d. Comments
3. The nurse demonstrates respect for the client by doing which of the following?
   a. Giving the client a special nickname
   b. Calling the client an endearing name
   c. Addressing the client by the formal name
   d. Avoiding the use of the surname
4. In order for the nurse to fully understand the caregiver's concerns, the nurse should listen to which of the following?
   a. Child's verbalizations
   b. Physician's documentation
   c. Experience and intuition
   d. Caregiver's gestures
5. The nurse's 1-year-old client cries each time the child's crib is approached. The nurse should do which of the following?
   a. Avoid approaching the child's crib unless absolutely necessary
   b. Combine care and procedures to prevent upsetting the infant
   c. Only work with the child when the mother is in attendance
   d. Bring a windup toy that is brightly colored
6. The nurse should avoid touching the heads of children who belong to which of the following cultural group?
   a. European Americans
   b. Chinese
   c. Vietnamese
   d. Puerto Ricans
7. The nurse should limit touching in the care of people of which of the following cultural group?
   a. Japanese
   b. Filipino
   c. African American
   d. Puerto Ricans
8. When an interpreter is not available, the nurse understands that the most appropriate way of communicating is to:
   a. Postpone contact until an interpreter is available.
   b. Use phrase books and flash cards on one topic.
   c. Smile, speak loudly and in an expressive tone.
   d. Use slang words from the client's language.
9. The nurse can use which of the following to bridge communication gaps when the child is fearful?
   a. Positive criticism
   b. Silence
   c. Humor
   d. Half-truths
10. Third-party communication can be used by a nurse to direct the child's attention away from their fears. The most appropriate third party is which of the following?
    a. "His or her" or "a" sibling
    b. A pacifier
    c. "His or her" or "a" parent
    d. A stuffed toy

REFERENCES

Albertson, L. (2007). Improved teacher and toddler communication through the use of American Sign Language. Thesis (M.A.)—Pacific Oaks College.

Andrews, M. M., & Boyle, J. S. (2007). *Transcultural concepts in nursing care* (4th ed.). Philadelphia: Lippincott.

Arnold, E., & Boggs, K. U. (2007). *Interpersonal relationships: Professional communication skills for nurses* (5th ed.). St. Louis, MO: Saunders/Elsevier.

Baby Einstein Music Box Orchestra & Weisbach, B. (2008). *Sing & Play*. Burbank, CA: Walt Disney Records.

Burnard, P., & Gill, P. (2008). *Culture, communication, and nursing*. Harlow, England: Pearson Education.

Estes, M. E. Z. (2010). *Health assessment & physical examination* (4th ed.). Clifton Park, NY: Delmar Cengage Learning.

Gardner, R. (1986). *Therapeutic communication with children: The mutual storytelling technique*. New York: Science Books.

Grover, G. (2008). Language development; Speech and hearing assessment. In C. Berkowitz, (Ed.). *Pediatrics: A primary care approach*. (3rd ed.). Philadelphia, PA: Saunders, pp. 95–100.

Hamama, L., & Ronen, T. (2009). Children's drawings as a self-report measurement. *Child and Family Social Work, 14*, 90–102.

Johnston, C. C., Fillon, F., Campbell-Yeo, M., Goulet, C., Bell, L., McNaughton, K., Byron, J., Aita, M., Findlay, G. A., & Walker, C. D. (2008). Kangaroo mother care diminishes pain from heel lance in very preterm neonates: A crossover trial. *BMC Pediatrics, 8*, 13.

Lefevre, M. (2004). Playing with sound: The therapeutic use of music in direct work with children. *Child and Family Social Work, 9*, 333–345.

Lester, B. M., Masten, A. S., & McEwen, B. S. (2006). Resilience in children. *Annals of the New York Academy of Sciences, 1094*. Boston, MA: Blackwell Publishing.

Marquis, B. L., & Huston, C. J. (2008). *Leadership roles and management functions in nursing: Theory and application* (6th ed.). Philadelphia, PA: Lippincott, Williams & Wilkins.

Martin, J. N. (2009). *Intercultural communication in contexts*. New York: McGraw-Hill.

Martin, R. A. (2007). *The psychology of humor: An integrative approach*. Amsterdam: Elsevier Academic Press.

May, L. (1999). "I've got tummy ache in my head": Communicating with sick children. *Pediatric Nursing, 11*, 21–23.

McDonald, H., & Rushforth, H. (2006). Children's views of nursing and medical roles: Implications for advanced nursing practice. *Pediatric Nursing, 18*, 32–36.

Munoz, C., & Luckman, J. (2005). *Transcultural communication in nursing* (2nd ed.). Clifton Park, NY: Delmar Cengage Learning.

Neumark-Sztainer, D., Eisenberg, M. E., Fulkerson, J. A., Story, M., & Larson, N. I. (2008). Family meals and disordered eating in adolescents longitudinal findings from Project EAT. *Archives of Pediatrics & Adolescent Medicine, 162*, 17–22.

Ockelford, A. (2008). *Music for children and young people with complex needs*. Oxford Music Education Series. Oxford, England: Oxford University Press.

Puckett, M. B., Black, J. K., & Moriarity, J. (2007). *Understanding toddler development*. St. Paul, MN: Redleaf Press.

Pullen, R. (2007). Tips for communicating with a patient from another culture. *Nursing 2007, 37*, 48–49.

Smith, L. S. (2007). Speaking up for medical language interpreters. *Nursing 2007, 37*, 49.

Stuart, G. W. (2009). *Principles and practice of psychiatric nursing*. (9th ed.). St. Louis, MO: Mosby.

SUGGESTED READINGS

Butz, A. M., Walker, J. M., Pulsifer, M., & Winkelstein, M. (2007). Shared decision making in school age children with asthma. *Pediatric Nursing, 33*, 111–116.

Flores, N. (2008). Dealing with an angry patient. *Nursing 2008, 38*, 30–31.

Holte, L., Prickett, J. G., Van Dyke, D. C., Olson, R. J., Lubrica, P., Knutson, C. L., Knutson, J. F., Brennan, S., & Berg, W. (2006). Issues in the management of infants and young children who are deaf-blind. *Infants and young children, 19*, 323–337.

LeBlanc, N. M. (2008). Play with me!: A guide to building therapeutic relationships with children through child-centered play therapy project. James Madison University.

Levetown, M. (2008). Communicating with children and families: From everyday interactions to skill in conveying distressing information. *Pediatrics-Springfield 121*, 1037.

Malloch, S., & Trevarthen, C. (2009). *Communicative musicality: Exploring the basis of human companionship*. New York: Oxford University Press.

Meerwein, G., Rodeck, B., & Mahnke, F. (2007). *Color: Communication in architectural space*. Basel: Birkhauser Verlag.

Mullett, S. (2008). A helping paw. *RN, 71*, 39–44.

Olmon, K., & Rogers, J. (2009). *Baby signs*. New York: Orchard Books.

Recob, A. (2008). *Bibliography: When kids need books, a guide for those in need of reassurance*. Bloomington, Indiana: iUniverse.

Riley, J. B. (2008). *Communication in nursing* (6th ed.). St. Louis: Elsevier.

Scheffler, F., Vogel D., Astern R., Burgess J., Conneally T., & Salerno K. (2007). Screening for communication and cognitive disorders in infants and toddlers. *Pediatric Nursing, 33*, 473–480.

Smith, G. (2007). Communicating competence. *American Journal of Nursing, 107*, 13.

Spector, R. E. (2009). *Cultural diversity in health and illness* (7th ed.). Englewood Cliffs, NJ: Prentice Hall.

Talk it through: Communicating with the parents of sick children. (2008). *Nursing Standard, 22*(30), 22.

Thompson, R. H. (2008). The handbook of child life: A guide for pediatric psychosocial care. Springfield, IL: Charles H. Thomas.

Williams, C. L. (2008). *Therapeutic interaction in nursing*. Sudbury, MA: Jones & Bartlett.

Zoucha, R., & Broome, B. (2008). The significance of culture in nursing: Examples from the Mexican American culture and knowing the unknown. *Urologic Nursing, 28*, 140–142.

RESOURCES

Refer to the online student StudyWARE for Potts & Mandleco at http://www.CengageBrain.com for additional content and study aids.

Organization: **American Academy of Pediatrics**
Description: Offers general information related to child health, specific guidelines concerning many pediatric issues, information regarding AAP programs, activities, policies, guidelines, publications, and other child health resources.
Website/Resource: http://www.aap.org

Organization: **Child Development Institute**
Description: Provides current, relevant, and easy to attain parent education including readers' development, parenting, psychology, learning, and health/safety.
Website/Resource: http://www.childdevelopmentinfo.com

Organization: **Kids Health Organization**
Description: Provides advice about a wide range of physical, emotional, and behavioral issues that affect children and teens.
Website/Resource: http://www.kidshealth.org

Organization: **Minority Health Network (MHNet)**
Description: Web based information source for individuals interested in minority health; offers information about different minority groups, diseases, publications, and upcoming events.
Website/Resource: http://www.mhnet.org

Organization: **National Center for Cultural Competence**
Description: Offers access to articles about implementing cultural competency.
Website/Resource: http://www.culturalbroker.info

Organization: **National Center for Health Statistics (NCHS)**
Description: Compiles statistical information to guide actions/policies to improve health of Americans; website offers statistical reports concerning health employment, health data standards and much more.
Website/Resource: http://www.cdc.gov

Organization: **National Institutes of Health**
Description: Offers information regarding countless health topics, clinical trials, grants, health related news, and current medical research.
Website/Resource: http://www.nih.gov

Organization: **Public Broadcasting**
Description: Offers information about TV shows, TV schedules, and access to PBS programs and an online shop.
Website/Resource: http://www.pbs.org

Organization: **Talking with Kids**
Description: A resource offering parents tips about talking to children about tough issues including sex/relationships, drug/alcohol, violence, race, HIV/AIDS, and divorce.
Website/Resource: http://www.talkingwithkids.org

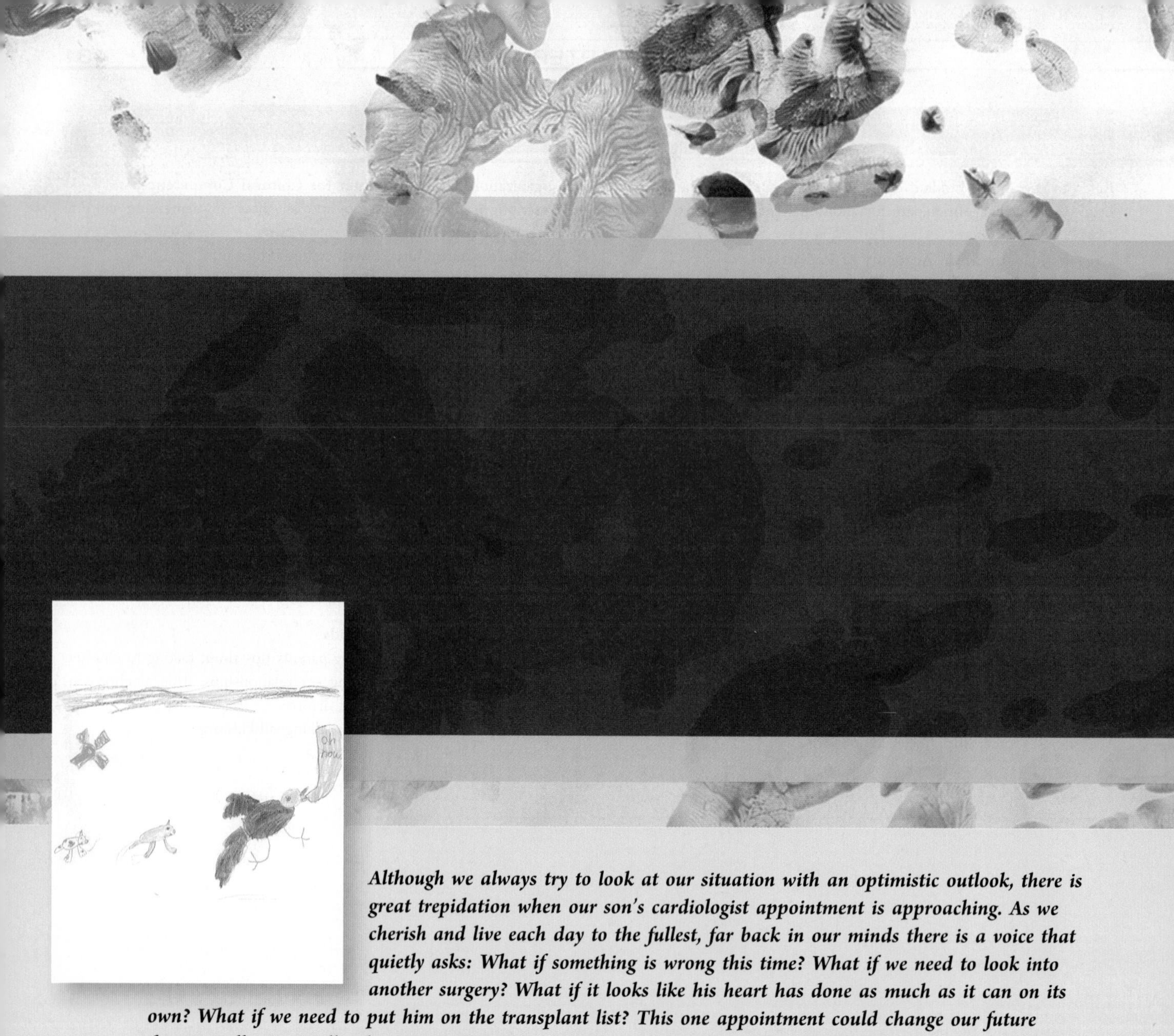

Although we always try to look at our situation with an optimistic outlook, there is great trepidation when our son's cardiologist appointment is approaching. As we cherish and live each day to the fullest, far back in our minds there is a voice that quietly asks: What if something is wrong this time? What if we need to look into another surgery? What if it looks like his heart has done as much as it can on its own? What if we need to put him on the transplant list? This one appointment could change our future dramatically. Ironically, the same appointment usually confirms that all is well, but this can never ease the nervousness. What is termed a simple appointment is actually a significant life-changing event for us every time.

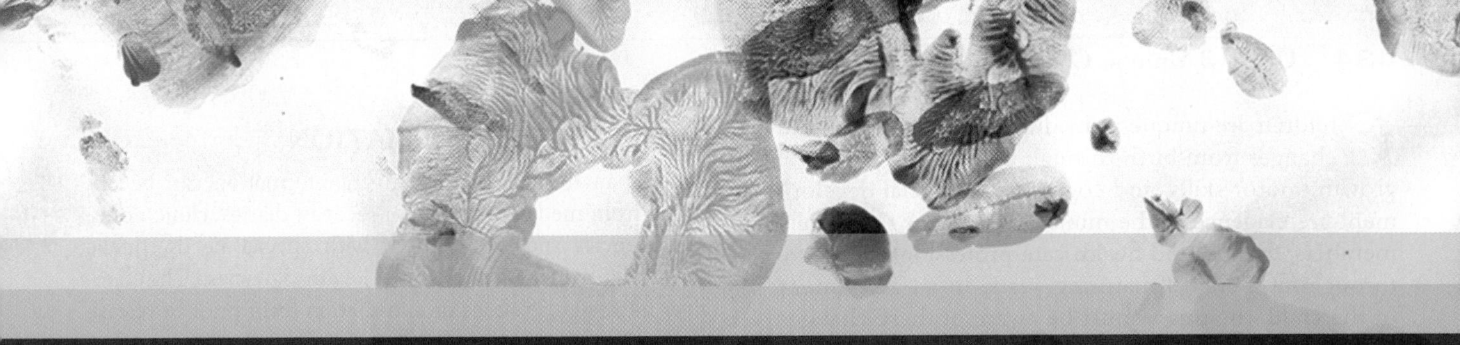

CHAPTER 14
Pediatric Assessment

KATHY MURPHY, RN, MSN, CS

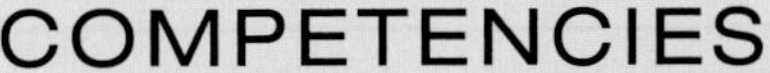

COMPETENCIES

Upon completion of this chapter, the reader will be able to:

- Elicit a complete health history from a child and caregiver using standard components of a pediatric health history.
- Discuss the purpose of a nutritional assessment and its components.
- Explain the purpose of a developmental assessment.
- Identify various techniques of approaching children at different developmental levels before initiating the physical assessment.
- Perform inspection, palpation, percussion, and auscultation in a head-to-toe assessment of a child.
- Identify normal and abnormal findings obtained during the physical assessment.
- Successfully complete the games and activities in the online student StudyWARE.

Children are unique individuals who undergo rapid changes from birth through adolescence. Physical growth, motor skills, and cognitive and social development are evidence of the numerous changes that family members, friends, and health care professionals observe throughout a child's maturing years. In an assessment of the child, the nurse must be aware of these changes while continually reassessing what is considered within normal limits.

PHYSICAL GROWTH

One important set of parameters required for pediatric health assessment is physical growth. The parameters of weight, length or height, and head circumference (dependent on age) are essential in serial physical growth measurements. Chest circumference is of less importance. For example, by plotting a child's growth on a chart (see Appendix B), the nurse is able to determine normal or abnormal growth curves according to the child's age.

HEALTH HISTORY

Because the historian in a pediatric history is less often the child and most likely the caregiver, it is very important to document the historian's relationship to the child. The child should be included in the history taking as is appropriate for her or his age and development.

BIOGRAPHICAL DATA

Child's Name

In addition to the child's name, obtain the full name of the legal guardian. Occasionally, the caregiver is not the legal guardian, such as when the child is a ward of the court or state.

Address and Phone Number

Obtain the address and phone number of the caregiver if different from those of the child.

> **NURSING TIP**
>
> **Adjusting Chronological Age**
>
> **For the infant born prematurely, you will need to adjust the chronological age on the growth chart. For instance, the corrected age for a 6-month-old infant who was born 2 months prematurely would be 4 months. Plot the obtained weight and length on the growth chart under the child's corrected age, and mark above the weight "corrected." The corrected age rule applies until the child is 18–24 months old.**

Source of Information

Other than the child or caregiver, information can be obtained from medical and school records, diaries, clinic notes, and agencies such as children with special needs, public health departments, and home health agencies. The caregiver must sign a release of information form prior to release of records from a third party.

Chief Complaint

The caregiver is often the individual who seeks health care for the child and provides a description of the perceived problems, especially for infants, toddlers, and young preschoolers whose age and mental status prevent them from offering genuine descriptions of their problem. You must frequently rely on the caregiver's intuition in such cases. The caregiver is usually acutely aware of cues to the child's illness. For instance, changes in sleeping patterns (difficulty falling asleep, reversion to night waking), regression to outgrown behaviors (bedwetting, finicky eating, thumb sucking), and unusual physical complaints in an otherwise healthy child (headaches, stomachaches) are important signs that the child may be experiencing stress or illness, and warrant further investigation. The older preschooler, school-age child, and adolescent are able to provide verbal descriptions of their complaints.

PAST HEALTH HISTORY

Pertinent information should be elicited regarding the birth history, including prenatal, labor and delivery, and postnatal history.

Birth History

Obtaining the birth history may be one of the more sensitive topics of the past health history. You must feel comfortable and show sensitivity when inquiring about whether the pregnancy was planned, the date prenatal care was first sought, and birth order of pregnancy, taking into account miscarriages and abortions.

Prenatal

1. Did you plan your pregnancy for __________ (insert month)?
2. How many weeks after thinking that you were pregnant did you go to a health care provider for a check-up?
3. How many children have you carried to full term?
4. Were there any pregnancies that you were not able to carry to full term? What happened?
5. Did you take any prescribed or over-the-counter medications, including ibuprofen products?
6. Did you drink alcohol or caffeine or smoke cigarettes during pregnancy?
7. Did you take any drugs during pregnancy, such as marijuana, crack cocaine, amphetamines, or

hallucinogens such as LSD and mescaline? If so, what were the amounts and frequency of use?
8. Were there any problems or illnesses that either you or your health care provider were worried about during pregnancy (pregnancy-induced hypertension, preterm labor, gestational diabetes, Human Immunodeficiency Virus (HIV), Group B Streptococcus (GBS), TORCH infection [toxoplasmosis, rubella, cytomegalovirus, and herpes] or an abnormal finding on a prenatal ultrasound)?
9. Was the pregnancy conceived naturally?

Labor and Delivery

1. How many weeks did you carry the baby before delivering?
2. Was the labor spontaneous or induced?
3. How many hours long was the labor?
4. Was the baby delivered vaginally or by cesarean section? If by cesarean section, why?
5. Was any analgesia or anesthetic used?
6. Did you hold your baby immediately after delivery? (This question will provide information about the neonate's condition at delivery.)
7. Immediately following delivery, what was the baby's color?
8. What were the baby's Apgar scores at 1 and 5 minutes?
9. What were the birth weight and length of the baby?
10. Was the baby's father at the birth with you?
11. Where was the baby born (home, hospital, automobile, or other location)?

Postnatal

1. Did you and your baby go home together? (If answered no, inquire as to the reason for separate discharges.)
2. If hospital delivery, how long was the hospitalization for you and the baby?
3. Did the baby have any breathing or feeding problems during the first week?
4. To your knowledge, did your baby receive any medications during the first week?
5. How would you describe the baby's color at 1 week? (For the light-skinned baby, ask if the skin was pale, pale pink, blue, or yellow. For the dark-skinned baby, inquire about the color of the sclera, oral mucosa, and nailbeds.)
6. If male, was the baby circumcised?
7. Did you start breast- or bottle-feeding your baby?
8. Were there any problems with your choice of feeding?
9. Did you or the baby have a fever after delivery?
10. Did you have anyone to help you take care of the baby in the first few weeks after delivery?

Medical

Inquire about the circumstances and outcomes of any hospitalizations or emergency department visits. Keep in mind that some children's caregivers may use the emergency department or Urgent Care Center for episodic health care and may not have a primary care provider.

Injuries or Accidents

Determine if the child has a pattern of frequent injuries or accidents. Repeat trauma may indicate abuse.

Childhood Illnesses

Document past and current exposure to measles, mumps, rubella, pertussis, chickenpox, and respiratory syncytial virus (RSV).

Immunizations

Immunizations provide protection against many contagious diseases of childhood. Maternal antibodies pass through the placenta and breast milk, offering the baby limited protection from disease. A schedule of recommended childhood immunizations is located in Appendix C. Many health care providers follow the immunization schedule as a guide for well-child check-ups. A record of immunizations is essential for school admission and to avoid repeat vaccinations.

FAMILY HEALTH HISTORY

Inquire about age and health status (if deceased, age and cause of death) of the child's mother, father, siblings, grandparents, aunts, and uncles. Ask about diseases in the family that could affect the child's health, including heart disease, diabetes, mental retardation, seizures, allergies, asthma, congenital disorders, alcoholism, and attention deficit hyperactivity disorder (ADHD). Also ask about sudden infant death syndrome (SIDS).

SOCIAL HISTORY

Work Environment

Day care facilities and schools are the child's equivalent of a work environment. Inquire about the number of hours the child attends a day care facility per week. Inquire about the child's academic performance. In addition, ask if the child is home alone before or after school.

Home Environment

Ask about potential exposure to lead in chipping paint because lead is harmful to the developing brain and nervous system of fetuses and young children. Living in a home built prior to 1978 is a risk factor for exposure to lead paint.

Child's Personal Habits

1. Determine what activities the child enjoys.
2. Ask how the child copes with stress and if a security object (blanket, stuffed toy) helps calm the child.
3. Determine if the child is prone to temper tantrums and what type of discipline is used.

HEALTH MAINTENANCE ACTIVITIES

Sleep

Determine if the child takes naps and if the child shares a bedroom, because children's different sleep habits may lead to interrupted sleep.

Diet

Questions concerning diet need to be tailored to the child's developmental level. Refer to *Nutritional Assessment, Dietary History* for questions appropriate to each developmental level.

Safety

Childproofing the environment, especially for young children, is an essential practice. Box 14-1 lists questions to include in your interview.

■ NUTRITIONAL ASSESSMENT

Good nutrition is essential for optimal health and disease prevention. Educating a child early in life about the importance of healthy eating habits can play a role in safeguarding the child against future disease. Never has there been a time in our history where so much emphasis is being placed on health promotion and preventing diet-related diseases or deficiencies. Nutritional assessment enables the nurse to provide anticipatory guidance, identify at-risk individuals, and collaborate with the health care team for early referral of the child as needed. A variety of methods are employed to assess the child's nutritional status, including history of dietary intake, analysis of laboratory data, anthropometric data, and physical examination.

DIETARY INTAKE

There are numerous ways to determine if a child is receiving adequate nutrition. One vehicle for doing so is through a record of dietary intake. Dietary intake is elicited through a 24-hour recall, food diary, or food frequency questionnaire. As with all open-ended questions, an accurate response is variable. Accuracy is hard to obtain if the child has multiple caregivers. Involving the primary caregiver and extended caregivers will be an important task. When obtaining the 24-hour food recall, inquire about the previous 24 hours. Involve any family members present during your interview. Ask the individual to recall the amount and types of food eaten by the child, including the amount and type of liquids consumed during the past 24 hours. A food diary is quite similar to the 24-hour recall in that you are requesting the family to keep track of the same information for a 3- to 7-day time span. Instruct the caregiver to allow others such as day care providers to record the time, type, and amount of foods and liquids consumed directly on the diary. A food frequency questionnaire can be used during the interview to collect information about consumption of foods from all the food groups. Information collected includes what type, and the amount and frequency of consumed liquids and foods.

DIETARY HISTORY

Another important tool for assessing dietary risk factors is a diet history. Dietary histories can identify a host of nutritional and behavioral problems, and anticipatory guidance can be provided for deficient areas of nutritional health. The following questions concerning diet are divided into age groups:

A. Infant (0–12 months)
   1. Are you breast- or bottle-feeding? (Breastfeeding provides superior immunologic properties.)
   2. How many wet diapers does your baby have in a 24-hour period? (Infants should have at least six very wet diapers every 24 hours.)
   3. If bottle-feeding, is the formula iron-fortified?
   4. How much formula does your baby drink per day, or how often does your baby breastfeed and how long are the feedings? (Newborns to 1 month of age drink up to 32 ounces per day, 1- to 3-month-olds drink up to 42 ounces a day, 3- to 6-month-olds drink up to 40 ounces a day, 6- to 12-month-olds drink up to 32 ounces per day; breastfed babies may want to feed every 2 hours, and should take at least one breast and suck for 10 minutes to completely empty the breast.)
   5. How long does it take for your baby to finish a bottle? (Generally, an infant should complete a bottle within 15 to 20 minutes. An oral or motor dysfunction or congenital heart disease could be suspected if the infant is unable to complete a bottle within the normal time frame.)
   6. Does your baby go to bed with a bottle with milk, juice, or formula in the crib? (Allowing the baby to fall asleep or keep the bottle with anything except water in the crib may lead to dental caries.)
   7. Have you introduced iron-fortified cereal? (Iron-fortified cereal can be introduced between 4 and 6 months of age and should be continued until the second birthday. Often, the child's hematocrit will fall around 9 to 12 months of age.)

BOX 14-1
QUESTIONS ABOUT CHILDPROOFING THE ENVIRONMENT

1. Would you tell me how you have childproofed your home?
2. Do you have gates on the top and bottom of the stairs?
3. Are the slats on the crib less than 2 3/8 inches apart?
4. Have you taken the crib mobile down and taken out the bumper pads (applies to infants who are trying to pull up)?
5. Is all sleepwear flame retardant?
6. Is the hot water thermostat turned down to 48.4°C (120°F)?
7. Have you installed potty locks to keep the toilet lid down?
8. Do you keep curtain and blind strings out of reach?
9. Have you placed all sharp items such as razors and knives out of reach of the child?
10. Do you stay with your child in the bathtub?
11. Do you always drain the water in the tub after getting out?
12. Have you placed cushioned covering on the tub's water faucet and drain lever?
13. Do you use a nonskid bath mat in the tub?
14. Are there outlet covers on every outlet in the house?
15. When you are cooking, do you keep the pot or pan handles turned in?
16. Have you taken tablecloths off all tables?
17. Do you keep the phone cord out of reach?
18. Is the slack taken up on all electrical appliance and lamp cords?
19. If you have a raised hearth, have you covered it with bumpers, pads, or towels?
20. Are all of your plants out of reach?
21. Are slip protectors under all rugs?
22. If you have a pool in the yard, is it fenced in, is there a protective cover on top, or is there a functional alarm system for the pool?
23. Do you empty pails that contain liquid after using them?
24. Are medications, cosmetics, pesticides, gasoline, cleaning solutions, paint thinner, and all other poisonous materials out of the child's reach?
25. Do you have your local poison control telephone number next to each phone?
26. Do you have smoke detectors close to or in the child's bedroom, and on each floor of the house? Do you have carbon monoxide detectors on each level of your house?
27. Do you have a fire extinguisher on each floor?
28. Have you devised and practiced an escape route plan in case of fire?
29. Are you CPR trained?
30. What would you do in case of an emergency?
31. Where do you place your child's car seat—in the front or back seat, facing front or rear? Do you place your child in the car where an airbag is supplied?
32. Does your child use protective gear such as a helmet or knee and elbow pads if participating in an activity in which injuries may occur?
33. Do you keep plastic dry cleaner overwraps, latex balloons (unattended by a caregiver), plastic trash bags, and grocery bags out of the child's reach?
34. Do you have a dog? Is the dog child-friendly? Do you keep the dog chained on a leash when other children are visiting your home?
35. Are firearms unloaded and locked up?

8. Do you give your baby honey? (Honey should not be given to children younger than 1 year of age because of the risk of botulism.)
9. Have you started solid foods? (Readiness cues include sitting without support, extrusion reflex present, being able to lean forward indicating desire for more, and turning away to indicate refusal of food.)
10. If solid foods have been started, how often do you introduce a new food? (Introduce one new food every 3–5 days in order to differentiate food allergies. Many pediatricians recommend starting vegetables first to avoid a "sweet tooth" phenomenon, then following with fruits, and starting meats at about 8–9 months of age.)

11. Do you give your baby fruit juices? (Excessive use of fruit juices can leave the baby feeling full and not wanting to take adequate amounts of formula.)

B. Toddler (1–3 years old)
 1. Have you started your child on whole milk? (Whole milk can now be safely substituted for formula. The caregiver is encouraged to switch from whole to 2% milk at 2 years of age.)
 2. How much milk does your child drink? (The recommended amount of milk per day is 16 ounces, with a maximum of 1 quart.)
 3. Is your child drinking from a cup? (Transitioning the child from bottle to cup occurs at or before 1 year of age. An early transition helps prevent dental caries. If the child is filling up on milk via a bottle, a variety of foods are not being taken in.)
 4. Have you transitioned your child to soft table foods? (Generally, at about 12 months of age, a child is able to chew soft food.)
 5. Are you present in the room while your child is eating? (Supervising the child is important to prevent choking.)
 6. Does your family include the child during mealtimes? (Starting family meals at an early age has many positive benefits such as establishing routines and communication between family members.)
 7. Is your child starting to feed him- or herself? (During the later phase of infancy and early toddlerhood, the child will begin to take an interest in self-feeding.)
 8. Do you let your child eat any of the following foods: nuts, popcorn, whole hot dogs, grapes, raw vegetables, or hard candy? (These foods and snacks may present a choking hazard.)
 9. Do you offer your child at least two healthy snacks per day? (Offering small nutritious snacks throughout the day will help provide the toddler with adequate nutrition not achieved at mealtimes.)
 10. Is your child eating foods from all food groups? (A good rule of thumb for determining the right amount of food for a child is ensuring the child eats 1 tablespoon of each food group per age in years; thus, a 2-year-old would need to eat 2 tablespoons of vegetables.)

C. Preschooler (3–5 years)
 1. How much milk does your child drink per day? (The preschooler needs to drink at least 20 ounces of milk per day.)
 2. How much juice does your child drink? (Limiting juice to no more than 8–12 ounces per day will help the child take more food at meals and snacks.)
 3. Does your child eat a variety of foods from all food groups? (Utilize the same rule of thumb for adequate food intake as described for toddlers.)
 4. Many of the same questions for the toddler group apply to the preschooler (questions 5, 6, and 9).

D. School-age child (6–12 years)
 1. How many servings of milk does your child drink per day? (School-age children should receive 800 mg of calcium per day, which is equivalent to about 21 ounces of milk.)
 2. Has your child switched from 2% to skim milk? (At the age of 6, children should switch to skim milk.)
 3. Is your child eating three meals per day? (Children often skip breakfast because of early morning time constraints.)
 4. Does your family sit down together for at least one meal per day? (Meals at this age tend to occur on the run because of extracurricular activities planned for dinnertime.)
 5. Does your child eat a hot lunch at school? (A school lunch will provide approximately one-third of the total recommended daily allowance.)
 6. Does your child brush his or her teeth at least two times per day? (Caregivers are encouraged to brush their child's teeth at least once a day until the child has mastered cursive writing. You can foster autonomy by allowing your child to brush his or her teeth in the morning.)
 7. Does your child eat sugary snacks? (Limit sugar intake to prevent dental caries and avoid empty calories.)
 8. Do you allow your child to sit in front of the television and eat a meal? (Obesity is on the rise, and spending excessive time watching television seems to contribute to decreased physical activity.)
 9. How often does your child eat fast food per week? (Incidence of obesity increases with frequent consumption of fast food.)

E. Adolescent (13–18 years): The same questions asked during the school-age child's interview can be used, but asking the questions of the adolescent directly may yield important information.

ASSESSMENT OF OBESITY

Sixty-seven percent of all Americans are defined as overweight with 40% considered obese by body mass index (BMI) standards (LaFontaine, 2008). Although genetics play a role in the U.S. obesity problem, environmental factors ultimately predispose youth to obesity. Factors include excess media usage leading to sedentary lifestyles, little to no physical education opportunities in schools, consumption of larger portions of food, and children being driven to school resulting in decreased walking or bike riding (Sothern, 2008). Long-term effects of childhood obesity are manifested by co-morbidities including hyperlipidemia, hypertension, type 2 diabetes, polycystic ovary syndrome, metabolic syndrome, and obstructive sleep apnea.

Tools to assess childhood obesity and those children at risk are now completed at each yearly visit to a child's primary health provider. Growth charts were revised in 2000 by the National Center for Health Statistics (NCHS), the National Center for Chronic Disease Prevention and Health Promotion (NCCDPHP), and various other experts. One addition, the body mass index for age percentile charts, is utilized to determine if a child's weight is appropriate for her or his height. The body mass index (BMI) growth chart is available for males and females 2 to 20 years of age (NHCS, 2000). To derive a child's BMI, the child's weight in kilograms is divided by the child's height in meters squared. In plotting the growth of a 9-year-old boy whose BMI is 19.4, this would indicate his BMI is higher than approximately 90% of 9-year-old boys in the United States. A child with a BMI at the 85th to 94th percentile is considered overweight. Obese is defined by a BMI at or above the 95th percentile.

LABORATORY EVALUATION

Data gathered during a nutritional assessment will give the interviewer an indication of at-risk factors. Inadequate caloric intake is a nutritional problem. Two commonly ordered laboratory tests are serum albumin and prealbumin. Both tests reflect adequate calorie and protein intake. A serum albumin reflects the previous month's food intake. The prealbumin reflects a shorter period of time, which is the previous 1 week of intake. A complete blood cell count, which includes hemoglobin, hematocrit, and red cell indices, provides an indication of adequate iron status. Cholesterol (low density lipoprotein, high density lipoprotein, triglyceride level and total cholesterol) screenings have become more frequently ordered in children whose family history predisposes them to elevated cholesterol levels or their BMI level warrants screening for hyperlipidemia.

ANTHROPOMETRIC DATA

Anthropometric measurements refer to the science of measuring the human body as to height, weight, and size of component parts, including skinfolds. Anthropometric data provides information about growth patterns and the nutritional status of children. Measurements of skinfold thickness and arm circumference are important indicators of body fat stores, nutritional status, and skeletal muscle mass.

Skinfold thickness is a more reliable indicator of body fat than is weight. The most common measurement site is over the tricep muscle in the child. This measurement may be threatening for the child. To alleviate anxiety let the child sit in the caregiver's lap. While the child's arm is dangling at her or his side in a fully relaxed position, lift the fold of subcutaneous tissue and skin away from the triceps muscle. Place the calipers on the skin next to the fingers, while lifting the fold of skin. Hold the skinfold in place while measuring the triceps skinfold. Repeat this step two more times and average the three readings to obtain the skinfold thickness value.

Arm circumference is measured at the midpoint of the upper arm. To locate the midpoint of the upper arm, have the child flex the arm at a 90° angle. Measure from the **acromion process** (the lateral extension of the spine of the scapula, forming the highest point of the shoulder) to the **olecranon process** (a proximal projection of the ulna that forms the point of the elbow) and mark the midpoint with a washable ink pen or marker. Ask the child to hold his or her arm in a relaxed position at the side. Using a tape measure, measure the circumference.

PHYSICAL EXAMINATION

The physical examination of nearly all body systems can identify nutritional deficiencies. Examination techniques are described throughout this chapter. Table 14-1 summarizes physical signs and symptoms of poor nutritional status.

EVALUATION OF DATA

Utilizing the diet history, compare and contrast this information with the new MyPyramid diet guidelines (Figure 14-1). Determine if the child is receiving the recommended amount and variety of food per day. The evaluation involves piecing together data obtained from the dietary history and physical examination, and extrapolating information to define the child's nutritional status. A referral to a specialist is made if suspected nutritional inadequacy exists.

■ DEVELOPMENTAL ASSESSMENT

Evaluation of developmental functioning is an essential component of any health assessment. A developmental assessment has several purposes: (1) validation that a child is developing normally; (2) early detection of problems; (3) identification of concerns of caregivers and child; and (4) provision of an opportunity for anticipatory guidance and teaching about age-appropriate expected behaviors. Several screening tests are currently available for developmental assessment (Table 14-2). These tests evaluate a variety of aspects, including fine and gross motor skills, social and language skills, behavior, temperament, cognition, and memory. Screening procedures using these measures quickly and reliably identify a child whose development is below normal and may also be used to monitor developmental progress. Some developmental assessment instruments can be administered in a variety of settings with a minimal amount of preparation, whereas others require proper training and supervision. Caution should always be taken to guarantee that administration is accurate; directions and

Table 14-1 Physical Signs and Symptoms of Poor Nutritional Status

	SUBJECTIVE	OBJECTIVE
General appearance	Fatigue, poor sleep, change in weight, frequent infections	Dull affect, apathetic, increased or decreased weight
Skin	Pruritis, swelling, delayed wound healing	Dry, rough, scaling, flaking, edema, lesions, decreased turgor, changes in color (pallor, jaundice), petechiae, ecchymoses, xanthomas (slightly elevated yellow nodules)
Nails	Brittle	Dry, splinter hemorrhages, spoon-shaped, pale
Hair	Easily falls out, brittle	Less shiny, dry, changes in color pigment
Eyes	Vision changes, night blindness, eye discharge	Hardening and scaling of cornea, conjunctiva pale or red
Mouth	Mouth sores	Lips: cracked, dry, swollen, fissures around corners Gums: recessed, swollen, bleeding, spongy Tongue: smooth, beefy red, magenta, pale, fissures, sores, increased or decreased in size, increased or decreased papillae Teeth: missing, caries
Head and neck	Headaches, decreased hearing	Xanthelasma (creamy, yellow plaque on eyelid due to hypercholesterolemia), irritation and crusting of nares, swollen cheeks (parotid gland enlargement), goiter
Heart and peripheral vasculature	Palpitations, swelling	Cardiac enlargement, changes in blood pressure, tachycardia, heart murmur, edema
Abdomen	Tender, changes in appetite, nausea, changes in bowel habits	Edema, hepatosplenomegaly
Musculoskeletal system	Weakness, pain, cramping, frequent fractures	Muscle tone is decreased, flabby muscles, bowing of lower extremities
Neurological system	Irritable, changes in mood, numbness, paresthesia	Slurred speech, unsteady gait, tremors, decreased deep tendon reflexes, loss of position and vibratory sense, paresthesia, decreased coordination
Female genitalia	Changes in menstrual pattern	None

Courtesy of Estes, M. E. Z. (2010). *Health assessment & physical examination* (4th ed.). Clifton Park, NY: Delmar Cengage Learning.

explanations to caregivers and children need to be clear and concise. Following administration, it would be helpful to ask caregivers if the child's performance was typical, since retesting may be necessary if the behavior was atypical. All results should carefully be communicated to caregivers so that misunderstandings and misinterpretations are kept to a minimum. Before administering any measure, it is essential to read and follow instructions carefully.

The most widely used developmental screening tool for assessing development of a child from birth through 6 years of age is the Denver Developmental Screening Test (DDST) and its revision, the DDST-R. These two tests have been revised, restandardized, and renamed the Denver II (Frankenburg & Dodds, 1992). The test is composed of four sections: personal-social, fine motor-adaptive, language, and gross motor. There are a total of 125 items described on the test. Some items can be accomplished easily by observing the child without commands from the observer. For instance, the child may be smiling spontaneously, saying words other than "mama" or "dada," or sitting with his or her head held steady. Certain items can be given an automatic pass mark if the caregiver indicates that the child is able to accomplish the corresponding item, such as drinking from a cup, washing and drying hands, or dressing without help.

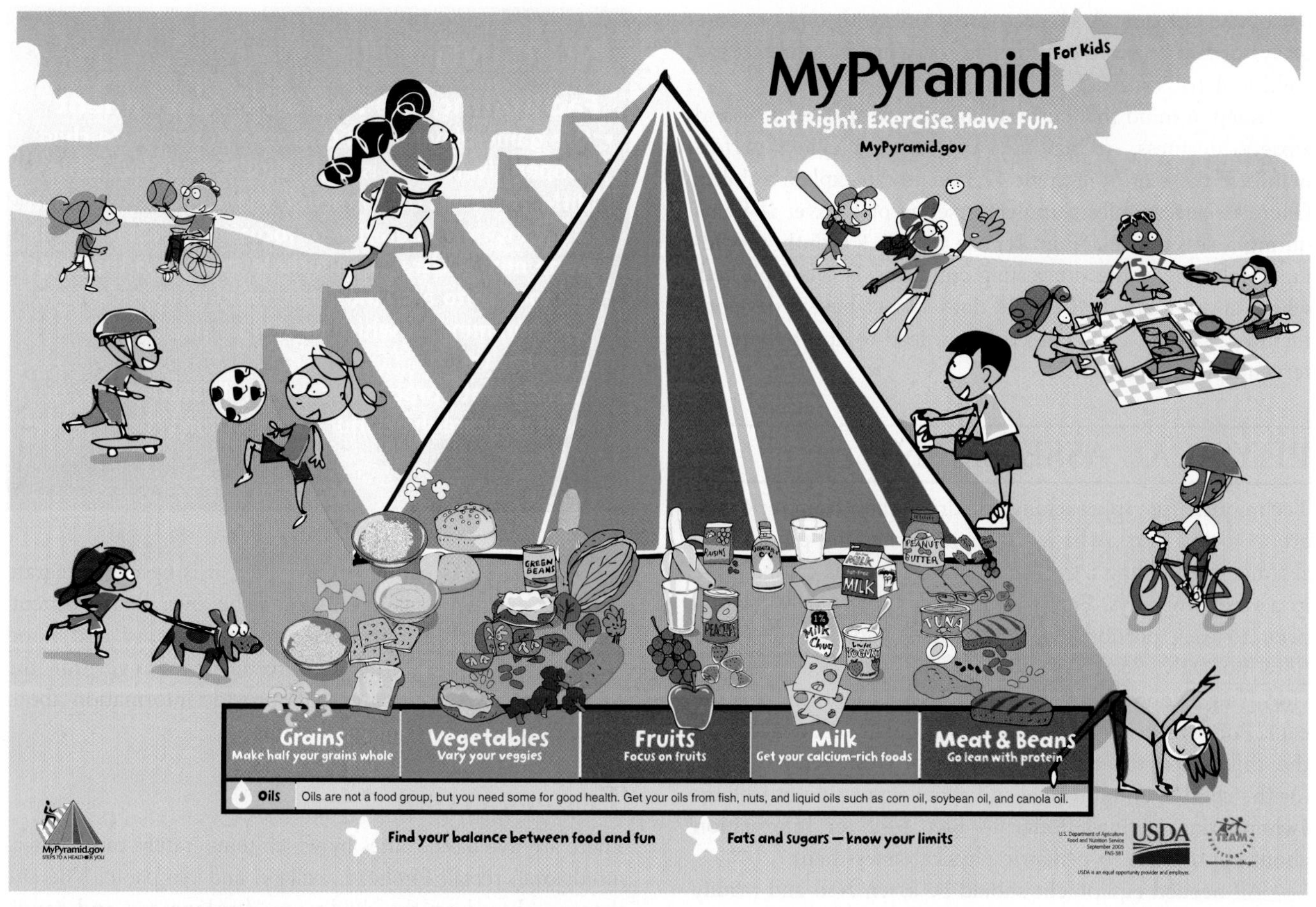

FIGURE 14-1 **MyPyramid for Kids.** COURTESY OF U.S. DEPARTMENT OF AGRICULTURE, 2005.

Documentation is reflected by using a "P" for pass, "F" for fail, "R" for refuses, and "no" for no opportunity. Give up to three trials before documenting the particular item's score on the Denver II. At the end, complete the five Test Behavior questions. A normal test consists of no delays and a maximum of one caution. A caution is failure of the client to perform an item that has been achieved by 75–90% of children the same age. A delay is a failure of any item to the

TABLE 14-2 Developmental Assessment Measures for Infants and Children

TEST NAME	AGES	FEATURES EVALUATED
Carey-Revised Infant	4 to 8 months	Temperament, patterns of feeding, sleeping, elimination, responses to different situations
Denver Articulation Screening Exam	2.5 to 6 years	Intelligibility; articulation of 30 sound elements
Denver II	Birth to 6 years	Personal-social, fine motor-adaptive, language, gross motor
Developmental Profile II	Birth to 9 years	Physical, self-help, social, academic, communication skills
Early Language	Birth to 3 years	Auditory expressive and receptive, visual components of speech
Goodenough-Harris Drawing Test	5 to 17 years	Child's drawing of a person; analyzed for body parts, clothing, proportion, perspective
McCarthy Scales of Children's Abilities	2.5 to 8.5 years	Intellectual and motor development, memory, quantitative, perceptual-performance, general cognition

left of the age line. A suspect test is one with one or more delays or two or more cautions; in these instances, retest the child in 1 to 2 weeks.

Keep in mind that current illness, lack of sleep, fear and anxiety, deafness, or blindness can affect a child's performance. If these or other logical rationale can explain a child's failure to successfully complete a series of Denver II items during a session, re-administer the test in 1 month, providing resolution of the preexisting condition is accomplished, where appropriate. If the child does in fact have a developmental disability, early detection can lead to appropriate intervention and assistance.

PHYSICAL ASSESSMENT

Techniques for approaching children vary from one age group to the next. A basic principle during any physical assessment is building a trusting relationship; this can be done in a variety of ways. First, always explain what will be done prior to each portion of the assessment and answer questions honestly. Second, praise the child for positive behaviors (e.g., cooperating during assessment of the middle ear). Portraying a caring attitude will greatly influence both the child's and the caregiver's sense of trust. Show respect for the child as an individual and allow expression of feelings (whimpering, crying). Refer to Box 14-2 for information about approaches to pediatric physical assessment.

All needed equipment should be assembled and readily available. The following items are recommended for a physical examination on a child:

- Clean gloves
- Scale (infant or stand-up)
- Appropriately sized blood pressure cuff
- Disposable centimeter tape measure
- Snellen E eye chart
- Allen cards
- Otoscope and speculum (2.5 or 4.0 mm) with pneumatic attachment
- Ophthalmoscope
- Pediatric stethoscope
- Thermometer
- Growth charts
- Skinfold calipers
- Marking pen
- Peanut butter or chocolate
- Small bell
- Brightly colored object
- Denver II materials

VITAL SIGNS

The act of measuring vital signs is often disturbing to a young child. Past experiences influence the degree of cooperation you will encounter. Vital signs may be obtained at the beginning of the assessment or during the assessment of a certain system.

NURSING TIP

Facilitating the Pediatric Assessment

- **Use game-playing and distraction to increase child cooperativeness. It is important to have available different items of distraction that can be used when a child is uncooperative or focusing on what will be done next. Distractions include small toys that easily hook onto a stethoscope, wind-up musical toys, and humming or whistling. Finger puppets are popular, too.**
- **Demonstrate procedures on a doll, stuffed toy, or even the caregiver prior to performing them on the child.**

If the child is particularly anxious, it is best to integrate the assessment of vital signs into the overall assessment. Vital signs include temperature, respiration, pulse, and blood pressure, which are compared to normal ranges for the child's age. These measurements provide information about the child's basic physiological status.

TEMPERATURE

There are five basic routes by which temperature can be measured: oral, rectal, forehead, axillary, and tympanic. The site chosen is based on the child's age, development, and condition. The oral route is convenient and accessible, but an accurate measurement is difficult to obtain in most toddlers and preschoolers because the child must be cognitively capable of following instructions for safe use. Therefore, the oral route is usually reserved for children ages 5 to 6 years and older. A rectal temperature is considered the most accurate and can be taken in children of all ages. However, it is not appropriate in all instances, for example, in the child who presents with a history of diarrhea or the child with neutropenia.

The infrared forehead thermometer has been shown to be more accurate than all the rest. It is by far the least distressing and the easiest to use, and is even being used with

NURSING TIP

Integrating Vital Signs into the Pediatric Examination

1. **An apical heart rate can be obtained during the cardiac assessment.**
2. **The respiratory rate can be obtained when auscultating the lungs.**
3. **Blood pressure and rectal temperature measurements are more threatening and should be performed toward the end of the assessment, preferably before using the otoscope.**

BOX 14-2
GENERAL APPROACHES TO PEDIATRIC PHYSICAL ASSESSMENT

1. Assess the child in a warm, quiet room. To prevent hypothermia, always keep infants under the age of 6 months warm during the examination.
2. Use natural lighting, if available, during the assessment. Fluorescent lighting makes assessing varying degrees of cyanosis and jaundice difficult.
3. To help reduce anxiety and uncooperativeness (especially when assessing young children), have a familiar caregiver present during the assessment.
4. Talk to the child in a soothing voice; even an infant who cannot understand your words will take comfort in a calm and supportive approach.
5. Explain all procedures and allow older infants, toddlers, preschoolers, and younger school-age children to manipulate medical equipment.
6. To promote the child's feeling of security, allow the infant who cannot sit up and the younger child to sit on the caregiver's lap for as much of the examination as possible.
7. Until the infant or toddler is comfortable, maintain eye contact with the caregiver while the assessment is taking place. Maintaining eye contact with the child who experiences anxiety in the presence of strangers can interfere with completing the examination. Maintain eye contact with the caregiver if other means of alleviating the fears are not successful.
8. Interview the older school-age child or adolescent separately, without the caregiver. Talking to the individual without the caregiver present may yield important information not gained during a group interview (e.g., that the child is using drugs or is sexually active).
9. Respect the child's modesty.
10. Warm your equipment (e.g., stethoscope).
11. Avoid making abrupt movements because these may startle a child.
12. If the child is sleeping, take advantage of the situation by performing simple procedures (length, head circumference) and system assessments that require a quiet room (such as the cardiac and respiratory assessments) first.
13. Perform all invasive or uncomfortable procedures (ear inspection, hip palpation) last because they may cause discomfort, crying, fear, and increased heart rate.
14. Always provide comfort measures following pain. It is especially helpful to allow the caregiver the opportunity to provide supportive measures. This shows the child that you are genuinely concerned about his or her feelings.
15. To prevent falls, always keep one hand on any infant who is placed on the examination table.
16. Prior to completing the examination, ask the caregiver and child what questions they have.

infants in some hospital settings. The technology is somewhat new, but its usage will be expanding.

An axillary temperature is safe, noninvasive, and can be taken in all age groups. This route may be contraindicated when accuracy is especially critical or in the initial stages of fever, when the axilla may not be sensitive to early temperature changes. When taking an axillary temperature, have the child sit or lie on the caregiver's lap to free your hands for other observation or to prepare for the next area of assessment. Explain to the child that this type of temperature measurement does not hurt. To pass the time, ask the caregiver to read the child a story. The thermometer is held in place with the arm held securely in position for five minutes.

A tympanic thermometer is convenient, safe, and noninvasive. The electronic tympanic measurement involves placing a small ear probe slightly into the opening of the external ear canal and directing the probe towards the tympanic membrane. The nearly instantaneous reading is taken by measuring heat of the tympanic membrane through infrared light. However, there are a couple of drawbacks to tympanic thermometry. Otitis media and cerumen within the ear canal may interfere with accurate readings.

Children dislike having a rectal temperature taken, so your approach to explanation should be matter of fact: "I need to measure your temperature in your bottom. You need to hold very still while I do this. Your mommy [or other appropriate person] will be right here with you." Caution is required in children less than 2 years of age due to risk of rectal perforation. Place the child in either a side-lying or a prone position on the caregiver's lap or place the child on the back on the examination table and firmly grasp the feet with your nondominant hand. After lubricating the tip of the thermometer, insert it gently into the child's rectum: 1/2 inch for newborns, 3/4 inch for infants, and 1 inch for preschoolers and older children. Hold the thermometer firmly between your fingers to avoid accidentally inserting it too far (Figure 14-2).

Normal body temperature (afebrile) varies with the age of the child (Table 14-3). A temperature above 38.6°C

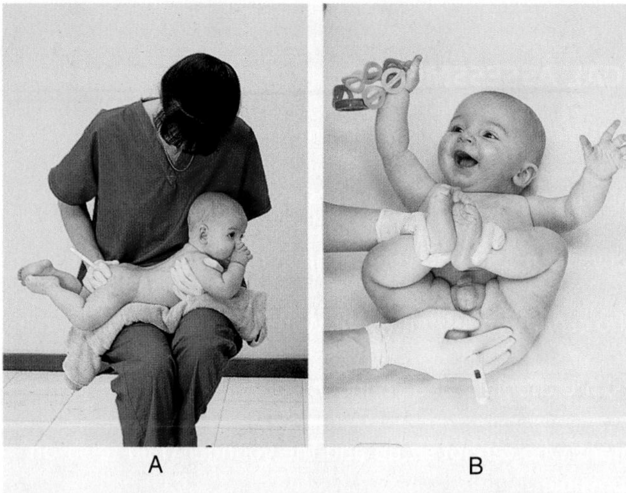

FIGURE 14-2 Rectal Temperature. (A) Infant in Prone Position (B) Infant in Supine Position. DELMAR CENGAGE LEARNING.

TABLE 14-3 Body Temperature: Normal Range According to Age

AGE	CENTIGRADE	FAHRENHEIT
Newborn to 1 year	37.5–37.7°	99.4–99.7°
3 to 5 years	37.0–37.2°	98.6–99.0°
7 to 9 years	36.7–36.8°	98.1–98.3°
10 years and older	36.6°	97.8°

(101.5°F) is interpreted as hyperthermia. An elevated body temperature can be related to severe illnesses such as meningitis, or common childhood illnesses such as otitis media and streptococcus pharyngitis, or heat exposure. In contrast, hypothermia is a body temperature below 35.0°C (95.0°F). A low body temperature can be related to sepsis, ambient cold exposure, or submersion cold injury.

RESPIRATORY RATE

Try to obtain the respiratory rate early in the assessment, when the child is most cooperative and not crying. If the child is crying, the measurement will not be accurate and should be retaken. Remember to observe the expansion of the abdomen in infants and toddlers. Table 14-4 lists the normal respiratory rates for children.

PULSE

An apical pulse should be taken on neonates, infants, and young children (under 2 years of age) and on all children with cardiac problems or taking digitalis preparations. To determine the heart rate, place the diaphragm (flat piece) of your stethoscope over the child's **precordium**, which is the part of the front of the chest wall that overlays the heart, great vessels, pericardium, and some pulmonary tissue. A radial pulse can be obtained on children over 2 years of age. An elevated heart rate or tachycardia is indicative of sepsis, fever, anxiety, dysrhythmia, congestive heart failure, or medications. A slow heart rate or bradycardia would suggest a surgically induced or congenital heart block, digoxin toxicity, or hypothermia (example, cold submersion injury). Table 14-5 depicts ranges for normal pulse rates by age.

TABLE 14-4 Respiratory Rate

AGE	RESTING RESPIRATORY RATE	AVERAGE
Newborn	30–50	40
1 year	20–40	30
3 years	20–30	25
6 years	16–22	19
10 years	16–20	18
14 years	14–20	17
18 years	16–20	18

Courtesy of Estes, M. E. Z. (2010). *Health assessment & physical examination* (4th ed.). Clifton Park, NY: Delmar Cengage Learning.

BLOOD PRESSURE

The most important aspect of obtaining a blood pressure is choosing the correct cuff size. The bladder of the cuff width should be 40% of the arm's circumference measured midway between the olecranon and acromion. Using a cuff too large

TABLE 14-5 Pulse Rate: Normal Range According to Age

AGE	RESTING PULSE RATE (BEATS/MINUTE)	AVERAGE
Newborn	100–170	140
1 year	80–170	120
3 years	80–130	110
6 years	70–115	100
10 years	70–110	90
14 years	60–110	85–90
18 years	60–100	72

Courtesy of Estes, M. E. Z. (2010). *Health assessment & physical examination* (4th ed.). Clifton Park, NY: Delmar Cengage Learning.

RESEARCH Highlight

Compare Methods of Newborn Temperature Measurement

STUDY PURPOSE

To (1) compare newborn temperature measurements obtained by digital disposable, electronic, and tympanic thermometers with glass mercury thermometers, and (2) compare the financial implications of each method.

METHODS

In this correlational study, 12 perinatal and neonatal nurses obtained temperature measurements of 184 newborns between 1 and 168 hours of age. The sample—stratified and convenience—was selected using medical records numbers. Instruments for measuring temperature included glass, tympanic, electronic, and digital thermometers. Data were analyzed by Pearson *r* coefficients, mean, standard deviation, and range using an SPSS statistical package.

FINDINGS

The glass, electronic, and digital thermometer temperature readings were highly correlated (0.748–1.0). The tympanic thermometer had a low correlation coefficient (0.35). Use of the glass thermometer was the most costly, whereas the tympanic thermometer was the most cost-effective.

IMPLICATIONS

In healthy newborns, the use of electronic and digital thermometers is appropriate if there is a concern about using glass thermometers. However, these results cannot be extrapolated to sick infants. Although tympanic thermometers had the lowest cost, their lack of correlation with the gold standard glass thermometers makes them a poor choice for healthy newborns.

REFERENCE

Sganga, A., Wallace, R., Kiehl, E., Irving, T., & Witter, L. (2000). A comparison of four methods of normal newborn temperature measurement. *American Journal of Maternal Child Nursing*, 25(2), 76–79.

for the child's arm results in an underestimation of blood pressure. Inversely, a small cuff size produces overestimation of blood pressure. The cuff bladder should cover 80–100% of the arm circumference (National Institutes of Health, & NHLBI, 1996; see Figure 14-3). Place the cuff on the upper extremity. Locate the brachial pulse with your finger. Place the stethoscope over the antecubital fossae. Manually inflate the cuff. As you are releasing the air, observe the dial and listen to record the systolic and diastolic numbers. You may need to palpate the blood pressure in the infant and toddler.

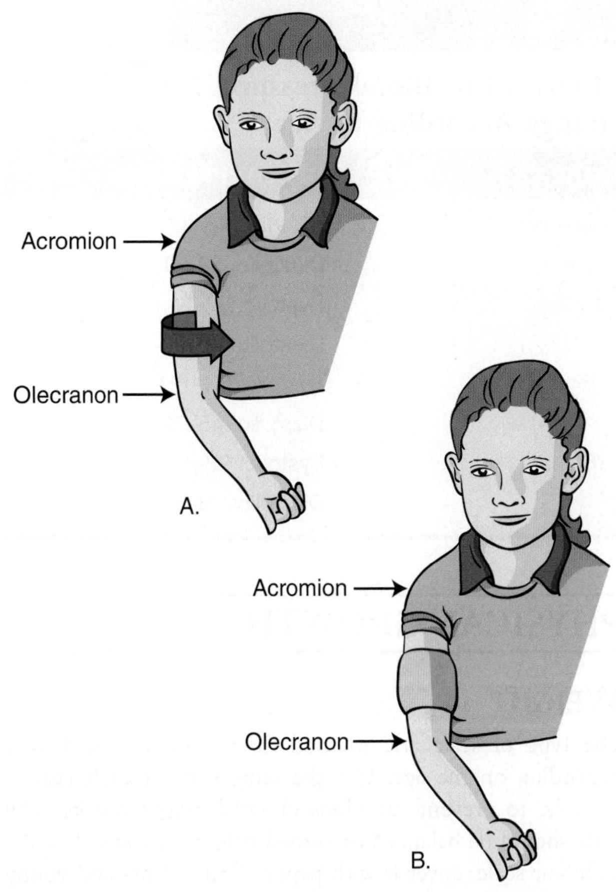

FIGURE 14-3 Determination of Proper Blood Pressure Cuff Size. (A) The cuff bladder width should be 40% of the circumference of the arm measured midway between the olecranon and acromion. (B) The cuff bladder covers 80–100% of the arm's circumference. DELMAR CENGAGE LEARNING.

Record the systolic number. Etiologies of hypertension are numerous. Renal disease, coarctation of the aorta, stress, and medication can result in hypertension. In adolescents prehypertension is defined as a blood pressure reading 120/80 or greater. In order to confirm a diagnosis of hypertension, blood pressure should be recorded at more than one visit (Falkner, Gidding, Portman, & Rosner, 2008). Causes of hypotension include hemorrhage, sepsis, septic shock, and medications. The average blood pressure readings for children at various ages are listed in Table 14-6.

NURSING TIP

Determining Normal Systolic Blood Pressure

In children 1 year of age and older, an easy rule of thumb for determining normal systolic blood pressure is: normal systolic BP (mm Hg) = 80 + (2 X age in years). Normal diastolic blood pressure is generally two-thirds of systolic blood pressure.

TABLE 14-6 Blood Pressure: Normal Range According to Age

AGE	BLOOD PRESSURE
Newborn	Systolic: 46–92
	Diastolic: 38–71
3 years	Systolic: 72–110
	Diastolic: 40–73
10 years	Systolic: 83–121
	Diastolic: 45–79
16 years	Systolic: 93–131
	Diastolic: 49–85

PHYSICAL GROWTH

WEIGHT

The type of scale and method for obtaining weight vary depending on the age. Use the same scale at each visit, if possible, to prevent variations in serial weight checks. The scale should be balanced or zeroed before weighing. If using an infant scale, cover it with paper. Place infants and young toddlers nude on the scale (Figure 14-4). Always keep one hand on the child to prevent falls and lift your hand slightly when obtaining the actual weight reading. Children who can stand without support can be weighed on a standard platform scale, wearing underpants. Weight should be noted, recorded, and plotted on a standardized growth chart. Neonates may lose up to 10% of birth weight by the third or fourth day after birth, and then regain it by 2 weeks of age. This expected change in weight is called physiological weight loss, and it is due to a loss of extracellular fluid and **meconium**.

LENGTH AND HEIGHT

Recumbent length is measured for children younger than 2 years old. Position the measuring board flat on the examination table. Place the child's head at the top of the board and the child's heels at the foot of the board, making sure the legs are fully extended. If a board is not available, place the child in a supine position and mark lines on the paper at the tip of the head and at the heel (Figure 14-5a), making sure the legs are fully extended. Measure between the lines and record. Height for all other age groups can be measured in the same fashion as for an adult. Figure 14-5b shows a preschooler's height being measured. Length and height should be plotted on a standardized growth chart (see Appendix B). A height below the 5th or above the 95th percentiles warrants investigation, as does the child who falls two standard deviations below his or her own established curve. Any such finding is abnormal.

HEAD CIRCUMFERENCE

Head circumference is measured in all children less than 2 years of age or in children with known or suspected

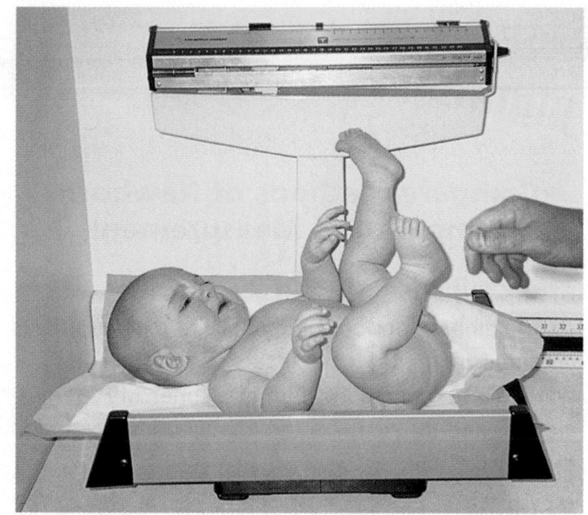

FIGURE 14-4 Measuring Weight in an Infant. DELMAR CENGAGE LEARNING.

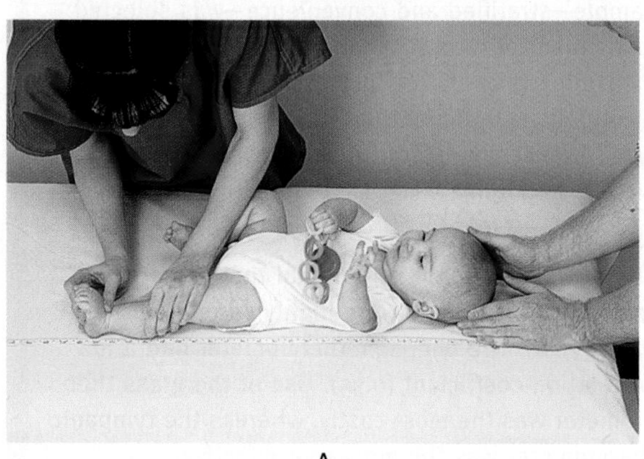

A

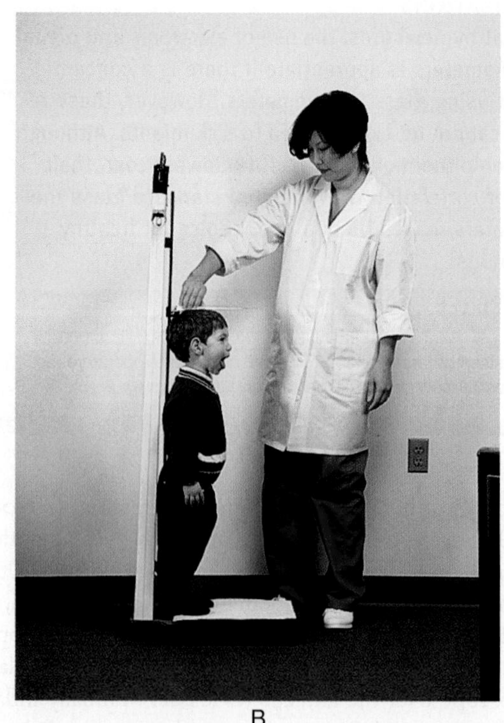

B

FIGURE 14-5 Measuring Length and Height in Children. (A) Recumbent Length in Infant (B) Height in Preschooler. DELMAR CENGAGE LEARNING.

CRITICAL THINKING

A Child Below the Third Percentile

You obtain the weight and height on a 2-year-old girl and plot these measurements on the appropriate growth chart. She is in the third percentile. What would you do about this?

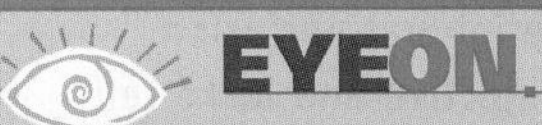

Variations in Height

Children of different races vary in height. African-American and Caucasian children are the tallest, followed by Native-American children, who are similar or a little shorter. Next in height are Mexican-American children, followed by the shortest group—Asian Americans. Within the same racial group, children from families with higher socioeconomic status are taller than those from lower socioeconomic status families. Obese children are taller than lean children (Seidel, Ball, Dains, Flynn, Solomon, & Stewart, 2011).

microcephaly or hydrocephalus. Serial measurement of head circumference is invaluable for the infant with suspected cessation of brain growth. Place the child in a sitting or supine position. Using a tape measure, measure anteriorly from just above the eyebrows and around posteriorly to the occipital protuberance (refer to Figure 14-6; also see Appendix B, head circumference for girls and boys birth to 36 months). Normal average head growth is 1.0–1.5 cm per month during the first year. Premature infants often have small head circumferences.

Microcephaly, a congenital anomaly characterized by a small brain with a resultant small head and a mental deficit, is an abnormal finding. Another abnormality, **hydrocephalus**, is an enlargement of the head without enlargement of the facial structures.

Chest Circumference

Chest circumference is measured up to 1 year of age. It is a measurement that, by itself, provides little information but is compared to head circumference to evaluate the child's overall growth. Measure the chest circumference by placing the tape measure around the chest at the nipple line (Figure 14-7). Measure at the end of exhalation. From birth to about 1 year, the head circumference is greater than the chest circumference. At 1 year, the head circumference is equal to the chest. After age 1, the chest circumference is greater than the head circumference. A measured chest circumference below normal limits is abnormal. A below-normal chest circumference for age can be attributed to prematurity.

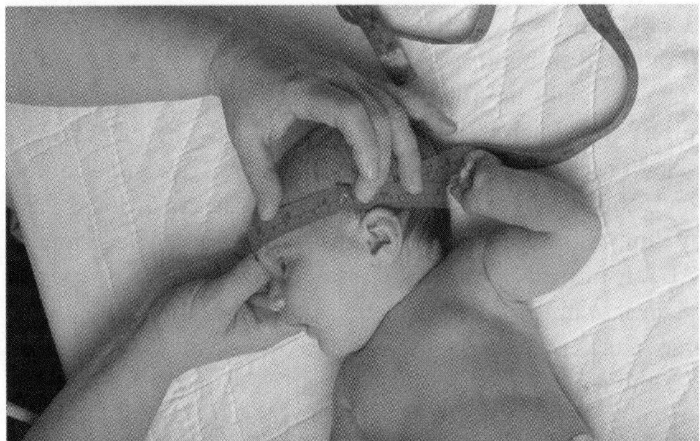

Figure 14-6 Measuring Infant Head Circumference. DELMAR CENGAGE LEARNING.

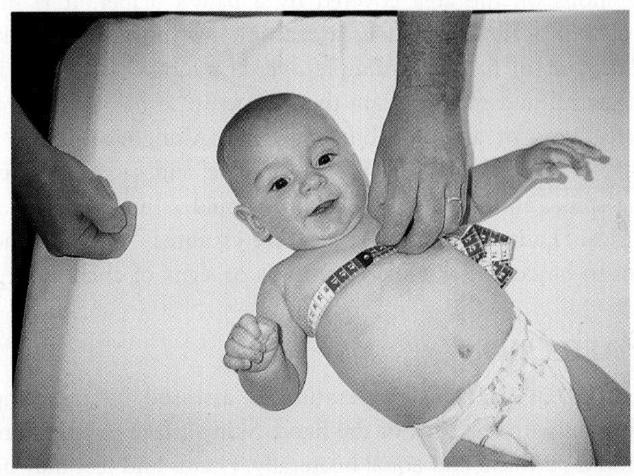

Figure 14-7 Measuring Chest Circumference. DELMAR CENGAGE LEARNING.

NURSING TIP

Obtaining Length and Height in Children under 2 Years of Age

1. If measuring a recumbent length, always plot on the birth-to-36-month chart.
2. If measuring height, plot the measurement on a birth-to-36-month growth chart and subtract 1 centimeter, or plot on a 2-to-18-year chart.

SKIN

Inspection

Color Observe the color of the body, especially at the tip of the nose, the external ear, the lips, the hands, and the feet. These areas are prominent locations for detecting cyanosis or jaundice.

Lesions Inspect the skin for lesions, noting the anatomic location, distribution, shape, color, size, and exudate. No skin lesions should be present except for freckles, birthmarks, or moles (nevi), which may be flat or elevated. Several abnormal skin conditions are associated with lesions. Eczema or atopic dermatitis (AD) is a common skin disorder involving inflammation of the epidermis and superficial dermis. The lesions of AD are usually symmetrical, scaly, erythematous patches or plaques with possible exudation and crusting. Inhaled allergens such as pollens, molds, dust mites, or food allergens are thought to induce mast-cell responses that cause AD. Erythema toxicum, a benign rash whose cause is unknown, appears as small, erythematous, maculopapular lesions that erupt on the newborn. Another lesion is **telangiectatic nevi**, commonly known as stork bites. Diaper dermatitis is characterized by diffuse redness, papules, vesicles, edema, scaling, and ulcerations on the area covered by a baby's diaper. It is the result of a bacteria and urea reaction on the skin. A dark-black tuft of hair or a dimple over the lumbosacral area is abnormal and may indicate that the neonate has a vertebral defect known as spina bifida occulta. Mongolian spots, a deep-blue pigmentation over the lumbar and sacral areas of the spine, buttocks, upper back, or shoulders in newborns of African, Latino, or Asian descent, are extremely common and not to be confused with ecchymosis or signs of child abuse.

PALPATION

Temperature Temperature is assessed by palpating the skin with the back of the hand. Skin surface temperature should be warm and equal bilaterally. Hands and feet may be slightly cooler than the rest of the body. Generalized hyperthermia may be indicative of a febrile state, hyperthyroidism, or increased metabolic function caused by exercise. Generalized hypothermia may be indicative of shock or some other type of central circulatory dysfunction.

Texture Use the finger pads to palpate the skin. The technique of palpating the skin of a younger child can be accomplished by playing games. For example, use the finger pads to walk up the abdomen and touch the nose. The skin of a child normally is smooth and soft. A common variation occurring in the infant is **milia**, which are small, white papules on the cheeks, forehead, nose, and chin due to sebum that occludes the opening of the follicles. Milia resolve spontaneously within a few weeks. Newborns may also have **vernix caseosa**, a thick, cheesy, protective, integumentary deposit that consists of sebum and shed epithelial cells.

Turgor Skin turgor or elasticity reflects the child's state of hydration. It is assessed by pinching a small section of the child's skin between your thumb and forefinger and quickly releasing it. The abdomen is the best location to assess skin turgor. Good turgor and adequate hydration is evidenced when the skin rapidly returns to its original contour after it is released. Decreased skin turgor, a sign of dehydration, is present when it slowly returns to its original contour or remains pinched or "tented" after it is released.

RESEARCH Highlight

Comparing Three Methods of Assessing Peripheral Perfusion in Critically Ill Children

STUDY PURPOSE

Qualitative assessment of foot temperature in the Pediatric Intensive Care Unit (PICU) is standard practice when evaluating peripheral perfusion. Although this method is subjective and lacks reliability, this standard practice continues to be utilized. This study describes correlation of foot warmth assessment, measured foot temperature and perfusion indicator value.

METHODS

The study was conducted in a 26-bed multispecialty PICU. Study participants included 39 critically ill patients between the ages of 1 month to 18 years. Simultaneous measurements of foot warmth, measured foot temperature, and perfusion indicator were made on all 39 patients. To measure perfusion indicator a pulse oximeter probe was placed on the patient's great toe to record the pulse oximetry signal. Measured foot temperature was assessed by placement of a skin temperature probe placed below the level of the pulse oximeter probe on the great toe. Lastly, the bedside RN documented foot warmth every two hours. The bedside RN was blinded to measured perfusion and probe foot temperature as these values were later retrieved from stored bedside data and matched to the RN's qualitative assessment of warmth.

FINDINGS

The researchers found a positive correlation between all three measurement values but a large variability between the three measurement groups.

IMPLICATIONS

The researchers concluded assessment of foot warmth as an indicator of perfusion is helpful as a screening examination but should not be relied on when subtle changes are needed for perfusion assessment in the sick ICU patient.

REFERENCE

Ridling, D. A. & Kroon, L. (2009). Comparing three methods of assessing peripheral perfusion in critically ill children. *Pediatric Nursing*, *35*(1), 11–15.

Edema Edema, an accumulation of fluid in the interstitial spaces, is assessed by pressing the thumb into an area of the body that appears puffy or swollen. Edema is most evident in dependent parts of the body (arms, hands, legs, ankles, feet,

REFLECTIVE THINKING

Suspecting Child Abuse

A young mother of five children brings her 2-year-old child, who is wheezing and having difficulty breathing, into the emergency department. The mother tells you she was up all night with the child. On auscultation of the posterior lung fields, you note three 4-mm rounded areas on the upper back that appear to be second-degree burns. There is erythema and tissue destruction surrounding the borders of each area.

1. What would be your first reaction?
2. How would you proceed with the assessment? What questions would you ask the mother?
3. Do you know your institution's policy and your state's laws on reporting suspected child abuse?
4. Are you, as a nurse, a mandated reporter?

and sacrum). Periorbital edema may be observed in children on the eyelids. Normally the skin surface stays smooth. If pressure leaves an indentation, pitting edema is present.

HAIR

To evaluate the scalp for lesions or signs of infestations, don gloves and lift the scalp hair by segments. Note the scalp's color, which should be similar to the child's skin. There should be no signs of lesions or infestations. Seborrheic dermatitis (cradle cap), caused by increased production of sebum, looks like yellow, greasy-appearing scales and crusts on the scalp of a light-skinned infant. In dark-skinned infants, the scaling is light gray. Head lice (pediculosis capitis) may be seen crawling within the hair.

HEAD

INSPECTION

Shape and Symmetry With the child sitting upright either in the caregiver's arms or on the examination table, observe the symmetry of the frontal, parietal, and occipital prominences. Normally, the shape of a child's head is symmetrical without depressions or protrusions. The anterior fontanel may pulsate with every heart beat. The infant of Asian descent generally has a flattened occiput, more so than infants of other races. A flattened occipital bone with resultant hair loss over the same area is abnormal and is usually caused by the infant being in the supine position for prolonged periods of time.

Head Control Head control is assessed when the infant is in a sitting position. With the head unsupported, observe the infant's ability to hold the head erect. At 4 months of age, most infants are able to hold the head erect and in midline. To evaluate for head lag, pull the infant by the hands from a supine to a sitting position. Again by 4 months of age, the head should stay in line with the body when being pulled forward. Documented prematurity, hydrocephalus, and illnesses causing developmental delays are possible causes of head lag. Significant head lag after 6 months of age may indicate brain injury and should be further investigated.

PALPATION

Fontanel Place the child in an upright position. Using the second or third finger pad, palpate the anterior fontanel at the junction of the sagittal, coronal, and frontal sutures. Palpate the posterior fontanel at the junction of the sagittal and lambdoidal sutures. Assess for depression, bulging, pulsations, and size. Crying will produce a distorted, full, bulging appearance. The anterior fontanel is soft and flat. Size ranges from 4 to 6 centimeters at birth. The fontanel gradually closes between 9 and 19 months of age. The posterior fontanel is also soft and flat. The size ranges from 0.5 to 1.5 centimeters at birth. The posterior fontanel gradually closes between 1 and 3 months of age. It is normal to feel pulsations related to the peripheral pulse.

If palpation reveals a bulging, tense fontanel, this is abnormal and indicates increased intracranial pressure. A sunken, depressed fontanel occurs with dehydration. A wide anterior fontanel in a child older than 2½ years is an abnormal finding. An anterior fontanel that remains open after 2½ years of age may indicate disease such as rickets. In rickets, there is a low level of vitamin D relative to decreased phosphate level. A posterior fontanel greater than 1.5 cm in diameter is abnormal and occurs with congenital hypothyroidism.

Suture Lines With the finger pads, palpate the sagittal suture line, which runs from the anterior to the posterior portion of the skull in a midline position. Palpate the coronal suture line, which runs along both sides of the head, starting at the anterior fontanel. Palpate the lambdoidal suture. The lambdoidal suture runs along both sides of the head, starting at the posterior fontanel. Ascertain if these suture lines are open, united, or overlapping. Grooves or ridges between sections of the skull are normally palpated up to 6 months of age. Suture lines that overlap or override one another, giving the head an unusual shape, warrant further investigation. **Craniosynostosis** is premature ossification of suture lines, whereby there is early formation and fusion of skull bones. Craniosynostosis may be caused by metabolic disorders or may be a secondary consequence of microcephaly. Figure 14-8 illustrates a superior and lateral view of an infant's head.

Surface Characteristics With the finger pads, palpate the skull in the same manner as the fontanels and suture lines. Note surface edema and contour of the cranium. Normally, the skin covering the cranium is flush against the skull and without edema. A softening of the outer layer of the cranial bones behind and above the ears combined with a ping-pong ball sensation as the area is pressed in gently

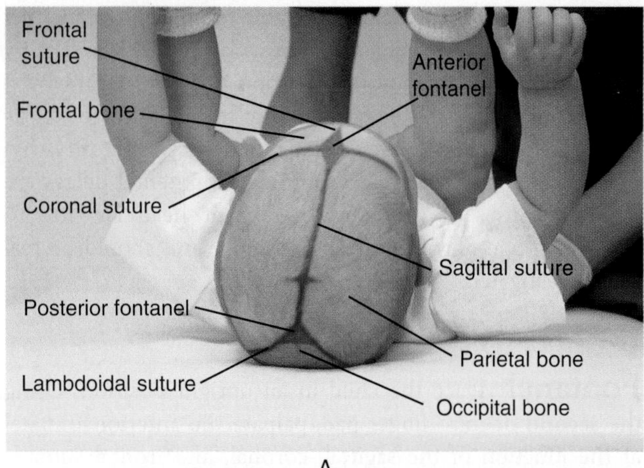

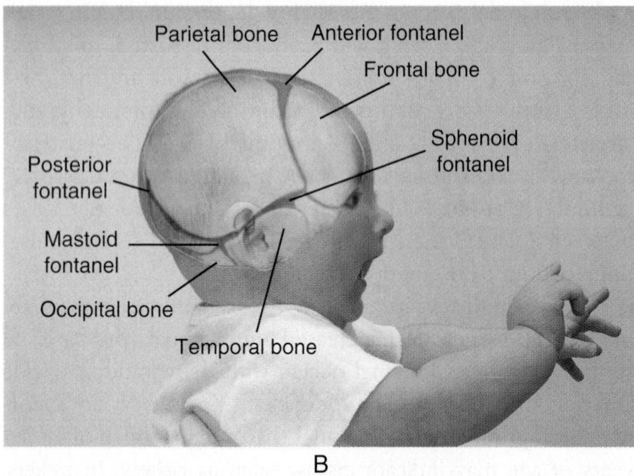

FIGURE 14-8 Infant Head Structures. (A) Superior View (B) Lateral View. DELMAR CENGAGE LEARNING.

with the fingers is indicative of **craniotabes**, an abnormal finding. Craniotabes is associated with rickets, syphilis, hydrocephaly, or hypervitaminosis.

Another abnormal finding in a newborn is a cephalohematoma, or a localized, subcutaneous swelling over one of the cranial bones.

Another variation in the newborn that causes the shape of the skull to look markedly asymmetric is known as **caput succedaneum** or swelling over the occipitoparietal region of the skull. A newborn's head may also feel asymmetric due to molding of the cranial bones as a result of induced pressure during delivery.

EYES

GENERAL APPROACH

From infancy through about 8 to 10 years, you should assess the eyes toward the end of the assessment, with the exception of testing vision, which should be done first. Remember that the child's attention span is short, and attentiveness decreases the longer you evaluate. Young children generally are not cooperative for eye, ear, and throat assessments. Place the young infant, preschooler, or school-age or adolescent child on the examination table. The older infant or the toddler can be held by the caregiver.

VISION SCREENING

General Approach Several screening tests are available to evaluate visual acuity in children including the adult Snellen, Snellen E, and Allen. The child's age and developmental level determine the measures used. The adult Snellen chart can be used on children as young as 6 years, provided they are able to read the alphabet. The Snellen E chart, which shows the letter "E" facing in different directions, is used for a child over 3 years of age or any child who cannot read the alphabet. Test every 1 to 2 years through adolescence. If the child resists wearing a cover patch over the eye, make a game out of wearing the patch. For example, the young child could pretend to be a pirate exploring new territory. Use your imagination to think of a fantasy situation. The Allen test (a series of seven pictures on different cards) can be used with children as young as 3 years of age (American Academy of Pediatrics, Committee on Practice and Ambulatory Medicine, Section on Ophthalmology, 2003).

Snellen E Chart Ask the child to point an arm in the direction the E is pointing. Observe for squinting. Vision is 20/40 from 2 to approximately 6 years of age, when it approaches the normal 20/20 acuity. The test is abnormal if results are 20/40 or greater in a child 3 years of age or 20/30 or greater in a child 6 years or older, or if results are different in each eye.

Nearsightedness or myopia is the result of congenital cataracts, retinal trauma, or a tumor.

Allen Test With the child's eyes open, show each card to the child and elicit a name for each picture. Do not use any pictures with which the child is not familiar. Place the 2- to 3-year-old child 15 feet from where you will be standing. Place the 3- to 4-year-old child 20 feet from you. Ask the caregiver to help cover one of the child's eyes. Show the pictures one at a time, eliciting a response after each showing. Show the same pictures in different sequence for the other eye. To record findings, the denominator is always constant at 30, because a child with normal vision should see the picture on the card (target) at 30 feet. To document the numerator, determine the greatest distance at which three of the pictures are recognized by each eye, for example, right eye 5 = 15/30, left eye 5 = 20/30. The child should correctly identify three of the cards in three trials. Two- to 3-year-old children should have 15/30 vision. Three- to 4-year-old children should be able to achieve a score of 15/30 to 20/30. Each eye should have the same score. If the scores for the child's right and left eyes differ by 5 feet or more or either or both eyes score less than 15/30, refer the child to an ophthalmologist.

NURSING TIP

Pseudostrabismus

Some infants have an epicanthal fold that gives the false appearance of strabismus. This situation is termed **pseudostrabismus**. However, in these infants the corneal light reflex is normal.

NURSING TIP

Lid Eversion in Children

Lid eversion is not performed in children unless you are assessing for an infection or foreign body. If performed, the technique is the same as for an adult.

Strabismus Screening

The Hirschberg test (corneal light reflex) and the cover-uncover test screen for strabismus. The latter is the more definitive test.

Hirschberg Test Hold a pen light by the side of your head with one hand so the light is facing straight ahead. The pen light should be approximately 12 inches from the child's head. Using your other hand turn the child's head so the light is in the midline position toward the child's eyes. Make a general observation of the light reflection relative to both cornea noting symmetry and central location. The reflected light should be seen symmetrically in the center of both corneas.

Esotropia, thought to be congenital, occurs when the light reflection is displaced to the outer margin of the cornea as the eye deviates inward. Some theories suggest that neurological factors contribute to its development. **Exotropia** occurs when the light reflection is displaced to the inner margin of the cornea as the eye deviates outward. This abnormality can result from eye muscle fatigue or can be congenital.

Cover-Uncover Test This test is performed on infants greater than 6 months of age through school-age. Stand 2 feet in front of the child. Place the child in a seated position on the examining table or caregiver's lap. Ask the child to focus attention on the pen light by the side of your head. Place a cover card or your hand over one eye. Wait until the uncovered eye focuses, then remove the occluder and evaluate the eye just uncovered for focusing movement.

The normal finding is neither eye moves when the occluder is being removed. Infants younger than 6 months of age display strabismus due to poor neuromuscular control of eye muscles. It is abnormal for one or both eyes to move to focus on the pen light during assessment. Assume strabismus is present. Strabismus after 6 months of age is abnormal and indicates eye muscle weakness.

Inspection

Eyelids Sit at the child's eye level. Observe for symmetrical **palpebral fissures** (opening between the margins of the upper and lower eyelids) and position of eyelids in relation to the iris. Normally, the palpebral fissures of both eyes are positioned symmetrically. The upper eyelid covers a small portion of the iris, and the lower lid meets the iris. Epicanthal folds are normally present in children of Asian descent. An epicanthal fold is an excess skinfold over the angle of the inner canthus of the eye. It is abnormal for a portion of the sclera to be seen above the iris as it is in children with hydrocephalus. As the forehead becomes prominent, the eyebrows and eyelids are drawn up, creating a setting sun appearance of the child's eyes. Children with Down syndrome have a fold of skin covering the inner canthus and lacrimal caruncle. During embryonic development, the fold of skin slants in a downward direction toward the nose.

Lacrimal Apparatus If lacrimal duct obstruction is suspected, use the index finger to lightly palpate the lacrimal sac area while bracing the child's head with the other hand. Note drainage from the lacrimal duct orifice. The child's caregiver reports that the child is unable to produce tears, an abnormal finding. The lacrimal ducts should be open by 3 months of age. **Dacryocystitis** is an infection of the lacrimal sac caused by obstruction of the lacrimal duct. It is characterized by tearing and discharges from the eye.

Anterior Segment Structures

Sclera The sclera is observed mainly to determine its color. Normally, the newborn exhibits a bluish-tinged sclera related to thinness of the fibrous tissue. The sclera is white in light-skinned children and a slightly darker color in some dark-skinned children. A yellowish color to the sclera indicates jaundice, which is due to hemolysis of red blood cells, nonfunctioning liver cells, or obstruction of bile in the common or hepatic duct.

Iris Using the light source on the ophthalmoscope, observe the iris for lesions and color. Up to about 6–12 months of age, the color of the iris is blue or slate gray in light-skinned infants and brownish in dark-skinned infants. By 12 months of age, complete transition of iris color has occurred. Small white flecks, called Brushfield's spots, noted around the perimeter of the iris are abnormal. Brushfield's spots are found on the iris of the child with Down syndrome. The spots develop during embryonic maturation.

Pupils The pupils should be inspected for size, shape, equality, and response to light. Pupils should be equal in size. To test for pupillary light reflex, dim the room lights.

> **NURSING TIP**
>
> **Recording Pupillary Response**
>
> The normal response of the pupils is recorded as PERRLA, which means the Pupils are Equal in size, Round in shape, and React to Light and Accommodate.

Position the child according to age. Move the lighted instrument in from the side and observe the change in the size of the pupils. The pupils should react equally and accommodate to light. An abnormality is suspected if one or both pupils are nonreactive. Any central nervous system insult (e.g., head injury, meningitis, seizures) may cause an abnormal response.

Utilize the pupillary reflex to elicit an optical blink reflex in the newborn. When the pupils' reaction to light is assessed, a newborn will normally blink and flex the head closer to the body. This is called the optical blink reflex.

Posterior Segment Structures

General Approach Observe the red reflex, retina, and optic disc. The assessment is easier to accomplish if the infant or toddler is lying supine on an examination table. The assistance of another individual, such as the caregiver, to hold the child in position is essential. The older child may be allowed to sit, if cooperative.

Inspection

Red Reflex Turn the ophthalmoscope to 0 diopters. Stand 10–12 inches from the client and observe the pupil through the ophthalmoscope's window. Note the color of the reflex within the eye. In children, the red reflex appears as a brilliant, uniform red glow. In newborns and infants, the red reflex will appear lighter. In many darker-skinned individuals, the reflex will appear darker. Black spots or opacities within the red reflex are abnormal and may indicate a cataract. Chromosomal disorders, intrauterine infections, and ocular trauma are possible causes of cataracts in newborns. A yellowish or white light reflex (cat's eye reflex) is also abnormal and may indicate retinoblastoma, a malignant glioma located in the posterior chamber of the eye.

Retina Assess the retinal background for color. Divide the retina into four quadrants and follow the retinal arteries and veins from the disc to periphery. Note the size and distribution of retinal arteries and veins. The retina's background is generally pink but may be lighter in some Caucasians and darker in African-American individuals. There is no difference in normal vasculature among children and adults. A red to dark-red color is abnormal. Some areas may be rounded or flame shaped. Hemorrhage is seen in trauma. Bleeding into the optic nerve sheath is found in children who have been physically shaken.

Optic Disc At a 15° lateral position to the eye, move in closer to the eye approximately 1 inch from the child. Move the diopter to −5 to 0. Locate a vessel and move medially (nasal side) to locate the disc. Observe the color of the disc along with margin definition. The disc is creamy yellow to salmon in color. The disc is lighter in an infant. It measures about 1.5 mm in diameter and is round in shape. The margins of the disc are regular and clearly defined. If abnormal, the margins are blurred. In papilledema, the optic disc margins are abnormal. The margins are poorly defined (blurred) related to increased intracranial pressure.

EARS

Auditory Testing

General Approach Perform auditory testing at about 3 to 4 years of age or when the child can follow directions. Newborn hearing tests are available for use and mandated in some states. Prior to 3 years of age, the following are a few parameters for evaluating hearing:

1. Does the child react to a loud noise?
2. Does the child react to the caregiver's voice by cooing, smiling, or turning eyes and head toward the voice?
3. Does the child try to imitate sounds?
4. Can the child imitate words and sounds?
5. Can the child follow directions?
6. Does the child respond to sounds not directed at him or her?

External Ear

Inspection of Pinna Position Position the child on the caregiver's lap or examining table. Draw an imaginary line from the outer canthus to the top of the ear. The top of the ear should be at or a little above the imaginary line. An abnormal finding occurs when the top of the ear is below the imaginary line drawn from the outer canthus to the top of the ear. Kidneys and ears are formed at the same time in embryonic development. If a child's ears are low set, renal anomalies must be ruled out. Low-set ears can also occur in Down syndrome.

Internal Ear

A cooperative child may be allowed to sit for the assessment. A young child may be held as shown in Figure 14-9a. Restrain the uncooperative young child by placing him or her supine on a firm surface (Figure 14-9b). Instruct the caregiver or assistant to hold the child's arms up near the head, embracing the elbow joints on both sides of either arm. Restrain the infant by having the caregiver hold the infant's hands down (Figure 14-9c).

With your thumb and forefinger grasping the otoscope, use the lateral side of the hand to prevent the head from

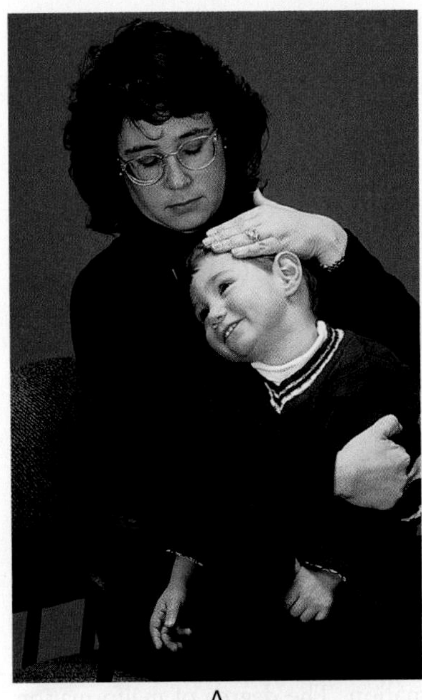

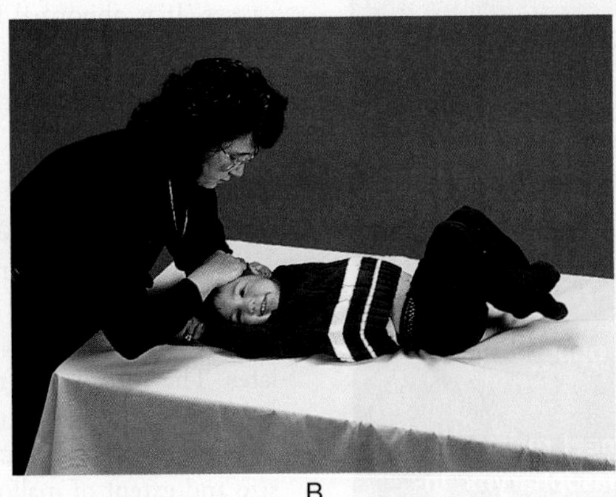

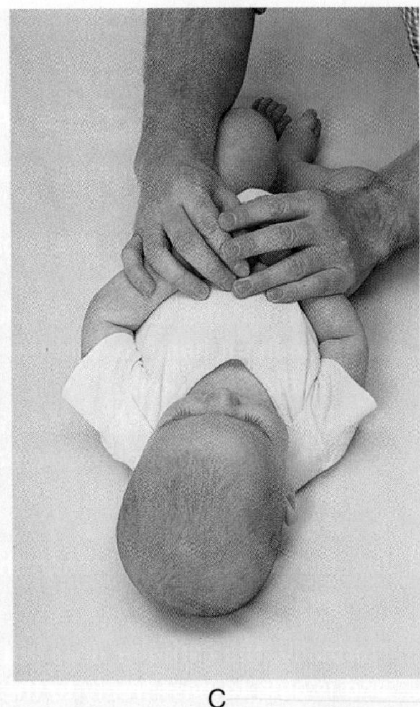

FIGURE 14-9 Restraining the Child for the Otoscopic Examination. (A) Preschooler in a Sitting Position (B) Preschooler in a Supine Position (C) Infant. DELMAR CENGAGE LEARNING.

jerking. Your other hand can also be used to stabilize the child's head. Pull the lower auricle down and out to straighten the canal. This technique is used in children up to about 3 years of age. Use the adult technique after age 3. Insert the speculum about 1/4 to 1/2 inch, depending on the child's age. Suspected otitis media must be evaluated with a pneumatic bulb attached to the side of the otoscope's light source. Select a larger speculum to make a tight seal and prevent air from escaping from the canal. If a light reflex is present, focus on the light reflection. Gently squeeze the bulb attachment to introduce air into the canal. Some nurses prefer to gently blow air through the tubing rather than squeezing air into the canal. Observe the tympanic membrane for movement.

The tympanic membrane is transparent and pearly gray to light pink in color. The membrane is smooth and continuous. Light from the otoscope is reflected off the membrane. The tympanic membrane moves when air is introduced into the canal.

CULTURAL CONSIDERATION

Ear Examination

Upon examining the middle ear of an Asian child, the examiner may note tiny white flecks within the canal. This is considered a normal finding representing dead skin cells.

NOSE

Observe the size and shape of the external nose, which should be symmetric and positioned in the center of the face. A short and small, large, or flattened nose may indicate congenital anomalies. Observe the external nose for flaring, discharge, or odor. Nasal flaring indicates respiratory distress. Purulent yellow or green discharge accompanies an infection. Clear, watery secretions may indicate allergic rhinitis, the common cold, Respiratory Syncytial Virus (RSV), or a foreign body. A foul odor may indicate a foreign body lodged in the nasal cavity. In an infant and young child, the nasal cavity can be visualized by tilting the head back and pushing the tip of the nose upward. The nasal mucosa should be firm and pink.

Patency of the nares must be determined at birth because newborns are obligatory nose breathers. With the infant's mouth closed, block one nostril and then the other. Observe the respiratory pattern. If total obstruction exists, the infant will not be able to inspire or expire through the

NURSING TIP

False Impressions of Otitis Media

If the child is screaming and crying, a flush or erythema on the tympanic membrane will be present. After allowing the caregiver to comfort the child, attempt to reassess. The flush or erythema can give false impressions of otitis media.

NURSING TIP

Assessing for Choanal Atresia

1. Select an appropriately sized catheter (10–12 French).
2. Place the newborn in a supine position on the examination table.
3. Stand at the newborn's side, and use the nondominant hand to hold the newborn's head in a midline position.
4. Use the dominant hand to insert the catheter through the nasal passage and into the nasopharynx.
5. Remove the catheter.
6. Perform the test through the opposite nare to evaluate patency.

Normally, the catheter does not meet resistance and is able to pass freely to the nasopharynx. Inability to insert the catheter into the nasopharynx coupled with symptoms of snorting respirations, feeding problems, and cyanosis are indicators of choanal atresia.

uncompressed nostril. If obstruction is suspected, an assessment for choanal atresia should be performed. In **choanal atresia**, there is a unilateral or bilateral bony or membranous septum between the nose and the pharynx.

MOUTH AND THROAT

INSPECTION

Lips Observe if the lip edges meet, which is normal. Cleft lip is seen as a separated area of lip tissue. It involves the upper lip and sometimes extends into the nostril. A cleft lip is an obvious finding during a newborn assessment. It occurs mainly on the left side and is more frequently found in males. A cleft lip develops during the fifth to sixth week after fertilization. Genetics plays a small role in etiology. Poor nutrition during pregnancy is likely (cleft lip is seen more frequently in poverty-stricken areas of the world).

Oral Mucosa If the child is unable to open the mouth on command, use the edge of a tongue blade to lift the upper lip and move the lower lip down. The mucous membranes are pink, moist, and smooth. Thrush, a thick, curdlike coating on the buccal mucosa or tongue, is abnormal. It can be acquired when a newborn passes through the vagina during delivery.

Teeth Count the number of teeth present on the gum line. Observe the condition of teeth surface for caries or chips. Infants cut their first tooth between 5 and 8 months. By one year of age there are normally eight teeth. Between 5 and 6 years of age, a child will shed the lower central incisors. About 1 year after deciduous shedding, the first permanent teeth erupt. A lack of visible teeth coupled with roentgenographic findings revealing absence of tooth buds is abnormal. Absence of deciduous teeth beyond 16 months of age signifies an abnormality most commonly related to genetic causes. It is abnormal for the teeth to turn brownish black, possibly with indentations along the surfaces of the teeth. These brownish black spots may be caries (cavities), which can be caused when a child falls asleep with a bottle in the mouth (Jones, Berg, & Coody, 1994).

Hard or Soft Palate Observe the palate for continuity and shape. For infants, you will need to use a tongue depressor to push the tongue down. Infants usually cry in response to this action, which allows visualization of the palates. The roof of the mouth is continuous and has a slight arch. It is abnormal if the roof of the mouth is not continuous. This anomaly is called cleft palate. Cleft palates vary greatly in size and extent of malformation. The degree of malformation is classified into two groups. A midline malformation may involve the uvula or extend through the soft or hard palates or both. If associated with cleft lip, the malformation may extend through the palates and into the nasal cavity. Cleft palates form between the sixth and tenth week of embryonic development, during fusion of the maxillary and premaxillary processes. Genetics plays a small role in etiology.

Epstein's pearls in the newborn appear on the hard palate and gum margins and are abnormal. The pearls are small, white cysts that feel hard when palpated. These cysts result from fragments of epithelial tissue trapped during palate formation.

Oropharynx Observe the position and color of the uvula. Observe the color and size of tonsillar tissue in the oropharynx. The tonsils are part of the lymphatic system and normally are hypertrophied in early childhood. Beginning at age 10 years, they gradually shrink in size. Tonsillar size ranges from 1+ to 4+ (Figure 14-10). Up to the age of 10 years, a tonsil grade of 2+ is considered normal. Tonsils should not

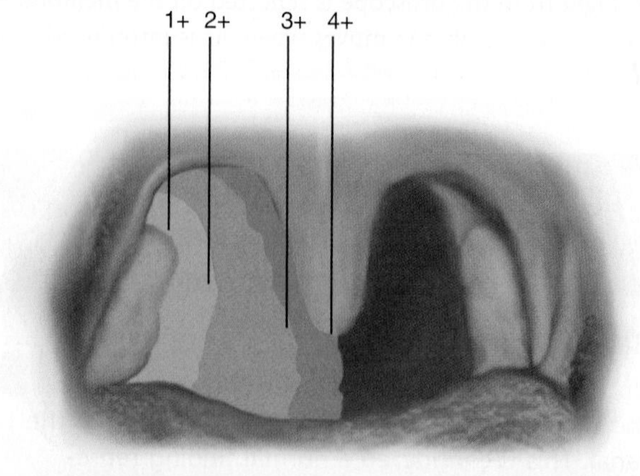

FIGURE 14-10 Grading of Tonsils. DELMAR CENGAGE LEARNING.

interfere with the act of breathing. Group A beta-hemolytic streptococcus (GABHS) causes pharyngeal or tonsillar inflammation or exudate. GABHS is responsible for 15–30% of all acute pharyngitis in children (Choby, 2009). Excessive salivation is an early sign of a tracheoesophageal fistula (TEF). Drooling is accompanied by choking and coughing during the child's feeding. The esophagus failed to develop as a continuous passage during embryonic formation.

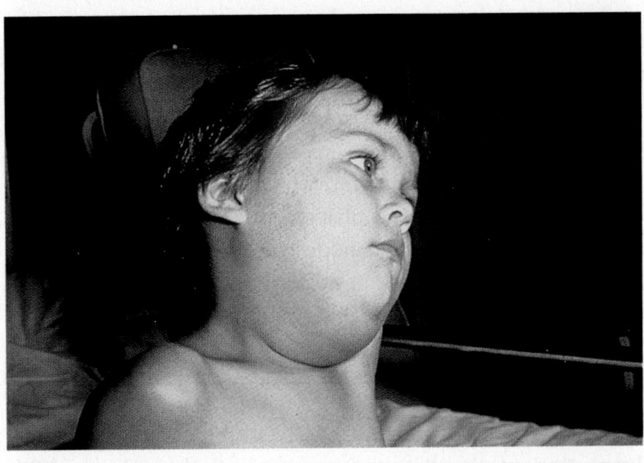

FIGURE 14-11 Parotitis (Mumps). COURTESY OF THE CENTERS FOR DISEASE CONTROL AND PREVENTION.

NECK

INSPECTION

General Appearance Observe the neck in a midline position while the child is sitting upright. Note shortening or thickness of the neck on both right and left sides. Note any swelling. Normally, there is a reasonable amount of skin tissue on the sides of the neck and no swelling. Unilateral or bilateral swelling of the neck below the angle of the jaw is abnormal (Figure 14-11). Enlargement of the parotid gland occurs in parotitis or mumps, an inflammation of the parotid gland. There is pain and tenderness in the affected area.

PALPATION

Thyroid Use the first two finger pads to palpate the thyroid gland and its lobes. Have the younger child who is unable to swallow on command take a drink from a bottle. Upon palpation, note any tenderness, enlargement, or masses. An enlarged thyroid gland can be indicative of hyperthyroidism.

Lymph Nodes Because of the infant's short neck, you must extend the chin upward with your hand before proceeding with palpation. With the finger pads, palpate the submental, submandibular, tonsillar, anterior cervical chain, posterior cervical chain, supra-clavicular, preauricular, posterior auricular, and occipital lymph nodes (Figure 14-12). Use a circular motion. Note location, size, shape, tenderness, mobility, and associated skin inflammation of any swollen

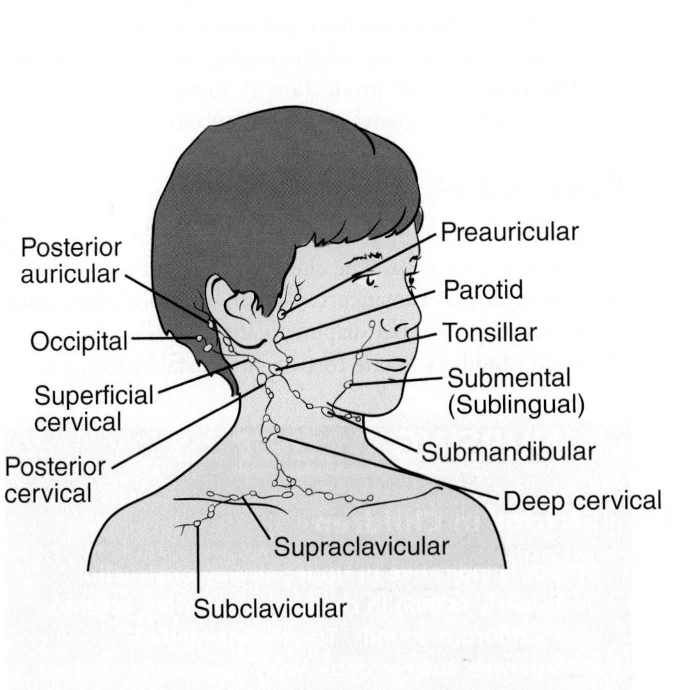

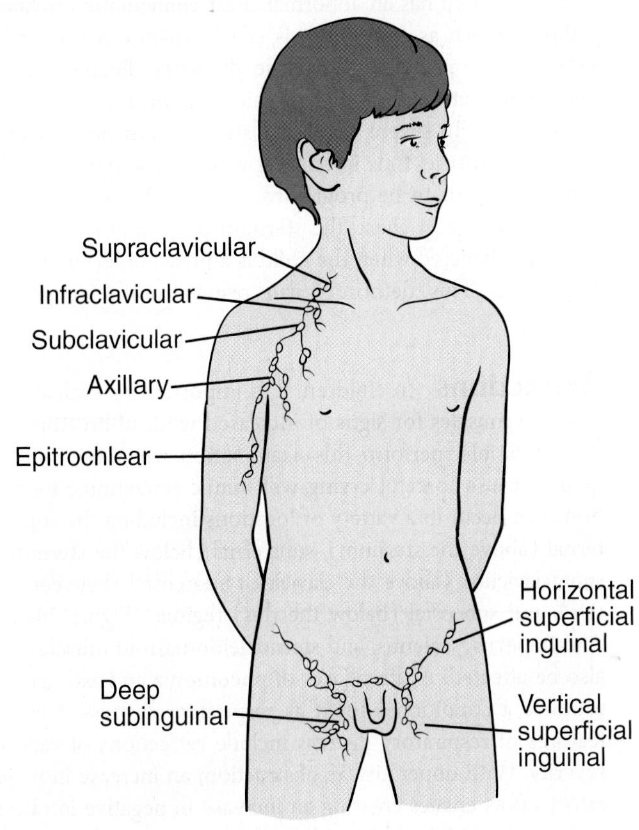

FIGURE 14-12 Lymph Nodes. DELMAR CENGAGE LEARNING.

nodes palpated. Lymph nodes are generally not palpable. Children often have small, movable, cool, nontender nodes referred to as "shotty" nodes. These benign nodes are related to environmental antigen exposure or residual effects of a prior illness and have no clinical significance. Enlargement of the anterior cervical chain, which is abnormal, occurs in bacterial infections of the pharynx, such as strep throat. Enlargement of the occipital nodes or posterior cervical chain nodes is abnormal. This can occur in infectious mononucleosis, tinea capitis, and acute otitis externa.

BREASTS

Inspection of the breasts is performed throughout childhood. Palpation is not usually performed on the child until puberty, unless otherwise indicated.

THORAX AND LUNGS

INSPECTION

Shape of Thorax Observe the configuration of the thorax noting bony structures and musculature. Note the anterior-posterior to lateral diameter and shape of the sternum. The infant has a rounded thorax with the anterior-posterior and transverse diameters approximately equal. By age 6, the chest attains the adult configuration of a lateral diameter greater than the anterior-posterior diameter. If a school-age child has an abnormal chest configuration, suspect pathology such as cystic fibrosis (CF), which can lead to an altered anteroposterior-transverse diameter. Pectus excavatum or funnel chest is a depression in the lower body of the sternum. In severe cases, the sternum can press against the right ventricle, thus interfering with cardiac function. The deformity tends to be progressive from birth. In pectus carinatum, or pigeon chest, the sternum projects forward. This is usually detected when the child is a preschooler or at early school-age. This deformity can result from a congenital anomaly.

Retractions In children, it is important to evaluate intercostal muscles for signs of increased work of breathing. If at all possible, perform this examination when the child is quiet because forceful crying will mimic retractions. Retractions can occur in a variety of locations including the suprasternal (above the sternum), substernal (below the sternum), supraclavicular (above the clavicles), intercostal (between the ribs), and subcostal (below the ribs) regions (Figure 14-13). The trapezus, scalenus, and sternocleidomastoid muscles can also be affected. Acute phases of pneumonia and asthma can produce a condition known as respiratory distress. Clinical features of respiratory distress include retractions of varying severity. With upper airway obstruction, an increase in respiratory effort ensues creating an increase in negative intrathoracic pressure. The net result is retractions.

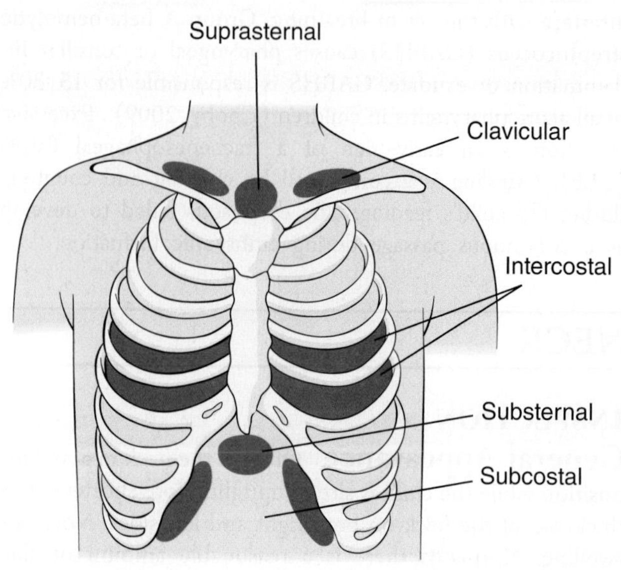

FIGURE 14-13 **Location of Retractions.** DELMAR CENGAGE LEARNING.

PALPATION

Tactile Fremitus Fremitus is easily felt when a child cries. If the infant or young child is not crying, it is advisable to defer this procedure until later in the assessment, perhaps after the throat and ear examinations, which usually produce crying. With the child in the same position as inspection, instruct the older child to repeat "99." As the child is crying or repeating "99," use both hands to palpate the chest simultaneously. Repeat the procedure until the anterior, posterior, and lateral sides are assessed, comparing the contralateral side. A soft vibration over the chest wall is normal. Increased sound production is caused by consolidation, as in pneumonia. Decreased sound production is caused by conditions such as pulmonary edema or pleural effusions.

PERCUSSION

Percussion is performed to further assess the underlying structures of the thorax. The chest is percussed to determine dullness or hyperresonance caused by consolidation, fluid, or air trapping. Normal diaphragmatic excursion in infants and young toddlers is one to two intercostal spaces.

NURSING ALERT

Stridor in Children

Stridor is indicative of upper airway obstruction, particularly edema in children. Inspiration accentuates stridorous sounds. To prevent medical emergencies such as occur with epiglottitis, prompt attention must be sought for children who present with stridor.

Auscultation

Breath Sounds Use the same assessment techniques as for an adult. Sometimes it is difficult to differentiate the various adventitious sounds because a child's respiratory rate is rapid; for example, differentiating expiratory wheezing from inspiratory wheezing can be difficult. Mastering the technique takes time and practice. Of the three types of breath sounds—bronchial, bronchovesicular, and vesicular—the bronchovesicular are normally heard throughout the peripheral lung fields up to 5–6 years of age because the chest wall is thin with decreased musculature. Lung fields are clear and equal bilaterally.

The common terms used to describe adventitious breath sounds are crackles (formerly called rales), rhonchi, and wheezes. Crackles may be caused by conditions such as bronchiolitis, CF, and bronchopulmonary dysplasia. Children with asthma and bronchiolitis may present with wheezing. Stridor is a high-pitched inspiratory crowing sound occurring with croup and acute epiglottitis.

HEART AND PERIPHERAL VASCULATURE

General Approach

The cardiovascular physical assessment has two major components: (1) assessment of the precordium and (2) assessment of the periphery. It is best to perform the cardiac assessment near the beginning of the examination, when the infant or young child is relatively calm. Do not get discouraged during the assessment. The novice nurse is not expected to identify a murmur and location within the cardiac cycle. Be patient because skill will come only with practice. Cardiac landmarks change when a child has **dextrocardia**. In this condition, the apex of the heart points toward the right thoracic cavity; thus, heart sounds are auscultated primarily on the right side of the chest.

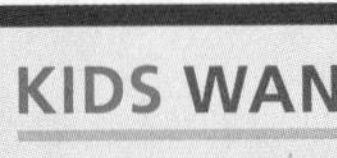

KIDS WANT TO KNOW

Why does the nurse have to listen to my heart in so many places?

Meredith is 8 years old and is curious about why the nurse puts the stethoscope in different locations on her chest. The nurse replies "your heart has valves like a door that open to allow blood to flow in and close to stop the flow. I am listening for sounds that let me know the valves are working OK."

Inspection

Apical Impulse With the child's entire chest exposed, look diagonally across the chest for the apical impulse. In infants and young children, the heart lies more horizontally in the chest than in an adult; therefore, the apical impulse is located at the fourth intercostal space and just left of the midclavicular line. The apical impulse of a child 7 years or older is at the fifth intercostal space and to the right of the midclavicular line. The impulse may not be visible in all children, especially in those who have increased adipose tissue or muscle. If the apical impulse is shifted toward the left side or downward expect pathology. Cardiac enlargement or a pneumothorax can cause the location of the apical impulse to deviate. The apical pulse moves laterally with cardiac enlargement. A pneumothorax shifts the apical impulse away from the area of the pneumothorax, which occurs when air enters the pleural cavity from a perforation, commonly as a result of injury to the chest wall.

Precordium Observe the precordium for any movements other than the apical impulse, which is normally visible. Movements other than the apical impulse are abnormal, and, if noticed, they should be described in terms of type, location, and timing in relation to the cardiac cycle. Another abnormality is a **heave**, or a lifting of the cardiac area secondary to an increased workload and force of the left ventricular contraction. A child with congenital heart disease is at risk for developing congestive heart failure (CHF) with associated volume overload and may have heaves. Large left-to-right shunt defects, such as a VSD, cause right ventricular volume overload.

Palpation

Thrill A **thrill** is a vibration that is similar to what one feels when a hand is placed on a purring cat. It is most commonly produced by blood flowing through a narrow opening from one chamber to another such as in a septal defect. Palpate as for an adult or use the proximal one-third of each finger and the areas over the metacarpophalangeal joints. Place the hand vertically along the heart's apex and move the hand toward the sternum.

Place the hand horizontally along the sternum, moving up the sternal border about 1/2 to 1 inch each time. When at the clavicular level, place the hand vertically and assess for a thrill at the heart's base. Use the finger pads to palpate a thrill at the suprasternal notch and along the carotid arteries. A thrill is not found in the healthy child. A thrill's anatomic location corresponds to a particular structural abnormality within the heart. For example, a thrill in the pulmonic area is felt at the second and third intercostal space on the upper left sternal border. A thrill at the second intercostal space on the right upper sternal border is attributed to pathology in the aorta.

Peripheral Pulses Use the same finger to assess each peripheral pulse. The sensation of one finger pad versus another can be different. Use the finger pads to palpate each pair of peripheral pulses simultaneously, except for the carotid pulses. The carotid pulses should not be palpated together because excessive stimulation can elicit a vagal response and slow down the heart. Palpating both carotid pulses at the same time could also decrease circulation to the child's head. Palpate the brachial and femoral pulses simultaneously. Pulse qualities are the same in the adult and the child. A brachial-femoral lag, when femoral pulses are weaker than brachial pulses when palpated simultaneously, is abnormal and occurs in a cardiac defect know as coarctation of the aorta (COA). COA is due to a narrowing of the aorta before, at, or just beyond the entrance of the ductus arteriosus, which causes reduced blood flow to the lower body.

If coarctation of the aorta is suspected (as when a brachial-femoral lag is present), obtain all four extremity blood pressures and compare the right upper extremity and left lower extremity readings. Remember to use an appropriately sized cuff. Refer to the section *Vital Signs: Blood Pressure* for information about determination of proper cuff size. Take the upper extremity blood pressure in the right arm. Because weak or absent leg pulses accompany coarctation, leg blood pressure measurements are difficult to obtain. Use a Doppler transducer to intensify the sound of the pulse. Until you feel proficient, the Doppler technique requires two people for accurate measurement; have the caregiver hold the child's leg still while you assess the pulse. Locate the posterior tibial pulse with the Doppler transducer and make an "X" with a pen where the pulse is felt or heard. Place an appropriately sized cuff on the lower right leg. The lower edge of the cuff should be 1/2 inch to 1 inch above the presumed posterior tibial pulse location. Apply a small amount of ultrasound gel to the area surrounding the presumed pulse. Turn the Doppler transducer on and adjust the volume control while the attached probe is locating the pulse. When a pulse is identified, proceed with the blood pressure measurement. Only the systolic number is obtained with this technique. Repeat the steps on the left side of the body.

Normally, upper and lower extremity blood pressures are equal. If the systolic blood pressure in the leg is lower than that in the arm and femoral, popliteal, posterior tibial, or dorsalis pedis pulses are weak or absent, you can assume coarctation of the aorta is present. If undiagnosed, as the child becomes older, the upper extremity pulses are bounding.

Auscultation

Heart Sounds Auscultating the infant's or the young pediatric child's heart is difficult because the heart rate is rapid and breath sounds are easily transmitted through the chest wall. Have the child lie down. If this position is not possible, the child should be held at a 45° angle in the caregiver's arms. A quiet environment and child is optimum in order to properly listen to the heart (Figure 14-14). Use the Z pattern to auscultate the heart. Place the stethoscope in

Reflections from Families

My 2-year-old son is always so frightened and upset when he goes in for his well-child checkup. I was so relieved during his last visit because the nurse practitioner knew exactly how to help him calm down. She kneeled down so she was on his level and talked with him before the exam. She allowed him to handle some of the equipment, like the stethoscope, before using it on him. At no time was he completely undressed. He was so cooperative and never cried. The whole experience was better than it had ever been.

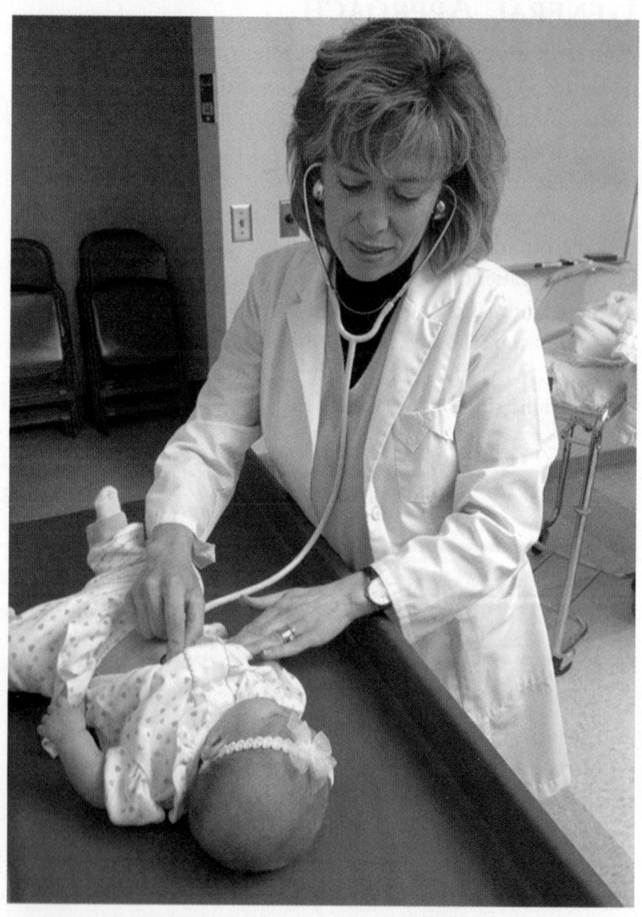

Figure 14-14 Auscultation of the heart requires a quiet infant. DELMAR CENGAGE LEARNING.

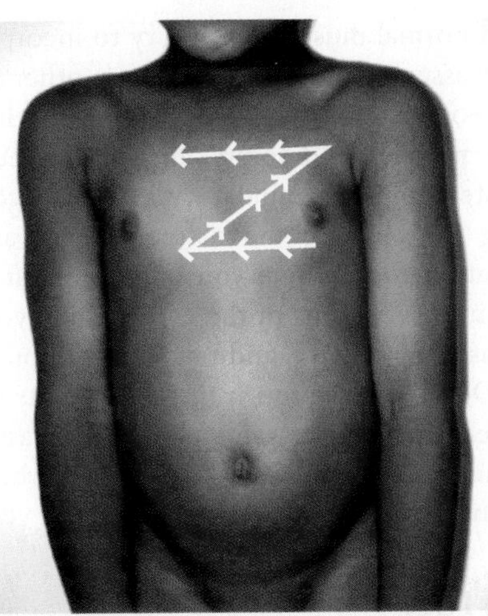

FIGURE 14-15 Z Auscultation Pattern for Young Children.
DELMAR CENGAGE LEARNING.

the apical area and gradually move it toward the right lower sternal border and up the sternal border in a right diagonal line. Move gradually from the child's left to the right upper sternal borders (Figure 14-15). Perform a second evaluation with the child in a sitting position.

Fifty percent of all children develop an innocent murmur at some time in their lives. Innocent murmurs are not associated with pathology and are accentuated in high cardiac output states such as fever, anxiety, or exercise. When the child is sitting, a murmur is heard early in systole at the second or third intercostal space along the left sternal border and is musical in quality, disappearing when the child lies down. Be aware of sinus arrhythmias during auscultation of the heart's rhythm. Sinus arrhythmia is normal in many children. On inspiration, the pulse rate speeds up, and the pulse rate slows with expiration. To determine if the rhythm is normal, ask the child to hold his or her breath while you auscultate the heart. If the heart rate variability stops, then a sinus arrhythmia is present.

S_1 is best heard at the apex of the heart, left lower sternal border. S_2 is best heard at the heart base. A fixed split S_2 that does not vary with respiration is abnormal, and you can suspect an atrial septal defect (ASD). In children, S_2 physiologically splits with inspiration and becomes single with expiration. This phenomenon is due to a greater negative pressure in the thoracic cavity. In children, S_3 often sounds like the three syllables of the word "Kentucky," especially when accompanied by tachycardia. A loud third heart sound may be present in children with CHF or VSD.

ABDOMEN

GENERAL APPROACH

If possible, ask the caregiver to refrain from feeding the infant prior to the assessment because palpation of a full stomach may induce vomiting. Children who are physically able should be encouraged to empty the bladder prior to the assessment. The young infant, school-age child, or adolescent should lie on the examination table. For the toddler or preschooler, have the caregiver hold the child supine on the lap, with the lower extremities bent at the knees. If the child is crying, encourage the caregiver to help calm the child before you proceed with the assessment. Observe nonverbal communication in children who are not able to verbally express feelings. The order of abdominal assessment is inspection, auscultation, and palpation. Auscultation is performed second because palpation can alter bowel sounds. During palpation, listen for a high-pitched cry and look for a change in facial expression or for sudden protective movements that may indicate a painful or tender area.

> **NURSING TIP**
>
> **Assessing for Umbilical Hernias in Children**
>
> **If the child is upset and crying, assess the umbilicus for an outward projection, which is indicative of an umbilical hernia. If an umbilical hernia is present, palpate the area to determine if the hernia reduces easily. Approximate the size of the inner ring (the diameter of the hernia).**

INSPECTION

Observe the abdomen for a distinct separation of the rectus muscles with a visible bulge along the midline known as **diastasis recti**. Normally the abdominal musculature is continuous. A separated abdominal muscle that lies vertically is abnormal. The gap between the two edges may range from 1 to 5 centimeters. Diastasis recti is more common in African-American infants and usually disappears by early childhood.

Peristaltic Wave Observe the abdominal wall below the xiphoid process and above the symphysis pubis for wave-like movements. Peristalsis is not normally visible. Visible peristaltic waves seen moving across the epigastrium from

> **NURSING TIP**
>
> **Measuring the Abdomen in Children**
>
> **If abdominal distention is seen during inspection, evaluate its circumference. Place the tape measure around the abdomen at the level of the umbilicus. If serial abdominal circumference measurements are to be taken, use a marking pen to indicate the location where the tape measure was placed.**

left to right are abnormal and may occur in the gastrointestinal disorder pyloric stenosis. In this condition, the pyloric muscle hypertrophies, resulting in obstruction at the pyloric sphincter.

Auscultation

After performing auscultation of the lungs, it is helpful to proceed to auscultating the abdomen because doing so allows you to complete a good portion of auscultation all at once. If the child is not cooperating, a simple distracting phrase such as "I can hear your breakfast in there" is helpful during auscultation.

Palpation

General Palpation Perform the same technique and sequence of light and deep palpation as done with the adult. On palpation, an olive-shaped mass felt in the epigastric area and to the upper right of the umbilicus is abnormal and is indicative of pyloric stenosis. Abdominal distention coupled with palpable stool over the abdomen and the absence of stool in the rectum is abnormal. An aganglionic segment of the colon is responsible for Hirschsprung's disease, which produces these abnormal gastrointestinal (GI) findings. A sausage-shaped mass that produces intermittent pain when palpated in the upper abdomen is abnormal. This is a manifestation of another GI disorder called intussusception. Bowel sounds heard in the thoracic cavity, a scaphoid abdomen, an upward displaced apical impulse, and signs of respiratory distress are abnormal findings in the newborn and suggest a diaphragmatic hernia.

Liver Palpation For infants and toddlers, use the outer edge of your right thumb to press down and scoop up at the right upper quadrant. For the remaining age groups, use the same technique as for an adult. The liver is not normally palpated, although the liver edge can be found 1 cm below the right costal margin in a normal, healthy child. The liver edge is soft and regular. It is abnormal for the liver edge to be palpated more than 2 cm below the right costal margin and be full with a firm, sharp border. Hepatomegaly occurs in several disease states such as viral or bacterial illnesses, tumors, congestive heart failure, and fat and glycogen storage diseases. Viral and bacterial illnesses and tumors cause liver cells to multiply in number, creating an enlarged liver. In heart failure, the hepatic veins and sinusoids enlarge from congestion, resulting in hemorrhage and fibrosis of the liver. In fat and glycogen storage diseases, fat and glycogen accumulate within the liver, and fibrosis ensues.

MUSCULOSKELETAL SYSTEM

General Approach

The extent or degree of assessment depends greatly on the child's or caregiver's complaints of musculoskeletal problems. Be aware that, during periods of rapid growth, children complain of normal muscle aches. Try to incorporate musculoskeletal assessment techniques into other system assessments. For instance, while inspecting the integument, inspect the muscles and joints. Inspecting the musculoskeletal system in the ambulatory child is accomplished by allowing the child to move freely about and play in the examination room while you inquire about the health history. Your observations of the child enable you to assess posture, muscle symmetry, and range of motion of muscles and joints. Do not rush through the assessment. Throughout the assessment, incorporate game playing that facilitates evaluation of the musculoskeletal system. Observe range of motion and joint flexibility as the child undresses.

Inspection

Muscles Assessment of the muscles includes examination of muscle mass (size), muscle tone, muscle strength, gross and fine motor ability, and involuntary movements.

Muscle Mass (Size) Note the symmetry and alignment of muscle mass by comparing one side of the body with the other. Muscles should have a firmness when palpated. In most instances muscle size and firmness will be equal. Muscles should be measured if hypertrophy or atrophy is suspected.

Muscle Tone Muscle tone is best evaluated by observation of active range of motion. Note any resistance, rigidity, spasticity, hypotonia, flaccidity, or paralysis as the child performs range of motion of the neck, spine, and extremities. Increased muscle tone (spasticity) is abnormal and may indicate cerebral palsy (CP), which results from a nonprogressive abnormality in the pyramidal motor tract. One of the more common contributing factors, perinatal asphyxia, causes abnormal posture, gross motor development, and varying degrees of abnormal muscle tone.

Muscle Strength To evaluate the strength of the infant's shoulder muscles, place your hands under the axillae and pull the infant into a standing position. The infant should not slip through your hands. Be prepared to catch the infant if needed. Evaluate the infant's leg strength in a semi-standing position. Lower the infant to the examination table so the infant's legs touch the table. Place the infant older than 4 months in a prone position. Observe the infant's ability to lift the upper body off the examination table using the upper extremities.

In children beyond infancy note the symmetry of strength by testing muscles with and without your resistance. To test hand strength, ask the child to squeeze your fingers hard. To test upper extremity strength, have the child flex each of her or his arms while you attempt to pull the forearm into extension. To test lower extremity strength, ask the child to keep the legs extended straight while you attempt to push each into flexion. Another method of testing the legs involves asking the child to stand, rising from a supine position. The child with good muscle strength is able to rise to a standing position without using the arms for leverage. The inability to rise from a sitting to a standing position is abnormal and occurs in the child with Duchenne's muscular dystrophy (MD) due to generalized muscle weakness.

Gross and Fine Motor Ability Assessment of gross motor function determines the child's ability to move large muscles in a coordinated and integrative manner. The status of gross motor function may be noted through observation of the coordination of the body in walking, sitting, and other activities that require the use of large muscles and joints. Fine motor function is assessed by determining the child's ability to coordinate small muscles. These types of movements require more precision and refinement in execution and in the visual-perceptual integration. Examples of these skills include grasping, holding, manipulating, and releasing objects. Use the Denver II to screen gross and fine motor skills that are appropriate for the child's specific age.

Involuntary Movements Normally, no involuntary movements occur. If they are present, note their location, frequency, rate, and amplitude. Note if the movements can be controlled at will. Abnormalities include tremors, tics, twisting, and jerking and irregular movements.

Joints and Spine Observe the medial, lateral, toe, and heel aspects of both shoes for signs of abnormal wear. Compare one shoe to the other for signs of excessive wear. Ask the ambulatory child to walk at least 10 feet. Note the scapula's position and symmetry. Note the flexibility of the radiocarpal, elbow, shoulder, hip, tibiofemoral, and tibiotalar joints while the child is walking. Inspect the joints from head to toe. The infant's spine is C-shaped. Head control and standing create the normal S-shaped spine of the adult. Lordosis, an exaggerated lumbar curvature of the spine, is normal as the child begins to walk. A toddler's protruding abdomen is counterbalanced by an inward deviation of the lumbar spine. Lordosis is abnormal after 6 years of age. It can be attributed to bilateral developmental dislocation of the hip or postural factors such as progression of congenital kyphosis, or can occur secondary to contractures of hip flexors. The spine should also be assessed for scoliosis.

Count the fingers and toes. **Polydactyly**, extra fingers or toes, may be found in certain congenital syndromes. A fusion between two or more digits, called **syndactylism**, is abnormal. It is also associated with certain congenital syndromes. It is abnormal for a young male (usually 2–12 years old) to present with a painless limp from the affected hip. The limp is accompanied by limited abduction and internal rotation, muscle spasm, and proximal thigh atrophy. These are manifestations of Legg-Calvé-Perthes disease, also called coxa plana. It is caused by an interruption in the blood supply to the capital femoral epiphysis with avascular necrosis of the femoral head resulting.

> **NURSING TIP**
>
> **Palpating Muscle Strength in Children**
>
> Playing games will assist you if the child is resistant to formal examination. For example, you can test plantar flexion by asking the child to pretend that the feet are pushing the brake on a car while you bear the force with your hands.

Tibiofemoral Bones Instruct the child to stand on the floor with the medial condyles together. Measure the distance between the two medial malleoli. Measure the distance between the two medial condyles. Normally, the distance between the medial malleoli is less than 2 inches (5 cm). The distance between the medial condyles is less than 1 inch (2.5 cm). If the distance between the medial condyles is less than 1 inch (2.5 cm) and the distance between the medial malleoli is more than 2 inches (5 cm), the child has knock-knee, or genu valgum. This is common between 2 and 4 years of age. Genu valgum persisting after 6 years of age is abnormal. If the measured distance between the two medial condyles is greater than 1–2 inches, bowleg or genu varum is present. Genu varum is a common finding in infants and toddlers until walking has been firmly established. Genu varum persisting after 2 years of age is abnormal and may be caused by rickets.

PALPATION

Joints Palpate the joints for heat, tenderness, and swelling. Joint flexibility values are within the same range as an adult. Findings are the same as the adult. Swollen, inflamed, painful joints, seen in juvenile rheumatoid arthritis (JRA), are abnormal. JRA causes synovial inflammation and degeneration of the joint. Its cause is unknown.

Feet Stand in front of the child. Hold the right heel immobile with one hand while pushing the forefoot (medial base of great toe) toward a midline position with the other hand. Observe for toe and forefoot adduction and inversion. Repeat on the left foot.

Normal findings are that the toes and forefoot are not deviated. Metatarsus varus (clubfoot) is characterized by medially adducted and inverted toes and forefoot. Clubfoot usually results from an abnormal intrauterine position of the fetal foot. Heredity also plays a role in the etiology.

Hip and Femur Approximately one in 85 live births are at risk for developmental dysplasia of the hip (DDH) (Cady, 2008). The hips should be evaluated to detect DDH to treat and prevent dislocation. One method, the Ortolani maneuver, should be performed by a trained individual at the very end of the assessment because it may produce crying. The test is performed on one hip at a time. Evaluate the hips up until 12–18 months of age or the child is an established walker. Place the infant supine on an examination table with the feet facing you. Stand directly in front of the infant. With the thumb, hold the lesser trochanter of the femur and with the index and middle fingers, hold the greater trochanter (Figure 14-16a). These two fingers should rest over the hip joint. Slowly press outward and abduct until the lateral aspects of the knees nearly touch the table (Figure 14-16b). The tips of the fingers should palpate each femoral head as it rotates outward. Listen for an audible clunk, which indicates a positive Ortolani's sign. With the fingers in the same locations, adduct the hips to elicit a palpable clunk (Ortolani's sign). As each hip is adducted, it is lifted anteriorally into the acetabulum. Abnormal findings indicating DDH include a positive Ortolani's sign; a sudden, painful cry during the test; asymmetrical thigh skin folds; uneven knee level; and limited hip abduction. Epidemiology of DDH is related to familial factors, maternal hormones associated with pelvic laxity, firstborn children, breech presentations, and **oligohydramnios** (an abnormally small amount or absence of amniotic fluid).

NEUROLOGICAL SYSTEM

The neurological examination includes evaluation of function within six major areas: (1) the cerebrum, (2) cranial nerves, (3) the cerebellum, (4) the motor system, (5) the sensory system, and (6) reflex status.

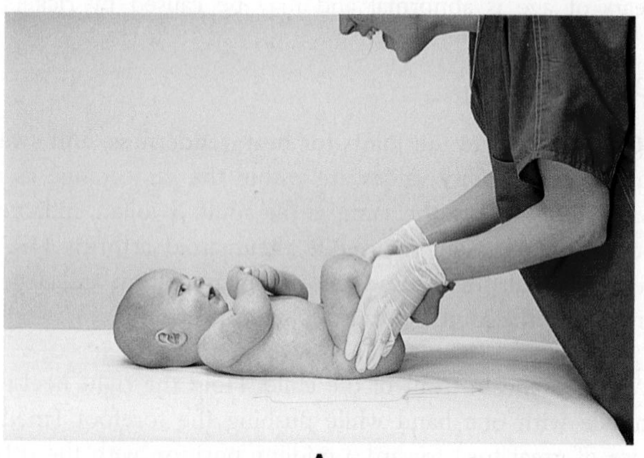

A

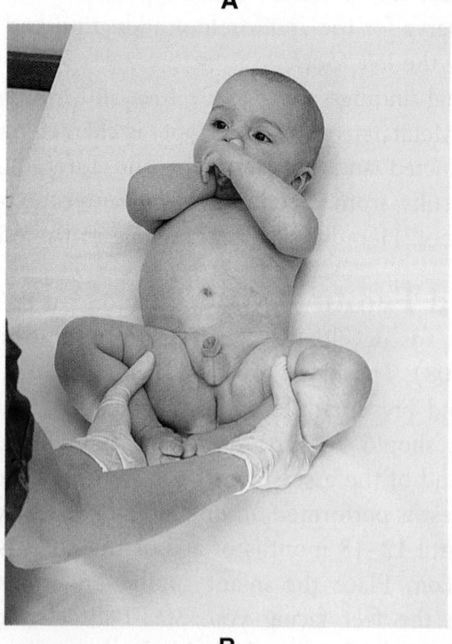

B

FIGURE 14-16 Ortolani Maneuver. (A) Hand Placement (B) Hip Abduction. DELMAR CENGAGE LEARNING.

CEREBRAL FUNCTION

Cerebral function is tested through an evaluation of behavior and mental status and includes appearance, judgment, memory, thought processes, language and speech, mood and affect, and orientation. An infant functions mainly at the subcortical level. Memory is about three-fourths developed by 2 years of age, when cortical functioning is acquiring dominance. Level of consciousness is also assessed as a function of the central nervous system. Because the infant cannot verbally express level of consciousness, instead assess the newborn's ability to cry, level of activity, positioning, and general appearance.

CRANIAL NERVES

A thorough assessment of cranial nerve function is difficult to perform on the infant less than 1 year old. Difficulty is also encountered with toddlers and preschoolers because they often cannot follow directions or are not willing to cooperate. Testing for the school-age child or the adolescent is carried out in the same manner as for an adult.

Infant (Birth to 12 Months)

To test cranial nerves (CNs) III (oculomotor), IV (trochlear), and VI (abducens), move a brightly colored toy along the infant's line of vision. An infant older than 1 month responds by following the object. Also evaluate the pupillary response to a bright light in each eye. CN V (trigeminal) is tested by assessing the rooting or sucking reflexes. CN VII (facial) is tested up until 2 months by assessing the sucking reflex and by observing symmetrical sucking movements. After 2 months of age, an infant will smile, allowing assessment of symmetry of facial expressions. A positive Moro reflex in an infant less than 6 months old is evidence of normal functioning of CN VIII (acoustic). CNs IX (glossopharyngeal) and X (vagus) are examined by using a tongue blade to produce a gag reflex. Do not test if a positive response was already elicited by using a tongue blade to view the posterior pharynx. To test CN XI (accessory), evaluate the infant's ability to lift the head up while in a prone position. CN XII (hypoglossal) is assessed by allowing the infant to suck on a pacifier or a bottle, abruptly removing the pacifier or bottle from the infant's mouth, and observing for lingering sucking movements.

Toddler and Preschooler (1 to 6 Years)

The older preschooler is able to identify familiar odors. Most children readily identify the smell of peanut butter and chocolate. Test CN I (olfactory) one side at a time by asking the child to close the eyes and to identify the smell of peanut butter and chocolate. Test each nostril with different substances while occluding the other nostril with your finger. Test vision (CN II [optic]) using Allen cards. CNs III, IV, and VI are tested in the same fashion as for the infant. CN V is tested by giving the child something to eat and evaluating chewing movements. Sensory responses to light and sharp touch are still not easily interpreted in these age

NURSING ALERT

Allergic Reaction to Inhaled Substances

Be aware of the child's allergies prior to testing CN I. For example, even the smell of peanut butter can cause a severe allergic reaction in some children. In such cases, use a different aromatic source when testing CN I.

groups. Observe facial weakness or paralysis (CN VII) by making the child smile or laugh. An older preschooler may cooperate by raising the eyebrows, frowning, puffing the cheeks out, and closing the eyes tightly on command. To evaluate CN VIII, ring a small bell out of the child's vision and observe the response to unseen sounds. Test CNs IX and X in the same manner as for the infant. CN XII is difficult to assess in this particular age group.

Cerebellar Function

Tests for cerebellar function mainly involve evaluation of posture, balance, and coordination. General evaluation of function includes observation of the child's body posture, stance, and gait; watching the child walk heel-to-toe, jump, skip, hop, and throw. The Romberg test is administered to evaluate balance by having the child stand with feet together, arms at side, and eyes open and then closed. If the child falls, loses balance, or leans to one side, the result is positive and indicates cerebellar dysfunction.

Motor System

Motor system function usually is evaluated as part of the musculoskeletal system examination and was discussed in that section.

Sensory System

Sensory function involves the body's response to various types of stimulation and usually is assessed during testing of cranial nerve function.

Reflex Status

Assessment of reflex status includes deep tendon reflexes (DTR), superficial, and newborn (often referred to as infant) reflexes.

Deep Tendon Reflexes Measurement of the DTRs reveals the intactness of the reflex arc at specific spinal levels and are tested in the same manner as with an adult. The following reflexes are routinely tested: upper extremities—biceps, triceps, and brachioradialis; lower extremities—patellar and Achilles. DTRs are evaluated for strength and symmetry of right and left sides, which should be equal. The tendon is slightly stretched and tapped with a reflex hammer. The expected response is contraction of the muscle.

Superficial Reflexes With superficial reflexes the receptors are in the skin rather than the muscles as in the DTRs. Superficial reflexes that are tested include the abdominal, cremasteric (testes), gluteal (buttocks), and plantar. They are elicited by stimulating the skin.

Newborn (Infant) Reflexes During infancy, examination includes identification of the presence or absence of newborn reflexes, which must be lost before motor development can proceed.

FEMALE GENITALIA

General Approach

Place the up-to-preschool-age child on the caregiver's lap or examination table. Ask the caregiver to assist by holding the legs in a froglike position. Place the child older than 4 years on the examination table in a semilithotomy position, without the feet in stirrups. Reserve the lithotomy position with the feet in stirrups for the older adolescent. Explain the procedure prior to the assessment. Never ask the caregiver of the infant or young school-age child to leave the room during this portion of the examination because the caregiver is a source of comfort to the child. Before the genitalia examination, the child should be told that it is all right for the provider to touch the genitals with the caregiver present. Explain that it is not appropriate for anyone else to do so for any reason. Drape the older-than-preschool-age child.

A vaginal or pelvic exam is not routinely performed on young females; however, it is warranted when signs of possible sexual abuse are present. The assessment is undertaken by a health care provider who is trained to perform pediatric vaginal examinations and can evaluate these problems. Any female who has reached menarche needs to be evaluated for a pregnant uterus.

Inspection

Perineal Area Stand directly in front of the child. Assess Tanner's stage (see Appendix D). Use the thumb and forefinger to separate the labia. Identify the labia majora and minora, clitoris, urethral meatus, hymen, and vaginal orifice. Observe color, size, and discharge from structures. Observe intactness and scarring of the hymen and vaginal orifice. The infant's labia minora are sometimes larger than the labia majora. The hymen is sometimes intact up until the point of sexual activity. It is abnormal for the female infant to display a rudimentary penis in the clitoral area, which is a finding in ambiguous genitalia. Genital ambiguity occurs during embryonic development as a consequence of genetic causes or androgens or androgen inhibitors that reverse genital characteristics. A bloody discharge noted at the vaginal opening or on the diaper is abnormal. It is not uncommon to note pseudomenstruation in an infant less than 2 weeks of age. Maternal hormones such as estrogen are the cause. Observe the perineal area for presence of genital warts. Human papillomavirus (HPV) is the most prevalent STD in the United States (Dempsey, Gebremariam, Koutsky, & Manhart, 2008).

MALE GENITALIA

GENERAL APPROACH

Female nurses may encounter difficulty assessing a reluctant adolescent. Be firm when explaining that this portion of the assessment is a required part of his examination. Infants and toddlers do not object to the assessment. In case the infant or toddler urinates during the examination, have a diaper or disposable cloth available to catch the stream of urine. The older school-age child and the adolescent should be draped in order to maintain modesty. Assess Tanner's stages during inspection.

Penis Note the position of the urethral meatus. Note the size of the penis. If you are not able to determine circumcision status, ask the caregiver if the child was circumcised. The meatus is normally found on the tip of the penis. A disappearing penis phenomenon occurs normally in infants with increased adipose tissue in the area surrounding the penis. Reassure the caregiver that this is normal and will resolve after adipose tissue is lost. It is abnormal for the urethral meatus to be located behind or along the ventral side of the penis, a condition known as hypospadias. During the third month of fetal development, the urethral meatus fails to move toward the glans penis. Mothers who take phenytoin (Dilantin) for epilepsy are at greater risk for having children with hypospadias. Another abnormality is epispadius in which the meatal opening is on the dorsal surface of the penis. During the third month of fetal development, the urethral meatus fails to move toward the glans penis.

Scrotum Evaluate scrotal size and color. Note if the testes are seen in the scrotal sac. The scrotum may appear underdeveloped if the testes have not been in the scrotal sac (Cakan & Kamat, 2009). The scrotum appears proportionately large in size when compared to the penis. The sac color is brown or black in dark-skinned children and pink in light-skinned children. Two testes should be present, but, in infants, they may retract into the inguinal canal or abdomen due to various stimuli, including cold and palpation.

PALPATION

Scrotum Place the infant in a supine position on the examination table. Instruct the young child to sit cross-legged to inhibit the **cremasteric reflex** (retraction of the testes from the scrotum) from occurring. The older child may be allowed to stand for this portion of the examination. Locate each testis within the scrotal sac by using the fingers of one hand in a milking motion to descend the testes. Palpate and note the size, shape, and mobility of each testis. Both testicles are palpated in the scrotum. They are smooth, round, or oval shaped and freely movable. It is abnormal to be unable to palpate the testes. **Cryptorchidism** is a failure of the testis to descend into the scrotal sac. One or both testes failing to descend within the inguinal canal occurs during embryonic development. Cryptorchidism is seen in about 3% of all newborn full-term males (Cakan & Kamat, 2009). An enlargement of the scrotum is abnormal and is seen in a congenital hydrocele, which results from failure of the fetal male reproductive tract to develop properly. This mass will transilluminate.

> **NURSING TIP**
>
> **Anal Reflex and Sexual Abuse**
>
> Anal trauma, such as occurs in sexual assault, manifests as poor anal sphincter control. Consider sexual abuse if a child exhibits an absent or slow anal reflex.

Hernia Place the infant supine on the examination table. All other children should stand during the examination. Use your little finger for the infant's exam and the index finger for the younger child's. Follow the inguinal canal as is done on an adult male. If possible, perform the assessment on a crying infant. Have preschoolers and early school-age children attempt to blow up a balloon while you palpate the inguinal areas. Palpate the inguinal areas while the older school-age child or adolescent coughs. No swelling or masses are palpated. A hernia palpated above the inguinal ligament is an abnormal finding. Indirect inguinal hernias occur during embryologic development as a result of persistent patency of the processus vaginalis testis.

ANUS

As a rule, rectal assessments are not performed on children unless you detect a problem or suspect abuse. In these cases, refer the child for further evaluation if you are not trained specifically for this procedure, and follow your institution's guidelines.

> **IN THE REAL WORLD**
>
> As a nursing student I was completely overwhelmed by the numerous sounds that the heart made. I could not always tell if I was listening to an infant's second or third heart sound because the heart was beating so rapidly. How was I going to describe the murmur? One of the pediatricians I worked with told me not to worry. He further said it had taken him at least a thousand settings of auscultating hearts before he could differentiate various sounds in pediatrics.

INSPECTION

Ask the child to lie on the abdomen. Gently separate the buttocks to allow direct visualization of the anal opening. Observe for bleeding, fissures, prolapse, skin tags, hemorrhoids, lesions, and pinworms. During separation of the buttocks, observe any movement of the anus. Stroke the perianal area with your finger, and note any movement. This is called the anal reflex or anal wink. No bleeding, fissures, prolapse, skin tags, hemorrhoids, lesions, or pinworms should be present. An anal reflex normally is observed. An absent anal reflex is abnormal. Conditions such as a spinal cord lesion, trauma, and tumors that interrupt nervous innervation to the anal sphincter cause this finding.

KEY CONCEPTS

- The parameters of weight, length or height, and head circumference (dependent on age) are essential for assessing physical growth. Using standardized growth charts, these measurements are used in determining normal and abnormal patterns.
- A pediatric health history includes biographical data, past health history, family health history, social history, and health maintenance activities.
- A nutritional assessment enables the nurse to provide anticipatory guidance, identify at-risk individuals, and collaborate with the health care team for early referral of the child as needed.
- A developmental assessment has several purposes: (1) validation that a child is developing normally or detects problems early, (2) identification of concerns of caregivers and child, and (3) provision of an opportunity for anticipatory guidance and teaching about age-appropriate expectations.
- In performing the physical assessment, techniques for approaching children vary from one age group to the next. However, a basic principle during any physical assessment is building a trusting relationship.
- Vital signs include temperature, respiration, pulse, and blood pressure, which are compared to normal ranges for the child's age. These measurements provide information about the child's basic physiological status.
- The skin is observed for color and lesions and palpated to determine temperature, texture, turgor, and edema.
- The head is inspected for shape, symmetry, and control, and the fontanels, suture lines, and surface characteristics are palpated.
- Examination of the eyes includes vision and strabismus screening, and assessment of the anterior and posterior segment structures.
- The thorax and lungs are examined using inspection, palpation, percussion, and auscultation.
- Assessment of the heart and peripheral vasculature consists of inspection (apical impulse, precordium), palpation (thrills, peripheral pulses), and auscultation of heart sounds.
- The order of abdominal assessment is inspection, auscultation, and palpation.
- The extent or degree of musculoskeletal assessment depends on the caregiver's and child's complaints of problems.
- A neurological examination includes assessment of infant reflexes (depends on age) and cranial nerves.

REVIEW ACTIVITIES

1. Describe the components of a health history for a child. What information is gathered in the following areas: (a) past health history, (b) social history, and (c) health maintenance activities?
2. List two environmental problems that put a child at risk for illness or death.
3. What is the purpose of a nutritional assessment?
4. What information is included in a nutritional assessment?
5. Describe factors that could lead to invalid results from a developmental screening test?
6. State an easy rule of thumb for determining normal systolic blood pressure in children older than 1 year.
7. How would the nurse obtain a height and weight for a 12-month-old child?
8. Describe the sequence for assessing the abdomen.
9. Describe the cranial nerve assessment of an infant and a toddler.

STUDY QUESTIONS

1. Childhood obesity predisposes an individual to which of the following comorbidities?
   a. Skeletal fractures and ligament sprains
   b. Hyperlipidemia, hypertension, and type 2 diabetes
   c. Emphysema and reactive airway disease
   d. Cognitive impairment
2. A rectal temperature should not be taken on a child with which of the following conditions?
   a. Emesis
   b. Fever of unknown origin
   c. A nasogastric tube
   d. Neutropenia
3. Which factor is most important when taking a blood pressure?
   a. Asking the caregiver to hold the child still
   b. Double checking the blood pressure reading after initial measurement
   c. Choosing the appropriate cuff size
   d. Holding the extremity at the level of the heart
4. Deviating from the normal adult head-to-toe sequence of physical examination is often necessary during a pediatric examination. Which system is often examined out of sequence?
   a. Integument
   b. Heart and peripheral vasculature
   c. Neurological
   d. Musculoskeletal
5. When plotting anthropometric data such as weight, a finding that warrants further evaluation is:
   a. A weight that has remained steady at the 50th percentile for two years.
   b. A weight at the 75th percentile that follows a jump from the 50th percentile one year earlier.
   c. A weight that has recently fallen below the 3rd percentile from the exam two months earlier.
   d. A weight that has risen to the 25th percentile from an exam one year earlier.
6. Cardiac landmarks change when a child has dextrocardia. Where would you place your stethoscope to auscultate heart sounds if dextrocardia is known?
   a. Over the left posterior chest wall
   b. Over the left anterior chest wall
   c. Over the right posterior chest wall
   d. Over the right anterior chest wall
7. A cardiac thrill palpated along the left upper sternal border (LUSB) correlates to pathology in the:
   a. Aortic area.
   b. Pulmonic area.
   c. Mitral area.
   d. Tricuspid area.
8. An enlarged liver or hepatomegaly is an abnormal physical finding. In children the liver is normally palpated:
   a. Two centimeters below the right costal margin.
   b. Two centimeters below the left costal margin.
   c. At the right costal margin, no more than one centimeter below the right costal margin.
   d. At the left costal margin, no more than one centimeter below the left costal margin.
9. Developmental dysplasia of the hip (DDH) is evaluated by which test?
   a. Allen test
   b. Ortolani maneuver
   c. Denver Developmental II
   d. Cover-uncover test
10. To test cranial nerves III, IV, and VI in an infant greater than 1 month the evaluator would:
    a. Move a brightly colored toy along the infant's line of vision.
    b. Stroke the infant's cheek to elicit a rooting response.
    c. Allow the infant to suck on a pacifier.
    d. Elicit the Moro reflex.

REFERENCES

American Academy of Pediatrics, Committee on Practice and Ambulatory Medicine, Section on Ophthalmology. (2003). Eye examination in infants, children, and young adults by pediatricians. *Pediatrics, 111*(4), 902–907.

Cady, R. B. (2008). Developmental dysplasia of the hip. Program and abstracts of the American Academy of Pediatrics 2008 National Convention and Exhibition, October 11, 2008: Boston, Massachusetts. Session A1072.

Cakan, N., & Kamat, D. (2009). Cryptorchidism: Primary care evaluation and management. *Consultant for Pediatricians, 8*(2), 46–50.

Choby, B. A. (2009). Management of streptococcal pharyngitis reviewed. *American Family Physician, 79*, 383–390.

Dempsey, A. F., Gebremariam, A., Koutsky, L.A., & Manhart, L. (2008). Using risk factors to predict human papillomavirus infection: Implications for targeted vaccination strategies in young adult women. *Vaccine, 26*(8), 1111–1117.

Estes, M. E. Z. (2010). *Health assessment & physical examination* (4th ed.). Clifton Park, NY: Delmar Cengage Learning.

Falkner, B., Gidding, S. S., Portman, R., & Rosner, B. (2008). Blood pressure variability and classification of prehypertension and hypertension in adolescence. *Pediatrics, 122*, 238–242.

Frankenburg, W. K., & Dodds, J. B. (1992). *Denver II screening manual.* Denver, CO: Denver Developmental Materials.

Jones, K. F., Berg, J. H., & Coody, D. (1994). Update in pediatric dentistry. *Journal of Pediatric Health Care, 8*(4), 160–167.

LaFontaine, T. (2008). Physical activity: The epidemic of obesity and overweight among youth: Trends, consequences, and interventions. *American Journal of Lifestyle Medicine, 2*(1), 30–36.

National Center for Health Statistics. (2000). Pediatric growth charts. Retrieved April 17, 2005, from http://www.cdc.gov/growth charts.

National Institutes of Health, National Heart, Lung, and Blood Institute. (1996). Update on the Task Force Report [1987] on high blood pressure in children and adolescents: A working group report from the National High Blood Pressure Education Program. Bethesda, MD: NIH pub. no. 96-3790.

Ridling, D. A., & Kroon, L. (2009). Comparing three methods of assessing peripheral perfusion in critically ill children. *Pediatric Nursing, 35*(1), 11–15.

Seidel, H., Ball, J., Dains, J., Flynn, J., Solomon, B., & Stewart, R. (2011). *Mosby's guide to physical examination* (7th ed.). St. Louis, Mo: Mosby.

Sganga, A., Wallace, R., Kiehl, E., Irving, T., & Witter, L. (2000). A comparison of four methods of normal newborn temperature measurement. *American Journal of Maternal Child Nursing, 25*(2), 76–79.

Sothern, M. (2008). Obesity prevention in children: Physical activity and nutrition. *Nutrition, 20*(7), 704–708.

U.S. Department of Agriculture Food and Nutrition Service. (2005). *Food Guide Pyramid for Kids.* U.S. Department of Agriculture, Author.

SUGGESTED READING

McCance, K. L., & Huether, S. E. (2010). *Pathophysiology: The biologic basis for disease in adults and children* (6th ed.). St. Louis, MO: Mosby.

RESOURCES

Refer to the online student StudyWARE for Potts & Mandleco at http://www.CengageBrain.com for additional content and study aids.

Organization: **American Academy of Pediatrics**

Description: The American Academy of Pediatrics is an organization of 60,000 pediatricians committed to the attainment of optimal physical, mental, and social health and well-being for all infants, children, adolescents, and young adults. This website offers general information related to child health as well as specific guidelines concerning many pediatric issues. In addition, the reader can access information regarding the Academy's many programs, activities, policies, guidelines, publications, and other child health resources.

Website/Resource: http://www.aap.org

Organization: **Centers for Disease Control and Prevention**

Description: The Centers for Disease Control and Prevention (CDC) serves as the national focus for developing and applying disease prevention and control, environmental health, and health promotion and health education activities designed to improve the health of the people of the United States. The CDC website offers readers information regarding current disease conditions, emergency preparedness and response, life stages and populations, healthy living, workplace environment and health, traveler's health, and much more.

Website/Resource: http://www.cdc.gov

Organization: **Denver Developmental Materials, Inc.**

Description: The Denver Developmental Materials are for providers of direct care to children. With procedures which are simple and quick, they can be used in a busy setting by both professionals and paraprofessionals. The procedures are designed to further the optimal development of children from birth to 6 years of age through guidance and identification of those who may require additional evaluation. The website offers users information regarding training sessions, orders, and articles.

Website/Resource: http://www.denver2.com

Organization: **Kids Health Organization**

Description: KidsHealth is the most-visited site on the Web for information about health, behavior, and development from before birth through the teen years. In addition to offering basic health facts, the KidsHealth website is part of The Nemours Foundation's Center for Children's Health Media. Therefore, KidsHealth provides families with perspective, advice, and comfort about a wide range of physical, emotional, and behavioral issues that affect children and teens.

Website/Resource: http://www.kidshealth.org

Organization: **Medem, Inc.**

Description: Medfusion has recently acquired the iHealthRecord service from Medem. Medfusion has been providing online patient-provider communication solutions to physicians for over ten years, and today Medfusion physicians are using its solutions to communicate with over 1.5 million patients. The website offers links for clients and access to an online demo.

Website/Resource: http://www.medem.com

Organization: **U.S. Department of Health and Human Services Office of Disease Prevention and Health Promotion Office of Public Health and Science, Office of the Secretary**

Description: The Department of Health and Human Services (HHS) is the United States government's principal agency for protecting the health of all Americans and providing essential human services, especially for those who are least able to help themselves. The HHS website offers users access to a health encyclopedia as well as access to other sources of health information.

Website/Resource: http://www.healthfinder.gov

Organization: **U.S. National Library of Medicine**

Description: Medicine is a goldmine of good health information from the world's largest medical library, the National Library of Medicine. Health professionals and consumers alike can depend on it for information that is authoritative and up to date. There are directories, a medical encyclopedia and a medical dictionary, easy-to-understand tutorials on common conditions, tests and treatments, health information in Spanish, extensive information on prescription and nonprescription drugs, health information from the media, and links to thousands of clinical trials.

Website/Resource: http://www.medlineplus.gov

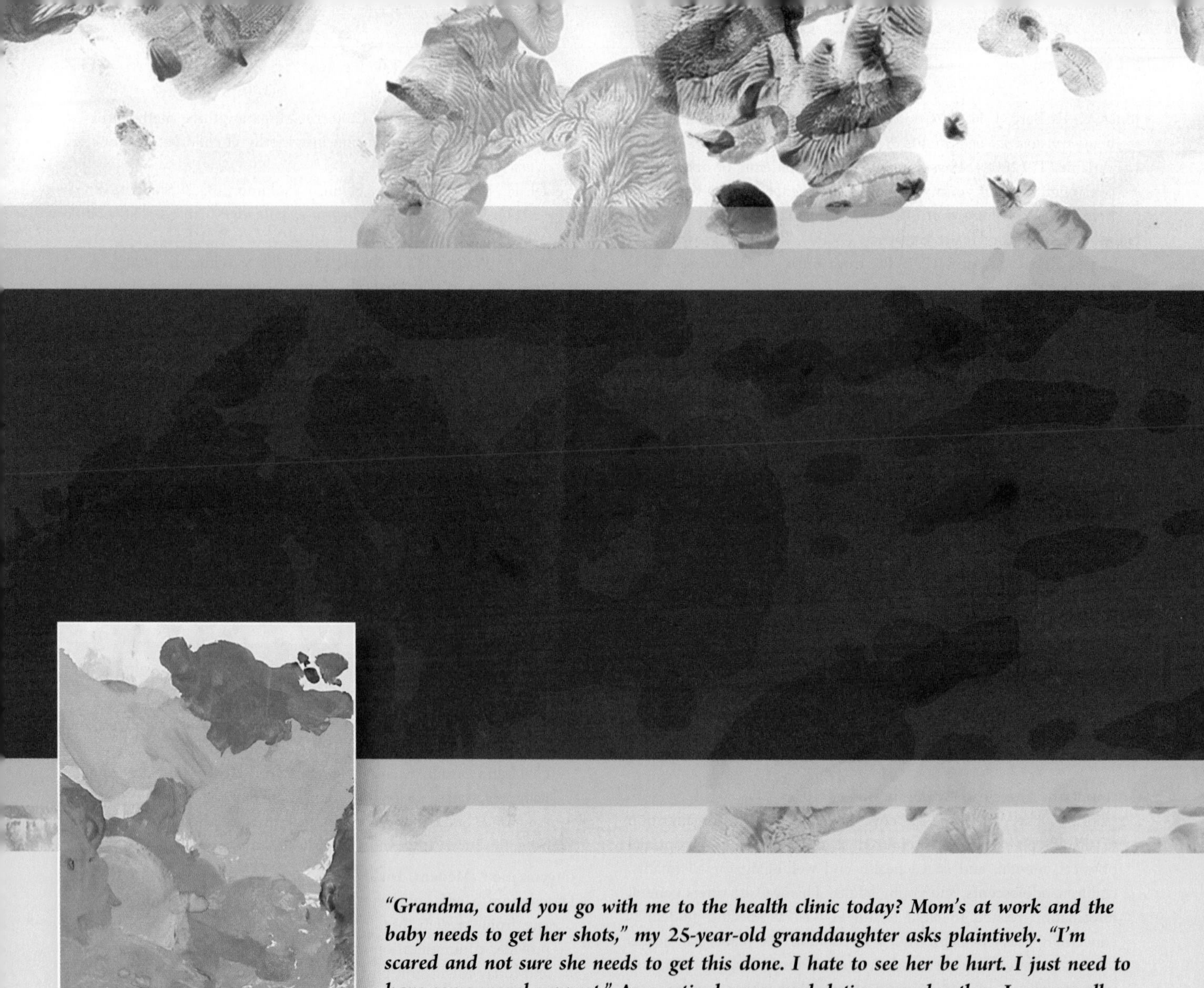

"Grandma, could you go with me to the health clinic today? Mom's at work and the baby needs to get her shots," my 25-year-old granddaughter asks plaintively. "I'm scared and not sure she needs to get this done. I hate to see her be hurt. I just need to have some moral support." As a retired nurse and doting grandmother, I am usually consulted when health issues arise.

I can understand my granddaughter's concern. Immunizations are not without controversy, but I can reflect as well about the progress made in preventing the childhood diseases through immunization. I remember my mother's stories of growing up in the early 20th century. Of the eight children born to her parents, only three survived into adulthood. Infectious diseases took their toll in her family by causing the deaths of five children, each one under the age of 4. As a child in the early 1930s, I suffered the throes of several infectious diseases without any consequences other than the inconvenience of being ill and feeling miserable. Immunizations came into practice as I was having children, yet during their childhood there was no protection against measles, mumps, rubella, or chickenpox. Polio was the scourge when my children were young. My children and grandchildren benefited from vaccines. Now my baby great-granddaughter is ready to begin that process. With the history of how my family has been affected by infectious diseases, I prepare to stand by my granddaughter and her baby as they keep their appointment.

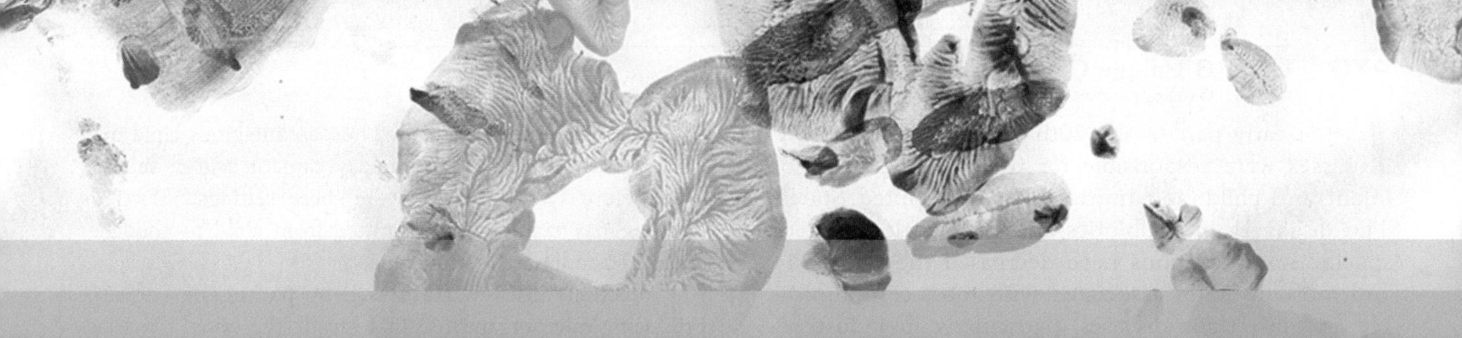

CHAPTER 15
Infectious Diseases

Becky Bunn, RNC, MSN
Barbara S. Kiernan, APRN, BC, PhD

COMPETENCIES

Upon completion of this chapter, the reader will be able to:

- Describe the mode of infectious disease transmission.
- Discuss how a child's developmental level affects the transmission of infectious disease.
- Discuss the impact of day care and school settings on the incidence of infectious diseases.
- Describe the etiology, clinical manifestations, treatment, and nursing management of common infectious diseases.
- Identify measures used to prevent common infectious childhood diseases, including immunizations.
- Identify the educational needs of families whose child has an infectious disease.
- Discuss the importance of adhering to the laws and policies related to infectious diseases, including immunizations.
- Successfully complete the games and activities in the online student StudyWARE.

In the early part of the 20th century, infectious illnesses were responsible for the high incidence of infant and childhood mortality in the United States. The discovery of antibiotics and the development of specific immunizations have decreased the morbidity and mortality rates associated with most communicable and infectious diseases, particularly in industrialized countries. Yet resistance to antibiotics and the emergence of new infections continue to plague the global community. The prevention of disease, disability, and death from infectious diseases, including those prevented by vaccines, is a major goal for ensuring the health care of all people in every stage of life, according to the Health Protection Goals and Objectives by the Office of Strategy and Innovation of the Centers for Disease Control and Prevention (CDC, 2007b).

Throughout the years from infancy to adolescence, children will be exposed to a number of infectious diseases. An **infectious disease** is any disease caused by invasion and multiplication of microorganisms in the body. It may or may not be communicable. A **communicable disease** is a disease caused by an infectious agent that is transmitted to a person by direct or indirect contact, vehicle or vector, or airborne route. Infectious diseases are common occurrences during infancy, childhood, and adolescence. For purposes of this chapter, the term *infectious disease* will be used. During the first year of life, most children who either attend day care or come from large families will experience several infectious illnesses. These include both respiratory and gastrointestinal infections. Although the majority of infectious illnesses are not life-threatening, some illnesses may cause serious lifelong disabilities or even death.

Many of these illnesses are preventable by receiving immunizations or by health promotion practices that avoid exposure to certain pathogens. Nurses play an important role in health promotion and education by intervening with children and their caregivers at all levels and in many environments. Awareness about developmental stages and anticipated behavior plus knowledge of disease processes enable nurses to be more effective in promoting children's health and wellness. This chapter provides an overview of the common infectious diseases that are prevalent during childhood and adolescence, including specific risk factors based on developmental age. Guidelines for current immunizations recommended are discussed. Risk reduction measures are provided to decrease the incidence of illnesses for which no vaccinations are available.

ANATOMY AND PHYSIOLOGY

Children experience higher incidences of infectious diseases than adults because of an immature immune system and developmental and biological variances. Maternally acquired antibodies decrease as the infant grows and develops. Children gradually develop immunity after exposure to diseases or through immunizations. Because young children are unable to verbalize that they do not feel well, a disease may be advanced before it is detected. Thus, a contagious child may inadvertently expose others in day care or school settings even before symptoms occur. In these settings, infectious diseases may readily be transmitted from child to child because of handling common objects.

Infectious diseases are caused by **pathogens** (disease-producing microorganisms) that invade the body. Once established they reproduce and multiply, creating a wide variety of symptoms and disease states. The seriousness of the disease is dependent upon several factors, including the microorganism, the method of transmission, the concentration of pathogens, and the environment. Infectious microorganisms or pathogens include bacteria, viruses, fungi, and parasites. Illness may be manifested by local cellular injury, secretion of toxins, or antigen-antibody reaction.

The transmission of disease is dependent upon six factors, which are referred to as the chain of infection (Figure 15-1). They include infectious agent, reservoir, portal of exit, mode of transmission, portal of entry, and susceptible host.

1. **Infectious agent:** The specific pathogen must be present in sufficient numbers to cause disease. Some organisms have a greater **virulence** (the degree or power of microorganisms to cause disease) than others and can be more devastating, depending on the age of the child and the development of the immune system.
2. **Reservoir:** A place where pathogens can survive without multiplication. Reservoirs can be animate (living), such as humans, animals, and insects, or inanimate (not living), such as soil, water, other environmental sources, and medical equipment (intravenous [IV] solutions and urine collection devices).
3. **Portal of exit from reservoir:** Pathogens can leave the reservoir through the blood or body secretions such as urine, feces, respiratory secretions, and saliva.
4. **Mode of transmission:** Pathogenic organisms are spread by direct contact from person to person through saliva, droplets from the respiratory tract, body contact, blood, and body fluids in the urinary, gastrointestinal, and reproductive systems. Pathogens can also be transmitted on objects, in contaminated water or food, or by **vectors** (animals or insects that carry the infectious organism from one host to another).
5. **Portal of entry to the host:** Pathogens can enter the body through the respiratory tract, the gastrointestinal tract, the urinary tract, the skin and mucous membranes, and across the placenta.
6. **Susceptible host:** Pathogens cause illness when the individual lacks immunity to specific organisms or when the immune system is dysfunctional.

Other factors that support the development of disease include: (1) the ability of the pathogens to survive in the environment; (2) the asymptomatic or carrier state; and (3) the dose of the pathogen. Regarding the first factor, many organisms remain viable from hours up to several weeks on environmental surfaces such as toys or changing

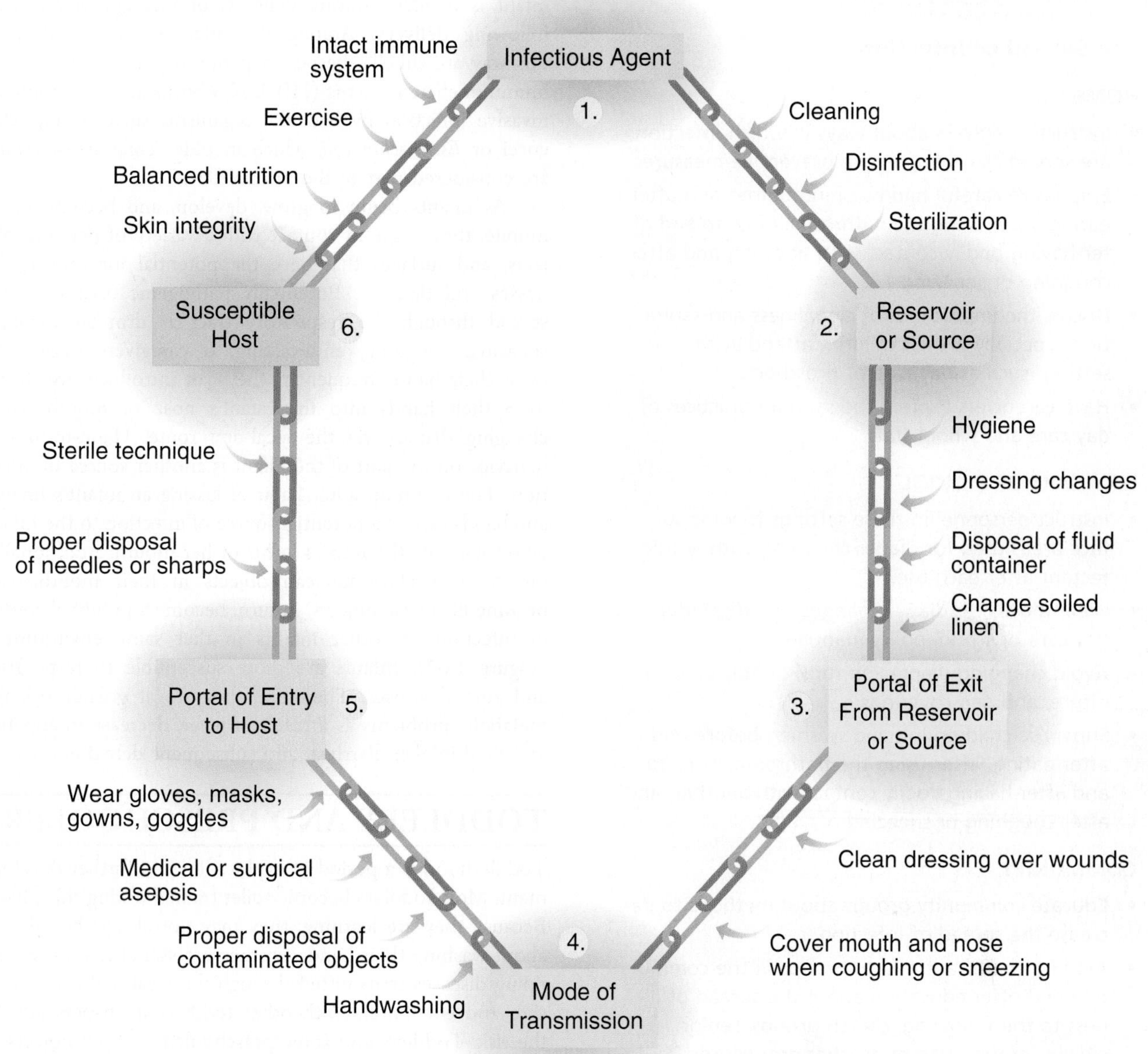

FIGURE 15-1 Chain of infection is the process by which organisms are transmitted from the environment to a host, invade the host, and cause an infection. Preventive measures for breaking the chain follow each link. DELMAR CENGAGE LEARNING.

tables in a day care center. Children put fingers and toys in their mouths during play time, thus increasing the possibility of infection if the environment is not cleaned properly. Examples include hepatitis A, rotavirus, and *Giardia* cysts (American Academy of Pediatrics [AAP], 2009).

Regarding the second factor, many children may remain asymptomatic but are able to transmit pathogens before they become ill. For example, children exposed to the varicella virus, which causes chickenpox, are contagious the day prior to becoming ill but may exhibit none of the characteristic lesions at that time. Others may be **carriers** (persons who can harbor and spread the organism to others without becoming ill).

Regarding the third factor involved in developing disease (the dose of the pathogen), the concentration of pathogens in a particular sample of fluid or blood determines whether or not infection occurs after a single exposure.

DEVELOPMENTAL STAGES AND THE RISK OF INFECTION

As children pass through each developmental stage they are susceptible to certain organisms because of psychosocial and physiological changes that occur during specific periods of life. At every stage, children are uniquely at risk of

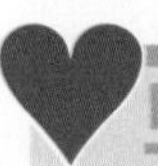

FAMILY**TEACHING**

The Spread of Infection

HOME

- Instruct caregivers about ways in which infections are spread as well as simple preventive measures.
- Emphasize careful handwashing before and after eating, after using the bathroom, prior to and after having bodily contact with another, and after coughing or sneezing.
- Discuss the importance of cleanliness and sanitation especially if their children attend institutional settings such as day care or preschool.
- Have caregivers explore the sanitary practices of day care and school staff.

DAY CARE OR SCHOOL

- Instruct personnel in these settings to wipe surface areas used for diaper changing with a disinfectant after each use.
- Wear gloves for diaper changes as indicated in day care or school policy manuals.
- Avoid changing diapers on rugs, upholstered furniture, and bed coverings.
- Supervise children in hand washing before and after eating, after using the bathroom, prior to and after having bodily contact with another, and after coughing or sneezing.

COMMUNITY

- Educate community groups about methods to decrease the spread of infection.
- Act in a consultant role to groups in the community and offer education about the spread of illness to the following: church groups, senior citizens groups, parent–teacher groups, and youth groups.
- Discuss the importance of keeping immunizations up to date for children as well as adults and senior citizens.
- Promote yearly immunizations against influenza for groups that are susceptible to being exposed.

developing certain infections beginning *in utero* and extending through adolescence.

INFANCY

During prenatal life, the developing fetus is susceptible to a number of illnesses through maternal infections that are potentially life threatening. The process of transmitting a disease from one generation to another is known as **vertical transmission**. It can occur through the placenta while the infant is *in utero,* during delivery, or through breast milk following delivery. Among the infections transmitted in this way are rubella, herpes, hepatitis B and C, and human immunodeficiency virus (HIV). Newborns are susceptible to invasive infection by bacterial organisms such as staphylococci or *Escherichia coli,* which in older children or adults are considered part of the normal flora.

As infants begin to grow, develop, and become more mobile, they come in contact with a variety of persons, objects, and surfaces that have the potential for causing illnesses and diseases. Potentially pathogenic organisms are spread through the respiratory tract as droplets through sneezing, coughing, and talking. If caregivers neglect to wash their hands frequently, they can introduce organisms from their hands into the infant's nose or mouth while changing diapers via the fecal-oral route. Hand-to-mouth behavior on the part of the infant is another source of infection. The common adult habit of kissing an infant's fingers and hands can be a potential source of infection to the infant who then puts the fingers in his or her mouth. Additionally, infants who place unclean objects in their mouths can become ill. These objects, in turn, become a potential source of infection for other infants in that same environment (Figure 15-2). Infants are more susceptible to respiratory and enteral viruses. Therefore, they are at greater risk for metabolic problems as a result of fever, decrease in appetite and fluid intake, diarrhea, and subsequent dehydration.

TODDLERS AND PRESCHOOLERS

Toddlerhood is a period of exploration and further development. Most toddlers become toilet trained during this phase. Because they are learning, they may not always be diligent about washing their hands, so they are still at risk for developing diseases transmitted through the fecal-oral route. Day care and encounters with other toddlers in diapers add to the risk. Toddlers and some preschoolers still put objects in

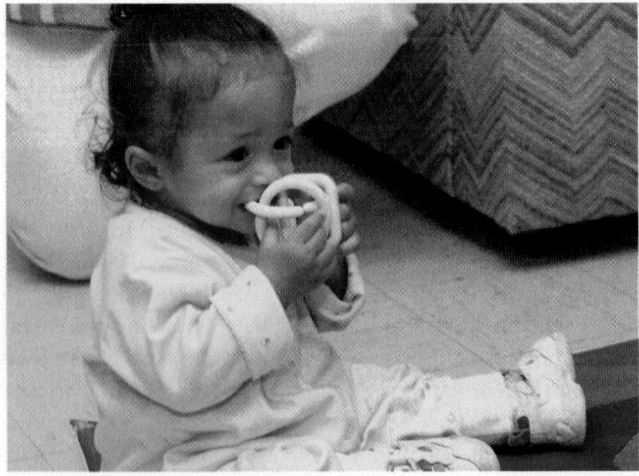

FIGURE 15-2 Infants learn through hand and mouth exploration. DELMAR CENGAGE LEARNING.

NURSING ALERT

Avoid Use of Aspirin

Caregivers should not use aspirin to treat the pain and fever of viral illnesses such as influenza and varicella (chickenpox) in children less than 13 years of age. The use of acetylsalicylic acid has been linked to the subsequent development of Reye's syndrome, which is a disorder combining both encephalopathy and fatty degeneration of the liver (see Chapter 32). Acetaminophen or ibuprofen are the drugs of choice for febrile illness in infants and children.

their mouths. It may be difficult to break the cycle of infection if sanitary conditions in these situations are lax.

Some toddlers and preschoolers enjoy encounters with small animals such as dogs or cats; however, their inquisitiveness places them at risk for being scratched or bitten. Organisms present in animal saliva or on their bodies can cause illness in any child who is scratched or bitten. Playing with infected animals may cause tinea corporis (ringworm of the body, or cat scratch fever).

The following school-age children section contains some information that is true of toddlers and preschoolers in day care centers.

SCHOOL-AGE CHILDREN

Schools are a perfect breeding ground for the spread of infection. Many children are lax in hygienic practices such as washing hands before eating and after using the bathroom. Some schools may operate on strict schedules; therefore, children are not given the opportunity to wash up when they should. Same-sex friendships are common in school-age children and frequently result in the mutual sharing of items of clothing, grooming devices, food, and toys. Children may spend the night together at each others' homes or on camping trips. Sharing beds and linens as well as personal items such as combs can result in outbreaks of head lice, scabies, pinworms, tinea corporis, and tinea capitis.

The leading cause of pneumonia for this age group is *Mycoplasma pneumoniae* and can be found where children are grouped together. This infection is highly contagious and can result in illness ranging from inflammation of the trachea and bronchioles to pneumonia. Behaviors exhibited among some schoolchildren such as not covering one's mouth while coughing or sneezing and not washing hands afterwards are contributing factors. Another common illness, *erythema infectiosum* or Fifth's disease, has a characteristic lacy rash and is highly contagious. The illness is caused by parvovirus B19. By the time the rash erupts, children are no longer contagious, but the epidemic nature of this disease and the uniqueness of the rash (intensely red with a slapped-cheek appearance) can give caregivers cause for concern.

NURSING TIP

Family Teaching about Disease Transmission

Each encounter with children and their caregivers is an opportunity for you to review the principles of disease transmission. It is important to assess basic knowledge about disease transmission. You may find that caregivers as well as children have misconceptions about the cause of illness such as going out in cold weather without a coat. Education should focus on personal hygiene, ways of staying healthy, and the basics of nutrition that support the immune system. You can use children's literature that reviews germ theory and illness prevention to illustrate important concepts. As caregivers are encouraged to take responsibility for the sex education of their children, you need to remind them to include open and frank discussion about sexually transmitted diseases.

ADOLESCENTS

Adolescents present unique challenges regarding the spread of infectious diseases. Adolescence is generally thought of as a period of wellness with the individual seeking health care for sports physicals, minor acute illnesses or conditions related to sexuality, sexually transmitted diseases (STDs; also known as sexually transmitted infections, or STIs), or pregnancy. During these visits, the health care provider should be aware of immunization updates for the adolescent. Adolescents need to receive booster doses of vaccines to maintain high levels of immunity. Rates of immunization against measles, mumps, rubella, and hepatitis B are increasing with the adolescent between the ages of 13 to 15 at or very near the *Healthy People 2010* goal for those diseases (goals for *Healthy People 2020* are being developed). However, approximately 15% of older adolescents remain unprotected against hepatitis B, a virus that can be acquired through sexual contact (Jain, Stokley, and Yankey, 2008). The prevalence of sexual intercourse as well as the rate of STDs has increased among adolescents. Factors associated with the increase in STDs in this age group include frequent unprotected sex, biological susceptibility to disease, and difficulty in accessing and utilizing confidential health care. Those at high risk for disease include intravenous drug users, sexually active heterosexuals, and male homosexuals (CDC, 2006).

Many adolescents do not believe that they are at risk for becoming infected or pregnant. The majority of adolescents who are having sexual intercourse are doing so without protection against pregnancy or sexually transmitted diseases.

NURSING TIP

Adolescent Immunizations

Assess for immunization status each time an adolescent is seen for a health encounter. Adolescents need a booster dose of tetanus and diphtheria vaccine (Td) about ten years after their last dose received prior to starting kindergarten. They may also need a booster dose of measles-mumps-rubella vaccine (MMR). The hepatitis B series should be started in adolescence if the adolescent did not receive it in infancy or early childhood. The hepatitis A series may be indicated for adolescents in certain high-risk categories. Varicella vaccine is recommended for adolescents who have not received the immunization or who have an unreliable history of having had chicken pox. Older adolescents should receive the two doses of the vaccine given 4 weeks apart (CDC, 2007a). Some states may allow adolescents to consent for their own immunizations. Nurses need to be familiar with the laws of the state in which they work.

College-bound adolescents and their families should receive information about the importance of vaccination against meningococcal disease. This group of adolescents is at particular risk for the development of meningitis, especially if they plan to live in dormitories or residence halls. The vaccine is effective for approximately three to five years.

Thus, the early introduction to sexual activity, with an increase in the frequency of activity with multiple partners, places them at higher risk (CDC, 2006). Intercourse can cause microscopic tears in both the vaginal and anal mucosa, thus creating a portal for the entry of pathogenic organisms.

Unprotected sexual intercourse and injection drug use have been linked to an increased rate of STDs. Adolescents who are engaged in these risk-taking behaviors increase their risk not only for STDs but also HIV (CDC, 2008b). Currently, the rate of adolescents who become newly infected with the HIV virus is rising.

Preadolescents and adolescents should be seen alone, apart from their caregivers, during a portion of the interview to assess their knowledge about disease transmission, especially STDs. Adolescents may be concerned about changes in their body, which may or may not be significant as they relate to infectious diseases. Nurses can assess whether adolescents are sexually active and if their behaviors are placing them at risk for sexually transmitted diseases. The majority of states have provisions that allow adolescents to consent to the confidential diagnosis and treatment of STDs without parental knowledge and consent. Other states may allow adolescents to obtain HIV counseling and testing without consent.

Reflections from Families

I have just been diagnosed with chlamydia and I am taking some medication to treat it. I have had sex with both of my girlfriends during the past year and am too embarrassed to tell them so they can get tested. I didn't use condoms because they're too inconvenient. I guess I really don't need to tell them because we didn't have sex often enough for them to be infected.

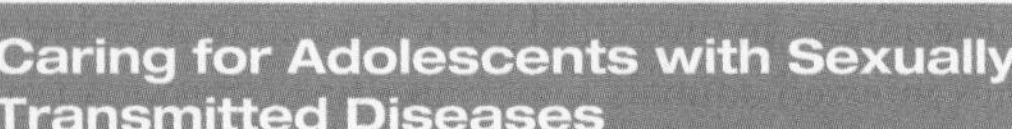

REFLECTIVE THINKING

Caring for Adolescents with Sexually Transmitted Diseases

To increase self-awareness and comfort level in discussing the care and treatment of STDs with adolescents, ask yourself:

1. How comfortable do I feel about asking adolescents personal questions about their sexual practices?
2. How knowledgeable am I about the extent and types of STDs affecting adolescents?
3. Can I be nonjudgmental when discussing health promotion practices that decrease the risk of illness?
4. Am I comfortable enough about my own sexuality and sexual behavior to be able to deliver care in a positive manner?

Still other states permit adolescents to obtain necessary vaccinations without parental consent (CDC, 2006). Nurses need to be familiar with the laws and regulations in their own states to provide the correct information to families.

INFECTIOUS DISEASES IN DAY CARE AND SCHOOL SETTINGS

Many children under the age of five years receive care in out-of-home child care settings. These children are at an increased risk for acquiring antimicrobial resistant organisms and other infectious diseases. There are several factors that can influence the incidence of infection as young infants and children are cared for in out-of-home settings such as day care and school, including the following (AAP, 2009):

- Personal hygiene and immunization status of the caregiver
- Personal hygiene and immunization status of the children
- Sanitation of the environment
- Specific procedures for toileting and diaper changing
- Procedures for the handling and preparation of food
- Caregiver-to-child ratio
- Quality and physical space of the facility
- Specific exclusion criteria for children with potentially infectious illnesses
- Good lines of communication with parents
- Access to qualified health consultants and public health personnel

FAMILY TEACHING

Nurses can make an impact in the decision-making process by acting as resources to caregivers who are considering the placement of their children in day care or preschool. Caregivers need to know about the characteristics of optimal day care as they relate to the health of the children. One topic concerns the facility policies related to illness. Will they allow a child with a temperature of 101°F (38.3°C) to attend? How many days after a fever subsides can the child return? If a child appears with a red, watery eye, what is the center's protocol? Many centers will provide caregivers with a written illness policy. Some programs may have facilities to care for children with minor illnesses. Another topic concerns sanitation. Caregivers need to ask about changing facilities if the children are still in diapers. Are children who are toilet trained separated from those who are not? Does the staff use frequent handwashing? When staffing is less than adequate, practices regarding handwashing may be relaxed. What about food preparation? Is it performed in an area separate from areas where diapers are changed? Nurses can help caregivers prepare a list of questions to ask when evaluating prospective child care facilities.

In addition to teaching the family, nurses who work in a day care or school setting should be resources to staff and students about the prevention of common illnesses as well as managing outbreaks of illness as they occur during the school year. Providing materials and references to teachers and caregivers may help reduce the anxiety that sometimes accompanies episodic illness.

Children who spend the better part of their day in out-of-home settings are exposed to respiratory tract and enteric pathogens. Enforcing hygienic measures and ensuring current immunizations are important factors in infection control that should be instituted in all child care facilities.

Many out-of-home facilities, whether they are private homes, licensed centers, or schools, have policies regarding the admission of ill children. Children who have fever, diarrhea, irritability, open mouth sores, rashes, and purulent conjunctivitis are excluded until the illness is treated appropriately or resolves. Other diseases, including tuberculosis, scabies, head lice, hepatitis A, streptococcal pharyngitis, impetigo, varicella, mumps, measles, and pertussis, require

RESEARCH Highlight

Measles, Mumps, and Rubella Vaccine Link to Autism

STUDY PURPOSE

In 1998 in the United Kingdom a report linked the measles-mumps-rubella (MMR) vaccination (specifically the measles component) with the development of autistic enterocolitis, a new form of Autistic Spectrum Disorder (ASD). Claims of this association have persisted despite epidemiologic evidence to the contrary. To determine any linkage between the measles-mumps-rubella (MMR) vaccination and autistic enterocolitis (ASD), this study was conducted to determine the presence of the measles virus nucleic acids. If the genetic material from the measles virus persisted, the link was assured.

METHODS

Blood samples for mononuclear cells were isolated from 54 children with ASD and 34 developmentally normal children. Specific assays targeting nucleoproteins and genes of the measles virus were run on the blood samples of both groups. Positive reactions were thoroughly evaluated and anti-measles antibody titers were measured using enzyme immunoassay.

FINDINGS

After rigorous testing and evaluation, no sample from either the ASD or control group was found to contain nucleic acids from the measles gene. And, further assessment found that there was no difference in the anti-measles titers between the groups.

IMPLICATIONS

This study shows no evidence of the persistence of the measles virus in the peripheral cells of children diagnosed with ASD. The researchers feel that there is no significant epidemiologic evidence proving the link between the MMR vaccination and the development of autism and that the arguments against immunizing children with the MMR vaccine undermine the success of immunization programs.

REFERENCE

D'Souza, Y., Fombonne, E., & Ward, B. (2006). No evidence of persisting measles virus in peripheral blood mononuclear cells from children with autism spectrum disorder. *Pediatrics*, *118*, 1664–1675.

specific treatments and time periods during which the disorder becomes noninfectious. Most of these children need physician proof of no longer being contagious in order to return to school or day care (AAP, 2009).

IMMUNIZATIONS

Immunizations are an important part of health promotion and disease prevention for all children. The vaccines used for immunizing against diseases are prepared from microorganisms or genetically engineered antigens, and introduced into the body to evoke an immune response. The term *immunization* often is used interchangeably with *vaccine*. The majority of vaccines are administered by injection, though some vaccines are given by the oral route and others are given by aerosol.

SCHEDULE OF IMMUNIZATIONS

Immunization schedules change periodically based on knowledge about the safety and efficacy of current as well as newly developed vaccines. In general, recommendations for childhood immunizations are based on the consensus of the Advisory Committee on Immunization Practices (ACIP) of the Centers for Disease Control and Prevention (CDC), the American Academy of Pediatrics (AAP), and the American Academy of Family Physicians (AAFP). The current recommended childhood immunization schedule is updated annually (Figure 15-3 and 15-4). It is important that nurses who work with families of growing children keep abreast of the latest immunization schedules and related research and information (see Research Highlight on previous page) so they can address questions and concerns those caregivers may have. Nurses should assess for immunization status at every opportunity when children enter any part of the health care system so that immunizations can be kept current. Caregivers often are aware of the importance of immunizations but find that inaccessible or appointment only clinics, long waiting times, and the expense of the immunizations are barriers to receiving scheduled immunizations. Additionally, factors such as illness, caregiver mobility, language barriers, and lack of caregiver knowledge about the importance of immunizations may also contribute to incomplete immunization records. Clinic staff who remind families of keeping immunization appointments can facilitate adherence to immunization guidelines.

When a child receives only one or two doses of vaccine and does not receive the remaining vaccines according to the recommended schedule, the series does not need to be restarted. Instead, only the missed doses need to be given according to the recommended immunization schedule for children not immunized during the first year in Figure 15-5. Nurses can help plan the remaining schedule with the family according to what the child has already received. Those who administer vaccines routinely should have the most up-to-date copy of the vaccine schedule on hand for reference.

REFLECTIVE THINKING

How Many Injections Will an Infant Receive?

The average infant who is immunized by the age of 2 according to current national guidelines will receive approximately 22 injections if each vaccine is given separately. On some visits, a child may receive multiple injections. This is based on using inactivated polio vaccine (IPV) as recommended for the series as well as pneumococcal conjugate vaccine (PCV). Current standards recommend the use of yearly influenza vaccine for infants from 6 to 23 months prior to the onset of the influenza season. Using some combination vaccines such as DTaP, hepatitis B, and IPV may reduce the number to 15. How do you feel when caregivers ask about the necessity for so many injections? What do you tell them? What can you do to alleviate the discomfort of the caregivers and the children being immunized? How can you prepare children and caregivers to decrease the discomfort from immunizations?

Many practitioners recommend a variety of methods to determine children's immunization status to avoid missed opportunities. The combination of caregiver-linked and provider-validated methods is the gold standard for measuring immunization status. Caregivers are asked to identify all those who provided immunizations to their children and contact them for validation. All immunization records are combined into one record. A copy can be given to the caregivers for reference. The ultimate goal is for the implementation of computer-based immunization registries for all children.

All states require children to be immunized prior to entry into licensed child care or school. Many states also have regulations requiring immunization of children in upper grades and those entering college. State immunization requirements may be obtained from state and local health departments. Since specific requirements for entry level programs vary, it is important that nurses become familiar with the immunization requirements of the state in which they practice.

COMBINATION VACCINES

Because of the number of injections that some infants and children may be receiving at one appointment, vaccine manufacturers have been researching ways to combine vaccines into a single dose. The diphtheria-tetanus-pertussis injection is an example of a combination vaccine. The present vaccine (DTaP) now contains acellular pertussis, which prevents many of the side effects of the whole-cell pertussis vaccine (DTwP). Other examples include measles-mumps-rubella

Recommended Immunization Schedule for Persons Aged 0 Through 6 Years—United States • 2010

For those who fall behind or start late, see the catch-up schedule

Vaccine ▼ Age ►	Birth	1 month	2 months	4 months	6 months	12 months	15 months	18 months	19–23 months	2–3 years	4–6 years
Hepatitis B[1]	HepB	HepB			HepB						
Rotavirus[2]			RV	RV	RV[2]						
Diphtheria, Tetanus, Pertussis[3]			DTaP	DTaP	DTaP	see footnote[3]	DTaP				DTaP
Haemophilus influenzae type b[4]			Hib	Hib	Hib[4]	Hib					
Pneumococcal[5]			PCV	PCV	PCV	PCV				PPSV	
Inactivated Poliovirus[6]			IPV	IPV	IPV						IPV
Influenza[7]					Influenza (Yearly)						
Measles, Mumps, Rubella[8]						MMR		see footnote[8]			MMR
Varicella[9]						Varicella		see footnote[9]			Varicella
Hepatitis A[10]						HepA (2 doses)				HepA Series	
Meningococcal[11]										MCV	

Range of recommended ages for all children except certain high-risk groups

Range of recommended ages for certain high-risk groups

This schedule includes recommendations in effect as of December 15, 2009. Any dose not administered at the recommended age should be administered at a subsequent visit, when indicated and feasible. The use of a combination vaccine generally is preferred over separate injections of its equivalent component vaccines. Considerations should include provider assessment, patient preference, and the potential for adverse events. Providers should consult the relevant Advisory Committee on Immunization Practices statement for detailed recommendations: **http://www.cdc.gov/vaccines/pubs/acip-list.htm**. Clinically significant adverse events that follow immunization should be reported to the Vaccine Adverse Event Reporting System (VAERS) at **http://www.vaers.hhs.gov** or by telephone, **800-822-7967**.

1. **Hepatitis B vaccine (HepB).** (Minimum age: birth)
   At birth:
   - Administer monovalent HepB to all newborns before hospital discharge.
   - If mother is hepatitis B surface antigen (HBsAg)-positive, administer HepB and 0.5 mL of hepatitis B immune globulin (HBIG) within 12 hours of birth.
   - If mother's HBsAg status is unknown, administer HepB within 12 hours of birth. Determine mother's HBsAg status as soon as possible and, if HBsAg-positive, administer HBIG (no later than age 1 week).

   After the birth dose:
   - The HepB series should be completed with either monovalent HepB or a combination vaccine containing HepB. The second dose should be administered at age 1 or 2 months. Monovalent HepB vaccine should be used for doses administered before age 6 weeks. The final dose should be administered no earlier than age 24 weeks.
   - Infants born to HBsAg-positive mothers should be tested for HBsAg and antibody to HBsAg 1 to 2 months after completion of at least 3 doses of the HepB series, at age 9 through 18 months (generally at the next well-child visit).
   - Administration of 4 doses of HepB to infants is permissible when a combination vaccine containing HepB is administered after the birth dose. The fourth dose should be administered no earlier than age 24 weeks.
2. **Rotavirus vaccine (RV).** (Minimum age: 6 weeks)
   - Administer the first dose at age 6 through 14 weeks (maximum age: 14 weeks 6 days). Vaccination should not be initiated for infants aged 15 weeks 0 days or older.
   - The maximum age for the final dose in the series is 8 months 0 days
   - If Rotarix is administered at ages 2 and 4 months, a dose at 6 months is not indicated.
3. **Diphtheria and tetanus toxoids and acellular pertussis vaccine (DTaP).** (Minimum age: 6 weeks)
   - The fourth dose may be administered as early as age 12 months, provided at least 6 months have elapsed since the third dose.
   - Administer the final dose in the series at age 4 through 6 years.
4. ***Haemophilus influenzae* type b conjugate vaccine (Hib).** (Minimum age: 6 weeks)
   - If PRP-OMP (PedvaxHIB or Comvax [HepB-Hib]) is administered at ages 2 and 4 months, a dose at age 6 months is not indicated.
   - TriHiBit (DTaP/Hib) and Hiberix (PRP-T) should not be used for doses at ages 2, 4, or 6 months for the primary series but can be used as the final dose in children aged 12 months through 4 years.
5. **Pneumococcal vaccine.** (Minimum age: 6 weeks for pneumococcal conjugate vaccine [PCV]; 2 years for pneumococcal polysaccharide vaccine [PPSV])
   - PCV is recommended for all children aged younger than 5 years. Administer 1 dose of PCV to all healthy children aged 24 through 59 months who are not completely vaccinated for their age.
   - Administer PPSV 2 or more months after last dose of PCV to children aged 2 years or older with certain underlying medical conditions, including a cochlear implant. See *MMWR* 1997;46(No. RR-8).
6. **Inactivated poliovirus vaccine (IPV)** (Minimum age: 6 weeks)
   - The final dose in the series should be administered on or after the fourth birthday and at least 6 months following the previous dose.
   - If 4 doses are administered prior to age 4 years a fifth dose should be administered at age 4 through 6 years. See *MMWR* 2009;58(30):829–30.
7. **Influenza vaccine (seasonal).** (Minimum age: 6 months for trivalent inactivated influenza vaccine [TIV]; 2 years for live, attenuated influenza vaccine [LAIV])
   - Administer annually to children aged 6 months through 18 years.
   - For healthy children aged 2 through 6 years (i.e., those who do not have underlying medical conditions that predispose them to influenza complications), either LAIV or TIV may be used, except LAIV should not be given to children aged 2 through 4 years who have had wheezing in the past 12 months.
   - Children receiving TIV should receive 0.25 mL if aged 6 through 35 months or 0.5 mL if aged 3 years or older.
   - Administer 2 doses (separated by at least 4 weeks) to children aged younger than 9 years who are receiving influenza vaccine for the first time or who were vaccinated for the first time during the previous influenza season but only received 1 dose.
   - For recommendations for use of influenza A (H1N1) 2009 monovalent vaccine see *MMWR* 2009;58(No. RR-10).
8. **Measles, mumps, and rubella vaccine (MMR).** (Minimum age: 12 months)
   - Administer the second dose routinely at age 4 through 6 years. However, the second dose may be administered before age 4, provided at least 28 days have elapsed since the first dose.
9. **Varicella vaccine.** (Minimum age: 12 months)
   - Administer the second dose routinely at age 4 through 6 years. However, the second dose may be administered before age 4, provided at least 3 months have elapsed since the first dose.
   - For children aged 12 months through 12 years the minimum interval between doses is 3 months. However, if the second dose was administered at least 28 days after the first dose, it can be accepted as valid.
10. **Hepatitis A vaccine (HepA).** (Minimum age: 12 months)
    - Administer to all children aged 1 year (i.e., aged 12 through 23 months). Administer 2 doses at least 6 months apart.
    - Children not fully vaccinated by age 2 years can be vaccinated at subsequent visits
    - HepA also is recommended for older children who live in areas where vaccination programs target older children, who are at increased risk for infection, or for whom immunity against hepatitis A is desired.
11. **Meningococcal vaccine.** (Minimum age: 2 years for meningococcal conjugate vaccine [MCV4] and for meningococcal polysaccharide vaccine [MPSV4])
    - Administer MCV4 to children aged 2 through 10 years with persistent complement component deficiency, anatomic or functional asplenia, and certain other conditions placing tham at high risk.
    - Administer MCV4 to children previously vaccinated with MCV4 or MPSV4 after 3 years if first dose administered at age 2 through 6 years. See *MMWR* 2009;58:1042–3.

The Recommended Immunization Schedules for Persons Aged 0 through 18 Years are approved by the Advisory Committee on Immunization Practices (**http://www.cdc.gov/vaccines/recs/acip**), the American Academy of Pediatrics (**http://www.aap.org**), and the American Academy of Family Physicians (**http://www.aafp.org**).

Department of Health and Human Services • Centers for Disease Control and Prevention

CS207330-A

FIGURE 15-3 Recommended Immunization Schedule for Persons Aged 0 Through 6 Years-United States-2010. COURTESY FOR CENTERS OF DISEASE CONTROL AND PREVENTION.

Recommended Immunization Schedule for Persons Aged 7 Through 18 Years—United States • 2010

For those who fall behind or start late, see the schedule below and the catch-up schedule

Vaccine ▼ Age ►	7–10 years	11–12 years	13–18 years
Tetanus, Diphtheria, Pertussis[1]		Tdap	Tdap
Human Papillomavirus[2]	*see footnote 2*	HPV (3 doses)	HPV series
Meningococcal[3]	MCV	MCV	MCV
Influenza[4]		Influenza (Yearly)	
Pneumococcal[5]		PPSV	
Hepatitis A[6]		HepA Series	
Hepatitis B[7]		Hep B Series	
Inactivated Poliovirus[8]		IPV Series	
Measles, Mumps, Rubella[9]		MMR Series	
Varicella[10]		Varicella Series	

Range of recommended ages for all children except certain high-risk groups

Range of recommended ages for catch-up immunization

Range of recommended ages for certain high-risk groups

This schedule includes recommendations in effect as of December 15, 2009. Any dose not administered at the recommended age should be administered at a subsequent visit, when indicated and feasible. The use of a combination vaccine generally is preferred over separate injections of its equivalent component vaccines. Considerations should include provider assessment, patient preference, and the potential for adverse events. Providers should consult the relevant Advisory Committee on Immunization Practices statement for detailed recommendations: **http://www.cdc.gov/vaccines/pubs/acip-list.htm.** Clinically significant adverse events that follow immunization should be reported to the Vaccine Adverse Event Reporting System (VAERS) at **http://www.vaers.hhs.gov** or by telephone, **800-822-7967.**

1. **Tetanus and diphtheria toxoids and acellular pertussis vaccine (Tdap).** (Minimum age: 10 years for Boostrix and 11 years for Adacel)
   - Administer at age 11 or 12 years for those who have completed the recommended childhood DTP/DTaP vaccination series and have not received a tetanus and diphtheria toxoid (Td) booster dose.
   - Persons aged 13 through 18 years who have not received Tdap should receive a dose.
   - A 5-year interval from the last Td dose is encouraged when Tdap is used as a booster dose; however, a shorter interval may be used if pertussis immunity is needed.
2. **Human papillomavirus vaccine (HPV).** (Minimum age: 9 years)
   - Two HPV vaccines are licensed: a quadrivalent vaccine (HPV4) for the prevention of cervical, vaginal and vulvar cancers (in females) and genital warts (in females and males), and a bivalent vaccine (HPV2) for the prevention of cervical cancers in females.
   - HPV vaccines are most effective for both males and females when given before exposure to HPV through sexual contact.
   - HPV4 or HPV2 is recommended for the prevention of cervical precancers and cancers in females.
   - HPV4 is recommended for the prevention of cervical, vaginal and vulvar precancers and cancers and genital warts in females.
   - Administer the first dose to females at age 11 or 12 years.
   - Administer the second dose 1 to 2 months after the first dose and the third dose 6 months after the first dose (at least 24 weeks after the first dose).
   - Administer the series to females at age 13 through 18 years if not previously vaccinated.
   - HPV4 may be administered in a 3-dose series to males aged 9 through 18 years to reduce their likelihood of acquiring genital warts.
3. **Meningococcal conjugate vaccine (MCV4).**
   - Administer at age 11 or 12 years, or at age 13 through 18 years if not previously vaccinated.
   - Administer to previously unvaccinated college freshmen living in a dormitory.
   - Administer MCV4 to children aged 2 through 10 years with persistent complement component deficiency, anatomic or functional asplenia, or certain other conditions placing them at high risk.
   - Administer to children previously vaccinated with MCV4 or MPSV4 who remain at increased risk after 3 years (if first dose administered at age 2 through 6 years) or after 5 years (if first dose administered at age 7 years or older). Persons whose only risk factor is living in on-campus housing are not recommended to receive an additional dose. See *MMWR* 2009;58:1042–3.
4. **Influenza vaccine (seasonal).**
   - Administer annually to children aged 6 months through 18 years.
   - For healthy nonpregnant persons aged 7 through 18 years (i.e., those who do not have underlying medical conditions that predispose them to influenza complications), either LAIV or TIV may be used.
   - Administer 2 doses (separated by at least 4 weeks) to children aged younger than 9 years who are receiving influenza vaccine for the first time or who were vaccinated for the first time during the previous influenza season but only received 1 dose.
   - For recommendations for use of influenza A (H1N1) 2009 monovalent vaccine. See *MMWR* 2009;58(No. RR-10).
5. **Pneumococcal polysaccharide vaccine (PPSV).**
   - Administer to children with certain underlying medical conditions, including a cochlear implant. A single revaccination should be administered after 5 years to children with functional or anatomic asplenia or an immunocompromising condition. See *MMWR* 1997;46(No. RR-8).
6. **Hepatitis A vaccine (HepA).**
   - Administer 2 doses at least 6 months apart.
   - HepA is recommended for children aged older than 23 months who live in areas where vaccination programs target older children, who are at increased risk for infection, or for whom immunity against hepatitis A is desired.
7. **Hepatitis B vaccine (HepB).**
   - Administer the 3-dose series to those not previously vaccinated.
   - A 2-dose series (separated by at least 4 months) of adult formulation Recombivax HB is licensed for children aged 11 through 15 years.
8. **Inactivated poliovirus vaccine (IPV).**
   - The final dose in the series should be administered on or after the fourth birthday and at least 6 months following the previous dose.
   - If both OPV and IPV were administered as part of a series, a total of 4 doses should be administered, regardless of the child's current age.
9. **Measles, mumps, and rubella vaccine (MMR).**
   - If not previously vaccinated, administer 2 doses or the second dose for those who have received only 1 dose, with at least 28 days between doses.
10. **Varicella vaccine.**
    - For persons aged 7 through 18 years without evidence of immunity (see *MMWR* 2007;56[No. RR-4]), administer 2 doses if not previously vaccinated or the second dose if only 1 dose has been administered.
    - For persons aged 7 through 12 years, the minimum interval between doses is 3 months. However, if the second dose was administered at least 28 days after the first dose, it can be accepted as valid.
    - For persons aged 13 years and older, the minimum interval between doses is 28 days.

The Recommended Immunization Schedules for Persons Aged 0 through 18 Years are approved by the Advisory Committee on Immunization Practices (**http://www.cdc.gov/vaccines/recs/acip**), the American Academy of Pediatrics (**http://www.aap.org**), and the American Academy of Family Physicians (**http://www.aafp.org**).

Department of Health and Human Services • Centers for Disease Control and Prevention

CS207330-A

FIGURE 15-4 Recommended Immunization Schedule for Persons Aged 7 Through 18 Years-United States-2010. COURTESY FOR CENTERS OF DISEASE CONTROL AND PREVENTION.

Catch-up Immunization Schedule for Persons Aged 4 Months Through 18 Years Who Start Late or Who Are More Than 1 Month Behind—United States • 2010

The table below provides catch-up schedules and minimum intervals between doses for children whose vaccinations have been delayed. A vaccine series does not need to be restarted, regardless of the time that has elapsed between doses. Use the section appropriate for the child's age.

Vaccine	Minimum Age for Dose 1	Minimum Interval Between Doses: Dose 1 to Dose 2	Dose 2 to Dose 3	Dose 3 to Dose 4	Dose 4 to Dose 5
PERSONS AGED 4 MONTHS THROUGH 6 YEARS					
Hepatitis B[1]	Birth	4 weeks	8 weeks (and at least 16 weeks after first dose)		
Rotavirus[2]	6 wks	4 weeks	4 weeks[2]		
Diphtheria, Tetanus, Pertussis[3]	6 wks	4 weeks	4 weeks	6 months	6 months[3]
Haemophilus influenzae type b[4]	6 wks	**4 weeks** if first dose administered at younger than age 12 months **8 weeks (as final dose)** if first dose administered at age 12–14 months **No further doses needed** if first dose administered at age 15 months or older	**4 weeks[4]** if current age is younger than 12 months **8 weeks (as final dose)[4]** if current age is 12 months or older and first dose administered at younger than age 12 months and second dose administered at younger than 15 months **No further doses needed** if previous dose administered at age 15 months or older	**8 weeks (as final dose)** This dose only necessary for children aged 12 months through 59 months who received 3 doses before age 12 months	
Pneumococcal[5]	6 wks	**4 weeks** if first dose administered at younger than age 12 months **8 weeks (as final dose for healthy children)** if first dose administered at age 12 months or older or current age 24 through 59 months **No further doses needed** for healthy children if first dose administered at age 24 months or older	**4 weeks** if current age is younger than 12 months **8 weeks** **(as final dose for healthy children)** if current age is 12 months or older **No further doses needed** for healthy children if previous dose administered at age 24 months or older	**8 weeks (as final dose)** This dose only necessary for children aged 12 months through 59 months who received 3 doses before age 12 months or for high-risk children who received 3 doses at any age	
Inactivated Poliovirus[6]	6 wks	4 weeks	4 weeks	6 months	
Measles, Mumps, Rubella[7]	12 mos	4 weeks			
Varicella[8]	12 mos	3 months			
Hepatitis A[9]	12 mos	6 months			
PERSONS AGED 7 THROUGH 18 YEARS					
Tetanus, Diphtheria/ Tetanus, Diphtheria, Pertussis[10]	7 yrs[10]	4 weeks	**4 weeks** if first dose administered at younger than age 12 months **6 months** if first dose administered at 12 months or older	**6 months** if first dose administered at younger than age 12 months	
Human Papillomavirus[11]	9 yrs	Routine dosing intervals are recommended[11]			
Hepatitis A[9]	12 mos	6 months			
Hepatitis B[1]	Birth	4 weeks	8 weeks (and at least 16 weeks after first dose)		
Inactivated Poliovirus[6]	6 wks	4 weeks	4 weeks	6 months	
Measles, Mumps, Rubella[7]	12 mos	4 weeks			
Varicella[8]	12 mos	**3 months** if person is younger than age 13 years **4 weeks** if person is aged 13 years or older			

1. **Hepatitis B vaccine (HepB).**
   - Administer the 3-dose series to those not previously vaccinated.
   - A 2-dose series (separated by at least 4 months) of adult formulation Recombivax HB is licensed for children aged 11 through 15 years.
2. **Rotavirus vaccine (RV).**
   - The maximum age for the first dose is 14 weeks 6 days. Vaccination should not be initiated for infants aged 15 weeks 0 days or older.
   - The maximum age for the final dose in the series is 8 months 0 days.
   - If Rotarix was administered for the first and second doses, a third dose is not indicated.
3. **Diphtheria and tetanus toxoids and acellular pertussis vaccine (DTaP).**
   - The fifth dose is not necessary if the fourth dose was administered at age 4 years or older.
4. ***Haemophilus influenzae* type b conjugate vaccine (Hib).**
   - Hib vaccine is not generally recommended for persons aged 5 years or older. No efficacy data are available on which to base a recommendation concerning use of Hib vaccine for older children and adults. However, studies suggest good immunogenicity in persons who have sickle cell disease, leukemia, or HIV infection, or who have had a splenectomy; administering 1 dose of Hib vaccine to these persons who have not previously received Hib vaccine is not contraindicated.
   - If the first 2 doses were PRP-OMP (PedvaxHIB or Comvax), and administered at age 11 months or younger, the third (and final) dose should be administered at age 12 through 15 months and at least 8 weeks after the second dose.
   - If the first dose was administered at age 7 through 11 months, administer the second dose at least 4 weeks later and a final dose at age 12 through 15 months.
5. **Pneumococcal vaccine.**
   - Administer 1 dose of pneumococcal conjugate vaccine (PCV) to all healthy children aged 24 through 59 months who have not received at least 1 dose of PCV on or after age 12 months.
   - For children aged 24 through 59 months with underlying medical conditions, administer 1 dose of PCV if 3 doses were received previously or administer 2 doses of PCV at least 8 weeks apart if fewer than 3 doses were received previously.
   - Administer pneumococcal polysaccharide vaccine (PPSV) to children aged 2 years or older with certain underlying medical conditions, including a cochlear implant, at least 8 weeks after the last dose of PCV. See *MMWR* 1997;46(No. RR-8).
6. **Inactivated poliovirus vaccine (IPV).**
   - The final dose in the series should be administered on or after the fourth birthday and at least 6 months following the previous dose.
   - A fourth dose is not necessary if the third dose was administered at age 4 years or older and at least 6 months following the previous dose.
   - In the first 6 months of life, minimum age and minimum intervals are only recommended if the person is at risk for imminent exposure to circulating poliovirus (i.e., travel to a polio-endemic region or during an outbreak).
7. **Measles, mumps, and rubella vaccine (MMR).**
   - Administer the second dose routinely at age 4 through 6 years. However, the second dose may be administered before age 4, provided at least 28 days have elapsed since the first dose.
   - If not previously vaccinated, administer 2 doses with at least 28 days between doses.
8. **Varicella vaccine.**
   - Administer the second dose routinely at age 4 through 6 years. However, the second dose may be administered before age 4, provided at least 3 months have elapsed since the first dose.
   - For persons aged 12 months through 12 years, the minimum interval between doses is 3 months. However, if the second dose was administered at least 28 days after the first dose, it can be accepted as valid.
   - For persons aged 13 years and older, the minimum interval between doses is 28 days.
9. **Hepatitis A vaccine (HepA).**
   - HepA is recommended for children aged older than 23 months who live in areas where vaccination programs target older children, who are at increased risk for infection, or for whom immunity against hepatitis A is desired.
10. **Tetanus and diphtheria toxoids vaccine (Td) and tetanus and diphtheria toxoids and acellular pertussis vaccine (Tdap).**
    - Doses of DTaP are counted as part of the Td/Tdap series
    - Tdap should be substituted for a single dose of Td in the catch-up series or as a booster for children aged 10 through 18 years; use Td for other doses.
11. **Human papillomavirus vaccine (HPV).**
    - Administer the series to females at age 13 through 18 years if not previously vaccinated.
    - Use recommended routine dosing intervals for series catch-up (i.e., the second and third doses should be administered at 1 to 2 and 6 months after the first dose). The minimum interval between the first and second doses is 4 weeks. The minimum interval between the second and third doses is 12 weeks, and the third dose should be administered at least 24 weeks after the first dose.

Information about reporting reactions after immunization is available online at **http://www.vaers.hhs.gov** or by telephone, **800-822-7967**. Suspected cases of vaccine-preventable diseases should be reported to the state or local health department. Additional information, including precautions and contraindications for immunization, is available from the National Center for Immunization and Respiratory Diseases at **http://www.cdc.gov/vaccines** or telephone, **800-CDC-INFO** (800-232-4636).

Department of Health and Human Services • Centers for Disease Control and Prevention

CS207330-A

FIGURE 15-5 Catch-up Immunization Schedule for Persons Aged 4 Months Through 18 Years Who Start Late or Who Are More Than 1 Month Behind-United States-2010. COURTESY FOR CENTERS OF DISEASE CONTROL AND PREVENTION.

vaccine (MMR) and trivalent (three strains) inactivated polio vaccine (IPV). New combination vaccines that are currently available include hepatitis B (HepB) and hemophilis influenza B (Hib); tetanus toxoid (T) and hemophilis influenza B (Hib); diphtheria and tetanus toxoids with acellular pertussis (DTaP) combined with hepatitis B (HepB) and inactivated polio vaccine (IPV); and diphtheria and tetanus toxoids plus acellular pertusssis combined with hemophilis B (Hib) and tetanus toxoid (T). Combination vaccines currently under study include DTaP, IPV, and Hib; DTaP, IPV, HIB, and hepatitis B; measles-mumps-rubella (MMR), and varicella (Var); and DTaP, Hib, IPV, hepatitis A, and hepatitis B.

Combining vaccines is subject to the U.S. Food and Drug Administration (FDA) approval. Combination vaccines have some drawbacks. Some of the difficulties encountered with combination vaccines include side effects such as febrile seizures associated with the MMRV (MMR and varicella) combined vaccines. These risks have caused the Advisory Committee on Immunization Practices to issue new recommendations for the MMRV (CDC, 2008a). Additionally, vaccine combinations that require different schedules may result in confusion when they are administered by several providers who use different products. However, combination vaccines might improve current immunization coverage as well as provide catch-up for children who are delayed in their immunizations. Reducing fear of needles and pain plus ensuring safety and efficacy should be a prime concern of all personnel involved with providing immunizations. As these new vaccines debut, nurses need to update their knowledge base about these preparations.

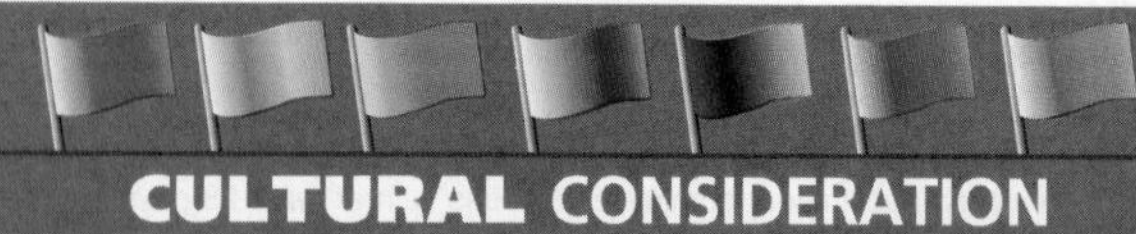

CULTURAL CONSIDERATION

Re-emergence of Polio

In 2003 the polio virus was confined to six countries—Nigeria, Niger, Pakistan, Egypt, Afghanistan, and India. In the summer of 2003, the leaders of northern Nigeria stopped polio inoculations after rumors spread that the vaccine could transmit AIDS and leave girls infertile. By 2008, 1,625 children had contracted acute flaccid paralysis in those countries. This represents a 150% increase over the number of cases reported in those countries in 2007. This increase has created the re-emergence of polio as one of the deadliest infections. In 2008 polio cases were detected in 14 countries and, as of 2009, polio remains endemic to India, Pakistan, and Afghanistan (Warraich, 2009). Nurses must also be aware that certain groups in the United States, for religious or other reasons, will not agree to have their children immunized.

Nurses are the primary administrators of vaccines in health care settings. In addition to immunization requirements, nurses must be familiar with the appropriate site for injectable vaccines, the appropriate storage of vaccines, the specifications of the National Childhood Vaccine Injury Act of 1986, expected reactions to various vaccines, reportable vaccine-related events, and contraindications to specific vaccine use.

VACCINE HANDLING AND STORAGE

Inappropriate handling or storage of vaccines can result in a decrease in vaccine potency and ineffective immunization. Some vaccines are sensitive to heat while others are affected by freezing. The most current recommendations for the handling and storage of vaccines can be obtained from the package insert. With the rapid development of new immunizations, it is imperative that package inserts be reviewed. The Centers for Disease Control and Prevention's National Immunization Program website provides the most current additional information on vaccine storage.

THE NATIONAL CHILDHOOD VACCINE INJURY ACT

The National Childhood Vaccine Injury Act of 1986 was established in response to concerns about serious vaccine-related injuries and deaths. It is a system in which persons who have suffered an injury or death as a result of vaccines may seek compensation. No negligence must be proven, and the program provides an alternative to civil litigation. The act requires every child to have a personal immunization record that is maintained in a permanent medical record. It mandates that the following information be recorded at the time of each immunization:

- Month, day, and year of administration
- Vaccine administered
- Manufacturer
- Lot number and expiration date
- Site and route of administration
- Name, address, and title of the health care provider administering the vaccine

Caregivers are asked to read and sign consent forms granting permission before any immunization is administered. Information regarding immunizations is presented to caregivers verbally and in writing. Most health care settings where immunizations are administered require written consent. Nurses must ensure that caregivers understand the information provided. Some may be reluctant to reveal that they cannot read or understand the written handouts. If the nurse assesses that the caregiver cannot read, then the contents of the consent form must be explained in terms that are understood. When working with non-English-speaking populations, nurses need to be aware of and use consent forms written in

NURSING TIP

Importance of Immunization Records

Caregivers should be given a copy of their child's immunization record. You need to stress the importance of keeping this record in a safe place and bringing it with them to each visit to the health provider. Telling caregivers that this record is "the child's passport to day care or school" places importance on the value of knowing their child's immunization status.

that particular language as well as seeking the assistance of an interpreter as indicated.

PRECAUTIONS AND CONTRAINDICATIONS

Although immunization is generally considered safe and effective, some children will have reactions ranging from minor to life-threatening, while others will not receive the level of protection from disease that is expected. Nurses must be aware of the relatively few contraindications to immunizations so that children are not prevented from receiving protection against possible life-threatening, preventable diseases. There are only two true, permanent contraindications to vaccination: (1) a history of severe anaphylactic reaction to a vaccine or its component; and (2) encephalopathy within seven days of administration of DTP/DTaP. Mild common illnesses such as otitis media, upper respiratory infections, colds, and diarrhea are *not* contraindications to immunizations. Precautions must be taken when administering live vaccines such as measles, mumps, and rubella as well as varicella to adolescent girls and women of childbearing age to make certain that they are not pregnant at the time of vaccination.

Despite the availability of vaccines to prevent the majority of communicable diseases, it cannot be assumed that every child has been immunized at the recommended age. Some children and adolescents may be exposed to certain viruses or bacteria and may not be fully immunized or may have inadequate levels of immunity to these organisms (CDC, 2009).

NURSING MANAGEMENT

Caregivers often look to nurses for guidance and counseling regarding the care of their children when an infectious disease occurs. Nurses are often asked questions such as, "My child has been exposed to chickenpox. What are her chances of getting it? When will that happen?" or "Several children at school have Fifth's disease. Should I worry about my child catching it?" Nurses need to be knowledgeable about the clinical manifestations, etiology, incidence, and incubation period, as well as the therapeutic management of each disease. Table 15-1 presents some of the more common infectious diseases seen in children, with recommendations for treatment and prevention.

NURSING TIP

Immunization History

Before giving vaccines, ask the caregivers about the child's response to the last dose. Ask them to recall what vaccine was given and where. That way, you will be able to assess if the reactions were normal or not. You can choose an alternate site for the present vaccine. Make sure that all immunizations are recorded on the child's record. Document both the amount of vaccine used and the sites of the injections.

EYE ON...

What Happened to Polio Drops?

Most families who have young children receiving immunizations have been immunized themselves when they were infants and children. Many caregivers recall receiving oral polio vaccine either as sugar cubes or as drops. When told by health care providers that their children will be immunized with a polio vaccine given as an injection, they may wonder and ask, "I thought polio has been eradicated, why does my child need this immunization?" Health care providers must be prepared to answer their questions. It is important to let caregivers know that, although polio has been eliminated in the United States, there is still a need for immunization against polio. The infection still exists in many parts of the world, and there is a possibility that the virus could be introduced accidentally, thus leading to an epidemic.

The first type of polio vaccine developed by Jonas Salk was licensed in 1955. It was a killed, inactivated vaccine, or IPV, that induced immunity through the blood system but was incapable of causing paralytic polio. The oral form of polio vaccine developed by Albert Sabin soon followed and was licensed in 1961. The oral preparation of polio vaccine (OPV) contained live but weakened virus, which acts in the intestines to produce immunity. It is capable of producing paralytic polio. Infants who receive their first dose orally (live virus) are susceptible to developing paralytic polio, although the chance is small. Weighing all of the variables, it remains imperative to continue vaccination against polio but with the killed virus, which is only available by injection.

Table 15-1 Infectious Diseases in Children

DISEASE	CLINICAL MANIFESTATIONS	ETIOLOGY	INCIDENCE/INCUBATION/ CONTROL	THERAPEUTIC MANAGEMENT
Cytomegalovirus (CMV)	Most CMV infections are asymptomatic; most infants with congenital CMV infection are asymptomatic; however, 5% have significant manifestations of fetal damage (intrauterine growth retardation, jaundice, hepatitis, hepatosplenomegaly; brain damage, petechial rash, retinitis) **Diagnosis**: viral culture specimens from urine, pharynx, cervical secretions, human milk, semen, peripheral blood leukocytes; presence of IgM CMV antibodies in cord blood identifies congenitally infected infants; polymerase chain reaction detects CMV DNA in tissues **Complications**: psychomotor retardation, microcephaly, hearing loss, seizures, learning disabilities	Cytomegalovirus, a member of the herpes family of viruses **Transmission**: direct person-to-person contact with virus-containing secretions and from mother to infant before, during, or after birth	**Incidence**: CMV infection is distributed worldwide; most humans have become infected by the time they reach adulthood; CMV causes congenital infection in 1–2% of all live births **Incubation**: unknown for person-to-person transmission **Control**: at greatest risk are susceptible pregnant women exposed to urine and saliva of CMV-infected children who attend day care centers; handwashing and simple hygienic measures should be reinforced in this population	Administer ganciclovir, an antiviral drug, to treat life-threatening CMV infections in immunocompromised hosts (individuals with AIDS and recipients of bone marrow, heart, and kidney transplants) and to treat retinitis.
Diphtheria	Low-grade fever; gradual onset of membranous nasopharyngitis, obstructive laryngotracheitis **Diagnosis**: nose and throat cultures **Complications**: thrombocytopenia, myocarditis, vocal cord paralysis, ascending paralysis	*Corynebacterium diphtheriae* bacillus **Transmission**: intimate contact with discharges from the nose, throat, eye, and skin lesions	**Incidence**: more frequent in fall and winter; most common and most severe in unimmunized or inadequately immunized individuals **Incubation**: usually 2–7 days or could be longer **Control**: universal immunization with diphtheria toxoid; prophylactic treatment of frequent close contacts with erythromycin or benzathine penicillin G; notification of public health officials	Administer single dose of equine antitoxin IV after sensitivity testing. Administer erythromycin orally or penicillin G IM or IV. Initiate strict isolation of hospitalized individuals until two sequential nose and throat cultures are negative. Monitor respiratory status. Assess for signs of complications. Offer comfort measures such as rest, fluids, and fever management.

(Continues)

TABLE 15-1 Infectious Diseases in Children (*Continued*)

DISEASE	CLINICAL MANIFESTATIONS	ETIOLOGY	INCIDENCE/INCUBATION/ CONTROL	THERAPEUTIC MANAGEMENT
Erythema infectiosum (Fifth's disease) 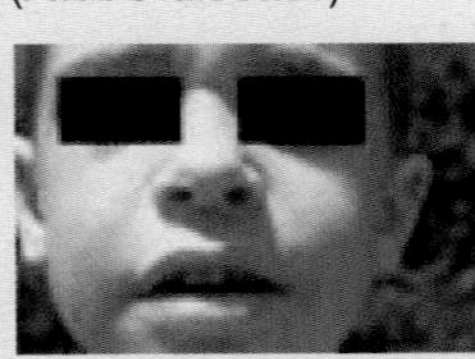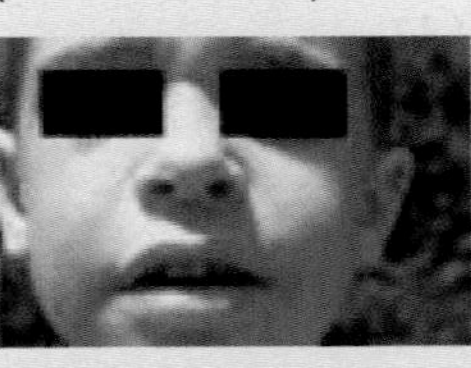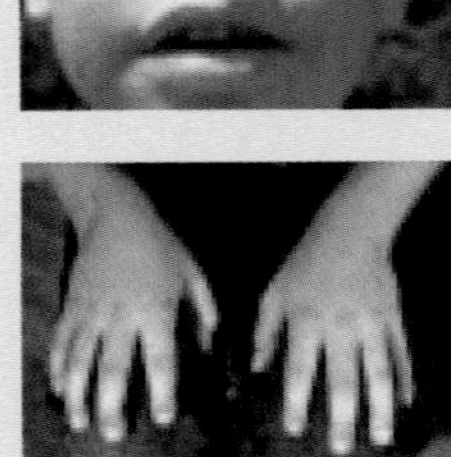 COURTESY OF THE CENTERS FOR DISEASE CONTROL AND PREVENTION (CDC).	Mild systemic symptoms, occasional fever, red facial rash giving a "slapped cheek" appearance, circumoral pallor, and symmetric lacy rash on trunk and limbs; rarely seen in dark skinned individuals; rash can recur for weeks with exposure to heat or sun **Diagnosis**: by clinical findings **Complications**: arthralgia, arthritis	Human parvovirus B19 **Transmission**: contact with respiratory secretions, blood or blood products; contagious before onset of illness	**Incidence**: often has outbreaks in elementary or junior high schools during late winter and early spring **Incubation**: 4–14 days; can be as long as 21 days **Control**: good hygiene practices including handwashing and disposal of tissues contaminated with respiratory secretions	Manage fever and offer comfort measures if needed. Allow children to attend school since they are not contagious after appearance of rash.
Infectious mononucleosis	Fever, fatigue, exudative pharyngitis, lymphadenopathy, hepatosplenomegaly; atypical lymphocytosis; occasional rash **Diagnosis**: usually confirmed by monospot or heterophile antibody blood tests **Complications**: aseptic meningitis, encephalitis, Guillain-Barré syndrome; rare: splenic rupture, thrombocytopenia, agranulocytosis, hemolytic anemia, orchitis, myocarditis	Epstein-Barr virus, a herpes virus (EBV) **Transmission**: contact with respiratory tract excretions and close personal contact	**Incidence**: common in group settings of adolescents, also found in children, no seasonal pattern **Incubation**: estimated to be 30–50 days **Control**: good hygiene practices including handwashing and disposal of tissues contaminated with respiratory secretions	Steroids may be considered when complications are present. Encourage rest. Manage fever. Maintain fluid intake with cool, nonacidic fluids, gelatin, popsicles. Suggest saline gargles for older children. Strongly advise avoidance of contact sports until splenomegaly resolves. If EBV is suspected, do not administer ampicillin or amoxicillin because they may cause a morbilliform nonallergic rash.

(Continues)

TABLE 15-1 Infectious Diseases in Children (*Continued*)

DISEASE	CLINICAL MANIFESTATIONS	ETIOLOGY	INCIDENCE/INCUBATION/CONTROL	THERAPEUTIC MANAGEMENT
Lyme Disease COURTESY OF THE CENTERS FOR DISEASE CONTROL AND PREVENTION (CDC).	Early stage: rash (erythema migrans), begins as a small papule and spreads peripherally; characterized by raised, red margin and clearing in the center at the site of the tick bite; fever; malaise; fatigue; headache; stiff neck; arthralgia. Late stage: arthritis of large joints, especially the knee, beginning months after the initial infection **Diagnosis**: based on history and serologic testing **Complications**: rare in children: involvement of neurological and cardiac systems	*Borrelia burgdorferi,* a spirochete **Transmission**: to humans through the bite of infected tick, especially deer or black-legged tick; person-to-person is not possible	**Incidence**: has been reported in 49 states to date; is highest in children 5—10 years of age **Incubation**: from tick bite to appearance of lesions (range 1–32 days) **Control**: avoid tick-infested areas; use tick repellent with DEET; wear light-colored long-sleeve top and pants (light color makes tick identification easier); inspect clothing and body daily after possible tick exposure; remove ticks from body immediately; immunize persons over 15 years of age who reside or recreate in geographical areas of high risk	Antibiotics—doxycycline (Vibramycin) or amoxicillin (Augmentin) for 14–21 days.
Mumps	Mild systemic symptoms, swelling of the salivary glands, meningeal signs in 10–30% of cases **Diagnosis**: complement-fixation test **Complications**: encephalitis, orchitis **Rare**: arthritis, renal involvement, thyroiditis, mastitis, pancreatitis, hearing impairment	Paramyxovirus **Transmission**: direct contact with respiratory secretions	**Incidence**: late winter and spring; peak incidence in 10- to 14-year-olds **Incubation**: usually 16–18 days; may be as long as 25 days **Control**: universal immunization of children; good hygiene practices including handwashing and disposal of tissues contaminated with respiratory secretions	Manage fever and comfort measures. Exclude from school until 9 days after onset of parotid swelling.

(Continues)

TABLE 15-1 Infectious Diseases in Children (*Continued*)

DISEASE	CLINICAL MANIFESTATIONS	ETIOLOGY	INCIDENCE/INCUBATION/ CONTROL	THERAPEUTIC MANAGEMENT
Pertussis (whooping cough)	Begins with mild upper respiratory symptoms known as the catarrhal stage; progresses to severe paroxysms of cough, often with a characteristic inspiratory whoop followed by vomiting; apnea is common in infants under 6 months **Diagnosis**: nasopharyngeal culture **Complications**: seizures, pneumonia, encephalopathy, death	*Bordetella pertussis* bacillus **Transmission**: close contact with respiratory secretions; most contagious during mild respiratory symptoms	**Incidence**: occurs in unimmunized or partially immunized infants and children; adolescents and adults are a major source; no seasonal pattern **Incubation**: 7–10 days (range 5–21 days) **Control**: universal immunization; erythromycin prophylaxis for household and other close contacts; good hygiene practices including handwashing and disposal of tissues contaminated with respiratory secretions	Infants under 6 months and other clients with severe disease are usually hospitalized. Administer erythromycin orally for 14 days. Observe respiratory isolation for 5 days after initiation of antibiotic treatment. Maintain airway. Maintain fluid intake. Provide a restful environment. Offer supportive care for respiratory distress and feeding difficulties. Support anxious parents by explaining about the illness and the nature of the cough. Without treatment, pertussis can last 6 to 10 weeks.
Polio	Nonspecific illness with low-grade fever and sore throat **Diagnosis**: throat and stool culture **Complications**: aseptic meningitis; rapid onset of asymmetric acute flaccid paralysis and residual paralytic disease involving the motor neurons; paralysis of respiratory muscles	Enterovirus **Transmission**: fecal-oral and possibly respiratory	**Incidence**: more common in infants and young children; most common in summer and fall; all endemic cases since 1979 have been associated with oral polio virus vaccine **Incubation**: 3–6 days **Control**: universal immunization; good hygiene practices including handwashing and handling of diapers	Offer comfort measures and supportive treatment depending on extent of complications present. Refer for physical therapy if required.

(Continues)

Table 15-1 Infectious Diseases in Children (*Continued*)

DISEASE	CLINICAL MANIFESTATIONS	ETIOLOGY	INCIDENCE/INCUBATION/CONTROL	THERAPEUTIC MANAGEMENT
Rocky Mountain spotted fever COURTESY OF THE CENTERS FOR DISEASE CONTROL AND PREVENTION (CDC).	Fever, headache, myalgia, nausea, vomiting, anorexia, confusion, erythematous and macular rash on ankles and wrists (may spread to rest of body) **Diagnosis**: history and serologic tests **Complications**: CNS disease; multisystem organ failure; disseminated intravascular coagulation (DIC); shock, and death	*Rickettsia rickettsii* **Transmission**: to humans through the bite of infected tick. **Reservoir**: dogs, wild rodents	**Incidence**: occurs in spring and summer; disease is widespread in United States; most cases reported in south Atlantic, southeastern, and south central states **Incubation**: 1 week (range of 2–14 days) **Control**: same as Lyme disease	Doxycycline (Vibramycin) is the drug of choice. Chloramphenicol (chloromycetin) is an alternative.
Roseola (human herpesvirus 6) COURTESY OF THE CENTERS FOR DISEASE CONTROL AND PREVENTION (CDC).	High fever for 3–5 days followed by a red maculopapular rash lasting up to several days **Diagnosis**: by clinical presentation **Complications**: seizures, encephalitis	Human herpesvirus 6 **Transmission**: contact with respiratory secretions	**Incidence**: highest in children between 6 and 24 months of age; rare before 3 months and after 4 years of age; no seasonal pattern **Incubation**: estimated to be about 9 days **Control**: good hygiene practices including handwashing	Manage fever. Manage fluid intake. Offer comfort measures.
Rotavirus	Diarrhea, usually preceded or accompanied by vomiting and low-grade fever; in severe cases, isotonic dehydration, electrolyte imbalances, and acidosis **Diagnosis**: history and clinical presentation; immunoassays **Complications**: death	*Rotaviruses* **Transmission**: fecal-oral route; possibly respiratory	**Incidence**: most common in infants and children under 2 years of age and in day care centers **Incubation**: 1–3 days **Control**: good hygiene; children in whom diarrhea cannot be contained by diapers or toilet use should be excluded from day care centers until diarrhea ceases; immunization with RV5 vaccine.	Prevention and treatment of dehydration; no antiviral therapy is available.

(Continues)

Table 15-1 Infectious Diseases in Children (*Continued*)

DISEASE	CLINICAL MANIFESTATIONS	ETIOLOGY	INCIDENCE/INCUBATION/ CONTROL	THERAPEUTIC MANAGEMENT
Rubella (German measles) 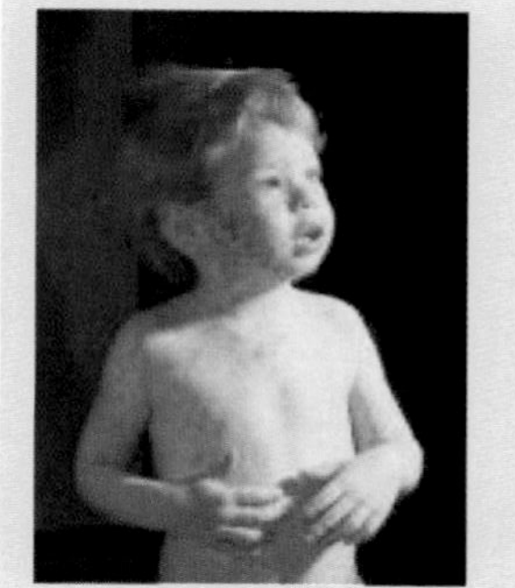 COURTESY OF THE CENTERS FOR DISEASE CONTROL AND PREVENTION (CDC).	Slight fever, red maculopapular discrete rash, lymphadenopathy; 25–50% of cases are asymptomatic; first day of rash: head and upper torso heavily covered with rash; by third day lower half is heavily covered with rash with upper part lessening in rash severity **Diagnosis**: nasal secretion culture; acute and convalescent antibody titers **Complications**: transient polyarthralgia and polyarthritis. **Rare**: encephalitis, thrombocytopenia teratogenic effect on fetus if client is pregnant	Rubella virus **Transmission**: direct or droplet contact with nasopharyngeal secretions	**Incidence**: peaks in late winter and early spring **Incubation**: 14–23 days **Control**: universal immunization; good hygiene practices including handwashing and disposal of tissues contaminated with respiratory secretions; isolate children from women who are pregnant or may be pregnant	Initiate isolation and school exclusion for 7 days after onset of the rash. Offer supportive care and comfort measures.
Rubeola (measles) 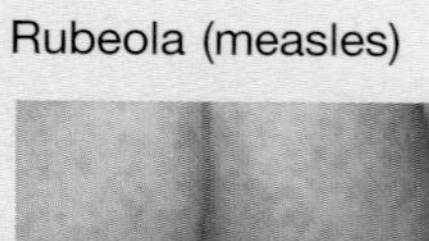 Kopliks spots appearing on the lingual and buccal mucosa in Rubeola. They are small red spots with bluish-white centers. COURTESY OF THE CENTERS FOR DISEASE CONTROL AND PREVENTION (CDC).	Acutely ill with fever, cough, coryza, conjunctivitis, Kopliks spots; rash begins light on upper body and head on first day; by third day the upper body rash has increased and progressed to lower body **Diagnosis**: viral tissue culture from nasopharyngeal secretions; acute and convalescent antibody titers **Complications**: otitis media, bronchopneumonia, croup, diarrhea, encephalitis resulting in permanent brain damage, death	Morbilli-virus **Transmission**: direct contact with infectious droplets; occasionally by airborne spread	**Incidence**: peaks in winter and spring, primarily in unimmunized individuals **Incubation**: 8–12 days **Control**: universal immunization; good hygiene practices including handwashing and disposal of tissues contaminated with respiratory secretions	Initiate respiratory isolation for 4 days after onset of rash. Consider administration of vitamin A if deficiency is suspected. Encourage hospitalization of infants and children with severe cases or complications. Observe fever control measures. Offer comfort measures, including dimming the lights in the presence of photophobia.

(Continues)

TABLE 15-1 Infectious Diseases in Children (*Continued*)

DISEASE	CLINICAL MANIFESTATIONS	ETIOLOGY	INCIDENCE/INCUBATION/ CONTROL	THERAPEUTIC MANAGEMENT
Scarlet fever 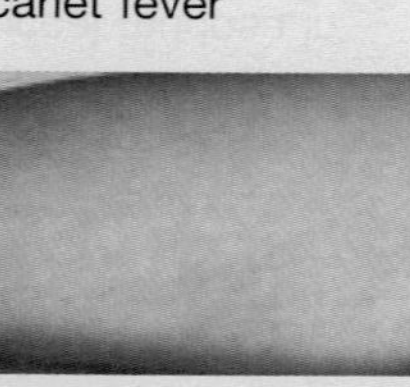 COURTESY OF THE CENTERS FOR DISEASE CONTROL AND PREVENTION (CDC).	Acute fever, sore throat, rhinitis, headache, red sandpaper-like rash prominent in creases, white strawberry tongue (day 1), flush cheeks, red strawberry tongue (day 2), pharynx and tonsils edematous and erythematous, enlarged and tender anterior cervical nodes **Diagnosis**: throat culture **Complications**: otitis media, sinusitis, peritonsillar and retropharyngeal abscesses, cervical adenitis, rheumatic fever, acute glomerulonephritis	Group A beta-hemolytic streptococci (GAS) **Transmission**: contact with respiratory secretions	**Incidence**: most frequent among school-aged children in late fall, winter, and spring **Incubation**: 2–5 days **Control**: prompt treatment; good hygiene practices including handwashing and disposal of tissues contaminated with respiratory secretions	Administer antibiotics for 10 days (penicillin, erythromycin, amoxicillin, cephalosporins). Encourage school exclusion for at least 24 hours after initiation of treatment and until afebrile. Manage fever. Maintain fluid intake with cool, nonacidic fluids, gelatin, popsicles. Suggest saline gargles for older children. Offer comfort measures. Provide anticipatory guidance regarding possible desquamation of skin.
Tetanus	Early signs—headache, restlessness, followed by spasms of masticatory (chewing) muscles, difficulty opening mouth (**trismus**), dysphagia; eventually, **opisthotonos** (severe spasm of back muscles causing back to arch acutely, head to bend back on neck); seizures; dysuria and urinary retention; bowel incontinence; and fever **Diagnosis**: based on clinical presentation **Complications**: airway obstruction and asphyxiation due to laryngeal and respiratory muscle spasms; death	*Clostridium tetani*—spore-forming bacillus produces a neurotoxin that affects the central nervous system (spinal cord and brain stem) **Transmission**: to humans through wound in skin from contact with soil contaminated with animal feces	**Incidence**: worldwide; prevalent in nonimmunized populations; mortality rate is high; spores, found in soil, dust, and intestinal tracts of humans and animals, especially horse and cattle **Incubation**: 3–21 days (average 8 days) **Control**: active immunization with tetanus toxoid; tetanus prophylaxis should be followed as part of wound management; prompt surgical cleansing and debridement of wounds	Administer human tetanus immune globulin (TIG) to neutralize the neurotoxin in the child's system in order to stop continuation of the infectious process. Administer penicillin G, IV initially, for 10–14 days. Surgically cleanse and debride wound. Administer diazepam (Valium) to reduce muscle spasms and control seizures. Respiratory support and intervention as needed. Provide quiet environment since muscle spasms are aggravated by external stimuli.

(*Continues*)

Table 15-1 Infectious Diseases in Children (*Continued*)

DISEASE	CLINICAL MANIFESTATIONS	ETIOLOGY	INCIDENCE/INCUBATION/CONTROL	THERAPEUTIC MANAGEMENT
Varicella (chickenpox) 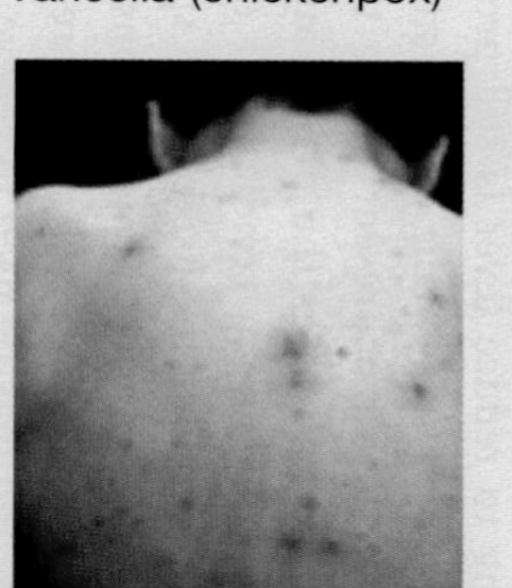 COURTESY OF THE CENTERS FOR DISEASE CONTROL AND PREVENTION (CDC).	Mild fever and systemic symptoms; generalized pruritic, vesicular rash **Diagnosis**: usually by clinical findings **Complications**: bacterial superinfection of lesions, thrombocytopenia, arthritis, hepatitis, encephalitis, meningitis, glomerulonephritis, Reye's syndrome, shingles later in life	Varicella-zoster virus, a herpes virus **Transmission**: highly contagious; direct contact and airborne spread from respiratory secretions	**Incidence**: most often in children under 10 years of age; most common in late winter and early spring **Incubation**: 10–21 days **Control**: universal immunization; good hygiene practices including handwashing and disposal of tissues contaminated with respiratory secretions	Oral acyclovir may be given in some cases, but is not recommended for routine treatment of uncomplicated cases in otherwise healthy children. Manage fever (aspirin is contraindicated since it increases risk of Reye's syndrome). Observe strict isolation for at least 5 days in hospitalized clients. Manage pruritus with oral antihistamine (Benadryl), baking soda or oatmeal baths, and calamine lotion to keep child cool. Maintain fluid intake with cool, non-acidic fluids, gelatin, popsicles. Prevent secondary infection by controlling pruritus and keeping child's fingernails clean and short. School exclusion until all lesions are dry and crusted over.

Adapted from Committee on Infectious Diseases, American Academy of Pediatrics. (2009). *2009 Red book: Report of the committee on infectious diseases* (28th ed.). Elk Grove Village, IL: American Academy of Pediatrics; and Centers for Disease Control and Prevention.

Several excellent resources are available for information about immunizations and vaccine recommendations. The main sources are publications and the Internet, which include the following:

- *Red Book: Report of the Committee on Infectious Diseases* of the AAP. This text is updated every three years and may be purchased from the AAP's website at www.aap.org.
- *Morbidity and Mortality Weekly Report (MMWR)* of the CDC. This is a weekly newsletter and is available from the CDC's website at www.cdc.gov.
- Statements and recommendations of the ACIP of the CDC.
- The National Immunization Program website at www.cdc.gov/nip is updated frequently and provides information for health care professionals, parents, the public, the media, and travelers.
- The Immunization Action Coalition website at www.immunize.org works to prevent disease and increase immunization rates by creating and distributing educational materials for the public and health professionals.

Nurses can refer to these resources when giving anticipatory guidance and instructing caregivers on the care and management of children with infectious diseases. Nurses must seize the opportunity to educate caregivers about routine immunizations and the potential consequences of nonadherence to recommended schedules.

The majority of children who experience infectious or communicable diseases are managed at home. Home is the ideal environment because the spread of the infection is limited to those in the immediate environment. A small percentage of children may need to be hospitalized because of complications or secondary infection. Still other children may require respiratory or nutritional support. When these children are hospitalized, isolation procedures may need to be instituted depending on the etiologic agent and the method of transmission. The hospital's infection control department is the best resource in directing the parameters of the isolation and precautions associated with the particular illness. Even at home, caregivers may want to isolate the ill child from well siblings to prevent the spread of infection.

NURSING ALERT

MMR Vaccine in Adolescent Females

When administering MMR vaccine to adolescent females, it is important to assess for the possibility of pregnancy. The vaccine is a teratogen (any substance or process that interferes with normal prenatal development) and can cause developmental abnormalities in the fetus when given during the first trimester. If the vaccine is given, nurses need to caution the adolescents against pregnancy for at least three months.

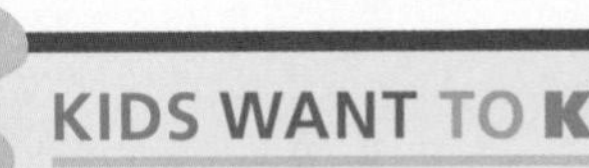

Can my classmates get chickenpox from me?

Martina, a 10-year-old, has chickenpox and has not been at school for the past 7 days. She returned 8 days after the onset of the rash. Her classmates are afraid to get near her because of all the lesions on her face, arms, and legs. The nurse explains that the infectious period is 1–2 days before the eruption of the rash to 6 days after the onset of the lesions, when crusts have formed. Although she has many lesions, they have all crusted over. Therefore, Martina can tell the other kids that they cannot get chickenpox from her.

CRITICAL THINKING

Implementing a Plan for Lapsed Immunizations

As the nurse in a pediatric clinic, you interview Ms. Cooper, the parent of 2-year-old Leslie. According to Leslie's immunization record, she has had the first and second hepatitis B vaccines plus the first diphtheria-tetanus-pertussis and polio vaccines. Ms. Cooper relates that "This is all she has ever received," and asks, "Will she have to start over again?" What will you tell Ms. Cooper about Leslie's current immunization status? What vaccines need to be administered today? How will you plan the remainder of Leslie's immunizations so that her mother knows when to return to the clinic?

Caregivers treating their children at home need education regarding supportive care and comfort measures. Many caregivers may be unfamiliar with the types of treatment that will promote their children's comfort while restoring them to health. Others may rely on home remedies, some of which may be harmful to children. For example, the use of alcohol sponging to reduce fever is still promoted by some family members but can be dangerous to small infants and children.

Fever is often present during the earliest stage of the illness, also known as the **prodrome** (the earliest phase or sign of a developing condition or disease). Fever management may include the use of tepid sponges, dressing in cool clothing, and antipyretic medications such as acetaminophen or ibuprofen. These medications are analgesic as well as antipyretic and may be used to relieve the discomfort of other

NURSING ALERT

Use of Acetaminophen

Acetaminophen (Tylenol) is available in liquid, tablet, and suppository form in a variety of strengths. Nurses will need to discuss the variation in concentration with caregivers to ascertain which particular form will be used. This will prevent either underdosing or overdosing of the medication. Regardless of the form of the acetaminophen, the recommended dose for infants and children is 10–15 mg/kg/dose every 4 hours, but not more than five times a day. The major toxicity from overdose is liver damage. Many over-the-counter cold remedies contain acetaminophen. Caregivers may not be aware of this and want to use a combination product in addition to acetaminophen. Instruct caregivers to read labels carefully to prevent overdosing, and keep this and all medications out of reach of children in the household.

accompanying symptoms such as headache, malaise, sore throat, or muscular aches and pains.

Some illnesses may be accompanied by vomiting or diarrhea. Caregivers will need to know the signs and symptoms of dehydration, as well as how to prevent dehydration and manage fluid intake (see Chapter 21). Some viral diseases that cause mouth lesions, such as varicella (chickenpox), may make oral intake difficult. Fluids that are soothing such as gelatins or popsicles should be offered. Some forms of oral rehydration solution come in ready-to-freeze packets for use as Popsicles. Once children begin to recover, they gradually may progress to their normal diets.

Children who manifest pruritic lesions may be treated with antihistamines such as diphenhydramine hydrochloride (Benadryl) or hydroxyzine hydrochloride (Atarax). Baking soda, oatmeal, or colloid preparations in bath water may assist in relieving discomfort. Topical drying agents such as calamine can be used to decrease itching. Fingernails should be cut short and kept clean to prevent secondary infections. Covering an infant's hands with cotton mittens or socks may inhibit the tendency to scratch, especially during periods of sleep.

Many respiratory illnesses may be accompanied by coughing, which may be **paroxysmal**, or severe, in character. Children may need extra humidification; this can be accomplished by room humidifiers or by placing the child in the bathroom with the mist from a shower. A mist tent can be constructed by draping a sheet over the crib or bed and directing the humidifier at the head of the bed. Sick children may need quiet activities to occupy their time during the convalescent period. Soft music, reading to children, and age-appropriate games and videos may provide some comfort and diversion to children and their families.

Caregivers will need to know approximately how long the illness will last, the period of communicability, plus the appropriate time for children to return to school or day care. All of these factors are specific to the etiology of the illness. Although the incidence of complications from childhood infectious diseases is rare, caregivers will need to know what signs and symptoms indicate problems. Neurological signs such as severe headache, irritability, stiff neck, altered levels of consciousness, and seizures may indicate viral encephalitis, an inflammation of the brain, which is a rare sequela of chickenpox, measles, mumps, or rubella infection. A disease that affects the respiratory system such as pertussis may cause respiratory distress and apnea. Part of the educational process should be directed to an understanding of the pathophysiology of the disease, the rationale for the therapy, and monitoring for signs of complications.

The infectious diseases that adolescents experience are most frequently related to their sexual activity. Adolescent behavior regarding sexuality has been discussed here and in Chapter 12. Table 15-2 lists some of the common sexually transmitted diseases experienced by adolescents. Nurses need to be aware that diseases thought of as being sexually transmitted may be seen in younger children. Some of these such as chlamydia, gonorrhea, syphilis, and HIV (other than perinatally transmitted) can be suggestive of sexual abuse. If sexual abuse is suspected, it must be reported (see Chapter 36).

Intestinal parasites including parasitic worms and protozoa are described in Table 15-3.

Many infectious diseases are reportable by law to local and state health departments who, in turn, must report them to the CDC. At the CDC, information about the occurrence and nature of such diseases is collected. With this data, the CDC monitors trends of disease, evaluates the effectiveness of disease-focused interventions, and makes recommendations to health care agencies for infection control and prevention. Some of the diseases discussed in this chapter are among those required to be reported (Box 15-1). The list of reportable infectious diseases may change based on suspected prevalence of particular diseases. It is important that the pediatric nurse be familiar with the current list of reportable infectious diseases.

FUTURE DIRECTIONS

Since the introduction of immunization practices for children began in the 1940s, the recommendations and requirements for vaccines continue to evolve. Researchers continuously engage in the practice of seeking treatments and cures for disease, with a primary goal of prevention through vaccine development. As newer vaccines are developed, they must undergo strict research and FDA approval before their release. There is renewed development of a vaccine for rotavirus to replace the previous vaccine made from rhesus recombinant rotavirus that was withdrawn from the market due to an association with intussusception. As of May 2008, no association between RV5 vaccine for rotavirus and the risk for intussusception has been identified (AAP, 2009).

TABLE 15-2 Sexually Transmitted Diseases in Adolescents (*Continued*)

DISEASE	CLINICAL MANIFESTATIONS	ETIOLOGY	INCIDENCE/INCUBATION/ CONTROL	THERAPEUTIC MANAGEMENT
Gonorrhea 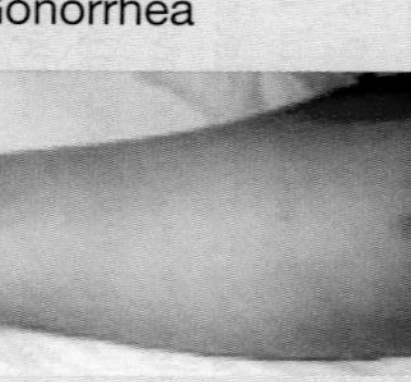 COURTESY OF THE CENTERS FOR DISEASE CONTROL AND PREVENTION (CDC).	**Female**: purulent discharge, urethritis, endocervicitis, pelvic inflammatory disease (PID) **Male**: purulent discharge, urethritis **Both sexes**: pharyngitis, conjunctivitis, proctitis **Neonates**: infection of the eyes; scalp abscess related to fetal monitor probe **Diagnosis**: Gram stain **Complications**: acute epididymitis, acute PID, arthritis, dermatitis, meningitis, disseminated gonococcal infection, infertility	*Neisseria gonorrhoeae* *a gram-negative diplo-coccus* **Transmission**: intimate contact, sexual intercourse, sexual abuse (sexual abuse should be considered when a diagnosis of gonorrhea is made in any child who is not sexually active), perinatal	**Incidence**: 132/100,000 in United States Highest rate reported in adolescents 15–19 years of age **Incubation**: 2–7 days **Control**: obtain an endocervical culture as part of prenatal care; evaluation for other sexually transmitted diseases; treatment of contacts; notification of public health officials	Administer ceftriaxone IM or cefixime PO in a single dose plus doxycycline twice a day for 7 days or azithromycin PO in a single dose. Evaluate for other STDs including syphilis, HIV, chlamydia, hepatitis B. Chlamydia occurs in 45% of cases of gonorrhea and should be treated. Encourage abstinence until treated and symptom free. Offer education regarding medication administration and importance of adherence to treatment regimen. Avoid sexual contact until cured. No need to return for test of cure one week after completing therapy unless symptoms persist.

(Continues)

Table 15-2 Sexually Transmitted Diseases in Adolescents (*Continued*)

DISEASE	CLINICAL MANIFESTATIONS	ETIOLOGY	INCIDENCE/INCUBATION/ CONTROL	THERAPEUTIC MANAGEMENT
Syphilis 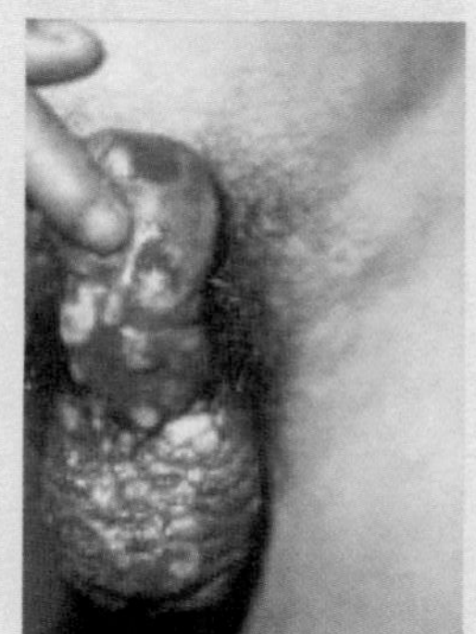 COURTESY OF THE CENTERS FOR DISEASE CONTROL AND PREVENTION (CDC).	**Congenital**: Stillbirth, prematurity, hydrops fetalis, multisystem sequelae including hepatosplenomegaly, mucocutaneous lesions, lymphadenopathy, thrombocytopenia **Acquired**: **Primary stage**: one or more painless ulcers of mucous membranes and skin usually on genitalia **Secondary stage**: maculopapular rash on palms and soles, fever, enlarged lymph glands, sore throat, headache, splenomegaly, arthralgia **Tertiary stage**: neurosyphilis, skin, bone or visceral changes, aortitis **Diagnosis**: serologic testing: VDRL, RPR **Complications**: if left untreated, client can experience manifestations of secondary and tertiary syphilis	*Treponema pallidum* spirochete **Transmission**: congenital; transplacental during pregnancy or at time of delivery **Acquired**: intimate contact, sexual intercourse, sexual abuse (sexual abuse should be considered when a diagnosis of acquired syphilis is made in any child who is not sexually active)	**Incidence**: 2.6 per 100,000 **Incubation**: 3 weeks with a range of 10–90 days **Control**: screen women early in pregnancy and at delivery; education and treatment of sexual contacts with reporting to public health authorities	**Congenital**: Administer aqueous crystalline penicillin GIV q12h for 7 days then q8h for 3 additional days for a total of 10 days or single dose of procaine penicillin G IM daily for 10 days. **Early acquired syphilis**: Primary, secondary, or tertiary of < 1 years duration. Administer single dose of benzathine penicillin G IM once. **Pregnancy**: Benzathine penicillin G IM two doses one week apart. **Penicillin allergy**: Administer tetracycline twice a day for 14 days or doxycycline twice a day for 14 days (this does not apply to clients who are pregnant). Offer education regarding the importance of adherence to medication administration. Advise client to refer sexual contacts for evaluation and treatment. Advise to avoid sexual activity until cured. Encourage follow-up to monitor serology as recommended. Instruct to use latex condoms to prevent further reinfection.

(Continues)

TABLE 15-2 Sexually Transmitted Diseases in Adolescents (*Continued*)

DISEASE	CLINICAL MANIFESTATIONS	ETIOLOGY	INCIDENCE/INCUBATION/ CONTROL	THERAPEUTIC MANAGEMENT
Chlamydia	Symptomatic or asymptomatic **Female**: mucopurulent cervicitis, urethritis, salpingitis, and proctitis **Male**: nongonococcal urethritis **Diagnosis**: chlamydia culture enzyme immunoassay for screening **Complications**: pelvic inflammatory disease, infertility, ectopic pregnancy **Neonates**: ophthalmia neonatorum, chlamydial pneumonia	*Chlamydia trachomatis* bacterial agent **Transmission**: sexual transmission In neonates, contact with infected genital tract during delivery	**Incidence**: 236/100,000 Most common STD in adults less than 25 years old Rate in pregnancy: 6–12% Rate during adolescence: as high as 37% **Incubation**: about a week **Control**: refer sexual contacts for evaluation and treatment Screen for infection during routine gynecological and prenatal exams	Administer doxycycline BID for 7 days or azithromycin 1 gram in a single dose or erythromycin QID for 7 days. Encourage abstinence until treated and symptom free. Offer education regarding medication administration and importance of adherence to the treatment regimen. Advise to avoid sexual contact until cured. Instruct in the use of latex condoms to prevent further reinfection.
Herpes genitalis (HSV-2) COURTESY OF THE CENTERS FOR DISEASE CONTROL AND PREVENTION (CDC).	Characterized by periods of latency between initial outbreak and recurrence **Primary infection**: itching or intense burning at site of outbreak; may be accompanied by flu-like symptoms; inguinal lymphadenopathy Initial lesions are painful raised vesicles Recurrent lesions are less painful and resolve more quickly Virus can be shed when client is asymptomatic and is contagious	*Herpes Simplex type 2* virus **Transmission**: in neonates, acquired during pregnancy through the placenta or contact with infected genital tract during delivery Sexual intercourse	**Incidence**: 1 out of 5 adults over age 12 30,000,000 cases annually **Incubation**: 2 days to 2 weeks **Control**: abstinence during outbreak; use of condoms at other times since transmission has been noted without evidence of lesions	No effective cure **Primary lesions**: administer oral acyclovir within 6 days of onset to shorten median duration of viral shedding from primary lesion and signs and symptoms by 3–5 days. **Recurrent lesions**: administer oral acyclovir within 2 days of symptom onset to shorten clinical course. Oral acyclovir decreases frequency of recurrence (6 or more episodes per year).

(Continues)

TABLE 15-2 Sexually Transmitted Diseases in Adolescents (*Continued*)

DISEASE	CLINICAL MANIFESTATIONS	ETIOLOGY	INCIDENCE/INCUBATION/ CONTROL	THERAPEUTIC MANAGEMENT
	Diagnosis: viral culture **Complications**: in newborns, generalized systemic infection including CNS and liver involvement; infections of skin, eyes, and mouth; high mortality rate in neonatal herpes infection			Valacyclovir and famciclovir can also be used. Counsel about asymptomatic viral shedding and potential for recurrent outbreaks. Keep lesions clean and dry. Encourage abstinence during active stage when lesions are present. Advise use of latex condoms to prevent infection in sexual partners.
Human papilloma-virus (HPV) 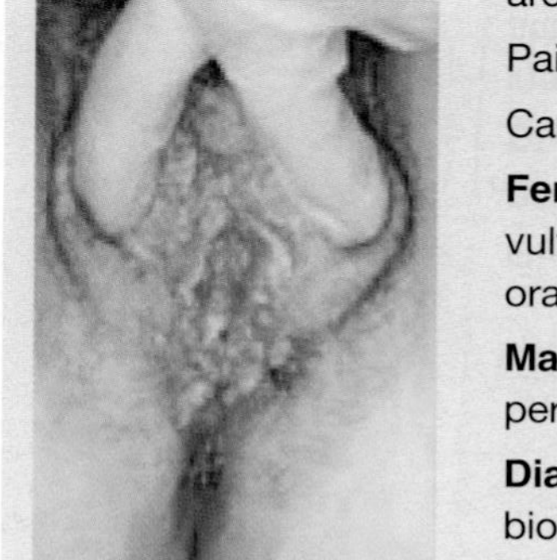 COURTESY OF THE CENTERS FOR DISEASE CONTROL AND PREVENTION (CDC).	Soft, fleshy, single or multiple papules which occur in the anogenital area and are known as genital warts Pain, pruritus Can be asymptomatic or subclinical **Female**: warts located on perineum, vulva, cervix, vagina, urethra, anus, oral cavity **Male**: warts located on penis, perineum, anus, oral cavity **Diagnosis**: clinical presentation; biopsy **Complications**: cervical, anal, or vaginal dysplasia Can lead to cervical cancer Reoccurrence	*Human papillomavirus* Over 20 types; most common types 6 or 11 **Transmission**: direct sexual contact; perinatal contact during delivery	**Incidence**: 50 per 100,000 population—3,000,000 cases annually **Incubation**: 3 months to several years **Control**: encourage sexual partner to be examined Counseling sex partner of client with HPV Cervical cancer screening for female partner of client with HPV Immunization of females ages 11–12 years with HPV4 vaccine is recommended.	Treatment depends on the location of the lesions. **Client application**: instruct client in self-application of Podofilox 0.5% solution or gel RID for 3 days, or Imiquimod 5% cream for 16 weeks. **Provider application**: Administer cryotherapy with liquid nitrogen every 1–2 weeks. Apply odophyllin resin 10–25% application to lesions every week. Apply trichloroacetic acid to lesions weekly. Assist in surgical removal by excision or laser surgery.

(Continues)

TABLE 15-2 Sexually Transmitted Diseases in Adolescents (*Continued*)

DISEASE	CLINICAL MANIFESTATIONS	ETIOLOGY	INCIDENCE/INCUBATION/CONTROL	THERAPEUTIC MANAGEMENT
	Laryngeal papilloma in newborn			Provide client with patient education regarding need for periodic screening for cervical cancer as well as examination of sexual partners for presence of warts.
Hepatitis B (HBV)	General fatigue, muscle and joint pain, loss of appetite **Diagnosis**: history of illness including sexual history, IV drug use, hepatitis panel **Complications**: chronic carrier state Chronic persistent hepatitis Progressive liver disease with cirrhosis or hepatocellular carcinoma	*Hepadnavirus* **Transmission**: contact with infected blood or body fluids; sexual contact, perinatal transmission	**Incidence**: 10,258 new cases 5–10% become chronic carriers **Incubation**: average 90 days with a range of 45–160 days Infected person can infect others approximately 4–6 weeks before symptoms appear **Control**: prenatal screening; universal precautions; immunoprophylaxis with hepatitis B vaccine Condom use for sexual activity	No specific treatment. Symptomatic management. Administer interferon alpha-2b antiviral medication, which is 40% effective in eliminating chronic HBV infection. Administer hepatitis B immune globulin when exposed to HBV. Offer counseling for clients who are chronic carriers of hepatitis B.
Human immunodeficiency virus (HIV type 1, more common in United States; HIV type 2, more common in West Africa)	Symptomatology of acute retroviral syndrome including fever, sore throat, skin rash, lymphadenopathy, malaise, arthralgia, myalgia, headache, nausea, and vomiting **Diagnosis**: HIV RNA PCR test in infants less than 18 months of age HIV antibody test in infants and children greater than 18 months of age and Western blot HIV culture	*Retrovirus, RNA virus* **Transmission**: contact with infected blood or body fluids; sexual contact, perinatal transmission	**Incidence**: 40,000–80,000 new infections annually **Incubation**: signs and symptoms may appear 2–12 weeks after infection; seroconversion (the ability of antibodies to HIV to be detected in the blood) may not occur until 4–12 weeks or longer after infection; the period when antibodies remain undetected is known as the "window period"	No known cure. Informed consent necessary to obtain HIV testing. Pre-and posttest counseling by trained professionals is essential to discuss the options for treatment if a test is positive.

(Continues)

TABLE 15-2 Sexually Transmitted Diseases in Adolescents (*Continued*)

DISEASE	CLINICAL MANIFESTATIONS	ETIOLOGY	INCIDENCE/INCUBATION/ CONTROL	THERAPEUTIC MANAGEMENT
	Complications: progression to AIDS as late manifestation (in 85% of cases within 17 years after infection) Opportunistic infections such as *Pneumocystis carinii pneumonia* (PCP), Kaposi's sarcoma (KS), *Mycobacterium avium complex* (MAC), AIDS		**Control**: avoid sex with individuals having multiple partner use; consistent use of latex condoms; avoid needle sharing; offer testing to HIV positive women during pregnancy; offer rapid HIV testing at time of delivery if HIV status is unknown	Treatment assists to slow the decline of the immune system. Current treatment includes highly active antiretroviral therapy (HAART) consisting of four classifications of medications: nucleoside reverse transcriptase inhibitors; nonnucleoside reverse transcriptase inhibitors; protease inhibitors; and fusion inhibitors. Treatment is individualized based on the clients' immune status and sensitivity to the specific drug. Treatment goals include maintaining high CD4 counts and decreased viral loads. Counseling, social support, behavioral change, referral for care.

Adapted from American Academy of Pediatrics (2009). *2009 Red Book: Report of the committee on infectious diseases* (28th ed.). Elk Grove Village, IL: Author; and Centers for Disease Control and Prevention (CDC). (2006). 2006 guidelines for treatment of sexually transmitted diseases. *Morbidity and Mortality Weekly Report, 55(RR11)*, 1–94.

Table 15-3 Intestinal Parasites (including Helminths [parasitic worms] and Protozoa)

DISEASE	CLINICAL MANIFESTATIONS	ETIOLOGY	INCIDENCE/INCUBATION/ CONTROL	THERAPEUTIC MANAGEMENT
Giardia	May be asymptomatic; chronic or relapsing diarrhea (may be watery or greasy, foul-smelling); crampy abdominal pain; anorexia leading to weight loss and failure to thrive; flatulence **Diagnosis**: identification of cysts in fecal sample or enzyme immunoassay to detect *G. intestinalis* antigens **Complications**: lactose intolerance	*Giardia intestinalis,* a protozoan **Transmission**: humans are main reservoir, but the organisms can infect dogs, cats, beavers, and other animals; animals can contaminate water with feces containing cysts; direct transmission: hand-to-mouth transfer of cysts from feces of infected person; indirect: ingestion of cyst-contaminated water or food	**Incidence**: more common in children than adults; endemic in areas of world with poor sanitation; associated with day care centers and residential institutions for the mentally retarded **Incubation**: 1–4 weeks **Control**: improved sanitation and personal hygiene in day care centers; good hand washing, especially after diapering infants and toileting; exclude infected child from day care centers until diarrhea resolves; educate families who camp and hike to avoid drinking water from streams	Drug of choice furazolidone (Furoxone); other drugs available: quinacrine hydrochloride (Atabrine) and metronidazole (Flagyl).
Pinworms (enterobius)	Nocturnal anal itching, sleeplessness **Diagnosis**: direct visualization of worms or microscopy; eggs detected on transparent tape pressed against perianal region in morning before child has a bowel movement **Complications**: movement of worm to appendix, female genital tract, and peritoneal cavity	*Enterobius vermicularis* **Transmission**: fecal-oral; ingestion or inhalation of eggs of worm; eggs are transmitted by fingers and hands from scratching anal area; eggs remain infective in indoor environment for 2–3 weeks and contaminate anything they contact such as shared toys, bedding, clothing, toilet seats, baths, and food	**Incidence**: most common helminth infection in United States; occurs frequently in preschoolers and school-age children, crowded conditions, institutions, and families **Incubation**: 1–2 months **Control**: good handwashing after contact with infected child, bed linens, clothes, after toileting and before eating; keep child's fingernails short to minimize chance of eggs collecting under nails from scratching	Drug of choice: mebedazole (Vermox) or pyrantel pamoate (Antiminth); all household members are treated simultaneously.

(Continues)

TABLE 15-3 Intestinal Parasites (including Helminths [parasitic worms] and Protozoa) (*Continued*)

DISEASE	CLINICAL MANIFESTATIONS	ETIOLOGY	INCIDENCE/INCUBATION/ CONTROL	THERAPEUTIC MANAGEMENT
Ascariasis	Mild infection: asymptomatic; moderate infection: abdominal pain, distention, enlarged abdomen, anorexia, weight loss, fever **Diagnosis**: eggs can be detected by microscopic stool examination **Complications**: intestinal obstruction, pulmonary involvement (pneumonitis) with cough and blood-stained sputum, perforation of intestines by migration of worms resulting in peritonitis, obstruction of common bile duct by migration of worms	*Ascoris lumbricoides,* a roundworm **Transmission**: ingestion of eggs via contact with contaminated soil, food, fingers, and toys; food can be contaminated wherever human feces are used as fertilizer	**Incidence**: most common in warm climates, in areas of poor sanitation; most prevalent in young children ages 1–4 years **Incubation**: prolonged, as the life cycle of the worm is 4–8 weeks, and feces contain eggs About 2 months after ingestion of embryonated eggs **Control**: sanitary disposal of feces; treatment of human feces before use as a fertilizer; vegetables cultivated in areas where human feces fertilizer is used must be thoroughly cooked or soaked in a dilute iodine solution before eating	Mebedazole (Vermox) or pyrantel pamoate (Antiminth); reexamination of stools 3 weeks after therapy to determine if worms have been eliminated; if partial or complete intestinal obstruction due to large number of worms, administer piperazine citrate (Piperazine) via NG tube which paralyzes worms and allows them to be passed easier

Adapted from American Academy of Pediatrics. (2009). *2009 Red Book: Report of the committee on infectious diseases* (28th ed.). Elk Grove Village, IL: Author.

BOX 15-1
SELECTED INFECTIOUS DISEASES THAT MUST BE REPORTED TO THE CENTERS FOR DISEASE CONTROL AND PREVENTION

- Acquired immunodeficiency syndrome (AIDS)
- Anthrax
- Chancroid
- *Chlamydia trachomatis,* genital infections
- Diphtheria
- Encephalitis, post chickenpox and mumps
- Gonorrhea
- Hepatitis A, B, and C
- Human immunodeficiency (HIV) infection, adult and pediatric
- Lyme disease
- Measles
- Meningococcal disease
- Mumps
- Paralytic polio
- Pertussis
- Rocky Mountain spotted fever
- Rubella
- Syphilis, all stages
- Tetanus
- Tuberculosis
- Varicella deaths

Adapted from American Academy of Pediatrics. (2009). *2009 Red book: Report of the committee on infectious diseases* (28th ed.). Elk Grove Village, IL: American Academy of Pediatrics.

A new vaccine, pneumococcal conjugate (Prevnar), has been developed for pneumococcus (*Streptococcus pneumoniae*), the most common cause of sepsis, sinusitis, pneumonia, otitis media, and meningitis in children under the age of 2. Previously, a form of vaccine, pneumococcal polysaccharide (Pneumovax, Pnu-Imune), was shown to be effective for children over 2 years of age and given to those who had chronic illnesses such as HIV infection and sickle cell anemia. It was not recommended for younger children (younger than 2 years of age) and infants because of poor antibody response. However, the new vaccine, Prevnar, has proven to be highly effective at inducing the desired response and preventing infection in children under 2 years old and infants. Therefore, it is recommended that all children receive it at the 2, 4, 6, and 12–15 months visits (AAP, 2009).

Although deaths from infectious diseases decreased markedly during the past century, there has been an increase in mortality over the past two decades, attributable in part to the emergence of new pathogens, specifically HIV. Influenza continues to re-emerge periodically and cause epidemics. *Mycobacterium tuberculosis,* which includes new drug-resistant strains, has made a comeback and is especially devastating to those infected with the HIV virus. Drug resistance due to the overuse of antibiotics has presented some distinct challenges, as noted by the growing incidence of penicillin-resistant *Streptococcal pneumoniae,* vancomycin-resistant enterococci, and methicillin-resistant *Staphylococcus aureus.* There are several factors that have contributed to this phenomenon, including population growth and crowding; increased use of day care and community living centers; destruction of natural habitats; increasing numbers of persons who are immunosuppressed; aging of the

CASE STUDY / CARE PLAN

A CHILD WITH PERTUSSIS

Marcus is a 3 ½ month old African-American male who lives with his mother and father and 4-year-old brother Jerome. Marcus and his brother attend a day care center while both of their parents work. Both boys have returned home from day care today and their mother notices that Marcus has a cough, nasal congestion and secretions, and a slight elevation in temperature to 99 degrees F. Jerome is asymptomatic. Marcus' mother cooks supper for the family and proceeds to breastfeed Marcus. She notes that Marcus is coughing more, is not interested in breastfeeding, and is irritable. Later in the evening, Marcus' cough becomes worse and his mother notes that on occasion he is cyanotic. She calls the patient advisory nurse at the pediatric clinic and the nurse advises her to take Marcus to the ER immediately. At the ER a history and physical are done including immunizations. Marcus is up-to-date on all immunizations, but because of his age he is not fully immune to pertussis. After testing, it is determined that Marcus has pertussis and is admitted to the pediatric unit for treatment. Marcus' mother is concerned about her other son and whether he will develop pertussis as well. The nurse assures her that since Jerome's immunizations are current for his age he is probably protected. However, for Jerome, his parents and any other close contacts, it is recommended that they receive chemoprophylaxis to limit secondary transmission regardless of immunization status (AAP, 2009). The day care center and all personnel will be notified of Marcus' illness and appropriate treatment will be given. Marcus will remain in the hospital for at least five days and will be placed in droplet isolation and will receive O_2 by nasal cannula as needed and Azithromycin for five days.

(Continues)

CASE STUDY / CARE PLAN (Continued)

ASSESSMENT

The nurse should obtain a history of Marcus' exposure to pertussis whooping cough. Marcus' immunization status needs to be determined; in other words, if and when he was given the DTaP vaccine. Ask about his current symptoms. During the physical examination, note the respiratory symptoms and any complications. Obtain his vital signs. Assess for associated manifestations such as apnea, cyanosis, and poor feeding.

NURSING DIAGNOSIS 1

Ineffective breathing pattern related to inflamed bronchial passages and coughing.

EXPECTED OUTCOMES

1. Marcus will have oxygen saturations that support the ability to breathe with comfort.
2. Marcus will demonstrate a breathing pattern that will support blood gas results within normal parameters.
3. Marcus will not have any prolonged apneic or cyanotic episodes.

NOC: Respiratory Status: Airway Patency, Ventilation, Vital Signs
NIC: Airway Management; Respiratory Monitoring

INTERVENTIONS/*RATIONALES*

1. Place Marcus on continuous cardiac-respiratory monitoring. *To assess for changes in cardiopulmonary status.*
2. Monitor respiratory rate, depth, and ease of respirations and assess for use of accessory muscles and retractions. *To assess for signs of worsening respiratory condition.*
3. Monitor oxygen saturation on a continuous basis as ordered. *To assess for hypoxia (oxygen saturation of less than 93%).*
4. Monitor arterial blood gases as ordered by physician. *To assess for acidosis/alkalosis.*

EVALUATION

Marcus' respiratory rate is 70 per minute and he has mild subcostal retractions. He is on oxygen at 1 L/minute by nasal cannula and his SaO_2 is 93%. He has had no episodes of apnea or cyanosis.

NURSING DIAGNOSIS 2

Ineffective airway clearance related to excessive nasal and tracheobronchial secretions.

EXPECTED OUTCOMES

1. Marcus will maintain a patent airway at all times.
2. Marcus will demonstrate clear breath sounds after suctioning.
3. Parents will demonstrate understanding of use of bulb syringe for suctioning for home use.

NOC: Respiratory Status: Airway Patency, Gas Exchange, Ventilation
NIC: Airway Management, Airway Suctioning, Cough Enhancement; Teaching Treatment

INTERVENTIONS/*RATIONALES*

1. Auscultate breath sounds every one to two hours and suction as necessary. *To assess for increased mucus in airways and lungs.*
2. Monitor respiratory pattern including rate, depth, and effort every two hours. *To assess for changes in ease of respirations.*
3. Teach Marcus' mother to suction his nose and mouth using a bulb syringe for home use. *To prepare for discharge to home.*

(Continues)

CASE STUDY / CARE PLAN (Continued)

EVALUATION

Marcus requires frequent suctioning of his nasopharynx because of excess secretions. His mother and father have been taught the use of a bulb syringe for suctioning Marcus after discharge from the hospital. They demonstrate correct technique and understand the rationale for bulb syringe suctioning.

EVIDENCE-BASED PRACTICE

Use of Oral Erythromycin in the Treatment of Pertussis in Infants Younger Than One Month of Age

CLINICAL PROBLEM

Is there an association between orally administered erythromycin and infantile hypertrophic pyloric stenosis?

BEST CLINICAL PRACTICE

Prevention. Pertussis is a vaccine preventable disease (caused by the Bordetella Pertussis virus) with a declining incidence related to the increased use of pertussis vaccine in children and adolescents. Erythromycin has been the drug of choice for treatment of pertussis or for chemoprophylaxis for close contacts of the patient with pertussis.

Treatment. There is some evidence, in a cohort study, that orally administered erythromycin to infants younger than one month of age is associated with infantile hypertrophic pyloric stenosis (IHPS). The American Academy of Pediatrics recommends the use of azithromycin as the drug of choice for infants younger than one month of age for treatment or prophylaxis of pertussis.

IMPLICATIONS FOR NURSING

- Nurses should encourage families to have all children, adolescents, and adults immunized against pertussis.
- Nurses need to identify children less than one month of age who are at risk for development of pertussis secondary to incomplete immunization status. Nurses should be aware of infants less than one month of age who are prescribed erythromycin for pertussis and inform caregivers of the risks of IHPS.

Reference: Centers for Disease Control and Prevention. (2005). Recommended antimicrobial agents for the treatment and postexposure prophylaxis of pertussis: 2005 CDC guidelines. *Morbidity and Mortality Weekly Report, 54*(RR14), 1–16.

population; use of antimicrobial drugs; and globalization of food distribution, commerce, and travel. Influenza vaccine should be administered to children who have chronic illnesses and are susceptible to respiratory disease and pneumonia. In addition, infants and small children between 6 and 23 months should receive influenza vaccine, as they are more likely to have severe respiratory illness due to influenza.

Other advances include research in the development of vaccines for human immunodeficiency virus, herpes simplex virus, and respiratory syncytial virus. Another study is exploring the use of nasal routes for vaccines against organisms that are transmitted via this method. Currently, the influenza vaccine is available as a nasal preparation.

A new approach to adolescent immunization is under consideration that includes not only hepatitis B vaccine, but also protection against meningococcal meningitis, pertussis, and hepatitis A. Nurses who interact with adolescents must be aware of the changes to educate their clients and families to increase protection against these particular infectious diseases.

As a consequence of the events of September 11, 2001, the world has been awakened to the threat of new terrors from infectious diseases such as smallpox and anthrax. Re-education about the dangers of these diseases must be ongoing. Health care clinicians have a heightened awareness of the use of biologic agents to create public health havoc and the Centers for Disease Control and Prevention (CDC) continue to increase preparedness in case of potential outbreaks.

The interplay of infectious diseases and the normal course of growth and development in humans is evident. Nurses have a unique opportunity to intervene at many levels and in many ways. The broad-based education of professional nurses gives them the foundation for

IN THE REAL WORLD

Quote from a veteran nurse with over 15 years of working in ambulatory pediatrics: "When I first became a nurse, the recommendations for immunizations were relatively simple. Now, if it weren't for the continued updates, I would be lost. As newer vaccines are developed, I have to keep abreast of all of the latest requirements. It keeps you on your toes and alert to assessing every child at every instance in order to keep up the level of protection."

assessment, planning, intervention, and education. The information regarding infectious diseases is constantly changing as new vaccines and drug therapy are developed. Health professionals have a better understanding of the distinctive properties of infectious agents and can better inform the public as to ways of prevention and treatment so that these illnesses may be kept to a minimum and eventually eradicated.

KEY CONCEPTS

- The transmission of disease is dependent upon six factors, which are referred to as the chain of infection.
- The development of children's immune systems begins early in fetal life. The intrauterine environment does not always protect children from contracting infectious illnesses.
- Handwashing is the best defense against the spread of infectious disease.
- The transmission of many infectious diseases can be traced to the developmental stage of children. Certain behaviors make children more vulnerable to infectious illnesses at different ages.
- Immunizations play a major role in the prevention of illness, and in reducing morbidity and mortality. Caregivers need to be instructed in the importance of this preventative health care measure.
- Health care personnel who administer immunizations must be knowledgeable about the rationale, care and handling, administration, and effects of each specific vaccine.
- Treatment of infectious disease is aimed at the reduction of symptomatology. Pharmacological therapy such as antibacterial, antiviral, and antifungal medications may be prescribed depending upon the etiology of the illness.
- The prevalence of sexual intercourse as well as the rate of sexually transmitted diseases (STDs) has increased among adolescents.
- Adolescents need to be assessed for the possibility of STDs.
- Caregivers can adequately care for children with infectious diseases at home. Most caregivers can be taught how to provide supportive care for their children.
- It is important for the nurse to understand the laws and policies related to communicable disease including reporting the incidence of certain diseases.

REVIEW ACTIVITIES

1. Explain why infants and children are more prone to infection than adults.
2. When should caregivers be instructed about immunizations?
3. Identify strategies to facilitate adherence to immunization schedules from infancy through adolescence.
4. Identify the common ways in which infants and children facilitate the spread of infectious disease.
5. Explain why acetaminophen is the drug of choice when treating viral illnesses.
6. What should be included in a plan to teach the staff of a day care center how to prevent the spread of illness?
7. What factors are associated with the spread of STDs in adolescents?
8. Explain why adolescents with herpetic lesions may be at risk for developing HIV infection.
9. Discuss the rationale for reporting certain infectious diseases to the proper health authorities.

STUDY QUESTIONS

1. Which of the following is described as the time from exposure to an infectious disease to the appearance of the first symptom?
   a. incubation period
   b. communicable period
   c. prodromal period
   d. desquamation period
2. Primary prevention of a communicable disease results from which of the following?
   a. strict hand washing
   b. immunizations
   c. early diagnosis and treatment
   d. isolation

3. A child who is receiving chemotherapy for leukemia has been exposed to chicken pox at school. The nurse should recommend which of the following?
   a. no precautions are necessary
   b. Varicella-Zoster immune globulin (VZIG) to prevent chicken pox
   c. Acyclovir (Zovirax) to minimize symptoms of the virus
   d. stopping chemotherapy
4. Which factor places an adolescent at the highest risk of contracting an STI?
   a. protected sexual intercourse
   b. multiple sexual partners in a short duration
   c. low income level
   d. smoking
5. What is the single most important factor in decreasing transmission of infection in a day care center?
   a. separation of children who are ill
   b. washing all toys daily
   c. meticulous hand hygiene
   d. outdoor playtime
6. In treating pain or fever associated with a viral illness, caregivers should be instructed to use which medication(s)?
   a. aspirin
   b. acetaminophen
   c. ibuprofen
   d. either acetaminophen or ibuprofen
7. Which of the following is an appropriate intervention to relieve itching associated with chicken pox?
   a. application of a thick coat of calamine lotion
   b. frequent warm baths
   c. give an antipruritic medication such as diphenhydramine (Benadryl)
   d. give aspirin or acetaminophen
8. When should caregivers be instructed about immunizations?
   a. at the time of an infant's birth
   b. at the first clinic visit for the newborn (approximately 2 weeks of age)
   c. only if the caregiver has questions about the immunization
   d. before any immunization is administered
9. An important role of the ambulatory care nurse or school nurse is the identification of communicable diseases for treatment and the prevention of the spread of the disease. An important component is the recognition of which aspect of the disease?
   a. the source
   b. the prodromal stage
   c. the causative agent
   d. the constitutional symptoms
10. A mother tells the nurse that she does not want her infant immunized because of the discomfort associated with the injections. The nurse should explain that:
    a. infants do not feel pain like older children and adults do.
    b. there is nothing that can be done about the pain and it does not last long.
    c. this is not a good reason to refuse immunizations.
    d. a topical anesthetic such as EMLA cream can be used before the injection.

REFERENCES

American Academy of Pediatrics. (2009). *2009 Red Book: Report of the Committee on Infectious Diseases* (28th ed.). Elk Grove Village, IL: American Academy of Pediatrics.

Centers for Disease Control and Prevention. (2005). Recommended antimicrobial agents for the treatment and postexposure prophylaxis of pertussis: 2005 CDC guidelines. *Morbidity and Mortality Weekly Report, 54*(RR14), 1–16.

Centers for Disease Control and Prevention. (2006). 2006 guidelines for treatment of sexually transmitted diseases. *Morbidity and Mortality Weekly Report, 55*(RR11), 1–100.

Centers for Disease Control and Prevention. (2007a). Prevention of varicella recommendations of the advisory committee on immunization practices (ACIP). *Morbidity and Mortality Weekly Report, 56(RR04)*, 21.

Centers for Disease Control and Prevention (2007b). *Health protection goals and objectives.* Retrieved June 13, 2009, from http://www.cdc.gov/osi/goals/people/index.html.

Centers for Disease Control and Prevention. (2008a). Update: Recommendation from the Advisory Committee on Immunization Practices (ACIP) Regarding administration of combination MMRV vaccine. *Morbidity and Mortality Weekly Report, 57*(10), 258–260.

Centers for Disease Control and Prevention. (2008b). Trends in HIV- and STD-related risk behaviors among high school students—United States, 1991–2007. *Morbidity and Mortality Weekly Report, 57*(30), 817–822.

Centers for Disease Control and Prevention. (2009). *Epidemiology and prevention of vaccine-preventable diseases* (11th ed.). Atlanta, GA: U.S. Department of Health and Human Services.

D'Souza, Y., Fombonne, E., & Ward, B. (2006). No evidence of persisting measles virus in peripheral blood mononuclear cells from children with autism spectrum disorder. *Pediatrics, 118*, 1664–1675.

Jain, N., Stokley, S., & Yankey, D. Centers for Disease Control and Prevention. (2008). Vaccination coverage among adolescents aged 13–17 years—United States 2007. *Morbidity and Mortality Weekly Report, 57*(40), 1100–1103.

Warraich, H. J. (2009). Religious opposition to polio vaccination (letter). *Emergency Infectious Disease.*

SUGGESTED READINGS

Bulechek, G., Butcher, H., & Dochterman, J. (2008). *Nursing interventions classification (NIC)* (5th ed.). St. Louis, MO: Elsevier Health Sciences.

Centers for Disease Control and Prevention. (2006). Update: Guillain-Barré syndrome among recipients of Menactra meningococcal conjugate vaccine, United States, June 2005–September 2006, *Morbidity and Mortality Weekly Report, 55*(41), 1120–1124.

Hognig, M., Briese, T., Buie, T., Bauman, M., Lauwers, G., Siemetzki, U., Hummel, K., Rota, P. A., Bellini, W. J., O'Leary, J. J., Sheils, O., Alden, E., Pickering, L., & Lipkin, W. I. (2008). Lack of association between measles viral vaccine and autism with enteropathy: A case control study. *PLoS One 3*(9), e3140.

Moorhead, S., Johnson, M., Maas, M., & Swanson, E. (2008). *Nursing outcomes classification (NOC)* (4th ed.). St. Louis, MO: Elsevier Health Sciences.

Rupp, R., Rosenthal, S., & Middleman, A. (2006). Vaccination: An opportunity to enhance early adolescent preventative services. *Journal of Adolescent Health, 39*, 461–464.

Schecter, N., Zempsky, W., & Cohen, L., McGrath, P., McMurtry, M., & Bright, N. (2007). Pain reduction during pediatric immunizations: Evidence-based review and recommendations. *Pediatrics, 119*(5), e1184–e1198.

Smith, M., Ellenberg, S., Bell, L., & Rubin, D. (2008). Media coverage of the measles-mumps-rubella vaccine and autism controversy and its relationship to MMR immunization rates in the United States. *Pediatrics, 21*(4), e836–e843.

Vessey, J., Sherwood, J., Warner, D., & Clark, D. (2007). Comparing hand washing to hand sanitizers in reducing elementary school students' absenteeism. *Pediatric Nursing, 33*(4), 368–372.

SUGGESTED READINGS FOR CHILDREN

Bakalar, N. (2007). *Where the germs are.* New York: John Wiley & Sons, Inc.

Karlen, A. (2008). *Biography of a germ.* New York: Pantheon Books.

Kornberg, A., & Alaniz, A. (2007). *Germ stories.* Sausalito, CA: University Science Books.

Verdick, E., & Heilnlen, M. (2006). *Germs are not for sharing.* Minneapolis, MN: Free Spirit Publishing Co., Inc.

RESOURCES

Refer to the online student StudyWARE for Potts & Mandleco at http://www.CengageBrain.com for additional content and study aids.

Organization: **Association for Professionals in Infection Control and Epidemiology**
Description: APIC's mission is to improve health and patient safety by reducing risks of infection and other adverse outcomes. APIC's members include nurses, epidemiologists, physicians, quality and patient safety professionals, health care executives, microbiologists, clinical pathologists, laboratory technologists, and public health practitioners. The website offers users information regarding membership services, education, certification, research, and guidelines/standards.
Website/Resource: http://www.apic.org

Organization: **Centers for Disease Control and Prevention**
Description: The Centers for Disease Control and Prevention (CDC) serves as the national focus for developing and applying disease prevention and control, environmental health, and health promotion and health education activities designed to improve the health of the people of the United States. The CDC website offers readers information regarding current disease conditions, emergency preparedness and response, life stages and populations, healthy living, workplace environment and health, traveler's health, and much more.
Website/Resource: http://www.cdc.gov

Organization: **Immunization Action Coalition**
Description: The Immunization Action Coalition (IAC) works to increase immunization rates and prevent disease by creating and distributing educational materials for health professionals and the public that enhance the delivery of safe and effective immunization services. The Coalition also facilitates communication about the safety, efficacy, and use of vaccines within the broad immunization community of patients, parents, health care organizations, and government health agencies. The website offers users information regarding publications, subscriptions, news, photos, and videos.
Website/Resource: http://www.immunize.org

Organization: **National Immunization Program**
Description: *The Pink Book—Epidemiology and Prevention of Vaccine-Preventable Diseases* can be downloaded from the CDC website.
Website/Resource: http://www.cdc.gov/vaccines

Organization: **National Vaccine Injury Compensation Program**
U.S. Department of Health and Human Services Health Resources and Services Administration
Description: The National Vaccine Injury Compensation Program (VICP) was established to ensure an adequate supply of vaccines, stabilize vaccine costs, and establish and maintain an accessible and efficient forum for individuals found to be injured by certain vaccines. The VICP is a no-fault alternative to the traditional tort system for resolving vaccine injury claims that provides compensation to people found to be injured by certain vaccines. The website offers users information regarding covered vaccines and filing a claim.
Website/Resource: http://www.hrsa.gov/vaccinecompensation/

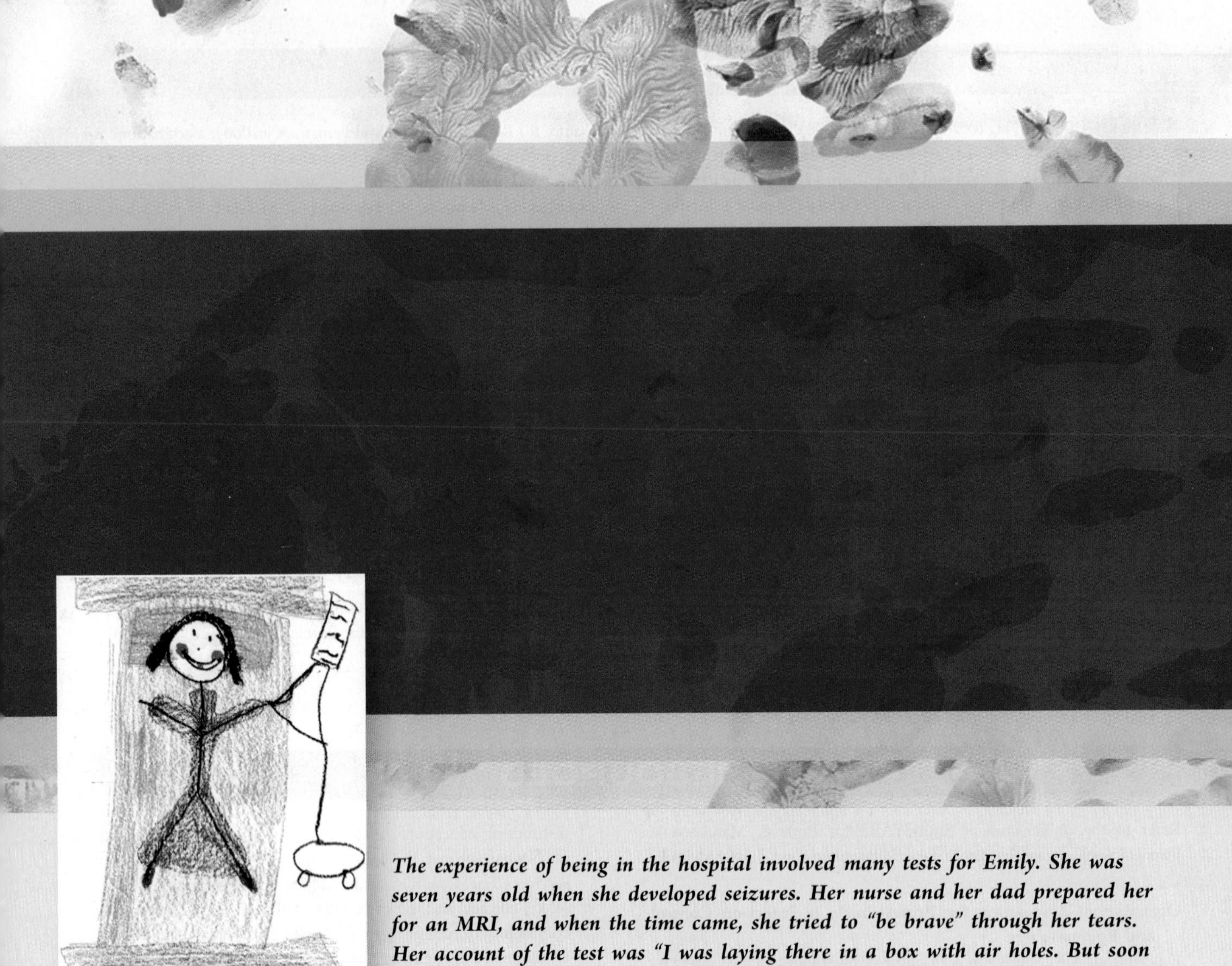

DRAWING BY E. SUMNER (PUBLISHED WITH PERMISSION OF MASSGENERAL HOSPITAL FOR CHILDREN)

The experience of being in the hospital involved many tests for Emily. She was seven years old when she developed seizures. Her nurse and her dad prepared her for an MRI, and when the time came, she tried to "be brave" through her tears. Her account of the test was "I was laying there in a box with air holes. But soon there was a sound like a fire alarm. I cried but if you move your head you have to do the test all over again … if you are still scared, whoever takes you can hold your hand."

—Sumner, 2006

CHAPTER 16

Care of Children Who are Hospitalized

E. Ann Sheridan, RN, MS, EdD
Sheila Q. Rucki, RN, PCNS, BC, PhD

COMPETENCIES

Upon completion of this chapter, the reader will be able to:

- Discuss the effects of illness and hospitalization on children, their caregivers, and their families.
- Discuss contributions of theorists and nurse researchers in understanding phenomena and intervention efforts related to the experiences of children and families during illness and hospitalization.
- Apply the factors that help children cope with illness and hospitalization to practice.
- Apply family-centered and participative nursing models to the care of hospitalized children and their families.
- Discuss the strengths and attributes which facilitate coping and healing processes for children and their caregivers and how nurses might apply that information to the care of hospitalized children.
- Discuss how caregiver attitudes and coping skills affect children's responses and abilities in regards to illness and hospitalization; apply that information to the care of hospitalized children.
- Apply knowledge of growth and development to appropriate nursing interventions that reduce stress and promote coping.
- Discuss the importance of delineating clear clinical outcomes related to the psychosocial health of children and evaluating these outcomes to determine the effectiveness of nursing interventions.
- Successfully complete the games and activities in the online student StudyWARE.

Millions of children under 17 years of age are hospitalized each year in the United States. Whether planned or unplanned, it is a time of stress and challenge for children and families because they are thrust into experiences of unknowns, uncertainties, and discontents. Some children and families are simultaneously coping with other untoward circumstances and recent disruptions in their lives such as ongoing physical, behavioral, or learning problems; recent losses or separations; and other major changes or difficulties in relationships. At this time of crisis, pediatric nurses play a vital role in establishing and maintaining trusting relationships with children and their families and responding to their needs for competent, compassionate care and guidance. When assuming this professional responsibility, it is essential to have learned the art and science of caring for ill and hospitalized children and the philosophy of family-centered care.

Developing the attributes of the expert pediatric nurse begins with understanding the nature and culture of childhood in a multicultural society, stages of growth and development, and mastery of basic knowledge and skill in the care of ill and injured children. Simulation learning laboratories and extensive supervised clinical experiences provide opportunities to apply this information to practice, thereby allowing nurses to gain confidence and competence in the field (Figure 16-1). The most difficult aspect of learning is the process of using reflective, critical thinking skills to select those facts, concepts, principles, and research findings relevant to individual situations and then to make reasoned decisions in the implementation and evaluation of nursing care.

Pediatric nursing is dynamic and challenging, owing to the increasing complexity and intensity of this sphere of nursing practice. There is continuous generation of knowledge and expansion of understanding about the nature of child development and the experience of childhood illness/hospitalization. Current practices, policies, and curricula in the care of children in hospitals have evolved over several decades. Pediatric nursing as a specialized area is inextricably bound to the leaders/events of the past. Therefore, it is initially important to understand how the history of pediatrics and pediatric nursing has led to refinement in the care of children in hospitals.

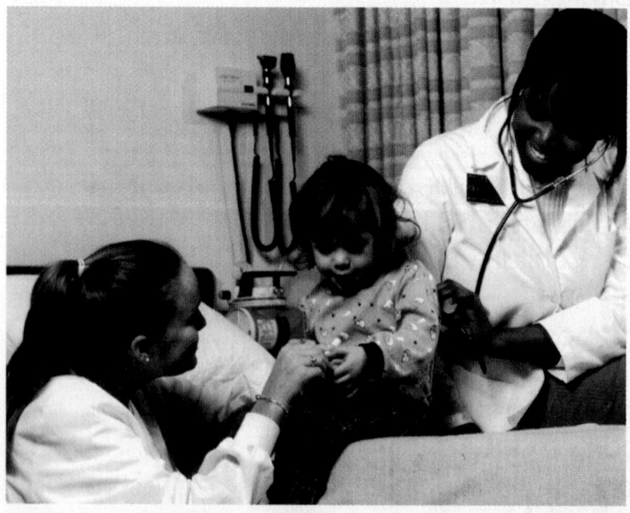

FIGURE 16-1 Pediatric nurses develop skill in minimizing the fears of children during physical examinations. REPRINTED WITH PERMISSION OF UNIVERSITY OF MASSACHUSETTS AMHERST SCHOOL OF NURSING.

HISTORY AND TRENDS IN PEDIATRICS AND PEDIATRIC NURSING

Until the 19th century, children were generally regarded as small adults, and there was limited recognition of childhood illnesses, physiological/psychosocial differences, individuality, or other attributes that directly affected care, treatment, and outcomes. For many years, they were admitted to adult units in hospitals. In 1860, Dr. Abraham Jacobi, the "father of American pediatrics," began to study and teach about special diseases of childhood, prevention of illness, parent education, and social activism for children's rights (Connolly, 2005). His contemporary, Dr. Thomas Rotch, proposed that growth and development needed to be understood in order to apply anatomic and physiologic principles properly to children (Scipien, Barnard, Chard, Howe, & Phillips, 1986). These ideas led to expanded interest in the health and welfare of children and the emergence of pediatrics as a specialty.

In 1885, Children's Hospital of Philadelphia was founded as the first U.S. hospital exclusively for children, following the lead of Grand Ormand Street Hospital in England which had pioneered the treatment of children separately from adults. Special instruction of nurses in the care of children roughly paralleled the development of separate units for children, first in foundling homes, then in children's hospitals, and finally in pediatric units within general hospitals. The early hospital schools of nursing, devoted to the "training" of nurses in the care of sick children, were associated with the earliest children's hospitals including those in Philadelphia, Denver, Boston, and New York (Blake, Wright, & Waechter, 1970).

Advances in the field of pediatrics occurred with the development of many organizations including the American Pediatric Society in 1888, Children's Bureau in 1912, and the American Academy of Pediatrics in 1930. In the 20th century, researchers focused on the welfare of infants and children, the aftermath of children who were orphaned by war, and those with prolonged institutionalization and separation from families. The pioneering work of Spitz (1954) and Bowlby (1965): demonstrated the deleterious effects of separation and loss on children. Their work was the basis for further research by Robertson (1958), whose now-classic films *A Two-Year-Old Goes to Hospital* (1952) and *Going to Hospital with Mother* (1958) graphically depicted the remarkable emotional changes of children even after short-term separations. These films were highly instrumental in changing practices about visiting children in hospitals and also provided a theoretical basis for understanding the effects of hospitalization, particularly at very young ages. As theorists and crusaders, Bowlby and Robertson were extremely influential in bringing about changes in the way children were cared for in hospitals and other institutions (Alsop-Shields & Mohay, 2001).

Prior to the study of the emotional impact of hospitalization on children, it was believed limited visiting was in their best interest because the intense physical and emotional reactions to separation at the time of leave-taking were detrimental to recovery. Caregivers abided by these practices even though they were often distraught when leaving their ill children. Many other reasons for these practices were pervasive, including hazards of infection from outside sources, disruption of the work of the staff, interference with the child's rest, and confidentiality of information (Giganti, 1998).

The issuance of the Platt Report in England was historic in describing existing policies and practices in the care of hospitalized children, how these practices adversely affected child development and recovery, and the kind of changes necessary for child-centered pediatric care and education (Platt, 1959). The changes were slowly implemented and, by the early 1960s, liberal visiting policies, rooming-in practices, and focus on families gradually became standards in many hospitals (Bradley, 2001). The adaptation from visiting for a few hours a day, or once a week in some hospitals (particularly long-term care facilities), to liberal visiting and staying with children required advanced understanding of the impact of hospitalization and focus on family-centered care. Although the benefits have been documented, restricted visiting practices, particularly in intensive care units, continued to exist until 1994 (Giganti, 1998).

In the latter part of the 20th century, pioneers in pediatric nursing generated new knowledge and understanding of children during periods of separation, trauma, and stress. With the advent of advanced educational programs, nurse educators and researchers carefully studied the responses of children in hospitals to gain a deeper understanding of the meaning of behavior and ways to alleviate their fears and anxieties (Blake, 1954a; Erickson, 1958). These theorists documented the significant contributions of nursing to the health and welfare of children, families and the community of health professionals. (Refer to Box 16-1 for a summary of the invaluable contributions of nurse leaders in pediatric nursing.) Through their research and collaboration, new policies and practices have enhanced direct care of children and families as well as innovations including play therapy and volunteer programs. These early leaders created the knowledge base from which subsequent research has been conducted and their methods influenced validation/application of evidence–based practices in pediatric nursing.

The American Association for the Care of Children in Hospitals, formed in 1965 by nurses, caregivers, and others interested in providing the best possible facilities and care for children, published informational materials, pamphlets, and films, and sponsored nationwide conferences devoted to the quality of child care. As the psychological and emotional impact of hospitalization was further studied, nurses began to integrate mental health principles in helping children manage the stress of hospitalization and treatment. Of particular importance was the work of Petrillo (1968; Petrillo & Sanger, 1980) who, as a nurse-consultant to the pediatric staff at New York Hospital, demonstrated and documented the essential role of nurses in the emotional care of children in hospitals. With advances in the field several pediatric nursing associations were formed. (See Chapter Resources.)

Graduate study in pediatric nursing started in the fourth decade of the 20th century (Blake et al., 1970), and by the end of the 20th century, most university schools of nursing had developed master's programs to prepare nurses for advanced practice as clinical nurse specialists in pediatric nursing and pediatric nurse practitioners. Doctoral programs had also developed, some with an emphasis on maternal–child health (University of Pittsburgh). With a focus on developing nursing theory and research, those with advanced degrees in the field conducted studies of nursing practice and published findings in nursing and medical journals. Early examples of published research reports included studies by Visintainer (1977), who explored pre-hospital preparation, and Fagin and Nasbaum (1978), who examined parental visiting in pediatric units.

Many important changes in pediatrics took place during the latter part of the 20th century, including the emergence of pediatric intensive care units and pediatric trauma units; concurrent complexities in medical care, procedures, and equipment; and pharmacological advances. These innovations and the implementation of family-centered care have influenced the expansion of pediatric nursing and furthered the development of comprehensive care for children and families.

As the 21st century began, a dramatic shift occurred in the acuity and extent of childhood illness and trauma: the length of hospitalization has been shortened, alternatives to inpatient care (same-day surgery, specialized clinics) have reduced the number of admissions, and increasing numbers of children are transferred from local hospitals to regional Children's hospitals. In addition, many children with complex health care needs are cared for at home, the need for rehabilitation facilities for children has become increasingly evident, and hospice and palliative care for children has expanded (Davies, Collins, Steele, Pipke, & Cook, 2003; Malloy, Ferrell, Virani, Wilson, & Uman, 2007). With the advent of more complex diagnostic and treatment protocols and expansion of pediatric intensive care units, the need for nurses with advanced education and specialized skills has become more acute. These changes are occurring at a time when the current shortage of nurses is predicted to become more acute (Buerhaus, Staiger, & Auerbach, 2008).

BOX 16-1
LEADERS IN PEDIATRIC NURSING

- **Gladys Sellew** (1887–1977): a nurse, nurse educator, sociologist, and humanitarian. Her work in the tenements, ghettoes, and settlements of Cincinnati, Cleveland, Chicago, and Washington, D.C., brought richness, reality, and a community dimension to the field of pediatric nursing. Her thesis on black families was the first research in nursing to be based on an original investigation that used participant observation as its methodology (Hawkins, 1988). Early in her career, she conducted a study of the time required for nursing care in a pediatric ward, and in 1926, she wrote a text, *Pediatric Nursing,* that was translated into several languages.
- **Florence G. Blake** (1907–1982): the first nurse to systematically study how children and caregivers cope with hospitalization and document the effectiveness of nursing in allaying the fears and concerns of hospitalized children. She published extensive case studies in national and international journals and wrote an early textbook entitled *The Child, His Parents and the Nurse* (1954a) and at least nine editions of the textbook *Nursing of Children.* She was the first to identify the importance of understanding the experience of illness and hospitalization from the child's perspective, applying knowledge of growth and developmental theory, using play in caring for hospitalized children, and involving family in pediatric care (1954b). Her belief that children can "grow" by managing crises successfully was a revolutionary idea in the field of child care in hospitals. She was an esteemed university professor who is also credited with designing and implementing two of the earliest graduate programs in pediatric nursing in the United States at the University of Chicago (1946) and the University of Wisconsin-Madison (1963).
- **Florence H. Erickson** (1914–2002): a professor and researcher in the field of nursing and child development. She started the masters program in the Nursing of Children in the late 1950s and the first Ph.D. program in Nursing in the 1970s, both at the University of Pittsburgh. She published an important monograph, *Play Interviews for Four-Year-Old Hospitalized Children* (1958), which was the impetus for extensive study on the benefits of using hospital equipment during play sessions with children to help them express feelings and understand their experience. This was influential in initiating the therapeutic advantages of using play in hospitals, a practice that evolved into the current Child Life Programs. Dr. Erickson cofounded the *Maternal-Child Nursing Journal* (*MCN*) and *The American Journal of Maternal-Child Nursing.*
- **Dorothy Marlow** (1921–1992): a nurse educator, administrator, author, and director of the Maternal-Child Health Master's Program at the University of Pennsylvania, wrote *Textbook in Pediatric Nursing,* which paralleled the major medical text *Nelson Textbook of Pediatrics* (Vaughn, McKay, & Behrman, 1959, originally authored by Waldo E. Nelson, MD). Her unique contribution was to arrange the content of child care by age groups with concurrent concepts and theories of growth and development, and the most common short- and long-term conditions of that age group, followed by children's responses to illness and ways to assist children during these developmental periods.
- **Eugenia Waechter** (1925–1982): a pioneer in both pediatric nursing and nursing research. She conducted the first controlled study done directly with children, *Death Anxiety in Children with Fatal Illness* (1958). Her writings about the care available to children and families guided the development of a theoretical base in pediatric nursing. With Blake, she authored two later editions of the text *Nursing Care of Children.*

EXPERIENCES OF CHILDREN IN HOSPITALS AND THEIR RESPONSES

Children are hospitalized for acute or chronic conditions; some require treatment before birth, while others are born with conditions incompatible with life but amenable to surgical correction. Accidents continue to be a major cause of death in children. Genetic and environmental factors and general vulnerability, particularly in situations of poverty and stressful living conditions, influence both the incidence and severity of illness in children. Both the nature of illness in children and their responses are different than in adults, owing primarily to stages of development, and physiological, psychological, and life experiences.

Many factors contribute to the distress of young children during hospitalization, and existing fears and emotions may be intensified with prolonged hospitalization (Figure 16-2). Their logic may be illogical; many have not developed a concept of time and they have fantasies that are real to them as they try to explain the unknown. Vessey (2003) described three major foci that contribute to children's psychological responses to hospitalization: maturational and cognitive variables (developmental level, experience, coping style); ecological factors (family and hospital milieu); and biological variables (inborn factors and pathophysiology).

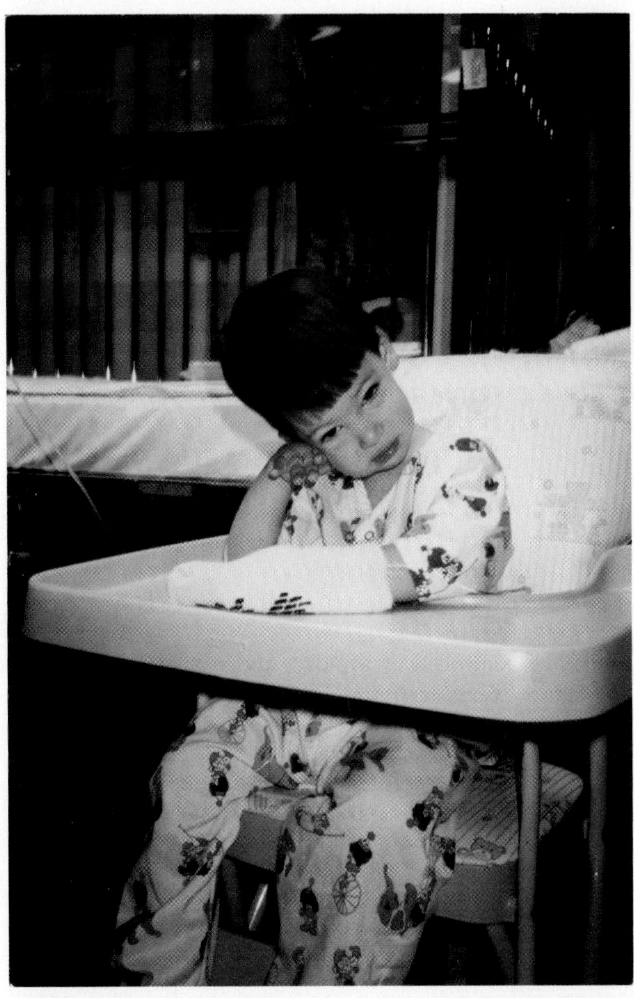

FIGURE 16-2 **Young children with serious illnesses are often sad and tired during hospitalization.** PUBLISHED WITH PERMISSION OF BAYSTATE CHILDREN'S HOSPITAL.

Children become anxious and normal fears are exacerbated when they think about being in pain, harmed, or mutilated in some way or being separated from caregivers (Algren & Algren, 1997). Regardless of the cause of illness or hospitalization, high levels of anxiety are also generated by fears and uncertainties of those responsible for their care. They often perceive a threat to basic needs for love and protection, control and independence, and fulfillment of basic physiological needs. Some fear they may die (Lamontagne, Hepworth, Byington, & Chang, 1997). To allay these fears, children need the constant support of their caregivers and nurses directly responsible for their protection and guidance (Figure 16-3).

The developmental level of children and their perceptions and interpretations of experiences are important. Their limited life encounters and immature intellectual capacities contribute to difficulty in comprehending what is happening. This is particularly true when there are physical intrusions into their bodies. For them, the intactness of their bodies is important; they feel the distress of exposure and intrusion acutely. The impact of hospitalization is also affected by the

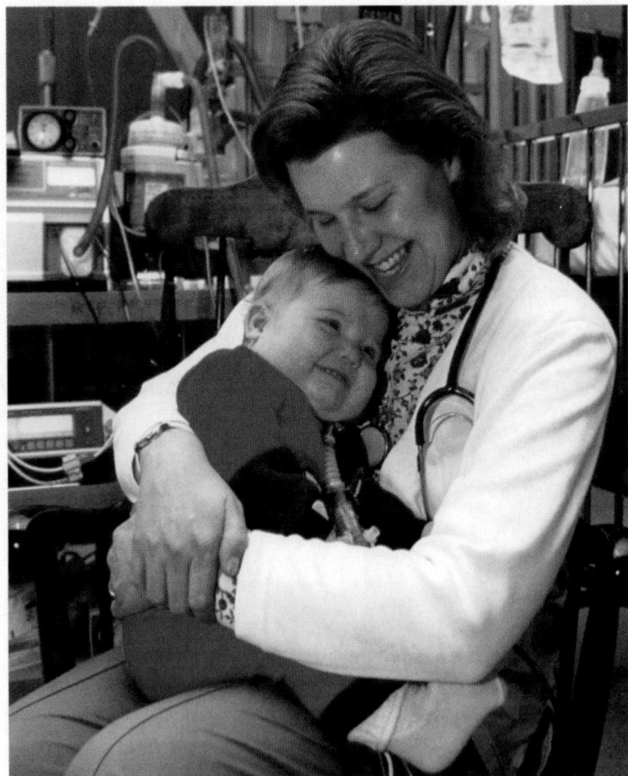

FIGURE 16-3 **Contact comfort increases a child's sense of security and contentment.** REPRINTED WITH PERMISSION OF ALFRED I DUPONT HOSPITAL FOR CHILDREN, WILMINGTON, DELAWARE. PHOTOGRAPHER: CYNTHIA BRODOWAY.

nature and severity of the health problem, the condition, and the degree to which activities and routines differ from those of everyday life.

Children's anxieties are also due to separation from caregivers and familiar persons and environments; the presence of strangers; equipment that looks ominous; the distress of other children; and the pain/discomfort of intrusions and interventions. Although age, maturity, vulnerability to anxiety, and previous experiences make a difference in the intensity of stress responses, there are many stressors pervading the hospital experience for children of all ages. The primary fears producing stress are lack of control, fear of intrusions and "hurt," and separations from the significant persons in their lives.

The cultural variations of families, their values and practices related to illness, general responses to stress, and attitudes regarding child rearing also have a significant influence on the child's behavior and responses. Refer to Chapter 3 for information about various cultural groups and their beliefs and values related to health and illness. The potentially negative impact of illness and hospitalization may be modified by a variety of factors, including age, developmental level, anxiety level of caregivers, individual characteristics and temperament of the child, child and caregiver coping skills, caregiver–family–child relationships, religion, previous hospital or surgery experiences, ethnic and cultural beliefs, and the type and quality of preparation for hospitalization or surgery (Fox, 2002).

Reflections from Families

Most of the time, someone was within calling distance, but when our 5-year-old, Karl, was first brought from the emergency room in a cast, he had to "go to the bathroom," so he put on his light as instructed to do when he "needed anything." Over the intercom, he heard a voice ask, "What do you want?" Perplexed, Karl looked all around, wondering where the person was, and then he said, "What do you say to a wall?" I went for the nurse directly. Karl then did not want us to leave because he was afraid of having an "accident" if someone didn't come right away.

Although there may be similarities in responses to hospitalization, children and their families each have different life situations, giving rise to the importance of understanding children and caregivers as individuals as well as their roles and relationships to each other. Youngblut & Brooten (1999) concluded some of the potentially negative effects of hospitalization for preschool children might be moderated by previous experiences with alternate child care. This is due, in part, to having had positive experiences with separation from mother, a peer group to talk about the experience, or actual instruction about being in the hospital while in preschool settings.

Children fear the unknown, and unfamiliar environments and situations where control is difficult to maintain. It is also distressing when language is heard but not understood. Children notice and become anxious when they see ominous-looking apparatus and strangers in unusual attire (surgical caps, masks, and garb), when they hear unfamiliar noises, or smell strange odors. They become distressed when they hear or see other children crying and wonder what may happen to make them cry also. They are also uncertain about how they will fulfill their essential needs if no one is nearby.

For many children, hospitalization is necessary for the treatment of acute phases of chronic illness, thus imposing additional stress. In a meta-analysis of nursing research on the stressors, coping responses, and health outcomes of children and adolescents living with chronic illness, Stewart (2003) concluded the most common stressors for children with chronic illnesses were: "rigorous treatment regimens that create intrusive medical and self-care demands; disruptions in everyday activities, self-and-peer awareness of physical differences; and varying degrees of social stigma" (p. 225). Stewart described how children use many strategies for coping with chronic illness including: "accessing supportive social resources; solving problems in response to illness and social demands; using cognitive, behavioral, and emotional strategies for ameliorating the aversive consequences of stressors that cannot be controlled or avoided; and relying on spirituality and faith in a positive future" (p. 229).

ALLEVIATING THE ANXIETIES OF CHILDREN

To lessen the anxieties of children, it is important to understand the common situations creating distress and then intervene to minimize or eliminate the source of stress. Those procedures involving any bodily intrusion or perceived pain are most feared, as are those involving equipment and technology (Figure 16-4). It is particularly stressful when injections or darkness is involved.

Children become apprehensive and frightened when they anticipate or experience pain. Therefore, it is important

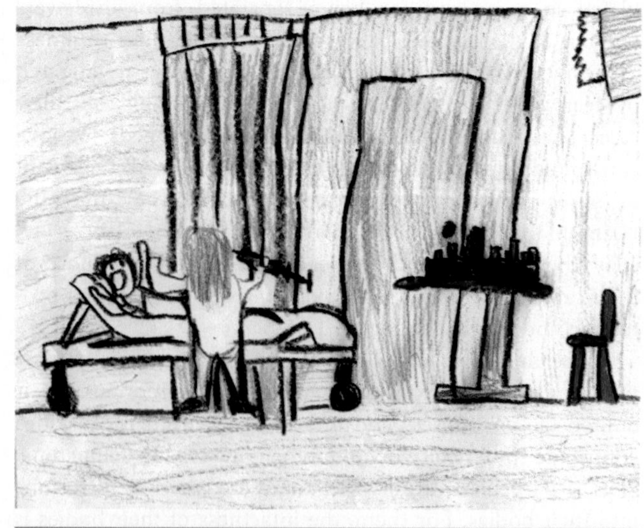

FIGURE 16-4 Drawing of a 10-year-old reveals the fear of being hurt by injections. DELMAR CENGAGE LEARNING.

to use age-appropriate assessment and pain management to create a pain-free environment (see Chapter 18). When children have severe cognitive impairment, the use of advanced assessment is recommended (Solodiuk & Curley, 2003). Success in this endeavor will prevent adverse consequences that may affect clinical and developmental outcomes when pain is not prevented or promptly alleviated (Walker & Wagner, 2003).

Newer pharmacological methods of effectively preventing and moderating pain are the use of topical anesthetics (Rogers & Ostrow, 2004) and conscious sedation (Basset, Anderson, Pribble, & Guenther, 2003; Barclay & Murata, 2008). In the care of neonates, oral glucose pacifiers have been deemed effective in minimizing procedural pain; the analgesic mechanism may be related to the release of endorphins or may be a local effect related to the sweet taste (Gradin, Eriksson, Holmqvist, Holstein, & Schollin, 2002).

Stress-point nursing helps children cope by using both procedural information (description of the treatment and sequence of steps) and sensory information (how this might feel) (Kauffman, Harrison, Burke, & Wong, 1998; Wolfer & Visintainer, 1975). This approach is most effective when there are new tasks and when interventions are focused on issues of greatest concern to the family (Burke, Kauffman, Harrison, & Wiskin, 1999). The combination of sensory preparation, topical anesthesia cream, and parental involvement has been effective in allaying the fears of young children undergoing venipuncture (Kolk, van Hoof, Fiedeldij Dop, 2000). When children feel they have some level of control in a situation, their apprehensions decrease.

NURSING ALERT

Psychological First Aid in Times of Stress

Although many stressful situations are foreseeable and untoward reactions preventable, children may exhibit acute responses even when the cause is not clear (e.g., crying, outbursts of emotion, and covers over head). Whenever there are signs or symptoms of obvious emotional distress, psychological "first aid" should be applied immediately. The specific interventions are situation-specific and most effective when nurses know and understand the individual child, and his or her unique circumstances and developmental level. Effective interventions may include holding, explanation or reassurance related to fears or concerns, and play activities. The child with an outburst of anger or frustration could be helped by carefully listening, clarifying misconceptions, playing out, or using hand puppets to express feelings. Consultation with the psychological team may be beneficial in an acute situation.

Even those situations that may appear minor to an adult are frightening to a young child. For example, when children are being transported to another area of the hospital for tests they may become anxious and resist, fearing that their caregivers may not be able to find them. Simply making a sign on the door, so the child could be "found" is reassuring. In a similar situation, children may not want to leave their room with anyone other than their caregiver because they fear getting lost. Reassurance of always being with someone and having a picture of an animal or cartoon character (different for each room) on the wall inside and outside the room helps children feel more confident about their place. To strengthen children's sense of feeling secure, it is important for nurses to let them know when they are leaving for the day, say good-bye, and tell them the name of their new nurse and when they will return.

MAJOR FACTORS IN SUPPORT OF COPING DURING ILLNESS AND HOSPITALIZATION

During illness, there are several dominant factors influencing the child's ability to cope and learn to use coping methods. These include the inner strengths, talents, and attributes of the child and external determinants such as the expertise of the nurse, the support of families, the quality of the partnership between the nurse and the family, the supportiveness of the environment, and the effectiveness of support through play.

INNER STRENGTHS, TALENTS, AND ATTRIBUTES OF THE CHILD

Each child is a unique individual with different temperaments and capacities for managing adverse situations. Inner strengths include the ability to cope developed from past episodes of getting through difficult situations with the assistance of adults in their world. Some children, however, may appear to be more resilient than they are because they want to appear strong or stoic. Other inner strengths include the abilities to express thoughts and fears, seek information in order to understand situations and expectations, and then feel the success of mastery. The temperament of children and their spirituality may also affect strength in coping (Feudtner, Haney, & Dimmers, 2003).

Another strength children have is their ability to form ideas and opinions about nurses and their manner of caring for them. It is helpful to encourage expression of their perceptions about the actions and attributes of nurses in order to understand what is helpful from the child's point of view. (See Research Highlight.)

Children's talents also help in coping. For example, through drawing, writing prose or poetry, and other creative activities, children not only express their thoughts and feelings, but also use these media to cope. Others may have a curiosity about how things work and seek information and

RESEARCH Highlight

Knowledge about Hospitalized Children's Perceptions of Nurses and Their Behaviors

STUDY PURPOSE

The purpose of this study was to contribute knowledge concerning hospitalized children's perceptions of nurses and nurse behaviors based on the words of children.

METHODS

A qualitative design was used to elicit responses from 63 hospitalized children, between the ages of 5 and 18. Eight experienced pediatric nurses used a semi-structured interview with children at a time when they were not in discomfort. Younger children responded orally or wrote responses if able. Using content analysis, themes were delineated and validated, which were then reviewed by an outside researcher.

FINDINGS

Seven themes were identified: positive attitude/affect (children appreciated nurses who smiled and used kind words); physical comfort (took measures to reduce pain); entertainment/humor (provided age-appropriate diversion and lighthearted conversation); advocacy (promoted positive well-being and a sense of security); basic needs (provided food and medicine); acknowledgment (interacted with them as an individual); and reassurance (provided comfort and support). Examples of responses on advice to nurses to make hospitalization easier were: "take an extra second before any procedure to make sure you have everything you need," "if all of you would wear your name tag ... since I might forget your name," "listen more," and "say it's alright if we're scared." In reference to the time of admission one commenter wrote, "she told me I don't have to be scared because she isn't going to hurt me, and we are going to take good care of you." Children did not appreciate nurses who failed to provide eye contact or verbal interaction while in their presence.

IMPLICATIONS

- Remember to enter a child's room with a smile and establish eye contact.
- Ask children directly how they feel and what they need.
- Do not assume that because a child's parent caregiver is present, the need for individualized sensitive nursing care and presence is diminished on previous page.
- Acknowledge children with each interaction by using each child's name and engaging them in conversation about their concerns related to hospitalization.
- Provide age-appropriate diversion and friendly interaction.
- Provide basic needs in a gentle, organized manner.
- Step into a child's room frequently, even if only for a brief moment, to assure the child's safety and well-being.
- Remember that older children continue to need physical comfort, reassurance, and conversation, and they appreciate the advocacy roles that nurses assume.
- Children/teens respect professionalism in their nurse and want to be respected as individuals.
- Make special efforts at the time of hospital admission to explain the role of the nurse to children inexperienced with hospitalization.
- Provide children with age-appropriate explanations of treatments, timely care, truthful responses, and privacy.
- Ensure that other health care providers deliver care that reflects the child's needs.

REFERENCE

Schmidt, C., Bernaix, L., Koski, A., Weese, J., Chiappeta, M., & Sandrik, K. (2007). Hospitalized children's perceptions of nurses and nurse behaviors. *MCN, Journal of Maternal Child Nursing*, *32*, 336–331.

opportunities to discuss their condition and experiences, or use computers. Some have the kind of personality, charm, and ability to interact and communicate in a way that attracts others to them.

EXPERTISE OF THE NURSE

The expert nurse understands nursing practice as a discipline requiring constant attention to changes and unpredictable signs and symptoms. Depth of knowledge about nursing as an art and science, growth and development, and family theory is the source of wise and effective clinical judgments and interventions. With extensive study and experience, nurses become experts in understanding the verbal and nonverbal behavior of ill children, discerning the meaning intended, and responding skillfully and accurately. They are versatile in using individualized methods such as swaddling, massage, and holding to assure comfort and contentment.

Expert nurses identify the strengths of each child and use them to design, implement, and evaluate nursing care, lend their own strengths to children/caregivers, and understand and manage the exigencies of illness successfully. These nurses also understand that the emotional and physical comfort of the child is more important than any personal satisfactions gained when children and their caregivers like them or express appreciation for their care.

All the nurse's senses are critical in identifying and meeting children's needs since illness is often so acute that children are unable to communicate their needs. It is important not only to look, but to see; not only to listen, but to hear; not only to touch, but to feel; and not only to smell and to taste, but to discriminate and be aware of verbal and nonverbal clues. It is also essential to see subtle changes indicating early signs of dehydration, or brow bulge or eye squeeze to indicate pain, and facial/body indicators of fear and sadness; to hear the sounds of distress, including changes in breathing, or cries of pain and misery; and to feel the muscular tension of anxiety. Nurses have detected acute illness through the odor of the acetone breath of a child not previously known to have diabetes, the unique cry of an infant with a neurological syndrome, or through the salty taste a grandmother described on the face of an infant subsequently diagnosed with cystic fibrosis. The highest level of skill is attained when nurses accurately identify the immediate needs of the child or family for help, validate the need, use knowledge and all resources available to meet this need, and then evaluate the outcomes. This is, in essence, the classic, dynamic nurse–patient relationship first iterated by Orlando (1961).

The experienced nurse may also be described as a nurse–artist because of the sensitivity and care exemplified in grasping the meaning of behavior in light of past and evolving events and the creative, skillful actions that reflect depth of understanding and commitment to attending to each child and family in unique ways. This nurse is thoroughly familiar with current knowledge and evidence-based practices and research in the field, and is highly successful in working in collaboration with colleagues. Nurses have an expanded repertoire of advanced assessment methods to determine physiological status as well as skill in a wide variety of interventions such as therapeutic play and the use of the arts and humanities (e.g., music, art, drama, and movement therapy) (Clatworthy, Simon, & Tiedeman, 1999).

SUPPORT OF CHILDREN BY CAREGIVERS

The support of families is a critical factor in the way children respond to and cope with illness (Institute for Family Centered Care, 2009; Lamontagne et al., 1997; Melnyk, Crean, Feinstein, & Alpert-Gillis, 2007; Wolfer & Visintainer, 1975). The anxieties of caregivers are transmitted to children and this has an effect on negative post-hospital behavior as well as behavior during hospitalization (Small & Melnyk, 2006).

With the turn of the century, the differences and complexities of family life are more evident, and many caregivers have difficulty being physically and emotionally available. Stress may be intensified by existing problems or recent changes (e.g., world events, job loss, moving, divorce, newly blended or foster families, and adoption). Family members may also be experiencing serious physical or mental health problems. Therefore, it is helpful to have a network of friends and family able to offer their resources, time, and assistance. The support of caregivers is dependent upon the empathic responses, assistance, and cooperation rendered by nurses, physicians, and other family members, as well as their own strengths in managing stressful situations. A focus on family-centered care enhances the ability of caregivers to support their children.

The presence of caregivers is of paramount importance particularly for infants and young children, yet the issues surrounding the ability to stay with children and facilities to accommodate caregivers are considered in light of the needs of the family and the child. The critical importance of caregiver presence in the hospital may need to be explained to families because young children are often cared for by others during the day, and the impact of separation in a strange environment may not be fully understood. There is growing recognition of the different ways fathers cope and

NURSING TIP

The Importance of Caregivers and Family Members

Nurses are able to minimize the anxiety of caregivers by preserving their ability to care for and comfort their children; coaching them as they learn new skills and ways of helping their children to cope; and encouraging them to take time to care for themselves. Anxiety is mediated when caregivers feel their thoughts/responses are acknowledged and that they are doing everything possible for their child during hospitalization. Addressing caregivers first and then the child is one way of continuous assessment of how caregivers are managing during their child's hospitalization.

Reflections from Families

When my daughter, Mary, was 2½ years old, there was a serious accident, and she suffered severe burns on her face. She was hospitalized for several days, and I will never forget her sweet face, covered with bandages and tears, and how my feelings of guilt, anxiety, and sadness felt so overwhelming. Each day in the hospital, Mary clung to me and said over and over, "Me go home," and it was heart wrenching for me to leave her. The doctor consented to early discharge if I would do the dressings at home, and this was one of the hardest things I have ever had to do.

participate in care and the value of involving them more deliberatively in children's care (Ahmann, 2006).

Some children are alone in the hospital for many hours and even days due to many factors. Children with severe burns, severe traumatic injuries, or those requiring highly specialized treatments or surgery may receive care many miles from home. In some situations children are sole survivors of accidents or children of single caregivers who need to care for siblings. In a retrospective study, Zengerie-Levy (2006) described the supportive roles of pediatric nurses to help these children heal holistically: being a parent-minded nurse; sustaining human connections; receiving the patient as a child; and renewing the spirit of the child.

Usually, there are choices of accommodations: rooming-in; caregiver sleeping rooms within the pediatric unit; or day-visiting and home-sleeping. There are many practices and provisions during this time (Stremier, Wong, & Parshuram, 2008). The selection of arrangements is complex, but whenever possible, rooming-in is of the highest priority for infants and young children. Parent bed space in pediatric intensive care units is a new trend that has many positive benefits. In a study by Smith and Hefley (2007) one learns that although caregivers are still stressed by changes in their role as comforters and protectors, having the opportunity to be continually present appears to decrease the stress of the parental role alteration—unless they experience sleep deprivation (McCann, 2008).

Whatever arrangements are chosen, caregivers need assurance children will receive support and comfort, particularly during times of discomfort and discontent. They also need to know that, if they are unable to be present, other supportive adults (e.g., grandparents, other significant adults) could take their place. Many hospitals also enlist the skills of volunteers for rocking, cuddling, reading to, and providing comfort and companionship for children. Children of all ages are best able to cope with and learn from experiences with supportive adults "by their side."

CULTURAL CONSIDERATION

Hispanic Beliefs about Illness and Health Practices

Hispanic beliefs about illness and health practices are based on old traditions and customs. For example, *susto,* whose symptoms include nervousness and loss of appetite and sleep, is believed to be caused by a frightening experience. The evil eye, *mal de ojo,* results from an individual looking at or admiring a child who suddenly develops a fever, vomits, has diarrhea, or loses his appetite. The evil eye can be prevented by touching the child while admiring the child and requires a *curandera* (traditional healer) for treatment. Maintaining good health requires establishing temperature equilibrium; some illnesses are considered "hot," such as fever, and others "cold," so the "hot" and "cold" qualities of illness may be taken into account during treatment. For example, a child with a fever should be bundled up and not exposed to cold, which can aggravate the condition.

When Hispanic children are ill, caregivers may consult both a physician and a *curandera,* who both offer treatment. A *yerbero,* who grows herbs and instructs people in their use and cures, may also be consulted. If a Hispanic family does have insurance, infants may be taken to see a doctor at the slightest sign of an ailment, such as a heat rash or minor cold. When a Hispanic child is hospitalized, the extended family, if living close by, may visit often. Most Hispanics believe in prescription medications, especially antibiotics. When a physician prescribes medication it indicates to the family they are being taken seriously and treated well. Doctors who do not prescribe drugs may be perceived as not being good doctors.

RELATIONSHIP BETWEEN NURSES AND FAMILIES

In developing helping relationships with caregivers the concept of identifying family strengths enhances the nurses' ability to work with families (Sittner, Hudson, & Defrain, 2010).

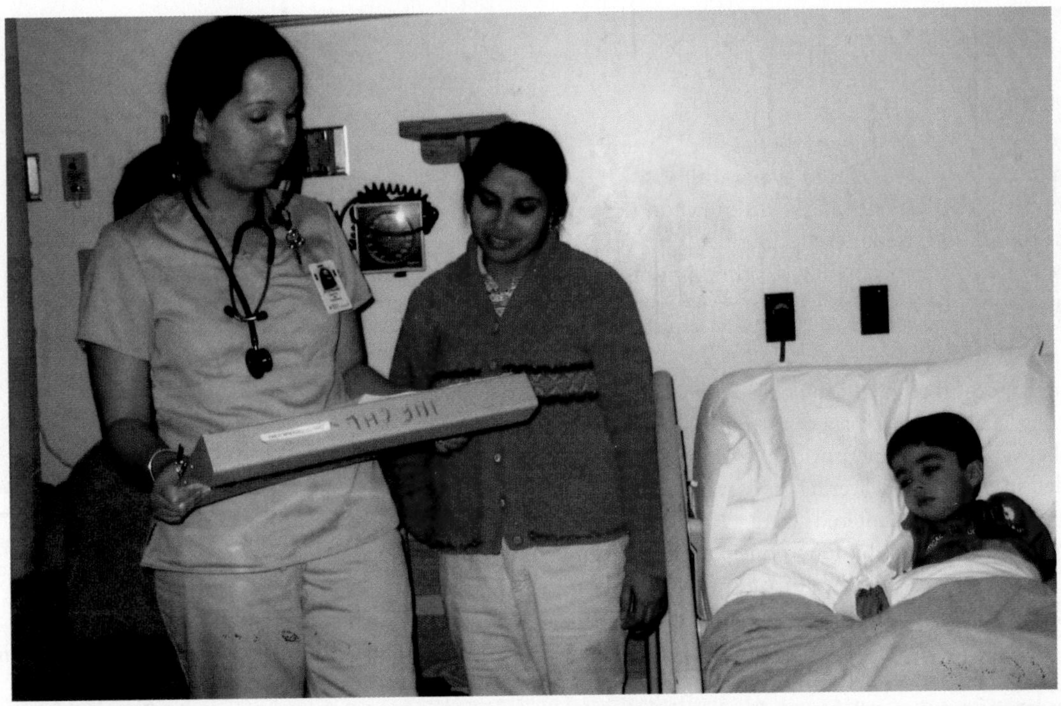

FIGURE 16-5 **Engaging caregivers in the care of their children provides opportunities to use both nurse and parent strengths.**

PUBLISHED WITH PERMISSION OF BAYSTATE CHILDREN'S HOSPITAL.

The quality of collaborative relationships and interactions between nurses and caregivers is fundamental to facilitating a child's coping ability. One highly successful design is based on the philosophy presented by the **nursing mutual participation model of care** (NMPMC) used by Brody (1980) in outpatient pediatric settings and Curley (1988, 1997) in children's hospitals. This model was designed to alleviate stress and empower caregivers to maintain their role during their child's acute illness and recovery. Here, caregivers are equal partners in planning, implementing, and evaluating care. In order for this model to be effective, however, it is essential for the nurse to value the presence and support of families as essential for optimal healing, recovery, and prevention of additional trauma. Rather than a hierarchical relationship, where the nurse and other health professionals assume an authoritarian role, caregivers and nurses form a partnership, where each lends their talent and expertise to promote the well-being of the child (Figure 16-5). In a review of parent participation Power and Franck (2008) reported that the attitudes of health care professionals are both barriers and facilitators in relationships.

Nurses who use an interactive, participative model of practice engage in a deliberative method of establishing and maintaining helping relationships with caregivers by creating a caring, trusting atmosphere for discussion and exploring needs and issues of concern. This is best accomplished by consistently identifying and validating immediate needs for help and exploring how these can best be met. Mutuality in the relationship is nurtured by honesty, openness, sensitivity, and commitment to fostering a healing environment for the child.

NURSING TIP

Working with Families

Parent–nurse conversation during direct care is an effective way of drawing attention to learning. Some examples are saying, "Notice how this adhesive bandage is applied so that it can be tied in place instead of removing the tape each time the dressing is changed" or "Look at how quickly his toenail returns to a pink color after I press it, this is how it should be" or "The reason the drainage bag is kept low is to prevent backflow and the possibility of infection" or "Applying skin cream lightly over the rash preserves the breathing function of the skin."

This model also assumes the nurse understands the changes occurring in families when children are hospitalized and recognizes the needs of caregivers as well as children. Working cooperatively minimizes the detrimental effects of illness experiences and requires considerable skill on the part of the nurse. This kind of nurse–parent participation was developed further into a conceptual framework for professional nursing practice (Curley, 2004). Mullen and Ascher (2007) explained the model thus: when the nurse competencies are driven by and match patient characteristics and needs, improved outcomes result for the patient and family, the clinical unit, and the health care system. **Family-centered care** is

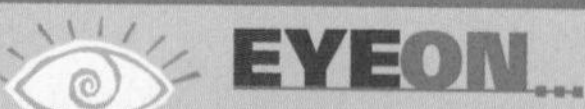

Asian families

The ideal Asian family is the extended family: a tightly knit group involving at least three generations. Parents, children, and grandchildren often live in the same household or in the same neighborhood. When a child of Asian descent is hospitalized, grandparents as well as parents may be involved in caring for the child.

the underlying concept that guides the collaborative nature of pediatric nursing. This approach suggests mutually beneficial partnerships between health care providers, children, and families are needed in planning, delivering, and evaluating health care (Institute for Family-Centered Care, 2009). Further, family-centered care is guided by four principles: people are treated with dignity and respect; health care providers communicate and share complete and unbiased information with patients and families in ways that are affirming and useful; patients and family members build on their strengths by participating in experiences that enhance control and independence; and collaboration among patients, family members, and providers occurs in policy and program development and professional education, as well as in the delivery of care (Institute for Family-Centered Care, 2009).

As one gains competence in participative models and family-centered care, a maturational process occurs in reaching a level of confidence in relating to children and their caregivers. There is also a gradual transition from the role of novice to the expert who has developed the skills and insights necessary for sensitive, evidence-based nursing practice. It is a continuous process of learning by consistently and critically reflecting on actions and reactions, routinely examining research literature, and being aware of one's own process of learning.

Siblings of Hospitalized Children

Interactions of pediatric nurses extend to other members of the child's family, particularly siblings who are also affected by the event of hospitalization (Figure 16-6). Sibling visitation has become a well-established practice in pediatric units because of the considerable benefits to the child, sibling, and family with minimal risks such as infections (Andrade, 1998). However, before siblings visit they may be screened for infectious diseases and their immunization status verified. Siblings have fears and fantasies about what is happening to their sister or brother, and seeing them helps alleviate concerns, since siblings may fear they may have caused illness or injury by something they did or didn't do. Many think they might get sick too.

Child-siblings who may find it most difficult are those who are emotionally close or those who feel distanced from caregivers. Older siblings may take on adult responsibilities and become the "perfect child" so as not to burden their caregivers, but secretly worry if normalcy will ever return (O'Brien, 2002). Helping caregivers understand the reactions of siblings and implementing ways to help them manage the crisis of illness is also within the purview of family-centered care. Many hospitals have sibling programs to respond to questions and help them understand the hospital experience. Books for siblings of children having illness or disability are also recommended (Ahmann, 1997) (Figure 16-7).

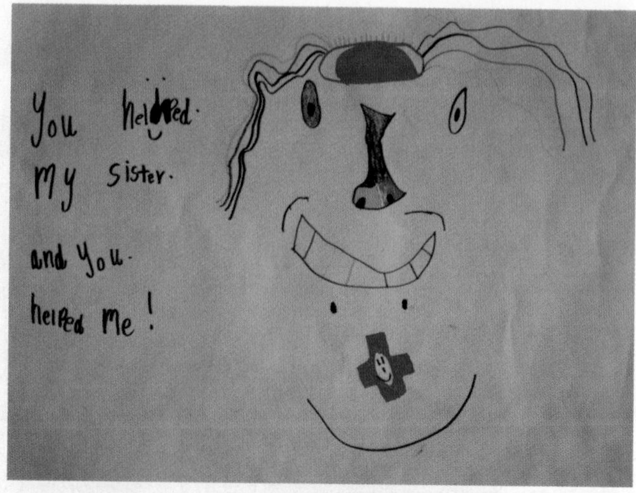

FIGURE 16-6 A drawing by a sibling is an expression of how she was helped to cope with her sister's hospitalization. PUBLISHED WITH PERMISSION OF BAYSTATE CHILDREN'S HOSPITAL.

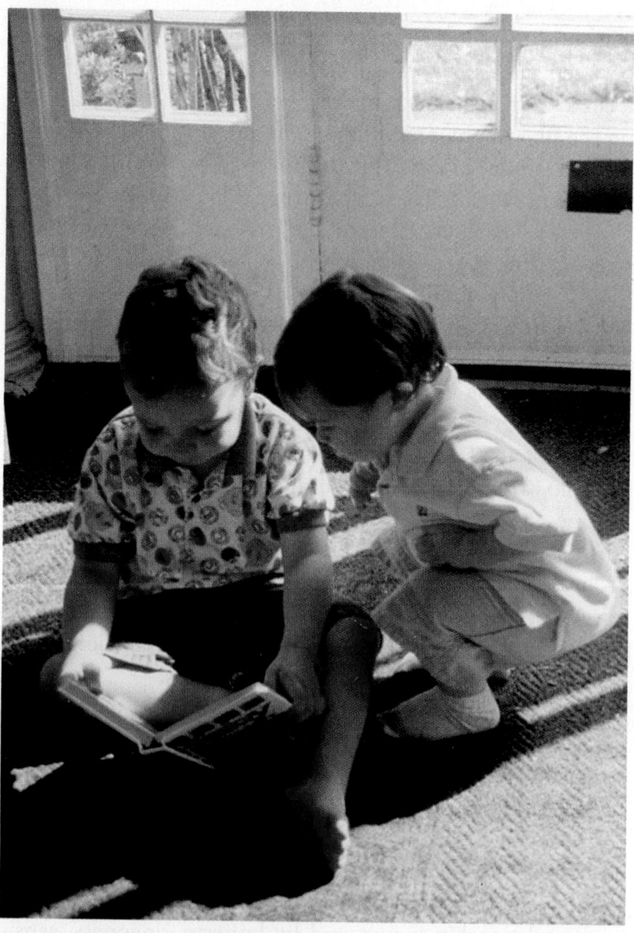

FIGURE 16-7 Children with close relationships would feel the loss of companionship if a sibling is hospitalized. DELMAR CENGAGE LEARNING.

CLIMATE OF THE PEDIATRIC UNIT AS A SUPPORTIVE ENVIRONMENT

As a place of healing, the environment of the pediatric unit should be conducive to feelings of well-being, safety, and security (Figure 16-8). This is often difficult when sights and sounds are strange and unfamiliar. Although it is essential to have aesthetically pleasing surroundings, sensitivity to the decor and child-centered accoutrements is secondary to the expertise, morale, satisfaction, and quality of the working relationships between and among the staff. Most critical is the conscious attention to the philosophy of family-centered care, where all contribute their talents and expertise to the health and welfare of those entrusted to their care. Because children sense the anxieties of adults, attending to the needs of adults, including health professionals is important. The mental and physical health of nurses is vital to creating an environment where children and caregivers experience the comfort, knowledge, and strength that prevails when nurses use themselves as instruments for healing.

Each child should have a place for personal possessions and mementos, including favorite things, regardless of the often well-worn appearance, such as a skinned, well-loved, stuffed animal or the remains of other transitional objects such as blankets and items of clothing. Shoes should be in sight because these are symbols of mobility and reminders of going home; these are to the child what a hat may be to an elderly gentleman in a similar situation—a symbol of life outside the hospital.

The demeanor, attitude, and kindliness of those caring for children are thought to be far more influential in children's responses than their attire. Although the latter has been the subject of much controversy, colored or patterned clothing is often worn in pediatric units because children like bright colors and many believe children may associate white clothing with fear of being hurt. However, there are some aspects related to attire that may be of consequence (e.g., long fingernails or rings which may harbor harmful organisms or cause injury; hoop earrings, which small fingers might pull; or designs on clothing that may be frightening, like large animal prints). Conversely, a small, fuzzy, animal figure attached to a stethoscope and other equipment or pleasant distractions help reduce children's fears.

Every pediatric unit needs a playroom as a safe haven where no painful treatments or scenes are encountered; a place where children are empowered to cope with stressful events on a day-to-day basis. The inclusion of play is so important that children should be brought to the playroom by any means possible (carts, wheelchairs, beds) and, when not feasible, play activities should be brought to the bedside. Play is the work of children, their source of learning and, as such, is an integral component of the plan of care for each child.

The environment needs to be flexible enough to accommodate family needs both for visiting and staying through the night; one that provides the amenities needed for families' rest, comfort, and nourishment. Consideration of visits from siblings, grandparents, and significant others may be critically important to some children.

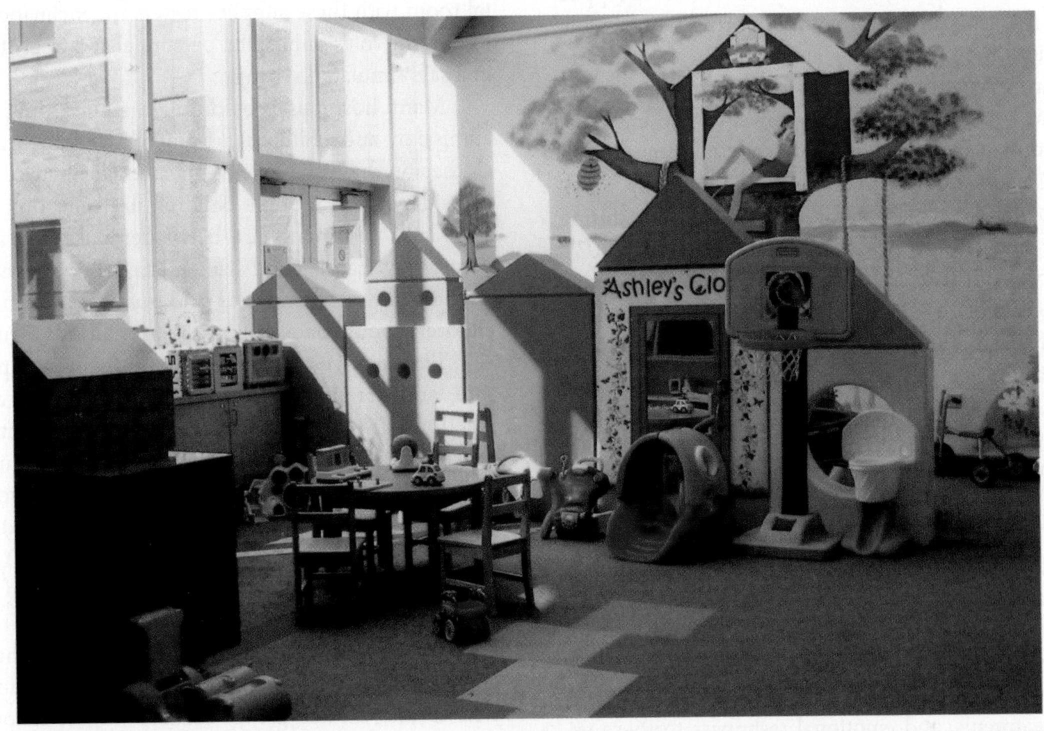

FIGURE 16-8 A colorful playroom is a haven for children and the site of therapeutic and creative play to reduce tension and anxiety. PUBLISHED WITH PERMISSION OF BAYSTATE CHILDREN'S HOSPITAL.

Reflections from Families

Our daughter Madison was 4 and had been hospitalized for several days following multiple seizures. She was born with serious delays in mental and physical development and while in the hospital she didn't want to look at anyone, eat, or drink. She was mostly silent except for saying, "Noah's comin." How could Madison understand that her brother couldn't come to visit her because he had an eye infection? I left pictures of him, but she just pointed and said again, "Noah's comin." In a few days, Noah visited and when she saw him, she opened her eyes wide, smiled, and said, "Here's Noah." That day she ate all her lunch and drank the "juicy" he brought for her.

PLAY AS THERAPEUTIC IN FACILITATING COPING

An early expert in child development defined play as any voluntary activity engaged in for the purpose of enjoyment (Hurlock, 1978). Play fosters the development of cognitive, psychomotor, language, and psychosocial skills. As early as 1954, Blake proposed that children gain mastery of fears and relief from tensions through play.

An active child life program, an attractive, well-equipped playroom, and a schoolroom provide opportunities for children to engage in play activities and learning designed to avert untoward effects of hospitalization. **Child life specialists** have the role of promoting optimal development of children, maintaining normal living patterns, and minimizing psychological trauma. They supervise diversional play activities and help prepare children for and assist them during medical tests and procedures (Child Life Council, 2003). Because play is critical to the emotional health of children, nurses assume major responsibility for determining the kind of play beneficial for individual children and ways to integrate this in the plan of care.

Children benefit from the opportunity to engage in play activities designed to promote expression of thoughts and feelings about situations that are difficult to understand or accept. Observation of play helps nurses gain insight about the meaning of behavior and ways to guide children in specific situations. It is advantageous for nurses to create their own small, readily available box or basket that contains dolls representing children, nurses, doctors and caregivers; a few hand-puppets; and frequently used clinical items. Play provides opportunities to assess a child's understanding of illness, procedures, treatments, and emotional responses to these experiences. For example, puppet dialogue could be about a recent experience: "I was crying today." "What happened?" "They put me in a box to see my insides." "Did it hurt?" "No, but I was scared." "What was it that scared you?"

Therapeutic play is a highly effective, nondirective way of assisting children to use hospital equipment and toys to express reactions to stressful events (Kuntz et al., 1996). This kind of play is stimulated by presenting doll figures (nurse, doctor, adult, anatomically correct child dolls, crying dolls, etc.), hospital equipment (e.g., stethoscope, catheters, IV materials, etc.) and clothing (gowns, masks, gloves), and observing or conversing with children as they play (Figure 16-9). A miniature hospital room with these supplies fosters the inclination of children to don the roles of hospital personnel and treat "their patients" in a safe simulated setting.

Many hospitals provide plain stuffed dolls shortly after admission and children are encouraged to draw faces and clothes on them to make them special (Gaynard, Goldberger, & Laidley, 1991). Some children use their doll when procedures and treatments are being demonstrated and in therapeutic play. Large, child-sized cloth dolls with visible layers of abdominal organs, muscles, and bones are helpful in teaching children about specific illnesses or injuries (Figure 16-10).

The creative arts including music, drama, poetry, literature, and drawing are other ways to express emotion and reactions. In using mini-drama a child can act the part of the nurse who says, "It won't hurt much," and when the nurse acting as child cries and says, "Ouch, you're hurting me," the responses of the child can be observed followed by discussion about what could be done so it won't hurt or help make it better. When art is used, it is helpful to ask children to "draw a picture of yourself in the hospital" and then to tell a story about their painting or drawing, thus providing an opportunity for expression, explanation, and discussion. Diaries and stories are a valuable way of helping children cope with their experiences. Most hospitals have a resource library with books to be read by or to children. Some

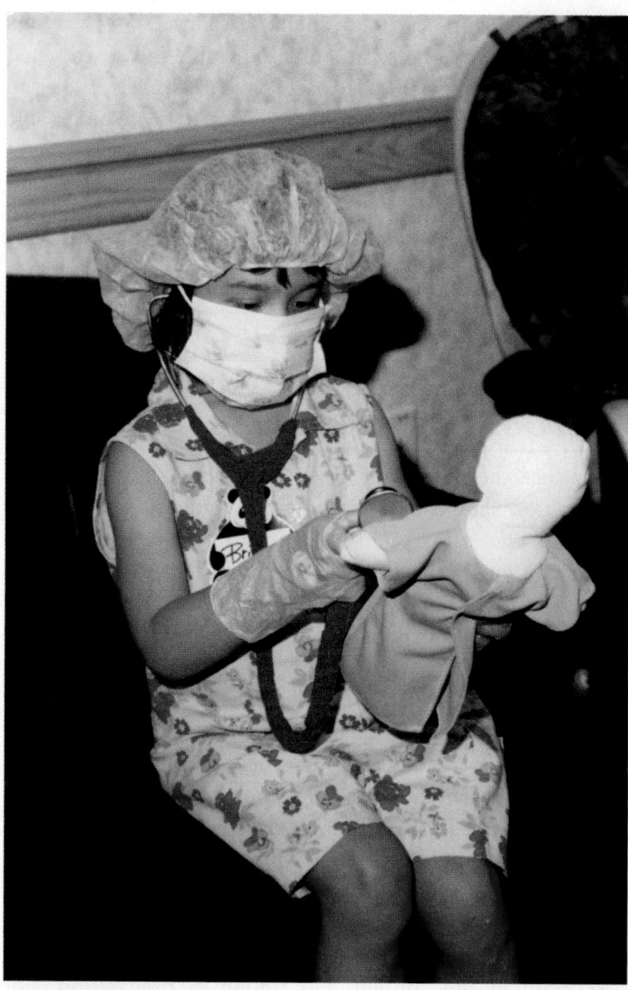

FIGURE 16-9 **Children learn and express feelings about hospital experiences by using dolls and equipment.** DELMAR CENGAGE LEARNING.

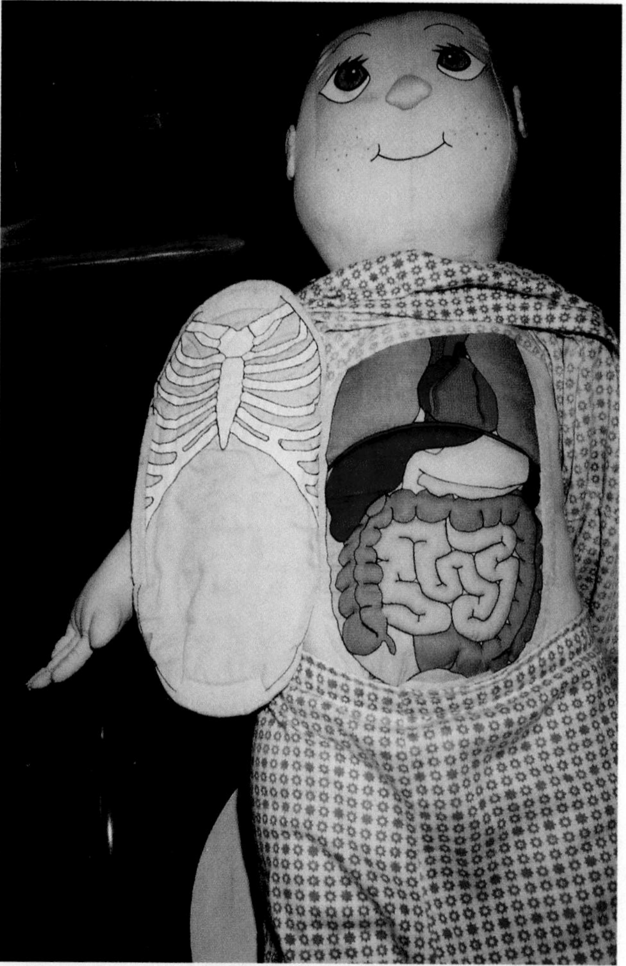

FIGURE 16-10 **Teaching dolls are an effective way of helping children learn about their bodies.** PUBLISHED WITH PERMISSION OF MASSGENERAL HOSPITAL FOR CHILDREN.

NURSING TIP

Play is Therapy

Play materials can be used to encourage deep-breathing exercises postoperatively; for example, a "party blower" or a pinwheel are effective alternatives to an incentive spirometer.

children write books which are beneficial for them and for others (see Resources at the end of the chapter).

Play mediates reactions to stress and has beneficial physiological benefits as well (Zahr, 1998). For example, anger and pent-up energy can be released through physical activities such as pounding boards, punching bags or balls, and throwing beanbags into containers. Play situations are created, but the child chooses the items and decides on the way to use these according to his or her level of comfort and readiness. Play materials can also be used to encourage strengthening exercises.

Involvement in using board games, video games, puzzles, and group activities helps children engage in familiar

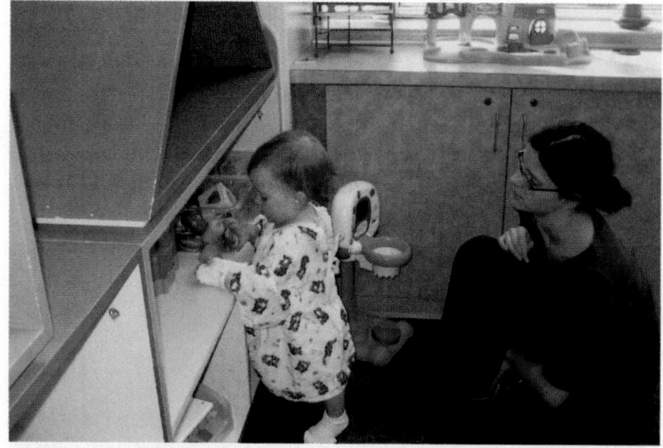

FIGURE 16-11 **Providing creative materials and guidance in the playroom provides diversion for children.** PUBLISHED WITH PERMISSION OF BAYSTATE CHILDREN'S HOSPITAL.

kinds of play. Materials like clay, finger-paints, and craft materials provide opportunities for learning as well as a change from hospital routines (Figure 16-11). It is difficult for children to resist play, but for those who have difficulty

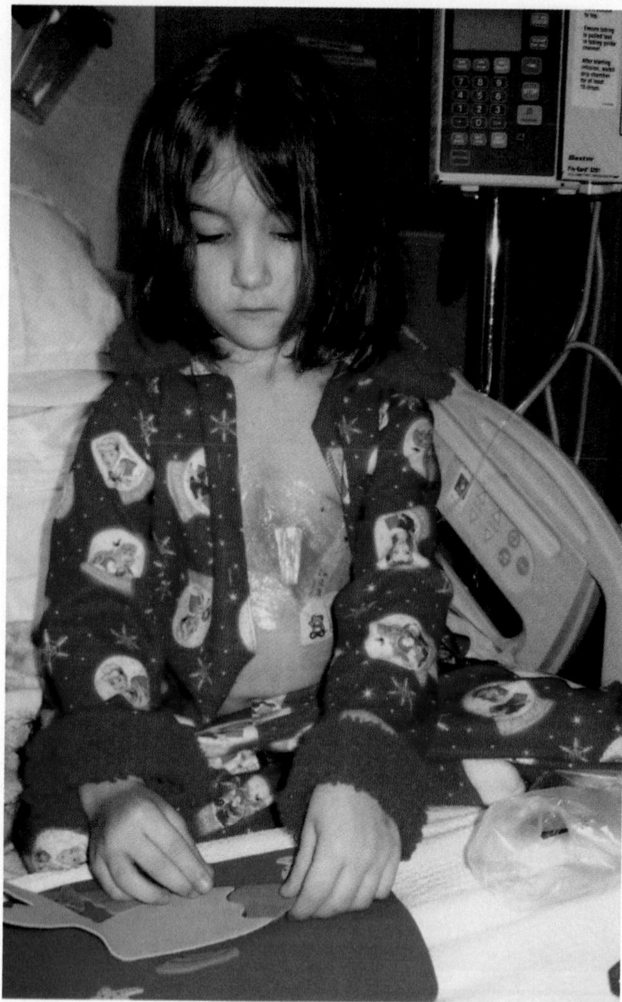

FIGURE 16-12 **When children are unable to go to the playroom, toys and play sessions at the bedside provide opportunities for learning and enjoyment.** PUBLISHED WITH PERMISSION OF BAYSTATE CHILDREN'S HOSPITAL.

engaging in active play due to fatigue, immobility, or diminished readiness, there are many ways of providing vicarious involvement (e.g., observing the play of other children, puppet shows, or play at the bedside) (Figure 16-12).

NURSING TIP

Play Interviews or Sessions with Young Children in Hospitals

Conducting therapeutic play interviews and play sessions with young children requires depth of understanding and skill in this technique. It is wise for novices to learn therapeutic play as an intervention from experts; then plan opportunities to observe therapeutic play, practice this intervention with supervision on several occasions, and receive feedback on this practice.

Sufficient time each day should be allocated for play experiences, particularly for immobilized children who are often in a "state of waiting and increased vigilance" (Gillis, 1989). In expanding their focus beyond their illness, they are better able to manage their perceptions of the slowness of the passage of time and engender positive feelings toward themselves and others. Creating environments and situations where children laugh and have fun is important to the recovery process.

PREPARATION OF CHILDREN AND FAMILIES FOR HOSPITALIZATION

To reduce the potentially adverse effects of hospitalization, preparation should take place prior to admission whenever possible. The primary purposes are to provide information, encourage emotional expression, establish trusting relationships, and teach coping strategies. These goals are met best when the age and experiences of the child and honesty and responsiveness to concerns and questions characterize the preparation process. Most children's hospitals have programs designed to prepare children for hospital experiences, day-stay surgery, and diagnostic procedures. Preparation materials and presentations are most helpful when these reflect the learning needs of children of different ages and stages of development, and accurately depict the sights, smells, sounds, policies, and procedures of the actual setting (Figure 16-13).

Cognitive development and language skills are key factors, both in the content and timing of preparation. For infants, the best approach is to prepare caregivers. By allaying caregiver fears and concerns they will be better able to communicate a sense of calmness and well-being to their infants. For planned admissions, the age of the child should be a guide to timing for preparation for hospitalization or surgery: 1- to 2-year-olds, the day or evening before or day of admission or surgery; 2- to 3-year-olds, 2–3 days before;

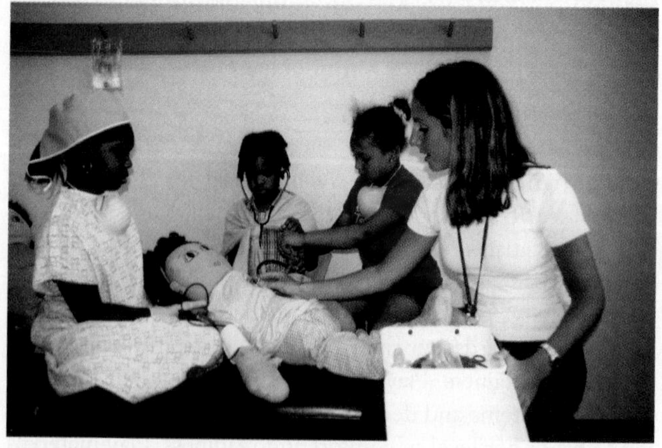

FIGURE 16-13 **Preparation for treatments is facilitated when children use dolls and play equipment.** PUBLISHED WITH PERMISSION OF MASSGENERAL HOSPITAL FOR CHILDREN.

4- to 7-year-olds, 4–7 days; and over 7 years, a few weeks before admission or surgery (Fox, 2002). Through tours, use of puppets, medical play, children's literature, and audiovisual media, children learn about the experience and their role in the recovery process. Whenever possible, children should have the opportunity to actively participate, (e.g., handling equipment such as blood pressure apparatus, stethoscope, and IV fluid tubing).

Group preparation is often effective for school-age children. Adolescents need opportunities to explore the meaning and consequences of the experience in addition to explanations relevant to preparation for surgery or hospitalization. Additionally, they need time to discuss fears, concerns, options, and alternatives. Although it is important for children and adolescents to understand as much as possible about the experience, it is equally important for caregivers to have information that will help them maintain their parental role. When caregivers have accurate information and feel confident, they can transmit a sense of security to their children.

Unexpected hospitalizations of young children under the age of 6 constitute most admissions to pediatric units. When caregivers and children are not prepared for sudden changes and stresses, higher anxiety levels and a higher risk for negative outcomes both during and after hospitalization occur (Melnyk, 1994; Melnyk et al., 2004). At the time of admission, children need to know about the new environment, routines, and expectations, and also ongoing, simultaneous explanations about what is occurring and the rationale. The family needs to know essential information to cope with the immediacy of the situation. This is best accomplished by anticipating needs and responding to questions and concerns as these arise.

CARE OF CHILDREN DURING ADMISSION TO A HOSPITAL

The process of admission begins with establishing a helping, trusting relationship with the child and caregivers. The first greeting of welcome should include a smile with the message of expecting their arrival followed by introductions. Shaking hands with caregivers and children (when age-appropriate) is a symbolic gesture of beginning the relationship (Figure 16-14). At this time the formal name and title of the nurse is followed by a brief discussion of the name each person prefers to be called. When young children are admitted to the hospital, the nurse should first establish a relationship with caregivers. As children see their caregivers trust the nurse, it is easier for them to engage in a relationship with the nurse. Being at eye level and having eye contact while talking to children facilitates positive responses.

During this time, it is also advisable to explain the pattern of staffing and names of other nurses who may be involved in the child's care. Knowing the role, responsibilities, and length of time the nurse will be caring for the child is helpful information, as are the names of health care practitioners, other nurses, and personnel who will be involved during the first day (a process that should be repeated each day). This is followed by a brief description of the general policies and sequence of activities. Preferably, the nurse during the initial orientation phase will be the primary nurse or one who will provide care during hospitalization.

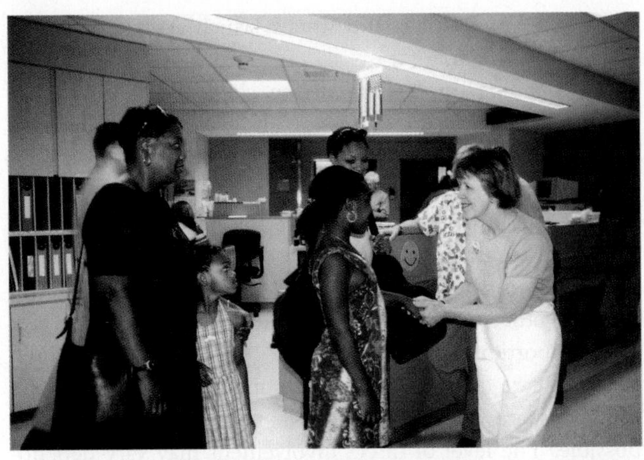

FIGURE 16-14 Welcoming children and families to the hospital by words and handshaking is an effective way to begin helping relationships. PUBLISHED WITH PERMISSION OF MASSGENERAL HOSPITAL FOR CHILDREN.

Admission routines include detailed history taking and complete assessment. In many children's hospitals a predefined pediatric nursing assessment is an integral part of the electronic medical record. A parent's guide is a helpful way of sharing the philosophy of care, children's developmental stages and reactions to hospitalization, and ways of working together as partners in a family-centered environment (see Resources at the end of the chapter).

In addition to obtaining information about the child's routines, reactions to stress, and understanding about the reason for hospitalization, it is important to obtain information about prior experiences with illness and hospitalization, including significant recent illness experiences of others in the child's home and school environment. Some children may have had recent experiences with the hospital as a place of birth or death. The association may be quite direct, for example when a child has a "heart problem" and experienced the hospitalization and death of someone who had a "heart attack." There also needs to be explicit clarification of the reason for hospitalization so perceptions can be clarified. The importance of accuracy in communication and careful interpretation of verbal and nonverbal behavior cannot be overemphasized.

When children with chronic illnesses are admitted, they need to know how this hospitalization is different than other experiences. With younger children, it is helpful for caregivers to write the home routine for feeding, exercises, and elimination. One mother of a toddler with cystic fibrosis had a plan that she entitled, "the care and feeding of one Nicholas Francis," a detailed account of his daily activities, routines, treatments, and medications. This kind of written plan provides an excellent source of information for consistency of routines and rituals, which are so reassuring to young children.

Depending on the age of the child and the acuity of illness at the time of admission, it is helpful to have an orientation to the unit stressing those areas of greatest relevance (e.g., play room and toilet facilities). The time of admission is also the time to explore the needs and desires of caregivers regarding their comfort, their involvement in the direct care of their child, and how the nurse and staff will work together during the child's hospitalization. It is a unique opportunity to explain the philosophy of family-centered care and the participative model of practice where caregivers are integral partners in providing the best care possible. The level of direct involvement may vary depending on a variety of circumstances. Establishing helping, supportive relationships at this time influences the way nurses and caregivers work harmoniously in caring and healing.

An initial **nursing interview** with caregivers provides an opportunity to establish helping relationships while learning essential information about the child/family and discovering ways of working together for the benefit of the child. Many hospitals have forms for this interview with sections for the child's growth and development and for the medical and immunizations history, which caregivers can complete separately. It is also helpful to have a separate interview with the child or adolescent in order to understand their perceptions related to illness and hospitalization. In addition to interview and data collection forms, most pediatric units have written guides with answers to frequently asked questions and helpful information. Usually included are explanations about philosophy of family-centered care, hospital procedures and resources, policies and practices of the pediatric unit, suggestions for helping children and siblings cope, and safety measures. Informational booklets are prepared by individual hospitals.

PREPARATION OF CHILDREN AND THEIR FAMILIES FOR SURGERY

When children are to be admitted for surgical procedures or examinations requiring anesthesia, both the timing and the content of the child's and family's preparation should be considered. Generally, children are prepared close to the time of the surgical procedure and the dialogue, audio, and visual materials should be age appropriate and relevant to the child's cognitive development. Prior to instruction, it is helpful to ascertain what they know and how they feel (Lamontagne et al., 1997; Lamontagne, 2000). Therapeutic play intervention has been shown to be effective and appropriate in preparing children for surgery (Li & Lopez, 2008).

Preparing caregivers helps improve the child's understanding and ease in asking questions, since family concerns and anxieties strongly influence the child's reaction to preoperative experience. (Noble, Micheli, Hensley, & McKay, 1997) Children's fears focus mainly on the unfamiliar environment, pain, mutilation, and separation from caregivers; parental presence may alleviate these fears (Algren & Algren, 1997). For example, in uncomplicated preoperative situations where caregivers are prepared and able, in their presence during induction of anesthesia is reassuring to children and minimizes the stress of separation. The need for heavy sedation decreases with parent-present induction (PPI), promoting more rapid recovery from anesthesia (LaRosa-Nash & Murphy, 1997) (Figure 16-15).

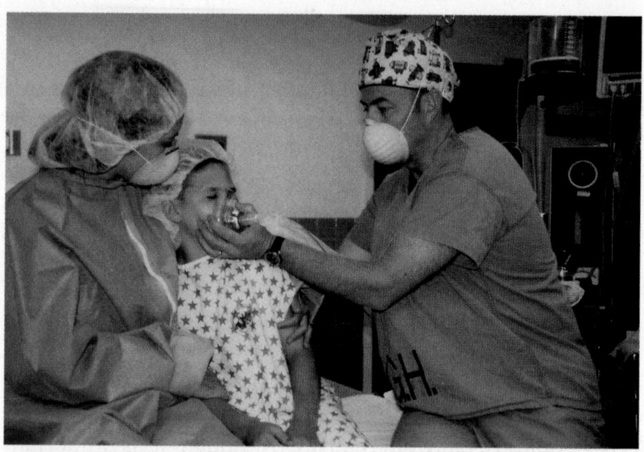

FIGURE 16-15 Children are more relaxed during the induction phase of anesthesia with a supportive person at their side.
PUBLISHED WITH PERMISSION OF MASSGENERAL HOSPITAL FOR CHILDREN.

Most hospitals have well-established protocols and resources to prepare children and caregivers for different kinds of surgery and some have multidisciplinary teams to provide a program that reflects culturally sensitive and multimodality preparation (Justus et al., 2006). These include tours of the facility, the use of films and puppets, as well as discussions (Figure 16-16). Age-related books to prepare children for surgery are available in libraries and websites. (See Chapter Resources.) When children are admitted for same-day surgery, there are fewer negative behavior changes at home after surgery when play with hospital equipment is integrated into preparation and care (Ellerton & Merriam, 1994; Schmidt, 1990).

Most children want to know if it will hurt and may be afraid something will go wrong or they will wake up during the operation. It is reassuring to speak with the "anesthesia doctor" and to know that he/she is always there during the surgery. Explanations regarding anesthesia need to be carefully considered. For example, the phrase "put to sleep" may be frightening, particularly when this has been used in reference to a euthanized pet. Among alternatives to reduce this kind of fear may be a phrase like, "a special kind of sleep like a nap" and adding, "you will be awakened when it's over and come back here where (person in family) will be waiting for you."

During a child's immediate preparation for surgery, every effort should be made to minimize stress. Young children who do not understand the rationale for withholding food and fluids need to be carefully observed so they do not take food or fluids inadvertently. When children of young ages have same-day surgery, it is advisable for caregivers to "snack-proof" the house on the evening before and not have anything to eat in the presence of the child on the day of surgery. Using a matter of fact approach rather than emphatic denials of food requests avoids an association of

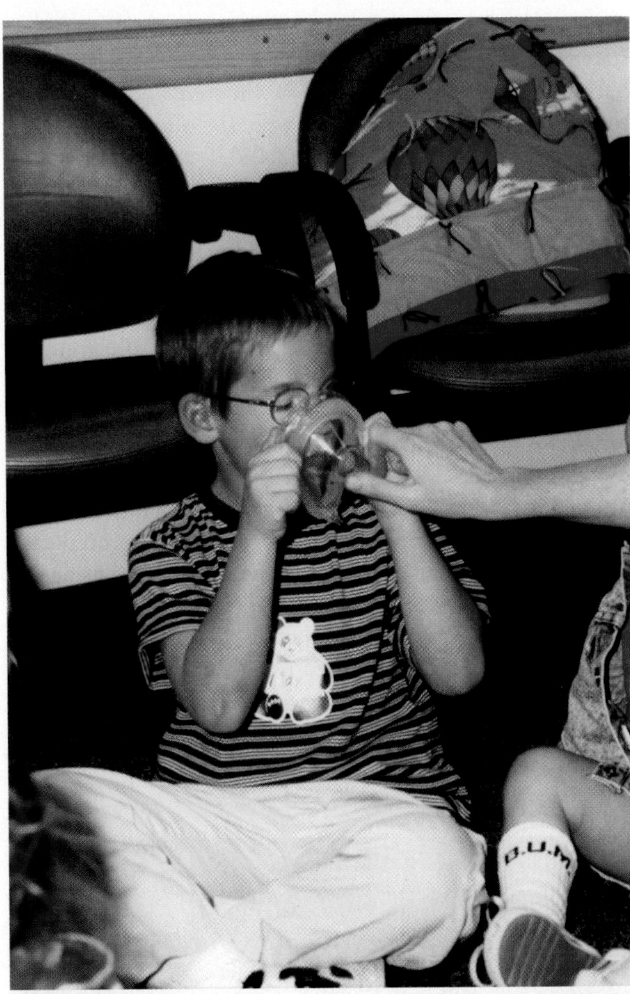

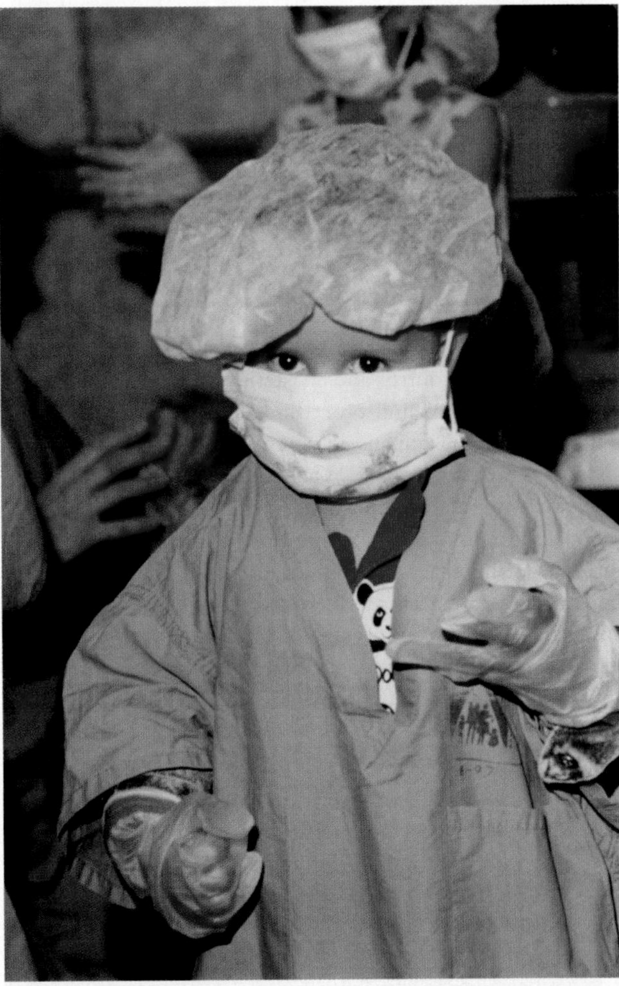

FIGURE 16-16 "Trying out" equipment and donning surgical garb preoperatively helps children prepare for the new experience of surgery.
DELMAR CENGAGE LEARNING.

food deprivation and disapproval. Saying, "Remember the nurse said that all children having surgery (or this test) are allowed to eat and drink only after their operation (test) but not before, so you will feel better faster," is more encouraging during the waiting period.

To prevent fear associated with preoperative injections, non-injectable medications should be used whenever possible. In transporting young children to the surgical suite, it is unwise to use their crib or bed, because doing so may precipitate postoperative fears related to sleep (e.g., the young child may reason that if you fall asleep, you may be taken away again). For example, for several days after surgery, 3½-year-old Marco was "awake all night" and only fell asleep when he was on the sofa in the playroom or sitting on his mother's lap. In play, he took several dolls and aggressively put them in and then took them out of their "hurt beds"—he then used buses and trucks to take them outside the room so no one could find them. In subsequent play sessions, his fears were expressed and misconceptions explained, following which he gradually returned the dolls to their beds and resumed more restful nighttime sleep.

The goal for optimal preoperative preparation is to provide and reinforce information for children and caregivers,

CRITICAL THINKING

Preparation of a Child and Family for Surgery

Think of a preschooler you know. Imagine that he or she is to be admitted to the hospital for repair of a ventricular septal defect in a week.

- What are the strengths of this child and family in preparing for hospitalization and surgery and for coping with these experiences?
- What would you include in a teaching plan for this child and caregivers?
- If you were the nurse at the time the child was going to surgery, describe the sequence of activities during the immediate preparation to the time that anesthesia is given.
- If this child were to be hospitalized for five days, describe the nursing interventions that would most likely be effective in helping this preschooler and caregivers cope with this experience. What behaviors would indicate difficulty in coping?

encourage emotional expression of fear, and teach coping strategies while minimizing intrusive, distressing, and painful procedures.

FACILITATING COPING WITH EXPERIENCES OF DIAGNOSTIC OR THERAPEUTIC PROCEDURES

When children know what to expect, there is greater potential for maintaining control and mastering fears during uncomfortable and frightening procedures. Although time may be limited, as often happens in acute illnesses, an explanation should always come first. When caregivers understand the procedure, they are better able to enhance the explanation by making comparisons to previous experiences or using terms most familiar to the child. However, they should not be expected to participate in restraining. There may be circumstances where they are unable or prefer not to participate in which case a supportive staff member may then assume this role. The presence of supportive caregivers and nurses during treatments and procedures cannot be overemphasized. As stated earlier, the use of sedation for pain free procedures is becoming an expected practice in children's hospitals. This requires experienced providers who are often members of pediatric sedation teams (Davis, 2008).

Because infants and toddlers are in the formative stage of developing language and cognitive skills, the presence of caregivers with their gentle handling and soothing words decreases the pain and anxiety of procedures. The role of adults during and after is also critical in alleviating the emotional and physical discomforts experienced. Preschoolers benefit most from the use of demonstrations and role-play using play equipment (e.g., using a doll or animal to apply a cast, change a dressing, or start intravenous fluids). The child should choose the object for the procedure as many do not like to use their favorite doll or toy animal. Box 16-2 describes various components of preparing children and caregivers for treatments and procedures.

During procedures, the nurse should consider using distraction techniques to help manage fear, anxiety, and pain (Cohen & Baster, 2008). In addition, the child should continue to be guided and coached using soft, reassuring words and giving praise intermittently for cooperation and following directions (e.g., "it's real hard to stay still, but you're doing this very well") (Figure 16-17). It is inadvisable to

BOX 16-2

CONSIDERATIONS IN PREPARING CHILDREN FOR PROCEDURES

- Assess the cognitive level, previous experiences with the particular procedure, and readiness for learning.
- Explain honestly and simply, using terms understandable to the child—include what will happen and associated sensations.
- Use the least aggressive language (e.g., "fixing the bandage or making it better" rather than "taking it off or taking it out").
- Include brief rationale and ways the child can safely participate (e.g., holding the adhesive tape).
- Offer opportunities to manipulate the equipment in advance of the procedure when possible (rehearsal is helpful).
- Practice alternate ways of maintaining control during the procedure (e.g., guided imagery, holding or squeezing a hand or a favorite toy, or counting).
- At the conclusion of the initial preparation, ask the child to explain what is going to happen during the procedure and clarify areas of misunderstanding.
- Decide on an activity or comforting measure when the treatment/procedure is over (e.g., read a story, drink a glass of juice, go to the playroom, or have a play activity).

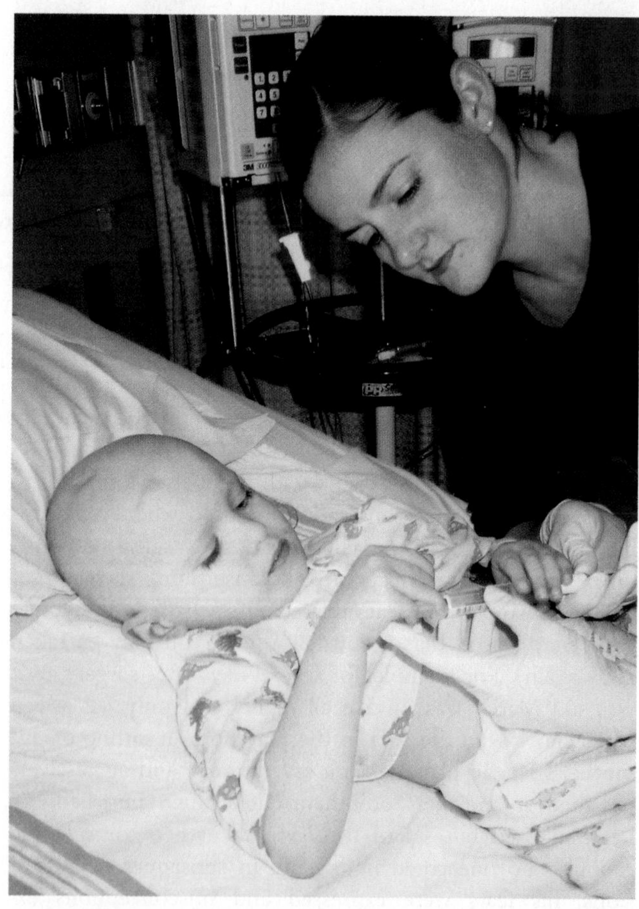

FIGURE 16-17 When nurses involve children in their own care, they are able to gain a sense of control and mastery. PUBLISHED WITH PERMISSION OF MASSGENERAL HOSPITAL FOR CHILDREN.

EVIDENCE-BASED PRACTICE

Should Caregivers Stay with Children During Invasive Procedures?

CLINICAL PROBLEM

There is strong evidence to support the importance of caregivers staying with their children during hospitalization, but the presence of caregivers when children are undergoing invasive procedures remains an issue of controversy and hesitancy. Decisions about whether or not caregivers should be present become increasingly difficult for caregivers, nurses, and physicians when highly invasive procedures are involved (e.g., placement of chest tubes or central lines, intubation, resuscitation). Often these procedures are performed in emergency situations when time for decision making is limited.

BEST CLINICAL PRACTICE

- Parents of children undergoing one or more invasive procedures in a pediatric intensive care unit found their presence to be helpful to their child, to themselves, and to the medical staff. Their presence also decreased personal anxiety and procedure-related anxiety. Nurses found parent presence to be helpful to the child; most parents would repeat their choice to be present.
- While there have been numerous studies to support the presence of caregivers during invasive procedures, the issue remains controversial. Further research and evidence-based practice protocols are needed.

IMPLICATIONS FOR NURSING

The decision about caregiver presence during highly invasive procedures requires discussion between caregivers who are informed about the nature of the procedure and the nurse–physician team who have responsibility for the care and treatment of the child. The role of the nurse is to assess the immediacy of the procedure and, in the time available, facilitate wise decisions based on individual circumstances, the exigencies of the moment, ethical–legal implications, and the comfort level of all involved. When caregivers are able to be present and helpful, there are benefits to both the child and caregiver. Future research could focus on analyzing decisions about caregiver presence during highly invasive procedures and those less invasive in order to provide a more extensive knowledge base to guide this process and to develop guidelines for practice.

References: Egemen, A., Ikizoglu, T., Darapnar, B., Cosar, H., & Karapnar, D. (2008). Parental presence during invasive procedures and resuscitation: Attitudes of health care professionals in Turkey. *Pediatric Emergency Care, 22*(4), 230–234; Piira, T., Sugiura, T., Champion, G. D., Donnelly, N., & Cole, A. S. J. (2005). The role of parental presence in the context of children's medical procedures: A systematic review. *Child-Care, Health, & Development, 31*(2), 233–243; Pruitt, L. M., Johnson, A., Elliot, J. C., & Polley, P. (2008). Parental presence during pediatric invasive procedures. *Journal of Pediatric Health Care,* (22)2, 120–127.

use phrases like "You're a good girl/boy," particularly for young children who may associate this experience with punishment. At the conclusion of treatments, offer a simple apology if the child experienced discomfort or pain (e.g., "I'm sorry if I hurt you"). Follow-up includes the fun activity or comfort measure agreed on in advance, encouraging expression or description of how the child experienced the procedure through conversations, and play. Considerable insight can be gained by asking children and caregivers what could have been done to make the experience easier to manage. Questions like "Now that this is over, what helped you the most in getting ready [or during] the procedure?" or, "What should I be sure to tell other children about what it is like and how it feels when they have their bandages changed?" may help with future explanations.

COMMUNICATING WITH CHILDREN AND FAMILIES

Talking directly to children is important in the process of caring and comforting (Figure 16-18). Sometimes words are confusing and cause distress. For example, a child was in her room crying and stopped long enough to ask "Is this tomorrow?" to which the nurse replied "No, it's today." Her crying escalated and the nurse discovered that the day before, the doctor said that she "could go home tomorrow." When the nurse assured her this was "tomorrow," the child was much relieved and could prepare for going home.

Children often do not understand the different language of the hospital setting or may misinterpret what is said to them or to others. To be effective, communication should be clear, honest, and understandable to the child. A prime example is when children are told they are to have "a shot"; even though this is commonly used to describe an injection, the child may conjure up visions of being maimed or harmed beyond the pain of the injection. They may think they will "be shot." Often, children hear, "it will only hurt a little," or "this won't hurt," when something is known to be painful. A more effective explanation is the truth in coping with and managing hurtful experiences. Sometimes words used are frightening and evoke fantasies of doom. One example is the shriek response of a child when the technician said she would put in dye for a test. The child reacted so vehemently because he thought, "I might die."

Nurses also need to know the words children commonly use for toileting and other vital needs and ways of communicating when they are unable to express themselves verbally. Some children have difficulty understanding because of hearing, cognitive, or neurological impairments, and others may not understand or have the ability to express their needs because of language, cultural differences, or fear. In a situation of a 4-year-old girl who understood only her native language, her mother left three cards with her when she had to leave, each one of a different color. On the yellow, it was written "I have to go to the bathroom," on the blue, "I want a drink of water," and on the red "I need to call my mother."

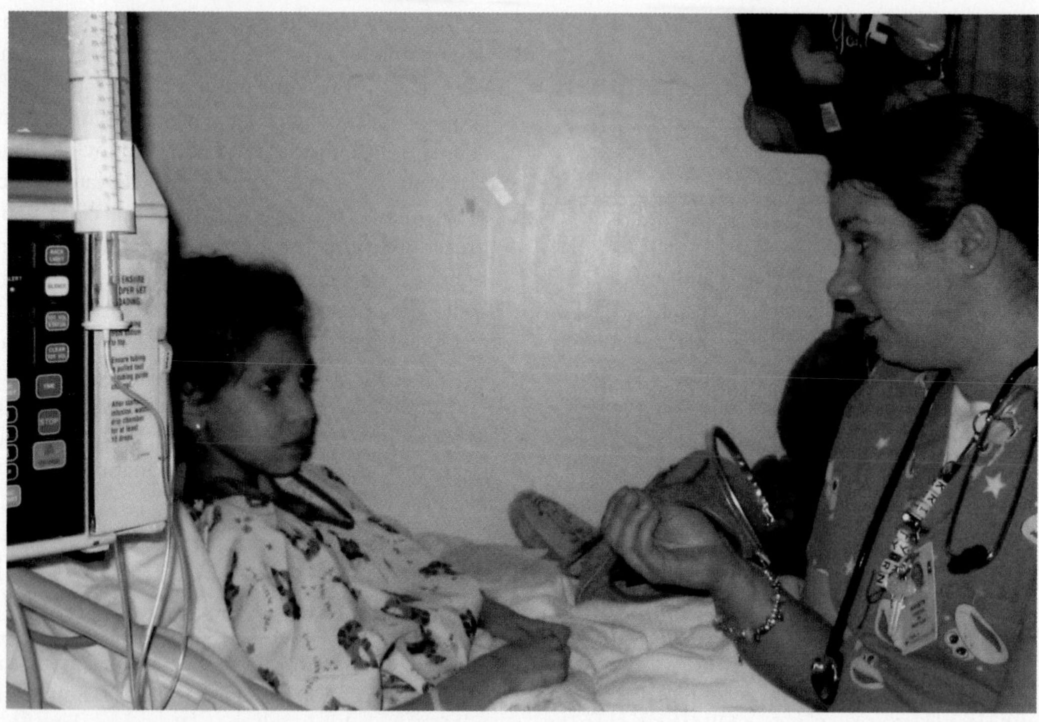

FIGURE 16-18 Talking directly to children is reassuring and comforting. PUBLISHED WITH PERMISSION OF BAYSTATE CHILDREN'S HOSPITAL.

NURSING TIP

How much do Children Know About their Diagnosis?

At the time of diagnosis, it is important to plan time for explanations and questions. A helpful approach is to ask caregivers or the child what they know or have heard about the diagnosis and respond to immediate concerns and reactions. Encourage writing questions for further discussion and clarification.

In communicating with children, the use of their preferred name is important. A 6-year-old whose name was Charles Brown was admitted to the hospital for a spinal cord injury following an automobile accident in which he had been hit by a car. (When asked, "What happened?" he said, "I didn't run fast enough.") The staff nurses amusingly called him "Charlie Brown" from the time he was admitted until one nurse asked him, "What do your caregivers call you?" to which he answered, "Chuckie." When his own nickname was used, there were notable changes in the way he engaged in exercises, and he talked more openly about his family and school.

The language used in reference to children is also important. To refer to children as "kids" or to an individual child as "this kid" minimizes the dignity of children. Even though these terms are commonly used in everyday conversation to refer to children as a group or to a child as an individual, the appropriateness in professional nursing practice is questionable. Similarly, one should be aware of the detrimental effects of labeling or stereotyping children or caregivers. Instead of saying "He's a diabetic," the phrase "He is a child with diabetes" emphasizes he is a child with a health problem and not one who is identified by a disease.

Honesty in explanations, responses to questions, and general information helps children to be trustful of others. This should be considered in minor situations as well, so when nurses say, "I'll be right back," they should return promptly because situations like this are symbolic of trusting relationships.

NURSING CARE AND GUIDANCE OF INFANTS

Newborns and infants during the first year of life may be hospitalized at a time of rapid growth and development. Some are hospitalized for long periods after birth, with transitions from newborn intensive care units to pediatric units, home, and return to hospital for surgery, diagnostic tests, and so forth. Others are admitted for congenital and adventitious conditions requiring short or long-term care. Their healthy attachment to caregivers and their progress toward optimal development are of paramount concern during these times.

SPECIAL NEEDS OF INFANTS

From the time of birth, infants depend on others for nurturance and protection. Gaining a sense of trust is facilitated

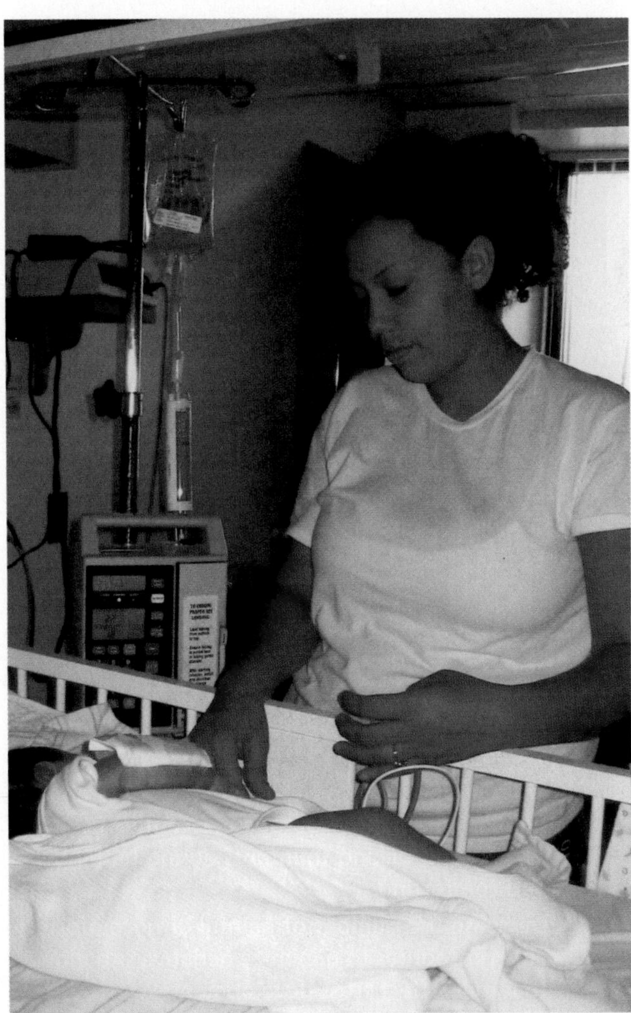

FIGURE 16-19 **Caregiver presence is comforting for both infant and caregiver.** PUBLISHED WITH PERMISSION OF BAYSTATE CHILDREN'S HOSPITAL.

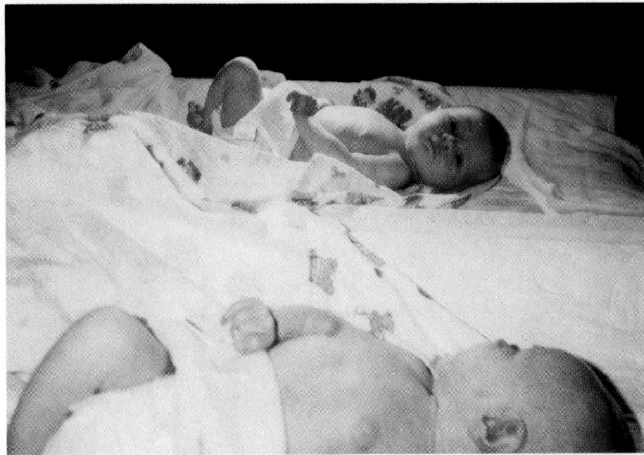

FIGURE 16-20 **Babies are visually stimulated and entertained by their own image.** DELMAR CENGAGE LEARNING.

when needs for bonding, contact comfort, and nutritional sustenance are fulfilled, and when rhythmical, reciprocal patterns develop. Infants need the kind of security predisposing them to restful sleep, satisfaction of oral and nutritional needs, relaxation of the body and body systems, and spontaneity in response to communication and gentle environmental stimuli.

Caregiver–infant attachment is critical to psychological health. Infants need their primary caregiver during illness. Infants beyond the age of 5–6 months are acutely aware of the absence of their primary caregiver and, within a few months, develop stranger anxiety and become fearful of unfamiliar persons. For hospitalized infants, it is essential not only to support caregivers in their role, but to also assure consistency in sensitive, responsive, and interactive nursing care.

The basic source of infant satisfaction is through satiation of oral needs. During illness, there is often disruption in the consistency of feeding patterns, contact comfort, sleeping, elimination, and stimulation. Nurses should be particularly aware of the effects of situations that interfere with the gratification of oral needs (e.g., oral surgery, vomiting, distasteful medications, withholding food and fluids, as well as periods of non-oral feedings). When oral satisfaction is threatened, it is difficult for infants to maintain pleasure through sucking, swallowing, digesting, and eliminating. An example is when tube feeding is required; the use of a pacifier during the time of feeding helps the infant develop the relationship between oral pleasure and the feeling of fullness and satiation when hunger is relieved.

DIRECT CARE OF INFANTS

Nurses have many responsibilities in securing optimal health for infants both in teaching caregivers and families and in providing direct care. For consistency, the patterns of care at home are a helpful guide to planning care in the hospital. For first-time mothers of young infants, the nurse is often a model for baby care.

Infants learn through sensorimotor experiences (Figure 16-20). Talking to infants slowly, singing lullabies, moving them gently and carefully, and rocking and cuddling are ways to help infants reduce tension. Smooth, continuous movements, gentle stroking, and holding confidently are additional methods to reduce stress responses. In some hospitals, grandmothers and other volunteers often provide comfort by rocking and cuddling, particularly for those children with prolonged hospitalizations (Figure 16-21). External stimuli, such as pictures, mirrors, music, and mobiles, provide the kind of visual stimulation needed for growth.

Infant massage is an intervention used by nurses who are prepared to use this technique to soothe infants and provide physical stimulation (Field, 1995; Lindrea & Stainton, 2000). Swaddling by wrapping the infant snugly in a soft blanket is a practice used by many cultural groups to promote infant comfort and security. See Box 16-3 for more suggestions on caring for infants.

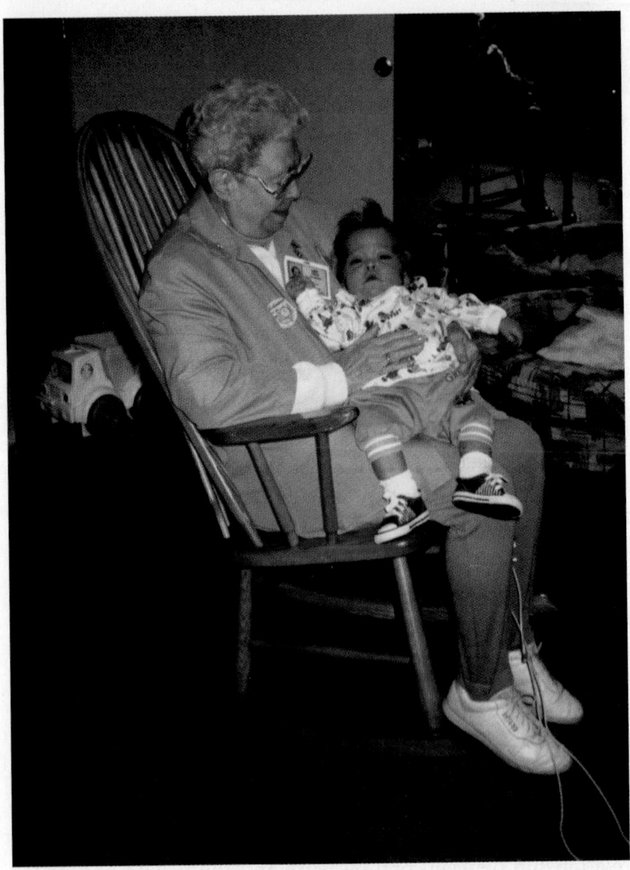

FIGURE 16-21 **Volunteer grandmothers provide relaxing moments for hospitalized infants and children.** PUBLISHED WITH PERMISSION OF BAYSTATE CHILDREN'S HOSPITAL.

BOX 16-3
POINTS OF EMPHASIS IN CARING FOR INFANTS

Safety

- Always have at least one hand on the infant when the crib sides are down.
- Place the child on the opposite side of the crib when lowering the crib sides.
- Put crib sides up all the way when the infant is in a crib, and push against the crib side when it is up to be sure that it is held securely in place.
- Avoid leaving harmful objects or objects small enough to be swallowed in the crib or within reach.
- Examine toys for safety and washability.

Other

- Be aware of both obvious and subtle signs of discomfort and discontent (crying, furrowed brow, body tension, wringing hands), and respond to needs.
- Assume open face position while feeding and holding infants—encourage eye contact by smiling and talking to infants during bathing and comforting.
- Decrease the number of painful or uncomfortable procedures to minimize negative situations that may affect trust development.
- After painful or distressing experiences, comfort infant by holding and using soothing tones and movement.
- Supporting caregivers is the primary way to support infants coping with tension.
- When it is difficult for caregivers to be present during procedures, their wishes should be respected and supported with reassurance.

NURSING CARE AND GUIDANCE OF TODDLERS

From babyhood to toddlerhood, children develop remarkable skills in all aspects of growth and development. They are now their own person as demonstrated by their awareness of self as a being with the power to use words and actions to express their will. They learn how their behavior affects others as they become individuals, while at the same time being conscious of the need for care and protection by others. When toddlers are hospitalized, preservation of the protective relationships of caregivers continues to be critical to their healthy development and healing (Neal, Frost, Kuhn, & Green, 2007).

SPECIAL NEEDS OF TODDLERS

Hospitalization or surgery imposes movement restrictions and changes that undermine beginning confidence in skill development. While in the midst of learning to feed themselves or learning sphincter control with all the praise and affirmation usually accorded these efforts, there may be little attention paid to these accomplishments in the hospital. Putting diapers on a child who has mastered toileting diminishes the sense of competence and control. To preserve developing autonomy and minimize shame and doubt, it is important to know the accomplishments of individual toddlers and maintain mastery insofar as possible. With different routines, separations from caregivers, misinterpretations of language and behavior, and being prevented from moving, enjoying, and controlling their bodies, toddlers become perplexed and may respond with regression, aggression, or withdrawal. Of great concern is the actual separation from caregivers in an unfamiliar environment when family members are not able to stay. When there are short separations, and toddlers have become familiar with a primary nurse, adaptation is facilitated.

However, in the hospital, everything is different and unpredictable. The presence of caregivers, especially during critical times of procedures, treatments, and before and after surgery, is essential. It is advisable for each child to have a family member present throughout the hospital stay. The primary goals in planning care for a toddler who is hospitalized are to sustain child–family bonds, to preserve their sense of autonomy by assuring opportunities to exercise their will, and to strengthen their ability to mature in cognitive and psychomotor skills. Effective nurse–caregiver relationships and consistency of care provide the kind of secure environment toddlers need to cope with the changes of illness and hospitalization.

EFFECTS OF PROLONGED SEPARATION ON TODDLERS

One of the most serious consequences of hospitalization is the response that occurs when prolonged hospital stays are combined with the inability of caregivers to spend extended time with their toddler. If caregivers leave and consistently return after short periods, toddlers can regain security, but if they do not reappear for long periods and children need them desperately, separation anxiety poses a serious threat to healthy development. The literature is replete with the progressive and potentially long-term effects of this kind of crisis. Bowlby (1965) was one of the first to study the psychological distress of children separated from their families during World War II. Spitz (1954) documented the effects of prolonged separation on infants in foundling homes, observing that many infants succumbed even though adequate physical care was provided.

Robertson (1958) studied the effect of separations of young children from their parents due to hospitalization and described three phases of response: protest, despair, and denial. In the initial stage of **protest**, toddlers cry loudly and desperately when parents leave, making every effort to bring them back. They are inconsolable and constantly look in the direction of where their parent departed. This way of communicating their displeasure is often misinterpreted by caregivers and nurses. Parents may think they should stay away so the child will not become upset, and nurses may try to encourage the child to be "good and not cry," instead of understanding this as a healthy and appropriate expression of emotion.

If separations continue, withdrawal, refusals of food, diminished communication, and general loss of interest in the environment occurs. During this **despair** phase, children may lie quietly and come to others, yet their internal distress is such that they do not express their feelings easily. When parents return, the toddler may look away or focus on toys or objects as if to ignore parents who disappointed them by going away. If separation is further extended, the child enters a phase of **denial**, or detachment, having lost hope for permanent reunion. There is an outward appearance of indifference and the toddler appears to be settled in, compliant, "adjusted," and indiscriminate in relationships with others and to the situation. This denial of emotion is often misinterpreted as coping well with their plight. Although these developments are now rare because of comparatively short hospitalizations, constant vigilance is necessary to prevent these severe responses (Figure 16-22). In the eyes of a child, even short separations during times of stress can be perceived as much longer than they really are.

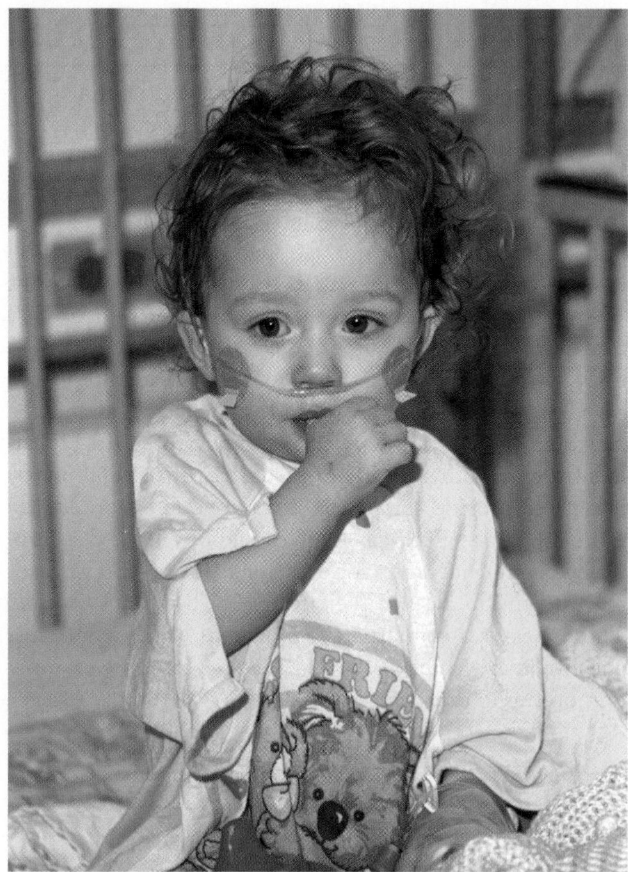

FIGURE 16-22 It is important to monitor toddlers closely to prevent severe responses to hospitalization. DELMAR CENGAGE LEARNING.

CRITICAL THINKING

A Toddler Who Is Immobilized

Timothy, a healthy, active child of 20 months, has been admitted to the hospital and is placed in traction for treatment of a fractured femur. A hip spica cast will be applied within a few days, and an individualized nursing plan of care has been developed regarding his unique needs, care in traction, care after the cast is applied, and discharge instructions. He is the youngest of four children and is rarely cared for by adults other than his caregivers. His mother plans to stay with him throughout the hospital stay except for brief periods of a few hours each day.

- What kind of assessment data at the time of admission would assist you in understanding the effects of this child's experience on the child and family? What strengths of a child of this age would facilitate coping? What strengths of the family would facilitate coping?
- What are ways of helping this child to manage immobility, diminished control, and brief separations?

DIRECT CARE OF TODDLERS

There are many constructive ways of applying knowledge of growth and development during hospitalization. For example, understanding autonomy in toddlers and the negativism that is part of this task is evident with choices for a toddler. If the nurse asks, "Do you want to take a nap now?" this implies a choice that is not age-appropriate and often precipitates a negative response. If, however, one were to say, "It's time for a nap now—do you want Pooh Bear or Clifford to come with you?" the toddler has the opportunity to exert autonomous behavior and cooperation is more likely.

To maintain areas of comfort, the child's bed and the playroom should not be used for painful procedures. Treatment rooms, with supportive persons (caregiver and nurse) present to provide comforting during and after procedures, is a better place. Each day, time should be allocated to providing comfort measures for each child, like rocking or reading to them, to balance the stressors of being hospitalized. Those measures comforting to individual children are most effective in alleviating stress. See Box 16-4 for more information on caring for toddlers.

BOX 16-4
POINTS OF EMPHASIS IN CARING FOR TODDLERS

Safety

- Assess crib safety and minimize the possibility of climbing out and possible injury (hospital cribs with extended protection, e.g., Springfield model, have been designed to prevent injuries from climbing out of the crib).
- Child should always be supervised by an adult when out of bed.
- Be aware of any hazardous objects or situations (e.g., sharp objects, materials, toxic substances, and electrical outlets).
- Avoid hard candies, balloons, plastic bags, or food or other material that may cause choking or suffocation.

Other

- Observe verbal and nonverbal behavior for signs of sadness or discontent.
- Explain the response of protest when caregivers must leave for short periods, and encourage them to leave an article of clothing such as a scarf, cap, or small purse so the child will have an object belonging to the person as a symbol of returning. Also explain it is not wise to leave when the child is sleeping, but at a time when the nurse is present. Then, even though it may be hard, encourage the child to wave and say good-bye.
- Play games of peek-a-boo or a variation of hide and seek with dolls to reinforce going away and coming back.
- Provide home routines and as much independence as possible in eating and mobility.
- Ascertain the way the toddler likes to be comforted when in distress.
- Provide for as much mobility and activity as possible.
- Take care of special toys or transitional objects such as blankets or worn toys.
- Keep a picture of the toddler and members of family close by and talk about family.
- Observe behavior closely for regression and aggression.
- Maintain locomotion even when walking is limited (e.g., stroller, cart, or moving the bed to the playroom).
- Provide simple directions and appropriate choices.

NURSING CARE AND GUIDANCE OF PRESCHOOL CHILDREN

Preschool children are hospitalized for a variety of reasons, including injuries, infectious or inflammatory processes, surgical procedures, and long-term illnesses. Although they are naturally curious, have facility with language and other skills, and enjoy the beginning independence that comes during these years, preschoolers are also acutely aware of their need for the presence and support of the adults in their lives (Figure 16-23).

SPECIAL NEEDS OF PRESCHOOL CHILDREN

Preschoolers learn best through observation and manipulation of objects (Figure 16-24). Abstractions or things not seen are difficult to understand. Many have not yet learned correct anatomical terms and most have had limited experience in learning about the body. They may think the skin holds them together and any disruption in integrity threatens their sense of being. They often think that, with intrusive procedures, their "insides may come out" or "they will lose all their blood and die." They are often distressed when urine or stool samples are obtained because this is a private matter, and vomiting or diarrhea is perplexing and disturbing because of their perceived loss of control.

Seeing blood or "taking blood" is frightening because of its symbolic nature. To many children, "Red is the color of hurting" (Shore, 1965). Children need explanations about their body organs and functions, and Band-Aids to cover any wounds, either by accident or by others, both physical and psychological.

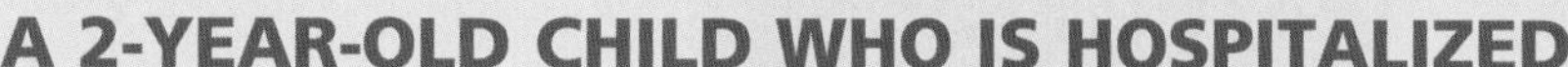

CASE STUDY / CARE PLAN

A 2-YEAR-OLD CHILD WHO IS HOSPITALIZED

Camden is a 3-year-old female who was initially admitted to the pediatric unit from the emergency room in acute respiratory distress several days ago. Since being on the unit, her respiratory distress has disappeared, but whenever the nurse comes in the room, Camden now seems fearful and displays signs of regression (she was toilet trained before being hospitalized).

NURSING CARE PLAN

ASSESSMENT

Camden manifests behaviors suggesting fear and regression

NURSING DIAGNOSIS 1

Fear related to lack of exposure to the hospital experience and being exposed to new personnel.

EXPECTED OUTCOME

1. Camden no longer displays behaviors suggestive of regression or is fearful of health care providers.

NOC: Illness Care

NIC: Environment Comfort

INTERVENTIONS/*RATIONALES*

1. Ascertain the way she likes to be comforted when in distress, *Child can be comforted similar to how caregivers comfort her at home.*
2. Encourage parents to leave an article of clothing such as a scarf, cap, or small purse when they leave. *Child she will have an object belonging to the person as a symbol of returning.*
3. If undergoing painful procedures, be sure to provide comfort during and after procedures. *Gives the child an opportunity to be nurtured and comforted after undergoing the procedure.*
4. Provide comfort measures (rocking or reading) each day. *To balance the stressors of being hospitalized.*

EVALUATION

Child will show signs of being comforted by parent and nurse (decreased crying and irritability).

NURSING DIAGNOSIS 2

Anxiety (parental) related to inexperience with hospitalization and observance of child's apparent regressive behaviors.

EXPECTED OUTCOME

1. Camden's mother will understand the regression is temporary and after the child returns to a familiar environment she will be able to be toilet trained again.

NOC: Knowledge; Illness Care

NIC: Learning Facilitation

INTERVENTIONS/*RATIONALES*

1. Provide information to caregivers regarding how toddlers cope with hospitalization. *With improved knowledge they will be less stressed.*
2. Allow Camden's mother to participate in her care as much as possible and as she is able and wants to participate. *When if caregivers participate in the care of their children the children will be less stressed and fearful.*

EVALUATION

Child's mother will verbalize understanding that toilet training can resume once hospitalization is concluded.

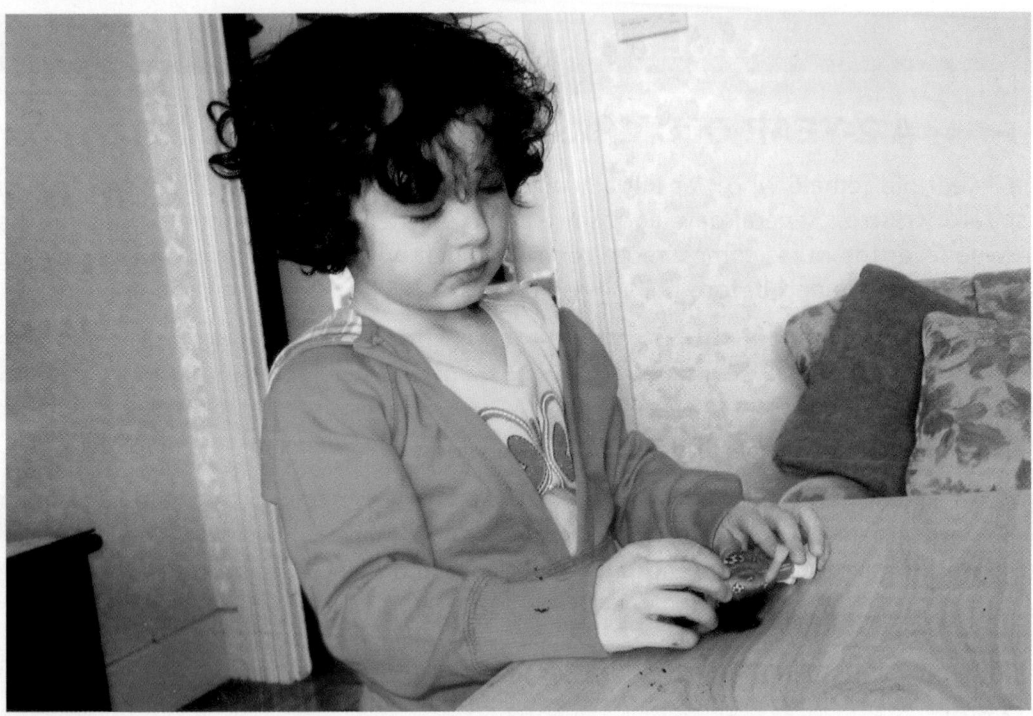

FIGURE 16-23 Young children develop a sense of autonomy through play activities. DELMAR CENGAGE LEARNING.

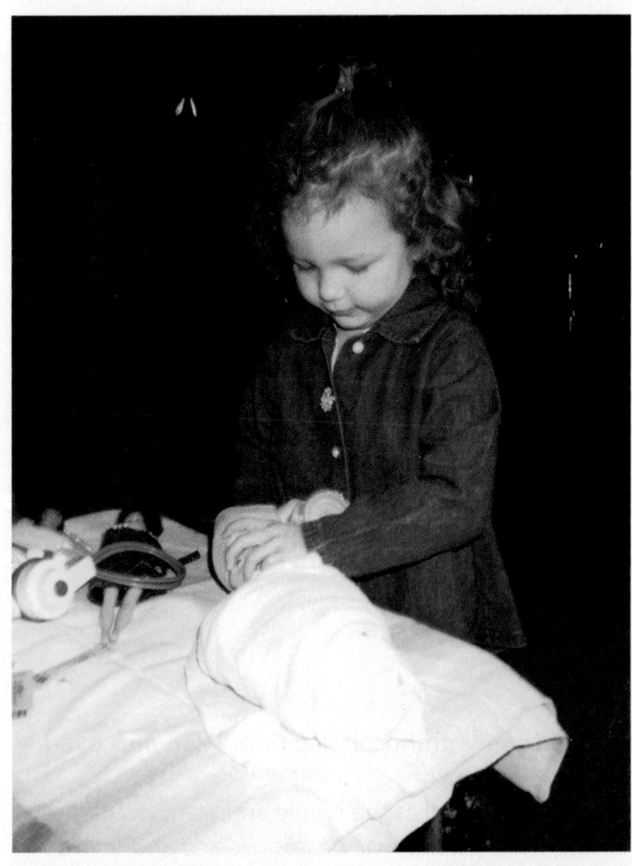

FIGURE 16-24 Children are serious about using dolls to "play hospital." DELMAR CENGAGE LEARNING.

Children of this age also need caregivers present to protect them from their fears and fantasies, and to explain events in terms they understand. They also need to know the sequence of what is to be done in tests or procedures and to carefully prepare using play equipment followed by therapeutic play after stressful events. Even though they explore their environment through intrusion, their greatest fears are related to intrusion into their bodies.

DIRECT CARE OF PRESCHOOL CHILDREN

To foster a sense of initiative, preschool children need to be as involved as possible in all aspects of their care and have opportunities for choices. They often experience illness and hospitalization as a consequence for misdeeds and it is essential they understand painful procedures are not punishment. Additionally, they may fear if they are not good or if they cry, further harm will ensue. It is helpful to tell preschoolers it is all right to cry, and to say "I'm sorry" when pain is incurred. Young children also benefit from learning active methods of coping such as guided imagery (Ott, 1996). Providing opportunities for playing out stressful events helps avoid feelings of being victimized.

Teaching is also a primary intervention in the care of preschoolers. This is most likely to be successful when children have adequate time to learn, but not too much time to worry. Continued teaching throughout procedures with opportunities for involvement when possible (e.g., hand the

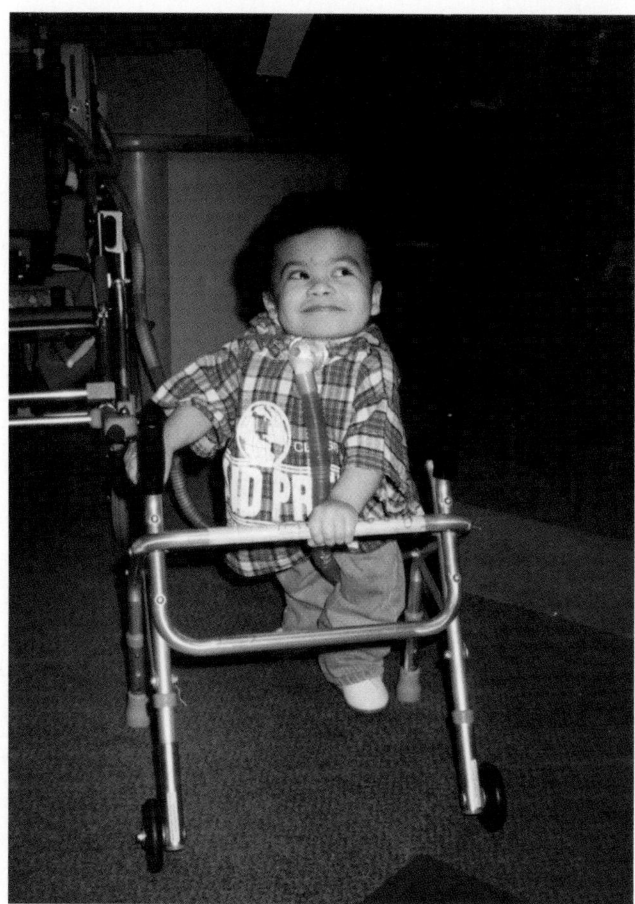

FIGURE 16-25 **For young children, mobility is important for developing a sense of autonomy.** PUBLISHED WITH PERMISSION OF BAYSTATE CHILDREN'S HOSPITAL.

tape for a dressing) and an explanation after the procedure to clarify any misconceptions is important. Follow-up opportunities for play complete a cycle for learning.

Preschoolers are usually sociable, and group play and activities are often successful. Sometimes when children are having difficulty taking fluids, a tea party, or playing restaurant when "drinks" are ordered, is more helpful than frequent encouragement to take fluids. It is advisable for children to have meals at a table or in an area with other children whenever possible and to maintain mobility (Figure 16-25). Children need praise for cooperation, regardless of their coping ability. Building on strengths is a key concept in fostering the ability to cope. See Box 16-5 for more information on caring for preschoolers.

BOX 16-5

POINTS OF EMPHASIS IN CARING FOR PRESCHOOL CHILDREN

Safety

- Anticipate stressful situations, and observe for behavior indicating signs of distress.
- Encourage adults to accompany preschool children.
- Keep environment free of harmful objects and equipment.
- Have child wear shoes instead of slippers when ambulating.

Other

- Understand fears of unfamiliar environment, abandonment, and punishment, and fears related to body integrity and deprivation.
- Have the picture of an animal or object outside and inside the door of each hospital room, so that the child can easily identify his or her place.
- Encourage involvement in learning to maintain a sense of initiative.
- Provide play activities and materials as a means of coping with stressful situations. Tell child the nurse's name and how to call for help.
- Being familiar with common television shows and movies for children facilitates conversation.
- Explore child's perceptions and understanding of the illness and treatments.
- Emphasize treatments are not punishment by explaining reason these are necessary.

NURSING CARE AND GUIDANCE OF SCHOOL-AGE CHILDREN

The school years are perhaps the healthiest of all ages; however, children are hospitalized during this time for many reasons (e.g., accidents, infections, autoimmune, and oncological conditions). Their developing confidence and self-esteem brought about by success in meeting challenges, competence in learning, and skill in relating to adults and peers are often strengths (Figure 16-26). During hospitalization, every effort needs to be put forth to help those whose primary focus is school-related to continue to learn and maintain their individual strengths.

SPECIAL NEEDS OF SCHOOL-AGE CHILDREN

The anxiety of illness, diagnostic tests, and therapeutic interventions is expressed in many ways and there are many factors involved in the success of school-age children in managing the stressors of hospitalization. Some children do not express distress openly, and an outwardly calm child may not be coping successfully. In fact, hospitalized children who were admitted for acute illnesses were more likely to perceive their coping as effective than those with chronic illnesses, and children with low anxiety as a trait were

KIDS WANT TO KNOW

Frequent Questions about Hospitalization

- What is an MRI (or CAT scan or chest X-ray)? Where will I go? Will it hurt? Will it be dark? How long will it take?
- Why are you here? What's next? What does that machine do? Is that for me?
- Can I talk to my friend on the computer? Can my dad go with me? Can my mother stay?
- Where are the video games? Where is the bathroom? Where are the toys?
- Who will take care of me when my caregivers leave? Can my friends come to visit?
- What did they say about me? What if I wake up during the operation? When can I go home?

Response

When children ask direct questions, it is helpful to respond with short, age-appropriate answers and encourage additional questions. Example: What's a chest X-ray? A chest X-ray is a picture of your chest taken with a large camera called an X-ray machine. It takes a few minutes of being in a room with very dim light. It won't hurt and will be over quickly when the picture has been checked by the person who took it; you will come back to your room. Children often do not ask the questions they are thinking about; or there may be a question behind the question being posed. It is helpful to clarify communication by asking, "Is there something else you really want to know or talk about?" or "Sometimes children wonder about (topic). Are you thinking about this, too?"

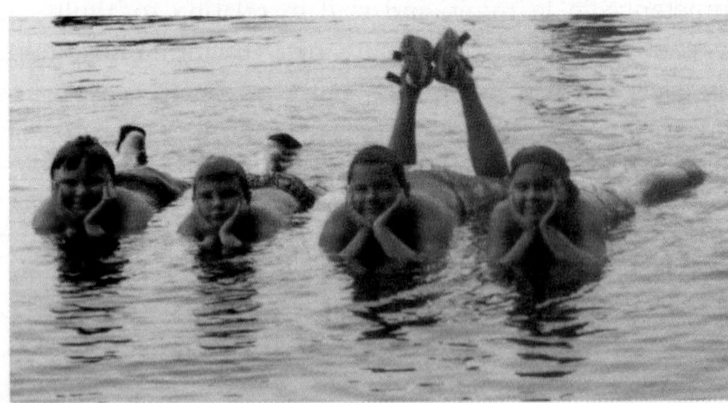

FIGURE 16-26 "Having fun" with peers helps school-age children develop social relationships and self-esteem. DELMAR CENGAGE LEARNING.

more likely to describe their coping behaviors as effective than those with high trait anxiety (Bossert, 1994).

There is an additional stressor when illness or surgery produces changes in appearance or threatens success in developing or maintaining friendships. For some, there is fear other children "will make fun of me," "tease," or "not like me anymore," especially when children have overt changes in appearance due to medications such as corticosteroid therapy, loss of hair or limbs, or scarring. In some situations, it is advisable to seek consultation with psychologists or clinical nurse specialists in psychiatric–mental health for ongoing counseling.

DIRECT CARE OF SCHOOL-AGE CHILDREN

For some school-age children, the ability to master the stress of hospitalization may be a source of accomplishment that increases their confidence in coping and mastering other difficult situations. Continuous, deliberative support, positive relationships, and coaching during stressful times are some measures leading to success in mastery and learning coping skills.

A brief description of some methods used effectively is in Table 16-1. Other alternative methods are aromatherapy, biofeedback, self-hypnosis, dance therapy, prayer, meditation, therapeutic touch, humor, and pet therapy. Pet-facilitated therapy helps children feel pleasure in seeing and reacting to animals. Children who have pets at home are particularly enthusiastic and smile spontaneously when specially trained dogs are brought to the hospital (Figure 16-27). In a research

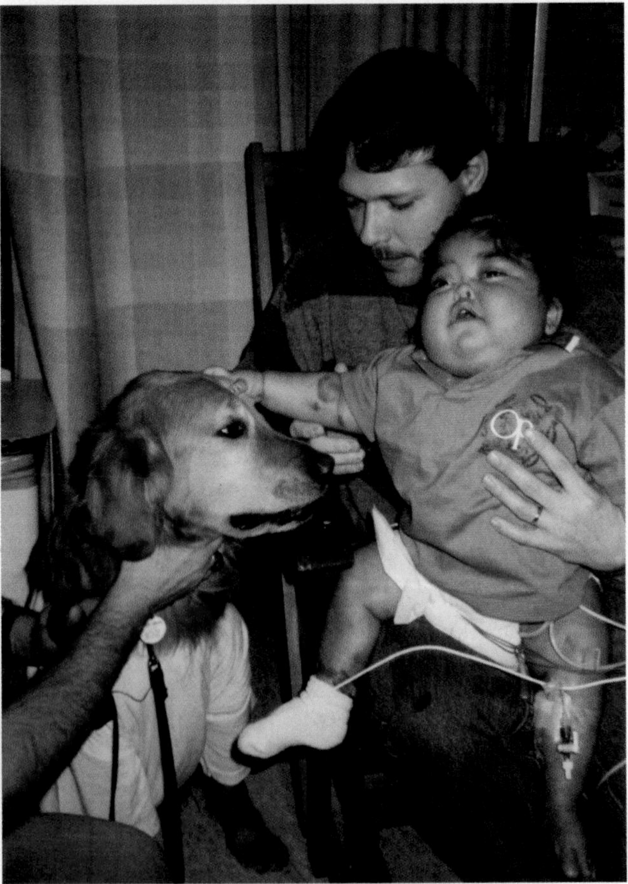

FIGURE 16-27 Pet therapy is a way of engendering positive emotions during hospitalization. PUBLISHED WITH PERMISSION OF BAYSTATE CHILDREN'S HOSPITAL.

TABLE 16-1 Alternative Ways of Helping Children Cope during Hospitalization

THERAPY	DEFINITION
Art therapy	A variety of art forms to encourage children to express thoughts and feelings (e.g., drawings of self and hospital experiences, use of clay, finger-painting, etc.). Also used as adjunctive mental health treatment (*Mosby's dictionary of medicine, nursing & health professions*, 2009).
Creative art and crafts	Paper, crayons, paint, pencils, and other materials for release of creative potential. Conscious interaction promotes expression of imagination, development of self-esteem, and contributes to sense of accomplishment (Ward, 1998).
Focused breathing	Rhythmic breathing to manage or reduce stress by attending to the process of inhaling and exhaling.
Guided imagery	Guiding imagination and visualization to facilitate (creative imagery) relaxed, focused concentration on images and scenes of pleasurable activity during tests and treatments as a way of empowering children and promoting coping abilities (Huth, Broome, & Good, 2003; Ott, 1996; Ward, 1998; Poikki, Pietila, Vehrilainen-Julkunen, Laukkala, & Kiviluomaki, 2008).
Interactive technology	Use of creative, interactive computer programs designed to help children cope with experience of illness and share experiences with others (e.g., Starbright World—see Resources).
Massage	Effleurage (stroking), petressage (kneading), rubbing, or tapping soft tissues of the body to increase circulation, improve muscle tone, and promote relaxation (Field, 1995; Ward, 1998).
Music therapy	Use of music as background or active child involvement (e.g., singing, sing-along) during play or during invasive procedures as a calming or distracting influence (Berlin, 1995; Kouretas, 1999).
Progressive muscle relaxation	Alternately tensing and relaxing muscle groups sequentially.
Written expression	Poetry, journals, diaries, composing songs or lyrics, letters to friends (or imaginary friends or pets) to reflect and express thoughts, feelings, or responses to illness experiences.

study by Kaminski, Pellino, & Wish, (2002) it was reported that seeing and interacting with animals increased emotional comfort, decreased loneliness and anxiety, and provided a source of self-esteem. In general, the well-being of children was enhanced and anxiety reduced. To extend the repertoire of alternative methods, nurses need to study each adjunctive technique thoroughly and feel confident in using these to help children and caregivers learn new ways of coping. Assessment of the appropriateness of using any particular method and evaluating the effectiveness of the method are essential components of these interventions.

When children are hospitalized, the important events in their lives and ongoing problems should be understood, particularly at times of prolonged hospitalization. If children are isolated because of communicable disease or for low immunity, every effort should be made to help them manage this confinement by minimizing the potential for sensory deprivation and the experience of being separated from others. They also need to clearly understand the reason and length of time (Figures 16-28 and 16-29).

School-age children who have developed reading skills benefit from books as well as Internet sources to understand their experiences. Most children's units have literature and instructions available to access these resources. Because their writing skills have been developed, there are several creative ways to express thoughts and feelings (described in Table 16-1). If hospitalized for an extended period, contact with schoolmates, teachers, and resuming schoolwork is

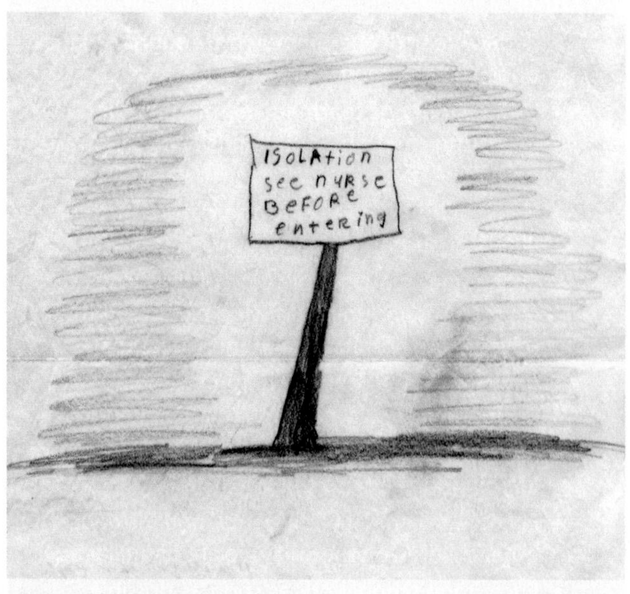

FIGURE 16-28 Being protected from infection is an isolating experience for a 12-year-old. DELMAR CENGAGE LEARNING.

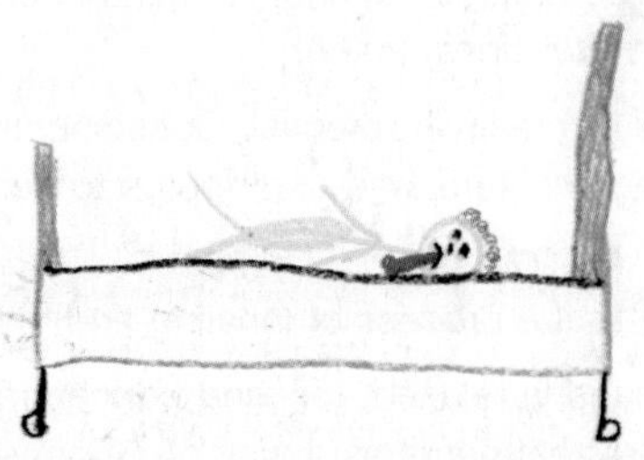

FIGURE 16-29 The art of an 11-year-old depicts his impression of what it is like to be in a hospital. DELMAR CENGAGE LEARNING.

recommended as soon as possible. To preserve their sense of industry, children should be complimented for learning during hospitalization. See Box 16-6 for more information on the care of school-age children.

BOX 16-6

POINTS OF EMPHASIS IN CARING FOR SCHOOL-AGE CHILDREN

Safety

- Be cognizant of responses to stress and methods of coping.
- Explain rules to prevent injury (e.g., hospital is not a place for running).

Other

- Reduce fear of the unknown through explanations and teaching.
- Use a variety of teaching–learning methods in preparing children—visual aids and stories are helpful.
- Help children understand the nature of their illness or surgery.
- Encourage creative expression of responses to experiences, including drawing pictures of themselves in the hospital and writing in journals.
- Use humor and jokes to help in coping and reducing anxiety.
- Be explicit in helping children see what they are learning in the hospital.
- Encourage contact with friends, and introduce other children on the unit who are of similar ages.
- Encourage schoolwork as soon as possible.

CRITICAL THINKING

A School-Age Child Being Discharged

At the time of discharge, Jose, a 12-year-old boy with advanced cystic fibrosis, hospitalized for seven days for treatment of bilateral lung infection, said, "I wish I didn't have to go back to school" and then hesitatingly said, "It's so embarrassing to be coughing all the time." You responded with encouragement: "All your friends will be glad to see you ... so will your teachers, and besides there are only a few months left." His father soon arrived to drive him home, and said, "You look great, let's go." Later, you recalled these interactions and reflected about your response in this situation. What assumptions were made that prompted your response to his comment about school? What were your thoughts or feelings about his comment? In recapturing and analyzing this situation, construct alternative responses and the rationale for any changes. Consider what his response "It's so embarrassing" meant.

NURSING CARE AND GUIDANCE OF ADOLESCENTS

During adolescence, developing a sense of identity is a primary task in development (Figure 16-30). The concerns and anxieties of adolescents are often masked by the appearance of sophistication, maturity, and what may be described as bravado. Their confidence and insecurities are often juxtaposed in such a way that hospitalization experiences are often perplexing and difficult. Their need for communication, understanding, and being understood by

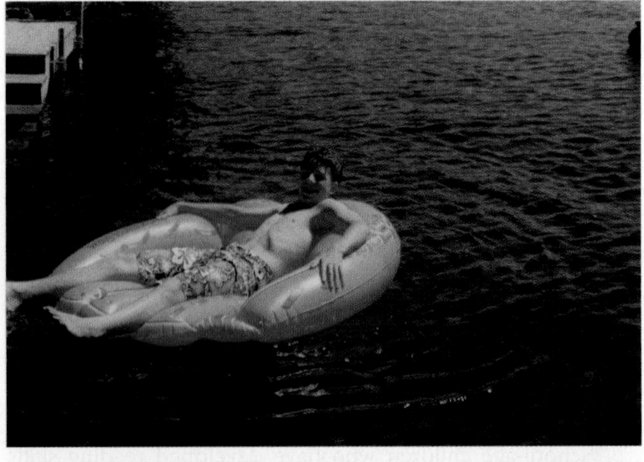

FIGURE 16-30 Early adolescence is a time for developing a sense of identity. DELMAR CENGAGE LEARNING.

adults and peers is important in meeting the challenges of their experiences and decisions related to illness and hospitalization.

SPECIAL NEEDS OF ADOLESCENTS

Adolescents who become ill are often in the midst of conflicts and struggles to establish a sense of identity as social and sexual beings. They are admitted to hospitals for many reasons, including severe body injury due to accidents or violence, an acute phase of a long-term illness, or surgical procedures. Regardless of the kind of health problem, adolescents fear disfigurement, changes in body image, and loss of body control. Having gained some measure of mental, physical, and social competence, they may be threatened by the stress of illness, treatments, and surgery. At a time when they have become more independent, there may be needs for dependence that lead to feelings of frustration, anger, and ambivalence about the situation and about those who provide assistance.

Adolescents who are hospitalized adapt best when they are with other adolescents in a separate unit where they have privacy and the opportunity to participate in the governance of their space. The environment should reflect their needs for such accouterments as mirrors, refrigerators, telephones, computers, areas of privacy, and a place for valuable possessions, including their own clothes.

DIRECT CARE OF ADOLESCENTS

Nurses with special preparation and interest in caring for adolescents are most successful in helping them cope with the exigencies of illness at a time when self-esteem and self-control are major aspects of development. Even though there may be ambivalent feelings toward adults, it is helpful when caregivers understand adolescents' need for coaches and opportunities to talk through situations of concern (e.g., impending surgery, diagnostic tests). Viewing the nurse and other health care professionals as high-status friends rather than persons in authoritarian roles facilitates their ability to engage in open, trusting relationships.

Nothing is more important than talking to adolescents and listening carefully to what they say and how they say it. Their need for uninterrupted time is very important to the process of developing coping skills. Adolescents are quick to identify those who have a genuine interest in them, and are equally sensitive when interest is feigned or when a person doesn't have time. Adolescents respond positively to those who have a sense of humor and are spontaneous and honest in their responses to questions and concerns. Attention to symptoms or explanations about treatments is not enough for adolescents to feel understood and cared for.

Establishing helping relationships may be difficult because adolescents are seeking independence from adults. However, it is within this kind of relationship that adolescents feel free to express their thoughts and feelings about situations they confront, and are more inclined to discuss personal issues not discussed with adults in their lives. They are also better able to cope with the problems they face during illness and hospitalization (Figure 16-31). When the nurse senses there are difficult questions, responses like, "Other teens with this problem wondered about or asked about ... and this is how I usually answer these questions" may help in discussing concerns.

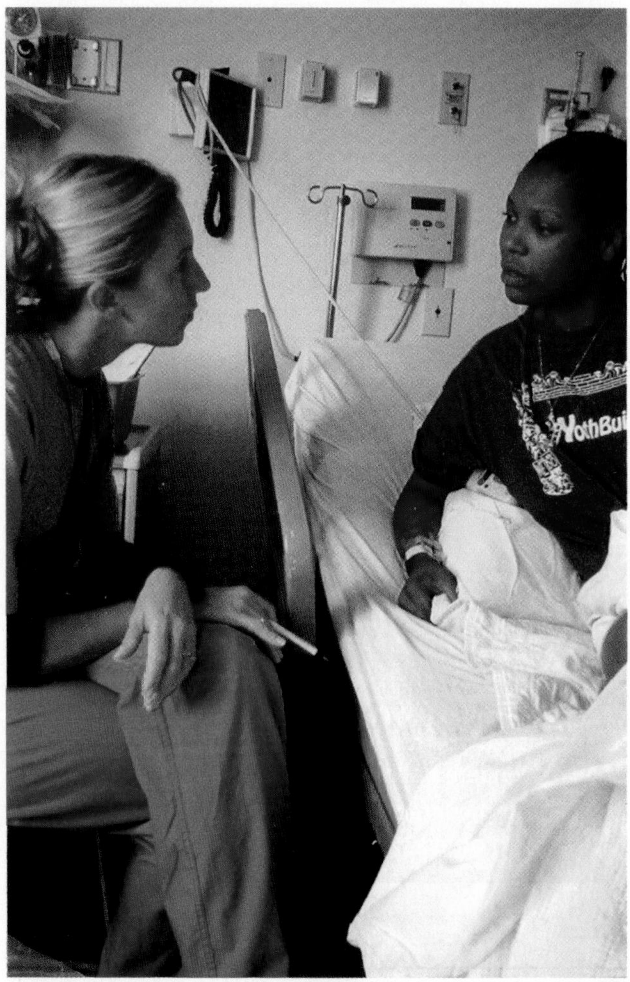

FIGURE 16-31 Careful listening and responding is helpful in establishing and maintaining helping relationships with adolescents. PUBLISHED WITH PERMISSION OF BAYSTATE CHILDREN'S HOSPITAL.

Adolescents may also develop crushes on nurses as a part of the process of developing a sense of identity and testing one's self in the formation of sexual identity. This often occurs with young nursing staff and students who need to understand this kind of response is related to developmental issues. Sometimes adolescents are openly curious about the personal lives of others as they seek to clarify their own lives and activities. In these situations, it is helpful to be direct and honest in setting boundaries, while understanding the need for working out relationships with others. See Box 16-7 for more information on caring for adolescents.

BOX 16-7
POINTS OF EMPHASIS IN CARING FOR ADOLESCENTS

- Plan uninterrupted time to teach and discuss responses.
- Encourage communication and involvement in decision making.
- Do not assume coping is effective if adolescent appears indifferent or full of bravado.
- Encourage reflective journals and creative means of expression (e.g., drawing, poetry).
- Use correct language and explain unfamiliar terms; a discussion rather than lecture format is usually more effective.
- Review recommended reading materials in advance; emphasize areas of greatest relevance—encourage writing questions and reflections each day as a basis for discussion.
- Refer to others who have had similar problems, and say, "Other teens in a situation like yours asked about … is this something that you wondered about?"
- Use the Internet and texting to communicate with others with similar conditions.

Reflections from Families

In my journey as a mother of a child on home parenteral and enteral nutrition (HPEN), I have gathered some wisdom worth sharing with the clinicians who take care of Luke and others like him. We want you to know that:

- *At times, we could be tired mentally and physically.*
- *We crave tangible empathy for our children.*
- *We want to understand everything you say and may ask you to explain it a number of different ways.*
- *There is a bigger picture than what you see in the hospital. There are siblings to deal with, a marriage to keep alive, and the mental stress of watching your child handle his situation daily.*
- *We need you to listen to what we have observed about the situation. We have become our child's homecare nurse and know him best.*
- *Our children like it when you talk to them. It makes them feel like they are the most important person around.*
- *We understand the stresses you are under, but will take faked compassion over no compassion.*
- *It may take a lot of work, both mentally and physically, to move an inch in our children's care, and that it is frightening, at times, to see the enormous mile ahead.*

A. Vohsing, 2004

EXPECTATIONS AND NEEDS OF CAREGIVERS DURING HOSPITALIZATION OF CHILDREN

From the time of admission, caregivers expect collegial relationships with health care professionals. What they need and what they need to know may differ from the health care professionals' assumptions. When difficulties arise, usually due to discrepant expectations, they may cause significant difficulties for caregivers relative to therapeutic goals, expectations about hospitalization, and perspectives about family involvement. There may also be misunderstandings about expectations regarding the amount of time spent with their child and the degree of participation in care.

During the crisis of hospitalization, caregivers need to have accurate and timely information, to trust the competence of physicians and nurses, and to know their child is comfortable and free from pain. They also need health professionals to trust them (Graves & Hayes, 1996). Although the priorities of caregivers may vary, common needs are for information, assurance, and proximity to their children when critically ill. Through developing a helping relationship with caregivers, these needs and concerns can be prioritized and incorporated into the plan of care. Caregivers also need to feel cared for in the social sense in order to feel more positive about their experiences and better able to cope. Future studies related to caregiver needs should focus on different ethnic and cultural groups as well as the needs of the family.

The complexity of relationships between children, caregivers, and nurses requires extensive understanding. In addition, there is potential for difficulties in communication and the development of adversarial relationships. Sometimes, nurses may not realize they subtly compete for the child's positive responses and must be cautious that their need for approval and self-satisfaction does not supersede their responsibilities.

In situations where children are hospitalized for extended periods of time, support groups for caregivers are an effective way of creating an environment to express concerns and strengthen coping abilities. Support groups in the community are also available for caregivers of children with special needs and for those whose children have succumbed to illness or injury. Each hospital has information about these resources.

CHILDREN WITH CHRONIC ILLNESS

A survey sponsored by Health Resources and Service Administration's (HRSA) Maternal Child Health Bureau (MCHB) and carried out by the Centers for Disease Control and Prevention's National Center for Health Statistics provides detailed information concerning children with special health care needs (CSHCN). One survey shows that 13.9% of U.S. children have special health care needs, and 21.8% of households with children include at least one child with a special health care need. Children with chronic illness are those "who have or are at increased risk for a chronic physical, developmental, behavioral, or emotional condition and who also require health and related services of a type or amount beyond that required by children generally" (HRSA, 2005–2006). Children with long-term and often complex health problems are well acquainted with diverse health care settings, and each new experience is framed within the context of previous experiences. Moreover, their caregivers, who deal with the challenges of parenting a child with chronic illness, have become experts in and can offer valuable information regarding interactions and requisite interventions (Coffey, 2006). When school-age children are repeatedly hospitalized, they experience the major stressors of invasive procedures, fear of death, loss of control, and isolation. Family and friends who have provided care in both the home and the community as a whole are very important in helping them cope. In fact, they describe health professionals as facilitating coping if they explain procedures, afford privacy, are patient and gentle, and have a sense of humor. When health professionals do not exhibit these qualities, the family's ability to "carry the burden of care is hindered and they live worried" (Coffey, 2006, p. 58). Furthermore, when health professionals do not partner with the child and the family and collaborate to meet the ongoing needs, anxiety, frustration, dissatisfaction, and mistrust occur.

Caregivers of these children are often experts about disease processes and treatments on a day-to-day basis and the children themselves become increasingly competent in self-care as they get older. However, at the same time ongoing access to needed services may be lacking. Nurses also become highly skilled as advocates and coordinators of family-centered care and assume roles of coordinator, leader, teacher, team member, and primary care provider. Continuity of care as well as care conferences to promote caregiver–professional collaboration are an excellent medium for planning when children have been hospitalized for long periods of time (McClain & Bury, 1998). These conferences prevent fragmentation of care and affirm the family as experts, managers, and sometimes pioneers as they provide for the child's care. Without adequate support and resources families sometimes "give up."

The field of pediatric rehabilitation nursing has evolved over the past 25 years to become a specialty committed to the care of families and children with disabilities and other chronic conditions (Edwards, Hertzberg, Hays, & Youngblood, 1999). Pediatric rehabilitation facilities as well as clinics and community agencies are sites for offering extensive services by interdisciplinary teams of health care providers and specialists to meet the needs associated with these children's complex, long-term health problems, including developmental, educational, economic, mobility, psychosocial, and vocational services. Attention also needs to be paid to ongoing services in community and school settings as well in order that the child's potential is maximized. As children grow and develop over time, individual and family needs change and the intensity of care may increase, requiring many adaptations and transitions to different health care facilities or health care personnel.

EMERGENCY CARE

To place the nature of pediatric emergencies in perspective, Peterson-Smith (2000) reported important statistics: infants and children account for 30% of all emergency department visits; the most critically ill children are under 6 years of age with central nervous system or respiratory emergencies; trauma is the reason for approximately 40% of all pediatric emergencies; and injuries account for almost one-half of all pediatric deaths annually and are the most frequent cause of death in children older than 1 year. Children often arrive in the emergency departments in the arms of caregivers or other adults. When they are treated in emergency rooms, unique challenges are presented because of high anxiety, fears, and uncertainties, intertwined with other serious and often life-threatening situations. The emotions of caregivers or accompanying adults are often overwhelming and communication may be difficult. When there are language and cultural differences, it is important to have a staff of interpreters.

In emergency care, pediatric nurses need to be highly skilled in immediate interventions. Because children are different from adults both anatomically and physiologically, it is critical to understand the nature of the differences that affect successful treatment (Peterson-Smith, 2000). In addition to body dimensions, differences of clinical significance include: small upper and lower airways, which are more easily obstructed; differences in breathing, circulation, neurological function, body surface, and immunity; and ability to metabolize pharmacological agents (Jundt & Whitefield, 2000).

With the urgency of treatment, time for preparation and explanations of procedures and progress is limited. It is essential, however, to explain events and prepare children to the degree possible and to create the opportunity for caregiver involvement as they desire and are able. Most caregivers want to be present to support their children whenever possible, and particularly want to participate in the decision about their presence (Boie, Moore, Brummett, & Nelson, 1999). If a caretaker chooses to be with his or her child during lifesaving procedures like resuscitation, it is important a support person from the staff be available also (Linder, Suddahy, & Mowery, 2004). Decisions about caregiver presence during highly invasive or life saving procedures are often difficult for all involved.

The prevention of emergencies and information about immediate care in the event of a sudden illness or injury is a critical component of the care of children in everyday settings. Extensive literature is available through local health departments and federal agencies. Persons responsible for the direct care of children should have vital information about each child including: body dimensions, existing health problems, allergies, immunizations, and telephone numbers for emergencies (911, caregivers, physician, poison control center). They need to know the techniques of cardiopulmonary resuscitation and the Heimlich maneuver in addition to knowledge and references for immediate action in the event of acute illness or injury.

PEDIATRIC INTENSIVE CARE UNITS

The pediatric intensive care unit (PICU) is a special environment because of the crisis orientation of care and the potential for sensory overload and sensory deprivation.

Pediatric intensive care (PICU) units were created in the 1960s in response to the increased acuity of illness and childhood trauma requiring advanced diagnostic tests, surgical procedures, pharmacological therapy, and lifesaving treatments. Common medical–surgical conditions encountered in PICU include: acute respiratory failure, multiple organ dysfunction, multiple trauma, sepsis and shock syndromes, neurological diseases, and complex postoperative surgical recovery. Advanced treatments in many units include negative pressure ventilation, ECMO (extracorporeal membrane oxygenation), and high-frequency oscillatory ventilation. Many conditions are life threatening and pose serious medical and ethical dilemmas. Most children are transferred to pediatric units as they progress in recovery. When there is transition from curing to palliative care, wisdom, skill, compassion, and the support of all members of the team are integral to compassionate end-of-life care for children and families.

In PICU, a cohesive team of nurses, advanced practice nurses, physicians, and specialized therapists is essential to provide the kind of critical care sensitive to the developmental and psychosocial needs of vulnerable infants, children, and families. Guidelines and levels of care describe the dimensions and standards of practice in PICU (Rosenberg & Moss, 2004; Truog et al., 2001). Family-centered care in PICU values the inclusion of caregivers in the process of direct care and decision making. Understanding parent responses to experiences such as highly technical therapy is important in helping caregivers cope (Curley & Meyer, 2003).

Although research in nursing has influenced the success of treating children in these environments, this experience is profound and the effects may be long-lasting both for children and their families (Balluffi et al., 2004). Infants and children in PICU are at higher risk for developing persistent psychological sequelae post-discharge, particularly when exposed to high numbers of invasive procedures (Rennick et al., 2004). The effects for some children and caregivers are similar to post-traumatic stress (Ward-Begnoche, 2007). Attention to the experiences of these children and their caretakers is of the highest priority and every effort should be made to prevent emotional and physical pain (Bouve, Rozmus, & Giodano, 1999; Small, 2002). The recent creation of bed spaces for caregivers in intensive care units has been found to reduce their stress (Smith & Hefley, 2007). When children no longer require intensive care, transition to a different level of care may cause a renewed increase in parental anxiety.

Reflections from Families

"As you watch your beloved child inch back from the edge of a steep precipice, the support of those who help him rings with bell-like clarity through the fog of pain and fear"

Mother of a teenager hospitalized for severe trauma (Massachusetts General Hospital, 2002)

HOME CARE

With technological innovations and changes in health care system financing and administration, children are usually hospitalized for very short periods of time and return home with complex, multisystem health problems. Examples of children previously cared for in hospitals or long-term care facilities, who are now cared for at home, include those who are respirator-dependent; require parenteral nutrition; or have severe physical and cognitive impairment. Extensive coordination is required to provide respite care, day care, and schooling. There are many community resources available to create environments most conducive to the health and welfare of these children and their families.

DISCHARGE AND POST-HOSPITAL EFFECTS

Throughout hospitalization, children and caregivers need to be prepared for discharge, post-hospital or post-surgical care, and the effects of this experience. This often involves extensive teaching and preparation for the transition, especially when there has been prolonged hospitalization, painful treatments and procedures, or changes in body image. With shortened hospital stays every opportunity for teaching both children and families should be used to the greatest advantage. It is important to prepare teachers, and other significant persons for the child's return to home, school, and community life.

The kind of preparation is dependent on the continued needs of the child and family for care and support in coping with fears and anxieties. In those situations where there is a change in appearance or mobility, the transition from hospital to home may be difficult. Some may benefit from spending brief periods with family and friends outside the hospital during the rehabilitation process to adapt gradually (e.g., those who have had an amputation or visible, physical changes). Peers may also need to be prepared by using discussions and films. Teachers and school nurses are valuable resources in helping children in classrooms to understand about hospitalization and changes to expect when a classmate returns to school.

Changes in behavior post-hospitalization are most evident in children between 6 months and 6 years of age. These include changes in eating, sleeping, and elimination, and in psychosocial behavior such as regression, clinging to parents, or becoming more aggressive, withdrawn, or fearful. The intensity and duration of these responses are dependent on many factors including the impact of the illness and hospitalization, frequency of intrusive procedures, level of cognitive development and maturity, previous experiences, and perceptions about being comforted in the process of coping with stressful events. When caregivers of children younger than 5 who spent a day in ICU were interviewed about their child's behavior, they reported changes related to regressive behaviors and withdrawal, aggression and demanding behavior, and fears and anxieties about sleeping and separation (Youngblut & Shiao, 1993).

Most changes in behavior occur after 2–3 days of hospitalization because children encounter multiple tests, treatments, and separations from those who provide support. This is also a time when caregivers are anxious and may be less able to give psychological support (Thompson & Vernon, 1993). Moderate lengths of stay involving more than minimal separation from home, yet insufficient time for accommodation, may place children at greater risk for post-hospital distress than longer or shorter stays.

There are many considerations in teaching caregivers about the potential changes in behavior after hospitalization. In addition to responding to illness and hospitalization, children may react to previous home sleeping arrangements, particularly when the caregiver has slept closely adjacent to the child while in the hospital. Therefore, for some children, it may be helpful for the caregiver to sleep in a separate room from the child for a few nights prior to discharge.

As the time for discharge approaches, caregivers may feel relief about resuming family life, yet also feel apprehensive about caring for the child at home. In addition to preparing the family for physical aspects of care, it is also important to know of the potential for the child's behavioral changes in response to the hospital experience. Therefore, it is advantageous to first ask caregivers how they think their child will respond to this experience of illness and hospitalization at home. Their responses are helpful as a basis for an individualized teaching plan using considerations suggested in the Family Teaching box.

PREPARATION FOR CLINICAL NURSING IN THE CARE OF CHILDREN AND THEIR FAMILIES

In learning about the care of ill children, it is important to reflect on one's own experiences and strengths, review theories about child growth and development, and realize, even through the trauma and stress of illness and hospitalization, children continue to grow physically, emotionally, socially, and spiritually. The predominant goal is to identify and preserve the strengths of children while trying to enhance their growth in the midst of stress and intrusions into their bodies, their space, and their very being. To do this successfully takes an understanding of the lives of individual children and their families and the courage and commitment to accurately discern and meet their emerging needs. Introspection, reflection, and understanding of personal styles and journeys in learning make it possible for nurses to mature in the transition from novice to expert.

Articulating a personal philosophy about the care of children in hospitals provides a foundation of beliefs that underlie practice. In doing so, it is helpful to consider the relationships between and among nurses, children, caretakers, and other health professionals. Identifying one's own strengths and talents, and delineating personal goals, are important steps in developing confidence and competence in pediatric nursing practice.

In the preparatory phase, it is important to review and validate previous knowledge including: theory and characteristics of child growth and development at each stage of the life cycle through young adulthood; stress, adaptation, and coping theory; family development theory; concepts and principles of teaching and learning; and cultural dimensions of nursing practice. The unique features of calculating and administering medications to children, infant and child

FAMILY TEACHING

Preparing Caregivers for Potential Behavior Changes of Infants and Young Children Post-Hospitalization

- Infants and young children may continue to react to hospitalization for a few weeks after discharge and gradually resume their developmental patterns and routines.
- Young children whose caregivers have roomed-in may have difficulty adapting to sleeping in a room alone or with siblings.
- Changes in behavior may include clinging behaviors and crying even if a parent goes to another room; whining; tearfulness at bedtime and wakefulness during the night; intensified protest when leaving the child in care of another person; resistance to changing clothes or diapers; outbursts of anger, frustration, or aggression in the form of temper tantrums or aggressive play; regression to earlier behaviors (thumb-sucking, changes in use of language); or withdrawal.
- Understanding guidance, consistency, and complimentary responses for positive behaviors are helpful during the transition from hospital to home.
- Siblings need to understand behavioral changes (their own and their sibling's) and be helped and helpful in reestablishing family routines and relationships.
- Telling a story about a child who was in the hospital and learned a lot about hospitals, nurses, and doctors may also be helpful. Tips on helping alleviate fear and how children learn to help themselves when they need to do things but feel afraid, are also beneficial.

safety, and relevant areas of screening and health promotion are also aspects to be reviewed. It is enlightening to become aware of the environment of a pediatric unit before clinical assignments begin. Viewing the environment of a pediatric unit from different perspectives is a way of understanding the impact of surroundings on thoughts, feelings, and reactions.

After initial orientation to pediatric nursing, the direct care of children and families requires considerable thought and preparation. Learning roles and responsibilities is a process facilitated by consistently raising questions and being aware of assumptions prior to and during direct care. The questions in Box 16-8 are designed to direct the kind of inquiry that will lead to accuracy and effectiveness in providing nursing care that is sensitive to the developmental and experiential needs of children and caregivers. These are in addition to those questions directly related to the assessment process and the ongoing, specific plan of care.

NURSING ALERT

Identification of Children at Risk Following Hospitalization or Surgery

Nurses studying the outcomes of children following hospitalization and surgery are able to identify several situations where children are at greatest risk for less than positive outcomes. According to Eldridge (1997) they include:

- Young children between the ages of 6 months and 6 years or children with developmental delays
- Moderate hospital stay of 4–8 days or prolonged hospital stay (longer than 8 days)
- More serious illnesses or trauma, especially those resulting in pain or painful procedures
- Hospitalizations that necessitate isolation of the child from the family
- Caregivers who exhibit high anxiety or limited skills in coping
- Insufficient preparation of the child and caregivers for hospitalization or surgery
- Children who have had multiple hospital or surgical experiences or who have had previous, unresolved negative experiences

With the guidance of mentors in the field, novices become experts in pediatric nursing over time. It is a continuous process of learning in all areas of relevance to this sphere of nursing practice and appreciating the concept of using one's self as an instrument of healing. The most significant attributes in the process of maturation to excellence are: commitment to evidence-based practice within the context of family-centered care; continuous learning about the art and science of pediatric nursing; and time for reflection and renewal of personal strengths, creativity, and aspirations.

TRENDS AND CHALLENGES IN PEDIATRIC NURSING PRACTICE

Trends in health care and changes in pediatric nursing practice lead to many challenges in the field. The ultimate goal is to be cognizant of these changes and to implement new knowledge and evidence-based practices, which will continuously improve the care of children who are hospitalized. The following trends are relevant:

- Increase in number of children transferred from local hospitals to children's hospitals.
- Implementation of Millennium goals with emphasis on both global and local initiatives to reduce poverty and increase equity in child care.

BOX 16-8

GUIDING QUESTIONS TO ADDRESS IN PLANNING NURSING CARE FOR A CHILD WHO IS HOSPITALIZED

- What child characteristics including age, gender, and cultural background will have a bearing on the plan of care (e.g., body dimensions for determining the appropriateness of dosages of medications, level of cognitive development)?
- What is the nature of the caregiver–nurse partnership during the hospital experience? What activities do caregivers want to assume in providing direct care (e.g., bathing, feeding)?
- What is the history of the illness, sequence of symptoms, or conditions of the injury? Are there other existing health problems or recent stressful experiences?
- What emergency measures or remedies have been used? How recent were treatments and medications given?
- What is the current status of the illness (e.g., is the condition improving or worsening)? Examine the progress and sequence of events during the past 24 hours.
- How does the child respond to treatments?
- What are the child's and caregivers' perceptions and understanding of the nature of the health problem, therapeutic measures, and plans for care?
- What are the strengths of the child and family in coping with stressful situations (e.g., ways of comforting one's self and being comforted by others)? Does the child have a transitional object or favorite toy that provides comfort?
- What are the usual routines at home (e.g., daily activities, care giving patterns, play or school, sleeping, eating, and elimination routines)?
- What are the most significant relationships in the child's life?
- What are the caregivers' greatest concerns surrounding the hospital stay?
- With the implementation of the plan of care, what are the predictions regarding outcomes?
- At the conclusion of your time with the child and family how will nursing care and patient outcomes be evaluated?

REFLECTIVE THINKING

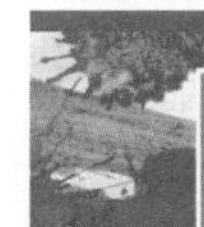

Viewing a Pediatric Unit from Different Perspectives

First, from the perspective of a child:

Enter the pediatric unit as if you were a young child being admitted to the hospital for the first time. Be aware of the sights, smells, and sounds, and the conversations of others. Use your imagination to identify thoughts, feelings, and anxieties that come to mind as you experience this process. Make a few notes as you proceed. For 10–15 minutes, walk around the unit and into a child's room as if this were to be your room. Be aware of the questions you would ask and the fears you may have. Continue to "look around the unit" absorbing the general atmosphere and responses to you from children or staff. Take another 15 minutes to reflect on this experience and to record your reflections to share with colleagues.

Second, from one's own perspective:

Tour the unit again, and take this opportunity to introduce yourself to members of the staff, a caregiver, and a child. Be aware of your own thoughts and feelings as you spend about 20 minutes becoming acquainted with personnel and the general environment. Then reflect on this experience, writing about your impressions and your thoughts about how you feel as you begin to assume responsibility for learning about the care of children and caregivers. Discuss these reflections with colleagues.

- Attention to child and caregiver health literacy; that is, the ability to understand and implement into practice healthy behaviors and lifestyle.
- Increase in formation of collaborative teams of nurses, physicians, and social workers before, during, and post hospitalization.
- Parent councils and advisory groups of caregivers in pediatric units and children's hospitals.
- Changes in educational methods for nurses, caregivers and children, to include simulations, role-playing and mentoring.
- Creation of healing environments in the design of children's units and hospitals with gardens, artwork, privacy, and individualized educational resources.
- Greater efforts for consistency of nurses and health care teams in family-centered care.
- Use of universal health records and electronic forms for assessment and treatment.
- Research in pediatric nursing more inclusive of ethnically diverse families.
- Inclusion of fathers more deliberatively in child care in hospitals.
- Identification of areas for assessment and promotion of health during hospitalization (e.g., dental, vision, nutrition, exercise, and harmful substances and habits).
- Increased focus on utilization of nursing research to implement evidence-based practices.

- Increased use of nanotechnology in the direct care and treatment of children as well as improved record-keeping.
- New graduate participation in pediatric internships in preparation for practice in the care of children and families.

Of great importance is the current shortage of nurses at a time when many researchers recognize the potential for post-traumatic stress and prolonged negative effects for both caregivers and children, especially after pediatric intensive care unit hospitalization (Rennick et al., 2004). The complex emotional support and learning needs of children and families in crisis require considerable expertise to prevent the untoward effects of severe illness, surgery, or life-threatening conditions and to heal psychological and bodily wounds. It is predicted that the care available to children identified as "vulnerable" will be further stressed and those subgroups at risk for poor outcomes will be adversely affected first (Shelton, 2003). The challenge is to recruit, educate, and mentor pediatric nurses for clinical and advanced practice, teaching, leadership, and research.

> **IN THE REAL WORLD**
>
> In pediatric nursing, one of the greatest challenges is to reach out beyond the physical and emotional strengths that exist and build on all the cultural assets a child, his family, and his social group may possess. There is so much to be learned from respectful observation and conversation.

The authors acknowledge with appreciation the support of Mary Ann Westcott, RN, Clinical Manager, and the nursing staff, Baystate Children's Hospital, Springfield, MA.

KEY CONCEPTS

- A primary goal in the nursing of children is to help them and their families grow during experiences of adversity and stress and learn meaningful ways of coping.
- The history of caring for children in hospitals and research related to the effects of hospitalization on children have influenced the development of current philosophies, policies, and practices in pediatric units and children's hospitals.
- During hospitalization children are more vulnerable to experiences of separation, loss of control, pain, body intrusions, changes in body image and integrity, uncertainty, and other situations which have meaning for them or their caretakers.
- Responses of infants, children, adolescents, and caretakers are influenced by many factors, including their perceptions of events, development and cognitive levels, previous experiences, and coping methods.
- Children in hospitals often regress to earlier behaviors as they learn to manage changes and feelings of insecurity.
- When caretakers are helped to reduce their stress through teaching, preparation for potentially stressful experiences, communication, and exploration of anxieties and needs, they are better able to assist their children to cope with the stressors of hospitalization.
- Play is the work of children and is integral to the developmental process, both as recreation and creativity, and as a means of expressing and exploring thoughts and feelings about events and experiences in their lives.
- Physical and psychosocial environments of pediatric units have a profound influence on the effectiveness of the care and comfort of children and caretakers.
- Transition from being a client or caretaker in a pediatric hospital to home or other facilities requires preparation for changes that may occur in reactions and behavior.
- Collaboration and communication with other health care professionals are essential to the care and well-being of children and caretakers before, during, and after hospital experiences.
- Models of nursing where nurses engage caretakers in a partnership for their children empower them to gain skill and confidence in coping with their stressors and those of their children.
- Family-centered care embraces the concerns and care of siblings in order to minimize their stressors in response to the illness experiences of their sister or brother.
- Learning the role and responsibilities of the nurse in minimizing stressful experiences of children and caretakers and maximizing the use of successful coping is a complex process and is enhanced by applying knowledge from the arts, sciences, and humanities; astute observations of the behavior of children and caretakers; and reflective nursing practice where situations are consistently reviewed for effectiveness and possible alternatives.
- The philosophy of the nurse about the nature of caretaker–nurse–child relationships influences the quality of child care.
- The role of the nurse in supporting the psychological well-being of children and their caregivers and

helping them grow during the crisis of illness is a critical and complex contribution to recovery and health.

- Students and novices in the field of pediatric nursing learn best when clinical practice is preceded by: understanding the philosophy of caring for children who are hospitalized and one's own philosophy about nursing; reflection on one's own strengths; studying extensively and preparing thoroughly for the care of each child and family; and reviewing the process of learning with a teacher or mentor.
- Expert clinicians, advanced practice nurses, and those in leadership, teaching, and research have had a significant positive influence on the quality of care for ill and hospitalized children and their families.

REVIEW ACTIVITIES

1. Compare and contrast how hospitalization affects infants, toddlers, preschoolers, school-age children, and adolescents.
2. Discuss the various factors affecting a child's reaction to a hospital experience.
3. Describe how the relationship between nurses and families of hospitalized children can be strengthened.
4. Describe how play can be used in helping hospitalized children cope with their experiences.
5. Discuss appropriate nursing interventions for hospitalized children of various ages.
6. Discuss the behaviors caregivers might see in a child after the child is discharged from the hospital.

STUDY QUESTIONS

1. Your 18-month-old patient has been brought to the treatment room for insertion of an IV. Her mother is upset and her eyes are filled with tears as she carries her infant down the hall. She asks if she can stay with her infant. Your best response is:
   a. "You can stay but if you become upset your toddler may become more frightened and uncooperative."
   b. "I notice you are very upset. It may be best if you wait outside. I will be quick and get you as soon as we are finished."
   c. "That will be helpful as you can help hold your infant still during the procedure."
   d. "You can stay close to your infant and help me and my team calm her as I start the IV."
2. You are assigned to care for a child who is well known to staff. Many staff members describe mom as very involved in and knowledgeable about her child's care. As you begin the child's care for the day you ask:
   a. "What time do you want to offer your child breakfast and give your child a bath?"
   b. "Would you like me to organize the items you will need for morning care?"
   c. "What care would you like me to provide for your child today?"
   d. "Your child has a busy day ahead of her. Would you like to bathe her early?"
3. It is time to administer 10 pm oral medications to your sleeping 3-year-old patient, who is all curled up and looks very comfortable. Mom is reading by his bedside. You should:
   a. Ask mom what the child's name is and encourage her to wake her child to give the oral medication.
   b. Leave the medication with mom and instruct her to give the medication when her child wakes up.
   c. Check the child's name band and wake the child to administer the medication.
   d. Reschedule the medication so the child's sleep does not need to be disturbed.
4. You note that your 6-year-old patient from the western part of the state is not visited regularly by family. You know the family is very worried about the child but transportation is problematic. Your best action is:
   a. Schedule a patient care team conference to update them regarding the child's status when the family visits.
   b. Designate a time each day when you can call the family to discuss the plan for the day.
   c. Provide the family with the names and contact information of the care team and advise them to call at any time.
   d. Encourage them to use the Internet in their town library and email daily questions to the primary nurse and chief resident.

5. Your 8-year-old patient remains hospitalized following a skiing accident. At the time of the injury he was with his 5-year-old sister. She has not visited her brother since he was taken away by ambulance to a regional tertiary care center and she is afraid her brother will not get better. Your best action is to:
   a. Assist the brother in emailing his sister to let her know he is ok.
   b. Schedule a daily telephone call so they can talk together.
   c. Speak with parents about the need for the child to see her brother.
   d. Enlist the assistance of child life so the sister can explore her fears.
6. A 5-year-old boy named Johnny has recently been diagnosed with acute leukemia. Consequently, the family is in turmoil and family friends are calling frequently for updates related to the child's condition. Many friends are visiting and bringing the child presents when they visit. His 3-year-old sister has begun to have accidents and his 7-year-old brother is acting out. Your best action is to:
   a. Advise parents to ask their extended family to spend extra time with the siblings so they can stay with Johnny.
   b. Advise parents to bring the presents home to share some of Johnny's gifts with his brother and sister.
   c. Advise parents to tell their extended family and friends not to visit and bring presents to Johnny.
   d. Advise parents to arrange special time with Johnny's siblings and ask other family members to stay with Johnny.
7. An adolescent with cystic fibrosis confides that he is so embarrassed by his frequent episodes of coughing when he is class. In order to help him address this concern you should:
   a. Speak with each of his teachers so he can leave class when he feels like he might begin to cough.
   b. Arrange for private school based tutorial sessions so he will not feel embarrassed in the classroom.
   c. Ask him if he would like help in speaking with his classmates about his disease.
   d. Speak with his class about the signs, symptoms, and treatment of cystic fibrosis.
8. A preschooler is scheduled for the operating room for surgery. Mom indicates she wants to accompany her child to the OR but the transport team has come for the child before mom has arrived. You should:
   a. Send the child with the team and wait on the unit to bring mom to the OR when she arrives.
   b. Tell the team they need to wait as mom is on the way and should be here shortly.
   c. Tell the child you will stay with him while he waits for the doctor.
   d. Using words familiar to the child, explain why they need to leave immediately for the OR.
9. A 7-year-old is scheduled to have a *porta cath* implanted and the procedure has not been explained. You should:
   a. Tell the child what the device looks like and how the device will look after the procedure.
   b. Use a specially-designed doll to demonstrate what is involved with pre- and post-procedure care.
   c. Allow the child to manipulate a demonstration *porta cath* and provide a needleless syringe to practice flushing.
   d. Provide a simply written page of instructions so the child and mother will learn about the procedure and postprocedure care.
10. A 10-year-old has had a sledding accident while on a school field trip and has been brought to the emergency room. His parents have been called but they live more than two hours away. He is frightened and needs to go to CAT scan for further evaluation. You should:
    a. Wait for his parents so you can explain what has happened and assure them that he will be fine.
    b. Accompany the child as you have become a familiar and trusted figure.
    c. Ask a volunteer to stay with him and to report back to you if he seems upset.
    d. Reassure the child that he will be okay and that you will tell his parents that he is okay.
11. A 24-month-old toddler has just returned home from a week's stay in the hospital. Mom calls very upset that her child is now fussy, irritable, and continually throwing her toys around. What would you say to reassure her that her child's behavior is usual posthospitalization behavior?
    a. "It's just a phase she's going through to let you know she is mad at you for bringing her to the hospital."
    b. "This behavior is not uncommon following hospitalization as she is regaining autonomy and trust."
    c. "Don't leave her for a few days so she will know you care about her."
    d. "Encourage visitors to stop by to provide diversion and extra attention."
12. The mother of a child you are caring for indicates she might lose her job because she has stayed with her sick child in the hospital. Your best response is:
    a. Have her employer call the child's doctor and explain why her child was hospitalized.
    b. Provide a note at the time of discharge that includes the dates of the child's hospitalization.

c. Tell the child's mother that her boss can call you on the unit and you will answer his questions.
d. Provide written information about the child's condition so she can hand it to her boss.

13. In the care of hospitalized children you observe that some parents report the use of complementary and alternative therapies for their children. Which of the following approaches is *most* appropriate?
    a. Discourage the use of these practices in the hospital.
    b. Routinely ask parents if their children use herbs or other supplements.
    c. Understand that most parents do not know about alternative health practices.
    d. Explain to parents that practices which vary from conventional medical treatments are harmful to children.

14. Nurse researchers have confirmed parents' desire and expectations to participate in their child's care. Which of the following statements best describes the effectiveness of this practice?
    a. Parents should stay with their children during the entire hospital stay in order to work with the nurse.
    b. The attitudes and activities of the nurse are both barriers and facilitators to parent participation.
    c. The nurse should have the primary relationship with the child and enlist the cooperation of the parent.
    d. Let the parents know how they should care for their child during the hospital stay.

15. Which of the following best indicates understanding of the importance of cultural awareness in the care of children and caregivers?
    a. Ask another member of the family to interpret for a parent when translation is needed.
    b. Say "If I do something that offends you, it is not my intent."
    c. Explain to caretakers that the way things are done in the hospital is in the best interest of the child.
    d. Provide a medical dictionary so that caregivers can learn the meaning of words used in the hospital.

REFERENCES

Ahmann, E. (1997). Family matters: Books for siblings of children having illness or disability. *Pediatric Nursing, 23*(5), 500–502.

Ahmann, E. (2006). Supporting father's involvement in children's health care. *Pediatric Nursing, 32*(1), 88–90.

Algren, C. L., & Algren, J. T. (1997). Pediatric sedation: Essentials for the perioperative nurse. *Nursing Clinics of North America, 32*(1), 17–30.

Alsop-Shields, L., & Mohay, H. (2001). John Bowlby and James Robertson: Theorists, scientists, and crusaders for improvements in the care of children in hospitals. *Journal of Advanced Nursing, 35*(1), 50–58.

Andrade, T. M. (1998). Sibling visitation: Research implications for pediatric and neonatal patients. *On-line Journal of Knowledge Synthesis, 5*(6).

Balluffi, A., Kassam-Adams, N., Kazak, A., Tucker, M., Dominquez, M. D., & Helfaer, M. D. (2004). Traumatic stress in parents of children admitted to the pediatric intensive care unit. *Pediatric Critical Care Medicine, 5*(6), 547–553.

Barclay, L., & Murata, P. (2008). AAP addresses use of complementary and alternative medicine. Retrieved January 24, 2010, from http://www.medscape.com/viewarticle/586271.

Bassett, K. E., Anderson, J. L., Pribble, C. G., & Guenther, E. (2003). Protocol for procedural sedation for children in the emergency department. *Annals of Emergency Medicine, 42*(6), 773–782.

Berlin, B. K. (1995). Music therapy with children during invasive procedures: Our emergency department's experience. *Journal of Emergency Nursing, 24*(6), 607–608.

Blake, F. G. (1954a). *The child, his parents and the nurse.* Philadelphia: Lippincott.

Blake, F. G. (1954b). *Open heart surgery in children: A study of nursing care.* Washington, DC: U.S. Government Printing Office.

Blake, F. G., Wright, F. H., & Waechter, E. H. (1970). *Nursing care of children* (8th ed.). Philadelphia: J. B. Lippincott Company.

Boie, E. T., Moore, G. P., Brummett, C., & Nelson, D. (1999). Do parents want to be present during invasive procedures performed on their children in the emergency department? A survey of 400 parents. *Annals of Emergency Medicine, 34*(1), 70–74.

Bossert, E. (1994). Factors influencing the coping of hospitalized school-age children. *Journal of Pediatric Nursing, 9*(5), 299–306.

Bouve, L. R., Rozmus, C. L., & Giodano, P. (1999). Preparing parents for their child's transfer from the PICU to the pediatric floor. *Applied Nursing Research, 12,* 114–120.

Bowlby, J. (1965). *Child care and the growth of love* (2nd ed.). Baltimore, MD: Penguin Books.

Bradley, S. (2001). Suffer the little children: The influence of nurses and parents in the evolution of open visiting in children's wards 1940–1970. *International History of Nursing Journal, 6*(2), 44–51.

Brody, D. S. (1980). The patient's role in clinical decision making. *Annals of Internal Medicine, 93,* 718–722.

Buerhaus, P. I., Staiger, D. O., & Auerbach, D. I. (2008). The future of the nursing workforce in the United States: Data, trends, and implications. Sudbury, MA: Jones & Bartlett Publishers Inc.

Burke, S. O., Kauffmann, E., Harrison, M. B., & Wiskin, N. (1999). Assessment of stressors in families with a child who has a chronic condition. *MCN American Journal of Maternal Child Nursing, 24*(2), 98–106.

Child Life Council. (2003). *Child life position statement.* Rockville, MD: Author.

Clatworthy, S., Simon, K., & Tiedeman, M. E. (1999). Child drawing: Hospital—an instrument designed to measure the emotional status of hospitalized school-age children. *Journal of Pediatric Nursing, 14*(1), 2–9.

Coffey, J. (2006). Parenting a child with chronic illness: A metasynthesis. *Pediatric Nursing, 32*(1), 51–59.

Cohen, L. L., & Baster, A. L. (2008). Distraction techniques for procedural pain in children. Posted on Medscape CME/CE. Retrieved

January 24, 2010, from http://cme.medscape.com/viewprogram/17791.

Connolly, C. (2005). Growth and development of a specialty: The professionalization of child health care. *Pediatric Nursing 31*(3), 211–215.

Curley, M. A. Q. (1988). Effects of the nursing mutual participation model of care on parental stress in the pediatric intensive care unit. *Heart & Lung, 17*(6), 682–688.

Curley, M. A. Q. (1997). Mutuality—An expression of nursing presence. *Journal of Pediatric Nursing: Nursing Care of Children and Families, 12*(4), 208–213.

Curley, M. A. Q., & Meyer, E. A. (2003). Parent experience of highly technical therapy, survivors and nonsurvivors of extracorporeal membrane oxygenation support. *Pediatric Critical Care Medicine, 4*, 214–219.

Curley, M. A. (2004). The state of synergy: Excellence in nursing knowledge. Retrieved January 24, 2010, from http://www.nursingknowledge.org/portal/main.aspx?pageid=3507&ContentID=55889.

Davies, B., Collins, J., Steele, R., Pipke, I., & Cook, K., (2003). The impact on families of a children's hospice program. *Journal of Palliative Care (Canada), 19*(1), 15–26.

Davis, C. L. (2008). Does your facility have a pediatric sedation team? If not, why not? *Pediatric Nursing, 34*(4), 308–309, 318.

Edwards, P. A., Hertzberg, D. L., Hays, S. R., & Youngblood, N. M. (1999). *Pediatric Rehabilitation Nursing*. Philadelphia: Saunders.

Egemen, A., Ikizoglu, T., Darapnar, B., Cosar, H., & Karapnar, D. (2008). Parental presence during invasive procedures and resuscitation: Attitudes of health care professionals in Turkey. *Pediatric Emergency Care, 22*(4), 230–234.

Eldridge, T. M. (1997). Preparation for painful procedures, hospitalization and surgery. In Ellerton, M. L., & Merriam, C. (1994). Preparing children and families psychologically for day surgery: An evaluation. *Journal of Advanced Nursing, 19*, 1057–1062.

Ellerton, M. L. (1994). Preparing kids and parents for surgery. *The Canadian Nurse, 90*(10), 25–27.

Erickson, F. H. (1958). Play interviews for four-year-old hospitalized children. *Monograph, 23*(3). Lafayette, IN: Society for Research in Child Development.

Fagin, C. M., & Nasbaum, J. G. (1978). Parental visiting privileges in pediatric units: A survey. *Journal of Nursing Administration, 8*(3), 24–27.

Feudtner, C., Haney, J., & Dimmers, M. S. (2003). Spiritual care needs of hospitalized children and their families: A national survey of pastoral care providers' perceptions. *Pediatrics, 111*(1), 67–72.

Field, T. (1995). Massage therapy for infants and children. *Developmental and Behavioral Pediatrics, 16*(2), 105–111.

Fox, J. A. (2002). *Primary health care of infants, children, and adolescents* (2nd ed.). St. Louis: Mosby-Year Book.

Gaynard, L., Goldberger, J., & Laidley, L. N. (1991). The use of stuffed body-outline dolls with hospitalized children and adolescents. *Children Health Care, 20*(4), 216–224.

Giganti, A. W. (1998). Families in pediatric critical care: The best option. *Pediatric Nursing, 24*(3), 261–265.

Gillis, A. J. (1989). The effect of play on immobilized children in hospital. *International Journal of Nursing Studies, 26*(3), 261–269.

Gradin, M., Eriksson, M., Holmqvist, F., Holstein, A., & Schollin, J. (2002). Pain reduction at venipuncture in newborns: Oral glucose compared with local anesthetic cream. *Pediatrics, 12*(110), 1053–1057.

Graves, C., & Hayes, B. E. (1996). Do nurses and parents of children with chronic conditions agree on parental needs? *Journal of Pediatric Nursing: Nursing Care of Children and Families, 11*(5), 288–299.

Hawkins, M. E. (1988). In M. Kaufman (Ed.). *Dictionary of American nursing biography*. New York: Greenwood Press.

HRSA (2005). The national survey of children with special health care needs chartbook, 2005–2006. Retrieved January 24, 2010, from http://mchb.hrsa.gov/cshcn05/.

Hurlock, E. B. (1978). *Child development* (6th ed.). New York: McGraw-Hill.

Huth, M. M., Broome M. D., & Good, M. (2003). Imagery reduces children's post-operative pain. *Pain, 110*, 439–448.

Institute for Family-Centered Care. (2009). *Family-centered care: Questions & answers*. Bethesda, MD. Retrieved January 24, 2010, from http://familycenteredcare.org/faq.html.

Jundt, D., & Whitefield, J. (2000). The art of assessing urgent and emergent problems in the pediatric setting. *Program and Abstracts of the 25th Primary Care Nurse Practitioner Symposium*, July 13, 2000; Keystone, CO.

Justus, R., Wyles, D., Wilson, J., Rode, D., Walther, V., & Lim-Sulit, N. (2006). Preparing children and families for surgery: Mount Sinai's multidisciplinary perspective. *Pediatric Nursing*, (32)1, 35–43.

Kaminski, M., Pellino, T., & Wish, J. (2002). Play and pets: The physical and emotional impact of child-life and pet therapy on hospitalized children. *Children's Health Care, 31*(4), 321–335.

Kauffman, E., Harrison, M. B., Burke, S. O., & Wong, C. (1998). Family matters: Stress point intervention for parents of children hospitalized with chronic conditions. *Pediatric Nursing, 24*(4), 362–366.

Kolk, A. M., van Hoof, R., & Fiedeldij Dop, M. J. C. (2000). Preparing children for venipuncture: The effect of an integrated intervention on distress before and during venipuncture. *Child: Care, Health Development, 26*, 251–260.

Kouretas, D. (1999). More on music therapy with children during invasive procedures (letter). *Journal of Emergency Nursing, 25*(3), 157.

Kuntz, N., Adams, J. A., Zahr, L., Kellen, R., Cameron, K., & Wassen, H. (1996). Therapeutic play and bone marrow transportation. *Journal of Pediatric Nursing, 11*(6), 359–367.

Lamontagne, L. (2000). Children coping with surgery: A process-oriented perspective. *Journal of Pediatric Nursing, 15*(5), 307–312.

Lamontagne, L. L., Hepworth, J. T., Byington, K. C., & Chang, C. Y. (1997). Child and parent emotional responses during hospitalization for orthopedic surgery. *MCN: American Journal of Maternal Child Nursing, 22*(6), 299–303.

LaRosa-Nash, P., & Murphy, J. M. (1997). An approach to pediatric perioperative care. *Nursing Clinics of North America, 32*(1), 183–199.

Li, H. C. W., & Lopez, V. (2008). Effectiveness and appropriateness of therapeutic play intervention in preparing children for surgery: A randomized controlled trial study. *Journal for Specialists in Pediatric Nursing, 13*(2), 63–73.

Linder, C. M., Suddahy, E. C., & Mowery, B. D. (2004). Parental presence during resuscitation: Help or hindrance. *Pediatric Nursing, 30*(2), 126–127.

Lindrea, D. B., & Stainton, M. B. (2000). A case study of infant massage outcomes. *MCN: The American Journal of Maternal-Child Nursing, 25*(2), 95–99.

Malloy, R., Ferrell, B., Virani, R., Wilson, K., & Uman, G. (2007). Palliative care education for pediatric nurses. *Pediatric Nursing 32*(5), 555–561.

Massachusetts General Hospital. (2002). *Caring headlines*. Boston: Massachusetts General Hospital.

McCann, D. (2008). Sleep deprivation is an additional stress for parents staying in hospital. *Journal for Specialists in Pediatric Nursing, 13*(2), 111–122.

McClain, C., & Bury, J. (1998). Family matters: The heart of the matter: Care conferences to promote parent–professional collaboration. *Pediatric Nursing, 24*(2), 151–154.

Melnyk, B. M. (1994). Coping with unplanned childhood hospitalization: Effect of informational interventions on mothers and children. *Nursing Research, 43*(1), 50–55.

Melnyk, B. M., Alpert-Gillis, L., Feinstein, N. F., Crean, H. F., Johnson, J., Fairbanks, E., Small, L., Rubenstein, J., Slota, M., & Corbo-Richert, B. (2004). Creating opportunities for parent empowerment: Program effects on the mental health/coping outcomes of critically ill young children and their mothers. *Pediatrics, 113*(6), 597–607.

Melnyk, B. M., Crean, H. F., Feinstein, N. F., & Alpert-Gillis, L. (2007). Testing the theoretical framework of the COPE program for mothers of critically ill children: An integrative model of young children's post-hospital adjustment behaviors. *Journal of Pediatric Psychology, 32*(4), 463–474.

Mosby's dictionary of medicine, nursing & health professions (8th ed.). (2009). St. Louis: Mosby.

Mullen, J. E., & Ascher, L. M. (2007). Implementation of a nursing professional practice model of care in a pediatric hospital. *Pediatric Nursing, 33*(6), 449–504.

Neal, A., Frost, M., Kuhn, J., & Green, A. (2007). Family-centered care within an infant-toddler unit. *Pediatric Nursing, 33*(6), 481–486.

Noble, R., Micheli, A. J., Hensley, M. A., & McKay, N. (1997). Perioperative considerations for the pediatric patient: A developmental approach. *Nursing Clinics of North America, 32*(1), 1–16.

O'Brien, M. D. (2002). The other victims of pediatric trauma: Parents and siblings. *Caring Headlines.* Boston: Massachusetts General Hospital.

Orlando, I. J. (1961). The dynamic nurse–patient relationship: Function, process and principles. Philadelphia: J. P. Putnam's Sons.

Ott, M. J. (1996). Imagine the possibilities! Guided imagery with toddlers and preschoolers. *Pediatric Nursing, 22,* 34–38.

Peterson-Smith, A. (2000). A clinical assessment of urgent and emergent pediatric problems: A summary of Jundt, D., & Whitefield, J., *The art of assessing urgent and emergent problems in the pediatric setting. Program and Abstracts of the 25th Primary Care Nurse Practitioner Symposium,* July 13, 2000; Keystone, CO.

Petrillo, M. (1968). Preventing hospital trauma in pediatric patients. *American Journal of Nursing, 68*(7), 1468–1473.

Petrillo, M., & Sanger, S. (1980). *Emotional care of hospitalized children* (2nd ed.). Philadelphia: J. B. Lippincott.

Piira, T., Sugiura, T., Champion, G. D., Donnelly, N., & Cole, A. S. J. (2005). The role of parental presence in the context of children's medical procedures: A systematic review. *Child-Care, Health, & Development, 31*(2), 233–243.

Platt, H. (1959). *The welfare of children in hospital.* London: Ministry of Health Central Health Services Council.

Poikki, T., Pietila, A. M., Vehrilainen-Julkunen, K., Laukkala, H., & Kiviluomaki, K. (2008). Imagery-induced relaxation in children's post-operative pain relief: A randomized pilot study. *Journal of Pediatric Nursing, 23*(3), 217–224.

Power, N., & Franck, L. (2008). Parent participation in the care of hospitalized children: A systematic review. *Journal of Advanced Nursing, 62*(6), 622–641.

Pruitt, L. M., Johnson, A., Elliot, J. C., & Polley, P. (2008). Parental presence during pediatric invasive procedures. *Journal of Pediatric Health Care,* (22)2, 120–127.

Rennick, J. E., Morin, I., Kim, D., Johnston, C. C., Dougherty, G., & Platt, R. (2004). Identifying children at high risk for psychological sequelae after pediatric intensive care unit hospitalization. *Pediatric Critical Care Medicine, 5*(4), 358–363.

Robertson, J. (1952). *A two-year-old goes to the hospital: A scientific film record.* London: Tavistock Publications Ltd.

Robertson, J. (1958). *Going to hospital with mother.* London: Tavistock Publications Ltd.

Robertson, J. (1958). *Young children in hospitals.* New York: Basic Books.

Rogers, T. L., & Ostrow, C. L. (2004). The use of EMLA cream to decrease venipuncture pain in children. *Journal of Pediatric Nursing, 19*(1), 33–39.

Rosenberg, D. I., & Moss, M. M. (2004). Guidelines and levels of care for pediatric intensive care units. *Critical Care Medicine, 32*(10), 2117–2127.

Schmidt, C., Bernaix, L., Koski, A., Weese, J., Chiappeta, M., & Sandrik, K. (2007). Hospitalized children's perceptions of nurses and nurse behaviors. *MCN, Journal of Maternal Child Nursing. 32,* 336–331.

Schmidt, C. K. (1990). Pre-operative preparation: Effects on immediate pre-operative behavior, post-operative behavior and recovery in children having day surgery. *Maternal-Child Nursing Journal, 19*(4), 321–330.

Scipien, G. M., Barnard, M. U., Chard, M. A., Howe, J., & Phillips, P. J. (1986). *Comprehensive pediatric nursing* (3rd ed.). New York: McGraw-Hill.

Shelton, D. (2003). The nursing shortage: Its impact on the care of children. *Newborn and Infant Nursing, 3*(1), 27–31.

Shore, M. F. (Ed.). (1965). *Red is the color of hurting.* Rockville, MD: U.S. Department of Health and Human Services, Public Health Service, National Institute of Mental Health.

Sittner, B., Hudson, D. B., & Defrain, J., (2007). Using the concept of family strengths to enhance nursing care. *MCN The American Journal of Maternal Child Nursing, 32*(6), 353–357.

Small, L. (2002). Early predictors of poor coping outcomes in children following intensive care hospitalization and stressful medical encounters. *Pediatric Nursing, 28*(4), 393–401.

Small, L., & Melnyk, B. M. (2006). Anxiety in the mother affects the long-term coping of a child in PICU. *Research in nursing & health, 29,* 622–635.

Smith, A., & Hefley, G. C., (2007). Parent bed spaces in the PICU: Effect on parental stress. *Pediatric Nursing, 33*(3), 215–221.

Solodiuk, J., & Curley, M. A. (2003). Pain assessment in nonverbal children with severe cognitive impairments: The Individualized Numeric Rating Scale (INRS). *Journal of Pediatric Nursing, 18,* 295–299.

Spitz, R. A. (1954). Hospitalism: An inquiry into the genesis of psychiatric conditions in early childhood. *Psychoanalytic Study of the Child, 1,* 53.

Stewart, J. L. (2003). Children living with chronic illness: An examination of their stressors, coping responses, and health outcomes. *Annual Review of Nursing Research, 21,* 203–243.

Stremier, R., Wong, L., & Parshuram, C. (2008). Practices and provisions for parents sleeping overnight with a hospitalized child. *Journal Pediatric Psychology, 33*(3), 292–297.

Sumner, E. (2006). *My MRI.* Boston: Partners Health Care, Massachusetts General Hospital.

Thompson, R. M., & Vernon, D. T. (1993). Research on children's behavior after hospitalization: A review and synthesis. *Journal of Developmental and Behavioral Pediatrics, 14*(3), 28–35.

Truog, R. D., Cist, A. F., Brackett, S. E., Burns, J. P., Curley, M. A., Danis, M., DeVita, M. A., Rosenbaum, S. H., Rothenberg, C. M., Sprung, C. L., Webb, S. A., Wlody, G. S., & Hurford, W. E. (2001).

Recommendations for end-of-life care in the intensive care unit: The Ethics Committee of the Society of Critical Care Medicine. *Critical Care Medicine, 29,* 2332–2348.

Vaughn, V. C., McKay, R. J., & Behrman, R. E. (1959). *Nelson Textbook of Pediatrics* (11th ed.). Philadelphia, PA: W. B. Saunders Co.

Vessey, J. A. (2003). Children's psychological responses to hospitalization. *Annual Review Nursing Research, 21,* 173–201.

Visintainer, M. (1977). The effects of pre-admission psychological preparation on children's stress responses and adjustment following hospitalization for minor surgery. *Nursing Research Reports, 12*(5), 3–5.

Vohsing, A. (2004). *What it's like to be Luke's mom.* Cincinnati Children's Hospital. Retrieved November 9, 2004, from http://www.o4isr.com/oley/lifeline/luke.html.

Waechter, E. (1958). *Death anxiety in children with fatal illness.* Unpublished Doctoral Dissertation. Stanford University.

Walker, P. C., & Wagner, D. S. (2003). Treatment of pain in pediatric patients. *Journal of Pharmacy Practice, 16*(4), 261–275.

Ward, S. L. (1998). Caring and healing in the 21st century. *Journal of Maternal Child Nursing, 23*(4), 210–215.

Ward-Begnoche, W. (2007). Posttraumatic stress symptoms in the pediatric intensive care unit. *Journal for specialists in pediatric nursing. 12*(2), 84–92. Published on line March 19, 2007.

Wolfer, J., & Visintainer, M. A. (1975). Pediatric patients' and parents' stress responses and adjustment. *Nursing Research, 24,* 244–255.

Youngblut, J. M., & Brooten, M. (1999). Alternate child care, history of hospitalization and preschool child behavior. *Nursing Research, 48*(1), 29–34.

Youngblut, J. M., & Shiao, S. P. (1993). Child and family reactions during and after pediatric ICU hospitalization: A pilot study. *Heart & Lung: Journal of Critical Care, 22*(1), 46–54.

Zahr, L. K. (1998). Therapeutic play for hospitalized preschoolers in Lebanon. *Pediatric Nursing, 23*(5), 449–454.

Zengerie-Levy, K., (2006). Nursing the child who is alone in the hospital. *Pediatric Nursing, 32*(3), 226–231.

SUGGESTED READINGS

Barclay, L., & Murata, P. (2008). AAP Addresses use of complementary and alternative medicine. *CME Medscape,* December 5, 2008.

Betz, C. L. (2008). Pediatric nursing: Scope and standards of practice: A unified professional effort. *Journal of Pediatric Nursing, 23*(2), 79–80.

Betz, C. L., Ruccione, K., Meeske, K., Smith, K., & Chang, N. (2008). Health literacy: A pediatric nursing concern. *Pediatric Nursing, 34*(3), 231–239.

Blake, F. G. (1965). A search for Kathy's problem. *International Journal of Nursing Studies, 2,* 125–136.

Bowlby, J. (1951). *Maternal care and infant health.* Geneva: World Health Organization.

Bricher, G. (2000). Children in the hospital: Issues of power and vulnerability. *Pediatric Nursing, 20*(3), 277–282.

Campbell, H., Duke, T., Wever, M., English, M., Carai, S., & Tamburlini, G. (2008). Global initiatives for improving hospital care for children: State of the art and future prospects. *Pediatrics. 121*(4), 984–992.

Chabra, A., & Chavez, G. F. (2000). A comparison of long pediatric hospitalizations in 1985 and 1994. *Journal of Community Health, 25*(3), 199–210.

Erikson, E. H. (1963). *Childhood and society.* New York: Norton.

Freda, M. C. (Ed.). (2008). A new day for pediatric nurses. *MCN The American Journal of Maternal Child Nursing, 33*(2), 70.

Levetown, M. A. (2004). A call for change: Recommendations to improve the care of children living with life-threatening conditions. Alexandria, VA: National Hospice and Palliative Care Organization.

London, F. (2004). How to prepare families for discharge in the limited time available. *Pediatric Nursing, 30*(3), 212–214, 227.

Melnyk, B. M., Small, L., & Carno, M. A. (2004). The effectiveness of parent-focused interventions in improving coping/mental health outcomes of critically ill children and their parents: An evidence base to guide clinical practice. *Pediatric Nursing, 30*(2), 143–148.

Pediatric Nursing: Scope & Standards of Practice. (2008). Silver Spring, Maryland: American Nurses Association.

Prugh, D. G., Staub, E., Sands, H., Kirschbaum, R., & Lenihan, E. (1953). A study of the emotional responses of children and families to hospitalization and illness. *American Journal of Orthopsychiatry, 23,* 70.

Tedder, J., Register, N. (2007). The "HUG": An innovative approach to pediatric nursing care. *MCN The American Journal of Maternal Child Nursing: 32*(4), 210–204.

Tiedeman, M. E. (1997). Anxiety responses of parents during and after the hospitalization of their 5- to 11-year-old children. *Journal of Pediatric Nursing, 12*(2), 110–119.

Wilkstrom, B. M. (2005). Communicating via expressive arts: The natural medium of self-expression for hospitalized children. *Pediatric Nursing, 31*(6), 480–485.

FOR CAREGIVERS:

Kelleher, M. L. (2003). *Helping your child cope with pain: An informational book for caregivers.* Boston: Massachusetts General Hospital.

Kelleher, M. L. (2004). *The ABC's of hospitalization: A parent's guide.* Boston: Massachusetts General Hospital for Children.

FOR CHILDREN:

Cork, B. (2002). *Katie goes to the hospital (First Experiences).* McGraw-Hill Children's Publishing.

Hatkoff, J. L., Hatkoff, C., & Mets, M. (2001). *Goodbye tonsils!* Viking Children's Books.

Jawarski, A. M., & Ball, L. (1998). *My brother needs an operation.* Babyhearts Press.

Karu, T., & Karu, T. (1999). *Henry & the white wolf.* New York: Workman Publishing.

Pace, B., & Hutton, K. (2003). *Chris gets ear tubes.* Kendall Green Publications.

Rey, M., & Rey, H. A. (1996). *Curious George goes to the hospital.* Houghton Mifflin, Co.

Rogers, F., & Judkis, J. (1988). *Mr. Rogers hospital.* Putnam Publishing.

RESOURCES

Refer to the online student StudyWARE for Potts & Mandleco at http://www.CengageBrain.com for additional content and study aids.

Organization: **American Academy of Pediatrics**
Description: Offers general information related to child health, specific guidelines concerning many pediatric issues, information regarding AAP programs, activities, policies, guidelines, publications, and other child health resources.
Website/Resource: http://www.aap.org

Organization: **Band-Aids & Blackboards**
Description: Offers children who are suffering from chronic illnesses and their parents opportunities to share their experiences.
Website/Resource: http://www.lehman.cuny.edu

Organization: **Child Life Council**
Description: Offers information about certification, career centers, a bookstore, the annual conference and much more.
Website/Resource: http://www.childlife.org

Organization: **Children's Hospice International (CHI)**
Description: Offers information about CHI's programs and resources as well as donation information.
Website/Resource: http://chionline.org

Organization: **Children's Hospice and Palliative Care Association**
Description: Offers general information about improving child health care and a special link for families.
Website/Resource: http://www.childrenshospice.org

Organization: **Children's Project on Palliative/Hospice Services (ChiPPs)**
Description: Offers users links and resources pertaining to child palliative care.
Website/Resource: http://www.nhpco.org

Organization: **Institute for Family-Centered Care**
Description: Offers information about Institute for Family-Centered Care services, resources for advancing practice, and events.
Website/Resource: http://www.familycenteredcare.org

Organization: **Institute for Family-Centered Care**
Description: Offers information about Institute for Family-Centered Care services, resources for advancing practice, and events.
Website/Resource: http://www.familycenteredcare.org

Organization: **National Information Center on Children and Youth with Disabilities**
Description: Offers information about child disabilities for families/communities, early intervention providers, school/administration, and state agencies.
Website/Resource: http://www.nichcy.org

Organization: **Net Wellness**
Description: Offers information regarding various health topics, health centers as well as access to a reference library.
Website/Resource: http://www.netwellness.org

Organization: **Starbright Foundation**
Description: Offers information about program actions, partners, news and social networks for children with chronic and life-threatening illnesses and life-altering injuries.
Website/Resource: http://www.starbright.org

Organization: **Starbright World**
Description: An online social network where 13 to 20 year olds with serious medical conditions, and siblings of seriously ill teens, can connect with each other via moderated chat rooms, games, bulletin boards, videos, etc.
Website/Resource: http://www.starbrightworld.org

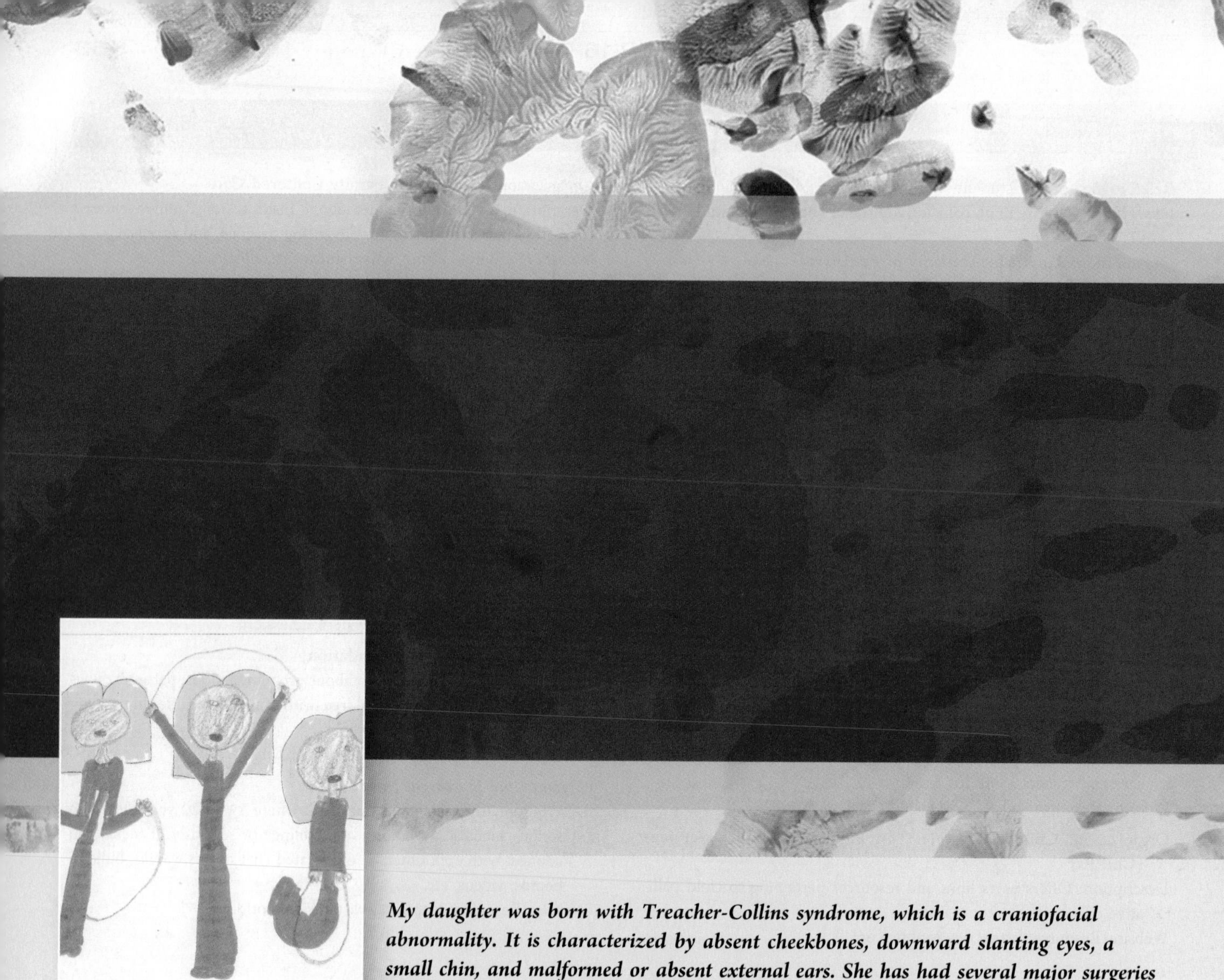

COURTESY EBONY S., AGE 8

My daughter was born with Treacher-Collins syndrome, which is a craniofacial abnormality. It is characterized by absent cheekbones, downward slanting eyes, a small chin, and malformed or absent external ears. She has had several major surgeries and will require more in the future to build the bones in her face and repair her external ears. She has a trach and wears hearing aids. We met a lot of resistance when I tried to enroll her in school. The trach scared the teacher, principal, and staff. I finally took Lisa to a meeting with the school personnel, and she showed them how to suction. They couldn't fight much once they saw this child could do that by herself. Sometimes I get so tired of having to fight for everything for Lisa. She's not really different from other kids. She even wants to get her ears pierced—as soon as the ears are done.

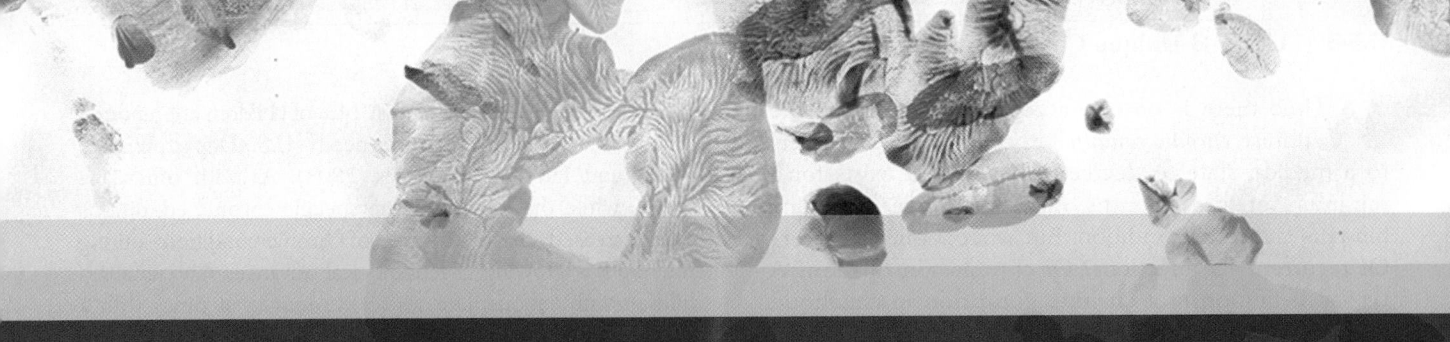

CHAPTER 17
Chronic Conditions

COURTNEY BROWNING, RN, MSN, CPN; Pam Schlomann, RN, PhD
JOAN SCHMITKE, ARNP, FNP, BC, DSN

COMPETENCIES

Upon completion of this chapter, the reader will be able to:

- Identify dimensions of childhood chronic conditions.
- Discuss the major focus of the deficit-orientation and health-orientation models used to understand childhood chronic conditions.
- Describe aspects of living with childhood chronic conditions from the perspective of the child, caregiver, and siblings.
- Explore the impact of cultural values on the child with a chronic condition and on those who interact with the child.
- Discuss the nursing management of children with chronic conditions.
- Successfully complete the games and activities in the online student StudyWARE.

While there is no one accepted definition of the phrase *chronic condition,* the term typically refers to a medical state or degree of health that exists for a minimum of three months. All would agree that spina bifida is a chronic condition. But what about hay fever? Or recurrent ear infections? Or chronic constipation? A typical definition of a **chronic condition** in childhood is a physical, psychological, or cognitive condition that places limitations on day-to-day functioning or requires reliance on special treatments and is expected to last a significant period of time (van der Lee, Mokkink, Grootenhuis, Heymans, & Offringa, 2007). Research about childhood chronic conditions has tended to focus on the more severe conditions while ignoring the mild ones.

Disability and *handicap* are two words that are frequently mentioned with chronic health conditions. **Disability** refers to a functional limitation that prevents or interferes with a person's ability to perform age-expected activities. In contrast, a **handicap** is a barrier imposed by society, the environment, or one's self in response to perceived differences. For example, lower extremity paralysis from spina bifida results in a disability when the child is unable to walk. By itself, this is not a handicap. However, a handicap would exist if the child is excluded from playing basketball, if a park is not wheelchair accessible, or if the child does not participate in activities because of the erroneous belief that the disability prevents participation. Recently, critical analysis of disability suggests that the notion of disability is socially constructed, much like handicap, and serves to restrict and stigmatize individuals. Furthermore, some have suggested that communication and attitudes of nurses often reinforce the negative experience of being handicapped or disabled (Boyles, Bailey, & Mossey, 2008). Think of times you have observed this happening.

A wide diversity in concepts and definitions for childhood chronic conditions produces a wide variability in reported prevalence rates. Depending on the definition used, the estimated prevalence of childhood chronic conditions has ranged from as little as 0.22% to as high as 44% (van der Lee et al., 2007). Almost 14% of children are reported to have a special health care need (U.S. Department of Health and Human Resources, 2008). As with other age groups, while the rates of some specific chronic conditions have decreased, the overall rate of chronic conditions during childhood is growing. Technological advances have enabled children with serious illnesses to live longer, at times with a newly acquired chronic condition. Furthermore, technology at times results in **iatrogenic** (treatment-induced) chronic conditions. Additionally, a rapid increase in obesity, with its associated chronic conditions, has developed in response to societal lifestyle changes. Environmental exposure may also contribute to increased rates of chronic conditions. Clearly, millions of children and their families live with chronic conditions. In addition to increasing prevalence, health care providers are concerned with growing disparities in the prevalence of chronic conditions (Perrin, Bloom, & Gortmaker, 2007). Nurses need to develop skills to effectively manage the care of these clients. This chapter discusses the dimensions of childhood chronic conditions and appropriate nursing management.

CRITICAL THINKING

Disability vs. Handicap

A 10-year-old child who is wheelchair dependent attends the local elementary school. The child is often excluded from participating in gym class and recess because appropriate activities are not available. The parents have informed the school that there are many activities, such as basketball and playing catch, that the child enjoys. Does this child have a disability or a handicap? What could the school do to improve this situation?

DIMENSIONS OF CHILDHOOD CHRONIC CONDITIONS

A disease-specific approach to childhood chronic conditions may not be the most helpful way of understanding them. As an alternative, clinicians have attempted to identify dimensions of chronic conditions and to understand how these affect the child's and the family's adjustment to the condition. For instance, knowing that a child has cerebral palsy might not be as important as knowing whether the condition affects mobility and the ability to care for one's self and that the condition is not life-threatening or progressive. Important dimensions of chronic conditions include:

1. Nature of onset: Was it a congenital condition or did it begin after a period of relative health? How do the child and family explain the cause of the condition?
2. **Trajectory** or progression of the condition: Will it get better, worse, or stay the same? Does it have episodic exacerbations or crises or is it stable? Is it terminal?
3. Effects on appearance: How visible is the condition? If visible, what is affected—the face, limbs, behavior?
4. Effects on daily functioning: Is the child able to do age-appropriate tasks? Is lifelong dependence anticipated?
5. Effects on behavior and ability to relate to others: Is the child's behavior and ability to relate age-appropriate and socially appropriate?
6. Care required: Does it require special procedures or equipment? Constant vigilance? Frequent hospitalizations or surgeries? Frequent visits to medical facilities? Time required? Discomfort of care?
7. Discomfort of symptoms: Is pain involved? Nausea? Fatigue? Difficulty breathing?

As researchers have attempted to uncover the significance of these dimensions, some unexpected, and many conflicting, findings have emerged. One unexpected finding in a number of studies is that the less visible the condition, the greater the difficulties the child, caregivers, and siblings often have in adjusting to it. Visibility involves both functional status and appearance. Various explanations have been offered to explain this finding. An early study explained it with the concept of **marginality**: a condition which is less visible to others results in ambiguity about whether an individual is different from or like others (McAnarney, Pless, Satterwhite, & Friedman, 1974). This leads to a conflict between "normal" (age-appropriate and socially appropriate expectations) and "different," which affects how others relate to the child and the expectations that are placed on the child. For example, a child with an invisible condition, such as diabetes, may be treated as if no condition existed, and therefore, be subjected to unrealistic expectations. The child and family also may experience stress from the fear of consequences of the condition becoming known and struggle with when and how to tell others about the condition. More negative responses to lower visibility have also been explained with the concept of **uncertainty**. Uncertainty exists as to whether the child is "normal" or has a limiting condition. Uncertainty may exist regarding many other aspects of childhood chronic conditions: diagnosis, prognosis, treatments, unpredictable symptoms, and so forth. Uncertainty, or ambiguity about what can be expected, creates a sense of limited control. This may lead to both child and parental psychological distress and subsequently to physical symptoms. Helping families gather, manage, and share information is one way to minimize uncertainty (Carpentier, Mullins, Wagner, Wolfe-Christensen, & Chaney, 2008; Holm, Patterson, Rueter, & Wamboldt, 2008).

Another counterintuitive finding is that the severity of the child's condition has little relationship to family functioning (Rodriguez & Patterson, 2007) or the child's quality of life (Walker, Winkelstein, Land, Lewis-Boyer, Quartey, Pham, & Butz, 2008). Early studies also suggested that the need to do special procedures in the care of a child with a chronic condition had no bearing on the child's and family's adjustment, but more recent findings have challenged this. Over time, the degree of care that is provided by family members has increased. Family members may be responsible for 24-hour-per-day care of children who require constant observation and are dependent on sophisticated equipment such as ventilators. Some caregivers have reported that the constancy of care contributes to the burden of that care and can be overwhelming and isolating (MacDonald & Callery, 2007; Yantzi, Rosenberg, & McKeever, 2006). The relationship between childhood chronic conditions and family/child functioning is complex and an ever-changing landscape.

REFLECTIVE THINKING

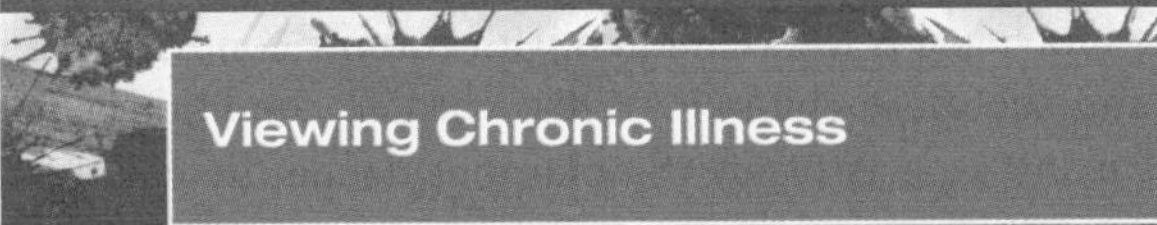

If you were to be diagnosed with a chronic condition, which would you least like to have and why? A condition like diabetes for which you would be required to do frequent monitoring and needle sticks? A condition like cerebral palsy for which you would have to use a walker in order to be mobile? A seizure disorder for which you would have to take daily medications? A condition that would not allow you to be independent, such as quadriplegia from a spinal cord injury? A condition like sickle cell anemia in which you would experience severe bouts of pain?

LIVING WITH CHRONIC CONDITIONS

A variety of models has been used to understand childhood chronic conditions and their influence on other's perceptions of and interactions with people living with chronic conditions. These models are helpful in framing the child's, caregiver's, and sibling's perspectives on living with the chronic condition. The effects of cultural and societal backgrounds are also considered.

MODELS OF CHRONIC CONDITIONS

Historically, chronic conditions were thought of as pathological states with major negative consequences in all aspects of life. This approach is an example of a **deficit-orientation model**, which assumes that people with chronic conditions are lacking important aspects of life, and thus clinicians look for abnormalities and problems in these individuals. According to this model, if a child indicates that a major disability does not affect self-esteem, the child is considered maladjusted or in denial. Although deficit-oriented models continue to be influential, **health-orientation models** have emerged that portray chronic conditions as variations in life. These models tend to be critical of professionals who make negative appraisals such as depicted above. These negative appraisals are viewed as misplaced projections of the health care professional's discomfort with disabilities. Health-orientation model proponents do not deny that children with chronic conditions and their families may be maladjusted, but focus on positive aspects of the individual's life rather than assuming maladjustment (Figure 17-1). The **ordinary model** is an example of a research-based health-orientation model which depicts the child's changing awareness of the chronic condition as the child goes through the developmental sequence. The chronic condition does not assume a central or relevant role in the development of identity or in activities of daily life. Instead, those with chronic conditions view themselves as "ordinary people coping with extraordinary situations" caused both by their condition and society's responses to

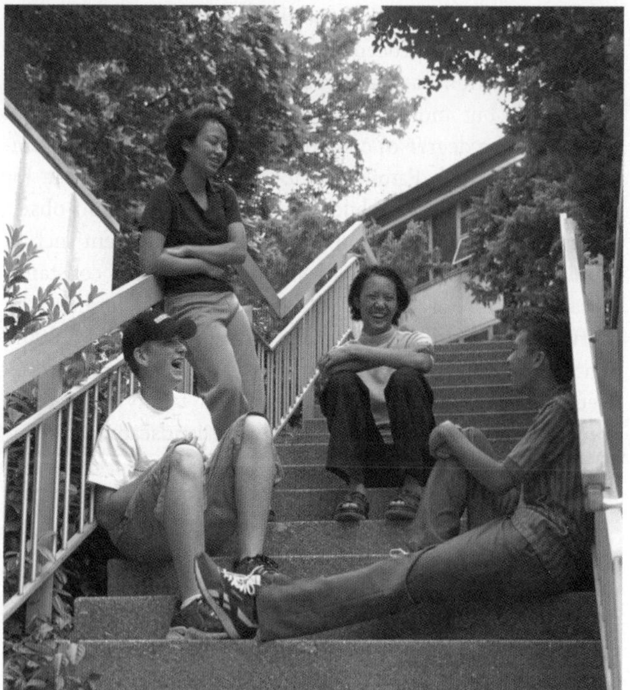

FIGURE 17-1 **Some chronic conditions are not readily apparent. As you look at this group of adolescents, would you be able to discern which adolescent has a chronic condition?**
DELMAR CENGAGE LEARNING.

that condition (Admi, 1996; Admi & Shaham, 2007). A social movement that opposes the deficit-orientation perspective has developed. Using **critical-orientation models** has shifted the focus to examining the ways in which the physical and social environment stigmatizes and excludes individuals with health issues. While this has been helpful, the critical-orientation model tends to emphasize the environment to the exclusion of the challenges of living with chronic conditions.

In addition to determining how professionals view individuals with chronic conditions, the model that one uses has implications for how the individual interacts with and what role she or he assumes with clients with chronic conditions. The deficit-orientation models tend to establish the professional as "the expert" who has the authority to diagnose and treat the client's illness. Some believe that this approach results in dehumanizing and paternalistic modes of interactions. In contrast, health-orientation models portray the relationship between client and professional as a partnership, with each individual bringing a different type of expertise to the situation. Families are central in the relationship and decision making. Focus shifts from treatment to prevention. The professional's role is to empower and enable clients to achieve their self-selected goals for self-identified concerns. Health-orientation models encourage approaches to the management of chronic conditions that are more holistic and consistent with nursing values. This is accomplished by nurses effectively using their knowledge and skills, approaching caregivers with compassion and caring, respecting

CRITICAL THINKING

Discharge Teaching for a Child with Cystic Fibrosis

A nurse is providing discharge teaching for a child with cystic fibrosis and his family. The nurse explains the changes to his medication and chest physiotherapy regimen. These changes include increased frequency and duration of treatments. The nurse tells the child and his family that he will need to change his after-school activities to accommodate the prescribed treatment regimen. The child becomes very upset and says that he will just quit doing his treatments so that he can be like his friends. What model of chronic conditions did the nurse use in her interactions with this family? How could the use of a different model have changed this interaction?

families and acknowledging their capabilities, and involving caregivers in joint decision making. Critical-orientation models also focus on empowerment and partnerships but tend to limit their focus to policy initiatives.

An early review of the literature on childhood chronic illness identified six major themes, representing 20 conceptual categories (Dluhy, 1995). These six themes continue to capture the literature. The current literature has increased coverage of responses of siblings and fathers as well as transitioning to adulthood. These six themes will provide the framework for a discussion of living with chronic conditions in the remainder of this chapter (Table 17-1).

THE CHILD'S PERSPECTIVE

"Mostly I'm just like other kids, but sometimes I have to take my nebulizer with me to gymnastics."—7-year-old with cystic fibrosis.

Discussions about living with chronic conditions can focus so much attention on the condition that the essence of the individual is lost. Children with chronic conditions are first and foremost children. While chronic conditions may affect many aspects of life, they do not define the children.

DEMANDS AND CHALLENGES

A growing body of literature sheds light on the child's perspective in managing a chronic condition. Since much of the research has been done in other countries, one must consider if the experience of individuals in the United States is the same. Common stressors noted by children with chronic conditions include dealing with the symptoms, treatment modalities, and the response of others. These are the things that restrict typical daily activities and which create, for self and others, a sense of being different. Even relatively common things such as publicly taking medications have been described by children as embarrassing (Smith, Taylor,

Table 17-1 Themes and Concepts in Chronic Illness

THEMES	CONCEPTUAL AREAS
• Demands and challenges	• Fatigue; dyspnea; pain; uncertainty; stress or adaptation
• Emotional and cognitive responses	• Defense mechanisms; control/mastery; coping or adaptation; attributions
• Day-to-day tasks of living with a chronic condition	• Life management/normalizing symptoms
• Having a chronic condition in the culture of a healthy society	• Role transitions; disability; stigma; social definitions of illness
• Changing interactional patterns	• Social support; relationship with health care providers
• Potential life outcomes	• Quality of life; meaning in illness; redefining the illness situation

Used with permission from Dluhy, N. (1995). Mapping knowledge in chronic illness. *Journal of Advanced Nursing*, 21, 1055.

Newbould, & Keady, 2008). One could imagine that health care professionals might not generate the same list of concerns as would children, or would prioritize entries differently. By listening to the children's perspectives professionals can learn from them and provide more effective care.

Management of symptoms is often condition specific. For spina bifida, the child may be concerned about incontinence. For asthma, the child may be concerned about limitations in sporting activities. Developmental issues are also a factor that affects the child's concerns. At one developmental stage, children with a given condition may tend to be concerned with one set of symptoms, while at a different age they may identify other symptoms. For example, younger children tend to identify pain more while adolescents are more likely to be concerned with things that interfere with their social life.

Children with a chronic condition must learn to manage the treatments associated with the condition as well as its symptoms. Waters (2008) referred to the work of managing everyday life with a chronic disease as "illness labor." It often requires vigilance, skill, and commitment. Again, developmental issues affect how children deal with this. Because of concrete thought processes and limited ability to understand disease processes, younger school-age children may question or resist treatments. The school-age child may not understand why treatments are necessary during symptom-free periods or when the benefits are not immediately apparent. They may respond to treatments with manipulative behavior or testing of boundaries. For example, a child may refuse to do physical therapy activities or do them in such a way as to minimize their effectiveness. Nevertheless, during school age, children, both by necessity and often desire, begin to assume more responsibility for managing their health condition.

Adolescence can be a difficult period for children with chronic conditions. During early adolescence understanding increases but youth still receive a lot of direction from caregivers. Middle adolescence may be a time of pushing boundaries, resisting direction, and resistance to treatment. In late adolescence, most youth develop a more balanced, responsible position with more flexible approaches to treatment management (Taylor, Gibson, & Franck, 2008). Time constraints, the mundaneness of treatments, and the impact of treatments on one's social life may lead the older adolescent to modify treatment (Badlan, 2006). The flexibility allows them to balance treatment and other life interests. Health professionals often may view this flexibility as noncompliance. Use of peer support groups and Internet-based support may be helpful to improve self-management among adolescents (Sawyer, Drew, Yeo, & Britto, 2007).

In dealing with the demands and challenges of chronic conditions, children attempt to create a sense of "normalcy." They do this by attempting to control the disease, emphasizing their abilities, and trying to decrease the centrality of the disease in their lives (Badlan, 2006; Guell, 2007; Protudjer, Kozyrskyj, Becker, & Marchessault, 2009; Van Staa, Jedeloo, Latour, & Trappenburg, 2008). This includes modifying treatments to fit their life and controlling or limiting information given to others, including peers, family members, and professionals.

Nurses need to be cognizant of developmental issues and the child's perspective as they are involved in managing

NURSING TIP

Child's Perspective

Use open-ended, nonjudgmental questions to explore how the child is managing the condition and its treatment. For example, "What kind of things have you tried? Has that worked? Were there problems with it?" Based on your knowledge of potential problem areas at different developmental stages, use statements that give the child permission to talk about these issues. For example, "Some children your age who have asthma don't like to use their inhalers in front of other kids. How has it been for you?"

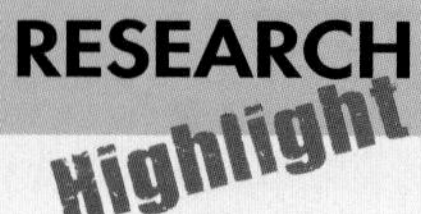

Normalization Strategies Used by Children Who Have Asthma

STUDY PURPOSE

To gain an understanding of how children with asthma develop strategies to normalize their lives.

METHODS

Using a qualitative design, 22 children, 11-years-old, were interviewed. Themes were derived from the transcribed interviews. Findings were related to the research question and literature.

FINDINGS

Children used the following strategies to normalize their lives: minimizing the health impact, stressing normality, emphasizing abilities, making adaptations, and managing symptoms.

IMPLICATIONS

Assisting youth to utilize the identified strategies to normalize life may enhance holistic care to this population.

REFERENCE

Protudjer, J., Kozyrskyz, A., Becker, A., & Marchessault, G. (2009). Normalization strategies of children with asthma. *Qualitative Health Research*, *19*, 94–104.

chronic conditions and as they facilitate movement of the child toward assuming increasing responsibility. Nurses can facilitate this process by listening and giving voice to the child. Rather than making assumptions about what is of concern to the child, professionals should ask open-ended, age-appropriate questions to elicit this information. Children need to be directly involved in developing treatment plans. Nurses may need to reframe flexible approaches to treatments as adaptive rather than noncompliant. Children also need an opportunity to learn about and role-play situations regarding telling others about their condition and responding to the reactions of others.

Emotional and Cognitive Responses

Most of the early research on living with chronic conditions from the child's perspective has dealt with emotional and cognitive responses. Children with and without chronic conditions have been compared based on various psychosocial measures of adjustment, such as measures of self-esteem, anxiety, and depression. While there is some indication that children with chronic conditions, as a group, are at greater risk for maladjustment, results have been inconsistent and have tended to show that most of the children are well-adjusted.

Children use various coping strategies to deal with their chronic conditions. As already mentioned, viewing oneself as "normal" is one strategy. Additionally, social support from family members, peers, and professionals is an important strategy. Some children with chronic conditions use less-adaptive coping strategies such as withdrawal, blaming themselves or others for their condition, negativity, and irritability. Extreme attempts at normalization can result in denial of symptoms and treatment nonadherence.

Asking the child about coping strategies that are utilized and about their effectiveness is an important aspect of assessment. If those strategies are inadequate, the child should be assisted to develop different ones. While the effectiveness of interventions to facilitate coping in children with chronic conditions has not been well studied, there are indications that support groups and educational programs may be effective.

Day-to-Day Tasks of Living with a Chronic Condition

Two important factors of day-to-day living for children are developmental issues and school issues. These factors are also important for children with chronic conditions.

Developmental Issues While the development pattern of children with chronic health conditions may be somewhat complicated by their condition, these children have the same developmental tasks as any other child. Additionally, they experience the same common childhood illnesses and demonstrate similar age-dependent behaviors, such as the "terrible twos." Little is known about how various symptoms or treatments of chronic conditions affect development. Based on developmental theories, one might speculate that various aspects of conditions affect a child's ability to master different developmental tasks. For example, conditions that affect sensations (such as sight or hearing impairment) or mobility would decrease a toddler's ability to explore the environment. According to Piaget's theory, one might expect that this would hamper the child's cognitive development. Similarly, a complicated medical regime may hinder an adolescent's attempts at establishing independence; or differences in physical appearance or function may affect the youth's ability to develop a positive body image. According to Erikson's theory, both of these could be problematic for the psychosocial development of the adolescent. These speculations obviously reflect a deficit model of chronic conditions. Rather than focusing on this aspect, one might consider creative ways in which children with chronic conditions and their caregivers can maximize development. For example, a child who uses a wheelchair may not achieve a sense of athletic accomplishment from playing football, but may do so from doing wheelies or playing wheelchair basketball (Figure 17-2).

School Issues One critical aspect of day-to-day living for children with chronic conditions is school, including attendance and performance. School attendance and accomplishment are typically viewed as essential aspects of

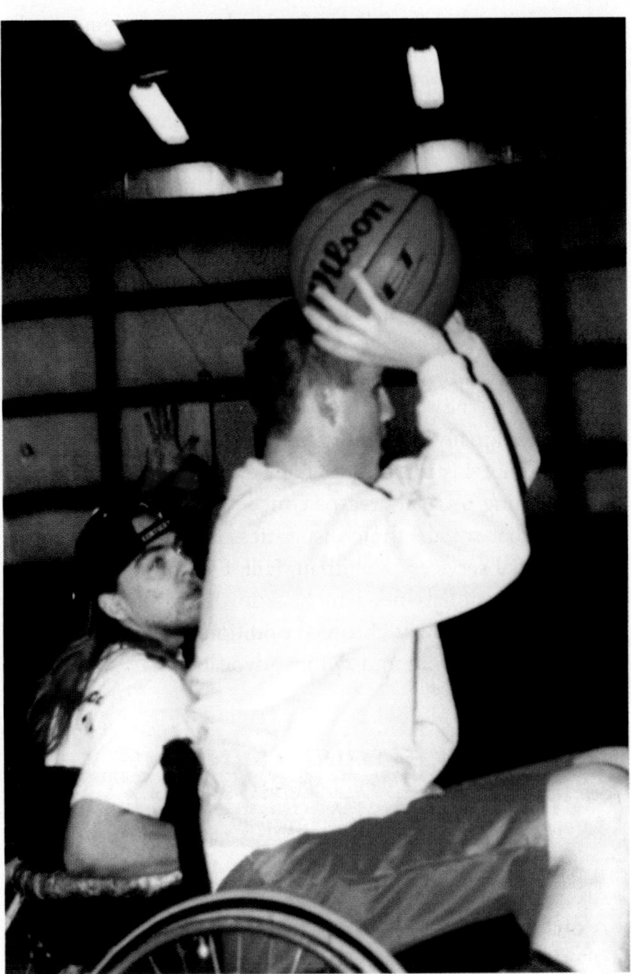

FIGURE 17-2 **By playing wheelchair basketball, adolescents can achieve a sense of athletic accomplishment.** DELMAR CENGAGE LEARNING.

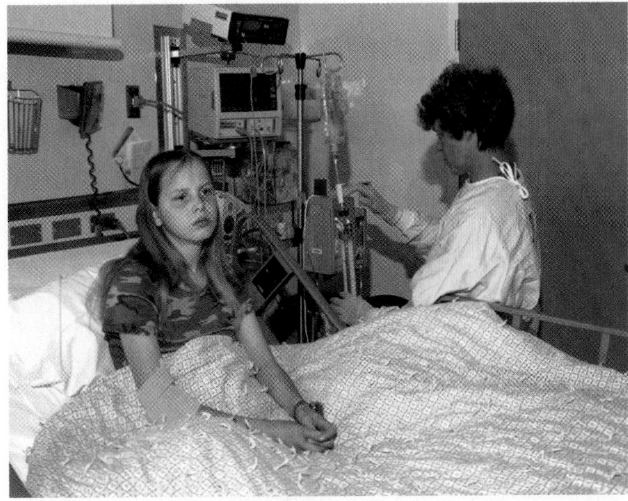

FIGURE 17-3 **When a child with a chronic condition has to return to the hospital, peers often question why their friend is not in school and when she will be back.** DELMAR CENGAGE LEARNING.

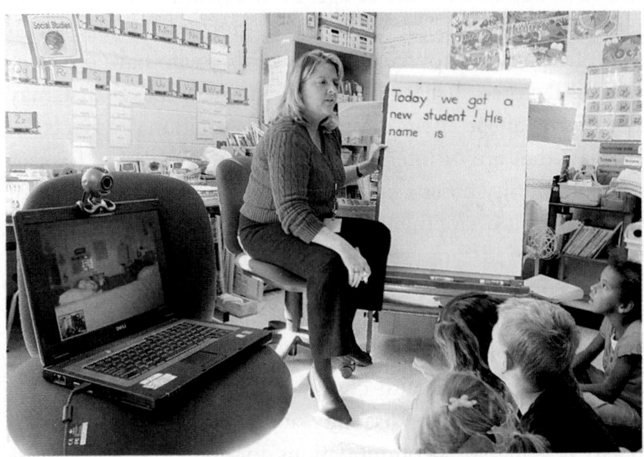

FIGURE 17-4 **New technologies enable children with chronic conditions to maintain contact with peers and school.** PHOTO BY NANCY TAGGART.

normalizing life and promoting healthy development. Nevertheless, school attendance may be negatively affected by illness exacerbations, protective caregivers, the response of the child to the condition, and by the school's response to the child and medical appointments (Figure 17-3). Emerging technologies have the potential to maximize children's participation (Figure 17-4). Children with chronic conditions tend to experience more academic problems than their healthy peers.

A series of federal laws mandates that appropriate education be provided to all children. Public Law 94-142, the Education for All Handicapped Children Act of 1975, requires a free, appropriate public education for all children ages 5–18 years regardless of the severity of the disability. This education must be provided in the least restrictive environment that is appropriate for the child, which can range from a regular classroom placement to the child's home. This stipulation has led to the placement of children with chronic conditions in settings that permit more interactions with others without chronic conditions. This concept has been referred to as **mainstreaming**. The benefits of the inclusive classroom for both groups of students have been well documented (Figure 17-5). In young children, however, interactions are limited unless teachers plan specific activities to facilitate social integration. This law also requires schools, at no cost to the family, to provide related services that would facilitate the child's development and capacity to benefit from the educational experience. Related services include a variety of offerings such as special transportation; speech, occupational, and physical therapy; counseling; and certain health-related services.

Part H of Public Law 102-119, the Individuals with Disabilities Education Act (formerly P.L. 99-457, Education for the Handicapped Amendments of 1986), first extended the components of Public Law 94-142 to children ages 3 to 5 who are handicapped or at risk for later delay, and then to the age period from newborn to 3 years. It later extended

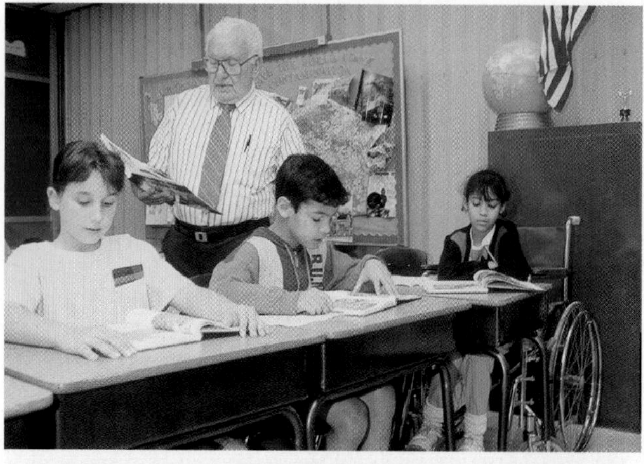

FIGURE 17-5 **Teachers report that when children with special needs are included in regular classes, they become part of the class without their disability being their most important characteristic.** DELMAR CENGAGE LEARNING.

the coverage to 21 years of age. Early identification of at-risk children is critical. "At risk" includes not only children with identified health problems, but also those who have environmental factors (such as poverty or homelessness) that may negatively affect their development. Additional aspects of this law that are of interest to nurses are that it: (1) focuses on community-based, early intervention with the hope of maximizing development and preventing problems; (2) has family-centered care as an integral component; and (3) dictates a coordinated, interdisciplinary approach.

Another law, the Americans with Disabilities Act of 1990, has an impact on the educational experience of children with chronic health conditions. The law prohibits discrimination based on disability and requires institutions to make reasonable accommodations for individuals with disabilities. Accessibility and accommodations can be denied only if they would create an undue financial burden on the institution or would create a public health or safety risk (e.g., a contagious disease). One application of this law has been to require educational facilities, including family day care, day care centers, and preschool programs, to accept children who have chronic conditions, including those who are HIV positive.

The Individuals with Disabilities Education Act (IDEA), most recently reauthorized in 2004, expanded upon these previous laws. The purpose of this law was to raise expectations for children with disabilities, increase parental involvement in the education of these children, improve teacher training, increase funding for schools and for early intervention programs, and decrease disparities among racial and ethnic groups. The No Child Left Behind Act of 2002 is another law which has an educational impact for children with chronic conditions. This law attempts to reform public education to ensure that ALL children perform well in reading and math and to decrease the achievement gap for at-risk children, including those with disabilities. The law increases accountability and flexibility of school systems, requires the use of evidence-based practice, has a greater emphasis on academics for children with disabilities, and gives families more choice and influence. While the intention of the law is typically praised, its implementation, especially in reference to children requiring special education, has been frequently criticized.

While these laws have made major changes in the lives of children with chronic health conditions, they are not a panacea. Attitudes cannot be mandated; they take time to change. Additionally, laws do not necessarily supply adequate resources to carry out the mandates. Therefore, compliance with the laws may be difficult, and sometimes impossible. Finally, the effort that families often have to exert to require institutions to comply with the law may be overwhelming. A final area of concern is that there is some evidence that racial/ethnic disparities exist in use of school-based special services (Kuhlthau, Hill, Fluet, Meara, & Yucel, 2008). Professionals need to be knowledgeable about laws affecting children with chronic conditions and, when appropriate, to act as child and family advocates.

REFLECTIVE THINKING

Education for All Handicapped Children Act

A child with multiple disabilities is in the first grade in a small rural community. The caregivers have requested that the school purchase an expensive computer system that will facilitate the child's communication. The school's very limited budget would be significantly affected by this purchase. This would affect the education of all children in the school. What are the requirements of P.L. 94-142 in relation to this situation? Is it appropriate that this child's needs be placed above the educational needs of other children? Explain your answer.

REFLECTIVE THINKING

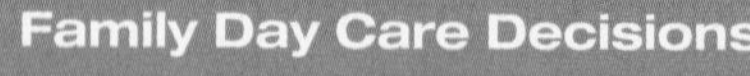

Family Day Care Decisions

You are the parent of a 3-year-old child who attends a family day care. Your day care provider has informed you that she has been mandated to accept a 2-year-old child who is HIV positive. How would you feel about your child attending the same family day care as the 2-year-old HIV positive child? How would you feel if you were the family day care provider? Explain your answer.

Having a Chronic Condition in the Culture of a Healthy Society

Having a chronic condition while living in the culture of a "healthy" society poses some potential challenges for a child. The children must navigate both the responses of others and their own evaluation of self relative to the norms of society.

As already indicated, while some children are at risk for a negative impact on their self-concept and self-esteem, overall they do well. Children have reported both rejection and acceptance from others. One of the main challenges is dealing with negative responses such as stares, comments, misinformation, and stereotypic expectations. The children sometimes experience difficulties with others being wrongly concerned that their conditions are contagious or fatal. They may be teased for taking medications, looking different, or acting differently. Fears and ignorance may result in their being excluded from activities. In addition, inaccessibility of some public places may limit full participation. Some health conditions, such as AIDS and obesity, are much stigmatized, which heightens the potential for negative consequences.

How children respond to these situations is a very complex process. Children and their families must learn how to manage condition-related information and be able to determine what and how much to tell to whom, when, and where. They need an opportunity to discuss and role-play responses to teasing, stares, and stereotypic characterizations. While caregivers have a major role in coaching children about managing questions about their condition, nurses can also help by listening and providing developmentally appropriate information. Support groups with other children who have chronic conditions may help by providing a safe environment in which the children can discuss feelings and problem-solve responses. School nurses can educate other children about health conditions and work to decrease stigma and misinformation. Finally, nurses can act as advocates and work to decrease barriers.

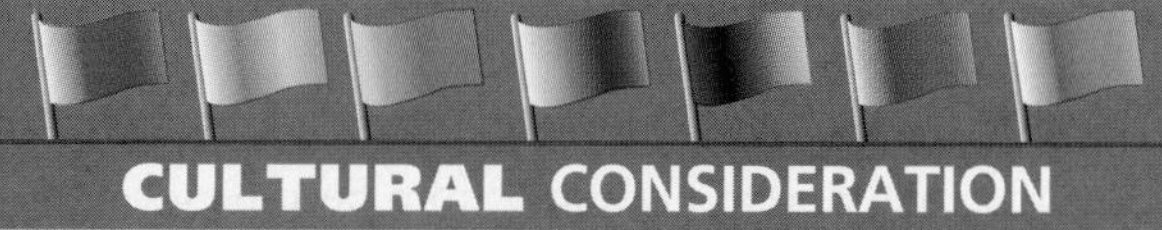

CULTURAL CONSIDERATION

Laws and Morality

Educational practices, such as mainstreaming, and public laws addressing education for children with disabilities, including admission of children with HIV to day care centers and schools, are policies based on beliefs and judgments of right and wrong. Our sense of ethics and morality is tied to our cultural background and experiences. Be sensitive to the possibility that parents and children from different cultures may hold beliefs that differ from those in common practice in the United States. Ensure that as a nurse you are ready to help these families understand the laws and how they may impact their child's care and development.

REFLECTIVE THINKING

Age-Related Responses to Chronic Conditions

Visualize a child with cerebral palsy walking with an unsteady gait through a shopping mall. What responses to a stranger's stares would you anticipate from a child who is 4 years old and a child who is 14 years old? Using the same ages, what differences would you anticipate in their responses to questions about their chronic conditions?

Changing Interactional Patterns

Very little is known about children with chronic conditions and their interactional patterns with health care providers. What is known, though, gives important insight for health care professionals and identifies interactional patterns as an area for further study. As already mentioned, health care providers often express frustration about nonadherence to treatment plans, especially by adolescents. On the other side, youth with chronic conditions have expressed frustration at being defined solely by a health problem, judgmental attitudes, and lack of understanding. Flexible, respectful, holistic care is needed (Taylor, Gibson, & Franck, 2008).

Peer relationships are considered a vital aspect to the healthy development of children with chronic conditions, just as it is with other children. While many children with chronic conditions develop positive peer relations, some have difficulties and experience a sense of isolation. Older children have indicated that talking with another child with the same condition is one of the best coping strategies available and decreases the sense of isolation. Electronic support groups may be beneficial in connecting some of these children. Nevertheless, a normalization strategy of some youth is to limit contact with others who have the same condition (Van Staa, Jedeloo, Latour, & Trappenburg, 2008).

Chronic conditions are often conceptualized as requiring dependence. This may affect not only immediate but also long-term expectations, hopes, and dreams for the child. A growing emphasis is to develop a mindset and resources that enable individuals with chronic conditions to be contributing members of society as adults. The challenges facing youth with chronic conditions as they transition into adulthood is receiving increased attention. Youth have described this as a time with heightened uncertainty, lack of continuity of services including loss of trusted relationships (Kirk, 2008), and inadequate resources. The transition does not include just service transition but also individual transition to greater independence. Youth have expressed concerns

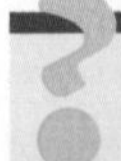

KIDS WANT TO KNOW

What should I do when people stare at me?

Stares and stigmatizing responses are common problems for individuals with chronic conditions. Stares, fears about touching, assumptions about abilities, and so forth are common reactions to which children must respond. Following are tips you can use in responding to the child:

- Anticipate occurrences (when a child is going into a new situation or has experienced a change in appearance or function).
- Listen to and explore the child's concerns. Give the child an opportunity to talk about negative responses of others.
- Coach children about how to react to negative responses; role-play situations with the child:
    1. Frontal approach: When other children are staring at you, ask them if they have a question.
    2. Indirect approach: Underscore your strengths without directly addressing stigmatizing responses. For example, you said the kids on the baseball team tease you and say you can't play because of your asthma. They said you have to stop too often to use your inhaler. You can reply with a statement that emphasizes your strengths such as, "Although I can't play this time, I know all the rules of baseball and can be the scorekeeper."
    3. Ignore: Affirm right to choose what to tell to whom.
- Facilitate the interaction of children with chronic conditions so they can support one another.
- At all times (not just in response to a negative situation), counter the stigmatizing message with one that affirms the child's value, appearance, and abilities.

EVIDENCE-BASED PRACTICE

Chronic Illness in Adolescence

CLINICAL PROBLEM

What is the experience of living with a chronic illness during adolescence? How can we use that information to improve practice?

BEST CLINICAL PRACTICE

- Developing and maintaining friendships was the most important aspect identified by the youths.
- As adolescence progressed, being "normal" gained heightened importance.
- Parents are an important source of support but can be overprotective.
- Attitudes toward treatment changed as the youth developed; mid-adolescence was the most difficult time.
- School often presented challenges because of absences, feeling different, and inadequately supportive teachers.
- Youth expressed a need to be valued as who they were rather than being defined by their health condition.
- Overall, the adolescents viewed themselves similarly as their healthy peers did.

IMPLICATIONS FOR NURSING

Providing developmentally appropriate care which focuses on wellness is important when addressing the health issues of adolescents with chronic conditions. Teaching parents and teachers ways to promote coping and normality would also be beneficial.

Reference: Taylor, R., Gibson, F., & Franck, L. (2008). The experience of living with a chronic illness during adolescence: A critical review of the literature. *Journal of Clinical Nursing, 17*, 3083–3091.

about the interplay of their conditions with career choices, moving away from home, and having children (Taylor, Gibson, & Franck, 2008). Reviews of self-management support studies fairly consistently demonstrate that these interventions can improve health outcomes and quality of life (Sawyer, Drew, Yeo, & Britto, 2007). Expansion of these services and development of an infrastructure to meet the needs of youth with chronic conditions is needed.

Potential Life Outcomes

As emphasized earlier, children with chronic conditions are *children* with a chronic condition. The condition, while a part of the child's identity, is not typically focal. In fact, these children exert some degree of effort to maintain the boundaries of the condition to prevent it from becoming central in their lives. Interestingly, and contrary to expectations, this is true even when the condition is a terminal illness. Adolescents with terminal illnesses often acknowledge the terminal nature of the illness and plan optimistically for the future. They need permission both to acknowledge the illness and to maintain an optimistic outlook. Quality of life and finding meaning in the chronic illness are dependent on maintaining a balance that puts boundaries on risk-taking behaviors while not allowing the reality and treatment routine of the condition to encroach on all aspects of life. For example, an adolescent with diabetes may occasionally choose to go to a fast food restaurant with his peers, even though this will interfere with control of his blood sugar.

Understanding and defining a chronic condition follows a developmental path for children. As expected, with increasing age, children are able to understand more complex and

REFLECTIVE THINKING

Dependence or Independence?

What does it mean to be independent? Dependent? Interdependent? Is "depending" on glasses to read different than "depending" on a wheelchair to get around? Is "depending" on someone for assistance with dressing different than "depending" on a hair dresser to style one's hair? What is "a contributing member of society"?

abstract descriptions of the disease process and treatment. Because of their experiences, children with chronic conditions may have more sophisticated explanations than expected for their developmental stage. Health care providers must learn the child's particular perspective.

THE CAREGIVER'S PERSPECTIVE

The caregivers of children with chronic conditions also face demands and challenges, emotional and cognitive responses, and changing roles within the family and society related to living with the condition. Each of these has the potential of adding different dimensions to typical parenting experiences.

DEMANDS AND CHALLENGES

The initial challenge of parenting a child with a chronic condition often revolves around finding out what is ailing the child. This time period preceding and surrounding diagnosis can be stressful. While some express relief in finally knowing what is wrong (Cashin, Small, & Solberg, 2008), many express feelings of being overwhelmed. Uncertainty and strong emotions are common (Coffey, 2006). Professionals who listen, with respect, to caregivers' concerns and who provide open, direct information help caregivers navigate this time. Facilitating a sense of hope is also important.

In addition to the variation in the amount of time between the onset of symptoms and learning about the diagnosis, chronic conditions vary in severity and in the amount of care required. Caring for a child with a chronic condition that is mild or does not have significant limitations is quite different than caring for a child whose condition requires the constant presence of a caregiver. Whatever the condition, however, one of the caregiver's challenges is to learn the skills required to care for the child. For example, the caregiver of a child with diabetes must learn how to test the blood for the presence of glucose (Figure 17-6) and how to calculate and inject the appropriate amount of insulin. The caregiver of a child with short gut syndrome may have to learn how to give parenteral or tube feedings. If a child is dependent on a ventilator, the caregiver will learn

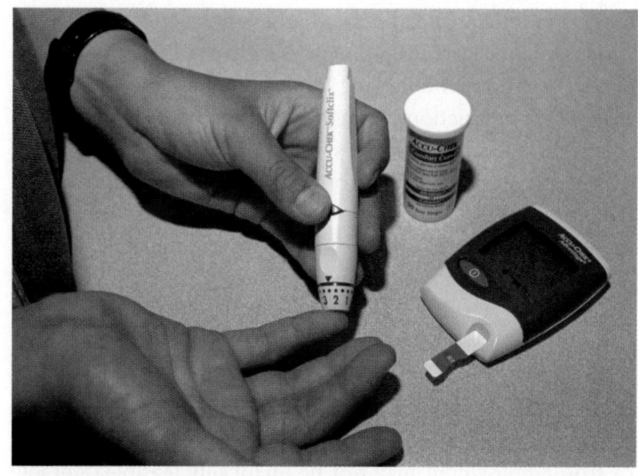

FIGURE 17-6 As the child becomes older, he will take on responsibilities of managing the condition. DELMAR CENGAGE LEARNING.

how to suction the child and, when the machine is malfunctioning, how to identify the problem. For all skills, in addition to learning to handle the technology, the caregiver must learn to look at the child and ascertain impending difficulties such as signs of hypoglycemia or signs of respiratory distress. Vigilance and worrying are common themes in the literature (Cashin, Small, & Solberg, 2008; Coffey, 2006; Woodgate, Ateah, & Secco, 2008). One parent described this as, "Always waiting for the other shoe to drop" (Murphy, Christian, Caplin, & Young, 2006). For a child who will not be independent as an adult, worrying about the future is a huge concern. Initially, caregivers have a steep learning curve and typically experience a lot of fear and self-doubt. Support and encouragement during this time is helpful. Establishing short-term goals is useful. Also, appropriately affirming the caregiver's growing expertise and primary role is important. Caregivers have repeatedly expressed frustration that professionals often undermine their role and do not give them adequate respect and recognition.

In addition to learning management skills themselves, caregivers must negotiate with the child regarding when and how to shift responsibility for care to the child. The child's age, developmental level, and interest are factors that are considered in the negotiation process. For example, a child diagnosed with diabetes as a toddler should assume increasingly greater responsibility for independent management of the condition. Initially, the caregiver will do all insulin adjustments. As the child reaches preschool age, the caregiver will verbalize the need for more insulin or food. During the early school-age time, the caregiver will verbalize specific amounts and rationale for insulin adjustments. Gradually, the child will be expected to verbalize this information with opportunity for correction and affirmation by the caregiver. By the end of elementary school, many children will be independently making these decisions. Throughout the process caregivers must walk a fine line between adequate supervision and overprotection. The final steps in the transition often entail conflict between caregiver and child. This may be a difficult time as the child assumes greater independence and the caregiver disagrees with decisions or feels a need to continue monitoring the child. Throughout the transition, nurses function as teachers and coaches. They have a role in supporting caregivers in gaining confidence in their own management skills in order for the caregiver to begin the transition process. They can help caregivers recognize the child's readiness to assume more responsibility. They teach negotiating skills during the final stages.

Another challenge for the caregiver is time management. Providing the care needed by the child and taking her or him to various appointments while working outside the home may produce stress or be impossible (Yantzi, Rosenberg, & McKeever, 2006). The decision for the caregiver to stop employment may not be financially feasible. Suitable day care for children with chronic conditions is extremely limited and often very expensive. Finding time for other family members, particularly siblings of the child with a chronic condition may also present a challenge to time management. The caregiver's effort to minimize the perceived harmful effects on siblings is an additional challenge. Time management issues are especially critical when the child is technologically dependent and requires constant monitoring. This typically requires a very structured routine and has a greater impact on all family members. Some of the challenges of caregiving involve adjustment to a new role, changing roles within the family, and the necessity of regular contact with the health care system. Particularly during the adjustment to caregiving responsibilities, caregivers may become frustrated with themselves because the intensity of their emotional responses to a given incident seems out of proportion. Lack of sleep for the caregiver may decrease coping abilities, heighten emotional responses, and increase conflict within the family.

The term **caregiver burden** has been used to describe the effect of the challenges and demands of caring for a child with a chronic condition. Most often, mothers assume the primary responsibility of caregiver and are at greatest risk for caregiver burden. However, the assumption should not be made that this is always the situation; others may have this role. The long-term implications of caregiving may be poor health for the caregiver (Burton, Lethbridge, & Phipps, 2008; Murphy, Christian, Caplin, & Young, 2006). Health care providers have a role in facilitating involvement of others. However, care must be taken in doing this to ensure that recommendations are acceptable to the family.

Respite care involves having a person relieve the usual caregiver of caregiving responsibilities for a period of time. It is one way to decrease caregiver burden. To those caring for a child who requires care 24 hours a day, it may be essential. The substitute may provide care in the home of the child with a chronic condition or may provide care for the child in another home or institution. Some caregivers have a substitute on a regular basis; for example, the substitute may care for the child two afternoons each week. Other families prefer to have a substitute less frequently, but for a longer time period; for example, a substitute may provide respite care while the rest of the family goes on vacation each year. Additionally, the length and type of respite needed often changes during the life course of the child (MacDonald & Callery, 2007). Respite care has been associated with many positive benefits: decreased stress and increased coping for families; delayed or prevented institutionalization for children; and increased opportunities for socialization for children. Nevertheless, respite care tends to be underutilized. Unavailability of competent, affordable care is the major problem. Caregivers find the hassles of training respite workers are not worth the benefits. Lack of trust and conflict with respite workers can increase stress rather than giving caregivers a break. In spite of needing the break, caregivers may have difficulty relinquishing control to others (Eaton, 2008). Some children fall between the cracks—requiring too low a level of care to qualify for respite, but too complex for a regular babysitter. Nurses can assist in a variety of ways. They can assess families' need for, use of, and problems with respite care and then respond appropriately. Caregivers may need to be encouraged to use respite care. Additionally, as professionals, nurses need to be active in increasing accessibility to respite care. This will include lobbying to secure more funding for respite care and helping to educate respite providers.

CRITICAL THINKING

Respite Care: What's in a Name?

A caregiver of three small children needs a break from child care responsibilities and hires a babysitter. Caregivers of a child with a chronic condition also need a break and arrange respite care. What are the implications of calling these services by different names?

Emotional and Cognitive Responses

Early research on childhood chronic conditions tended to focus on documenting the stress encountered by parents, especially mothers. More recently, the experience of fathers has been explored. While families with children with chronic conditions do not typically have more psychosocial problems than families with healthy children, there is evidence that many experience stress, social isolation, fatigue, and worries about the welfare of all family members. Caregivers also report the positive impact both the child with a chronic condition and caring for that child has on them and other family members (Coffey, 2006; Murphy, Christian, Caplin, & Young, 2006). Seriousness of disease does not tend to be predictive of the caregivers' experience.

Most caregivers effectively cope with the stressors of living with a child with a chronic condition and typically

REFLECTIVE THINKING

Caregiver Responsibilities

Imagine that you have just become the caregiver of a child with a severe disability. The child requires constant supervision, as she is dependent on a ventilator. How would your life change? How would your plans and dreams for the future change? What supports would you have available? What role might a nurse have in helping you adjust to the situation?

say they "just have to." They use a variety of coping strategies including: (1) information-seeking; (2) mastering skills and knowledge; (3) balancing "taking charge" and "letting go"; (4) social supports; (5) focusing on the positive and **downward comparisons** (assuming another's situation is worse than one's own); (6) brief breaks and relaxation; and (7) religion (Coffey, 2006; Murphy, Christian, Caplin, & Young, 2006; Wong & Heriot, 2008; Woodgate, Ateah, & Secco, 2008).

Adjustment to having a child with a chronic condition has been described as similar to the grief process, which includes the stages of shock and denial, anger, guilt, and finally acceptance. An alternative way of viewing the adjustment process is as one of **chronic (cyclic) sorrow**, a concept developed to explain the experience of parents with developmentally delayed children, and later applied to other chronic conditions. The notion is that the adjustment process and grief experience do not happen just once with a final resolution as suggested by the stage perspective. Instead, they reoccur at often predictable times and, perhaps with increasing intensity, during the child's life. Examples of those times include unmet or delayed developmental milestones, such as walking, learning to read, and getting a driver's license. Other problematic times are: (1) when younger siblings achieve expected milestones before the older sibling with a chronic condition; (2) at culturally defined celebrations and age-dependent rites-of-passage, such as reaching age 18 or 21 in mainstream U.S. culture, or age 13 in the Jewish culture; and (3) during exacerbation of symptoms. They may also occur at unexpected moments, triggered by thoughts about the future. In addition to grief, caregivers often experience heightened stress at these milestones. For instance, when the child first goes to school the caregiver may have safety concerns (Coffey, 2006). Caregivers have indicated that learning to cherish and celebrate their child's milestones, even if experienced differently from other children, is an important life strategy (Woodgate, Ateah, & Secco, 2008).

Nurses should assess the effectiveness of coping strategies used by caregivers and suggest additional strategies as necessary. Anticipatory guidance, based on knowledge of trigger events, and acknowledgment of the difficulties involved in caring for their child may also be beneficial to the caregivers. At the same time, maintaining a sense of hope and acknowledging the unique milestones of the child may be beneficial.

Day-to-Day Tasks of Living with a Chronic Condition

As part of the adjustment to caring for a child with a chronic condition, the family rearranges life schedules and routines to include long-term care of the child. In this process, there is an emphasis on continuous efforts to facilitate day-to-day normalization of life for the child and the family. **Normalization** is defined as cognitive and behavioral strategies used by a family of a child with a chronic condition in order to view it as normal. While the caregiver acknowledges the condition and its impact on the child and family, effort is made to define the situation as normal, to maintain important aspects of their pre-illness lifestyle, and to interact with others based on this perspective. They work to control the total situation—the disease and its impact on the child and family. Therefore, they both adjust their lifestyle to meet treatment regimens and adjust treatment regimens to fit into their lifestyle. Sometimes this can mistakenly be labeled as "noncompliance." As part of normalization, caregivers also may focus on positive aspects of their child and be labeled as "in denial." Efforts are made to continue usual involvement in family and outside activities for siblings and the child with a chronic condition.

Having a Chronic Condition in the Culture of a Healthy Society

Coming to terms with the realization that the child with a chronic condition is not going to be cured through the efforts of the professional is one of the most difficult aspects of the caregiver's role. Additionally, caregivers must deal with the responses and expectations of others. Caregivers of severely disabled children have indicated that health care professionals often treat their children with disrespect. They have suggested that professionals need to be sensitive to the humanity of all children.

Changing Interactional Patterns

The relationship of the parents of children with chronic conditions has received much attention. While early studies, based on deficit-orientation models, attempted to demonstrate negative consequences on their relationship, research has not typically supported this. Parents often describe their spouse as their strongest support. Nevertheless, the stress of caregiving as well as lack of time, different coping styles, and different approaches to parenting can lead parents to experience high stress (Waite-Jones & Madill, 2008b). Elevated stress in any relationship can lead to higher rates of separation and divorce.

Time issues, physical challenges, and stigmatizing and fearful responses can also result in caregivers feeling socially isolated from friends and extended family (Coffey, 2006; Yantzi, Rosenberg, & McKeever, 2006). Some have described this as "living in a world of our own" and as undermining hope (Woodgate, Ateah, & Secco, 2008).

Caregivers report that relationships with professionals, health care and educational, are both helpful and harmful. While professionals can be a source of support, often they are not. Negative comments by caregivers generally address professionals': (1) disregard for the caregivers' knowledge and interests; (2) interactions which are insensitive, uncaring, or undermining hope; or (3) inadequate information or skill. Health care professionals need to have a more collaborative interaction style which is based on mutual respect and is empowering to caregivers. Acknowledging caregivers' expertise, role, and concerns is a critical first step. Being more relational and validating caregivers' feelings is also helpful.

Potential Life Outcomes

While living with a child who has a chronic condition has many challenges, caregivers typically make sense of and find meaning in the situation. They often discover positive outcomes in their experiences of caring for a child with a chronic condition. For example, family relationships may be strengthened as a result of working together. As caregivers come into contact with other caregivers of children with chronic conditions, they become aware of situations that are worse than their own. This process of downward comparison enables them to view their own situation in a more favorable light. Networking with other caregivers also helps them to obtain information and to receive emotional support. Many caregivers find networking most effective at an individual, informal level rather than through support groups because caregiving responsibilities make formal support group attendance difficult. Internet contacts are also a potentially powerful resource for caregivers.

In addition to identifying the positive outcomes in the process of finding meaning and making sense of their situation, caregivers also identify the strains of caring for a child with a chronic condition. Caregivers of children with severe chronic conditions often ask questions such as "But when do I get on with *my* life?" For some families, the burden (financially, emotionally, physically, socially) is excessive and compromises individual and family integrity.

NURSING TIP

Caregiver-Professional Partnership

Discuss with caregivers strategies for developing effective partnerships with health care professionals such as:

- Make a list of questions to be asked and information to be provided prior to appointments.
- Ask for immediate clarification of any terminology, information, or technology with which you are unfamiliar.
- Know your rights in any given circumstance. Federal laws protect you and your child.
- Expect your expertise to be respected. As caregiver, you know your child and your family best. You know what has worked, what hasn't worked, and have insight into how new approaches might be integrated into your situation.
- In situations in which you feel uncomfortable or adversarial, take a support person (e.g., nurse, social worker, clergy, friend, representative from Protection and Advocacy). Discuss with the support person, prior to the situation, what your concerns are and what you hope to achieve.
- Directly express frustration and confront discounts of your expertise with statements such as, "When you [professional's problem behavior or communication], I feel like [you are discounting me as caregiver, you are discounting my knowledge]."

CRITICAL THINKING

Caregiver Assessment

Parents are scheduled to visit your clinic with their 2-year-old child who was recently diagnosed with cystic fibrosis. They also have a 4-year-old child. What areas or issues would you explore when assessing the caregivers in this situation? How would you phrase questions to address these assessment areas? Reflect on those questions. Will they empower and affirm the caregivers? Will they help you identify strengths as areas where growth or assistance might be needed?

THE SIBLING'S PERSPECTIVE

The perspectives of siblings of children with chronic conditions are increasingly being addressed in research and in practice. The assumption is that being the sibling of a child with a chronic condition has a profound impact on the well-sibling's emotional, psychological, and social development. Researchers have explored the sibling's knowledge about the chronic condition, age, gender, self-esteem, peer relationships, adjustment, attitudes, family socioeconomic status and interactions, and support systems. Current research shows that having a sibling with a chronic illness has both negative and positive consequences for the healthy sibling. Parent reports of the impact on the healthy sibling tend to be significantly more negative than the siblings' self-reports (Waite-Jones & Madill, 2008a).

Demands and Challenges

The healthy sibling must live with the emotional responses of the others in the home and usually receives less attention because of increased demands on the caregiver (Waite-Jones & Madill, 2008a). Research has shown that siblings often assume greater responsibilities for activities such as housework and caring for younger family members. Parents report placing greater expectations on the healthy siblings due to the demands they face in caring for the ill child. They often expect the healthy child to decrease time spent with peers or in after-school activities in order to accommodate the needs of the family (Branstetter, Domian, Williams, Graff, & Piamjariyakul, 2008).

Emotional and Cognitive Responses

Although siblings of children with chronic conditions experience many negative emotions, including ambivalence, resentment, anger, fear, and sadness, they often have a positive self-perception and speak positively of their chronically ill sibling and family (Bellin, Kovacs, & Sawin, 2008). Many siblings feel protective of their ill sibling and are empathetic to the challenges their siblings face. The caregiver's ability to tune into the sibling's attitudes and perceptions facilitates adjustments. Nurses can encourage caregiver awareness of the attitudes and experiences of the sibling of a child with a chronic condition.

Most caregivers feel that their children receive different amounts of attention, particularly when the child with the chronic condition experiences an exacerbation. Some caregivers report a positive change in the sibling's attitude when explanations are provided about the necessity of the attention or treatment for the child with the chronic condition (Branstetter et al., 2008). Siblings report a desire for more information, involvement, and support from their parents and health care providers (Batte, Watson, & Amess, 2006).

Day-to-Day Tasks of Living with a Chronic Condition

Siblings' schedules are often tied to the needs of the child with a chronic condition. The sibling may be required to accompany the caregiver and the child with a chronic condition to frequent therapy sessions or health care appointments. These visits and other caregiving activities may limit the sibling's participation in sports, school, or religious activities. Siblings of children with chronic illnesses often report participating in caring for their ill sibling. Children report participating in activities such as dressing their sibling, helping lift and transfer their sibling, and assisting with physical therapy. These well-siblings report feeling that they have more responsibilities than their peers and feeling that they are forced to mature earlier (Bellin et al., 2008).

> **NURSING TIP**
>
> **Helping Siblings Cope**
>
> **Encourage siblings of children with chronic conditions to participate in sibling support groups in which they can gain knowledge, share feelings and emotions, and find help in coping with the sibling's condition. Support groups are often available at city-based children's hospitals, but more need to be started in rural areas.**

Having a Chronic Condition in the Culture of a Healthy Society

Because of close identification between siblings, characteristics of the chronically ill child may be associated with the siblings. Therefore, the sibling may share some of the stigma faced by the ill child. Children are more likely to feel socially stigmatized if their sibling has an obvious physical disability. Well-siblings often report feeling that they and their families are seen as being "different" from other children and families. Many children and adolescents feel that they are being stared at or judged by strangers when they visit public places with their chronically ill siblings. These siblings report various peer responses, including pity and teasing, as well as feelings of exclusion and isolation (Bellin et al., 2008). Like the child with the chronic condition, the siblings may benefit from coaching and role-playing to explore ways to respond to peers. For example, the siblings of a child with cystic fibrosis who plays on a baseball team may be asked why his brother has a tube coming out of his nose or why he coughs so much. Coaching the siblings to provide simple explanations that the tube helps him breathe and the coughing is not contagious would be appropriate.

Changing Interactional Patterns

Siblings have identified being able to be involved in the child's care and experiencing an increased sense of closeness with other family members as positive changes, while the lack of attention from caregivers is considered a negative aspect. Children and parents report feelings of dysfunctional communication within the family. Children often are afraid to express their fears or other feelings and feel that their parents do not have enough time to listen (Batte et al., 2006). Parents suggest that because of their children's maturity and increased contact with adults that they are often more comfortable interacting with adults than with their peers (Branstetter et al., 2008).

Potential Life Outcomes

Potential life outcomes for siblings have seldom been researched. Siblings worry about the possible death of the brother or sister. In addition, they may worry about their own future if the brother or sister lives to adulthood but is unable to function independently as an adult. The siblings may be expected and groomed to assume the caregiver role at some point in the future when the present caregivers can no longer meet the needs of the child with the chronic condition. The anticipation and preparation for this role or the exploration of alternative options have a significant effect on the well-siblings' life experiences.

CULTURAL ISSUES

Health care workers seek to provide culturally sensitive and culturally appropriate care to those with chronic illness and their families. With limited research-based knowledge regarding the interactions between ethnicity, culture, and illness, particularly chronic illness, stereotypes prevail. In addition to inhibiting communication between people of different cultures, stereotypes prevent intra-group differences from being taken into account. The global nature of health care and the multiethnic, multicultural composition of people in the United States requires that sensitivity be embraced in all health care interactions. Communication among the chronically ill child, the child's caregivers, and the health care professional regarding key aspects of care may be compromised by linguistic and cultural barriers. In addition, caregivers do not have the power base from which to access available services for their child, and the problem can be compounded if the family is part of a minority group.

One advantage of health-oriented models is intercultural applicability. In this model, the child, caregiver, and professional are seen as partners in identifying and proposing solutions to problems. The knowledge and expertise of each partner and an attitude of mutual respect are assumed. This foundation promotes an increased sensitivity to the cultural aspects of care and views the child in context of the family. By combining a partnership approach and sensitivity to the culture, health care professionals and caregivers are able to propose solutions that conform to the value system of the family. If proposed solutions do not conform to the value system or culture of the family, they are not likely to be followed.

One caution must be mentioned in utilizing the health-oriented model interculturally. For some cultures, the professional is viewed as the expert and the client is viewed as the passive recipient. In this situation, caregivers could perceive requests for their input as evidence that the professional lacks knowledge. Culturally sensitive role negotiations are necessary for an ongoing effective relationship.

Height and weight charts are used in health care settings to provide objective measurements of appropriate physical growth in children. The measurements in these charts are based on "normal" growth parameters for mainstream U.S. children. However, children from other backgrounds may be larger or smaller than the parameters designated on these growth charts. Children with chronic conditions are often smaller than their age mates. When a child with a chronic condition is also part of an ethnic group that is typically of short stature, the child may be deemed ever

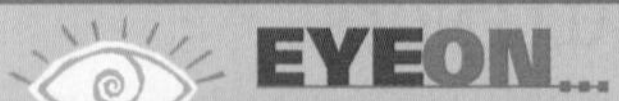

Differences in Developmental Expectations Across Cultures

In addition to being sensitive to the cultural values of the caregivers, the professional should take into account the differences in normal developmental or age-appropriate expectations between cultures. For example, in some cultures, the child is carried until approximately the age of 1 year. At that point, there is a celebration, a foot-touching-the-ground ceremony. Without considering cultural perspectives, a professional could interpret consistently carrying around an 11-month-old child as "babying" the child. If the child has a chronic condition, such as cystic fibrosis, the caregiver may be labeled as overprotective. However, recommendations to put the child down would not make sense to these caregivers.

further outside the "normals." The health care professional may advise the caregivers that the child is extremely small, when in reality, the individual may be only slightly smaller than age mates of the same ethnic heritage. Interpreting growth charts in light of the parents' stature will help minimize this problem.

In order to effectively care for people from other cultures, professionals need to examine their own ethnocentrism, particularly as this relates to health and illness. **Ethnocentrism** is the tendency for all individuals and cultures to believe their values are the best and the most correct. Ethnocentrism prevents professionals from learning from people of other cultures or perhaps even from seeing that other cultures have anything worth learning. In reality, professionals could learn a great deal about ways of conceptualizing illness and identifying and solving problems as they work with people from other cultures. For example, health care professionals in the United States are now beginning to shift from a deficit orientation to a health orientation. This perspective has been present in some other cultures for a long time. An openness to learn from children with chronic conditions and their caregivers, particularly those from other cultures, will facilitate effective care.

SOCIETAL ISSUES

Children with chronic conditions are often viewed in terms of their cost to society. This is not totally without basis. Total health care costs for children with chronic illnesses are approximately three times the health care costs of other children. The use of nonphysician health professionals, home health services, medication prescriptions, and inpatient hospitalization is five times higher in children with chronic illnesses than those without (Newacheck & Kim, 2005). This does not include the cost of special services at school, cost of special equipment, loss of employment for caregivers, or intangible costs to families.

In spite of the many resources used by children with chronic conditions, their level of care and access to health care are often inadequate and frequently distributed unevenly throughout society. Children with chronic conditions are more likely to be behind on immunizations and basic health screenings than other children because of illness, hospitalization, or relative lack of importance. The emergence of managed care has had a further impact on accessibility and quality of care for children with chronic conditions. There is a potential for positive effects, such as more comprehensive, coordinated, community-based care with an emphasis on prevention. However, there is also a potential for negative effects, such as discontinued relationships with current providers, limited access to specialty providers, and financial incentives to limit the use of expensive services (Davidoff, Hill, Courtot, & Adams, 2008). Monitoring is necessary to validate these potential effects.

Access to health care is a major problem for low-income children and this problem is even greater if the child has a chronic condition. While most of the children with chronic conditions were insured, approximately one-third of the insured families report that the insurance does not adequately meet their child's needs. This is often because the insurance does not have the appropriate benefits to meet their child's needs, the charges are unreasonable, and they do not have access to specialty providers (U.S. Department of Health and Human Services, 2008). There are a higher proportion of children with disabilities living in rural poverty than those in urban areas or those not living in poverty. If the child living in a rural community has a severe disability, the situation is critically complicated because of limited access to specialty care. Universal access to comprehensive health care is needed to provide adequate care to children with chronic conditions and to prevent the occurrence of many conditions.

Caring for children with chronic conditions is expensive; for those with severe, chronic conditions, the costs can be staggering. In light of recent trends in health care management, more children with severe, chronic conditions are being cared for at home rather than in institutions. Although this arrangement is less expensive, society must consider the potential harm being done to families if caring for the child at home is the only option available to them. There are few available institutional placements for children with severe disabilities. Besides having a long waiting list or being of questionable quality, the facility may be located at a great distance from the family's home. This creates a burden for the family because it becomes difficult for them to remain involved in the child's life. Society must decide if decisions about home versus institutional placement of children with severe, chronic conditions will be exclusively driven by economic issues. As family and child advocates, nurses have a major role in the development of policies that provide for adequate resources for these families.

NURSING MANAGEMENT OF CHILDREN WITH CHRONIC CONDITIONS

Children with chronic conditions and their caregivers have frequent, ongoing contacts with health care professionals, especially nurses. Nursing care may take place in an acute care setting, a clinic, school, home, or other community facility. Because of the chronic nature of the child's condition, communication and collaboration between professionals in all settings and with the child and caregiver are crucial to effective nursing care.

DEMANDS AND CHALLENGES

Nurses, caregivers, and children tend to perceive the experience of living with childhood chronic conditions differently. Nurses often focus on the illness and the technical skills required to manage the illness. They tend to dwell on deficits and negative aspects of the situation. While knowledge of potential problems a caregiver may encounter is useful, nurses must realize that each family's experience with chronic conditions is unique. Nursing assessment should include identifying strengths and areas for growth from the caregivers' perspectives. Affirming and building on the caregivers' strengths is an effective strategy in providing information and in collaboratively planning for the child's care. Nurses can assist the family in dealing with the demands and challenges of caring for a chronically ill child by including the family in decision making, helping to maintain communication between the family and health care providers, and providing information about treatments, treatment options, and treatment programs and services (Nolan, Orlando, & Liptak, 2007).

Nurses often teach the child and caregivers about the chronic condition and its potential trajectory. Before beginning to teach the child and caregivers, the nurse needs to thoroughly assess the family's current level of knowledge, skills, and resources. The family may have cared for the child for a number of years and may know more than the nurse about these areas. In this situation, the nurse can acquire valuable information from the family.

If the condition has been recently diagnosed, the family needs information about the condition in order to provide appropriate care, to decrease uncertainty, and to hold realistic expectations for the child. They may also need to acquire complex skills and knowledge about how to access resources. Although the information is needed, it may overwhelm the family. Nurses need to assess the readiness of caregivers to learn and will need to adjust the pace and the amount of information based on that assessment. In addition, nurses should be sensitive to the responses of caregivers to the teaching and to assess their understanding of the information by asking appropriate questions or by having them demonstrate a newly acquired skill.

RESEARCH Highlight

Asthma Care of Children in Clinical Practice: Do Parents Report Receiving Appropriate Education?

STUDY PURPOSE

To document parent perceptions of asthma education received from their child's health care provider.

METHOD

The study was part of a larger cross-sectional study that involved a one-time, semi-structured home interview. The sample included 228 parents of children with asthma and nearly half of the families represented poor and minority populations. The measures used included a structured questionnaire that used NAEPP criteria to evaluate asthma severity and an interviewer-administered parent report of asthma education received from the health care provider (PRAER) questionnaire.

FINDINGS

Parents reported an overall score of 61% for items fully discussed; therefore, approximately 40% of the items considered critical to asthma management had not been fully discussed with the family. Items most frequently discussed were those related to acute symptoms, such as how to use a metered dose inhaler, how to manage an asthma attack, and advice regarding the effects of smoking. The items discussed with the least frequency were those related to ongoing management and care planning, including discussing the child's feelings, talking about goals in management, and providing written guidelines and plans. The items that were discussed less than 50% of the time included those items that are associated with a health care provider/parent partnership that develops through open communication.

IMPLICATIONS

Nursing education provided to parents and families should focus on managing the ongoing aspects of chronic illness, as well as the acute symptoms. Pediatric nurses can provide education and develop partnerships with families that involve open communication in order to improve child and family adherence and satisfaction with care.

REFERENCE

McMullen, A., Yoos, H. L, Anson, E., Kitzmann, H., Halterman, J. S., & Arcoleo, K. S. (2007). Asthma care of children in clinical practice: Do parents report receiving appropriate education? *Pediatric Nursing*, *33*(1), 37–44.

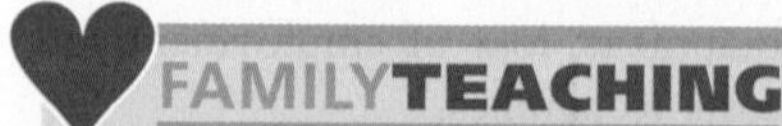

Caring for the Family of a Child with a Chronic Condition

HOME

- Supply the family with information about the child's chronic condition, its trajectory, and its therapies.
- Provide educational sessions and materials for caregivers to learn skills needed to provide optimum care.
- Educate the family about the normalcy of feelings of denial, anger, grief, and so forth, related to having a child with a chronic condition.
- Assist caregivers to talk with siblings about the child's condition and to assess their needs and concerns. Make a referral to groups for siblings with children who have a similar condition.
- Arrange frequent care conferences with the caregivers and the health care team. Encourage caregivers to take an active role in discussions about their child's condition and care.
- Encourage caregivers to identify support systems (i.e., other family members, friends, clergy, and community support groups).
- Encourage interaction with other families who have a child with a similar chronic condition.
- Refer family to social services for respite care, financial assistance.

SCHOOL

- Communicate with school personnel about the child's functional potential and needed modifications in the child's activities.
- Communicate to teachers when homebound or hospital education is needed.
- Promote the child's participation in school and after-school social activities.
- Reinforce with caregivers the importance of regular communication with the school nurse.
- Teach school personnel about the use and maintenance of medical or adaptive equipment to be used by the child.

COMMUNITY

- Involve the family in social and recreational activities sponsored by disease-related organizations.
- Provide a referral to a visiting nurse or a home care nurse for assistance in complex care.
- Make a referral to a community health nurse to provide reinforcement of teaching conducted in acute care settings.

EMOTIONAL AND COGNITIVE RESPONSES

In working with families, nurses need to be careful not to assume that: (1) emotional or psychosocial problems exist for the child, the caregivers, or the siblings just because a child in the home has a chronic condition; (2) the nurse's and the family's perceptions of what constitutes a problem are the same; and (3) the problems encountered by the child, caregiver, or siblings are fewer or less significant because the condition is less visible or involves fewer functional impairments. By consciously decreasing assumptions and by listening to and understanding the family's perspectives, nurses can facilitate coping for the child and family.

Initially and periodically, nurses need to assess the family's coping and psychosocial needs. This assessment should include the nurse's observations of coping strategies, family interactions, and attitudes, as well as their responses to direct questions. Nurses should ask specifically about caregiver burden, their perceptions of the efficacy of coping strategies, their sense of control or mastery of the situation, and problems encountered. Nurses should provide support through active listening and referrals to community agencies and support groups (Hallstrom & Elander, 2007). Families also need to know that negative emotions are normal and should be expressed in appropriate ways rather than suppressed. Caregivers should be taught to encourage the child with the chronic condition and siblings to express emotions. Support groups provide an avenue for the expression of thoughts and feelings and can be helpful for the entire family.

DAY-TO-DAY TASKS OF LIVING WITH A CHRONIC CONDITION

Many of the day-to-day tasks include efforts at normalization in physical and emotional development and in daily activities. Nurses can monitor the child's developmental progress and use anticipatory guidance in making suggestions for facilitating development. For example, the nurse can encourage the caregivers of a toddler to find creative play activities that encourage exploration of the environment, which in turn facilitates independence in the child. For adolescents, the nurse can encourage the development of relationships with peers of both genders. Sexuality develops in children with chronic conditions just as it does in children without those conditions. Nevertheless, children with chronic conditions are often treated as asexual and also know less about sexuality-related topics than other children do. This aspect of development needs to be considered when working with children with chronic conditions. The child and family need information and opportunities to discuss puberty, reproduction capacity, safe sex practices, and intimate relationships. Key times for explaining these topics include after diagnosis, prepubescence, mid-puberty, and prior to transfer to the adult health care system.

Nurses can also play a role in normalizing day-to-day living by working with the family in getting the child into an appropriate school placement. The nurse can educate teachers and other personnel in order to facilitate the child's reentry into school. Depending on the situation, the child's peers may also be prepared for the child's placement or return to school. There are many barriers that affect the chronically ill child's ability to attend school, including a lack of resources for health care within the school, lack of clarity of school policies, lack of health education for school staff, and poor systems of communication between families, health care providers, and educators (Wales & Crisp, 2007). The Healthy Learner Model provides a bridge between the medical setting, home setting, and the school that fosters both the health status and academic success of children with chronic conditions. This model combines the elements of leadership, evidence-based practice, capacity building, a resource nurse, the healthy learner (a chronically ill child well enough to attend school), partnerships with families, and partnerships with health care providers. This model has been shown to be effective in the community-based management of asthma, diabetes, life-threatening allergies, and mental health (Erickson, Splett, Mullett, & Heiman, 2006).

The day-to-day tasks of living with a chronic condition most often take place in the child's home where the child and caregivers have developed routines for providing daily

NURSING TIP

Developing Partnerships

Nurses can use the interview time to develop the parent-provider partnership by acknowledging the parents' expertise in caring for their child and seeking their opinions in developing the plan of care.

CRITICAL THINKING

Minimizing the Effects of Hospitalization

You are the nurse admitting a 6-year-old child who has cerebral palsy. While taking the nursing history her mom describes to you her regular home regimen, including the physical therapy schedule and the times and methods that she uses for giving medications and gavage feedings. You realize that the home schedule varies greatly from the standard schedule used by the physicians and nurses on your unit. How will this affect your plan of care? How will you incorporate the family's home routine into your care plan?

care. However, when the child is hospitalized, these routines are frequently interrupted and may cause frustration for everyone. Nurses need to help facilitate the implementation of these day-to-day routines in the acute care setting.

HAVING A CHRONIC CONDITION IN THE CULTURE OF A HEALTHY SOCIETY

One way that nurses can facilitate a positive self-concept in a child with a chronic condition is to promote normalcy by emphasizing what the child can do and encouraging involvement in age and developmentally appropriate tasks. Nurses may be involved in the decisions as to when and how the caregiver can begin to shift the responsibility for care to the child. Observations by the nurse and the caregiver's opinions about the child's readiness to assume responsibility for care are crucial to a successful transition.

As the child and family interact with others, they may be subject to discrimination, stares, and inappropriate questions and advice. The child may encounter mocking from other children. Assessment should periodically include questions about the child's and family's experiences as they interact with others. Not all situations can be prevented; however, the nurse, the child, and the caregiver will need to develop acceptable ways to respond to negative responses from others. Examples of coping strategies include getting involved in support groups of other children with similar conditions, communicating directly and providing information about the condition and its limitations, ignoring responses of others, and emphasizing capabilities of the child.

CHANGING INTERACTIONAL PATTERNS

In the process of caring for a child with a chronic condition, caregivers and sometimes siblings redefine their roles. For the caregiver of a child with a newly diagnosed chronic condition, the nurse may use anticipatory guidance in facilitating role transition. Periodic, ongoing assessment of family interaction patterns will be necessary, particularly as the child and the family go through times of change such as the addition of a family member or the beginning of school. The nurse can listen and suggest ways to reframe role expectations or to make transitions.

Interactions with professionals also change as caregivers become more knowledgeable about the effects of the condition on the child, more competent in working with the child, and more confident in their abilities to serve as an advocate. Nurses should be aware that the child's care can best be customized and provided when nurses, parents, and children work in cooperation with each other. Parents describe good communication as both receiving the information they need from staff, as well as the staff recognizing that the parents are the experts concerning their child's care and asking for their opinions and knowledge (Hallstrom & Elander, 2007). For the nurse, viewing the caregiver as a partner may reemphasize the importance of listening intently to others' perspectives and suggestions, being willing to learn as well as teach, being sensitive to cultural differences, and being flexible and willing to try different approaches. These attitudes are crucial to an effective partnership with the caregiver and the child.

Transitioning from pediatric health care providers to adult health care providers can be a difficult process for many adolescents with chronic illness. These adolescents are not only transitioning care providers and frequently insurance sources, but they are also transitioning into adulthood and learning to take more responsibility for themselves. In a recent survey, less than half of youth with special health care needs met core performance outcomes for transition. Those who were African-American, Hispanic, lower income, and having more serious health needs were less likely to have their transition needs met (Lotstein et al., 2009). Nurses can help ease this transition by assessing children for individual readiness and maturity and preparing children early. The nurse can

IN THE REAL WORLD

I am a school nurse at an elementary school. We have several students who have chronic conditions. In September, a new child was enrolled in a second grade class. Rory suffers from seizures at least one to two times a day. During the second week of school, Rory had a seizure. The students—some with looks of fear, horror, and puzzlement—watched as the aides quickly took measures so Rory would not injure himself. When the seizure was over and the room settled down, the children had many questions regarding what had happened. Rory's parents, Rory, myself, and the second grade teacher decided to meet with the students and discuss seizures, why they happen, and what to do when they happen.

The discussion took place the very next day. The students were very inquisitive as we provided an explanation. They seemed to have absorbed the information quite quickly. They felt comfortable with information and the events that will take place when Rory has a seizure.

The next time Rory had a seizure the students knew to clear the area of items that he may injure himself with while the teacher and aides placed him on his side. After the seizure was over, the students asked Rory how he was and then resumed their normal activities. Rory felt better emotionally that his classmates knew about his condition and that he was still needed and wanted as a friend without a moment's hesitation.

help plan the transition and serve as a liaison between the pediatric and adult services. Familiar nurses are a good source of support for adolescents during this transition (Baines, 2009).

POTENTIAL LIFE OUTCOMES

Nurses have the privilege of working closely with caregivers and children as they struggle to make sense of their situations, to adjust to the child's illness, and to maintain some sort of normalcy for these families. Nurses will be involved with the families in times of encouragement and optimism, in times of discouragement and grief, and in the struggle to make sense of the situation in the context of their lives. This provides opportunities for nurses to create new meanings for themselves as they reflect on their own lives.

KEY CONCEPTS

- Childhood chronic conditions include a variety of physical, emotional, and cognitive problems that last for at least three months and may prevent the child from accomplishing age-appropriate physical, intellectual, psychological, and sociocultural developmental functions. The conditions may range in severity from mild to severe.
- Dimensions of childhood chronic conditions include nature of onset, trajectory of the condition, effects on appearance, effects on daily functioning, effects on behavior and ability to relate to others, and the kind and amount of care required.
- A chronic condition requires the child, siblings, and caregivers to adjust to the changes in roles and responsibilities, to learn new skills, to deal with the uncertainty regarding the impact of the condition, and to attempt to normalize life.
- The child's age and developmental level affect the coping strategies used by the child with a chronic illness.
- The adaptive tasks that have been identified for caregivers include: accepting the condition, managing the condition, meeting the child's developmental needs, meeting the developmental needs of other family members, coping with stress and crisis, assisting family members to manage feelings, educating others about the condition, and establishing a support system.
- Meeting the needs of a child with a chronic condition may lead to caregiver burden, a sense of being overwhelmed with the responsibilities at hand. This can be exacerbated by chronic fatigue, a constant state of vigilance, and the demands of caregiving.
- The psychosocial well-being and information needs of well-siblings need to be considered in planning care.
- Nurses play a major role in listening, mutual problem identification and solving, and teaching, thereby empowering the child and the family and helping them achieve a sense of control.

REVIEW ACTIVITIES

1. Discuss the potential effects of the visibility of a chronic condition on the child, the family, and others who come into contact with the child.
2. Describe the implications of lifelong dependency for a child with a chronic condition on the child, siblings, and caregivers.
3. The caregivers of a child with a newly diagnosed chronic condition meet with a nurse to discuss the care of their child. Describe the approach that would be used if the nurse followed the deficit-orientation model of chronic conditions. Describe the approach that would be used if the nurse followed a health-orientation model of chronic conditions.
4. Give an example of the way in which the developmental level will affect a child's response to having a chronic condition. How might a chronic condition affect a child's development?
5. Discuss the impact of federal laws on the educational rights of children with chronic conditions.
6. Describe some of the challenges faced by caregivers of children with chronic conditions.
7. Describe the impact of managed care on the care received by children with chronic conditions.
8. What would be an appropriate response for the nurse when a caregiver tells a sibling of a child with a chronic condition never to get angry with the child?

STUDY QUESTIONS

1. A nurse is caring for a 12-year-old child who has cerebral palsy. While taking her history and physical the nurse focuses on questions which identify how the child views her chronic illness and how this has affected her identity and ability to perform activities of daily living. This nurse is practicing within which of the following models?
   a. Deficit-orientation model
   b. Health-orientation model
   c. Ordinary model
   d. Critical-orientation model
2. You are the nurse who is providing discharge teaching for a 15-year-old adolescent who has spina bifida. You are aware that adolescents with chronic illnesses favor flexibility in learning to self-manage their illness. Which of the following is the best way to foster self-management behaviors in this adolescent client?
   a. Encourage him to attend care planning conferences where he can provide input related to his treatment regimen.
   b. Inform him of the necessity of following the prescribed treatment regimen exactly as it is ordered.
   c. Tell him that if he is noncompliant his mother will resume responsibility for his care.
   d. Provide him with only simple, necessary information about his treatments so that he is not overwhelmed.
3. The mother of a chronically ill child tells the nurse that she is physically, emotionally, and mentally exhausted and doesn't feel like she can continue to provide the constant 24-hour-per-day care that her child requires. The *best* response by the nurse would be:
   a. "It sounds like you probably need to talk to someone about your concerns."
   b. "You don't have a choice when it comes to caring for your child so you will have to find a way to deal with it."
   c. "You need to develop better time-management skills so that you will have more time to rest."
   d. "I believe that you would benefit from respite care. I can give you more information on local respite care providers."
4. You are the nurse caring for the family of an 8-year-old child who was diagnosed with type 1 diabetes mellitus four days ago. You notice that during all of the teaching sessions the parents are actively involved but the 4-year-old sibling sits in the corner of the room and appears quiet, scared, and withdrawn. The most appropriate action would be which of the following?
   a. Ask the child why he does not want to learn about his brother's diabetes.
   b. Engage the sibling in the teaching by explaining what you are doing directly to him and asking him if he has any questions.
   c. Ignore the sibling because he is too young to understand what is happening to his brother.
   d. Encourage one of the parents to take the sibling into the playroom during teaching sessions so that he will not be scared.
5. The 13-year-old sibling of a chronically ill child expresses feelings of embarrassment and isolation in relation to her sibling's visible deformities. Appropriate actions by the nurse would include all but which of the following?
   a. Refer the child to a sibling support group.
   b. Work with the child to brainstorm ways to respond to her peers' stares and comments.
   c. Ensure the child that her feelings are normal.
   d. Tell the child that it will be easier to deal with when she gets older.
6. Which of the following laws requires institutions to make reasonable accommodations for individuals with disabilities and prohibits discrimination based on the individual's disability?
   a. Education for All Handicapped Children Act of 1975
   b. Individuals with Disabilities Education Act
   c. Americans with Disabilities Act of 1990
   d. No Child Left Behind Act
7. A condition which is less visible to others resulting in ambiguity about whether an individual is different from or like others is referred to as which of the following?
   a. Marginality
   b. Uncertainty
   c. Disability
   d. Handicap
8. Which of the following statements about children with chronic illnesses is NOT true?
   a. Children with chronic illness have the same developmental tasks as any other child.
   b. Children with chronic illness are more likely to have negative self-esteem and to remain dependent on their parents.
   c. Children with chronic illness attempt to remain "normal" by emphasizing their abilities and decreasing the role illness plays in their life.
   d. Children with a chronic illness are more likely to experience academic problems than their peers.

9. Many parents of children with a chronic illness will experience recurring periods of grief and stress at predictable times throughout their child's life, such as when the child does not meet a developmental milestone or during an exacerbation of symptoms. This is often referred to as which of the following?
   a. Caregiver burden
   b. Trajectory of illness
   c. Chronic (cyclic) sorrow
   d. Normalization

10. Nursing management of a child with a chronic illness and his or her family should include which of the following?
   a. Focusing on the technical skills required to treat the illness
   b. Making important medical decisions for the child and family whenever possible
   c. Providing education that is focused on the acute aspects of illness exacerbations
   d. Recognizing the child and family's expertise by asking questions and seeking their opinions

REFERENCES

Admi, H. (1996). Growing up with a chronic health condition: A model of an ordinary lifestyle. *Qualitative Health Research, 6*(2), 163–183.

Admi, H., & Shaham, B. (2007). Living with epilepsy: Ordinary people coping with extraordinary situations. *Qualitative Health Research, 17*(9), 1178–1187.

Badlan, K. (2006). Young people living with cystic fibrosis: An insight into their subjective experience. *Health and Social Care in the Community, 14*, 264–270.

Baines, J. M. (2009). Promoting better care: Transition from child to adult services. *Nursing Standard, 23*(19), 35–51.

Batte, S., Watson, A. R., & Amess, K. (2006). The effects of chronic renal failure on siblings. *Pediatric Nephrology, 21*, 246–250.

Bellin, M., Kovacs, P. J., & Sawin, K. J. (2008). Risk and protective influences in the lives of siblings of youths with spina bifida. *Health & Social Work, 33*(3), 199–209.

Boyles, C., Bailey, P., & Mossey, S. (2008). Representations of disability in nursing and healthcare literature: An integrative review. *Journal of Advanced Nursing, 62*, 428–437.

Branstetter, J. E., Domian, E. W., Williams, P. D., Graff, J. C., & Piamjariyakul, U. (2008). Communication themes in families of children with chronic conditions. *Issues in Comprehensive Pediatric Nursing, 31*, 171–184.

Burton, P., Lethbridge, L., & Phipps, S. (2008). Children with disabilities and chronic conditions and longer-term parental health. *Journal of Socio-Economics, 37*, 1168–1186.

Carpentier, M., Mullins, L., Wagner, J., Wolfe-Christensen, C., & Chaney, J. (2008). Examination of the cognitive diathesis-stress conceptualization of the hopelessness theory of depression in children with chronic illness: The moderating influence of illness uncertainty. *Children's Healthcare, 36*, 181–196.

Cashin, G., Small, S., & Solberg, S. (2008). The lived experience of fathers who have children with asthma: A phenomenological study. *Journal of Pediatric Nursing, 23*, 372–385.

Coffey, J. (2006). Parenting a child with chronic illness: A metasynthesis. *Pediatric Nursing, 32*, 51–59.

Davidoff, A., Hill, I., Courtot, B., & Adams, E. (2008). Are there differential effects of managed care on publicly insured children with chronic health conditions? *Medical Care Research and Review, 65*(3), 356–372.

Dluhy, N. M. (1995). Mapping knowledge in chronic illness. *Journal of Advanced Nursing, 21*, 1051–1058.

Eaton, N. (2008). "I don't know how we coped before": A study of respite care for children in the home and hospice. *Journal of Clinical Nursing, 17*, 3196–3204.

Erickson, C. D., Splett, P. L., Mullett, S. S., & Heiman, M. B. (2006). The healthy learner model for student chronic condition management – Part 1. *Journal of School Nursing, 22*(6), 310–318.

Guell, C. (2007). Painful childhood: Children living with juvenile arthritis. *Qualitative Health Research, 17*, 884–892.

Hallstrom, I., & Elander, G. (2007). Families' needs when a child is long-term ill: A literature review with reference to nursing research. *International Journal of Nursing Practice, 13*, 193–200.

Holm, K., Patterson, J., Rueter, M., & Wamboldt, F. (2008). Impact of uncertainty associated with a child's chronic health condition on parents' health. *Families, Systems and Health, 26*, 282–295.

Kirk, S. (2008). Transitions in the lives of young people with complex healthcare needs. *Child: Care, Health and Development, 34*, 567–575.

Kuhlthau, K., Hill, K., Fluet, C., Meara, E., & Yucel, R. (2008). Correlates of therapy use and expenditures in children in the United States. *Developmental Neurorehabilitation, 11*(20), 115–123.

Lotstein, D., Ghandour, R., Cash, A., McGuire, E., Strickland, B., & Newacheck, P. (2009). Planning for health care transitions: Results from the 2005–2006 National Survey of Children with Special Health Care Needs. *Pediatrics, 123*, e145–e152.

MacDonald, H. & Callery, P. (2007). Parenting children requiring complex care: A journey through time. *Child: Care, Health and Development, 34*, 207–213.

McAnarney, E., Pless, I., Satterwhite, B., & Friedman, S. (1974). Psychological problems of children with chronic juvenile arthritis. *Pediatrics, 53*(4), 523–527.

McMullen, A., Yoos, H. L., Anson, E., Kitzman, H., Halterman, J. S., & Arcoleo, K. S. (2007). Asthma care of children in clinical practice: Do parents report receiving appropriate education? *Pediatric Nursing, 33*(1), 37–44.

Murphy, N., Christian, B., Caplin, D., & Young, P. (2006). The health of caregivers for children with disabilities. *Child: Care, Health and Development, 33*, 180–187.

Newacheck, P. W., & Kim, S. E. (2005). A national profile of health care utilization and expenditures for children with special health care needs. *Archives of Pediatrics and Adolescent Medicine, 159*, 10–17.

Nolan, K., Orlando, M., & Liptak, G. (2007). Care coordination services for children with special health care needs: Are we family-centered yet? *Families, Systems & Health: The Journal of Collaborative Family HealthCare, 25*(3), 293–306.

Perrin, J., Bloom, S., & Gortmaker, S. (2007). The increase of childhood chronic conditions in the United States. *Journal of the American Medical Association, 297*, 2755–2759.

Protudjer, J., Kozyrskyj, A., Becker, A., & Marchessault, G. (2009). Normalization strategies of children with asthma. *Qualitative Health Research, 19*, 94–104.

Rodriguez, N., & Patterson, J. (2007). Impact of severity of a child's chronic condition on the functioning of two-parent families. *Journal of Pediatric Psychology, 32*(4), 417–426.

Sawyer, S., Drew, S., Yeo, M., & Britto, M. (2007). Adolescents with a chronic condition: Challenges living, challenges treating. *The Lancet, 369*, 1481–1489.

Smith, F., Taylor, K., Newbould, J., & Keady, S. (2008). Medicines for chronic illness at school: Experiences and concerns of young people and their parents. *Journal of Clinical Pharmacy and Therapeutics, 33*, 537–544.

Taylor, R., Gibson, F., & Franck, L. (2008). The experience of living with a chronic illness during adolescence: A critical review of the literature. *Journal of Clinical Nursing, 17*, 3083–3091.

U.S. Department of Health and Human Resources. (2008). *The national survey of children with special health care needs chartbook 2005–2006.* Retrieved January 13, 2008, from http://mchb.hrsa.gov/cshcn05/.

van der Lee, J., Mokkink, L., Grootenhuis, M., Heymans, H., & Offringa, M. (2007). Definitions and measurement of chronic health conditions in childhood: A systematic review. *Journal of the American Medical Association, 297*(24), 2741–2751.

Van Staa, A., Jedeloo, S., Latour, J., & Trappenburg, M. (2008). A normal life with an unhealthy body: Self-identity in adolescents growing up with chronic illness. *Pediatrics, 121*(S2), S103.

Waite-Jones, J., & Madill, A. (2008a). Amplified ambivalence: Having a sibling with juvenile idiopathic arthritis. *Psychology and Health, 23*(4), 477–492.

Waite-Jones, J., & Madill, A. (2008b). Concealed concern: Fathers' experiences of having a child with juvenile idiopathic arthritis. *Psychology and Health, 23*(4), 585–601.

Wales, S., & Crisp, J. (2007). The views of nurses on adherence in school-aged children with a chronic illness. *Neonatal, Pediatric, and Child Health Nursing, 10*(2), 5–10.

Walker, J., Winkelstein, M., Land, C., Lewis-Boyer, L., Quartey, R., Pham, L., & Butz, A. (2008). Factors that influence quality of life in rural children with asthma and their parents. *Journal of Pediatric Health Care, 22*, 343–350.

Waters, A. (2008). An ethnography of a children's renal unit: Experiences of children and young people with long-term renal illness. *Journal of Clinical Nursing, 17*, 3103–3114.

Woodgate, R., Ateah, C., & Secco, L. (2008). Living in a world of our own: The experience of parents who have a child with autism. *Qualitative Health Research, 18*, 1075–1083.

Wong, M., & Heriot, S. (2008). Parents of children with cystic fibrosis: How they hope, cope, and despair, *Child: Care, Health and Development, 34*, 344–354.

Yantzi, N., Rosenberg, M., & McKeever, P. (2006). Getting out of the house: The challenges mothers face when their children have long-term care needs. *Health and Social Care in the Community, 15*, 45–55.

SUGGESTED READINGS

Center for Disability Information and Referral (http://www.iidc.indiana.edu/CEDIR/). Kid's Corner page has summaries of books and other resources with interactive sections for children with special health care needs.

Meyer, D., & Vadasy, P. (2007). *Sibshops: Workshops for siblings of children with special needs.* Baltimore: Paul H. Brookes Publishing.

Rissman, R. (2009). *Disabilities and differences series.* Chicago: Heinemann Library.

Wolvier, R. (2008). *Alphabet kids—From ADD to Zellweger Syndrome: A guide to developmental, neurobiological and psychological disorders for parents and professional.* London: Jessica Kingsley Publisher.

RESOURCES

Refer to the online student StudyWARE for Potts & Mandleco at http://www.CengageBrain.com for additional content and study aids.

Organizations and Websites

Organization: **Access to Respite Care Help (ARCH)**

Description: The mission of the ARCH National Respite Network is to assist and promote the development of quality respite and crisis care programs; to help families locate respite and crisis care services in their communities; and to serve as a strong voice for respite in all forums. The website offers readers access to fact sheets, products, memberships, and respite locators.

Website/Resource: http://www.archrespite.org

Organization: **American Association of People with Disabilities (AAPD)**

Description: The American Association of People with Disabilities (AAPD), the country's largest cross-disability membership organization, organizes the disability community to be a powerful voice for change—politically, economically, and socially. The website offers users information regarding programs, membership, and advocacy.

Website/Resource: http://www.aapd.com

Organization: **Center for Disability Information and Referral**

Description: This website has a lending library of videos and books, a blog, and other resources on disability. While primarily intended for Indiana residents, it is still a good resource for information.

Website/Resource: http://www.iidc.indiana.edu/CEDIR

Organization: **Children with Special Needs**

Description: Sponsored by the Seattle Children's Hospital, this website offers parents information about children with special needs. The website also offers additional information regarding clinics, programs, and helpful classes.

Website/Resource: http://kidshealth.org

Organization: **Family Village: Global Community of Disability-Related Resources**

Description: The Family Village is a global community that integrates information, resources, and communication opportunities on the Internet for persons with cognitive and other disabilities, for their families, and for those that provide them services and support. The website provides links to disability-related resources including disease-specific information, chat rooms, educational information, recreational opportunities, and spiritual resources.

Website/Resource: http://www.familyvillage.wisc.edu

Organization: **Federation for Children with Special Needs**

Description: The Federation for Children with Special Needs provides information, support, and assistance to parents of children with disabilities, their professional partners, and their communities. The website provides users with valuable information regarding health care, early childhood, education, and special needs.

Website/Resource: http://www.fcsn.org

Organization: **Films Involving Disabilities**

Description: This website catalogues feature films and documentaries on disabilities It includes access to reviews or summaries.

Website/Resource: http://www.disabilityfilmfestival.eu

Organization: **Kids on the Block**

Description: Kids on the Block is an organization that uses puppets as an educational aid to teach children to have healthy attitudes about disability. Readers have access to information regarding program curriculum and available puppet programs.

Website/Resource: http://www.kotb.com

Organization: **National Early Childhood Technical Assistance Center**

Description: The National Early Childhood Technical Assistance Center (NECTAC) is supported by the U.S. Department of Education's Office of Special Education Programs (OSEP). NECTAC's mission is to strengthen service systems to ensure that children with disabilities (birth through five years) and their families receive and benefit from high quality, culturally appropriate, and family-centered supports and services. The website offers users access to information regarding helpful contacts, topic pages, conferences, and publications.

Website/Resource: http://www.nectac.org

Organization: **National Father's Network**

Description: The National Father's Network's mission is to celebrate and support fathers and families raising children with special health care needs and developmental disabilities. The website provides users with links to network news, photos, stories, and helpful resources.

Website/Resource: http://www.fathersnetwork.org

Organization: **National Dissemination Center for Children with Disabilities**

Description: The National Dissemination Center for Children with Disabilities provides access to information regarding disabilities in children and youth, programs and services for infants, children, and youth with disabilities, IDEA (the nation's special education law), No Child Left Behind (the nation's general education law) and research-based information on effective practices for children with disabilities. The website has specific links for families, early intervention providers, schools, and state agencies.

Website/Resource: http://www.nichcy.org

Organization: **Parents Helping Parents: The Family Resource Center**

Description: Parents Helping Parents (PHP) is a non-profit, community-based, parent-directed family resource center. PHP provides lifetime guidance, supports, and services to children with any special need, their families, and the professionals who serve them. The website provides users with links to PHP services, volunteer information, and helpful resources.

Website/Resource: http://www.php.com

Videos

Father's Voices: A Journey of the Heart

(Tells the story of how the lives of four fathers were changed by raising children with special needs. Produced by the National Fathers' Network. Visit: http://www.fathersnetwork.org.)

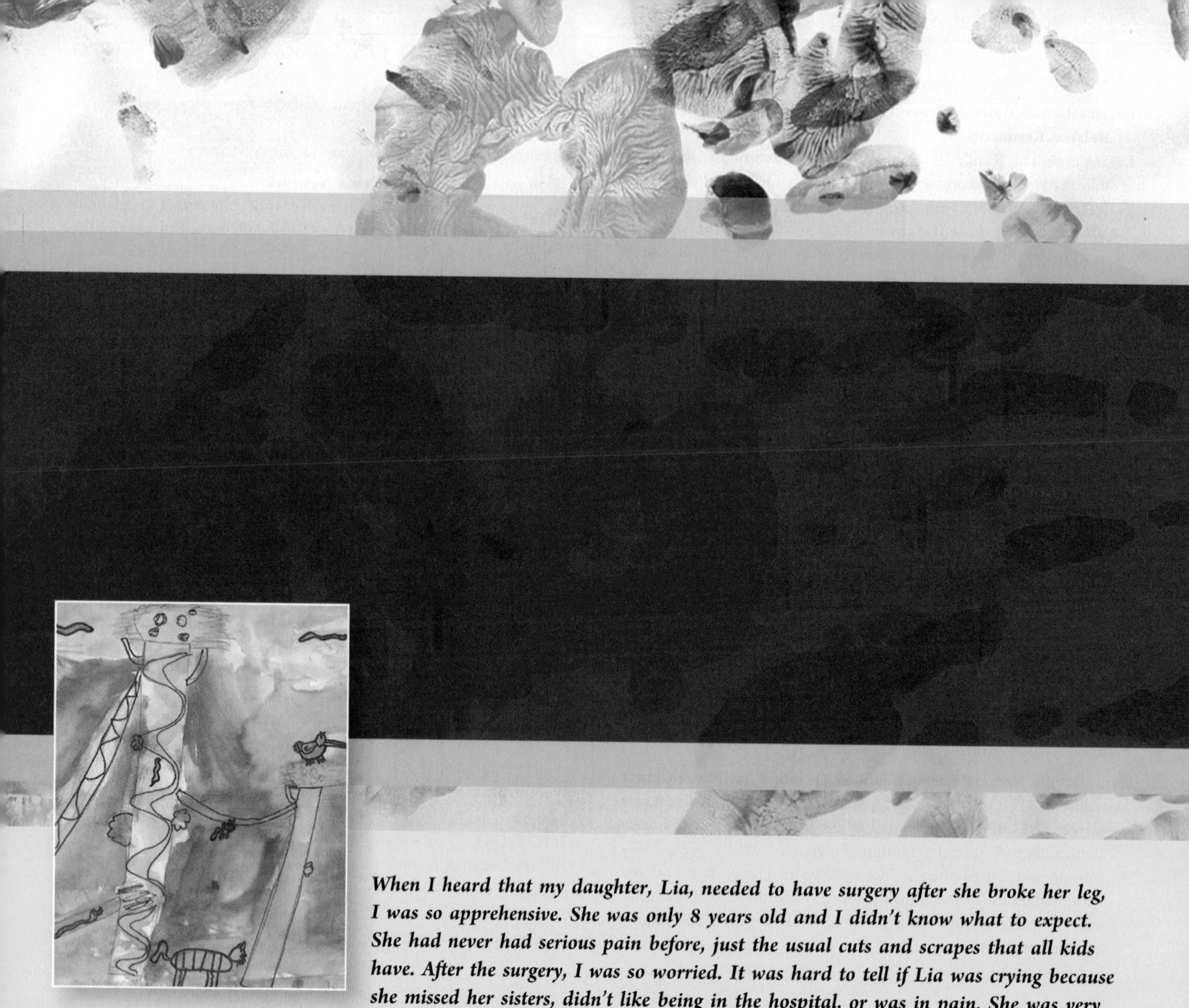

When I heard that my daughter, Lia, needed to have surgery after she broke her leg, I was so apprehensive. She was only 8 years old and I didn't know what to expect. She had never had serious pain before, just the usual cuts and scrapes that all kids have. After the surgery, I was so worried. It was hard to tell if Lia was crying because she missed her sisters, didn't like being in the hospital, or was in pain. She was very quiet, which was so different from the chatterbox Lia we were used to, and she wouldn't even look at me when I tried to talk to her. The nurses were really helpful, though. They suggested that we give Lia the pain medicine when it was time for it even if she wouldn't tell us she was in pain. The nurses said that some children act withdrawn when something hurts. They were right. Lia perked up and was much more like her usual self after she got the morphine.

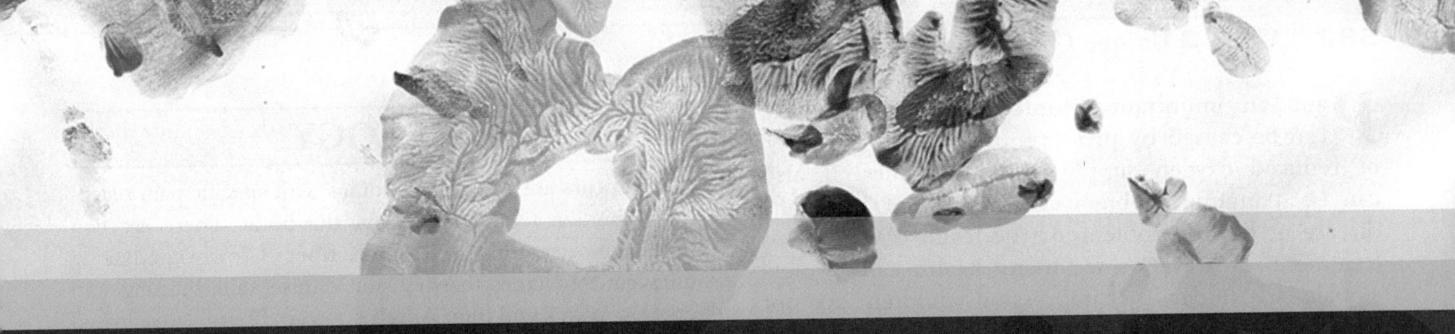

CHAPTER 18

Pain Management

Jennifer Obrecht, RN, MS, ARPN
Vicki Ann Andreoni, RN, MS, CPNP

COMPETENCIES

Upon completion of this chapter, the reader will be able to:

- Describe the physiology of pain, including the gate control theory.
- Discuss common pain misconceptions.
- Discuss developmental differences in pain behavior and assessment strategies.
- Describe various pediatric pain assessment scales and their application to children of varying developmental and cognitive levels.
- Describe nonpharmacologic techniques for pediatric pain management.
- Discuss the uses, age-appropriate doses, and side effects of opioid and nonopioid pain medications.
- Differentiate acute from chronic pain.
- Discuss information families need to know when caring for a child experiencing pain at home.
- Successfully complete the games and activities in the online student StudyWARE.

Pain, an important symptom seen in children, can be caused by pressure, overstretching, injury, or reduced oxygen supply to body tissues. It also can be a unique problem, a symptom of a specific disease or health problem, or the result of disease or treatment. However, since many health care professionals are under the impression children do not experience pain or are less sensitive to pain than adults, understanding pediatric pain management and related strategies is essential to delivering holistic, effective care.

Appropriate pain relief is important for physiological as well as psychological reasons. For example, male infants circumcised without any type of anesthesia showed more distress during immunizations later in infancy than infants who received anesthesia or those who were not circumcised (Brown-Trask, Van Sell, Carter, & Kindred, 2009). This resulted in evidence-based practice guidelines that address pain management during circumcision (AAP, 2005). Timely and effective pain management also promotes wound healing and decreases the length of hospital stay. Therefore, infants and children treated throughout the health care spectrum should be afforded the opportunity for effective **analgesia**—pain relief using medications or other interventions.

This chapter discusses the pediatric pain experience. The text provides information about the developmental implications of pediatric pain, especially in the age groups that generally cannot describe their pain. **Acute pain**, pain generally lasting three to five days, and attributed to a specific cause such as surgery or an injury, is differentiated from **chronic pain**, or pain that lasts for long periods of time or comes and goes frequently over long periods of time. Treatment options for all pain problems are reviewed and appropriate assessment techniques for pediatric clients, including formal assessment scales, a review of physiological pain indicators, and a description of pediatric pain behaviors, are included. The importance of nursing care and advocacy for children in pain is stressed throughout the chapter (Figure 18-1).

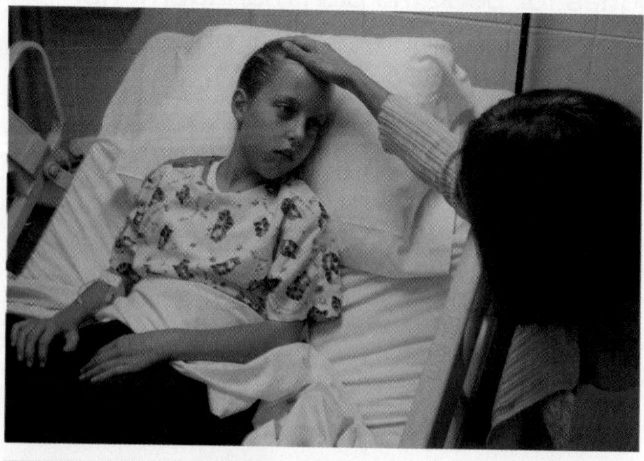

FIGURE 18-1 **This child is in pain, manifested as seriousness and sadness rather than as crying.** DELMAR CENGAGE LEARNING.

PAIN PHYSIOLOGY

Nociceptors are free nerve endings with specific pain receptors found in tissue throughout the body. There are two types of nociceptors, the **C-nerve fibers** (slowly conducting unmyelinated axons that transmit diffuse, dull, burning, and chronic pain) and the **A-delta nerve fibers** (myelinated nerves that fire impulses more rapidly and transmit sharp, well localized pain). A pain impulse starts when these receptors are stimulated by noxious stimuli (mechanical, chemical, or thermal) provoking an electrical activity, called **transduction**. Transduction leads to **transmission** whereby the pain impulse moves along peripheral sensory nerves to the spinal column and then to the brain (Helms & Barone, 2009) (Figure 18-2).

The intensity and duration of the pain impulses are modified by neural activity and chemical factors, termed **modulation**. Specifically, the prolonged firing of the C-fibers causes a chemical cascade that stimulates the **N-methyl-D-asparate (NMDA) receptors**, causing the spinal column receptors to be more responsive to pain. The release of chemical mediators such as **substance P**, a neuropeptide, sensitizes the nerve endings and increases the rate of firing. Investigating the role and composition of these chemical mediators may lead to new understanding and treatment of pain.

The **perception** of pain completes the transmission cascade. Perception takes place in the cerebral cortex where meaning or recognition of the pain impulse occurs. Until recently, the primary role of pain was thought to be passive.

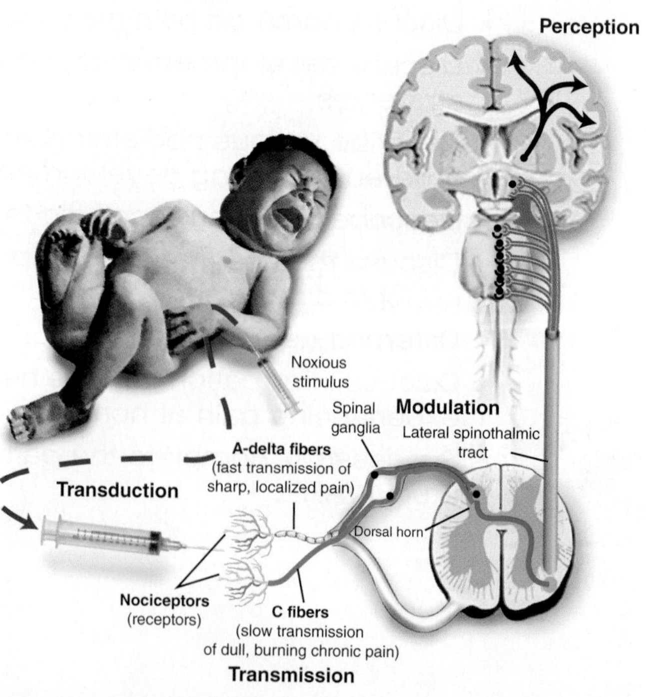

FIGURE 18-2 **Physiology of Pain.** DELMAR CENGAGE LEARNING.

However, studies over the past decade have shown that an extensive central pain network including the thalamus and some somatosensory structures exist. With a better understanding of the mechanism of the pain cascade, new information about treatment and pharmacologic management emerges.

GATE CONTROL THEORY

The classic **gate control theory** of pain explains how pain impulses travel and are interpreted in the body (Melzack & Wall, 1965). At the level of the dorsal horn, a gating mechanism opens and closes to permit or hinder the passage of pain impulses. The input of large fibers closes the gate (inhibits pain sensations) and the input of small fibers opens the gate (allows pain sensations to travel to the brain). However, stimulating the larger afferent nerves that carry the pain impulses, such as rubbing an injured finger or applying cold or heat to an injury, can also blunt pain sensations. The gate's ability to open and close is influenced by stimulation, emotion, anxiety, distraction, sensation, and memory. This physiologic response supports assessing and treating pain by using both physiological and psychological techniques.

PEDIATRIC PAIN RESEARCH

Early description of pediatric pain focused on inadequate analgesia in children with acute or postoperative pain. Often, comparisons with adults experiencing pain after similar procedures were described (Hamunen, Maunuksela, & Olkkola, 2008). The role of the nurse, physician, and parent in treating a child's pain was the focus, and research was generally conducted with hospitalized children.

Anand and Hickey (1987) performed a now classic study which described the phenomenon of pain in infants. This double-blind controlled study compared the effect of pain management in infants to postoperative morbidity and mortality. The infants in the control group received no anesthesia or pain medication for thoracotomy, as was the standard of care at the time. The experimental group received general anesthesia as well as postoperative pain management and demonstrated remarkable improvement in postoperative morbidity and mortality.

Research has also been conducted on pain assessment and the development and testing of a variety of scales for use in children (Bailey, Bergeron, Gravel, Daoust, 2007; Bijur, Latimer, & Gallagher, 2003; Schiavenato et al., 2008; von Baeyer, Spagrud, McCormick, Choo, Neville, & Connelly, 2009). Researchers have also described the ability of children to quantify and accurately describe their pain response. More recent studies have examined methods to assess pain in cognitively impaired children and congruence between children's and parents' pain ratings (Johansson & Kokinsky, 2009; Zhou, Roberts, & Horgan, 2008). Children of different age groups and developmental cognitive levels assess their pain using numbers, colors, faces, or drawings. (See Assessment Measures for more details.)

A growing body of research examines alternative or adjunct therapies for treating cancer, procedural, and immunization pain in children. For example, pediatric patients listening to music during painful procedures had a decreased pain rating after the procedure and fewer vital sign changes during the procedure than those who did not listen to music (Beebe & Wyatt, 2009). Similar responses have also occurred when behavioral therapies such as guided imagery, hypnotism, and relaxation techniques were used.

Other researchers have explored the nurse's perceptions of pain. Educational level, personal pain experience, and the number of years in practice play a role in nurses' decisions to medicate or not medicate a child for pain. Findings indicate many nurses let personal pain perceptions influence their assessment and selection of treatment modalities for clients in pain (Gimbler-Beglund, Ljusegren, & Enskar, 2008; Vincent, 2007). In addition, accurate assessment and improvement in consistent pain treatment correlate with nurses' education about pain and years of nursing experience. Other researchers have examined children's and parents' preoperative pain education needs (Zhou, Roberts, & Horgan, 2008) and safety and efficacy of interventions for neonatal pain (Hall & Shbarou, 2009).

A general rule of thumb regarding pain in children is if an intervention would hurt an adult it will also hurt a child. As the nurse caring for the pediatric client, it may be effective to consider this when deciding whether it is appropriate to implement pain management strategies.

Refer to Table 18-1 for common pain misconceptions.

CHILD DEVELOPMENT AND PAIN

Children interpret and perceive pain within the context of their unique cognitive and development levels. Their perceptions and understanding of the world around them affect their behavior and response to pain (Table 18-2).

INFANTS

Historically, it was felt that infants did not feel pain, or perhaps experienced it in a less distressing way than older children and adults due to their immature nervous system. Research over the past three decades has shed new light on our knowledge of early human pain experiences. Fetuses and infants can perceive and respond to painful stimuli. The neonate can experience acute, constant, and chronic pain through a complex process whereby the pain system is activated and modulated. Unremitting pain may lead to permanent alterations in the pain system so that processing of signals at the spinal and supraspinal levels is distorted. This may lead to increased pain sensitivity (Anand et al., 2006).

Table 18-1 Pediatric Pain Misconceptions

MISCONCEPTION	SCIENTIFIC RESEARCH SHOWS
Infants and young children do not experience, feel, or remember pain.	The human fetus is capable of transmitting pain impulses at 30 weeks' gestation. Infants respond to repeated noxious stimuli (Howard, 2003).
Infants and older children are more sensitive than adults to opioid pain medication.	When receiving weight-appropriate doses, children are not more susceptible than adults to undesired opioid effects such as respiratory depression or hypotension.
Pain is to be endured and can be a character-building experience.	Pain interrupts sleep, play, and appetite. The child experiencing pain from hospitalization, injury, or illness would benefit from treatment.
The risk of opioid addiction prohibits appropriate pain treatment.	The risk for opioid addiction from analgesics is low in these age groups (Box 18-1).
Children who are sleeping, playing, or can be distracted are not experiencing pain.	Most children will engage in developmentally appropriate play or distraction, including sleep, when in pain. The client should be regularly assessed for pain and treated according to his or her pain rating.

BOX 18-1
PAIN MANAGEMENT TERMINOLOGY

Addiction: The psychological and physical need to use a medication for nonprescribed purposes. The desired effect is usually the euphoric feeling or "high" associated with opioid analgesics.

Tolerance: The physical need for an increasing dose of a medication over time to achieve the desired effect. The body adapts to the presence of the medication so the analgesic effect is lessened.

Physical dependence: Physical adaptation to the presence of the medication in the bloodstream. Clients should be weaned from the medication rather than stop receiving it abruptly to avoid symptoms of withdrawal.

A full-term newborn can localize and purposefully withdraw from painful stimuli. Infants have a distinctive cry when experiencing acute pain, characterized as high-pitched and shrill, and followed by a period of apnea, then several short gasps or bursts of crying. Often, this cry is thought to be a response to other noxious stimuli, such as hunger or cold, but the distinct nature of this cry should alert the nurse to the presence of pain. Pain intensity has been found to correlate with cry intensity (Bellieni, Sisto, Cordelli, & Buonocore, 2004). A facial expression of pain, known as the primal face of pain, may also accompany the cry. Here, the brow is furrowed, the mouth opening is squarish and the tongue is taut during the cry. The primal face of pain has been found to cross gender and sociocultural lines (Schiavenato et al., 2008). The primal face of pain is shown in Figure 18-3.

Table 18-2 Developmental Stages and Pain Responses

PHASE	DEVELOPMENTAL TASK	UNIQUE PAIN RESPONSE
Infancy	Trust vs. mistrust Sensorimotor	Cry, withdraw, furrowed brow, taut mouth.
Toddlerhood	Autonomy vs. shame and doubt Sensorimotor; Preoperational thought	Cry, scream, protest, withdraw.
Preschooler	Initiative vs. guilt Preoperational thought	Cry, localize body part, anticipate painful procedures. Body image concerns.
School-age	Industry vs. inferiority Concrete operations	Body image concerns, may assume pain is punishment.
Adolescent	Identity vs. role confusion Formal operations	Assume pain will be treated, can conceptualize pain relief.

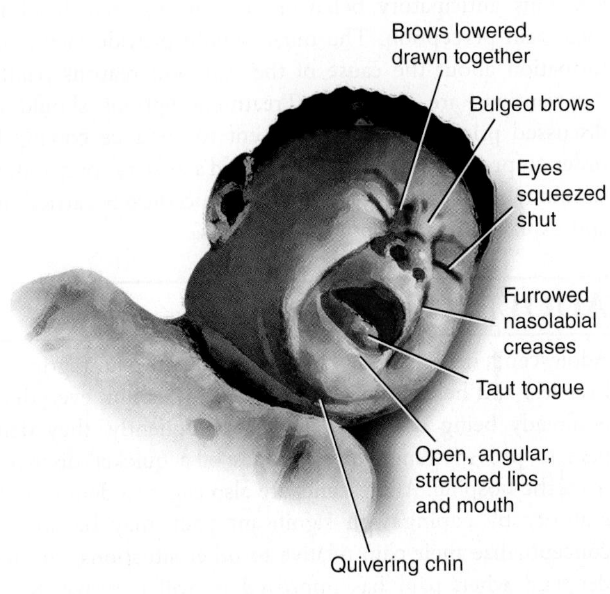

FIGURE 18-3 Facial Characteristics of Infant Pain Expression.
DELMAR CENGAGE LEARNING.

TODDLERS

Hospitalization or other interactions with health care providers (i.e., visits to the physician's office) are new and challenging experiences for a toddler. Often, exposure to a painful procedure is associated with separation from parents or primary caregivers, heightening the toddler's anxiety and exacerbating the pain. Therefore, the toddler's age-appropriate protest to unpleasant or noxious stimuli may be confused with an indication of pain. It is easy to identify when toddlers are in pain, but difficult to assess the degree of pain, as all painful stimuli may be met with the same degree of intensity.

PRESCHOOLERS

The pain response may be subdued or less physical than expected for this age group, and lack of physical activity may indicate the preschooler is experiencing pain, because preschoolers, when healthy, are not capable of sitting or lying for long periods of time. The child of this age who does not readily run, jump, or wiggle may be in pain. Preschoolers also may not be capable of describing the location of pain, and use a general term like *stomach* or *belly*. However, they may not accurately differentiate what part of their "midsection" hurts, that is, chest, torso, back, or abdomen.

Preschoolers benefit from medical play prior to a painful procedure. Touching and exploring the unfamiliar medical equipment may help decrease their anxiety, and,

EVIDENCE-BASED PRACTICE

Pain in Children

CLINICAL PROBLEM

Children of all ages frequently experience pain when hospitalized. Although pain scales using self report are well accepted as a reliable means of assessing pain in adults, health care providers are much more reticent to believe a child's self report of pain due to children's limited verbal and cognitive abilities. Health care providers have a moral obligation to listen to children's perceptions of their pain experiences and children have an ethical right to receive adequate pain treatment. Pain is a subjective experience, and regarding children as experts on their pain only increases options for pain management, decreases their anxiety, and minimizes potential negative effects of an unpleasant hospitalization. Children between 4 and 11 years old, a normally challenging group to assess, were able to explain what they thought would help their pain, the type of help they thought would be effective, and who could provide the help they needed when asked open-ended questions.

BEST CLINICAL PRACTICE

Children are adept at using self-help strategies including sensory/physical and cognitive/ behavioral methods to relieve their pain. Information giving and receiving is helpful as they experiment with methods to alleviate their pain. Children expect competence and empathy from nurses and sometimes will demand pain control if it is not provided as expected. If nurses are trusted, children will allow them to engage in pain relieving activities with them, but many times, parents or significant others are the preferred helpers. Some children cannot engage in self-help methods effectively and have a fatalistic attitude towards pain.

IMPLICATIONS FOR NURSING

- Take time to develop rapport with the child and his or her family. This will aid in determining the child's expectations as well as the most effective interventions for the child.
- Demonstrate a genuine interest in helping the child cope with his or her pain.
- Develop an awareness of specific cultural factors that influence the child's pain experience.
- Realize that pain at or above moderate levels can be physically and psychologically harmful and that health care providers have a duty to provide pain relief to children.
- Believe the child's self report of pain and use developmentally appropriate tools to measure pain.
- Provide suggestions on ways family members can support the child in pain and augment the child's self help strategies.

Reference: Korteslauoma, R., Nikkonen, M., & Serlo, W. (2008). "You just have to make the pain go away"—Children's experiences of pain management. *Pain Management Nursing, 9*(4), 143–149.

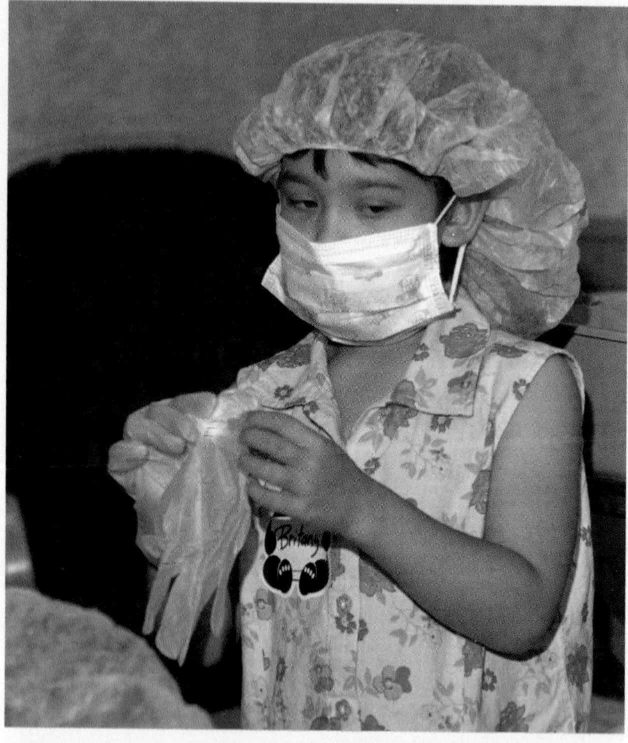

FIGURE 18-4 Medicinal play prior to procedures provides familiarity to help children cope with a painful experience. DELMAR CENGAGE LEARNING.

subsequently, the pain they experience (Figure 18-4). However, the playing preschooler can be deceiving as many youngsters play despite pain, because this is normal and helps distract them from their pain. Play also helps these children cope with pain as some preschoolers use play to exhibit pain. For example, drawing or acting out the situation may help preschoolers express their feelings without specifically saying they hurt or something is painful.

SCHOOL-AGE

School-age children are concrete thinkers, learning cause and effect, and often experience pain in an "all or nothing" phenomena. When prompted, school-age children can recall that today's hurt may be less intense than yesterday's, but in response to open-ended questions about pain, often maintain the pain continues at the same intensity until it is completely gone. Some school-age children may have preconceived ideas about pain and its treatment. School-age children also have body image concerns and some fear their insides will leak out after receiving an injection or undergoing surgery. Therefore, covering all wounds can decrease their anxiety and help decrease their pain perception. School-age children need to gain some control over their environment and should also be given choices whenever possible. Allowing a child to choose the limb for a painful procedure, or breaking down the procedure into several smaller steps if possible, highlighting that only one small part is painful, may help. In addition, children may view their pain as punishment or something they caused by bad behavior. This anticipatory behavior and anxiety may heighten their pain perception. The nurse should provide factual information about the cause of the pain and reasons painful interventions are necessary. Treatment options should be discussed prior to the painful event to enhance coping. In order to prevent heightening the child's anxiety, preparation should take place shortly before the procedure is carried out and explained in age-appropriate terms.

ADOLESCENTS

Adolescents may feel they need to hide their pain ("grin and bear it") and hesitate to report pain if they think everything is already being done to relieve it. Frequently, they deny pain to prove strength or in hopes of a quicker discharge from the hospital. Adolescents are also eager to demonstrate maturity by coping with significant pain, may be able to conceptualize their pain relative to other situations, and understand when pain has improved or will improve. Some adolescents deny pain because they are concerned that taking medications for pain will lead to addiction. In addition, cultural or family values regarding the use of drugs can strongly influence how an adolescent experiences pain and how the pain is treated. Therefore, in caring for adolescents in pain, the nurse should acknowledge and frequently assess their pain. Although adolescents crave independence, it is important to include parents or family members in discussions regarding effective pain treatment.

Adolescents may also cope with their pain by watching videos, listening to audiotapes, playing games, or sleeping. The lack of interest in discussing pain does not mean adolescents do not have pain, because distraction is a powerful pain management strategy. The adolescent should be included in discussions about which techniques effectively reduce their pain and consulted regarding treatment options.

PAIN ASSESSMENT

Complete and accurate assessment of a child's pain can lead to better and more effective intervention. The following discussion identifies several strategies and tools used in pediatric clients.

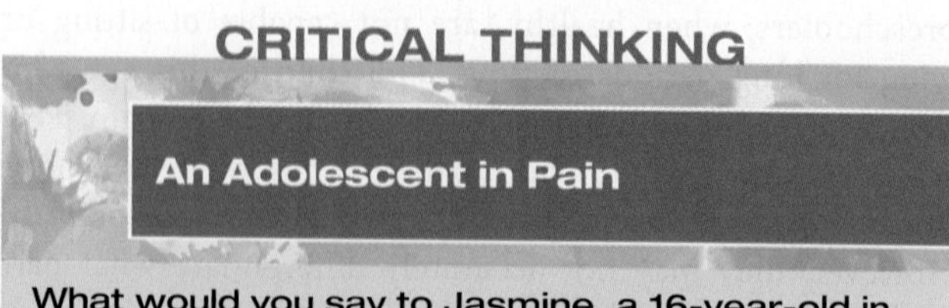

CRITICAL THINKING

An Adolescent in Pain

What would you say to Jasmine, a 16-year-old in obvious pain who refuses medications because she fears addiction? What if her family agreed and supported her decision?

PAIN INTERVIEW AND HISTORY

The initial assessment includes a pain history and comprehensive information about the child's past pain experiences, treatment strategies, and preferences. The nurse queries the child and caregiver about interventions and coping strategies that have helped in the past. The PQRST format (Box 18-2) prompts the nurse to interview both the parent or primary care provider and the child, and then the child is given the opportunity to describe and rate his or her pain using a self-rating scale. A systematic means of obtaining a pain history can lead to a more comprehensive assessment.

Caregivers are also interviewed about the child's pain. For children developmentally or cognitively unable to describe or discuss their own pain, parent information should be valued as if the client had responded. Table 18-3 lists questions the nurse can use in obtaining a pain history.

BOX 18-2
THE PQRST PAIN ASSESSMENT

P—presence of pain: "Are you hurting today?"

Q—quality: "What words describe your pain?" (i.e., sharp, burning, tingling ...)

R—radiation or location: "Where is your pain? Does it shoot or radiate anywhere else?"

S—severity: "Give me a number between 0—10 for your pain."

T—timing: "How long have you had this pain? How long does it last when the pain comes?"

ASSESSMENT MEASURES

A number of assessment measures have been developed to quantify a child's pain. They are divided into two categories: objective measures used by the observer to score client behavior or physiologic parameters associated with a painful response such as heart rate and blood pressure, and self-reporting instruments designed so children may rate their own pain.

OBJECTIVE MEASURES

Objective pain measures are ideal for the infant, preverbal child, or developmentally delayed child who is not able to self-rate his or her pain. Most objective rating measures score behaviors and physiological changes to determine the intensity of pain experienced. Most are used to measure acute pain since reliability and validity are less well established for long-term pain. Objective pain assessment measures are most effective when combined with self-reporting tools for children and adolescents because they are able to report or score their own pain. Objective measures are also a useful method of documenting improvements in pain intensity over time, especially postoperatively (refer to Figure 18-5 for an example of an objective measure of pain in neonates). The FLACC scale (Figure 18-6) and the COMFORT (Figure 18-7) pain measure are two commonly used objective pain scales.

SUBJECTIVE (SELF-RATING) MEASURES

In all types of pain, the most information can be gained when children measure the pain themselves. Several methods assist children in rating their own pain. The choice

TABLE 18-3 Pain History Questions

CHILD QUESTIONS	CAREGIVER QUESTIONS
Tell me what pain is to you.	What words does your child use to describe pain?
Tell me about times you have hurt before today.	Describe the pain experiences your child has had.
Who do you tell if you hurt?	Who does your child tell when he or she hurts?
What do you do for yourself when you hurt?	How do you know when your child is in pain?
What do you want others to do for you when you hurt?	How does your child usually react when he or she is in pain?
What don't you want others to do for you when you hurt?	What do you do to help your child when he or she is hurting?
What helps the most to take your pain away?	What does your child do to help himself or herself when he or she hurts?
	What works best to decrease or relieve your child's pain?
Is there anything else you want to tell me about when you hurt? (If yes, describe.)	Is there anything special you would like me to know about your child's pain? (If yes, describe.)

Adapted from Hester, N.O. & Barcus, C.S. (1986). Assessment and management of children in pain. *Pediatrics: Nursing Update, 1*, 2–8.

Parameter	Score		
Facial expression	0—relaxed	1—grimace	
Cry	0—no cry	1—whimper	2—vigorous
Breathing pattern	0—relaxed	1—change in breathing	
Arms	0—relaxed or restrained	1—flexed or extended	
Legs	0—relaxed or restrained	1—flexed or extended	
State of arousal	0—sleeping or awake	1—fussy	

FIGURE 18-5 Neonatal Infant Pain Scale (NIPS). USED WITH PERMISSION FROM LAWRENCE, J., ALCOCK, D., MCGRATH, P., KAY, J., MACMURRAY, S. B., & DULBERG, C. (1993). THE DEVELOPMENT OF A TOOL TO ASSESS NEONATAL PAIN. *NEONATAL NETWORK*, 12(6), 59–66.

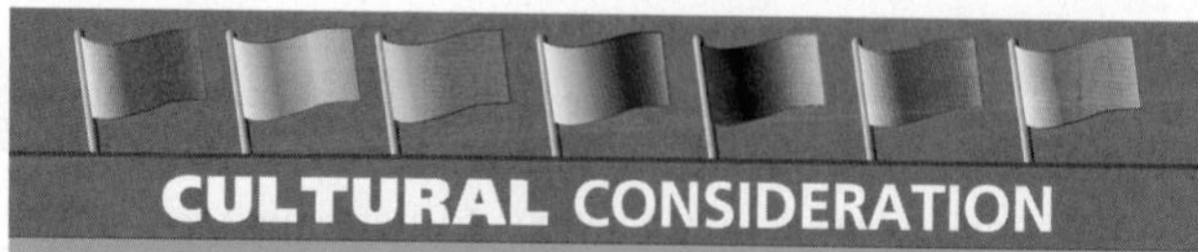

CULTURAL CONSIDERATION

Pain and Culture

Pain is a universal experience. However, there is inequality in the pain experience not only between individuals but also between individuals in cultural groups. One's culture socializes individuals on how to act when in pain and what behavior is acceptable to others when in pain. Culture also affects pain assessment. For example, Amish children are taught not to say much about pain; thus if they experience pain accompanying appendicitis, for example, care providers may not know they are in pain and sick. These children may also wince and tighten up even before an abdominal assessment but not complain of pain during the assessment.

Effective nursing care for pediatric clients in pain from varying cultures includes:

1. Being aware of cultural differences in the expression of pain. Some cultures are stoic; others are emotive;
2. Being sensitive to varying communication styles in relation to pain; nonverbal and verbal messages need to be considered when assessing and asking pediatric clients about their pain ("pain," "hurt," and "ache" may mean similar or different things to Hispanic, American Indian, African-American, and Caucasian clients);
3. Using pediatric pain assessment instruments developed for various cultures (the Wong-Baker FACES scale has been translated into Japanese, Chinese, French, Italian, Spanish, Vietnamese, Romanian, and Portuguese);
4. Being aware of and appreciating the meaning of pain in a particular culture (for example, many Hispanics and individuals of Latin American descent are Catholic and may relieve or endure their pain by attending mass, praying, or receiving a blessing or communion from a priest. Using this religious context, many of these patients may see pain as a punishment and suffering as part of life that must be endured in order to enter Heaven);
5. Recognizing some cultures may not believe it is acceptable to communicate that one is having pain, or feel asking for help or assistance is seen as weak (for example, some cultural groups may view asking for a pain medication as a sign of weakness; a Chinese client may view asking for a pain medication as taking the nurse away from much more important duties);
6. Becoming aware of one's own values and beliefs that may affect one's response to pain (for example, if the care provider sees pain as part of life that needs to be endured, he or she may not provide appropriate pain management to a child in pain);
7. Being aware that biological variations affect pain (for example, there are differences in drug metabolism, therapeutic response, side effects, and dosing requirements in ethnic and racial groups).

Source: Davidhizar, R., & Giger, J. (2004). A review of the literature on care of clients in pain who are culturally diverse. *International Nursing Review*, *51*, 47–55.

of a specific measure should be based on the child's developmental level and preferences, institutional policies, and instrument availability (Figures 18-8, 18-9, and 18-10). A quantifiable measure of pain also adds to validity when discussing pain treatment with members of the health care team because reporting a child's pain by numbers or measures is more credible than saying "She says she hurts." However, the limitation to all instruments is their availability and consistency of use when accurately assessing pain.

For the verbal child, the pain assessment scale of 0 to 10 or 0 to 5 may be the simplest and best understood. Here, the nurse asks the child to rate pain on a scale where "zero is no pain at all" and the higher number is "the worst pain ever you can imagine" (Figure 18-10). The scale points should be documented when recording the child's measure of pain

Categories	Scoring		
	0	1	2
F Face	No particular expression or smile	Occasional grimace or frown, withdrawn, disinterested ***appears sad or worried***	Frequent to constant frown, clenched jaw, quivering chin ***distress-looking face: expression of fright or panic***
L Legs	Normal position or relaxed	Uneasy, restless, tense ***occasional tremors***	Kicking, or legs drawn up ***marked increase in spasticity, constant tremors or jerking***
A Activity	Lying quietly, normal position, moves easily	Squirming, shifting back and forth, tense ***mildly agitated (eg. head back and forth, aggression); shallow, splinting respirations intermittent sighs***	Arched, rigid, or jerking ***severe agitation, head banging, shivering (not rigors); breath-holding, gasping or sharp intake of breath; severe splinting***
C Cry	No cry (awake or asleep)	Moans or whimpers, occasional complaint ***occasional verbal outburst or grunt***	Crying steadily, screams or sobs, frequent complaints ***repeated outbursts, constant grunting***
C Consolability	Content, relaxed	Reassured by occasional touching, hugging, or being talked to, distractable	Difficult to console or comfort ***pushing away caregiver, resisting care or comfort measures***

FIGURE 18-6 FLACC Behavioral Pain Scale.

(i.e., "rates pain 5 out of 10" rather than "rates pain a 5"). Drawing a 10-centimeter line and asking the child to point to the level of pain on the line may also be effective (Figure 18-11).

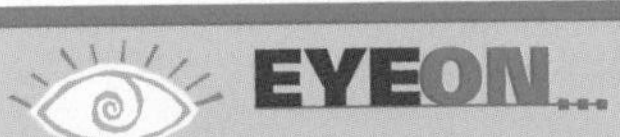

Perception of Pain

Culture determines the way persons derive meaning from their lives and appropriate behaviors. One's cultural upbringing teaches behaviors, including those exhibited when in pain. People from different cultures use different types of words to describe pain (for example, in sensory or emotional terms). These differences should not be ignored, but the nurse also needs to be careful not to prejudge a client based on cultural background or ethnicity. Due to the unique experience of pain, people will exhibit individualized behaviors even though they are influenced by cultural upbringing.

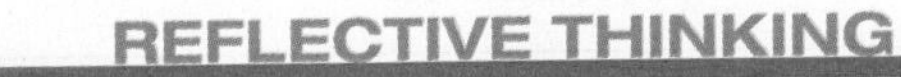

Two Boys: Differences in Pain Perception

You are caring for two young boys of approximately the same age who underwent the same operative procedure on the same day. Abraham is walking in the hall three times per day, playing video games, and talking on the phone. Joshua lies in bed moaning, is reluctant to walk, and is not interested in any activities. Both children have the same pain rating by objective or subjective measure. Would you discount one rating based on a comparison of the children's behaviors? Would your perceptions affect the care you deliver or pain medication given to relieve each child's pain?

COMFORT Behavior Scale and Scoring Form

Patient Sticker

Date ______ Time ______

Observer ______

Alertness	• Deeply asleep (eyes closed, no response to changes in the environment)	❑ 1
	• Lightly asleep (eyes mostly closed, occasional responses)	❑ 2
	• Drowsy (child closes his or her eyes frequently, less responsive to the environment)	❑ 3
	• Awake and alert (child responsive to the environment)	❑ 4
	• Awake and hyperalert (exaggerated responses to environmental stimuli)	❑ 5
Calmness–Agitation	• Calm (child appears serene and tranquil)	❑ 1
	• Slightly anxious (child shows slight anxiety)	❑ 2
	• Anxious (child appears agitated but remains in control)	❑ 3
	• Very anxious (child appears very agitated, just able to control)	❑ 4
	• Panicky (child appears severely distressed, with loss of control)	❑ 5
Respiratory response (score only in mechanically ventilated children)	• No spontaneous respiration	❑ 1
	• Spontaneous and ventilator respiration	❑ 2
	• Restlessness or resistance to ventilator	❑ 3
	• Active breathing against ventilator or regular coughing	❑ 4
	• Fighting against ventilator	❑ 5
Crying (score only in children breathing spontaneously)	• Quiet breathing, no crying sounds	❑ 1
	• Occasional sobbing or moaning	❑ 2
	• Whining (monotone)	❑ 3
	• Crying	❑ 4
	• Screaming or shrieking	❑ 5
Physical movement	• No movement	❑ 1
	• Occasional (3 or fewer) slight movements	❑ 2
	• Frequent (more than 3) slight movements	❑ 3
	• Vigorous movements limited to extremities	❑ 4
	• Vigorous movements including torso and head	❑ 5
Muscle tone	• Muscles totally relaxed, no muscle tone	❑ 1
	• Reduced muscle tone, less resistance than normal	❑ 2
	• Normal muscle tone	❑ 3
	• Increased muscle tone and flexion of fingers and toes	❑ 4
	• Extreme muscle rigidity and flexion of fingers and toes	❑ 5
Facial tension	• Facial muscles totally relaxed	❑ 1
	• Normal facial tone	❑ 2
	• Tension evident in some facial muscles (not sustained)	❑ 3
	• Tension evident throughout facial muscles (not sustained)	❑ 4
	• Facial muscles contorted and grimacing	❑ 5
	Total Score	
VAS (Visual Analogue Scale) Put a mark on the line below to indicate how much pain you think the child has **at this very moment.** no pain ├──────┤ worst pain	**VAS Score**	
Treatment details		
Details of child's condition		
Assessments made *(before or after medication or standard assessment)*		

FIGURE 18-7 COMFORT Behavioral Scale and Scoring Form. USED WITH PERMISSION FROM VAN DIJK, M., PETERS, W. B., VAN DEVENTER, P., & TIBBOEL, D. (2005). THE COMFORT BEHAVIOR SCALE. *AMERICAN JOURNAL OF NURSING, 105*(1), 33–35, 37. DR. MONIQUE VAN DIJK AT M.VANDIJK.3@ERASMUSMC.NL.

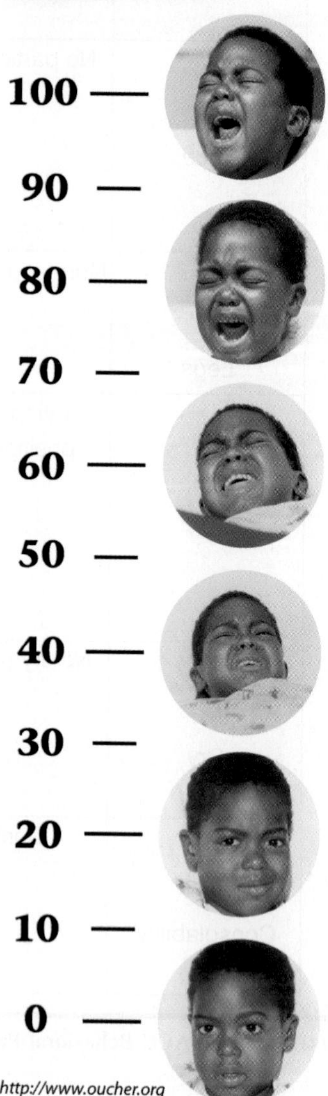

FIGURE 18-8 The Oucher Pain Assessment Tool for Use with Children 3–12 Years of Age. Caucasian, Hispanic, and African-American versions are available. THE AFRICAN-AMERICAN VERSION OF THE OUCHER, DEVELOPED AND COPYRIGHTED BY JUDITH E. BEYER, RN, PHD, 1983. USED WITH PERMISSION.

MANAGEMENT OF ACUTE PAIN

Every child has the right to appropriate and safe pain relief. Interventions that may cause pain are sometimes an unavoidable consequence of health care encounters. A variety of methods are available for use by trained personnel to decrease or eliminate the pain of needlesticks and other painful treatments. Nurses play a major role in assessing, treating, and managing a child's pain.

GOALS OF ACUTE PAIN MANAGEMENT

Pain associated with an injury, surgical procedure, or a specific disease state is described as acute pain. The intensity of acute pain fades predictably over a few days to a week, and many hospitalized children experience a phase of acute pain that is nearly resolved or easily managed with oral analgesics by discharge.

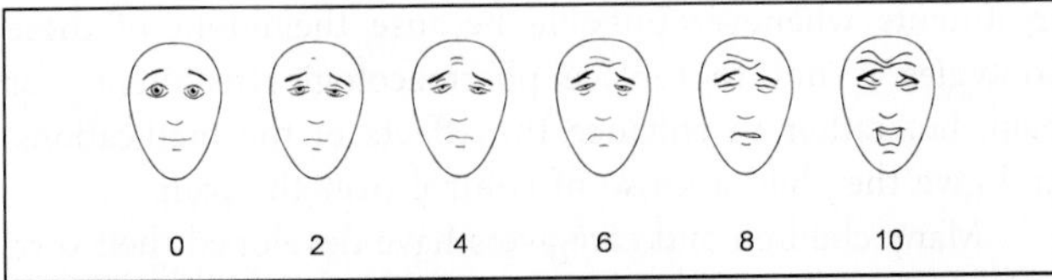

FIGURE 18-9 **Hicks, C. L., von Baeyer, C. L., Spafford, P., van Korlaar, I., & Goodenough, B. Faces Pain Scale—Revised: Toward a Common Metric in Pediatric Pain Measurement. *PAIN* 2001, 93, 173–183.** USED WITH PERMISSION FROM HICKS, C. L., VON BAEYER, C. L., SPAFFORD, P., VAN KORLAAR, I., GOODENOUGH, B. FACES PAIN SCALE - REVISED: TOWARD A COMMON METRIC IN PEDIATRIC PAIN MEASUREMENT. PAIN 2001; 93, 173-183. THIS FIGURE HAS BEEN REPRODUCED WITH PERMISSION OF THE INTERNATIONAL ASSOCIATION FOR THE STUDY OF PAIN® (IASP®). THE FIGURE MAY NOT BE REPRODUCED FOR ANY OTHER PURPOSE WITHOUT PERMISSION.

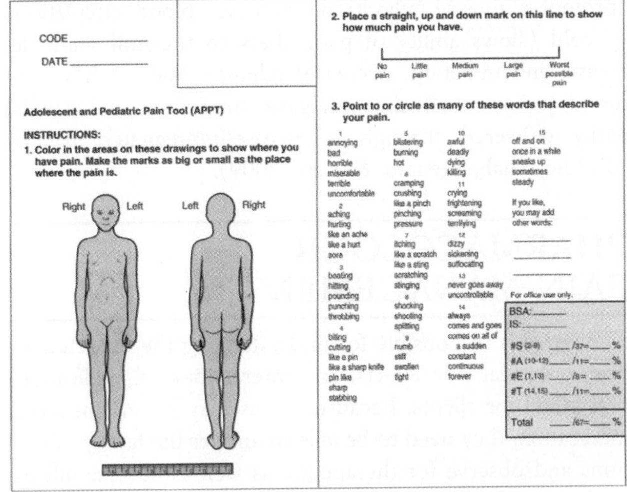

CODE ____________

DATE ____________

Adolescent and Pediatric Pain Tool (APPT)

INSTRUCTIONS:

1. Color in the areas on these drawings to show where you have pain. Make the marks as big or small as the place where the pain is.

Right Left Left Right

2. Place a straight, up and down mark on this line to show how much pain you have.

No pain | Little pain | Medium pain | Large pain | Worst possible pain

3. Point to or circle as many of these words that describe your pain.

1: annoying, bad, horrible, miserable, terrible, uncomfortable

2: aching, hurting, like an ache, like a hurt, sore

3: beating, hitting, pounding, punching, throbbing

4: biting, cutting, like a pin, like a sharp knife, pin like, sharp, stabbing

5: blistering, burning, hot

6: cramping, crushing, like a pinch, pinching, pressure

7: itching, like a scratch, like a sting, scratching, stinging

8: shocking, shooting, splitting

9: numb, stiff, swollen, tight

10: awful, deadly, dying, killing

11: crying, frightening, screaming, terrifying

12: dizzy, sickening, suffocating

13: never goes away, uncontrollable

14: always, comes and goes, comes on all of a sudden, constant, continuous, forever

15: off and on, once in a while, sneaks up, sometimes, steady

If you like, you may add other words:

____

____

____

For office use only.

BSA: ________

IS: ________

#S (2-9) ____ /37= ____ %

#A (10-12) ____ /11= ____ %

#E (1,13) ____ /8= ____ %

#T (14,15) ____ /11= ____ %

Total ____ /67= ____ %

FIGURE 18-10 **Adolescent and Pediatric Pain Tool.** FROM SAVEDRA, M., TESLER, M., HOLZEMER, W., & WARD, J. (1992). UNIVERSITY OF CALIFORNIA, SAN FRANCISCO, SCHOOL OF NURSING, SAN FRANCISCO, CA 94143-0606. COPYRIGHT © 1989, 1992. USED WITH PERMISSION.

The impact of effective pain treatment for children cannot be underestimated. Pain has serious physical and psychological consequences, such as increased oxygen uptake in the blood and alteration in blood glucose metabolism. Therefore, the benefits of aggressive pain treatment before, during, and after surgery or invasive procedures are far reaching. Prevention is better in treating acute pain because pain that has already occurred and is severe is difficult to control. Children and their families should be told effective pain treatment is available and an expected part of their care as they recover.

Goals and expectations of pain management should also be discussed with the child and family as they can be involved in choosing assessment strategies and developing pain management techniques. Whenever possible, the child and family should be prepared for pain associated with a procedure or surgical intervention. Finally, the preparation and discussion should include treatment options. The main goals of effective pain management are to relieve pain, maximize function, and minimize side effects.

RESEARCH *Highlight*

Nurses' Perception and Pediatric Postoperative Pain Management Practices

PURPOSE

To determine whether a nurse's perception of pain management impacts individual pain management practices.

METHODS

Nurses were observed while taking care of patients on a pediatric ward. The delivery of pediatric pain management was observed. The nurses also completed a questionnaire outlining their pain management beliefs and practices.

FINDINGS

By comparing the questionnaire responses with pain practices, it was determined that the perception of how important an aspect of pain management care was did not impact the likelihood of a nurse's performing the task.

IMPLICATIONS

Nurses do not always accurately treat or respond to children's pain. Several factors are attributed to this lack of adequate pediatric pain management. Per the results of this study, perceived importance of the task is not one of the factors.

REFERENCE

Twycross, A. (2008). Does the perceived importance of a pain management task affect the quality of children's nurses' post-operative pain management practices? *Journal of Clinical Nursing, 17*, 3205–3216.

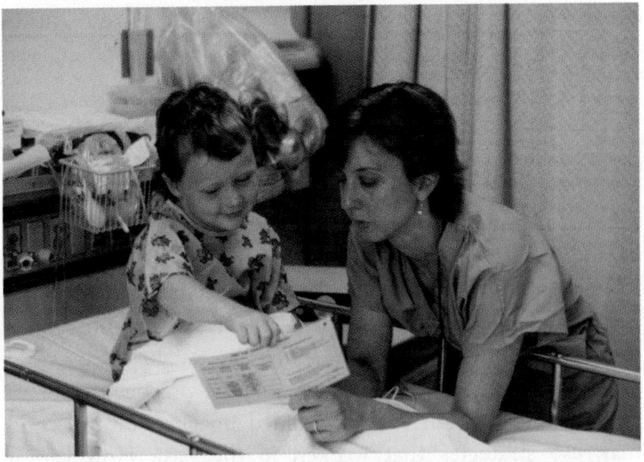

FIGURE 18-11 **Nurse and child review a pain rating scale prior to the child experiencing pain so he is familiar with it.** DELMAR CENGAGE LEARNING.

NURSING TIP

Pain Assessment Measures

Many institutions where children are cared for agree on a consistent pediatric pain assessment measure. Recommend a measure of your choice if there is not one consistently used where you practice.

Relieve Pain

The chosen treatment should first and most importantly improve or relieve the pain. However, it may not be practical or possible to relieve all the pain without rendering the child unconscious. Children and their families need to understand the limitations of effective pain management.

Maximize Function

Effective pain treatment allows the child the opportunity to walk, eat, and otherwise participate in the recovery process. Adequate pain control may contribute to a shorter hospital stay, promote quicker return to normal functioning, and lead to a more positive hospital experience.

Minimize Side Effects

All medications have side effects; some are unpleasant, others are dangerous. Most commonly prescribed pain medications also have the potential for unpleasant or harmful side effects, but these drugs are dosed or delivered so side effects are minimized. For example, a patient-controlled device may deliver intravenous opioids so the client receives the benefit of the prescribed medication with few side effects. If side effects do occur, most can be adequately treated with adjunct medications that promote pain relief while relieving unpleasant effects.

NONPHARMACOLOGIC PAIN MANAGEMENT

A strong nurse-client-family relationship promotes accurate reporting of pain as the client learns to trust pain will be relieved. An understanding of methods to comfort the child, in addition to receiving analgesics, can assist caregivers in managing their child's pain. Several specific pain management modalities, which are most effective when introduced prior to the anticipated pain, should be taught to the child and caregivers. Some techniques may be practiced prior to the painful situation such as guided imagery, or the child may use strategies that worked in the past. However, it may not be practical or effective to use more than one modality at a time. In addition, nonpharmacologic techniques should be used in conjunction with pharmacologic treatments whenever possible because the intent of these strategies is not to replace pharmacologic treatments for pain, but rather to enhance the effects of the medications, and give the child a sense of control over the pain.

Many children and caregivers have developed their own independent strategies to cope with painful procedures. The nurse should always explore these individualized strategies of pain management with the child and family and communicate them to members of the health care team. All attempts should be made to promote and continue these strategies in the acute care setting. Specific nonpharmacologic pain management strategies are described in Table 18-4.

Successful nonpharmacologic interventions include biofeedback, caregiver involvement, hypnosis, cutaneous stimulation (rubbing, massaging, holding), and applying heat (promotes muscle relaxation, increases blood circulation) or cold (slows ability of pain fibers to transmit pain, decreases inflammation, decreases edema). Sucrose has been found to be an effective analgesic for infants and can be easily delivered through a sucrose-impregnated pacifier (Taddio, Shah, Atenafu, & Katz, 2009).

PHARMACOLOGIC PAIN MANAGEMENT

The nurse is responsible for understanding the expected action, potential side effects, and interactions of medications prescribed for clients. Because nurses may be administering medication, they need to be able to answer the family's questions and observe for therapeutic as well as adverse effects. With appropriate dosing, the medications can be used for children of all ages. A general description of the classifications of analgesics follows.

Opioid Analgesics

Opioid analgesics are a class of medications derived from the opium plant for the specific purpose of relieving pain. Used alone or in combination with other medications, opioids are among the strongest pain medications and the cornerstone of management for moderate to severe pain, including acute pain (e.g., postoperative pain) and long-term chronic pain (e.g., cancer pain). The use of opioids for pain relief is unlikely to result in addiction even when used for the long term.

Opioid analgesics are effective when administered in small, frequent doses. The technique of delivering small doses of the medication until the desired effect (pain relief) is observed is called **titration**. Titrating the dose up or down may be necessary in order to obtain adequate analgesia with minimal side effects. Opioids are unique in that they have no **ceiling dose** (that is, there is no point after which they are no longer effective). In the most severe pain situations, opioid analgesics can be titrated to extremely high doses if needed to achieve adequate analgesia with minimal side effects.

Morphine is the gold standard of opioids, and the effectiveness, cost, and uses of other opioids are compared to

TABLE 18-4 Nonpharmacologic Pain Management Techniques for Children

NAME OF INTERVENTION	STEP-BY-STEP DESCRIPTION	USES
Distraction	1. Ask the family or child to identify the child's favorite activities, toys, and so forth. 2. Consider incorporating audio- or videotapes, television, music. 3. Promote play as the child would in his or her usual state of health. 4. Encourage interactions with same age and developmental level children.	All age groups. Strategies are good for ongoing acute pain (i.e., after surgery) or for procedural pain (i.e., phlebotomy or IV catheter insertion).
Preparation	1. Explain in developmentally appropriate terms what the child can expect to see, feel, hear, smell, or taste. Confirm the child understands the explanation. 2. Give realistic time frames for each sensation. 3. The younger the child, the closer to the time of the procedure preparation should occur. Prepare the child for what to expect and be honest about pain. 4. Encourage the child to safely play with equipment and act out the procedure on a doll or toy.	Most effective for preschool, school-age, or adolescent patients. Limited use in toddlers, not appropriate for infants. Should occur prior to a procedure expected to cause pain.
Relaxation	1. Position the child in a comfortable position. 2. Ask the child to take a deep breath, relaxing as he or she breathes in and out. 3. Starting with the toes, instruct the child to progressively relax body parts until the head is reached. 4. Decrease as much outside stimulation as possible.	For school-age or adolescent clients. Ideally, the instructions should be made prior to the pain. Useful for chronic or episodic pain. May be used as frequently as desired.
Cutaneous stimulation	1. Rub affected area in a consistent manner. 2. Apply ice or heat as warranted and desired to affected area or contralateral area. 3. Apply consistent gentle pressure to site of pain. 4. Use of a TENS (transcutaneous electrical nerve stimulator) also possible.	Useful for all age groups as tolerated. Combining techniques (i.e., heat and rubbing) is of maximum benefit.
Self exercises	1. *Positive Thinking*—Gives the child a positive focus "I will get better soon." 2. *Thought Stopping*—Memorize and repeat a statement focusing on positives of situation. "Short procedure, nice nurse, go home soon." 3. *Guided Imagery*—Formal exercises to help children through painful situations. Ask the child to envision a pleasant situation (real or imagined). Encourage the child to "go there" whenever the pain occurs. The child may need to develop a script of pleasant places and record it or write it down. When needed, the script may be played or read to the child. Details about the experience (sounds, smells, colors, textures) are included. Encourage the child to concentrate on the pleasant experience whenever pain is felt.	Most appropriate for older children. Encourage creativity and parent input. Good for children with chronic or cancer pain.
Hypnosis	Focused attention, altered state of consciousness (Specially trained personnel should induce hypnotic state).	Used with sequential painful procedures, such as burns, sickle cell disease, anticipated nausea, and vomiting associated with cancer treatment.

Table 18-5 Selected Opioid Pain Medications for Children

MEDICATION	INITIAL (STARTING) DOSING GUIDELINES	COMMENTS
Morphine	Parenteral: 0.05-0.1 mg/kg q 3–4 hours Oral: 0.3-0.5 mg/kg q 4 hrs	Oral formulation in elixir and tablets. Elixir ideal for younger children who cannot swallow tablets. Parenteral: oral conversion = 1:3.
Fentanyl	Parenteral: 0.5-2 mcg/kg q 1–2 hours Transmucosal or transdermal: 10–15 mcg/kg	Unique side effect with parenteral dosing is chest wall rigidity. (Reversed with naloxone Narcan.) Transmucosal (Fentanyl Oralet) for single-dose administration. Transdermal not recommended in children unless high opioid requirement (e.g., cancer pain).
Meperidine	Parenteral: 1 mg/kg q 3–4 hours Oral: 1–1.5 mg/kg q 6 hours	Not recommended for pain relief in children as metabolite accumulation (normeperidine) may cause CNS irritability and seizures.
Methadone	Parenteral/Oral: 0.1–0.2 mg/kg q 8–12 hours	Parenteral to oral conversion is 1:1. Oral formulation available as elixir or tablets.
Hydromorphone	Parenteral: 0.015 mg/kg q 3–4 hours Oral: 0.02 mg/kg q 3–4 hours	Often associated with less itching, nausea, or vomiting than other opioids.
Codeine	Parenteral: not recommended because of poor and painful site absorption and high occurrence of side effects Oral: 1 mg/kg q 3–4 hrs	Available as elixir and tablets combined with acetaminophen. This form is less expensive than codeine alone.
Oxycodone	Parenteral: not available Oral: 0.1 mg/kg q 4–6 hours	Available as elixir and tablets combined with acetaminophen.
Hydrocodone	Parenteral: not available Oral: 0.1-0.2 mg/kg q 4–6 hours	Available as elixir and tablets combined with acetaminophen or ibuprofen.

Adapted from Agency for Health Care Policy and Research. (1992). Acute pain management in infants, children, and adolescents: Operative and medical procedures. Clinical practice guidelines. (AHCPR Publication No. 92-0020). Rockville, MD; Author; American Pain Society (2008). ***Principles of analgesic use in the treatment of acute pain and cancer pain*** (6th ed.), Glenview, IL: Author.

morphine. For children, opioids are dosed by weight. Neonatal doses are reduced by one-third to one-quarter to account for their immature liver function and differences in metabolism. (See Table 18-5 for specific dosing recommendations.) Larger children (greater than 50 kilograms) may receive adult doses. Appropriate dosing is an important aspect of pain management and care should be taken to appropriately individualize the dose so as to promote adequate analgesia and minimize side effects. Most intravenous opioids can also be converted to oral doses of the same or similar opioids. Side effects of opioids are most commonly nausea, vomiting, constipation, and pruritus.

Rather than discontinue the use of opioids, side effects should be treated as long as the analgesic is effective. If a child is experiencing severe side effects from an opioid analgesic and not receiving adequate pain relief, a nonopioid pain medication should be added to the pain management protocol to augment pain relief while minimizing opioid side effects. Adjuvant medications such as antihistamines or a low dose intravenous infusion of naloxone are effective in treating pruritus, while antiemetics can be used to treat nausea and vomiting (Miaskowski, Bair, Chou, D'Arcy, Hartrick, & Huffman, 2008).

Respiratory depression and hypotension are rare and dangerous side effects of opioid analgesics treated with the opioid antagonist naloxone at a dose that reverses respiratory depression but does not reverse analgesic effects. Dosing of naloxone is given in Box 18-3.

Opioids should be dosed at regular intervals; commonly, they are on a PRN schedule and administered when pain is assessed or reported. However, this type of dosing is inappropriate for children. First, PRN dosing places the onus to request medication for pain on the child and many children do not report their pain. Second, children may fear the treatment

NURSING ALERT

Fentanyl

Fentanyl has a unique, additional side effect: chest wall rigidity. The client is unable to breathe because of ineffective movement of the chest wall muscles, and manual ventilation is difficult. Carefully monitor clients for this side effect, which is reversible with naloxone. Slow IV administration of the medication will also decrease the potential side effect.

NURSING TIP

Reverse PRN Method

When using the reverse PRN method, prompt children by informing them pain medication is available and will be available again. For example, "It is time for your pain medication. Would you like it now?" The children can make their own decisions regarding accepting or declining the medication. For infants and toddlers, perform a pain assessment when it is time to administer the medication and administer as warranted.

for pain will be an injection. Third, despite repeated instructions, children may forget the pain medication is available upon request. Finally, very young children are not able to request pain medication because of undeveloped language and cognitive skills. Therefore, an alternative to PRN dosing is "reverse PRN" medication delivery. Here, the nurse asks about or assesses the client's pain at the prescribed time interval the medication may be administered. Medication is then administered if pain is present. Often children respond favorably to this method.

Analgesics may also be administered using an around-the-clock dosing schedule. Here, the child receives pain medications at preset intervals. The effects of the medication should be continually reassessed to assure the child is receiving adequate analgesia. The presence of side effects, level of analgesia, and level of consciousness are also continually monitored. If side effects appear, the medication may be titrated, discontinued, or a substitute analgesic given.

Nonsteroidal Anti-Inflammatory Drugs (NSAIDs)

Nonsteroidal anti-inflammatory drugs (NSAIDs) may be used independently to treat mild to moderate pain or in conjunction with opioids to treat more severe pain. NSAIDs work by inhibiting prostaglandins at the site of the pain. The most common NSAIDs are ibuprofen, naproxen, and ketorolac. Aspirin, another NSAID, is rarely used in children because of its association with Reye's syndrome. These drugs are beneficial because of their anti-inflammatory, antipyretic, and analgesic effects. Table 18-6 reviews dosing for this class of medications.

Another class of NSAID analgesics is the cyclooxygenase-2 (COX-2) inhibitors. These drugs inhibit only one part of the prostaglandin pathway, resulting in fewer adverse hematologic, gastrointestinal, and renal effects (American Pain Society, 2008). Celecoxib is the most commonly used drug in this class. Research suggests that COX-2 inhibitors may not negatively impact bone healing as seen with traditional NSAIDs (American Pain Society, 2008). This may allow for use of these medications in clients with postoperative orthopedic pain. Adverse cardiovascular effects may also occur with COX-2 inhibitors, so patients should be carefully monitored while receiving these drugs.

Other Drugs

Acetaminophen is not an anti-inflammatory drug because it has no effect on prostaglandin synthesis. The drug of choice for fever in children, acetaminophen is also effective for relieving mild to moderate pain, and may be used in conjunction with opioids or NSAIDs for moderate to severe pain. Another useful analgesic is tramadol hydrochloride, a synthetic analog of codeine which acts by binding to the

BOX 18-3

NALOXONE (NARCAN) DOSING

Children: 0.005 – 0.01 mg/kg. May repeat every 2 – 3 minutes up to 3 doses. Repeat dosage at 1 to 2 hour intervals as necessary.

American Pain Society (2008). *Principles of analgesic use in the treatment of acute pain and cancer pain* (6th ed.). Glenview, IL: Author.

NURSING ALERT

Opioid-Induced Respiratory Depression

Opioids can have a cumulative effect. The drugs may accumulate in a client's system due to slow acetylation or decreased end organ function. Monitor clients on an around-the-clock dosing schedule for oversedation leading to respiratory depression.

Table 18-6 Selected Nonsteroidal Anti-Inflammatory Pain Medications

MEDICATION	INITIAL DOSING GUIDELINES	COMMENTS
Ibuprofen	5-10 mg/kg po q 6–8 hours. Maximum: 40 mg/kg/day	Associated with gastric irritation. Administer with food or milk. Available as solution or chewable or oral tablets. Do not administer with other NSAIDs.
Acetylsalicylic acid (Aspirin)	10-15 mg/kg po q 4 hours Maximum daily dose: 75 mg/kg/day up to 4 gm/day	Associated with Reye's syndrome. Do not administer to any child with viral illness within the last four weeks.
Ketorolac	Oral dose (Adult): 10 mg/dose. Parenteral: 0.5 mg/kg q 6 hours Maximum single dose: 30 mg Maximum daily dose: 120 mg/day	Do not administer for longer than five consecutive days because of increased incidence of gastric bleeding, renal insufficiency. Do not administer with other NSAIDs.
Naproxen	5-10 mg/kg po q 12 hours Maximum dose: 1.5 gm/day	Available as solution or tablets. Do not administer with other NSAIDs.

Adapted from Agency for Health Care Policy and Research. (1992). Acute pain management in infants, children and adolescents: Operative and medical procedures; American Pain Society (2008). ***Principles of analgesic use in the treatment of acute pain and cancer pain*** (6th ed.), Glenview, IL: Author.

Mu opioid receptor in the central nervous system and inhibiting the reuptake of the neurotransmitters serotonin and norepinephrine (American Pain Society, 2008). Tramadol is an effective analgesic alone or as an adjunct to other analgesics for pain of mild to moderate intensity. Adverse effects are generally mild; nausea and vomiting were found to be no more common with Tramadol than with morphine (Chu, Lin, Hsieh, Chan, & Tsou, 2006).

PATIENT-CONTROLLED ANALGESIA

Patient-controlled analgesia (PCA) is a computer-operated pump that allows the patient to self-administer pain medication. By pushing a button on the pump, children as young as 5 or 6 years old may self-administer intravenous opioids to relieve pain. Patient-controlled analgesia is available to most children in the acute care setting and may also be administered at home. The PCA dosing regimen allows for a steady drug state and more consistent analgesia while avoiding the undesired side effects associated with delivering relatively large doses of bolus analgesics. The delivery of small frequent doses of opioids provides better pain relief without sedation. By maintaining a steady amount of the analgesic, the child receives better pain control with less risk of untoward effects (Figure 18-12).

PCA pain relief offers several advantages over traditional treatment modalities. Aside from the already mentioned advantages of superior analgesia and safer drug delivery, PCA offers the child the ability to quickly and independently relieve his or her pain. For many school-age children and adolescents, having a sense of control over their treatment is an important element of care. The dose is tailored to the patient's weight and easily titrated for a child's changing pain control needs. Several medications are available for delivery via a PCA pump: morphine, fentanyl, hydromorphone and Tramadol.

PCA pumps offer several programming options. The pump may be programmed in "PCA only" mode, where doses of the medication are delivered only when the client

Reflections from Families

My son, D'andre, has Sickle Cell Disease. He gets bad pain in his arms or legs when the weather changes. When he hurts a lot, I take him to the hospital and they give him the PCA. That usually helps his pain. Since we come in so often, D'andre has his favorite nurses. They are the ones who talk to him about his pain and ask him how he is feeling and what can they do to make his pain less. The other thing that helps him is playing video games, because it takes his mind off his pain.

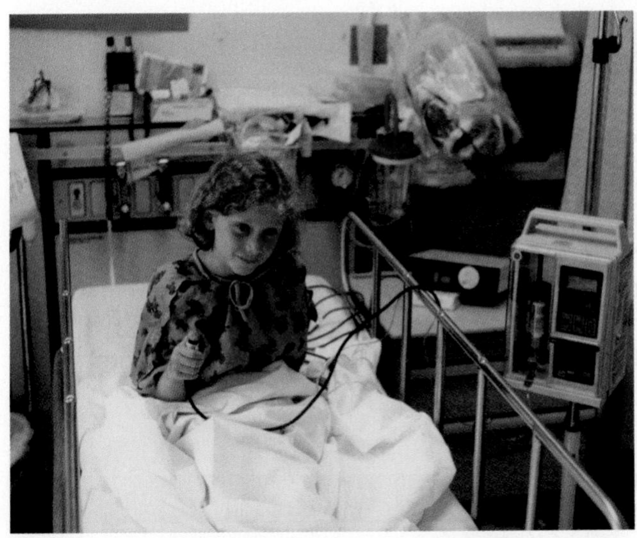

FIGURE 18-12 This child is using her PCA pump. DELMAR CENGAGE LEARNING.

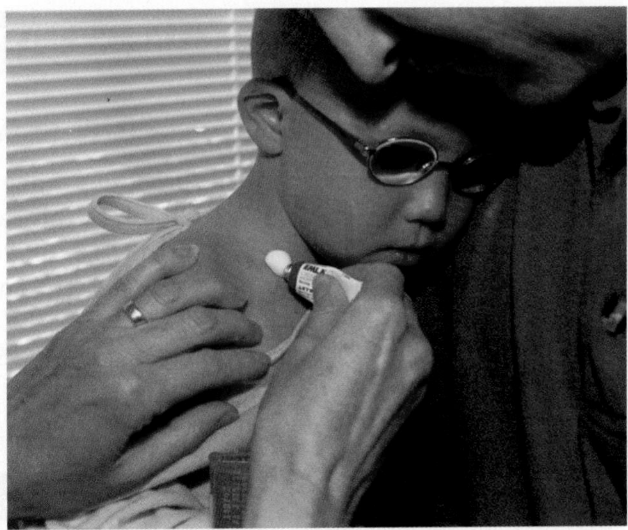

FIGURE 18-13 EMLA Application. DELMAR CENGAGE LEARNING.

requests a dose by pushing the button. In the "PCA plus (1) continuous" mode, the pump delivers a preprogrammed background infusion of the analgesic and administers additional medication according to patient request. The PCA (1) continuous mode is especially effective for young children who are often remiss or do not realize they need to push the button to administer their analgesic. The use of different modalities should be tailored to the child's ability to push the PCA button, considering developmental level and the anticipated pain management needs (Figure 18-12). A somewhat controversial but sometimes effective practice is that of parent- or nurse-assisted analgesia. When a child is too ill to participate in his or her care or developmentally incapable of understanding the concept of PCA, a parent or nurse can serve as the authorized agent by operating the PCA button for the child. Education of the authorized agent is critical since operation of the button by an individual other than the client puts the client at greater risk for oversedation. It is recommended the authorized agent be trained in proper use of the device and interpretation of pulse oximetry and pediatric pain assessment (Wuhrman, Cooney, Dunwoody, Eksterowicz, Merkel, & Oakes, 2007).

LOCAL OR REGIONAL ANESTHESIA

Several techniques are now available to relieve pain using local or regional anesthesia. The area of the body where pain is expected may be numbed by using a local or regional anesthetic injection with or without an opioid. Procedural pain (lumbar puncture, bone marrow aspiration) may also be ameliorated by using a local anesthetic cream such as eutectic mixture of local anesthetics (EMLA, composed of prilocaine and lidocaine) or LMX (lidocaine in a liposomal vehicle). Both are applied to the skin prior to the procedure (EMLA up to three hours), covered with an occlusive dressing, and can eliminate the pain of the initial injection for most children (Figure 18-13). ELA-max (lidocaine topical local anesthetic) has the advantage of faster onset of analgesia (30 minutes) and no need for an occlusive dressing (Cregin, Rappaport, Montagnino, Sabogal, Moreau, & Abularrage, 2008).

Regional anesthesia is applied to a region of the body, usually in association with a surgical procedure by blocking or numbing specific nerves or nerve segments prior to the surgical procedure to prevent the pain sensation. Some surgeries or procedures are performed using only local or regional anesthesia. In such cases, the area may be numb for a period of time (2–12 hours) following the procedure. Once the block has worn off, the client will need an alternate pain management plan.

EPIDURAL OR INTRASPINAL ANALGESIA

Opioids, local anesthetics, or a combination of the two can also be administered via the epidural or intraspinal route. This method of delivery provides complete analgesia for surgery or postoperatively, when medications are delivered via a single injection that lasts 2–12 hours or by an indwelling catheter that remains in for 1 to 5 days. The catheter is generally removed before the fifth postoperative day, because risk of infection increases with each day the catheter remains in place. The catheter exit site should be assessed at regular intervals to detect any signs of infiltration or infection and should be covered with an occlusive transparent dressing.

SEDATION AND ANALGESIA FOR PROCEDURES

Many hospitalized and ill children require analgesia and sedation to control motion and anxiety during necessary

CASE STUDY / CARE PLAN

PAIN MANAGEMENT

Ryan is a 2-year-old boy who had surgery to repair a congenital hip problem 12 hours ago. He is in a full body cast. Ryan cries constantly and grabs at his cast. He weighs 40 lbs (18 kg) and has no known drug allergies. His vital signs are T 37.2 ax, HR 140, RR 28, BP 94/64. The night shift nurse is concerned Ryan's pain is not adequately controlled on his current analgesic regime of 2 mg morphine every 4 hours PRN and acetaminophen 240 mg rectally every 6 hours. Ryan is scheduled to go home in the morning with his grandmother, Mary, who is his primary caregiver. She, too, is concerned about his current pain and how she will manage his pain at home.

NURSING CARE PLAN

ASSESSMENT

- Toddler with restricted mobility
- Elevated heart rate
- Fear related to medical procedures
- Inability to communicate about how he is feeling
- Pain related to surgical procedure

NURSING DIAGNOSIS

Pain related to surgical procedure.

EXPECTED OUTCOMES

1. Ryan will have adequate pain control as evidenced by normal vital signs, less crying, ability to sleep, ability to tolerate position changes, and engagement in pleasurable activities.
2. Grandmother will verbalize signs that indicate pain versus frustration in Ryan.
3. Grandmother will verbalize appropriate action to take when child exhibits pain.

NOC: Pain Control—Adequate

NIC: Pain Management

INTERVENTIONS/*RATIONALES*

1. Assess Ryan's pain using an objective pain scale such as FLACC. *Child is too young to self-rate pain.*
2. Administer morphine every 4 hours. *Child is too young for PRN dosing, cannot request pain medication.*
3. Reassess pain within 30 minutes of analgesic. *Will provide information about adequacy of morphine dose.*
4. Request order for oral acetaminophen if tolerated. *Deliver analgesics via least traumatic route.*

(Continues)

CASE STUDY / CARE PLAN (Continued)

5. Use cold packs over surgical site. *Cold minimizes inflammation.*
6. Incorporate familiar toys and security objects from home. *Decreases anxiety and provides distraction.*
7. Incorporate input from grandmother. *She is most familiar with his reactions to stress and pain.*

EVALUATION

Ryan's grandmother stated he is normally a very active child and was upset about the restricted mobility imposed by the cast. He received morphine for a FLACC score of 7. Thirty minutes after receiving morphine, Ryan's FLACC score was 0 and he was able to sleep for 3 hours. In the morning, the grandmother was able to put Ryan in a cart so he could go to the playroom where he enjoyed watching other children playing with trucks. Continue to monitor Ryan's pain regularly using the FLACC scale and provide analgesics as necessary.

KIDS WANT TO KNOW

Numbness

"I can't feel my foot. Is it still there?" Peter asks after receiving a local anesthetic.

- Assure Peter the feeling of numbness is temporary from medication and will subside.
- Show Peter his foot by moving blankets, using a mirror, or repositioning.
- Tell Peter he may experience tingling or "pins-and-needles" in the affected area as sensation returns.

FAMILY TEACHING

Chronic Pain

Household activities should not revolve around the child's pain. Advise caregivers not to question the child every day regarding the pain, so as not to emphasize the experience or promote secondary gains. The child should be asked to only discuss pain if there is a significant change in the pain experienced.

medical procedures (i.e., bone marrow aspiration, burn or wound dressing care, endoscopy, or radiological procedures). The goal of this type of sedation, called **conscious sedation** or sedation and analgesia, is to safely prevent the child from experiencing pain while also decreasing memory of the procedure. This depressed state of consciousness, usually achieved by administration of intravenous sedatives and analgesics, leaves protective reflexes intact. The child continues to breathe spontaneously. Clients receiving such sedation need to have their heart rates, respiratory rates, and blood oxygen levels electronically monitored and have an independent observer who watches the client but does not participate in the procedure. Commonly used sedative medications include chloral hydrate, fentanyl citrate, midazolam hydrochloride, ketamine hydrochloride, and propofol. It is important to note that midazolam can be reversed with the benzodiapine antagonist Flumazenil, but ketamine and propofol have no such reversal agents (Dolansky, Shah, Mosdossy, & Rieder, 2008).

HEADACHE PAIN

Migraine or cluster headaches are intense and often associated with nausea or photophobia (light sensitivity). They tend to involve the frontal or temporal regions of the head or are localized retro-orbitally (Winner, 2008). The child can often predict the onset of a migraine headache by an **aura**, or premonition of its beginning. These headaches last from several hours to days and can be very debilitating. Often, there is a positive family history of migraines. Several medications have been effective in treating migraine headaches, including Fiorinal, Midrin, and sumatriptan (Imitrex). Biofeedback and relaxation therapy as well as prophylactic treatment with propanolol (Inderal), phenobarbital, and amitriptyline (Elavil) have also proven successful (Winner, 2008).

Chronic tension headaches are most often seen in adolescents or older school-age children. They tend to involve the temporal or occipital regions bilaterally, are diffuse, extend to the neck, and are continuous during the day. Stress in the child's life is a contributing factor in this type of headache and steps should be taken to identify the stressors. Often, these children become accustomed to having a headache and can no longer identify the inciting triggers or

EVIDENCE-BASED PRACTICE

Parent's Assessment and Management of a Child's Postoperative Pain

CLINICAL PROBLEM

Even though same day or minor surgery is beneficial to children, pain continues to be an issue parents need to manage after discharge. Parents are expected to assess and treat their child's pain at home and also be involved in the care of their children postoperatively, especially when the child is discharged. However, the increasing number of outpatient surgeries children experience may be pushing the boundaries of family-centered care, especially if parents are unprepared to assess and manage postoperative pain in these children.

BEST CLINICAL PRACTICE

Evidence suggests families are willing and able to effectively manage a child's pain, especially if they are supported and provided with information about the analgesic administered and other methods of pain relief (distraction, breathing exercises, body massage). Parents may also sometimes have difficulty detecting pain in a child, could be concerned about addiction, and receive most of their advice about pain management from nurses. Use of a simple checklist including guidelines for administering pain medication as well as other methods of pain relief (see above as well as appropriate positioning and handling of the child) can be helpful. Follow up with written instructions after an oral discussion may also be useful, especially if the discharge teaching relative to pain management is timely and relevant. Family members need information about resources or actions when the prescribed analgesics does not reduce the child's pain. Phone contact from health care professionals after discharge may also allay parent's anxiety and provide opportunities for questions to be answered.

IMPLICATIONS FOR NURSING

- Provide parents whose child will be discharged after having surgery or other painful procedure with comprehensive written and oral instructions on the analgesic ordered (dose, importance of administering medication regularly instead of when the child complains of pain). Written materials should be in a language familiar to the parents and at an appropriate literacy level.
- Begin to prepare parents for home care before admission to the hospital.
- Provide parents with assessment and treatment strategies appropriate to the child's age for use at home. Include information on how to assess pain in children.
- Educate parents about nonpharmacologic measures for pain control.
- Provide parents with adequate medication upon discharge.
- Provide information regarding places to go for answers to postdischarge questions relative to pain management.
- Provide postdischarge support by contacting families by telephone within 24–48 hours after discharge.

Reference: Wilson, M. E., & Helgadóttir, H. L. (2006). Patterns of pain and analgesic use in 3- to-7-year-old children after tonsillectomy. *Pain Management Nursing, 7*(4), 159–166.

IN THE REAL WORLD

I used to worry about giving these kids such strong medication but I have never seen a serious problem. They are happy to have their pain relieved so they can go to the playroom. The kids are different than adults on the med-surg floor who never got out of bed and slept all the time after surgery.

situations. Children suffering from chronic tension headaches are best treated with a program combining stress management, behavior management, and individual and family therapy (Hershey, Winner, Kabbouche, & Powers, 2007).

ABDOMINAL PAIN

Abdominal pain is another common chronic pain complaint in children. It is classified as visceral (dull or crampy and poorly localized), somatic (reflects peritoneal inflammation, is localized to the area of the involved viscera), or referred (caused by local irritation and referral along the organ's innervation pathway). An organic cause of a child's abdominal pain should always be explored because it may indicate colic, food allergy, intussusception, appendicitis, Meckel's diverticulum, peritonitis, urinary tract infection, or other pathology.

Periumbilical pain is often associated with functional abdominal pain disorder, a common childhood disorder affecting children between the ages of 5 and 19 years of age that is severe enough to affect activities. The pain rarely occurs at night and does not interrupt sleep. Sometimes, constipation is associated with functional abdominal pain. Nursing care for the child with chronic abdominal pain consists of support, education about coping techniques, assurance the experience is common and probably will be outgrown, and, if applicable, a bowel program regime.

HOME CARE OF THE CHILD IN PAIN

Many children with pain conditions are now managed at home. Whether the source of the pain is a chronic condition, a pain syndrome, or following a surgical or invasive procedure, caregivers should be instructed in the home care of the child experiencing pain. Medications, including route, doses, actions, and the administration schedule are taught to the caregivers and child, if appropriate. The family is also encouraged to use specific home remedies or their own nonpharmacologic interventions to relieve the child's pain. Some families may wish to use herbal or folk remedies. However, caregivers should be cautioned that when ingesting herbal remedies, dosing information, safety, and drug interactions might not be known. Families wishing to utilize such remedies should consult their health care provider and every effort should be made to investigate the safety of such interventions.

KEY CONCEPTS

- Pain physiology involves transmission, transduction, modulation, and perception.
- The gate control theory is the most common pain theory.
- Misconceptions of pain in children include: infants do not feel pain, infants and children are more sensitive to opioids than adults, pain is character building, children and adolescents will become addicted to opioids if used, and children who are playing, sleeping, or can be distracted are not in pain.
- Children experience pain in the context of their developmental level, social and psychological experiences, and their environment.
- Several objective and subjective measures are available to determine a child's pain experience or responses to treatment.
- Nonpharmacologic pain treatment can be used as an alternative to or in conjunction with pharmacologic pain treatment.
- For moderate to severe pain, opioids are the treatment of choice with doses tailored to the child's height, weight, and individual analgesic needs.
- Nonopioid pain medications, such as topical preparations, NSAIDs, and acetaminophen, may be used to treat mild to moderate pain or given in conjunction with opioids to treat more severe pain.
- Local or regional anesthesia, used before, during, or after a procedure, is an appropriate method of treating pain in children.
- Chronic pain, including headaches and abdominal pain, is a unique and difficult-to-treat problem with specific treatment regimes for long-term management.
- In caring for the child at home, families can incorporate their own treatments for pain with prescribed pharmacologic and nonpharmacologic interventions. However, home or folk remedies, including herbal treatment, should be carefully reviewed for possible drug interactions or dangerous side effects.

REVIEW QUESTIONS

1. Describe the physiology of pain. Chart or diagram the cycle of the pain impulse through the nervous system; include the components of the gate control theory.
2. Describe common pediatric pain misconceptions. Delineate scientific information correcting the misperceptions.
3. How do infants experience pain? What indicates an infant is experiencing pain?
4. What unique pain behaviors do toddlers exhibit? Preschoolers? School-age children?
5. What differentiates an adolescent's pain experiences from those of adults?
6. Describe the components of a complete pain assessment.
7. Choose three common pediatric pain assessment tools. Describe their implementation. For what age child is each appropriate?
8. How are opioids dosed in children? How is patient-controlled analgesia used in children?
9. How are opioid side effects managed in children? (Specify side effect and management.)
10. Describe regional analgesia.
11. What are the characteristics of chronic pain in children? How is chronic pain treated?
12. What would you include in a home treatment pain management plan? What treatments would you caution a family to use at home?

STUDY QUESTIONS

(Questions 1 and 2) A new graduate nurse is caring for 2-year-old Timmy, who is postoperative day #1 S/P surgery for a ruptured appendix. At 8:00 a.m., the nurse notes that Timmy is sleeping and that no pain assessment has been recorded since 9:00 p.m. the previous evening, just prior to receiving a dose of 2 mg. Morphine I.V.

1. The nurse does not want to disturb Timmy since he is sleeping. Select the statement that best describes an evidence-based plan of care:
   a. Timmy should not be awakened until he awakens naturally.
   b. Timmy should not be awakened because he cannot be experiencing pain if he is sleeping.
   c. Timmy should be awakened to assess his pain and level of consciousness.
   d. Timmy should be awakened because he is unlikely to have significant pain.
2. Which pain scale would be most appropriate to use to assess Timmy's pain if he is developmentally and cognitively normal for his age?
   a. Numeric Pain Rating Scale
   b. Faces Pain Scale
   c. The Oucher
   d. Face, Legs, Arms, Cry, and Consolability (FLACC)

(Questions 3 through 7) You are caring for 7-year-old Tatanesha, who is receiving treatment for sickle cell pain. Tatanesha is receiving a weight-appropriate dose of morphine via PCA (0.3mg/hr., 0.3 mg q 8 minutes). She rates her pain 8/10 on the Faces pain scale. Her mother thinks Tatanesha's pain is not that high, probably more like a 4 or 6.

3. Select the most accurate statement regarding pain assessment in this situation:
   a. When a discrepancy between the child's and parent's pain rating exists, the parent's rating is usually more accurate.
   b. Tatanesha is vying for attention since she is receiving an adequate opioid dose to relieve her pain.
   c. Self-report is the best method to assess pain in this situation.
   d. The nurse should validate Tatanesha's pain rating using a second scale.
4. Tatanesha begins to complain of her face, neck, and chest itching. No skin changes are noted. What is the most appropriate action for the nurse to take?
   a. Stop the morphine PCA and call the physician.
   b. Obtain an order for a medication to counteract the itching.
   c. Change the sheets on Tatanesha's bed to hypo-allergenic sheets.
   d. Suggest that the PCA drug be switched to hydromorphone.
5. Tatanesha complains of 8/10 pain and asks for an increase in her morphine. Her mother says, "No, baby. The more of that medicine you take, the more addicted you're going to be." How would you respond?
   a. "I can see that you are concerned about the effects of the pain medication. However, it's unlikely that Tatanesha will become addicted since she is using the medication to relieve severe pain."
   b. "Although addiction is a concern, Tatanesha must continue taking the medication or she will not get better."
   c. "Would you like to speak to the doctor about changing Tatanesha's medication to something less addicting?"
   d. "Don't worry, I'm sure everything will be just fine."
6. What other therapies might you suggest to help relieve Tatanesha's pain?
   a. Physical therapy
   b. Addition of a scheduled nonsteroidal anti-inflammatory agent (NSAID)
   c. Frequent ambulation
   d. Addition of an oral opioid
7. Tatanesha weighs 26 kg. By day 3 of her pain crisis, she is receiving morphine 0.9 mg per hour and 0.9 mg q 8 minutes via PCA. She is currently rating her pain 2/10, is alert and talkative. The dose of morphine she is receiving is:
   a. Too high for her age and weight
   b. Too low because her pain is not yet 0
   c. Appropriate
   d. Likely to cause renal failure
8. Darnell, 11 years old, has chronic pain that has been diagnosed as functional abdominal pain. Which strategy would be least helpful?
   a. Encourage consistent attendance at school
   b. Expectation that he will continue to do his daily chores
   c. Asking him to rate his pain regularly and record it in a diary
   d. Reassurance that the pain will get better
9. Three months after Darnell begins treatment, he is going to school on most days and tells his parents when his pain is worse than usual, although he still complains about doing his chores. How would you assess Darnell's behavior?
   a. He is coping well.
   b. His pain has resolved.

c. His pain was due to anxiety.
d. He is a chronic complainer.

10. Julia, 2 years old, had outpatient surgery for an umbilical hernia. Intra-operatively, she received a single dose of epidural local anesthetic. She appears comfortable during her stay in the post-anesthesia recovery unit. Select the most important item to teach Julia's parents:
a. Do not give Julia pain medication until she requests it or shows nonverbal signs of pain.
b. Mix the liquid analgesic in at least four ounces of juice.
c. An oral analgesic will not be necessary because she received a block.
d. The local anesthetic will wear off about six hours after it was given. Oral analgesics should be started before this happens.

REFERENCES

Agency for Health Care Policy and Research. (1992). Acute pain management in infants, children, and adolescents: Operative and medical procedures. Clinical practice guidelines. (AHCPR Publication No. 92-0020). Rockville, MD; Author.

American Academy of Pediatrics. (2005). Circumcision Policy Statement. *Pediatrics, 103*(3), 686–693.

American Pain Society (2008). Principles of analgesic use in the treatment of acute pain and cancer pain (6th ed.), Glenview, IL: Author.

Anand, K., Aranda, J., Berde, C., Buckman, S., Capparelli, E., & Carlo, W. et al., (2006). Summary proceedings from the neonatal pain-control group. *Pediatrics, 117*(3), S9–S22.

Anand, K., & Hickey, P. (1987). Pain and its effect on the human fetus and neonate. *New England Journal of Medicine, 317*, 1321–1329.

Bailey, B., Bergeron, S., Gravel, J., & Dauost, R. (2007). Comparison of four pain scales in children with acute abdominal pain in a pediatric emergency department. *Annals of Emergency Medicine, 50*(4), 379–383.

Beebe, L., & Wyatt, T. (2009). Guided imagery and music: Using the Bonny method to evoke emotion and access the unconscious. *Journal of Psychosocial Nursing and Mental Health Services, 47*(1), 29–33.

Bellieni, C., Sisto, R., Cordelli, D., & Buonocore, G. (2004). Cry features reflect pain intensity in term newborns: An alarm threshold. *Pediatric Research, 55*(1), 142–146.

Bijur, P., Latimer, C., & Gallagher, E. (2003). Validation of a verbally administered numerical rating scale of acute pain for use in the emergency department. *Academic Emergency Medicine, 10*(4), 390–392.

Brown-Trask, B., Van Sell, S., Carter, C., & Kindred, C. (2009). Circumcision care. *RN, 72*(2), 22–28.

Chu, Y., Lin, S., Hsieh, Y., Chan, K., & Tsou, M. (2006). Intraoperative administration of tramadol for postoperative nurse controlled analgesia resulted in earlier awakening and less sedation than morphine in children after cardiac surgery. *Anesthesia and Analgesia, 102*, 1668–1673.

Cregin, R., Rappaport, A., Montagnino, G., Sabogal, G., Moreau, H., & Abularrage, J. (2008). Improving pain management for pediatric patients undergoing nonurgent painful procedures. *American Journal of Health-System Pharmacy, 65*(8), 723–727.

Davidhizar, R., & Giger, J. (2004). A review of the literature on care of clients in pain who are culturally diverse. *International Nursing Review, 51*, 47–55.

Dolansky, G., Shah, A., Mosdossy, G., & Rieder, M. J. (2008). What is the evidence for the safety and efficacy of using ketamine in children? *Paediatric Child Health, 13*(4), 307–308.

Gimbler-Beglund, I., Ljusegran, G., & Enskar, K. (2008). Factors influencing pain management in children. *Paediatric Nursing, 20*(10), 21–24.

Hall, R., & Shbarou, R. (2009). Drugs of choice for sedation and analgesia in the neonatal ICU. *Clinics in Perinatology, 36*(1), 15–26.

Hamunen, K., Maunuksela, E., & Olkkola, K. (2008). Interpretation of the large red-and-white visual analog scale by children compared with adults. *Journal of Pediatric Nursing, 23*(2), 142–144.

Helms, J., & Barone, C. (2009). Physiology and treatment of pain. *Critical Care Nurse, 28*(6), 38–49.

Hershey, A., Winner, P., Kabbouche, M., & Powers, S. (2007). Headaches. *Current Opinions in Pediatrics, 19*(6), 663–669.

Hester, N. O., & Barcus, C. S. (1986). Assessment and management of children in pain. *Pediatrics: Nursing Update, 1*, 2–8.

Hicks, C. L., von Baeyer, C. L., Spafford, P., van Korlaar, I., & Goodenough, B. (2001). Faces Pain Scale-Revised: Toward a common metric in pediatric pain measurement. *Pain, 93*, 173–183.

Howard, R. (2003). Current status of pain management in children. *JAMA—Journal of the American Medical Association, 290*(18), 2464–2469 (November 12, 2003).

Johansson, M., & Kokinsky, E. (2009). The COMFORT behavioural scale and the modified FLACC scale in paediatric intensive care. *Nursing in Critical Care, 14*(3), 122–130.

Kortesluoma, R., Nikkonen, M., & Serlo, W. (2008). "You just have to make the pain go away"—Children's experiences of pain management. *Pain Management Nursing, 9*(4), 143–149.

Lawrence, J., Alcock, D., McGrath, P., Kay, J., MacMurray, S. B., & Dulberg, C. (1993). The development of a tool to assess neonatal pain. *Neonatal Network, 12*(6), 59–66.

Melzack, R., & Wall, P. (1965). Pain mechanisms: A new theory. *Science, 150*, 971–979.

Miaskowski, C., Bair, M., Chou, R., D'Arcy, Y., Hartrick, C., & Huffman, L. (2008). Principles of analgesic use in the treatment of acute pain and cancer pain. Glenview, IL: *American Pain Society.*

Savedra, M., Tesler, M., Holzemer, W., & Ward, J. (1992). *Adolescent pediatric pain tool: User manual.* San Francisco: University of California.

Schiavenato, M., Byers, J., Scovanner, P., McMahon, J., Xia, Y., Lu, N., & He, H. (2008). Neonatal pain facial expression: Evaluating the primal face of pain. *Pediatrics, 138*(2), 460–471.

Taddio, A., Shah, V., Atenafu, E., & Katz, J. (2009). Influence of repeated painful procedures and sucrose analgesia on the development of hyperalgesia in newborn infants. *Pain, 144*(1–2), 43–48.

Twycross, A. (2008). Does the perceived importance of a pain management task affect the quality of children's nurses' post-operative pain management practices? *Journal of Clinical Nursing, 17,* 3205–3216.

Van Dijk, M., Peters, W. B., Van Deventner, P., & Tibboel, D. (2005). The comfort behavior scale. *American Journal of Nursing, 105*(1), 33-35, 37.

Vincent, C. (2007). Nurses' perceptions of children's pain: A pilot study of cognitive representations. *Journal of Pain and Symptom Management, 33*(3), 290–301.

von Baeyer, C. L., Spagrud, L. J., McCormick, J. C., Choo, E., Neville, K., & Connelly, M. (2009). Three new datasets supporting use of the Numerical Rating Scale (NRS-11) for children's self-reports of pain intensity. *Pain, 143*(3), 223–227.

Wilson, M. E., & Helgadóttir, H. L. (2006). Patterns of pain and analgesic use in 3- to 7-year-old children after tonsillectomy. *Pain Management Nursing, 7*(4), 159–166.

Winner, P. (2008). *Pain Management Nursing.* (3), 316–322.

Wuhrman, E., Cooney, M. F., Dunwoody, C. J., Eksterowicz, N., Merkel, S., & Oakes, L. L. (2007). Authorized and unauthorized ("PCA by Proxy") dosing of analgesic infusion pumps. *Pain Management Nursing, 7*(4), 136.

Zhou, H., Roberts, P., & Horgan, L. (2008). Association between self-report pain ratings of child and parent, child and nurse, and parent and nurse dyads: Meta-analysis. *Journal of Advanced Nursing, 63*(4), 334–342.

SUGGESTED READINGS

American Academy of Pediatrics. (2001). The assessment and management of acute pain in infants, children, and adolescents. *Pediatrics, 108,* 793–797.

Anderson, B. J., & Palmer, G. M. (2006). Recent developments in the pharmacological management of pain in children. *Current Opinion in Anaesthesiology, 19*(3), 285–292.

Bursch, B., Tsao, J. C., Meldrum, M., & Zeltzer, L. K. (2006). Preliminary validation of a self-efficacy scale for child functioning despite chronic pain (child and parent versions). *Pain, 125*(1-2), 35–42.

Connelly, M., & Rapoff, M. A. (2006). Assessing health-related quality of life in children with recurrent headache: Reliability and validity of the PedsQLTM 4.0 in a pediatric headache sample. *Journal of Pediatric Psychology, 31*(7), 698–702.

Ellis, J. A., McCleary, L., Blouin, R., Dube, K., Rowley, B., MacNeil, M., & Cooke, C. (2007). Implementing best practice pain management in a pediatric hospital. *Journal of Specialty in Pediatric Nursing, 12*(4), 264–277.

Latimer, M. A., Johnston, C., Ritchie, J., Clarke, S., & Gillin, D. (2009). Factors affecting delivery of evidence-based procedural pain care in hospitalized neonates. *Journal of Obstetric, Gynecologic, and Neonatal Nursing, 38*(2), 182.

Logan, D. E., Catanese, S. P., Coakley, R. M., & Scharff, L. (2007). Chronic pain in the classroom: Teachers' attributions about the causes of chronic pain. *Journal of School Health, 77*(5), 248–256.

MacLaren, J. E., Cohen, L. L., Larkin, K. T., & Shelton, E. N. (2008). Training nursing students in evidence-based techniques for cognitive-behavioral pediatric pain management. *Journal of Nursing Education, 47*(8), 351–358.

Mowery, B. D., Suddaby, E., Kang, K. A., & Cooper, L. (2008). The art of procedural sedation and analgesia. *Pediatric Nursing, 34*(6), 490–492.

Von Baeyer, C. L., & Spagrud, L. J. (2007). Systematic review of observational (behavioral) measures of pain for children and adolescents aged 3 to 18 years. *Pain, 127*(1–2), 140–150.

RESOURCES

Refer to the online student StudyWARE for Potts & Mandleco at http://www.CengageBrain.com for additional content and study aids.

Organization: **American Pain Society**

Description: Offers information regarding membership in the American Pain Society, education, publications, advocacy, and much more.

Website/Resource: http://www.ampainsoc.org

Organization: **AstraZeneca, Corp.**

Description: Offers information regarding new medicines designed to improve the health and quality of life of patients around the world; research; and careers.

Website/Resource: http://www.astrazeneca.com

Organization: **Children's Hospice International (CHI)**

Description: Offers information about CHI's programs and resources as well as donation information.

Website/Resource: http://chionline.org

Organization: **Children's Hospice and Palliative Care Association**
Description: Offers general information about improving child health care and a special link for families.
Website/Resource: http://www.childrenshospice.org

Organization: **Children's Project on Palliative /Hospice Services (ChiPPs)**
Description: Offers users links and resources pertaining to child palliative care.
Website/Resource: http://www.nhpco.org

Organization: **Pediatric Pain: Science Helping Children**
Description: Provides information related to professional research, pediatric pain sourcebook of protocols/policies/pamphlets, and access to a self help link.
Website/Resource: http://pediatric-pain.ca

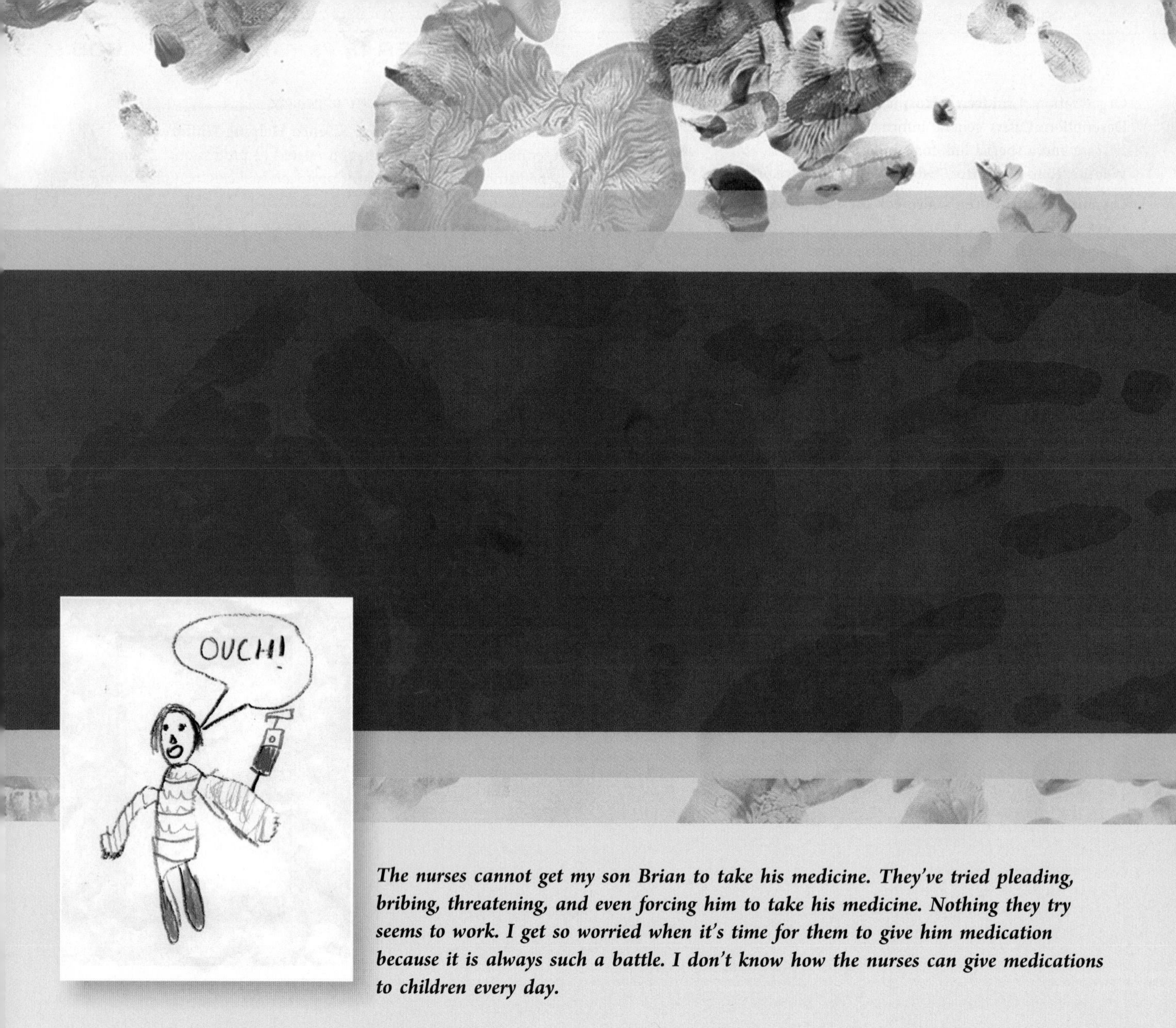

The nurses cannot get my son Brian to take his medicine. They've tried pleading, bribing, threatening, and even forcing him to take his medicine. Nothing they try seems to work. I get so worried when it's time for them to give him medication because it is always such a battle. I don't know how the nurses can give medications to children every day.

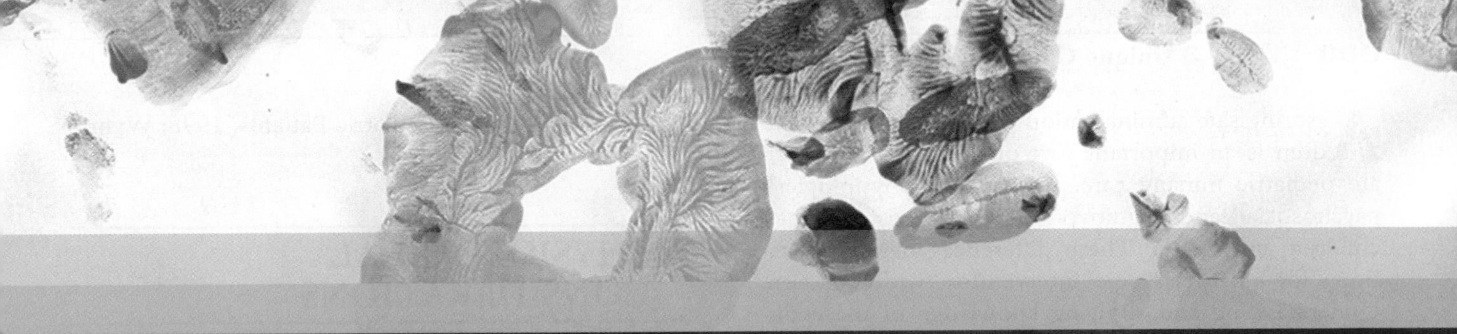

CHAPTER 19

Medication Administration

Karlen E. Luthy, DNP, FNP; Amanda Orme, MS, FNP;
Mary Tiedeman, RN, PhD

COMPETENCIES

Upon completion of this chapter, the reader will be able to:

- Describe pharmacokinetic and pharmacodynamic processes.
- Discuss age-related differences in pharmacokinetic and pharmacodynamic processes.
- Explain the impact of psychosocial and cognitive development on giving medications to infants and children.
- Discuss special considerations and approaches for safely administering medications to infants and children.
- Discuss appropriate methods for calculating a pediatric medication dose.
- Explain age-appropriate techniques for administering medications to children via the oral, enteral, intravenous, intramuscular, subcutaneous, rectal, ophthalmic, otic, nasal, inhaled, and topical routes.
- Describe the advantages and disadvantages of each route of pediatric medication administration.
- Successfully complete the games and activities in the online student StudyWARE.

Assuring safe administration of medications to children is an important part of providing appropriate pediatric nursing care. Anatomical, physiological, psychosocial, and cognitive differences exist between children and adults. These differences have implications for pharmacologic intervention with children. Understanding and applying knowledge of these differences is essential to safely administering medication to children (Adams, Josephson, & Holland, 2005; Karch, 2010; Lehne, 2010; Wynne, Woo, & Olyaei, 2007). Because there is limited research on pharmacologic intervention with children, it is particularly important to understand these developmental differences. Until recently, children have been excluded from drug trials due to ethical constraints related to informed consent and research risks. Since most medications have not been adequately tested in the pediatric population, there is a relative lack of information on drug safety and efficacy in infants and children. Therefore, infants and children are at risk for adverse reactions, including age-specific adverse reactions or ineffective treatment. While in the past decade the Food and Drug Administration (FDA) has issued new laws and regulations which increase pediatric drug research, it will be some time before we have the information necessary for safe and effective medication use in young clients (American Academy of Pediatrics, 2007; Anley & Siu, 2005; Best Pharmaceuticals for Children Act, 2002; Deveaugh-Geiss et al., 2006; Gracely-Kilgore, 2005; Herrman, 2009; Lehne, 2010; Regulations Requiring Manufacturers to Assess the Safety and Effectiveness of New Drugs and Biological Products in Pediatric Patients, 1998; Wynne et al., 2007).

PHYSIOLOGICAL CONSIDERATIONS

In general, physiological differences between children and adults make children more sensitive to medications and increase the risk of adverse reactions. Differences in body size and composition, and the immaturity of various organ systems, account for some of these differences. Of particular significance are body fluid composition and differences in cardiovascular, gastrointestinal, renal, and neurological system functioning. These age-related physiological differences, which change as children grow and develop, are responsible for alterations in pharmacokinetic and pharmacodynamic processes (Hedaya, 2007; Herrman, 2009; Karch, 2010; Lehne, 2010; Potter & Perry, 2005; Wynne et al., 2007). Table 19-1 defines several terms commonly used when discussing medication administration.

Pharmacokinetics involves the movement of drugs throughout the body by the processes of absorption, distribution, biotransformation, and excretion. Basically, pharmacokinetics affects how drugs enter the body, how they reach their site of action and in what concentration, and how they are eliminated. Thus, the pharmacokinetics of any drug may be altered depending on physiological differences between clients (Adams et al., 2005; Bauer, 2008; LaMattina & Golan, 2007; Lehne, 2010; Pepper, 2005; Potter & Perry, 2009).

Absorption is the process whereby drugs move from the site of administration into the bloodstream. The rate

TABLE 19-1 Medication Administration Terminology

Pharmacokinetics: The movement of drugs throughout the body by the processes of absorption, distribution, biotransformation, and excretion.

Absorption: The process whereby drugs move from the site of administration into the bloodstream.

Bioavailability: The portion of a drug that reaches general circulation and is available to exert its effect at its site of action.

Distribution: The process whereby a drug moves from the blood to interstitial spaces of tissues and from there into cells.

Biotransformation (Metabolism): The transformation/alteration of chemical structures from their original form.

Half-life: The time required for 50% of the administered dose of a drug to be eliminated from the body.

First-pass Effect: Effect of biotransformation of a drug by the liver before reaching systemic circulation.

Excretion: The process whereby drugs, active metabolites, and inactive metabolites are moved from the tissues back into the circulation and then to the organs of elimination.

Pharmacodynamics: The biochemical and physiological effects of drugs and their mechanisms of action within the body by the processes of absorption, distribution, biotransformation, and excretion.

Injection Sites: Identified sites for injections based on muscle development and the amount of fluid to be injected.

and extent of absorption determine how soon the effects of the drugs begin and the intensity of those effects. Absorption is a major determinant of **bioavailability** (i.e., the portion of a drug that reaches general circulation and is available to exert its effect at its site of action) (Adams et al., 2005; Bauer, 2008; Lehne, 2010; Pepper, 2005; Tozer & Rowland, 2006; Wynne et al., 2007). Normal physiological differences in the gastrointestinal (GI) tract, muscle mass, and body surface area (BSA) between infants and children affect the process of absorption (Burton, Shaw, Schentag, & Evans, 2005).

Gastric emptying time and pH are two factors influencing the absorption of orally administered drugs (Hedaya, 2007; Herrman, 2009; Karch, 2010; Wynne et al., 2007). Gastric emptying time is slower in neonates and infants (up to 6-8 hours) but progressively increases until it reaches adult values (2 hours) around 8 months of age. Delayed gastric emptying interferes with drugs designed to be absorbed from the intestine. Therefore their absorption and therapeutic effect are postponed when gastric emptying is delayed or when peristalsis is slowed (Gracely-Kilgore, 2005; Herrman, 2009; Lehne, 2010; Nahata & Taketomo, 2008; Wilson, 2009).

Alterations in absorption also occur for drugs absorbed primarily in the stomach. Gastric pH is higher (more alkaline) in the newborn and gradually decreases (becomes more acidic) to reach adult levels around 1 year of age. Acidic drugs are better absorbed from an acidic environment; alkaline drugs are better absorbed from an alkaline environment. Therefore, in infancy, alkaline medications will be more readily absorbed from the stomach, and acidic drugs will be less well absorbed from the stomach when compared to older children and adults (Aschenbrenner & Venable, 2008; Herrman, 2009; Lehne, 2010).

Intestinal transit time also influences the absorption of orally administered drugs. With a more rapid transit time (such as with diarrhea), less medication will be absorbed; with slower transit time (such as with constipation), more drug will be absorbed. Peristalsis, the constant wave of contraction responsible for GI motility, is both irregular and unpredictable in the neonate and infant. Therefore, the amount of drug absorbed in the small intestine of a neonate or infant may be unpredictable (Hedaya, 2007; Lehne, 2010; Nahata & Taketomo, 2008).

In addition, infants have lower levels of some transport substances, such as enzymes, needed for absorption and transport of certain medications. For example, premature neonates have little lipase and no alpha-amylase. The activity of pancreatic enzymes continues to be low in neonates and infants up to 4 months of age. Overall, variations in the gastrointestinal system result in slower, more irregular absorption of orally administered drugs during the first 6 months of life (Herrman, 2009; Lehne, 2010; Nahata & Taketomo, 2008).

Absorption of drugs administered intramuscularly is affected by muscle mass and perfusion. Neonates and infants have less muscle mass than older children or adults (25% of body weight compared to 40% of body weight in adults). The smaller muscle size results in less volume capacity and less absorptive surface; there is also decreased muscle tone and lower muscle oxygenation in this age group. In addition, neonates and infants have vasomotor instability with diminished and unpredictable peripheral blood flow. Thus, absorption of drugs administered intramuscularly is slower and less reliable in this age group. Perfusion to the area also influences the absorption of drugs administered subcutaneously. When there is diminished blood flow, absorption is delayed. However, when perfusion is adequate, the subcutaneous route can facilitate the rapid absorption of nonirritating, lipid-soluble drugs (Gracely-Kilgore, 2005; Karch, 2010; Lehne, 2010; Nahata & Taketomo, 2008; Ricci, Kyle, & Kyle, 2008).

There is more rapid absorption of topical medication in infants and children due to greater BSA to weight ratio. The skin of neonates, infants, and children is also thinner and more permeable (Herrman, 2009; Lehne, 2010; Nahata & Taketomo, 2008; Wynne et al., 2007). Absorption is further increased if skin integrity is compromised, there is prolonged contact time, or an occlusive dressing is applied. These factors necessitate careful attention to instructions for using topical medication, especially since plastic-coated diapers can be considered an occlusive dressing (Gracely-Kilgore, 2005; Herrman, 2009; Lehne, 2010; Wynne et al., 2007).

Distribution is the process whereby a drug moves from the blood to interstitial spaces of tissues and from there into cells. Simply stated, distribution involves the movement or transport of drugs throughout the body. Factors influencing drug distribution in the body include body composition and fluid distribution, protein binding, blood flow to the tissues, and special membrane barriers (Adams et al., 2005; Herrman, 2009; Kee, Hayes & McCuistion, 2009; Lehne, 2010; Pepper, 2005).

Body water distribution and amounts vary with age. Neonates, infants, toddlers, and preschoolers have a higher percentage of body water than adults (75–85% in a neonate, approximately 85% in an infant, compared to 50–60% in an adult), with a greater portion of this water in the extracellular fluid. Because the proportion of body water is so much higher in the neonate and infant, water-soluble medications are diluted to a greater degree. As a result, neonates and infants may have a decreased serum concentration of water-soluble medications. This is most pronounced in children under 2 years of age and may require higher mg/kg doses of water-soluble drugs in order to achieve therapeutic levels (Aschenbrenner & Venable, 2008; Gracely-Kilgore, 2005; Herrman, 2009; Luedtke, 2006; McCance & Huether, 2010).

Body fat percentage varies by age and gender as well as between individual children. Fat comprises 15–16% of the body weight of a neonate. Although, for the premature neonate the percent of body weight comprised of fat may be as little as 1%. The percentage of body fat peaks around 9 months of age and then decreases between 1 and 5 years to between 8–12%. It increases again around adolescence, with girls having a higher percent than boys. The percentage of body fat influences drug distribution throughout the body and affects the concentration of medications in the circulatory system and at the site of action. Lipid-soluble drugs have a high affinity for adipose tissue and can be stored which can then leave lower levels of drug available in circulation and at the site of action. Thus, with lipid-soluble drugs, body fat must be saturated before drug blood levels begin to rise, requiring different mg/kg dosages, depending on the amount of body fat, to achieve therapeutic levels. An individual with a higher percentage of body fat requires a higher mg/kg dose of a lipid-soluble drug than an individual with a lower percentage of body fat (Blackburn, 2007; Herrman, 2009; Maples, James, & Stowe, 2005).

Immaturity of the liver in neonates and infants results in lower serum protein levels and fewer protein binding sites. In addition, albumin also has a lower binding capacity for certain drugs during infancy. With drugs that tend to bind to protein, decreased protein binding increases the serum level of unbound drugs. Since the unbound drug exerts an effect, decreased protein binding intensifies the drug's effect, potentially leading to toxicity. Drugs excreted in their active form (not biotransformed but excreted unchanged) may be more rapidly eliminated from the body since it is the unbound portion of a drug that can be excreted. Due to the increased serum levels and more rapid excretion, some drugs may require a decreased dose but an increased frequency of administration (Herrman, 2009; Lehne, 2010; Maples et al., 2005).

Certain drugs also compete with endogenous substances, such as free fatty acids, bilirubin, or steroids, for protein-binding sites. Since the number of binding sites is already limited in young children, competition for binding sites may lead to higher levels of unbound drug necessitating lower drug doses or higher levels of the endogenous substances. In neonates, competitive drug binding may lead to increased concentrations of unbound, unconjugated bilirubin leading to kernicterus or bilirubin encephalopathy (Herrman, 2009; Lehne, 2006; Maples et al., 2005).

A large number of drugs are bound to plasma proteins which serve as the transport vehicle for the medication. Because proteins are large structures, usually these substances are unable to cross into the brain. However, the immature blood-brain barrier in children under 2 years of age allows relatively easy access to the central nervous system (CNS), making these children more sensitive to drugs that act on the brain, thus increasing the risk of CNS toxicity. Therefore, lower doses of certain drugs may be required to protect young children from undesired effects (Aschenbrenner & Veneble, 2008; Gracely-Kilgore, 2005; Herrman, 2009; Lehne, 2010).

Biotransformation, also called metabolism, refers to the transformation or alteration of chemical structures from their original form. This transformation facilitates the eventual excretion of the substance via the renal system. Most biotransformation of drugs occurs in the liver (Adams et al., 2005; Herrman, 2009; Lehne, 2010; Pepper, 2005).

Due to liver immaturity, the drug-metabolizing capacity of premature infants and neonates is low. Although liver function develops rapidly during the first few months after birth, complete maturation of hepatic enzyme activity is not reached until 1 to 2 years of age. During this time, drugs metabolized by the liver have a longer **half-life** (time required for 50% of administered dose of a drug to be eliminated from the body) and there is an increased risk of toxicity. This requires reducing the dosages of some drugs and adjusting the frequency of administration. During early childhood, children have higher metabolic rates, causing drugs to be metabolized more rapidly, necessitating higher doses or more frequent administration. This is especially pronounced between 2 to 6 years of age but continues until 10 to 12 years of age (Blackburn, 2007; Herrman, 2009; Lehne, 2010; Peterson, 2005).

Temperature, which may have dramatic fluctuations in infants and young children, also impacts drug metabolism. Any increase or decrease in temperature alters the metabolic rate, resulting in alteration of drug half-life and duration of therapeutic effect. This is an especially important consideration during febrile illness since any drug given when the child has an elevated temperature may be metabolized faster than if the temperature was normal (Gutierrez, 2003).

Some metabolism of drugs may occur in the gastrointestinal tract where microflora alter physiochemical property. Since infants have lower levels of gastrointestinal flora, there is less metabolism of these drugs in the gastrointestinal tract. For example, digoxin-reducing microorganisms do not reach adult levels until approximately 2 years of age, so the dose of that medication should be watched closely (Herrman, 2009; Pepper, 2005).

Some biotransformation of orally administered drugs occurs before the drug reaches the general circulation. For example, drugs absorbed from the stomach and small intestine pass through the portal circulation where some biotransformation occurs before the drug reaches the general circulation. This phenomenon, known as **first-pass effect**, decreases the bioavailability of orally administered medications. Therefore, drugs administered orally may require larger mg/kg doses for therapeutic effect than drugs administered by other routes. Drugs that are highly cleared by the liver may undergo considerable biotransformation via first-pass effect. Examples of such drugs are opioids such as morphine and meperidine, certain tricyclic antidepressants such as nortriptyline, and antiarrhythmics such as propanolol (Adams et al., 2005; Algren, 2005; Herrman, 2009; Kee et al., 2009; Lehne, 2010; Pepper, 2005).

Excretion is the process whereby drugs, active metabolites, and inactive metabolites are moved from the tissues back into the circulation and then to the organs of elimination. Drugs and their metabolites are excreted from the body in urine, bile, sweat, saliva, and expired air (Adams et al., 2005; Herrman, 2009; Lehne, 2010; Pepper, 2005).

The kidneys are the primary route of drug excretion. The kidneys are immature at birth with decreased renal blood flow, glomerular filtration, and tubular secretion.

CRITICAL THINKING

Medication Administration to a Child with Impaired Renal Function

Three-year-old Marc, with renal failure secondary to trauma, is receiving a morphine injection for pain. What concerns do you have regarding giving morphine? What adjustments might be needed in dose and administration?

Renal function increases rapidly during infancy, especially in the first few weeks of life, and peaks by 6 to 12 months of age. Reduced renal excretion during infancy results in a longer drug half-life and increases the risk of toxicity to drugs that are excreted primarily by the renal system. Therefore, reduced dosages are required during infancy, especially during the neonatal period. By 3 years of age the glomerular filtration rate surpasses the adult rate and drugs are eliminated more rapidly. Therefore, a drug's half-life may be shorter in toddlers than in older children and adults (Aschenbrenner & Venable, 2008; Herrman, 2009; Lehne, 2010; Wynne et al., 2007).

Pharmacodynamics describes the drug's concentration and effect once it reaches the site of action. That is, how the drug affects the body. Drug action may involve nonspecific modification of the cellular environment, as for example when altering the pH of the surrounding body fluid. Drug action also occurs at the cellular level through an interaction of the drug and cellular components. Most drugs are thought to act at the cellular level by attaching to receptors on the cells where they mimic or block the action of endogenous regulatory molecules. For example, propranolol blocks beta-adrenergic receptors, thus decreasing heart rate, whereas albuterol stimulates beta-adrenergic receptors, thus producing bronchodilation (Adams et al., 2005; Bauer, 2008; Hedaya, 2007; Karch, 2010; Kee et al., 2009; Pepper, 2005).

Even though the mechanism of action of a drug remains the same in all individuals, infants and children may demonstrate variations in drug effects related to the immaturity of target organs and receptor sensitivity. Therefore, an infant or child may require a lower or higher dose of a drug when compared to an older person. In general, infants and children have heightened sensitivity to drugs (Aschenbrenner & Venable, 2008; Lehne, 2010; Potter & Perry, 2009).

DEVELOPMENTAL CONSIDERATIONS

Administering medications to children requires an understanding of all aspects of growth and development and its impact on the approach to giving medications. Of particular importance is the child's psychosocial and cognitive development. Physical and motor development are also important (e.g., ability to swallow tablets and size of muscles) and will be discussed in relation to their impact on the various routes of administering medication.

Infants are developing trust and are helped by consistency, both in caregivers and in approaches to nursing care. In later infancy, stranger anxiety may make the infant less receptive to care by the nurse. Involving caregivers in medication administration can make this experience less stressful for infants. Caregivers can administer oral medications and they can hold and comfort the infant when medication is administered by other routes (Gracely-Kilgore, 2005).

Toddlers are developing autonomy and attempting to control their environment. If the toddler is unsuccessful at controlling the environment, negative behaviors such as temper tantrums may occur. Following rituals and routines can give toddlers some sense of control and may enhance cooperation in taking medications. Giving choices and allowing toddlers to handle equipment also fosters a sense of control and may enhance cooperation. At this age, choices should be kept simple, that is, a choice between two things. For example, "Do you want mommy or the nurse to give you your medicine?" As with infants, toddlers can benefit

CULTURAL CONSIDERATION

Cultural Concerns with Nursing Care

Those with an Asian, Latino, African-American, Arabic, Muslim, or Caribbean cultural background may ascribe to the theory of humoral health, which focuses on balance or harmony with nature. The cultural belief is that if there is imbalance with nature, the result can be illness or disease; the treatment of disease with hot or cold substances restores the body's humoral balance. To restore this balance for their children, parents may ask the nurse to support their cultural beliefs by providing hot or cold substances, including hot or cold drinks, depending on the child's illness.

Nurses should also recognize that there are many variations regarding the humoral health theory within cultural groups and that individuals may have health practices that differ from the larger cultural group. Nurses striving to provide culturally competent care should always question which cultural practices are personally relevant to each individual. Refer to Chapter 3 for more information relative to cultural group beliefs related to health care.

References: Hunt, R. (2008). *Introduction to community-based nursing* (4th ed.). Philadelphia: Lippincott, Williams, & Wilkins; Andrews, M. M., & Boyle, J. S. (2007). *Transcultural concepts in nursing care* (5th ed.). Philadelphia: Lippincott, Williams, & Wilkins.

from caregiver participation in medication administration (Gracely-Kilgore, 2005; Potter & Perry, 2009). Toddlers should be approached in a positive manner conveying a belief in their ability to accomplish the needed behavior (e.g., successfully taking the medication). When giving medications to toddlers, administer them promptly, restrain as needed, and reward positive behavior. Toddlers should not be told or given the message they are bad when not able to fully cooperate in taking medications (Bowden & Greenberg, 2007; Gracely-Kilgore, 2005).

Preschoolers are developing initiative, and benefit from the opportunity to play with equipment and respond positively to explanations and comforting. To help foster a sense of control, choices should be offered when possible. However, the number of choices should be limited (e.g., "Do you want to take the pink medicine or the white medicine first?" or "Do you want water or juice with your medicine?"). Care should be taken not to inadvertently offer a choice that does not really exist (e.g., "Do you want to take your medicine?"). Preschoolers can also benefit from caregiver involvement in medication administration. Giving suppositories may be upsetting to preschoolers because of their fears of bodily intrusion and mutilation. As with toddlers, preschoolers should not be given the message they are bad when not able to fully cooperate with medication administration (Gracely-Kilgore, 2005; Herrman, 2009; Wynne et al., 2007).

School-age children are developing industry. They benefit from explanations regarding the purpose of medications and can be active participants in their care. School-age children are generally cooperative in taking medication. However, a reward system may serve as an effective feedback mechanism for school-age children, thus enhancing their cooperation. Play activities also can help with coping. School-age children also should be given choices; older school-age children can handle a broader range of choices (e.g., "What do you want to drink with your medication?") (Gracely-Kilgore, 2005; Herrman, 2009; Wynne et al., 2007).

Adolescents may be approached in the same manner as adults. A more detailed discussion of growth and development of the specific age groups can be found in Chapters 7 through 12.

One situation nurses may encounter with psychosocial implications is when caregivers use the threat of needles or "shots" to influence children's behavior. Such a situation can be a challenge for the nurse who needs to assure the child painful or frightening interventions are not a consequence of behavior, while still fostering trust between the child and caregiver. The nurse needs to tactfully provide the caregivers with factual information regarding growth and development, children's fears and anxiety with regard to hospitalization, and suggest or role model alternative ways of dealing with undesired behavior. At the same time, the nurse must acknowledge and accept the caregivers' feelings and frustrations regarding their child's behavior. In intervening with children, the nurse must use age-appropriate teaching approaches regarding illness and treatment while being careful not to convey negative feelings about caregivers' behaviors.

MEDICATION ADMINISTRATION

Administration of medications to pediatric patients requires special considerations, unique approaches, and skilled technique. Special considerations include preparation for safe administration, dosage determination, and routes of delivery. Infants and children require unique approaches that are based on their growth and development level. Whatever the route, it is important to be skilled in each route of medication delivery (oral, intravenous, intramuscular, subcutaneous, rectal, ophthalmic, otic, nasal, inhaled, and topical).

GENERAL CONSIDERATIONS

Children are unique with respect to medication delivery, and a variety of techniques is required to successfully administer medications to children. Prior to administering any medication, it is important to consider general nutritional status, size, medical status, and use of other prescription or nonprescription drugs (Turkoski, 2007). Prior to administering the medication, explanations should be given to the child and caregivers using age appropriate language that explains why the child needs the medication, what the child will experience, the method of delivery, what is expected of the child, and how the caregivers can participate and help support their child. This explanation may include description of tastes, exploring coping strategies (counting, singing, music, or movies), or positioning for comfort during the administration of the medication. A caregiver's role in the procedure needs to be defined prior to beginning the delivery of medication. Be truthful and use nonthreatening words to describe what the child will do, feel, taste, see, smell, and hear while receiving their medications. For example, "This medicine may taste different than anything you have tasted before" rather than saying, "This medicine tastes bad." Age appropriate comfort should be provided as needed after the medication has been administered.

PREPARATION FOR SAFE ADMINISTRATION

Medication administration traditionally adheres to the five rights: right medication, right dose, right patient, right route, and right time. It has been proposed that adding a sixth right may be appropriate: the right technique in medication preparation or the right documentation (Stein, 2006). Another may be the right approach in actually administering it to a pediatric patient.

Children are less able to protect themselves from errors that may occur in the medication administration process (Cahill, 2009). Check medications received from the pharmacy against the written order and the transcribed or computer-generated medication administration record (MAR). Determining the right dose in the pediatric population requires more than verifying that the dose delivered is

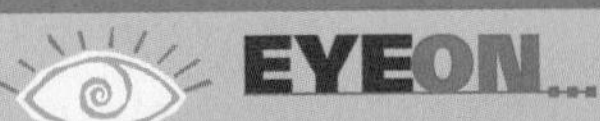

Possibility of Herbal and Medication Interactions

Always ask patients and their caregivers if they are taking any herbal remedies or vitamin supplements prior to any medication administration. The active ingredients in herbs and vitamins can cause unexpected reactions when used with medications. The effect may be in the drug distribution, metabolism, or excretion of the medication and can lead to drug toxicity (Kemper et al., 2008).

the same as the dose ordered by the physician. The nurse must also verify that the ordered dose is within the recommended dosage range for each patient. This varies depending on the patient's age, weight, and medical condition.

Correct identification of a pediatric patient begins with correct placement of identification bracelets at the time of admission. Nurses should check identification bracelets at the beginning of each shift and prior to giving medications. The nurse cannot expect a child to correctly self-identify. As adolescents change they may find it fun to misidentify themselves to authority figures. It is known that the adolescent's ability to adhere to medication schedules independently is decreased (Matsui, 2007). Patient identifiers include the patient's name, birthday, and medical record number. Using specific patient identifiers will assist the nurse in correctly identifying the right patient. Verification of right drug, right dose, right route, and right time is a basic safety measure.

In addition to the five rights of medication administration, the nurse has the responsibility to check the appropriate formulation and concentration of a medication (Ince, Saskia, Tibboel, Danhof, & Knibbe, 2009). High alert medications must be double-checked by a second nurse prior to administration to patients; these medications have critical responses and a higher risk of death if given in error (Raja Lope, Boo, Rohana, & Cheah, 2009). Often high alert medications that need a double check prior to administration are listed in an institution's policies and procedures manual. Some examples of such medications may include narcotics, insulin, digoxin, heparin, pressors, blood products, or total parenteral nutrition (TPN).

Reflections from Families

Seven-year-old Stephanie, who received an injection earlier in the day, states: "My mom and nurse told me it wouldn't hurt. It did. I wish they had told me the truth."

DOSAGE DETERMINATION

Examining medication dosing for children is necessary to determine therapeutic range, appropriate dose, and developmental interactions. Through the FDA Modernization Act (1997) and the Best Pharmaceuticals for Children Act (2002), incentive programs were made available to drug manufacturers to support and supply pediatric clinical trials. A third legislative act, the Pediatric Research Equity Act (2003), combined with the other two legislative acts have increased the information available about pediatric drug labeling, proper dosing, and possible risks of therapy (Rodriguez et al., 2008).

Nurses must ensure that the right dose has been calculated. This may be done by referencing a pediatric dosing handbook or online resource. Take note that pediatric medications are often prescribed in unit per kilogram of body weight per day or per dose; sometimes, although less commonly, the calculations are determined by using the body surface area (BSA). It is critical that nurses understand how to correctly calculate a medication dose and avoid medication errors (Wright, 2008). There are many calculation techniques available to help accurately calculate medication doses for pediatric patients (Andrew, Salamonson, & Halcomb, 2009).

When calculating appropriate medication dosages for an individual child it is essential that the correct recommended dosage be used in the calculation since recommendations differ based on age, route of administration, and purpose (Box 19-1). Most dosage recommendations are for a 24-hour period (mg/kg/24 hours). However, some dosage recommendations are for a single dose (mg/kg/dose). It is important the nurse differentiate between these when doing calculations.

BOX 19-1
CALCULATING RECOMMENDED PEDIATRIC DOSE FROM MG/KG/DAY

Example: The child you are caring for has an order for Amoxicillin 400 mg PO BID. Begin by checking the dose against the pediatric drug dosing handbook. The child's weight is 10 kg. You note that the appropriate dose for Amoxicillin is 80 mg/kg/day divided BID. Set up the equation by multiplying the recommended dose by the child's weight. Divide the dose calculated (80 x 10 = 800) by the number of doses recommended (800 / 2 = 400). So, an appropriate dose for a 10 kg child would be 400 mg per dose, two times per day.

ORAL MEDICATION

Preparation

Oral medications come in several forms—liquid, powder, tablets, and capsules. Liquid medications also include syrups, elixirs, and suspensions, which may contain undissolved particles suspended in a liquid. Suspensions require shaking before administration to distribute the medication evenly throughout the liquid so an appropriate dose is administered each time. Since children under 5 years of age generally are unable to swallow tablets or capsules, it may be necessary to crush tablets or open capsules to remove the powder or liquid. Before crushing a tablet or opening a capsule it is essential to determine if this will interfere with the pharmacokinetics of the drug (e.g., enteric coated or timed release tablets should not be crushed). Crushed tablets or capsule contents generally have a bitter taste. Therefore, to make the medication more palatable it can be mixed with a pleasant tasting liquid or nonessential food before administering, such as flavored syrups provided by the pharmacy, jelly, pudding, ice cream, or applesauce. The medication should not be mixed with formula or other essential foods since the child might associate the medicine taste with the food. Chilling a liquid medication is another way of making it more palatable. Whatever method is used to make oral medications more palatable, care must be taken to preserve integrity (Mennella & Beauchamp, 2008).

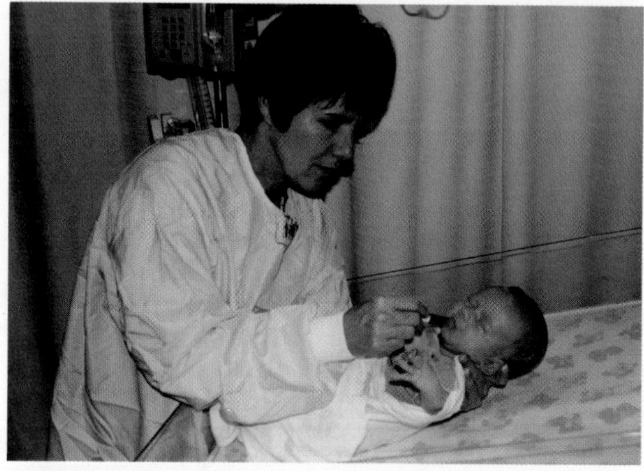

Figure 19-1A Using a syringe to administer oral medications to an infant. DELMAR CENGAGE LEARNING.

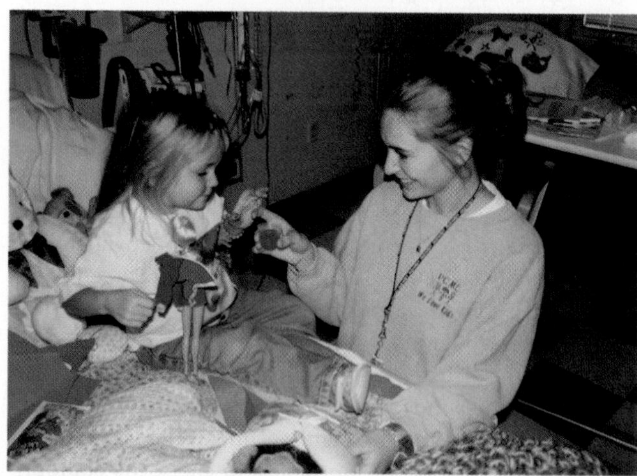

Figure 19-1B Toddlers and preschoolers will often take their oral medications cheerfully if placed in a small cup. DELMAR CENGAGE LEARNING.

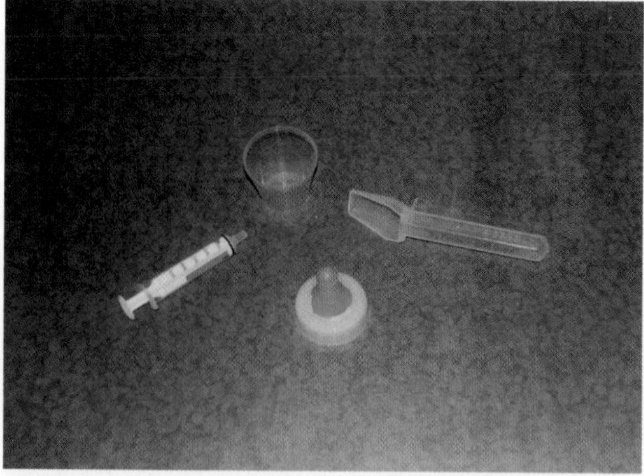

Figure 19-1C Oral medications can be administered to children through a variety of devices: cup, syringe, dropper, nipple, or medicine spoon. DELMAR CENGAGE LEARNING.

Administration

The administration of oral medications in the pediatric population may be a challenge since the appearance, smell, or taste of the medications may make children reluctant to accept them. Therefore, a firm, matter-of-fact approach, based on developmental level and ability, usually results in cooperation. For example, ask children to administer the oral drug to themselves or use the syringe to squirt the medicine into their mouth (Anand, Kataria, Kukkar, Saharan, & Choudhury, 2007; Mennella & Beauchamp, 2008; Turkoski, 2007).

Liquid medication can be administered in a medicine cup, a measured medicine spoon, an oral syringe, a dropper, or through a nipple without the bottle attached. A dropper or oral syringe can be used to administer liquid medication

NURSING ALERT

Giving Oral Medications When the Child Is Not Cooperative

Never pinch the nose or force a screaming child to swallow medication. This increases the risk of aspiration.

to infants and young children. The liquid is directed posterior and to the side of the mouth and given slowly in small quantities (0.2-0.5 mL), allowing the child to swallow before more medication is placed in the mouth. A nipple also may be used for administering liquid medication to infants (Purswani et al., 2009). The medication is placed directly in the nipple; care should be taken to keep the nipple filled with medication so the infant does not suck air while taking the medication. However, some nurses may hesitate to use a nipple for medication administration for fear the infant may associate the nipple with medication and refuse to feed. To avoid aspiration, the infant or child should be placed in an upright position, and never flat (Anand et al., 2007; Mennella & Beauchamp, 2008; Turkoski, 2007). Older children are able to take liquid from a medicine cup or measured medicine spoon. Toddlers and preschoolers may enjoy using an oral syringe to "squirt" medicine into their mouth. See Figure 19-1A.

As children mature, they learn to swallow tablets or capsules. The nurse can facilitate learning this skill by having children practice by placing the medication in a small amount of food such as ice cream and then having the child swallow the spoonful of food. The child should be told medication is in the food. This helps the child learn a new skill (Garvie, Lensing, & Rai, 2007).

For some pediatric clients, oral medications are administered via a nasogastric, a gastrostomy, or a nasojejunal tube. Before administering oral medications in this manner it is essential to determine proper placement of the tube. In addition, medications that act directly on the stomach (e.g., liquid antacids) will be ineffective if given via a nasojejunal tube. A syringe is used to flush the tube before administering the medication. The medication is then put through the tube using a syringe, followed by a sufficient amount of water to ensure the medication enters the gastrointestinal system rather than remaining in the tube (Williams, 2008).

NURSING ALERT

Use of Spoons in Administering Liquid Medication

Do not substitute an ordinary teaspoon or tablespoon or kitchen measuring spoons for a measured medication spoon. Such spoons are not consistently calibrated and may alter the dose of medication that a child receives.

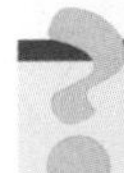

KIDS WANT TO KNOW

What will the medicine taste like?

Beth, a 4-year-old, is receiving a liquid antibiotic for an ear infection. She asks "What does it taste like?" and "Does it taste bad?" Be honest in your reply. If you don't know what it tastes like, you can say "Some children tell me it tastes like cherry. You can tell me what it tastes like to you." Another response could be "It smells like cherry. You can tell me what it tastes like to you." If you have tasted the medicine, you may say "It tastes like cherry to me." Remember that what one person thinks tastes okay, another person may think tastes bad. You should give descriptions of taste or smell rather than labeling the taste good or bad. Both children and their caregivers will benefit from further research and understanding of children's acceptance of medicines (Mennella & Beauchamp, 2008).

INTRAVENOUS MEDICATION

Intravenous (IV) administration of medication improves the therapeutic blood level of the medication and eliminates the discomfort associated with repeated intramuscular or subcutaneous injections. Since the medication is placed directly into the bloodstream where it can have an immediate effect, the nurse must follow guidelines related to concentration of medication, rate of delivery, and compatibility of solutions to help ensure the safety of the patient when using this method of administering medications.

PREPARATION

Before administering IV medications, the nurse should consult pharmacologic references for the recommended time of infusion, maximum concentration of the drug in solution, and compatibility of the drug with IV solutions and other IV medications administered concurrently. The nurse should check the IV site just before giving the medication to ensure the IV is patent without swelling, redness, or tenderness at the site. This will ensure the medication is given intravenously, not into the surrounding tissue, and not given into an inflamed and irritated vein. In addition, the nurse must be sure the medication is completely dissolved and does not contain any particles which can be seen. If possible, the medication should be ready for administration before entering the child's room to avoid causing unnecessary anxiety. Necessary labels also should be prepared to ensure safe delivery.

Figure 19-2 illustrates venous access sites in infants.

ADMINISTRATION

IV medication can be administered in several ways—by syringe infusion pump, solution administration set (Metriset, Buretrol, or Soluset), piggyback, IV push, or retrograde. Factors to consider when selecting an appropriate method of delivery include: (1) volume of solution necessary to dilute

FAMILY**TEACHING**

Safe Administration of Oral Medications

HOME

Teach caregivers:

- Generic and brand names of medications.
- The purpose of medications, why they are necessary, and their expected effects.
- Potential side effects of medication and what to do if they occur.
- How to give medication (amount, frequency, length of time to be given). Provide a demonstration and allow caregivers to give a return demonstration.
- About acceptable measuring devices for liquid medications, for example, oral syringes, measured medicine spoons, or medicine droppers calibrated for a specific medication.
- Medication can be mixed with small amounts of food, such as pudding or ice cream.
- What to do if child vomits following medication administration or if a dose is forgotten; it should be made up at the next scheduled dosage.
- To inform health care provider of any over-the-counter medications or herbal preparations being given.

SCHOOL

Teach caregivers:

- To be aware of and follow local school policy regarding medications taken at school.
- To inform appropriate school personnel of the medication the child is taking including the purpose, how long the child will be taking the medication, and any special precautions or considerations needed while taking the medication.

COMMUNITY

- Encourage caregivers to inform other community caretakers of needed information for administering the medication safely.

the medication; (2) volume of solution tolerated by child; and (3) agency policies and procedures. Whatever method is used, the amount of fluid used for the medication and flushes must be included in the child's daily fluid intake.

Syringe infusion pumps, allowing medications to be delivered in a small volume of fluid over a prescribed period of time, are appropriate when larger fluid volumes are contraindicated. Tubing used with syringe infusion pumps is generally low volume (less than 5 mL, some as small as 0.5 mL) so only a small amount of solution is needed to flush the

CRITICAL THINKING

Assuring Administration of an Appropriate Medication Dose

Six-year-old Daniel is receiving IV gentamicin for an infection. He weighs 18.5 kg. The recommended dose is 2–2.5 mg/kg/dose every 8 hours. The order is for 30 mg every 8 hours. Consider whether this is an appropriate dose and what actions, if any, you need to take.

medication through the tubing and the entire dose is received by the patient. The tubing for the syringe infusion pump is primed with IV solution, and then the syringe containing the medication is attached to the tubing. The syringe is then placed in the infusion pump and the pump is programmed to deliver the medication in the prescribed amount of time. Once the syringe is empty, the tubing is flushed. The tubing or syringe should be clearly labeled to indicate the presence of medication or flush.

Medications that can be placed in a larger volume of solution may be administered via a solution administration set (Metriset, Buretrol, or Soluset). After cleansing the

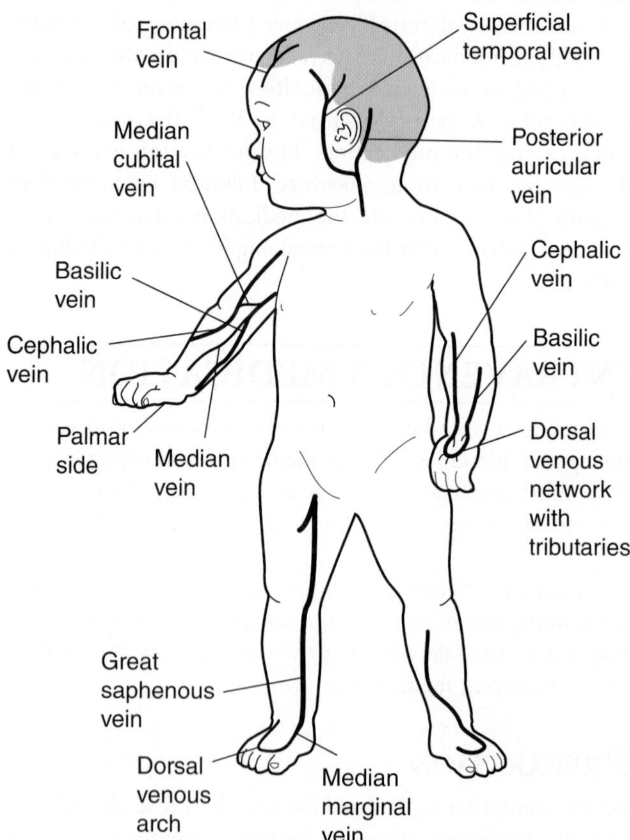

FIGURE 19-2 Venous Access Sites in Infants. DELMAR CENGAGE LEARNING.

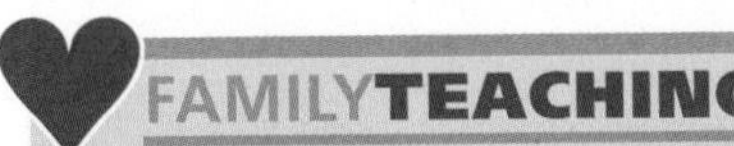

Safe Storage, Use, and Disposal of Oral Medications

HOME

Teach caregivers:

- To store all medications out of reach of children, in a locked place if possible.
- Not to remove labels from medications or to store medications in other than the original container.
- To dispose of outdated medications or medications which are no longer needed.
- Not to save medication to give at a later time.
- Not to give medication that has been prescribed for another individual even if the illness is similar.
- Not to refer to medicine as candy.

SCHOOL

Teach:

- Caregivers to check school policy regarding medications at school.
- Children not to share their medications with others.
- Children not to accept medications from others.

COMMUNITY

- Provide caregivers with phone number of local poison control center, and caution against use of syrup of ipecac.
- Have caregivers educate other care providers, such as grandparents and day care center staff, regarding safe storage, use, and disposal of medications.

injection port, the medication is placed in the administration set and the IV rate is set to allow infusion of the medication in the prescribed amount of time. A larger volume of fluid is required to flush the tubing (up to 20 mL) after the administration of the medication. The flush must run at the same rate set for the infusion of the medication. Once the flush is completed, the IV rate is returned to its ordered rate, or the IV may be locked as ordered. When medication is in the administration set it should be clearly labeled or flagged in some way so the IV rate is not changed and no additional fluid is added to the chamber until the medication has completely infused. There also should be a method to indicate the flush is running so the rate of the IV is not changed, resulting in the child getting the portion of the medication in the tubing too rapidly or too slowly.

Larger volumes of medication also can be administered via piggyback. Here, the medication is diluted in 50- or 100-mL

EVIDENCE-BASED PRACTICE

Pediatric Medication Safety

CLINICAL PROBLEM

Medication errors can occur at any point along the medication administration process. Of particular concern are the challenges of calculating correct pediatric doses combined with the challenge of multiple health conditions and developmental concerns. In April 2008, The Joint Commission issued a *Sentinel Event Alert: Prevent Pediatric Medication Errors.* This report focused attention on strategies that will reduce the risk of errors to children. The errors occur as a result of events in the dosage calculation (from premature infants to adolescents), unexpected effects of medication (due to immature physiology), less predictable rate of metabolism (compared with older children and adults), and lack of available dosing formulations. Not all providers, nurses, or even pharmacists have education specific to pediatric medication safety. Not only are children less able to participate directly in strategies to ensure their safety with medication, but also parents can be a source of medication administration error in the home as well.

BEST CLINICAL PRACTICE

- The formation of clinical teams with members from all disciplines including nursing, pharmacy, medicine, and families to address strategies for avoiding medication errors in pediatrics.
- Review all facility specific medication error rates and compare them with the national data.
- Use a pediatric formulary, pediatric specific pharmacy group, and when available always use pediatric compatible devices for the administration of medication to children.
- Using medication processes such as an order set review, computerized physician order entry, or preprinted orders have shown to provide more team input and improve pediatric patient safety resulting in fewer medication errors.

IMPLICATIONS FOR NURSING

- Nurses must devote a significant amount of time to record keeping, record review, transcription, reconciliation, preparation, dispensing, and administration of medications to children.
- Adequate number of staff is required to care for children in intensive care units, including: neonatal, pediatric, and emergency settings.
- Provide education of parents and involve children in learning appropriate information about taking medications, recognizing adverse drug reactions, and correctly administering medications.

Reference: Cahill, M. (2009). Pediatric medication safety: The power of the team. *Nursing Administration Quarterly*, 33(1), 38–47.

RESEARCH Highlight

Nurses' Knowledge of Pharmacology

STUDY PURPOSE

To determine if nurses had adequate pharmacology knowledge of the medications they commonly administer.

METHODS

The study used a descriptive survey design with a convenience sample of 42 nurses working in surgical wards of a foundation hospital in the North of England. Data were gathered during structured interviews when questions were asked about specific drugs commonly given and by having participants complete questionnaires related to knowledge about those drugs.

FINDINGS

The majority of nurses (57.2%) had inadequate knowledge of the mechanism of action and drug interactions of the medications they were administering. In addition, those with less experience had less knowledge about the medications they were administering.

IMPLICATIONS

Nurses in a clinical setting need supplementary pharmacology education, focusing on common medications they administer. This will increase nurses' knowledge and confidence in drug administration and safe management of medication.

REFERENCE

Ndosi, M. E., & Newell, R. (2009). Nurses' knowledge of pharmacology behind drugs they commonly administer. *Journal of Clinical Nursing, 18*(4), 570–580.

bags, usually 5% dextrose and water (D5W) or normal saline (NSS). The IV tubing is primed, attached to the bag with the medication, and then connected into the primary IV line. These small IV bags can be infused using gravity or via an IV pump, which will monitor the rate and volume. Since gravity infusion is subject to the child's movements, which can alter drip rate, the nurse must assess the infusion frequently to maintain appropriate flow rate. Caregivers and children should be instructed not to tamper with the IV rate or level of fluid in the administration set.

Some medications may be delivered by direct, slow IV push into the injection port closest to the child. These medications are generally of small volume and can be administered over a period of several minutes (e.g., 3–5 minutes). The nurse must carefully time the administration of the medication to be evenly spaced over the recommended time. For example, when giving 5 mL over a period of 5 minutes, each 1 mL should be administered slowly over a 1-minute period of time. Further details related to intravenous administration can be found in a nurses drug handbook or online.

NURSING TIP

Cleaning IV Injection or Access Ports

The procedure for cleaning injection or access ports on a vascular access device (VAD) may differ from that of peripheral IV lines. Check your agency or unit procedure manual before injecting medications into a VAD.

A final method for administering IV medication is the retrograde method. The IV line to the client is clamped off, and the medication is injected into the injection port that has been cleaned. The medication goes up the tubing toward the IV bag. The line is then opened and the medication flows into the client with the IV solution. Tubing should be labeled to indicate the presence of medication in the IV line.

INTRAMUSCULAR MEDICATION

Intramuscular (IM) injections are often associated with discomfort and distress and therefore, the least preferable route used to administer medications to children. However, at times, it may be necessary to administer medication by this route. Selection of needle size and **injection sites** as well as techniques of administration are important considerations.

Selecting Needle Size

Needle length and gauge are selected based on the child's size, amount of subcutaneous tissue over the injection site, and viscosity of the medication. Age-based guidelines for selecting needle length and gauge can be found in Table 19-2, although each child and situation must be assessed individually. Viscous solutions require a larger gauge needle (i.e. 20 gauge). The nurse should use the smallest gauge needle that will effectively deposit the medication in the muscle.

Table 19-2 Age-Based Guidelines for Selecting Needle Length and Gauge

AGE GROUP	NEEDLE LENGTH	NEEDLE GAUGE
Infant	5/8 inch	25–27
Toddler or Preschool	1 inch	22–23
School-age or adolescent	1–1½ inch	22–23

Injection Sites

Injection sites are determined primarily on muscle development and the amount of medication to be injected. The preferred injection site for infants and toddlers is the vastus lateralis. The rectus femoris is also an acceptable site and may be used as an alternative or to rotate injection sites. The ventrogluteal muscle may be used for children older than 3 years of age who have been walking for several years. The deltoid muscle is generally used only in children over 4-5 years of age due to the small muscle mass. However, it may be used for immunizations in children over 1½ years of age since only a small amount of fluid is administered. Figure 19-3 illustrates injection sites.

The amount of solution safely injected intramuscularly varies according to the age of the child and the specific muscle. Age-based guidelines for the amount of solution injected can be found in Table 19-3.

Administration

Before administering IM injections, the skin at the injection site should be cleaned with alcohol or an antiseptic solution and allowed to dry. The nurse should insert the needle into the skin at a 90-degree angle, aspirate, and inject the medication. Positioning the infant or child to relax the muscle being used for the injection may lessen the degree of discomfort experienced. For example, flexing the knee may promote relaxation of the vastus lateralis, while lying on the side and flexing the top leg at the knee may relax the ventrogluteal muscle.

When administering the IM injection, the infant and young child should be securely restrained to avoid injury or giving the injection at the wrong site. It is best to have two adults help hold the child when giving IM medications to toddlers and preschoolers. The school-age child also may need some help to remain still. It is also necessary to have a firm grip on the lower portion of the syringe to ensure safety should the infant or child move. Figure 19-4 illustrates two methods of restraining an infant when giving an IM injection.

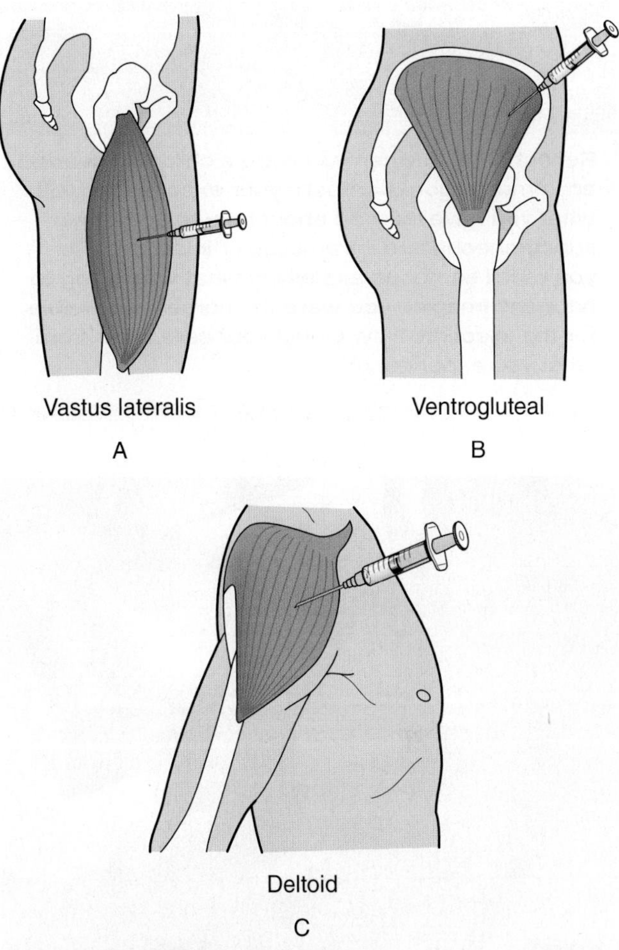

Figure 19-3 **Intramuscular injection sites. (A) Vastus lateralis: Identify the greater trochanter. Place hand at the lateral femoral condyle. The injection site is in the middle third and anterior to the lateral aspect. (B) Ventrogluteal: Place palm of the left hand on right greater trochanter so the index finger points toward the anterosuperior iliac spine. When middle finger is spread to form a V, the injection site is in the middle of the V. (C) Deltoid: Locate the lateral side of the humerus. One finger width below the acromion process is the deltoid.** DELMAR CENGAGE LEARNING.

Table 19-3 Age-Based Guidelines for Amount of Solution to Be Injected Intramuscularly

	AGE GROUP				
MUSCLE	INFANT	TODDLER	PRESCHOOLER	SCHOOL-AGE CHILD	ADOLESCENT
(Age in years)	0–1.5	1.5–3	3–6	6–15	≥15
Vastus lateralis or rectus femoris	0.5–1 mL	*1 mL	1.5 mL	1.5–2 mL	2–2.5 mL
Dorsogluteal	*	*1 mL	1.5 mL	1.5–2 mL	2–2.5 mL
Ventrogluteal	**	*1 mL	1.5 mL	1.5–2 mL	2–2.5 mL
Deltoid	**	*0.5 mL	0.5 mL	0.5 mL	1 mL

** Not recommended; **Not recommended unless other sites are not available.*

REFLECTIVE THINKING

Getting a "Shot"?

Reflect back to when you were a child and needed an immunization. Compare your experiences with what you have learned about how to administer subcutaneous and intramuscular injections. Do you recall someone explaining what was going to happen? Imagine you were the nurse responsible for the injection. How would your care differ from what you experienced?

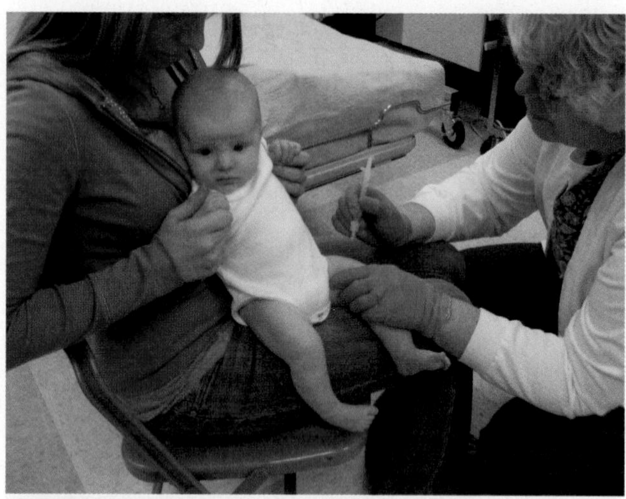

FIGURE 19-4A Restraining an Infant on the Mother's Lap when administering an intramuscular injection. DELMAR CENGAGE LEARNING.

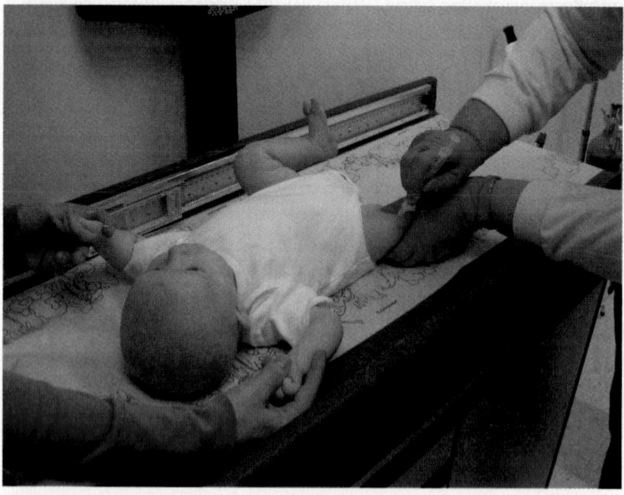

FIGURE 19-4B Restraining an infant's leg for an intramuscular injection when the infant is on a bed. DELMAR CENGAGE LEARNING.

NURSING ALERT

Giving IM Medication to a Combative Child

It may require more than two adults to safely restrain a child who is combative. Using a matter-of-fact approach, the child should be gently but firmly restrained and the procedure accomplished as quickly as possible.

SUBCUTANEOUS MEDICATION

Medication administered subcutaneously (SC) is placed in the subcutaneous fat layers of the body. Fat deposits differ between infants or children and adults, and must be considered when administering medication by this route. The anterior thigh, buttocks, upper arms, and abdomen are the preferred sites for injection. Pinching the subcutaneous layer isolates the site and prevents injection into a muscle, especially when the infant or child has little subcutaneous tissue. The infant or child should be restrained as necessary.

RECTAL MEDICATION

Rectally administered drugs may be erratic and unpredictable in their absorption and are not the most desirable route of medication administration for pediatric clients. However, this route of administration may occasionally become the route of choice if the child is vomiting or NPO. This invasive procedure may be extremely upsetting to toddlers and preschoolers because of age-related fears; school-age children and adolescents may be embarrassed by this procedure. Therefore, age-appropriate explanation and reassurance are needed, as is proper restraint. The suppository, the most common form of drug used rectally, is lubricated with a water-soluble lubricant and inserted in the rectum beyond the rectal sphincter. The fifth finger is used in infants and children under 3 years of age. The index finger can generally be used in children over 3 years of age. After inserting the suppository, the buttocks should be held together for several minutes or until the child loses the urge to defecate to prevent expulsion of the suppository. If the child has a bowel movement within 10-30 minutes after administration of a suppository, examine the stool for the presence of the suppository. If it is seen, notify the health care provider since the medication may need to be readministered.

RESEARCH Highlight

Barcode Medication Administration Systems and Adverse Drug Events

STUDY PURPOSE

To determine the effect of barcode medication administration systems in reducing adverse drug events in a Neonatal Intensive Care Unit.

METHODS

The study used a prospective, observational method to detect adverse drug events in an inpatient neonate population over the course of 50 weeks.

FINDINGS

A total of 92,398 medication doses were administered to 958 subjects. The use of a barcode medication administration system significantly reduced adverse drug events by 47%.

IMPLICATIONS

Neonatal intensive care unit patients are at a relatively high risk of harm from medication errors. Barcode administration medication systems may reduce the occurrence of adverse drug events in children. However, barcode administration medication systems cannot prevent all potential medication errors. Additionally, there are many barcode administration medication systems available, but they may not all be equally effective at reducing medication errors.

REFERENCE

Morriss, F. H., Abramowitz, P. W., Nelson, S. P., Milavetz, G., Michael, S. L., Gordon, S. N., Pendergast, J. F., & Cook, E. F. (2009). Effectiveness of a barcode medication administration system in reducing preventable adverse drug events in a neonatal intensive care unit: A prospective cohort study. *Journal of Pediatrics*, *154*, 363–368.

OPHTHALMIC MEDICATION

Administering ophthalmic medication requires special consideration in the pediatric population. Age-related concerns cause young children to fear having anything placed in their eyes and even infants may close their eyelids so tightly it is difficult for the nurse to open them. Proper restraint is necessary to control the head, keep the child's hands from interfering, and prevent injury to the eye. Children who are old enough to comprehend the procedure should be given an age-appropriate explanation, which may help gain their cooperation. If possible, avoid giving ophthalmic medications when the child is crying since this limits contact of medication with the eye and decreases its therapeutic effect (Kyle & Kyle, 2007).

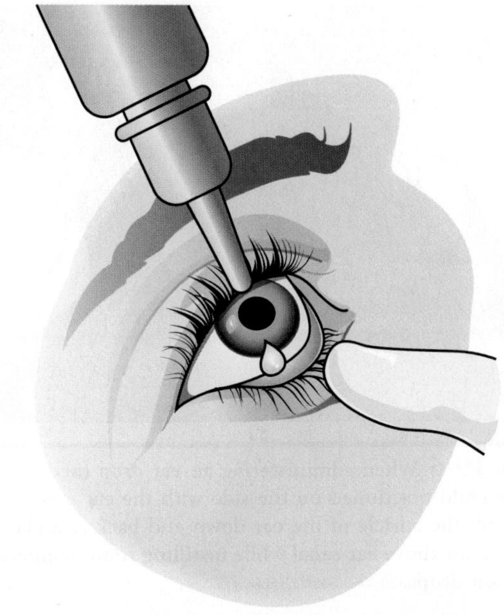

FIGURE 19-5 **When administering an eye medication, gently press the lower lid down and have the child look upward while you instill the drops into the lower conjunctival sac.** DELMAR CENGAGE LEARNING.

To administer eye drops or ointment, the child should be placed in a supine position. Hyperextension of the neck with the head lower than the body may help disperse the medication over the cornea. The hand used to instill the medication should be stabilized by resting the heel of the hand on the child's forehead with the dropper or tube of ointment held with the forefinger and thumb. This is a safety precaution to help prevent injury to the eye, and it also helps ensure the medication goes in the eye and not on the face. The lower eyelid should be retracted and the medication placed in the conjunctival sac while not letting the dropper touch the sac. Ointment should be placed in the sac from the inner canthus outward. The dropper or tube of ointment should not touch the eye lashes or the eye, ensuring sterility as well as protecting the eye. Once the medication has been instilled, the child who is old enough to cooperate should be asked to gently close the eyes to allow greater contact of the medication with the conjunctival area (Figure 19-5).

OTIC MEDICATION

Age-related fears are also a concern when administering otic medications to young children. The younger child may need to be restrained to prevent movement of the head during instillation of the medication. An explanation may help the older child cooperate with the procedure. The child should be placed in a side-lying position with the affected ear exposed. For children under 3 years of age the pinna is pulled downward and back. For the child older than 3 years, the pinna is pulled up and back as with adults. After instillation of the medication, the child should remain in the side-lying position for several minutes. If cotton is placed in the ear

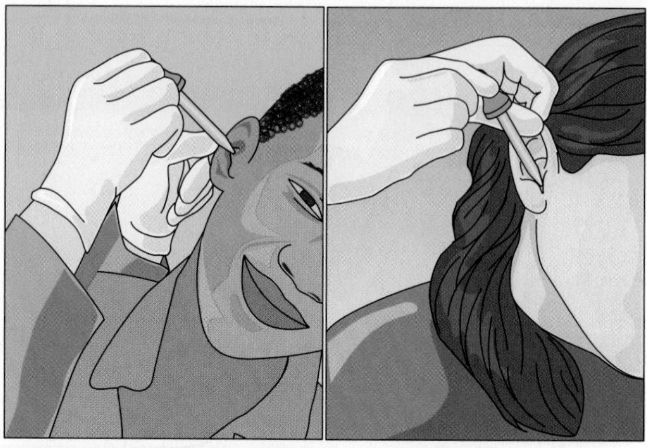

FIGURE 19-6 When administering an ear drop medication, have the child positioned on the side with the ear exposed. Gently pull the auricle of the ear down and back and place dropper 1 cm above ear canal while instilling room temperature medication drops. DELMAR CENGAGE LEARNING.

canal, it needs to be loose enough to allow discharge of any drainage (Figure 19-6).

NASAL MEDICATION

The infant and young child may react negatively to nose drop instillation and proper restraint is necessary to safely accomplish the procedure. The infant or child is placed in a position with the head hyperextended. This can be accomplished by extending the head over the caregiver's lap, the bed, or an examining table. The child should remain in that position for at least 1 minute following the instillation of the nose drops (Figure 19-7).

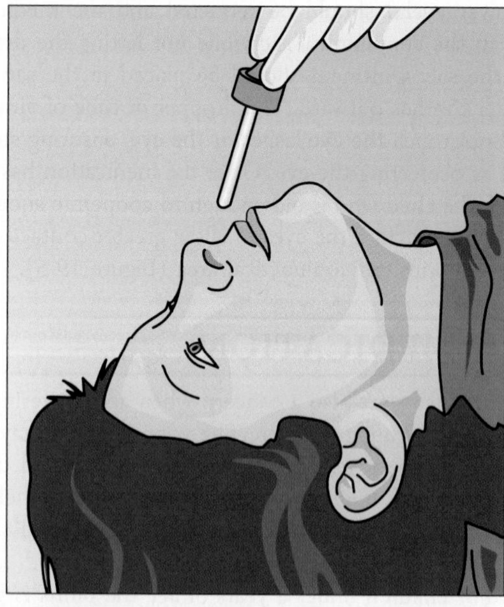

FIGURE 19-7 When instilling nose drops, the child should be placed on his or her back with the head tilted down or over the side of the bed. This will allow the medication to reach the back of the nose. DELMAR CENGAGE LEARNING.

INHALED MEDICATION

Administering inhaled medication to children through a nebulizer has the advantage of delivering a medication directly to the needed site of action. Advantages of administering inhaled medication with appropriate technique show an improvement in the onset of action, and a decrease in the dose needed. The standard inhaler consists of a pressurized canister, a plastic holder, and a cap. Often a spacer or special tube that attaches to the inhaler is used to increase the amount of medication delivered to the lungs per spray. A spacer has either a mouthpiece or a mask for ease of administration and is specific to the child's developmental need. A spacer also acts as a medication holding chamber so that a child can take several breaths to obtain one dose of inhaled medication (Figure 19-8).

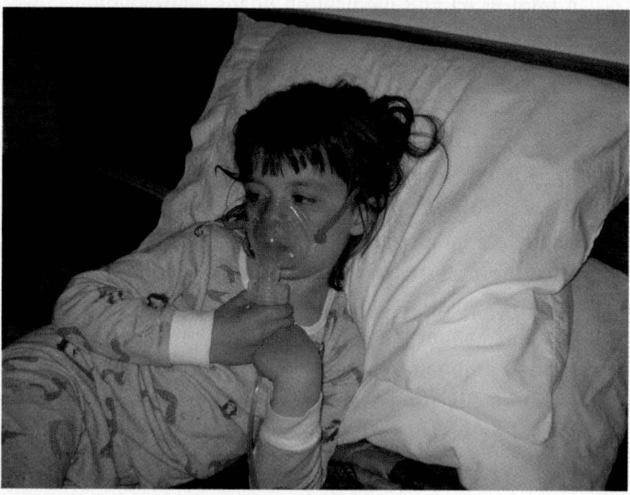

FIGURE 19-8A This child is receiving her medication through a face mask. DELMAR CENGAGE LEARNING.

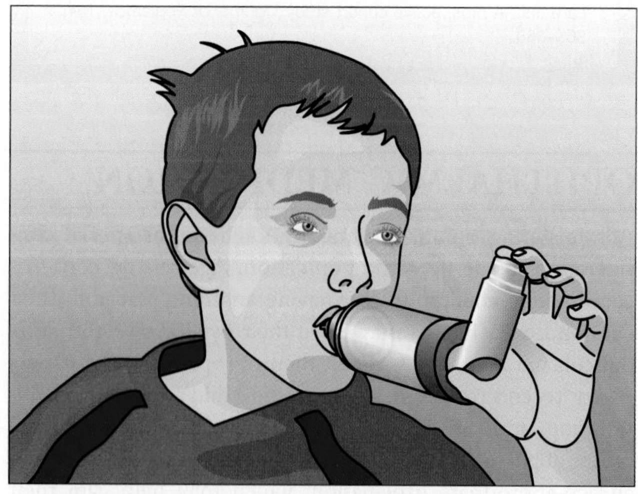

FIGURE 19-8B When administering an inhaled medication, a child should hold the spacer in the upright position and allow 3-4 seconds to inhale the medication after it is dispensed into the spacer. DELMAR CENGAGE LEARNING.

Preparation

Prepare to give inhaled medication by removing the cap from the inhaler and spacer as needed. Prime the inhaler by squirting a puff of medication into the air if the canister is new or has not been used in the last 48 hours. If a spacer is used, insert the inhaler's mouthpiece into the rubber end of the spacer. Shake the inhaler immediately before each puff.

Administration

To administer an inhaled medication using a metered-dose inhaler with spacer, begin by placing the mouthpiece fully into the mouth between the teeth. Hold the inhaler in the upright position and close the lips around the mouthpiece. Press down on the canister to dispense the medication into the spacer. Instruct the patient to breathe deeply for 3–5 seconds through the mouth, and then hold the breath for 10 seconds. Remove the spacer from the mouth and breathe out slowly. A patient should rinse the mouth out with water after each use of inhaled steroids to help prevent oral infections, and the spacer should routinely be washed with warm soapy water and air dried. Teach families to consistently use proper technique with their children. Often young children resist the mask when it is first introduced; however, with consistent practice eventually they will cooperate when they realize the parent is serious about giving their medications effectively.

TOPICAL MEDICATION

Administering topical medication to children is the same as for an adult. If the skin is broken, sterile technique is required. The biggest challenge for the nurse administering topical medication to infants and children may be preventing the child from scratching an irritated or infected area. The child's finger nails should be kept short and clean, and the child's hands may need to be covered with mittens.

IN THE REAL WORLD

As a student, I felt overwhelmed when I first started administering medications to infants and children. There were all these calculations needed to determine a therapeutic dose range and the amount (volume, number of pills) of medication to be given. Often the amount given was small and required transferring liquids into smaller syringes or cutting pills in half in contrast with my experience when caring for adults. In addition, at times I had to crush pills, and it was sometimes challenging to get them dissolved in a medium that the child would accept. As I progressed through my pediatric nursing experience, the supervised practice I received in giving medications to children increased my skills and my confidence in my ability to perform this task safely and efficiently.

KEY CONCEPTS

- Most drugs have not been adequately tested in the pediatric population; therefore, standardized doses have not been established, and children may be at risk for adverse reactions or ineffective treatment.
- Physiological differences between children and adults make children more sensitive to drugs and increase the risk of adverse drug reactions.
- Age-related physiological differences are responsible for alterations in pharmacokinetic and pharmacodynamic processes and determine the method, dose, and frequency of drug administration.
- Safe drug administration in a pediatric population requires an understanding of physiological differences and their impact on pharmacokinetic and pharmacodynamic processes.
- Approaches to children and techniques of medication administration must be based on growth and development, including physical, psychosocial, and cognitive development.
- Children should be given developmentally appropriate and truthful explanations about medication administration.
- The form of oral medication administered and the method of administration should be developmentally appropriate.
- Intravenous administration of medication improves the therapeutic blood level of medication and eliminates the discomfort associated with repeated injections.
- Injections are not the preferred route in children since they are painful and distressing. In addition, physiological factors make this a less effective route in infants.
- When injections are necessary, care should be taken to select the appropriate injection site and size of needle based on the child's size. The needle size selected should be the shortest and smallest gauge possible.
- Administration of rectal, ophthalmic, otic, and nasal medications are invasive procedures that may elicit fears in toddlers and preschool-age children.

REVIEW ACTIVITIES

1. What are the four pharmacokinetic processes?
2. How does gastric emptying time influence the absorption of orally administered drugs? What are the implications for administering medications to infants and children?
3. How does protein binding influence distribution of a drug? What are the implications for administering medications to infants and children?
4. What physiological factors influence the half-life of drugs administered to infants and children?
5. What are two psychosocial or cognitive aspects of toddler growth and development that influence the administration of medication to this age group? How would you approach giving medication to this age group based on your knowledge of these aspects of growth and development?
6. What actions should the nurse take before administering a medication when there is a discrepancy between the ordered dose and the recommended dose?
7. A 3-year-old has an order for Cefazolin 300 mg IV every 8 hours. The child weighs 21.6 lbs (9.8 kg). The recommended dose for Cefazolin is 50–100 mg/kg/24 hours. Calculate the recommended dosage range for this child and compare it with the ordered dose. Is the ordered dose appropriate? If not, why not?
8. What are two methods for administering an oral liquid medication to an infant? How would you administer the medication using each method, including any safety precautions?
9. The nurse is administering an intravenous (IV) medication to a child and has verified the five rights of medication administration, as well as comparing the ordered dose with the recommended dose. What additional information is needed in order to safely administer the IV medication?

STUDY QUESTIONS

1. Anatomic and physiological factors that affect orally-administered drug absorption in the infant include:
   a. Increased transit time of drugs through the lower gastrointestinal tract.
   b. Decreased gastric emptying, thus increasing the time medications remain in the stomach.
   c. Increased gastric acidity that affects the way tablets dissolve.
   d. Increased digestive enzymes that metabolize medications more rapidly.
2. The nurse has an IM medication order for an infant. Which of the following is true?
   a. Infant muscles have a high level of oxygenation which can increase the absorption of medication.
   b. Medication solutions that are less viscous require a larger gauge needle.
   c. Infants have vasomotor instability with diminished and unpredictable peripheral blood flow.
   d. The rectus femoris is the first choice of injection site for infants.
3. The nurse is familiar with special considerations of topical medications in the infant population and knows that which of the following is false?
   a. Because infants have a greater body surface area to weight ratio, topical medications are absorbed rapidly.
   b. Absorption of topical medications is increased if the infant's skin integrity is compromised where the topical medication is to be applied.
   c. If the infant's skin is compromised, sterile technique is required to apply the topical medication.
   d. There are differences in technique when administering topical medication for infants and adults.
4. The nurse would evaluate that the parents correctly understand the care of their infant based on which of the following parent comments?
   a. "I will give the liquid medication through a nipple without the bottle attached to get my baby to take the medicine."
   b. "I can use an oral syringe and let the baby suck the medication from the end of the syringe."
   c. "I can administer the medication while my baby is lying in her crib, awake and not crying."
   d. "When measuring the liquid medication, it is important to use a teaspoon."
5. A 3-year-old patient seen in the Emergency Department needs an oral medication administered. The nurse knows that in this age group:
   a. The drug's half-life may be shorter than in infants or adults.
   b. The renal system is immature and may affect the excretion of the medication in urine.

c. Children are generally cooperative in taking oral medications as long as they are given choices and control over their environment.
d. If the child is resistant to taking the medication, the nurse will be more successful if the parent leaves the room.

6. The nurse needs to calculate the dose of Augmentin (amoxicillin/clavulanate) for a 6-year-old child with otitis media. The child has an order for Augmentin 45 mg/kg/day PO divided BID. Augmentin is available as 400 mg/5 mL. If the 6-year-old child weighs 55 pounds, how much would each individual dose be?
   a. 10 mL
   b. 5 mL
   c. 7 mL
   d. 3 mL
7. When a child is receiving an IV medication, which of the following should be given the highest priority?
   a. Parents should be instructed not to tamper with the IV.
   b. The medication should be administered over several minutes.
   c. The IV should be running at a stable rate.
   d. Consultation of pharmacologic references for recommended concentration of medication and IV compatibility.
8. The nurse is using a syringe infusion pump to administer an IV pain medication to an 8-year-old child who has recently undergone surgery. The nurse should consider all of the following except:
   a. Total volume of medication to be administered.
   b. Flushing the IV tubing with D5 ½ NS solution.
   c. Programming the pump to infuse medication in prescribed amount of time.
   d. Labeling the tubing or syringe with name of medication.
9. The nurse needs to administer an ophthalmic medication to a 5-year-old child with bilateral bacterial conjunctivitis. The nurse should consider all of the following except that:
   a. Restraining the child may be necessary, with special effort to control the child's legs to keep them from kicking.
   b. Children typically fear having anything placed in their eyes.
   c. Administration should be avoided, if possible, while the child is crying.
   d. Medication should be placed in the conjunctival sac using sterile technique.
10. The nurse is teaching a newly diagnosed 8-year-old child with asthma how to properly use his inhaler with a spacer. Which of the following statements indicates that the patient has understood the nurse's teaching?
   a. "When I use my spacer, I can breathe my medication all in one deep breath. Then I need to hold my breath for ten seconds."
   b. "I should not drink anything after using my inhaler."
   c. "I know I need to first shake the inhaler and squirt a puff of medication into the air if I haven't used it for awhile."
   d. "I should take three deep breaths before using my inhaler."

REFERENCES

Adams, M. P., Josephson, D. L., & Holland, L. N. (2005). *Pharmacology for nurses: A pathophysiologic approach.* Upper Saddle River, NJ: Prentice-Hall.

Algren, C. (2005). Family-centered care of the child during illness and hospitalization. In K. Gutierrez & S. F. Queener (Eds.), *Pharmacology for nursing practice.* St. Louis, MO: Mosby, pp. 33–43.

American Academy of Pediatrics. (2007). Pediatric Research Equity Act of 2007. (Public Law 110-85). Retrieved April 27, 2009, from http://www.aap.org/advocacy/washing/Therapeutics/docs/bpcapreasidexside.pdf.

Anand, V., Kataria, M., Kukkar, V., Saharan, V., & Choudhury, P. K. (2007). The latest trends in the taste assessment of pharmaceuticals. *Drug Discovery Today, 12*(5-6), 257–265.

Andrew, S., Salamonson, Y., & Halcomb, E. J. (2009). Nursing students' confidence in medication calculations predicts math exam performance. *Nurse Education Today, 29,* 217–223.

Andrews, M. M. & Boyle, J. S. (2007). *Transcultural concepts in nursing care* (5th ed.). Philadelphia: Lippincott, Williams, & Wilkins.

Anley, P., & Siu, A. (2005). Principles of pharmacotherapy in pediatrics. In V. P. Arcangelo, & A. M. Peterson, *Pharmacotherapeutics for advanced practice* (2nd ed.). Philadelphia: Lippincott, Williams, & Wilkins, pp. 40–48.

Aschenbrenner, D. S., & Venable, S. J. (2008). *Drug therapy in nursing* (3rd ed.). Philadelphia: Lippincott, Williams, & Wilkins.

Bauer, L. A. (2008). *Applied clinical pharmacokinetics* (2nd ed.). New York: McGraw-Hill.

Best Pharmaceuticals for Children Act (Public Law 107-109) (2002). Retrieved April 30, 2009, from http://www.fda.gov/opacom/laws/pharmkids/pharmkids.html.

Blackburn, S. T. (2007). *Maternal, fetal, & neonatal physiology: A clinical perspective* (3rd ed.). Philadelphia: Elsevier Health Sciences.

Bowden, V. R., & Greenberg, C. S. (2007). *Pediatric nursing procedures* (2nd ed.). Philadelphia: Lippincott, Williams, & Wilkins.

Burton, M. E., Shaw, L. M., Schentag, J. J., & Evans, W. E. (2005). *Applied pharmacokinetics & pharmacodynamics: Principles of therapeutic drug monitoring.* Philadelphia: Lippincott, Williams, & Wilkins.

Cahill, M. (2009). Pediatric medication safety: The power of the team. *Nurse Administration Quarterly, 33*(1), 38–47.

Deveaugh-Geiss, J., March, J., Shapiro, M., Andreason, P. J., Emslie, G., Ford, L. M. et al. (2006). Child and adolescent psychopharmacology in the new millennium: A workshop for academia, industry, and government. *Journal of the American Academy of Child & Adolescent Psychiatry, 45*(3), 261–270.

Garvie, P. A., Lensing, S., & Rai, S. N. (2007). Efficacy of pill-swallowing training intervention to improve antiretroviral medication adherence in pediatric patients with HIV/AIDS. *Pediatrics, 119*, e893–e899.

Gracely-Kilgore, K. A. (2005). Pediatric issues. In Youngkin, E. Q., Sawin, K. J., Kissinger, J. F., & Israel, D. S., *Pharmacotherapeutics: A primary care clinical guide* (2nd ed.). Upper Saddle River, NJ: Pearson Prentice-Hall, pp. 173–188.

Gutierrez, K. (2003). Pediatric pharmacotherapeutics. In K. Gutierrez & S. F. Queener (Eds.). *Pharmacology for nursing practice.* St. Louis, MO: Mosby, pp. 33–43.

Hedaya, M. A. (2007). *Basic pharmacokinetics.* Boca Raton, FL: CRC Press.

Herrman, J. W. (2009). Pediatric pharmacology. In J. L. Kee, & E. R. Hayes, *Pharmacology: A nursing process approach* (6th ed.). St. Louis, MO: Saunders, pp. 187–196.

Hunt, R. (2008). *Introduction to community-based nursing* (4th ed.). Philadelphia: Lippincott, Williams, & Wilkins.

Ince, I., Saskia, N., Tibboel, D., Danhof, M., & Knibbe, C. (2009). Tailor-made drug treatment for children: Creation of an infrastructure for data-sharing and population PK-PD modeling. *Drug Discovery Today, 14*(5-6), 316–320.

Karch, A. M. (2010). *Focus on nursing pharmacology* (5th ed.). Philadelphia: Lippincott, Williams, & Wilkins.

Kee, J. L., Hayes, E. R., & McCuistion, L. E. (2009). *Pharmacology. A nursing process approach* (6th ed.). St. Louis, MO: Saunders.

Kemper, K. J., Vohra, S., Walls, R., The Task Force on Complementary and Alternative Medicine, & The Provisional Section on Complementary, Holistic, and Integrative Medicine. (2008). The use of complementary and alternative medicine in pediatrics. *Pediatrics*, 122, 1374–1386.

Kyle, T., & Kyle, T. (2007). *Essentials of pediatric nursing.* Philadelphia: Lippincott, Williams, & Wilkins.

LaMattina, J. C., & Golan, D. E. (2007). In D. E. Golan, A. H. Tashjian, E. J. Armstrong, & A. W. Armstrong, *Principles of pharmacology.* Philadelphia: Lippincott, Williams, & Wilkins, pp. 31–48.

Lehne, R. A. (2010). *Pharmacology for nursing care* (7th ed.). Philadelphia: Saunders.

Luedtke, S. A. (2006). Pediatric and neonatal therapy. In R. A. Helms, E. T. Herfindal, D. J. Quan, & D. R. Gourley, *Textbook of therapeutics* (8th ed.). Philadelphia: Lippincott, Williams, & Wilkins, pp. 325–337.

Maples, H. D., James, L. P., & Stowe, C. D. (2005). Special pharmacokinetic and pharmacodynamic considerations in children. In M. E. Burton, L. M. Shaw, J. J. Schentag, & W. E. Evans, *Applied pharmacokinetics & pharmacodynamics* (4th ed.). Philadelphia: Lippincott, Williams, & Wilkins, pp. 213–227.

Matsui, D. (2007). Current issues in pediatric medication adherence. *Pediatric Drugs, 9*(5), 283–288.

McCance, K. L. & Huether, S. E. (2010). *Pathophysiology: The biologic basis for disease in adults and children* (6th ed.). St. Louis, MO: Elsevier Mosby.

Mennella, J. A., & Beauchamp, G. K. (2008). Optimizing oral medications for children. *Clinical Therapeutics, 30*(11), 2120–2132.

Morriss, F. H., Abramowitz, P. W., Nelson, S. P., Milavetz, G., Michael, S. L., Gordon, S. N., Pendergast, J. F., & Cook, E. F. (2009). Effectiveness of a barcode medication administration system in reducing preventable adverse drug events in a neonatal intensive care unit: A prospective cohort study. *Journal of Pediatrics, 154*, 363–368.

Nahata, M. C., & Taketomo, C. (2008). Pediatrics. In J. T. DiPiro, R. L. Talbert, G. C. Yee, B. G. Matzke, & L. M. Posey, *Pharmacotherapy: A pathophysiologic approach* (7th ed.). New York: McGraw-Hill, pp. 47–56.

Ndosi, M. E., & Newell, R. (2009). Nurses' knowledge of pharmacology behind drugs they commonly administer. *Journal of Clinical Nursing, 18*(4), 570–580.

Pepper, G. A. (2005). Pharmacokinetics and pharmacodynamics. In E. Q. Youngkin, K. J. Sawin, J. F. Kissinger, & D. S. Israel, *Pharmacotherapeutics: A primary care clinical guide* (2nd ed.). Upper Saddle River, NJ: Pearson Prentice-Hall, pp. 7–41.

Peterson, A. M. (2005). Pharmacokinetic basis of therapeutics and pharmacodynamic principles. In V. P. Arcangelo, & A. M. Peterson, *Pharmacotherapeutics for advanced practice: A practical approach* (2nd ed.). Philadelphia: Lippincott, Williams, & Wilkins, pp. 13–26.

Potter, P. A. & Perry, A. G. (2009). *Fundamentals of nursing* (7th ed.). St. Louis, MO: Mosby.

Purswani, M. U., Radhakrishnan, J., Irfan, K. R., Walter-Glickman, C., Hagmann, S., & Neugebauer, R. (2009). Infant acceptance of a bitter-tasting liquid medication: A randomized controlled trial comparing the Rx medibottle with an oral syringe. *Archives of Pediatric Adolescent Medicine, 163*(2), 186–188.

Raja Lope, R. J., Boo, N. Y., Rohana, J., & Cheah, F. C. (2009). A quality assurance study on the administration of medication by nurses in a neonatal intensive care unit. *Singapore Medicine Journal, 50*(1), 68–72.

Regulations Requiring Manufacturers to Assess the Safety and Effectiveness of New Drugs and Biological Products in Pediatric Patients: Final Rule Fed Reg. *Vol. 63*, No. 231, pp. 66631–66672 (December 2, 1998) (FR Doc 98-31902 Filed 11-27-98).

Ricci, S. S., Kyle, T., & Kyle, T. (2008). *Maternity and pediatric nursing.* Philadelphia: Lippincott, Williams, & Wilkins.

Rodriguez, W., Selen, A., Avant, D., Chaurasia, C., Crescenzi, T., Gieser, G., et al. (2008). Improving pediatric dosing through pediatric initiatives: What we have learned. *Pediatrics, 121*, 530–539.

Stein, H. G. (2006). Glass ampules and filter needles: An example of implementing the sixth "R" in medication administration. *MEDSURG Nursing, 15*(5), 290–294.

Tozer, T. N., & Rowland, M. (2006). *Introduction to pharmacokinetics and pharmacodynamics: The quantitative basis of drug therapy.* Philadelphia: Lippincott, Williams, & Wilkins.

Turkoski, B. (2007). Medicating young or very young patients—Part I. *Orthopaedic Nursing, 26*(2), 134–139.

Williams, N. T. (2008). Medication administration through enteral feeding tubes. *American Journal of Health Systems Pharmacology, 65*, 2347–2357.

Wilson, D. (2009). Health promotion of the newborn and family. In M. J. Hockenberry, & D. Wilson, (Eds.) *Wong's Essentials of Pediatric Nursing* (8th ed.). St. Louis, MO: Elsevier Mosby.

Wright, K. (2008). Drug calculations part 1: A critique of the formula used by nurses. *Nursing Standard, 22*(36), 40–42.

Wynne, A. L., Woo, T. M., & Olyaei, A. J. (2007). *Pharmacotherapeutics for nurse practitioner prescribers* (2nd ed.). Philadelphia: F. A. Davis Company.

SUGGESTED READINGS

Bindler, R. C, & Ball, J. W. (2008). *Clinical skills manual for pediatric nursing: Caring for children* (4th ed.). Upper Saddle River, NJ: Prentice-Hall.

Mandleco, B. L. (2005). *Pediatric nursing skills & procedures.* Clifton Park, NY: Delmar Cengage Learning.

Rising, D. L. (2008). *Pharmacology for nursing practice.* Philadelphia: Lippincott, Williams, & Wilkins.

Taketomo, C. K., Hodding, J. H., & Kraus, D. M. (2006). *Pediatric dosage handbook* (13th ed.). Hudson, OH: Lexi-Comp.

The Johns Hopkins Hospital, Robertson, J., & Shilkofski, N. (2005). *The Harriet Lane handbook* (17th ed.). St. Louis, MO: Mosby.

RESOURCES

Refer to the online student StudyWARE for Potts & Mandleco at http://www.CengageBrain.com for additional content and study aids.

Organization: **How to Dispose of Unused Medicines**
Description: This article informs clients about how to dispose of unused household medications.
Website/Resource: http://www.fda.gov/ForConsumers/ConsumerUpdates/ucm101653.htm

Organization: **Find Your Local Poison Center**
Description: Users of this website can access their local poison center by entering their zip code.
Website/Resource: http://www.aapcc.org/dnn/Resources/FindLocalPoisonCenters/tabid/130/Default.aspx

Organization: **Kids Health Understanding Medications and What They Do**
Description: This article has three main sections: what are medications, different types of medications, and taking medications.
Website/Resource: http://kidshealth.org/PageManager.jsp?dn=primarychildrens&article_set=30269&lic=292&cat_id=20120

Organization: **National Association of School Nurses (NASN)**
Description: Offers information regarding continuing education, helpful resources, education campaigns, policy/advocacy, and research, as well as professional information to active school nurses.
Website/Resource: http://www.nasn.org

Organization: **National Association of School Nurses Position Statement: Medication Administration in the School Setting**
Description: The article discusses current implementations of delegating medication administration to unlicensed assistive personnel.
Website/Resource: http://www.nasn.org/Default.aspx?tabid=230

Organization: **Safer Healthcare for Kids: 20 Tips to Help Prevent Medical Errors in Children**
Description: This article is directed towards parents and discusses 20 tips to prevent medical errors in children.
Website/Resource: http://www.aap.org/saferhealthcare/files/5907_20tipkid.pdf

Organization: **Society of Pediatric Nurses (SPN)**
Description: Offers access to information regarding SPN committees, conventions, chapters, awards/scholarships, and much more.
Website/Resource: http://www.pedsnurses.org

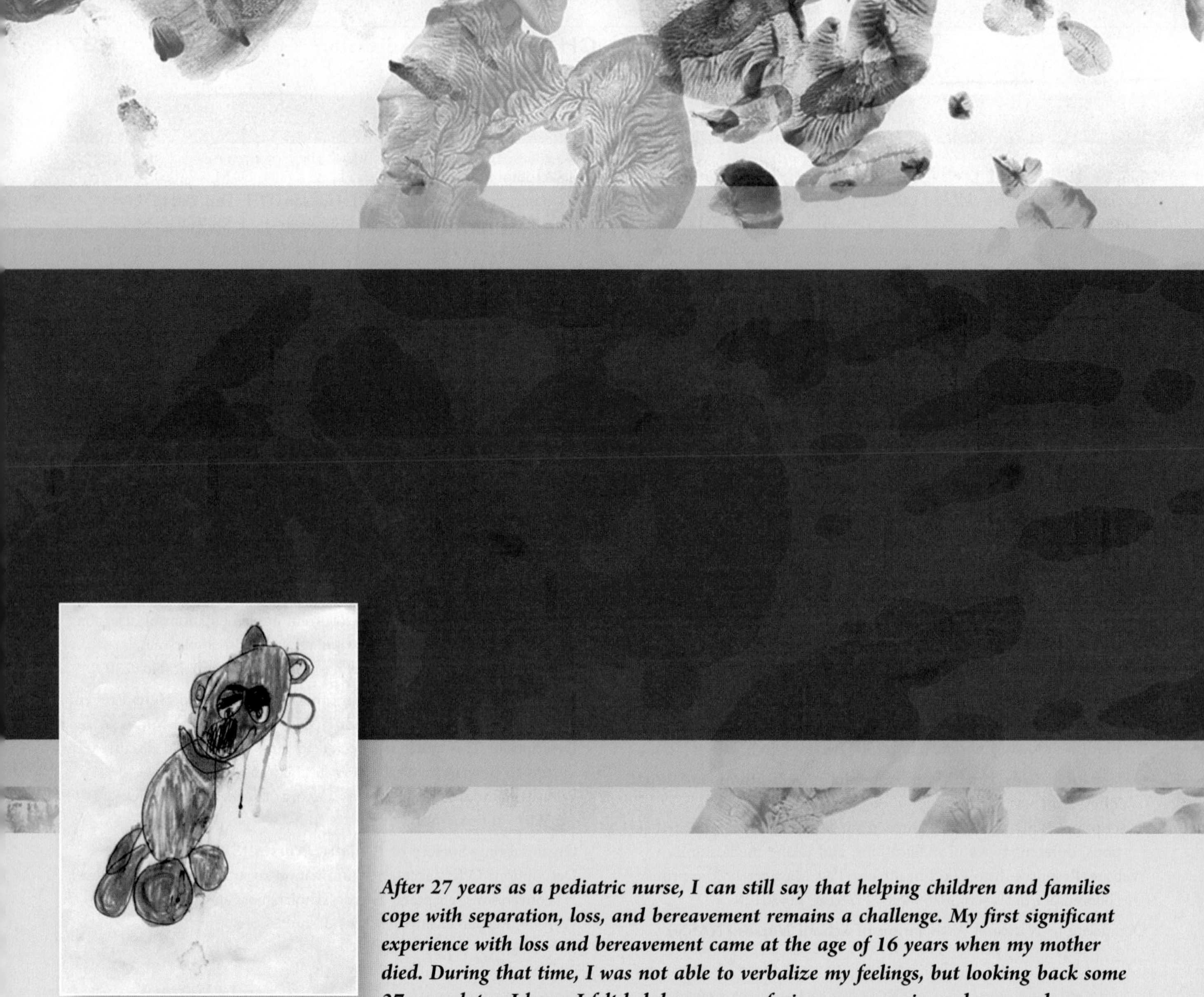

After 27 years as a pediatric nurse, I can still say that helping children and families cope with separation, loss, and bereavement remains a challenge. My first significant experience with loss and bereavement came at the age of 16 years when my mother died. During that time, I was not able to verbalize my feelings, but looking back some 37 years later, I know I felt helplessness, confusion, anger, pain, sadness, and even relief. Some years later I experienced the death of my pet dog Akidu. I experienced some of those same feelings, mainly sadness and anger. These 27 years have also taught me children experience loss and separation not only related to a person but to pets and objects as well; and as adults grieve, so do children.

When caring for children experiencing loss, I try to incorporate the knowledge gained from my experience. At the same time, I try to remember many factors influence how an individual copes with loss, and there is no prescriptive way a person responds to loss. I also teach students that in order to assist clients to cope with loss and bereavement, we must recognize and acknowledge the feelings of the individual which may be both verbal and nonverbal.

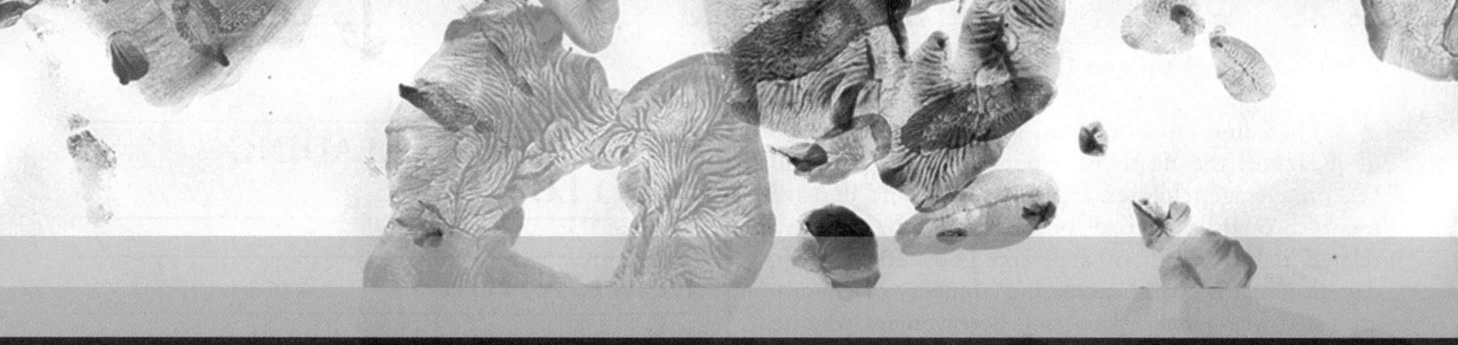

CHAPTER 20

Loss and Bereavement

Hazel M. Sanderson-Marcoux, RN, EdD

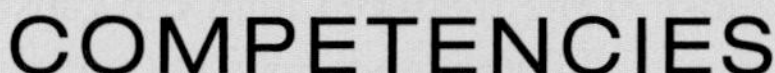

COMPETENCIES

Upon completion of this chapter, the reader will be able to:

- Describe common situations that can lead to feelings of loss and separation in children.
- Explain how children of various ages conceptualize death.
- Apply the process of grief and bereavement to practice.
- Discuss factors that influence children's reactions to loss.
- Apply the common responses of children to loss to practice.
- Explain how children respond to the death of a parent or sibling.
- Discuss strategies to help communities cope with loss due to disaster or traumatic events.
- Discuss the role of the nurse in providing care to families experiencing a life-threatening illness of a child.
- Explain why hospice might be a good alternative to hospital care for the terminally ill child.
- Discuss the importance of self-care for nurses caring for the terminally ill child.
- Apply evidence-based nursing findings related to loss and bereavement in children.
- Successfully complete the games and activities in the online student StudyWARE.

When one thinks of loss, separation, or bereavement, the death of a person comes to mind; yet, on average, children experience loss and bereavement through a myriad of situations that are not related to the death of a person (Box 20-1). Every day around the world increasing numbers of children are faced with issues of loss and bereavement whether it is the loss of someone through divorce, death, abandonment, relocation, or incarceration. Today's children are coping with various types of losses at much earlier ages.

These early experiences are important and help shape an individual's ability to cope with loss later in adult life. Lynch (2008) tells us that initially these losses are often more real to children than the loss of a parent and that providing help and support at these times can help prevent problems later in life.

BOX 20-1

COMMON SITUATIONS LEADING TO FEELINGS OF LOSS AND SEPARATION IN CHILDREN

- Relocation
- Loss of a possession
- Pet loss
- Parental separation or divorce

SITUATIONS LEADING TO LOSS

RELOCATION

Today's economic climate has made it likely that the average family will move to a different home at least once. The effects of relocation may initiate feelings of anxiety and loss for children. Relocation may be a positive or negative experience based on the circumstances. Relocation for adults may mean a new job, better finances, and larger living space; it may be the result of a need to be close to elderly parents; or it may be the result of a disruption in a family such as divorce. However, for young children, such a move may be seen as a loss of comfortable and familiar things, people, and surroundings; moving to a new school or even starting a new grade may trigger feelings of anxiety and loss.

LOSS OF A POSSESSION

Children at an early age develop attachments to objects such as toys and items of clothing. Such objects may bring about a sense of relaxation, security, and comfort. A blanket snuggled close to the body during naptime or while crying may be soothing and reassuring. A favorite toy that accompanies the child to the babysitter, to the child care center, or to the health care provider helps maintain a sense of security and belonging. The loss of the treasured item can cause feelings of anxiety in young children and may be a child's initial experience with loss and separation.

Reflections from Families

I don't remember how old I was when we moved to another state. My mother said I was five years old. I know I was sad because my aunt and uncles were not moving with us. I remember crying and telling my mother that I did not want to go. My aunt kept saying "I'm going to miss you." I could not sleep in my bed any longer, I did not like being by myself. I slept with my mother or one of my uncles. I know I was afraid, but I don't know what I was afraid of. I am now 24 years old and am preparing to go away to college. I have a small box with three items in it—a trophy, a cap, and a little wooden house. These items were given to me by my uncles and aunt the day my mother and I left. They told me to choose one item from each of them to take with me. Now I am going off to college and my family will not see me as often. I will give everyone an item of mine. My father will get one of my caps, my mother will get a tee-shirt. I don't know what I will give my two little brothers, but I think I will let them choose something from my room.

PET LOSS

To understand pet loss, it is important to understand the significance of pet ownership. Most pet owners view their pets as members of the family and attribute human characteristics to them. Field, Orsini, Gavish, & Packman, (2009) state that people become emotionally close and committed to pets and that the human-pet attachment bond is quite similar to that between humans. Many relationships between pets and children are positive; they learn to share, care, be empathetic and to communicate socially. A pet may be the friend who understands the child's feelings when the child feels no one else does (Figure 20-1.) A pet may provide unconditional love and acceptance, and children will generate increased feelings of self-worth when they successfully care for the pet's needs. Hence, the loss of a pet may be of great significance to a child. Because children view pets as friends, the loss of the pet (death, lost from running away, or stolen) may be the child's first real experience with loss, separation, and grieving. Pet loss may be anticipated (old age or terminal illness) or unexpected. Regardless of the reason, children tend to feel much the same way about the loss (Figure 20-2). Therefore, the manner in which adults interact with children after the loss of a pet can greatly impact how children learn to cope with separation and loss later in life. Brodkin (2007) recommends that it is best to be honest about the death of a pet and that honoring the pet's life is important.

Reflections from Families

Sparky was old, 18 years old. He was almost blind and could hardly get upstairs. He was smart; he would wait at the bottom of the stairs and just bark until I came to get him. He was my "Sparky" for all my life. My parents got him for me when I was only 6 months old. He was like my brother. I miss him; I keep his ashes in my room. I don't know if I want another dog. I love him and miss him a lot.

PARENTAL SEPARATION OR DIVORCE

Divorce, an extremely stressful event in the life of a family, is a leading cause of separation experienced by families. However, even though many children adjust well after parental divorce, others suffer adjustment problems requiring therapeutic interventions This is because parental divorce may disrupt not only ties between partners and between parents and children but also relationships among the children themselves (Poortman & Voorpostel, 2008). But most children of divorced parents do not have long-term negative outcomes (Lansford, 2009).

Two major factors in children's reaction to loss are the child's age at the time of the loss and the child's cognitive development. Children's adjustment to divorce is related to many interconnected factors such as: age at time of divorce, parents' well-being/psychosocial state, reasons for divorce, and child support and child custody issues (Lansford, 2009). Children at different developmental stages exhibit behaviors differently. For example, preschoolers who are able to sense the conflict in the house tend to feel confused and bewildered though they may have a limited understanding

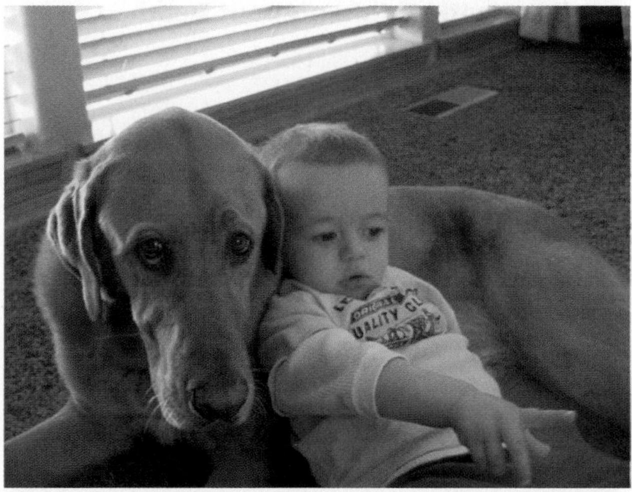

FIGURE 20-1 Pets often afford children unconditional love and acceptance, and demonstrate this by being patient and willing to let children spend time with them, even if it means being used as a pillow. DELMAR CENGAGE LEARNING.

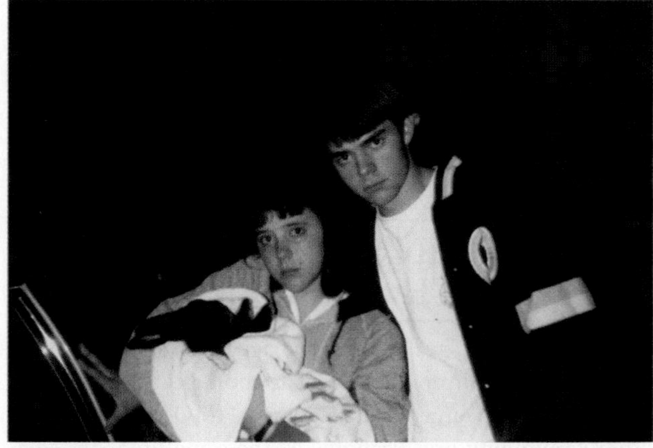

FIGURE 20-2 Children grieve when their pets become ill or die. DELMAR CENGAGE LEARNING.

about what is taking place. Children at this age perceive divorce as one parent moving away or leaving. The child often assumes he or she did something wrong. This in turn causes the child to fear abandonment by the custodial parent. Children who are afraid of being abandoned tend to manifest clinging or hanging-on behaviors with the custodial parent. These children may temporarily lose any independence recently acquired, and return to bedwetting, thumb sucking, or even bottle feeding. Preschoolers may experience nightmares or sleep disturbances and their play may become aggressive as they attempt to act out their feelings of confusion. Lansford et al. (2006) suggest that parental divorce occurring from kindergarten to fifth grade exerted more adverse effects on internalizing (sadness, withdrawal) and externalizing (aggression, acting out) problems than did parental divorce occurring between sixth and tenth grade, whereas parental divorce occurring between sixth and tenth grade exerted more adverse effects on grades.

School-age children may believe their parents' emotional distress is related to how they have been behaving and can perceive the divorce as a rejection, resulting in feelings of guilt. Fear of being replaced may exist along with low self-esteem. Children in this age group may have fantasies of reunification of parents and family, and may lie in an attempt to make this fantasy come true. Children between 9 and 12 years of age may experience conflicts with loyalty and also exhibit outbursts of anger toward either or both parents. **Parentification**, which is assuming the caregiver (parent) role, is common in this age group. These children may also manifest their distress in anger, somatic complaints, and social withdrawal. Parentification is also common in adolescents, especially when daily activities of the home are neglected and the adolescent must take the role of the absent parent by preparing meals or doing the laundry. Adolescents may also distance themselves from one or both parents, or may be openly critical, or display both behaviors. Antisocial behaviors such as delinquency, becoming physically violent, smoking, alcohol abuse, or truancy may occur. For some adolescents, school may become a refuge from turmoil at home, and they may spend all their energies in school activities to avoid thinking about the situation at home. An emotional attachment to a member of the opposite sex may provide some form of compensation for family life, whereas other adolescents may sever any newly formed relationships they have just entered (Amato & Afifi, 2006; Sobolewski & Amato, 2007).

CHILDREN'S AWARENESS OF DEATH

Rapid changes in health care management have expanded the nurse's role from traditional to nontraditional settings such as schools, urgent care centers, HMOs, shelters, and other community organizations. At the same time, our society witnessed an increase in accidental deaths, violent crimes, terrorist acts, and natural disasters. In addition, we began to enjoy advancement in technology that brought every new event directly into our living rooms via the Internet and television. Information once shielded from young children, such as death and violence, is now readily discussed in playgrounds, school yards, and neighborhoods.

Nurses caring for children now face the challenges of caring for children and families affected by death. In order to provide competent care to children it is important for nurses to understand how children perceive the concept of death at various stages of development.

CONCEPT OF DEATH

Children's understanding of the concept of death takes place over time. The development of the death concept stems from children's communication with parents and experiences with death in the social environment, for example, the death of a pet. Four distinct components of the concept of death have been explored and include universality, irreversibility, nonfunctionality, and causality (Hunter & Smith, 2008). **Universality** refers to the notion that all things die, death is all inclusive, and comes to every living thing; death is inevitable. **Irreversibility** means when the physical body dies it cannot come back to life—death is permanent. **Nonfunctionality** means when a person or living thing dies, all functions that make the being alive stop. **Causality** refers to the notion that death has an internal and external cause. These causes may be natural, unnatural, good, or bad.

The statement that "children are not small adults" must be understood when discussing grief and loss. Children experience distress and anguish but often manifest it in developmentally different ways. Younger children are more likely than older children to state that death is avoidable and

FAMILY TEACHING

Talking with Children About Death

IN THE HOME

- Allow the child to grieve.
- Provide the child with quiet time according to the child's age and development.
- Communicate how you feel.
- Provide opportunities for all members of the family to share their grief.
- Provide avenues for the child to express feelings such as drawing, singing, or writing a poem or letter.

IN SCHOOL

- Provide opportunities for children to talk about their feelings.
- Offer supportive counseling.
- Provide related books and resources.

occurs in the future. In essence, it is temporary and reversible. This thinking is reinforced in cartoons and particularly in video games where characters die temporarily. The notion of "quit, pause, restart" are that of this new generation of "techno" children. Also, words adults use to describe death to younger children may reinforce this thinking. For example, oftentimes phrases such as *at rest, is asleep,* and *took a final journey* indicate the state is reversible. Himebauch, Arnold, & May, (2008) state that the two most important predictive factors of a child's successful outcome after suffering a loss are the availability of a significant adult and a safe physical and emotional environment.

UNDERSTANDING DEATH—A DEVELOPMENTAL PROCESS

The literature on children's understanding of death reveals on average, children under the age of four have little to no understanding of the concept of death. Yet, quite early in infancy, children develop a sense of cause and effect, learning that when they cry the caregiver provides some form of comfort. It is in these early years that children first experience and react to separation, even though it is temporary. Between infancy and early toddlerhood, children experience separation anxiety and learn to overcome it. Children also master the concept of object permanence and no longer cry when the caregiver leaves the room or them at school. It is theorized these early experiences and losses later in life may be a precursor to an individual's ability to cope with separation. For example, a preschooler in child care cries when left by the caregiver. The child does not want the parent to leave, and the day is spent crying and sometimes clinging to the teacher. This may continue for a while until the child learns a routine of the day, knowing that at a particular time the caregiver will return.

Piaget's theory of cognitive development (1969) provides a theoretical basis for conceptualizing the process of how children perceive and understand death (Table 20-1).

Infants and children are in the first stage (sensorimotor) of cognitive development and have no understanding of death. The second stage of cognitive development, which according to Piaget occurs between the ages of 2 and 7, is the preoperational stage, and incorporates egocentricity and tangible thinking. Here, children begin to explore the world around them and begin to question, share, and interact with others. Between the ages of 3 and 4 years, children begin to question the sequence of time and events, and develop a limited understanding of death, which often is viewed as a reversible process. The limited understanding of death is illustrated in the preschooler who, after being told a loved one has died, initially feels sad and cries, and then in a short time asks when the deceased will return. By the age of 5, children's definition of death is more focused on function. People die when they are unable to breathe, eat, talk, and walk, for example. These two examples of functionality or the cessation of function raise the question of whether young children define nonfunctionality as the cause or the outcome of death.

Concrete operations, Piaget's third stage of cognitive development, occurs between the ages of 7 and 11. Here, children begin to develop skills necessary for organizing and sorting information and problem solving. Children of this age are no longer governed by egocentricity and develop

Reflections from Families

Four-year-old Avery is attending the funeral of her grandfather who died after a long time battle with emphysema. She looks at the body in the casket and says to her mother, "Look mommy, now papa is dead he is breathing better, see, he does not need his oxygen."

TABLE 20-1 Theoretical Basis of Understanding the Concept of Death

AGE	PIAGET	BEHAVIORAL MANIFESTATION	UNDERSTANDING OF DEATH
0–2 years	Sensorimotor	Egocentric	None
2–4 years	Preoperational	Egocentric	Reversible, temporary
5–6 years	Preoperational	Egocentric	Avoidable
7–11 years	Concrete operations	Completion of task	Causality
12–17 years	Formal operations	Role confusion and intimacy	Selective universality (does not include self)

the ability to deal with different views of a situation and consider another person's point of view. It is during this time concrete thinking and inductive reasoning develops. Formal operation, the final stage of Piaget's cognitive development, includes the age group of 12–17; here, the individual learns to achieve emotional separation from parents; strives toward mastery, control, and competence; and later establishes intimacy and commitment. Although the adolescent is capable of understanding and conceptualizing death as permanent and universal, often there is an exclusion of the self from this concept. In other words, there is the notion "it won't happen to me." Adolescents tend to participate in high-risk activities such as driving at high speeds, rollerblading between traffic, and other activities that place them at high risk for injury and death.

GRIEF AND BEREAVEMENT

Grief, an individual's response to loss, is viewed as a natural and healthy reaction and an ongoing process across development (Heath et al., 2008). It is a complex range of feelings, cognitions, and behaviors that an individual has in reaction to a loss. **Bereavement** is seen as an adaptation to a loss, and **mourning** is the process one goes through on his or her way to adaptation. To help clarify these terms, one can describe grief as the reaction an individual has to a loss, and bereavement as the behaviors one exhibits after the loss. Each person's response to loss and bereavement is influenced by cognitive development, age of the individual, religious/ethnic/cultural influences, and personal and family experiences.

GRIEVING AND MOURNING

Kubler-Ross (1969) identified five distinct stages of the grieving process (Table 20-2). Grieving, an individual's reaction to a loss, is viewed as a passage of time through which an individual may progress at different rates, sometimes moving in and out of the various stages.

Denial is a time of shock and disbelief. Like all phases of the grieving process, it is a healthy reaction to a shock but may become detrimental when individuals are unable to move past the disbelief and accept support to help them with their feelings. When the grieving person experiences feelings of **anger** (feelings of rage, envy, and resentment) over a loss, the anger may be directed toward God—for taking away the loved one, or at the custodial parent or both parents, as seen in divorce.

Bargaining is seen at times when there is impending loss. The loss does not have to be limited to death, but may include loss of good health, an appendage, or even a way of life. **Bargaining** is an attempt to postpone the occurrence of the event, as the griever bargains with family and health care providers for one more chance to complete a task, or may wish to make a deal with God. In the event of divorce, children may bargain with parents. For example, the child might begin completing household tasks in the event the good behavior might keep the family intact. **Depression** is a time when the reality of the situation is subconsciously beginning to take hold. The individual becomes confused, irritable, and sometimes sad. It is a time when a great deal of support is needed to assist the griever in making sense of what is happening.

Acceptance is a time when the griever is consciously aware of what has happened or what is most likely to occur. If the griever is the terminally ill individual, he/she may be ready to participate in health care activities prescribed by the health care providers, or may choose palliative care with the aid of a health care proxy or living will. If the child is experiencing separation from a parent because of divorce, he/she may be concerned with developing avenues whereby contact with the noncustodial parent is maintained.

Walter and McCoyd (2009) cite the work of Worden as a view of mourning which is a process an individual must undergo in order to adapt to a loss. The process includes four stages which are discussed in the following paragraph.

Task 1. Accept the Reality of the Loss

Before children can deal with the loss, they must believe the deceased is dead and will not return to life. To negotiate this task, Worden (1996) suggests children should be told about

Table 20-2 Understanding the Grieving Process According to Kübler-Ross

STAGE	RESPONSES TO LOSS FROM SEPARATION OR DIVORCE	DEATH
1. Denial	"I don't believe you."	"It is not so."
2. Anger	"I hate you."	"I don't like God anymore."
3. Bargaining	"Will daddy come back if I behave?"	"I'll be a good boy, don't take my mother away."
4. Depression	"Don't leave me."	"Don't leave."
5. Acceptance	"Please call me every day."	"My daddy is living in heaven."

the death in appropriate age-related language. The information may need repeating depending on the age of the child.

Task 2. Experience the Pain or Emotional Aspects of the Loss

This task requires that behaviors and feelings of children are recognized and acknowledged. A child's ability to process the pain of loss will be influenced by observing an adult's experience of the loss.

Task 3. Adjust to an Environment in Which the Deceased Is Missing

Adjustment is closely related to the roles and relationships the deceased held in the child's life as well as the family. Worden (1996) states this adjustment goes on over time, and mourning for a childhood loss can be revived at any point in life. For example, the loss of a parent during childhood may be revived again when the individual has accomplished a significant task. A graduation from college, marriage, or birth of a child may revive the loss, as the individual may wish the parent could be there to share the joy.

Task 4. Relocate the Dead Person's Memory within One's Life and Find Ways to Memorialize the Person

The author states this involves finding a new and appropriate place for the deceased in one's emotional life. For example, the deceased's memory might be relocated to a special place in the heart or the mind, or a tree might be planted in memory of the deceased.

In order to assist an individual in adapting to a loss, the four tasks must be facilitated (Table 20-3).

Understanding How Children React to Loss

Children's response to grief is influenced by many factors as listed in Box 20-2.

Children may have long periods when they are overcome with grief which is then followed by an interval when they do not seem to be affected by the loss. For example, within a few

BOX 20-2

FACTORS INFLUENCING CHILDREN'S REACTION TO LOSS (SEPARATION OR DEATH)

- Developmental level
- Concept of loss (death)
- Relationship with the deceased or grieved
- Circumstances surrounding the loss
- Caregiver's ability to communicate and provide emotional support
- Emotional reaction to separation
- Support from peers and others
- Prior experience with loss
- Availability of one significant adult
- Safe physical and emotional environment
- Religious and cultural belief systems

Heath, M. A., Leavy, D., Hansen K., Ryan, K., Lawrence, L., & Sonntag, A. G. (2008). Coping with grief: Guideline and resources for assisting children. *Intervention in School and Clinic, 43*(5), 259–269; Himebauch, A., Arnold, R., & May, C. (2008). Grief in children and developmental concepts of death # 138. *Journal of Palliative Medicine, 11*(2), 243–244; Hunter, S. B., Smith, D. (2008). Predictors of children's understandings of death: Age, cognitive ability, death experience and maternal communicative competence. *Omega, 57*(2), 143–162.

Table 20-3 Understanding Worden's Four Tasks of Mourning with Helpful Strategies

WORDEN'S FOUR TASKS OF MOURNING	STRATEGIES TO FACILITATE THE TASK
1. Accept the reality of the loss	• Tell the child about the death in appropriate age-related language. • Depending on the child's age, repetition may be needed. • Use related books to help child understand the loss.
2. Experience the pain or emotional aspects of the loss	• Allow child to express feelings-allow various forms of expression. • Acknowledge child's feelings or behaviors associated with the loss.
3. Adjust to an environment in which the deceased is missing	• Help the child determine the relationship that the deceased person played in the child's life.
4. Relocate the dead person within one's life and find ways to memorialize the person	• Help the child find a place in his or her heart for memories of the deceased.

Used with permission from Worden, J. W. (1996). *Children and grief: When a parent dies.* New York: Guilford Press.

Reflections from Families

All my life I have heard how much I resemble and behave like my mother. She died in her mid-forties. I was a teenager then, so many people "complimented" me on how I reminded them of her. From that day forward, I believed that I would become ill like my mother and die in my mid-forties. Ever since I lived beyond my mid-forties, I acknowledge my birthday as a "celebration of life."

weeks after the death of a close relative, the child who was depressed and upset may seem to have forgotten about the loss and resume activities without any mention of the deceased. Nurses must help grieving caregivers understand the child's behavior is a normal process of grieving since children do not grieve the same as adults, and the manner in which a child responds is highly influenced by socialization (Heath et al., 2008). A major factor influencing how children react to grief is the relationship with the deceased. For example, a child may have little reaction to the death of an older sibling where there has been little contact or interaction, yet may react significantly to the loss of the after-school care provider where there was a close relationship.

Children's reactions to loss, whether it be due to separation or death, are also related to their personality, family structure, cultural and religious affiliation, age, and cognitive development. Reactions may be manifested in both physical and psychosocial ways (Table 20-4).

Although young children may have little comprehension of death and separation, they manifest behaviors indicative of what they are sensing. Preschool children often manifest sleep disturbances, including nightmares, bedwetting, or fear of falling asleep. They may also demonstrate clinging behaviors such as holding on to caregivers, crying, or not wanting to be left alone or separated from loved ones. Other behaviors in this age group are temper tantrums and regression. School-age children may experience feelings of guilt about what they thought or said about the deceased person. They may also take on the role of caregiver (parentification), where they assume responsibilities such as looking after siblings, organizing household chores, or taking care of their caregiver. Other behaviors could include psychosomatic symptoms such as headaches, abdominal pain, and overall feelings of not feeling well (Heath et al., 2008). The adolescent years are usually times of turmoil, finding a direction for self, forging one's own independence, selecting friends, and developing a sense of self-confidence. Bereaved and grieving adolescents may be angry and depressed but may not share their feelings with relatives and keep their feelings hidden inside. Parents and significant others may interpret these behaviors as signs of uncaring, but it is usually adolescents' way of maintaining their individuality. The adolescent may also act out angry feelings in activities such as consuming alcohol, using drugs, dropping or staying out of school, isolating themselves from peers, and severing recently formed relationships.

Table 20-4 Common Responses of Children to Loss

AGE GROUP	PHYSICAL RESPONSES	PSYCHOSOCIAL RESPONSES
Preschooler	Decreased activity Decreased appetite Regression such as bedwetting	Irritability Fear Anxiety
School age	Physical complaints such as not feeling well, abdominal pains, headaches, body aching, nausea, joint and muscle pains	Depression Fear of being rejected Fantasies of parental reunification
Adolescent	Decreased appetite Decreased or increased activity Increase in smoking, alcohol, substance abuse	Feelings of betrayal Anger Distancing self from parents or family Increase or decrease in school activities Withdrawal

CHILDREN'S RESPONSES TO DEATH

DEATH OF A CAREGIVER

The death of a parent is an extremely traumatic experience and a major crisis in the life of a child. Nearly 5% of American children experience the death of a parent before they are 16 years old, and that translates to approximately 1.5 million children in the United States living in a single-parent home because of the death of one parent.

The death of a parent and its consequences in the home and family change the very core of the child's existence (Haine, Ayers, Sandler, & Wolchik, 2008). In fact few events hold as much potential to disrupt a child's family pattern of life and place the child at risk for enduring psychological stress as the death of a parent. Children's reaction to the loss of a parent is often influenced by how the surviving parent and other adult family members react to the loss. When the surviving parent expresses feelings, openly grieves, and is able to spend time talking to the children about the loss in a positive and loving manner, children may openly express their feelings in age-appropriate ways. When a grieving child reaches out to the surviving parent and is scolded or dismissed, but comforted by another adult relative, the child may become confused about how to feel or react to the loss.

The death of the mother may bring about a change in the roles of family members. Routines, schedules, and responsibilities may change. For example, an older sibling might now be responsible for caring for younger siblings. Additional caregivers may be introduced into the family such as a babysitter, grandparent, or aunt, who now carries out activities and chores that were once done by the mother. The death of the mother, the primary caregiver in most families, may leave grieving children with feelings of anxiety as their refuge for comfort and security is gone. The loss of a father, oftentimes the principal financial provider in a two-parent family, may bring concerns about financial issues. Children of single-parent families whose parent dies experience additional hardships as the entire home environment changes. Children may be placed with relatives or foster parents. These children lose their parent, their haven, and their home.

Although children grieve differently than adults, they also need support, encouragement, a listening ear, a lap or a shoulder, and arms to hold them. When working with families experiencing the loss or the impending loss of a parent, nurses must be aware of the needs of the children who are sometimes removed from the immediate environment, which more often than not is their home.

Heath et al. (2008) emphasize that the key elements of grief interventions include listening, giving accurate information, and adapting information to the child's age and developmental level. Therefore, when providing support for the surviving parent, support measures should be considered for the children also. The way children are informed of the death of a parent often remains indelible in their minds forever (Box 20-3). The role of parental and other emotional support both at the time of the death and subsequently may be crucial to the child's response (Brown et al., 2008).

DEATH OF A SIBLING

Death of a sibling is usually due to an illness (acute and chronic) or an increase in sudden and traumatic deaths.

Reflections from Families

Don, a 36-year-old male, and his seven siblings talk about the impending death of their father. Don tells his siblings that he must tell his 6-year-old daughter, Grace, that her grandfather will die soon. When questioned about the urgency of his actions, Don states he will not allow Grace to go through what was done to him and his younger siblings when their mother died when he was 10 years old. Don tells his siblings that he can still remember how frightened he felt that morning, sensing something had happened but no one was responding to his request for an answer to what had happened. He still remembers that morning, sitting with his two younger brothers all huddled together in one chair. There seemed to be an eerie silence, followed by a great deal of activity, yet no one informed them that their mother had died, even though they suspected something terrible had happened.

EVIDENCE-BASED PRACTICE

Parentally Bereaved Children and Their Families

CLINICAL PROBLEM

Parental death is one of the most traumatic events that occurs in childhood. It can have a significant negative impact on children's self-esteem and has been associated with greater mental health issues. Parentally bereaved children can feel helplessness and believe they have less internal control over events happening to them than their nonbereaved peers. These children can benefit when they hear that their living parent will be able to manage his or her own distress. They should not focus on trying to "take care" of the surviving parent, but rather focus on tasks such as going to school, completing assignments, and spending time with their friends. The authors emphasize the need to understand the role culture may play in a child's adaptation to the death of a parent.

BEST CLINICAL PRACTICE

Providers should focus both on the creation of a safe environment for parentally bereaved children to mourn and on cognitive/behavioral skill building. Effective interventions provide both an open environment for parentally bereaved children to understand and experience their grief as well as provide a set of skills children can use to handle the life challenges that accompany the death of a parent.

IMPLICATIONS FOR NURSING

- Work with surviving parents to ensure they do not rely on their children for emotional or practical support.
- Encourage parents to find "adult ears" to listen to their own problems.
- Assist children to develop/improve their own coping skills.
- Support adaptive expressions of emotion children may wish to express.
- Facilitate positive parent-child relationships.
- Encourage parents to increase their use of positive reinforcement when interacting with their children.
- Promote parent–child communication and parent/child staff communication.
- Use good listening skills when interacting with bereaved children and/or families.
- Be aware that the nature of children's reactions to the death of a parent changes over time.

Reference: Haine, R. A., Ayers, T. S., Sandler, I. N., & Wolchik, S. A. (2008). Evidence-based practices for parentally bereaved children and their families. *Professional Psychology: Research and Practice*, *39*(2), 113–121.

BOX 20-3
PREPARING A CHILD FOR THE DEATH OF A PARENT

When planning to discuss with parents and other caregivers what and how much information should be told about the death of a parent or other significant person, you should base your plan on the knowledge that children should be given accurate information, in a clear manner, using age-appropriate language. The information should be given by an individual whom the children trust and feel comforted by. Children should be allowed to express their feelings (verbal, nonverbal, games, role-play, letter writing) and be provided with bereavement support, nurturing, and continuity. The physical and emotional availability of the surviving parent are important to the child's adjustment after the loss, and talking about the deceased is important. Finally, children should be included in activities related to funeral and burial rites when appropriate. Nurses must respect the cultural and religious needs of the bereaved family at all times.

Regardless of the cause, a child's death can have a profound and lasting effect on surviving siblings, and the roles of surviving siblings may change immediately. This is because sibling relationships are the most consistent and frequently the longest ongoing relationships one has in life, as well as the source of a number of emotions and experiences: love, caring, sharing, protecting, comforting, envy, and blaming. Siblings are also peers, friends, rivals, mentors, protectors, and teachers. To parents, children are the hopes, dreams, and future of a family; when a child dies, not only is the child lost, but also the hopes tied to that child, which is often also felt by the surviving sibling.

However, often following the death of a child, surviving siblings are overlooked, as support is generally provided to grieving parents. For example, when a parent, grandparent, or child dies, support is initially directed toward the adult—the surviving spouse, adult child, or parent. Children are sometimes sent to neighbors or relatives while support is provided to the grieving adult. Regardless of the cause of death or who dies, siblings should be allowed to grieve and be supported in their grief. A surviving sibling may experience not only sorrow at the loss of a brother or sister, but also guilt about something that was thought or said about the deceased. Surviving siblings may also experience guilt about being alive, regrets and guilt about previous bad behavior, ongoing connections with deceased sibling, and questions related to their own belief and faith (National Child Traumatic Stress Network Traumatic Grief Committee, 2009). Guilt or ambivalent feelings can have an impact on how the surviving sibling copes with the loss. The closer the relationship was before death, the more behavior problems the surviving siblings demonstrate afterward. Also, emotional closeness that existed between siblings prior to the death of one tends to be related to the outcome of the surviving child's grieving process, which may resurface at different times during the life span of the surviving child.

When a child dies, the surviving sibling loses not only a brother or a sister but the functional loss of the grieving parent since frequently parents are likely to experience their own difficulties coping with loss, which impairs their ability to parent or assist their children (Owens, 2008). Depending on the circumstances of the death, siblings may feel guilty, angry, or sad. Some of the emotions expressed and experienced by the surviving siblings may be characterized by universal ambivalence. After the death of a sibling, surviving siblings may experience a sense of increased vulnerability, anger at parents for not protecting the deceased, or on the other hand, protectiveness of parents. Behaviors seen in surviving siblings may be related to the emotional unavailability of parents, the surviving sibling's lack of connectedness with the world after the loss of their brother or sister, and limited communication that can occur in families after the death of one of its members. Therefore, it is important for nurses to understand because grieving parents may be emotionally unavailable to the surviving children and because support is generally directed toward parents, siblings are often the most neglected family members when a child dies (Brown et al., 2008). Box 20-4 offers some facts to remember when helping children cope with sibling loss.

BOX 20-4

FACTS TO REMEMBER WHEN HELPING CHILDREN COPE WITH SIBLING LOSS

- Remember that children have a need to grieve.
- Be prepared to answer loaded questions.
- Expect behavioral changes and responses.
- Allow children to express their feelings.
- Be aware parents might be emotionally unavailable to surviving children.
- Inform the school community of the child's loss.
- Provide peer support groups.

CRITICAL THINKING

When a Child Is Dying

You are in your pediatric clinical rotation in a hospice unit and assigned to 13-year-old Harrison in the terminal stage of an acute illness.

- What would you say to the child and family about dying and death?
- What would you do or say if the client says the following: "I don't want to die"?

DISASTERS OR TRAUMATIC EVENTS

The rise in violent crimes committed by children in generally safe environments such as schools, playgrounds, and homes has propelled this generation of children to a new level and kind of unprecedented risk. Children may suffer the effects of a disaster regardless of whether they are directly involved or were witnesses (McNess, 2007). Events such as the Columbine school shooting of 1999, the terrorist attacks on the United States in 2001, the tsunami disaster of 2004, and the hurricanes of 2005 will have long-term effects on children as well as adults. The effects of the disaster or traumatic events may have long-term consequences, interfering with the child's ability to engage in productive behavior and adequately function socially, academically, and professionally (Feigelman, Jordan, & Gorman, 2009; Haine et al., 2008). See Box 20-5 for the long-term consequences of traumatic loss in children.

In addition to grieving the loss of classmates, friends, peers, or significant others such as teachers or other adults, children have to cope with the experience of the trauma. In other words, not only did someone die, but it is the circumstances under which the individual or individuals died or became injured that are traumatic. Children who experience traumatic losses often have the same reactions, but in addition, may exhibit rage, suffer sleep disturbances, repeatedly have thoughts about the incident, experience an increased alertness to dangers, and fear attending school or any other environment similar to the traumatic incident

When prioritizing supportive care to children who experienced a violent and traumatic incident, it is important to note that such incidents occur against and have ramifications for a community and not just individuals. For example, the consequences of a shooting occurring in a school are felt by everyone in the community and beyond, and have ramifications nationwide. When support is provided it must be provided to the community at large. Box 20-6 lists some ideas to help communities cope with traumatic incidents.

BOX 20-5

LONG-TERM CONSEQUENCES OF TRAUMATIC LOSS

- Cognitive dysfunction (emotional regression)
- Health disturbances (depression)
- Altered personality trait (may appear uneasy)
- Disruption in moral development
- Attempts at masking emotions

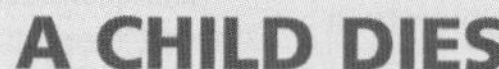

CASE STUDY / CARE PLAN

A CHILD DIES

Noah, 12 years old, is in the final stage of a terminal illness. His immediate family keeps vigil at his bedside. Noah is no longer alert.

NURSING DIAGNOSIS 1

Anticipatory grieving by family related to child's terminal illness.

EXPECTED OUTCOME

The family will be given opportunities to begin the grieving process.

NOC: Family Coping

NIC: Grief Work Facilitation; Family Support

INTERVENTIONS/*RATIONALES*

1. Allow family private time to spend with Noah; limit visitors according to family wishes. *Provides privacy and opportunities to gather and grieve as a family.*
2. Provide family with private space to meet and grieve. *Helps family maintain a sense of control and belonging as a family without the interruption and intrusion of others.*
3. Provide opportunities for family to express feelings to each other and to the staff. *Provides support and allows time to clarify feelings and concerns as well as providing psychosocial support where appropriate.*
4. Provide support for family. *Allows family members to grieve and to understand and accept individual style of grieving.*
5. Encourage family to participate in Noah's care. *Promotes dignity, respect, and self-worth of all individuals.*
6. Minimize the number of health care personnel providing information to family. *Decreases the risk of overwhelming and confusing family members. Allows for more accurate identification of family's needs.*
7. Maintain optimum care to Noah. *Helps family maintain a sense of control and belonging.*

NURSING DIAGNOSIS 2

Anticipatory grieving by staff related to child's terminal illness.

EXPECTED OUTCOME

The staff will express grief in a positive manner.

NOC: Caregiver Emotional Health

NIC: Emotional Support

INTERVENTIONS/*RATIONALES*

1. Provide peer support to staff members. *Peer support allows staff members to express feelings, to exchange ideas and experiences, and to teach and learn from each other.*
2. Encourage staff to discuss their feelings. *Discussion of feelings helps minimize fears and clarify issues and misconceptions.*
3. Maintain supportive working environment. *Promotes physical and mental health of the individual and the team.*
4. Maintain optimum care to Noah. *Fosters dignity, respect, and self-worth of individuals.*

EVALUATION

Two days later Noah dies; his family was at his bedside. The nurse stayed late to say her final good-bye to Noah and to provide post-mortem care. Information about the funeral was sent to the nursing unit; a number of nursing staff attended the funeral.

(Continues)

CASE STUDY / CARE PLAN (Continued)

One month later, Maggie, the 7-year-old sister of Noah, is admitted to the hospital with acute abdominal pains. Her parents are extremely nervous, and Maggie is visibly afraid and crying. She clings to her mother and becomes hysterical when left alone. Maggie tells her mother she is afraid she will die like her brother.

NURSING DIAGNOSIS 3

Anxiety (caregiver) related to hospitalization of child.

EXPECTED OUTCOME

Family will report decreased anxiety related to hospitalization of child.

NOC: Anxiety Control

NIC: Anxiety Reduction

INTERVENTIONS/*RATIONALES*

1. Provide opportunities for caregivers to express their feelings. *Provides support for caregivers to express their feelings.*
2. Provide key personnel to communicate information to caregivers. *Decreases the risk of overwhelming and confusing family members. Allows for more accurate identification of family's needs.*
3. Keep caregivers informed about child's condition. *Helps family maintain a sense of belonging and control.*
4. Involve caregivers in plan of care. *Helps family maintain a sense of belonging and control.*
5. Provide support services for family. *Helps maintain the physical and psychological health of the family.*

NURSING DIAGNOSIS 4

Increased anxiety related to hospitalization and recent death of sibling.

EXPECTED OUTCOME

The sister will report a decreased level of anxiety related to hospitalization and recent death of sibling.

NOC: Anxiety Control

NIC: Anxiety Reduction

INTERVENTIONS/*RATIONALES*

1. Encourage caregiver to remain with child. *Promotes a sense of safety and belonging for the child and decreases anxiety.*
2. Allow Maggie to express feelings. *Helps to understand child's perceptions, and to provide appropriate interventions.*
3. Minimize the number of staff interacting with Maggie. *Decreases the risk of overwhelming the child.*
4. Explain procedures and treatment in age-appropriate language. *Helps promote child's understanding of events taking place.*
5. Refrain from using words and terminology that can be misconstrued. *Decreases the chances of misunderstanding, decreases anxiety.*
6. Encourage caregiver involvement in Maggie's care. *Helps child and caregivers maintain a sense of control and normalcy.*
7. Encourage self-care. *Helps promote sense of independence and control.*
8. Provide Maggie with avenues to express herself (drawing, painting, writing, puppet play). *Helps staff and family to understand how the child feels and to provide appropriate interventions.*

EVALUATION

Three days later, Maggie is discharged home. The interdisciplinary team recommends the family continue to receive counseling to help deal with the two stressful events.

RESEARCH Highlight

Parental Perspectives of Initial End-of-Life Care Communication

STUDY PURPOSE

To examine parents' perspectives of what was helpful or harmful when health care providers introduce or discuss palliative and end-of-life care options for the dying child.

METHODS

Twenty-eight parents were interviewed in this retrospective descriptive study. The interviews were audio-taped and transcribed verbatim.

FINDINGS

- Major primary health care provider was the physician.
- Introduction to end-of-life option was done spontaneously late in the child's dying process and done without the supportive presence of a nurse, a social worker, and/or a hospital chaplain.
- Parents vividly remembered the circumstances when the end-of-life option was introduced. These circumstances were both positive and negative in nature.
- Positive memories about the end-of-life topic included the health care provider being very informative and compassionate and that the transition to hospice care was easier.
- Negative memories about the end-of-life topic included the health care provider being uncaring and uncomfortable and that they were not informed of available supportive services. These parents also stated that their child did receive compassionate care while in hospice care.

IMPLICATIONS

Nurses and other health care providers can learn a great deal from the information provided by family members/parents regarding the end-of-life care of a dying child. Methods of communication remain important along with professional compassionate and caring nursing practice.

REFERENCE

Hendricks-Ferguson, V. (2007). Parental perspectives of initial end-of-life care communication. *International Journal of Palliative Nursing, 13*(1), 522–531.

BOX 20-6

HELPING COMMUNITIES COPE WITH VIOLENT TRAUMATIC INCIDENTS

- Provide counselors from within and outside the community (Red Cross, other agencies). Counselors and other health care providers who live in the community may be dealing with their own sense of loss in regards to the incident.
- Encourage discussion at community board meetings. This helps identify the needs of the community.
- Educate the community about how children grieve.
- Allow children to grieve.
- Facilitate grieving of children—allow them to see and hear how adults are dealing with the traumatic loss, which will help them express their feelings.
- Listen to the children, and provide opportunities such as acting in plays, writing, drawing, dancing, and listening to music. Listening helps adults understand how children are feeling about the incident. The use of other avenues of expression will provide opportunities for children to express their feelings both verbally and nonverbally.
- Involve school nurses in providing interventions to help children grieve

REACTIONS OF FAMILY TO A CHILD WITH A LIFE-THREATENING OR TERMINAL ILLNESS

Children are supposed to lead strong and healthy lives, and outlive their parents and other caregivers. However, children may suffer from a variety of life-threatening illnesses, from congenital to acquired—including heart defects/disease, cystic fibrosis, accidents, cancer, and AIDS. The anguish a family experiences from the time of diagnosis to the final outcome can only be described as excruciatingly painful—a time when life instantly becomes chaotic and unpredictable.

The experience of coping with a life-threatening illness presents many challenges to both the family and the health care providers. Refer to Table 20-5 for helpful information as to phases and behaviors one goes through when a child experiences a life-threatening illness as well as appropriate nursing care.

LOSS OF A NEWBORN

Loss of a newborn remains a stressful and traumatic event for parents, families, nurses, and others regardless of the reason for

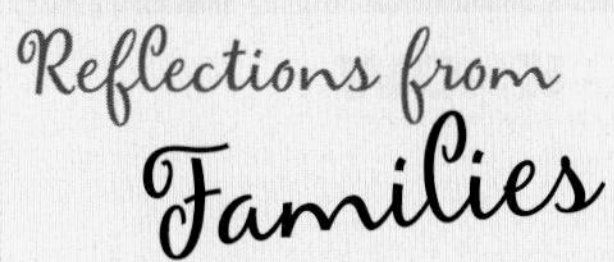

It's been 15 years since the accident. Whenever I think about the morning they told me she might not survive, I get that numb but tight feeling in my throat. Sophia was only 8 years old and was happily riding her bike when she was hit by a car. I was confused and dazed for a very long time. I don't remember events of the hospitalization; probably I don't want to remember. I believe I woke up out of my confusion when Sophia was placed in rehab and had to learn to walk and eat again. It's something I pray will not happen to another parent.

TABLE 20-5 Nursing Care of Families Experiencing Life-Threatening Illness of a Child

PHASE	DEFINITION	BEHAVIORS OR TASK	NURSING CARE
Prediagnostic	From suspicion to time of medical attention.	Guilt. What did I do wrong? Increase in anxiety about the unknown.	• Allow family members to express feelings. • Provide information to family in a timely manner.
Diagnostic or acute phase	Period when tests and studies to determine the diagnosis occur.	Afraid. Feeling of uncertainty and helplessness. Family life at a standstill. Overwhelmed with information in regards to the diagnosis. May seek second or third opinions.	• Continue to allow family members to express feelings and ask questions. • Assess need for psychological and spiritual support. • Maintain communication among members. • Provide information to family in a timely manner.
Chronic phase	Treatment in progress.	Family's anxiety level may be decreased slightly. Parents and others may be physically exhausted. May question therapies and seek opinions or alternate forms of treatment.	• Continue supporting the expression of feelings. • Assess parents' need for rest. • Provide information about therapies. • Encourage other health team members to provide information to family in a timely manner. • Assess siblings' need for additional support since parents may be physically and mentally exhausted.
Terminal phase	Recovery is not an option.	Family must prepare for death of child. Parents may have difficulty accepting treatment modality that is more palliative.	• Provide support to family. • Assist family in communicating their wishes to the interdisciplinary team. • Minimize the number of personnel providing information to family. • Provide appropriate support for decision making regarding hospice care, hospital care, home care, DNR, and other therapies.
Recovery phase	May include living with long-term consequences of the illness.	Family must now learn to live with the effects of the death. May include a change in previous lifestyle for family.	• Provide avenues for discussion of feelings, fears, concerns. • Provide family teaching regarding care of child. • Provide information regarding support services for family and child.

REFLECTIVE THINKING

Personal Experiences with Death

Have you ever experienced the death of a close family member, friend, or a pet? If yes, how has that shaped your view of dealing with loss? If no, how do you imagine you will deal with a future loss?

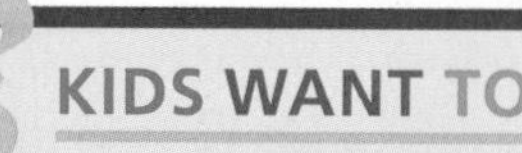

Am I going to die?

One day Ronnie, a 7-year-old with a terminal illness, said to the nurse, "I don't feel better any more, am I going to die? Everyone is acting kind of weird."

- Do not trivialize Ronnie's comments.
- Determine what Ronnie knows about his current status.
- Discuss with parents, family, caregivers, and the health care team what Ronnie needs to know, who will tell him, and what is being told.

the loss. When preparing the deceased newborn for viewing by the parents, it is important the newborn be washed and dressed appropriately. This helps parents see their deceased newborn as their child. Clothing the infant in an outfit and wrapping the newborn in a blanket selected by the parents helps the family takes ownership of the deceased and the loss. The area for viewing the deceased newborn should be clean, quiet, and in an area appropriate for the family to grieve. The manner in which nurses prepare the deceased newborn for viewing can have a major impact on how parents and relatives remember the event. Therefore, the deceased newborn should be placed in a bassinette, fully clothed and swaddled in a blanket. Chairs should be provided. Parents should be allowed to hold the baby and to stay as long as they choose. A nurse should present the baby to the parents just as if the newborn were alive.

HOW MUCH SHOULD THE CHILD BE TOLD?

Dunlop (2008) states that when a child is dying, he/she may not be told the truth regarding his/her condition. Consequently, the amount of information provided to the terminally ill and dying child is unsettled. Some parents and caregivers, in their desire to protect, may not want the child to know many details about the diagnosis. It is imperative the interdisciplinary team and caregivers discuss what and how much information the child should receive. Also, there should be discussions about the information given to siblings. Attempts to protect children from illness and death are often futile, and by middle childhood children are exposed to information about diseases and many have already experienced loss of some kind. Usually, children can sense something is wrong by the way adults treat them. Since there is often a tendency to walk away from the child when issues are being discussed, this behavior suggests to the child something is wrong. Therefore, in efforts to protect children from knowing they are ill, nonverbal behaviors may alert the child that something is wrong and cause increased anxiety.

WHAT SHOULD THE CHILD BE TOLD?

Children as early as preschool age should be told they are ill. Information should be concise, clear, and simple. For example, a young child (5–9 years old) with leukemia can be told blood cells in the body are not strong enough to fight off infection, and the medicines and treatments will help strengthen those cells. An older child (10–12 years old) may need to know more about leukemia and the reasons for specific therapies. Today, children have many avenues to obtain information such as books, television, and the Internet; however, not all the information available is accurate; therefore, it is important the family and health care team collaborate to provide appropriate and accurate information.

WHO SHOULD TELL THE CHILD?

When planning to discuss who will be responsible for informing a child about his or her illness, caregivers and the interdisciplinary team should discuss the matter. No rule exists on who should inform a child about illness, but a small group of individuals who will be primary care providers are the best. The small group may consist of parents or caregivers, a nurse, and the physician or primary health care provider. An older sibling or another family member with whom the child has a significant relationship should be included. A number of caring and loving individuals with whom the child has a trusting relationship, as well as members of the interdisciplinary team with whom a relationship will or has developed, help the child maintain a sense of security, love and trust, and belonging. Nurses can play a pivotal role in maintaining a sense of security and a trusting relationship with the ill child.

DECISIONS ABOUT HOSPICE

Just as caregivers are given options for types of treatment for the ill child, they should also be given options and opportunities to plan where and how the child will spend the final chapter of life. Children's hospice care, a growing alternative to hospital care for the dying child and family, incorporates a holistic approach providing psychosocial, spiritual, and physical support to the child and family. In this setting, the parent and child are the primary decision makers with the interdisciplinary team functioning in a more supportive role. Hospice can be provided at home, the hospital, or in a facility for hospice care. Professional support to the family continues long after the child's death. The support team for the child in hospice includes the family, significant support individuals, and the interdisciplinary hospice team. Hospice provides physical, respite, and bereavement care to the child and family. The primary focus of physical care is to maintain a comfortable and pain-free environment for the child through the implementation of pain management programs. Parents and other caregivers also have the opportunity to provide physical care for the child, and the child is allowed the right and dignity to be a child, and cared for by a parent or other family members.

Hospice service also provides respite care to allow family members to take a break or time off for themselves before resuming the primary care of the child. Hospice personnel are also trained to recognize the signs of anticipatory grieving in the child or family, and to support them through this healthy process.

CULTURAL CONSIDERATION

Is there racial disparity in the utilization of hospice care?

Hospice offers a comprehensive program of services specifically designed to meet the need for end of life care of terminally ill clients with cancer. This article suggests African-American clients are less likely than white clients to use hospice. Is this due to African-Americans delaying enrollment in hospice because of the requirement that they forgo further "curative" treatments? Do African-American clients view hospice care as a death sentence rather than "end of life" care? The authors believe a variety of factors exclude these clients, and cultural beliefs may play only a small part. The restriction that clients should be in the last six months of life and give up curative treatment may be a major obstacle as many people may want to "fight to the end." The authors also state the hospice eligibility criteria for Medicare and other insurers requiring clients to give up cancer treatment contribute to racial disparities in hospice care.

Reference: Fishman, J., O'Dwyer, P., Lu, H., Henderson, H., Asch, D., & Casarett, D. (2008). Race, treatment preferences, and hospice enrollment: Eligibility criteria may exclude patients with the greatest needs for care. *Cancer*, February 1, 689–697.

ORGAN AND TISSUE DONATION

The discussion of tissue donation is a very sensitive and uncomfortable topic for many health care providers, since the possible hope for life/living for one person means the death of another. It is an awkward time for the health care providers, whose actions may seem cruelly intrusive on a grieving family. Therefore, the timing for discussion must be planned and well coordinated. Most large hospitals and acute care settings have established programs with well-trained health care personnel who are responsible for discussing tissue and organ donation with families.

Nurses caring for the dying child are aware of the total plan of care for their clients, at a pivotal position to evaluate family concerns about the issue, and provide avenues for family members to openly discuss their concerns with the transplant team. In order to maintain the rights and dignity of a dying child and family, specific steps are usually taken to obtain tissue and organs, which may vary according to individual health care agencies.

AUTOPSY

The decision to perform an autopsy is a requirement of law when death is caused by unnatural causes such as murder or suicide, if it occurs within 24 hours of hospitalization, or if death occurs at home or in an institution when a person has not been under the care of a health care provider. Nurses can only emphasize to the family the decision to perform the autopsy is not a decision based on hospital policy, but a requirement of state law. If a child does have an autopsy, it may be important for the family to see the child after the procedure, and this information should be obtained before the autopsy is performed.

CARE FOR NURSES WORKING WITH TERMINALLY ILL CHILDREN

The idea of dying is not easily discussed in U.S. society, as it represents the end of life as we know it and fear of the unknown. The association between death and children is paradoxical because children represent life and future. When children are terminally ill and expected to die, all individuals involved in the care of the child are emotionally affected. Nurses, the primary caregivers to the child and the family, often experience emotional battles within themselves as they attempt to provide the best care to the child and family and put their own feelings aside. Nurses providing physical and emotional care to others oftentimes neglect their own need for support and place themselves at risk both physically and emotionally.

The care of terminally ill children is often provided in specialty areas, units, or institutions, where the majority of the clients are at high risk of dying. Therefore, the atmosphere of the environment may be stressful, with various levels of anxiety apparent among staff and families. Just as the ill child and family have special needs, so do the nurses; unfortunately the needs of the nurses often go unmet. One reason for this is the nursing staff may not recognize they too are grieving the loss. When nurses do not tend to their need to grieve, they may feel anger, frustration, and depression, manifested by sick calls, breakdown in communication at work and at home, feelings of not being appreciated, and sometimes guilt.

When death involves a child, the acceptance and acknowledgment of the death is more difficult to understand. At times, nurses who are experiencing those feelings begin to question the technology, the profession, and even their faith. During this time, these nurses are not able to appropriately attend to the needs of the dying child or the family, must come to terms with their own feelings about dying and death, and must allow themselves to grieve so they can help others. To do so, nurses must seek assistance.

To maintain the physical, emotional, and psychological integrity of the nursing staff, institutions should provide a caring or health promoting environment with an emphasis on wellness and the promotion of health. Assistance programs for employees or staff are examples of such services. Nurses and other health care providers may be given the opportunity to use mental health days or recharge time when they can seek the assistance of providers such as psychologists and psychiatrists to assist them in dealing with their concerns and feelings. Some institutions have support groups established, while others initiate support services when the psychological integrity of the staff is being threatened. Interventions should be ongoing, where nurses can meet individually, privately, or in groups to discuss their needs and concerns.

Nurses caring for terminally ill children and their families must actively focus on promoting their own health. The following questions should be kept in mind and attempts should be made to answer them and to seek help when needed:

1. How do I feel about the concept of dying?
2. Am I comfortable caring for the needs of the dying child?
3. Can I cope with the family's needs also?
4. Am I becoming overwhelmed with caring for this child and family?
5. Who can assist me in finding ways to deal with my needs and concern?
6. How can I preserve my own health and well-being?

Nurses should be given opportunities to share the answers to their questions with other health care professionals, with the goal being these feelings and concerns are only human experiences and concerns.

THE NURSE AND TERMINALLY ILL CHILD

The nurse providing care to the terminally ill child is involved in caring for physical, psychosocial, and spiritual needs. The child may be alert and responsive at some times, and at other times may be weak and uncomfortable. The plan of care should not only be individualized and realistic, but also based on the immediate needs of the child. When the terminally ill child is dying, the nurse must cope with the additional needs of the child and the family.

RESPONDING TO THE PHYSIOLOGICAL NEEDS OF THE DYING CHILD

A primary goal at this time is keeping the child comfortable and pain free. Maintaining a clean environment, providing hair and oral care, and other aspects of daily hygiene can help maintain the dignity of the human experience and promote the psychological integrity of the family. The administration of therapies to reduce pain, promote comfort, maintain hydration and nutrition, and promote respiratory and circulatory integrity remains important. Nurses must continue to provide care to these clients with the same enthusiasm even when they question the purpose of their interventions.

EYE ON...

Cultural Practices Related to Death and Dying

Ragda, a young girl from a Middle Eastern country, is in the process of dying. Her parents ask the nurses to allow Ragda to be prepared for death. To do this, the child must be dressed daily in a specific garment and her head adorned with a specific head dress. Since the parents cannot do this every day, they teach the nurses how to apply the garment and head dress. The nurses respectfully apply the apparel under the watchful eyes of family members. Regardless of the time the family visited, Ragda was properly attired. Although Ragda was comatose, the parents were relieved to know that when death occurred she was ready.

RESPONDING TO THE PSYCHOSOCIAL NEEDS OF THE DYING CHILD

Psychosocial needs are more difficult and taxing for nurses to fulfill, particularly when the nurse may be psychologically uncomfortable with personal feelings about dying and death. Many individuals, upon hearing of the death of an older adult, are more accepting of the outcome since the older person most likely lived a full life. However, when death involves a child, acceptance and acknowledgment is more difficult to understand. When providing care to terminally ill children nurses must:

- Revisit their own thoughts and feelings about dying and death
- Understand the process of grieving
- Talk to children in age-appropriate language
- Help children verbalize their feelings about dying and death
- Be consistent in care provided
- Be honest in discussions

During the time of death, nurses must also uphold and respect the cultural and religious beliefs and rituals of the family.

ATTENDANCE OF NURSING STAFF AT FUNERALS

Questions arise about the attendance of nurses at the funeral of a child cared for. Although there is no hard and fast rule, it may be a venue for nurses to acknowledge their loss and to put closure to the experience. At times, the request for the attendance of nursing staff at the funeral is made by the family through announcement of funeral arrangements sent to the unit. Nurses need to determine for themselves on an individual basis what works best.

IN THE REAL WORLD

I feel nurses should talk with families about the treatment options and use empathy skills. I have seen decision making in situations of life and death be emotionally charged and extremely complicated. I believe it is within nurses' stewardship to help families understand information and access resources necessary for making the wisest choices. I also realize once decisions are made, nurses have an obligation to respect families' choices and continue providing the best care possible regardless of personal opinions.

KEY CONCEPTS

- Children may experience feelings of loss and separation (divorce, moving to a new neighborhood, changing schools) long before they experience the death of a loved one.
- Four components of the concept of death are universality, irreversibility, nonfunctionality, and causality.
- Understanding the concept of death is a gradual process related to the individual's age, cognitive development, culture, religious belief, and psychological development.
- Children grieve differently than adults; their responses are both physical and psychosocial.
- Children's reaction to the death of a loved one is often influenced by the relationship the child had with the deceased and ways those around them react to the loss.
- After the death of a sibling, children may experience a sense of increased vulnerability, anger, survivor guilt, and parent overprotectiveness.
- Hospice care incorporates a holistic approach providing psychosocial, spiritual, social, and physical support to the terminally ill child and family.
- Nurses must come to terms with their own feelings about dying and death, and allow themselves to grieve in order to help others.

REVIEW ACTIVITIES

1. What information should the nurse give to parents to assist them in explaining to their 6-year-old child that a grandfather has died?
2. How can the school nurse assist children in coping with the death of a classmate?
3. How are children's reactions to parental separation or divorce similar to that of death?
4. What factors influence a child's response to death?
5. How can the nurse help a terminally ill child and family prepare for impending death?
6. How can nurses help a community cope with a traumatic event?
7. What are the benefits of hospice care for the terminally ill child and family?
8. Why is caring for self important for nurses caring for the terminally ill child?

STUDY QUESTIONS

1. The mother of a terminally ill child tells the nurse that she wants to take her child home to die. The best response by the nurse at this time is which of the following?
   a. Ask the mother if she knows any parent whose child recently died at home.
   b. Ask the mother if she discussed this with the health care team.
   c. Ask the mother what she knows about hospice care.
   d. Ask the mother to tell you why she wants to do this.
2. The school nurse notes that a 7-year-old boy who has asthma has been experiencing increasing need for his inhaler pump at school. The nurse interviews the child to determine what could be precipitating his respiratory discomfort. Which of the following statements made by the child to the nurse is most likely the precipitating factor?
   a. "I have to walk to school with my younger sister."
   b. "I hurt my leg so I am not running around."
   c. "My father no longer lives with us."
   d. "My mother has a job now."
3. A pediatric client has been admitted to hospice care. The nurse notes that the family is wearing garments that seem to be of a religious nature. When planning to interview the relatives, which of the following questions would be appropriate to ask?
   a. "Is there any custom or tradition that I/we need to be aware of?"
   b. "How many relatives will be visiting on a daily basis?"
   c. "What language do you speak?"
   d. "To whom should I address my questions?"
4. A nurse is caring for a terminally ill preschooler. The child is irritable and tells the nurse that he is afraid. In order to provide safe and effective care to this child, which of the following is not appropriate?
   a. Knowledge of the child's growth and development
   b. Talking to the child in age appropriate language
   c. Evading the child's questions about his condition
   d. Providing consistent care
5. The nurse overhears the parent of a critically injured child who is praying at the child's bedside say "I will stop drinking and smoking". The nurse understands that the parent is in which stage of the grieving process?
   a. Denial
   b. Acceptance
   c. Bargaining
   d. Anger
6. The nurse is aware that a person's response to loss and bereavement is influenced by many factors. Which of the factors below is not one of those?
   a. Cognitive development
   b. Time of the day and day of the month
   c. Religious/ethnic beliefs
   d. Previous experiences with loss

7. Mrs. Smith's husband is dying. She tells the nurse that she needs "to be strong" for her teenage children and she does not want them to see her fall apart. The nurse's response to Mrs. Smith should be based on the knowledge that:
   a. When adults express their grief it is interpreted as a sign of weakness by their children.
   b. Teenagers are better adapted to deal with loss than younger children.
   c. Support measures during loss should be considered for the entire family.
   d. Teenagers expect that a surviving parent needs to be strong.
8. Many situations may trigger feelings of separation and loss in individuals. Which of the following would most likely not trigger feelings of loss and separation?
   a. A birthday
   b. Financial instability
   c. Decline in health
   d. Winning the lottery
9. The nurse in the bereavement center is speaking to a group of bereaved parents. A parent smiles and tells the nurse that her deceased daughter's memory is a special place in her heart where no one can reach. The nurse understands that the parent is in which task of mourning?
   a. Acceptance of the death
   b. Experiencing the aspects of the loss
   c. Adjusting to the loss
   d. Relocating the loss
10. Which of the following factors plays a significant role in a nurse's ability to provide safe and effective care to terminally ill children?
   a. Knowledge of advanced psychomotor skills
   b. Understanding of the dying process
   c. Experience with terminally ill adults
   d. Acknowledgement of own feelings about dying and death

REFERENCES

Amato, P., & Afifi, T. (2006). Feeling caught between parents: Adult children's relations with parents and subjective well-being. *Journal of Marriage and Family, 68*(1), 222–235.

Brodkin, A. (2007). Saying goodbye to a pet. *Scholastic Parent & Child, (Oct.)*, 41–42.

Brown, E. J., Amaya-Jackson, L., Cohen, J., Handel, S., Thiel De Bocanegra, H., Goodman, R. F., & Mannarino, A. (2008). Childhood traumatic grief: A multisite empirical examination of the construct and its correlates. *Death Studies, 32*, 899–923.

Dunlop, S. (2008). The dying child: Should we tell the truth? *Paediatric Nursing, 20*(6), 28–31.

Feigelman, W., Jordan, J., & Gorman. B. (2009). How they died, time since loss, and bereavement outcomes. *Omega, 58*(4), 252–273.

Field, N. P., Orsini, L., Gavish, R., & Packman., W. (2009). Role of attachment in response to pet loss. Death Studies, 33, 334–355.

Fishman, J., O'Dwyer, P., Lu, H., Henderson, H. H., Asch, D., & Casarret, D. (2008). Race, treatment preferences, and hospice enrollment: Eligibility criteria may exclude patients with the greatest needs for care. *Cancer*. February 1, 689–697.

Haine, R. A., Ayers, T., Sandler, I., & Wolchik, S. (2008). Evidence-based practices for parentally bereaved children and their families. *Professional Psychology: Research and Practice, 39*(2), 113–121.

Heath, M. A., Leavy, D., Hansen K., Ryan, K., Lawrence, L., & Sonntag, A. G. (2008). Coping with grief: Guideline and resources for assisting children. *Intervention in School and Clinic, 43*(5), 259–269.

Hendricks-Ferguson, V. (2007). Parental perspectives on initial end-of-life care communication. *International Journal of Palliative Nursing, 13*(11), 522–531.

Himebauch, A., Arnold, R., & May, C. (2008). Grief in children and developmental concepts of death # 138. *Journal of Palliative Medicine, 11*(2), 243–244.

Hunter, S. B., & Smith, D. (2008). Predictors of children's understandings of death: Age, cognitive ability, death experience and maternal communicative competence. *Omega, 57*(2), 143–162.

Kubler-Ross, E. (1969). *On death and dying*. New York: MacMillan.

Lansford, J. E., Manole, P. S., Castellino, D. R., Dodge, K. A., Pettit, G. S., & Bates, J. E. (2006). Trajectories of internalizing, externalizing, and grades for children who have and have not experienced their parents' divorce. *Journal of Family Psychology, 20*, 292–301.

Lansford, J. E. (2009). Parental divorce and children's adjustment. *Perspectives on Psychological Science, 4*(2), 140–152.

Lynch, E. (2008). Murky waters: The death of someone close can affect children in many ways and it may be difficult to support them. The Candle Project could help. *Nursing Standard, 22*(36), 18.

McNess, A. (2007). The social consequences of "how the sibling died" for bereaved young adults. *Youth Studies Australia, 26*(4), 12–20.

National Child Traumatic Stress Network Traumatic Grief Committee (2009). Sibling loss fact sheet: Sibling death and childhood traumatic grief: Information for families. Los Angeles, CA and Durham NC: National Center for Child Traumatic Stress.

Owens, D. A. (2008). Recognizing the needs of bereaved children in palliative care. *Journal of Hospice and Palliative Nursing, 10*(1), 14–17.

Piaget, J. (1969). *The theory of stages in cognitive development.* New York: McGraw-Hill.

Poortman, A., & Voorpostel, M. (2008). Parental divorce and sibling relationships: A research note. *Journal of Family Issues, 30*(74), 74–91.

Solbolewski, J. M., Amato, P. R. (2007). Parents' discord and divorce, parent-child relationships and subjective well-being in early adulthood: Is feeling close to two parents always better than feeling close to one? *Social Forces, 85*(3), 1105–1124.

Walter, C. A., & McCoyd, J. L. M. (2009). Grief and loss across the lifespan: A biopsychosocial perspective. New York: Springer Publishing Co.

Worden, J. W. (1996). Children and grief: When a parent dies. New York, NY: Guilford Press.

SUGGESTED READINGS

Black, S. (2005). From 9/11 to Katrina: Helping students grieve. *American School Board Journal, 192,* 28–30.

Jaffe, S., & LaFleur, J. (2008). *For the grieving child: An activity manual* (2nd ed.). Self-published.

Levinson, N., Baskette, P., & Caruso, L. (2007). Remembering my pet: A kid's own spiritual remembering workbook for when a pet dies. Woodstock, VT: Skylight Paths Publishing.

Oedfern, S., & Gilbert, S. (2008). The Grieving Garden: Living with the death of a child. Newburyport, MA: Hampton Roads Pub. Co.

RESOURCES

Refer to the online student StudyWARE for Potts & Mandleco at http://www.CengageBrain.com for additional content and study aids.

Organization: **A Time to Grieve**
Description: Provides links to resources for those dealing with loss, including loss of a parent, bereavement, dealing with grief, and sign and symptoms of depression.
Website/Resource: http://www.atimetogrieve.net

Organization: **Association for Pet Loss and Bereavement**
Description: Provides users information regarding free chat rooms, aftercare, and newsletters related to pet loss and bereavement.
Website/Resource: http://www.aplb.org

Organization: **Candlelighters Childhood Cancer Foundation**
Description: Provides information/awareness for families/children/adolescents with cancer; advocates for and supports research.
Website/Resource: http://www.candlelighters.org

Organization: **Center for Loss & Life Transition**
Description: Dedicated to "companioning" grieving people as they mourn transitions/losses; provides information to trainings/bookstores/newsletters, and about program director Dr. Alan Wolfelt.
Website/Resource: http://www.centerforloss.com

Organization: **Children and Pet Loss**
Description: Provides information about childhood developmental stages, how stages are linked to pet death, the types of questions children may ask, and how to help them memorialize pets.
Website/Resource: http://www.aplb.org/services/children

Organization: **Children's Hospice International (CHI)**
Description: Offers information about CHI's programs and resources as well as donation information.
Website/Resource: http://www.chionline.org

Organization: **Children's Hospice and Palliative Care Association**
Description: Offers general information about improving child health care and a special link for families.
Website/Resource: http://www.childrenshospice.org

Organization: **Children's Project on Palliative/Hospice Services (ChiPPs)**
Description: Offers users links and resources pertaining to child palliative care.
Website/Resource: http://www.nhpco.org

Organization: **The Compassionate Friends for Bereaved Parents and Siblings**
Description: Provides information regarding local chapters, news/events, and helpful resources related to grief following the death of a child.
Website/Resource: http://www.compassionatefriends.org

Organization: **Elder Hope**
Description: Offers access to forums, downloads, articles, and a blog related to care and comfort for the dying and the bereaved; and to support the bond between the elderly and all caregivers.
Website/Resource: http://www.elderhope.com

Organization: **Grief Counseling for Kids**
Description: Offers information regarding bereavement centers, events, media, and volunteers.
Website/Resource: http://www.aCaringHand.org

Organization: **Grief Net for Children**
Description: A place to deal with feelings in e-mail support group, to share and view artwork and stories, and for parents and kids to ask questions and find answers.
Website/Resource: http://www.kidsaid.com

Organization: **Grief Recovery Online**
Description: Offers message boards, resource listings, and secure chat rooms to help people find partners in pain sharing their experience and strength.
Website/Resource: http://www.groww.org

Organization: **Kid Source Online**
Description: Online community allowing parents to share values and goals in raising, educating and providing for children; access to parenting, education, recreation, organizations, and product information.
Website/Resource: http://www.kidsource.com

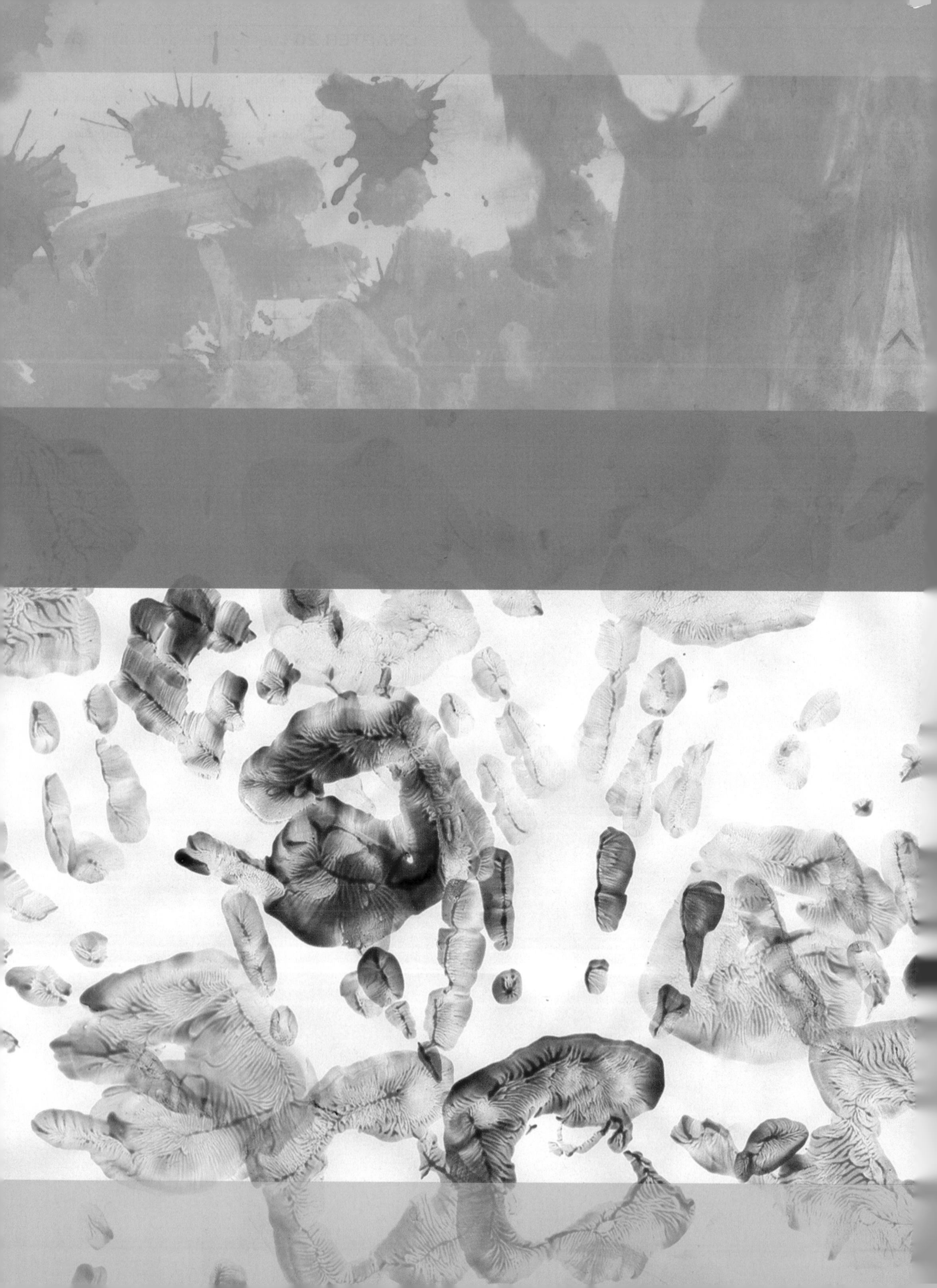

UNIT 4 Alterations in Nutrition and Elimination

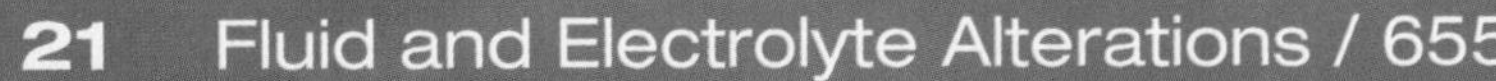

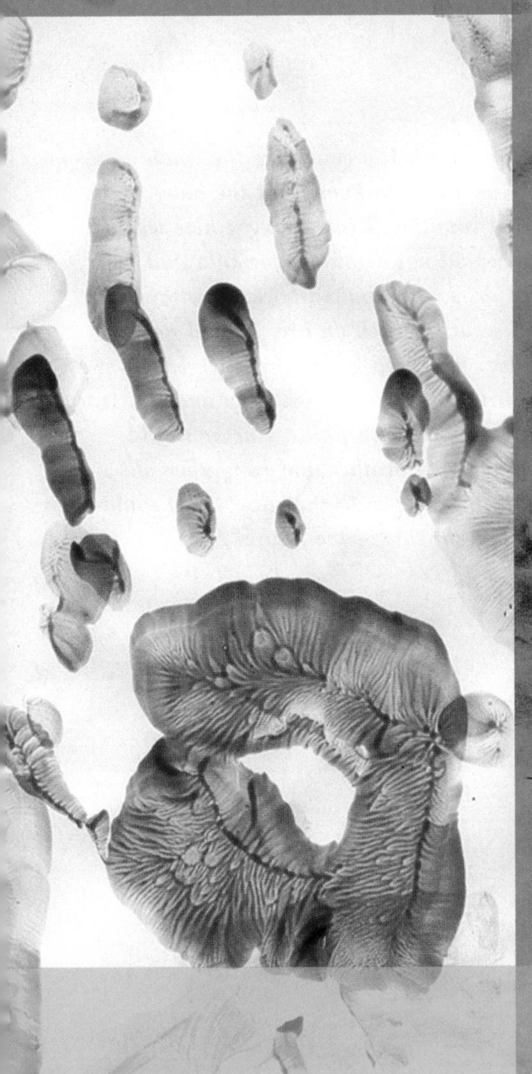

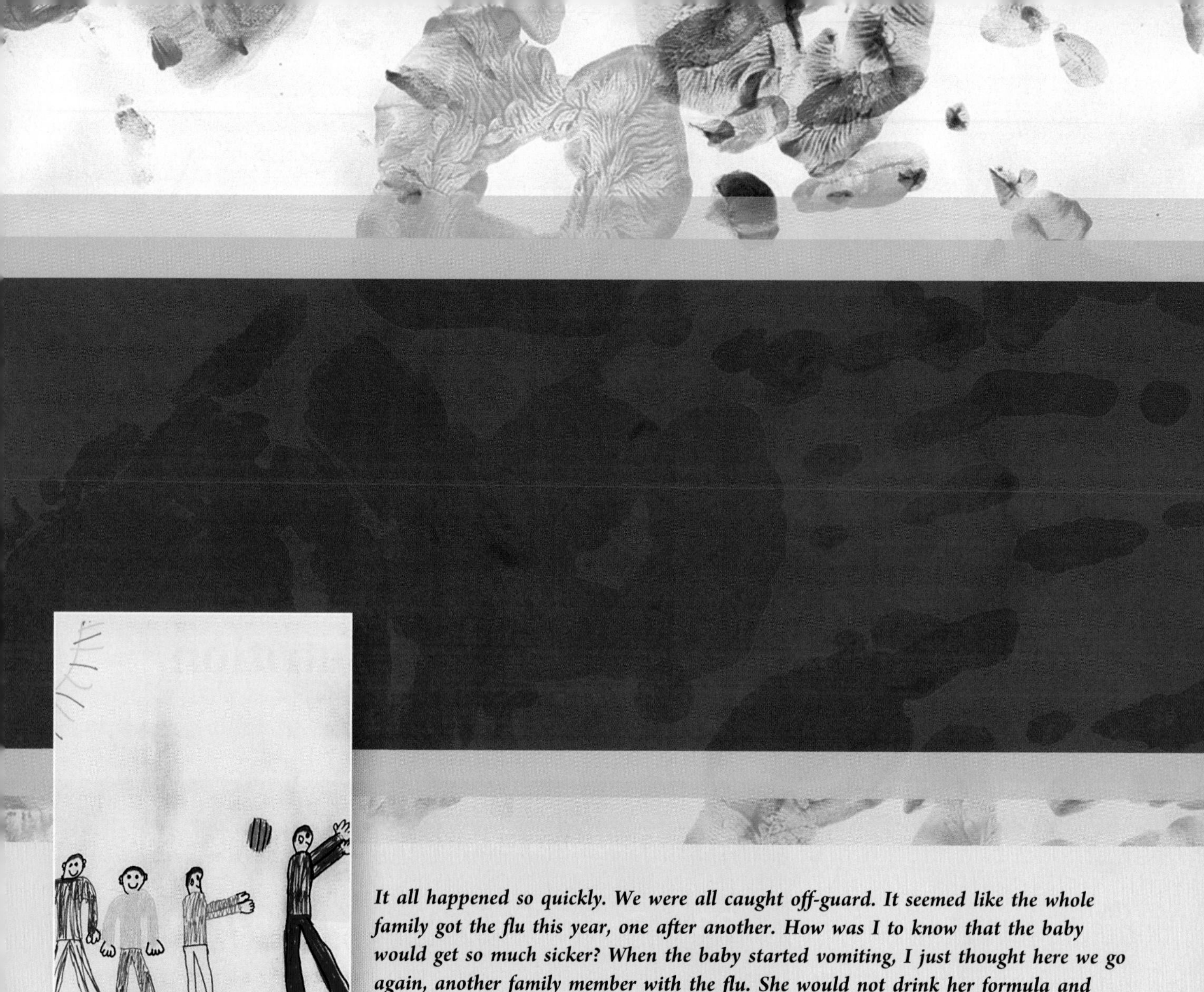

It all happened so quickly. We were all caught off-guard. It seemed like the whole family got the flu this year, one after another. How was I to know that the baby would get so much sicker? When the baby started vomiting, I just thought here we go again, another family member with the flu. She would not drink her formula and would not take clear liquids. Everything she did drink she vomited back up within 15 minutes. She was very fussy, so I put her to bed. Four hours later when I went to check on her, I could not wake her up. She was very limp and felt hot. I knew she was in big trouble. We raced her to the emergency room, and the nurses started an IV immediately. As the fluids ran in her arm, she began to wake up and cry. It was amazing how quickly her condition changed for the worst and then got better with fluids. I never would have thought that the baby would have gotten this sick so quickly. Her 5-year-old brother and her father all seemed to do fine, even though they also had the same symptoms. Why did this happen to the baby? How could I have gotten her to drink when she pushed the bottle away? How can I prevent this in the future?

CHAPTER 21

Fluid and Electrolyte Alterations

Jane H. Lassetter, RN, PhD
Elaine R. Graf, RN, PNP, NE-BC, PhD

COMPETENCIES

Upon completion of this chapter, the reader will be able to:

- Identify differences among adults, children, and infants related to fluid requirements, fluid therapy, and electrolytes.
- Calculate daily maintenance fluid requirements for children of various ages.
- Explain the principles of acid-base imbalances.
- Explain the causes and clinical manifestations of the four major types of acid-base imbalances.
- Compare mild, moderate, and severe dehydration.
- Describe the treatment of the child with gastroenteritis based on the degree of dehydration.
- Discuss common types of burn injuries in children and their prevention.
- Describe the treatment and nursing management of the child with a major burn injury.
- Successfully complete the games and activities in the online student StudyWARE.

An understanding of body fluids, electrolytes, and acid-base **buffers** (a substance that either releases or absorbs hydrogen ions to maintain a stable blood pH) is essential in the treatment of many childhood illnesses. Alterations in electrolytes, fluids, and acid-base metabolism can occur quickly in children and, as a result, can be life threatening. Any illness that alters a child's intake, elimination, or need for water and electrolytes has the potential to cause imbalances. The child's survival hinges on the ability of health care providers to accurately assess at-risk situations, diagnose the alteration, initiate the appropriate treatment plan, and implement prevention strategies (Holliday, Ray, & Friedman, 2007).

This chapter begins with an introduction of the principles associated with the movement of fluids and electrolytes within a child's body, followed by a discussion of how the body buffers these fluids in order to maintain a stable body pH. Next is a discussion of the common alterations, including dehydration, acute gastroenteritis, edema, and burns, that cause fluid shifts to occur in children. Emphasis is placed on the nurse's ability to quickly recognize these alterations and implement an appropriate plan of care.

ANATOMY AND PHYSIOLOGY

The complex chemical and physiological processes that sustain life depend on the presence of water and the body's ability to maintain **homeostasis**, a dynamic equilibrium of the body that is maintained by processes of feedback and regulation. The most abundant body fluid is water. Four key physiological factors are responsible for the fluid and **electrolyte** (a charged particle found in body fluid) differences between children and adults. These include: (1) percentage and distribution of body water, (2) body surface area, (3) rate of basal metabolism, and (4) status of kidney function (Besner & Otabor, 2009; Crellin, 2008; D'Anci, Constant, & Rosenberg, 2006; Roberts, 2005).

Body water volumes are estimates based on age, size, activity, hydration and other factors. Infants have a higher percentage of body water than adults. Because of this, infants require proportionately greater fluid intake than adults and are more vulnerable to dehydration when illness strikes. At birth, total body water is 80 mL/kg. By approximately 6 months of age, it decreases to adult levels of 60-65 mL/kg where it remains constant (Crellin, 2008). Percentage of total body water also changes with age. Water constitutes 50% to 60% of an adult's weight compared to 70% to 75% of a neonate. The percentage declines during the first year of life, and more changes occur during puberty with increased adipose tissue, which has relatively lower water content (D'Anci et al., 2006; Roberts, 2005). These differences, in addition to their inability to independently meet their own hydration needs, help explain why infants are more susceptible to dehydration than adults.

It is important to note that total body water (TBW) estimates of infants and children from previous decades are now thought to overestimate total body water in today's children, especially in infants and girls. Changes in diet and activity habits have led to increased average body fat content, which contributes to these overestimations (Wells, Fewtrell, Davies, Williams, & Cole, 2005).

The body's water is found in two main fluid compartments: within the cell (intracellular, or ICF) and outside the cell (extracellular, or ECF). **Intracellular fluid** is body fluid that is located inside the cells and contains large amounts of potassium, phosphate, sulfate, and proteins. **Extracellular fluid** includes **interstitial fluid** (the fluid between the cells and outside the blood and lymph vessels), **intravascular fluid** (within the blood vessels, e.g., plasma), and **lymphatic fluid** (Schweer, 2008). Extracellular fluid is predominately saline because it contains large amounts of sodium, chloride, and bicarbonate (Figure 21-1).

Distribution of water between the intracellular and extracellular compartments changes with age. Infants have a higher proportion of their total body water in extracellular fluid; therefore, fluid volume deficits can rapidly intensify in them. It also helps explain why signs of cardiovascular compromise become evident more quickly in dehydrated infants than in dehydrated older children and adults (Roberts, 2005; Schweer, 2008). At approximately 3 to 6 months of age, the extracellular/intracellular fluid distribution becomes similar to that of an adult (Crellin, 2008; Roberts, 2005). During illness states (vomiting, diarrhea, or hemorrhage), fluid that is located in the extracellular compartment is lost first. Therefore, infants are more at risk for fluid alterations because a higher percentage of their body weight is water, and more of that water is located in the extracellular compartment (Holliday et al., 2007). The second factor accounting for fluid and electrolyte differences is that infants and children have a relatively greater body surface area than does an adult. Therefore, insensible water losses through the skin and lungs are higher for children, and any situation that results in an increase in loss of water and electrolytes alters the body fluid balance to a greater degree than in an adult (D'Anci et al., 2006). Additionally, infants and young

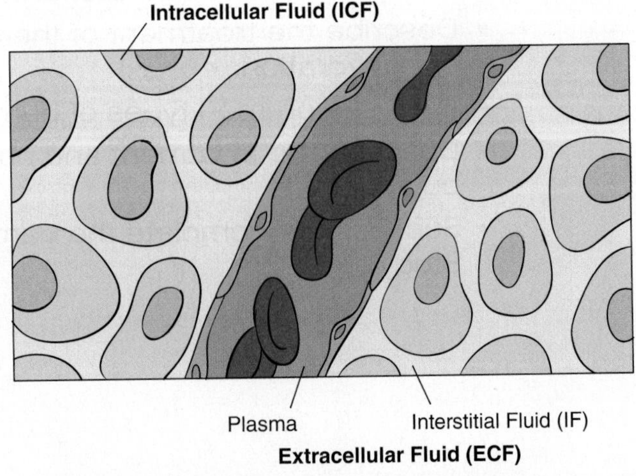

FIGURE 21-1 Body Fluid Compartments. DELMAR CENGAGE LEARNING.

children will lose water more quickly than adults because they have a higher basal metabolic rate (BMR). Due to their higher BMR, the fluid intake per kilogram of body weight per day must exceed the per kilogram fluid requirements of an adult.

Further, infants cannot regulate homeostatic changes as quickly as adults due to immature kidneys and buffering systems. They need more water to excrete a given amount of solute. Compared to adults, infants have less blood flow to the kidneys and a lower glomerular filtration rate. Infants are less able to acidify and concentrate urine than adults; thus, infants' kidneys are unable to respond aggressively to hypovolemia, dehydration, or reduced cardiac output (Crellin, 2008).

The distribution and movement of body fluids between the ICF and ECF compartments are affected by the amount and type of solutes present, the type of membrane to be crossed, and changes in the permeability of the capillary beds. A **solute** is a substance that is dissolved in a solution (e.g., a teaspoon of salt dissolved in a glass of water is an example of a solute). Solutes found in the human body include electrolytes, such as potassium, sodium, and calcium; nonelectrolytes, such as glucose, urea, and creatinine; and large molecules, such as plasma proteins (Holliday et al., 2007; Silva et al., 2008).

Fluids and solute move as a result of diffusion, filtration, osmosis, and active transport (Table 21-1). These processes account for the movement of fluid between intracellular and extracellular spaces. The concentration of a solute in a fluid creates a type of pressure called **osmotic pressure** (a force within the capillary beds that tends to pull water into the capillaries). Osmotic pressure is determined by the type and thickness of the capillary membrane and the size and concentration of circulating molecules.

Oncotic pressure is caused by the amount of plasma proteins present in the vascular system and holds fluids in the capillaries. A decrease in plasma proteins would allow fluid to escape into interstitial spaces. Capillaries are normally impermeable to plasma proteins. However, in certain illnesses, such as sepsis and burns, capillary permeability increases, allowing proteins to move into interstitial spaces along with water, resulting in the formation of edema. Finally, another pressure within the body that is responsible for the movement of fluids is hydrostatic pressure. **Hydrostatic pressure** is the pressure of blood against the capillary walls generated when the heart contracts. Hydrostatic pressure within the capillary bed pushes fluid across capillary membranes into the interstitial space and is balanced by osmotic pressures. It is measured by blood pressure and is important in maintaining the fluid balance within the vascular system.

During various illness states (e.g., shock, burns, dehydration), it becomes important to maintain osmotic pressure within the body. This is often accomplished by giving intravenous solutions at a rate sufficient to replace the loss of fluids. If the child is not able to tolerate fluids orally, the rate also needs to include fluids to cover the daily maintenance requirements. While administering intravenous fluids, it is important to decide the type of solution based on the intended need and to determine the appropriate rate (Holliday et al., 2007). Table 21-2 provides a classification of common intravenous fluids.

ELECTROLYTE IMBALANCES

Serum electrolyte concentrations within the ICF and ECF vary slightly between adults and children. Although many electrolytes are found in the body, all serving vital functions, sodium and potassium are the major electrolytes that influence fluid balance (Roberts, 2005). Normal serum levels of these electrolytes are listed in Table 21-3. Electrolytes influence the formation and retention of water in the ICF and ECF, and can have a dramatic effect on the function of vital organs (D'Anci et al., 2006; Roberts, 2005).

TABLE 21-1 Movement of Fluids and Solutes

CONCEPT	DEFINITION
Osmosis	Fluid moving across a semipermeable membrane from a lower solute concentration to a higher solute concentration.
Diffusion	Particles moving through a solution or gas from a high concentration area to a lower concentration area until equilibrium is reached. The diffusion rate depends on the concentration gradient, occurring more quickly when the concentration rate is great.
Filtration	Fluid and solute moving from an area of high hydrostatic pressure to an area with lower hydrostatic pressure.
Active Transport	Movement of particles against a concentration gradient, a process requiring energy. The sodium-potassium pump is an example.

Adapted from Roberts, K. E. (2005). Pediatric fluid and electrolyte balance: Critical care case studies. *Critical Care Nursing Clinics of North America 17*, 361–373.

TABLE 21-2 Intravenous Fluid Classifications

HYPERTONIC SOLUTIONS	ISOTONIC SOLUTIONS	HYPOTONIC SOLUTIONS
10% glucose in water	Ringer's lactate (RL)	Water
Dextrose 5% in 0.45 normal saline	Normal saline (NS)	
Dextrose 5% in Ringer's lactate	Dextrose 5% in 0.2% NS	
	Dextrose 5% in water	

Adapted from Diehl-Oplinger, L., & Kaminski, M. F. (2004). Choosing the right fluid to counter hypovolemic shock. *Nursing 2004, 34*(3): 52–54.

TABLE 21-3 Normal Serum Concentration for Sodium, Potassium, and Chloride

Sodium	136–146 mEq/L (newborns only)
	139–146 mEq/L (infant)
	135–148 mEq/L (child)
	135–146 mEq/L (adult)
Potassium	3.0–6.0 mEq/L (newborns only)
	3.5–5.0 mEq/L (infants to adults)
Chloride	97–110 mEq/L (infant)
	98–111 mEq/L (child)
	95–106 mEq/L (adult)

CRITICAL THINKING

Selecting IV Fluid with Proper Tonicity

This experiment will illustrate the importance of selecting IV fluid with the proper tonicity for the child's circumstance.

1) Completely cover three eggs in white vinegar and set them aside until the outer shell completely dissolves (about three days). The eggs without shells are comparable to human cells.
2) Remove the eggs from the vinegar and rinse with water. Weigh the eggs and measure their circumference. Record measurements.
3) Place each egg in a clear glass container. Using equal amounts of fluid, cover one egg with distilled water (hypotonic), one with corn syrup (hypertonic), and one in a normal saline mixture (isotonic; 2 teaspoons of salt in 1000 mL of water).
4) Leave the eggs in their respective fluids for four days. Remove the eggs to weigh them, measure their circumference, and record the amount of fluid in the container when the egg is removed.
5) Consider the following questions:
   a. Which egg is the largest? Why?
   b. Which egg is the smallest? Why?
   c. Why did the amounts of fluid in the containers vary?
   d. How does this relate to selecting IV fluid for a pediatric patient?

SODIUM IMBALANCE

Sodium, the major extracellular electrolyte, is responsible for establishing and maintaining the **osmolarity** (the concentration of solute within a solution measured by the number of moles per liter of water) and fluid balance of ECF. Hyponatremia is a decreased serum sodium concentration (<135 mEq/L). When serum sodium decreases, water shifts from ECF to ICF to equalize the **osmolality** (the concentration of solute within a solution measured by the number of moles per kilogram of water) between compartments. This can lead to generalized edema and cerebral edema, which can result in brain herniation and death. Hyponatremia can be caused by excessive administration of sodium bicarbonate or baking soda, diarrhea, vomiting, nasogastric suctioning, diuretics, water intoxication, malnutrition, excessive sweating, burns, diabetic ketoacidosis, renal disease, and cystic fibrosis. Children with cystic fibrosis lose excess salt when they sweat, making them susceptible to hyponatremic dehydration and metabolic alkalosis. Recently researchers have encouraged health care providers to investigate the possibility of cystic fibrosis when children present with unexplained hyponatremic dehydration (Ballestero et al., 2006). Signs and symptoms of hyponatremia are irritability, disorientation, lethargy, seizures, headache, muscle cramps, abdominal cramps, oliguria, and cerebral edema. Care for hyponatremia includes treating the underlying cause, carefully replacing fluid with a hypertonic saline IV fluid, frequently assessing the patient's neurological status, and monitoring serum sodium levels (Roberts, 2005).

Hypernatremia is an increased serum sodium concentration (>145 mEq/L). When serum sodium levels are elevated, fluid moves from the ICF to the ECF, causing cells to shrink. It is caused by an excessive intake of sodium or an increased water loss. Conditions related to hypernatremia include diabetes mellitus, diabetes insipidus, diarrhea, increased insensible water loss, and dehydration. Symptoms in infants and children include extreme thirst, agitation, a high-pitched cry, flushed skin, lethargy, muscle weakness and twitching, seizures, and coma. Under normal circumstances, an elevation in serum sodium causes antidiuretic hormone (ADH) to be released and stimulates thirst. Critically ill children may not be able to respond effectively to these compensatory mechanisms. Care for hypernatremia includes treating the underlying cause, strictly monitoring intake and output, frequently assessing the patient's neurological status, slowly correcting the fluid deficit, and monitoring serum sodium levels (Roberts, 2005).

POTASSIUM IMBALANCE

Potassium is the major electrolyte in the ICF with a concentration of 160 mEq/L inside cells. However, potassium is readily measured in serum, an ECF, where the normal concentration is 3.5–5.0 mEq/L. It has vital roles in the body, including maintenance of osmolality and acid-base balance, transmission of nerve impulses, electrical conductivity, and contractions of skeletal and cardiac muscles (Roberts, 2005). Any potassium imbalance will greatly affect heart muscle contraction. For example, an elevated serum potassium can cause cardiac irritability, which can lead to **ventricular fibrillation** (disorganized electrical impulses leading to improperly timed lower heart muscle contractions). Cardiac irritability associated with an elevated or decreased serum potassium can be seen on an electrocardiogram (ECG). In addition, potassium is necessary for transmission of glucose into cells.

NURSING TIP

Assessing Daily Maintenance Fluid Requirements and Minimum Urine Output

Maintenance of homeostasis requires that the child ingest adequate amounts of fluids and excrete adequate amounts of urine. The following formulas are used to calculate these requirements and also to assess intake and output status (Crellin, 2008).

Maintenance fluid requirements for 24 hours

WEIGHT	*FLUID REQUIREMENT*	*EXAMPLES*
1–10 kg	100 mL/kg	2.5-kg infant = 250 mL
		10-kg infant = 1,000 mL
10–20 kg	1,000 mL + 50 mL/kg over 10 kg	11-kg infant = 1,050 mL
		13-kg infant = 1,150 mL
		20-kg infant = 1,500 mL
>20 kg	1,500 mL + 20 mL/kg over 20 kg	21-kg toddler = 1,520 mL
		30-kg child = 1,700 mL

Minimum urine output by age group

Infant	2mL/kg/hr
Children	1 mL/kg/hr
Adults	½ mL/kg/hr

CRITICAL THINKING

What Does Serum Sodium Indicate?

Identify if the following serum sodium levels are normal, too low, or too high. What effect will these serum sodium levels have on the body's fluid distribution?

140 mEq/L from a 6-year-old child
120 mEq/L from an infant
168 mEq/L from a newborn

Hypokalemia is a decreased serum potassium concentration (<3.5 mEq/L) that results from a true potassium deficit or a potassium shift from the intravascular space to ICF. True potassium deficits can occur with a loss of gastric or intestinal fluids, excessive renal secretion, extreme diaphoresis, or inadequate intake. Potassium shifts from the intravascular space to ICF as a result of alkalosis, excess secretion, or administration of insulin. Symptoms of hypokalemia include lethargy, irritability, nausea/vomiting, abdominal distention, paralytic ileus, arrhythmias, decreased blood pressure, and ECG changes (flattened T waves, ST wave depression, and premature ventricular contractions). Care for hypokalemia includes treating the underlying cause, replacing potassium loss, monitoring serum potassium levels and serum pH, monitoring ECG, and frequently assessing neuromuscular changes (Roberts, 2005).

Hyperkalemia is an increased serum potassium concentration (>5.0 mEq/L) that can result from crushing injuries, burns, tissue necrosis, hemolysis, renal failure, severe dehydration, or a rapid infusion of IV potassium. Metabolic acidosis shifts potassium from ICF to ECF. Although this does not change the overall content of potassium in the body, it creates a hyperkalemic state in the serum. Clinical manifestations of hyperkalemia include abdominal cramps, nausea, vomiting, diarrhea, muscle weakness, hyperreflexia, confusion, apnea, arrhythmias, and ECG changes (tall peaked T waves and a widened QRS complex), and will lead to cardiac arrest if not treated quickly. Care for hyperkalemia includes treating the underlying cause; holding medications and fluids that contain potassium; monitoring ECG changes; carefully administering insulin and glucose (to move potassium into cells), IV calcium, or Kayexalate; and monitoring serum pH and potassium levels (Roberts, 2005).

HORMONES

Hormones can also affect fluid balance in the body. Two major hormones that affect fluid balance are the antidiuretic hormone (ADH) and aldosterone. ADH is secreted by the posterior pituitary when serum osmolality increases, causing the renal tubules of the kidneys to reabsorb water. ADH is secreted when a person is hypovolemic. It causes an immediate increase in vascular volume and a decrease in urine output (D'Anci et al., 2006). However, it is important to remember that renal immaturity of infants limits their capacity to concentrate urine (Crellin, 2008). Aldosterone is a mineralocorticoid produced by the adrenal cortex, which causes the distal renal tubules in the kidneys to reabsorb sodium and excrete potassium. Aldosterone is excreted when the body needs to retain fluids, because increased sodium retention leads to increased water reabsorption. Table 21-4 provides a summary of common disturbances in water, potassium, and sodium balances.

TABLE 21-4 Disturbances in Fluid and Electrolyte Balances

TYPE/CAUSES	SIGNS AND SYMPTOMS	NURSING MANAGEMENT APPROACHES
Water Loss		
Failure to intake or absorb water	Thirst	Calculate replacement needs based on losses and maintenance fluid needs
Inappropriate ADH secretion	Dry skin and mucous membranes	
Diabetes (glycosuria)	Poor skin turgor	Measure intake and output
Fluid loss from gastrointestinal tract	Weight loss	Assess for electrolyte imbalances
• Diarrhea	↓ Pulse pressure, urine output	Assess vital signs
• Vomiting	Slow capillary refill	Monitor urine specific gravity
• Nasogastric suctioning	Fatigue	
• Gastrointestinal fistula	Tachycardia	
Excessive perspiration	↑ Urine specific gravity > 1.020	
Prolonged fever	↑ Hct, BUN, serum osmolarity	
Impaired skin integrity (burns)		
Hemorrhage		
Overuse of diuretics		
Inadequate fluid management		
Water Excess		
Intake > output	Edema	Take full history to determine cause
Excessive water intake	Pulmonary edema, rales	Monitor urine specific gravity
Hypotonic fluid overload	Weight gain	Limit fluid intake
Use of plain water enemas	↑ Venous pressure	Administer diuretics and monitor for effects
↑ Output with normal intake	↓ Urine specific gravity	Monitor vital signs
Kidney failure	↓ Hct, serum electrolytes	Assess for electrolyte imbalances
Congestive heart failure		
Formula prepared with excess water		
↓ Potassium (hypokalemia)		
Poor food intake	Muscle cramping, weakness	Determine cause and treat appropriately
Malabsorption	Irritability, fatigue	Monitor vital signs and ECG
Diuresis	Cardiac arrhythmias	Administer potassium
Fluid loss from gastrointestinal tract	Hypotension	IV: give slowly, only after assured of adequate urine output
Diabetes mellitus	Ileus	
Nephritis	↓ Serum potassium ≤3.5 mEq/L	Oral: give high potassium food and fluids
Corticosteroid use or administration		If giving oral KCL—mix in juice

(Continues)

TABLE 21-4 Disturbances in Fluid and Electrolyte Balances (*Continued*)

Overuse of thiazide diuretics	Abnormal ECG findings	Assess for acid-base imbalances
Alkalosis	Flattened T waves	
	↓ ST segment, ↑ PVCs	
↑ Potassium (hyperkalemia)		
Renal disease and failure	Muscle weakness, twitching	Determine cause and treat appropriately
Addison's disease	↑ Reflexes	Monitor vital signs and ECG
Dehydration	Oliguria	Monitor serum potassium levels
Burns (cellular destruction)	Ventricular fibrillation or arrest	Administer calcium gluconate, as ordered (used to alter cardiac effects)
Hemolysis	↑ Serum potassium ≥5.5 mEq/L	
↑ Intake of potassium foods	Abnormal ECG findings	Administer IV insulin, sodium bicarbonate, or glucose (causes K to move into cells)
Improper IV potassium administration	Flat P wave, tall peaked T wave	Assess for acid-base imbalances
Metabolic acidosis	Widened QRS complex, ↑ PR interval	
↓ Sodium (hyponatremia)		
↓ Sodium intake	Cerebral edema	Determine cause and treat appropriately
Inappropriate ADH syndrome	Muscle weakness	Monitor serum electrolyte levels
Loss of gastrointestinal fluids	Abdominal cramps	Monitor vital signs
Diuretics	Weight loss	Administer IV fluids, as ordered
DKA	Headaches	
Renal disease	Lethargy	
Excessive sweating	Oliguria	
Liver failure	Dehydration	
Low sodium diet	↓ Serum sodium <130 mEq/L	
Cystic fibrosis	Seizures	
↑ Sodium (hypernatremia)		
Excessive intake or retention of sodium	Dry, sticky mucous membranes	Determine cause and treat appropriately
	Thirst	Measure intake and output
Diabetes insipidus	Flushed skin	Monitor neurologic status
Use of mineralocorticoid	Firm skin turgor	Monitor laboratory studies
Hyperglycemia	Disorientation, irritability	Administer fluids as ordered
↑ Insensible water losses	Convulsions	Monitor vital signs
Fever	↑ Serum sodium ≥150 mEq/L	
	↑ Plasma volume	
	Alkalosis	

ACID-BASE BALANCE AND IMBALANCE

Homeostasis in body fluids is also affected by acid-base metabolism. The balance of free acids and bases within the body is regulated by the respiratory and renal systems and must be maintained within a very limited range in order to sustain life. The acidity of body fluids is affected by the concentration of hydrogen ions in the blood, or blood pH. Blood pH is best measured by an arterial blood gas (ABG). Normal blood pH ranges from 7.35 to 7.45. A blood pH below 6.80 or higher than 7.80 is incompatible with life. **Acidosis** is indicated by a blood pH below 7.35, while **alkalosis** is indicated by a blood pH above 7.45 (Lynch, 2009).

The respiratory system controls acid-base metabolism by retaining or releasing carbon dioxide (CO_2), thereby causing a shift in the bicarbonate-carbonic acid buffering system. The amount of dissolved carbon dioxide in the blood (pCO_2) is measured by an ABG, and ranges from 35 to 45 mm Hg. Carbonic acid (H_2CO_3) is a weak, unstable acid, formed when carbon dioxide combines with water (H_2O), that will dissociate into bicarbonate and one hydrogen ion ($HCO_3 + H^+$). The free hydrogen ions will combine with oxygen to form water. Bicarbonate and water can then be released or retained by the kidneys in order to maintain the necessary balance. Bicarbonate levels are measured by an ABG and range from 22-26 mEq/L. The ability of the kidneys to excrete hydrogen ions and bicarbonate can be inferred from the blood bicarbonate level obtained from an ABG.

To maintain a stable acid-base balance, the body will try to maintain a 20:1 ratio between bicarbonate and carbonic acid, and an equilibrium of the carbonic acid and dissolved carbon dioxide found in blood. The lungs will compensate for pH changes caused by metabolic disorders (e.g., diabetes, vomiting, and diarrhea) by controlling the carbon dioxide level in the blood. Hyperventilation or deep rapid breathing (Kussmaul respirations) will occur in an attempt to blow off carbon dioxide. The kidneys will compensate for pH changes caused by respiratory problems or a buildup of metabolic acids (e.g., lactic acid, hydrochloric acid, pyruvic acid, sulfuric acid) by controlling hydrogen ion and bicarbonate levels in the blood. However, renal compensation is much slower than respiratory compensation and often requires days to restore balance. **Compensation** is a body process to restore blood pH to normal by changing the partial pressure of carbon dioxide (pCO_2) or the bicarbonic ion concentration. (Figure 21-2 illustrates acid-base balance and imbalance.)

Related to Respiratory Function | Related to Metabolism of the Body

Balance

H_2CO_3 (Acid) | HCO_3^- (Bicarbonate)

Imbalance

Respiratory Acidosis | Acidosis | Metabolic Acidosis

Excess H_2CO_3 (Acid) pH↓ $PaCO_2$↑ | Deficit HCO_3^- (Bicarbonate) pH↓ HCO_3↓ Serum CO_2↓

Respiratory Alkalosis | Alkalosis | Metabolic Alkalosis

Deficit H_2CO_3 (Acid) pH↑ $PaCO_2$↓ | Excess HCO_3^- (Bicarbonate) pH↑ HCO_3^-↑ Serum CO_2↑

FIGURE 21-2 Acid-Base Balance and Imbalance. DELMAR CENGAGE LEARNING.

Acid-base imbalances are common in children and fall into four categories: respiratory acidosis, respiratory alkalosis, metabolic acidosis, and metabolic alkalosis. The body will compensate for these disturbances by using a renal or a respiratory buffering mechanism. These responses are monitored by ABG analysis. Table 21-5 lists the causes, clinical manifestations, and management of the four acid-base disturbances.

RESPIRATORY ACIDOSIS

Respiratory acidosis can be caused by any condition that decreases a child's respiratory effort. Slowed or shallow respirations will result in a buildup of carbon dioxide, which combined with water forms carbonic acid and leads to acidosis (↓ pH, ↑ pCO_2). Many clinical conditions can cause respiratory acidosis and are listed in Box 21-1.

Acidosis causes central nervous system depression. As a result, the child will be lethargic, confused, and disoriented, may complain of a headache, and, if not treated, may become comatose. Efforts to improve ventilation help correct the underlying cause of respiratory acidosis. Without correction, the body, via the kidneys, will retain bicarbonate to help neutralize the increased acid. However, the kidneys' attempt to compensate is slow and does not correct the underlying respiratory problem.

RESPIRATORY ALKALOSIS

Respiratory alkalosis occurs when the carbon dioxide level is too low. This most commonly occurs from conditions that cause the child to hyperventilate (e.g., anxiety, pain, meningitis, gram-negative septicemia, early response to salicylate

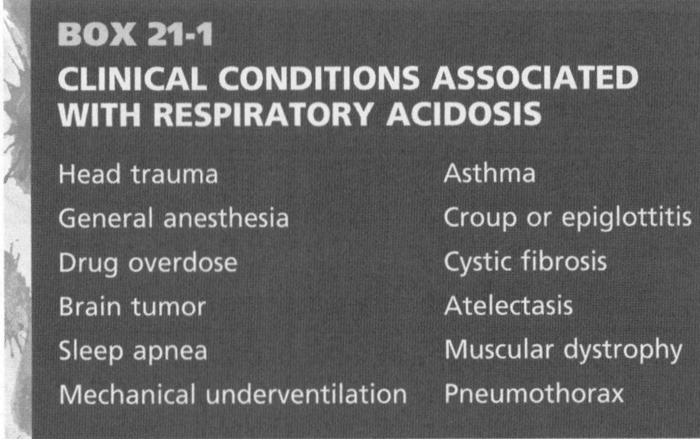

BOX 21-1
CLINICAL CONDITIONS ASSOCIATED WITH RESPIRATORY ACIDOSIS

Head trauma	Asthma
General anesthesia	Croup or epiglottitis
Drug overdose	Cystic fibrosis
Brain tumor	Atelectasis
Sleep apnea	Muscular dystrophy
Mechanical underventilation	Pneumothorax

TABLE 21-5 Comparative Analysis of Acid-Base Disturbances

CONDITION/PRIMARY CAUSE	CLINICAL MANIFESTATIONS	MANAGEMENT APPROACHES
Respiratory Acidosis		
Alveolar hypoventilation: ↑ pCO_2	Dyspnea	Monitor blood gases
Chronic respiratory disease	↑ Use of accessory muscles	Improve ventilation
Depression of CNS	Cyanosis	Give oxygen, consider intubation
Inadequate mechanical ventilation	CNS depression	Administer sodium bicarbonate
Pneumothorax	↑ Intracranial pressure	Monitor vital signs
Neuromuscular disease	Tachycardia	
Respiratory Alkalosis		
Alveolar hyperventilation: ↓ pCO_2	Tachypnea	Monitor blood gases
Anxiety	Numbness, tingling of toes and fingers	Encourage slow ventilation
Sepsis	Lightheaded, dizzy	Use rebreathing oxygen masks or bag
Heart failure	Syncope	Administer sedative, if ordered
Hepatic failure	Diaphoresis	Monitor vital signs
Fever or hypermetabolic states		
Salicylate poisoning		
Overzealous mechanical ventilation		
Metabolic Acidosis		
↑ Body acids or ↓ HCO_3	Confusion	Correct underlying problem
Diabetic ketoacidosis (DKA)	Lethargy	Administer sodium bicarbonate
Alcoholic ketoacidosis	Deep, rapid respirations	Administer oxygen
↑ Intake of acids (salicylates)	Acetone odor to breath	Correct DKA with insulin or glucose
Diarrhea	Tachycardia	Monitor vital signs
Renal failure	Cold, clammy skin (mild acidosis)	
Starvation	Warm, dry skin (severe acidosis)	
Shock		
Metabolic Alkalosis		
↓ Body acids or ↑ HCO_3	Slow, shallow respirations	Correct underlying problem
Vomiting	Tremors, muscle twitching	Administer sodium NaCl and KCl
Prolonged NG suctioning	Disorientation	Replace loss of fluids
Overuse of antacids	Seizures	Take seizure precautions
Hypokalemia		Monitor intake and output
Diuretics		Monitor electrolyte status

poisoning, mechanical overventilation). The child will often feel numbness or tingling in toes and fingers, lightheadedness, and confusion, and may faint. Renal compensation for respiratory alkalosis is rarely seen clinically because the underlying condition is often corrected before the kidneys have time to respond. However, if seen, the kidneys would retain free hydrogen ions and excrete bicarbonate. The child's urine pH would increase as a result of the increased bicarbonate excretion.

METABOLIC ACIDOSIS

Metabolic acidosis is most commonly caused by a loss of bicarbonate in the stool or an increase in ketone bodies (e.g., acetoacetic acid, acetone, beta-hydroxybutyric acid) in the blood. These conditions most frequently result from diarrhea and diabetic ketoacidosis. Children are often confused, lethargic, and tachycardic. The body compensates by

NURSING ALERT

Electrolyte Shift in Metabolic Acidosis

Metabolic acidosis causes an electrolyte shift: hydrogen and sodium ions move into the cell, and potassium moves into the ECF, increasing serum potassium. Hyperkalemia may cause ventricular fibrillation and death.

CRITICAL THINKING

Respiratory Buffer Response to Metabolic Acidosis

Consider the answers to the following questions related to metabolic acidosis:

1. What effect does metabolic acidosis have on the pH of blood?
2. What is the underlying imbalance (carbon dioxide, bicarbonate, hydrogen ion)?
3. What does the body accomplish by increasing the rate and depth of respiration?

increasing the depth and rate of respirations in order to blow off carbon dioxide, thus decreasing pCO_2 and carbonic acid.

METABOLIC ALKALOSIS

Metabolic alkalosis occurs as a result of bicarbonate retention or hydrogen ion loss. It is most commonly seen in children with prolonged vomiting as emesis is acidic stomach contents. It can also occur with ingestion of large quantities of bicarbonate antacids, massive blood transfusions, loss of nasogastric fluids due to gastric suction, and hypokalemia. A child experiencing metabolic alkalosis is often weak and dizzy and may complain of muscle cramps. The respiratory response would be to increase pCO_2 by decreasing the rate and depth of respirations (hypoventilation).

DEHYDRATION AND HYPOVOLEMIA

The terms dehydration and hypovolemia are often thought to be synonymous, but they are not. Hypovolemia is a decrease in the circulating blood volume, and dehydration is a deficit of total body water. Severe dehydration can lead to hypovolemia, hypovolemic shock, end organ failure, and even death (Crellin, 2008). As previously stated, children, particularly infants, are more susceptible to dehydration than adults. Therefore, early recognition and treatment of dehydration and hypovolemia in children is important.

Clinical manifestations of hypovolemia and dehydration have some overlap. The most definitive sign of dehydration is weight loss. Clinical dehydration is classified as mild (<3% weight loss), moderate (3–9% weight loss), or severe (>9% weight loss) (Centers for Disease Control and Prevention, 2008). However, this is often difficult to determine because many parents do not know their children's baseline weights accurately enough to determine how much weight may have been lost before they sought health care (Crellin, 2008). In addition, based on understanding of renal physiology, an elevated urine specific gravity has long been used as an indicator of dehydration in children; however, there is evidence that this is not a helpful test to determine dehydration in children with gastroenteritis, a common cause of dehydration (Steiner, Nager, & Wang, 2007). Therefore, other symptoms need to be considered. The three signs found to be most indicative of dehydration are poor skin turgor, prolonged capillary refill, and an abnormal respiratory pattern. Other indications of dehydration include a recent history of diarrhea and/or vomiting, parental report of the child experiencing decreased urine output and/or poor fluid intake, decreased or absent tears, dry mucous membranes, tachycardia, sunken eyes, sunken fontanel (in infants), cool extremities, and a generally ill appearance. Children vary considerably in how they exhibit dehydration. When assessing the severity of children's dehydration, it is helpful to consider how many signs of dehydration they have rather than relying on a single indicator (Crellin, 2008). Table 21-6 lists the clinical manifestations associated with the degree of dehydration.

Evidence of poor end organ perfusion and compensatory effort indicate hypovolemia. In the early stages of hypovolemia, increased heart rate and evidence of vasoconstriction, such as skin pallor and mottling, indicate that compensatory mechanisms are at work to improve cardiac output and end organ perfusion. As hypovolemia worsens, the child's condition will deteriorate, and evidence of other compensatory mechanisms will be seen, such as tachypnea to combat metabolic acidosis. Left uncorrected, significant hypovolemia will result in diminished perfusion to vital organs. A child in this state will exhibit prolonged capillary refill time, decreased urine output, altered state of consciousness, increased respiratory rate, metabolic acidosis, and decreased blood pressure. Recognition of the early signs of hypovolemia and appropriate intervention are essential because declining blood pressure of infants and children is a late and ominous sign that does not occur until the circulating blood volume has been reduced by approximately 30% (Crellin, 2008).

TYPES OF DEHYDRATION

There are three types of dehydration: isotonic, hypotonic, and hypertonic. The most common type is isotonic, accounting for about 80% of dehydration cases. Hypotonic and hypertonic dehydration each account for approximately

TABLE 21-6 CDC's Summary of Clinical Manifestations According to Degree of Dehydration

SYMPTOMS	DEGREE OF DEHYDRATION		
	Minimal or none (<3% loss of body weight)	**Mild to moderate (3–9% loss of body weight)**	**Severe (>9% loss of body weight)**
Mental status	Well; alert	Normal, fatigued or restless, irritable	Apathetic, lethargic, unconscious
Thirst	Drinks normally; might refuse liquids	Thirsty; eager to drink	Drinks poorly; unable to drink
Heart rate	Normal	Normal to increased	Tachycardic; bradycardic in severe cases
Quality of pulses	Normal	Normal to decreased	Weak, thready, or impalpable
Breathing	Normal	Normal; fast	Deep
Eyes	Normal	Slightly sunken	Deeply sunken
Tears	Present	Decreased	Absent
Mouth and tongue	Moist	Dry	Parched
Skin fold	Instant recoil	Recoil in <2 seconds	Recoil in >2 seconds
Capillary refill	Normal	Prolonged	Prolonged; minimal
Extremities	Warm	Cool	Cold; mottled; cyanotic
Urine output	Normal to decreased	Decreased	Minimal

From Centers for Disease Control and Prevention. (2008). Information for healthcare providers: Guidelines for the management of acute diarrhea. Retrieved March 1, 2009, from http://www.bt.cdc/gov/disasters/hurricanes/pdf/dguidelines.pdf.

CRITICAL THINKING

Why Would Vomiting, Hypokalemia, Cystic Fibrosis, Loss of Nasogastric Fluids, or Blood Transfusions Cause Metabolic Alkalosis?

Consider the above alterations. Explain why they can lead to metabolic alkalosis. How can a nurse prevent metabolic alkalosis in the above illness states?

5–10% of the cases (Huang, Anchala, Ellsbury, & George, 2008). The type of dehydration a child has depends on the ratio of water loss to salt loss. As long as the child's homeostatic mechanisms are able to maintain normal sodium concentrations, as might be the case with a short bout of diarrhea, **isotonic dehydration** results. In this state, serum sodium values are normal because water and sodium are lost in equal proportions (Petersen-Smith & McKenzie, 2009). Fluid is lost equally from both intravascular and extravascular spaces (Huang et al., 2008).

Hypotonic dehydration occurs when sodium loss is greater than water loss, resulting in the serum sodium falling below 130 mEq/L. Hypotonic dehydration can occur when there is a substantial loss of water and salt in stool, and only water is ingested (Petersen-Smith & McKenzie, 2009). It can also result from inappropriate IV therapy, gastroenteritis, nephrosis, adrenal insufficiency, or not replacing gastric secretions. In hypotonic dehydration, intracellular fluid becomes more concentrated, and the body responds by moving fluid from extracellular spaces to intracellular spaces. While this response helps reestablish osmotic equilibrium within the body, it also exaggerates the intravascular loss in comparison to total body water loss (Huang et al., 2008).

Hypertonic dehydration occurs when water loss is greater than sodium loss. This might occur when infants or children experience vomiting and diarrhea with reduced water intake (Petersen-Smith & McKenzie, 2009) or when they have diabetes insipidus or are treated for diarrhea with fluids containing high concentrations of electrolytes. In hypertonic dehydration, serum sodium rises above 150 mEq/L, and serum osmolarity increases. In the presence of high serum sodium, extravascular fluid moves to the intravascular compartment to minimize the intravascular loss compared to total body water loss (Huang et al., 2008). This makes shock less apparent. However, it is the most dangerous type of dehydration because the fluid replacement strategy is much more difficult to determine and manage.

INCIDENCE AND ETIOLOGY OF DEHYDRATION

Although the exact incidence of dehydration is unknown, it can be caused from many common illnesses or prolonged NPO status in preparation for many hospital procedures. Infants and children under 5 years of age are most at risk for developing dehydration. Morbidity and mortality are associated with the severity of dehydration and the rapidness of treatment initiation. When oral or intravenous rehydration is initiated quickly and appropriately, recovery is usually complete. Nevertheless, diarrhea associated with dehydration remains a significant cause of childhood mortality worldwide (Huang et al., 2008).

NURSING TIP

Assessing Fluid, Electrolyte, and Acid-base Alterations

Assessing a child who has an alteration in fluid, electrolytes, or acid-base balance requires an understanding of developmental norms for vital signs and behavior and excellent observation skills. Ask yourself the following questions:

- Has the child been ill recently?
- What are the presenting symptoms?
- Is the child's intake and output balanced?
- How many times has the child voided in the last 24 hours?
- Has the child gained or lost weight recently, or as a result of this illness?
- Are the child's vital signs within normal limits for age?
- Does the child's skin reflect a dehydrated state or an edematous state?
- Are the child's mucous membranes dry?
- Are the fontanelles flat, sunken, or bulging?
- Does the child have tears when crying?
- What is the child's general appearance and behavior?
- What does the child's urine specific gravity reflect?
- What does the child's lab work for electrolytes and blood gases reflect?

The answers to these questions will help in determining if the child has a fluid and electrolyte problem, and in confirming the correct nursing diagnosis.

CRITICAL THINKING

Water Intoxication

Although not as common as isotonic dehydration, water intoxication can also be a serious condition in children. What would you teach a low-income mother who is diluting her infant's formula to make it stretch farther?

CRITICAL THINKING

Heart and Kidney Responses to Extracellular Fluid Losses

Draw a picture of the body's response to an extracellular fluid loss. Describe the effects of epinephrine, antidiuretic hormone, and the renin-angiotensin system. Why is venous constriction and sodium retention beneficial to a child with an extracellular fluid loss? How would you describe these compensatory mechanisms to a caregiver?

PATHOPHYSIOLOGY OF HYPOVOLEMIA

The body compensates for extravascular fluid losses in very specific ways. A decrease in the fluid circulating in the vascular system lowers cardiac output and can lead to hypotension (a decrease in blood pressure). Blood pressure sensors in the heart, kidneys, and brain react quickly to increase cardiac output and increase sodium and water retention. Any decrease in blood pressure triggers sensory nerves in the aortic arch to stimulate the sympathetic nervous system, causing the fight-or-flight response or a release of epinephrine. Epinephrine improves cardiac output by increasing heart rate, cardiac contractility, and venous constriction. This compensatory mechanism helps to circulate the remaining blood faster but does not increase the circulating volume. Compensatory mechanisms within the kidneys activate the renin-angiotensin system, which improves circulating fluid volume by increasing sodium retention. Additionally, blood pressure sensors in the brain respond by releasing ADH, which stimulates thirst and retention of water by the kidneys. These compensatory mechanisms are the body's first line of defense but are only temporary. Without prompt recognition and treatment, cardiac ischemia and arrhythmias will develop.

UNDERLYING CAUSES OF DEHYDRATION AND HYPOVOLEMIA

Determining the cause of dehydration and/or hypovolemia is often essential to effective treatment. Gastroenteritis is the most common cause of dehydration, and, in this case, dehydration is primarily caused by fluid loss. If the child is vomiting and experiencing diarrhea, the severity of the dehydration can quickly intensify. Other illnesses can lead to dehydration by decreasing a child's willingness to eat and drink. For instance, pain in the mouth or throat from illnesses, such as stomatitis,

NURSING TIP

Diarrhea is not a Disease

Diarrhea is an indication of a gastrointestinal disturbance, not a disease. It can be caused by a variety of problems, including infection and malabsorption. Diarrhea is defined as "an abnormal increase in stool liquidity, stool frequency, and stool weight" (Sabol & Carlson, 2007). Diarrhea lasting 7 to 14 days is acute. When diarrhea continues beyond 2 to 3 weeks, it is considered chronic. Acute diarrhea is most frequently caused by infection, and chronic diarrhea is most frequently associated with irritable bowel syndrome (Sabol & Carlson, 2007).

tonsillitis, or pharyngitis, may discourage the child from eating and drinking. Likewise, any febrile illness increases insensible water loss and can cause irritability and diminished appetite. Some causes of dehydration require rather complex treatment. For example, if dehydration is the result of diabetic ketoacidosis, rehydration has to be carefully orchestrated to avoid poor neurologic outcomes. In such cases, if rehydration is too aggressive, cerebral edema can result. Fluid loss from burns can be extreme and requires aggressive fluid management. If dehydration is from cystic fibrosis, the child is at risk for severe hypotonic dehydration from excess sodium loss. If the child has diabetes insipidus, the risk for hypertonic dehydration is great from excessive output of extremely dilute urine (Gharahbaghian, Lotfipour, McCoy, Hoonpongsimanont, & Langdorf, 2008; Huang et al., 2008; Schulman & King, 2008). Thus, determining the underlying cause of dehydration can have a significant impact on the course of treatment.

CARING FOR CHILDREN WITH DEHYDRATION

Treatment of dehydration depends upon the severity of dehydration. See Table 21-7 for the CDC's recommended treatment based on degree of dehydration. The focus is on correcting the fluid and electrolyte imbalances and treating the underlying cause. If nausea and vomiting are the cause of dehydration, oral ondansetron may reduce vomiting and improve the

TABLE 21-7 CDC's Recommended Rehydration Based on Degree of Dehydration

DEGREE OF DEHYDRATION	REHYDRATION THERAPY	REPLACEMENT OF ONGOING LOSSES	NUTRITION
Minimal or none (<3% loss of body weight)	Not applicable	<10 kg body wt.: 60–120 mL oral rehydration solution (ORS) for each diarrheal stool or vomiting episode >10 kg body weight: 120–240 mL ORS for each diarrheal stool or vomiting episode	Continue breastfeeding or resume age-appropriate normal diet after initial rehydration, including adequate caloric intake for maintenance
Mild to moderate (3–9% loss of body weight)	ORS, 50–100 mL/kg body weight over 3–4 hours	Same	Same
Severe (>9% loss of body weight)	Lactated Ringers solution or normal saline* intravenously in boluses of 20 mL/kg body weight until perfusion and mental status improve, then administer 100 mL/kg body weight ORS over 4 hours or 5% dextrose ½ normal saline intravenously at twice maintenance fluid rates * In severe dehydrating diarrhea, normal saline is less effective for treatment because it contains no bicarbonate or potassium. Use normal saline only if Ringers lactate solution is not available, and supplement with ORS as soon as the patient can drink. Plain glucose in water is ineffective and should not be used.	Same: if unable to drink, administer through nasogastric tube or administer 5% dextrose ¼ normal saline with 20 mEq/L potassium chloride intravenously	Same

From Centers for Disease Control and Prevention. (2008). Information for healthcare providers: Guidelines for the management of acute diarrhea. Retrieved March 1, 2009, from http://www.bt.cdc/gov/disasters/hurricanes/pdf/dguidelines.pdf.

chances of success with oral rehydration (Freedman, Adler, Seshadri, & Powell, 2006). Dehydrated breastfed infants should breast feed more frequently and for less time than their normal routine. For other dehydrated infants and children, rehydration solutions should be initiated without a period of gut rest and given frequently (every 5–10 minutes) in small (even as little as 5–10 mL) amounts. Volume can be increased and given less frequently as vomiting subsides (Koslap-Petraco, 2006; Petersen-Smith & McKenzie, 2009). Oral rehydration is time-intensive and requires patience; nurses should encourage caregivers and praise their efforts to rehydrate children.

The United Nations Children's Fund and the World Health Organization (UNICEF & WHO, 2006) recommend **oral rehydration solution** (ORS) as the first-line therapy for mild to moderate dehydration. Appropriate oral rehydration solutions such as Pedialyte, Lytren, Infalyte, and Resol are available commercially. Some children will tolerate ORS better if it is frozen. For children who refuse to drink ORS, diluted fruit juices or soft drinks (one part to four parts water) can be used as an alternative. Diluting these drinks by one part to four parts reduces their osmolarity, making them similar to the ORS osmolarity recommended by the UNICEF and WHO (Crellin, 2008).

When children with moderate to severe dehydration refuse to drink or are not tolerating oral fluids, other methods of rehydration are needed. In such cases, rehydrating through nasogastric tubes is often successful (Crellin, 2008). However, when dehydration is severe or vomiting is uncontrollable, intravenous (IV) therapy should be initiated. In the event that venous access is unobtainable, intraosseous (IO) administration of fluids is a viable option. IO access involves inserting a needle into the bone marrow cavity, usually with insertion devices, such as injection guns or drills. Once IO access is obtained, fluids and medications can be given as they would through an IV, except fluids will not run by gravity and must be pumped with pressure into the patient (Crellin, 2008; de Caen, 2007; Horton & Beamer, 2008). The rate of IV or IO fluid replacement depends on the child's degree of dehydration and the presence of cardiac, pulmonary, or renal problems. The volume of fluid to be given is based on the child's weight and clinical signs and symptoms. Boluses of 20mL/kg are usually recommended (Crellin, 2008).

The type of IV solution used varies with the type of dehydration. Generally, isotonic dehydration (most common type in children) is treated with **isotonic fluids** (fluids that have the same concentrations as normal body fluid),

NURSING ALERT

Fluid Losses Due to Hemorrhage

Hemorrhage that results in external losses of blood and fluid is fairly easy to assess. However, an internal hemorrhage causing blood to accumulate in a third-space compartment, such as the thoracic or peritoneal cavity, is often very difficult to detect because the blood loss is not outwardly visible. Based on the child's history, a nurse must consider if the child is at risk for an internal hemorrhage and then assess for signs and symptoms, such as decreases in blood pressure, hematocrit, and pulse rate. A child with an internal hemorrhage has the same risk for hypovolemic shock as a child with an external hemorrhage. Signs and symptoms of hypovolemic shock such as hypotension, bradycardia, weak peripheral pulses, and decreased urine output will be the same for both internal and external hemorrhages, except that a child with an internal hemorrhage will not lose weight.

NURSING ALERT

Dehydration from Diarrhea as a Leading Cause of Morbidity and Mortality

Dehydration from diarrhea remains a leading cause of childhood morbidity and mortality throughout the world. In fact, diarrhea is currently the second leading cause of death in children (WHO, 2006). In developing countries, the use of ORS in recent years has helped manage diarrhea in children. Mostly due to the promotion and use of ORS, an estimated 1 million lives per year were saved in the 1990's. In developing countries, the mortality rate associated with acute diarrhea in children less than 5 years of age dropped from 4.5 million in 1979, before the introduction of ORS, to 1.9 million in 2005 (UNICEF & WHO, 2004; WHO, 2006). Although this is an impressive improvement, acute diarrhea and dehydration continue to exact a high toll. In addition, there are indications of declining knowledge and use of ORS in countries at highest risk (UNICEF & WHO, 2004).

Problems associated with diarrhea and dehydration are not limited to developing countries; they are also problematic in the United States. Children under 5 years of age in the United States average two episodes of gastroenteritis per year. Children of all ages with dehydration in the United States make more than 2 million office visits to health care providers and account for 220,000 hospitalizations (10% of hospital admissions for children) and $2 billion in direct medical costs yearly. In addition, 400 children in the United States die each year from diarrhea and dehydration (Huang et al., 2008; Steiner et al., 2007).

FAMILY TEACHING

Dehydration

Teach caregivers to watch for the signs and symptoms of dehydration:

- fewer wet diapers, especially none for more than 6–8 hours
- rapid breathing (respiratory rate will vary with the child's age)
- prolonged capillary refill time (blanching of skin on an extremity that lasts 3-4 seconds after applying pressure and releasing it)
- poor skin turgor (slow recoil of skin when gently pinched)
- inside of mouth dry or parched
- reduction or lack of tears when crying if older than 2–4 months of age
- irritable or lethargic (difficult to arouse or awaken)
- sunken fontanel
- pale, gray, or mottled skin color

hypotonic dehydration with **hypertonic fluids** (fluids that are more concentrated than normal body fluid), and hypertonic dehydration with **hypotonic fluids** (fluids that are less concentrated than normal body fluid). (refer to Table 21-1.) Common intravenous rehydration solutions are Ringer's lactate (RL) and normal saline (NS), including one-fourth and one-half strength.

NURSING ALERT

ORS Saves Lives: Improved ORS May Save Even More Lives

For over a quarter of a century, UNICEF and WHO have advocated the use of ORS to prevent and treat dehydration from diarrhea. The result has been a dramatic decline in the global mortality from diarrhea. In an effort to further improve outcomes, they researched the use of reduced osmolarity ORS solution to help avoid hypertonicity and its adverse impact on net fluid absorption. By decreasing the concentrations of glucose and salt, researchers reduced the osmolarity from 311 mOsmol/L in the original formula to 245 mOsmol/L. They found improved efficacy with their lower osmolarity formula compared to the original formula, including a 33% reduction in the need for supplemental intravenous fluid therapy, a 30% reduction in vomiting, and a 20% reduction in stool output (UNICEF & WHO, 2004). Based on these findings, UNICEF and WHO (2004) recommend the following electrolyte concentrations be used to manufacture ORS solutions: 2.6 grams/liter sodium chloride; glucose, anhydrous 13.5 grams/liter; potassium chloride 1.5 grams/liter; trisodium citrate, dihydrate 1.9 grams/liter. Nurses should encourage caregivers to look at product labels and make sure that the rehydration fluid they choose has the prescribed electrolyte concentrations.

NURSING MANAGEMENT

Assessment

When assessing hydration status, the nurse should assess the color, warmth, and turgor of the child's skin. Color indicates the state of perfusion and will turn from pink to pale, dusky, or gray as perfusion decreases. Perfusion is also reflected in the temperature of the skin. The skin will feel cool, and the child may complain of cold fingers and toes with decreased perfusion. Capillary refill time will also be prolonged (3–4 seconds or more) as perfusion decreases. Extracellular fluid losses will cause the skin to become dry and loose, referred to as a loss of skin turgor. Decreased skin turgor results in a tenting of the skin when pinched and indicates a decreased fluid state. Additional measures of the adequacy of systemic perfusion include assessment of heart rate, blood pressure, and peripheral pulses (Petersen-Smith & McKenzie, 2009).

Nurses should assess mucous membranes for the presence of dry, sticky mucus and note the presence or absence of tears. Tears should be present if the child is crying. In a child less than 18 months of age, it is also important to check the anterior fontanel. The fontanel should be even with the contour of the skull. When the child is dehydrated, the fontanel is often depressed or sunken in appearance. Weight is a critical indicator of the child's fluid status and should be compared with a pre-illness weight, if available, or the weight from the previous day (Petersen-Smith & McKenzie, 2009).

NURSING TIP

Calculating Fluid Loss from Weight Loss

Fluid loss can be calculated according to weight lost. One kilogram of body weight equals 1 L of water. Therefore, each kilogram of weight lost is equal to 1,000 mL of fluid loss.

Intake and output should also be assessed. An assessment of output should include measurements of urine, stools, emesis, wound drainage, and an estimate of insensible fluid loss. The child's urine should be observed for amount, color, and odor. Note the presence of blood or mucus in the stools. Watery stools should also be measured or estimated and documented as output. If the child has any draining wounds, the dressings should be weighed to estimate fluid loss. Finally, excessive perspiration may require estimating fluid loss by weighing clothing or linens. The use of radiant warmers or warming lights can also increase insensible fluid losses in small infants and should be monitored. Several behavioral changes may also be present in children with dehydration. These include decreased activity levels, loss of interest in their environment, restlessness, irritability, lethargy, and a high-pitched, weak cry. The last assessment should include a review of serum electrolyte results (Petersen-Smith & McKenzie, 2009).

Nursing Diagnosis

Nursing diagnoses appropriate for a child with dehydration may include:

1. *Deficient fluid volume* related to excessive fluid volume loss or inadequate fluid intake.
2. *Risk for injury (fall)* related to weakness and possible orthostatic (postural) hypotension.
3. *Deficient knowledge (caregiver)* related to lack of exposure to information about preventing or detecting dehydration.

Outcome Identification

1. The child will receive sufficient fluids to replace losses.
2. The child will exhibit signs of adequate hydration.
3. The child will not fall or sustain other injuries while hypotensive or lethargic.
4. Caregivers will demonstrate understanding of conditions that can lead to dehydration and of the early signs and symptoms.

Planning and Implementation

Nursing interventions include administration of IV or IO fluids, assessment of daily weight, vital signs, and maintenance of accurate intake and output records. Nurses can prevent injury from falls by making sure that the side rails of the bed are raised, assessing level of consciousness, and monitoring the serum sodium level. An elevation in serum sodium will cause the brain cells to dehydrate and result in a loss of consciousness if not corrected quickly. An informed nurse will be able to recognize the signs and symptoms of dehydration as they develop and quickly initiate an appropriate plan of care.

Evaluation

Evaluation is accomplished by assessing for a decrease or absence of the defining characteristics of dehydration or electrolyte imbalance, which is achieved with continued reassessments. To evaluate the effectiveness of the nursing interventions, explore the answers to the following questions: Is the child able to take in adequate fluids and food? Is the child gaining weight? Are the child's electrolytes within normal limits? Is the child alert and interactive? Does the family understand how to manage the child's care at home?

NURSING ALERT

Adding Potassium to Intravenous Solutions

- Be sure that the child is able to void (1–2 mL/kg/hr) before adding potassium to the IV. Children who are dehydrated are oliguric and can become anuric. An anuric child will not be able to excrete electrolytes that are in the IV solution; therefore, IV fluids containing potassium can elevate serum potassium, which can cause cardiac irritability and ventricular fibrillation.
- Always check the dose and dosage calculations prior to giving. Never give more than 40 mEq/L at a rate not to exceed 1 mEq/kg/hr.
- After adding potassium to an IV bag, shake it to ensure the potassium is equally distributed.
- Never give potassium by IV push.

FAMILY TEACHING

Nurses should recommend rehydration fluids and discuss how to administer them. Dehydration can often be managed at home if caregivers are well informed and prepared. They need to know the signs of dehydration and should watch for lethargy or changes in their child's normal behavior. They should also be alert to changes in their child's urine output: How often has the child voided? How much with each void? Is the urine dark or concentrated? Help them to be able to make accurate decisions as to when to contact a health care provider (no improvement after 4 hours of rehydration fluid, inability to retain fluids, decreasing urine output, and change in mental alertness).

ACUTE GASTROENTERITIS

Acute gastroenteritis is a disease that causes inflammation of the mucous membranes of the stomach and intestines. Symptoms vary somewhat depending on the causative agent, but generally include nausea, vomiting, diarrhea, fever, abdominal pain, headache, and electrolyte imbalances. Most cases of gastroenteritis are self-limited; however, more severe or prolonged illnesses can result in dehydration with significant morbidity and mortality (Koslap-Petraco, 2006). Children who attend day-care centers, schools, institutions, and other facilities are especially susceptible to episodes of gastroenteritis.

INCIDENCE AND ETIOLOGY

Gastroenteritis is caused by a variety of viruses, bacteria, and parasites. Table 21-8 lists the pathogens of acute gastroenteritis. One of them, rotavirus, is the most common cause of diarrhea in children throughout the world, and gastroenteritis from rotavirus is generally more severe than gastroenteritis caused by other pathogens. Gastroenteritis from rotavirus most commonly afflicts children with distribution peaking in children aged 6 to 24 months (Albano et al., 2007). By 5 years of age, 70% of children in the United States become ill from rotavirus at least once. Many children become ill from rotavirus infections several times before they develop a broad immunity to rotaviruses. One reason for this is that there are several rotavirus groups and serotypes that can infect humans. The immunity developed against one serotype provides only partial protection against subsequent infections. Immune protection seems to build with each new exposure, reducing the severity of illness. Another reason that infants and children are particularly vulnerable is that rotavirus spreads quickly through fecal-oral transmission. A lone rotavirus can cause infection, and it can live on clothing, toys, and other surfaces for several days. Most ordinary disinfectants and hand soaps are not strong enough to destroy rotavirus. Disinfectants containing chlorine and hand soaps with chlorine dioxide are the most effective in halting rotavirus (Koslap-Petraco, 2006). These complexities associated with rotavirus combine to create an estimated "3.5 million episodes of diarrhea, 500,000 physicians' visits, 50,000 hospitalizations, and 20 deaths each year among children younger than 5 years" in the United States (Koslap-Petraco, 2006).

Although rotavirus is particularly challenging, other pathogens that cause gastroenteritis create their own havoc. Norwalk viruses primarily affect older children and are a major cause of epidemic gastroenteritis worldwide, especially in developing countries. Several pathogens (*Shigella, Salmonella,* and *Campylobacter*) are responsible for bacterial infection. *Shigella* is spread by person-to-person contact, fecal-oral transmission, or by ingestion of contaminated food. House flies can spread it by transporting the bacteria from infected feces (Sureshbabu, Venugopalan, Abuhammour, & Burny, 2008). *Salmonella* is transmitted through contact with infected animals, such as pet turtles, iguanas, or other reptiles, and from contaminated food products, such as poultry, produce, eggs, and milk (Chatterjee, O'Keefe, & Varman, 2009). *Giardia* and *Cryptosporidium* are the most common intestinal parasites that produce disease. *Giardia* is transmitted through ingestion of cysts either from contact with an infected individual or from food or water contaminated with infected feces. It is endemic in some areas, with a very high occurrence rate in day-care centers (Hökelek & Nissen, 2008).

TABLE 21-8 Pathogens that Cause Acute Gastroenteritis

VIRUSES	BACTERIA	PARASITES
Rotavirus	*Shigella*	*Giardia lambia*
Norwalk	*Salmonella*	*Cryptosporidium*
Adenovirus	*Campylobacter*	*Entamoeba*
	Escherichia coli	*Histolytica*
	Clostridium difficile	
	Yersinio	

PATHOPHYSIOLOGY

The pathophysiological process of viral infection is poorly understood; however, it is hypothesized that the virus destroys or damages the epithelial cells and brush border lining the intestines, interfering with absorption of electrolytes (Prescilla, 2009a). Viral illness is self-limiting, and recovery involves regeneration of these cells. There are three processes that produce bacterial gastroenteritis (Box 21-2).

BOX 21-2
PATHOPHYSIOLOGY OF BACTERIAL GASTROENTERITIS

- The bacteria destroy the mucosal cells of the villi in the small intestines, resulting in decreased surface area and less capacity to absorb fluid and electrolytes.
- The bacteria penetrate the mucosa and submucosa of the intestines, causing damage to the cells, necrosis, and ulceration. Eventually, the organism may reach systemic circulation. Diarrhea ensues and is often mixed with red and white blood cells (e.g., *Shigella, Campylobacter*).
- The bacteria produce enterotoxins that stimulate secretion of fluid and electrolytes from the primary secretory cells in the small intestines. Action of the enterotoxin also interferes with the absorptive function of the surface area of the upper small intestines. Thus, the imbalance between fluid secretion and absorption leads to the loss of water in the stool. Diarrhea associated with this process is profuse and watery, leading to dehydration and acidosis (e.g., *Shigella*, enterotoxigenic *E. coli*).

DIAGNOSIS

Diagnosis is based on the history, physical exam, and laboratory studies focused on evaluating the child's hydration status and identifying the causative agent. The history should include the following data:

- recent exposure to infectious agents
- travel history, especially if outside the United States
- exposure to contaminated food and water supplies
- exposure to turtles, iguanas, other reptiles, roaches, flies, and mice
- attendance at a day-care center

The child's hydration status is evaluated, including a history of fluid intake, such as types, amounts, and tolerance of fluid intake. The stooling pattern, frequency, and volume, as well as urination frequency, amount, and color, are also investigated. Current weight compared to pre-illness weight is useful in determining fluid loss (Prescilla, 2009b).

Generally, if no systemic manifestations are present (fever, lethargy, and malaise) and if dehydration is absent, diagnostic laboratory tests are not indicated. Stool cultures are generally done only for children with bloody diarrhea, a history of immunocompromise, or severe dehydration. Finding leukocytes in the feces should prompt further investigation to rule out invasive bacterial disease as this most commonly occurs in *E coli* and *Shigella* and *Campylobacter infections*. Rotavirus can be diagnosed by testing the stool using a commercially available kit or electron microscopy. In cases where a parasitic infection is suspected, the stool is examined for ova and parasites (Prescilla, 2009b).

If dehydration is present, additional tests may be performed to evaluate hydration status, such as CBC, urinalysis, blood urea nitrogen (BUN), and electrolyte studies. If the child is dehydrated, the hemoglobin, hematocrit, and BUN will be elevated (Prescilla, 2009b). The presence of ketones in the urine reflects increased fat metabolism due to caloric deprivation. Metabolic acidosis is common with severe dehydration and diarrhea.

CARING FOR CHILDREN WITH GASTROENTERITIS

Treatment for acute gastroenteritis focuses on fluid replacement and correction of electrolyte disturbances, and is dependent on the degree of dehydration. Review the section Caring for Children with Dehydration for further information.

In addition to addressing issues associated with dehydration, further steps are needed when children have gastroenteritis. It is important to teach care providers how to minimize the spread of gastroenteritis with an emphasis on the need for good hand washing (especially after changing diapers or using the bathroom and before preparing or eating food), cleansing of children's environment and food preparation areas with appropriate cleaning products, and isolating ill children as much as possible from other children and family members. These actions should be modeled by nurses caring for children hospitalized with gastroenteritis. In addition, care providers need information about when they should seek care. Children with suspected gastroenteritis should be seen by a health care provider if they are less than 6 months old, weigh less than 18 pounds, or have an estimated weight loss greater than 5%. Other symptoms that warrant a visit to a health care provider include persistent and substantial diarrhea or vomiting, inability to ingest ORS, mental status changes, or a fever above 38°C (100.4°F) for infants less than 3 months old or 39°C (102.2°F) or higher for infants and children 3–36 month (Koslap-Petraco, 2006).

Caregivers should be instructed to change diapers frequently to prevent irritation to the skin. Wash perineal area with mild soap and water after each diarrheal stool. Apply a protective ointment to buttocks.

Teach caregivers how to monitor intake and output: record amount of fluids taken; frequency, consistency, and color of stools; frequency and characteristics of vomitus; number of wet diapers per day; weighing wet diapers; and number of voids per day.

Most cases of bacterial or viral gastroenteritis are self-limited and do not require medical therapy. Determination to treat with antibiotics depends on the causative pathogen and the child's immune state. Antibiotics are not generally given to treat bacterial gastroenteritis. Probiotics, such as *Lactobacillus* GG, may shorten the duration of diarrhea. Antimotility medications are not used in most cases (Bonheur, Arya, Frye, & Tamer, 2009). Vomiting and diarrhea are the body's method of eliminating the infecting organism, and these drugs can decrease the speed at which this is accomplished.

NURSING ALERT

The BRAT Diet for Gastroenteritis

The traditionally recommended BRAT diet, consisting of bananas, rice, applesauce, and toast or tea/clear liquids, is needlessly restrictive and offers no advantage over an age appropriate diet. Foods to avoid are those with high simple sugar content, such as gelatin (Koslap-Petraco, 2006).

NURSING TIP

Preventing Gastroenteritis

The most effective treatment for gastroenteritis is prevention, specifically good hand washing with an effective soap (after defecation or diapering and before food preparation and consumption) and proper diaper disposal.

The Impact of Rotavirus Gastroenteritis on the Family

STUDY PURPOSE

To determine the emotional, social, and economic impact of having a child with rotavirus gastroenteritis on family functioning.

METHOD

Researchers used a mixed methods design, including qualitative interview and focus groups and quantitative questionnaires. Parents were invited to participate in a focus group or interview and complete a questionnaire if they sought care at the study locations (an outpatient clinic and emergency room) for their rotavirus-positive children (2 to 36 months of age) who had experienced diarrhea and/or severe vomiting within 3 days. Seventeen parents participated in a focus group or an in-depth interview and completed a questionnaire.

FINDINGS

Participants expressed fear about the severity of their children's illness and worry about dehydration. The sick children's behavior, which ranged from whining to extreme lethargy, was very concerning and sometimes terrifying to participants. They were exhausted and frustrated at their inability to help their children feel better. Having a child with rotavirus gastroenteritis substantially disrupted sleep, complicated tasks of daily living, such as housecleaning and food preparation, and caused them to be absent from their employment. Parents were motivated by illness severity to bring their children to a health care provider and expressed little or no prior knowledge of rotavirus. Participants' opinions varied on the economic impact of the illness on their families, but they mentioned expenses associated with additional diapers and laundry, ORS, and antipyretic medications.

IMPLICATIONS

Rotavirus gastroenteritis negatively impacts the health and well-being of the infected children and their parents. Nurses should be aware of the parental concerns identified in this study and focus on these areas when teaching caregivers about rotavirus gastroenteritis. Fears can be eased as nurses discuss the usual course of the disease. Nurses can empower parents to help prevent the spread of rotavirus by teaching them about proper hand washing, cleaning, and containing the spread of the illness by limiting symptomatic children's interactions with other children in the family and neighborhood.

REFERENCE

Mast, T. C., DeMuro-Mercon, C., Kelly, C. M., Floyd, L. E., & Walter, E. B. (2009). The impact of rotavirus gastroenteritis on the family. *BMC Pediatrics*, *9*(11), 1–9. Retrieved April 25, 2009, from http://www.biomedcentral.com/content/pdf/1471-2431-9-11.pdf.

Note: This study was funded by Merck Research Laboratories.

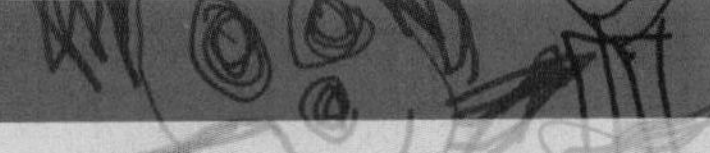

CASE STUDY / CARE PLAN

THE CHILD WITH ACUTE GASTROENTERITIS

Hannah Torres is a 23-month-old Chilean infant brought by her mother to a local emergency room at 8 P.M. with a history of persistent diarrhea and vomiting for the past 36 hours. Mrs. Torres states that Hannah was seen earlier in the day by their primary doctor who felt she had a viral infection and should be given Pedialyte and allowed to rest. Mrs. Torres became concerned when Hannah continued to have diarrhea and vomiting and was difficult to wake up.

ASSESSMENT

Initial assessment should include the child's hydration status since there is a potential for hypovolemic shock developing from dehydration. Skin turgor, capillary refill time, and respiratory status should be

(Continues)

CASE STUDY / CARE PLAN (Continued)

assessed. The onset, frequency, color, and amount of stools is obtained. If the child is vomiting, assess the frequency, amount, and characteristics of the vomitus. The child's intake and tolerance for fluids and solids should be assessed, and current weight should be compared to the child's last known weight.

NURSING DIAGNOSIS 1

Deficient fluid volume related to losses associated with diarrhea.

EXPECTED OUTCOMES

1. Child will exhibit signs of rehydration.
2. Child will be free from fluid and electrolyte deficits.
3. Child will maintain weight within normal parameters.

NOC: Fluid Balance

NIC: Fluid Management

INTERVENTIONS/*RATIONALES*

1. Administer oral rehydration solution. *To replace essential fluids and electrolytes.*
2. Administer and monitor IV fluids as prescribed. *IV therapy is based on degree of dehydration and the child's response to oral rehydration.*
3. Monitor and record intake and output. *To evaluate hydration status and effectiveness of fluid replacement.*
4. Check urine specific gravity every 8 hours. *Increasing specific gravity indicates increasing dehydration.*
5. Weigh child daily on same scale at the same time of day. *To assess for dehydration. Weight is an important indicator of fluid status.*
6. Assess for signs of dehydration to evaluate effectiveness of fluid replacement: decreased or absent tearing, dry mucous membranes, loss of skin turgor, and prolonged capillary refill time.

EVALUATION

Child has signs of normal hydration such as presence of tears, improved skin turgor, moist mucous membranes, and urine output of at least 1–2 mL/kg/hr.

NURSING DIAGNOSIS 2

Impaired skin integrity related to moisture (irritation) from frequent stools.

EXPECTED OUTCOME

1. Child will maintain intact skin in perineal and perianal areas.

NOC: Tissue Integrity: Skin

NIC: Skin Care: Topical Treatments

INTERVENTIONS/*RATIONALES*

1. Change diaper frequently. *To minimize exposure of skin to stool.*
2. Clean diaper area with water and mild soap after each stool. *To remove diarrheal stool, this is acidic and very irritating to the perineum. Commercial baby wipes contain alcohol and may cause further irritation.*
3. Leave diaper area open to air as often as possible. *To promote healing.*
4. Apply creams and ointments (A&D Ointment, zinc oxide, Desitin, petroleum jelly). *To provide a protective barrier from frequent stools.*

EVALUATION

The child's skin remains intact and pink.

EDEMA

Edema is an excess accumulation of interstitial fluid that usually results from a disturbance in the fluid exchange between capillaries and interstitial spaces.

INCIDENCE AND ETIOLOGY

Edema is associated with many illnesses. Heart failure, renal failure, and acute pulmonary edema cause an increase in blood hydrostatic pressure that results in the formation of edema. A loss of blood protein or albumin (often seen with liver disease, nephrotic syndrome, or malnutrition) will cause a shift of fluid into interstitial spaces due to a decrease in blood osmotic pressure. Burns, allergic reactions, and inflammation alter the integrity of the capillary membrane, resulting in the movement of fluid and blood proteins into interstitial spaces. Hypothyroidism and tumors that obstruct the lymphatic system cause an increase in interstitial osmotic pressure that will pull fluid into the interstitial space, resulting in the formation of edema.

PATHOPHYSIOLOGY

Edema develops as a result of changes in normal capillary dynamics. Normal capillary dynamics are maintained by balancing hydrostatic and osmotic pressures both within the capillaries and within the surrounding interstitial spaces. Hydrostatic pressures tend to push fluid out of a compartment, and osmotic pressures pull fluid into a compartment. Edema may be caused by four mechanisms: increased blood hydrostatic pressure, decreased blood osmotic pressure, increased interstitial fluid osmotic pressure, and impaired lymphatic drainage.

Increased Blood Hydrostatic Pressure

Blood hydrostatic pressure is the pressure of blood against the capillary walls that tends to push fluid out of the capillaries into the interstitial spaces. When this pressure is increased (as in increased capillary flow) excess fluid may enter the interstitial area. The result is edema. Venous congestion may also increase the blood hydrostatic pressure by back pressure, as seen in congestive heart failure.

Decreased Blood Osmotic Pressure

Severe and widespread edema may occur when the serum albumin is decreased. Albumin normally contributes to the inward pull of blood osmotic pressure. With decreased numbers of albumin particles, this inward pull diminishes and fluid leaks out into the interstitial area. A decrease in serum albumin may be caused by either albumin loss or diminished albumin synthesis. The most common condition associated with massive albumin loss is nephrotic syndrome. Decreased albumin synthesis accompanies severe protein-calorie malnutrition.

Increased Interstitial Fluid Osmotic Pressure

Normally the interstitial fluid osmotic pressure is small compared to the blood osmotic pressure because of the absence of large amounts of protein in the interstitial fluid. If protein leaks into this fluid, increased interstitial fluid osmotic pressure results, and edema develops. The major cause of this process is increased capillary permeability due to major burns and locally with inflammation (sprained ankle) and hypersensitivity reactions (bee sting).

Impaired Lymphatic Drainage

The lymph vessels normally drain small amounts of fluid and protein from the interstitial spaces and return them to the capillaries. However, if the lymph drainage is impaired through obstruction by a tumor or surgery, fluid and proteins accumulate in the interstitial area, causing edema.

CLINICAL MANIFESTATIONS

Edema results in swelling, either localized or general. In most cases, edema in children is manifested initially periorbitally or dependently. If the child is ambulatory, dependent edema will be evident in the ankles. Children on bed rest will have edema in the sacral area. Pitting edema is always a clear sign of an extracellular fluid excess. It is assessed by pushing a finger gently into the edematous tissue and observing for an indentation on the skin. The degree of edema is rated on a five-point scale:

+0 = No persisting indentation
+1 = 1/4″ (< 6.35 mm) indentation (mild)
+2 = 1/4 − 1/2″ (6.35 − 12.7 mm) indentation (moderate)
+3 = 1/2 − 1″ (12.7 − 25.4 mm) indentation (severe)
+4 = greater than 1″ (> 25.4 mm) indentation (very severe)

Edematous areas may also appear shiny and full. Additional signs may include a sudden weight gain, an elevation in blood pressure, a bounding pulse, neck vein distention, and dyspnea.

DIAGNOSIS

A diagnosis of edema is determined based on the clinical manifestations that are identified during the history and physical examination. It is important to determine the underlying cause so that appropriate treatment is initiated.

TREATMENT

Treatment for edema is focused on correcting the underlying condition and often includes the use of diuretics and restriction of sodium and fluid intake. Diuretics are given to promote fluid excretion through the kidneys. Since most diuretics cause potassium loss, it is extremely important to monitor serum potassium levels and provide potassium supplements as necessary. Edema that is due to an inflammatory response, such as an injury or allergic reaction, can be treated by applying cold compresses to reduce blood hydrostatic pressure through decreasing capillary blood flow.

NURSING MANAGEMENT

Nursing management begins with a thorough history and physical assessment. Note the location and extent of the edema. The caregiver may note that the child complains of tight shoes by the end of the day; eyes may appear puffy due to periorbital edema; or the child may complain that his fingers are swollen or feel like sausages. The child may also voice concerns about looking fat. Assess for alterations in body image. Ask if the edema is causing any pain or restriction of movements.

The nurse must maintain accurate measurements of intake and output as well as body weight, which should be measured on the same scale at the same time each day. When diuretics are used, blood electrolytes should be monitored for potassium depletion. If daily measurements of an edematous limb or abdomen are performed, it should be taken at the exact location with the same measuring tape. Double check any measurement that shows a dramatic increase or decrease. Edematous limbs should also be checked for circulation integrity by assessing peripheral pulses. Elevating the limb on a pillow will also help the reabsorption of extracellular fluids. Vital signs are important to monitor, especially blood pressure and respiratory rate. An increasing blood pressure reflects an increased loss of fluids into extracellular spaces; an increased respiratory rate, along with the presence of rales, often reflects pulmonary edema. Consider elevating the head of the bed if pulmonary edema is suspected.

FAMILY TEACHING

Prevention of skin breakdown is paramount. Teach caregivers the importance of good skin care for their child. Edematous tissue is very fragile and, if not kept dry and free from friction, it can easily break down. Special care must be taken to keep the diaper area clean and dry. An infant or child on bed rest should be turned every 2 hours to prevent pressure sores. If the child is on a potassium-depleting diuretic, encourage caregivers to include potassium-rich foods and fluids in the diet such as bananas, apricots, cantaloupe, dates, tomato juice, orange juice, peaches, potatoes, raisins, and figs. Older children may need to be reassured that the edema will be temporary.

BURNS

Significant research-based advances in fluid therapy, wound care management, and respiratory, metabolic, and nutritional support have improved the survival rate of children with burns (Gore et al., 2007). In 1940, half of the children in the United States who experienced burns over 30% of their bodies died, but in 2000 one study found no children in the United States died from burns covering up to 59% of their bodies (Peden et al., 2008). Although these advances are noteworthy, burns still result from accidents that, for the most part, could have been prevented. Health care providers need to be concerned not only with burn management but also with burn prevention (Peden et al., 2008).

Appropriate care of burns is essential, beginning with early stabilization. The goals of early stabilization are to cool the burn with cool water and prevent further burn and contamination. On arrival at an acute care facility, care focuses on assessment and stabilization of airway, breathing, circulation and pain management (Peden et al., 2008). The delivery of ideal burn care requires a team of health care providers working together, carefully assessing and timing the treatments necessary for survival. The team must establish a communication system that includes the child's family so that they can be fully informed of current care and prepared for future treatments.

INCIDENCE AND ETIOLOGY

Children are at high risk for burns. In 2004 an estimated 310,000 people died as a result of a fire-related burns, 96,000 of whom were under 20 years of age. In fact, fire-related burns are the 11th leading cause of death for children aged 1 to 9 years; infants have the highest global death rate from this cause of any age group. Globally the death rate of children from fire-related burns is 3.9 per 100,000, with low-income and middle-income countries having a fire-related death rate that is eleven times higher than high-income countries, 4.3 per 100,000 compared to 0.4 per 100,000 (Peden et al., 2008).

It is difficult to determine the morbidity associated with burns because global data on nonfatal burn injuries are not readily available. However, it appears that electrical and chemical burns are relatively rare in children, but contact burns and scalds contribute significantly to fire-related disabilities in children (Peden et al., 2008). In fact, the majority of burn-related injuries in the United States that required hospitalization in children under 4 years of age were from scalds (65%) and contact burns (20%) (Lucile Packard Children's Hospital at Stanford, 2008). Among the leading causes of scald injuries in children are hot tap water and hot soup (Palmieri et al., 2008; Peden et al., 2008; Lucile Packard Children's Hospital at Stanford, 2008). Some consequences of burns are long lasting and include hypertrophic scarring, contractures, keloid formation, and the need to amputate a limb. Physical disfiguration that results from burn

NURSING ALERT

Preventing Burns in Kitchens

An estimated 65% of burns in children occur in and around the home, most frequently in the kitchen. Children are naturally curious and sometimes physically awkward, making them prone to upsetting pans on a stove or being in the proximity of hot oil when it splashes (Peden et al., 2008). Care providers should be taught to turn pan handles inward so children cannot readily grab them.

Smoke detectors in homes have been shown to reduce the risk of fire-related deaths by 70% (Peden et al., 2008). Most homes in the United States (96%) have at least one smoke detector; however, only 75% have a smoke detector that works (Lucile Packard Children's Hospital at Stanford, 2008). The smoke detectors that do not work are likely the result of people either removing the batteries to avoid false alarms or failing to check the batteries monthly and change them every six months (Peden et al., 2008).

injuries challenges the self-esteem of the involved children. When children suffer a significant burn, they and their parents can experience post-traumatic stress disorder (Peden et al., 2008).

There are four major types of burns: thermal (most common in children), electrical, chemical, and radiation. Thermal burns occur from flames, flash, inhalation, scalds, or contact with hot objects. Flame injuries are caused by ignition of combustible materials and contact with the fire; household or residential fires are responsible for most flame burns. Flash injuries are caused by explosions, especially of combustible fuels such as gasoline, kerosene, and charcoal lighter. Inhalation burns occur when children breathe superheated gases, steam, or hot liquids which burn their airways and lungs. Smoke inhalation, often from house fires, is a major determinant of mortality associated with burns. Scald burns occur when hot liquids spill on a child or from hot tap water. Contact burns result from touching a hot object such as an oven, hot irons, and radiators.

As children become more mobile and curious, they are exposed to additional household burn hazards, such as electricity. Inserting objects into electric sockets or chewing on electrical wires can cause electrical burns. These burns are often not highly visible, but internal damage may be extensive. For example, burns from chewing on wires can harm growth of teeth, mandible, and maxilla. Chemical burns occur when children ingest or are exposed to caustic agents such as household cleaning products. Radiation burns commonly result from overexposure to the ultraviolet rays of the sun (Peden et al., 2008).

It is difficult to know how many burns in children result from child abuse. "Although the reported incidence of child abuse by burn ranges from 4 to 39%, less than one-half are substantiated" (Ojo, Palmer, Garvey, Atweh, & Fidler, 2007). In general, child abuse by burns is thought to be underreported because of difficulty determining the cause of burn injuries (Ojo et al., 2007). Health care providers should be alert to the possibility of a non-accidental trauma by burning when:

1. the child is very young and lacks verbal skills,
2. physical findings are inconsistent with the reported history or are incompatible with the child's motor ability,
3. the history of the injury is unclear,
4. care providers delayed seeking treatment, or
5. stories conflict about how the burn occurred.

Additionally, certain types of burn wounds are common in child abuse cases: scald burns from immersion in hot liquid (i.e., stocking and glove burns with a clearly demarcated line on the buttocks, perineum, ankle, or wrist) or burns from a cigarette or an iron. Burns to the extremities are particularly suspicious if they are symmetrical. Information about the burn should be documented thoroughly. If abuse is suspected, health care providers are legally obligated to notify the police or child protective services. Figure 21-3 illustrates an immersion burn of a child's hand.

PATHOPHYSIOLOGY

The impact of a burn can range from a minor local injury to multisystem involvement when a major burn is sustained.

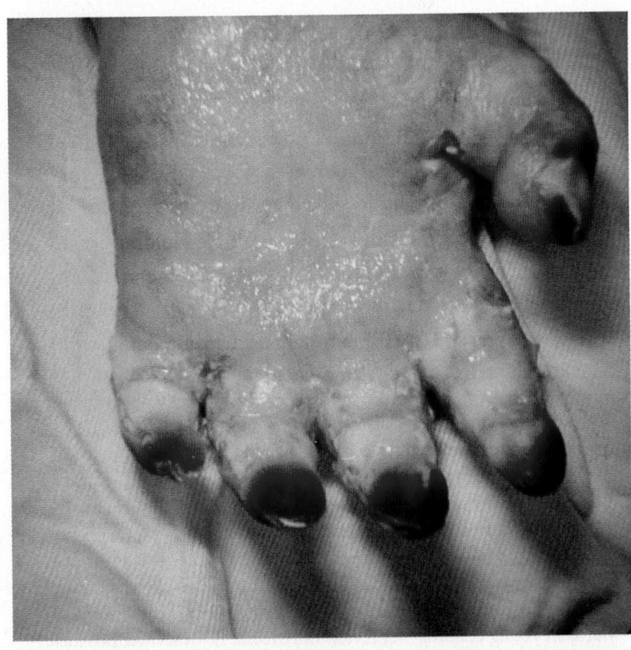

FIGURE 21-3 Immersion Burns of a Child's Hand. COURTESY OF DR. ROBERT ARENSMAN, PEDIATRIC SURGERY, UNIVERSITY OF ILLINOIS, CHICAGO.

EVIDENCE-BASED PRACTICE

Preventing Unintentional Scald Burns

CLINICAL PROBLEM

Scald burns are the most common type of burn in children. Over half of emergency department visits for children less than 5 years of age are to treat scalds. Current scald prevention strategies are aimed at adjusting the temperature settings on hot water heaters to no more than 120° F. While this is a worthy effort, likely reducing the number of this type of scald burn, other types of scald burns are prevalent. What are the prevalent mechanisms of injury in childhood scald burns? How can they be prevented?

BEST CLINICAL PRACTICE

- 80–90% of scald burns occurred during activities involving food preparation or consumption.
- Common mechanisms of scald burns were: (1) children pulling a cup, bowl, or cookware containing a hot substance onto themselves, (2) other people spilling a hot substance on the children, (3) children climbing to reach a hot substance, and (4) children scalding themselves when they opened a microwave oven, removed a hot substance, and spilled it on themselves.
- Prepackaged instant soups prepared in their original packaging in microwave ovens were involved in many scald burns.
- Children in low-income families with multiple children accounted for many of the scald victims in the two studies that included these demographic data.
- The number of Hispanic children burned was higher than expected based on the population in the two studies that reported ethnicity.

IMPLICATIONS FOR NURSING

- Advocate for modification of microwave oven doors so that they are childproof.
- Advocate for modification of prepackaged instant soup containers from tall and narrow to wide and flat, making them more stable and less likely to tip over.
- Target low-income families with multiple children in prevention efforts that specifically discuss safe preparation of instant soups in microwave ovens.
- Expand prevention efforts to target Hispanic families in culturally sensitive ways in Spanish.

References: Lowell, G., Quinlan, K., & Gottlieb, L. J. (2008). Preventing unintentional scald burns: Moving beyond tap water. *Pediatrics, 122*(4), 799–804; Palmieri, T. L., Alderson, T. S., Ison, D., O'Mara, M. S., Sharma, R., Bubba, A., Coombs, E., & Greenhalgh D. G. (2008). Pediatric soup scald burn injury: Etiology and prevention. *Journal of Burn Care & Research, 29*(1), 114–118; Rimmer, R. B., Weigand, S., Foster, K. N., Wadsworth, M. M., Jocober, K., Matthews, M. R., Drachman, D., & Caruso, D. M. (2008). Scald burns in young children—A review of Arizona Burn Center pediatric patients and a proposal for prevention in the Hispanic community. *Journal of Burn Care & Research, 29*(4), 595–605.

When a burn covers more than 15 to 20% of a child's body surface area, the inflammatory response extends beyond the injury site, and multiple organs and body systems are affected. If fluids are not administered quickly enough, the child's blood pressure can plunge to a critically low level, and the child can go into shock and die. Even if resuscitation fluids are quickly and appropriately administered and the child survives the first 48 hours, the risk of death remains high because the skin barrier has been compromised, making the child susceptible to infection (Peden et al., 2008). Table 21-9 lists the alterations of the cardiovascular, renal, respiratory, gastrointestinal, and central nervous systems and changes in metabolism.

CLINICAL MANIFESTATIONS

The severity of the burn is determined by how deeply the damage extends into the tissue and the total body surface area involved. In the past, burns were classified as first, second, third, and fourth degree. However, currently burns are categorized according to the depth of tissue destruction into the following categories: superficial, partial-thickness, and full-thickness (Besner & Otabor, 2009; Oliver, Spain, & Stadelmann, 2006; Sidor, Benson, Schwartz, Desposito, & Lucchesi, 2006). Both classification systems are still used in many clinical settings. Figure 21-4 illustrates the tissues involved with different depths of injury.

Superficial burns (first-degree) involve only the epidermis. A minor sunburn without blistering is an example

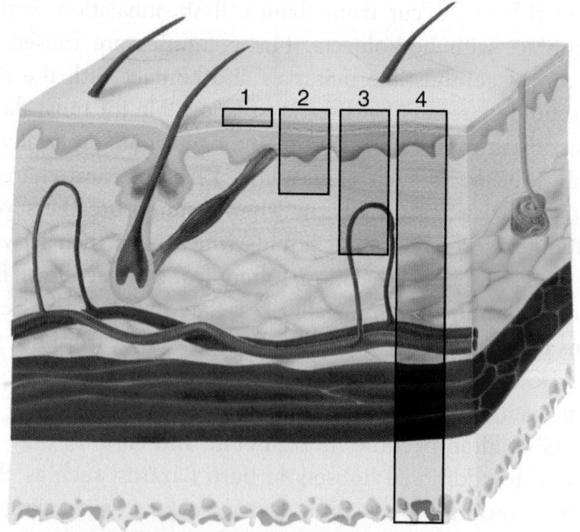

FIGURE 21-4 Depths of Burns and Corresponding Tissues Involved. DELMAR CENGAGE LEARNING.

Table 21-9 Body System Manifestations after a Major Burn

RESPONSE	TREATMENT
Cardiovascular System	
First 24–48 hrs postburn	
↓ Cardiac output resulting from ↑ capillary permeability and vasodilation	Adequate fluid replacement Monitor vital signs, especially BP
↑ Metabolic acidosis hematocrit	Assess blood gases
48–72 hrs postburn	
Capillary permeability is restored	Monitor vital signs
Interstitial fluids move back into bloodstream	Monitor urine output
↓ Hematocrit	↓ IV fluids
↓ Platelet count	Monitor PTT
Renal System	
Reduced blood flow to kidneys leads to ↓ urine output	Monitor I/O
Potential for acute renal failure	Administer IV fluids at a rate that maintains urine output of 1–2 cc/kg/hr
↑ BUN, ↑ Creatinine	
With fluid remobilization, ↑ urine output as interstitial fluid is mobilized and eliminated	Anticipate fluid remobilization Assess BP
Respiratory System	
Upper airway edema and obstruction from inhaling heated gases	Monitor respirations
Lower airway obstruction and pneumonia from smoke inhalation	Assess for rales, wheezes
Carbon monoxide poisoning and hypoxia from inhaling end products of combustion causes mucosal erythema and edema	Assess depth of respirations Monitor blood gases
Atelectasis and respiratory failure	Assess for equal respirations
Pulmonary edema from too vigorous fluid replacement	
Restriction of chest excursion from edema and eschar formation with circumferential burns	Notify health care provider and prepare client for escharotomy
Gastrointestinal System	
↓ Perfusion of GI tract and liver due to ↓ blood flow	Monitor bowel sounds
↓ Gastric acid production for 48–72 hrs followed by	Assess liver enzymes
↑ acid production and risk of stress ulcers	Assess NG drainage for evidence of blood
↓ GI motility	Place NG tube for decompression of stomach
Central Nervous System	
Burn-related encephalopathy due to hypoxemia, hypovolemia, and septicemia	Monitor fluids and blood gases Assess signs of infection
Manifestations include:	Assess neurologic status frequently
Hallucinations, personality changes, delirium, seizures, and coma	Initiate seizure precautions
Metabolism	
↑ Metabolic rate from nitrogen losses and stress of injury	Monitor intake of calories
↑ Heat losses through damaged skin	Give parenteral nutrition as needed
Rapid protein breakdown and muscle wasting	Give diet high in proteins
↑ Blood glucose levels due to insulin resistance and breakdown of glycogen stores	
Delayed growth and maturation from need to use energy to repair burned tissues	Give multivitamin, ↑ vitamins C and A

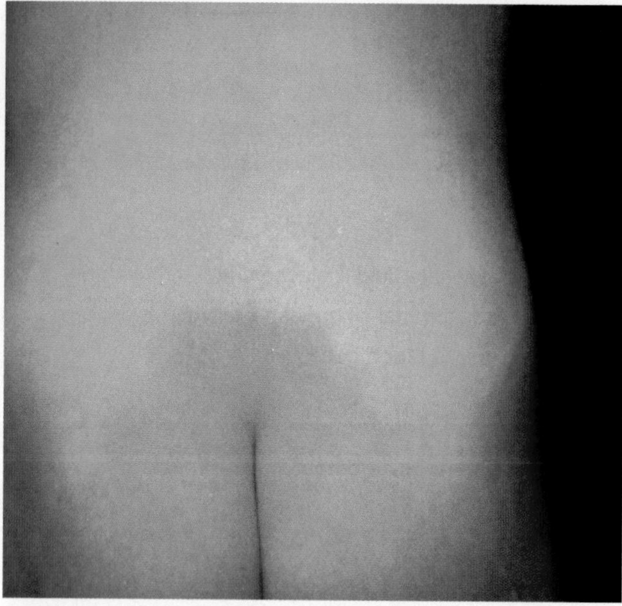

FIGURE 21-5 **Child with a Superficial-Thickness (First-Degree) Burn.** COURTESY OF DR. ROBERT ARENSMAN, PEDIATRIC SURGERY, UNIVERSITY OF ILLINOIS, CHICAGO.

of a superficial burn. (Figure 21-5 is a photograph of a superficial-thickness burn.) Typically they are somewhat painful for 48 to 72 hours and heal spontaneously without scarring in 5 to 10 days. **Partial-thickness burns** (second-degree) are divided into superficial partial thickness, involving the epidermis and superficial dermis, and deep partial thickness burns, involving the epidermis and deeper dermis. **Superficial partial-thickness burns** blister and are erythematous, moist, and painful. Typically they heal spontaneously without scarring in 1 to 3 weeks. (Figure 21-6 is a photograph of a superficial partial-thickness burn.) **Deep partial-thickness burns** appear white with less erythema noted as the injury extends deeper into the dermis.

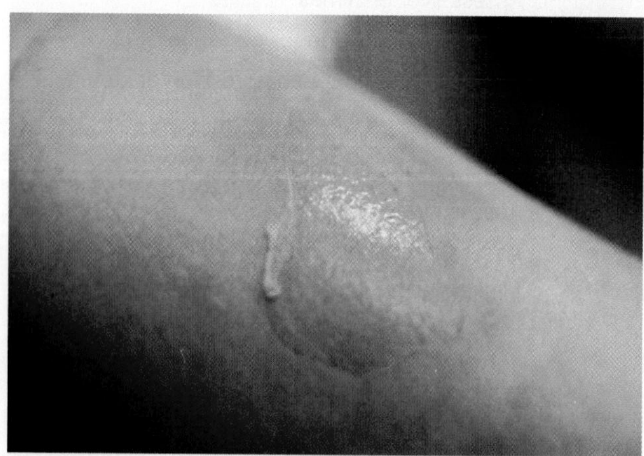

FIGURE 21-6 **Child with a Partial-Thickness (Second-Degree) Burn with a Blister.** COURTESY OF DR. ROBERT ARENSMAN, PEDIATRIC SURGERY, UNIVERSITY OF ILLINOIS, CHICAGO.

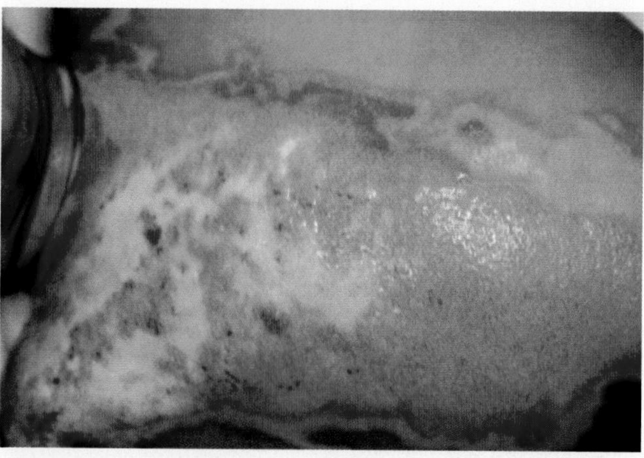

FIGURE 21-7 **Child with a Full-Thickness (Third-Degree) Burn.** COURTESY OF DR. ROBERT ARENSMAN, PEDIATRIC SURGERY, UNIVERSITY OF ILLINOIS, CHICAGO.

Sensation is usually diminished, and capillary refill is prolonged. The amount of scarring is associated with how long it takes the burn wound to heal, usually a minimum of 3 to 4 weeks. Skin grafting is often needed for satisfactory healing. **Full-thickness burns** (third-degree) involve the epidermis and the entire dermis and can extend into the subcutaneous tissue (Figure 21-7). They can be white, black, or brown. These burns do not heal spontaneously unless they are small, and then they heal with contraction. The eschar that develops has a leathery texture and diminished sensation. Skin grafting is usually performed on these burns. Most **devastating full-thickness burns** (fourth degree) are lethal. They extend into the muscle, fascia, and bone (Besner & Otabor, 2009; Oliver et al., 2006; Sidor et al., 2006).

The extent of the burn injury is usually expressed as the percentage of the total body surface area (TBSA) affected. In children, the most accurate method of determining the area burned is by mapping the injured areas on a Lund and Browder–like body chart, taking into account the proportional changes that occur during growth. Figure 21-8 is an example of a chart for estimating the extent of burns on a child. If such a chart is not available, the palm of the child's hand, representing 1% of body surface area, can be used to estimate the extent of the burn. Calculation of the percent of body surface area burned is important in determining fluid resuscitation needs (Sidor et al., 2006).

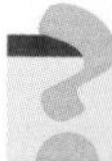

KIDS WANT TO KNOW

When will my burn scars disappear?

When a scar develops from a burn, it never completely disappears. Scars can be altered through plastic surgery or camouflaged with makeup so they are less noticeable. The red appearance of the scar decreases as the wounds mature.

Burn Estimate and Diagram
Age vs Area

Initial Evaluation

Cause of burn ____________

Date of Burn ____________

Time of Burn ____________

Age ____________

Sex ____________

Weight ____________

Date of Admission ____________

Signature ____________

Date ____________

Burn Diagram

Color Code

Red - 3°
Blue - 2°

Area	Birth 1 yr.	1-4 yrs.	5-9 yrs.	10-14 yrs.	15 yrs.	Adult	2°	3°	Total	Donor Areas
Head	19	17	13	11	9	7				
Neck	2	2	2	2	2	2				
Ant. Trunk	13	13	13	13	13	13				
Post. Trunk	13	13	13	13	13	13				
R. Buttock	2 1/2	2 1/2	2 1/2	2 1/2	2 1/2	2 1/2				
L. Buttock	2 1/2	2 1/2	2 1/2	2 1/2	2 1/2	2 1/2				
Genitalia	1	1	1	1	1	1				
R.U. Arm	4	4	4	4	4	4				
L.U. Arm	4	4	4	4	4	4				
R.L. Arm	3	3	3	3	3	3				
L.L. Arm	3	3	3	3	3	3				
R. Hand	2 1/2	2 1/2	2 1/2	2 1/2	2 1/2	2 1/2				
L. Hand	2 1/2	2 1/2	2 1/2	2 1/2	2 1/2	2 1/2				
R. Thigh	5 1/2	6 1/2	8	8 1/2	9	9 1/2				
L. Thigh	5 1/2	6 1/2	8	8 1/2	9	9 1/2				
R. Leg	5	5	5 1/2	6	6 1/2	7				
L. Leg	5	5	5 1/2	6	6 1/2	7				
R. Foot	3 1/2	3 1/2	3 1/2	3 1/2	3 1/2	3 1/2				
L. Foot	3 1/2	3 1/2	3 1/2	3 1/2	3 1/2	3 1/2				
						Total				

FIGURE 21-8 Estimation of the Extent of Burns in Children. COURTESY OF THE SHRINERS BURN HOSPITAL; CINCINNATI, OHIO.

DIAGNOSIS

A diagnosis of burns is determined from the clinical manifestations identified during the history and physical examination.

CARING FOR CHILDREN WITH MAJOR BURNS

When caring for children with major burns, emphasis is on respiratory management, fluid resuscitation, pain management, wound care, prevention of impaired mobility, nutritional support, and psychological support (Sidor et al., 2006). As with many patients, the major initial focus is on airway, breathing, circulation, and pain management (Oliver, Spain, & Stadelmann, 2006).

RESPIRATORY MANAGEMENT

Initial treatment consists of assessing for airway patency, establishing it, if needed, and maintaining it. Pulmonary complications are a leading cause of death in thermal burns. Anticipate respiratory involvement if the burn occurred in an enclosed space or the child was found unconscious. Any child with a significant burn should receive supplemental oxygen titrated to keep oxygen saturation above 90%. ABGs (arterial blood gases) provide evidence of smoke inhalation and the adequacy of gas exchange. Most children with extensive burns require prompt intubation and ventilation (Figure 21-9). Children who experience less extensive burns may initially have a patent airway but develop stridor from edema that occurs within a few hours of the injury. They may need intubation and ventilation at that time. In addition, narcotics given to control pain will depress the respiratory drive, further compromising the respiratory system (Oliver, Spain, & Stadelmann, 2006). In addition, placing a nasogastric tube to empty stomach contents and decompress it will reduce the likelihood of vomiting and aspiration, which would create further respiratory problems (Sidor et al., 2006).

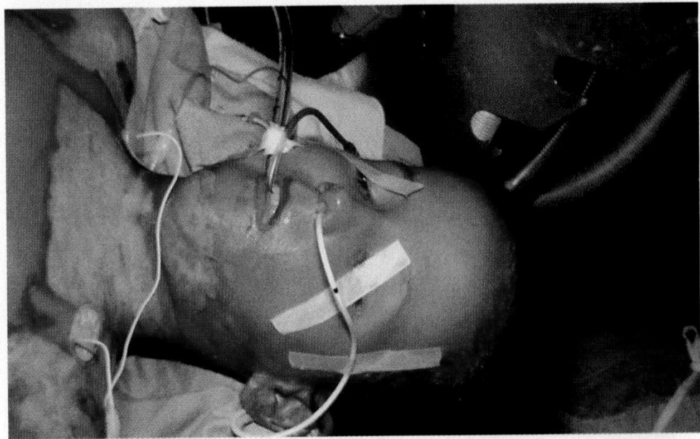

FIGURE 21-9 A Girl Who Was Wearing Flame-Retardant Pajamas with Burns from a House Fire. COURTESY OF DR. ROBERT ARENSMAN, PEDIATRIC SURGERY, UNIVERSITY OF ILLINOIS, CHICAGO.

FLUID RESUSCITATION

In the early stages following a major burn injury, promptly establishing adequate IV/IO access and beginning fluid resuscitation are essential to the child's survival. Whenever possible, the IV should be placed away from the burn. It is difficult to secure an IV in the area of the burn, and the edema that develops could dislodge the IV, causing extravasation (Oliver, Spain, & Stadelmann, 2006).

All burn injuries alter capillary permeability and, if severe enough, require fluid replacement. Fluid resuscitation is a major focus of seriously burned children during the initial treatment period in order to prevent hypovolemic shock. The goal is to infuse intravenous fluids (usually Lactated Ringer's solution) at a sufficient rate and volume to compensate for increased capillary permeability and the loss of intravascular fluids. A large-bore central venous catheter is used in order to administer massive fluid loads. A variety of formulas are available as guidelines for fluid volume and rate of administration; however, each is based on the relationship between body weight and total body surface area burned. The Parkland formula (Box 21-3) is one that is frequently used to determine initial fluid resuscitation requirements (Sidor et al., 2006).

Formulas to calculate fluid requirements are generally 2–4 mL times the child's weight in kg times the percentage of body surface area that is burned (See Box 21-3 for the

BOX 21-3

PARKLAND FORMULA FOR FLUID RESUSCITATION

4 mL Lactated Ringer's solution × kg of body weight × % total body surface area burned

- One-half of the total is given in the first 8 hours postburn.
- One-fourth of total is given in the second 8 hours postburn.
- One-fourth of total is given in the third 8 hours postburn.

Note: Time is calculated from the time of the injury, not the time of admission to the hospital.

Parkland formula). These formulas are only guidelines to resuscitation, and actual fluid administration rates are based on the child's response. Certain patient populations, such as those with inhalation burns, require more fluid than suggested by these formulas, up to 5.7 mL times weight in kg times the percentage of the body surface area that is burned (Hansen, 2008; Oliver, Spain, & Stadelmann, 2006). Adequacy of the resuscitation is reflected in: urine output of 1 mL/kg/hr for a child who weighs more than 30 kg or 1-1.5 mL/kg/hr for a child who weighs less than 30kg; stable vital signs; and an alert and oriented mental status. A Foley catheter is inserted to facilitate urine output measurement. If the urine output falls below the amounts as described above, the child is not receiving adequate fluids and may develop renal tubular obstruction if not corrected quickly (Sidor et al., 2006).

After initial fluid resuscitation, capillary permeability is regained. At this time, the child's urine output will increase dramatically because interstitial fluids are pulled back into the bloodstream. Intravenous fluids should be decreased to maintenance levels to prevent fluid overload and pulmonary edema. The type and amount of fluid used will be based on the results of blood electrolyte tests (Oliver, Spain, & Stadelmann, 2006).

Pain Management

The pain following a burn is both acute and chronic. Thermal destruction of tissue results in one of the most severe and prolonged types of pain. Pain from the injury is compounded by performing procedures on the wound, especially dressing changes. Other factors, such as fear and anxiety, contribute to children's perceptions of pain. Pain management is an essential element of quality care for burned children because it promotes their comfort, eases their breathing, and has a sedating effect. For children with major burns, intravenous narcotics, such as morphine sulfate, are indicated. Intramuscular injections should be avoided because blood flow to the tissues may be diminished and repeated injections can increase muscle damage (Sidor et al., 2006).

NURSING ALERT

Cool the Burn

WHO recommends teaching immediate application of cool (not ice cold) water to burns as a highly effective first-aid practice. Researchers in Vietnam found that children who received immediate cooling with water after a burn required 32% less skin grafting than children who did not receive this important first-aid measure (Peden et al., 2008). It should be noted that traditional practices, such as applying butter, toothpaste, sugar water, or honey, can be harmful because they can cause skin to slough off, exposing the lower layers and increasing vulnerability to infection (Peden et al., 2008).

For children with minor burns, oral pain medications, such as acetaminophen with codeine, can be given. Children should always be assessed for pain using appropriate assessment tools for their age, and pain medications should be given prior to all painful procedures. Children also respond well to behavioral interventions, such as imagery, relaxation therapies, and hypnosis.

Wound Care

The overall goal of burn care is to close the wound as quickly as possible, either by allowing the wound to heal on its own (secondary intention) or surgically grafting the wound. Burn care has evolved to the point that small, deep, secondary burns can be managed well enough that the result is cosmetically pleasing with little, if any, lasting morbidity. Treatment of such burns involves excising the wound and then covering it with a synthetic or biological wound covering. However, large, deep secondary or tertiary burns continue to be very challenging to treat. Excising and grafting these wounds are associated with a high blood loss, and care of the child undergoing excision and grafts requires a highly skilled team of physicians, nurses, and occupational and physical therapists (Peden et al., 2008).

Initial wound care is started after the child has been stabilized. Care should be taken to use aseptic techniques when cleaning the burned areas and to medicate the child prior to the procedure. The wounds are gently cleaned and debrided. **Debridement** is the removal of dead tissue from the burn site and is associated with severe pain. This procedure is performed by soaking the wound for about 10 minutes to soften the tissue. The wound is then washed from the inner to outer edges using a firm, circular motion. Any loose or dead tissue is removed by gently lifting it up with forceps and cutting it away. After the wound and surrounding areas are cleaned, an antimicrobial cream, such as silver sulfadiazine (Silvadene), is applied to minimize bacterial

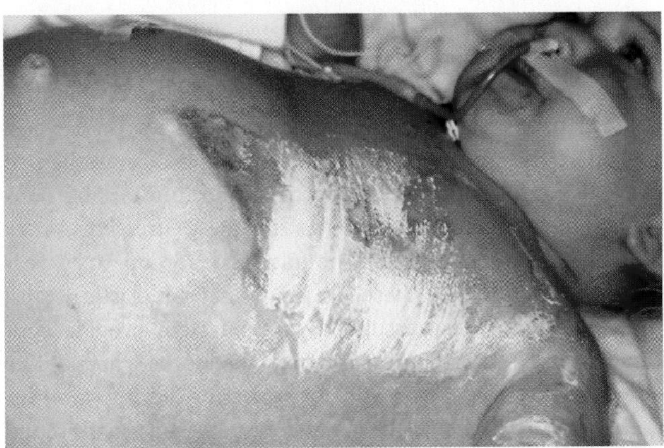

FIGURE 21-10 A Child Having Silvadene Applied to a Scald Burn of the Chest. COURTESY OF DR. ROBERT ARENSMAN, PEDIATRIC SURGERY, UNIVERSITY OF ILLINOIS, CHICAGO.

CULTURAL CONSIDERATION

Burns are the only unintentional injury that occurs more frequently in females than males. The disparity is particularly noteworthy in adolescence (15 to 19 years of age) and is likely due to cultural practices that involve teaching females their gender roles. In low-income countries, while the males are outdoors, many females learn to prepare food, which often involves cooking by open fire and hot liquids. Risks for burns are increased if loose-fitting clothing is a cultural norm because dangling material can more easily ignite. These differences in gender roles place females at increased risk for burns (Peden et al., 2008).

proliferation and prevent infection. Some type of dressing is then applied. Figure 21-10 shows a child having Silvadene applied to a burn wound.

Hydrotherapy is used to soften dead tissue to help in the debridement process and to improve circulation to the wound. The experience is very painful and scary for all burn clients (Hoffman et al., 2008). Children should be medicated prior to hydrotherapy and dressing changes. It is helpful if caregivers can be present to comfort and distract the child. Figure 21-11 shows a child in a whirlpool bath.

Once the wounds have been debrided and begin to heal, various temporary skin grafts can be used to facilitate the healing process. These include homografts (cadaver skin), heterografts (pig skin), and synthetic skin coverings (Ruszczak, Schwartz, Joss-Wichman, & Wichman, 2009). Homografts can remain in place until donor site tissues are available. Typically, homografts will begin to slough off around 14 days. Pigskin dressings are replaced daily or every other day. They are often used in children with scald burns of the hands and face because they allow free movement and reduce risk of contracture formation. Temporary grafts accelerate wound healing by creating an environment that promotes epithelial growth in the form of granulation tissue. Adequate granulation tissue must be present before the child can be permanently grafted. Figure 21-12 demonstrates a child's hand with red granulation tissue.

Extensive full-thickness burns will require a permanent skin graft, an autograft, to fully heal. The skin for an autograft is taken from an unburned area of the child's own skin. Once an autograft is placed on the wound, the area must be immobilized. This is often difficult in children

EYE ON...

Virtual Reality Pain Control during Burn Wound Debridement in the Hydrotank

Many patients with burn injuries rate their pain during wound debridement as severe to excruciating despite pain medication, and some report that the pain during debridement reminds them of the pain experienced at the time the burn occurred. Nurses often perform this wound care for patients in hydrotanks during the early phases of recovery. Recently, researchers investigated the possibility of reducing debridement pain by using water-friendly virtual reality helmets and headphones to distract patients and block out the sights and sounds of the hospital environment. The patient is able to interact with the virtual world by moving a joystick. Patients reported that this intervention reduced their pain intensity, pain unpleasantness, and the time they spent thinking about their pain during the procedure (Hoffman et al., 2008).

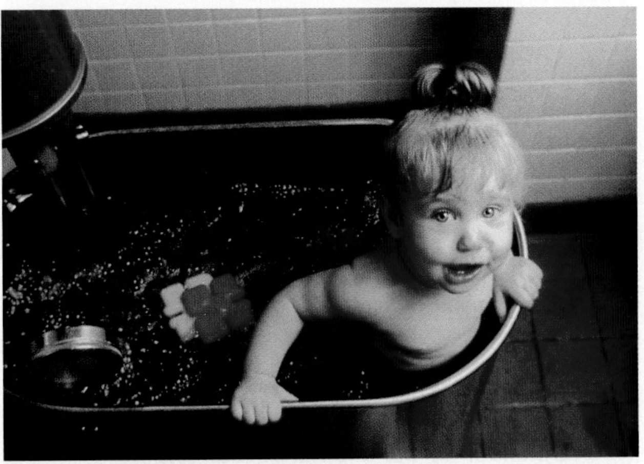

FIGURE 21-11 A Child with Burns on the Legs in a Whirlpool. COURTESY OF DR. ROBERT ARENSMAN, PEDIATRIC SURGERY, UNIVERSITY OF ILLINOIS, CHICAGO.

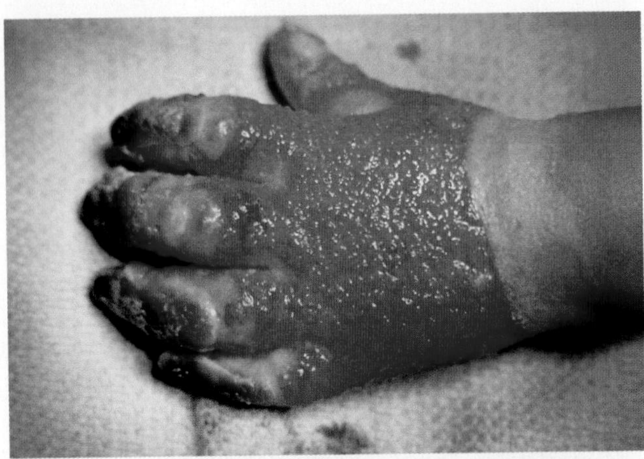

FIGURE 21-12 A Child's Hands with Red Granulation Tissue. COURTESY OF DR. ROBERT ARENSMAN, PEDIATRIC SURGERY, UNIVERSITY OF ILLINOIS, CHICAGO.

requiring the use of splints or casts. Splints are used less frequently than they were in the past, and a properly preformed splinting program can help avoid contractures (Sheridan, 2008).

After the grafts heal, pressure dressings are applied to prevent the formation of contractures and to minimize scarring. To maximize effectiveness of these dressings, they should be worn almost 24 hours a day for up to 1 year (Sidor et al., 2006). These dressings may be elastic wraps, pressure splints, or pressurized garments that provide continuous and uniform pressure over the burned areas. The elasticized garments are usually worn for several months, and therefore, need to be altered or replaced as the child grows.

Prevention of Impaired Mobility

Children are at risk for impaired mobility and the development of contractures due to prolonged bed rest, muscular atrophy and shortening, and stiffening of burned tissues. It is essential to implement appropriate positioning strategies to prevent deformities and an exercise program to maintain muscle strength and joint mobility. When joints are not being exercised, they should be maintained in maximal extension using splints if needed. Particular attention should be paid to the hands and neck since these are the most prone to rapid contractures (Sheridan, 2008). Early exercise is encouraged and compliance can be improved with judicious use of analgesics. Range of motion exercises are performed actively at least three times a day. Active range of motion of muscles is possible in infants and toddlers by using familiar toys; however, most of the joints will require passive range of motion exercises. Caregivers can support and encourage older children to participate in active range of motion.

Nutritional Support

The nutritional needs of burned children are vitally important to their recovery. Protein catabolism after a burn can be

NURSING TIP

Calculating Maintenance IV Fluid Rate Using the 4:2:1 Rule

To calculate the hourly IV rate, first determine the child's daily maintenance fluid requirement, then divide that number by 24. In practice, this process can be simplified by using the 4:2:1 rule without sacrificing accuracy. Try it out.

IV rate = 4 mL/kg for each kg of weight up to 10 kg
+ 2 mL/kg/hr for each kg of weight between 10 and 20 kg
+ 1 mL/kg/hr for each kg over 20 kg

Example: Daily IV fluid rate for a 45-kg child who is NPO would be:
40 mL + 20 mL + 25 mL = 85 mL/hr

REFLECTIVE THINKING

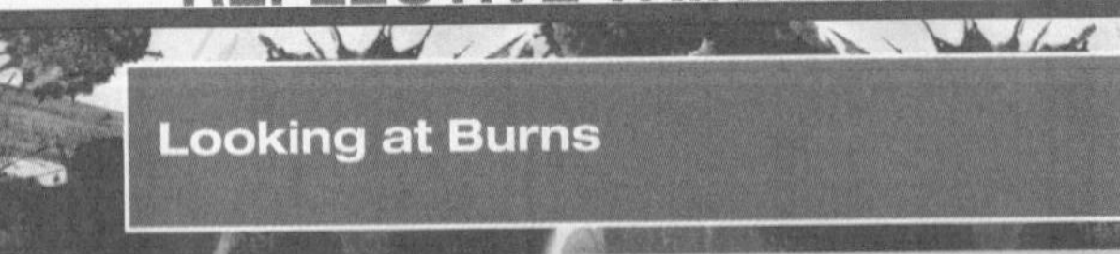

Looking at Burns

Burns are often difficult to look at.

How would you feel about working with a child who has been severely burned? How could you move past the way burns look to deliver adequate care?

Consider verbal and nonverbal language. What message would you hope to convey as you work with the child and family?

NURSING ALERT

Fireworks—Danger Alert!

Fireworks are used for religious and national holidays throughout the world, and many burn related injuries occur at these celebrations. Children, especially adolescent boys, are at particular risk for this type of injury. In Greece, boys aged 10 to 14 years account for 70% of the firework burn injuries. Most of these boys had set the fireworks off by themselves. Most of the girls injured by fireworks were bystanders. The WHO recommends strict laws regulating the manufacture and sale of fireworks (Peden et al., 2008).

Reflections from Families

At first I was in shock. How could this have happened to my child? Will he be all right? Will he have scars? I worried about the way his face was going to look and I constantly watched all of his machines, looking for signs of improvement. It takes time to put everything in order. I could not remember simple things. I often asked the same questions over and over. I just could not seem to concentrate. The accident disrupted our whole family life. If it wasn't for the compassionate care that the nurses gave to my son and their understanding of my anxieties and stress, I do not know how I would have gotten through this ordeal.

KIDS WANT TO KNOW

What do I tell people who stare at me?

Sometimes people stare to figure out what it is that looks different, not bad or ugly. Sometimes they stare when they really have questions they want to ask you. When this happens, you can ask them kindly if they have a question you could answer. You can also ask that they please stop staring because it makes you feel uncomfortable. It is also important for you to have someone with whom you can freely discuss your feelings. Many kids find it helpful to talk with another child who has experienced burns and has a similar frustration with people staring. Most communities have support groups for burn survivors.

severe, and burned children's basal metabolic rates (BMR) can increase to more than twice normal. As a general rule, children's caloric intake should increase in proportion to the percentage of their body that is burned. For instance, if a child sustains burns over 50% of her body, she requires at least 50% more calories than she normally would (Sidor et al., 2006). Children should be offered a variety of foods and be allowed to choose meals when they feel better. They will often eat more if they have their meals with other children or family members. Most children with major burns are unable to meet their nutritional requirements orally; therefore, it is necessary to use enteral feedings. Changes in stools (increased stooling, diarrhea) may indicate that the child is not tolerating the feedings.

Psychological Support

Anxiety for the child and caregivers can be overwhelming. Play therapy is used to help the child deal with the frustrations of burn therapy. It encourages the child to move and actively participate in activities with other children.

Nurses in burn units find it essential to gain the trust of the family and the child to create a healing environment in the midst of such a stressful situation. Once a trusting relationship is established, the nurse can then build the caregivers' confidence in their abilities to continue care after the child is discharged by modeling proper care and involving them in the care of their child. When a child will survive a burn injury, nurses can help the patient, caregivers, and families grieve the loss of what the child was prior to the burn injury and learn to love and accept the child, forever changed, that will go home with them. As recovery continues, counseling with various support services may be implemented to foster the child's self-esteem. When a child does not survive, nurses can cry with families and provide much needed support and referrals to support groups (Zengerle-Levy, 2006).

Research on the long-term adjustment of children and families has found that they adjust well to school and their communities with the support of teachers and social workers. Earliest possible return to school and/or activities of daily living are critical to burned children's overall recovery (Sidor et al., 2006).

FAMILY TEACHING

The home care needs of the family should be addressed long before the child is ready for discharge. Discharge teaching often includes nutrition and diet requirements, daily dressing changes and skin care, application of elasticized garments,

CASE STUDY / CARE PLAN

A CHILD WITH MAJOR BURNS

Jorge Santiago, a 6-year-old Hispanic boy, sustained 40% partial- and full-thickness scald burns to his hands, chest, and both thighs. He was helping his big sister who was cooking macaroni and cheese for lunch. He tried to take the pot of boiling macaroni to the sink, but it was heavier than he thought. It slipped out of his hands, and the boiling water splashed on him. When he arrived at the emergency department, he was alert but crying.

NURSING CARE PLAN

ASSESSMENT

During the immediate hours following the injury, nursing assessment focuses on respiratory, cardiac, and renal status and includes monitoring airway, breathing, circulation, vital signs, infusion of fluids, and urine output. The nurse should also assess for additional injuries that may have occurred at the time of the burn. The history should include the following:

- Description of how and where the burn occurred, including the agent of injury and length of time in contact with the skin
- When the injury occurred
- Circumstances surrounding injury
- Initial treatment of the burn

After the initial period (48 hours after the injury), physical assessment findings are directed to maintenance of the cardiovascular and respiratory systems.

NURSING DIAGNOSIS 1

Risk for deficient fluid volume related to increased capillary permeability, extracellular fluid shift, and fluid losses through the burn wounds.

EXPECTED OUTCOME

1. Jorge will remain hydrated

NOC: Fluid Balance

NIC: Fluid/Electrolyte Management

INTERVENTIONS/*RATIONALES*

1. Assess for signs or symptoms of fluid volume deficit: hypotension, tachycardia, pale or cool skin, decreased urine output, change in mental status (restlessness, disorientation). *Decreases the risks associated with hypovolemic shock.*
2. Monitor lab values for abnormal electrolyte values. *To identify fluid and electrolyte disturbances.*
3. Monitor vital signs. *Fluid excess or deficit can cause changes in vital signs.*
4. Monitor intake and output. Measure specific gravity of urine. Report if urine output is < 1–2 mL/kg/hr. *Assures prompt recognition and treatment of hypovolemia. Urine output is the most sensitive indicator of cardiac output and tissue perfusion.*
5. Administer IV fluids as prescribed and maintain patency. *Restores adequate intravascular volume and replaces ongoing fluid losses.*
6. Monitor daily weight to assess for fluid retention or diuresis. *Weight is an indicator of hydration status.*

(Continues)

CASE STUDY / CARE PLAN (Continued)

EVALUATION

Jorge remains well hydrated as evidenced by the following:

Electrolyte values remain within normal ranges.

Urine output remains adequate for weight with a specific gravity ranging between 1.005–1.025.

NURSING DIAGNOSIS 2

Ineffective tissue perfusion due to edema or circumferential injuries to extremities.

EXPECTED OUTCOMES

1. Jorge will maintain adequate tissue perfusion as evidenced by:
   Absence of complaints of numbness or tingling in the extremities.
   Presence of peripheral pulses with good capillary refill.
2. Jorge will be able to move all extremities and digits.

NOC: Tissue Perfusion: Peripheral

NIC: Peripheral Sensation Management

INTERVENTIONS/*RATIONALES*

1. Question Jorge regarding sensation in extremities and fingers. *To ascertain adequacy of circulation.*
2. Assess peripheral pulses and capillary refill frequently. Notify health care provider of any changes in distal pulses. *To assess adequacy of circulation.*
3. Assist with performing escharotomies as needed. *Eschar can constrict peripheral circulation.*
4. Position carefully to prevent compromising the blood flow to the extremities. *Enhances circulation and promotes venous return.*

EVALUATION

Jorge maintains adequate sensation, circulation, and movement in all extremities and digits.

NURSING DIAGNOSIS 3

Impaired gas exchange/ineffective airway clearance related to airway obstruction, pulmonary edema, and hypoventilation.

EXPECTED OUTCOMES

1. Jorge will demonstrate a normal spontaneous respiratory rate, effort, depth, and adequate air movement.
2. Jorge will have normal arterial blood gases (ABGs).
3. Jorge will exhibit an absence of adventitious breath sounds or pulmonary edema.

NOC: Respiratory Status: Gas Exchange/Airway Patency

NIC: Respiratory Status: Monitoring/Airway Management

INTERVENTIONS/*RATIONALES*

1. Monitor respiratory rate and effort and assess for hoarseness. *Increased respiratory rate and effort and developing hoarseness are indications of airway obstruction.*

(Continues)

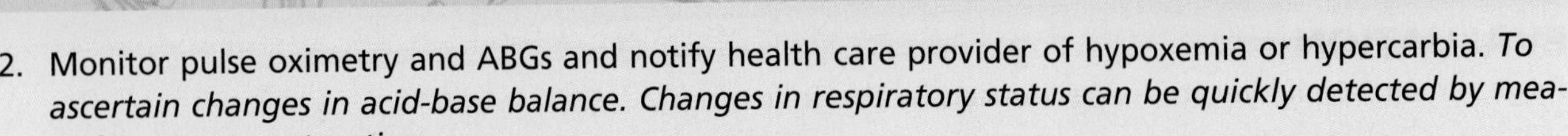

CASE STUDY / CARE PLAN (Continued)

2. Monitor pulse oximetry and ABGs and notify health care provider of hypoxemia or hypercarbia. *To ascertain changes in acid-base balance. Changes in respiratory status can be quickly detected by measuring oxygen saturation.*
3. Provide oxygen therapy as needed and monitor response. *Enhances respiratory effort.*
4. Encourage turning, coughing, and deep breathing. *Promotes lung expansion, facilitates mucus clearing, and prevents development of pneumonia.*
5. Be prepared to assist with intubation and mechanical ventilatory support as needed. Make sure that emergency equipment is close by. Prophylactic intubation may be performed in children with known facial burns. *Maintenance of patient airway is essential to recovery.*

EVALUATION

Jorge's respiratory status remains stable as evidenced by normal rate, effort, and ease of breathing.

NURSING DIAGNOSIS 4

Acute pain related to tissue destruction, debridement, dressing changes, and exercise of burned extremities.

EXPECTED OUTCOMES

1. Jorge will indicate reduction or elimination of pain.
2. Jorge and family will express satisfaction with pain control measures.
3. Jorge will be able to tolerate activities of daily living and care.

NOC: Pain Control

NIC: Pain Management

INTERVENTIONS/*RATIONALES*

1. Assess level of pain frequently and as needed using an age-appropriate assessment tool. *Provides consistent measurement of pain.*
2. Administer pain medication IV on a scheduled basis rather than PRN. *Pain associated with burns is severe.*
3. Assess factors that aggravate or alleviate pain and modify care appropriately. *Individualizes treatment to child's needs.*
4. Ensure adequate analgesia before all painful procedures such as wound care and dressing changes. *Helps ease the pain.*
5. Provide diversionary activities as additional method of pain relief. *Techniques such as relaxation, distraction, and therapeutic touch can help alleviate pain.*

EVALUATION

Jorge's level of pain is reduced or eliminated as indicated and quantified by decreased scores on pain assessment tools.

NURSING DIAGNOSIS 5

Risk for infection due to tissue destruction and prolonged use of invasive therapies (indwelling catheters, central venous catheters).

EXPECTED OUTCOMES

1. Jorge's burned skin areas and graft sites will heal within appropriate time intervals.
2. Jorge will demonstrate no signs of systemic sepsis.

(Continues)

CASE STUDY / CARE PLAN (Continued)

NOC: Risk Control

NIC: Infection Protection

INTERVENTIONS/*RATIONALES*

1. Monitor for signs of infection (increasing temperature, increasing WBC, purulent foul smelling drainage from wounds, redness or swelling around invasive lines) and of sepsis (fever, ileus, disorientation, tachypnea, tachycardia). *Monitoring allows prompt recognition and treatment.*
2. Monitor lab values as ordered (CBC, wound cultures, blood cultures). *Assesses for potential complications and ascertains any changes in wound flora growth.*
3. Maintain sterile or aseptic techniques, as appropriate, with invasive procedures and dressing changes. *Minimizes exposure to infectious agents.*
4. Administer tetanus toxoid as indicated. *Prevents Jorge from acquiring tetanus.*
5. Administer intravenous or topical antibiotics per order. *Controls bacterial growth.*
6. Ensure good hand washing technique by all members of health care team before and after contact with child. *Minimizes exposure to infections.*

EVALUATION

Jorge has no signs of systemic infection as evidenced by stable vital signs and normal wound culture.

NURSING DIAGNOSIS 6

Imbalanced nutrition: Less than body requirements related to increased basal metabolic rate and reduced caloric intake.

EXPECTED OUTCOMES

1. Jorge will show steady weight gain prior to discharge.
2. Jorge's wounds will heal appropriately.

NOC: Nutritional Status: Nutrient Intake

NIC: Nutritional Management

INTERVENTIONS/*RATIONALES*

1. Provide a high-calorie, high-protein diet. *Avoids protein breakdown and meets additional caloric requirements.*
2. Monitor ability to tolerate oral, tube, or parenteral feedings by assessing for abdominal distention, vomiting, diarrhea, reflux, or increasing gastric residuals. *Avoid feeding intolerances.*
3. Measure and record weight weekly. *Monitors nutritional status.*
4. Provide oral hygiene each shift and as needed. *Encourages appetite.*
5. Involve Jorge in food selection and encourage the family to provide child's favorite foods. *Stimulates the appetite and meets nutritional requirements.*
6. Allow adequate uninterrupted time for meals that encourages socialization with family or other children on the unit. *Meets nutritional requirements by providing a homelike environment.*
7. Monitor and record intake and output. *Allows evaluation of sufficiency of intake.*

EVALUATION

Jorge consumes an appropriate amount of nutrients and has restored weight to preburn status.

(Continues)

CASE STUDY / CARE PLAN (Continued)

NURSING DIAGNOSIS 7

Deficient knowledge (caregivers) regarding home management.

EXPECTED OUTCOME

1. Caregivers will express and demonstrate confidence regarding home care needs.

NOC: Knowledge: Treatment Regimen

NIC: Teaching: Procedure/Treatment

INTERVENTIONS/*RATIONALES*

1. Plan discharge teaching based on assessment of Jorge and family's level of cognition, psychosocial, and physical needs. *Assures comprehension of knowledge taught.*
2. Record response to all discharge teaching. *To document progress and facilitate further education by other health care providers.*
3. Encourage questions and return demonstrations of all procedures that will need to be done at home. *Assures full understanding and ability to do psychomotor skills.*
4. Provide written and verbal home instructions and indications for contacting health care provider. *Written instructions provide family with documents to refer to when questions arise at home.*
5. Arrange for follow-up appointments and referrals. Provide family with phone numbers and office locations. *To provide continuity of care.*

EVALUATION

The caregivers demonstrate confidence in Jorge's home care needs and know who, when, and how to contact if questions arise.

IN THE REAL WORLD

As a student, I wondered if nurses really had to interpret their client's fluid and electrolyte status. Wasn't this what the physician did? I found it very difficult to remember how to differentiate acidosis from alkalosis and memorize lab values. Understanding fluid and electrolyte physiology and pathophysiology is not easy. There is no anatomical model to pull apart and put back together. It just seemed like a set of disjointed facts to memorize and study for the next test. As a practicing nurse, I no longer wonder if this is important information to know. I use it every day on all my clients to assess if their fluids are balanced. Are they dehydrated or fluid overloaded? What do their electrolyte values tell me about their response to treatment? What information is critical that the physician should be notified of immediately? Being able to interpret a child's fluid and electrolyte status is the foundation on which my assessment begins and from which my critical thinking about my client's condition begins.

application of splints, and daily range of motion exercises. Discharge teaching books are often helpful for families to refer to as they learn. However, these books must take into consideration the educational, ethnic, and language backgrounds of the caregivers. Caregivers need support and encouragement to perform these treatments appropriately. Remember, most of these daily routines will be painful for the child. If not done well, the child's wounds will not heal appropriately. Caregivers, who may feel guilt because of the child's burns, often have trouble doing painful procedures without support. Home care should emphasize returning the child to as many independent tasks as possible. Home tutors may be necessary to help the child catch up/keep up with school. Support is often needed to help the child and school personnel prepare for the child's return to the classroom. Encourage all involved to explore their feelings and be supportive of the child's return to the community.

KEY CONCEPTS

- Forty percent of an infant's body water is located in extracellular spaces. ECF is the first to be lost during illnesses, putting infants at a greater risk for dehydration.
- Body fluids move as a result of the type of membrane to be crossed, changes in the permeability of capillaries, and the amount and type of solutes present.
- The respiratory system compensates for changes in blood pH caused by metabolic conditions by retaining or releasing carbon dioxide.
- The kidneys compensate for changes in blood pH caused by respiratory problems or a buildup of metabolic acids by controlling hydrogen ion and bicarbonate levels in the blood.
- Renal compensation is much slower than respiratory compensation.
- Urine output should be maintained at 1–2 mL/kg of body weight per hour.
- Nursing management for the child with acute gastroenteritis includes assessing fluid and electrolyte status, administering ORS or IV therapy for severe dehydration, providing an appropriate diet, and giving perineal skin care.
- Burns alter the integrity of the capillary membrane, resulting in the easy movement of fluid and blood proteins into interstitial spaces.
- Immediately following a major burn, body fluids shift from intravascular to interstitial spaces due to increased capillary permeability and cause hypovolemic shock if not corrected quickly.
- Pain management should be integrated into the plan of care based on frequent assessments using an age-appropriate pain scale. Children should not have to experience severe pain after a burn injury. Medicate based on child's need, not the comfort level of the health professional.
- Family involvement is essential for the child to cope with body image and self-esteem issues that arise as a result of a burn.

REVIEW ACTIVITIES

1. Differentiate between the concepts of diffusion, filtration, and osmosis.
2. What are the normal serum concentrations for sodium, potassium, and chloride?
3. Describe what would happen within the body if there were an excess or a depletion of sodium or potassium.
4. Describe the effects that antidiuretic hormone and aldosterone have on the body. Under what conditions would the body release these hormones?
5. Describe how the body compensates for metabolic acidosis.
6. What signs and symptoms would you expect to see if a child was experiencing respiratory acidosis? What clinical situations might cause respiratory acidosis?
7. What clinical situations might cause metabolic alkalosis?
8. How does the body compensate for acid-base imbalances?
9. Outline the treatment and nursing management for a child with dehydration.
10. What would you include in a discharge teaching plan for caregivers of a child recovering from dehydration?
11. Discuss the treatment of the child with acute gastroenteritis who has diarrhea and vomiting, and moderate dehydration.
12. What nursing interventions will achieve the goal of maintaining skin integrity in an edematous child?
13. Outline the treatment and nursing management for a child during the first 24 hours postburn.
14. Describe how you will determine if the child is receiving adequate IV fluids.
15. What is the most appropriate way to administer pain medication to a burned child? Give the rationale behind your answer.
16. What nursing interventions would you include in a plan of care for a child experiencing a burn dressing change? What role would the caregivers play? How would you facilitate their involvement?
17. Differentiate between the various types of skin grafts.

STUDY QUESTIONS

1. A mother brings her 9-month-old infant to the emergency department and explains to the nurse that she is concerned because her child has been irritable and seems to have abdominal discomfort. She had been breast feeding until a week ago when her milk "dried up." Since then she began feeding the infant formula. To save money she has been adding twice the amount of water specified in the package instructions so that it will "go further." Which of the following conditions does the infant most likely have?
   a. lactose intolerance
   b. gastroenteritis
   c. hyponatremia
   d. appendicitis
2. A young child is admitted to the pediatric unit with a history of nausea/vomiting for four days and abdominal distention and lethargy for the last few hours. When you place the cardiac monitor on the child, you notice that the T waves are flat. You are concerned that she might be hypokalemic, and talk to the physician, who orders an electrolyte panel. When you draw the blood, you have to massage around the site to get enough blood to fill the tube. When the results are available, you find that the potassium level is 5.8mEq/L. Which of the following is most likely?
   a. The massaging you did to get enough blood caused hemolysis.
   b. You were right. the child is hypokalemic.
   c. You must have missed something. The child is hyperkalemic.
   d. There must be something else going on because the potassium level is normal.
3. An 8-year-old girl is admitted to the pediatric unit with a seven day history of diarrhea. When you assess her, you notice that she seems confused and tired. You learn from her father that she is normally very alert and active; her current behavior is abnormal and concerns him. When you check her vital signs, you note that her heart rate is 150 beats/minute, respiratory rate is 35 breaths/minute, temperature is 37.9°C, and her blood pressure is 100/65. Which of the following acid-base disturbances is most likely?
   a. respiratory acidosis
   b. respiratory alkalosis
   c. metabolic acidosis
   d. metabolic alkalosis
4. A 6-month-old infant has been vomiting for two days and has poor skin turgor and prolonged capillary refill time. The infant's urine output is 2mL/kg/hr. Which of the following most likely explains the urine output?
   a. The urine output is low and is consistent with the other symptoms of dehydration.
   b. The urine output is normal, suggesting that the infant's condition is stable or improving.
   c. The urine output is high, suggesting that the infant's condition has a renal origin.
   d. The infant's kidneys are immature and cannot concentrate urine.
5. A 1-year-old child has a three-day history of vomiting and diarrhea. Which of the following recommendations is based on current research?
   a. Feed the child a BRAT diet to help settle the stomach and provide needed nutrients.
   b. Encourage the child to drink ORS and eat his or her normal diet for age as tolerated.
   c. Begin intravenous rehydration and do not give the child anything by mouth for 24 hours.
   d. Initiate oral rehydration with high-glucose clear liquids like soda pop and gelatin.
6. When a moderately dehydrated child's vomiting is uncontrollable and no venous access is obtainable after multiple attempts, which of the following is the best choice?
   a. Insert a nasogastric tube and slowly administer fluids.
   b. Make the child NPO for four hours to allow the gut to rest before restarting oral rehydration.
   c. Continue to administer small amounts of fluid orally so the child will have some hydration.
   d. Obtain intraosseous access and rehydrate through this access.
7. When teaching the parents of a child with rotavirus, which of the following is correct to teach?
   a. Rotavirus can survive on countertops, toys, and clothing for several days, making proper disinfection essential.
   b. Rotavirus spreads easily because it is an air-borne pathogen, making it possible to inhale the virus and become ill.
   c. Washing your hands with ordinary soap and water will prevent the spread of the illness.
   d. Once a child has had rotavirus, he/she will develop immunity and never get it again.
8. Many dehydrated/hypovolemic children have elevated hematocrits. Which of the following explains this?
   a. The body produces more red blood cells to help deliver oxygen to the cells. Once oxygenation improves, red blood cell production will return to normal.

b. The concentration of red blood cells is higher. Once rehydrated, the hematocrit will return to normal.
c. The body produces more red blood cells to help fight infection. Once the infection is resolved, red blood cell production will return to normal.
d. In dehydration, the life cycle of red blood cells is prolonged to help with tissue oxygenation. This results in more red blood cells in circulation than normal.

9. Children who experience burns may initially have a patent airway but develop airway challenges within a few hours. Which of the following explains why this occurs?
a. The burn causes increased capillary permeability which results in pulmonary edema and stridor.
b. Stress and fear increase as the child remembers what has happened and begins to hyperventilate.
c. If untreated, pain from the burn can cause the child to hyperventilate.
d. The burn results in decreased fluid volume and difficulty oxygenating the cells, which eventually causes orthopnea.

10. Evidence-based practice indicates the appropriate first-aid for a burned child should include which of the following?
a. Immediately apply butter to moisturize the site.
b. Immediately apply ice cold water to the site.
c. Immediately apply cool water to the site.
d. Immediately apply warm water to the site.

REFERENCES

Albano, F., Bruzzesse, E., Bella, A., Cascio, A., Titone, L., Arista, S., et al. (2007). Rotavirus and not age determines gastroenteritis severity in children: A hospital-based study. *European Journal of Pediatrics, 166*, 241–247.

Ballestero, Y., Hernandez, M. I., Rojo, P., Manzanares, J., Nebreda, V., Carbajosa, H., Infante, E., & Baro, M. (2006). Hyponatremic dehydration as a presentation of cystic fibrosis. *Pediatric Emergency Care, 22*(11), 725–727.

Besner, G. E., & Otabor, I. A. (2009). Burns: Surgical perspective. Retrieved April 30, 2009, from http://emedicine.medscape.com/article/934173-overview.

Bonheur, J. L., Arya, M., Frye, R. E., & Tamer, M. A. (2009). Gastroenteritis, bacterial: Treatment & medication. Retrieved April 29, 2009, from http://emedicine.medscape.com/article/176400-treatment.

Centers for Disease Control and Prevention. (2008). Information for healthcare providers: Guidelines of the management of acute diarrhea. Retrieved March 1, 2009, from http://www.bt.cdc.gov/disasters/hurricanes/pdf/dguidelines.pdf.

Chatterjee, A., O'Keefe, C., & Varman, M. (2009). Salmonella infection. *Emedicine*. Retrieved April 28, 2009, from http://emedicine.medscape.com/article/968672-overview.

Crellin, D. (2008). Fluid management for children presenting to the emergency department: Guidelines for clinical practice. *Australasian Emergency Nursing Journal, 11*, 5–12.

D'Anci, K. E., Constant, F., & Rosenberg, I. H. (2006). Hydration and cognitive function in children. *Nutrition Reviews, 64*(10), 457–464.

de Caen, A. (2007). Venous access in the critically ill child when the peripheral intravenous fails! *Pediatric Emergency Care, 23*(6), 422–427.

Diehl-Oplinger, L., & Kaminski, M. F. (2004). Choosing the right fluid to counter hypovolemic shock. *Nursing 2004, 34*(3), 52–54.

Freedman, S. B., Adler, M., Seshadri, R., & Powell, E. C. (2006). Oral ondansetron for gastroenteritis in a pediatric emergency department. *New England Journal of Medicine, 354*, 1698–1705.

Gharahbaghian, L., Lotfipour, S., McCoy, C. E., Hoonpongsimanont, W., & Langdorf, M. (2008). Central diabetes insipidus misdiagnosed as acute gastroenteritis in a pediatric patient. *Canadian Journal of Emergency Medical Care, 10*(5), 488–492.

Gore, D. C., Hawkins, H. K., Chinkes, D. L., Chung, D. H., Sanford, A. P., Herndon, D. N., et al. (2007). Assessment of adverse events in the demise of pediatric burn patients. *Journal of Trauma, Injury, Infection, and Critical Care, 63*(4), 814–818.

Hansen, S. L. (2008). From cholera to "fluid creep": A historical review of fluid resuscitation of the burn trauma patient. *Journal of Burn Care & Research, 23*(4), 258–265.

Hoffman, H. G., Patterson, D. R., Seibel, E., Soltani, M., Jewett-Leahy, L., & Sharar, S. R. (2008). Virtual reality pain control during burn wound debridement in the hydrotank. *Clinical Journal of Pain, 24*(4), 299–304.

Hökelek, M., & Nissen, M. D. (2008). Giardiasis. Retrieved April 28, 2009, from http://emedicine.medscape.com/article/998168-overview.

Holliday, M. A., Ray, P. E., & Friedman, A. L. (2007). Fluid therapy for children: Facts, fashion, and questions. *Archives of Disease in Childhood, 92*, 546–550.

Horton, M. A., & Beamer, C. (2008). Powered intraosseous insertion provides safe and effective vascular access for pediatric emergency patients. *Pediatric Emergency Care, 24*(6), 347–350.

Huang, L. H., Anchala, K. R., Ellsbury, D. L., & George, C. S. (2008). Dehydration. *Emedicine* Retrieved April 27, 2009, from http://emedicine.medscape.com/article/906999-print.

Koslap-Petraco, M. B. (2006). Homecare issues in rotavirus gastroenteritis. *Journal of the American Academy of Nurse Practitioners, 18*, 422–428.

Lowell, G., Quinlan, K., & Gottlieb, L. J. (2008). Preventing unintentional scald burns: Moving beyond tap water. *Pediatrics, 122*(4), 799–804.

Lucile Packard Children's Hospital at Stanford. (2008). Fire Safety and Burns—Injury Statistics and Incidence Rates. Retrieved December 20, 2008, from http://www.lpch.org/DiseaseHealthInfo/HealthLibrary/safety/firestat.html.

Lynch, F. (2009). Arterial blood gas analysis: Implications for nursing practice. *Pediatric Nursing, 21*(1), 41–44.

Mast, T. C., DeMuro-Mercon, C., Kelly, C. M., Floyd, L. E., & Walter, E. B. (2009). The impact of rotavirus gastroenteritis on the family. *BMC Pediatrics, 9*(11), 1–9.

Ojo, P., Palmer, J., Garvey, R., Atweh, N., & Fidler, P. (2007). Pattern of burns in child abuse. *American Surgeon, 73*(3), 253–255.

Oliver, R. I., Spain, D., & Stadelmann, W. (2006). Burns, resuscitation and early management. Retrieved April 30, 2009, from http://emedicine.medscape.com/article/1277360-overview.

Palmieri, T. L., Alderson, T. S., Ison, D., O'Mara, M. S., Sharma, R., Bubba, A., Coombs, E., & Greenhalgh D. G. (2008). Pediatric soup scald burn injury: Etiology and prevention. *Journal of Burn Care & Research, 29*(1), 114–118.

Peden, M., Oyegbite, K., Ozanne-Smith, J., Hyder, A. A., Branche, C., Rahman, A. K. M. F., Rivara, F., & Bartolomeos, K. (2008). World report on child injury prevention. Retrieved January 3, 2009, from http://whqlibdoc.who.int/publications/2008/9789241563574_eng.pdf.

Petersen-Smith, A. M., & McKenzie, S. B. (2009). Gastrointestinal disorders. In C. E. Burns, A. M. Dunn, M. A. Brady, N. B. Starr & C. G. Blosser (Eds.), *Pediatric primary care* (4th ed.). St. Louis, MO: Saunders Elsevier.

Prescilla, R. P. (2009a). Gastroenteritis. Retrieved April 28, 2009, from http://emedicine.medscape.com/article/964131-overview.

Prescilla, R. P. (2009b). Gastroenteritis: Differential diagnoses & workup. Retrieved April 28, 2009, from http://emedicine.medscape.com/article/964131-diagnosis.

Rimmer, R. B., Weigand, S., Foster, K. N., Wadsworth, M. M., Jocober, K., Matthews, M. R., Drachman, D., & Caruso, D. M. (2008). Scald burns in young children—A review of Arizona Burn Center pediatric patients and a proposal for prevention in the Hispanic community. *Journal of Burn Care & Research, 29*(4), 595–605.

Roberts, K. E. (2005). Pediatric fluid and electrolyte balance: Critical care case studies. *Critical Care Nursing Clinics of North America, 17*, 361–373.

Ruszczak, Z., Schwartz, R. A., Joss-Wichman, E., & Wichman, R. (2009). Surgical dressing. Retrieved May 1, 2009, from http://emedicine.medscape.com/article/1127868-overview.

Sabol, V. K., & Carlson, K. K. (2007). Diarrhea: Applying research to bedside practice. *AACN Advanced Critical Care, 18*(1), 32–44.

Schulman, C. I., & King, D. R. (2008). Pediatric fluid resuscitation after thermal injury. *Journal of Craniofacial Surgery, 19*(4), 910–912.

Schweer, L. (2008). Pediatric trauma resuscitation: Initial fluid management. *Journal of Infusion Nursing, 32*(2), 104–111.

Sheridan, R. L. (2008). Burns, rehabilitation and reconstruction. Retrieved May 1, 2009, from http://emedicine.medscape.com/article/1277235-overview.

Sidor, M., Benson, B. E., Schwartz, R. A., Desposito, F., & Lucchesi, M. (2006). Burns, thermal. Retrieved April 30, 2009, from http://emedicine.medscape.com/article/926015-overview.

Silva, A. M., Heymsfield, S. B., Gallagher, D., Albu, J., Pi-Sunyer, X. F., Pierson, R. N., Wang, J., Heshka, S., Sardinha, L. B., & Wang, Z. (2008). Evaluation of between-methods agreement of extracellular water measurements in adults and children. *American Journal of Clinical Nutrition, 88*, 315–323.

Steiner, M. J., Nager, A. L., & Wang, V. J. (2007). Urine specific gravity and other urinary indices. Inaccurate tests for dehydration. *Pediatric Emergency Care, 23*(5), 298–303.

Sureshbabu, J., Venugopalan, P., Abuhammour, W., & Burny, I. (2008). Shigella infection. Retrieved April 28, 2009, from http://emedicine.medscape.com/article/968773-overview.

United Nations Children's Fund (UNICEF) & World Health Organization (WHO). (2004). Clinical management of diarrhea. *WHO/UNICEF Joint Statement.* Retrieved January 1, 2009, from http://www.afro.who.int/cah/documents/intervention/acute_diarrhoea_joint_statement.pdf.

United Nations Children's Fund (UNICEF) & World Health Organization (WHO). (2006). Oral Rehydration Salts. Production of the new ORS. Retrieved January 1, 2009, from http://whqlibdoc.who.int/hq/2006/WHO_FCH_CAH_06.1.pdf.

Wells, J. C. K., Fewtrell, M. S., Davies, D. S. W., Williams, J. E., & Cole, T. J. (2005). Prediction of total body water in infants and children. *Archives of Disease in Childhood, 90*(9), 965–971.

World Health Organization. (2006). Improved formula for oral rehydration salts to save children's lives. Retrieved January 1, 2009, from http://www.who.int/mediacentre/news/releases/2006/pr14/en/index.html.

Zengerle-Levy, K. (2006). The inextricable link in caring for families of critically burned children. *Qualitative Health Research, 16*(1), 5–26.

SUGGESTED READINGS

Allen, K. (2007). The vomiting child. What to do and when to do it. *Australian Family Physician, 36*(9), 684–687.

Black, R. E., Morris, S. S., & Bryce, J. (2003). Where and why are 10 million children dying every year? *Lancet, 361*, 2226–2234.

Blumetti, J., Hunt, J. L., Arnoldo, B. D., Parks, J. K., & Purdue, G. F. (2008). The Parkland formula under fire: Is the criticism justified? *Journal of Burn Care & Research, 29*(1), 180–186.

Diggins, K. C. (2008). Treatment of mild to moderate dehydration in children with oral rehydration therapy. *Journal of the American Academy of Nurse Practitioners, 20*, 402–406.

Hanson, M. D., Gauld, M., Wathen, N., & MacMillan, H. L. (2008). Nonpharmacological interventions for acute wound care distress in pediatric patients with burn injury: A systematic review. *Journal of Burn Care & Research, 29*(5), 730–741.

Hardy, A., Harrell, D., Tran, K., Smith, S., Mattingly, R., Zins, B., Zaeske, K., Thomas, J., Sharp, P., & Annan, L. (2007). Exploring the effects of wound dressings and patient positioning on skin integrity in a pediatric burn facility. *Ostomy Wound Management, 53*(6), 67–74.

Lam, N. N., & Dung, N. T. (2007). First aid and initial management for childhood burns in Vietnam—An appeal for public and continuing medical education. *Burns, 34*, 67–70.

MacDonald, S. E., Moralejo, D. G., & Matthews, M. K. (2007). Maternal understanding of diarrhea-related dehydration and its influence on ORS use in Indonesia. *Journal of Public Health, 19*(1), 34–39.

Paut, O., & Lacroix, F. (2006). Recent development in the perioperative fluid management for the paediatric patient. *Current Opinion in Anesthesiology, 19*, 268–277.

Sullivan, S. R., Ahmadi, A. J., Singh, C. N., Sires, B. S., Engrav, L. H., Gibran, N. S., Heimbach, D. M., & Klein, M. B. (2006). Elevated orbital pressure: Another untoward effect of massive resuscitation after burn injury. *Journal of Trauma, Injury, Infection, and Critical Care, 60*(1), 72–76.

RESOURCES

Refer to the online student StudyWARE for Potts & Mandleco at http://www.CengageBrain.com for additional content and study aids.

Organization: **American Burn Association**

Description: The American Burn Association (ABA) and its members dedicate their efforts and resources to promoting and supporting burn-related research, education, care, rehabilitation, and prevention. Members include physicians, nurses, occupational and physical therapists, researchers, social workers, firefighters, and hospitals with burn centers. ABA's website offers users access to information regarding advocacy, burn prevention, and center verification.

Website/Resource: http://www.ameriburn.org

Organization: **American Society for Parenteral and Enteral Nutrition**

Description: The American Society for Parenteral and Enteral Nutrition (A.S.P.E.N.) is an interdisciplinary organization whose members are involved in the provision of clinical nutrition therapies, including parenteral and enteral nutrition. A.S.P.E.N.'s website summarizes the parenteral/enteral nutrition standards and provides access to professional resources.

Website/Resource: http://www.nutritioncare.org

Organization: **Burn Prevention Foundation: Prevention Through Education**

Description: The mission of the Burn Prevention Foundation is to provide burn injury prevention education to and advocacy for those at greatest risk. The Foundation's primary service area is in Eastern Pennsylvania, although many of their programs and products are utilized worldwide. The website offers users access to the Burn Prevention Foundation's programs, services, and products.

Website/Resource: http://www.burnprevention.org

Organization: **International Medical Education Foundation: Burnsurgery.org—Educating Burn Wound Professionals Worldwide**

Description: Burnsurgery.org is a website designed to provide a comprehensive, up-to-date educational tool for burn care professionals throughout the world. The website offers burn care professionals to a series of educational modules aimed at improving care to burn victims.

Website/Resource: http://www.burnsurgery.org

Organization: **International Shriners Headquarters**

Description: Shriners International is a fraternity based on fun, fellowship, and the Masonic principles of brotherly love, relief, and truth. Shriners International supports Shriners Hospitals for Children, an international health care system of 22 hospitals dedicated to improving the lives of children by providing specialty pediatric care, innovative research, and outstanding teaching programs. Shriners International website provides readers access to information regarding temples (chapters) and programs.

Website/Resource: http://www.shrinershq.org

Organization: **National Safety Council**

Description: The National Safety Council saves lives by preventing injuries and deaths at work, in homes and communities, and on the roads, through leadership, research, education, and advocacy. The website offers readers information regarding safe practices at work, home and on the road. In addition, the website offers information concerning current safety news/resources and safety products.

Website/Resource: http://www.nsc.org

Organization: **Oley Foundation**

Description: The Oley Foundation is a national, independent, nonprofit organization that provides up-to-date information and emotional support to people who are receiving home intravenous or tube-fed nutrition. Information is provided in Spanish, French, and Dutch.

Website/Resource: http://www.oley.org

Organization: **Shriners Burn Care Hospitals**

Description: The Shriners Hospitals for Children specializing in burns have been leaders in burn care and research since opening in the mid-1960s. Treatment is provided for burn injuries and related scarring, along with physical and emotional rehabilitation. The website provides the location of the Shriners Hospitals that specialize in burn care.

Hospital Locations:

Boston
Cincinnati
Galveston
Sacramento

Website/Resource: http://www.shrinershq.org/Hospitals

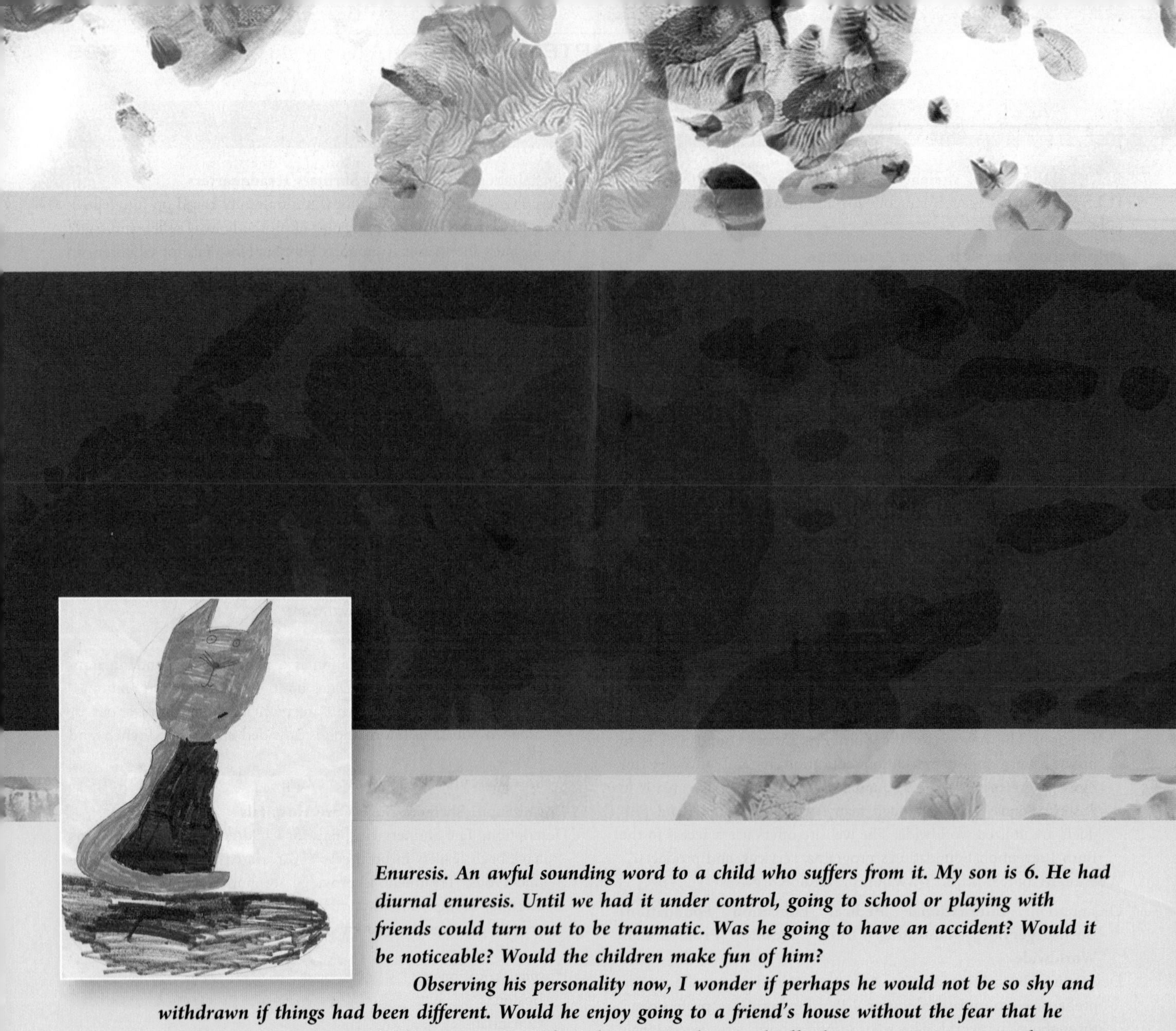

Enuresis. An awful sounding word to a child who suffers from it. My son is 6. He had diurnal enuresis. Until we had it under control, going to school or playing with friends could turn out to be traumatic. Was he going to have an accident? Would it be noticeable? Would the children make fun of him?

Observing his personality now, I wonder if perhaps he would not be so shy and withdrawn if things had been different. Would he enjoy going to a friend's house without the fear that he would have a reoccurrence of enuresis? My wife and I support him and offer him encouragement. Is that enough?

CHAPTER 22

Genitourinary Alterations

Carole Kenner, RNC-NIC, FAAN, DNS; Maribeth Moran, RN, MSN, CPN, CNE; Kerry Fitzgerald Zebold, RN, MSN, PNP; Barbara J. Keating, RN, MSN; and Stephanie Rockwern Amlung, RN, PhD

COMPETENCIES

Upon completion of this chapter the reader will be able to:

- Identify the anatomy and physiology of the pediatric urinary tract.
- Describe the etiology, clinical manifestations, treatment, and nursing management of urinary tract infections (UTI) in children.
- Explain the causes of enuresis and differentiate the disorder from incontinence.
- Describe the etiology, treatment, nursing support, and management of common genitourinary alterations.
- Describe the etiology, clinical manifestations, treatment, and nursing management of common congenital malformations of the urinary tract and external genitalia in children.
- Identify the educational needs of families and children with genitourinary alterations.
- Explain the types of renal failure and their treatment.
- Successfully complete the games and activities in the online student StudyWARE.

The genitourinary system is responsible for the maintenance of homeostasis of the body (water and electrolytes) and for the excretion of waste products. Homeostasis is essential for creating an optimal environment for many other functions of the body. In the male client the urinary system also has a reproductive role and, hence, is critical in a child's development past the phase of toilet training. Because of these essential functions, any alteration in the kidneys and other urinary system organs can pose a major threat to the child's health. Such alterations include infections, structural disorders, and disease processes.

Problems involving the genitourinary system can range from the simple, such as urinary tract infections and enuresis, to the complex, such as renal failure and exstrophy of the bladder. This chapter will discuss infections of the urinary tract, the voiding disorder enuresis, structural defects (vesicoureteral reflux, hypospadias, cryptorchidism, inguinal hernia, hydrocele), glomerular disorders (acute glomerulonephritis, nephrotic syndrome, hemolytic uremic syndrome), and renal failure.

> **NURSING TIP**
>
> **Calculating Bladder Volume**
>
> Bladder capacity in ounces = Age of child in years + 2
> Example: A 3-year-old child has a bladder capacity of approximately 5 ounces (3 years of age + 2 = 5 ounces or 150 mL).

ANATOMY AND PHYSIOLOGY

The genitourinary system is composed of the kidneys, ureters, bladder, and urethra (Figure 22-1). The kidneys are situated posterior on the abdominal wall behind the intestines. The medulla and nephrons of the neonatal kidney are functional at birth; however, the peripheral tubules are small and immature. These will slowly mature, so that by adolescence, the kidneys are of mature size and weight. The bladder presents itself in young children close to the anterior abdominal wall, and with growth, lowers into the pelvis. For these reasons it is easy to palpate a full bladder on infants and young children.

Anatomically, the kidneys are a pair of symmetrically shaped organs located in the posterior abdominal cavity adjacent to the lumbar spinal column. The right kidney is slightly lower than the left. The kidneys are partially protected by the ribs and are further protected by a tough outer capsule embedded in adipose tissue and supported by the renal fascia. The kidneys produce urine and transport it via the ureters into the bladder where it is stored until it exits the body via the urethra. The weight of the kidney is less in the child than in the adult. However, in the infant and young child the kidney makes up a larger proportion of the child's total body weight. The kidneys are less protected in the child compared with an adult because of unossified ribs, less fat padding, and the larger size proportional to the abdomen. Therefore, they are more susceptible to trauma from compression force to the abdomen.

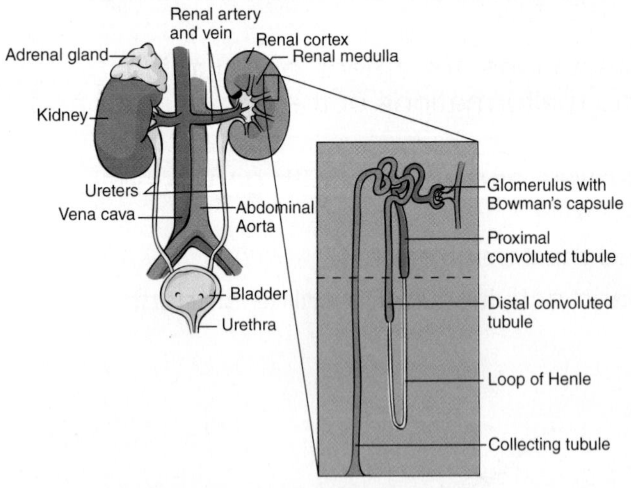

FIGURE 22-1 Anatomy of the Genitourinary System with Inset of a Nephron. DELMAR CENGAGE LEARNING.

To control homeostasis, the kidneys have both excretory and nonexcretory functions. Excretory functions include the kidneys' ability to clear the body of wastes such as urea, creatinine, uric acid, phosphates, sulfates, nitrates, and phenols, along with excess fluids and electrolytes. It is this fine-tuning that maintains the volume and osmolarity of extracellular and intracellular fluids. The kidneys also play a role in the excretion of some drugs and hormones. Nonexcretory functions include the secretion of renin, erythropoietin, metabolism of carbohydrates, and regulation of vitamin D. The fetal kidney begins to develop before many women realize they are pregnant. By the seventh week of gestation, **nephrogenesis**, or development and growth of the kidney, begins and continues to 32 to 36 weeks. Urine production begins in the third month and by the fifth month the collecting tubules and renal pyramids have formed.

At birth the kidney suddenly assumes the role of the placenta, and its response to this change is largely influenced by the gestational age of the baby at delivery. Renal blood flow increases dramatically at birth. Urine production is readily established. Ninety-nine percent of newborns void within the first 48 hours post delivery. Serum creatinine levels, which are maternally influenced at birth, decrease by 50% during the first week of life. At birth the amount of fluid that is filtered by the glomeruli (**glomerular filtration rate**) (GFR) is lower than in adults. The GFR reaches adult levels by 2 years of age. The ability to concentrate urine is not well developed in the newborn for several months and even more restricted in the premature infant (specific gravity of 1.001 to 1.015). The neonate's excretory units are

NURSING TIP

Calculating Minimal Urine Output for Infants

To determine the minimal urine output for an infant, apply the following formula:

1 mL/kg/hour

Example: If an infant weighs 4.4 kg (about 10 pounds), at 1 mL/kg/hour, the minimal urine output must be 4.4 mL/hour (4.4 X 1 mL = 4.4 mL per hour).

underdeveloped and cause disruption in reabsorption of amino acids and bicarbonate, thus causing the infant to be in a state of mild acidosis (plasma pH of 7.11 to 7.36).

CULTURAL CONSIDERATION

Ethnic Differences in Urinary Tract Infections

Caucasian and Hispanic children are more likely to be diagnosed with urinary tract infections than are African-American children during the first two years of life. The evidence supports the findings that these girls are affected much more frequently with urinary tract infections than African-American girls. It is hypothesized that this ethnic difference in incidence may be due to differences in blood group antigens on the surface of uroepithelial cells that may affect *E. coli* adherence (Baker, 2006).

URINARY TRACT INFECTION

Urinary tract infection (UTI) is an infection of one or more structures of the urinary tract and can be classified as lower urinary tract (cystitis, urethritis) or upper urinary tract (pyelonephritis). The most common site is the bladder (**cystitis**) with infection confined to the urethra called **urethritis** and to the kidneys (**pyelonephritis**). Pyelonephritis is usually considered more severe and is accompanied by an increase in the severity of symptoms. Identification of the site of infection is important in determining the treatment.

INCIDENCE AND ETIOLOGY

UTI is the most common disorder of the genitourinary tract. The incidence of UTI in infants is about 40 per 1,000 with the rates being equal among sexes until 3 months of age. At that point the risk for UTI is 4 times greater in the female (Mistry & Gorelick, 2007). This change is due to the increase in bacterial UTIs (Mistry & Gorelick, 2007). Boys who are uncircumcised are more likely to have UTI than those who are circumcised (Mistry & Gorelick, 2007). The highest rates of UTI occur in uncircumcised males under 3 months of age and in females under 1 year (Shaikh, Morone, Bost, & Farrell, 2008).

The most common bacteria organism that infects the urinary tract is *Escherichia coli,* likely because of its presence in the gastrointestinal tract and perianal skin. Less commonly seen colonization occurs from *Klebsiella pneumonia, Enterobacter, Proteus* species, and *Pseudomonas.* The latter four are usually associated with more complicated UTI often seen in children with chronic conditions that alter the urinary tract, such as neurogenic bladder in individuals with spina bifida. Virus and fungi, particularly *Candida* species, may also cause UTI.

PATHOPHYSIOLOGY

In infancy, bacteria frequently enter the urinary tract through the blood and cause infection. After infancy, almost all UTI occur when bacteria enter the urinary tract by ascending through the urethra. Females are especially at risk for infection because of the structure of the lower urinary tract, the short urethra. Males are less susceptible to UTI because of a longer urethra and secretions from the prostate that have antibacterial properties. Therefore, when UTI is found in males, it is important to investigate for urinary tract anomalies. Structural anomalies and abnormal function of the urinary tract have an important role in the pathogenesis of UTI. Such anomalies include vesicoureteral reflux and neurogenic bladder, which is common in children with spina bifida. Other factors that predispose a child to infection include urinary stasis, congenital anomalies of the urinary tract, an obstruction in the urinary tract, and urinary catheters. Urinary stasis increases the risk of UTI. Normally, emptying the bladder frequently completely washes out any organisms. Stasis may be caused by reflux, dysfunction of the voiding mechanism, and infrequent voiding.

CLINICAL MANIFESTATIONS

The presenting signs and symptoms of UTI are often vague, especially in young children. Symptoms in the older child generally include malodorous urine, **dysuria** (difficult or painful urination), urinary frequency, fever, vomiting, diarrhea, irritability, poor feeding, or loss of appetite. Table 22-1 lists the clinical manifestations of UTI in children of various ages. Typically, cystitis is distinguished from pyelonephritis, a syndrome involving fever often greater than 101°F (38.3°C), chills, and back pain. Children with pyelonephritis will also appear to be quite ill.

TABLE 22-1 Clinical Manifestations of Urinary Tract Infections in Children of Various Ages

INFANTS	PRESCHOOLERS	SCHOOL-AGE AND ADOLESCENTS
Malodorous urine	Malodorous urine	Malodorous urine
Malaise	Malaise	Malaise
Irritability or colic	Hematuria	Hematuria
Fever	Fever	Fever and chills
Vomiting and diarrhea	Vomiting and diarrhea	Vomiting and diarrhea
Jaundice in neonates	Dysuria	Dysuria
Poor feeding	Frequency	Frequency
Poor weight gain	Abdominal pain	Abdominal pain
	Flank pain	Flank pain
	Costovertebral angle tenderness	Costovertebral angle tenderness
		Avoidance of urination

DIAGNOSIS

A urinalysis (UA) and urine culture with sensitivity (urine C&S) will be performed to diagnose UTI. The means by which a urine sample is obtained has great impact on the interpretation of results. Urine specimens obtained by collection bag methods in non-toilet-trained children have been widely utilized for initial evaluation of UTI. The American Academy of Pediatrics (AAP), in an evidence-based practice parameter on UTIs in febrile infants and young children (Roberts, 2000), recommended that, due to possible contamination of collection bag specimens and routine urinalysis, it was best to use ultrasonography and a lower urinary tract study if a UTI was suspected. However, in practice many health care practitioners will still opt for this method of collection because it is the least traumatic. While this parameter is several years old it is still followed. Shah, Mandlik, Kumar, Andaya, & Patamasucon (2008) conducted a study to determine compliance with this AAP parameter. They found 70% compliance with urine collection and 97% adherence to the urinalysis, but the follow-up was only 61% (Shah et al., 2008). In any case, if repeated infections develop, it is prudent to perform either sterile catheterization or suprapubic aspiration of urine to evaluate true infection status. More research is needed to determine the best noninvasive method of screening and diagnosis.

An adequate specimen, usually 5–10 cc of urine (may differ among institutions), must be obtained prior to any antimicrobial therapy to avoid affecting the bacterial count and to ensure an accurate diagnosis. The presence of bacteria (**bacteriuria**) and white blood cells (**pyuria**) in the urine confirm the diagnosis of a UTI. Laboratory confirmation of a positive urine culture indicates the presence of greater than 100,000 colony forming units (CFU)/mL of a urinary tract

EVIDENCE-BASED PRACTICE

Treatment of Nocturnal Enuresis in Children

CLINICAL PROBLEM

Nocturnal enuresis is the involuntary loss of urine at night at an age when a child could reasonably be expected to be dry (5 years old). Nocturnal enuresis is a complaint that affects many families. The prevalence is 5% to 20% of 5-year-olds. It may bring social and emotional stress and inconvenience for both the child and their families. The child may experience teasing, parental disapproval, and repeated treatment failures, thus, possibly leading to low self-esteem. This review of research studies was conducted to assess the effectiveness of the medication desmopressin (DDAVP) and to compare it with other interventions.

BEST CLINICAL PRACTICE

- Desmopressin rapidly reduced the number of wet nights per week, but only for as long as the drug was used.
- Tricyclic drugs (imipramine or Tofranil and amitriptyline or Elavil) had effects similar to DDAVP but are associated with more side effects (Table 22-2).
- Children treated with alarms took longer to achieve dryness at night, but their effect may persist longer than treatment with DDAVP.
- In 2007 it was recognized that DDAVP may put some children at risk for hyponatremia. Children during acute illnesses or who have a history of hyponatremia or water intoxication should not take this medication (FDA, 2007).
- The intranasal spray delivery system is no longer recommended (FDA added a black box warning). The preferred

(Continues)

EVIDENCE-BASED PRACTICE *(Continued)*

DDAVP delivery mechanism is the sublingual, fast-melting oral formulation (Lane & Robson, 2009).

IMPLICATIONS FOR NURSING

- If a child is treated with DDAVP, nurses need to teach children and their families about the potential adverse effects of the drug (symptoms associated with water intoxication, i.e., headache, nausea, or vomiting demand discontinuation). In particular, DDAVP increases water reabsorption from the kidneys. Therefore, children should be advised to drink no more than 8 ounces of fluid before bedtime. Nurses need to teach parents to avoid administering DDAVP on nights when there is excess fluid intake (evening sports or social activities).
- Treatment with DDAVP is more expensive than tricyclics but has fewer adverse effects and less risk of fatal overdose.
- Alarm interventions are intermediate in cost and are more disruptive in the short term; however, they do not have side effects associated with drugs.

References: Lane, W. & Robson, M. (2009). Evaluation and Management of Enuresis. *New England Journal of Medicine, 360*(14), 1429–1436; Glazner, C. M., & Evans, J. H. (2002/2006). Desmopressin for nocturnal enuresis in children. *Cochrane Database of Systematic Reviews, 3*. Reassessed and supported 2006; Food and Drug Administration (FDA). (2007). Information for Healthcare Professionals Desmopressin Acetate (marketed as DDAVP Nasal Spray, DDAVP Rhinal Tube, DDAVP, DDVP, Minirin, and Stimate Nasal Spray). *U.S. Food and Drug Administration: Center for Drug Evaluation and Research*. Retrieved February 22, 2009, from http://www.fda.gov/CDER/DRUG/InfoSheets/HCP/desmopressinHCP.htm.

pathogen. If pyelonephritis is suspected, a serum sample may be required. The child with pyelonephritis usually presents with an elevated white blood cell count (WBC), an elevated erythrocyte sedimentation rate (ESR), and an increased C-reactive protein (CRP).

The health care provider may recommend renal scanning with dimercaptosuccinic acid or glucoheptonate to identify anatomic abnormalities that may be the cause of UTI. This study identifies both renal scarring and acute pyelonephritis but does not differentiate between the two. However, it is helpful in identifying children who require long-term follow-up and is more sensitive than the traditional intravenous pyelogram (IVP), which is still utilized to rule out urinary tract obstructions. Other testing that may be ordered includes a renal ultrasound and a voiding cystourethrogram (VCUG). A renal ultrasound may identify certain abnormalities, such as **hydronephrosis,** an abnormal swelling in the kidney, while the VCUG may identify urethral and bladder abnormalities, in particular vesicoureteral reflux. According to the AAP practice parameter for UTI, diagnosis and management suggests antibiotic coverage until appropriate screening has been performed (Roberts, 2000).

TREATMENT

Treatment for UTI includes: (1) eradicating the infection, (2) preventing reinfection by identifying contributing factors, (3) correcting underlying causes of infection, and (4) preserving renal function. Treatment depends upon a variety of factors, including the child's age, other existing medical conditions, and his or her ability to maintain hydration. Oral antibiotic therapy is used to treat UTI. Antibiotics

TABLE 22-2 Common Medications to Treat Enuresis

NAME OF MEDICATION	ACTIONS	ADVERSE REACTIONS
Oxybutynin chloride (Ditropan)	Anticholinergic used for children with small functional bladder capacity. Ditropan affects the bladder muscle by reducing uninhibited bladder contractions, inhibiting voiding, and increasing voluntary control of the urethral sphincter.	Facial flushing Dry mouth Constipation Heat intolerance Drowsiness Insomnia Blurred vision
Imipramine hydrochloride (Tofranil)	Tricyclic antidepressant. Decreases depth of sleep during latter part of the night.	Dry mouth Nervousness Insomnia Changes in personality
Desmopressin acetate (DDAVP)	A synthetic analog of vasopressin that works by increasing water retention and urine concentration in the renal tubules. By concentrating urine and decreasing the amount of urine produced, the child may not reach bladder capacity and therefore stays dry.	Headaches Nausea Nasal congestion Nose bleeds Hyponatremia

such as trimethoprim in combination with sulfamethoxazole (Bactrim, Septra), amoxicillin (Amoxil), a cephalosporin, or nitrofurantoin (Furadantin) are given for 7 to 10 days. A follow-up urine culture should be performed 48 to 72 hours after initiating treatment. For infants or young children 2 months to 2 years of age who are assessed as toxic, dehydrated, or unable to retain oral fluids, initial antibiotic therapy should be given intravenously and hospitalization should be considered (Roberts, 2000). Untreated UTI can lead to a variety of complications including renal scarring. Of those clients who develop scarring, some may develop kidney stones, hypertension, end stage renal disease, and possible complications of pregnancy. It is therefore imperative that urinary tract infections be evaluated and treated carefully. With appropriate management, many of these severe complications can be prevented.

EVIDENCE-BASED PRACTICE

Antibiotics for Acute Pyelonephritis

CLINICAL PROBLEM

The most severe form of UTI is acute pyelonephritis, which results in significant acute morbidity and may cause permanent renal damage. Published guidelines recommend treatment initially with intravenous antibiotic therapy followed by oral therapy for 7 to 14 days. There is concern about resistance to amoxicillin; the initial treatment should be with third or fourth generation cephalosporin. There is no consensus on the duration of either IV or oral therapy.

BEST CLINICAL PRACTICE

- Children with acute pyelonephritis can be treated effectively with oral cefixime or with short courses (2 to 4 days) of IV therapy followed by oral therapy. There are no real differences in outcomes between oral and IV.
- If IV therapy is chosen, single daily dosing with aminoglycosides is safe and effective. Trials are required to determine the optimal total duration of therapy and if other oral antibiotics can be used in the initial treatment of acute pyelonephritis.

IMPLICATIONS FOR NURSING

Oral antibiotics may be as effective as the combination of injection and oral antibiotics for kidney infections in children.

References: Arnoff, S. C., & McCoy, A. C. S. (2007). Pyleonephritis: Treatment & Medication. *Emedicine*. Retrieved January 27, 2009 from http://emedicine.medscape.com/article/968028-treatment; Bloomfield, P., Hodson, E., & Craig, J. (2005/2007). Antibiotics for acute pyelonephritis in children. *Cochrane Database of Systematic Reviews, 1*: CD003772. Assessed and updated 2007.

ENURESIS

Enuresis is defined as involuntary voiding of urine beyond the expected age at which voluntary control should be achieved after successful toilet training (Austin & Coplen, 2007). Enuresis differs from incontinence in that incontinence results from a structural abnormality, usually an anatomic malformation. Enuresis can be primary or secondary, diurnal or nocturnal, or both. A child who has never achieved a period of dryness for at least 3 months is referred to as a primary enuretic. Secondary enuresis occurs when a child has been dry for at least 3 to 6 months and then resumes wetting. Diurnal enuresis is wetting that occurs only during the daytime, and nocturnal enuresis is wetting that occurs only at night.

Enuresis can have a great impact on a child's life. Children with enuresis may avoid participating in activities with their peers. Social activities such as a sleepover or a camping trip can cause a great deal of stress for these children. Children with daytime wetting often face more problems. Staying dry during the school day can be a challenge and concealing wet clothing can be the largest obstacle of all. These children may also have problems with odor control.

INCIDENCE

Because the age at which urinary continence is achieved covers a wide range of normal, the incidence is difficult to determine. However, it is estimated that 15% to 20% among 5-year-olds and 5% among 10-year-olds suffer from enuresis. Most children have nocturnal enuresis, and most are primary enuretics. Primary nocturnal enuresis is more common in boys, whereas primary diurnal enuresis is more common in girls. In contrast to enuresis, incontinence is caused by a malformation of the urinary tract and is the least common cause of wetting, affecting about 1% to 3% of children.

ETIOLOGY AND PATHOPHYSIOLOGY

Enuresis is a symptom, not a disease, and many hypotheses have been proposed to describe its causes. Etiologic factors are classified as organic (having a physical basis) and nonorganic or functional (exogenous or with no physical disorder or disease). Organic factors should be ruled out before nonorganic ones are considered. Organic causes include:

- Neurologic developmental delay in which the child is unable to inhibit bladder contraction
- Urinary tract infections; a child with a urinary tract infection may involuntarily lose urine, but this is caused by the physiological response to the infection that makes the bladder sensitive to any stimulation
- Structural disorders of the urinary tract such as obstructive lesions and small bladder capacity; the child may not be able to hold the large volume of urine produced and therefore may experience urgency and the involuntary loss of urine

CASE STUDY / CARE PLAN

CHILD WITH URINARY TRACT INFECTION

Elena is a 3-year-old Canadian child who is brought to the clinic by her mother. She has been complaining of abdominal pain and nausea for the past three days. Her mother says her skin "felt hot to touch" although she did not take her temperature and that several days ago she was irritable and seemed uncomfortable. She complained of perineal irritation, although she did not complain of painful urination. This is the second time she has been seen in the clinic in three months for these same symptoms.

NURSING CARE PLAN

ASSESSMENT

Initial nursing assessment should begin with questions regarding the child's present illness in terms of onset, duration, intensity of symptoms, associated symptoms, patterns of intake and elimination, allergies, past medical history, and last visit to the clinic. The child's vital signs need to be taken, especially her temperature and blood pressure. Assessment needs to focus on her overall state of health and nutrition, as well as level of comfort. She needs to have a head-to-toe assessment with emphasis on abdominal and perineal areas. A clean-catch urine specimen needs to be obtained with careful instruction on how to provide it.

NURSING DIAGNOSIS 1

Risk for injury related to complications of infection (chronic renal disease and kidney damage).

EXPECTED OUTCOME

1. Elena will be free of infection and complications including recurrent UTI.

NOC: Infection Severity

NIC: Infection Control

INTERVENTIONS/*RATIONALES*

1. Collect urine specimens as ordered. *Organisms must be identified so that appropriate anti-infective drugs can be ordered. The nurse must ensure that the urine specimen is collected properly. Teaching regarding the collection may be necessary.*
2. Administer antibiotics as ordered. *Antibiotics are given to eradicate the infection. Caregivers need to be taught the importance of completing the full course of medication even if Elena begins to feel better.*
3. Teach mother ways to prevent UTI: wiping perineum from front-to-back; cleansing perineal area well during bathing; avoiding tight-fitting underwear or pants; wearing cotton panties instead of nylon; encouraging fluids, especially water; avoiding urinary retention. *These tips can help prevent recurrent UTI by keeping the perineal area clean and dry, diluting urine, and preventing stasis of urine in the bladder as a place for germs to grow.*
4. Teach mother to recognize signs of UTI: frequent urination; malodorous urine; incontinence in a toilet-trained child; itching, red, or painful perineal area; abdominal or flank pain; fever; nausea or vomiting. *By teaching the mother to watch for signs of UTI, early treatment can be obtained and complications can be avoided.*
5. Provide information about follow-up care if needed. *Because this is a recurring infection, it may be necessary that Elena be seen by a pediatric nephrologist. If this is needed, she and her family will need preparation regarding the consult and further diagnostic testing.*

(Continues)

CASE STUDY / CARE PLAN (Continued)

EVALUATION

Elena has no further recurrences of UTI and does not suffer from complications of UTI.

NURSING DIAGNOSIS 2

Risk for deficient fluid volume related to nausea, decreased intake, and fever.

EXPECTED OUTCOME

1. Elena will maintain fluid and electrolyte balance.

NOC: Fluid Balance

NIC: Fluid Monitoring

INTERVENTIONS/*RATIONALES*

1. Determine hydration status. *Monitoring fluid and electrolyte status will help ensure balance.*
2. Teach mother to take Elena's temperature. *Fever is usually a sign of infection and also increases fluid requirements.*
3. Administer antipyretics as prescribed. *Antipyretics will help control fever and associated discomfort.*
4. Teach mother alternative forms of temperature management when Elena runs a fever: using light clothing; keeping the environment cool. *These methods help promote surface cooling.*
5. Encourage favorite fluids by mouth in small amounts offered frequently. *Elena will be more likely to take fluids if she is offered small amounts of ones that she likes. Fluid intake will help control temperature as well as maintain blood flow to the urinary tract, dilute urine, and wash out bacteria.*
6. Teach mother to monitor fluid intake. *This will help ensure that Elena takes adequate fluids.*

EVALUATION

Elena maintains fluid balance.
Elena's temperature is within normal limits.

NURSING DIAGNOSIS 3

Acute pain related to UTI.

EXPECTED OUTCOME

1. Elena's pain will be diminished or absent.

NOC: Pain Control

NIC: Analgesic Administration

INTERVENTIONS/*RATIONALES*

1. Assess level of pain using an age-appropriate pain assessment tool. *This provides a consistent measurement of pain so that interventions can be tailored to her needs.*
2. Administer analgesics as ordered. *Mild pain relievers will help control Elena's pain.*
3. Apply warm moist heat to the abdomen. *Warm moist heat will help improve blood flow and decrease bladder spasms.*

EVALUATION

Elena's level of pain will be controlled and reduced.

(Continues)

CASE STUDY / CARE PLAN (Continued)

NURSING DIAGNOSIS 4

Deficient knowledge related to lack of information of disease process, diagnostic procedures, management, and prevention of UTI.

EXPECTED OUTCOME

1. Elena's mother will demonstrate an understanding of the disease process, diagnostic procedures, management and prevention of UTI.

NOC: Knowledge: Disease Process, Diagnostic Procedures, Management, Prevention of UTI

NIC: Teaching: Prescribed Medication/Treatment

INTERVENTIONS/*RATIONALES*

1. Assess understanding and educational level of Elena's mother. *In order to develop a teaching plan that meets the mother's needs, the nurse must first assess cognitive and educational levels including what she already knows about UTI.*
2. Develop a relationship with Elena and her mother. *In order to provide effective teaching, the nurse must first establish a caring relationship with the client and family.*
3. Provide individualized teaching regarding anatomy and physiology of the urinary tract, disease process, diagnostic procedures, stressing the importance of follow-up consultation and care. *There should be follow-up on the UTI. It is important that another urine specimen be obtained after completion of antibiotics to determine effectiveness of treatment. Also, it may be necessary to refer Elena to a pediatric nephrologist since this is a recurrent problem.*

EVALUATION

Elena's mother demonstrates confidence in managing Elena's UTI, preventing further recurrences, and following up with care as needed.

- Disorders that affect the concentrating ability of the kidneys such as chronic renal failure
- Diseases associated with an excessive production of urine (**polyuria**), as in diabetes mellitus and diabetes insipidus
- Chronic constipation

EYE ON...

Enuresis

There are many myths and misconceptions about children with enuresis. If a child is not successfully dry during the day and night by 4 to 5 years of age, it may reflect negatively on the child and caregivers. Our society considers nighttime wetting normal behavior for infants and toddlers, but it is not acceptable for school-age children. Families often view enuresis as a problem when their child is around 5 years of age.

Nonorganic or functional causes include:

- Sleep arousal pattern problems, that is, sleeping soundly so the child does not awaken in the night to void
- Sleep disorders such as enlarged tonsils, sleep apnea, and other upper respiratory problems (Aydil et al., 2008)
- Psychological stress and family disruptions such as divorce, death, or birth of a new sibling
- Family history of UTIs or diurnal voiding symptoms (DVS)
- Inappropriate toilet training, that is, early chronologic or developmental age, overly demanding or punitive caregivers

CLINICAL MANIFESTATIONS

Most children achieve urinary and bowel control between 2 1/2 and 3 1/2 years of age. The typical sequence for the development of bladder and bowel control is: (1) nocturnal bowel control, (2) daytime bowel control, (3) daytime

BOX 22-1
POSSIBLE CLINICAL MANIFESTATIONS OF ENURESIS

- Dribbling after voiding
- Urgent need to void (child may be seen leg-crossing, dancing, or holding genitals to avoid wetting)
- Constant dribbling with ineffective stream
- Infrequent and painful voiding
- Straining to void
- Incontinence when laughing

control of voiding, and (4) nighttime control of voiding. It is unclear why some children are not able to accomplish bladder control while other children of the same age have attained control. Any child who continues to experience nighttime wetting after the age of 5 warrants an evaluation for enuresis. Possible presenting clinical manifestations of a child with enuresis are presented in Box 22-1.

DIAGNOSIS

Physical examination and a careful family history are the hallmarks of determining a diagnosis of enuresis or incontinence. A thorough physical examination to distinguish between organic and nonorganic (functional) enuresis should be performed initially. The examination should include assessing the abdomen and genitals for any abnormalities. A neurologic exam of the peripheral reflexes, perianal sensation, anal sphincter tone, and inspection of the lower back to rule out any spinal defects should also be included.

Results of the history, voiding diary (keeping track of frequency and amount of void), and physical examination may determine which diagnostic tests are required for further evaluation. Some of the more frequently required tests include urinalysis, urine culture, renal ultrasound, and VCUG for children with a history of urinary tract infections. Urine flow rates determine voiding characteristics. One can determine if structural problems are present by measuring the amount of urine voided and the time it takes the child to void, as well as the force of his or her urine stream.

TREATMENT

The following treatments can be used separately or in combination to treat children with wetting problems: medication(s), bed-wetting alarms, motivational therapies, elimination diets, and bowel programs for children who are constipated. If the child is experiencing incontinence, the structural cause will need to be determined and treated. Successful treatment requires both the child and caregivers to commit to active involvement in an enuresis program. The most commonly used medications to treat enuresis are oxybutynin chloride (Ditropan), desmopressin (DDAVP), and imipramine hydrochloride (Tofranil) (Table 22-2). Medications are often used in conjunction with other treatments for the most effective outcomes. Medications for enuresis should not be considered a cure but as part of the treatment and solely symptom relief. Children with the best long-term outcomes for staying dry most often used a combination of treatments in conjunction with medications. Research is examining the use of a combination of behavioral and pharmacologic therapies to decrease enuresis. These may be physician or parent driven. Diaz Saldano et al. (2007) found that the remission of nocturnal enuresis was higher in the physician led intervention than the bowel, bladder, alarm, and medication protocol driven by parents. Behavioral therapy is aimed at supporting or building the child's self-esteem. Research aimed at examining physiologic factors such as small bladder and abnormal urodynamics regarding micturation along with treatments has found that behavioral therapy

NURSING ALERT

DDAVP

DDAVP should not be used for children who are hypersensitive or who have a potential for fluid and electrolyte imbalances (cystic fibrosis, renal disease) because of the potential for water intoxication and hyponatremia. DDAVP should not be used during acute illnesses or in those children with a history of water intoxication or hyponatremia (FDA, 2007; Health Canada, 2008). The Food and Drug Administration added a black box warning to the intranasal spray. The majority of reported episodes of hyponatremia were linked to the nasal spray due to its extended half-life. Consequently, the *intranasal spray* is no longer recommended (Lane & Robson, 2009).

NURSING ALERT

Warning for Imipramine Hydrochloride (Tofranil) Overdose

Fatal accidental overdoses caused by cardiac arrhythmias may occur from imipramine; therefore, labeling should include this information. Nurses should educate families that this medication should be stored in a childproof bottle in a secure place out of the reach of children. Imipramine must only be dispensed by adults.

when compared to pharmacologic intervention was more likely to produce remission and have less relapse as long as the urinary tract and urodynamics were normal (Sehgal, Paul, & Mohanty, 2007).

Bed-wetting alarms are widely used treatment for enuresis. Some models are meant to be placed under the bottom sheet of the child's bed (Figure 22-2). Most alarms consist of a moisture sensor that is attached to the child's underwear or pajamas (Figure 22-3A and 22-3B). The alarm starts to buzz as the first few drops of urine are detected. The sound of the alarm arouses the child, and the urinary flow is interrupted. The child is instructed to turn off the alarm and go to the bathroom to complete voiding. The alarm teaches the child to recognize bladder fullness and awaken before bed-wetting occurs. Long-term follow-up has been conducted in children ages 5 to 16 years who had monosymptomatic primary nocturnal enuresis. Of the 62 patients enrolled in the study and followed for on average 19.2 month, the researchers found that in general the enuretic alarms do produce positive long-term effects (Tuncel et al., 2008).

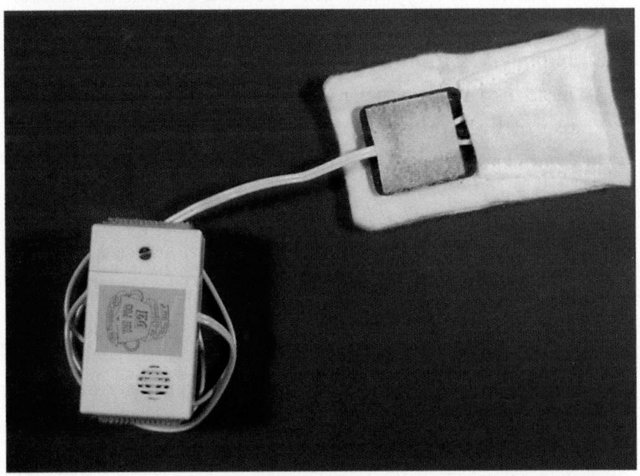

FIGURE 22-2 A bed-wetting alarm is often used to treat enuresis. COURTESY OF KERRY ZEBOLD.

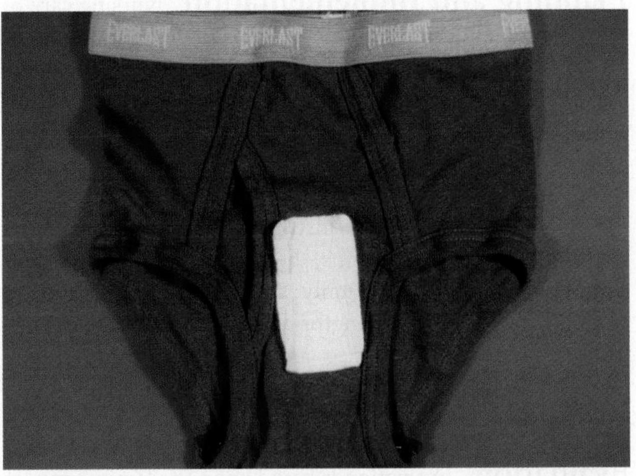

FIGURE 22-3A Proper Attachment of Bed-Wetting Alarm (male). DELMAR CENGAGE LEARNING.

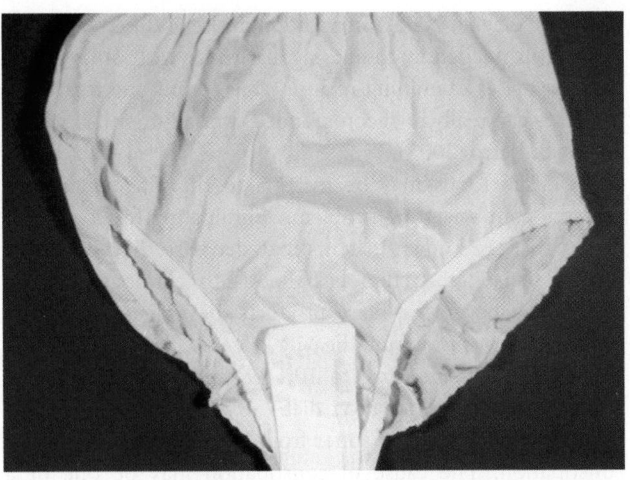

FIGURE 22-3B Proper Attachment of Bed-Wetting Alarm (female). DELMAR CENGAGE LEARNING.

Motivational therapies may include using star charts to record the child's progress during the treatment program (Figure 22-4). Rewarding the child for dry nights is effective because over time the behavior may be changed when the child feels proud of his or her accomplishments. The child should be included when designing a reward program. By rewarding children with special treats (stickers, collectable cards, etc.) or privileges that they value, it increases the chances that the rewarded behavior will occur again. Rewards are most effective if they are given to the child immediately after the desired behavior. However, reward programs should be used with caution: If a child consistently fails to receive rewards, it can decrease self-esteem and motivation to continue the program. More evidence is needed to support the use of alarms or motivational or cognitive therapies. To date many of the studies have been flawed or had small sample sizes so that no definitive conclusions can be drawn (Glazener,

NAME ______ MONTH ______

SUNDAY	MONDAY	TUESDAY	WEDNESDAY	THURSDAY	FRIDAY	SATURDAY
Diet Alarm	Diet Alarm	Diet Alarm	Diet Alarm	Diet Alarm	Diet Alarm	Diet Alarm
AM AS PM	AM AS PM	AM AS PM	AM AS PM	AM AS PM	AM AS PM	AM AS PM
Diet Alarm	Diet Alarm	Diet Alarm	Diet Alarm	Diet Alarm	Diet Alarm	Diet Alarm
AM AS PM	AM AS PM	AM AS PM	AM AS PM	AM AS PM	AM AS PM	AM AS PM
Diet Alarm	Diet Alarm	Diet Alarm	Diet Alarm	Diet Alarm	Diet Alarm	Diet Alarm
AM AS PM	AM AS PM	AM AS PM	AM AS PM	AM AS PM	AM AS PM	AM AS PM
Diet Alarm	Diet Alarm	Diet Alarm	Diet Alarm	Diet Alarm	Diet Alarm	Diet Alarm
AM AS PM	AM AS PM	AM AS PM	AM AS PM	AM AS PM	AM AS PM	AM AS PM
Diet Alarm	Diet Alarm	Diet Alarm	Diet Alarm	Diet Alarm	Diet Alarm	Diet Alarm

FIGURE 22-4 Behavior Modification Star Chart is often used to reward desired behavior in children with Enuresis. DELMAR CENGAGE LEARNING.

Evans, & Cheuk, 2005). In addition, more and better quality research is needed in comparing alarm use with other therapies as well as examining relapse rates before one treatment modality can really be recommended over another (Glazener, Evans, & Petro, 2005).

Certain foods may be irritants to the bladder and increase a child's wetting problems. Eliminating foods or beverages that are known irritants may decrease the number of wetting episodes a child has. Foods to eliminate include carbonated beverages, dairy products, beverages with artificial coloring, citric fruit, heavily sugared foods, and beverages with caffeine. Five to 10% of children with enuresis benefit from the elimination diet.

Many children who suffer from enuresis also experience constipation. The cause of constipation may be one or a combination of several factors such as insufficient fluid intake, low fiber diet, history of painful bowel movements and holding back of stool, changes in daily routine, lack of physical activity, and no routine for daily bowel movements. Stools may be infrequent, hard or large, and may be painful to pass. These children may not completely empty the colon of stool and further perpetuate the cycle of constipation. Treatment for enuresis may not be successful if constipation management is not addressed at the same time. Children may show improvement with wetting once they are on a successful bowel program. To assess for constipation a rectal exam, X-ray, or ultrasound of the abdomen can determine if the child has a large mass of stool.

BOX 22-2
ASSESSMENT QUESTIONS—ENURESIS

1. Has the child ever been toilet trained by day or night and at what age?
2. How frequently does the child have wetting episodes?
3. Does the child have a history of dysuria, polyuria, frequency, or urgency?
4. Has the child ever experienced urinary tract infections?
5. Is there a family history of enuresis or voiding problems?
6. Does the child have any sleep problems, such as deep sleep, snoring, or sleep walking?
7. Is there a history of constipation, fecal soiling, large bowel movements, or painful bowel movements?
8. How is the family currently handling the wetting problems?
9. Have they tried any treatments or medications for the wetting?
10. What are the child's and family's feelings or attitudes about enuresis?

NURSING TIP

Feeling Comfortable with the Alarm System

Have younger children practice using the alarm with a doll or stuffed animal to help them feel comfortable with the system.

Nursing Management

Assessment

In assessing a child who presents with enuresis, the history will provide important information for formulating a plan of care. Questions to cover during the assessment of the enuretic child are listed in Box 22-2.

Nursing Diagnosis

1. *Impaired urinary elimination* related to lack of bladder control.
2. *Impaired skin integrity* related to contact with urine.
3. *Disturbed sleep pattern* related to bed-wetting and the use of bed-wetting alarms.
4. *Low self-esteem* related to urinary incontinence or bed-wetting.
5. *Impaired social interactions* related to urinary incontinence.

Outcome Identification

1. The child will achieve bladder control.
2. The child will be free of skin irritation in the perineal area.
3. The child will have minimal disturbance during sleep.
4. The child will use expressions that indicate positive self-esteem.
5. The child will actively participate in age-appropriate social interactions.

Planning and Implementation

Nursing care of the enuretic child most often includes ongoing family education and support during a long treatment phase. The nurse can provide the child and family with information about the causes of enuresis and the variety of treatment options. The family should be involved in the decision about the treatment plan. As appropriate to the treatment, the child and family need instruction on the use of bed-wetting alarms, medications, behavior modification, and elimination diets. The family should be encouraged to emphasize the child's strengths and praise attempts at control to increase confidence and self-esteem. The nurse needs to assist the child and family to verbalize feelings of frustration.

Evaluation

Evaluation is based upon the family's report of the child's progress with the program. Families are instructed to follow up with the nurse by telephone one week after starting the program or sooner if problems develop. Monthly appointments may be necessary until the child achieves 14 consecutive dry nights.

FAMILY TEACHING

Nurses can provide children and caregivers with information on hygiene and treatment or prevention of skin breakdown caused by exposure of skin to urine. They will need education about the use of bed-wetting alarms. Explain to the caregivers that the child's sleep will be disrupted during the program, and that it may be beneficial to the child to have an earlier bedtime. Nurses can also educate children and caregivers on the use, schedule, and adverse reactions of medications prescribed as part of the enuresis program. Families and children need support and encouragement during the treatment for enuresis. Nurses should provide children with positive feedback for complying with the prescribed programs. The nurse needs to discuss with the child feelings of embarrassment or guilt as a result of the enuresis. The nurse should encourage keeping an extra set of clothes at school until enuresis is resolved.

STRUCTURAL DEFECTS

Structural defects include vesicoureteral reflux, hypospadias, cryptorchidism, inguinal hernia, and hydrocele.

VESICOURETERAL REFLUX

Vesicoureteral reflux (VUR) is defined as the backflow of urine from the bladder up the ureter to the kidney. VUR results when the **ureterovesical/vesicoureteral junction** (site where the ureter enters the bladder) fails to maintain a unidirectional flow of urine from the ureter to the bladder. Normally, urine is produced in the kidneys and travels down the ureters into the bladder for storage. In the normal bladder, the junction of the ureter into the bladder forms a one-way valve mechanism or flap valve that allows urine to flow into the bladder while preventing regurgitation back into the ureters or kidneys.

Incidence and Etiology

VUR is the most common anatomic disorder affecting the genitourinary tract. The exact incidence is unknown because routine screening of children without a history of urinary tract infection is not practiced. However, VUR has been estimated to occur in less than 1% of all healthy children, with most cases being in red-haired children, Caucasians, newborn males, and in females older than 1 year (Cendron, 2008). The incidence is much higher (40% to 50%) in those children diagnosed with UTIs (Cendron, 2008). Often it is diagnosed when the child is between the ages of 2 and 3 years. However, in some cases it may be diagnosed in older children or infants depending upon the underlying pathology. For example, children with spina bifida are usually screened for reflux as infants.

It is important to note that reflux has a genetic component but the exact mechanism is unknown (Cendron, 2008). Familial reflux is common and the role of genetics is being explored. Reflux is present in approximately one-third of siblings who have an affected brother or sister. Recent studies have also revealed a high incidence of transmission of reflux from parent to child (Cendron, 2008).

Pathophysiology

Anatomically, the ureter extends from its respective kidney downward to the top of the bladder **trigone** (a small triangular area at the base of the bladder where the ureters normally join the bladder). It then passes obliquely through the bladder wall for a distance that enables the ureter to act as a sphincter despite not having an anatomic sphincter. The ureter at this point functions as a one-way valve to prevent reflux. When this length is not sufficient, backward flow of urine, hence vesicoureteral reflux will ensue. With growth, the ureter tunneling through the bladder wall may elongate, and this increase in tunnel length will help promote the resolution of reflux.

Clinical Manifestations

The clinical manifestations of VUR usually are not directly apparent. However, persistent and repeated urinary tract infections are the most common indicator of reflux. Therefore, the child with repeated UTI should be evaluated. Other manifestations of reflux less commonly seen are enuresis, flank pain, and abdominal pain. However, these symptoms can be vague in children too young to describe and localize their symptoms and may be easily confused with other diagnoses.

Diagnosis

The diagnosis of VUR is made by radiographic evidence of backflow of urine on a **cystogram** (radiograph of bladder, urethra, and ureters), or **voiding cystourethrogram** (VCUG) (radiograph of bladder, urethra, and ureters during voiding). Reflux is graded to determine its severity on a scale of I to V. The degree to which contrast material from the bladder travels up the ureters to the kidneys is graded I to V, with I being the least severe and V the most severe.

Treatment

The medical treatment for vesicoureteral reflux is determined by the severity of the reflux and the fact that some degrees of reflux resolve spontaneously as the child grows. The less severe the reflux (grades I and II), the greater the likelihood of resolution. The goals of medical management for children with reflux include prevention of UTIs, prevention of kidney damage, and prevention of the subsequent complications of reflux and renal scarring. Currently, treatment options include long-term use of antibiotics to prevent UTI, and on occasion the use of anticholinergics. Anticholinergics such as oxybutynin chloride (Ditropan) are used to decrease bladder pressure.

Other treatment options include surveillance of the child over time to observe for signs of deterioration such as increase in incidence and severity of UTIs. Deterioration in a child would necessitate an advance in treatment, such as a change in prophylactic antibiotics and an increase in anticholinergic medication. Lastly, surgery to correct reflux is indicated when medical treatment options have failed. Indications of failure include breakthrough UTIs, particularly pyelonephritis, despite strict compliance to medical management and pharmacotherapy, or increased renal damage, which threatens the survival of the kidney. In general, medical versus surgical outcome differences are small unless medical therapy is failing to gain a response (Cendron, 2008).

Surgical management may be performed endoscopically or with traditional surgical techniques involving an abdominal incision. When kidney function is impaired and the ureters are massively dilated, a urinary diversion may be recommended to improve renal function and allow the dilated ureters to reestablish tone. This is usually a temporary measure to allow time to consider further reconstruction or reestablishment of the ureters into the bladder. Surgery involves reimplantation of the ureter into a position on the trigone that allows for sufficient submucosal length to prevent the reflux from recurring. There are several different surgical techniques that can be used. However, overarching consideration should be long-term outcomes and prevention of further complications (Cendron, 2008).

Nursing Management

Because the nonsurgical management for a child with VUR focuses on UTI prevention and management, an important aspect of nursing care focuses on education of the child and caregivers. The child and caregivers should be aware that the treatment may continue for years and compliance with the medication regimen is important. They must also maintain close contact with their health care provider and inform the individual when the goals are not being achieved (i.e., recurrent UTI), hence necessitating more aggressive management.

If surgery is necessary, the nurse provides the child and caregivers information about the surgical procedure and preoperative and postoperative care. Immediate postoperative care for a child after reimplantation of one or both ureters can be challenging. While managing the acute pain the child may be experiencing it is important to strictly monitor intake and output. The well-organized nurse will label all drainage devices and stents and note where they originate (i.e., ureter, bladder, or peritoneum). The nurse should assess the integrity of all tubes and drainage bags; breaks in tubing can increase risk for infection by introducing bacteria into the drainage system. Noting any kinks or disruptions will assure accurate I & O.

HYPOSPADIAS

Hypospadias is a common congenital malformation in which the urethral meatus is on the ventral surface (underside) of the penis (Figure 22-5). The position of the urethral opening may vary, occurring at any point along the ventral surface of the penis or on the scrotum or perineum.

Incidence and Etiology

Hypospadias occurs in 1 in 250 live male births in the United States (Gatti & Kirsch, 2007). Rates are increasing probably due to the increase in premature and low birthweight (Gatti & Kirsch, 2007). Rates are highest among Caucasians, lowest among Hispanics, and intermediate among African Americans. The exact etiology is unknown and may be multifactorial. Some affected boys have defects in testosterone metabolism or testosterone receptors, which suggests that hypospadias can result from an abnormality in endocrine factors that influence the development of the male genitalia. There is some genetic predisposition, as evidenced by a family history of another male with hypospadias. Studies are underway to examine a potential genetic

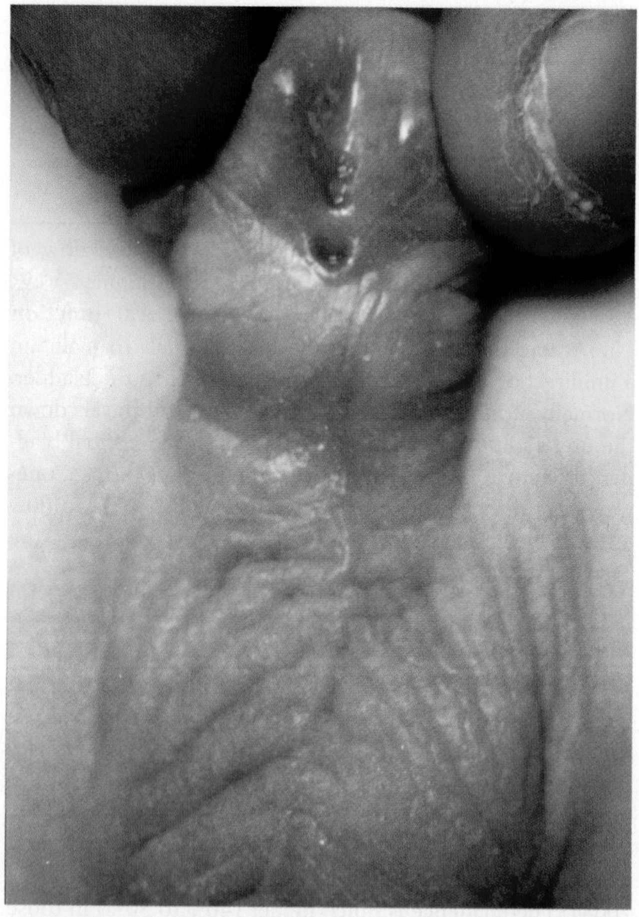

Figure 22-5 Hypospadias is a congenital anomaly in which the urethral meatus is on the ventral surface (underside) of the penis. PHOTO COURTESY OF CASIMIR FIRLIT, MD, PHD, WILLIAM E.KAPLAN, MD, MAX MAIZELS, MD, AND JEFFREY PALMER, MD, CHILDREN'S UROLOGY LTD.

linkage. It has been noted to have an eight-fold increase among monozygotic twins compared with singleton infants (Gatti & Kirsch, 2007). In addition, fathers with hypospadias produced infants with the disorder 8% of the time. Subsequent siblings of a male child with hypospadias were affected 14% of the time (Gatti & Kirsch, 2007). Hypospadias is also part of several syndromes that have a genetic component. There is also a potential linkage between ingestion of estrogen during pregnancy and the development of hypospadias (Gatti & Kirsch, 2007). Loratadine (Claritin) has also been implicated; however, Schwarz and colleagues (2008) conducted a systematic review and meta-analysis of risk and found no significant linkage.

Pathophysiology

Hypospadias is a congenital birth defect caused by altered embryogenesis or an insult to the developing fetus during the third through fifth months of gestation. In utero, the penile urethra develops from the urogenital sinus. By the twelfth week of gestation, the endodermal edges of the secondary urethral groove fuse to form a tube. The urethra fuses in a proximal to distal direction. Failure of this fusion results in the urethral meatus opening in a location other than the tip of the penis and failure of the foreskin to develop properly. The foreskin usually appears as a hood in children affected with hypospadias.

Clinical Manifestations

The **prepuce**, or skin forming a hood over the glans, is abnormally small ventrally and may be redundant dorsally. Many caregivers of infants with hypospadias claim it appears that their newborn son has already been circumcised. Associated conditions may include **chordee** (downward curvature of the penis and an incomplete foreskin), undescended testes, and inguinal hernia. In some cases the urinary stream may be deflected downward secondary to the ventral position of the meatus.

Diagnosis

Diagnosis is based on physical examination. Careful inspection of the external genitalia of all newborn males should be performed at birth.

> **NURSING TIP**
>
> **Testosterone Cream Side Effects**
>
> It is imperative to instruct caregivers about some of the side effects of the testosterone cream. Along with enlargement and growth of the male genitalia, localized acne and pubic hair may appear. Caregivers should be instructed that these side effects will resolve when the cream is discontinued.

Treatment

Treatment for hypospadias involves surgical correction of chordee and placement of the urethral meatus to the tip of the penis. Successful surgery will enable the child to void in a standing position, have a cosmetically normal appearing penis, and have a sexually adequate penis. Historically, surgery to correct hypospadias was performed in stages and involved lengthy hospitalizations and uncomfortable postoperative treatments and drains. Currently, because of advances in surgical technique, the surgery can be performed in one single outpatient procedure. In more severe cases a two-stage repair also may be performed.

Surgery is usually performed before the child is 18 months of age, prior to toilet training and the development of body image or gender identity, thus minimizing psychological trauma (Snodgrass, 2009a). Several surgical techniques are available and vary depending on the severity of the anomaly and the surgeon's preference. All techniques involve reconstruction to elongate the urethra, bring it to the tip of the penis, and straighten the chordee. The foreskin is frequently used as a graft whereby it is rolled into a tube and fashioned into a urethra. Hence, no neonatal circumcision should be performed on these infants. On occasion, the size of the penis is augmented preoperatively with testosterone cream or injections to allow for growth of the tissue and thus facilitate surgery.

Several types of dressings may be utilized postoperatively. Some may be as extensive as a compression-type dressing, most commonly a penile-wrap-type dressing, and still some others may have no application of a dressing at all. Postoperatively, a urethral stent or foley catheter may be used to facilitate urination and prevent obstruction of urine flow secondary to edema.

Nursing Management

Assessment Preoperatively, the nurse should assess the infant or child for evidence of other genitourinary defects such as undescended testes, inguinal hernia, or hydrocele. The caregivers' understanding of hypospadias, the surgical procedure, and their expectations of the appearance of the penis after surgery is investigated. The nurse needs to assess their response to having a newborn with a genital defect. Postoperatively, an assessment for adequate urinary output is essential. The nurse observes for signs of wound and urinary tract infection (e.g., penile incision for purulent drainage and excessive erythema, increase in temperature, cloudy urine with a foul odor). The infant or child is assessed for signs and symptoms of pain from incision and bladder spasms.

Nursing Diagnosis The nursing diagnoses for a child undergoing surgical hypospadias repair are similar to those for many urologic abnormalities. They include:

1. *Acute pain* related to surgical incision.
2. *Deficient knowledge (caregivers)* related to the diagnosis, surgery, postoperative care, and prognosis of hypospadias.
3. *Risk for infection* related to indwelling catheter or stents and surgical incision.

Outcome Identification

1. The child will have minimal to no pain postoperatively.
2. Caregivers will verbalize an understanding of the disorder, the surgical procedure, and prognosis, and will participate in postoperative care.
3. The child will be free of infection of the urinary tract and the incision.

Planning and Implementation Postoperative pain is usually minimal following repair of hypospadias. A dorsal or caudal nerve block provides adequate pain relief for most children; however, occasionally acetaminophen (Tylenol) may be helpful for a few days to alleviate incisional discomfort. Anticholinergics such as oxybutynin chloride (Ditropan) may be administered if ordered to alleviate bladder spasms while the urethral stent is in place. Caregivers should be informed that anticholinergic medication might cause facial flushing and dry mouth. The child should be encouraged to take in adequate fluids to maintain adequate urinary output and the patency of the stent.

Discharge instructions should include information regarding antibiotic use to prevent infections, timing of dressing and stent or Foley catheter removal, and anticipatory guidance for the caregiver and older child regarding postoperative appearance of the penis. They should understand that the penis will look bruised, wrinkled, and swollen because of the trauma, and that it will resolve in a few days to weeks.

These instructions may differ between surgeons. Some may remove the dressing in four to five days while others may maintain a larger compression dressing for longer periods depending on the severity of the hypospadias and surgical technique. If a small layered penile dressing is used, the caregiver will be instructed to have the child soak for 20 minutes in a bathtub filled to the child's waist with clear warm water prior to the appointment for removal. This allows the dressing to loosen and often fall off at home.

Complications of hypospadias repair can occur. Urethral fistula or an opening along the urethra that leaks urine to the skin surface, strictures at the anastomosis site, and retrusion of the urethral meatus to its original position have been reported. If the fistula does not resolve, repeat surgery may be indicated six months after the initial repair. However, newer surgical techniques are making a second surgery less likely (Snodgrass, 2009a).

Evaluation The child should be comfortable and participating in age-appropriate activities. The caregivers can explain the surgical intervention and the postoperative course and care involved. They are participating in their child's care. The child should not exhibit signs of UTI or incisional infection.

CRYPTORCHIDISM

Cryptorchidism or undescended testes (UDT) is defined as failure of one or both testes to descend through the inguinal canal into the scrotum (Figure 22-6). Further classification is based on whether the testis is retractable or ectopic. A retractile testis is one that has descended normally but readily retracts with physical stimulation and exam, and is often mistakenly diagnosed as UDT. An ectopic testis is one that is found outside the normal path of descent. It may be in the groin, perineum, or abdominal wall.

Incidence and Etiology

UDT is a common urologic problem. The incidence of UDT increases as the degree of prematurity increases. In full-term male newborns it is about 3% and in premature males the rate is 30% (Swierzewski, 2007). Incidence of cryptorchidism decreases with age so that by 3 months of age the incidence is 1% and 0.8% at 9 months of age. In many cases the testes descend spontaneously; however, after 1 year of age, spontaneous descent does not usually occur.

Pathophysiology

Sexually indifferent gonads are found at 3 to 5 weeks' gestation. During the seventh week of gestation the gonads begin to differentiate into a testis or ovary. A network of strands form into the seminiferous tubules; where spermatozoa are produced as the testes increase in size. During the third trimester, the testis begins its descent into the scrotum through the inguinal canal. Many theories attempt to explain the failure of the testes to descend into the scrotum including increasing abdominal pressure and hormonal influences. In the undescended testis, sperm production is decreased and may cause infertility. The child with UDT also has an increased risk for developing a malignant

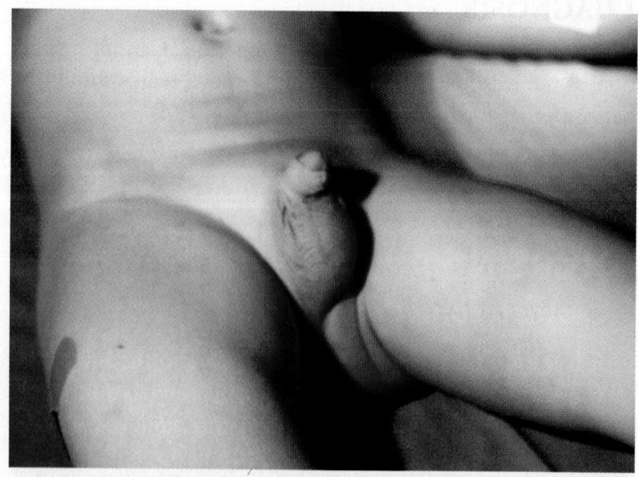

Figure 22-6 Cryptorchidism. PHOTO COURTESY OF CASIMIR FIRLIT, MD, PHD, WILLIAM E. KAPLAN, MD, MAX MAIZELS, MD, AND JEFFREY PALMER, MD, CHILDREN'S UROLOGY LTD.

testicular tumor in adulthood if not corrected. Studies are underway to determine the basis for this predisposition (Swierzewski, 2007).

Clinical Manifestations

UDT, which may be unilateral or bilateral, is unilateral in 85% of males and most often affects the right testis. One side of the scrotum (unilateral) or the entire scrotum (bilateral) appears flaccid, nonpendulous, and smaller than normal.

Diagnosis

The diagnosis of cryptorchidism involves primarily the physical examination in which the scrotum is palpated for the testis, a small nodule. It is important to perform the physical examination without stimulating the testicle to retract by the examiner having warm hands and the child being relaxed. If the testis is not palpable, ultrasound may be used to determine its location.

Treatment

Management of cryptorchidism may involve observation while awaiting spontaneous descent of the testis during the first year of life. Human chorionic gonadotropin (HCG) may also be used to stimulate testosterone production to help induce descent of the testis into the scrotum. Limited success with this technique has been reported. However, HCG does increase testicular vasculature and size thereby assisting in locating the testis either before or during surgery. Hormonal treatment may not be effective and may even preclude further ascent, thus indicating that surgery may be the better option (Snodgrass, 2009b). If the testis fails to descend spontaneously or with the administration of HCG, surgery, orchiopexy, is performed. The optimal timing for surgical correction is when the child is between 1 and 2 years of age. The goals of surgical correction are to bring the testis into the scrotum and secure it by scrotal fixation without damaging the testicle.

Nursing Management

Assessment

At birth and the first well-child visit the nurse can evaluate for the presence of both testes. By gently compressing both inguinal canals, a small nodule should be felt on both sides. The nurse should assess the caregivers' understanding of UDT and the importance of timely surgical correction.

Nursing Diagnosis

1. *Deficient knowledge (caregiver)* related to cryptorchidism and its treatment.
2. *Anxiety (caregiver)* related to the possible decreased fertility and increased risk of malignancy.

Outcome Identification

1. The caregivers will verbalize an understanding of the disorder and treatment.
2. The caregivers' anxiety will be decreased by explaining that the child should have appropriate referrals for fertility testing when appropriate and should perform testicular self-exam beginning at adolescence.

Planning and Implementation

Education of the caregiver should include clarification and reinforcement of information gleaned from the surgeon, including the use of HCG if ordered. Caregivers need simple explanations regarding how to prepare their child (if age-appropriate) for surgery and what to expect postoperatively. The issue of fertility is of great concern to the caregivers of children with UDT. Biopsies of these testes reveal histologic abnormalities including decreased number of germ cells. Sperm counts in a nondescended testis decrease proportionally with age after the second year of life. The contralateral testis even if normally positioned may also demonstrate abnormal histology. Even after successful orchiopexy, the testes may continue with decreased spermatogenesis (Snodgrass, 2009b).

Family Teaching

Nurses are helpful in teaching and preparing both the child and caregivers for surgery. If HCG therapy is utilized, the caregiver should be aware of the desired effects as well as secondary effects. For example, caregivers may express concern during this treatment when they observe increased penile growth and increased pigmentation of the scrotum as well as growth of pubic hair. Caregivers should be reassured that these side effects will dissipate after therapy is discontinued. They should also be instructed that their child will have discomfort postoperatively. Loose clothing is recommended so as not to apply pressure to the wounds immediately after surgery. Analgesics such as acetaminophen (Tylenol) and acetaminophen with codeine are routinely ordered. The child may appear to have difficulty walking related to tenderness, but this will resolve in a few days. The scrotum will appear quite edematous and ecchymotic. Caregivers need reassurance that all these are expected because of surgery but will resolve in a few days to several weeks.

Sutures and dressings are minimal. Usually dissolving sutures are utilized to close the groin and scrotal wound. Hence, the child does not require suture removal that may induce further fear and trauma. Tegaderm, or other clear plastic-type dressings, cover the groin wound and may be removed at home one week after surgery. Nurses must teach the caregiver to observe for signs of infection including increased pain, redness, swelling, and drainage from the incisions, along with fever. Frequent diaper changes and proper hygiene will reduce the risk of infections. Lastly, caregivers should be instructed to help the child avoid strenuous activity, sports, and riding toys that may be straddled until appropriate healing has taken place. The child should be instructed on testicular examination monthly once he reaches puberty to regularly evaluate and assist in early detection of tumors. Nurses are essential in assisting the caregiver to develop a supportive environment in which the child has opportunities to ask questions regarding sexuality and fertility as he becomes an adolescent.

INGUINAL HERNIA AND HYDROCELE

Inguinal hernia and hydrocele are similar disorders, both clinically and in their treatment. An inguinal hernia is a scrotal or inguinal swelling, or both, that includes the abdominal contents. A hydrocele is a collection of peritoneal fluid in the scrotal sac.

INCIDENCE

Inguinal hernias occur in children at a rate of approximately 10 to 20 per 1,000 live births (3.5% to 5% of term infants) and occur more frequently in boys than girls (ratio of 4:1) (Figure 22-7A). The incidence increases dramatically with other risk factors including prematurity and low birth weight (American Pediatric Surgical Association [APSA], 2009). The majority of infantile inguinal hernias are diagnosed in the first month of life. Hydroceles occur in approximately 6% of full-term infant boys (Figure 22-7B). Children who also present with ventriculo-peritoneal shunts and those receiving **dialysis** (treatment that acts as a filtration system outside the body to rid the body of waste products) are also at increased risk for development of hernias and hydroceles secondary to the persistence of increased intra-abdominal pressure (APSA, 2009).

ETIOLOGY AND PATHOPHYSIOLOGY

An inguinal hernia is caused by abdominal contents exiting the peritoneal cavity and protruding into the **processus vaginalis** (a fold of peritoneum that precedes the testicle as it descends through the inguinal canal into the scrotum). An incomplete or abnormal obliteration of the processus vaginalis at birth allows peritoneal fluid or abdominal contents to enter the scrotum, resulting in a hydrocele or inguinal hernia. The processus vaginalis follows the same descending pathway of the testes into the scrotum. Normally fusion of the processus vaginalis occurs spontaneously after the testis is in the scrotum (APSA, 2009).

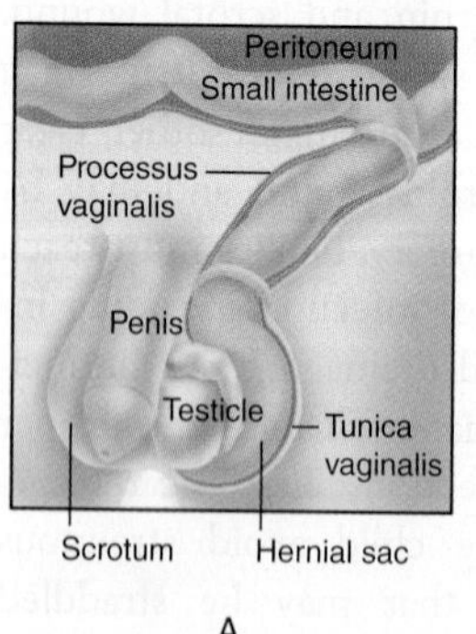

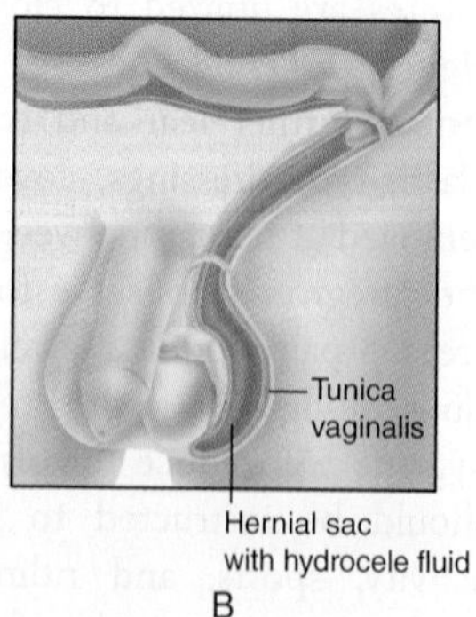

FIGURE 22-7 (A) An inguinal hernia is a scrotal or inguinal swelling, or both, that includes the abdominal contents. (B) A hydrocele is a collection of peritoneal fluid in the scrotal sac. DELMAR CENGAGE LEARNING.

CLINICAL MANIFESTATIONS

An inguinal hernia presents as a bulge or a swelling in the scrotum or groin whose size increases because of increased intra-abdominal pressure from crying or straining. Pain is usually not associated with the hernia unless it becomes strangulated. A hernia can become strangulated when the herniated intestines are trapped within the defect and become edematous and twisted. With strangulation, the blood supply to the herniated segment is cut off. There is ischemia and obstruction of the bowel, which can lead to necrosis and possible perforation. Clinical manifestations include scrotal color changes (redness), pain, intense inconsolable irritability, vomiting, abdominal distention, and tachycardia.

When a hydrocele is present, the scrotal swelling is painless and does not change in size and shape when the infant cries or coughs (Figure 22-8). It is not reducible (APSA, 2009).

DIAGNOSIS

The diagnoses of hernia and hydrocele are based on the physical examination of the scrotum and inguinal area. Differentiation between the two may be made on physical exam. Upon palpation a hernia may feel boggy and may be reduced by applying gentle upward pressure on the enlarged area of the hernia. In contrast, a hydrocele will be fluid-filled and feel more tense and is not reducible.

TREATMENT

The treatment of choice for an inguinal hernia is surgery (herniorrhapy), which is usually performed on an outpatient basis. The procedure is done through an incision in the

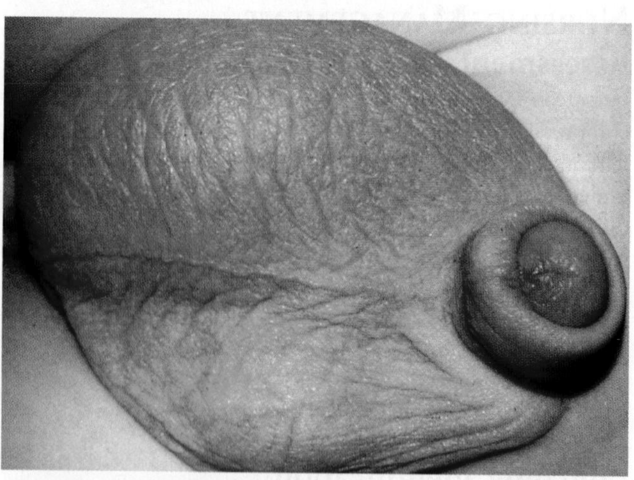

FIGURE 22-8 Hydrocele. PHOTO COURTESY OF CASIMIR FIRLIT, MD, PHD, WILLIAM E. KAPLAN, MD, MAX MAIZELS, MD, AND JEFFREY PALMER, MD, CHILDREN'S UROLOGY LTD.

inguinal crease, and the processus vaginalis is identified and ligated. The wound is often covered with a protective sealant after surgery. A hydrocele usually resolves by one year of age. However, if it does not resolve spontaneously by this time, it means a hernia is present and should be surgically repaired. The procedure is called a hydrocelectomy and is the same as for a hernia.

Nursing Management and Family Teaching

Nursing care for inguinal hernia and hydrocele focuses on teaching the caregivers about the surgical procedure, preoperative and postoperative care, and signs and symptoms of complications such as wound infection and strangulation (preoperatively). Preoperatively the nurse needs to be vigilant for signs of **incarceration** (strangulation of a portion of the bowel leading to circulation impairment and tissue necrosis). After surgery the surgical site is observed for bleeding, drainage, and recurrence of the hernia. The nurse instructs the caregivers that the infant requires frequent diaper changes to prevent infection, and that there are no activity or dietary restrictions. They should be instructed to observe the wound for signs of infection, that is, redness, elevated temperature, and drainage.

■ ACUTE GLOMERULONEPHRITIS

Acute glomerulonephritis (AGN) is an acute or sudden inflammation of the glomeruli within the kidney. This inflammation can result in acute renal failure. Because the inflammation results in damage to the glomeruli within the kidney, renal failure caused by glomerulonephritis is often referred to as intrarenal acute renal failure. It is classified further according to the exact site of the damage, for example, the glomerular capillaries or the membrane.

INCIDENCE AND ETIOLOGY

The exact incidence of AGN has been estimated at more than 470,000 cases per year with most of these cases occurring in developing countries (Carapetis, Steer, Mulholland, & Weber, 2005). AGN peaks at 7 years of age, is unusual in children younger than 3 years of age, and occurs more often in males with a ratio of 2:1. The etiology is usually an infectious agent that has been present in the body for at least two to three weeks prior to the clinical renal manifestations. There may have been other signs and symptoms that were more systemic prior to the onset of the renal manifestations.

The agents usually involved are bacterial or viral. The most common organism is group A beta-hemolytic streptococcus (GAS) (Baum, 2008). The primary site of infection is typically the throat or the skin, or in the case of Henoch-Schonlein nephritis (HSN) there is an upper-respiratory tract infection in many children that precedes the nephritis. In these cases the problem is related to an immunological response resulting in a nephritis-associated plasmin receptor (NAPlr), a GAS antigen that is present in the glomerular tissue (Rodriguez-Iturbe & Batsford, 2007). In cases following streptococcus infection the disease is referred to as acute post streptococcal glomerulonephritis (APSGN). Other causes of this condition are systemic or chronic diseases that eventually affect the glomeruli as the disease progresses, such as sickle cell anemia.

PATHOPHYSIOLOGY

Either a bacterial or viral agent invades the child's system. The immune system responds by trying to fight the infection and produces antibodies to attack the foreign antigens. This antibody-antigen reaction within the kidney glomeruli forms immune complexes against antigens such as GAS, and inflammation occurs. The end result is damaged or scarred glomeruli. Glomerular membrane permeability is altered by this immune response, thus allowing protein-including blood cells to leak into the urine. Sodium is retained within the serum along with water because of a decrease in the plasma filtration. The accumulation of water and sodium leads to edematous tissues, hypervolemia, and hypertension. The glomerular filtration rate (GFR) is slowed as the passage through the kidney gets narrower.

CLINICAL MANIFESTATIONS

The clinical manifestations of AGN are **hematuria** (presence of blood in urine), dependent and periorbital edema, diminished urinary output, proteinuria, hypertension, fatigue, diminished glomerular filtration rate, elevated serum sodium levels, and elevated potassium. Most patients have hypertension which is most likely due to fluid retention and vascular congestion (Ahn & Ingulli, 2008). All these symptoms are related to the inflammatory process, the changing permeability of the glomerular membrane, and progressive kidney damage. BUN and creatinine levels may also be elevated, and a low-grade fever may be present. Again these symptoms are related to inflammation, progressive kidney damage, and loss of protein. Urine may appear grossly bloody or just blood-tinged, smoky, or tea-colored because red blood cells are allowed to pass out of the blood into the filtrate. It is usually greatly reduced in volume depending on the degree of inflammation. Although hematuria is usually present, there is often a delay in diagnosis and treatment (Pais, Kump, & Greenbaum, 2008). If the patient is found to have proteinuria together with hematuria, there is a significantly increased likelihood of serious renal disease and prompt diagnosis is critical (Quigley, 2008).

DIAGNOSIS

The diagnosis is dependent upon the previously listed clinical manifestations including urine analysis which reveals hematuria, proteinuria, and increased specific gravity. Other diagnostic tests include the WBC with differential. This count may or may not be within normal limits depending on the length of the infection and its severity. Immunologic tests include: (1) serum complement (c3) test for complement cascade of the immune system (usually low); (2) antistreptolysin O titer which if elevated means that a streptococcal infection is or has been present; and (3) a culture of the primary site of infection such as the throat. If a culture is not possible or is negative, then the diagnosis is made on the renal symptoms, especially the presence of hematuria and the history of a prior streptococcal infection. The complement system is composed of about 20 serum proteins that assist the specific immune system to fight infection. Because there are so many proteins involved, the system responds in a cascade fashion to enhance the immune response. When infection is present, especially bacterial infection, the complement is depleted from the serum as it moves to create an inflammatory effect at the site of infection. Specific renal tests besides the serum chemistries, BUN, and creatinine might include a renal biopsy if there is no clear diagnosis from any other source of testing.

TREATMENT

Treatment depends in part on the degree of kidney damage and if the patient is symptomatic. The aims of the treatment are: to identify and treat the source of the inflammatory process, to maintain fluid and electrolyte balance, to maintain the blood pressure within the normal range, and to prevent complications. As the primary source of glomerulonephritis is usually not renal, a thorough physical examination must be done. A history of symptoms over the past few weeks must be taken. Areas to focus on include: exposures to other sick children or adults, treatment for any minor infections (including over-the-counter medications for fever or aches and pains), the respiratory system (especially the upper respiratory area), the throat for any redness or inflammation, any cough (productive or nonproductive), and respiratory difficulties that interfere with the child's normal sleep patterns.

Children with normal blood pressure and urine output can usually be managed at home. However, those with generalized edema, significant oliguria, hypertension, and gross hematuria should be hospitalized because of the possibility of developing acute renal failure, hypertensive encephalopathy, or pulmonary congestion. If the edema is generalized, it may be necessary to give diuretics. Antihypertensive agents are given for hypertension. Antibiotics are given only if there is an active bacterial infection. Dietary restrictions are based on the severity of the disorder, especially the extent of edema and hypertension. Sodium, potassium, and fluids may be restricted. The prognosis for children with APSGN is excellent, with most recovering completely.

FAMILY**TEACHING**

Home Care of the Child with Acute Glomerulonephritis

Caregivers need explanations regarding the prognosis for their child. The normal course of this disorder is one to three weeks of therapy without residual effects. They need to be taught:

- Signs of edema or worsening of the renal failure.
- Dietary and fluid restrictions such as a low sodium diet, which is essential for the care of this child if urinary output is compromised (low or absent) or edema is present.
- Skin integrity and the need for cleanliness. The caregivers are taught to observe for red areas, excessively dry areas, open areas, abrasions, or pressure areas that may appear red or bruised.
- Need to reposition the child or encourage the child's moving about at least every two hours.
- Elevation of lower extremities on a pillow when sitting in a chair. This position will decrease the chance of dependent edema and promote circulation.
- Rest periods during activities are important because the child will fatigue easily.
- Signs of dehydration and the importance of reporting them immediately to the health care provider.
- Signs of a worsening condition, which include grossly bloody urine, increased edema, increased lethargy or activity intolerance, restlessness, or any change in respiratory status. These signs would usually warrant hospitalization.

NEPHROTIC SYNDROME

Nephrotic syndrome (NS) is a clinical entity characterized by massive proteinuria and **hypoalbuminemia** (low levels of albumin in the blood) leading to edema and hyperlipidemia. NS can develop during the course of renal or systemic diseases and can be classified as either primary or secondary. Primary or idiopathic NS results from glomerular disease of the kidney. Secondary NS results in renal malfunctioning as a result of a systemic disease, drugs, or toxins such as liver malfunction, hepatitis, systemic lupus erythematosus, lead poisoning, childhood cancer or its therapies, or other diseases that ultimately put a stress on the renal system. The most common type of NS in children is primary.

INCIDENCE AND ETIOLOGY

The incidence of NS has been reported to be 2 to 7 cases per 100,000 children in the United States per year, but this

CASE STUDY / CARE PLAN

CHILD WITH NEPHROTIC SYNDROME

David is a 3-year-old Caucasian male, who was brought to the clinic by his grandmother. She reported that she and his mother have noticed that every morning his eyes are swollen and red. His hands and feet seem to be "puffy" as the day goes on. His appetite has been poor, but he has gained weight over the past few weeks according to their scale at home. His grandmother says that he has just not been acting like his usual cheerful, active self after an upper-respiratory infection four weeks ago. David appears pale and rather lethargic. Dependent and periorbital edema are evident. Vital signs are within normal limits. After a thorough physical examination and diagnostic tests, including urinalysis and blood work, it is determined he has nephrotic syndrome. Because of his edema and weight gain, he is hospitalized.

NURSING CARE PLAN

ASSESSMENT

The nursing assessment focuses on signs and symptoms of fluid overload. The child should be assessed for edema, especially in the lower extremities, genitals, and periorbital. His weight should be measured. David's skin needs to be checked for redness or other signs of pressure and breakdown, as well as for signs indicating hypovolemia or bleeding. His lungs should be auscultated for adventitious lung sounds, and increased work of breathing, indicating pulmonary fluid overload. Vital signs should be assessed, especially for elevated temperature and blood pressure.

NURSING DIAGNOSIS 1

Imbalanced fluid volume related to renal loss of protein resulting in decreased osmotic pressure and fluid shifts into interstitial spaces as evidenced by decreased urine output and edema.

EXPECTED OUTCOME

David will exhibit signs of returning fluid balance as evidenced by no proteinuria, normal serum albumin, normal urinary output, weight loss, and decreased edema.

NOC: Fluid Balance

NIC: Fluid Management

INTERVENTIONS/*RATIONALES*

1. Measure intake and output every 2 to 4 hours. *Comparisons of the intake and output will help to determine if the renal function is returning.*
2. Check urine for frothy appearance. *Frothy appearance of urine indicates proteinuria.*
3. Monitor serum and urine protein levels. *The amount of protein in the urine is an indicator of how well the kidneys are retaining protein and managing protein loss. The amount of proteinuria is also an indicator of how the disease is progressing. Serum protein levels are also helpful in monitoring progression or recovery.*
4. Weigh David daily on the same scale and with the same clothing on at the same time. *An increase in weight can indicate fluid retention in interstitial spaces. Loss of weight can mean the renal function is returning or the intake is less than body requirements.*
5. Monitor for increase in edema especially ascites and scrotal edema. Measure abdomen as indicated for changes in ascites. *Presence of edema indicates loss of protein in urine and poor renal function.*
6. Give corticosteroids as ordered. *Corticosteroids help decrease the inflammatory process that results in massive protein loss in urine. These drugs help normalize serum protein levels, restore osmotic (oncotic) pressure, and promote diuresis.*
7. Give diuretics as ordered. *Diuretics help rid the body of excess fluid.*

(Continues)

CASE STUDY / CARE PLAN (Continued)

EVALUATION

David's serum and urine protein levels moved back within normal limits. His urine output increased; his weight and edema decreased.

NURSING DIAGNOSIS 2

Imbalanced nutrition: Less than body requirements related to loss of protein in urine and by a decreased food intake.

EXPECTED OUTCOME

David will have adequate nutrition.

NOC: Nutritional Status: Food & Fluid Intake

NIC: Nutrition Management

INTERVENTIONS/*RATIONALES*

1. Offer small frequent, low sodium, well balanced meals. *Small frequent meals are more easily tolerated by sick children. Sodium restrictions may be necessary for children with nephrosis because of fluid retention, but they often make food less appealing.*
2. Give him some choices regarding foods he likes. *Giving the child some choices increases the chance he will eat.*
3. Encourage his mother and grandmother to bring low sodium foods from home. *Familiar foods are often accepted better than hospital food.*
4. Weigh the child on the same scale with the same type of clothing daily. *Daily weights will indicate if the child is losing water weight as well as weight from a decreased intake.*
5. Perform intake and output measurements every 2 to 4 hours. *Comparisons of intake and output will give an indication of how well the child is maintaining his fluid and electrolyte and nutritional balance.*

EVALUATION

David had a normal intake of food and fluids for his age and gained weight gradually according to norms after edema subsided.

NURSING DIAGNOSIS 3

Risk for infection related to impaired immunity from decreased proteins and as a side effect of corticosteroid administration.

EXPECTED OUTCOME

The child will exhibit no signs of infection as evidenced by the normal WBC count, normal vital signs including temperature.

NOC: Immune Status

NIC: Infection Protection

INTERVENTIONS/*RATIONALES*

1. Monitor for and report immediately signs of infection, such as an increase in WBC count, temperature above 101.5° F, tachycardia, and pulmonary congestion. *Careful monitoring and reporting allows for prompt treatment of infection.*

(Continues)

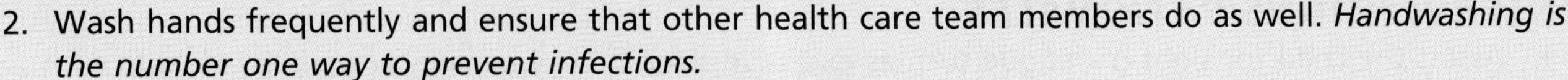

CASE STUDY / CARE PLAN (Continued)

2. Wash hands frequently and ensure that other health care team members do as well. *Handwashing is the number one way to prevent infections.*
3. Keep David away from crowds or sick individuals. *This will help prevent the spread of disease from someone with an illness to David, who is immunocompromised because of his nephrosis and treatment.*
4. Teach David's grandmother, mother and other family members to do these interventions. *David will be discharged from the hospital and his family will need to be sure and monitor for and prevent infection.*

EVALUATION

No signs of infection were noted.

NURSING DIAGNOSIS 4

Risk for impaired skin integrity related to edema and decreased activity.

EXPECTED OUTCOME

1. David will have no signs of impaired skin integrity as evidenced by no redness or other signs of skin breakdown.

NOC: Tissue integrity: Skin and mucous membranes

NIC: Skin surveillance

INTERVENTIONS/*RATIONALES*

1. Observe the skin for signs of redness or edema at least every four hours. *Assessing the skin frequently allows for early signs of impaired skin integrity to be discovered.*
2. Change position at least every two hours. *Changing the position keeps pressure sores from appearing.*
3. Give bath daily and cleanse skin as needed. *Attention to hygiene deters skin breakdown.*
4. Use lotions over areas of dry skin. *Lotions help add moisture to the skin to decrease the chance of skin breakdown.*
5. Use a support pillow under any edematous extremity. *A support pillow will increase circulation and decrease pressure points that might lead to skin breakdown.*

EVALUATION

David's skin remained intact with no signs of redness or tautness or skin breaks.

NURSING DIAGNOSIS 5

Fatigue related to disease process as evidenced by complaints of tiredness or of not wanting to play as reported by family members.

EXPECTED OUTCOME

1. The child will be able to play and engage in normal activities without complaints of fatigue.

NOC: Activity Tolerance

NIC: Exercise Promotion

(Continues)

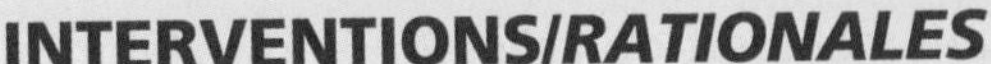

CASE STUDY / CARE PLAN (Continued)

INTERVENTIONS/*RATIONALES*

1. Assess the child for signs of fatigue such as excessive sleepiness, yawning, or inability to help with activities of daily living. *A child may show signs of fatigue in subtle ways such as sleeping more than usual, yawning, or reluctance to help with bath or feeding activities.*
2. Ask David what he wants to play with or what activities he wishes to engage in today. *A child 3 years of age usually wants to play no matter how sick he is. If he has some choice he may play more than if he was told what to do.*
3. Observe the child's ability to do activities even if these are bed games. *Observation will indicate the child's tolerance of an activity and level of fatigue.*
4. Plan for rest times throughout the day. *Scheduling in rest periods may help prevent fatigue in a child who may not be able to recognize overtiredness.*

EVALUATION

David began to show little or no signs of fatigue and was able to participate in activities as desired.

NURSING DIAGNOSIS 6

Pain related to edema as evidenced by wincing on movement.

EXPECTED OUTCOME

David's edema will subside; he will express that he is comfortable.

NOC: Comfort Level

NIC: Positioning, Calming Technique, Analgesic Administration

INTERVENTIONS/*RATIONALES*

1. Assess the child for signs of discomfort such as grimacing, crying, staying quiet, verbal complaints of pain, or reluctance to move. Use a pain scale (numbers or faces) to quantify pain. *Assessment of the child's pain level allows for early intervention to make the child more comfortable.*
2. Gently move and reposition the child every two hours if he is to remain in a bed or chair position. *Moving the child gently promotes circulation of the blood, lessens chance of pain, and helps comfort the child.*
3. Position an edematous extremity on a support pillow. *Supporting a swollen leg, arm, or scrotum will help decrease the discomfort.*
4. Keep the room quiet and at an even temperature. *A calm, moderate temperature room helps comfort the child.*

EVALUATION

David's edema subsided and he exhibited no signs of discomfort as evidenced by absence of nonverbal signs or verbal complaints.

statistic varies significantly by region. African-American, Native-American and Hispanic children have a higher incidence (Agraharkar, Gala, & Gangakhedkar, 2007). NS is slightly more common in males than females with a ratio that varies from study to study of 2:1 to 3:2 (Lane, 2008). It usually affects children between the ages of 2 and 6 years. The etiology of the primary form is believed to be an immune response. The immune response is to a glomerular disease or a systemic infection by the body that alters the structure of the glomerulus. It also results secondary to HIV infection—again relating to an immune response (Lane, 2008).

PATHOPHYSIOLOGY

Nephrotic syndrome results when there is a threat to the immune system and an inflammatory response is evoked.

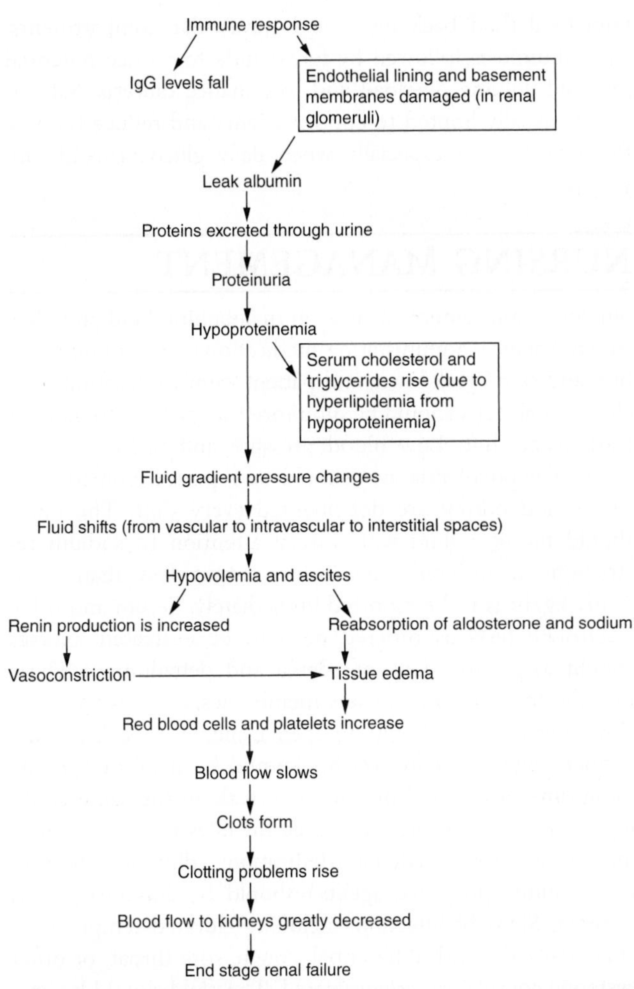

FIGURE 22-9 Pathophysiology of Nephrotic Syndrome. DELMAR CENGAGE LEARNING.

Figure 22-9 illustrates the pathophysiology of NS. The glomeruli become increasingly permeable to plasma protein resulting in massive urinary protein loss or proteinuria. Massive proteinuria is a hallmark sign resulting in hypoalbuminemia. When protein is lost, fluids shift from the intravascular to the interstitial spaces. The result is tissue edema, ascites or accumulation of fluids in the abdominal cavity, and hypovolemia. Once the volume diminishes in the vascular spaces, then renal blood flow declines and urine output diminishes. Renin production is stimulated to maintain volume and systemic pressure. The result is secretion of aldosterone which causes tubular reabsorption of sodium. Water follows the sodium leading to even more congestion and edema. Serum cholesterol and triglyceride levels rise from the stimulation of lipoprotein production in the liver in the face of hypovolemia and falling serum protein levels. This stimulation is an attempt to make up for the lost proteins and is seen in conditions of starvation. If immunoglobulin levels are monitored, IgG levels are diminished. As blood volume falls, hemoconcentration causes an increase in red blood cells and platelets. The net result is a slowing of the blood flow and ultimately the clumping or clotting of red blood cells and platelets. That coupled with protein losses puts the child at risk for coagulation or clotting problems.

CLINICAL MANIFESTATIONS

These children exhibit some of the same symptoms as any other child with renal failure. Edema is usually the first clinical feature (Lane, 2008). Initially, it is often mild, being periorbital in the early morning hours and becoming more generalized after the child has been ambulatory. Anorexia, abdominal pain or tenderness caused by the inflammation of the kidney, abdominal swelling, fatigue, history of recent respiratory infection, increased weight or rapid weight gain, and vital signs (initially including blood pressure) within the normal range may also be noted. Hyperlipidemia is also present and most likely due to increased hepatic lipid metabolism in response to hypoproteinemia (Tang et al., 2007).

DIAGNOSIS

The diagnosis is dependent upon proteinuria. Serum albumin levels are diminished (hypoalbuminemia). Laboratory evaluation includes urinalysis for protein, red blood cell casts, serum albumin (2.5 g/dl—hypoalbuminemia), serum cholesterol, triglycerides, hemoglobin, hematocrit, platelet count, electrolytes, BUN, and creatinine. Complement levels and antistreptolysin O (ASO) titer, are done to rule out other glomerular diseases. The presence of proteinuria and red blood cells indicates kidney inflammation. The rise in serum cholesterol, triglycerides (in the face of falling hemoglobin), hematocrit, and platelet count indicates some problem with hypoproteinemia in the serum. The serum electrolytes will be altered as renin and aldosterone levels change and sodium is reabsorbed. The BUN and creatinine rise if kidney function fails.

TREATMENT

Treatment focuses on reducing proteinuria, controlling edema, and preventing infection. The mainstay of treatment is corticosteroid therapy with prednisone and prednisolone (Prelone) in order to obtain a remission. Corticosteroids decrease the inflammation and the loss of proteins, thus restoring oncotic pressure and promoting diuresis. Oral preparations of prednisolone allow for accurate dosing and increased palatability in young children. A typical protocol is to start with a high dose of either drug (2 mg/kg/day; maximum of 80 mg/day). Treatment is continued until the child becomes free of proteinuria or for a period of at least three months (Hodson, Willis, & Craig, 2009a). The medication is gradually tapered over a period of several weeks and then stopped as long as the child remains asymptomatic. However, the rate of relapse is high, 60% to 70%, and is often triggered by viral upper respiratory infections. Relapse is

NURSING TIP

Terms Used to Define Response to Treatment

Remission is achieved when a urine dipstick measures negative or trace proteinuria for three days or urinary protein excretion is less than 4 mg/m²/hr. Relapse is defined as a urine dipstick measurement of 2 + proteinuria or more for three days or a child found to have 3 to 4 + proteinuria plus edema.

treated with a short course of high-dose daily steroids until the child is free of proteinuria for three days (Abeyagunawardena & Trompeter, 2008). Diuretics, although not always effective, can sometimes be used when edema is especially severe and causes respiratory compromise. When there is failure to respond to steroid therapy or when side effects are troublesome, other immunosuppressant medications are given. These include cyclophosphamide (Cytoxan), chlorambucil (Leukeran), or cyclosporin (Sandimmune) (Hodson, Willis, & Craig, 2009b). If an infection develops as a result of long-term steroidal use, an antibiotic is ordered. Other complications of treatment include thrombosis and renal failure (Lane, 2008).

Diuretics, such as furosemide (Lasix), should not be used to treat mild degrees of edema; however, they may be used if the child has severe edema. Because diuretics can precipitate hypovolemia, hyponatremia, and hypokalemia, electrolyte levels should be monitored closely. The use of potassium-sparing diuretics, such as spironolactone (Aldactone), may help limit hypokalemia (Lane, 2008). Albumin may be given if the edema is marked and causes the child to have decreased mobility, poor oral intake, or decreased urine output. Albumin helps to restore normal plasma oncotic pressure and promotes the movement of interstitial fluid back into the intravascular compartments. The albumin is followed by furosemide to reduce potential for fluid volume overload and to enhance diuresis. Salt intake is usually limited to control edema and reduce the risk for hypertension especially when daily glucocorticoids are given.

NURSING MANAGEMENT

Nursing management focuses on maintaining fluid and electrolyte balance, administering medications, preventing infection and skin breakdown, and patient/family education. The child's vital signs should be monitored every four hours or at least every shift. Low blood pressure and tachycardia are signs of hypovolemia and should be reported immediately. Intake and output are documented every shift. The nurse should monitor fluid with special attention to sodium restrictions if ordered. Any urine output less than 1 to 2 mL/kg/hr is to be reported immediately. Serum and urine electrolyte tests as ordered need to be evaluated. Nurses should assess for signs of edema and dehydration. These include dry skin, dry mucous membranes, poor skin turgor, slowed capillary refill, pitting edema, sunken eyeballs, or dependent edema. Daily weights should be measured at the same time of day and on the same scale in the same clothing. Assessment of breath sounds for rales or wheezes may indicate pulmonary edema. Medications (diuretics, steroids, or immunosuppressive agents) should be administered as ordered. Signs of infection, including elevated temperature, changing CBC with differential, cough, sore throat, or other systemic complaints, are evaluated. The child should be protected from visitors, personnel, or other clients who may have infections. Nurses should use good handwashing while caring for the child, and give antibiotics as ordered to prevent or treat infection. The child's skin needs to be protected from breakdown especially if edema is present. The child should be repositioned every two hours. The nurse should place an edematous extremity on a pillow or other support making sure the circulation is not impeded. Skin

Reflections from Families

We were so worried about the use of steroids with our son Adam, who is 4 years old. We had heard all the bad things that can happen with steroids. For example, his health care provider had talked about such things as depression of the immune system, which could put him at risk for infection, growth retardation, and bone demineralization. Will these drugs put Adam at risk for infection? Will they stop his bones from growing? Will his bones become brittle and break easily?

NURSING ALERT

The Appetite-Stimulating Effect of Steroids

A side effect of steroids in some children is a ravenous appetite, which causes them to gain a significant amount of weight. Nurses should provide explanations to caregivers and the child, if age-appropriate, about the appetite-stimulating effects of these medications. Recommendations should be made for a nutritious, relatively low-fat diet with age-adjusted daily allowances of protein, carbohydrates, and other components.

should be assessed for areas of redness or discoloration. For boys with edematous scrotums, padding and support to this area should be provided.

FAMILY TEACHING

Nurses should explain to caregivers what is known about nephrotic syndrome and its expected course. Caregivers should be allowed to ask questions and to express their feelings. Nurses must teach caregivers how to perform urine dipstick protein level measurements and the importance of measuring and recording the readings daily. They should be instructed to obtain daily weights for their child. The nurse needs to explain how important their role is in identifying relapses, the first signs of which are increases in weight and levels of protein in the urine. Caregivers should be taught about steroids and their immunosuppressive action and the need to protect their child against infection. They also need to know that steroids can increase appetite, and may benefit from having a nutritionist consultation prior to discharge to help with the child's diet.

Caregivers should be instructed to notify the health care provider if the child is exposed to chickenpox if he or she has not had the disease or the vaccine. Live viral vaccines should not be given to children receiving high doses of steroids or other immunosuppressive medications, and caregivers need to be cautioned about this.

HEMOLYTIC UREMIC SYNDROME

Hemolytic uremic syndrome (HUS), an acute renal disease, is the most frequent cause of acute renal failure (ARF) in children.

INCIDENCE AND ETIOLOGY

Though relatively uncommon, HUS gained attention after children acquired the disorder as a result of an *Escherichia coli* (*E. coli*) infection from eating contaminated beef. It is more prevalent in developing countries where sanitation and the undercooking of meats are a problem. It is most common in children younger than 2 to 3 years. The incidence in children under 5 years of age is highest (6.1 per 100,000) with an overall incidence (all ages) of 0.5 to 2.1 per 100,000. Incidence peaks in the summer and fall (Parmar, 2008). It occurs equally in both sexes. The exact etiology of HUS has not been determined, but it is thought to be associated with bacterial toxins, viruses, drugs, and especially chemotherapeutic agents (Camp-Sorrell, 2008) and chemicals. The organisms involved include *E. coli*, shigella, rickettsia, coxsackievirus, ECHO virus, adenovirus, pneumococci, and salmonella. There seems to be a genetic predisposition to some types.

PATHOPHYSIOLOGY

The pathophysiology of HUS is complex. The most frequently seen sequence is a bacterial invasion of the gastrointestinal tract leading to vomiting and diarrhea. The bacteria cling to the intestinal mucosa where they quickly multiply. Intestinal peristaltic action is slowed. An endotoxin is produced from the bacteria. An inflammatory response is created that leads to capillary wall damage and occlusion of the surrounding blood vessels by microthrombi. Hemolysis of red blood cells occurs. This same reaction occurs within the renal vasculature deep in the glomerular arterioles. The endothelial lining of the affected tissues swell, and platelets move to the injured site. This move results in clot formation and intravascular coagulation. In HUS, the platelet clot or aggregate slows the blood flow through the renal system. Renin production is stimulated resulting in systemic hypertension. The platelet count falls as these platelets are damaged in the same manner as the red blood cells and the result is thrombocytopenia (less than 100,000/mL) which lasts one to two weeks. When the vessels of the glomeruli are affected, the result is a lowered glomerular filtration rate; eventually urine output is lower, and acute renal failure with hypertension follows. Clot formation and the inflammatory process can occur in any organ of the body, although it is most common in the gastrointestinal, respiratory, and genitourinary systems.

CLINICAL MANIFESTATIONS

The clinical manifestations of HUS are a triad of symptoms, which include acute renal failure, thrombocytopenia, and anemia. The prodromal symptoms are gastrointestinal with diarrhea and vomiting or an upper respiratory infection. The history may include bloody diarrhea, decreased urinary output, and slight abdominal pain. Once the hemolytic process starts, it may last from a few days to two weeks. The child becomes progressively more irritable, lethargic, and anorectic. Soon the child experiences anemia, and as it worsens, pallor increases, the hematocrit falls, and urine output diminishes. As the platelet count falls, there is increased chance of bleeding, bruising, and purpura. As renal blood flow becomes more restricted with clot formation, renin is secreted and fluids are retained leading to hypertension. Upon physical examination, hepatosplenomegaly (the enlargement of the liver and spleen) may be present. Edema, hypertension, abdominal tenderness, and pain are the common manifestations. There may be altered levels of consciousness or seizure activities reported especially if calcium, phosphorus, and other serum electrolyte levels are outside normal limits. Toxins normally cleared from the kidneys build up and the tubular reabsorption or excretion of sodium and potassium are altered. The result is an adverse effect on the central nervous system leading to seizures and altered consciousness.

DIAGNOSIS

Mild proteinuria may be present. Serum creatinine and blood urea nitrogen levels are elevated. CBC will indicate anemia and thrombocytopenia. Other coagulation studies may be done. A stool culture may also be done to determine presence of *E. coli* and shigella bacteria (Parmar, 2008).

TREATMENT

Primarily the treatment is symptomatic. If the serum electrolytes are outside normal limits and renal failure is severe, hemo- or peritoneal dialysis or fluid restriction may be necessary to raise the serum sodium levels that have fallen because of dilutional or volume overload. Dialysis is most often reserved for those children who are **anuric** (without urine output) for 24 hours or have oliguria and are extremely hypertensive, hyperkalemic, or experiencing seizures. If the serum potassium level is high because of a decreased excretion of this ion by the renal system, a Kayexalate enema or nasogastric solution may be given. Serum glucose levels may also be low because of increased metabolic needs; therefore, dextrose or total parenteral nutrition must be given. If the pancreas has been affected by clot formation, the insulin production may be altered. Some children may develop hyperglycemia and must receive insulin therapy.

Calcium and phosphorous levels are affected with calcium falling and phosphorus rising. Calcium is excreted by the kidney and reabsorbed in the tubules. It is also dependent on intestinal function and transport across the epithelial tissue. In HUS these systems fail resulting in decreased calcium with the rebound of phosphorus, which is normally filtered by the kidney. Either calcium gluconate or calcium chloride can be given depending on institutional policy or health care providers' preference. Treatment for hypertension is accomplished with hydralazine (Apresoline) and captopril (Capoten). The child may also be in metabolic acidosis from the inability of the kidney to buffer acids normally produced in the body, and may require bicarbonate therapy. If there are central nervous system symptoms, such as altered consciousness or seizures, a central venous line may be placed for central venous pressure (CVP) monitoring. If the bleeding has been severe or the blood counts are low, then blood transfusions with fresh, packed red blood cells are given. Any time that fluids are given, even in the form of packed cells, fluid overload must be considered and prevented, if possible. Some institutions will give plasma products to these children to avoid the increased volume needed with packed red blood cells. Oral feedings may be resumed once the vomiting and diarrhea are controlled. More than 85% of children with HUS recover with normal renal function (Parmar, 2008). However, there is potential for the development of chronic renal failure.

NURSING MANAGEMENT

Nursing management focuses on maintaining renal function and fluid and electrolyte balance, and providing family support. Nurses should assess the child for signs of dehydration: increased temperature, pulse, respirations, falling blood pressure, decreased peripheral perfusion, dry skin and mucous membranes, decreased urine output with a rising urine specific gravity, and poor skin turgor. Intake and output should be documented at least every four hours. If the child is in intensive care, this may be done every one to two hours. Nurses should check weights daily and administer fluids as ordered. Serum electrolytes, BUN, creatinine, Hct, Hgb, WBC, and arterial blood gases should be monitored. If the child experiences any central nervous system symptoms, a central venous catheter may be placed to measure this pressure. If it measures 15 or greater, dialysis may be necessary. A cardiorespiratory monitor should be placed on the child. Attention should be paid to any changes in EKG tracings, such as a peaked T wave (related to potassium increase) and a widened QRS complex, or signs of heart block.

The child is assessed for signs of fluid overload: tachycardia, tachypnea, hypertension, visible edema, and increased pulmonary secretions. Upon auscultation of the lungs, rales or wheezes may be heard. Oxygen may be required to support ventilation. Chest X-rays should be done to determine any pulmonary edema or cardiomegaly.

The child is evaluated for signs of bleeding or injury related to thrombocytopenia, and any signs of petechiae, bleeding, excessive bruising, or rashes are documented. Any invasive procedures should be avoided when possible, such as injections and rectal temperatures. Nurses should monitor vital signs for changes from baseline, and assess neurologic status, including increasing restlessness, irritability, or lethargy; difficulty in arousal; or decreased sensation to touch or pain.

Nurses should assess the child for signs of possible increased intracranial pressure. These include: changes in level of consciousness; inability to respond appropriately to verbal cues, touch, or pain; bulging fontanels; and changes in movements of the extremities or a decreased muscle tone in one or all four extremities. Pupillary changes or seizure activity should be noted also. The head of the bed should be elevated at least 30 degrees, and the room should be quiet and without excessive lights. If the neurologic status is impaired and the central venous pressure is rising, hypotonic IV solutions should be avoided. Osmotic diuretics should also be avoided as they add to problems of hypervolemia caused by fluid shifts.

Nurses should assess for gastrointestinal disturbances, document any vomitus and stools and describe the characteristics, and auscultate for bowel sounds. If none are present, a nasogastric tube may need to be placed to assist with gastric decompression. Antacids are used if the gastric pH is less than 5. Once feeding can be tolerated, small frequent feedings should be started and increased as tolerated.

FAMILY TEACHING

The caregivers may feel guilty that they missed something and did not know their child was so sick. They need reassurance that the symptoms are very subtle. They should be told as much of the pathophysiology as is known and helped to understand the normal course of HUS. They should be encouraged to participate in their child's care.

RENAL FAILURE

Renal failure refers to a condition that adversely affects the kidney, resulting in decreased functioning of this organ system. It may take two main forms: acute or chronic.

ACUTE RENAL FAILURE

Acute kidney injury (AKI), formerly known as acute renal failure (ARF), is a sudden onset of impaired renal function. Most children with AKI regain renal function. AKI is classified according to the part of the renal system that is affected. Three main types of causes of AKI are prerenal, intrarenal, and postrenal.

Incidence

AKI is uncommon in children, but it can be life-threatening when it does develop. The exact incidence is unknown, but there does seem to be a rise in the number of hospitalized children who develop AKI (Andreoli, 2009). It is associated with many disorders such as ischemic insults, exposure to drugs, an underlying infection, or HUS. Although it can be reversible, some types progress to chronic kidney disease.

Etiology and Pathophysiology

AKI is characterized by reversible damage to the kidney that results in increased serum creatinine and urea nitrogen, both breakdown products of protein, and problems with fluid and electrolyte imbalance (Andreoli, 2009). Renal injury can be categorized into three types of renal failure: prerenal failure, intrarenal failure (intrinsic renal disease), or postrenal failure (obstructive uropathies).

Prerenal failure is characterized by a sudden decrease in renal blood flow or perfusion to the kidneys. This type of renal failure can result from dehydration, hypovolemia or shock, sepsis, burns, heart failure, renal artery obstruction, or perinatal asphyxia. *Intrarenal* failure is associated with damage to the tissues of the kidney. The causes are secondary to antibiotic therapy (aminoglycosides or other nephrotoxic medications), contrast dyes, glomerulonephritis, pyelonephritis, hemolytic uremic syndrome, or other infections that affect renal tissue. *Postrenal* failure results from an obstruction of urine at some point between the kidney and the urinary meatus. It is usually an outflow obstruction that causes a "back-up" of urine within the kidney, putting pressure on the endothelial lining and ultimately diminishing renal function. The causes of postrenal failure that can occur in utero or during postnatal life are:

- Posterior ureteral valves
- **Ureterovesical obstruction**—an obstruction at the junction of the ureters into the bladder
- **Ureteropelvic obstruction**—an obstruction at the junction of the ureters into the renal pelvis
- Neurogenic bladder, primarily one without innervation
- Wilms tumor—a nephroblastoma or solid mass, which is the most common renal tumor in children
- Renal calculi

Clinical Manifestations

The most common clinical manifestations are oliguria, fluid and electrolyte imbalance, metabolic acidosis, and signs of dehydration or edema that result from the kidneys' inability to maintain balance. Pallor, listlessness, lethargy, anorexia, vomiting, and in some cases seizures may also be observed. The child's vital signs may or may not be within normal limits depending upon the cause and duration of the renal dysfunction. The child may have dependent, pitting, or periorbital edema. There may be hypertension accompanying the edema. This hypertension is caused by volume overload and the buildup of edema. As the blood flow to the kidneys decreases, renin production increases leading to vasoconstriction. The heart works harder to pump the blood, thus raising the blood pressure. Pulmonary edema occurs in some children presenting with increasing respiratory distress.

Diagnosis

The diagnosis is based on history, laboratory evaluation, and physical examination. Anuria or a urine output of 1 mL/kg/hr is a potential finding, although some children will have a normal volume of urinary output. Renal serum panel usually reveals a rising BUN and creatinine; serum electrolytes, especially sodium and potassium, may also be elevated and life-threatening. As the renal blood flow falls, the glomerular filtration rate falls, and the amount of sodium that is filtered by the kidney diminishes. Although more research is needed, several genetic biomarkers show promise for earlier detection of AKI (Bunchman, 2008).

Treatment

The aims of the treatment for the child with acute kidney injury renal failure are to increase renal perfusion, to restore

NURSING TIP

Nephrotoxicity

Many medications including antibiotics, such as aminoglycosides (gentamicin and vancomycin), and nonsteroidal anti-inflammatory drugs, for example, are detoxified and excreted through the kidneys. These medications, when given in the presence of diminished renal function or dehydration, can be nephrotoxic (Patzer, 2008; John, Saroha, & Jones, 2008). Always question the health care practitioner or nurse practitioner when a medication should be given if renal output is low. Peak and trough levels of these medications must be monitored to determine if the levels are rising, indicating that renal clearance is impeded.

and maintain fluid, electrolyte, and acid-base balance, to minimize complications, and to promote nutrition (Andreoli, 2008). This treatment may be with or without renal replacement therapy (RRT). The treatment without RRT is as follows: If the sodium level is too high and edema is present, fluid and sodium restriction are necessary. If the potassium level is too high, then polystyrene sodium sulfonate (Kayexalate) orally or per rectum is given. This resin binds potassium in the intestine and removes it from the body. If metabolic acidosis is present, treatment is sodium bicarbonate to replace the lacking renal buffer. Sometimes diuretics are used to increase urine output and limit kidney damage (Andreoli, 2009).

If these interventions do not control the fluid and electrolyte balance, or pulmonary edema or heart failure is present, then RRT must be considered. Other indications for RRT are severe systemic hypertension, a BUN 0.120 mg/dl, hyperkalemia, increasing metabolic acidosis, or change in mental status. There are three main modalities of RRT: hemodialysis, peritoneal dialysis, and continuous hemofiltration (Andreoli, 2008; Bunchman, 2008).

Renal Replacement Therapy

Hemodialysis is an RRT using a hemofiltration system that occurs outside the body. An arteriovenous (AV) fistula, shunt, or external access device is required to be placed in a large vessel. This central line provides access to the circulatory system to pump the blood out from the body to an extracorporeal circuit and through a filtration system. This serves to remove the body's waste products that can no longer be effectively filtered through the kidneys. These access devices require surgical placement and the nurse must use aseptic techniques when caring for them. Hemodialysis can be performed on an intermittent time-cycled basis, either in a hospital, dialysis center, or home setting. It is usually a 3- to 4-hour procedure repeated three to four times per week. It is more efficient at removing nitrogenous wastes than any other form of dialysis.

Peritoneal dialysis requires the placement of a catheter into the peritoneal cavity for the purposes of removing excess fluids, solutes, and nitrogenous wastes (Figure 22-10). This placement may or may not require an open surgical procedure. It usually does not require a heparinized line. The treatment or filtration process involves the slow flow of fluid through the catheter into the peritoneal cavity until the desired fluid level has been administered. At that time a clamp is put in place allowing the fluid to dwell for a time in the peritoneal cavity to remove waste products. When the clamp is released, the fluid drains into the dialysis system. This cycle is repeated either automatically or manually four to five times per day. The procedure is usually repeated for several days and is normally done at home. Advantages of different types of continuous peritoneal dialysis over hemodialysis in children include less need for rigid fluid restriction, more food choices, and better ability to maintain

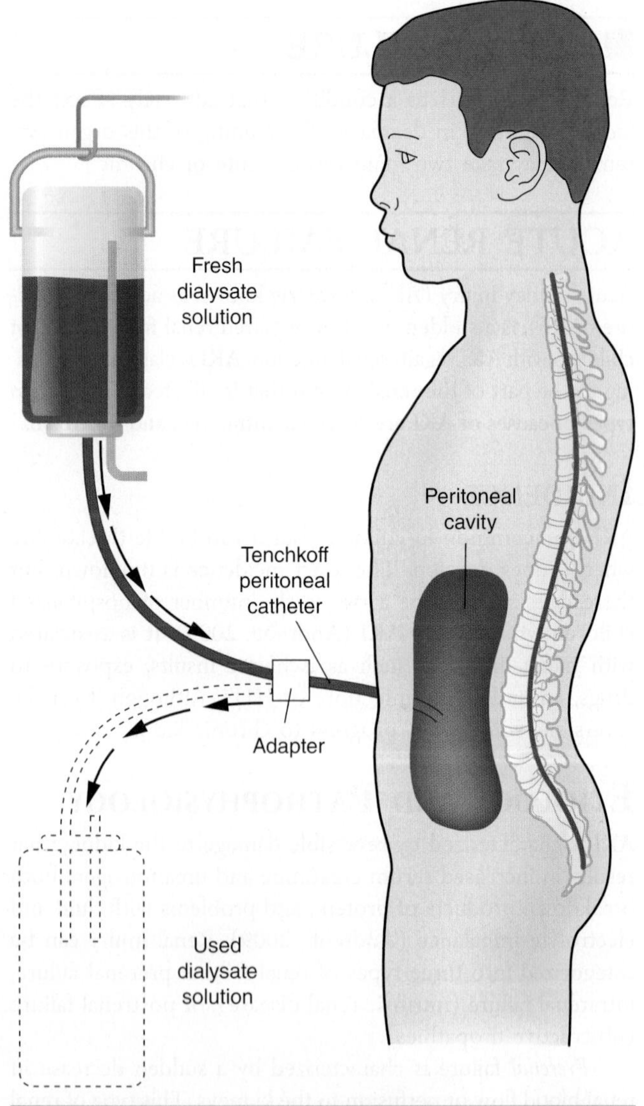

FIGURE 22-10 Peritoneal Dialysis Setup. DELMAR CENGAGE LEARNING.

normal activity levels. Peritoneal dialysis is problematic for infants requiring dialysis, as the clearance of toxic wastes, solutes, and fluids is slow. Their abdominal areas are small and, if the treatment is not successful, the hypervolemia may be worse, a condition not tolerated well by small infants.

Hemofiltration is a continuous form of dialysis. Continuous renal replacement therapy (CRRT), a form of hemofiltration, was developed because of disadvantages of traditional dialysis and has increased in use over the past few years (Bunchman, 2008). CRRT is used in patients who have difficulty handling large fluid and electrolyte shifts since its action is slower and gentler than hemodialysis. Several forms of CRRT exist including continuous arteriovenous hemofiltration (CAVH) and continuous venovenous hemofiltration (CVVH). All types of CRRT involve the cannulation of either arteries or veins providing vascular access through which blood is removed from the body, filtered, and then returned again. Outside the body, blood is gently and continuously filtered of excess fluid, electrolytes, and nitrogenous wastes using a semipermeable membrane. If an arteriovenous shunt is used (CAVH), the client's own blood pressure is enough to circulate the blood throughout the hemofiltration system. If two veins are used (CVVH), a pump is required to move the blood throughout the circuitry. Specially trained hemodialysis nurses are not needed to care for the child receiving CRRT, although the procedure is done in intensive care. Critical care nurses carefully monitor fluid and electrolyte balance and watch for problems such as hemorrhage, clotting, air embolism, and hypothermia. It has been the perception that continuous gentle filtering of blood is tolerated better by patients because they experience fewer episodes of hemodynamic instability than they do on hemodialysis. However, a recent literature review indicated that there were no significant differences in kidney tissue death or survival between intermittent hemodialysis and CRRT. More research is needed in this area related to long-term outcomes (Centre for Reviews & Dissemination, 2009). If rapid fluid, electrolyte, or toxin removal is necessary, hemodialysis or peritoneal dialysis is the method of choice. When any form of dialysis is used, there are risks. Morbidity and mortality for children on dialysis are most often related to bleeding, infection, or vessel blockage.

CRITICAL THINKING

Dialysis

1. What is the purpose of dialysis?
2. What are the differences among hemodialysis, peritoneal dialysis, and CRRT?
3. What are the advantages and disadvantages of each of these modalities?
4. Why is intraperitoneal bleeding a potential complication with peritoneal dialysis?

Nursing Management

This section will be divided into two parts. The first will be for the child and family that do not require dialysis but is experiencing acute renal failure. The second part will be for the child and family with acute renal failure who requires dialysis. The nursing care for both groups of children is aimed at restoring and maintaining fluid and electrolyte balance. In addition, for the child and family undergoing dialysis, the focus is also on maintaining the integrity of the circuit, protecting the child from bleeding at the shunt site, and preventing injury or infection. For both groups of children, a thorough history must be taken to elicit the underlying cause of the acute renal failure. Questions should focus on those conditions described as potential etiologies of prerenal, intrarenal, and postrenal acute renal failure, such as: have there been any previous periods of dehydration, urinary tract infections, episodes of low oxygen levels as with a premature infant, any antibiotic therapy, or renal stones? Physical examination, initially and subsequently, includes vital signs, weight, intake and output, urine specific gravity, and laboratory values, especially BUN and creatinine. The remainder of the nursing management is the same as that described for the child with nephrotic syndrome.

Family Teaching

Fear and anxiety are very real emotions for caregivers of a child with acute kidney injury. They need honest and thorough explanations about what is known about the cause and

REFLECTIVE THINKING

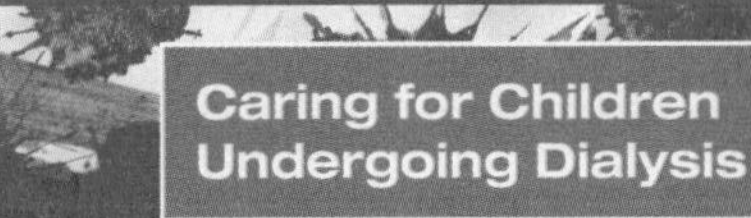

Caring for Children Undergoing Dialysis

To increase self-awareness about children undergoing dialysis, ask yourself:

1. How do I feel about caring for children undergoing dialysis?
2. Is my care affected by the child's appearance? (The child may be edematous with very shiny, taut skin, or have a moon face and be very pale.)
3. Do I spend less time interacting with these children because I feel uncomfortable?
4. How do I ensure that these children receive the same quality of care as those children who do not have a chronic illness or life-threatening disease?

KIDS WANT TO KNOW

What is a renal ultrasound and will it hurt?

A 10-year-old girl with a diagnosis of acute renal failure is scheduled for a renal ultrasound. Before the scan she asks, "What will the scan do to me? Will it hurt?"

The young girl is old enough to probably know what a computer scan is but may not have any concept of what or how a renal scan is done. You can reply by explaining that the scan will not hurt, how the picture is taken, and that the machine will move over her. She may be afraid she has to be sent through a machine for the picture to be taken. Honest answers may calm her fears.

the expected course of the illness. They need time to express their feelings. They may benefit from referrals to clergy or to support groups, especially if the treatment will be prolonged. Encourage them to participate in the child's care as they feel comfortable.

For the child and family undergoing dialysis, teaching regarding treatments, home care and what they will experience is essential. Family teaching should include the following:

- How to give medications (doses, times, methods of administration, what to do if a dose is missed).
- How to recognize signs of infection or the worsening of the renal problem and what to do about it (such as calling the health care provider). Signs to be reported would include weight gain caused by edema, headache that could indicate hypertension, changes in level of consciousness caused by retention of by-products of metabolism, flank pain, fever, sore throat, or flu-like symptoms that would indicate infection and decreased urine output that would indicate deterioration of renal function.
- How to maintain meticulously clean care of the catheter or graft site and to protect the child from infection, including teaching the child about good handwashing and to stay away from other children who have obvious colds, flu, or other infections.
- How to maintain the routine schedule or cycling of the dialysis, either at the clinic or in the home.
- Why it is necessary to have available telephone contact and running water if dialysis is to be done at home. The electric company as well as the police and fire departments need to be notified to make sure that power is restored immediately to this family in case of electrical failure. A backup generator should also be available in the home to be used until power can be restored in the event of a power outage.
- Why it is important for the child to eat a low-protein diet if this is to be maintained at home.
- How to incorporate activity for the child as tolerated each day.
- How to talk about the child's renal disease with teachers or friends.

If the child is school age, caregivers need to be encouraged to promote the child's discussion of fears, concerns about peers, and any self-esteem or body-image issues he or she may have. If the nurse notes signs of depression or severe anxiety in the child or caregivers, a mental health consultation may be necessary. This child and family will require a great deal of emotional support and referrals to resource groups such as the National Kidney Foundation or local support groups are quite helpful.

CHRONIC RENAL FAILURE AND END STAGE RENAL DISEASE

Chronic renal failure (CRF) is a progressive disease. The damage that is done to the renal system in some cases is irreversible. This condition is considered chronic when approximately 50% of the renal function remains or when the glomerular filtration rate is less than 60 mL/min (normal is 125 mL/min) and the condition has lasted for at least three months (Drawz & Mahboob, 2009). If it is considered to be permanent and irreversible, then it is classified as end stage renal disease (ESRD). All chronic renal failure will first progress to uremia. **Uremia** is a condition in which toxic nitrogenous waste products, blood urea, and creatinine buildup in the system. If this condition is not reversed, it progresses to ESRD.

Incidence and Etiology

The incidence of CRF has been estimated to be between 1.5 and 3.0 per million in the pediatric population; however, the exact figures are difficult to determine due to the multitude of underlying conditions that can result in CRF. The etiology of CRF and ESRD varies but may be caused by prematurity, use of nephrotoxic medications such as aminoglycosides, genetic syndromes with congenital urinary or renal obstructions, hemolytic uremic syndrome, glomerulonephritis, pyelonephritis, and other systemic infections. Some children experience CRF or ESRD as a result of immunologic dysfunction that causes actual injury to renal tissue. Others have chronic systemic diseases such as lupus or diabetes that lead to renal failure.

Pathophysiology

The exact pathophysiology depends on the etiology of the condition that began to disrupt the kidney function. In any case, eventually the renal system is compromised, as is renal blood flow through the kidney, leading to loss of oxygen to the tissues and ultimately to destruction of portions of the nephron. The nephron is the working unit of the kidney and functions to create urine, filter substances through the kidney, and reabsorb and excrete solutes in the body. The nephron is composed of the glomerulus and the renal tubule. Nephrons once destroyed cannot be regenerated. As portions of the nephrons die, renal function becomes less efficient. The remaining nephrons attempt to take over complete function so they hypertrophy. The glomerular pressure increases, as does the arterial pressure in the glomerular capillaries and renal arteries. Eventually the glomeruli sclerose and die. If this cycle is not stopped and the arterial pressure lowered, ESRD results.

Clinical Manifestations

As with acute renal failure, the main clinical manifestations of CRF and ESRD include fluid and electrolyte imbalance, dehydration or edema, metabolic acidosis, and systemic hypertension. The child may also experience anemia, pallor, fatigue, anorexia, vomiting, slowed linear growth, organic failure to thrive, and chronic kidney disease-mineral bone disorder. This new term is used to describe a systemic abnormality of bone and mineral metabolism and extra-skeletal calcification seen in children with chronic renal disease (Sanchez, 2008). Patients with CRF also frequently have alterations in lipid metabolism that result in dyslipidemia and can increase risk of cardiovascular disease (Kastarinen et al., 2009; Vaziri, 2006).

Diagnosis

The diagnosis is based on the history of either long-standing renal problems or growth problems accompanied by altered laboratory values. The child's presentation may be one of dehydration, edema, hypertension, electrolyte imbalance, altered calcium, phosphorus ratios, elevated serum BUN, creatinine levels, decreased creatinine clearance, low hematocrit and hemoglobin, and long bone X-rays revealing mineral bone disorder. Pallor, lethargy, anorexia, and vomiting may or may not be present.

Treatment

Treatment for the child with CRF and ESRD is aimed at restoring or maintaining fluid and electrolyte balance. If edema is present, then fluid restriction and sodium and potassium restriction may be necessary. Diuretics are used if edema is significant. Antihypertensive medications are given if hypertension is present. Protein intake may be restricted because of the kidney's inability to rid the body of waste products, although a recent review of research indicates that restricting protein in children with CRF does not significantly impact the progression of their disease to ESRD (Chaturvedi, 2007). Phosphorus is restricted in order to increase the calcium levels. If calcium levels are maintained, then there is less chance of bone disease that can result when calcium levels are low. Vitamin D supplementation may be given. The result is that vitamin D will be present to boost the calcium levels to prevent bone disease. Calcium-based phosphate-binders (Tums, PhosLo) may be given to bind with phosphorus and decrease the gastrointestinal absorption. Aluminum-based phosphate binders should not be used because aluminum levels can become high and result in seizures.

Other therapies include erythropoietin to combat anemia and growth hormone to boost linear growth. Immunosuppressive therapy is also used, especially if the child is going to require renal transplantation. While this immunosuppressive therapy is not experimental, the combination of medications (more than one immunosuppressive medication at a time) is undergoing research. For those children with ESRD, dialysis or renal transplantation are the only treatment options.

Renal transplantation is usually reserved for children in ESRD for whom medication and dietary management of fluid and electrolyte balance and hypertension have been unsuccessful. They may or may not have been maintained on dialysis for a long period of time prior to the transplant. Transplants can be performed on children of all ages including infants. The surgical team and the family make the determination of the candidate for a transplant. In some institutions an ethics committee also looks at quality of life issues to help in the decision-making process. The question they usually ask is: "What will the long-term quality of life be for this child if the transplant is done?" Unfortunately there are no guarantees with this type of surgery, although renal transplants have the highest success rates for all types of transplants in infants and children (Ikuta, 2007). In addition, children who receive a kidney transplant have a long-term survival advantage over children who are on the waiting list for a transplant (Gillen et al., 2009).

Reflections from Families

I was so angry when I learned that my son was acutely ill. I knew that he was going to have a renal transplant and I did not know if I was up to the challenge. I resented the fact that my life was going to dramatically have to change. What impact was this going to have on my younger daughter? I have never been so frightened in my life and so angry with myself for sounding so selfish!

Kidneys for transplantation are obtained either through living donors—usually close relatives—or cadavers. Tissue typing to determine a match requires meticulous tests similar to crossmatching for blood transfusions. Close relatives are most likely to be a very good tissue match, but even then there is a chance of graft (the transplanted kidney) or organ rejection. Cyclosporine, azathioprine (Imuran), and prednisone or other immunosuppressive drugs are used to suppress the natural immune response. Organ rejection is always a problem with transplantation. However, the danger of rejection can be minimized by careful donor/recipient tissue typing and matching of human leukocytic antigens (HLA). Most renal transplants are not lost by rejection but the tissue dies from vascular thrombus or clots in the renal vessels.

Transplantation is just one aspect of ESRD treatment. Post-transplantation, immunosuppressive medications are required for life. Protein intake may still be restricted. Medications for hypertension and diuretics may still be needed following surgery. These patients need frequent monitoring of serum and urine chemistries, immunologic examination for signs of rejection and aggressive infections, and growth and development follow-up care. As they are on immunosuppressive medication along with steroids to decrease the chance of rejection, these children must be followed for any side effects of the steroids.

There are several concerns about the long-term effects of steroid or cyclosporine therapy. Both of these medications increase the susceptibility to infection as previously mentioned. They both affect other glucocorticosteroids that in turn alter serum glucose and insulin levels. Other recognized serious adverse effects related to corticosteroid therapy include obesity, disruption of growth, and hypertension (Hodson, Willis, & Craig, 2009a). Cushing syndrome or round moon face and deposition of fat around the scapular region caused by the glucocorticosteroid effects have most often been associated with long-term steroid therapy, but can also come from cyclosporine use. Other effects from steroids are seen in bone mineralization and strength, which are concerns for a growing, active child. The effects on endogenous growth hormone of the renal disease itself are made worse by some of the therapies. Growth hormone used in children with CRF and growth retardation results in catch-up growth (Nissel, Lindberg, Mehls, & Haffner, 2008). All these issues need further research to either substantiate or refute clinical observations.

CRITICAL THINKING

Cushing Syndrome Secondary to ESRF

What is the physiological process involved in the development of Cushing syndrome when steroids are administered? What other effects may this child exhibit from steroid therapy? What is the nurse's role in working with the child and family in terms of teaching about steroids?

Nursing Management

This section will be divided into two parts. The first will be the management of the child and family with CRF or ESRD. The second part will be the management of the child and family undergoing a renal transplant. The goals of the nursing care are to restore and maintain fluid and electrolyte balance; restore and maintain nutrition and growth; and decrease the anxiety of the child and family. Most of the nursing management is the same as with acute renal failure. Other points of nursing management are discussed below.

Nurses should administer medications (diuretics, steroids, or immunosuppressive agents) as ordered, and assess for signs of infection: elevated temperature, changing CBC with differential, cough, sore throat, or other systemic complaints. The child should be protected from visitors or personnel who may have infections. Antibiotics are administered as ordered. Nurses should always consider if these medications are cleared through the kidney; if so,

NURSING ALERT

Recognizing Need for Dialysis

The signs or indicators for dialysis are BUN 0.120 mg/dL, increasing metabolic acidosis, hyperkalemia, fluid overload with pulmonary edema or congestive heart failure, and severe systemic hypertension.

peak and trough levels must be monitored as some medications are nephrotoxic.

If anemia is severe, blood transfusions with packed red blood cells may be administered, but this presents the danger of fluid overload. Newer therapies that are less risky than blood transfusion include the use of erythropoietin to boost the reticulocyte development. This therapy is used in the predialysis phase and is associated with delaying renal function deterioration. Erythropoietin boosts the hemoglobin and is used with iron therapy to treat anemia (Koshy & Geary, 2008). This child may also need dialysis and should be assessed for signs indicating the need for this form of treatment.

The posttransplant assessment and care remains the same as that described for the child and family with CRF and ESRD. These children are at risk for the development of vesicourethral reflux in the graft, which may lead to pyelonephritis. Signs of a kidney infection such as fever, flank pain, burning on urination, cloudy or blood-tinged urine, and sometimes abdominal cramping must be monitored, and the caregivers must be taught these signs as well.

Family Teaching

Because either CRF or ESRD is a chronic, lifelong problem, the family will have many learning needs, especially related to the need for meticulous follow-up care. They need to understand the etiology of the problem and the course of treatment. They will need to be taught about dietary restrictions, use and side effects of medications, signs of further deterioration of the renal function, and possibly how to perform dialysis in their homes. The side effects from steroids and immunosuppressive therapies include a depressed immune system so the child is more vulnerable to infection, growth retardation, and bone demineralization. There is a greater risk for fractures. Some children will feel hyperactive with high doses of steroids. If they take the steroids for a long time, they may develop a moon face, fat deposits along the shoulders, and generally gain weight. If the child is on diuretics, the individual may lose potassium and feel weak or faint or experience heart palpitations. Caregivers need to know that these side effects are possible but do not always occur.

Caregivers may benefit from financial counseling, as these are costly problems and are not always covered by health insurance policies or managed care contracts. They need to understand the impact that a chronic illness has on themselves and their child. They should be encouraged to take advantage of psychological counseling or participate in a support group. For the family whose child has undergone a transplant, additional teaching is needed. The family must be taught signs of rejection and a kidney infection. They must also understand the need for lifelong follow-up care and medications given on the established schedule. It will be necessary to arrange for home care and nursing follow-up in the home. Quality of life issues need to be addressed.

Families also need to know that generally childhood immunizations should be given, and that there is no adverse effect on the kidney. The rationale is that while these children may be immunosuppressed, their immune system still can respond to the vaccines in the immunizations. It is better to have the children challenged by a laboratory-controlled dose of the "disease" than to actually acquire the childhood disease itself. The misperceptions about immunizations and who should or should not receive them is an issue for concern and an opportunity for nurses to educate the lay public as well as colleagues.

NURSING ALERT

Signs of Renal Transplant Rejection

Acute rejection usually occurs within the first six months after transplantation.

Signs of rejection are:

- Fever, graft pain, decreased urine output, weight gain, and hypertension

Laboratory signs of rejection are:

- Increasing BUN and creatinine

REFLECTIVE THINKING

How Would You Feel If Your Child Had a Renal Transplant?

As nurses we must try to imagine what it is like for caregivers to face seeing their child first have a life-threatening disease such as chronic renal failure, then to have to choose a treatment that may or may not be effective. They also know that this treatment will have risks and change their child's life as well as their own forever. These are very emotionally-laden decisions and require a lot of empathy and support from health care professionals. Explore your feelings. What would you consider in making your decision?

BLADDER EXSTROPHY-EPISPADIAS COMPLEX

Bladder exstrophy-epispadias complex is a rare serious congenital anomaly affecting the urologic and musculoskeletal systems. In early fetal life the abdominal wall and underlying structures fail to fuse, producing an exposed bladder and urethra, pubic bone separation, and associated genital and anal abnormalities. This complex occurs in males more frequently than in females. Epispadias is considered a mild form of bladder exstrophy, and in more severe cases the

RESEARCH Highlight

Anemia and Risk of Hospitalization in Pediatric Chronic Kidney Disease

STUDY PURPOSE

To assess the prevalence of anemia in children with predialysis Chronic Kidney Disease (CKD) and examine the link between anemia and morbidity.

METHODS

This study used a retrospective cohort design. The sample consisted of 2,779 patients aged 2 to 20 years who had been diagnosed with CKD. These children had to be enrolled in the North American Pediatric Renal Trials and Collaborative Studies (NAPRTCS). The disease was staged as to I to V according to the glomerular filtration rate, presence of anemia set at <33%. Morbidity was defined as a hospitalization during one year of follow up after study enrollment.

FINDINGS

Upon examination of the anemia it was found that its prevalence increased from 18.5% in stage II to 68% in stage V. Not surprising the more severe the anemia the more likely the child was to be hospitalized at a level of 55% when other factors were controlled. These factors were race, height, albumin levels, and erythropoietin use. At the 36% anemia threshold or above resulted in a decreased rate of hospitalization or morbidity.

IMPLICATIONS

1. The clinical implications are that follow-up care and an examination and treatment of anemia is important if morbidity rates are decreased.
2. It must be acknowledged that this NAPRTCS is a voluntary registry and therefore the subjects included could represent a biased sample.
3. There were also a number of cases excluded from the final data analysis due to missing data or children lost to follow-up, again potentially biasing the sample.

REFERENCE

Staples, A. O., Wong, C. S., Smith, J. M., Gipson, D. S., Filler, G., Warday, B. A., Martz, K., & Greenbaum, L. A. (2008). Anemia and risk of hospitalization in pediatric chronic kidney disease. *Clinical Journal of the American Society of Nephrology, Dec., 3.* Retrieved on April 10, 2009, from http://www.anemia.org/professionals/reviews/content.php?contentid=000345§ionid=00014.

two coexist. In males, epispadias is characterized by the urethral opening on the dorsal side of the penis in contrast to hypospadias where it is on the ventral surface (Figure 22-11). Females with epispadias present with separation of the labia and a **bifid** (split into two parts) clitoris. Total incontinence results if the internal bladder sphincter is affected. In exstrophy the lower urinary tract is exposed, and the everted bladder appears bright red through the abdominal opening. There is also a widening of the symphysis pubis.

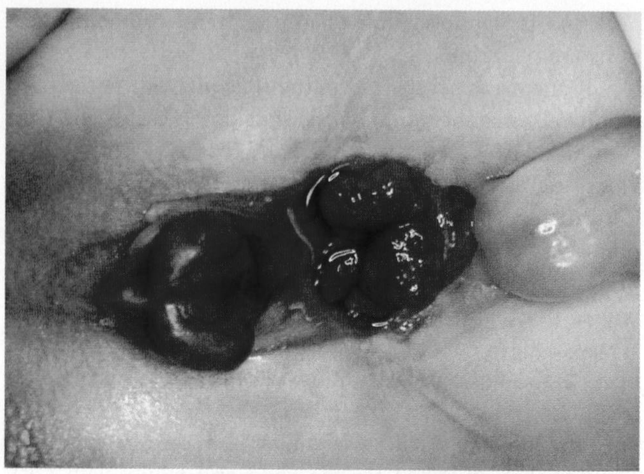

FIGURE 22-11 Bladder Exstrophy with Epispadias. PHOTO COURTESY OF CASIMIR FIRLIT, MD, PHD, WILLIAM E. KAPLAN, MD, MAX MAIZELS, MD, AND JEFFREY PALMER, MD, CHILDREN'S UROLOGY LTD.

IN THE REAL WORLD

As a student nurse, I found caring for a 2-year-old child with hemolytic uremic syndrome to be quite scary. I knew that the child might not recover or at the very least have some lifelong problems. The family was devastated as they were on a family vacation and had eaten at fast-food restaurants, where the child more than likely had contracted *E. coli.* While empathetic with the family and their situation, all I could think about was my own 2-year-old. I talked with a colleague about my mixed feelings about getting too close to this family. She suggested that rather than being scared of my feelings to let them help me work with the family as I would hope a nurse would if it were my child. This perspective gave me renewed strength so that instead of feeling anxious and guilty I could use this positive "energy" to be more empathetic with the family.

Musculoskeletal anomalies seen in these children include an outward rotation of the hips and widening of the pelvis. Male infants have a short penis with dorsal chordee, or upward curvature, and a ventral prepuce. Females present with a bifid clitoris and nonfused labia. At birth the bladder mucosa is thin, reddened, and susceptible to injury. Various techniques are utilized to protect the mucosa and preserve hydration.

Surgical management of bladder exstrophy is usually performed within the first 48 hours of life but may be deferred secondarily to the infant's stability or until further testing is performed. Goals of management include preservation of the primary bladder and abdominal wall and provision of an adequate pelvic structure to support the bladder. Other goals include the achievement of a functional bladder and cosmetic reconstruction to preserve kidney and bladder function (Retik, 2009). Initially, the bladder, abdominal wall, and symphysis are closed surgically.

Long-term care focuses on continence issues and social adjustment. In its severest forms continence may only be achieved through augmentation of the bladder to increase its storage capacity and in some cases a urinary diversion procedure. Issues of sexuality need to be addressed as the child approaches adolescence, including information regarding reproduction. Research indicates that most clients with exstrophy do not develop long-standing maladjustment and have a high level of sexual functioning. Reproductive options have increased for even those with severe exstrophy (Retik, 2009). Management of exstrophy is one of the most complex of all urologic disorders.

KEY CONCEPTS

- The genitourinary system of the infant and child is immature compared to an adult's; therefore, medications and therapies must be considered in terms of renal maturation.
- Embryologically, the genital and urinary systems are interrelated; hence, any insult during fetal development can have devastating consequences for the child and family.
- Common manifestations of genitourinary alterations in children include vague symptoms such as abdominal pain, nausea, vomiting, and diarrhea.
- Nursing assessment of the child with genitourinary alterations includes a history about diet and feeding or eating pattern, elimination pattern (stool and urine), growth pattern, gastrointestinal symptoms, and a physical examination.
- Untreated UTIs can lead to progressive infections with kidney involvement, subsequent renal scarring, and decreased kidney function.
- Enuresis is the involuntary voiding of urine in children over the age of 5 years without a structural defect. Incontinence is wetting that results from a structural defect or abnormality.
- Vesicoureteral reflux is the backflow of urine from the bladder into the upper urinary tract. Clinically these children may be diagnosed only after a full radiographic workup after UTI.
- Hypospadias is a congenital malformation and displacement of the urethra to the underside or ventral surface of the penis, requiring surgical repair.
- Cryptorchidism is synonymous with undescended testes. It may be unilateral or bilateral and is often treated before the age of 2 in an attempt to preserve spermatogenesis. Children with UDT must be followed through puberty and into adulthood secondary to issues regarding fertility and increased tumor potential.
- Hernias present as a bulge or a swelling in the scrotum or groin and may fluctuate with increased intra-abdominal pressure such as crying.
- Acute glomerulonephritis is an inflammation of glomeruli within the kidney caused by a viral or bacterial agent.
- Nephrotic syndrome manifests as massive proteinuria and hypoalbuminemia that leads to edema and hyperlipidemia.
- Hemolytic uremic syndrome, though rarely seen in children, has been found to be secondary to *E. coli* infection.
- The three types of acute renal failure are prerenal, intrarenal, and postrenal.
- Chronic renal failure is a progressive disease that can lead to end-stage renal failure.
- Nursing management of children undergoing urologic procedures generally involve extensive family education and anticipatory guidance preoperatively along with postoperative issues of accurate fluid management, care of various drainage tubes, and meticulous wound care and assessment.
- Teaching for the child and family undergoing dialysis must include dietary needs, infection control, and performing the dialysis. The nurse must also emphasize the signs and symptoms of worsening renal failure and the need for close follow-up.
- Nursing management for the child with a renal transplant is directed toward teaching the family about dietary needs, infection control, and signs and symptoms of rejection.

REVIEW ACTIVITIES

1. Identify the signs and symptoms of urinary tract infections including the standard clarification between cystitis or bladder infection and pyelonephritis.
2. Describe the necessary urologic workup for a child post-first-documented UTI and the rationale for this further testing.
3. Describe the differences between the terms *enuresis* and *incontinence*. What questions should be asked when obtaining a history for a child with wetting problems?
4. Describe the conservative medical management for a child with vesicoureteral reflux.
5. Describe the clinical manifestations of hypospadias in the newborn period and nursing interventions that should be instituted.
6. Develop a teaching plan regarding the importance of long-term follow-up for a boy with UDT.
7. Develop a teaching plan for caregivers regarding signs and symptoms of increasing problems and risk of incarceration in a child with hernias or hydrocele.
8. Describe the pathophysiology of hemolytic uremic syndrome.
9. What should the nurse advise caregivers about fluid restrictions and dietary restrictions for the child with acute or chronic renal failure?
10. List the clinical indicators for dialysis.

STUDY QUESTIONS

1. The nurse knows that the bladder capacity of a 5-year-old child is approximately what?
   a. 3 ounces
   b. 5 ounces
   c. 7 ounces
   d. 9 ounces
2. What is the best indication to the nurse that antibiotic treatment for a urinary tract infection in a 6-year-old girl is effective?
   a. Symptoms have subsided within 24 hours.
   b. The entire amount of prescribed antibiotic has been taken as ordered.
   c. Follow-up urine culture within 72 hours is negative.
   d. Mother states the child is voiding normally.
3. Which diseases are most often associated with polyuria and enuresis in a child?
   a. Diabetes mellitus and diabetes insipidus
   b. Vomiting and diarrhea
   c. Acute renal failure and kidney stones
   d. Glomerulonephritis and nephritic syndrome
4. Which drug is most likely prescribed for an 8-year-old who has enuresis?
   a. Prednisolone (Prelone)
   b. Imipramine hydrochloride (Tofranil)
   c. Furosemide (Lasix)
   d. Sodium sulfonate (Kayexalate)
5. The nurse knows that the most common anatomic disorder of the urinary tract in children is what?
   a. Hypospadias
   b. Glomerulonephritis
   c. Exstrophy of the bladder
   d. Vesicoureteral reflux
6. The nurse is teaching the family of a child with nephrotic syndrome about taking corticosteroids. What should be included in the teaching plan?
   a. Protect the child from sources of infection.
   b. Expect the drugs to suppress appetite.
   c. Ensure the child receives scheduled live virus vaccines.
   d. Be prepared for hair loss associated with these drugs.
7. The nurse is caring for a child with possible glomerulonephritis. What diagnostic tests should the nurse prepare the child and family to expect related to this diagnosis?
   a. Stool culture
   b. Anti-streptolyn O titer
   c. Blood cultures
   d. 24-hour urine collection
8. The nurse is caring for a child with pre-renal acute renal failure (ARF). What would be the most likely cause of this type of ARF?
   a. Vesicoureteral reflux
   b. Diagnostic studies involving contrast dye
   c. Heart failure
   d. Lupus erythematosus
9. Which type of primary acid base disorder is most likely seen in a child with renal failure?
   a. Respiratory acidosis
   b. Respiratory alkalosis

c. Metabolic alkalosis
d. Metabolic acidosis

10. The nurse is giving a child in chronic renal failure an injection of erythropoietin (Epogen). The mother of the child asks about the purpose of this drug. What information about the drug should the nurse give to the mother?
    a. Erythropoietin decreases inflammation.
    b. Erythropoietin removes excess potassium from the blood.
    c. Erythropoietin boosts linear growth.
    d. Erythropoietin combats anemia.

REFERENCES

Abeyagunawardena, A. S., & Trompeter, R. S. (2008). Increasing the dose of prednisolone during viral infections reduces the risk of relapse in nephrotic syndrome: a randomized controlled trial. *Archives of Disease in Childhood, 93*(3), 226–228.

Agraharkar, M., Gala, G., & Gangakhedkar, A. K. (2007). Nephrotic syndrome. *Emedicine.* Retrieved March 17, 2009, from http://emedicine.medscape.com/article/244631-overview.

Ahn, S. & Ingulli, E. (2008). Acute poststreptococcal glomerulonephritis: An update. *Current Opinion in Pediatrics, 20*(2), 157–162.

American Pediatric Surgical Association (APSA). (2009). Inguinal hernia and hydrocele. Retrieved March 1, 2009, from http://www.eapsa.org/parents/resources/inguinal.cfm.

Andreoli, S. P. (2008). Management of acute kidney injury in children: a guide for pediatricians. *Pediatric Drugs, 10*(6), 379–390.

Andreoli, S. P. (2009). Acute kidney injury in children. *Pediatric Nephrology, 24*(2), 253–263.

Arnoff, S. C., & McCoy, A. C. S. (2007). Pyleonephritis: Treatment & medication. *Emedicine.* Retrieved January 27, 2009, from http://emedicine.medscape.com/article/968028-treatment.

Austin, P. F., & Coplen, D. E. (2007). Enuresis and dysfunctional elimination. *Missouri Medical, 104*(5), 421–424.

Aydil, U., Iseri, E., Kizil, Y., Bodur, S., Ceylan, A., & Uslu, S. (2008). Obstructive upper airway problems and primary enuresis nocturna relationship in pediatric patients: Reciprocal study. *Journal Otolaryngology Head Neck & Surgery, 37*(2), 235–239.

Baker, C. L. (2006). Racial and ethnic differences in the rates of urinary tract infections in febrile infants in the emergency department. *Pediatric Emergency Care, 22*(7), 485–487.

Baum, M. (2008). Pediatric glomerular diseases. *Current Opinion in Pediatrics, 20*(2), 137–139.

Bloomfield, P., Hodson, E., & Craig, J. (2005/2007). Antibiotics for acute pyelonephritis in children. *Cochrane Database of Systematic Reviews, 3,* CD003772. Accessed and updated 2007.

Bunchman, T. E. (2008). Treatment of acute kidney injury in children: From conservative management to replacement therapy. *Nature Clinical Practice Nephrology, 4,* 510–514.

Camp-Sorrell (2008). Hemolytic uremic syndrome. *Oncology Nursing Forum, 35*(4), 593–595.

Carapetis, J. R., Steer, A. C., Mulholland, E. K., & Weber, M. (2005). The global burden of group A streptococcal diseases. *Lancet Infectious Diseases, 5,* 685–694.

Cendron, M. (2008). Vesicoureteral reflux. *Emedicine.* Retrieved March 1, 2009, from http://emedicine.medscape.com/article/439403-overview.

Centre for Reviews & Dissemination (2009). Acute renal failure in the intensive care unit: A systematic review of the impact of dialytic modality on mortality and renal recovery. *Database of Abstract of Reviews of Effects, 1,* 00125498.

Chaturvedi, S. (2007). Protein restriction for children with chronic renal failure. *Cochrane Database of Systematic Reviews, 4,* CD006863.

Diaz Saldano, D., Chaviano, A. H., Maizels, M., Yerkes, E. B., Cheng, E. Y., Losavio, J., Porten, S. P., Sullivan, C., Zebold, K. F., Hagerty, J., & Kaplan, W. E. (2007). Office management of pediatric primary nocturnal enuresis: A comparison of physician advised and parent chosen alternative treatment outcomes. *Journal of Urology, 178*(4 Pt 2), 1758–1762.

Drawz, P., & Mahboob, R. (2009). In the clinic: Chronic kidney disease. *Annals of Internal Medicine, 150*(3), 228–244.

Food and Drug Administration (FDA). (2007). Information for Healthcare Professionals Desmopressin Acetate (marketed as DDAVP Nasal Spray, DDAVP Rhinal Tube, DDAVP, DDVP, Minirin, and Stimate Nasal Spray). *U.S. Food and Drug Administration: Center for Drug Evaluation and Research.* Retrieved February 22, 2009, from http://www.fda.gov/CDER/DRUG/InfoSheets/HCP/desmopressinHCP.htm.

Gatti, J. M., & Kirsch, A. J. (2007). Hypospadias. *Emedicine.* Retrieved March 1, 2009, from http://emedicine.medscape.com/article/1015227-overview.

Gillen, D. L., Stehman-Breen, C. O., Smith, J. M., McDonald, R. A. Warady, B. A., Brandt, J. R., & Wong, C. S. (2009). Survival advantage of pediatric recipients of a first kidney transplant among children awaiting kidney transplantation. *American Journal of Transplantation, 8*(12), 2600–2606.

Glazener, C. M., & Evans, J. H. (2002/2006). Desmopressin for nocturnal enuresis in children. *Cochrane Database of Systematic Reviews, 3,* Reassessed and supported 2006.

Glazener, C. M., Evans, J. H., & Cheuk, D. K. (2005). Complementary and miscellaneous interventions for nocturnal enuresis in children. *Cochrane Database of Systematic Reviews, 2,* CD005230.

Glazener, C. M., Evans, J. H., & Petro, R. E. (2005). Alarm interventions for nocturnal enuresis in children. *Cochrane Database of Systematic Reviews, 2,* CD002911.

Health Canada. (2008). DDAVP Spray (Desmopressin Acetate Nasal Spray) and DDAVP Rhinyle (Desmopressin Acteate Nasal Solution) have been associated with an increased risk of hyponatremia—for the public. Retrieved February 22, 2009, from http://www.hc-sc.gc.ca/dhp-mps/medeff/advisories-avis/public/_2008/desmopressin_pc-cp-eng.php.

Hodson, E. M., Willis, N. S., & Craig, J. C. (2009a). Corticosteroid therapy for nephrotic syndrome in children. *Cochrane Database of Systematic Reviews, 1,* CD00956.

Hodson, E. M. Willis, N. S., & Craig, J. C. (2009b). Non-corticosteroid treatment for nephrotic syndrome in children. *Cochrane Database of Systematic Reviews, 1,* CD01650.

Ikuta, L. M. (2007). Newborn or infant transplant patient. In C. Kenner & J. W. Lott (Eds.). *Comprehensive neonatal care: An interdisciplinary approach* (4th ed.). St. Louis: Saunders/Elsevier, pp. 393–403.

John, C. M., Saroha, V., & Jones, C. (2008). Using nonsteroidal anti-inflammatory drugs in volume-depleted children can precipitate acute renal failure. *Pediatrics, 121,* S142.

Kastarinen, H., Horkko, S., Kauma, H., Karjalainen, A., Savolainen, M., & Kesaniemi, Y. (2009). Low-density lipoprotein clearance in patients with chronic renal failure. *Nephrology Dialysis Transplantation, (Feb. 5),* 1–5.

Koshy, S. M., & Geary, D. F. (2008). Anemia in children with chronic kidney disease. *Pediatric Nephrology, 23,* 209–219.

Lane, J. C. (2008). Nephrotic syndrome. *Emedicine.* Retrieved March 17, 2009, from http://emedicine.medscape.com/article/982920-overview.

Lane, W., & Robson, M. (2009). Evaluation and management of enuresis. *New England Journal of Medicine, 360*(14), 1429–1436.

Mistry, R. D., & Gorelick, M. H. (2007). Urinary tract infection in infants. In J. M. Baren, S. G., Rothock, J. Brennan, & L. Brown. *Pediatric Emergency Medicine.* Philadelphia: Saunders, pp. 299–305.

Nissel, R., Lindberg, A., Mehls, O., & Haffner, D. (2008). Factors predicting the near-final height in growth hormone-treated children and adolescents with chronic kidney disease. *Journal of Clinical Endocrinology & Metabolism, 93*(4), 1359–1365.

Pais, P. J., Kump, T., & Greenbaum, L. A. (2008). Delay in diagnosis in poststreptococcal glomerulonephritis. *Journal of Pediatrics, 153*(4), 560–564.

Parmar, M. S. (2008). Hemolytic-uremic syndrome. *Emedicine.* Retrieved March 18, 2009, from http://emedicine.medscape.com/article/201181-overview.

Patzer, L. (2008). Nephrotoxicity as a cause of acute kidney injury in children. *Pediatric Nephrology, 23,* 2159–2173.

Quigley, R. (2008). Evaluation of hematuria and proteinuria: How should a pediatrician proceed? *Current Opinion in Pediatrics, 20*(20), 140–144.

Retik, A. B. (2009). Exstrophy of the bladder. Retrieved March 1, 2009, from http://www.duj.com/exstrophy.html.

Roberts, K. B. (2000). The American Academy of Pediatrics practice parameter on urinary tract infections in febrile infants and young children. *American Family Physician, 62*(8), 1777–1778, 1780.

Rodriguez-Iturbe, B., & Batsford, S. (2007). Pathogenesis of post-streptococcal glomerulonephritis a century after Clemens von Pirquet. *Kidney International, 71,* 1094–1104.

Sanchez, C. P. (2008). Mineral metabolism and bone abnormalities in children with chronic renal failure. *Review of Endocrine Metabolic Disorders, 9,* 131–137.

Schwarz, E. B., Moretti, M. E., Nayak, S., & Koren, G. (2008). Risk of hypospadias in offspring of women using Loratadine during pregnancy: A systematic review and meta-analysis. *Drug Safety, 31*(9), 775–788.

Sehgal, R., Paul, P., & Mohanty, N. K. (2007). Urodynamic evaluation in primary enuresis: An investigative and treatment outcome correlation. *Journal of Tropical Pediatrics, 53*(4), 259–263.

Shah, L., Mandlik, N., Kumar, P., Andaya, S., & Patamasucon, P. (2008). Adherence to AAP practice guidelines for urinary tract infections at our teaching institution. *Clinical Pediatrics (Philadelphia), 47*(9), 861–864.

Shaikh, N., Morone, N. E., Bost, J. E., & Farrell, M. H. (2008). Prevalence of urinary track infection in childhood: A meta-analysis. *Pediatric Infectious Disease Journal, 27*(4), 302–308.

Snodgrass, W. (2009a). Hypospadias-surgery, symptoms, & treatment. Retrieved March 1, 2009, from http://www.childrens.com/Specialties/template.cfm?groupid=4&pageid=179.

Snodgrass, W. (2009b). Undescended testes (cryptochidism). Retrieved March 1, 2009, from http://www.childrens.com/healthlibrary/healthlibcontent.cfm?pageid=p03081.

Staples, A. O., Wong, C. S., Smith, J. M., Gipson, D. S., Filler, G., Warday, B. A., Martz, K., & Greenbaum, L. A. (2008). Anemia and risk of hospitalization in pediatric chronic kidney disease. *Clinical Journal of the American Society of Nephrology, Dec., 3.* Retrieved 10, 2009, from http://www.anemia.org/professionals/reviews/content.php?contentid=000345§ionid=00014.

Swierzewski, S. J. (Ed.). (2007). Pediatric urology: Undescended testicle, causes, diagnosis, treatment. *Urologychannel.* Retrieved March 4, 2009, from http://www.urologychannel.com/pediatric/udt.shtml.

Tang, J. H., Wen, Y., Wu, F., Zhao, X. Y., Zhang, M. X., Mi, J., & Cianflone, K. (2007). Increased plasma acylation-stimulating protein in pediatric proteinuric renal disease. *Pediatric Nephrology, 23*(6), 959–996.

Tuncel, A., Mavituna, I., Nacacioglu, V., Tekdogan, U., Uzun, B., & Atan, A. (2008). Long-term follow-up of enuretic alarm treatment in enuresis nocturna. *Scandinavian Journal of Urology & Nephrology, 42*(5), 449–454.

Vaziri, N. D. (2006). Dyslipidemia of chronic renal failure: The nature, mechanisms, and potential consequences. *American Journal of Physiology—Renal Physiology, 290,* F262–F272.

SUGGESTED READINGS

Bergmann, M., Corigliano, T., Ataia, I., Renella, R., Simonetti, G. D., Bianchetti, M. G., & von Vigier, R. O. (2009). Childhood extraordinary daytime urinary frequency: A case series and a systematic literature review. *Pediatric Nephrology 24*(4), 789–795.

Chen, J. S. (2009). A worldwide food safety concern in 2008—Melamine-contaminated infant formula in China caused urinary tract stone in 290,000 children in China. *Chinese Medical Journal, 122*(3), 243–244.

Jia, L. Q., Shen, Y., & Bhatnagar, V. (2009). Ultrasonographic diagnosis of urinary calculus caused by melamine in children. *Chinese Medical Journal, 122*(3), 252–256.

Jindal, B., Grover, V. P., & Bhatnagar, V. (2009). The assessment of lower urinary tract function in children with anorectal malformations before and after PSARP. *European Journal of Pediatric Surgery, 19*(1), 34–37.

Lee, M. D., Lin, C. C., Huang, F. Y., Tsai, T. C., Huang, C. T., Tsai, J. D. (2009). Screening young children with a first febrile urinary tract infection for high-grade vesicoureteral reflux with renal ultrasound scanning and technetium-99m-labeled dimercaptosuccinic acid scanning. *Journal of Pediatrics,* epub 2009/02/24.

Mukherjee, S., Joshi, A., Carroll, D., Chandran, H., Parashar, K., McCarthy, L. (2009). What is the effect of circumcision on risk of urinary tract infection in boys with posterior urethral valves? *Journal of Pediatric Surgery, 44*(2), 417–421.

Prais, D., Shoov-Furman, R., Amir, J. (2009). Is ritual circumcision a risk factor for neonatal urinary tract infections? *Archives of Disease in Childhood, 94*(3), 191–194.

Sureshkumar, P., Jones, M., Cumming, R. G., Craig, J. C. (2009). Risk factors for urinary tract infection in children: A population-based study of 2856 children. *Journal of Paediatrics and Child Health,* epub 2009/02/13.

Zegers, B. S., Winkler-Seinstra, P. L., Uiterwaal, C. S., de Jong, T. V., Kimpen, J. L. de Jong-de Vos van Steenwijk, C. C. (2009). Urinary tract infections in children with spina bifida: An inventory of 41 European centers. *Pediatric Nephrology, 24*(4), 783–788.

RESOURCES

Refer to the online student StudyWARE for Potts & Mandleco at http://www.CengageBrain.com for additional content and study aids.

Organization: **American Association of Kidney Patients**
Description: The American Association of Kidney Patients (AAKP) is a national non-profit organization founded by kidney patients for kidney patients. AAKP strives to educate and improve the health and well-being of chronic kidney disease (CKD) patients, those on hemodialysis, peritoneal dialysis and transplant recipients. The website offers readers a wealth of information regarding kidney conditions and patient outreach services.
Website/Resource: http://www.aakp.org

Organization: **American Nephrology Nurses Association**
Description: The mission of the American Nephrology Nurses' Association (ANNA) is to advance nephrology nursing practice and positively influence outcomes for individuals with kidney disease through advocacy, scholarship, and excellence. ANNA's website offers users access to information regarding local chapters, related nursing practice, and current health policies.
Website/Resource: http://www.annanurse.org

Organization: **American Society of Pediatric Nephrology**
Description: The American Society of Pediatric Nephrology is an organization of pediatric nephrologists and affiliated health care professionals. Their primary goals are to promote optimal care for children with kidney disease through advocacy, education, and research, and to disseminate advances in clinical practice and scientific investigation. The website offers readers access to general kidney information and highlighted articles of interest.
Website/Resource: http://www.aspneph.com

Organization: **The National Association for Continence**
Description: National Association For Continence is a national, private, nonprofit organization dedicated to improving the quality of life of people with incontinence, voiding dysfunction, and related pelvic floor disorders. NAFC's purpose is to be the leading source for public education and advocacy about the causes, prevention, diagnosis, treatments, and management alternatives for incontinence. NAFC's offers readers access to a wealth of information regarding bladder/bowel health.
Website/Resource: http://www.nafc.org

Organization: **National Institute of Diabetes & Digestive & Kidney Diseases (National Institutes of Health)**
Description: The National Institute of Diabetes and Digestive and Kidney Diseases (NIDDK) conducts and supports basic and clinical research on many of the most serious diseases affecting public health. NIDDK's website offers users information regarding clinical diseases and current NIDDK publications.
Website/Resource: http://www2.niddk.nih.gov

Organization: **National Kidney Foundation**
Description: The National Kidney Foundation (NKF), a major voluntary nonprofit health organization, is dedicated to preventing kidney and urinary tract diseases, improving the health and well-being of individuals and families affected by kidney disease and increasing the availability of all organs for transplantation. NKF provides vital patient and community services, conducts extensive public and professional education, advocates for patients through legislative action and supports kidney research to identify new treatments. The website offers links to information regarding transplants, common kidney diseases, upcoming new/events as well as specific links for patients and professionals.
Website/Resource: http://www.kidney.org

Organization: **United Network for Organ Sharing**
Description: The United Network for Organ Sharing (UNOS) is a nonprofit, scientific and educational organization that administers the nation's only Organ Procurement and Transplantation Network (OPTN), established by the U.S. Congress in 1984. Through the OPTN, the UNOS collects and manages data about every transplant event occurring in the United States, facilitates the organ matching and placement process using UNOS-developed data technology and the UNOS Organ Center, and brings together medical professionals, transplant recipients and donor families to develop organ transplantation policy. The UNOS website offers information regarding organ transplant recipients, donors, and patients still on the waiting list.
Website/Resource: http://www.unos.org

Anjan, a 6-year-old boy, has experienced daily fecal soiling in his underwear for the past three years. He has had a hard time moving his bowel since 1 year of age when he started drinking whole milk. He was toilet trained for urine at 3 years of age, but he was never completely trained for stool. His parents recall that he would often sit tight and stiffen his body to avoid using the toilet. Anjan has a bowel movement once every 1–2 weeks. The stools are hard and large in diameter, often plugging the toilet. Anjan complains of abdominal pain that is relieved with defecation. He admits to withholding stool because he is afraid it will hurt to defecate and wants to avoid passing stool in his underwear. His parents are frustrated. They do not understand why he does not know when he has soiled his underwear or why he does not smell it.

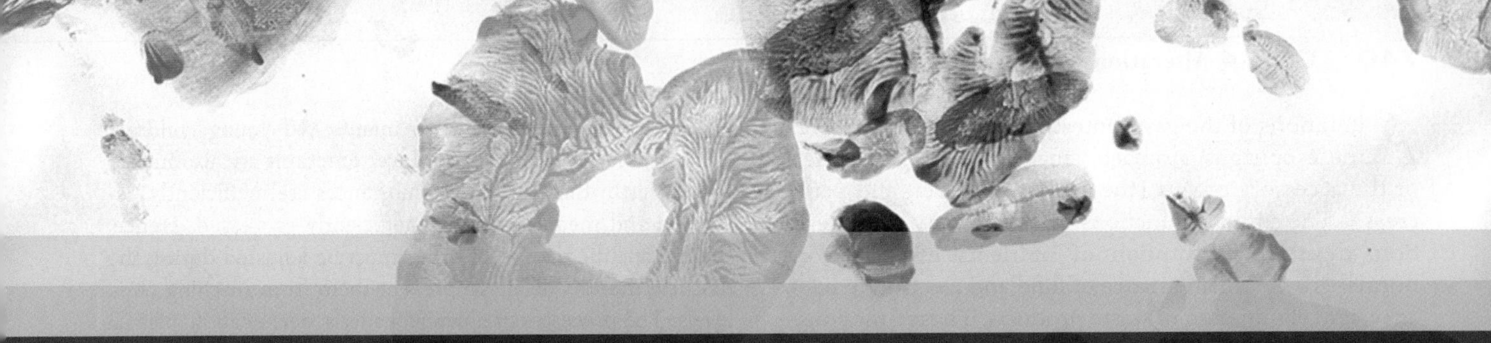

CHAPTER 23

Gastrointestinal Alterations

AMY MA, APRN, FNP-BC, DNP
MARY DOWELL, RN, BC, PhD

COMPETENCIES

Upon completion of this chapter, the reader will be able to:

- Describe the anatomy and physiology of the gastrointestinal (GI) system of the infant and child and how it differs from the adult GI system.
- Describe the etiology, pathophysiology, clinical manifestations, diagnosis, and treatment of common GI alterations.
- Explain how the pathophysiology is associated with the clinical manifestations of common GI alterations.
- Discuss nursing management and interventions appropriate for children requiring abdominal surgery for specific disorders.
- Identify the educational needs for families and describe appropriate content to be taught by the nurse.
- Successfully complete the games and activities in the online student StudyWARE.

Alterations of the gastrointestinal system can involve the esophagus, stomach, small and large intestine, or the accessory organs (the liver, gallbladder, and pancreas). The primary functions of the system are ingestion, digestion, absorption of nutrients essential for normal growth, maintenance of fluid and electrolyte balance, and elimination of waste products. These functions are vital for normal growth and development of infants and children. Gastrointestinal complaints are common in this age group. Alterations of function can be expressions of congenital anatomic abnormalities or alterations acquired after birth from disease, infection, or trauma. The severity of gastrointestinal problems ranges from minor illnesses causing inconvenience to severe, life-threatening disorders such as intestinal obstruction.

This chapter presents a discussion of the anatomy and physiology of the GI system and how it compares to the adult system and the most common GI alterations and disorders. These include upper and lower gastrointestinal alterations, alterations in motility, inflammatory disorders, malabsorption disorders, poisoning, and hepatic disorders.

ANATOMY AND PHYSIOLOGY

In comparison with adults, the newborn has a less effective gastrointestinal system because of its immaturity at birth. Sucking and swallowing are automatic reflexes at birth, gradually coming under voluntary control as the nerves and muscles develop by 6 weeks of age. The newborn's stomach capacity is only 60 mL, but expands rapidly to 200 mL by 1 month of age. **Peristalsis**, the coordinated, rhythmic, serial contraction of the smooth muscle of the GI tract, is stronger in the infant than in the older child. The emptying time of the stomach increases from 2 to 3 hours in the newborn to 3 to 6 hours by 2 months of age. These factors, the small stomach capacity, increased peristalsis, and increased stomach emptying rate, result in the need for small, frequent feedings of the newborn. The infant's metabolic rate is faster than an adult's, thus requiring approximately 100 calories per kilogram of body weight compared with 30 to 40 for an adult. Regurgitation is common in the infant because the lower esophageal sphincter tone is decreased.

The length of the small intestine is proportionately greater in an infant than an adult: six times the body length in infancy as opposed to four times the height of the adult. However, the infant's intestine is supplied with an adult's proportion of functional secretory glands per unit of area; therefore, an infant secretes proportionately more fluids and electrolytes into the intestine than does an adult. Similarly, the infant's small intestine has a larger surface for absorption relative to body size than does an adult's. Therefore, if diarrhea develops, more electrolytes will be lost from the intestinal secretions. In contrast, the large intestine of the infant is proportionately shorter than an adult's, resulting in less epithelial lining available for absorption of water from the feces. These two characteristics, more secretions and less absorption, are responsible for the soft, frequent stools of infants. In case of diarrhea in infants and young children, dehydration develops rapidly. Liver functions are also immature at birth; therefore, toxic substances are inefficiently detoxified and medications are inefficiently processed. Hence, the therapeutic dosage of drugs must be adjusted during the first few months of life to prevent them from reaching toxic levels. The processes of gluconeogenesis, deamination, plasma protein and ketone formation, and vitamin storage are immature during the infant's first year.

The infant is deficient in several digestive enzymes that are usually not sufficient until 4–6 months of age. The pancreatic enzyme *amylase,* responsible for the initial digestion of carbohydrates, is insufficient, resulting in an intolerance of starches. If cereals are given before 4–6 months, the infant may develop gas and diarrhea. The enzyme *lactase* breaks down or hydrolyzes lactose, the primary source of carbohydrates in infant formula and breast milk. Lactase levels are low in the preterm infant, increase in infancy, and decline after early childhood. This initial decreased level results in incomplete absorption of lactose, which can cause gas, abdominal distention, and diarrhea. Digestion and absorption of fats is impaired because of low levels of the enzyme *lipase.* Fat in breast milk is absorbed more readily than in formula because human milk contains lipase. Protein digestion and absorption are fairly efficient in the newborn and infant. The infant intestine is more permeable to proteins than the older child or adult, thus allowing passage into the bloodstream of cow's milk protein and other potential allergens. Therefore, infants ingesting formula instead of breast milk are more susceptible to food protein allergies. Breast-fed infants receive protective immunoglobulin proteins from human milk, whereas formula-fed infants do not. Figure 23-1 illustrates the gastrointestinal tract of the child.

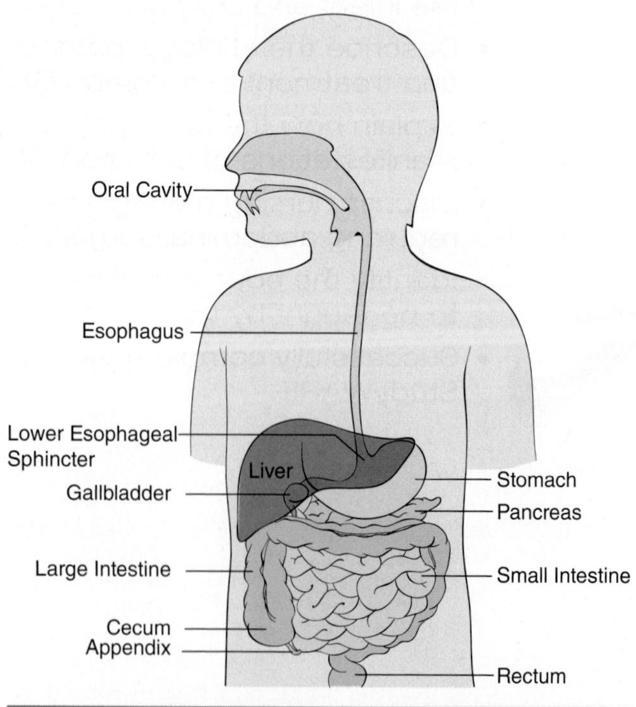

FIGURE 23-1 Gastrointestinal Tract of a Child. DELMAR CENGAGE LEARNING.

UPPER GASTROINTESTINAL ALTERATIONS

Upper gastrointestinal alterations in children include hypertrophic pyloric stenosis, cleft lip and cleft palate, esophageal atresia, and tracheoesophageal fistula.

HYPERTROPHIC PYLORIC STENOSIS

Hypertrophic pyloric stenosis (HPS) is the most common intra-abdominal condition requiring surgery during the neonatal period. Figure 23-2A illustrates a normal pyloric opening; Figure 23-2B shows pyloric stenosis.

Incidence and Etiology

HPS occurs in approximately 2 to 3.5 per 1,000 live births and affects four to six times as many males as females (To, Wajja, Wales, & Langer, 2005). First-born Caucasian males are the group most commonly affected. It is more common among Caucasians of Northern European ancestry, less common among African Americans, and rare in Asians. The exact cause is not known; however, several theories have been proposed to explain the etiology. Environmental factors, allergies, and pylorospasm are a few of the unproven etiologies. Genetic predisposition seems to increase the risk of HPS (To, Wajja, Wales, & Langer, 2005). A new theory proposed that persistent duodenal hyperacidity is created by an inherited high parietal cell mass and loss of gastrin control. These two factors produce pyloric stenosis through work hypertrophy from repeated pyloric contraction in response to hyperacidity (Rogers, 2006). The administration of oral **macrolide antibiotics** has been associated with infantile hypertrophic pyloric stenosis (Shoji et al., 2008). The use of macrolide antibiotics among women during late pregnancy or while breastfeeding is also associated with HPS (Sorensen et al., 2003).

Reflections from Families

My son, Robert, is three weeks old and had been healthy since he was born. I am breastfeeding him, and he feeds vigorously and has gained weight. All that changed two days ago when he began vomiting after every feeding. The vomiting has become more forceful, and it looks like curdled milk. He always seems hungry and eagerly sucks when I feed him. He feeds for about five minutes before he starts vomiting. He cried almost all night, and his diaper was dry this morning. He is my first child, I don't know what to do. I'm so upset and worried that something is seriously wrong with him. I feel so guilty because I can't console him for long. I can't even satisfy his hunger. What have I done to cause him to be so sick?

Pathophysiology

The pylorus is the opening through which food passes from the stomach to the intestines. This opening is surrounded by a muscular ring, the pyloric sphincter. In HPS the pyloric sphincter hypertrophies and increases to four times its normal width, resulting in a narrowed opening and gastric outlet

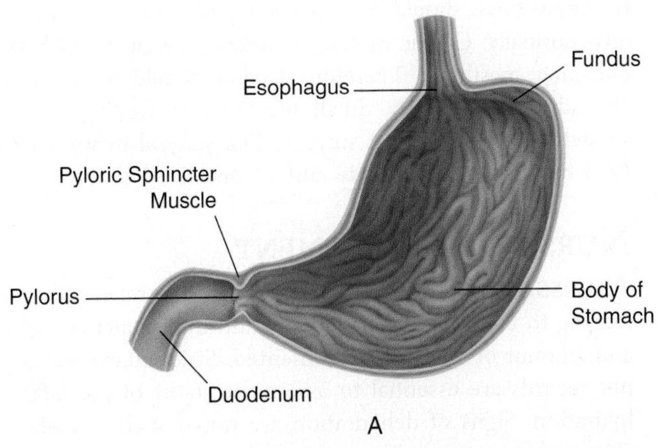

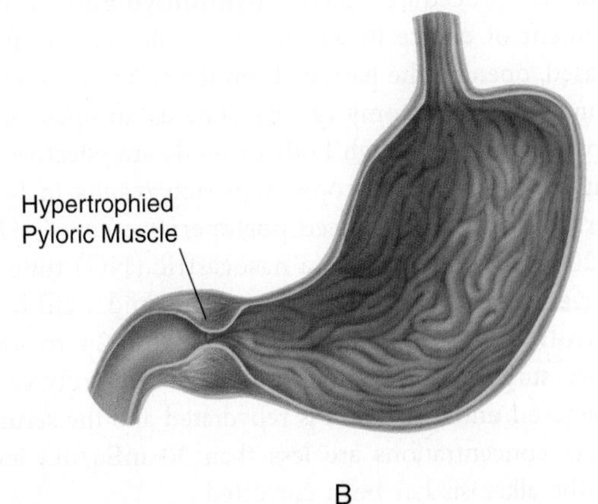

FIGURE 23-2 (A) Normal Pyloric Opening; (B) Pyloric Stenosis. DELMAR CENGAGE LEARNING.

obstruction. This obstruction prevents gastric contents from emptying into the duodenum.

Clinical Manifestations

Symptoms usually develop during the third and fourth weeks of life. Nonbilious vomiting beginning between the second and fourth week of life is the initial symptom. Because of the progressive nature of the obstruction, the vomiting increases in frequency and eventually becomes projectile with vomitus being propelled up to several feet. The emesis is not bile stained because the obstruction occurs above the outlet of the bile duct. The infant is hungry in spite of the vomiting and will usually feed again. Because food does not pass through the pylorus, bowel movements are small. As vomiting continues, there is loss of fluid, leading to dehydration, and hydrogen and chloride ions are lost, leading to hypochloremic metabolic alkalosis. Serum potassium levels are usually maintained, but there may be a total body potassium deficit. The infant has poor weight gain or experiences weight loss and becomes increasingly irritable and lethargic as dehydration and electrolyte imbalances worsen.

Diagnosis

Diagnosis may be made on history and physical identification of the hypertrophic pylorus, which can sometimes be palpated as an olive-shaped mass in the epigastrum, above and to the right (sometimes midline) of the umbilicus. In many cases the enlarged muscle cannot be felt and prompt diagnostic imaging is required for further evaluation. The diagnosis may be confirmed with a barium upper gastrointestinal (UGI) series or an abdominal ultrasound. The UGI, if positive, will reveal a delay in gastric emptying and a narrow, elongated pyloric channel. Ultrasonography is becoming the diagnostic method of choice because it is highly accurate (direct visualization of the muscle hypertrophy and the pyloric channel) and can be done without exposing the infant to radiation.

Treatment

A surgical procedure called a **pyloromyotomy** is often the treatment of choice in which the circular muscle fibers are released, opening the passage from the stomach into the duodenum. Pyloromyotomy can be done as an open or laparoscopic surgery. Although both methods are effective ways to treat HPS, the laparoscopic approach results in less postoperative pain and reduced postoperative emesis (Peter et al., 2006). Preoperatively, a nasogastric (NG) tube may be inserted, and the stomach emptied. Fluid, acid-base, and electrolyte losses must be corrected for 24 to 48 hours before surgery. Intravenous fluids and electrolytes are administered until the infant is rehydrated and the serum bicarbonate concentrations are less than 30 mEq/dL, indicating that the alkalosis has been corrected.

Sometimes medical management works and surgery is unnecessary. Antispasmodic medications before feedings (atropine/Phenobarbital) can be given to relax the stomach and pyloric sphincter muscle (Kawahara et al., 2005). Thickened feedings are recommended for babies on medical treatment.

Postoperatively, the NG tube should be removed, unless there is a reason to keep it in place, such as injury to or perforation of the duodenum. The blood glucose, electrolytes, and complete blood count (CBC) should be monitored. Intravenous fluids should be continued until the infant is able to feed normally. Gastric motility is delayed for up to 24 hours following anesthesia. Therefore, feeding should begin slowly and advance cautiously. Small and frequent feedings are resumed at 4–6 hours post surgery. The surgical treatment for HPS has a high success rate and is considered curative.

NURSING ALERT

Warning Signs of Hypertrophic Pyloric Stenosis

To prevent the infant from losing excessive fluid, nutrients, and calories, watch for early signs of HPS, which include:

1. The infant appears always hungry and wants to be fed again, in spite of feeding and vomiting.
2. The infant does not act or look sick otherwise.
3. The vomiting becomes more and more forceful, and sometimes is ejected several feet. This is the clue that it is structural in nature and not from other causes such as an infection.
4. The infant is not gaining weight.

NURSING TIP

Palpating the Olive-Shaped Mass

Successful palpation of the olive-shaped mass requires a relaxed abdominal musculature and an empty stomach. The abdominal muscles will relax by holding the infant, offering a bottle of warm sugar water, and elevating the baby's feet or flexing the knees and hips.

Nursing Management

Assessment In the nursing history the relationship of feeding to vomiting is determined, and the frequency, color, and amount of emesis is documented. Strict intake and output records are essential to assess the status of the infant's hydration. Signs of dehydration are noted such as inelastic skin turgor, crying without tears, dry mucous membranes, a depressed anterior fontanel, urine output <1 mL/kg/hr, increased pulse, decreased blood pressure, and weight loss. The infant is observed for evidence of pain or discomfort.

Nursing Diagnosis Nursing diagnoses for the infant with HPS include:

1. *Deficient fluid volume* related to the effects of frequent vomiting.
2. *Imbalanced nutrition: Less than body requirements* related to vomiting and gradual reintroduction of feedings.
3. *Acute pain* related to surgical trauma.
4. *Risk for infection* related to surgical incision.
5. *Deficient knowledge (caregivers)* related to care of infant after discharge.

Outcome Identification

1. The infant will demonstrate improved fluid and electrolyte balance.
2. The infant will tolerate feedings and will demonstrate adequate nutrition by maintaining or regaining preadmission weight.
3. The infant will experience minimal postoperative pain.
4. The infant's surgical incision will remain free of infection as evidenced by decreased swelling without redness or purulent discharge.
5. Caregivers will verbalize an understanding of incision care, feeding techniques, and signs and symptoms of complications (recurrent vomiting, wound infection, failure to gain weight).

Planning and Implementation Preoperative nursing care focuses on rehydration and correction of the electrolyte imbalance. Daily weights obtained at the same time of day using the same scale are the best indicator of extracellular deficient fluid volume. Because vomiting will continue until surgical correction, the infant is given nothing by mouth; thus, maintaining a patent intravenous infusion is essential. Monitoring the infusion, intake and output, are important nursing activities in fluid replacement. Family members need to be reminded to save diapers for weighing to measure urine output. If NG suction is used to decompress the stomach preoperatively, the nurse's responsibility is to maintain its patency and record the amount, color, and type of drainage. Laboratory data are assessed for electrolyte abnormalities. The nurse continually assesses the infant's hydration status.

Postoperative care includes maintaining fluid and electrolyte balance by: (1) monitoring intravenous infusion until oral fluids are tolerated; (2) monitoring infant's response to feedings by mouth; and (3) assessing for signs of dehydration. Appropriate analgesics are given for pain. The incision site is monitored for signs of infection, such as redness, inflammation, purulent drainage, or temperature of 101°F (38.3°C) or higher. Most surgeons remove the NG tube immediately after surgery and begin feeding within 4 to 6 hours if bowel sounds are normal. Initial feedings consist of small amounts of an electrolyte solution such as Pedialyte, and the volume is gradually increased. If greater volumes are tolerated without vomiting, formula or breast milk is offered. Most infants experience some vomiting in the first 24 to 36 hours after surgery; therefore, intravenous fluids are administered until full feedings are tolerated.

RESEARCH Highlight

Recovery after Open versus Laparascopic Pyloromyotomy for Pyloric Stenosis

STUDY PURPOSE

Laparoscopic approach to pyloromyotomy for infantile pyloric stenosis has gained popularity but its effectiveness remains unproven. The study compared outcomes after open or laparoscopic pyloromyotomy for the treatment of pyloric stenosis.

METHODS

A multicenter international, double-blind, randomized, controlled trial was done between June 2004 and May 2007 across six tertiary pediatric surgical centers. A total 180 infants were randomly assigned to open (n = 93) or laparoscopic pyloromyotomy (n = 87) with control for age, weight, gestational age at birth, bicarbonate at initial presentation, feeding type, preoperative duration of symptoms, and trial center. Infants with a diagnosis of pyloric stenosis were eligible. Primary outcomes were time to achieve full enteral feed and duration of postoperative recovery.

FINDINGS

Time to achieve full enteral feeding in the open pyloromyotomy group was about 5.5 hours longer than in the laparoscopic group (23.9 vs. 18.5); postoperative length of stay was longer too. Postoperative vomiting and intra-operative and postoperative complications were similar between the two groups.

IMPLICATIONS

Laparoscopy has advantages over open pyloromyotomy, and it is recommended that laparoscopic surgery should be done when the infant's condition permits and when the medical center has suitable laparoscopic experience.

REFERENCE

Hall, N. J., Pacilli, M., Eaton, S., Reblock, K., Gaines, B. A., Paster, A., Langer, J. C., Koivusalo, A. I., Pakarien, M. P., Stroedter, L., Beyerlein, S., Haddas, M., Clarke, S., Ford, H., & Pierro, A. (2009). Recovery after open versus laparoscopic pyloromyotomy for pyloric stenosis: A double-blind multicentre randomised controlled trial. *The Lancet*, *373*(9661), 390–398.

CASE STUDY / CARE PLAN

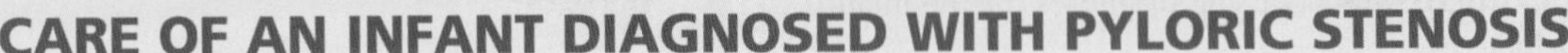

CARE OF AN INFANT DIAGNOSED WITH PYLORIC STENOSIS

Robert is a 3-week-old boy who comes to the pediatric unit after being diagnosed with pyloric stenosis. Robert was born healthy and has no other health problems. He started forceful vomiting three days ago and hasn't been able to tolerate feedings well since. He is admitted to the nursing unit for further work ups and monitoring for feeding status. No surgery has been scheduled. This is the first baby for Robert's parents and they express great concern for Robert's condition. They expressed guilt and appear anxious.

NURSING CARE PLAN

ASSESSMENT

Robert's color is pink. He is crying but has no tears. His pulse rate is 180 and respiratory rate is 36. His lips are slightly dry and his fontanel is flat. An IV is infusing into his left hand, and the site is patent without signs of infection and infiltration.

NURSING DIAGNOSIS 1

Deficient fluid volume related to vomiting and decreased oral intake as evidenced by dry lips and no tearing when crying.

EXPECTED OUTCOME

Robert will have proper hydration as evidenced by moist lips, positive tearing when crying, adequate urine output, flat fontanel, and stable vital signs.

NOC: Hydration, fluid balance

NIC: Fluid monitoring, fluid management, environmental management

INTERVENTIONS/*RATIONALES*

1. Assess and document behavioral and physiological signs of dehydration. Monitor vital signs for increase in heart rate and decreased blood pressure. Assess mental status, skin, mucous membrane, tearing, fontanel, and urination status. *Provides subjective and objective data.*
2. Administer IV fluid as ordered. *IV hydration is essential for patient with decreased oral fluid intake.*
3. Control the room temperature so the baby is comfortable but not sweating. *Can help to decrease water loss.*
4. Assess the urine for color and weigh the diaper at each change. *To determine the effectiveness of IV hydration.*
5. Maintain accurate record of daily intake and output. *I & O can help determine hydration status.*
6. Weigh the baby daily. Rapid *weight loss is often the result of poor hydration status.*

EVALUATION

Robert will have adequate hydration while waiting for surgery. He will be able to rest appropriately.

NURSING DIAGNOSIS 2

Risk for aspiration related to vomiting secondary to GI obstruction.

EXPECTED OUTCOME

Robert will be free from aspiration during hospital stay.

NOC: Aspiration prevention, electrolyte balance, nutritional status

NIC: Aspiration precautions

(Continues)

CASE STUDY / CARE PLAN (Continued)

INTERVENTIONS/*RATIONALES*

1. Feeding with thickened formulas or thickened breast milk. *Thickened feeding helps to prevent aspiration.*
2. Feed baby small amount and slowly. *Give baby time to empty the gastric content.*
3. Feed baby while placing baby on right side, upright by holding the baby, or put in the car seat. *These positions help to decrease abdominal pressure and facilitate gastric emptying.*
4. Burp baby upright gently and carefully after feeding. *Burping helps decrease gas and vomiting.*
5. Assess lung sound and vital signs every four hours. Obtain sample of aspirate for lab tests to eliminate pneumonia. *Elevated temperature can indicate lung infection.*
6. Minimal handling after feeding and refeed if vomiting occurs. (Some hospitals will not automatically refeed, but will wait for further orders or may reduce the amount to be fed.) *Ensure gastric emptying and adequate nutritional intake.*
7. Give antispamodic medication before feeding as ordered. *The medication may help relax the pyloric muscle and therefore facilitate adequate gastric emptying.*
8. Weigh the baby daily. *Weight is a good indicator of nutritional intake.*

EVALUATION

Robert is able to maintain his weight.

NURSING DIAGNOSIS 3

Knowledge deficit related to unfamiliar disease process and feeding regimen as evidenced by guilt and anxiety (parents).

EXPECTED OUTCOME

Robert's parents will be knowledgeable about HPS disease process and his care and treatment plan.

NOC: Knowledge: Treatment Regimen, knowledge: disease process

NIC: Teaching: Procedure/Treatment, teaching: disease process

INTERVENTIONS/*RATIONALES*

1. Assess parents' knowledge about HPS. *Establishing baseline knowledge can help formulate teaching plan.*
2. Explain to Robert's parents about the HPS and reassure that they are not at fault for Robert's condition. *Exact cause of HPS is unknown.*
3. Encourage parents to stay with the baby and assist in care and feeding. *Allows parents to care for and support child and continue parental role.*
4. Give the parents as much input in decisions about care and routines as possible. *Allows for more control over situation.*
5. Assess parent's ability to feed infant. Demonstrate feeding techniques, alternatives, and amount to be fed. Have them return demonstrate. Teach regarding indicators of weight gain and signs of adequate hydration and nutrition. *Infants with HPS have problems with nutritional intake before surgery. Teaching parents about signs of poor weight gain and dehydration can assure early and proper interventions.*
6. Explain to the parents that vomiting might still occur even when they are doing everything as directed. This is not their fault. Refeed the baby as needed. *Despite meticulous care, the baby might not tolerate the feeding well. Surgery is usually needed to correct the problem.*
7. Allow parents to vent concerns and ask questions about caring for a child with feeding problems. *Reinforce parents' normal feelings of concern for caring for child; can be a time to support and boost their confidence.*

EVALUATION

Parents understand the HPS disease process; understand and demonstrate correct care procedures; and express confidence in being able to maintain therapeutic regimen.

Evaluation Evaluation of nursing care is based on how effectively the identified outcomes were met. When feedings are resumed, the infant should be able to tolerate them without vomiting, and weight should be gained to the pre-illness level. The surgical incision should heal without signs of infection. The caregivers need to be able to demonstrate correct care of the incision, state plans for feeding and caring for the infant at home, and verbalize the signs and symptoms of complications and when to contact their health care provider.

Family Teaching

Caregivers often feel ineffective and powerless because their baby has been hungry and yet, they have not been able to satisfy this hunger. They may believe they have done something wrong. Nurses can support them by explaining that they are not at fault and the condition is caused by a structural defect. They need to be encouraged to be involved in caring for the baby before and after surgery. Prior to surgery the infant is irritable, hungry, and cries often. Caregivers can be involved by holding, rocking, and cuddling their baby. A pacifier may satisfy the infant's sucking needs.

Nurses should instruct caregivers about the care of the incision (if any is required) and signs of infection. The infant's response to feedings should be observed. Vomiting may still be present; however, if it persists beyond 48 hours, the health care provider should be notified.

CLEFT LIP (CL) AND CLEFT PALATE (CP)

A cleft is a fissure or elongated opening. A cleft of the lip, palate, or both is one of the most common congenital anomalies of newborns. Most afflicted will have both cleft lip and palate; some have only a cleft of the lip and others only of the palate. Any type of cleft interferes with the development of the normal anatomic structures of the lips, nose, muscles, and palate. The degree to which these structures are incomplete or malformed depends on the type, placement, and severity of the cleft(s).

Incidence and Etiology

The incidence of cleft lip or palate (CL/CP) is 1 in 700 births (de la Torre & Thurman, 2008). The incidence is highest in Asians, followed by Caucasians, and is lowest in African Americans. Clefts of the lip with or without cleft palate are more common in males, while clefts of the palate alone are more common in females.

Possible etiologies include genetic and environmental factors. If there is a family history of a cleft, the risk of other children also having a cleft is higher. Environmental factors have also been identified as a possible etiology of CL/CP including parental age, maternal intake of excessive alcohol, maternal drug exposure to phenytoin (Dilantin) or diazepam (Valium), and dietary factors such as folic acid and vitamin deficiencies. The incidence of CL among infants born to mothers who smoke during pregnancy is twice as high as the infants born to nonsmoking mothers (de la Torre & Thurman, 2008).

REFLECTIVE THINKING

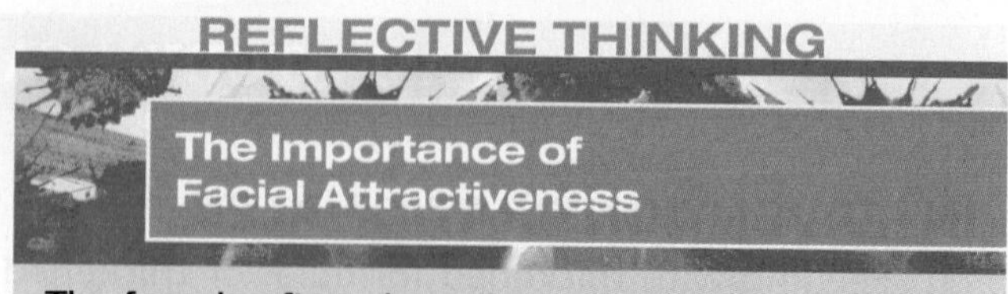

The face is often viewed as a "reflection of the self." The birth of an infant with a cleft lip and palate brings to the forefront just how much facial attractiveness is valued. Not only must caregivers deal with questions, stares, and comments from others, but eventually they must answer the child's questions, "What happened to my face? Why don't I look like everyone else?" How would you respond if it was your child? What types of emotions would you feel?

Pathophysiology

The hard palate is the bony front part of the roof of the mouth. The soft palate lies behind the hard palate and is composed of muscle and fibrous tissue. The flap of mucosa that hangs down from the soft palate is the uvula. Cleft lip is caused by a failure of the nasal and maxillary processes to fuse between the 5th and 8th week of gestation. The lip and palate develop independently; therefore, it is possible to have either a cleft of the lip or the palate separately or together. Cleft palate is caused by the failure of the palatine plates to fuse between the 7th and 12th weeks of gestation.

Clinical Manifestations

Cleft lip can occur as either unilateral (only on one side) or bilateral (both sides) and can vary from a slight notch in the red portion of the lip to a complete separation extending into the nostril. Cleft palate can occur in the hard or bony palate or in the soft palate, with or without a cleft lip being present (Figure 23-3A and 23-3B).

Diagnosis

Cleft lip and, in most cases, cleft palate are obvious at birth. Even a small cleft of the palate can be detected by visual inspection and palpation. When cleft palate is not diagnosed at birth, breast milk or formula coming from the nose may be the first sign. Both of these defects can be diagnosed in utero by ultrasound, and if present, the family will be referred to a multidisciplinary team at a cleft palate, craniofacial, or orofacial center.

Treatment

The treatment for a child with a cleft lip and palate is complex and involves many specialists, including a plastic

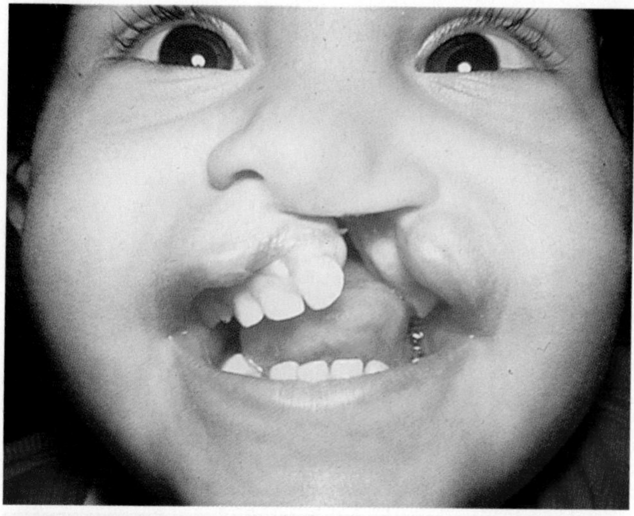

A

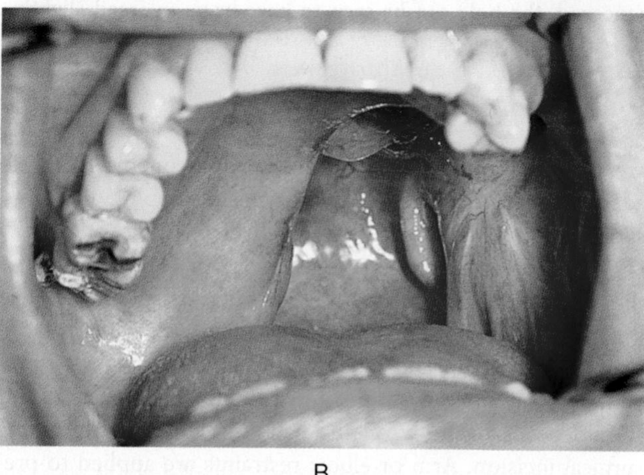

B

FIGURE 23-3 (A) **Cleft Lip.** (B) **Cleft Palate.** COURTESY OF DR. JOSEPH KONZELMAN, SCHOOL OF DENTISTRY, MEDICAL COLLEGE OF GEORGIA.

surgeon, neurosurgeon, orthodontist, otolaryngologist, pediatrician, nurse, speech pathologist, and audiologist. Reconstruction begins in infancy and can continue through adulthood. Wide variations exist in the timing and technique for surgical repair. Closure of the lip is usually performed when the infant is approximately 3 months of age or 12 pounds. The goal of surgery is to close the cleft so scarring will be minimal, and the face will have an increased chance to develop normally. Clefts of the hard or soft palate are surgically closed at approximately 1 year of age to assist feeding and to promote speech and language development. Additionally, good nutritional status and general health are essential factors influencing timing for surgery. Long-term consequences of cleft lip and palate may include speech difficulties, malocclusion problems (abnormal tooth eruption pattern), hearing problems from recurrent otitis media caused by abnormalities of the eustachian tube, and possible disrupted body image and self-esteem.

NURSING MANAGEMENT

Assessment A cleft of the lip and usually the palate are observable at birth. During the newborn assessment the nurse examines the palate by visualization and palpation with a gloved finger. A description of the location and extent of the defects is documented. The neonate's ability to suck, swallow, and feed are also noted. Nurses must also assess the caregiver's reactions, as the birth of a baby with a cleft may be devastating.

Nursing Diagnosis Preoperative nursing diagnoses for the infant with cleft lip or palate include:

1. *Imbalanced nutrition: Less than body requirements* related to feeding difficulties.
2. *Altered parenting* related to interruption in the bonding process.

Postoperative nursing diagnoses for the infant with cleft lip or palate include:

1. *Risk of injury and infection to the surgical site* related to surgical procedure.
2. *Acute pain* related to surgical correction of clefts.
3. *Deficient knowledge (caregivers)* related to the condition, treatment, and long-term care.

Outcome Identification

1. Infant will consume adequate nutrients.
2. Caregivers will demonstrate feeding techniques that provide adequate nutrients.
3. Caregivers will begin to adjust and bond to their infant.
4. Infant will maintain optimum comfort.
5. Infant's incision will heal without disruption or infection.
6. Caregivers will verbalize understanding of treatment plan, feeding and restraint techniques, surgical site care, and need for possible later surgeries and speech therapy.
7. Infant will demonstrate normal growth and development.

Planning and Implementation Preoperatively, nursing care focuses on providing support for the caregivers, preventing aspiration and infection, and ensuring adequate nutrition. The birth of a child is usually a time of joy and celebration; however, the birth of a child with a craniofacial anomaly has potentially devastating effects on a family. The initial reactions are shock, grief, feelings of isolation, and feelings of failure or inadequacy. Shock is usually followed by anger, guilt, frustration, and depression. Caregivers may become preoccupied with the baby's appearance and experience negative feelings toward the infant, which may disrupt or delay attachment. Nurses working with these families must realize that these are normal reactions and that they can aid in the bonding process by demonstrating acceptance of the baby and by encouraging the caregivers to hold and touch their infant. Fears may be allayed by seeing before and after photographs of successful surgical repairs. Providing an opportunity to talk with other families who have a child with a cleft is also important. Agencies such as the Cleft Palate Foundation provide information and support for children and their families (see Resources).

Once the initial shock has been dealt with, the caregivers usually have many questions pertaining to the child's condition. The four most frequently asked are:

1. Why did this happen?
2. Is this hereditary?
3. What can be done? Can anything be done right away?
4. What about our baby's future? Will my child be normal?

Feeding problems, such as poor or inadequate suction, prolonged feeding time, frequent nasal regurgitation, and inadequate weight gain, can be a frustrating and exhausting experience for many caregivers. Early teaching by nurses about the anatomy and functioning of the palate and successful feeding techniques can decrease caregiver anxiety. When an infant sucks, the soft palate rises up, closing off the nasopharynx from the oropharynx, thereby creating negative pressure. This mechanical vacuum draws liquid into the mouth and delivers it to the back of the throat where it is swallowed.

Breastfeeding an infant with a CL/CP is one option for the mother. The infant with only a CL will probably have no more difficulty than other babies in achieving effective breastfeeding. The breast itself tends to fill the opening in the lip because it has the capacity to mold to the shape of the oral cavity. It may be possible to breastfeed an infant with both CL and CP; however, if this method is unsuccessful, a breast pump may be used to express the milk and bottle feeding with special nipples should be used.

If the method chosen is bottle feeding, it is important for caregivers to initially try a regular nipple and bottle as some infants with small clefts may feed satisfactorily without special adaptations. One method using readily available standard nipples and bottles that is inexpensive and convenient is the ***E***nlarge, ***S***timulate, ***S***wallow, and ***R***est (ESSR) method. Enlarging the nipple hole by making a cross-cut allows the infant to receive formula in the back of the mouth for swallowing, thus bypassing the sucking problem. The next step, stimulate, refers to stimulating the sucking reflex by rubbing the nipple on the lower lip. The nipple is inserted into the mouth, and then the bottle is inverted. The infant swallows the fluid normally. The last step is a rest. Shortly before infants choke or gag, their facial expression will signal a need for a short break to finish swallowing formula already in their mouth. The signal consists of elevating eyebrows and wrinkling of the forehead. The nipple should be removed slowly and gently from the mouth. Frequent burping is needed. These steps are repeated until the infant has consumed normal amounts of formula, 3 or 4 ounces, in a normal amount of time, 15 to 30 minutes. Figure 23-4 illustrates a cross-cut nipple.

If standard nipples are ineffective for feeding, a variety of special nipples, for example, soft, "preemie," or elongated, are commercially available. If the infant is unable to ingest adequate milk using any of these types of nipples, an asepto syringe with a rubber tip may be effective.

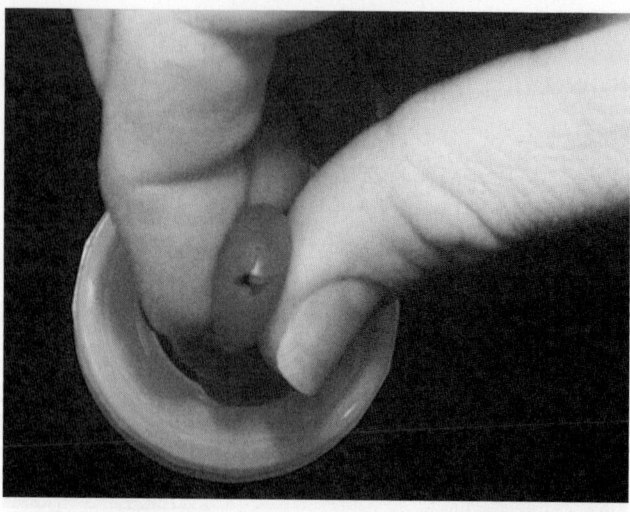

FIGURE 23-4 Cross-Cut in Nipple. When the nipple is squeezed, the hole can be seen to have been enlarged slightly.
FROM GOLDING-KUSHNER, K. J. (2001). THERAPY TECHNIQUES FOR CLEFT PALATE, SPEECH, & RELATED DISORDERS. CLIFTON PARK, NY: DELMAR CENGAGE LEARNING.

The major emphasis after surgery for cleft lip repair is the protection of the operative area. A small metal strip called a Logan bow or a butterfly adhesive may be placed over the upper lip and taped to the infant's cheeks to prevent tension on the suture line (Figure 23-5). The infant should be placed only on the back or side opposite of the surgical incision. Arm or elbow restraints are applied to prevent touching or pulling the site. These restraints should be removed periodically to exercise the arms (Figure 23-6). Adequate pain medication needs to be administered to minimize crying and stress on the suture line. In the postoperative

NURSING TIP

Caring for Families Whose Child Has a Cleft Lip or Palate

Help caregivers to understand this condition by explaining that:

1. Clefting occurs by the 35th day after conception, which is often before a woman knows she is pregnant.
2. The mother needs reassurance that she did nothing wrong during the pregnancy.
3. Many caregivers feel guilty about having a child with this disorder. Counsel caregivers appropriately.
4. Nothing is missing from their child's face. The pieces just need to be put together.

NURSING TIP

Breastfeeding an Infant with a Cleft Lip or Palate

The infant usually feeds best when the breast is full; therefore, teach the mother to place a warm washcloth on the breast to encourage the milk let-down prior to having the infant latch on.

REFLECTIVE THINKING

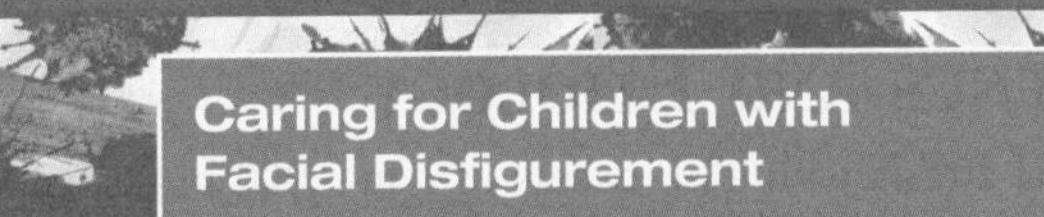

Caring for Children with Facial Disfigurement

To increase self-awareness about children with facial disfigurements, ask yourself:

1. How do I feel about caring for children with facial abnormalities?
2. Is my care affected by the child's appearance?
3. Do I unconsciously consider the disfigured child as less desirable?
4. Do I spend less time interacting with this child?
5. How can I ensure that children who have this anomaly receive the same quality health care as those who do not have this anomaly?

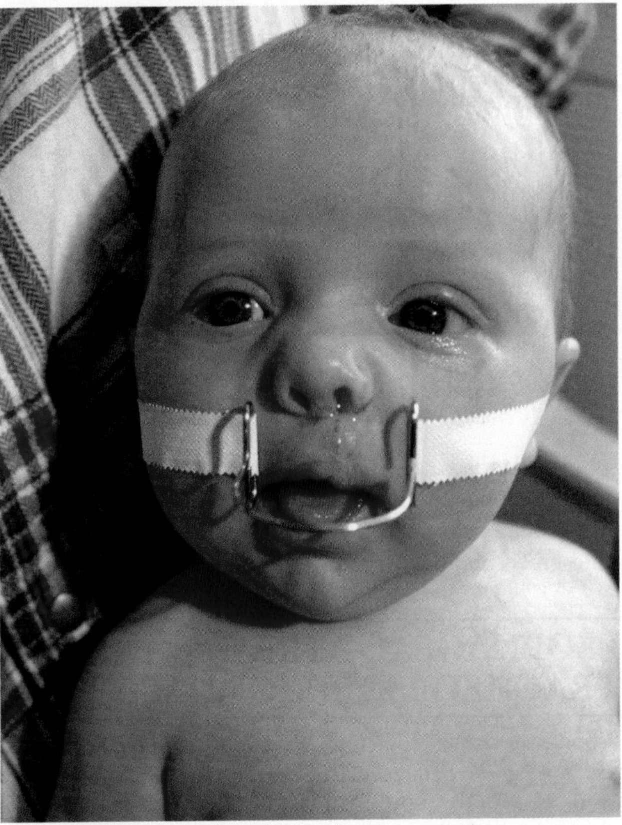

FIGURE 23-5 Infant with Logan Bow to Protect Suture Line After Repair of Unilateral Cleft Lip. DELMAR CENGAGE LEARNING.

period and for treatment in general, the nurse should consider referring the parents to occupational therapy for assistance in feeding techniques.

Evaluation Evaluation is based on how effectively the outcomes of nursing management are met. The infant consumes adequate nutrients and gains weight along a normal growth curve. Caregivers demonstrate increased feelings of confidence with feeding techniques and routine. Caregivers begin to bond with their infant by stroking, touching, and nurturing appropriately. The infant appears content while resting and displays behaviors consistent with comfort. Caregivers verbalize understanding of CL/CP pathology, treatment plan, home care, and long-term care.

FAMILY TEACHING

Family teaching includes information about feeding techniques and care of the operative site. Nurses should instruct caregivers to clean the suture line after feeding and as necessary with cotton-tipped applicators dipped in diluted hydrogen peroxide. Small amounts of water should be offered after feedings to rinse away any milk residue that could lead to bacterial growth. The elbow restraints should be removed one at a time several times each day for about ten minutes.

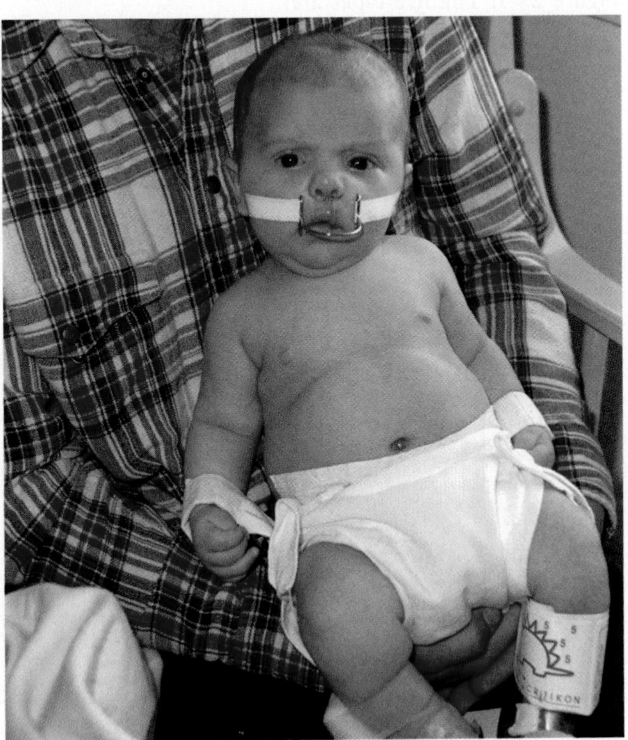

FIGURE 23-6 Infant with Arm Restraints to Prevent Injuring Operative Site. DELMAR CENGAGE LEARNING.

NURSING ALERT

Avoiding Hard Objects in the Oral Cavity

Hard objects such as thermometers, tongue depressors, straws, and forks should not be allowed in the child's mouth until healing has adequately progressed after repair of a cleft palate.

If the infant had a cleft lip repair, a side- or back-lying only position should be used. Nurses should discuss the possibility of additional surgeries on the lip, nose, and palate as the child grows and matures.

ESOPHAGEAL ATRESIA AND TRACHEOESOPHAGEAL FISTULA

Esophageal atresia (EA) and tracheoesophageal fistula (TEF) are congenital defects of the esophagus. They can each occur as a single entity, but usually occur together. EA is characterized by incomplete formation of the esophagus so it terminates before reaching the stomach. It is usually associated with a fistula between the trachea and the esophagus (TEF). Many anatomic variations of EA with or without TEF have been described and are illustrated in Figure 23-7. The five types are:

1. esophageal atresia with distal tracheo-esophageal fistula (upper segment of the esophagus ends in a blind pouch; lower segment is connected to the trachea by a fistula) (87%);
2. isolated or pure esophageal atresia (blind pouch of upper and lower segments of the esophagus without a connection to the trachea) (8%);
3. tracheoesophageal fistula without esophageal atresia (intact esophagus with fistula between the esophagus and trachea; "H-type") (4%);
4. esophageal atresia with proximal tracheoesophageal fistula (blind pouch at each end of the esophagus with a fistula from the trachea to upper segment of the esophagus) (<1%);
5. esophageal atresia with proximal and distal tracheoesophageal fistula (both upper and lower segments of esophagus connect to the trachea) (<1%).

INCIDENCE AND ETIOLOGY

Esophageal atresia with TEF occurs in 1 in 3,000 births, with an equal incidence in the sexes (Shaw-Smith, 2006). The birth weight of infants with this anomaly is significantly lower than average. Esophageal atresia has been associated with prematurity. Associated congenital anomalies occur in approximately one-half of infants with EA with TEF. The presence and severity of these anomalies are thought to be the most important factor influencing mortality. Cardiac anomalies, such as ventricular septal defect, patent ductus arteriosus, and tetralogy of Fallot, are encountered in approximately 30% of all cases. Gastrointestinal anomalies including imperforate anus and malrotation may occur in 25% of these infants. Musculoskeletal defects are also common and include vertebral malformations. The acronym VACTERL has been used to describe the condition of multiple anomalies in infants with tracheoesophageal defects (Spoon & Trotter, 2003):

V—**V**ertebral defect

A—**A**norectal malformation

C—**C**ardiac defects

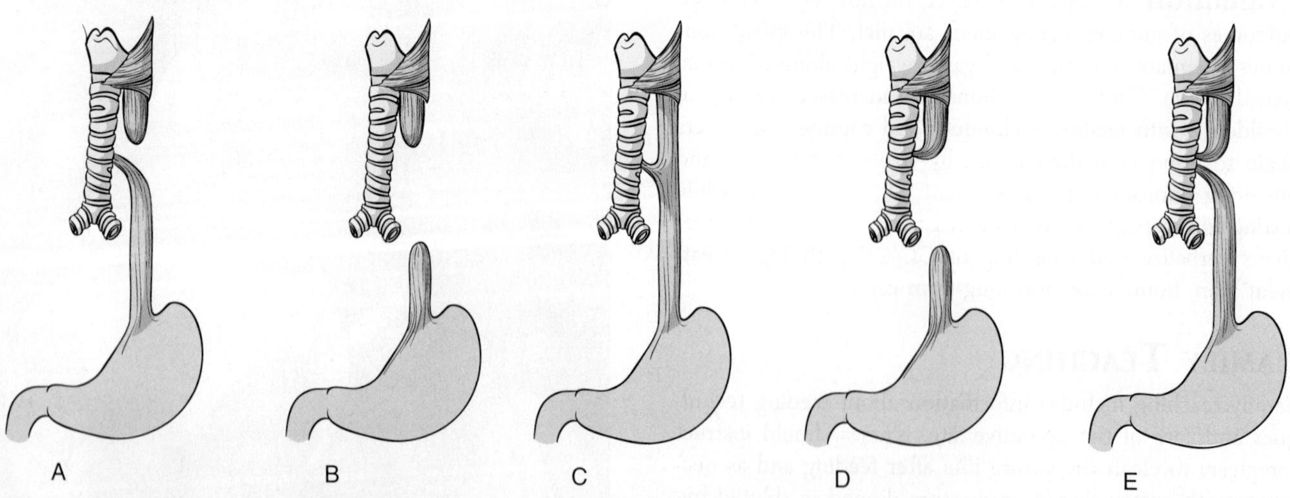

FIGURE 23-7 **Types of Esophageal Atresia and Tracheoesophageal Fistula. (A) Esophageal atresia with distal tracheoesophageal fistula; (B) Isolated or pure esophageal atresia; (C) Tracheoesophageal fistula without esophageal atresia; (D) Esophageal atresia with proximal tracheoesophageal fistula; and (E) Esophageal atresia with proximal and distal tracheoesophageal fistula.** DELMAR CENGAGE LEARNING.

T—Tracheoesophageal fistula

E—Esophageal atresia

R—Renal anomalies

L—Limb defects

Pathophysiology

The esophagus and trachea derive from the common primitive foregut (embryonic digestive tube from which the pharynx, esophagus, stomach, and duodenum form) during the fourth and fifth weeks of embryonic development. This foregut lengthens and separates the esophagus from the trachea during the sixth to eighth week. EA and TEF are caused by defective separation. EA as an isolated anomaly occurs rarely. The atresia is attributable to failure of the recanalization of the esophagus.

Clinical Manifestations

Typically, the neonate with EA/TEF presents with copious, fine, frothy bubbles of mucus in the mouth and sometimes the nose. These secretions may clear with aggressive suctioning but eventually return. The infant may have rattling respirations and episodes of coughing, choking, and cyanosis. These episodes may be exaggerated during feeding. If a fistula between the esophagus and the trachea is present, abdominal distention develops as air builds up in the stomach.

Diagnosis

A history of maternal **polyhydramnios**, an excessive amount of amniotic fluid, should suggest the possibility of a high gastrointestinal obstruction, which prevents the fetus from swallowing and absorbing the fluid. The inability to identify the fetal stomach bubble on a prenatal sonogram in a mother with polyhydramnios makes the diagnosis of EA more likely. If it is suspected, after birth a radiopaque nasogastric or feeding tube should be passed through the nose to the stomach. In infants with atresia, the tube typically stops at 10–12 cm. The normal distance is 17 cm (Spoon & Trotter, 2003). The type of esophageal abnormality is further determined by radiographic studies. When present, curling of the tube in the upper esophageal segment is shown on radiography. If TEF is present, air may be seen in the stomach if there is a fistula that connects the trachea with the distal esophagus. The absence of air in the stomach indicates EA without TEF.

Treatment

Before the performance of the first successful repair in 1939, this condition was fatal. However, over the past 50 years, refinements in neonatal surgical technique, preoperative support, anesthesia, and neonatal intensive care have improved the outcome. Treatment is aimed at preventing aspiration pneumonia until surgical repair of the defect is completed. Healthy infants without pulmonary complications or other major anomalies usually can undergo surgery in the first few days of life. The type of surgical correction depends on the esophageal abnormality. A one-stage repair to connect both ends of the esophagus and close the fistula is preferred in all infants with TEF.

Occasionally, the infant's condition (preterm, low birth weight, pneumonia, other major anomalies) requires that surgery be performed in stages. The first is closing of the fistula and inserting a gastrostomy tube for feeding. The second stage involves **anastomosis** (surgical connection of two tubular structures) of the two ends of the esophagus. Eight to ten days after this procedure, oral feedings are begun and usually tolerated.

Nursing Management

The goals preoperatively are prevention of aspiration of secretions from the upper esophageal pouch and prevention of regurgitation of stomach contents through the fistula into the trachea. Nursing care initially includes maintaining hydration status by allowing nothing by mouth and administering intravenous fluids. The infant is positioned supine with the head elevated to decrease pressure against the thoracic cavity and increase pooling of secretions in the bottom of the upper esophageal pouch. This position minimizes reflux of gastric secretions into the trachea and bronchi. Intermittent or continuous suction of the esophageal segment, if ordered before surgery, is essential.

In the postoperative period the nurse's goals are to maintain a patent airway and prevent trauma to the anastomosis. Suctioning must be performed gently to avoid trauma to the tissues to maintain the airway. The nurse observes the infant for early signs of airway obstruction, such as an anxious expression on the infant's face, tachypnea (increase in respiratory rate), and the presence of abnormal breath sounds. In the immediate postoperative period the gastrostomy tube is elevated to allow gastric secretions to flow into the small intestine and air to escape. A pacifier is offered to meet the infant's sucking needs and to prepare for oral feeding. The infant remains fluid restricted (NPO) until bowel sounds return and there is no danger of disturbing the surgical site. Nutrients are obtained through intravenous fluids. When the infant is begun on gastrostomy feedings glucose water is given and, if tolerated, followed by formula or breast milk.

Family Teaching

Infants who have the single-stage repair need to be observed for signs of esophageal stricture. The nurse explains and provides a written list of these and instructs the caregivers to contact their health care provider if any occur. Signs include dysphagia, inability or difficulty swallowing, increased drooling, and frequent coughing and choking that appear to be related to swallowing. The family of infants who require multiple stage surgery needs to learn how to perform the necessary procedures for gastrostomy feeding and care and oral feeding.

LOWER GASTROINTESTINAL ALTERATIONS

Lower gastrointestinal alterations in infants and children include obstructive disorders in which nutrients and secretions are unable to pass through the GI tract, and elimination disorders. The alterations that will be presented include intussusception, Hirschsprung's disease, and anorectal malformations.

INTUSSUSCEPTION

Intussusception is a common pediatric condition that occurs when one segment of the bowel telescopes into the lumen of an adjacent segment of intestine.

INCIDENCE AND ETIOLOGY

Intussusception is the most frequent cause of intestinal obstruction in infants and young children. The incidence is 1–4 in 1,000 live births with the peak in the third to ninth month of life and occurring two times more frequently in boys compared with girls. In most cases the cause cannot be identified. Approximately 75 percent of cases of intussusception in children are considered to be idiopathic because there is no clear disease trigger or pathological lead point. Idiopathic intussusception is most common in children between three months and five years of age (Kitagawa & Miqdady, 2008). In a minority of cases, a specific lesion, such as a polyp or foreign body, or a viral infection can be identified as a possible trigger. Figure 23-8 illustrates intussusception.

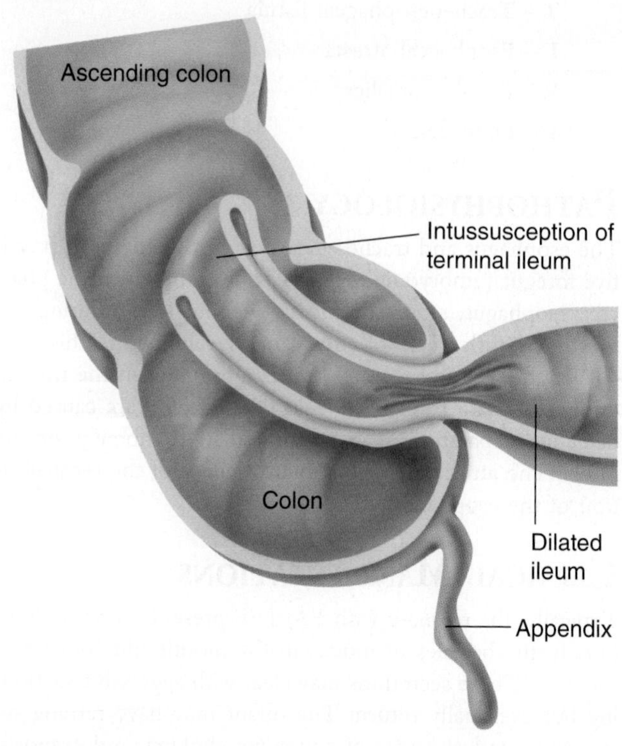

FIGURE 23-8 Intussusception of Terminal Ileum into the Ascending Colon. DELMAR CENGAGE LEARNING.

PATHOPHYSIOLOGY

Intussusception occurs most often near the ileocecal junction (ileocolic intussusception). Ileo-colic, jejuno-jejunal, jejuno-ileal, or colo-colic intussusception also have been reported. As one segment of the bowel telescopes or invaginates into another, the walls of the bowel press against each other and compromise the blood and lymph flow. The involved intestine becomes inflamed and edematous and bleeding occurs resulting in blood and mucus in the stool. Eventually, complete bowel obstruction develops producing abdominal distention and vomiting. If untreated, it may progress to necrosis and perforation (Huppertz et al., 2006).

CLINICAL MANIFESTATIONS

Five signs and symptoms are classically described in the infant with intussusception: colic, intermittent abdominal pain, crying while drawing the legs to abdomen, vomiting, and currant jelly-like stools. However, these are present in fewer than half of infants with the disease (Kuppermann, O'Dea, Pinckney, & Hoecker, 2000). Characteristically, a previously healthy, thriving infant has a sudden onset of severe and intermittent abdominal pain. Nonbilious vomiting is the predominate sign in neonates and is usually seen early in the illness. In the later phase the vomitus becomes bile stained. Blood and mucus appear in the stool, resulting in the red, currant jelly-like appearance. The abdomen is tender, and a sausage-shaped mass may be felt in the right upper quadrant. As the intussusception progresses, the infant becomes listless and lethargic. Eventually a shock-like state may develop with a weak and thready pulse, shallow respirations, and a marked elevation of body temperature.

DIAGNOSIS

An X-ray of the abdomen is nonspecific in the diagnosis; however, it will reveal intraperitoneal air if present, which indicates bowel perforation. The definitive test for diagnosing intussusception has been the barium or air contrast enema. Contrast enema is a safe procedure with minimal risk of bowel perforation. Nonetheless, it is invasive and presents the potential risk of radiation exposure. In addition, this test may be unnecessary if a less invasive technique can be used to accurately rule out intussusception. In recent years, abdominal ultrasound has been found to be a reliable and noninvasive screening tool for this disease (Kairam, Kaiafis, & Shih, 2009).

TREATMENT

The treatment of choice for intussusception is nonsurgical hydrostatic reduction using barium, a water-soluble contrast agent, or air enema. The water-soluble contrast and air **insufflation** (blowing air into a cavity) are believed to be safer than

NURSING TIP

Helping Families Visualize Intussusception

Comparing the anatomy of intussusception to a folding telescope may help caregivers and families understand the diagnosis. A rubber glove with one finger inverted into the glove can be used as a visual aid. To demonstrate the principle of reduction by hydrostatic pressure, fill the glove with water until the inverted finger resumes its normal position.

barium, with less risk of bowel perforation. Successful reduction rates have been reported as high as 90% for air and 65–85% for barium or the water-soluble contrast agent. If there is evidence of intestinal perforation, peritonitis, or shock, or if hydrostatic reduction is unsuccessful, prompt surgical intervention is indicated to manually reduce the intussuscepted bowel.

Nursing Management

Because the onset of this disorder is so abrupt, most caregivers need much reassurance regarding the effectiveness of treatment and excellent prognosis. Preparation for hydrostatic reduction involves placing the infant on NPO status, inserting a nasogastric tube that is connected to low suction, and administering intravenous fluids. The nurse monitors the infant's vital signs and mental status for changes that might indicate perforation, peritonitis, or shock; assesses for worsening abdominal pain; and examines and records all stools. The passage of normal stool may indicate spontaneous resolution of the obstruction. For a few hours after reduction, the child should remain in the hospital and be observed for the passage of stool and barium or water-soluble contrast, as indicated, and for the recurrence of the intussusception. Recurrence develops in about 10% of children following hydrostatic reduction. If hydrostatic reduction is unsuccessful, surgical treatment is indicated. For the child undergoing surgery, postoperative care is similar to that described in the nursing care plan for a child having an appendectomy.

Family Teaching

When the child is discharged, the nurse should instruct the caregivers to observe for signs of intestinal obstruction and recurrence. These include increasing abdominal pain, abdominal distention, blood in the stools, bile-stained vomiting, and decreased or absent stools, all of which should be reported to their health care provider.

HIRSCHSPRUNG'S DISEASE

Hirschsprung's disease (HD), also called congenital aganglionic megacolon, is a motility disorder of the bowel caused by the absence of parasympathetic ganglion cells in the large intestine. This absence prevents peristalsis and causes feces to accumulate proximal to the defect, leading to bowel obstruction. It is the most common cause of distal bowel obstruction in the newborn; however, it may not be diagnosed until infancy or childhood.

Incidence and Etiology

The incidence is 1 in 5,000 live births, with males affected three to four times more often than females; the racial distribution is equal. HD is not a hereditary condition, but an inherited predisposition is relatively strong. A family history is present in about 10% of cases, and the incidence in siblings is about 3.5%. Other associated congenital anomalies include imperforate anus, urinary tract abnormalities, cardiac defects, seizure disorders, and Down syndrome (McAlhany & Popovich, 2007; Swenson, 2002). Genetic mutations, predominantly RET proto-oncogene have been identified in patients with HD (Dasgupta & Langer, 2004).

Pathophysiology

The disease is caused by an absence of parasympathetic ganglion cells in the colon. The aganglionic segment is most frequently located in the rectosigmoid area. Defecation is controlled by the parasympathetic nervous system (the ganglion cells), to which the lower colon, the internal and external anal sphincters, and the anus respond in a coordinated manner. The affected bowel (absence of ganglion cells) is unable to transmit coordinated peristaltic waves and to pass fecal contents along its length, resulting in an accumulation of fecal material and distention proximal to the defect. The normal portion of the bowel becomes hypertrophied and dilated; hence, the name megacolon. Figure 23-9 illustrates the bowel in HD. The distention of the bowel wall may cause the intestinal distention and ischemia, which could lead to the development of enterocolitis (Dasgupta & Langer, 2004).

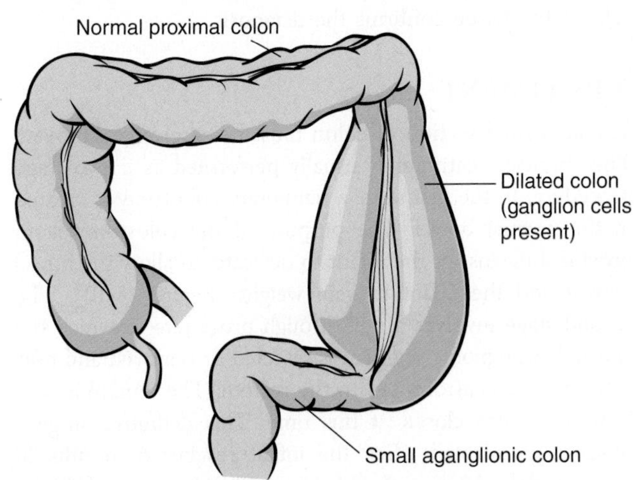

Figure 23-9 Hirschsprung's Disease with Dilation of the Colon Proximal to the Aganglionic Section. DELMAR CENGAGE LEARNING.

Clinical Manifestations

In the newborn the primary manifestations are failure to pass meconium (the first feces of the newborn) within 24 to 48 hours after birth, abdominal distention, bile-stained vomitus, refusal to feed, and intestinal obstruction. In older infants and children, the initial symptom is chronic constipation. Abdominal distention; episodes of explosive passage of stools; inadequate weight gain; ribbon-like or pellet shaped, foul-smelling stools; vomiting; and an easily palpable fecal mass may also be present.

The most ominous complication is **enterocolitis**, inflammation of the small intestine and colon. An otherwise well infant who has a history of constipation has an abrupt onset of foul-smelling diarrhea, abdominal distention, and fever. The illness may progress rapidly, with perforation of the bowel and sepsis, and may occur before, during, or after surgery. Enterocolitis and sepsis remain the most serious complication and major causes of death in HD, occurring in about 30% of cases (Swenson, 2002).

Diagnosis

Hirschsprung's disease is diagnosed in 15% of infants within the first month of life, in 60% by the third month, and in 80% by 1 year of age (Swenson, 2002). It can present with symptoms varying from complete intestinal obstruction with enterocolitis to simple constipation. In the neonate who does not pass meconium and has abdominal distention the diagnosis of HD is suspected. In older infants and children a history of chronic constipation should raise the question of HD. A rectal examination reveals the absence of stool in the rectum, and the internal anal sphincter is tight. A barium enema documents a transition zone between the narrowed aganglionic segment of the colon and the dilated, hypertrophied section. This sign may be absent in the first few weeks of life because it takes some time for normal ganglionic bowel to dilate with stool; therefore, the barium enema may not be diagnostic in newborns. For a definitive diagnosis, a rectal biopsy is required. The absence of ganglionic cells in the tissue confirms the diagnosis.

Treatment

The abnormal section of colon must be surgically removed. The surgical treatment is usually performed as a two-stage procedure. In the first stage a temporary colostomy is created in the normal bowel. The purpose of the colostomy is to provide a means for the infant to defecate, to allow the bowel to rest and the infant to gain weight (Figure 23-10). The second stage involves a pull-through procedure in which the affected, aganglionic segment is resected or removed and normal bowel is anastomosed to the rectum. The temporary colostomy is also closed at this time. This definitive surgical repair is performed when the infant reaches 6 months of age or weighs 20 pounds (McAlhany & Popovich, 2007).

In recent years, the treatment has been changing from a two-stage surgical repair to a one-stage pull-through without a temporary colostomy with excellent results. The timing of the definitive procedure also has been changing from approximately 12 months to early neonatal surgery. Benefits of the one-stage correction include avoidance of multiple operations, reduction in the number of hospital admissions and the cost of treatment, elimination of the problems in colostomy care, and completion of treatment at an earlier age.

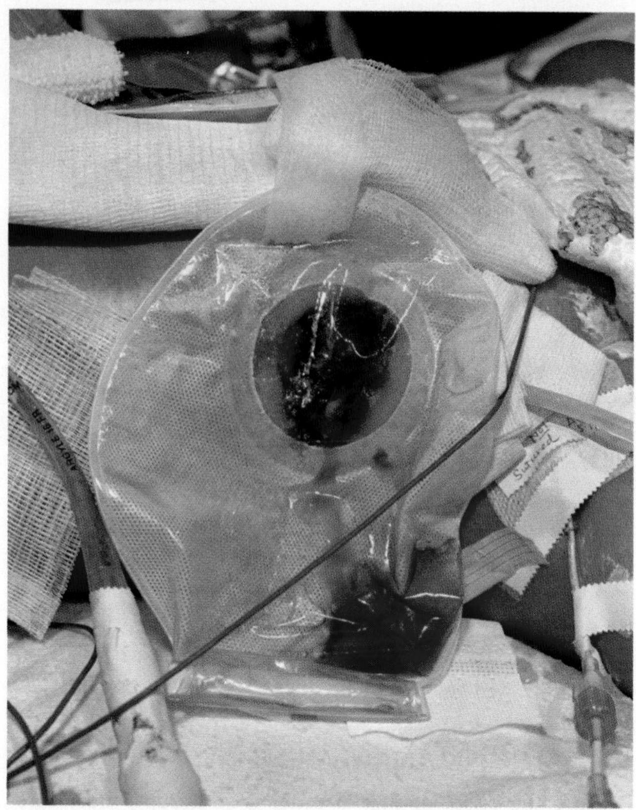

Figure 23-10 Colostomy After the First Stage of Surgical Repair of Hirschsprung's Disease. DELMAR CENGAGE LEARNING.

Another advancement in the treatment is a procedure called the laparoscopic-assisted pull-through. The laparoscope allows surgeons to enter the child's body through the anus and pull the affected segment of bowel through the opening, thereby eliminating major abdominal surgery. Because the laparoscope requires only a few small incisions, the length of hospital stay is decreased, the scar is minimal, and complications are reduced.

Nursing Management

Preoperative assessment of the infant's fluid and electrolyte status is essential because preparation for surgery involves extensive bowel cleansing with repeated saline enemas. The infant is NPO, and an NG tube is inserted. Intravenous fluids and electrolytes are administered to prevent dehydration and correct electrolyte deficiencies if they occur. Oral administration of antibiotics may be ordered in conjunction with antibiotic enemas to reduce intestinal flora.

Postoperative nursing care includes routine post-abdominal surgery interventions, such as maintaining patency of the NG tube, monitoring for abdominal distention, incision site care, and assessing for return of bowel sounds. The nurse measures and records the amount of colostomy and NG drainage. An enterostomal therapist (ET) fits the ostomy with an appropriate appliance and begins education with the family about colostomy care.

Family Teaching

The nurse explains to the caregivers about the need for the surgery and the temporary colostomy and how to care for it. Instructions include skin care, appliance application, and information about community resources for obtaining supplies. Referral to an ET is important for assistance if problems occur with the appliance or stoma. The nurse teaches the family signs and symptoms of complications such as enterocolitis and leaks or strictures at the site of the anastomosis. Signs of leaks are abdominal distention and irritability, and signs of strictures are constipation, vomiting, or diarrhea. These indications of complications should be reported to their health care provider. Families will usually require encouragement, understanding, and support, especially regarding the colostomy. They should be informed that with proper management their child can return to a normal lifestyle in a short time.

ANORECTAL MALFORMATIONS

Anorectal malformations are defined as an arrest of rectal descent resulting in absence of an anal opening and occur during the 4th–16th week of gestation. Examples of these malformations include anorectal agenesis (imperforate anus), rectal atresia, and anal agenesis.

Incidence and Etiology

Anorectal malformations occur in 0.2 in 1,000 live births and are more common in males (Haider & Fisher, 2007). The etiology is unknown; however, these defects are associated with several other congenital anomalies of the urinary tract, esophagus, and intestines. In some cases, environmental factors or drug exposure during pregnancy may play a role, but this is still unclear.

Pathophysiology

The origin of the anus and rectum is an embryonic structure called the cloaca, which is the precursor of the anorectal and genitourinary structures. Both the rectum and the urinary structures become completely separated by the 7th week of gestation. Any abnormality in the development of these systems results in anorectal and genitourinary malformations. Depending on the week of gestation when the embryonic development is disrupted and on the level to which the rectal pouch has descended, the anomaly will be either low or high. Low malformations occur between the 10th and 12th week; high ones occur during the 4th week. In low anomalies the rectal pouch has descended below the rectal sphincter muscle complex. For rectal continence to occur the rectum must descend to this point. In high defects the rectum terminates above the sphincter muscle complex, making continence more difficult to establish (Nisell, 2003).

Clinical Manifestations

Anorectal malformations are usually obvious at birth. Low defects vary from a normal appearing anus, to a thin translucent anal membrane, to a deep anal dimple. The anal dimple will demonstrate strong muscular contractions when pricked with a pin. High defects present as a flat perineum, absence of an anal dimple, and no muscular contraction to a pin prick. If meconium is noted in the urine, a fistula is present between the bowel and the urinary tract. Fistulas can also be present between the bowel and vagina in females.

Diagnosis

Diagnosis is made by physical exam of the anal features and by radiologic imaging of the abdomen. The level of the defect and presence and location of any fistulas are determined by these tests. During the abdominal X-rays the neonate is held in an inverted position for a few minutes to allow air to fill the blind colonic pouch and permit identification of the level of the defect. The presence of gas in the bladder or urethra during imaging indicates a fistula between these structures and the bowel.

Treatment

Treatment depends on the extent of the malformation. Anal stenosis is managed with repeated manual dilatation of the anus. All other defects require surgery. Low defects are corrected by creating an anal opening, followed by anal dilation to prevent stenosis. High malformations are treated with a two-stage repair, the first involving creation of a temporary colostomy. The second stage includes closure of the colostomy and a pull-through procedure in which the blind pouch of the rectum is anastomosed to the anus (Quinn & Shannon, 1996).

Nursing Management

During the newborn examination, the nurse assesses the patency of the anus by inserting a rectal thermometer. The defect is obvious when there is an absence of a normal anal opening. Nursing observations that should be documented and reported include failure of the neonate to pass meconium within the first 24 hours of life, inability to insert a rectal thermometer, and the presence of an anal dimple. Nursing care depends on the type of lesion corrected. For low defects with the anoplasty, the main focus is on preventing infection of the perineal and anal wounds. Because of the location of the surgical incisions, they are at high risk for infection from urine and stool; therefore, meticulous skin care is essential. For high lesions, postoperative care initially includes colostomy care, perineal wound care, IV fluid management, and NG tube maintenance. Oral feedings are begun when stooling has started through the stoma. Oral feedings following the pull-through are begun when peristalsis resumes, stooling occurs through the anus, and initial healing has taken place.

Family Teaching

Caregivers are instructed in colostomy care, perineal wound care, and anal dilations as appropriate. Prevention of constipation is stressed in family education. Adequate fluid, dietary fiber, and stool softeners or bulk agents help the child to achieve normal bowel activity. It is important to advise caregivers that toilet training may be delayed and children may have difficulty with this developmental task. Their patience and understanding of their child is essential. Encouraging the family and child during this stressful time is a key nursing intervention.

■ ALTERATIONS IN MOTILITY

Disorders discussed in this section include gastroesophageal reflux and constipation.

GASTROESOPHAGEAL REFLUX

Gastroesophageal reflux (GER) is the most common esophageal disorder of infants and the condition most frequently referred to a pediatric gastroenterologist (Arguin & Swartz, 2004). GER is defined as the return of gastric contents into the lower esophagus through the lower esophageal sphincter (LES). The LES is a distinct area formed by the union of the muscle fibers from the esophagus and stomach (Figure 23-11).

Physiological GER is a common occurrence in many healthy infants. About 50% of infants less than 2 months old are reported to have GER (Suwandhi, Ton, & Schwarz, 2006). Improvement is usually seen between 6 and 12 months of age as the infant matures. The esophagus elongates and the LES moves down below the diaphragm, decreasing the chance of reflux. Pathologic GER is reflux that manifests as respiratory disorders, esophagitis or its complication (strictures), and malnutrition (failure to thrive).

Incidence and Etiology

GER affects about 5% of otherwise healthy children (Pulsifer-Anderson, 2009). Boys are affected three times more frequently than girls. GER is more common in premature infants and those with neurologic impairment. The exact cause is unknown although it is thought to result from the delayed maturation of the lower esophageal neuromuscular function or impaired local hormonal control mechanisms. Infants living in an environment with tobacco smoke have a higher incidence of GER. It has been reported that some conditions, including neurologic impairment, hiatal hernia, repaired esophageal atresia, and morbid obesity predispose children to a high prevalence of GER (Suwandhi et al., 2006).

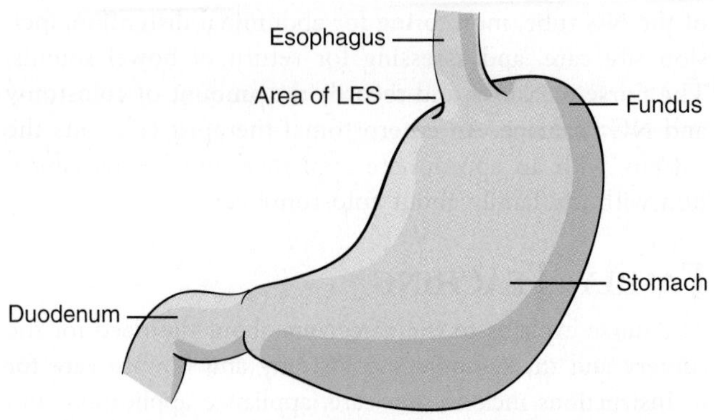

Figure 23-11 Stomach contents are refluxed into the esophagus through the lower esophageal sphincter (LES) in GER. DELMAR CENGAGE LEARNING.

Pathophysiology

The LES acts as a physiological barrier to reflux of stomach contents into the esophagus. It is innervated by the vagal nerves, so a defect in this nerve transmission may result in inappropriate relaxation of the LES. This allows the reflux of gastric contents into the esophagus. Delayed gastric emptying also occurs in infants caused by hypomotility or retrograde peristalsis of the duodenum (Suwandhi et al., 2006).

Clinical Manifestations

Vomiting and regurgitation are the most common symptoms. The regurgitated matter is typically nonbilious and consists of undigested formula and mucus. The infant displays excessive crying and irritability from esophagitis, which is caused by recurrent reflux of acidic gastric contents into the esophagus. Coughing occurs when aspiration is suspected. Refusal to feed may develop in infants with esophagitis as they learn to associate feeding with pain. Esophagitis can cause bleeding in the gastrointestinal tract, which produces anemia and is seen as blood in the stools. Insufficient caloric intake resulting from caregivers' hesitancy to feed infants who are repeatedly spitting up and nutrient losses in emesis contributes to malnourishment and growth retardation. Complications of GER include apnea, choking spells, recurrent aspiration pneumonia, and frequent other respiratory infections.

Diagnosis

The diagnosis of GER is established by taking a history, performing a physical examination, observing the infant's feeding habits, and conducting several diagnostic tests. The first goal is to rule out other possible causes for the symptoms such as gastrointestinal tract obstructions, neurologic disease, or metabolic disorders. Several diagnostic tests exist to help confirm GER. Initially an upper GI barium series is performed to eliminate anatomic abnormalities (esophageal stricture, pyloric stenosis, and intestinal malrotation) from consideration. Upper GI endoscopy allows direct visualization of the esophageal mucosa to detect inflammation and

CRITICAL THINKING

What's the Difference between Gastroesophageal Reflux and Hypertrophic Pyloric Stenosis?

Vomiting is a classic symptom of GER and HPS. Based on the clinical manifestations of each disorder, how would you distinguish between the two?

ulceration, which are indicative of esophagitis. Another test is the esophageal pH probe study. A small catheter is placed through a nostril into the distal third of the esophagus and is left in place for 18 to 24 hours (Suwandhi et al., 2006). The infant is fed a substance with a known pH such as unfiltered apple juice. The probe measures the pH of the distal esophagus, indicating the number of reflux episodes and the time it takes for acid to clear from the esophagus. Although a sensitive test, the pH probe is not needed for routine diagnosis. Because of the cost and the need for hospitalization, this test is best used for infants who have complicated courses or who present diagnostic dilemmas.

Treatment

Medical management involves dietary modifications, positioning, tobacco smoke avoidance, and medications. Nonpharmacologic therapies are beneficial to infants with GER (Sondheimer, 2008). Small, frequent feedings are recommended because of the probable relationship between gastric volume and reflux. This feeding method decreases the duration of reflux episodes. However, increased frequency causes more frequent stimulation of stomach acids. Therefore, the advantages must be weighed against the disadvantages. Many infants have benefited from this traditional approach. Another dietary adjustment that is recommended is the thickening of formula with cereal. This approach has major benefits for the regurgitating infant, particularly when there has been poor weight gain. These include increased caloric density; decreased time spent crying, and decreased episodes of emesis.

Controversy surrounds positioning therapy in the medical treatment for GER. Recommendations for positioning have changed from the upright or seated position prior to the early 1980s, to the 30-degrees prone or head elevated prone in the middle 1980s, to the flat prone in the early 1990s (American Academy of Pediatrics, 2000). One aspect of the controversy involves positioning to prevent sudden infant death syndrome (SIDS). The American Academy of Pediatrics recommends that infants be placed in the supine (on their back) position for sleep. Most of the SIDS deaths in the prone position are attributable to suffocation because of puffy bedding materials such as comforters. If these materials are eliminated from the infant's bed, the superiority of the prone position for GER is clear and has been recommended by the American Academy of Pediatrics (AAP, 2000). Currently, the National Digestive Diseases Information Clearinghouse (2006) recommends that infants with GER should usually sleep on their backs, as is suggested for all infants. Rarely, alternative sleep positions may be considered.

Persistent problems and complications of GER warrant pharmacological intervention. Pharmacologic management with the use of an acid suppressant is generally the first line of therapy. This group of medications includes histamine-2 receptor antagonists (H-2 blockers), proton-pump inhibitors (PPIs), and antacids. H-2 blockers competitively bind to histamine H-2 receptors on parietal cells in gastric glands; thereby inhibiting acid secretion elicited by histamine, but have no effect on acid secretion by gastrin. Ranitidine (Zantac), an H-2 receptor antagonist, is approved for use in infants and children. Other H-2 blockers such as cimetidine (Tagamet), famotidine (Pepcid), and nizatidine (Axid) are also used to treat the condition. PPIs decrease the secretion of gastric acid and are antagonists of the proton pump that stimulate the production of gastric acid. Use of a proton-pump inhibitor is indicated for infants with recurrent vomiting and failure to thrive or irritability, who have not responded to H-2 receptor antagonists. Two PPIs approved for pediatric use are: lansoprazole (Prevacid) and omeperazole (Prilosec). The use of antacids in pediatric GER is generally not recommended. Significant aluminum absorption from antacids can occur in infants approaching levels reported to cause osteopenia and neurotoxicity. The prokinetic, metoclopramide (Reglan), is used to improve gastric emptying and esophageal motor tone, but to date there are no studies supporting its use in managing symptoms of GER in infants and children.

The role of surgical treatment has decreased as pharmacotherapy has improved. Repeated episodes of pneumonia, failure to gain weight, recurrent esophagitis with stricture, severe apnea, and failure to respond to 4 to 6 weeks of medical management are indications for surgery. The Nissen fundoplication in which the fundus of the stomach is wrapped around the lower part of the esophagus is the procedure of choice. A temporary gastrostomy tube may be inserted to allow for venting of the stomach and initial feedings. The success rate with surgery is high, but recurrences are common. Less invasive fundoplication performed laparoscopically is available in a limited number of hospitals.

Nursing Management

Assessment An in-depth assessment of the infant's feeding pattern should include the amount, type, and frequency of feedings, and the timing of emesis afterwards. The nurse inquires about the positioning of the infant during feeding and the frequency of burping. It is important to obtain height, weight, and head circumference measurements and to plot them on a growth chart to assess current and potential growth problems. Infants with GER are at high risk for aspiration; therefore, assessment of a baseline respiratory status is imperative, such as lung sounds, respiratory rate, and effort.

Nursing Diagnosis

1. *Risk for aspiration* related to vomiting and reflux of gastric contents into the esophagus.
2. *Imbalanced nutrition: Less than body requirements* related to reduced nutrient intake and vomiting.
3. *Deficient knowledge (caregivers)* related to infant's condition and care including feeding, positioning, and home management.

Outcome Identification

1. Infant maintains normal respiratory status (respiratory rate appropriate for age, oxygen saturation within normal limits, clear, bilateral breath sounds).
2. Infant will maintain normal growth pattern and will ingest adequate number of calories.
3. Caregivers will verbalize or demonstrate understanding of GER, feeding and positioning of infant, and home care.

Planning and Implementation Nursing management focuses on caregiver education including dietary modifications, positioning, medication administration, and developmental needs of the infant, and on peri-operative care if surgery is performed. Dietary modifications include small, frequent feedings, thickened feedings, and avoidance of foods that irritate the GI tract. Small, frequent feedings can cause additional stress on caregivers; therefore, they need to know that higher volume and less frequent feedings can be tolerated as the infant grows. The infant should be burped frequently during feeding. Thickening of formula with rice cereal increases consistency and retention, and supplies needed calories for the infant who vomits frequently. If the health care provider has recommended the head elevated prone position after feedings and during sleep, maintaining this can be challenging for caregivers. This position can be achieved by using a wedge, sling, harness, and towel rolls, some of which are commercially available.

Nursing interventions related to the treatment of GER with pharmacotherapy include caregiver education about dosages, proper administration and scheduling, and potential side effects. Verbal information should be augmented by written material to assure proper understanding. The nurse can support the caregivers by encouraging them to identify and verbalize their fears and concerns. They often feel guilt and inadequacy because of the frequent vomiting of feedings and weight loss of the infant. They may feel overwhelmed with doubt and anxiety about their ability to adequately care for the child. Nurses can be instrumental in forming a network of caregivers of children with GER to provide support, share experiences, and foster confidence.

Evaluation The effectiveness of the nursing interventions is evaluated by the infant experiencing no respiratory difficulty or aspiration. A decrease in the frequency of vomiting and improvement in growth and development are also evaluated. Most important is the caregivers' comfort with the diagnosis and treatment plan, and their confidence in being able to care for the infant at home.

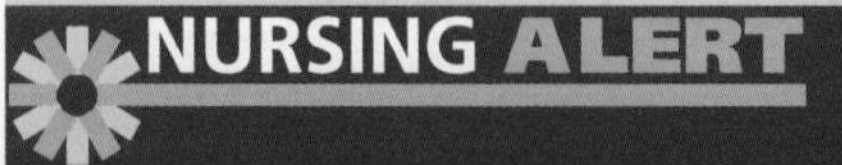

Infant Seats for Positioning

Infants with GER should not be placed in an infant seat as a mode of treatment. The reduced truncal tone in infants raises their intra-abdominal pressure and actually promotes reflux.

Family Teaching

Family teaching includes an explanation of the physiology of GER so caregivers understand their feeding technique is not the cause of the frequent vomiting. In order to accommodate the thickened feedings, the nurse should demonstrate how to enlarge the hole in the nipple. Caregivers need information about spicy and acidic foods and beverages to avoid feeding their infant because they increase secretion of gastric acid. These include citrus fruits and fruit drinks and tomato products such as tomato juice. Esophageal irritants such as chocolate and caffeine (tea, coffee, and colas) for older infants and children should also be avoided. Because of the infant's limited mobility, adequate stimulation becomes essential. Bright and colorful objects, wrist rattles, mobiles, and mirrors are all appropriate. Touching and stroking the infant provide tactile stimulation. Family teaching should also include an explanation about avoiding vigorous playing with their infant after feeding to prevent reflux.

CONSTIPATION

Constipation is the difficult passage of stool or infrequent passage of hard stool, associated with straining, abdominal pain, or withholding behaviors for more than 2 weeks. Children vary widely in the frequency with which they have a bowel movement; therefore, frequency alone is not a good diagnostic criterion (van den Berg, Benninga, & Di Lorenzo, 2006). Constipation is common in children and is usually without long-term consequences; however, it can diminish a child's quality of life, cause emotional problems, and create family stress. Rarely, constipation is a sign of a more serious health problem.

Incidence and Etiology

Constipation is common in children, accounting for 3–5% of office visits to pediatricians and 25% of visits to pediatric gastroenterologists (Coughlin, 2003). Constipation is the second most referred condition and accounts for as much as 25% of pediatric gastroenterology consultations. It is more common in males during early childhood; however, during adolescence it is seen more frequently in females. The cause of constipation can be organic or nonorganic, also called functional. Organic causes include:

1. Dietary (e.g., low fiber, inadequate fluid intake, excessive dairy intake)
2. Structural disorders of the gastrointestinal tract (e.g., Hirschsprung's disease, intestinal strictures)
3. Metabolic and endocrine disorders (e.g., hypothyroidism, diabetes mellitus, lead poisoning)
4. Neurogenic diseases (e.g., cerebral palsy, myelomeningocele)
5. Medications (e.g., opiates, antidepressants, anticholinergics, antacids)

For the majority of children, nonorganic or functional problems are the cause.

Constipation during infancy is rare and usually caused by excessive milk intake or the transition from formula to cow's milk. In toddlers, constipation is often caused by toilet training practices. Forced training may cause the child to withhold stool. Bowel and feeding issues are common manifestations of intense autonomy struggles with toddlers. Additionally, a previously painful bowel movement because of a hard stool or anal fissures can result in fear of having a bowel movement. Magical thinking is a characteristic of toddlers' cognitive development, which can result in their fear of the toilet and cause difficulty in having a bowel movement. For example, a 2-year-old boy who had developed a fear of having a bowel movement admitted he was worried that his "poo would drown." Another child wanted to know, "Do poos have brains?" Fear of the toilet may be initiated by television. Commercials for toilet cleaners, for example, contain images of "germs and monsters" climbing out of the toilet. This can seem very real in a young child's imagination.

The older toddler, preschooler, and school-age child may develop problems when starting nursery school, kindergarten, or first grade. Bathrooms in these settings may lack privacy and tend not to have soft toilet paper. As a result, the urge to defecate is suppressed during school hours. Continual suppression of defecation can lead to constipation.

Pathophysiology

Normal defecation occurs when stool moves into the rectum, causing rectal distention and relaxation of the internal anal sphincter. The conscious awareness of rectal distention results in contraction of the voluntary muscles of the external anal sphincter. Voluntary relaxation of the external sphincter and increased intra-abdominal pressure result in defecation. Constipation tends to be self-perpetuating. As stool is retained, the simultaneous process of stretching the rectal wall and decreasing sensory feedback leads to less frequent bowel movements, which result in further stool retention and larger stools. As water is reabsorbed, the stool becomes harder, and bowel movements may become painful. As this cycle progresses, the external and internal sphincters become compromised. Sensitivity to rectal distention and control of rectal evacuation diminish, and the child soon loses the urge to have a bowel movement.

Clinical Manifestations

The child who is constipated will have hard, small stools that may be passed at regular intervals or large masses of stool at intervals of days to weeks. Soiling of underwear in a child who is toilet trained is possible. Abdominal pain or distention develops as more stool accumulates in the bowel. The child often cries during toilet time. The child may become irritable and experience a loss of appetite. Often a palpable fecal mass is felt on physical exam.

Diagnosis

Diagnosis is based on the history and physical exam. When attempting to determine the cause, it is important to rule out any organic causes. A thorough dietary history is obtained. A description of stool pattern, such as frequency, consistency, and size of stools, and toilet training history is elicited. Certain medications can cause constipation; therefore, it is important to determine if the child is taking any of these. An abdominal X-ray shows a colon enlarged with stool and gas.

Treatment

Constipation is treated with a combination of therapies, which include cleansing the bowel, establishing a regular pattern of defecation, and modifying the diet. Cleaning the bowel of hardened or impacted stool is accomplished with enemas, oral medications, and suppositories. There are many types of oral medications that can be used. The choice depends on the child's age, the child's ability to take the medication, the ease of giving it, and how well it works. Stool-softeners such as docusate or lactulose may be used, and polyethylene glycol (PEG) 3350 without electrolytes (Miralax) is tolerated well by children because it can be mixed with beverages the child likes (Leoening-Baucke & Pashankar, 2006). Occasionally, if feces are impacted, they may need to be removed manually.

Modification of the diet includes increasing the intake of fiber and fluids. Establishing a regular pattern for defecation is largely a matter of caregiver education about normal defecation and bowel training techniques.

Nursing Management and Family Teaching

Nursing intervention focuses on education. Dietary modifications include increasing dietary fiber and fluids. The nurse should teach caregivers about high-fiber foods and diet planning. High-fiber foods include: whole grain breads and cereals; bran; high fiber snack bars; raw vegetables; fruits, especially raisins, prunes, cherries, and apricots; beans; popcorn; nuts; and seeds. In addition, caregivers need instruction in the appropriate way to administer an enema.

Establishing a regular pattern of defecation is accomplished by requiring the child to sit on the toilet after a meal for a reasonable amount of time, 5–10 minutes. Positive reinforcement with star charts or small prizes can be used to reward success and adherence with the toileting schedule and taking of medications.

The family needs to understand causes of constipation to be compliant with the treatment plan. Parents often continue to blame behavioral aspects on fecal soiling. These include laziness, carelessness, and emotional problems. The nurse needs to educate the family that this is often not the cause. Emotional support to the child is essential. Denial of fecal soiling is common in children. Shame and fear of punishment may contribute to this denial.

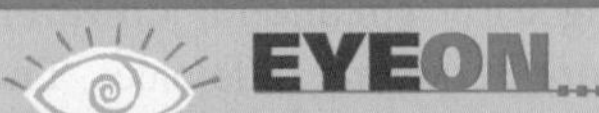

Empacho

Empacho is a Spanish word that means indigestion, stomach pains, and abdominal cramps. It is sometimes perceived as stomach or intestinal blockage. Some Hispanics believe these symptoms are caused by a ball of undigested food clinging to some part of the gastrointestinal tract and are due to one being forced to eat against one's will or lying about the amount of food eaten. Treatment is to massage and gently pinch the spine. This therapy can be problematic if the cause of symptoms is something serious such as appendicitis.

INFLAMMATORY DISORDERS

Disorders caused by chronic inflammation of the GI tract can occur at any age, newborns through adolescents. Some of these disorders are short term and readily resolved like appendicitis; others are chronic and affect growth and development. Appendicitis, inflammatory bowel disease (ulcerative colitis and Crohn's disease), peptic ulcers, and necrotizing enterocolitis will be discussed in this section.

APPENDICITIS

Appendicitis, the inflammation of the vermiform appendix or the small sac at the end of the cecum, is the most common condition requiring abdominal surgery in children. Although appendicitis was first described over 100 years ago, the vagueness of its signs and symptoms in children poses a continuing challenge for health care providers to arrive at a timely and accurate diagnosis. Failure to diagnose appendicitis is the third most frequent subject of malpractice suits and the most expensive source of claims for emergency department physicians.

INCIDENCE AND ETIOLOGY

Appendicitis is the most common condition requiring abdominal surgery in childhood, occurring at a rate of 4 per 1,000 children younger than 14 years of age, although it rarely happens to children less than 2 years of age (Zeller, Burke, & Glass, 2007). It is more common in summer, has a higher incidence in males than females, and Caucasians than non-Caucasians. Although the exact cause is poorly understood, the appendix usually becomes inflamed because of obstruction between the appendix and cecum or a systemic or enteric infection. Appendicitis is rare in third-world countries where diets are high in fiber; however, no causal relationship has been established between dietary fiber and the prevention of appendicitis.

PATHOPHYSIOLOGY

The appendix is vermiform (wormlike) in shape, with a diameter similar to a lead pencil. It rises from the wall of the cecum portion of the large intestine, below the ileocecal valve. However, its location can vary among individuals. As food passes through the cecum, the appendix also fills and empties. In 70% of cases, the lumen between the appendix and the cecum becomes obstructed with agents such as a **fecalith**, fecal matter that becomes petrified and stone-like, calculi, tumors, parasites, and foreign bodies. In the remaining 30% with no evidence of obstruction, the inflammation may be caused by a bacteria, virus, trauma, or postoperative fecal stasis (Pisarra, 2001).

CLINICAL MANIFESTATIONS

Abdominal pain is the first symptom in typical cases of appendicitis. Initially, the pain may be vague and poorly localized to the periumbilical area; gradually migrating to the right lower quadrant (RLQ). Anorexia and nausea with or without vomiting may also be present, but occur after the initial symptom of pain. The most reliable information gained from the history is the sequence of symptoms. Pain nearly always precedes anorexia, nausea, or vomiting. Nausea and vomiting that precede abdominal pain often indicate gastroenteritis. Additional clinical manifestations that may be present are constipation or diarrhea. The child's temperature is usually normal or slightly elevated. A temperature of 101°F (38.3°C) or higher suggests the presence of peritonitis.

NURSING TIP

Palpating the Abdomen for Pain

Children frequently tense their abdominal muscles when they are being examined. Warm your hands and stethoscope before touching their abdomens. Maintain eye contact with them while palpating their abdomens, and they will watch your face rather than your hands and relax. This technique provides more reliable information about the presence of pain.

NURSING TIP

Assessing for Appendicitis

When appendicitis is suspected, ask the child if she or he is hungry. If the answer is yes, chances of the child having appendicitis are less likely. In most cases, the child who has this disorder does not feel like eating from the onset of symptoms.

EVIDENCE-BASED PRACTICE

Nasogastric (NG) Tube Placement Verification

CLINICAL PROBLEM

Misplacement of NG tubes can cause significant problems for pediatric and neonatal patients such as pneumonia and pneumothorax. Little research exists regarding the verification of NG tubes in children. Several clinical studies and anecdotal reports questioned the reliability of using auscultation to verify NG tube placement. However, the vast majority of nurses continue to check NG tube placement by auscultation of air insufflation over the abdomen.

BEST CLINICAL PRACTICE

- Upon initial NG tube placement, an X-ray is recommended to confirm proper placement before initiation of feedings or medication administration.
- X-ray remains the only 100% reliable method to verify NG tube placement; however, getting an X-ray before each feeding is costly and impractical.
- Nurses should verify tube placement before each feeding and medication administration using the following methods: (1) confirming the mark on the tube is at the point it exits the nares; (2) aspirating gastric contents and assessing color (clear, light yellow, or light green); (3) measuring the pH of the aspirate from the stomach (pH = 1–4).
- Using more than one bedside assessment method to verify NG tube placement is superior to any single placement-verification method used alone.
- Auscultating over the abdomen for air insufflation into the NG tube is ineffective.

IMPLICATIONS FOR NURSING

An accurate and reliable evidence-based guideline on verifying NG tube placement can prevent complications caused by misplaced NG tube.

Reference: Farrington, M., Lang, S., Cullen, L., & Stewart, S. (2009). Nasogastric tube placement verification in pediatric and neonatal patients. *Pediatric Nursing, 35*(1), 17–25.

NURSING TIP

Assessment of Peritoneal Irritation

One way to check for peritoneal irritation in a toddler or preschooler is to have the child jump up and down with you. If the child does so several times without bending over in pain, you can confidently rule out peritoneal irritation.

Diagnosis

Appendicitis remains a diagnosis made largely on the basis of the history and physical examination. Diagnosis is challenging in children because the clinical manifestations can present atypically. Children who are misdiagnosed have an increased incidence of perforation, abscess, wound infection, and even mortality. Abdominal tenderness on palpation is a common, important, and reliable symptom. Tenseness of the muscles (muscle rigidity) over the tender area may be felt. Rigidity over the entire abdomen, accompanied by tense positioning and **guarding** (involuntary contraction of abdominal muscles caused by fear of impending pain), indicates a perforated appendix with peritonitis. **Rebound tenderness** describes a sensation of severe pain that occurs after deep pressure is applied and released and is indicative of peritonitis. However, many practitioners consider the elicitation of rebound tenderness to be a crude and unnecessarily painful technique. The resultant severe pain may adversely affect the element of trust with the child. Palpation with a stethoscope is a preferred method for children in order to identify areas of tenderness. Auscultation will likely reveal decreased bowel sounds.

Laboratory findings do not establish the diagnosis, but there is often a moderate elevation of the white blood cell (WBC) count, seldom higher than 15,000 to 20,000/mm3, with a "shift to the left" (an increased number of immature WBCs). However, some children with appendicitis have a normal white blood cell count. Abdominal computed tomography (CT) scan may reveal a fecalith or some other cause of obstruction. Other causes of acute abdominal pain must be ruled out, including severe constipation, urinary tract infection, acute gastroenteritis, pelvic inflammatory disease, and discomfort associated with ovulation. Abdominal ultrasound has been employed in an attempt to increase accuracy of appendicitis diagnoses. CT had a significantly higher sensitivity than did ultrasound in studies of children (Doria et al., 2006). However, it may be more appropriate in verifying other causes of abdominal pain than in diagnosing appendicitis.

Delay in diagnosing appendicitis in children is a factor contributing to perforation rates of 30% to 60%. Complications of the perforation are major abscess, phlegmon, enterocutaneous fistula, peritonitis, and partial bowel obstruction (Kwok, Kim, & Gorelick, 2004). Young children have a thinner appendiceal wall, so progress from inflammation to perforation

BOX 23-1
A MNEMONIC FOR PERITONITIS

P Pain: front, back, sides, shoulders
E Electrolytes fall, shock ensues
R Rigidity or rebound of abdominal wall
I Immobility
T Tenderness
O Obstruction
N Nausea and vomiting
I Increasing pulse, decreasing blood pressure
T Temperature falls, then rises
I Increasing girth of abdomen
S Silent abdomen (no bowel sounds)

From Katz, J. (2001). *Keys to nursing success*. Upper Saddle River, NJ: Prentice Hall.

is more rapid than in adults. Children also have a poorly developed omentum, so local perforation is not usually confineable, and peritonitis develops. The close proximity of abdominal and pelvic organs further favors the spread of peritonitis to other structures. The inflammatory process associated with perforation may lead to intestinal obstruction or paralytic ileus. The signs and symptoms of peritonitis can be remembered by using the mnemonic *PERITONITIS* (Box 23-1).

KIDS WANT TO KNOW

What will the scar look like after my appendectomy?

Maria, a 14-year-old girl, has been diagnosed with appendicitis and is going for an appendectomy. She asks her nurse "What will the scar look like? How big will it be? Will I still be able to wear my bikini swimming suit?" Because Maria's appendix has not perforated prior to surgery, a laparoscopic appendectomy has been scheduled. The nurse should explain that the surgical incisions will be three to four tiny cuts in the abdomen. She will be in the hospital for only about a day if no complications occur. With proper care, the incision sites heal quickly. There is minimal scarring and she should be able to wear her bikini. The nurse can further explain that if her appendix had ruptured and peritonitis had developed before surgery, the abdominal incision would be larger, and a drain would be placed in the abscess site. The incision may be closed only through the fascia with the skin left open and the wound packed to decrease the potential for infection or problems with healing.

NURSING ALERT

Treatments to Avoid in Suspected Appendicitis

Caregivers should be told to avoid giving their child laxatives or enemas and applying heat to the abdomen if appendicitis is suspected. These measures may stimulate bowel motility and increase the danger of perforation. Additionally, pain medication may be avoided because it can mask the signs of intraperitoneal inflammation.

TREATMENT

Once the diagnosis of appendicitis has been made, surgery is required as soon as possible. In an uncomplicated open appendectomy, an incision approximately 2–3 inches is made in the right lower quadrant. If perforation is suspected, has occurred, or the appendix is in an atypical position, the incision is larger. Current practice suggests that an uncomplicated appendectomy should be performed via laparoscopy. Laparoscopic surgery leads to fewer complications, such as hospital-related infections, and has a shorter recovery time. Preoperatively, the child is managed with an NPO status, intravenous fluids to replenish fluid volume and to correct electrolyte or acid-base imbalances, and pain medication. Postoperatively in an uncomplicated appendectomy, the child will receive antibiotics for 24 hours, remain NPO until intestinal peristalsis returns, and will be discharged in 2–3 days. If perforation occurred, drains may protrude from the incision site or the incision may remain open and allowed to heal by secondary intention to prevent infection. Figure 23-12 illustrates an incision healing by secondary intention after an appendectomy for a perforated appendix. Additional treatment includes IV antibiotics for 7–10 days, NPO status, NG tube suction, IV fluids, and pain medication. The child

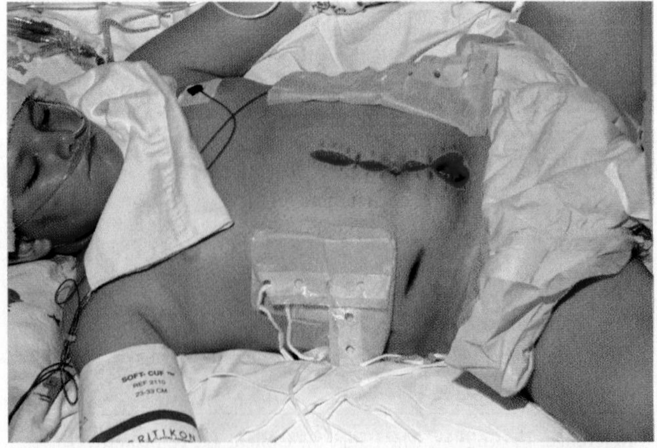

FIGURE 23-12 Incision Healing by Secondary Intention After Appendectomy for a Ruptured Appendix. DELMAR CENGAGE LEARNING.

CASE STUDY / CARE PLAN

A CHILD WITH APPENDICITIS

Maria is a 14-year-old girl who is being seen in the emergency department with a complaint of abdominal pain, vomiting, fever, and anorexia. Two days ago she awoke complaining of a dull stomach ache and not feeling well. She went to school but returned by noon and went back to bed. By early evening the pain was sharp and she could indicate the umbilical area as hurting. She refused to eat all day but did drink water and juices. The next morning she vomited yellow emesis, and the pain was periodically severe. Her temperature was 100.5°F (38.1°C), and she vomited several more times that day. In the middle of the night she awoke with pain so severe she was crying and would not stand up straight. She was diagnosed with acute appendicitis and admitted to the hospital for surgery.

NURSING CARE PLAN

ASSESSMENT

Because prompt and accurate diagnosis of appendicitis is important, nurses need to assess any child presenting with abdominal pain for the early signs and symptoms. Nurses in a variety of settings, such as emergency departments, school and school-based clinics, and ambulatory care clinics, are in an ideal position to recognize these early indicators of appendicitis. The nursing assessment should include detailed information about the child's pain (onset, location, intensity), changes in behavior (refusing to attend school or play outside, loss of appetite), and vomiting. If the symptoms of appendicitis are present, the child should be referred for further evaluation.

NURSING DIAGNOSIS 1

Acute pain related to inflamed appendix and postoperative surgical incision.

EXPECTED OUTCOME

1. Maria states or exhibits reduced pain.

NOC: Comfort Level; Pain Control; Pain: Disruptive Effects; Pain Level

NIC: Analgesic Administration; Medication Management; Pain Management; Patient-Controlled Analgesia (PCA) Assistance

INTERVENTIONS/*RATIONALES*

1. Use a pain assessment scale appropriate for child's developmental level to determine severity of pain. In this case, a 0-10 pain scale may be used. *The pain scale provides objective data and the child's input.*
2. Assess behavioral cues (crying, movement, facial grimace) that indicate discomfort or pain. *Behavior of child provides clues to pain experience.*
3. Use nonpharmacologic approaches such as distraction with games, TV, movies, or relaxing music. *Concentration on something other than pain directs the discomfort from conscious thought.*
4. Administer pain medication by continuous infusion or every 3–4 hours around the clock as prescribed. *Pain breakthrough occurs even during sleep; pain is continuous for 1–2 days post-op.*
5. Assist child to assume position of comfort. *Fowler's position with knees flexed avoids strain on the abdomen.*
6. Use pillow to splint when coughing, sneezing, and even laughing to decrease pain and pressure. *Splint prevents a sudden increase of the intra-abdominal pressure.*

EVALUATION

Maria will experience no pain or reduced pain as evidenced by relaxed body posture and facial expression; heart, respiratory rate and blood pressure within appropriate range for age; naps and sleeps appropriately for age undisturbed by pain; and ambulation without undue resistance.

(Continues)

CASE STUDY / CARE PLAN (Continued)

NURSING DIAGNOSIS 2

Risk for deficient fluid volume related to inadequate intake and losses secondary to vomiting, diarrhea, and NPO status.

EXPECTED OUTCOME

1. Maria will regain adequate hydration status.

NOC: Fluid Balance; Hydration

NIC: Fluid Management; Fluid Monitoring; Hypovolemia Management; Intravenous (IV) Therapy

INTERVENTIONS/*RATIONALES*

1. Administer IV fluids as prescribed. *Inadequate oral intake, vomiting, and diarrhea deplete total body water.*
2. Replace NG output with additional IV fluids as prescribed. *NG suction removes gastric contents that contain water, hydrochloric acid, and potassium.*
3. Maintain accurate intake and output; estimate wound drainage and include as output. *Provides an ongoing assessment of hydration status.*

EVALUATION

Maria has adequate fluid volume as evidenced by appropriate intake of IV and oral fluids and urine output (minimum of 1 to 2 ml/kg/hr); moist mucous membranes, elastic skin turgor, and normal vital signs for age.

NURSING DIAGNOSIS 3

Risk for infection related to possible or actual rupture of appendix and surgical incision.

EXPECTED OUTCOME

1. Maria will be free of infection.

NOC: Immune Status; Infection Status; Wound Healing: Primary Intention

NIC: Infection Control; Infection Protection; Incision Site Care

INTERVENTIONS/*RATIONALES*

1. Preoperative
   a. Assess child for clinical and laboratory manifestations of appendicitis. *Successful treatment is dependent on timely diagnosis of the disorder.*
   b. Assess for and immediately report symptoms of peritonitis (initial relief of pain at time of perforation followed by increased intensity, abdominal distention, guarding, decreased or absent bowel sounds, elevated temperature, and shock-like symptoms). *Perforation occurs in a high percentage of children with acute appendicitis, which greatly increases the risk of serious complications.*
2. Postoperative
   a. Monitor incision for signs of infection. *Postoperative infection may increase length and cost of hospitalization and prolong child's recovery time.*
   b. Maintain intact abdominal dressing, change or reinforce per hospital routine. *To prevent infection.*
   c. Monitor temperature every 4 hours and PRN; watch WBC count for leukocytosis. *Temperatures that exceed 101°F (38.3°C) and elevated WBC suggest the presence of infection.*

EVALUATION

The surgical incision is free from edema, excessive redness, warmth, or purulent drainage. The incision has minimal clear to serosanguineous drainage. Maria is afebrile with WBC within normal limits. Her heart rate is within an acceptable range for her age.

remains NPO until bowel function returns and is discharged when wound drainage is minimal and oral intake satisfactory. If a laparoscopic procedure was performed, the child may remain in the hospital overnight or be discharged on the day of surgery.

INFLAMMATORY BOWEL DISEASE

Inflammatory bowel disease (IBD) refers to a group of chronic disorders that cause inflammation or ulceration in the small and large intestine and include ulcerative colitis (UC) and Crohn's disease (CD). Ulcerative colitis involves inflammation of the mucosa and submucosa of the colon and rectum, while CD is an inflammation that may involve the entire gastrointestinal tract and all layers of the bowel wall (transmural).

Incidence and Etiology

Once considered rare in children and adolescents, IBD is now being recognized with increasing frequency in this age group. In fact, 20% of all individuals with UC and 25–30% of those with CD present before age 20. Peak onset is in late adolescence. With increasing recognition of IBD, it has become one of the most significant chronic diseases affecting children and adolescents.

The incidence of IBD is similar in males and females, is higher among the Caucasian population of developed Western countries, and lower among African Americans and Asians. The incidence of UC is 0.05 per 1,000; the incidence of CD is 0.04 per 1,000. The etiology of IBD is unclear; however, infectious agents, autoimmune, genetic, and environmental factors have been implicated. Current thinking suggests that a triggering factor, possibly a virus or an atypical bacterium, interacts with the body's immune system to induce an inflammatory reaction in the intestinal wall. About 15–20% of individuals with IBD have a close relative with one of these diseases, suggesting a genetic factor. Research indicates that individuals with a genetic predisposition have defective immunoregulation of the inflammatory response to bacteria or viruses in their GI tract (Silbermintz & Markowitz, 2006).

Pathophysiology

The bowel responds to an environmental trigger that the immune system identifies as dangerous and causes an injury resulting in vasoconstriction. This is followed by localized release of cellular mediators, including histamine, which produce a marked vasodilation. Capillaries become distended with blood and begin to contract, causing ruptures in the walls. The swollen engorged bowel is fragile and is, therefore, inclined to ulcerate, causing a break in the mucosal barrier. Digestive enzymes and intestinal bacteria act on this exposed tissue, causing further irritation, inflammation, ulceration, and bleeding. Ulcers can become fissures as they penetrate more deeply into the intestinal wall. Fistulas can occur into the bladder or vagina (more common in CD). Inflammatory exudate consisting of plasma proteins draws more fluid into the bowel resulting in diarrhea that may be bloody. Healing lesions result in scar tissue formation, and subsequent scarring of bowel may lead to strictures and bowel obstruction.

Clinical Manifestations

The most common symptoms of UC are rectal bleeding, diarrhea, and abdominal pain. Multiple patterns of presentation occur in children and adolescents. Mild disease is seen in 50–60% of cases. The onset of diarrhea is insidious, and there are no extraintestinal or systemic signs of fever, weight loss, or hypoalbuminemia. Thirty percent present with moderate disease characterized by bloody diarrhea, abdominal cramping and tenderness, and the urgency to defecate. These individuals have associated systemic signs such as anorexia, weight loss, low-grade fever, and mild anemia. Severe cases occur in 10% of clients. Clinical manifestations in these cases are more than six bloody stools per day, abdominal tenderness, fever, anemia, leukocytosis, and hypoalbuminemia. Occasionally, children with UC may have predominately extraintestinal manifestations such as growth failure, arthritis, and skin lesions (Rufo & Bousvaros, 2007).

In contrast to UC, CD may occur in any segment of the gastrointestinal tract. The clinical manifestations are determined primarily by the location and extent of disease involvement. The majority of children (50–70%) have disease involving the terminal ileum. In these children symptoms of malabsorption predominate including diarrhea, abdominal pain, anorexia, weight loss, and growth failure. CD that occurs in the colon may be indistinguishable from UC, with symptoms of bloody diarrhea, crampy abdominal pain, and urgency to defecate. Perianal involvement includes painful defecation, bright red rectal bleeding, skin tags, hemorrhoids, fistulas, and abscesses.

Growth failure occurs more frequently in children with CD than with UC. Children with either disorder tend to reduce dietary intake below that recommended for age to diminish symptoms induced by eating, which results in growth failure, characterized by an abnormally slow growth velocity. A major consequence of prolonged reduction in growth velocity is permanent short stature, frequently seen in adults who had CD during childhood (Ceballos, 2008). Additionally, delayed sexual development is frequently seen. More importantly, growth failure and delayed puberty are often debilitating symptoms for adolescents, potentially affecting their self-esteem, social interactions, and school performance. Children with severe disease and children of single parents are most at risk of low self-esteem (Lindfred, Saalman, Nilsson, & Reichenberg, 2008). Systemic or extraintestinal symptoms are more common in children with CD than UC. Some of these symptoms tend to be more severe in children than in adults. For example, children have higher fevers, more joint pain, nausea, and in general feel sicker than

TABLE 23-1 Comparison of Ulcerative Colitis and Crohn's Disease

PATHOLOGY	ULCERATIVE COLITIS	CROHN'S DISEASE
Area of involvement	Colon and rectum	May affect entire GI tract from mouth to anus
Bowel wall involvement	Superficial (mucosa and submucosa)	All layers of bowel wall (transmural)
Distribution of lesions	Symmetric, continuous	Asymmetric, segmented (disease-free skip areas)
CLINICAL MANIFESTATIONS	**ULCERATIVE COLITIS**	**CROHN'S DISEASE**
Alteration in bowel pattern	Severe diarrhea	Mild to moderate diarrhea
Abdominal pain	Mild, lower abdominal	Common, severe
Rectal bleeding	Common	Uncommon
Weight loss	Mild to moderate	Common, severe
Growth retardation	Mild	Often severe
Perianal disease	Rare	Common
Fistulas	Rare	Common

do adults with CD. See Table 23-1 for a comparison of UC and CD.

DIAGNOSIS

Presenting symptoms and clinical course of UC and CD are similar enough that they often elude a differential diagnosis, sometimes for years. Diagnosis is based on history and physical exam and endoscopic or radiologic examination of the colon to evaluate the character and location of lesions. Endoscopy includes either a sigmoidoscopy or a colonoscopy and biopsies of the mucosa are obtained and examined. Radiologic studies include a barium enema and an upper gastrointestinal contrast examination. Laboratory studies may indicate anemia, hypoproteinemia, fluid and electrolyte imbalances, and an elevated sedimentation rate.

TREATMENT

Treatment for inflammatory bowel disease involves pharmacologic, nutritional, and surgical approaches. The goals include controlling the disease, inducing remission and preventing relapses, providing adequate nutrition for growth and development, and assisting the child to function as normally as possible (e.g., school attendance, participation in sports). Pharmacotherapy is aimed at either decreasing inflammation or directly suppressing the immune system. Categories of medications include corticosteroids, aminosalicylates, antibiotics, and immunosuppressants. Corticosteroids are used during acute episodes for treating moderate to severe IBD. The aminosalicylate azulfidine (Sulfasalazine) acts directly on the bowel mucosa to reduce inflammation. Metronidazole (Flagyl), an anti-infective, has been helpful in the treatment of perianal complications in CD. Immunosuppressive medications such as cyclosporine have been useful in children with corticosteroid-resistant CD.

The goal of nutritional support is to replace lost nutrients and to provide adequate caloric intake for growth and normal metabolic functions. While no special diet has been proven effective for treating IBD, some individuals find their symptoms are aggravated by milk, highly seasoned foods, and fiber. The lactose in milk and milk products is usually poorly tolerated when IBD is active, resulting in bloating, pain, and increased diarrhea. This is a problem because dairy products constitute the largest source of calories and calcium in the diets of most children. Lactase hydrolyzed milk can be helpful in providing extra calories for lactose-intolerant children. High-calorie liquid nutritional supplements such as Ensure may be recommended for children with growth failure. Vitamins and minerals are often deficient and replacements are necessary. Since fats are digested and assimilated in the small intestine, children with CD have a deficiency of the fat-soluble vitamins, A, D, E, and K. Elemental formulas, which are almost completely absorbed in the small intestine and leave little residue, have been useful in inducing remission and improving nutritional status. These formulas can be given either by mouth or nasogastric tube feeding at night. Total parenteral nutrition (TPN) in children with severe CD can help to reverse growth failure. Most individuals with IBD find that a low-fiber, low-residue diet is therapeutic.

Another approach to treatment is surgery. When children experience severe complications of UC, surgery may be indicated. Severe complications are bowel perforation, hemorrhage, and conventional treatment failure. Surgical removal of the entire colon and rectum (proctocolectomy) provides a permanent cure. A permanent ileostomy is created at the same time. Indications for surgery in cases of CD are disease that is unresponsive to medical treatment, bowel strictures, obstruction, or perforation, and intractable bleeding or diarrhea. The diseased segment of the intestine is removed or resected, and the two ends of healthy intestine are reattached or anastomosed. CD is not cured with surgery because the lesions tend to recur in other parts of the bowel.

Nursing Management

The focus of nursing care includes medication and nutritional management, emotional support, and community referrals. An area for potential strife between the child and caregivers is the medication regimen. When IBD is in remission, the child may see no reason for taking medications. The concept that the disease is still present although no symptoms are evident is often difficult for children to understand. The nurse should emphasize continuation of medications despite the absence of symptoms. The nurse can provide information about medications used to treat IBD and their side effects, emphasizing that they be continued despite remissions of symptoms. The side effects of corticosteroids include increased appetite and weight gain, increased susceptibility to infections, increased risk for osteoporosis and aseptic necrosis of the hip, acne, rounding of the face, and personality changes. Side effects of azulfidine (Sulfasalazine) include gastric upset, nausea, vomiting, allergic reactions, **crystalluria** (crystals in the urine), and bone marrow suppression. The total dose of the medication should be given in evenly spaced doses and after meals to minimize gastrointestinal upset. The child should be encouraged to drink a full glass of water with each dose to prevent crystalluria.

Providing emotional support is an important nursing intervention in IBD. In addition to the expected effects of chronic illness, depression, anxiety, and low self-esteem appear to be more common in children and adolescents with IBD. Early detection of psychological problems is invaluable because appropriate referral and psychological therapy can help prevent further psychopathology. Often both the child and the family require counseling. Support groups are also

NURSING ALERT

Side Effects of Sulfasalazine

Warn the child and family that the child's urine or skin may be yellow-orange in color. Instruct caregivers to notify their health care provider if skin rash, fever, sore throat, mouth sores, bruising, bleeding, fatigue, or joint pain occur. These are signs and symptoms of blood dyscrasias resulting from bone marrow suppression, a serious side effect of Sulfasalazine.

FAMILY TEACHING

Inflammatory Bowel Disease

HOME

- Teach the child and family about medication regimen, side effects of drugs, and the need to continue drug therapy despite remission of symptoms.
- Instruct the child and family about the dietary plan. A low-fiber, low-residue diet generally provides some relief of symptoms such as diarrhea and abdominal pain.
- Teach caregivers methods to increase oral caloric intake such as: (1) eating three meals plus three "mini-meals" each day; (2) including a source of protein at each meal; (3) ingesting milk products as tolerated (yogurt with live cultures and aged, hardened cheeses are tolerated by many children with lactose intolerance); (4) using extra fats as tolerated, such as butter, margarine, vegetable oil, mayonnaise, cream, and cream cheese; and (5) limiting low-calorie foods and beverages.

SCHOOL

- Instruct the family that the child can be as active as she or he feels like being.
- Encourage caregivers to try giving the child the responsibility of determining whether she or he is able to go to school during flare-ups.
- Encourage the child to find practical ways of dealing with the illness in school, such as locating the nearest bathrooms, carrying extra underclothes, and visiting the school nurse as needed.
- Assess for school avoidance because of embarrassment of diarrhea. If the child is not active in school, some element of the program should be adjusted.
- Allow the child to make the decision whether to tell friends and teachers about the illness. If there are frequent hospitalizations or frequent absences from school, teachers and school administrators should be told about the illness.
- Have caregivers contact the school district to arrange for tutoring if extended absences from school become necessary.

COMMUNITY

- Refer the family to the Crohn's and Colitis Foundation of America (see Resources). This organization provides information and support that families may find helpful.
- Refer caregivers to social services, the visiting nurse association, and home health care agencies.

useful in helping the child and caregivers deal with the diagnosis and disease. The nurse should assess the impact of the disease as reflected by impaired social activities and school absences. School activities (e.g., gym and bathroom privileges) may need to be modified.

PEPTIC ULCERS

Peptic ulcers occur when there is erosion of the mucosal wall of the gastrointestinal tract. They develop most often in the stomach and duodenum. They are classified as primary or secondary, gastric or duodenal. Primary ulcers occur in the absence of another underlying disease and often in individuals with a family history of the disorder. Secondary or stress ulcers are associated with severe physiological stress of an underlying systemic disease or injury such as shock, sepsis, burns, or surgery. Certain drugs also contribute to secondary ulcers. Gastric ulcers are usually located at the junction of the fundus and the pylorus on the lesser curvature of the stomach. Duodenal ulcers occur in the pylorus or duodenum. Figure 23-13 illustrates the most common sites for peptic ulcers.

Incidence and Etiology

The true incidence of peptic ulcers in children is unknown; however, with the advent of endoscopy, more cases have been detected and diagnosed. Primary ulcers are most common in older children and adolescents. Up to the age of 6, most ulcers are secondary. Gastric ulcers are uncommon in children, whereas duodenal ulcers are seen most frequently. Males are affected with peptic ulcers more than females.

The exact etiology is unknown; however, several factors have been implicated. There is a close association between the bacilli *Helicobacter pylori* (*H. pylori*) and duodenal ulcers (Sgouros & Bergele, 2006). This organism is transmitted by the fecal-oral route and is more common in lower socioeconomic areas and in developing countries. Certain drugs contribute to peptic ulcers; for example, nonsteroidal anti-inflammatory agents such as aspirin and ibuprofen (Advil), corticosteroids, tobacco, and alcohol. For many years, diet and psychological factors were suggested as important etiologic factors; however, there is no conclusive evidence that they cause peptic ulcers.

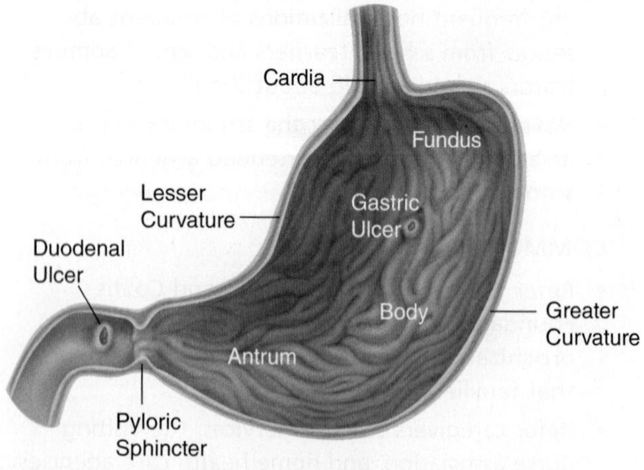

Figure 23-13 Most Common Sites for Peptic Ulcers. DELMAR CENGAGE LEARNING.

Pathophysiology

The parietal cells of the stomach secrete hydrochloric acid (HCL) in the digestive process; other cells secrete pepsinogen. Pepsinogen converts to pepsin when activated by HCL, which adds to the acidity of the stomach. Gastric epithelial cells secrete a mucus-bicarbonate barrier to provide protection from the acid and pepsin. Ulcers occur when a substance stimulates excessive HCL production, damages the mucus barrier, or decreases mucus production.

Clinical Manifestations

The signs and symptoms of peptic ulcers in children vary depending on their age. The clinical manifestations according to age are illustrated in Table 23-2.

Diagnosis

An upper GI barium series is often the initial test for a child suspected of having peptic ulcers. With this exam the ulcer crater is detected; however, the practitioner is not able to biopsy the mucosa to determine if *H. pylori* is present. A more definitive test is an endoscopy of the upper GI tract. The ulcer crater can be directly visualized, and a biopsy can be obtained to detect the organism. A blood test is also available that detects *H. pylori* antibodies. A stool exam for occult blood may be performed to diagnose GI bleeding. The C-urea breath test is used to screen for *H. pylori* by measuring bacterial colonization in the gastric mucosa. Other methods like polyclonal and monoclonal stool antigen tests are used for the initial diagnosis of *H. pylori* and for the confirmation of its eradication after treatment (Gisbert, de la Morena, & Abraira, 2006).

Table 23-2 Clinical Manifestations of Peptic Ulcers According to Age

AGE	CLINICAL MANIFESTATIONS
0–3 years	Primary ulcers: anorexia, vomiting, melena, hematemesis, crying after meals
	Secondary ulcers: hemorrhage and perforation
3–6 years	Primary ulcers: vomiting related to eating, periumbilical or generalized pain
	Secondary ulcers: melena, hematemesis, perforation
6–18 years	Melena, hematemesis, occult bleeding, anemia

TREATMENT

The goals of treatment are to relieve pain, hasten healing, and prevent complications. Medications are the primary method for managing ulcers. The rationale for medication therapy involves different mechanisms:

- neutralization or buffering of gastric acid (antacids)
- reduction of gastric acid secretions (histamine receptor antagonists)
- suppression and blockage of gastric acid secretions (proton-pump inhibitors)
- protection of the mucus barrier (mucosal barrier fortifiers) by decreasing the activity of pepsin and HCL
- treatment of *Helicobacter* infections (antibiotics and bismuth preparations)

Antacids decrease discomfort and pain but do not affect healing of the ulcer or prevent recurrence. A common antacid dosage schedule is 1 to 3 hours after each meal and at bedtime. Antacid is rarely used in young children. The most common histamine (H) receptor antagonists for peptic ulcers are ranitidine (Zantac), cimetidine (Tagamet), and famotidine (Pepcid), all of which have few side effects, primarily diarrhea or constipation, headache, and rash. In some cases, proton-pump inhibitors, which effectively suppress or block all gastric acid secretions, are used in children. Omeprazole (Prilosec), one of the most commonly prescribed proton-pump inhibitor, has minimal side effects that are similar to H-receptor antagonists. Mucosal barrier fortifiers such as sucralfate (Carafate) coat the stomach, adhere to the ulcer surface, and reinforce the mucosal protective coat of the stomach to prevent further digestive action of HCL and pepsin. It is administered on an empty stomach 1 hour before or 2 hours after meals and at bedtime and constipation is the more common side effect. Cure of peptic ulcers associated with *H. pylori* requires eradication of the organism. The optimal therapeutic regimen is still undetermined; yet, in children, the antibiotics metronidazole (Flagyl) and ampicillin in combination with bismuth salicylate (Pepto-Bismol) is most often prescribed. Diet therapy is not indicated in the treatment of ulcers because restriction of diet does not promote or accelerate healing. Surgery is rarely needed in children but is indicated if perforation, hemorrhage, or gastric outlet obstruction occurs.

NURSING MANAGEMENT AND FAMILY TEACHING

Because peptic ulcers are usually managed at home by caregivers, a major nursing intervention is caregiver education. Adherence with the medication regimen is important in healing the ulcer and preventing recurrences; therefore, the child and caregivers need to understand the rationale for each drug, the administration schedule, and side effects. The nurse explains that a special diet is not necessary, but the child should avoid substances that increase acid secretion such as caffeine-containing beverages (coffee, tea, cola). Any food or beverage that causes discomfort or pain needs to be avoided. Older children and adolescents need information about how alcohol and cigarette smoking cause gastric irritation and contribute to ulcer formation. It is important that caregivers know the signs and symptoms of ulcer complications, which must be reported to their health care provider immediately. **Melena** (black or tarry stool indicating presence of blood) or **hematemesis** (vomiting of blood) indicate hemorrhage; severe abdominal pain and a rigid abdomen may signal perforation.

The nurse can be instrumental in preventing secondary or stress ulcers that are due to physiological stress or certain medications by identifying infants and children who may be at risk for developing these ulcers. For critically ill individuals, maintaining gastric pH above 3.5 will help prevent ulcer formation. Thus, gastric pH values should be checked frequently and treated if too low. Additionally, histamine-2 blockers may be given as prophylaxis therapy in those identified at high risk for stress ulcers.

NECROTIZING ENTEROCOLITIS

Necrotizing enterocolitis (NEC), a life-threatening condition of preterm neonates, is characterized by necrosis of the mucosa of the small and large intestine, most frequently the distal ileum and proximal colon. It is the most common surgical emergency in this age group. The necrosis may be very superficial and only detectable microscopically, or it may be through the bowel wall. Mild disease may be completely reversible, but neonates with extensive involvement may not survive.

INCIDENCE AND ETIOLOGY

NEC commonly occurs in preterm, low birthweight neonates and is rarely seen in term infants. NEC occurs in up to 7% of very low birth weight infants (Lin, Nasr, & Stoll, 2008). It equally affects all races and both sexes. The incidence has been rising in recent years because of the improved survival of this high-risk group. The exact etiology of NEC is unclear; however, several factors are associated with its development. These risk factors include intestinal ischemia, bacterial colonization of the bowel, and the presence of hypertonic solutions in the intestinal lumen, usually formula (Lin et al., 2008). Perinatal asphyxia, respiratory distress syndrome, exchange transfusions, and umbilical artery catheters may all contribute to ischemia of the bowel. Controversy exists about various aspects of feeding practices as a possible etiologic factor. These include feeding neonates within the first 48 hours after birth, the use of formula rather than breast milk, and enteral feedings of hypertonic solutions, for example, formula.

PATHOPHYSIOLOGY

NEC appears to occur in preterm neonates whose bowel has experienced an injury, resulting in vascular compromise. This leads to decreased blood flow to the bowel and ischemia of the intestinal mucosa. The disruption of the intestinal mucosal barrier introduces significant vulnerability to infection. Then normal intestinal bacteria **hydrolyze** (to cause a substance to break down into its component parts by adding water) formula in the intestine, forming gas or air in the bowel wall called **pneumatosis intestinalis**. The bowel becomes edematous and distended. Progressive infiltration of the bowel wall with bacteria leads to more extensive tissue inflammation, destruction, and necrosis. Sepsis and perforation of the bowel may occur.

Clinical Manifestations

The classic clinical presentation of the neonate with NEC includes the symptom group of abdominal tenderness, distention, and erythema of abdominal wall, bloody stools, decreased bowel sounds, increased **gastric residuals** (feeding retained in stomach following tube feeding), and bilious vomiting after feeding. Manifestations of clinical deterioration include apnea and bradycardia, lethargy, temperature instability, decreased urine output, further abdominal distention, and evidence of shock (cool, mottled skin, pallor, decreased intensity of peripheral pulses). Hypotension is a late sign of deterioration. Acidosis, sepsis, and death may occur if NEC is not treated.

Diagnosis

Diagnosis is based on clinical findings and abdominal X-rays. Radiographic findings associated with NEC are dilated bowel loops and pneumatosis intestinalis. **Pneumoperitoneum**, free air in the peritoneal cavity, or air in the portal circulation indicate severe disease and perforation of the bowel.

Treatment

If NEC is diagnosed in its early stages and treatment is initiated promptly to prevent perforation, the infant may improve without surgical intervention. Initial treatment includes:

- Cessation of oral feedings
- Continuous gastric drainage and decompression via an NG tube
- Maintenance of oxygenation; ventilation if necessary
- Administration of IV fluid therapy for parenteral nutrition and broad spectrum antibiotics, and to restore acid-base and electrolyte balance
- Administration of probiotics and prebiotics

Probiotics are live microorganisms (in most cases, bacteria) that are similar to beneficial microorganisms found in the human gut. They are also called "friendly bacteria" or "good bacteria" (National Institute of Health, 2008). Prebiotics are nondigestible foods that make their way through the digestive system and help good bacteria grow and flourish. Prebiotics keep beneficial bacteria healthy. Frequent monitoring of laboratory data is essential in order to detect deterioration in the infant's condition. Commonly ordered tests include blood gases, white blood cell count, hematocrit, platelet count, electrolytes, and abdominal X-rays.

Despite appropriate medical treatment, surgical intervention becomes necessary in 20 to 60% of cases (Thompson & Bizzarro, 2008). Surgery is required if the infant demonstrates evidence of perforation, localized peritonitis, persistent metabolic acidosis, or clinical deterioration unresponsive to vigorous medical management (see Box 23-2).

BOX 23-2
INDICATIONS FOR SURGICAL INTERVENTION OF NECROTIZING ENTEROCOLITIS

1. Free intraperitoneal air (pneumoperitoneum)
2. Persistent and visible bowel loops
3. Radiographic evidence of peritonitis
   a. Increased free peritoneal fluid
   b. Increased bowel wall edema
4. Clinical deterioration despite medical treatment
   a. Irreversible metabolic acidosis
   b. Shock
   c. Respiratory failure

Resection of the necrotic bowel is necessary, and in cases of extensive removal, intestinal diversion is performed by creating a temporary ileostomy, jejunostomy, or colostomy. Postoperative complications include intestinal obstruction secondary to stricture of the ischemic portions of the bowel and short bowel syndrome characterized by malabsorption, malnutrition, and growth failure.

Nursing Management

The nurse has a major responsibility to be aware of and continually assess for early warning signs of NEC. Frequent measurement of abdominal girth is performed to assess for distention. Prior to feedings gastric residual contents are measured to determine if the volume is increasing, which indicates malabsorption. The presence of bowel sounds is also noted to evaluate for decreased intestinal activity, and all stools are tested for blood. When NEC is diagnosed, nursing interventions include accurate intake and output measurements, frequent assessment of vital signs, maintenance of IV therapy, and ongoing assessment for changes in the infant's condition. Vital signs are monitored for changes that may reveal impending sepsis or shock from perforation, peritonitis, and electrolyte imbalance. When oral feedings are restarted, the nurse must observe the infant's response and tolerance because NEC can recur. Breast feeding has been

NURSING ALERT
Warning Signs of NEC

- abdominal distention
- residual gastric contents
- feeding intolerance
- decreased bowel sounds
- bloody stools

shown to help prevent NEC (Lin et al., 2008). Nurses should educate parents of very low birth weight infants about initiating breast feeding as early as possible.

MALABSORPTION ALTERATIONS

Malabsorption occurs when there is a disruption in the digestive process causing insufficient assimilation of nutrients. Common causes of problems in absorption in infants and children that will be discussed are celiac disease and lactose intolerance.

CELIAC DISEASE

Celiac disease, also known as gluten-sensitive enteropathy, is a disorder caused by permanent intolerance to gluten, the protein component of wheat, barley, rye, and oats. It is second only to cystic fibrosis as the most common cause of malabsorption in children.

Incidence and Etiology

Celiac disease is a genetic disorder that occurs in all races but is more common in Caucasians. The incidence varies in different regions and is more common in Europe than the United States. The incidence has been reported to be 1 in 3000 white individuals in the United States. The disease coincides with the introduction of foods containing gluten (Telega, Bennet, & Werlin, 2008). The incidence is higher in children with type 1 diabetes, thyroid disease, Down syndrome, and family history of celiac disease.

Pathophysiology

Genetic predisposition is an essential factor in the development of celiac disease. A couple of genes located on the HLA region of chromosome 6 are found in almost 100% of those affected with celiac disease (Murdock & Johnston, 2005). The exact mechanism by which gluten damages the mucosa of the small intestine is unclear. One theory postulates that gluten toxicity results in an alteration in immunologic response. Gluten consists of two protein components, glutenin and gliadin. The harmful protein appears to be gliadin. Gliadin plays the role of antigen and causes an immune response that results in inflammation of and damage to the finger-like projections called villi in the small intestine. The villi flatten out and atrophy, leading to a decrease in the absorptive surface area. Initially, fat absorption is impaired, followed by protein, carbohydrates, and fat-soluble vitamins (A, D, E, K).

Clinical Manifestations

Early clinical manifestations of celiac disease are subtle and include anorexia, irritability, listlessness, and weight loss. As the disease progresses, abdominal distention and chronic diarrhea appear with large amounts of unabsorbed fats being excreted in the stools (**steatorrhea**). The stools are bulky, putty colored, foul-smelling, greasy, and often float because of the high fat content. Signs of progression include a protuberant abdomen, loss of subcutaneous fat, and muscle wasting secondary to hypoproteinemia. The child may appear pale because of anemia, and bruising may develop secondary to inadequate vitamin K absorption. Late signs include severe growth retardation, osteoporosis, and in the adolescent, delayed menses or puberty.

Diagnosis

Serologic tests to detect Immunoglobulin A antihuman tTG is commonly ordered. The immunofluorescence IgA endomysial antibody (EMA) test has equivalent diagnostic accuracy and is slightly more specific (Tully, 2008). Laboratory tests may be used to evaluate malabsorption and nutritional deficiencies. Use of more tests increases diagnostic accuracy (Gelfond & Fasano, 2006). If the serologic test is positive for tTG, the definitive diagnostic test is a small bowel biopsy, which will reveal atrophy of the villi and deep crypts on the intestinal mucosa. These characteristic lesions return to normal after dietary restriction of gluten, which helps confirm the diagnosis.

Treatment

Medical management consists of a lifelong adherence to a gluten-free diet. Education about the diet is the main goal of treatment and involves the health care provider, nurse, dietician, caregivers, other family members, and the child. All wheat, barley, rye, and oats are eliminated and substituted with rice, corn, and millet. Specific nutritional supplements may be used to correct deficiency states. The most common are supplements of iron, folate, calcium, and fat-soluble vitamins. The intolerance to gluten is permanent, and lack of adherence to a gluten-free diet can cause exacerbation of symptoms. Gluten avoidance is almost impossible in the American food industry, and even tiny amounts of gluten can cause symptoms.

Nursing Management and Family Teaching

The long-term goal of nursing care is to provide dietary education and supervision. The nurse explains to the caregivers the disease process, the signs and symptoms, and the rationale behind the gluten-free diet. A dietician should be involved in diet planning and nutrition education, and serves as a resource for gluten-free foods and recipes. Families are taught to read labels of all commercially prepared foods for the presence of gluten or gluten-containing additives such as hydrolyzed vegetable protein. Fats used to fry foods may contain gluten, and families must be cautious when consuming fast foods.

Children and their families often react to the necessity of a gluten-free diet with grief and may have a hard time accepting that something so fundamental to their diet could be injuring the child. Caregivers should be forewarned that many adolescents specifically have a difficult time accepting the dietary restrictions and may experiment with foods containing gluten. They may be motivated to adhere to the restrictions by the expectation of dramatic improvements in gastrointestinal symptoms such as bloating, abdominal pain, and diarrhea, and in their general well-being. Referrals to community resources for dietary and peer support organizations are important.

LACTOSE INTOLERANCE

Lactose intolerance is the inability to digest lactose, a sugar (disaccharide) present in human and cow's milk, standard infant formulas, and dairy products such as cheese and ice cream. Lactose is also added to many prepared foods, including bread and other baked goods, breakfast cereals, and mixes for cakes, cookies, pancakes, and biscuits. This disorder results from a deficiency or absence of lactase, an enzyme in the small intestine required for the digestion and absorption of lactose. Lactose intolerance can be congenital or acquired. In the congenital type, which is extremely rare, the newborn is born with a complete absence of lactase. Acquired lactose intolerance involves the gradual loss of lactase, is more common, and appears from early childhood to late adolescence.

Incidence and Etiology

The incidence appears to vary widely among different ethnic and racial groups. Low lactose levels are least common among northern and western Europeans and highest among populations from the Far East. In the United States the incidence is lowest in Caucasians and highest in Vietnamese-Americans, Native Americans, and African Americans. Lactose intolerance is most often secondary to other disorders. Diarrheal disease, particularly when caused by rotavirus, other infections of the small intestine, and acquired immune deficiency syndrome (AIDS), may decrease the activity of lactase. Another cause may be mucosal damage to the small bowel induced by dietary components such as gluten sensitivity (celiac disease), and sensitivity to soy protein and cow's milk. Lactose intolerance can develop following gastrointestinal infections, particularly in infancy, as a result of minor damage to the villi in the gut leading to an inability to digest milk. However, the gut usually heals in 6-12 weeks. Milk is then tolerated.

Pathophysiology

The absence or deficiency of lactase results in the inability of the small intestine to digest lactose. Subsequently, the undigested lactose moves into the colon where GI bacteria break down the lactose and release hydrogen, methane, and carbon dioxide. This process causes excessive gas production and abdominal bloating and pain. The undigested lactose also causes an increased number of solutes in the colon, resulting in an increase in the osmotic pressure. Therefore, water is drawn into the colon causing watery diarrhea.

Clinical Manifestations

Symptoms occur in response to ingestion of lactose and include explosive, watery diarrhea; abdominal distention; abdominal pain; and excessive flatus. Symptoms develop rapidly after the child ingests milk or foods containing lactose. Some children are able to tolerate small amounts of lactose without symptoms; yet, when larger amounts are consumed, severe symptoms occur.

Diagnosis

Diagnosis is usually made using a hydrogen-breath test that measures the amount of hydrogen left after fermentation of undigested and unabsorbed carbohydrates such as lactose. Or, it may be diagnosed by removing lactose from one's diet and observing for symptoms to disappear.

Treatment and Nursing Management

Treatment consists of reducing or eliminating lactose from the child's diet. In most cases, total elimination is unnecessary. For infants, switching to a soy-based formula (Isomil, Nutramigen, Prosobee) is effective. For older infants and children, when fluids or foods containing lactose are consumed, a commercial lactose preparation (Lact-Aid, Dairy-Ease) can be ingested or sprinkled on the items to improve tolerance. Additionally, milk products that have been commercially pretreated with microbial derived lactase are available.

■ POISONING

A poison is any substance that harms the body and interferes with the body's normal functioning. A poisoning can occur through ingestion, inhalation, skin exposure, eye contact, or any other mode that causes adverse effects. Ingestion accounts for the majority of poisonings.

INCIDENCE AND ETIOLOGY (PATHOPHYSIOLOGY)

Children under the age of 5 have the highest rate of nonfatal poison exposures at home compared to any other age group. Poisonings were the second leading cause of home injury fatality, resulting in approximately one-fourth of all home injury death (Runyan & Casteel, 2004). The American Association of Poison Control Centers reported approximately 1.2 million childhood poisonings in the United States in 2002 (Home Safety Council, 2004). There were an estimated 86,194 child poisoning incidents treated in US hospital emergency departments in 2004 (Franklin & Rodgers, 2008). Since many children with toxic ingestions are managed without contact with poison control centers or

Reflections from Families

My daughter, Maya, is 4 years old. She is a picky eater. I try to get her to take vitamins. She doesn't like it. My mother came to visit us and bought two bottles of Gummy Vitamins for Maya. She gave Maya one piece; Maya liked it a lot. Mom put the bottle on the dining table and started playing with Maya. I went to the basement for the laundry. After playing with grandma for a while, Maya started watching TV. My mom went to take a shower. I guess in between the commercials, Maya found her "candy". She always loves to eat her gummy candy. I was folding laundry in my basement. Maya came to tell me that she wants more gummy candy, with the empty Gummy Vitamins bottle in her hand. I threw the laundry on the floor and called the Poison Center right away... I then called 911. I thought my house was "child proof." We locked away all the medicine and cleaning chemicals. But this still happened.

emergency facilities, the total number of cases is much larger than the numbers reported by these centers. Poisoning is the leading cause of injury and the fourth leading cause of death in toddlers and preschoolers. In infants, their tendency to explore objects with their mouth puts them at high risk for accidental ingestion of toxic substances. In toddlers and preschoolers, poisoning is more often a result of curiosity. Older children may experiment with drugs and household products to produce euphoric and/or hallucinogenic effects (Dunn & Burns, 2004). Because ingestions in children under the age of 6 are most commonly accidental, they rarely ingest enough poison to cause death. In contrast, adolescents are less frequently exposed to poisons but their exposure is more commonly intentional and results in more fatalities than in younger children. The incidence of childhood poisoning has decreased significantly in the past fifty years because of federal regulation of products and product safety, child-resistant containers, and safe storage of toxic substances in the home and elsewhere.

Although the majority of poisonings occur in the home, incidents may occur anywhere medications and toxic substances are stored. Substances commonly ingested by children less than 6 years of age are listed in Table 23-3. Adolescents tend to ingest psychopharmacologic drugs such as tranquilizers, sedatives, and antidepressants.

CLINICAL MANIFESTATIONS

Clinical manifestations are dependent on the specific poison ingested. Table 23-4 lists the signs and symptoms associated with toxins that are frequently ingested or that cause significant mortality.

DIAGNOSIS

Identification of the type and amount of the exposure is important. Physical findings, a detailed history, and examination of the medication containers may suggest the type of toxin. In the history the following information should be obtained: who—the child's age and weight; what—the name and dosage of the medication or substance ingested; when—the time of ingestion; how—the route of poisoning (ingested, inhaled, absorbed, or injected); and why—whether intentional or unintentional. Information about signs and symptoms that have appeared since the poisoning, emergency care given, and whether vomiting was induced or occurred spontaneously should be determined. A detailed past medical history should also be obtained including previous poisonings, medical conditions, and medications currently taken that might affect the child's or adolescent's response to and metabolism or elimination of the toxic substance. Analysis of specimens such as emesis can be helpful in determining the type of poison. Laboratory evaluation may be performed when the poison is unknown, if the poison has the potential to produce moderate to severe toxicity, and if the ingestion was intentional (Powers, 2000).

TREATMENT

Treatment approaches vary with the type of poison, amount of exposure, time elapsed since exposure, and susceptibility of the child. Stabilization of the child is the first priority in managing toxic ingestions and should address the ABCs (airway, breathing, circulation). Vital body functions must be maintained regardless of the poison. Oxygen may be

TABLE 23-3 Agents Most Commonly Ingested by Children Less than 6 Years of Age

TYPE	EXAMPLES
Cosmetics and personal care products	• Perfume • Cologne • Aftershave lotion
Cleaning products	• "Household" bleach • Pine oil disinfectants
Plants	• Azalea • Buttercup • English ivy • Holly • Mistletoe • Philodendron
Foreign bodies, toys, and miscellaneous	• Thermometers • Bubble-blowing liquid
Hydrocarbons	• Gasoline • Kerosene • Lighter fluid • Turpentine • Paint thinner

Adapted from Bronstein, A. C., Spyker, D. A., Cantilena, L. R. Jr., Green, J. L., Rumack, B. H., & Heard, S. E. (2008). 2007 Annual Report of the American Association of Poison Control Centers' National Poison Data System (NPDS): 25th Annual Report. *Clinical toxicology (Philadelphia), 46*(10), 927–1057.

administered. Maintenance of respiratory function may require endotracheal intubation or mechanical ventilation.

Following stabilization of the individual, attention is directed toward gastric **decontamination** (decreasing absorption of the ingested poison from the GI tract). This includes use of gastric lavage, an absorbent agent (activated charcoal), or a cathartic agent (American Academy of Pediatrics (AAP), 2003). Gastric emptying with an emetic or lavage should not be used routinely in all oral poisonings because it is ineffective when used at a late stage, may delay more effective interventions, and may cause complications such as aspiration. Yet it is beneficial when used early in the treatment of potentially severe poisonings and is most effective when used within one hour of the ingestion (Criddle, 2007). The stomach may be emptied by gastric lavage. The American Academy of Pediatrics (AAP) recommends that syrup of ipecac to induce vomiting no longer be used routinely as poison treatment in the home and that clinicians advise caregivers to discard any ipecac they have in the house (AAP).

CRITICAL THINKING

Administering Activated Charcoal to a Toddler

You are preparing to administer a dose of activated charcoal to an older toddler. What strategies can you use to facilitate the toddler's compliance with drinking the charcoal?

GASTRIC LAVAGE

In most situations, gastric lavage is preferable to administration of ipecac, particularly in emergency departments where prolonged ipecac-induced vomiting may delay more effective interventions. Lavage is used for gastric emptying in the first 1 to 2 hours after the ingestion. It is indicated when the substance ingested is highly toxic (large ingestions or substances associated with high morbidity or mortality); when the toxin is not well absorbed by activated charcoal (i.e., lithium, iron, lead, methanol); or in children with the potential for a jeopardized airway (e.g., altered alertness). Contraindications to gastric lavage include ingestion of corrosives and ingestions by children with depressed gag reflexes who are not intubated. Complications of lavage are aspiration and perforation of the esophagus or bronchus. The procedure involves insertion of a nasal or orogastric tube and administration of small amounts of normal saline through the tube until the fluid returned is clear.

ACTIVATED CHARCOAL

Activated charcoal is effective for most oral poisonings when given alone or following the use of ipecac or gastric lavage. The use of activated charcoal decreases the amount of the toxic agent available for absorption by the gastric mucosa by up to 75%. It can be given when the ingestion has occurred up to 2 hours prior to treatment. The main concern with activated charcoal is vomiting, which occurs in approximately 15% of children and increases the risk of aspiration and pneumothorax. Superactivated charcoal products for gastric decontamination are more palatable and just as effective (Criddle, 2007).

CATHARTIC AGENTS

Administration of cathartic agents increases GI motility and hastens the expulsion of the toxin. Magnesium citrate and sorbitol are the two most commonly used agents.

ANTIDOTES

Antidotes are available for several of the common and dangerous poisons. They are typically given once the child has been stabilized, usually within a few hours of the ingestion. Examples of antidotes for some common toxins include:

Table 23-4 Clinical Manifestations of Commonly Ingested Poisonous Substances

SUBSTANCE	CLINICAL MANIFESTATIONS
Acetaminophen (Tylenol)	Nausea, vomiting, malaise, right upper quadrant abdominal pain, jaundice, confusion, somnolence; coma may develop later
Salicylates	Nausea, vomiting, hyperpnea, tinnitus, fever, disorientation, lethargy, coma, seizures, diaphoresis, abdominal pain
Cyclic antidepressants	CNS excitability, confusion, blurred vision, dry mouth, fever, mydriasis, seizures, coma, arrhythmias, hypotension, tachycardia, respiratory depression; physical condition can rapidly change
Benzodiazepines	Drowsiness, lethargy, dysarthria, ataxia, hypotension, hypothermia, coma, respiratory depression with severe overdoses
Cocaine	Anxiety, euphoria, nausea, headache, chest pain, fever, hypertension, tachypnea, tachycardia, vomiting, agitation, mydriasis, diaphoresis, twitching, confusion, hallucinations, abdominal cramps, seizures, hypotension, dysrhythmias, cardiopulmonary arrest
Narcotics	Drowsiness, nausea, vomiting, miosis, respiratory depression, cyanosis, coma, seizures, bradypnea, noncardiac pulmonary edema
Hydrocarbons	Coughing, gagging, and choking; altered level of consciousness; tachypnea, grunting, retractions, and cyanosis because of pulmonary aspiration; nausea, vomiting
Corrosives (toilet drain and oven cleaners; mildew remover; ammonia)	Severe chemical burns and burning in mouth, throat, and stomach; edema of lips, pharynx, and tongue; violent vomiting; difficulty swallowing; white, swollen mucous membranes

(1) N-Acetylcysteine (Mucomyst) for acetaminophen; (2) bicarbonate for tricyclic antidepressants; (3) deferoxamine (Desferal) for iron; (4) EDTA for lead; (5) ethanol for methanol and ethylene glycol; (6) flumazenil (Romazicon) for benzodiazepines; and (7) naloxone (Narcan) for narcotics such as opiates.

NURSING MANAGEMENT

The solution to the problem of childhood poisonings is prevention. The nurse can discuss various preventive measures. To facilitate protection of the child, the environment should be modified during infancy before she or he crawls. The nurse should teach caregivers to call the poison control center before instituting treatment if their child has been exposed to a toxic substance. Box 23-3 lists poison prevention guidelines to teach caregivers.

LEAD POISONING

Lead poisoning is defined as blood lead level (BLL) of 10 mcg/dL and above. Even though the median BLLs in children aged <5 years have declined 89% from 1976–1980 to 2003—2004, children continue to be exposed to lead, and it is still a major environmental health problem that could harm their health and impair their ability to learn (US Environmental Protection Agency (USEPA), 2008). An estimated 250,000 children remain at risk for exposure to harmful lead levels in the United States (USEPA). Children living in housing undergoing rehab and built before 1978, when lead-based paint was banned from residential use, and particularly those built before 1950, when concentrations of lead in paint were higher, are now at high risk for elevated BLLs. Children between 1 and 5 were more likely to have elevated BLLs if they were Hispanic, African American heritage, were poor, or lived in older housing.

Due to these statistics, CDC recommends state-based BLL screening (CDC, 2005). State health departments assess risk factors and local data on BLLs. The CDC also recommended screening children receiving Medicaid for lead unless "reliable, representative blood lead data that demonstrate the absence of lead exposure among this population" exists. Specifically, the recommendations to health care providers were to screen BLLs of all children between 1 and 2 years of age enrolled in Medicaid, refer children identified as having elevated BLLs to environmental and public health services, and provide medical management that is appropriate if the blood levels were elevated (CDC, 2005). Healthy People 2020 has made eliminating elevated lead levels in children a priority goal. In 2007, the extensive media coverage surrounding the U.S. Consumer Product Safety Commission recall of imported, lead-contaminated children's toys raised awareness of the dangers of lead.

BOX 23-3
POISON PREVENTION GUIDELINES

- Store potentially toxic substances such as household cleaning products, medications, and vitamins out of reach of children.
- Return toxic substances to safe storage immediately after use.
- Store products in their original containers. Never put potentially harmful products in food or beverage containers.
- Refer to medications by their proper names. Avoid calling them candy.
- Buy products with child-proof caps.
- Avoid having poisonous plants in the home.
- Keep the telephone number of the poison control center beside each phone.

HEPATIC ALTERATIONS

The liver performs a wide variety of vital functions; therefore, hepatic alterations can result in life-threatening severe illness. Viral hepatitis, the most common of these disorders, will be discussed.

HEPATITIS

Hepatitis is an acute or chronic inflammation of the liver caused by several viral or bacterial infections, fungal or parasitic infections, or chemical and drug toxicity. Five distinct viruses have been identified as causing hepatitis: hepatitis A virus, hepatitis B virus, hepatitis C virus, hepatitis D virus, and hepatitis E virus. In this section hepatitis A, B, and C will be discussed. Hepatitis D and E are very uncommon in children.

Hepatitis A causes only acute hepatitis, whereas hepatitis B and C cause chronic infections. Hepatitis viruses are classified as enteral or parenteral, in reference to their mode of transmission. The enteral form, hepatitis A, is transmitted by the fecal-oral route. Parenteral forms, hepatitis B and C, are transmitted via venous blood transfer or through intimate sexual contact. Currently vaccines are available to prevent hepatitis A and B.

Incidence and Etiology

Hepatitis A Hepatitis A (HAV) is responsible for most cases of hepatitis in children and occurs most frequently in children 5 to 14 years of age. It is caused by oral ingestion of the hepatitis A virus, which is found in the stool of infected individuals. Because the virus is transmitted via the fecal-oral route, it is easily spread in areas where there are poor sanitary conditions or where good personal hygiene is not observed. Employees and children in daycare settings are at high risk for developing the disease. The risk of spread and an outbreak in this setting is related to the number of infants and children in diapers (Steele, 2002). The source of infection is either contact with an infected person or direct contact with infected fecal material that has entered food or water supplies. Outbreaks have been related to sewage-contaminated water, infected food handlers (who do not wash their hands after defecating), and shellfish caught in waters contaminated by sewage. In children, HAV is characterized by either a mild course similar to that of stomach virus or is asymptomatic.

NURSING ALERT

Risk Factors for Hepatitis A

- overcrowded living conditions
- poor personal hygiene (poor handwashing especially after defecation)
- poor sanitation (sewage disposal)
- food and water contamination
- ingestion of shellfish caught in contaminated water
- frequent travel outside of the united states

Hepatitis B Hepatitis B (HBV), previously called serum hepatitis, is spread parenterally via direct contact with infected blood or body fluids. It can be an acute or chronic infection and is potentially lethal. Most cases of HBV in children are acquired perinatally from an infected mother during pregnancy or delivery. The disease can also be acquired from contaminated needles, especially affecting IV drug users, through sexual activity, and from blood transfusions. The clinical course of hepatitis B may be varied. It may have an insidious onset with mild or no symptoms, which is common in children, or it may result in serious complications such as fulminant or chronic hepatitis.

NURSING ALERT

Risk Factors for Hepatitis B

- perinatal transmission to infant from HBV-infected mother
- IV drug use with shared needles
- receipt of multiple transfusions of blood or blood products (hemophiliacs, oncology, and hemodialysis clients)
- heterosexual activity or sexual activity with homosexual males
- immigrant or refugee status

Hepatitis C Among children in the United States, the seroprevalence of HCV infection is 0.2% for those less than 12 years of age and 0.4% for those 12 to 19 years of age. Hepatitis C (HCV) in children has been observed most frequently after transfusion with blood and blood products; therefore, the incidence is highest in hemophiliacs. Similar to HBV, HCV can be transmitted perinatally. The average rate of HCV infection among infants born to HCV-positive mothers is 5–6%. Because HCV can be transmitted through blood transfusions or perinatally, the American Academy of Pediatrics recommends screening for the following groups: (1) infants born to HCV-infected mothers; (2) drug users (injecting); (3) recipients of one or more units of blood or blood products prior to 1990; (4) individuals receiving hemodialysis; and (5) individuals receiving clotting factor concentrates before 1987 when effective inactivation procedures were introduced. HCV can also be transmitted sexually; however, it does not appear to be acquired as easily by sexual contact as does HBV. In sexually promiscuous individuals, the risk of infection is related to the number of sexual partners.

Pathophysiology

After exposure to the hepatitis virus, the liver becomes inflamed, causing damage to the cells. As the liver becomes edematous, bile channels from the liver into the intestine become obstructed, causing biliary stasis and further destruction of cells. In most cases the disease is self-limiting and liver cells regenerate completely within 2–3 months. However, hepatitis B and C may be associated with continued degeneration of liver cells and chronic hepatitis. Chronic hepatitis is characterized by progressive liver failure, cirrhosis, or liver cancer. Fulminant hepatitis, a rare but often fatal complication of HBV and HCV, can also occur. It results from failure of the liver cells to regenerate, causing massive hepatic necrosis. Death can occur within 1–2 weeks.

Clinical Manifestations

The manifestations of viral hepatitis are similar. Generally, children have mild, nonspecific symptoms without jaundice or are asymptomatic. Initially, the child experiences nausea and vomiting, anorexia, slight fever, fatigue, headache, and abdominal pain in the epigastrium or upper right quadrant. These flu-like symptoms last approximately 1 week and may be so mild that they go unnoticed in infants and young children. Following this period, jaundice may develop, beginning with darkening of the urine and gray-colored stools, followed by yellowing of the skin and sclera. However, many children with acute hepatitis never develop jaundice. The liver usually is enlarged and tender to palpation. Children with HBV and HCV may also present with dermatologic symptoms such as rashes and pruritus or severe itching. Refer to Table 23-5 for a comparison of hepatitis A, B, and C.

Diagnosis

Diagnosis of hepatitis is based on history, specifically exposure to the hepatitis virus; physical examination; serologic testing for markers of hepatitis A, B, and C; and liver function tests. Diagnosis is confirmed by the presence of antigens or antibodies formed in response to specific hepatitis viruses. In hepatitis, liver enzymes are elevated, specifically ALT, AST, and serum total bilirubin, indicating liver damage.

Treatment

There is no specific treatment for hepatitis, which is generally supportive. The management for children is based on measures to rest the liver, promote cellular regeneration, and prevent complications. Rest is an essential focus of treatment to reduce the liver's metabolic demands and increase its blood supply. Treatment is aimed at maintaining comfort and providing adequate nutrition.

Once the diagnosis of hepatitis is made, attention should be directed to prevention. Vaccines have been developed to prevent HAV and HBV. Children who have been exposed to a person with HAV should receive standard immune globulin (IG) within two weeks of exposure. Immune globulin when given in this time period is 80–90% effective in preventing the disease. Hepatitis A vaccine is approved for children ages 1 through 18 years of age. The vaccine is routinely administered to all children aged 1 year. Two doses are administered at least six months apart. (AAP, 2009; MMWR, 2009).

Hepatitis B vaccine is recommended for all newborns as part of the routine childhood immunization schedule. All children who have not received the vaccine previously should be immunized by or before 11 to 12 years of age. Additionally, administration of hepatitis B immune globulin (HBIG) is recommended for individuals exposed to HBV. If given within two weeks of exposure, HBIG is effective in preventing the infection (AAP, 2003).

Nursing Management and Family Teaching

Nursing care is directed toward supportive care and education of the family about prevention measures. Most children with mild or uncomplicated hepatitis are cared for at home. Because fatigue and listlessness can last for weeks, children usually limit their own activity during the early stages of the disease. Anorexia is common; therefore, small, frequent meals and snacks are tolerated well. The nurse should instruct caregivers to contact their health care provider prior to administering over-the-counter medications since normal doses of many drugs may be toxic. A primary focus of education is prevention of the spread of the infection as delineated in Box 23-4. Additionally, the nurse should educate the family about the method of transmission of hepatitis and about the availability of immunoprophylaxis after exposure and of vaccines for HAV and HBV.

TABLE 23-5 Comparison of Hepatitis A, B, and C

TYPE	INCUBATION PERIOD	MODE OF TRANSMISSION	PREVENTION	POSSIBLE COMPLICATIONS
A	15–30 days	Fecal-oral through contaminated food or water	Immunization Education on proper food handling	
		Poor hygiene	Handwashing using clean water and soap Waterless hand cleaner	
B	45–180 days	Perinatally	Immunization Testing of pregnant females	Potential chronicity
		Unsafe sex	Education to practice safe sex and avoid body fluids	Cirrhosis
		Poor hygiene	Handwashing using clean water and soap Waterless hand cleaner	Liver cancer
		Blood transfusions		
		Body secretions	Avoid exposures to blood and body fluids	
		Contaminated needles	Needle exchange program Identification of carriers	
C	2 weeks–6 months	Blood transfusions IV drug use	Education to prevent exposure to blood and body fluids Needle exchange program Identification of carriers	Potential chronicity Cirrhosis Liver cancer

Adapted from Hitchcock, J., Schubert, P., & Thomas, S. (Eds.). (2003). *Community health nursing: Caring in action* (2nd ed.). Clifton Park, NY: Delmar Cengage Learning.

BOX 23-4
PREVENTION OF VIRAL HEPATITIS

- HAV and HBV vaccines.
- Wash hands carefully after changing diapers, using the toilet, and before food preparation and eating.
- Wash linen or clothing contaminated with stool or blood separately in hot water.
- Dispose of diapers, tampons, and sanitary napkins in plastic bags.
- Wear gloves to clean up a child's emesis, blood, or loose stool.
- Clean contaminated household surfaces with a solution of bleach and water (1/4 cup bleach to 1 gallon water).
- Avoid sharing personal items that can get contaminated with infected blood such as razors, pierced earrings, and toothbrushes.

ADDITIONAL GASTROINTESTINAL DISORDERS

The following disorders are rare in children; therefore, they are discussed briefly.

ABDOMINAL WALL DEFECTS: GASTROSCHISIS AND OMPHALOCELE

Omphalocele and gastroschisis are congenital abdominal wall defects that result in herniation of the peritoneal contents through the abdominal wall with (omphalocele) or without (gastroschisis) a membranous cover. The incidence of omphalocele and gastroschisis has been reported to increase two- to four-fold worldwide for the past three decades. Their incidence is 0.4 to 3 in 10,000 live births world wide (Lund, Bauer, & Berrios, 2007). In gastroschisis the defect in the abdominal wall permits extrusion of the abdominal contents, primarily the small and large intestines, without involving the umbilical cord. The defect is usually to the right of the umbilicus, and there is no protective sac covering the intestines. The etiology is unclear, although one theory explains gastroschisis as resulting from an incomplete lateral infolding of the embryonic disc, which allows herniation of the bowel.

An omphalocele is centrally located, includes the umbilical cord and the abdominal viscera, and is covered by a protective sac. Omphalocele results from failure of the intestines to re-enter the abdominal cavity at approximately the seventh week of gestation. The size of the defect is variable, ranging from one cm in diameter to a large mass containing all the abdominal contents.

Clinical Manifestations

In gastroschisis the bowel eviscerates into the amniotic cavity, and exposure to the amniotic fluid results in thickened, beefy-red, edematous intestines. The bowel is normal in appearance in the neonate with omphalocele; however, the abdominal cavity is small and underdeveloped.

Treatment

Goals of initial management of the newborn with either of these disorders are to prevent hypothermia, maintain a sterile environment, and maintain tissue perfusion. Two accepted surgical techniques for these defects are a primary and a staged repair. Primary repair is the procedure of choice if the exposed abdominal contents will fit into the abdominal cavity. If not, a staged repair is performed. A synthetic material is used to create a sac to cover the abdominal contents. The bowel is then gradually returned to the abdomen over 7–10 days. The abdominal wall is closed in the second surgery.

BILIARY ATRESIA

Biliary atresia is characterized by congenital absence or obstruction of bile ducts outside the liver (extra hepatic), thus preventing flow of bile from the liver to the intestines. There is no known cure for the disease. Females appear to be slightly more at risk for developing the disease than males. It is the single most frequent indication for liver transplantation in children. The cause is unknown; however, possible infectious, genetic, and immunologic etiologies have received much recent focus (Bassett & Murray, 2008).

Clinical Manifestations

The newborn with biliary atresia is asymptomatic at birth; however, between 2 weeks and 2 months of age, jaundice appears. The infant's urine is tea-colored because of the excretion of bilirubin and bile salts. Stools are light in color because of the absence of bile pigments. Hepatomegaly may be present from the pathologic processes occurring, such as fibrosis of the liver. Failure to thrive and malnutrition eventually develop.

Treatment

Treatment involves surgery to correct the obstruction and allow for drainage of bile from the liver directly into the intestines. Hepatic portoenterostomy, such as the Kasai procedure, may be performed, thereby attempting to slow the pathologic processes that occur in the biliary duct. This surgery is not a cure, and not all surgeries are successful in delaying biliary duct injury. Complications of liver disease continue to develop and eventually result in end stage liver disease. A liver transplant is required at this point. Parents, siblings or close relative may donate a portion of their liver to the child.

CIRRHOSIS

Cirrhosis is a pathologic condition of the liver that occurs secondary to liver disease or inflammation. Viral hepatitis, inborn errors of metabolism (galactosemia), congenital anomalies of the bile ducts (biliary atresia), and chronic diseases such as cystic fibrosis are the main disorders that cause severe liver disease and cirrhosis in infants and children. Cirrhosis is rare in the pediatric population. Fibrotic scar tissue develops in the liver as a result of chronic inflammation or disease, and the organ assumes an irregular, nodular appearance.

Clinical Manifestations

Clinical manifestations vary depending on the cause of cirrhosis. When the etiology is viral hepatitis, inborn errors of metabolism, or chronic disease, initially the child demonstrates vague symptoms of GI dysfunction, including lethargy, anorexia, and nausea. Steatorrhea is frequently present caused by disordered fat metabolism. In cases caused by biliary anomalies, ascites (accumulation of fluid in the peritoneal cavity) and portal hypertension develop. The most important sign of portal hypertension is splenomegaly, which produces anemia, leukopenia, thrombocytopenia, and often esophageal varices. The child may demonstrate easy bruising or epistaxis (nose bleeds), or GI hemorrhage. Jaundice, dark urine, and pruritis are other symptoms that occur with biliary malformations.

Treatment

Medical management focuses on preventing and treating the complications of cirrhosis. Nutritional treatment of malabsorption problems consists of a low-fat, low-protein diet and supplemental vitamins, especially fat-soluble ones. Ascites is treated with fluid restriction, decrease in sodium content of food, and diuretics. Hepatic encephalopathy is treated with reduction of protein intake and administration of lactulose (to control increased ammonia levels) and an antibiotic such as neomycin. Bleeding complications may necessitate administration of blood and blood products. Definitive treatment for cirrhosis and end stage liver disease is a liver transplant.

UMBILICAL HERNIA

An umbilical hernia results from incomplete closure of the umbilical ring, which allows the intestines to protrude through the defect, especially during crying or straining. It is most common in African American low birth weight females.

Clinical Manifestations

The size of the defect varies from less than 1 cm in diameter to as much as 5 cm; however, large ones are rare. It appears as a soft swelling covered by skin.

Treatment

The use of binders, tape, or other materials to flatten the protrusion do not aid in closing the defect. Most umbilical hernias disappear spontaneously by 1 to 3 years of age. If the hernia persists beyond this age; if it becomes strangulated; or if it grows larger, it is surgically corrected.

CONGENITAL DIAPHRAGMATIC HERNIA

Congenital diaphragmatic hernia (CDH) involves herniation of the abdominal contents through a defect in the diaphragm into the chest cavity and usually develops on the left side. All degrees of protrusion of the abdominal viscera through the diaphragmatic opening into the thoracic cavity may occur. The extent of herniation determines the severity and timing of the symptoms. The incidence is 1 of every 2,500-3,000 live births (Waag et al., 2008). Separation of the developing thoracic and abdominal cavities is accomplished during the eighth week of gestation by closure of the pleuroperitoneal (opening between the chest and abdomen) canal. CDH occurs when this canal fails to close.

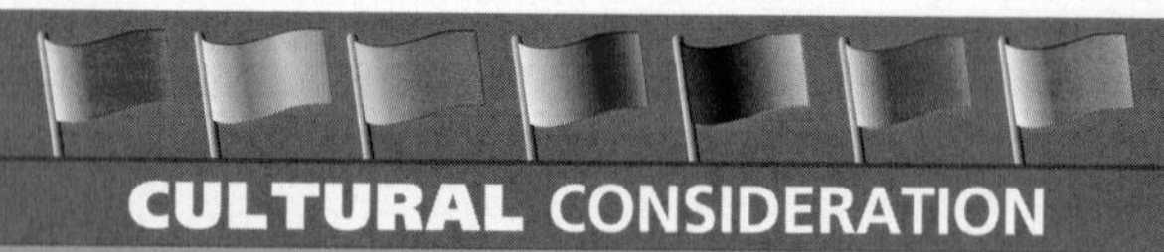

CULTURAL CONSIDERATION

Hernias

Umbilical hernias occur slightly more frequently in infants of African-American descent. There is no known prevention. Taping or "strapping" an umbilical hernia will not cause it to go away though it is culturally a common practice for some.

Clinical Manifestations

Newborns will have severe respiratory distress, cyanosis, tachypnea, and retractions at birth because the lung on the side of the defect is usually **hypoplastic** or underdeveloped. Breath sounds are decreased or absent on the affected side, and the chest is barrel-shaped. Heart sounds are shifted to the right. Bowel sounds may be heard over the chest. The abdomen is scaphoid.

Treatment

Mortality rate is high (up to 60%) despite advances in current treatment modalities (Waag et al., 2008). Some fetuses are diagnosed prenatally by ultrasound in which case surgical repair is performed in utero. If not diagnosed and repaired at this time, the newborn is stabilized before surgery. Ventilatory support is required to manage respiratory compromise. Metabolic acidosis is corrected with the administration of bicarbonate. If stabilization is not possible, extracorporeal membrane oxygenation is required in most cases. The surgery involves repositioning the abdominal contents into the abdomen and closing the defect.

MALROTATION AND VOLVUS

Malrotation is the incomplete normal rotation of the midgut during fetal development as it returns from the umbilical pouch to the abdominal cavity. During early gestation the midgut grows extensively and protrudes into the umbilical cord pouch until it lies completely outside the abdominal cavity. Eventually this cavity enlarges and the midgut returns to the intra-abdominal position. Malrotation occurs when the bowel fails to rotate normally as it returns to the abdominal cavity. Volvus, a complication of malrotation, occurs when the incompletely rotated bowel twists on itself, leading to arterial obstruction, ischemia, and necrosis.

Clinical Manifestations

Most infants with this anomaly experience symptoms of bowel obstruction, abdominal distention, and bilious vomiting in the first year of life. Diarrhea may be an early symptom in infants under the age of six months. If volvus occurs, bloody stools may be followed by perforation and peritonitis. Older children may have intermittent abdominal cramping, pain, vomiting, and diarrhea or constipation.

Treatment

Treatment for malrotation is surgical. The intestine is rotated and placed into the abdominal cavity with the cecum in the left lower quadrant. If volvus and bowel necrosis are present, the affected area is removed.

MECKEL'S DIVERTICULUM

Meckel's diverticulum, the most common congenital malformation of the GI tract, is a blind sac or pouch protruding from the wall of the ileum. It results when a duct connecting the embryonic yolk sac to the primitive gut fails to atrophy. It occurs in 2–3% of the population and is usually asymptomatic.

CLINICAL MANIFESTATIONS

Most symptomatic cases appear within the first two years of life. Painless rectal bleeding is the most common clinical manifestation. Bleeding occurs because the tip of the pouch of the ileum contains ectopic gastric mucosa rather than ileal mucosa. The gastric mucosa secretes acid and pepsin, causing irritation, ulceration, and eventually lower GI bleeding. Rectal bleeding is massive and dark or bright red in color.

TREATMENT

Treatment is surgical removal of the diverticulum or pouch to prevent hypovolemic shock from hemorrhage. In most cases, intestinal resection is not required, and the child recovers rapidly.

SHORT BOWEL SYNDROME

Short bowel syndrome (SBS) is a disorder characterized by inadequate surface area of the small intestine and usually occurs after surgical resection of the intestine in cases of necrotizing enterocolitis, volvus, or Crohn's disease. The small intestine may be congenitally short in conditions such as gastroschisis, omphalocele, and intestinal atresia. SBS may not be a permanent disorder because the intestine can grow and adapt. This process of adaptation is gradual, requiring months to years.

CLINICAL MANIFESTATIONS

The most common clinical manifestations are malabsorption, malnutrition, and diarrhea. Carbohydrate malabsorption and steatorrhea also occur. Fluid and electrolyte losses may lead to dehydration, hyponatremia, hypokalemia, and acidosis. Vitamins and minerals are lost and deficiencies occur. Skin irritation and breakdown on the buttocks and perineum are caused by the frequent loose, watery stools. Bacterial overgrowth in the remaining small intestine is common and occurs when the ileocecal valve is absent or when there is impaired motility in the bowel and stasis. This overgrowth leads to increased diarrhea and intestinal gas.

TREATMENT

Medical management of SBS focuses on maintaining optimum nutrition and preventing complications. Nutritional therapy initially includes total parenteral nutrition (TPN) via a central line and enteral feedings via an NG or gastrostomy tube. The main purpose of enteral nutrition is to stimulate the adaptive growth of the small intestine. Oral feedings are given when tolerated so the infant can learn to suck and swallow. Additionally, to maintain an interest in oral feeding and to stimulate sucking, a pacifier may be used. When enteral and oral feedings are increased, TPN is gradually decreased proportionately. Several complications may occur as a result of long-term use of TPN, including central catheter infection, occlusion, and thrombosis; liver disease; and **cholestasis** (interruption in the flow of bile). Therefore, when TPN is initiated and regularly used throughout therapy, certain laboratory values are obtained. These include liver and renal function tests, liver enzymes, calcium, magnesium, and phosphorus.

IN THE REAL WORLD

I was totally unprepared for what I saw when I cared for my first infant client with a bilateral cleft lip and palate. I was a new graduate working on a pediatric unit and had studied this defect in school. I had even seen pictures of it in my textbook. But what I saw horrified me. My client, a 2-month-old girl, had a gaping hole in the middle of her face. All I could feel was pity for this tiny baby. She would be stared at when her parents took her out in public. I then thought of them and how disappointed they must be because their daughter was imperfect. All parents hope for and expect a perfect baby. Neither of them was in the room when I entered, and I was glad I did not have to see them right then. I soon came to my senses and remembered I was a "real" nurse now and had to care for this infant. So I began my nursing assessment and was gradually able to look at her face without dreading it. Eventually I noticed her other features, like lots of beautiful black curly hair and sky blue eyes.

KEY CONCEPTS

- The gastrointestinal system of the infant and child is immature compared to an adult; therefore, feeding must be in smaller amounts, more frequent, and consist of a greater number of calories per kilogram of weight.
- Pyloric stenosis is characterized by projectile vomiting without loss of appetite, poor weight gain, dehydration, and a palpable olive-shaped mass in the epigastrium.
- Clefts of the lip and palate are some of the most common congenital anomalies. Initial reactions of caregivers to an infant with this defect include shock, grief, feelings of failure, inadequacy, and isolation.
- Nursing management for the infant with a cleft palate or lip focuses on adapting feeding methods, providing preoperative and postoperative care, educating caregivers, and providing emotional support.
- The typical presentation of an infant with esophageal atresia includes copious, fine, frothy bubbles of mucus in the mouth and sometimes the nose.
- Intussusception is one of the most common causes of intestinal obstruction in infancy and presents with severe abdominal pain, vomiting, and blood and mucus in stools.
- Hirschsprung's disease, the most common cause of distal bowel obstruction in the newborn, is treated with surgical removal of the aganglionic portion of the bowel.
- Anorectal malformations are usually noted at birth, and after surgical repair, these infants may have difficulty with toilet training.
- Nursing care for gastroesophageal reflux is directed toward teaching caregivers methods to prevent or reduce reflux by feeding and positioning.
- For the child with chronic constipation nursing management is directed toward cleansing the bowel, diet therapy, and establishing a regular elimination pattern.
- Signs and symptoms of appendicitis include abdominal pain that begins in the periumbilical area and migrates to the right lower quadrant, low-grade fever, nausea, and sometimes vomiting.
- Prompt and accurate diagnosis of appendicitis is essential to prevent perforation and peritonitis, which are common in children.
- Inflammatory bowel disease includes ulcerative colitis and Crohn's disease and is characterized by persistent diarrhea, abdominal pain, and growth failure. Treatment focuses on reducing the symptoms with medications, nutritional therapy, and often surgery.
- Nursing management for a child with a peptic ulcer includes teaching caregivers about medication therapy and dietary modifications.
- The nurse has a significant role in early detection of NEC, assessing for signs of complications, and providing emotional support for the family.
- For the child with celiac disease, nursing management focuses on education about the gluten-free diet and referral to community resources for emotional and dietary support.
- For a child with lactose intolerance, treatment and nursing management focuses on educating the child and caregivers about dietary needs.
- Nursing management for the child with hepatitis is directed toward teaching about dietary needs, infection control, and signs and symptoms of severely impaired liver function.

REVIEW ACTIVITIES

1. Differentiate between hypertrophic pyloric stenosis and gastroesophageal reflux.
2. Outline a teaching plan for caregivers related to feeding an infant born with bilateral CL/CP.
3. List the clinical manifestations of an infant with esophageal atresia and tracheoesophageal fistula.
4. Discuss the nonsurgical treatment for intussusception.
5. Explain the pathophysiology of Hirschsprung's disease.
6. Describe the nurse's role in detecting an anorectal malformation in a newborn infant.

7. Explain the American Academy of Pediatrics recommended sleeping position for the infant with gastroesophageal reflux.
8. Discuss why appendicitis in children frequently progresses to perforation.
9. List the clinical manifestations of appendicitis.
10. Compare ulcerative colitis and Crohn's disease in the following areas: (a) pathologic changes in intestine and (b) clinical manifestations.
11. Outline a plan for teaching the child with celiac disease and the child's family.
12. Identify strategies to enhance compliance with dietary restrictions for the child with celiac disease.
13. Compare the methods of transmission and clinical manifestations of hepatitis A, B, and C.

STUDY QUESTIONS

1. Which assessment would the RN do first when a child returns to the unit after an emergency appendectomy?
   a. Bladder distension
   b. Intravenous fluid infusion site
   c. Nasogastric tube function
   d. Surgical dressing
2. Which of these menus, if chosen by a parent of a child who has celiac disease, would indicate to a nurse that the parent understood the teaching about a gluten-free diet?
   a. Broiled steak, baked potato, and spinach
   b. Pork chop, egg noodles, and green peas
   c. Fried chicken, white roll, and mixed vegetables
   d. Baked macaroni with cheddar cheese and corn
3. The feeding of a baby who has a cleft lip and palate requires the use of a bulb syringe with sterile rubber tubing. The mother demonstrates correct feeding of the baby when she demonstrates which of these actions?
   a. She allows the baby to suck on the rubber-tipped syringe
   b. She aims the flow of liquid to the back of the throat
   c. She positions the tubing into the clefted palate
   d. She directs the flow of liquid to the side and back of mouth
4. Four hours ago an infant was returned to the unit after surgery to correct pyloric stenosis. Select the most important nursing intervention.
   a. Feed small amounts frequently and assess emesis.
   b. Keep the infant NPO and encourage parent to perform oral care.
   c. Monitor intake and output and administer medications.
   d. Monitor urine output and encourage parent to rest.
5. After surgery for a cleft lip repair, an infant is having difficulty breathing. Which nursing action would be most helpful in bringing relief?
   a. Raise the baby's head
   b. Turn the baby onto the abdomen
   c. Administer oxygen per mask
   d. Exert downward pressure on the infant's chin
6. A parent calls the pediatric clinic and is frantic about the bottle of cleaning fluid containing hydrocarbons that her child drank 20 minutes ago. Which of the following is the most important instruction the nurse can give the parent?
   a. "This too shall pass."
   b. "Take the child immediately to the ER."
   c. "Contact the Poison Control Center immediately."
   d. "Give the child syrup of ipecac."
7. The mother of a neonate with gastroschisis feels guilty because she believes she did something to cause the condition. You should explain that the cause of gastroschisis is
   a. Not clear.
   b. Hereditary.
   c. Caused by restricted movement in uterus.
   d. Caused by young pregnant age.
8. The nurse knows that a conclusive diagnosis of pyloric stenosis will be made by which of the following tests?
   a. A flat X-ray of the abdomen
   b. A colonoscopy
   c. An electrolyte panel
   d. An upper GI series

9. The nurse is assessing a child with a tentative diagnosis of appendicitis. The nursing assessment is most likely to reveal what characteristics concerning the pain?
   a. Rebounding tenderness in the right lower quadrant, associated with decreased bowel sounds and vomiting
   b. Gnawing pain, radiating through to the lower back, with severe abdominal distention
   c. Sharp pain with severe gastric distention, frequently associated with hemoptysis
   d. Pain on light palpation in midepigastric area, chronic low-grade fever, and diarrhea
10. What is the reason for positioning an infant with tracheoesophageal fistula supine with head and shoulders elevated prior to surgical repair?
   a. To reduce respiratory and cardiac workload
   b. To alleviate pressure of distended abdominal contents on the diaphragm
   c. To increase pooling of secretions in the bottom of the upper esophageal pouch
   d. To reduce gastric distention by allowing air bubbles from the fistula to escape

REFERENCES

American Academy of Pediatrics, Committee on Infectious Diseases. (2009). In Pickering, L. (Ed.). *Red book: Report of the committee on infectious diseases* (28th ed.). Elk Grove Village, IL: American Academy of Pediatrics.

American Academy of Pediatrics, Committee on Injury, Violence, and Poison Prevention. (2003). Poison treatment in the home. *Pediatrics, 112*(5), 1182–1185.

American Academy of Pediatrics, Task Force on Infant Sleep Position and Sudden Infant Death Syndrome. (2000). Changing concepts of sudden infant death syndrome: Implications for infant sleeping environment and sleep position. *Pediatrics, 105*(3), 650–656.

Arguin, A., & Swartz, M. (2004). Gastroesophageal reflux in infants: A primary care perspective. *Pediatric Nursing, 30*(1), 45–51.

Bassett, M. D., & Murray, K. F. (2008). Biliary atresia: Recent progress. *Journal of Clinical Gastroenterol, 42*(6), 720–729.

Bronstein A. C., Spyker, D. A., Cantilena, L. R., Jr., Green, J. L., Rumack, B. H., Heard, S. E. (2008). 2007 Annual Report of the American Association of Poison Control Centers' National Poison Data System (NPDS): 25th Annual Report. *Clinical toxicology (Philadelphia), 46*(10), 927–1057.

Ceballos, C. (2008). Growth and early onset inflammatory bowel disease. *Gastroenterology Nursing, 31*(2), 101–106.

Centers for Disease Control and Prevention. (2005). Preventing lead poisoning in young children: A statement by the Centers for Disease Control and Prevention. Retrieved March 15, 2009, from http://www.cdc.gov/nceh/lead/publications/prevleadpoisoning.pdf.

Coughlin, E. (2003). Primary care approaches: Assessment and management of pediatric constipation in primary care. *Pediatric Nursing, 29*(4), 296–301.

Criddle, L. M. (2007). An overview of pediatric poisonings. *AACN Advanced Critical Care 18*(2), 109–118.

Dasgupta, R., & Langer, J. C. (2004). Hirschsprung disease. *Current Problems in Surgery, 41*(12), 949–988.

de la Torre, M. A., & Thurman, M. A. (2008). Cigarette smoking and orofacial cleft development: Dental hygiene's role in education and prevention. *Access, 22*(1), 30–33.

Doria, A. S., Moineddin, R., Kellenberger, C. J., Epelman, M., Beyene, B., Schuh, S., Babyn, P. S., & Dick, P. D. (2006). US or CT for diagnosis of appendicitis in children and adults? A meta-analysis. *Radiology, 241*, 83–94.

Dunn, A., & Burns, C. (2004). Environmental health issues. In C. Burns, A. Dunn, M. Brady, N. Starr, & C. Blosser (Eds.), *Pediatric primary care: A handbook for nurse practitioners* (3rd ed.). Philadelphia: W. B. Saunders, pp. 1283–1309.

Farrington, M., Lang, S., Cullen, L., & Stewart, S. (2009). Nasogastric tube placement verification in pediatric and neonatal patients. *Pediatric Nursing, 35*(1), 17–25.

Franklin, R., & Rodgers, G. B. (2008). Unintentional child poisonings treated in United States hospital emergency departments: National estimates of incident cases, population-based poisoning rates, and product involvement. *Pediatrics, 122*(6), 1244–1251.

Gelfond, D., & Fasano, A. (2006). Celiac disease in the pediatric population. *Pediatric Annals 35*(4), 275–279.

Gisbert, J. P., de la Morena, F., & Abraira, V. (2006). Accuracy of monoclonal stool antigen test for the diagnosis of *H. Pylori* infection: A systematic review and meta-analysis. *American Journal of Gastroenterology 101*(8), 1921–1930.

Golding-Kushner, K. J. (2001). Therapy techniques for cleft palate, speech, and related disorders. Clifton Park, NY: Thomson Delmar Learning.

Haider, N., & Fisher, R. (2007). Mortality and morbidity associated with late diagnosis of anorectal malformations in children. *Surgeon, 5*(6), 327–330.

Hall, N. J., Pacilli, M., Eaton, S., Reblock, K., Gaines, B. A., Paster, A., Langer, J. C., Koivusalo, A. I., Pakarien, M. P., Stroedter, L., Beyerlein, S., Haddas, M., Clarke, S., Ford, H., & Pierro, A. (2009). Recovery after open versus laparoscopic pyloromyotomy for pyloric stenosis: A double-blind multicentre randomised controlled trial. *The Lancet, 373*(9661), 390–398.

Hitchcock, J., Schubert, P., & Thomas, S. (Eds.). (2003). *Community health nursing: Caring in action (2nd ed.).* Clifton Park, NY: Thomson Delmar Learning.

Home Safety Council. (2004). Retrieved April 10, 2009, from http://www.homesafetycouncil.org/resource_center/resourcecenter.aspx.

Huppertz, H. I., Soriano-Gaabarro, M., Grimprel, E., Franco, E., Mezner, Z., Desselberger, U., Smit, Y., Wolleswinkel-van den Bosch, J.,

De Vos, B., & Giaquinto, C. (2006). Intussusception among young children in Europe. *Pediatric Infectious Disease Journal, 25*(1), 22–29.

Kairam, N., Kaiafis, C., & Shih, R. (2009). Diagnosis of pediatric intussusception by an emergency physician-performed bedside ultrasound: A case report. *Pediatric Emergency Care, 25*(3), 177–180.

Katz, J. (2001). *Keys to nursing success.* Upper Saddle River, NJ: Prentice Hall.

Kawahara, H., Takama, Y., Yoshida, H., Nakia, H., Okuyama, H., Kubota, A., Yoshimura, N., Ida, S., & Okada, A. (2005). Medical treatment of infantile hypertrophic pyloric stenosis: Should we always slice the "olive"? *Journal of Pediatric Surgery, 40*(12), 1848–1845.

Kitagawa, S, & Miqdady, M. (2008). Intussusception in children. Retrieved March 14, 2009, from http://www.uptodate.com/patients/content/topic.do?topicKey=~WevvYJlLs9of0e&selectedTitle=1~63&source=search_result.

Kupperman, N., O'Dea, T., Pinckney, L., & Hoecker, C. (2000). Predictors of intussusception in young children. *Archives of Pediatric and Adolescent Medicine, 154,* 250–255.

Kwok, M. Y., Kim, M. K., Gorelick, M. H. (2004). Evidence-based approach to the diagnosis of appendicitis in children. *Pediatric Emergency Care 20*(10), 690–698.

Leoening-Baucke, v., & Pashankar, D. S. (2006). A randomized, prospective, comparison study of polyethylene glycol 3350 without electrolytes and milk of magnesia for children with constipation and fecal incontinence. *Pediatrics, 118*(2), 528-535.

Lin, P. W., Nasr, T. R., & Stoll, B. J. (2008). Necrotizing enterocolitis: Recent scientific advances in pathophysiology and prevention. *Seminars in Perinatology, 32*(2), 70–82.

Lindfred, H., Saalman, R., Nilsson, S., & Reichenberg, K. (2008). Inflammatory bowel disease and self-esteem in adolescence. *Acta Paediatrica. 97*(2), 201–205.

Lund, C. H., Bauer, K., & Berrios, M. (2007). Gastroschisis: Incidence, complications, and clinical management in the neonatal intensive care unit. *Journal of Perinatal & Neonatal Nursing, 21*(1), 63–68.

McAlhany, A., & Popovich, D. (2007). Hirschsprung disease. *Newborn and Infant Reviews, 7*(3), 151–154.

Morbidity and Mortality Weekly Report (MMWR). (2009). Recommended immunization schedules for persons aged 0 through 18 years—United States, 2009. *MMRW, 57*(52), q1–q4.

Murdock, A. M., & Johnston, S. D. (2005). Diagnostic criteria for celiac disease: Time for change? *European Journal of Gatroenterology & Hepatology, 17*(1), 41–43.

National Digestive Disease Information Clearinghouse. (2006). Gastroesophageal reflux in infants. Retrieved March 20, 2009, from http://digestive.niddk.nih.gov/ddiseases/pubs/gerdinfant/.

National Institute of Health, National Center for Complementary Medicine. (2008). An introduction to probiotics. Retrieved April 19, 2009, from http://nccam.nih.gov/health/probiotics/.

Nisell, M. (2003). International pediatric nursing: How a family is affected when a child is born with anorectal malformation: Interviews with three patients and their parents. *Pediatric Nursing, 18*(6), 423–432.

Peter, S. D. S., Holcomb III, G. W., Calkins, C. M., Murphy, J. P., Andrews, V., Sharp, R. J., Snyder, C. L., & Ostlie, D. J. (2006). Open versus laparoscopic pyloromyotomy for pyloric stenosis: A prospective, randomized trial. *Annals of Surgery, 244*(3), 363–370.

Pisarra, V. (2001). Recognizing the various presentations of appendicitis. *Dimensions of Critical Care Nursing, 20*(3), 24–27.

Powers, K. (2000). Diagnosis and management of common toxic ingestions and inhalations. *Pediatric Annuals, 296,* 330–342.

Pulsifer-Anderson, E. (2009). Helping families understand and manage pediatric gastroesophageal reflux. *Zero to Three, 29*(3), 50–59.

Quinn, D., & Shannon, L. (1996). Congenital anomalies of the gastrointestinal tract—Part III: The colon and rectum. *Neonatal Network, 15*(2), 63–67.

Rogers, I. M. (2006). The true cause of pyloric stenosis is hyperacidity. *Acta Paediatrica, 95*(2), 132–136.

Rufo, P. A., & Bousvaros, A. (2007). Challenges and progress in pediatric inflammatory bowel disease. *Current Opinion in Gastroenterology, 23*(4), 406–412.

Runyan, C. W., & Casteel, C. (Eds). (2004). *The state of home safety in America: Facts about unintentional injury in the home* (2nd ed.). Home Safety Council. Washington, DC. Retrieved March 22, 2009, from http://www.homesafetycouncil.org/state_of_home_safety/sohs_2004_p001.pdf.

Sgouros, S. N., & Bergele, C. (2006). Clinical outcome of patients with Helicobacter pylori infection: The bug, the host, or the environment? *Postgraduate Medicine Journal 82*(967), 338–342.

Shaw-Smith, C. (2006). Oesophageal atresia, tracheoesophageal fistula, and the VACTERL association: Review of genetics and epidemiology. *Journal of Medical Genetics 43*(7), 545–554.

Shoji, H., Suganuma, H., Daigo, M., Shinohara, K., Umezaki, H., Shiga, S., Shimizu, T., & Yamashiro, Y. (2008). Hypertrophic pyloric stenosis in mono-ovular extremely preterm twins after use of erythromycin. *Pediatrics International, 50*(5), 701–702.

Silbermintz, A., & Markowitz, J. (2006). Inflammatory bowel diseases *Pediatric Annals 355*(4), 268–274.

Sondheimer, J. (2008). Non-pharmacologic therapy may be effective for infants with gastroesophageal reflux. *Journal of Pediatric, 153*(3), 441–442.

Sorensen, H. T., Skriver, M. V., Pedersen, L., Larsen, H., Ebbesen, F., & Schonheyder, H. C. (2003). Risk of infantile hypertrophic pyloric stenosis after maternal postnatal use of macrolides. *Scandinavian Journal of Infectious Diseases 35*(2), 104–106.

Spoon, R., & Trotter, C. (2003). Neonatal radiology VATER association. *Neonatal Network: The Journal of Neonatal Nursing, 22*(3), 71–75.

Steele, R. (2002). Hepatitis A vaccine: Time for universal immunization. *Clinical Pediatrics, 41*(1), 1–3.

Suwandhi, E., Ton, M. N., & Schwarz. S. M. (2006). Gastroesophageal reflux in infancy and childhood. *Pediatric Annals, 35*(4), 259–266.

Swenson, O. (2002). Hirschsprung's disease: A review. *Pediatrics, 109*(5), 914–918.

Telega, G., Bennet, T. R., & Werlin, S. (2008). Emerging New Clinical Patterns in the Presentation of Celiac Disease. *Archive of Pediatric Adolescence Medicine, 162*(2), 164–168.

Thompson, A. M., & Bizzarro, M. J. (2008). Necrotizing enterocolitis in newborns: Pathogenesis, prevention and management. *Drugs, 68*(9), 1227–1238.

To, T., Wajja, A., Wales, P. W., & Langer, J. C. (2005). Population demographic indicators associated with incidence of pyloric stenosis. *Archives of Pediatrics & Adolescent Medicine, 159*(6), 159–520.

Tully, M. A. (2008). Pediatric celiac disease. *Gastroenterology Nursing, 31*(2), 132–140.

U.S. Environmental Protection Agency. (2008). America's children and the environment. Measure B1: Lead in the blood of children. Retrieved March 15, 2009, from http://www.epa.gov/envirohealth/children/body_burdens/b1-graph.htm.

van den Berg, M. M., Benninga, M. A., & Di Lorenzo, C. (2006). Epidemiology of childhood constipation: A systematic review. *American Journal of Gastroenterology, 101*, 2401.

Waag, K. L., Loff, S., Zahn, K., Ali, M., Hien, S., Kratz, M., Neff, W., Schaffelder, R., & Schaible, T. (2008). Congenital diaphragmatic hernia: A modern day approach. *Seminars in Pediatric Surgery, 17*(4), 244–254.

Zeller, J. L., Burke, A. E., & Glass, R. M. (2007). Acute appendicitis in children. *Journal of The American Medical Association, 298*(4), 482.

SUGGESTED READINGS

Beaumont, D. (2008). A study into weight gain of infants with cleft lip/palate. *Pediatric Nursing, 20*(6), 20–23.

Brown-Guttovz, H. (2007). Action stat. intussusception. *Nursing, 37*(2), 80.

Bulechek, G., Butcher, H., & Dochterman, J. (2007). *Nursing Interventions Classification (NIC)* (5th ed). St. Louis, MO: Mosby.

Feragen, K. B., Borge, A. I., and Rumsey, N. (2009). Social experience in 10-year-old children born with a cleft: Exploring psychosocial resilience. *Cleft Palate-Craniofacial Journal, 46*(1), 65–74.

Greenley, R. N., & Cunningham, C. (2009). Parent quality of life in the context of pediatric inflammatory bowel disease. *Pediatric Psychology, 34*(2), 129–136.

Higgins, R. (2009). Abdominal assessment and diagnosis of appendicitis. *Emergency Nurse, 16*(9), 22–24.

Montgomery D. F., Navarro F., Cromwell P. F., & Yetman, R. J. (2008). Practice guidelines. Management of constipation and encopresis in children. *Journal of Pediatric Healthcare, 22*(3), 199–204.

Moorhead, S., Johnson, M., & Maas, M. (2007). *Nursing Outcomes Classification (NOC)* (4th ed). St. Louis, MO: Mosby.

Moya, F. R., & Lally, K. P. (2005). Evidence-based management of infant with congenital diaphragmatic hernia. *Seminars in Perinatology, 29*(2), 112–117.

Murray, L., Hentges, F., Hill, J., Karpf, J., Kreutz, M., Woodall, P., Moss, T., & Goodacre, T. (2008). The effect of cleft lip and palate, and the timing of lip repair on mother-infant interactions and infant development. *Journal of Child Psychology & Psychiatry, 49*(2), 115–123.

Pai, M. S., Bhaduri, A., Jain, A. G., Kumar, V., Sethi, S., & Holaday, B. (2008). International pediatric nursing. The experiences of mothers of pediatric surgery children—A qualitative analysis. *Journal of Pediatric Nursing, 23*(6), 479–489.

Pelchat, D. (2004). Parental satisfaction with an early family intervention program. *Journal of Perinatal & Neonatal Nursing, 18*(2), 128.

Rocca, D. (2007). Minimizing the perils of appendicitis. *Nursing, 37*(1), 64hn1–64hn3.

Sandberg, D. (2002). Neonatal cleft lip and cleft palate repair. *Association of Perioperative Registered Nurses, 75*(3), 488, 490–491, 501.

Sims, R. J. M., & Woodgate, R. L. (2008). Managing chronic hepatitis B in children. *Journal of Pediatric Healthcare, 22*(6), 360–367.

Taylor, C. (2008). Primary care nursing, lactose intolerance in infants. *Nursing Times, 102*(17), 43–44.

Thapa, M., & Sze, R. W. (2005). Pediatric gastrointestinal emergencies. *Radiology, 34*(4), 8–10.

RESOURCES

Refer to the online student StudyWARE for Potts & Mandleco at http://www.CengageBrain.com for additional content and study aids.

Organization: **American Association of Poison Control Centers**
Description: This is the national leader in poison prevention, education, research and treatment. Its mission is to support and promote our members in their public health mission to provide quality poison control center services.
Website/Resource: http://www.aapcc.org

Organization: **American Liver Foundation**
Description: This foundation facilitates, advocates, and promotes education, support, and research for the prevention, treatment, and cure of liver disease.
Website/Resource: http://www.liverfoundation.org

Organization: **Celiac Disease Foundation**
Description: CDF promotes awareness and builds a supportive community for patients, families, and health care professionals. CDF is actively involved in advocating for patient concerns and networking with other national and international organizations.
Website/Resource: http://www.celiac.org

Organization: **Celiac Sprue Association/USA, Inc.**
Description: CSA is nonprofit organization dedicated to helping individuals with celiac disease and dermatitis herpetiformis worldwide through research, education, and support.
Website/Resource: http://www.csaceliacs.org

Organization: **The Cleft Palate Foundation**
Description: CPF provides the essential information and research that enhances the quality of life for individuals affected by cleft lip and palate and other facial birth defects.
Website/Resource: http://www.cleftline.org

Organization: **Crohn's and Colitis Foundation of America, Inc.**
Description: The Crohn's and Colitis Foundation of America is a nonprofit, volunteer-driven organization dedicated to finding the cure for Crohn's disease and ulcerative colitis. Its mission is to cure Crohn's disease and ulcerative colitis and to improve the quality of life of children and adults affected by these diseases.
Website/Resource: http://www.ccfa.org

Organization: **National Digestive Diseases Information Clearinghouse**
Description: NDDIC is an information dissemination service of the National Institute of Diabetes and Digestive and Kidney Diseases (NIDDK). The NIDDK is part of the National Institutes of Health (NIH), which is part of the U.S. Department of Health and Human Services. NDDIC was established in 1980 to increase knowledge and understanding about digestive diseases among people with these conditions and their families, health care professionals, and the general public.
Website/Resource: http://www.digestive.niddk.nih.gov

Organization: **Wound, Ostomy, and Continence Nurses Society**
Description: The WOCN Society is a professional nursing society that supports its members by promoting educational, clinical, and research opportunities to advance the practice and guide the delivery of expert health care to individuals with wounds, ostomies, and incontinence.
Website/Resource: http://www.wocn.org

Organization: **Hepatitis Foundation International**
Description: HFI is dedicated to the eradication of viral hepatitis, a disease affecting over 500 million people around the world. The organization seeks to raise awareness of this enormous worldwide problem and to motivate people to support this important–and winnable–battle.
Website/Resource: http://www.hepfi.org

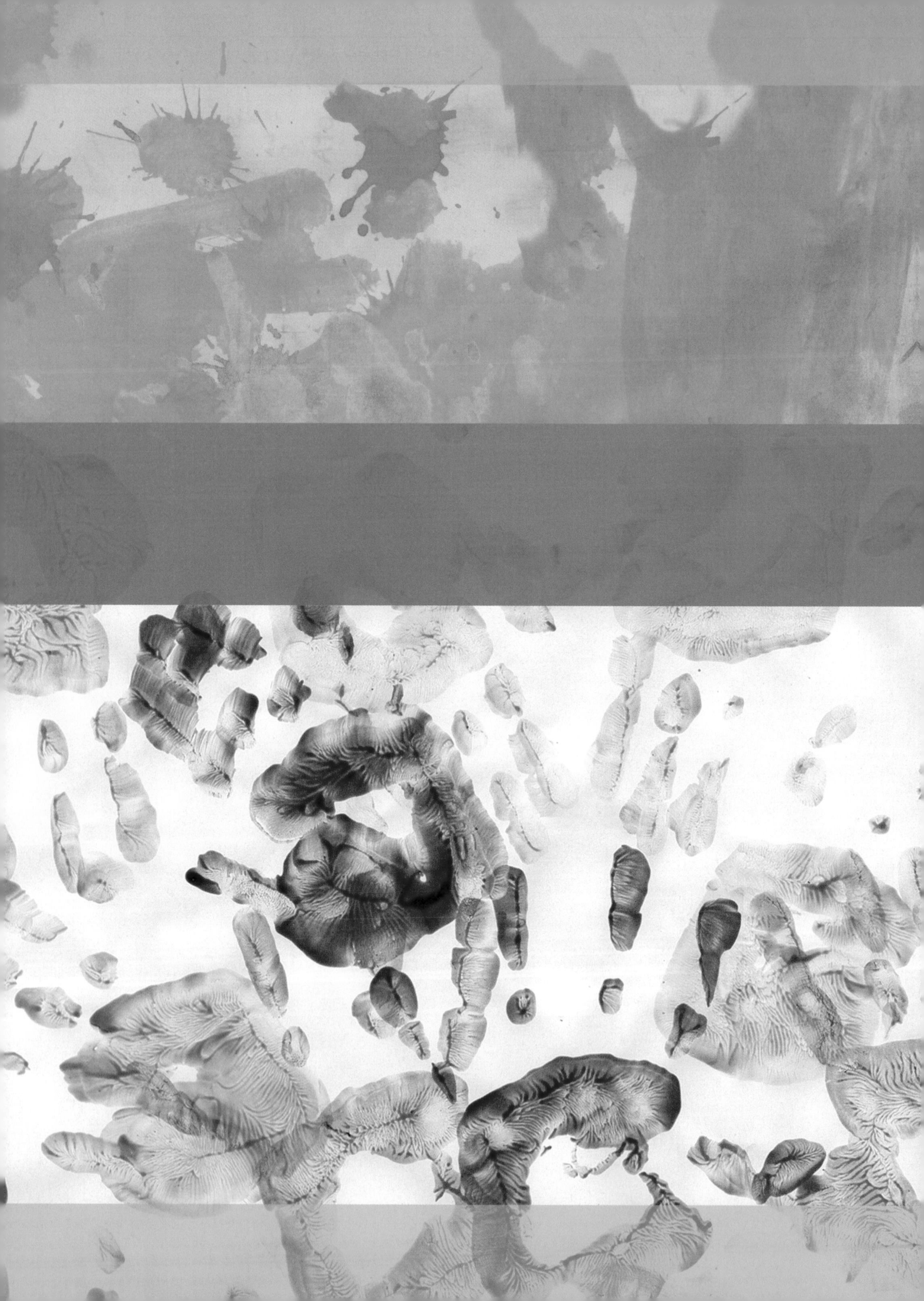

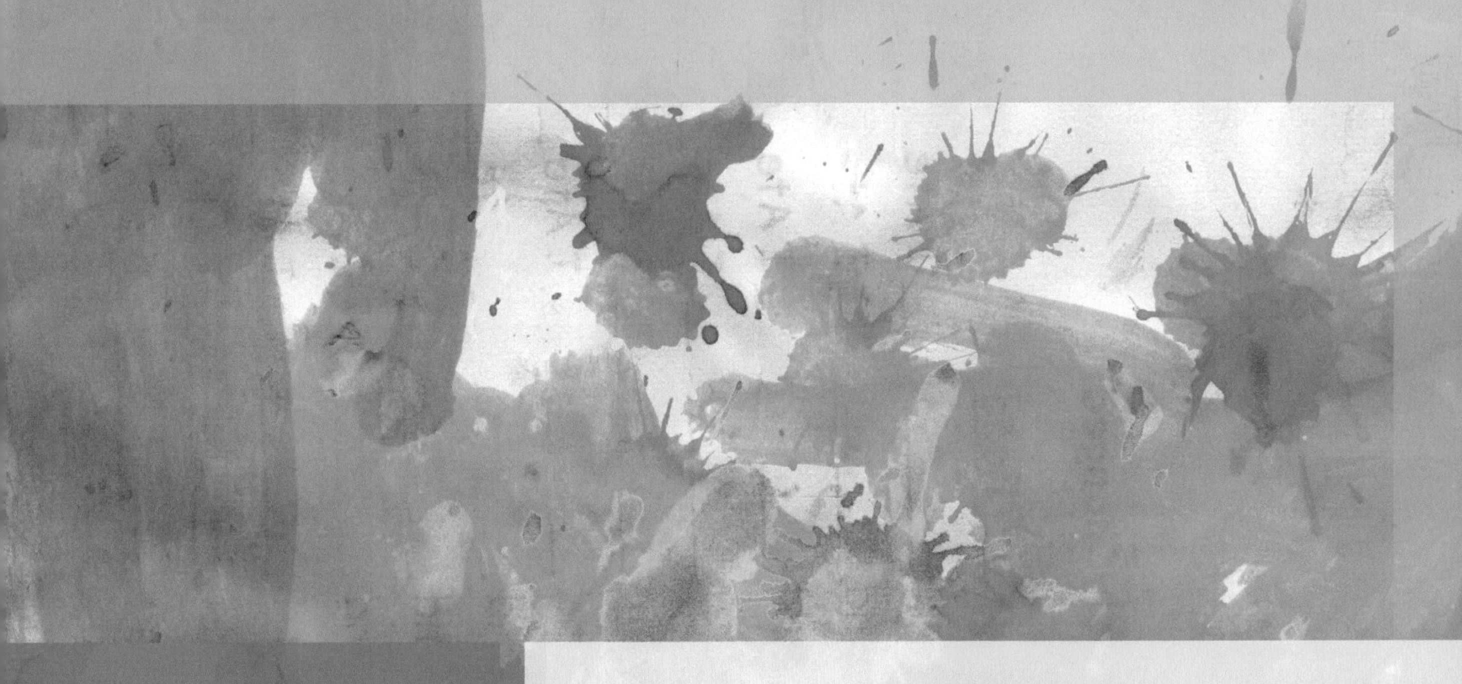

UNIT 5 Alterations in Oxygen Transport

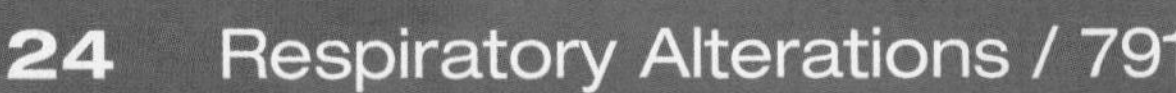

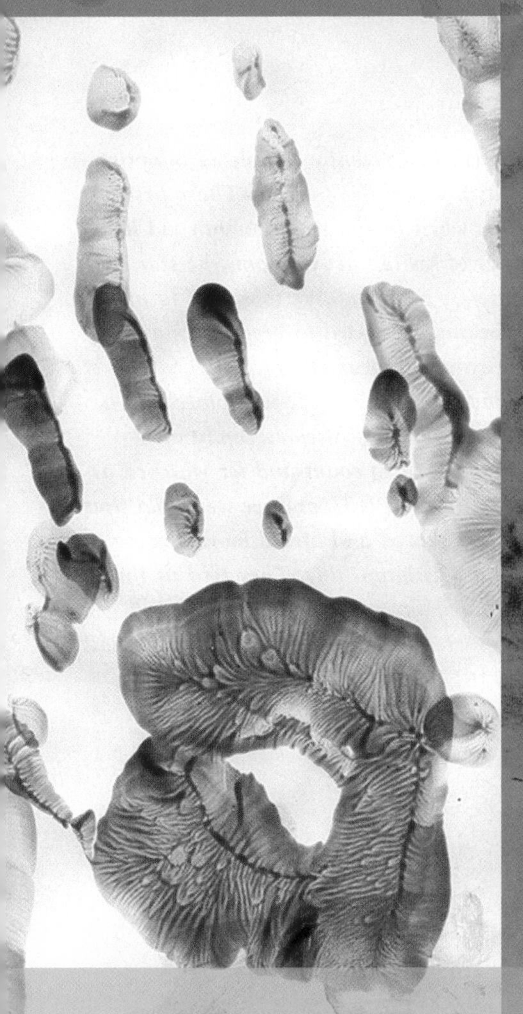

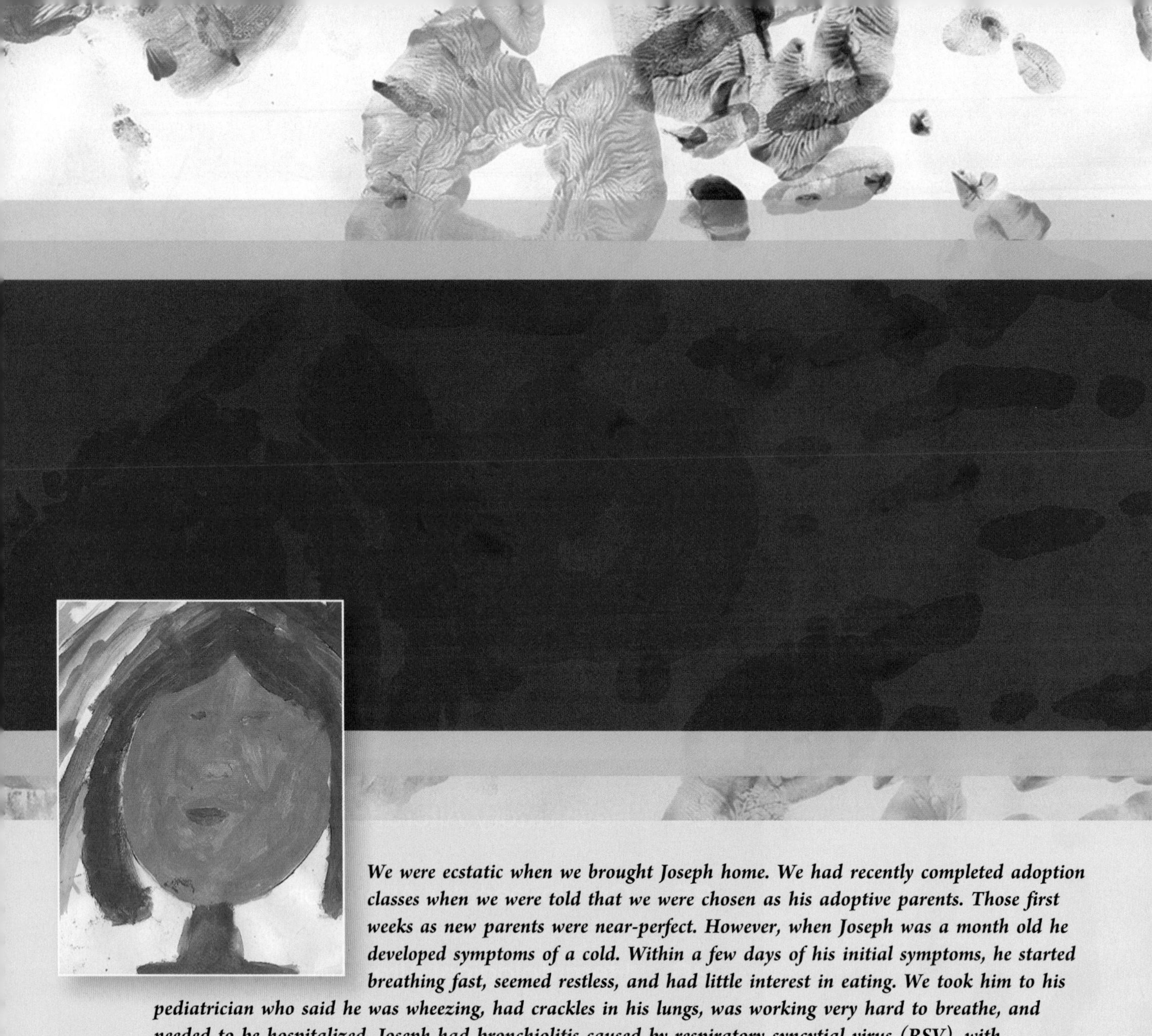

We were ecstatic when we brought Joseph home. We had recently completed adoption classes when we were told that we were chosen as his adoptive parents. Those first weeks as new parents were near-perfect. However, when Joseph was a month old he developed symptoms of a cold. Within a few days of his initial symptoms, he started breathing fast, seemed restless, and had little interest in eating. We took him to his pediatrician who said he was wheezing, had crackles in his lungs, was working very hard to breathe, and needed to be hospitalized. Joseph had bronchiolitis caused by respiratory syncytial virus (RSV), with pneumonia. He was started on intravenous fluids, antibiotics, and was placed on oxygen. He was placed on a machine that monitored his oxygen saturation and heart rate. Over the next 24 hours Joseph's condition worsened. His heart rate rose to over 200, his breathing rate so rapid it was hard to count and we watched as his oxygen saturation fell whenever the oxygen was removed. He was moved to the PICU, and we were told that he might need to be placed on a ventilator to help him breathe. We were very scared and afraid he was going to die. The nurses were so supportive, and kept us informed of everything that was happening. They told us that RSV is a common respiratory virus affecting young infants, but that with adequate support and time, most infants fully recover. It took almost a week but Joseph's condition finally started to improve and in time he had fully recovered and was back to his cute, happy self.

CHAPTER 24

Respiratory Alterations

JENNIFER BEIER, RN, MS, APN-CPNP
STACY VANDENBRANDEN, RN, MS, APN-CPNP, AE-C

COMPETENCIES

Upon completion of this chapter, the reader will be able to:

- Explain the anatomy, physiology, and functioning of the respiratory system of children.
- Describe the common assessment findings seen in children with a respiratory difficulty.
- Discuss measures to prevent respiratory alterations in children.
- Describe the pathophysiology, clinical manifestations, treatment, and nursing management of common acute respiratory alterations: nasopharyngitis, pharyngitis, tonsillitis, otitis media, croup, bronchiolitis, pneumonia, and sinusitis.
- Describe the pathophysiology, clinical manifestations, treatment, and nursing management of common chronic respiratory alterations: allergic rhinitis and asthma.
- Discuss the pathophysiology, clinical manifestations, treatment, and nursing management of less common respiratory alterations: cystic fibrosis, respiratory distress syndrome and tuberculosis.
- Discuss the manifestations and treatments of additional, rarely occurring respiratory alterations: foreign body aspiration and smoke inhalation injury.
- Discuss the most effective ways to prevent respiratory alterations in children.
- Successfully complete the games and activities in the online student StudyWARE.

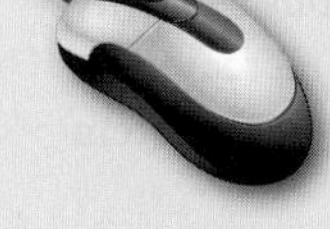

The primary function of the respiratory system is to facilitate gas exchange in the body. Several elements are necessary for this gas exchange to occur. Neurochemical controls, for example, regulate the rate, depth, and rhythm of breathing. These controls signal the respiratory muscles to contract and expand the thoracic cavity. This expansion creates negative pressure in the airways, which causes air to flow into the lungs. As the respiratory muscles relax, the chest falls, and air flows from the lungs. Oxygen is taken into the lungs during inhalation and carbon dioxide waste is removed from the body during exhalation. Another critical component of this gas exchange process is a patent airway. Other essential elements include sufficient alveolar-capillary diffusion, circulation, and gas transport (West, 2004).

A respiratory system dysfunction is a frequent health concern for individuals across the life span. Infants and young children are particularly vulnerable to respiratory related diseases because of specific age-related physical differences. The purpose of this chapter is to describe these physical differences, examine varying respiratory alterations that occur in infants and children, and explore the role of the nurse in optimizing the health of the pediatric population.

ANATOMY AND PHYSIOLOGY

Several developmental variations increase the pediatric population's risks for acquiring a respiratory system dysfunction. Small airways, fewer alveoli, and increased chest compliance are leading factors that predispose them to respiratory alterations. Figure 24-1 illustrates the pediatric respiratory tract.

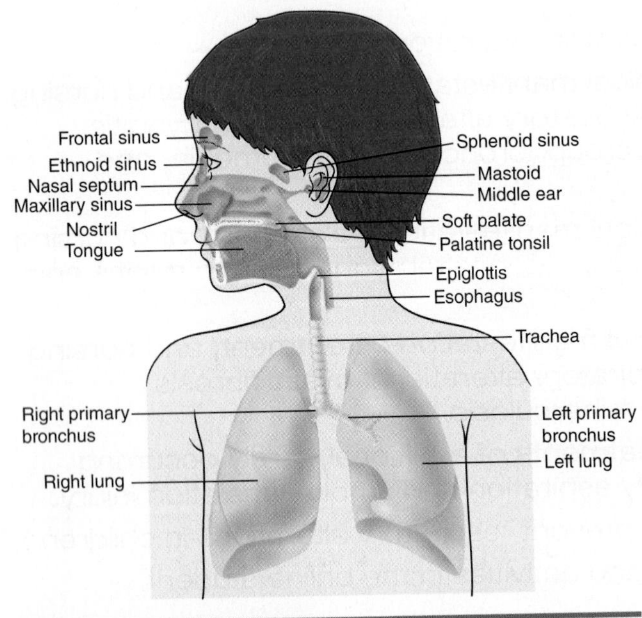

FIGURE 24-1 Pediatric Respiratory Tract. DELMAR CENGAGE LEARNING.

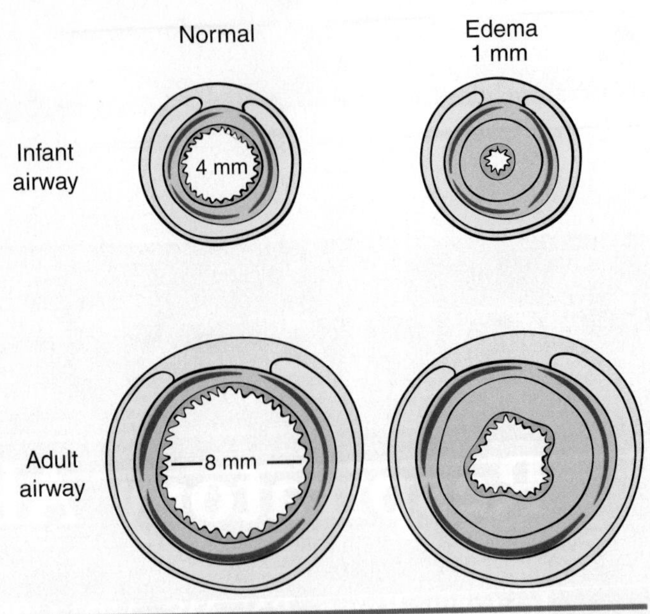

FIGURE 24-2 Comparison of Edema in Pediatric and Adult Airways. DELMAR CENGAGE LEARNING.

The size of an infant's trachea and lower airway are smaller than an adult's airway. Even small reductions in the lumen of an infant or young child's airway can significantly increase airway resistance and the work of breathing. Figure 24-2 provides a comparison of infant and adult airways that have become inflamed and edematous. The effect is similar when secretions collect in the airways. The negative impact of this structural difference decreases after early childhood as the lumen of the airway begins to increase in size.

The infant and young child's nose, nasopharynx, and pharynx are also smaller and more vulnerable to obstruction. Further, infants are typically nose breathers. This causes them to have difficulty breathing when their nasal passages become blocked by the edema and mucus associated with upper respiratory infections.

At birth the chest wall is soft and pliable and the infant's respiratory muscles are not fully developed. These factors lead to poor expansion of the chest, decreased lung volumes at the end of exhalation, and contribute to the respiratory distress infants experience with respiratory alteration. The pliable chest walls of infants in respiratory distress move inward instead of expanding. **Retractions** occur as the soft tissue surrounding the ribs and sternum move inward during inhalation. They are associated with increased respiratory effort and airway obstruction.

Other developmental factors may increase the pediatric population's risk for acquiring a respiratory alteration. Infants and young children have immature immune systems that make them more susceptible to a microorganism invasion. They also tend to be around other infants and children with respiratory infections. Further, hand-to-mouth activity characteristic of infants and young children may increase this population's opportunity for acquiring a respiratory system infection or injury.

Surfactant is made in the body of the fetus and present in high levels by 20 weeks' gestation, but does not reach the surface of the lungs until later. It can be found in amniotic fluid between 28 and 32 weeks' gestation. Preterm infants lack sufficient surfactant for effective lung functioning. Without adequate surfactant these infants are at high risk for developing respiratory distress syndrome and bronchopulmonary dysplasia. Treatment with exogenous surfactant therapy at birth effectively decreases the incidence of these respiratory alterations. Metabolic demands, and thus oxygen consumption, are greater in infants and young children than in adults. Additionally, infants and children have limited oxygen stores. For this reason, they tend to get hypoxic quickly and develop respiratory distress when their oxygen demand exceeds the supply.

THE CHILD WITH RESPIRATORY DIFFICULTY

Children with a respiratory alteration will demonstrate signs and symptoms that may be common to a variety of respiratory disease processes. Although specific conditions may have particular findings the nursing assessment should always include the following components:

Color: Children with respiratory problems may be pale or have cyanosis due to decreased oxygenation. Particular notice should be made of perioral cyanosis, a pale or bluish tinge around the lips and mouth.

Respiratory Effort: Observe the child's breathing. Is the child having difficulty breathing or exerting extra effort in breathing? Note if retractions or accessory muscles are used for breathing, or if nasal flaring is present.

Vital Signs: Observe the respiratory rate. A child with a respiratory problem often displays tachypnea. Is the heart rate elevated? Tachycardia will occur in response to decreased oxygenation, increased metabolic demand, infection or fever. Hyperthermia can indicate infection.

Auscultation of Lung Sounds: Is there good air flow in and out of all areas of the lungs? Are there any adventitious sounds? Wheezing? Crackles? Rhonchi? Are these sounds heard on inspiration and/or expiration? Are abnormal sounds only heard in one area of the lungs or are they scattered throughout the lung fields?

Assess respiratory effort by looking for retractions, and wheezing. Note frequency and quality of cough. Cough may be harsh, loose, dry, or barking. If the cough is productive and the child is old enough to expectorate sputum, describe its color and consistency. Also, is there nasal discharge or are the nasal passages blocked by mucus? Is the voice hoarse? Is there a sore throat? Observations need to be made of the entire oral cavity checking for redness, lesions, and the condition of the tonsils.

NURSING ALERT

Signs of Impending Respiratory Failure

Restlessness or anxiety, altered level of consciousness, **tachypnea**, tachycardia, diaphoresis, use of **accessory muscles** (neck, back, and abdomen), and retractions are signs of impending respiratory failure.

Children with some respiratory infections may have a fever, so their temperature should be checked. Some children may not be eating well when they have a respiratory problem so their feeding pattern needs to be assessed as well. In addition, some children experience vomiting and diarrhea when they have a respiratory problem.

Since parents and primary caregivers are highly involved when a child has a respiratory condition, they will be able to give a complete history of the child's illness. Be sure to ask about the immunization status of the child, since the lack of certain immunizations in a child with a respiratory problem may help diagnose a particular problem. Of special note should be the lack of DTaP (diphtheria-tetanus-pertussis) immunizations if a child has a severe cough (which could be pertussis or whooping cough) or the absence of an influenza vaccination history in a child with asthma or cystic fibrosis. Please refer to Chapter 15, "Infectious Diseases," for a complete discussion of immunizations for children.

Besides providing the history, caregivers also have common concerns. Mainly, the caregivers are usually quite anxious when a child has a respiratory problem. Nurses must be able to help the family cope with their child's illness. Box 24-1 summarizes the common symptoms of a child with a respiratory condition. For a complete discussion of respiratory assessment in children, see Chapter 14, "Pediatric Assessment."

CULTURAL CONSIDERATION

Respiratory Ailments

Children and families who have recently moved to the United States from other countries may be missing vaccinations and should be screened for potential communicable diseases. In addition, they may have been exposed to respiratory diseases in their homelands or during their travels. Nurses should assess all children and families for any respiratory symptoms so that they can be treated early in their disease.

BOX 24-1
COMMON SYMPTOMS OF RESPIRATORY PROBLEMS IN CHILDREN

- pale skin
- increased respiratory rate
- dyspnea
- stridor, wheezing, or crackles on auscultation
- fever
- cough
- nasal discharge or obstructed nasal passages
- pharyngitis
- anorexia
- vomiting or diarrhea
- anxiety or restlessness
- fatigue or lethargy

COMMON ACUTE RESPIRATORY ALTERATIONS

Pediatric respiratory alterations can be categorized as acute or chronic conditions. Common acute alterations include nasopharyngitis, pharyngitis, tonsillitis, otitis media, croup, bronchiolitis, and pneumonia. Common chronic alterations include allergic rhinitis and asthma and will be discussed in the next section.

NASOPHARYNGITIS (THE COMMON COLD)

Nasopharyngitis, also known as rhinosinusitis, is a frequently occurring pediatric respiratory alteration. Caused by an infectious agent, this respiratory condition is most prevalent in children in daycare and school, where children are in very close contact (National Institute of Allergy and Infectious Diseases [NIAID], 2007). The common cold is responsible for an estimated 70 million lost workdays each year in the US and an additional 140 million lost workdays due to caregivers staying home to take care of sick children (Kurugol, Bayram, & Atik, 2007).

Incidence and Etiology

Nasopharyngitis, one of the most frequently encountered complaints in ambulatory pediatric care, is almost always caused by a microorganism. Viruses are the etiologic agents most of the time, with rhinovirus being the most common. It is estimated that children have between six and ten colds per year, on average. Colds usually occur in the fall and winter months, as the viruses that cause colds survive best in nonhumid air (NIAID, 2007). Children have more upper respiratory illnesses than any other infection. As they get older, children get fewer colds per year. Adults average two to four colds each year (NIAID, 2007).

Pathophysiology

The nasopharynx is positioned behind the nasal cavities and is bordered by the soft palate and the skull. The infection causes an inflammation of the involved tissue. The inflammatory process is associated with tissue swelling and the formation of **exudate** (fluid, cells, or other substances released from the body). Nasal congestions caused by edema and secretions impede airflow through the nasal passages.

Clinical Manifestations

Manifestations of viral nasopharyngitis include nasal stuffiness, rhinitis, sneezing, nasal discharge, coughing, sore throat, fever, irritability, malaise, irritability, headache, and muscle aches (Kurugol et al., 2007). Infants may be unable to eat well and children may have poor appetites. Any child is also at risk for vomiting and diarrhea.

Diagnosis

Diagnosis of nasopharyngitis is based on client history and physical exam. The presence of associated manifestations leads to the diagnosis. Often times, a child's cold symptoms can resolve in 48–72 hours without the use of medications (Traynor, 2007).

Treatment

There is no specific treatment for viral nasopharyngitis. Management is supportive. Nonaspirin analgesics and antipyretics may be given to reduce fever and relieve discomfort. Saline nasal drops may be instilled every three to four hours, particularly before feeding infants, to relieve nasal congestion. Older children may find relief by gargling with a saline solution. Antihistamines tend to dry mucous membranes, so they are not used in the management of nasopharyngitis. Because colds are caused by viruses, antibiotics are not effective and are not indicated in the treatment of viral nasopharyngitis (Turkoski, 2007).

The use of over-the-counter cough and cold medications in young children is not recommended by the AAP (Turkoski, 2007). The Centers for Disease Control (CDC) reported that during 2004 and 2005, there were more than 1,500 children less than two years of age who presented to emergency departments for adverse effects associated with OTC cough and cold medications. Several sudden infant deaths were also reported related to these medications (CDC, 2007).

Nursing Management

Assessment The nursing assessment for a child with nasopharyngitis includes collecting information about the degree and duration of the child's signs and symptoms. Specifically, the nurse needs to know how well the individual has been drinking and eating and if the child has had a fever or cough. It is also important to note the amount and color of any nasal secretions and degree of discomfort the child has had. The physical examination includes assessing the character of nasal discharge, hydration status, and presence of any respiratory distress.

Nursing Diagnosis

1. *Ineffective airway clearance* related to inflammation of the nasopharynx.
2. *Deficient fluid volume* related to poor fluid intake caused by discomfort associated with nasal congestion, mouth breathing, and sore throat.
3. *Acute pain* related to inflammatory process and sore throat.

Outcome Identification

1. The child will have a patent airway and be free from signs of respiratory distress.
2. The child will consume fluids adequate to maintain balance as evidenced by moist mucous membranes and urine output of at least 1 mL/kg/hr.
3. The child will achieve an acceptable level of comfort when measured via a pain scale.

Planning and Implementation Children with viral nasopharyngitis are usually managed at home. The nurse's role related to these children's health care is to provide education and support to their caregivers. In addition to the treatments previously outlined, they may want to position the child with his or her head elevated. This position can ease the work of breathing. Nasal saline drops can be administered pre-feeds, and a bulb syringe can be used to suction secretions from infants' nares. Caregivers also need to ensure that their child consumes adequate fluids. Offering favorite beverages at regular intervals is a helpful strategy to ensure that hydration is not overlooked. Feeding young infants is particularly challenging because nasal congestion forces mouth breathing, which impedes the coordination of breathing, sucking, and swallowing. A calm approach and frequent rest periods during feedings are methods to maximize affected infants' fluid and nutrition intake.

Preventing the spread of the common cold is also an important health intervention. Facial tissues should be used when the child sneezes or when wiping away nasal secretions. Soiled tissues need to be discarded promptly to minimize the spread of the organisms to others in the home. Soiled handkerchiefs, if used, need to be contained until they can be washed. Regular hand washing following sneezing or nose blowing also deters the spread of the infection and is probably the most important preventive measure.

Evaluation Children with nasopharyngitis are typically managed in the home. Caregivers must have the requisite knowledge to care for the ill child in order for identified outcomes to be met.

Family Teaching

As discussed, caregivers and sometimes daycare providers are the primary care providers for children with nasopharyngitis. Providing comfort measures, ensuring adequate hydration, alerting the health care provider of complications, and preventing the spread of infection are the focus for family teaching.

TONSILLITIS AND PHARYNGITIS

Tonsillitis and pharyngitis are common comorbidities of childhood and are generally attributed to a viral infection. Bacterial infections, however, can also cause tonsillitis and pharyngitis and lead to serious health problems if left untreated.

Incidence and Etiology

Bacteria, primarily *group A beta-hemolytic streptococci* (GABHS), is the most common cause of bacterial pharyngitis and tonsillitis. Left untreated, GABHS can lead to complicated health issues for young children, including acquired heart disease. Bacterial sepsis caused by GABHS is an increasing cause of death in all age groups (Brook & Gober, 2008). Untreated streptococcal tonsillitis and pharyngitis infections may lead to health problems such as scarlet fever, otitis media, and **suppurative** (pus forming) infections of surrounding tissues. More serious complications of untreated streptococcal infections include acute glomerulonephritis, meningitis, and rheumatic fever (AAP Red Book, 2006).

Pathophysiology

Tonsils are lymphoid tissue located in the oropharynx that serve to protect the body from invading organisms. Figure 24-3 illustrates the location of tonsils in the pharyngeal cavity. Tonsillitis refers to an inflammation, and frequently an infection, of the palatine tonsils. Adenoiditis refers to inflammation or infection of the pharyngeal

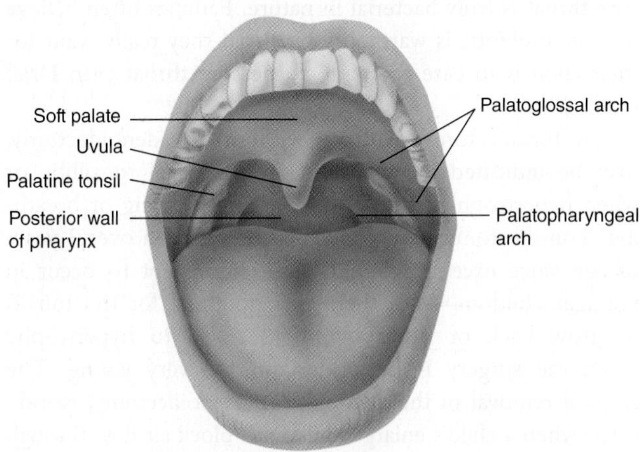

Figure 24-3 Tonsils are lymphoid tissue located in the pharyngeal cavity. DELMAR CENGAGE LEARNING.

tonsils, or adenoids. Children are prone to tonsillitis because they have a large amount of lymphoid tissue in the pharyngeal cavity, tend to have frequent upper respiratory tract infections, and are around other children who may be infected.

Clinical Manifestations

Manifestations of tonsillitis and pharyngitis include sore throat, difficulty swallowing, and fever. Nasal congestion that accompanies upper airway infections leads to mouth breathing and causes drying of the mucous membranes. This dryness further aggravates the pain associated with the tonsillitis and pharyngitis. Children with GABHS pharyngitis and tonsillitis may also experience a headache, abdominal pain, nausea, vomiting, and diarrhea. Inflamed tonsils and oropharynx, generally with exudate, will be evident with inspection. Cervical adenopathy (glandular enlargements in the neck) is also present (AAP Red Book, 2006).

Diagnosis

The diagnosis of tonsillitis and pharyngitis is based primarily on the child's symptoms and visual inspection of the throat. Throat cultures and rapid strep screening are used to determine etiologic agents. The rapid strep screening test became available in the 1980s and yields results within 5–10 minutes. The throat culture takes approximately 24–48 hours (Wright, Williams, & Ludeman, 2007).

Treatment

If a virus is the suspected cause of infection, the child is managed with supportive care. Warm saline gargles may be used to soothe the inflamed mucous membranes. Nonaspirin analgesics and antipyretics may be used to reduce pain and fever. If a bacterial source is identified as the etiologic agent, the child needs to be treated with an antibiotic such as penicillin or amoxicillin. If allergic to penicillin, the next drug of choice is erythromycin (AAP Red Book, 2006). It is very important to fully assess whether the cause of the sore throat is truly bacterial in nature. Families often believe that an antibiotic is warranted but what they really want for their child is to ease the pain of the sore throat (van Driel et al., 2006).

A tonsillectomy, with or without an adenoidectomy, may be indicated for recurrent streptococcal tonsillitis or when hypertrophied tonsils interfere with eating or breathing. Tonsillectomies are performed on children over 3 years of age since excessive blood loss is more apt to occur in younger children. Also, there is a potential for the tonsils to grow back or other lymphoid tissue to hypertrophy when the surgery is performed on the very young. The surgical removal of the adenoids, or adenoidectomy, is indicated when a child's enlarged adenoids block air flow through nasal passages. If a patient is a chronic carrier of Group A Strep, tonsillectomy may also be considered (AAP Red Book, 2006).

Nursing Management

Assessment

The nursing assessment for a child scheduled to have a tonsillectomy and adenoidectomy includes gathering information about the course of the child's illness and completing a physical exam. Clinical findings consistent with tonsillitis and pharyngitis include sore throat, difficulty swallowing, and fever. Postsurgical assessments include monitoring for bleeding and infection and assessing the child's pain level.

Nursing Diagnosis

1. *Risk for deficient fluid volume* related to decreased intake because of throat pain when swallowing.
2. *Acute pain* related to surgical excision of tonsils.
3. *Risk for injury: bleeding* related to surgical incision.

Outcome Identification

1. The child will have moist mucous membranes and elastic skin turgor.
2. The child will achieve an acceptable level of comfort and swallow without difficulty.
3. The child will be free from bleeding.

Planning and Implementation

As with other operative procedures, a complete history, physical, and baseline assessments should be obtained before a tonsillectomy or adenoidectomy is performed. Preoperative laboratory tests need to include clotting and bleeding times as the operative site is considerably vascular and prone to postoperative bleeding. Preoperative care also includes client and family education.

The nursing care following a tonsillectomy is centered on supportive care and ensuring client safety. Postoperatively, the child is positioned on the side to facilitate drainage of secretions. Once fully awakened, the child may sit up if so desired. The nurse reminds the child not to cough often or blow the nose, as this can disrupt an operative clot and cause bleeding. Secretions and emesis are examined for any sign of fresh bleeding. The family should be taught the difference between fresh and old blood. Old blood, dark-brown in color, is commonly in the mouth, nose, and emesis. Bright red or fresh blood suggests active bleeding and warrants further investigation. Although postoperative hemorrhage is uncommon, the health care provider is contacted if this is suspected.

> **NURSING ALERT**
>
> **Postoperative Caution**
>
> Frequent swallowing following tonsillectomy is the earliest manifestation of bleeding, as the child swallows more often because of trickling blood. The health care provider should be called immediately if bleeding is suspected.

Initially, cool noncarbonated, nonacidic liquids are encouraged. The liquids are soothing and help maintain hydration. Red and brown liquids are avoided as they interfere with assessment of bleeding. Straws are contraindicated because of the suction they require. A soft diet is indicated until the throat has healed. Healing of the operative site takes approximately three weeks. Cool humidification assists in moistening mucous membranes, which become dried during mouth breathing. Opioids are typically given in the early postoperative period in order to relieve the initial moderate to severe pain generally associated with the surgery. This intensity of pain generally decreases between 4–7 days. Acetaminophen is usually sufficient once the pain has diminished to a mild level.

Health care providers need to remember that children who are undermedicated are less likely to want to drink and eat. An ice collar may provide some pain relief. When fully alert, the child can be offered crushed ice or sips of water. Citrus juices are avoided since they cause discomfort to the operative site.

Evaluation The achievement of outcomes is dependent on the appropriate care by nurses and caregivers. Moist mucous membranes and elastic skin turgor indicate the child is adequately hydrated. Pain control is achieved when the level of comfort is such that swallowing occurs without difficulty and the child indicates that the level of comfort is acceptable. No postoperative bleeding is a critical outcome for these children because of the risk for hemorrhage following tonsillectomies. Evaluation of this outcome is made based on visual inspection of the operative site and the absence of frequent swallowing.

Family Teaching

Family teaching includes promoting adequate fluids and rest for the ill child, administering analgesics for discomfort and antipyretics for fever, and seeking medical attention if manifestations persist or signs of a bacterial infection are present. Preoperative education includes information related to the surgery and postoperative care. Discharge instructions include teaching the caregivers about the need for providing their child with appropriate fluids and diet, pain management, activity limitations, and potential complications of the postoperative period. A membrane that forms over the operative site during the first few hours after surgery begins to pull apart around 4–10 days. During this time the surgical site may hemorrhage. Caregivers and children need to be aware of this critical period and be ready to seek medical treatment as indicated.

For a patient with strep pharyngitis who does not undergo tonsillectomy, treatment is an oral antibiotic. The recommendation is to give penicillin, usually for a ten-day period. If the patient is allergic to penicillin products, erythromycin is the second antibiotic of choice. Care is also supportive, including acetaminophen for pain and fever along with rest and comfort measures (AAP Red Book, 2006).

OTITIS MEDIA

Incidence and Etiology

Otitis media accounts for millions of health care encounters every year. Acute otitis media (AOM) is the most common bacterial illness in children for which antibiotics are prescribed (Lieberthal et al., 2004). One estimate found that more than 30 million cases are reported in this country annually (Harrison, 2004). It is estimated that otitis media accounts for 20–40% of the pediatric office visits for children under the age of five years. Up to 90% of children will experience at least one episode of AOM in the first four years of life (Rosenfeld et al., 2004).

AOM is an infectious process most commonly caused by *Streptococcus pneumoniae, Haemophilus influenzae,* or *Moraxella catarrhalis,* although AOM can be caused by viruses and other bacterial pathogens. Most children with AOM will also have signs and symptoms of an upper respiratory infection. Associated clinical factors, other than upper respiratory infections, include allergic rhinitis, sinusitis, cleft palate, adenoidal hypertrophy, and immune deficiency. Environmental risk factors for AOM include passive smoke exposure, daycare attendance, and improper feeding techniques (bottle propping or sleeping with a bottle). Adherence to recommended immunizations and breastfeeding has been identified as preventive measures.

Pathophysiology

Children under the age of three years are especially vulnerable to OM as they have eustachian tubes that are wider, shorter, and straighter than those of older children and adults. Their eustachian tubes are also positioned horizontally. These anatomic differences allow microorganisms and nasopharyngeal secretions easy access into the middle ear. This invasion creates the right environment for inflammation and infection. The inflammatory process leads to an accumulation of exudate in the middle ear. This stagnant fluid impedes the middle ear's ability to transmit sound and creates an environment conducive to pathogen colonization. The fluid can also readily block the connection between the middle ear and the pharynx, interrupting the Eustachian tube's pressure equalizing function. Enlarged lymphoid tissue can further obstruct the flow of drainage from the middle ear. As the volume of fluid in the middle ear increases, the pressure rises. If unrelieved, this process can lead to a rupture of the tympanic membrane.

Clinical Manifestations

The primary symptoms of AOM are pain, fever, irritability and symptoms of an upper respiratory illness. Children with developed verbal skills can readily express their pain through oral communication. Nonverbal and preverbal children may express pain by tugging or pulling at their ears but this is an unreliable manifestation of AOM. All of the above symptoms except ear pain are nonspecific and can be part of any respiratory infection making the diagnosis of AOM difficult without clear physical findings. If the OM creates a conductive hearing impairment, the child may become inattentive to voices and other noises.

Diagnosis

A diagnosis of AOM is based on three criteria: rapid onset of illness, presence of fluid (effusion), and signs/symptoms of inflammation in the middle ear. The absence of any of these three criteria makes a clear diagnosis difficult. In addition, the tympanic membrane can be difficult to visualize in very young infants, uncooperative children or in children with impacted cerumen, which adds to the uncertainty in diagnosis (Lieberthal et al., 2004). Normally, the tympanic membrane (TM) is pearly gray with clearly visible bony landmarks and light reflex. Figure 24-4 demonstrates the middle ear landmarks. An otoscopic examination of a child with an AOM reveals a red and bulging TM. The short process and handle of the malleus are prominent and the light reflex is dull or absent. Purulent or serous fluid is visible behind the TM. Figure 24-5 shows a comparison of a normal tympanic membrane and AOM. Pneumatic otoscopic assessment of TM mobility reveals diminished movement with AOM and diminished or absent movement with chronic OM. In those instances where the tympanic membrane has ruptured a culture of ear fluid for antibiotic sensitivity testing can be done to guide antibiotic selection.

Treatment

The first option for treatment for an uncomplicated AOM in low-risk populations is a "watchful waiting" approach, observing for spontaneous resolution of symptoms without antibiotics (Spiro & Arnold, 2008; Lieberthal et al., 2004; Chao, Kunkow, Reyes, Licten, & Crain, 2008). Low-risk populations include children six months to two years of age without symptoms of severe illness and an uncertain diagnosis, and children over two years of age without severe disease or a certain diagnosis. In these situations it is prudent to instruct reliable caregivers to observe the child over a period of 48–72 hours while providing supportive symptomatic care with oral analgesics. A majority of children will have a decrease in symptoms and the infection will resolve with supportive care. Topical analgesic ear drops may be used although there is mixed evidence to support the use of this therapy (Bolt, Barnett, Babl, & Sharwood, 2008; Foxlee et al., 2006). There is no role for antihistamines and/or decongestants in the treatment of AOM (Griffen, Flynn, Bailey, & Schultz, 2006). In high-risk children, high-dose amoxicillin is the first-line antibiotic used to treat AOM. In cases where a child has severe symptoms (high fever or severe pain) or there is suspicion for antibiotic resistance high-dose

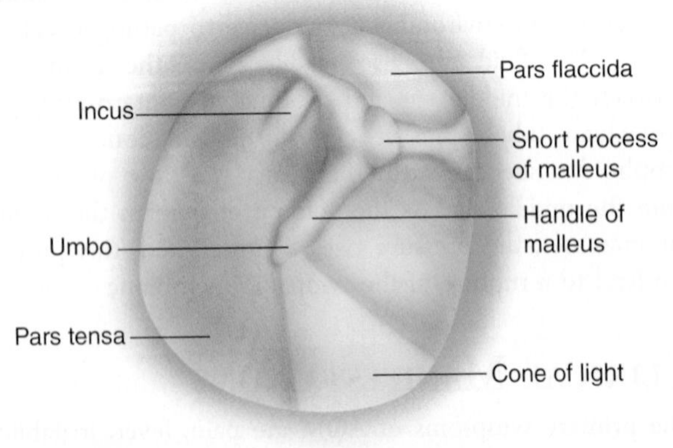

FIGURE 24-4 Middle Ear Landmarks. DELMAR CENGAGE LEARNING.

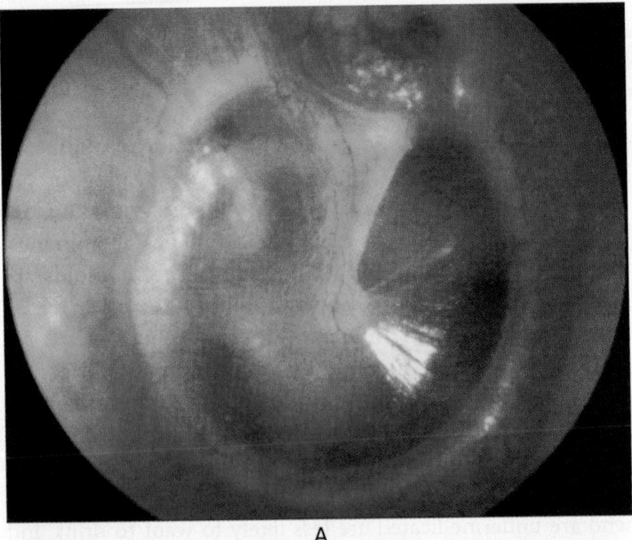

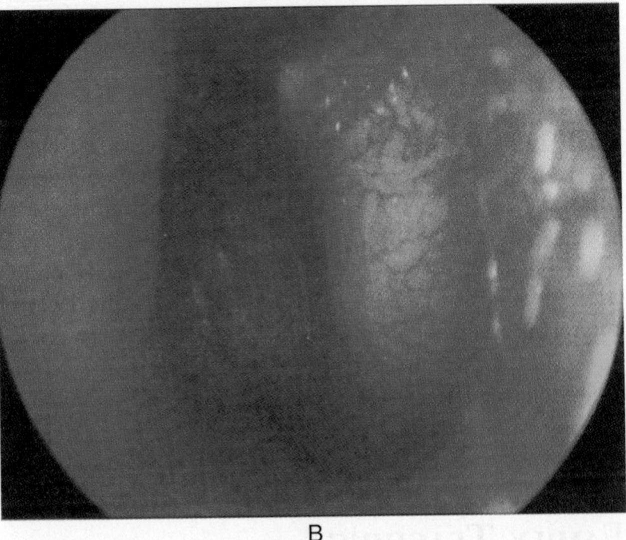

FIGURE 24-5 Comparison of (A) Normal Tympanic Membrane and (B) Acute Otitis Media. DELMAR CENGAGE LEARNING.

amoxicillin-clavulanate is prescribed. Other antibiotic choices include second and third generation cephalosporin, azithromycin, erythromycin, or sulfamethozaxole-trimethoprim which can also be used in the case of penicillin allergic patients or those with poor clinical response to the first line choices.

Most AOM begins to resolve within 2–3 days. However, the inflammation from an AOM may lead to the development of an otitis media with effusion (OME). Children less than two years of age with recurrent AOM are at greater risk to develop an OME. Effusions may take weeks to months to resolve. Antibiotics are not indicated during this resolution stage (Koopman et al., 2008).

The primary complication of OM is conductive hearing loss and related speech problems. Less common complications include abscess formation in the tissues adjacent to the middle ear, meningitis, and septicemia. Follow-up visits for children with AOM are scheduled 2–4 weeks post-treatment to evaluate the effectiveness of the antibiotic treatment and to determine if further treatment or testing is necessary. Follow-up visits should be earlier if complications arise.

A diagnosis of recurrent otitis media is made if a child has three or more episodes of AOM within a six-month period. Chronic OME treatment involves ongoing assessment and antibiotics with or without steroid treatment. Children with OME or recurrent AOM are often referred to an otolaryngologist for evaluation to see if myringotomy tube placement is warranted. **Tympanostomy** (surgical incision in the tympanic membrane for draining fluid) and myringotomy tube placement may be indicated if an episode of OME lasts for longer than 3–4 months or for recurrent AOM. Tympanostomy tubes allow for fluid drainage and middle ear ventilation, with resultant resolution of the effusion. The primary reason for treating children with chronic OME is to minimize the risks for hearing loss and related speech delays. Children with severe recurrent or chronic OM should also be followed by an audiologist for hearing evaluation.

Because myringotomy tubes create an opening between the external canal and middle ear, care should be taken to minimize the amount of water that accidentally enters the ear as long as the tubes are in place. Ear plugs are recommended when children with PE tubes swim or bathe.

Nursing Management

Assessment

The nursing assessment of OM begins by obtaining an accurate history from the primary caregiver regarding the child's signs and symptoms and their frequency and duration. It is important to assess for pain, fever, other respiratory symptoms as well as interventions tried to date. It is also important to ask if the child has had past ear infections, other medical conditions, and if they are up-to date with recommended immunizations. Identifying environmental risk factors such as day-care attendance, environmental tobacco smoke exposure, or bottle propping is also important. An otoscopic examination provides the definitive assessment data that leads to the diagnosis of OM.

Nursing Diagnosis

The nursing diagnoses for a child with OM include:

1. *Acute pain* related to middle ear inflammation and pressure on the eardrum.
2. *Infection* related to presence of infective organisms (AOM).
3. *Potential for delayed growth and development* related to hearing impairment.
4. *Potential for deficient fluid volume* related to decreased fluid intake and fever.

Outcome Identification

1. The child will be free from pain.
2. The child will be afebrile.
3. The child will maintain hearing function and normal speech development.
4. The child will have moist mucous membranes and elastic turgor.

Planning and Implementation

An important focus of nursing care for a child with OM is on family education. The ultimate goal of the education is for the child to meet identified outcomes. Alleviating the pain associated with OM is a primary concern for caregivers. Acetaminophen or ibuprofen are commonly used medications that reduce children's pain. Topical analgesic drops may be helpful in alleviating ear pain as well. Elevating the head and positioning children on the unaffected side may also help minimize pain. Individuals in pain from an OM are frequently uninterested in eating or drinking. Implementing pain relief measures promotes a child's willingness to drink and helps ensure adequate hydration, as well as comfort. Offering children their favorite liquids at regular intervals also encourages them to consume adequate fluids.

The importance of administering antibiotics as prescribed is a critical factor in the management of AOM. This includes completing the full course of antibiotics even if the OM symptoms resolve. The child's health care provider needs to be contacted if the OM symptoms have not lessened within the first 24–48 hours after initiation of an antibiotic or if manifestations of complications exist. Antipyretics may be used to reduce the child's fever. Children with chronic or recurring OM need to be observed for signs of impaired hearing. Hearing tests are suggested if a deficit is suspected. These children also need regular follow-up visits in order to evaluate the resolution of their OM.

Family Teaching

An assessment of caregivers' understanding about the prevention and management of OM is a fundamental component of family education. They need to recognize the benefits of controlling factors that increase their child's risk for developing an OM. For example, children exposed to secondhand smoke are at an increased risk for developing OM. Tobacco smoke irritates the eustachian tube. This irritation can cause an inflammatory process and resultant OM. Feeding practices also influence a child's risk for developing

EVIDENCE-BASED PRACTICE

Sharing Knowledge with Parents on the Management of Ear Pain in their Child

CLINICAL PROBLEM

Can providing anticipatory guidance to parents on the home management of ear pain reduce the need for acute care visits for mild ear complaints?

BEST CLINICAL PRACTICE

Acute care visits for parental concern about potential ear infections and ear pain in young children account for millions of health care encounters. Yet many mild ear infections and complaints of ear pain will resolve spontaneously regardless of medical intervention. It has been found that the simple and brief, yet effective nursing intervention of providing good anticipatory guidance on the management of ear pain to parents of toddlers can reduce unnecessary visits to the emergency department or urgent care for ear complaints. Parents/caregivers were provided with information that focused on three goals: how to identify ear pain, how to relieve ear pain (using acetaminophen, ibuprofen, and analgesic ear drops), and how to recognize symptoms of a serious illness requiring urgent medical attention. After this intervention, ED visits for ear pain decreased by 80%, urgent care visits by 40%, and primary care visits by 28%.

IMPLICATIONS FOR NURSING

Nurses are in a key role to provide education to empower parents and caregivers to triage a generally benign condition at home, reducing unnecessary burden on the health care system and both stress and cost to families.

Reference: McWilliams, D. B., Jacobson, R. M., Van Houten, H. K., Naessens, J. M., Ytterberg, K. L., & Berman, S. (2008). A program of anticipatory guidance for the prevention of emergency department visits for ear pain. *Archives of Pediatric and Adolescent Medicine, 162*(2), 151–156.

an OM. Horizontal positioning during bottle feedings allows formula to trickle into the eustachian tube, which can act as an irritant or block the tube. Either effect can lead to OM. Breastfeeding is beneficial because it provides maternal immune protection and facilitates a more upright feeding position.

CROUP

Croup is a broad term commonly used to describe several croup-like illnesses affecting infants and children. These are similarly characterized by a croupy or "barking" cough, inspiratory **stridor** and hoarseness (from swelling around the larynx), and some degree of respiratory distress. Croup is classified as spasmodic croup, acute laryngotracheitis, laryngotracheobronchitis, laryngotracheobronchopneumonitis (including bacterial tracheitis), and rarely laryngeal diphtheria. The majority of croup in children represents spasmodic croup and acute laryngotracheitis, and the term croup will be used synonymously with these illnesses for the purposes of this text (Cherry, 2008).

Incidence and Etiology

Croup usually occurs in children under 7 years of age, and most predominately between the ages of 6 and 36 months. It occurs more commonly in boys (Cherry, 2008). The primary etiologic pathogen is the parainfluenza virus, although other viral etiologies can cause croup including influenza A and B, respiratory syncytial virus, adenovirus and rhinovirus. Croup is diagnosed most commonly in late autumn (Cherry, 2008). Most children with croup are managed in the home.

Pathophysiology

The primary symptoms of croup result from swelling in the trachea just below the vocal cords or in the subglottic region, either with or without inflammation, secretions, and muscle spasms. Varying degrees of airway obstruction can occur because of the combined factors associated with the inflammatory process and the narrow lumen of a child's airway. Additionally, the glottis has a tendency to collapse during inspiration in response to edema and muscle spasms. This further obstructs the airway. The obstruction creates turbulence during inspiration causing the characteristic inspiratory

NURSING ALERT

Acute Epiglottitis Is a Life-Threatening Bacterial Infection

Acute epiglottitis, sometimes confused with croup, is a life-threatening bacterial infection that can lead to complete airway obstruction. Classic manifestations include respiratory distress, fever, sore throat, dysphagia, drooling (from edema or pain), agitation, and lethargy. The child prefers to sit upright and lean forward, supported by the arms. The chin is thrust out and the mouth is open to attain the best airway possible. Affected children generally have no spontaneous cough. ***Examination of the throat by depressing the tongue is contraindicated because it has the rare possibility of causing complete airway obstruction.*** Children with epiglottitis are managed with antibiotics, fluids, and supportive care. Necessary equipment should be on hand in the event that a child's condition progresses to the point of requiring an emergency tracheotomy. The incidence of epiglottitis has been decreased with the recommendation for vaccination with the HIB vaccine.

stridor associated with croup. Other signs of respiratory distress occur as the child works to inhale sufficient oxygen.

Clinical Manifestations

Manifestations of croup include a hoarse or "barking" cough, often sudden in onset and most often at night. The child can also have accompanying symptoms of an upper respiratory viral infection including nasal drainage, sore throat, and fever. Inspiratory stridor is a classic feature associated with croup. Depending on the severity of the airway obstruction, stridor may be audible with inspiration and expiration without the aid of a stethoscope. Retractions of the soft tissues of the neck, intercostal muscles, and sternum also may be present. Children can be classified as having mild, moderate, severe, or life-threatening croup, based on the degree of symptoms. While most children are not seriously ill, if untreated airway edema and the increased work of breathing can cause energy stores to become depleted and respiratory muscles to become fatigued. Endotracheal intubation and mechanical ventilation are indicated in the rare instance of impending respiratory failure.

Diagnosis

Croup is a clinical diagnosis based on a child's history and physical examination findings. Additional evaluations including a complete blood count, airway and chest radiographs can help distinguish between spasmodic croup, acute laryngotracheitis, and more serious illnesses like laryngotracheobronchitis or laryngotracheobronchopneumonitis.

Treatment

The mainstay of treatment for croup is systemic steroids given to reduce airway edema and inflammation. The current recommendation is for a single dose of dexamethasone (0.6 mg per kilogram of body weight) given orally or intramuscularly (Fifoot & Ting, 2007; Cherry, 2008). Nebulized epinephrine, a short acting bronchodilator is added in more severe cases to reduce airway inflammation (Bjornson & Johnson, 2008; Cherry, 2008). In addition, nursing care should focus on the following supportive care measures as needed:

1. Oxygen supplementation in children who are hypoxic (O_2 saturation less then 93%)
2. Assistance in maintaining hydration by offering oral liquids of the child's choosing in small but frequent amounts
3. Management of fever with the administration of antipyretics as ordered
4. Reduction of anxiety by allowing the child to assume a position of comfort (i.e., sitting on a parents lap)

Humidified air, once thought to be beneficial, has been demonstrated in several studies to lack any added treatment benefit (Carter, 2006; Moore & Little, 2007) although anecdotal parental reports repeatedly testify to the benefits of brief exposure to cool night air or cool mist showers in the home.

> **NURSING TIP**
>
> **Helping the Child to Drink the Needed Amount of Fluid**
>
> For many children, the amount of fluid necessary to loosen secretions seems overwhelming. The nurse can assist the child to reach the desired goal by offering a medicine cup full of liquid and then charting the data on a tracking board in her or his room. The intervention can be introduced as a game with the child ever trying to exceed the previous record. Stickers or other "prizes" may be awarded as records are broken.

BRONCHIOLITIS AND RESPIRATORY SYNCYTIAL VIRUS (RSV)

Bronchiolitis is an acute, typically viral, infection of the bronchioles. Occurring most often in young children, the infection causes inflammation in the bronchioles. **Wheezing** is a classic manifestation of bronchiolitis and is caused by airway obstruction from edema and secretions. Respiratory syncytial virus (RSV) is the most common cause of bronchiolitis and pneumonia in children less than a year of age (Robinson, 2008). Other viruses which can commonly cause bronchiolitis are influenza, parainfluenza, rhinoviruses, and adenoviruses (Smyth & Openshaw, 2006).

Incidence and Etiology

Bronchiolitis is an acute respiratory infection of the lower tract. It is commonly found to affect children less than two years of age. The peak incidence is typically at 6 months of age. (Sung et al., 2008). The most common cause of bronchiolitis is RSV. RSV is found to be the cause of bronchiolitis in approximately 75% of cases, with peak occurrence in the winter months from November to March (Scottish Intercollegiate Guidelines Network [SIGN], 2006). There are a few major factors that increase the risk of being infected with RSV. These include being born within six months prior to the onset of RSV season, being one of a multiple birth, not being breastfed, having siblings who attend school, attending daycare, exposure to tobacco smoke, and maternal education of grade 12 or less (Checchia, 2008).

Pathophysiology

The inflammation created by the infectious process leads to airway edema and the accumulation of mucous and cellular debris. The event that causes the edema is the infection of the epithelial cells in the lower respiratory tract (Smyth & Openshaw, 2006). These effects result in a narrowing or occlusion of the bronchioles. The occlusion causes air trapping, which leads to hyperinflation of some alveoli and **atelectasis** (collapse of lung tissue) in others.

Clinical Manifestations

Initially, children with bronchiolitis exhibit symptoms of an acute upper respiratory illness (URI) such as rhinorrhea, sneezing, decreased appetite, a low-grade fever, and coughing. After several days the symptoms worsen. Characteristic wheezing and tachypnea become apparent. Other manifestations include poor feeding, nasal flaring, retractions, wheezing, crackles, prolonged expiratory phase, and intermittent cyanosis. Complications are most likely to occur in children who have an underlying condition, including prematurity, chronic heart disease, or chronic lung disease (NIAID, 2008).

Diagnosis

The physical examination and medical history are the main diagnostic tools for bronchiolitis. The white blood cell count is typically normal. Chest films of children with bronchiolitis typically show patchy atelectasis and hyperinflation. Nasopharyngeal secretions may be obtained for culture or antigen assay to determine the etiologic agent. Most studies have shown that rapid antigen detection tests have an overall sensitivity of 80–90% (Smyth & Openshaw, 2006).

Treatment

The treatment of bronchiolitis is dependent upon the severity of the symptoms. The majority of children with bronchiolitis are managed in the home, but a significant number are hospitalized for supportive care (SIGN, 2006). The decision to admit a patient typically occurs in the emergency department (Smyth & Openshaw, 2006). Home management includes promoting rest, ensuring adequate fluid intake, and managing the child's fever and discomfort. Children who demonstrate signs of respiratory distress or who become dehydrated require hospitalization. Monitoring in the hospital may include measuring oxygen saturation, assessing hydration status, and observing work of breathing. Treatment instituted in the hospital setting generally includes humidified oxygen, suctioning, and intravenous fluids. Intubation and mechanical ventilation is indicated for children in respiratory failure (AAP Red Book, 2006).

Ribavirin (Virazole), the only specific therapy for RSV bronchiolitis, is an aerosol antiviral medication reserved for severely ill infants and children with underlying chronic conditions. The drug is restricted to this population for several reasons. The medication is extremely costly. It is also potentially quite toxic to exposed health care professionals, and the results of its effectiveness in clinical trials have led to controversy about the use of this drug. The decision to use this medication should be made on a case-by-case basis by the care provider (AAP Red Book, 2006).

One drug is currently available for prevention of RSV. It goes by the name palivizumab (Synagis). Synagis is a monoclonal antibody to treat RSV and is indicated for children at high risk for developing severe complications with RSV bronchiolitis. These children would include those born prematurely (especially prior to 32 weeks' gestation) and those with history of chronic lung disease (especially those with pulmonary hypertension). Synagis is administered monthly as an IM injection. The first dose is given prior to initiation of the RSV season with following doses administered monthly throughout the season.

REFLECTIVE THINKING

Parenting an Infant with an Upper Respiratory Infection

Upper airway viral infections are common in pediatric clients. These infections are of particular concern when they occur in infants. Imagine being a new mom of a 1-month-old with its first cold. What might you be thinking or worried about? What questions would you have? What information do you think you would need or want? How would you want your nurse to respond?

Nursing Management

Assessment

Ongoing and thorough respiratory system assessment, including oxygen saturation monitoring, is critical for children with bronchiolitis. Vigilant observation for these children allows for early recognition and treatment of increasing respiratory distress. Early intervention is important in minimizing the child's risk for developing respiratory failure.

Nursing Diagnosis

1. *Ineffective airway clearance* related to air trapping and increased mucus production.
2. *Deficient fluid volume* related to poor fluid intake and fever.
3. *Deficient knowledge (caregivers)* related to unfamiliarity with disease and its management.

Outcome Identification

1. The child will have clear lung sounds.
2. The child will have moist mucous membranes and a urine output of at least 1 mL/kg/hr.
3. The caregivers will verbalize an understanding of the disease and its management.

Planning and Implementation

Nursing care of the child managed in the home is focused on family teaching. In the acute care setting nursing care is focused on promoting adequate ventilation and fluid balance. Effective airway clearance is facilitated through nasopharyngeal suctioning with either a suction catheter or bulb syringe. Supplemental oxygen is administered through a nasal cannula. An oxygen hood may be used for young infants. Other strategies that foster adequate ventilation include raising the head of the bed, consolidating care, and encouraging caregiver involvement in the child's care. Raising the head of the bed allows for improved chest expansion, consolidating care provides the child with periods of rest, and caregiver presence reduces stress and the child's work of breathing.

Intravenous fluids are administered until the child can drink an adequate amount of oral fluids. While ill, a large portion of the child's energy is going towards his or her increased respiratory effort. Until the breathing is easier, IV fluids keep the child hydrated. Antipyretics may be ordered to reduce fever. Nursing management also involves ensuring that ordered nebulized pulmonary medications and chest physiotherapy have been implemented. Another most important aspect of care of children with RSV bronchiolitis is consistent hand washing, the most effective means of preventing the spread in health care facilities.

Evaluation The evaluation of the outcomes is a critical step in determining if the plan of care was effective in meeting the child's and family's needs. Visually looking at the child's respiratory effort is a large portion of the exam, assessing for tachypnea, nasal flaring, grunting, and retracting. Clear lung sounds is a primary criteria for evaluating the resolution of ineffective airway clearance. Moist mucous membranes and adequate urine output are measures of adequate fluid intake. Children in respiratory distress and those with fever are at risk for becoming fluid depleted. Finally, caregiver understanding of bronchiolitis and its management is a necessary step in their ability to provide appropriate care for their ill child.

Family Teaching

The nurse needs to provide information necessary for caregivers to understand their child's disease and the treatment plan. Specific information is dependent on the severity of the symptoms and whether the child is managed at home or in the hospital. Caregivers of children cared for at home are taught to alert the health care provider if signs of respiratory distress occur or if the child becomes dehydrated. Beyond being necessary for normal body functioning, fluids help liquefy thick airway secretions. Caregivers also need to know how to use a bulb syringe and to be advised of hygiene to prevent the spread of germs, as RSV is highly contagious.

PNEUMONIA

Pneumonia is an acute inflammation of the pulmonary **parenchyma** (the functional tissue of an organ as distinguished from supporting or connective tissue) associated with alveolar consolidation. Pneumonia can appear as a primary disease or a complication of another dysfunction.

Incidence and Etiology

Pneumonia affects children of all ages and continues to be a significant cause of childhood disease, with an even more significant contribution to mortality in underdeveloped countries (Barson, 2009). Most pneumonia in children occurs as community acquired pneumonia (CAP) and will be the focus of this text. CAP is defined as a pneumonia occurring in a previously healthy child with no underlying contributing disorder or disease, outside of the hospital setting. Less commonly occurring etiologies of pneumonia arise from aspiration disorders, neuromuscular disease, exposure to hospital acquired pathogens, or immune deficiencies.

S. pneumoniae is the most common pathogen in CAP across age groups, but other bacterial and viral pathogens can be the cause of pneumonia as well (Hale & Issacs, 2006). Certain pathogens are more common in specific age groups. In infants and preschool children, viral pathogens are more likely to be the cause of CAP and occur with greater frequency during the fall, winter, and spring, with RSV being the most common viral pathogen. In older children, bacterial causes are most likely the cause of CAP with more common sources being *S. pneumoniae, Chlamydia pneumoniae,* and *mycoplasma pneumoniae* in this age group.

Pathophysiology

The body has many defense mechanisms in place to protect individuals against pneumonia. These include the cough reflex, normal mucociliary action, phagocytosis by alveolar macrophages, as well as the inflammatory and immune response. In pneumonia a pathogen manages to invade a susceptible individual and releases toxins that stimulate secondary and tertiary defense mechanisms. The toxins and by-products of the body's defenses damage pulmonary mucous membranes and cause the accumulation of debris and exudate in the airways. These effects lead to **ventilation-perfusion ratio** (the ratio of alveolar ventilation to capillary perfusion) abnormalities. Pneumonia is frequently classified as lobar, interstitial, or bronchial (Brashers, 2004). Lobar pneumonia involves a major portion of one or more lobes of a lung. Interstitial pneumonia includes the alveolar walls and peribronchial and interlobular tissues. Bronchial pneumonia is more diffuse and involves the bronchi and lung fields.

Clinical Manifestations

Common manifestations of pneumonia include fever, hypoxia, and varying degrees of respiratory distress: tachypnea, cough, crackles, decreased breath sounds and increased work of breathing (Ostapchuk, Roberts, & Haddy, 2004). Pneumonia of bacterial etiology is more likely in children with a rapid onset of symptoms, fever >38.5°C (101.3°F), tachypnea, and retractions (Chetty & Thomson, 2007).

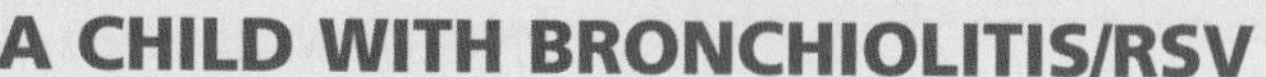

CASE STUDY / CARE PLAN

A CHILD WITH BRONCHIOLITIS/RSV

Madison is a 6-month-old little girl brought into the ED by her parents. She had been hospitalized in the NICU at birth for being born approximately eight weeks premature. She was intubated and ventilated for about five days, then received supplemental oxygen via nasal cannula for about one week and quickly improved. She was discharged home on room air. It is now the beginning of January when she is brought to the ED. Her parents are worried because they notice that she is breathing faster than normal and "some of her skin is pulling between her ribs when she breathes." She has not been taking her bottles well, has been irritable, and her diapers are not as wet as usual. She has had a cough for three days and some nasal congestion, as well. In the ED, her respiratory rate is 64 breaths per minute and she has some nasal flaring and subcostal retractions. Some circumoral cyanosis is noted and her SaO_2 is 92% on room air, with a heart rate of 160 and temp of 101° F.

NURSING CARE PLAN

ASSESSMENT

It is important when evaluating Madison to keep in mind the "ABC's" – airway, breathing, and cardiovascular. Madison's airway is patent but it is important to keep her as clear of secretions as possible. Her breathing is labored with a low oxygen saturation level, retractions, nasal flaring, and cyanosis. She is irritable, given her increased work of breathing, and likely dehydrated as all of her energy is going towards breathing, not eating nor drinking. With the help of the history from her parents, and observations by assessing her, better care can be taken to treat Madison appropriately.

NURSING DIAGNOSIS 1

Ineffective breathing pattern related to inflammation and congestion.

EXPECTED OUTCOMES

1. Respiratory rate will be within normal limits.
2. Madison will be breathing comfortably, with unlabored breaths and no retractions.
3. Madison's color will return to baseline and irritability will decrease.

NOC: Respiratory Status: Airway Patency

NIC: Airway Management

INTERVENTIONS/*RATIONALES*

1. Administer supplemental oxygen and humidity as ordered. *To relieve hypoxia, decrease distress, and keep airways from drying out; include humidity.*
2. Position Madison upright *to allow for maximum ventilation and lung expansion.*
3. Suction nasal and oral secretions as needed *to maintain a patent airway.*
4. Obtain nasal cultures, as ordered, to rule out RSV and influenza *in order to treat Madison as appropriately as possible.*
5. Administer nebulized or systemic corticosteroids as ordered *to help decrease inflammation in her airway.*
6. Have ER equipment close *in case intubation is necessary.*
7. Provide supportive environment *to decrease stress and create calming atmosphere.*

(Continues)

CASE STUDY / CARE PLAN (Continued)

EVALUATION

We want Madison to have a clear airway, decreased inflammation of her airway and adequate oxygenation and ventilation. As we implement our interventions, Madison should have decreased respiratory distress, more comfortable breathing, clear lung sounds, no retractions, and decreased irritability and anxiety.

NURSING DIAGNOSIS 2

Dehydration related to poor fluid intake and fluid loss from increased work of breathing.

EXPECTED OUTCOMES

1. Madison's respiratory distress will improve to the point where she will be able to take PO fluids again.
2. Until Madison can take PO fluids, she will be hydrated with IV fluids.
3. Madison will prove to be hydrated by producing urine at approximately 1–2mg/kg/hr.

NOC: Fluid Balance/Hydration

NIC: Fluid Resuscitation

INTERVENTIONS/*RATIONALES*

1. Administer and monitor IV fluids as ordered *to increase hydration status while in respiratory distress and unable to take PO fluids. Also, there is increased risk of aspiration with PO intake while in respiratory distress.*
2. Assess hydration status by documenting and watching intake and output, assessing mucous membranes, skin turgor, etc. *This can allow you to know whether methods to rehydrate have been effective.*
3. Once respiratory rate is decreased and respiratory failure is no longer a major risk, allow Madison to do trials of PO feeds. *Until Madison is able to feed normally, she cannot return home.*

EVALUATION

Madison will have moist mucous membranes, normal skin turgor, and decreased respiratory effort, which will allow her to take PO fluids willingly and safely. Urine output will return to baseline.

NURSING DIAGNOSIS 3

Fear/anxiety related to child's illness, increased respiratory effort, and fearing long hospitalization once again.

EXPECTED OUTCOMES

1. Parents will be less anxious after being educated on Madison's illness and reassured as she improves in the hospital.
2. Parents will be educated on how Madison's history of prematurity and ventilation as a newborn may put her at risk for episodes such as these.
3. Madison's parents' decreased anxiety will allow them to care for and comfort Madison, leading to her relaxation.

NOC: Anxiety

NIC: Anxiety Reduction

INTERVENTIONS/*RATIONALES*

1. Attempt to explain to parents the rationale and need for each procedure prior to doing it. *Fear of the unknown causes nervousness. The parents will have a better, more relaxed outlook if they know why procedures are being done.*

(Continues)

CASE STUDY / CARE PLAN (Continued)

2. Encourage parents to participate in Madison's care and remind them that she will sense their relaxation. Give parents a break as needed. *Participation will allow parents to become confident and truly involved in Madison's care and will comfort her, as well.*
3. Remind parents to bring Madison's favorite blankets or toys from home, *which will make them all feel more comfortable while in the hospital and add security to a foreign environment.*

EVALUATION

Madison will have decreased respiratory distress. She will have increased feeding and her parents will see her improving and feel more comfortable caring for her. Parents will be able to explain bronchiolitis and why treatment was needed. She will be taking good PO and not need supplemental oxygen prior to discharge.

DIAGNOSIS

The diagnosis of pneumonia is based on history, physical findings and, in most cases, chest radiographs (CXR). The CXR is helpful in determining the location and extent of disease and can identify complicating factors (pleural effusion, recurrence of disease in one area of the lung). Sputum cultures for bacteria are rarely used in the workup and diagnosis of pneumonia (Hale & Issacs, 2006). Viral cultures for RSV and influenza can be helpful in distinguishing between pneumonia of viral or bacterial etiology; however the diagnosis of a viral illness does not exclude a concurrent bacterial infection. The history should always include a careful review of any underlying conditions (pulmonary, cardiac, neuromuscular, or immune disease), possible foreign body aspiration or recent choking episodes, risk factors (environmental tobacco smoke exposure, daycare attendance, known sick contacts), immunization status, and other systemic symptoms (poor feeding, lethargy, gastrointestinal symptoms). The physical examination should include an assessment of vital signs, oxygen saturation, lung exam for adventitious lung sounds, respiratory signs (tachypnea, grunting, retractions, and nasal flaring), hydration, and overall well being.

TREATMENT

Treatment for CAP is based on the child's age and clinical symptoms. Antibiotics therapy should be initiated promptly in all children suspected of having bacterial pneumonia. The majority of children with CAP can be treated at home. However, any infant under 3 weeks of age or under 3 months of age with fever should be hospitalized for inpatient initiation of treatment. In addition, hospitalization should be considered in older children with any hypoxia or significant increase in the work of breathing.

NURSING MANAGEMENT

Assessment As with other respiratory alterations, a thorough respiratory assessment is a critical step in the

BOX 24-2
REVIEW OF THE VARIOUS TYPES OF ISOLATION

Standard Precautions

Used to prevent transmission of infection through contact with body fluids, skin openings, or mucous membranes.

Recommended for Standard Precautions:

1. hand hygiene
2. gloves
3. face mask/shield when risk of splashing of body fluids exists
4. gown

Transmission-Based Precautions – Airborne, Droplet, and Contact

When patients have an increased risk of spreading infectious agents

Recommended for Airborne Precautions:

1. single patient room, if possible
2. negative air-pressure ventilation, if possible
3. if TB is diagnosed or suspected, proper respiratory protective devices must be worn.

Recommended for Droplet Precautions:

1. single patient room, if possible
2. mask

Recommended for Contact Precautions:

1. single patient room, if possible
2. gloves
3. hand hygiene after gloves are removed
4. gowns for entrance into patient room, to be removed prior to exiting room.

nursing process. This includes monitoring for manifestations of pneumonia and signs that suggest increasing respiratory distress. Assessing for fever, pain, and hydration are also important when caring for children with pneumonia.

Nursing Diagnosis

1. *Impaired gas exchange* related to ventilation/perfusion abnormalities caused by pulmonary infection.
2. *Ineffective airway clearance* related to edema and exudate.
3. *Ineffective breathing pattern* related to an inflammatory infection of the lower airway.

Outcome Identification

1. The client will be well oxygenated with a normal heart and respiratory rate.
2. The client will have clear lung fields with good aeration throughout all lung fields.
3. The client will demonstrate a normal breathing pattern as evidenced by the absence of tachypnea, retractions, cough, wheezing, grunting, and nasal flaring.

Planning and Implementation The nursing care for children with pneumonia depends upon the severity of the symptoms and the etiologic agent. Supportive care should focus on maintaining adequate oxygenation with oxygen and airway clearance as prescribed, maintaining hydration with IV and/or oral fluids and reducing fever with antipyretics. If the pneumonia is thought to be caused by a bacterial agent, antibiotics are administered as prescribed. Additionally, pain assessment is an important nursing intervention in the child experiencing pleuritic pain with coughing or deep breathing. In an attempt to minimize pain, children with pneumonia may take shallow breaths and resist coughing. For these children, pain medications not only promote comfort, they also may facilitate deep breathing and airway clearance.

Evaluation As the pneumonia resolves, the child's respiratory assessment will also normalize and illness symptoms (fever, cough) will abate. CXR findings may not normalize for weeks to months; routine follow-up chest radiographs are not indicated in uncomplicated CAP.

Family Teaching

Most children with pneumonia are managed at home, and it is important that the nurse provide adequate instructions and teaching regarding the child's care. Caregivers should be educated regarding the need for good hydration and rest and taught the signs or symptoms that might require reevaluation. Offering small amounts of liquids more frequently can help promote hydration in the child reluctant to drink or eat. If the child is prescribed an antibiotic, the nurse needs to instruct the caregivers about the child's antibiotic, its administration, and the importance of completing the entire prescription even if symptoms have resolved. If symptoms are worsening, families should know who and when to call for additional evaluation and intervention. Finally it is important to stress that the child's energy level will be reduced until completely recovered.

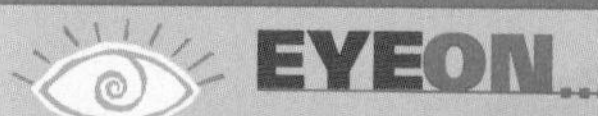

Herbal Remedies

Individuals in various cultures believe that diseases or conditions result from a cold or hot or wet or dry imbalance in the fluids of the body. They believe that the remedy for disease lies in restoring balance. Pneumonia, for example, is considered a "cold" disease that should be managed with "hot" treatments. Other respiratory illnesses also fall into this "cold" category. Herbal remedies may be used to achieve balance in the body. These remedies are used in different forms such as a poultice or tea. Some examples of herbs used to treat respiratory illnesses are:

- *Garlic*—treats coughs and serves as an antibiotic (eaten raw).
- *Eucalyptus*—clears stuffy nasal and sinus congestion; used for asthma, bronchitis, and tuberculosis (boil in water and breathe in steam).
- *Mullein*—soothes and relaxes the airway and relieves cough; used for asthma, tuberculosis, and as a cough suppressant (mixed with water and taken orally).

Health care professionals need to incorporate questions about the use of herbal remedies in their history taking. This is important because some of these remedies are not considered safe and others may have adverse interactions with prescribed medications.

SINUSITIS

Acute sinusitis is an inflammation of the sinuses due to a bacterial cause. Sinusitis is usually caused by an upper respiratory infection that causes inflammation in the nasal passages. The inflammation can cause trapping of bacteria. It is easy to confuse the common cold with sinusitis, for patients and health care providers, so a good health history is extremely important. In rare cases, if left untreated, sinusitis can lead to an infection in the brain or other serious complications (NIAID, 2007).

Incidence and Etiology

The most common bacterial agents associated with sinusitis are *Streptococcus pneumoniae,* and *H. influenzae.* Other possible causes include exposure to cigarette smoke, foreign bodies, and nasal polyps. Asthma also has a strong association with sinusitis, and people who have environmental allergies and hay fever are also at increased risk for nasal symptoms (NIAID, 2007).

Pathophysiology

Sinusitis is typically preceded by a rhinovirus, or common cold episode with runny nose and cough. Sinusitis occurs when thick mucus from an upper respiratory infection

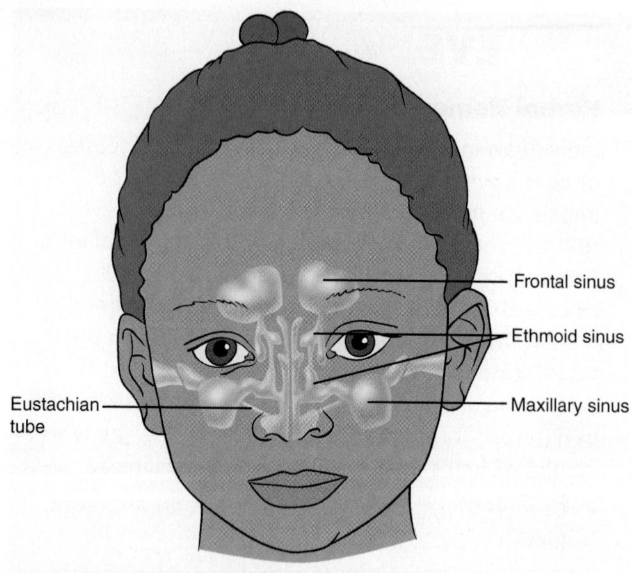

FIGURE 24-6 Diagram of Sinuses. DELMAR CENGAGE LEARNING.

impairs the ciliary action in the nasal passages. The cilia are unable to effectively clear the sinuses, and the passages become obstructed. An accumulation of mucus and foreign particulate in these passages can put people at risk for sinusitis. Also, with a cold, people tend to blow their nose more frequently, which causes the normally benign bacteria in their nasal passages to be forced up into the sinus cavities (NIAID, 2007). Figure 24-6 demonstrates the location of the sinuses.

Clinical Manifestations

One of the most common symptoms of sinusitis is facial pain. It can occur over the forehead, jaw, near the eyes or ears. The classic manifestations of sinusitis—headache, facial pain, and tenderness—may be more easily identified in older children. Younger children more often have postnasal drip, malodorous breath, and periorbital swelling. Rhinorrhea, which may range from clear to purulent, cough, fever, fatigue, headache, and a mild sore throat are other common manifestations (NIAID, 2007).

Diagnosis

The diagnosis of sinusitis is generally based on the child's medical history and physical examination. Clinical diagnosis of acute sinusitis with a bacterial etiology is based upon the presence of nasal discharge with no improvement for 10–14 days or temperature of over or equal to 39° C (102.2°F) with purulent nasal discharge for at least 3 days in an ill patient. Because the common cold can elicit sinus involvement on an X-ray, these should be used only in certain instances and should be read keeping this in mind (AAP Red Book, 2006).

Treatment

Typical treatment once sinusitis is diagnosed includes an antibiotic and pain reliever, along with palliative measures. Initial antibiotic treatment is typically a narrow-spectrum medication, such as amoxicillin (AAP Red Book, 2006) prescribed for 10–14 days. In a secondary analysis of data by De Sutter et al. (2006), it was found that it is not possible to predict which patients with sinus symptoms will benefit from antibiotic treatment. Saline drops and sprays can also be helpful in alleviating sinusitis symptoms. They help liquefy nasal secretions, which facilitates their movement and clearance out of the sinuses.

Nursing Management and Family Teaching

The nursing management of sinusitis is focused on family education. This teaching includes informing the family about sinusitis and their child's treatment regimen. This includes instructing them on the proper administration of any medications prescribed for the child. Families may need to be reminded that antibiotics are useful only for bacterial infections, and in the majority of patients, antibiotics are not needed (De Sutter et al., 2006). Although it is often unavoidable, parents and children should be educated that nose blowing can force mucus into the sinus cavities and further the spread of infection. Saline nasal sprays can help to keep the nose as moist as possible. Exposure to irritants such as tobacco smoke should be avoided (NIAID, 2007).

■ COMMON CHRONIC RESPIRATORY ALTERATIONS

Some respiratory alterations are chronic, requiring the nurse to give acute care to the child while in the hospital and coordinate long-term care with caregivers and other health professionals. These respiratory alterations are important from an epidemiologic standpoint because of the staggering numbers of children and families affected by the disorders and the exorbitant costs associated with treatment. The most common chronic alterations are allergic rhinitis and asthma.

ALLERGIC RHINITIS

Allergic rhinitis (AR), commonly referred to as hay fever, is the most common disease in the pediatric population and is increasing in prevalence (Meltzer, 2006). AR is frequently associated with other common chronic diseases including asthma, sinusitis, and recurrent otitis media. AR is often delineated further into two subgroups: seasonal allergic rhinitis (SAR) and perennial allergic rhinitis (PAR). SAR is generally related to outdoor allergens such as tree, grass, and weed pollens. PAR is most often related to sensitivity to indoor allergens such as dust mites and mold. Children may develop sensitivities to both outdoor and indoor allergens; the treatment approach to SAR and PAR is basically the same.

Incidence and Etiology

Allergic rhinitis affects 20–40% of children (Milgrom & Leung, 2004). It is significant in terms of morbidity because of its impact on quality of life, school performance and absenteeism, and the propensity for AR to cause exacerbations in other disease conditions such as asthma, sinusitis, or otitis media (Carr, 2008; Kaari, 2006).

Pathophysiology

Allergic rhinitis is caused by a type I allergic response to indoor and outdoor allergens. Pollens, dust mites, pet dander, and mold spores are examples of causative agents. Allergen exposure stimulates the release of IgE. The IgE binds to mast cells, which then become receptors for allergen antigens, a process that leads to mast-cell degranulation. During this process varying mast-cell products are released (Milgrom & Leung, 2004; Rote, Huether, & McCance, 2004). A primary mediator released is histamine. Histamine has varying effects, including increasing vascular permeability, which causes edema, increasing mucus production, and narrowing of the airway (Rote et al., 2004). Ongoing or repeated exposure of sensitized membranes to allergens may lead to chronic nasal congestion.

Clinical Manifestations

Manifestations of allergic rhinitis include chronic nasal congestion, sneezing, rhinitis, rhinorrhea, mouth breathing, snoring, and itching of the eyes, nose, and ears. An allergic salute is common in children with allergic rhinitis as they scratch their noses with the palms of their hands, which may lead to a transverse line across the child's nose. The child may also have allergic shiners, which are darkened areas under the eyes, as well as the observed mouth breathing. Additionally the child may have boggy or enlarged nasal turbinates.

Diagnosis

The diagnosis of allergic rhinitis is a clinical diagnosis based on symptoms obtained from the history and signs observed on physical examination. Additionally, the child may have evidence of other atopy with signs and/or symptoms of asthma, food allergies, or atopic dermatitis. Elevated serum IgE and eosinophil levels are nonspecific indicators of the presence of an allergic disorder. Skin tests may be helpful in identifying specific allergens that trigger allergic response in the child.

Treatment

Management of allergic rhinitis begins with allergen avoidance. Reducing exposure to environmental allergens can be aided by reducing dust mites in the home, with frequent cleaning of mattresses, linens, and floors, use of allergen barrier pillowcases and mattress covers, controlling mold counts through use of a dehumidifier, using air conditioners, and keeping windows closed during peak pollen seasons. Pharmacotherapy is the other mainstay of AR management.

The first line pharmacologic choices in the treatment of AR are intranasal steroids. The newer generation of intranasal steroids has minimal effect on growth and is well tolerated in the pediatric population (Carr, 2008; Kaari, 2006; Meltzer, 2006; Scadding, 2008). The second line choice of pharmacotherapy for AR is oral antihistamines, preferably the second generation antihistamines (ex: ceftirizine, loratidine), which do not have the negative sedating effects of first generation drugs. Another alternative in the treatment of AR is montelukast, an oral agent particularly useful in children with comorbid condition of asthma, as it is also indicated for treatment of airway inflammation in asthma and exercise induced asthma (Nayak & Langdon, 2007). Finally, nasal saline irrigation (Huabin et al., 2009) and probiotics (Vilagoftis, Kouranos, Betsi, & Falagas, 2008) have both been found to be useful adjunctive therapies in the treatment of AR. There is insufficient evidence that immunotherapy in any form has positive effects on symptoms in children and adolescents with allergic rhinoconjunctivitis (Roder, Berger, deGroot, & Van Wijk, 2008).

Nursing Management

Assessment Children with allergic rhinitis generally have a history of frequent or chronic nasal drainage, with accompanying sniffles, sneezing, and congestion. Nasal congestion may force children to be mouth breathers. The child's past medical history may reveal other allergic conditions, particularly asthma or eczema, which together with AR are referred to as the "allergic triad" being often seen together in one individual. Children with AR are at higher risk for sinusitis or otitis media as well, and should be assessed for manifestations of these conditions. An assessment of the family medical history will often reveal family members with allergic conditions, as there is a familial predisposition to developing allergies. Finally it is crucial that an assessment of the child's environment (both at home, school, and other care settings) be performed, focusing on allergens, such as pets, houseplants, mold, dust mites, and irritants such as chalk dust, wood-burning stoves, and cigarette smoking.

Nursing Diagnosis

1. *Impaired oral mucus membranes* related to mouth breathing.
2. *Deficient knowledge (caregiver)* related to child with environmental allergies.

Outcome Identification

1. The child's lips and oral mucous membranes will be moist and intact.
2. The child's caregivers will verbalize a commitment to reduce possible allergens in the environment.

Planning and Implementation Children with allergic rhinitis are managed in the home. Caregivers are taught ways to reduce the allergens in the home and to minimize the child's exposure to seasonal allergens. Box 24-3 lists strategies for reducing allergen exposure indoors and outdoors. Prescribed medications should be reviewed and the proper

BOX 24-3
REDUCING ALLERGEN EXPOSURE IN THE HOME AND OUTDOORS

In the Bedroom
- Encase mattress, box springs, and pillows in vinyl covering or other similar barrier.
- Tape over zippers of barriers of bedding covers.
- Launder curtains, blankets, mattress pads, and comforters every two weeks.
- Launder bed linens and favorite stuffed animals weekly.
- Maintain laundry water at 55°C (130°F).
- Avoid nonessential fabric items and those made with feathers.
- Wash down the bedroom and closet every couple of months.

Pets and Pests
- Keep animals outside the home.
- Clean the home thoroughly if animals have lived indoors.
- Keep the indoor pet in uncarpeted areas that are easily cleaned.
- Premedicate the child before visiting a home with an animal.
- Eradicate cockroach populations in the home.
- Clean the home thoroughly if cockroaches have been present.

Throughout the House
- Clean moldy surfaces with 1:10 solution of bleach and water.
- Use a dehumidifier to reduce mold growth in damp houses; keep humidity at 45%.
- If humidifier is used, change water regularly and clean with bleach solution.
- Avoid house plants.
- Damp mop and damp dust at least once per week.
- Vacuum carpets and upholstery at least once per week.
- Dry clean drapes and carpets.
- Remove carpeting and replace if possible with wood or vinyl.
- Replace furnace filters or use an electrostatic filter.
- Filter furnace vents.
- Close windows and use air conditioners when outdoor air quality is poor.
- Keep home a smoke-free environment (tobacco or wood).
- Avoid use of strong odors or sprays.

Outdoors
- Keep child from compost or leaf piles, woods, and other high mold areas.
- Keep child indoors when air quality is poor and when mold or pollen counts are high.
- Keep child from wood smoke, animals, and agricultural chemicals.
- Avoid exercise in cold, dry air.

administration of nasal steroids should be demonstrated. Adequate hydration should be encouraged to help maintain fluids lost through mouth breathing. Lip balm can be recommended to keep the child's lips from becoming chapped.

Evaluation The ultimate goal for the child with AR is to be asymptomatic with the right combination of allergen avoidance and pharmacotherapy. Ongoing evaluation should include changes of flare-ups in symptoms, adherence to medications and allergy avoidance, possible new allergen exposure, and other comorbid conditions that may arise.

Family Teaching

Allergic rhinitis is a chronic alteration that requires ongoing attention on the part of the child's caregivers. Environmental reduction of allergens is a critical factor in minimizing the affected child's symptoms. Families need to be able to identify possible sources for their child's allergies and how to reduce exposure to these.

ASTHMA

Asthma is a complex respiratory illness characterized by chronic inflammation, bronchoconstriction, and bronchial hyperresponsiveness. The primary manifestations of the disease—wheezing, coughing, and **dyspnea**—are caused by airway obstruction from edema, mucus, and bronchoconstriction. Among susceptible individuals, asthma ranges in severity but the common thread is the interplay between airway inflammation and clinical symptoms (National Asthma Education and Prevention Program [NAEPP], 2007).

Incidence and Etiology

Asthma is one of the most common pediatric chronic illnesses. As of 2007, 8 million children in the United States (between 5–17 years of age) had the highest prevalence rates of being diagnosed with asthma (American Lung Association, 2009). In America, approximately 22 million people, in total, have been diagnosed with asthma (NAEPP, 2007). Some estimates show that up to 300 million people in the world are affected by asthma (Fanta, 2009). Asthma is a huge burden to the patients and families causing lost work and lost school days, ED visits, and hospitalizations, not to mention the extreme cost of having a chronic illness (NAEPP, 2007).

Over several years, from 1980 to 1996, the incidence of asthma in Americans increased. Since 1999, however, things seem to be improving. Hospitalizations and mortality due to asthma seem to no longer be increasing in number. In 2007, asthma appeared to be more common in females than in males, affecting 13.4 million females in the U.S. and 9.5 million males in the U.S. However, when looking at children (under 18 years of age), asthma prevalence was 15% higher in males than in females (American Lung Association, 2009). Prior to puberty, more males than females are affected by the disease. However, postpuberty, more females than males are affected. Asthma is a disease that affects people from all races and ethnicities (Fanta, 2009). Asthma prevalence rates in the Hispanic population were lower than non-Hispanic blacks and non-Hispanic whites in 2007 (American Lung Association, 2009).

Pathophysiology

The inflammatory response associated with asthma is triggered by agents such as antigens, irritants (e.g., pollution, tobacco smoke, cold air), infection, medications (e.g., aspirin, nonsteroidal anti-inflammatory drugs), gastroesophageal reflux, foods and food preservatives, physical and emotional stress, and exercise. These triggers stimulate a cascade of events that affect the entire respiratory tract. Allergens stimulate an increase in circulating IgE, mast cells, and macrophages. These products cause the release of other substances such as histamine, basophils, eosinophils, neutrophils, platelets, T lymphocytes, and prostaglandins. The result of this inflammatory cascade is bronchoconstriction, mucosal edema, and an increased mucus production. Figure 24-7 illustrates the effects of this alteration on the airway. These effects cause airway obstruction and air trapping, which lead to ventilation-perfusion alterations, an increased work of breathing, hypercapnia, and hypoxemia. If left untreated, respiratory failure and death can result. A summary of this process can be seen in Figure 24-8.

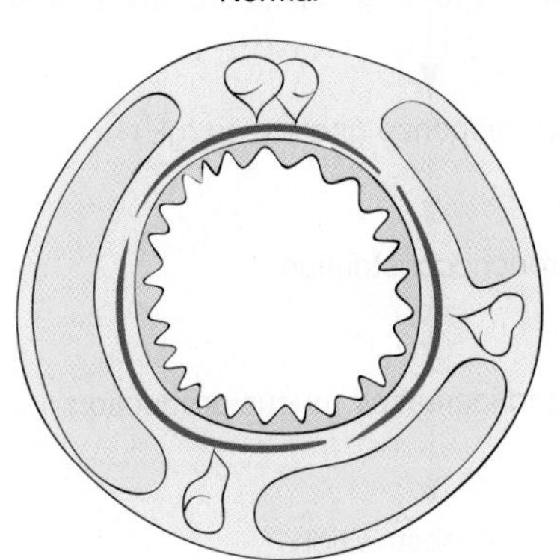

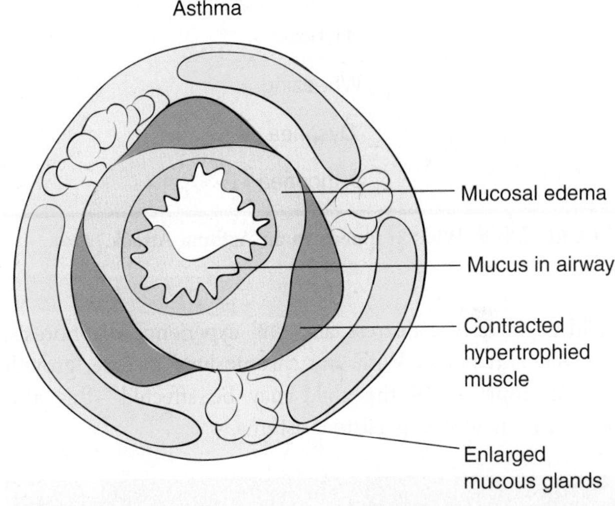

Figure 24-7 Pathophysiology of Asthma. DELMAR CENGAGE LEARNING.

Clinical Manifestations

A diagnosis of asthma usually comes after recurrent respiratory symptoms are noted. The most common symptoms associated with asthma are wheezing, recurrent cough, frequent episodes of difficulty breathing, or chest tightness. Any combination of these symptoms may be present and they are not all necessary to diagnose asthma. Oftentimes with asthma, there is a trigger which induces these symptoms. The most common triggers are environmental allergens, respiratory infections, exercise, and changes in the weather (NAEPP, 2007).

Older children may sit upright with shoulders in a hunched-over position with their arms braced (Figure 24-9).

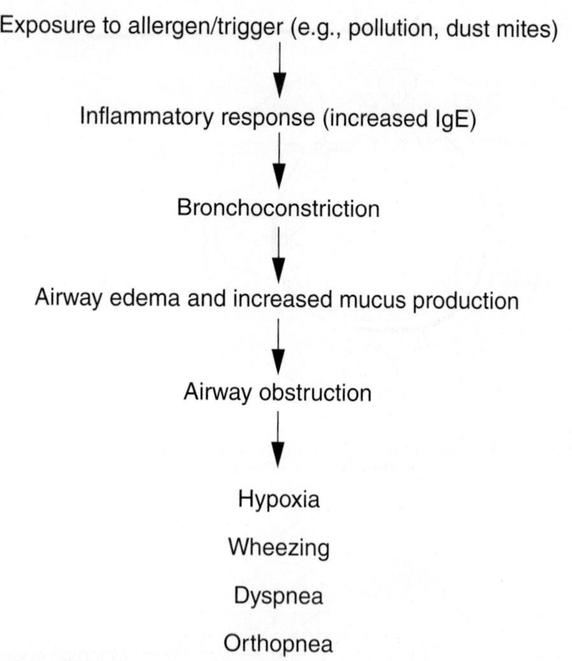

FIGURE 24-8 What Happens in an Asthma Attack. DELMAR CENGAGE LEARNING.

Children in severe distress also will experience diaphoresis, cyanosis, and pallor. With any chronic lung disease, growth and development of the child may be affected—this also holds true in severe, persistent asthma.

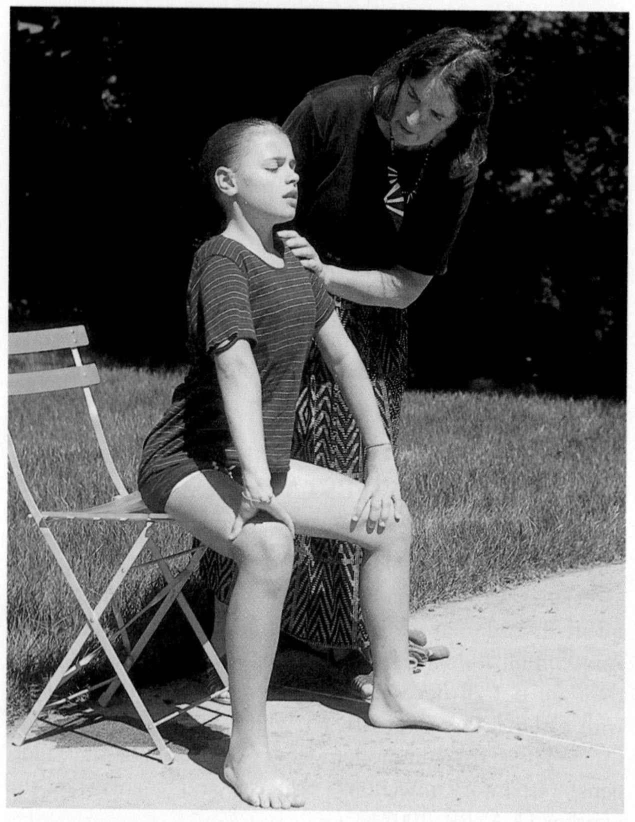

FIGURE 24-9 This position in an older child is a classic sign of an asthma episode. DELMAR CENGAGE LEARNING.

DIAGNOSIS

The diagnosis of asthma is made based on the client history, physical assessment findings, and pulmonary function studies. The medical history of a child with asthma should include a wide variety of questions. Inquiring about symptoms is necessary, including patterns: when symptoms present, duration, frequency, etc. Also, it is extremely important to discuss apparent triggers – viral illness, cold weather, exercise, etc. Chronological history of symptoms is another necessity, along with discussing when the exacerbations are most likely to occur. Family history, social history, and the patient and family's perception of the disease are also a quite significant portion of the history. The physical exam may or may not reveal the symptoms listed under the common clinical manifestations. The diagnosis of asthma cannot be ruled out based on physical exam alone, as the disease is variable and symptoms can be absent between exacerbations. With a history that points in the direction of an asthma diagnosis, the upper and lower respiratory tract exam (including ear, nose and throat) along with skin exam is very important. Spirometry is one of the mainstays of an asthma diagnosis. It can show evidence of obstruction in an objective way, as the history and physical exams can often vary. Spirometry is recommended in children who are 5 years of age or older, as it is not often reliable in younger children. It is more helpful then a peak flow meter in diagnosing asthma. The peak flow meters should be reserved for home use of the patient as a monitoring tool (NAEPP, 2007).

According to the most recent expert panel report on the Guidelines for the diagnosis and management of asthma (National Asthma Education and Prevention Program, 2007), the assessment and severity level should be based on various components (see Tables 24-1, 24-2, and 24-3 from the National Asthma Education and Prevention Program, Expert Panel Report 3). The impairment of the child and the risk the child is at should be taken into consideration when classifying their asthma severity level. In order to assess impairment, the child or caretaker is asked to recall the child's symptoms over the previous 2–4 weeks (see Tables 24-4, 24-5, and Table 24-6). The long-term management can then be based upon the severity level and response to treatment (see Tables 24-7, 24-8, and 24-9).

TREATMENT

The main goal of therapy in treating asthmatic patients is to keep the asthma under control. The patients should be able to live as normal a life as possible, and as care providers, we should work with the families to prevent chronic symptoms. Some other important goals would be for the patients to necessitate use of their rescue medications infrequently, maintain as normal pulmonary function as possible, and maintain normal activity levels and for the families to be satisfied and happy with their care. Avoidance of triggers, regular peak flow monitoring, medications including inhalation therapies, family education, ongoing follow-up, and rapid access to medical care are the chief components of

Table 24-1 Assessing Asthma Control and Adjusting Therapy in Children 0–4 Years of Age

Components of Control		Classification of Asthma Control (0–4 Years of Age)		
		Well Controlled	**Not Well Controlled**	**Very Poorly Controlled**
Impairment	Symptoms	≤2 days/week	>2 days/week	Throughout the day
	Nighttime awakenings	≤1x/month	>1x/month	>1x/week
	Interference with normal activity	None	Some limitation	Extremely limited
	Short-acting beta$_2$-agonist use for symptom control (not prevention of EIB)	≤2 days/week	>2 days/week	Several times per day
Risk	Exacerbations requiring oral systemic corticosteroids	0–1/year	2–3/year	>3/year
	Treatment-related adverse effects	Medication side effects can vary in intensity from none to very troublesome and worrisome. The level of intensity does not correlate to specific levels of control but should be considered in the overall assessment of risk.		
Recommended Action for Treatment		• Maintain current treatment. • Regular followup every 1–6 months. • Consider step down if well controlled for at least 3 months.	• Step up (1 step) and • Reevaluate in 2–6 weeks. • If no clear benefit in 4–6 weeks, consider alternative diagnoses or adjusting therapy. • For side effects, consider alternative treatment options.	• Consider short course of oral systemic corticosteroids, • Step up (1–2 steps), and • Reevaluate in 2 weeks. • If no clear benefit in 4–6 weeks, consider alternative diagnoses or adjusting therapy. • For side effects, consider alternative treatment options.

Key: EIB, exercise-induced bronchospasm

Notes:

- The stepwise approach is meant to assist, not replace, the clinical decisionmaking required to meet individual patient needs.
- The level of control is based on the most severe impairment or risk category. Assess impairment domain by caregiver's recall of previous 2–4 weeks. Symptom assessment for longer periods should reflect a global assessment such as inquiring whether the patient's asthma is better or worse since the last visit.
- At present, there are inadequate data to correspond frequencies of exacerbations with different levels of asthma control. In general, more frequent and intense exacerbations (e.g., requiring urgent, unscheduled care, hospitalization, or ICU admission) indicate poorer disease control. For treatment purposes, patients who had ≥2 exacerbations requiring oral systemic corticosteroids in the past year may be considered the same as patients who have not-well-controlled asthma, even in the absence of impairment levels consistent with not-well-controlled asthma.
- Before step up in therapy:
  – Review adherence to medications, inhaler technique, and environmental control.
  – If alternative treatment option was used in a step, discontinue it and use preferred treatment for that step.

Courtesy of National Heart, Lung, and Blood Institute, a part of the National Institutes of Health and the U.S. Department of Health and Human Services. Retrieved December 9, 2010, from http://www.nhlbi.nih.gov/guidelines/asthma.

Table 24-2 Assessing Asthma Control and Adjusting Therapy in Children 5–11 Years of Age

Components of Control		Classification of Asthma Control (5–11 Years of Age): Well Controlled	Not Well Controlled	Very Poorly Controlled
Impairment	Symptoms	≤2 days/week but not more than once on each day	>2 days/week or multiple times on day ≤2 days/week	Throughout the day
	Nighttime awakenings	≤1x/month	≥2x/month	≥2x/week
	Interference with normal activity	None	Some limitation	Extremely limited
	Short-acting beta$_2$-agonist use for symptom control (not prevention of EIB)	≤2 days/week	>2 days/week	Several times per day
	Lung function • FEV_1 or peak flow • FEV_1/FVC	>80% predicted/ personal best >80%	60–80% predicted/ personal best 75–80%	<60% predicted/ personal best <75%
Risk	Exacerbations requiring oral systemic corticosteroids	0–1/year	≥2/year (see note)	
		Consider severity and interval since last exacerbation		
	Reduction in lung growth	Evaluation requires long-term followup.		
	Treatment-related adverse effects	Medication side effects can vary in intensity from none to very troublesome and worrisome. The level of intensity does not correlate to specific levels of control but should be considered in the overall assessment of risk.		
Recommended Action for Treatment		• Maintain current step. • Regular followup every 1–6 months. • Consider step down if well controlled for at least 3 months.	• Step up at least 1 step and • Reevaluate in 2–6 weeks. • For side effects: consider alternative treatment options.	• Consider short course of oral systemic corticosteroids, • Step up 1–2 steps, and • Reevaluate in 2 weeks. • For side effects, consider alternative treatment options.

Key: EIB, exercise-induced bronchospasm; FEV_1, forced expiratory volume in 1 second; FVC, forced vital capacity

Notes:

- The stepwise approach is meant to assist, not replace, the clinical decisionmaking required to meet individual patient needs.
- The level of control is based on the most severe impairment or risk category. Assess impairment domain by patient's/caregiver's recall of previous 2–4 weeks and by spirometry/or peak flow measures. Symptom assessment for longer periods should reflect a global assessment such as inquiring whether the patient's asthma is better or worse since the last visit.
- At present, there are inadequate data to correspond frequencies of exacerbations with different levels of asthma control. In general, more frequent and intense exacerbations (e.g., requiring urgent, unscheduled care, hospitalization, or ICU admission) indicate poorer disease control. For treatment purposes, patients who had ≥2 exacerbations requiring oral systemic corticosteroids in the past year may be considered the same as patients who have persistent asthma, even in the absence of impairment levels consistent with persistent asthma.
- Before step up in therapy:
  - Review adherence to medications, inhaler technique, environmental control, and comorbid conditions.
  - If alternative treatment option was used in a step, discontinue it and use preferred treatment for that step.

Courtesy of National Heart, Lung, and Blood Institute, a part of the National Institutes of Health and the U.S. Department of Health and Human Services. Retrieved December 9, 2010, from http://www.nhlbi.nih.gov/guidelines/asthma.

TABLE 24-3 Assessing Asthma Control and Adjusting Therapy in Youths ≥12 Years of Age and Adults

COMPONENTS OF CONTROL		CLASSIFICATION OF ASTHMA CONTROL (≥12 YEARS OF AGE)		
		WELL CONTROLLED	NOT WELL CONTROLLED	VERY POORLY CONTROLLED
Impairment	Symptoms	≤2 days/week	>2 days/week	Throughout the day
	Nighttime awakenings	≤2x/month	1–3x/week	≥4x/week
	Interference with normal activity	None	Some limitation	Extremely limited
	Short-acting beta-2 agonist use for symptom control (not prevention of EIB)	≤2 days/week	>2 days/week	Several times per day
	FEV_1 or peak flow	>80% predicted/ personal best	60–80% predicted/ personal best	<60% predicted/ personal best
	Validated questionnaires ATAQ ACQ ACT	 0 ≤0.75* ≥20	 1–2 ≥1.5 16–19	 3–4 N/A ≤15
Risk	Exacerbations requiring oral systemic corticosteroids	0–1/year	≥2/year (see note)	
		Consider severity and interval since last exacerbation		
	Progressive loss of lung function	Evaluation requires long-term followup care		
	Treatment-related adverse effects	Medication side effects can vary in intensity from none to very troublesome and worrisome. The level of intensity does not correlate to specific levels of control but should be considered in the overall assessment of risk.		
Recommended Action for Treatment		• Maintain current step. • Regular followups every 1–6 months to maintain control. • Consider step down if well controlled for at least 3 months.	• Step up 1 step and • Reevaluate in 2–6 weeks. • For side effects, consider alternative treatment options.	• Consider short course of oral systemic corticosteroids, • Step up 1–2 steps, and • Reevaluate in 2 weeks. • For side effects, consider alternative treatment options.

*ACQ values of 0.76–1.4 are indeterminate regarding well-controlled asthma.

Key: EIB, exercise-induced bronchospasm; ICU, intensive care unit

Notes:

- The stepwise approach is meant to assist, not replace, the clinical decisionmaking required to meet individual patient needs.
- The level of control is based on the most severe impairment or risk category. Assess impairment domain by patient's recall of previous 2–4 weeks and by spirometry/or peak flow measures. Symptom assessment for longer periods should reflect a global assessment, such as inquiring whether the patient's asthma is better or worse since the last visit.
- At present, there are inadequate data to correspond frequencies of exacerbations with different levels of asthma control. In general, more frequent and intense exacerbations (e.g., requiring urgent, unscheduled care, hospitalization, or ICU admission) indicate poorer disease control. For treatment purposes, patients who had ≥2 exacerbations requiring oral systemic corticosteroids in the past year may be considered the same as patients who have not-well-controlled asthma, even in the absence of impairment levels consistent with not-well-controlled asthma.
- Validated Questionnaires for the impairment domain (the questionnaires do not assess lung function or the risk domain)
  ATAQ = Asthma Therapy Assessment Questionnaire© (See sample in "Component 1: Measures of Asthma Assessment and Monitoring.")
  ACQ = Asthma Control Questionnaire© (user package may be obtained at www.qoltech.co.uk or juniper@qoltech.co.uk)
  ACT = Asthma Control Test™ (See sample in "Component 1: Measures of Asthma Assessment and Monitoring.")
  Minimal Important Difference: 1.0 for the ATAQ; 0.5 for the ACQ; not determined for the ACT.
- Before step up in therapy:
  – Review adherence to medication, inhaler technique, environmental control, and comorbid conditions.
  – If an alternative treatment option was used in a step, discontinue and use the preferred treatment for that step.

Courtesy of National Heart, Lung, and Blood Institute, a part of the National Institutes of Health and the U.S. Department of Health and Human Services. Retrieved December 9, 2010, from http://www.nhlbi.nih.gov/guidelines/asthma.

Table 24-4 Classifying Asthma Severity and Initiating Treatment in children 0–4 Years of Age

Assessing severity and initiating therapy in children who are not currently taking long-term control medication

Components of Severity		Classification of Asthma Severity (0–4 Years of Age)			
			Persistent		
		Intermittent	Mild	Moderate	Severe
Impairment	Symptoms	≤2 days/week	>2 days/week but not daily	Daily	Throughout the day
	Nighttime awakenings	0	1–2x/month	3–4x/month	>1x/week
	Short-acting beta$_2$-agonist use for symptom control (not prevention of EIB)	≤2 days/week	>2 days/week but not daily	Daily	Several times per day
	Interference with normal activity	None	Minor limitation	Some limitation	Extremely limited
Risk	Exacerbations requiring oral systemic corticosteroids ←	0–1/year	≥2 exacerbations in 6 months requiring oral systemic corticosteroids, or ≥4 wheezing episodes/1 year lasting >1 day AND risk factors for persistent asthma		
		Consider severity and interval since last exacerbation. Frequency and severity may fluctuate over time. → Exacerbations of any severity may occur in patients in any severity category.			
Recommended Step for Initiating Therapy		Step 1	Step 2	Step 3 and consider short course of oral systemic corticosteroids	
		In 2–6 weeks, depending on severity, evaluate level of asthma control that is achieved. If no clear benefit is observed in 4–6 weeks, consider adjusting therapy or alternative diagnoses.			

Key: EIB, exercise-induced bronchospasm

Notes:

- The stepwise approach is meant to assist, not replace, the clinical decisionmaking required to meet individual patient needs.
- Level of severity is determined by both impairment and risk. Assess impairment domain by patient's/caregiver's recall of previous 2–4 weeks. Symptom assessment for longer periods should reflect a global assessment such as inquiring whether the patient's asthma is better or worse since the last visit. Assign severity to the most severe category in which any feature occurs.
- At present, there are inadequate data to correspond frequencies of exacerbations with different levels of asthma severity. For treatment purposes, patients who had ≥2 exacerbations requiring oral systemic corticosteroids in the past 6 months, or ≥4 wheezing episodes in the past year, and who have risk factors for persistent asthma may be considered the same as patients who have persistent asthma, even in the absence of impairment levels consistent with persistent asthma.

Courtesy of National Heart, Lung, and Blood Institute, a part of the National Institutes of Health and the U.S. Department of Health and Human Services. Retrieved December 9, 2010, from http://www.nhlbi.nih.gov/guidelines/asthma.

successful asthma management (NAEPP, 2007). Avoidance of triggers is the primary means for preventing the symptoms of asthma. Box 24-3 provides a listing of steps that can be taken to lower allergen exposure. Other preventive actions include warm-ups before exercising, short-term beta-2 agonist 20–30 minutes before exercising, and avoiding outdoor exercising when the air is cold and dry. Children with asthma need to have a good night's sleep and adequate nutrition. It is also important for them to avoid being around others with infections, particularly respiratory infections, although this is often impossible in the school setting and with school-aged siblings.

Regular monitoring of peak expiratory flow (PEF) provides a guide to how well the asthma is controlled. Lowered flow rates, along with clinical symptoms, should alert the child and family that the asthma symptoms are worsening.

The pharmacologic management of asthma depends on the severity and the frequency of the child's symptoms.

TABLE 24-5 Classifying Asthma Severity and Initiating Treatment in Children 5–11 Years of Age

Assessing severity and initiating therapy in children who are not currently taking long-term control medication

COMPONENTS OF SEVERITY		CLASSIFICATION OF ASTHMA SEVERITY (5–11 YEARS OF AGE)			
			PERSISTENT		
		INTERMITTENT	MILD	MODERATE	SEVERE
Impairment	Symptoms	≤2 days/week	>2 days/week but not daily	Daily	Throughout the day
	Nighttime awakenings	≤2x/month	3–4x/month	>1x/week but not nightly	Often 7x/week
	Short-acting beta$_2$-agonist use for symptom control (not prevention of EIB)	≤2 days/week	>2 days/week but not daily	Daily	Several times per day
	Interference with normal activity	None	Minor limitation	Some limitation	Extremely limited
	Lung function	• Normal FEV_1 between exacerbations • FEV_1 >80% predicted • FEV_1/FVC >85%	• FEV_1 = >80% predicted • FEV_1/FVC >80%	• FEV_1= 60–80% predicted • FEV_1/FVC=75–80%	• FEV_1 = <60% predicted • FEV_1/FVC <75%
Risk	Exacerbations requiring oral systemic corticosteroids	0–1/year (see note)	≥2/year (see note) →		
		← Consider severity and interval since last exacerbation. → Frequency and severity may fluctuate over time for patients in any severity category.			
		Relative annual risk of exacerbations may be related to FEV_1.			
Recommended Step for Initiating Therapy		Step 1	Step 2	Step 3, medium-dose ICS option	Step 3, medium-dose ICS option, or step 4
				and consider short course of oral systemic corticosteroids	
		In 2–6 weeks, evaluate level of asthma control that is achieved, and adjust therapy accordingly.			

Key: EIB, exercise-induced bronchospasm; FEV_1, forced expiratory volume in 1 second; FVC, forced vital capacity; ICS, inhaled corticosteroids

Notes:

- The stepwise approach is meant to assist, not replace, the clinical decisionmaking required to meet individual patient needs.
- Level of severity is determined by both impairment and risk. Assess impairment domain by patient's/caregiver's recall of the previous 2–4 weeks and spirometry. Assign severity to the most severe category in which any feature occurs.
- At present, there are inadequate data to correspond frequencies of exacerbations with different levels of asthma severity. In general, more frequent and intense exacerbations (e.g., requiring urgent, unscheduled care, hospitalization, or ICU admission) indicate greater underlying disease severity. For treatment purposes, patients who had ≥2 exacerbations requiring oral systemic corticosteroids in the past year may be considered the same as patients who have persistent asthma, even in the absence of impairment levels consistent with persistent asthma.

Courtesy of National Heart, Lung, and Blood Institute, a part of the National Institutes of Health and the U.S. Department of Health and Human Services. Retrieved December 9, 2010, from http://www.nhlbi.nih.gov/guidelines/asthma.

TABLE 24-6 Classifying Asthma Severity and Initiating Treatment in Youths $\geq$12 Years of Age and Adults

Assessing severity and initiating treatment for patients who are not currently taking long-term control medication

COMPONENTS OF SEVERITY		CLASSIFICATION OF ASTHMA SEVERITY $\geq$12 YEARS OF AGE			
			PERSISTENT		
		INTERMITTENT	MILD	MODERATE	SEVERE
Impairment **Normal FEV_1/FVC:** **8–19 yr 85%** **20–39 yr 80%** **40–59 yr 75%** **60–80 yr 70%**	Symptoms	$\leq$2 days/week	>2 days/week but not daily	Daily	Throughout the day
	Nighttime awakenings	$\leq$2x/month	3–4x/month	>1x/week but not nightly	Often 7x/week
	Short-acting $beta_2$-agonist use for symptom control (not prevention of EIB)	$\leq$2 days/week	>2 days/week but not daily, and not more than 1x on any day	Daily	Several times per day
	Interference with normal activity	None	Minor limitation	Some limitation	Extremely limited
	Lung function	• Normal FEV_1 between exacerbations • FEV_1 >80% predicted • FEV_1/FVC normal	• FEV_1 >80% predicted • FEV_1/FVC normal	• FEV_1 >60% but <80% predicted • FEV_1/FVC reduced 5%	• FEV_1 <60% predicted • FEV_1/FVC reduced >5%
Risk	Exacerbations requiring oral systemic corticosteroids	0–1/year (see note)	$\geq$2/year (see note) →		
		← Consider severity and interval since last exacerbation. → Frequency and severity may fluctuate over time for patients in any severity category. Relative annual risk of exacerbations may be related to FEV_1.			
Recommended Step for Initiating Treatment		**Step 1**	**Step 2**	**Step 3** and consider short course of oral systemic corticosteroids	**Step 4 or 5**
		In 2–6 weeks, evaluate level of asthma control that is achieved and adjust therapy accordingly.			

Key: FEV_1, forced expiratory volume in 1 second; FVC, forced vital capacity; ICU, intensive care unit

Notes:

- The stepwise approach is meant to assist, not replace, the clinical decisionmaking required to meet individual patient needs.
- Level of severity is determined by assessment of both impairment and risk. Assess impairment domain by patient's/caregiver's recall of previous 2–4 weeks and spirometry. Assign severity to the most severe category in which any feature occurs.
- At present, there are inadequate data to correspond frequencies of exacerbations with different levels of asthma severity. In general, more frequent and intense exacerbations (e.g., requiring urgent, unscheduled care, hospitalization, or ICU admission) indicate greater underlying disease severity. For treatment purposes, patients who had $\geq$2 exacerbations requiring oral systemic corticosteroids in the past year may be considered the same as patients who have persistent asthma, even in the absence of impairment levels consistent with persistent asthma.

Courtesy of National Heart, Lung, and Blood Institute, a part of the National Institutes of Health and the U.S. Department of Health and Human Services. Retrieved December 9, 2010, from http://www.nhlbi.nih.gov/guidelines/asthma.

TABLE 24-7 Stepwise Approach for Managing Asthma in Children 0–4 Years of Age

Intermittent Asthma	Persistent Asthma: Daily Medication. Consult with asthma specialist if step 3 care or higher is required. Consider consultation at step 2.					
Step 1 *Preferred:* SABA PRN	**Step 2** *Preferred:* Low-dose ICS *Alternative:* Cromolyn or Montelukast	**Step 3** *Preferred:* Medium-dose ICS	**Step 4** *Preferred:* Medium-dose ICS + either LABA or Montelukast	**Step 5** *Preferred:* High-dose ICS + either LABA or Montelukast	**Step 6** *Preferred:* High-dose ICS + either LABA or Montelukast Oral systemic corticosteroids	↑ Step up if needed (first, check adherence, inhaler technique, and environmental control) *Assess control* Step down if possible (and asthma is well controlled at least 3 months) ↓

Patient Education and Environmental Control at Each Step

Quick-Relief Medication for All Patients

- SABA as needed for symptoms. Intensity of treatment depends on severity of symptoms.
- With viral respiratory infection: SABA q 4–6 hours up to 24 hours (longer with physician consult). Consider short course of oral systemic corticosteroids if exacerbation is severe or patient has history of previous severe exacerbations.
- Caution: Frequent use of SABA may indicate the need to step up treatment. See text for recommendations on initiating daily long-term-control therapy.

Key: **Alphabetical order is used when more than one treatment option is listed within either preferred or alternative therapy.** ICS, inhaled corticosteroid; LABA, inhaled long-acting $beta_2$-agonist; SABA, inhaled short-acting $beta_2$-agonist

Notes:

- The stepwise approach is meant to assist, not replace, the clinical decisionmaking required to meet individual patient needs.
- If alternative treatment is used and response is inadequate, discontinue it and use the preferred treatment before stepping up.
- If clear benefit is not observed within 4–6 weeks and patient/family medication technique and adherence are satisfactory, consider adjusting therapy or alternative diagnosis.
- Studies on children 0–4 years of age are limited. Step 2 preferred therapy is based on Evidence A. All other recommendations are based on expert opinion and extrapolation from studies in older children.

Courtesy of National Heart, Lung, and Blood Institute, a part of the National Institutes of Health and the U.S. Department of Health and Human Services. Retrieved December 9, 2010, from http://www.nhlbi.nih.gov/guidelines/asthma.

Short-acting bronchodilators such as inhaled beta-2 agonists are typically the only treatment indicated for children with mild intermittent asthma. Inhaled corticosteroids are the most consistently effective long-term control medications for persistent asthma. Inhaled antiasthmatics (e.g., cromolyn, nedocromil) are used as an alternative, but not preferred, therapy for patients with mild persistent asthma. Long-acting beta-2 agonists (e.g., salmeterol and formoterol) can be used in conjunction with inhaled corticosteroids for children with moderate or severe persistent asthma, but are not used as monotherapy. They are often convenient as they last at least 12 hours after a single dose. Short-acting inhaled beta-2 agonists are used as needed to manage acute symptoms in children with mild persistent asthma (NAEPP, 2007). Table 24-10 gives common medications with usual dosages used to treat asthma in children. Table 24-11 compares low, medium, and high daily dosages for inhaled corticosteroids.

Inhaled medications are administered via a metered-dose inhaler (MDI). For instructions on using a MDI, read Nursing Tip: Proper MDI technique with spacer. Children are taught to use a spacer with their MDIs. Spacers make the administration of the inhaled medication easier and facilitate better distribution and inhalation of the medication. Spacers

Table 24-8 Stepwise Approach for Managing Asthma in Children 5–11 Years of Age

Intermittent Asthma	Persistent Asthma: Daily Medication. Consult with asthma specialist if step 4 care or higher is required. Consider consultation at step 3.				
Step 1	**Step 2**	**Step 3**	**Step 4**	**Step 5**	**Step 6**
Preferred: SABA PRN	*Preferred:* Low-dose ICS *Alternative:* Cromolyn, LTRA, Nedocromil, or Theophylline	*Preferred:* EITHER: Low-dose ICS + either LABA, LTRA, or Theophylline OR Medium-dose ICS	*Preferred:* Medium-dose ICS + LABA *Alternative:* Medium-dose ICS + either LTRA or Theophylline	*Preferred:* High-dose ICS + LABA *Alternative:* High-dose ICS + either LTRA or Theophylline	*Preferred:* High-dose ICS + LABA + oral systemic corticosteroid *Alternative:* High-dose ICS + either LTRA or Theophylline + oral systemic corticosteroid

Step up if needed (first, check adherence, inhaler technique, environmental control, and comorbid conditions)

Assess control

Step down if possible (and asthma is well controlled at least 3 months)

Each step: Patient education, environmental control, and management of comorbidities.

Steps 2–4: Consider subcutaneous allergen immunotherapy for patients who have allergic asthma (see notes).

Quick-Relief Medication for All Patients

- SABA as needed for symptoms. Intensity of treatment depends on severity of symptoms: up to 3 treatments at 20-minute intervals as needed. Short course of oral systemic corticosteroids may be needed.
- Caution: Increasing use of SABA or use >2 days a week for symptom relief (not prevention of EIB) generally indicates inadequate control and the need to step up treatment.

Key: **Alphabetical order is used when more than one treatment option is listed within either preferred or alternative therapy.** ICS, inhaled corticosteroid; LABA, inhaled long-acting beta$_2$-agonist, LTRA, leukotriene receptor antagonist; SABA, inhaled short-acting beta$_2$-agonist

Notes:
- The stepwise approach is meant to assist, not replace, the clinical decisionmaking required to meet individual patient needs.
- If alternative treatment is used and response is inadequate, discontinue it and use the preferred treatment before stepping up.
- Theophylline is a less desirable alternative due to the need to monitor serum concentration levels.
- Step 1 and step 2 medications are based on Evidence A. Step 3 ICS + adjunctive therapy and ICS are based on Evidence B for efficacy of each treatment and extrapolation from comparator trials in older children and adults—comparator trials are not available for this age group; steps 4–6 are based on expert opinion and extrapolation from studies in older children and adults.
- Immunotherapy for steps 2–4 is based on Evidence B for house-dust mites, animal danders, and pollens; evidence is weak or lacking for molds and cockroaches. Evidence is strongest for immunotherapy with single allergens. The role of allergy in asthma is greater in children than in adults. Clinicians who administer immunotherapy should be prepared and equipped to identify and treat anaphylaxis that may occur.

Courtesy of National Heart, Lung, and Blood Institute, a part of the National Institutes of Health and the U.S. Department of Health and Human Services. Retrieved December 9, 2010, from http://www.nhlbi.nih.gov/guidelines/asthma.

minimize large droplets from being deposited in the mouth which, in the case of corticosteroid MDIs, can cause candidal mouth infections. Children should be taught to rinse their mouth following MDI use. Figure 24-10 shows a child using a spacer with a mouthpiece. Mouthpieces require the child to be able to hold his or her breath for 5–10 seconds once the medication is released from the MDI canister. When a mask is used, the canister is activated, and the mask is left in place until the child has taken 5–6 breaths. Oral or intravenous corticosteroids and one or more hours of continuous short-acting beta-2 agonist nebulizer treatments may be used for children in severe distress. Inhaled ipratropium bromide, an anticholinergic drug that potentiates the action of beta-2 agonists, may also be used for the emergency management of symptoms. Children receiving continuous nebulizer treatments need close observation not only because of the degree of their respiratory distress, but also because of increased risks for side effects associated with the medications. Figure 24-11 illustrates a child at home receiving short-acting beta-2 agonist via a nebulizer.

TABLE 24-9 Stepwise Approach for Managing Asthma in Youths ≥12 Years of Age and Adults

Intermittent Asthma	Persistent Asthma: Daily Medication Consult with asthma specialist if step 4 care or higher is required. Consider consultation at step 3.				
Step 1 *Preferred:* SABA PRN	**Step 2** *Preferred:* Low-dose ICS *Alternative:* Cromolyn, LTRA, Nedocromil, or Theophylline	**Step 3** *Preferred:* Low-dose ICS + LABA OR Medium-dose ICS *Alternative:* Low-dose ICS + either LTRA, Theophylline, or Zileuton	**Step 4** *Preferred:* Medium-dose ICS + LABA *Alternative:* Medium-dose ICS + either LTRA, Theophylline, or Zileuton	**Step 5** *Preferred:* High-dose ICS + LABA AND Consider Omalizumab for patients who have allergies	**Step 6** *Preferred:* High-dose ICS + LABA + oral corticosteroid AND Consider Omalizumab for patients who have allergies

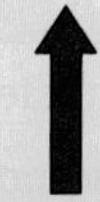

Step up if needed

(first, check adherence, environmental control, and comorbid conditions)

Assess control

Step down if possible

(and asthma is well controlled at least 3 months)

Each step: Patient education, environmental control, and management of comorbidities.

Steps 2–4: Consider subcutaneous allergen immunotherapy for patients who have allergic asthma (see notes).

Quick-Relief Medication for All Patients

- SABA as needed for symptoms. Intensity of treatment depends on severity of symptoms: up to 3 treatments at 20-minute intervals as needed. Short course of oral systemic corticosteroids may be needed.
- Use of SABA >2 days a week for symptom relief (not prevention of EIB) generally indicates inadequate control and the need to step up treatment.

Key: **Alphabetical order is used when more than one treatment option is listed within either preferred or alternative therapy.** EIB, exercise-induced bronchospasm; ICS, inhaled corticosteroid; LABA, long-acting inhaled beta$_2$-agonist; LTRA, leukotriene receptor antagonist; SABA, inhaled short-acting beta$_2$-agonist

Notes:

- The stepwise approach is meant to assist, not replace, the clinical decisionmaking required to meet individual patient needs.
- If alternative treatment is used and response is inadequate, discontinue it and use the preferred treatment before stepping up.
- Zileuton is a less desirable alternative due to limited studies as adjunctive therapy and the need to monitor liver function. Theophylline requires monitoring of serum concentration levels.
- In step 6, before oral systemic corticosteroids are introduced, a trial of high-dose ICS + LABA + either LTRA, theophylline, or zileuton may be considered, although this approach has not been studied in clinical trials.
- Step 1, 2, and 3 preferred therapies are based on Evidence A; step 3 alternative therapy is based on Evidence A for LTRA, Evidence B for theophylline, and Evidence D for zileuton. Step 4 preferred therapy is based on Evidence B, and alternative therapy is based on Evidence B for LTRA and theophylline and Evidence D for zileuton. Step 5 preferred therapy is based on Evidence B. Step 6 preferred therapy is based on (EPR—2 1997) and Evidence B for omalizumab.
- Immunotherapy for steps 2–4 is based on Evidence B for house-dust mites, animal danders, and pollens; evidence is weak or lacking for molds and cockroaches. Evidence is strongest for immunotherapy with single allergens. The role of allergy in asthma is greater in children than in adults.
- Clinicians who administer immunotherapy or omalizumab should be prepared and equipped to identify and treat anaphylaxis that may occur.

Courtesy of National Heart, Lung, and Blood Institute, a part of the National Institutes of Health and the U.S. Department of Health and Human Services. Retrieved December 9, 2010, from http://www.nhlbi.nih.gov/guidelines/asthma.

NURSING MANAGEMENT

Assessment A critical component of the nursing management of asthma is the recognition of common early symptoms associated with an exacerbation. Of particular importance is the identification of children at risk for severe or life-threatening attacks. To help assess the level of control that the patient has attained, some important questions to ask may include:

- Does your asthma ever wake you up during sleep?
- How often are you using your "rescue medication"?
- Have you had to go to urgent care or the emergency room for asthma symptoms?
- Are you able to take part in the physical activities that you enjoy?

Reference: (NAEPP, 2007)

TABLE 24-10 Usual Dosages for Asthma Medications

MEDICATION	DOSAGE FORM	ADULT DOSE	CHILD DOSE*	COMMENTS
Inhaled Corticosteroids *(See Table 24-11, Estimated Comparative Daily Dosages for Inhaled Corticosteroids.)*				
Systemic Corticosteroids			*(Applies to all three corticosteroids)*	
Methylprednisolone	2, 4, 8, 16, 32 mg tablets	7.5–60 mg daily in a single dose in A.M. or every other day as needed for control	0.25–2 mg/kg daily in single dose in A.M. or every other day as needed for control	• For long-term treatment of severe persistent asthma, administer single dose in A.M. either daily or on alternate days (alternate-day therapy may produce less adrenal suppression). If daily doses are required, one study suggests improved efficiency and no increase in adrenal suppression when administered at 3 P.M. • Short courses or "bursts" are effective for establishing control when initiating therapy or during a period of gradual deterioration. • The burst should be continued until patient achieves 80% PEF personal best or symptoms resolve. This usually requires 3–10 days but may require longer. There is no evidence that tapering the dose following improvement prevents relapse.
Prednisolone	5 mg tablets, 5 mg/5 mL, 15 mg/5 mL	Short-course "burst": to achieve control 40–60 mg per day as single or 2 divided doses for 3–10 days	Short-course "burst": 1–2 mg/kg/day maximum 60 mg/day for 3–10 days	
Prednisone	1, 2.5, 5, 10, 20, 50 mg tablets; 5 mg/mL, 5 mg/5 mL			
Long-Acting Inhaled Beta-2 Agonists				• **Should not be used for symptom relief or exacerbations. Use with corticosteroids.**
Salmeterol	MDI 21 mcg/puff	2 puffs q 12 hours	1–2 puffs q 12 hours	• May use one dose nightly for symptoms.
Formoterol	DPI 50 mcg/blister DPI 12 mcg/single-use capsule	1 blister q 12 hours 1 capsule q 12 hours	1 blister q 12 hours 1 capsule q 12 hours	• Efficacy and safety have not been studied in children <5 years of age. • Each capsule is for single use only; additional doses should not be administered for at least 12 hours. • Capsules should not be used only with the Aerolizor inhaler and should not be taken orally.

(Continues)

Table 24-10 Usual Dosages for Asthma Medications (*Continued*)

MEDICATION	DOSAGE FORM	ADULT DOSE	CHILD DOSE*	COMMENTS
Combined Medication				
Fluticasone/ Salmeterol	DPI 100 mcg, 250 mcg, or 500 mcg/50 mcg	1 inhalation BID; dose depends on severity of asthma	1 inhalation BID; dose depends on severity of asthma	• Not FDA approved in children <12 years of age. 100/50 for patient not controlled on low-to-medium dose inhaled corticosteroids. • 250/50 for patients not controlled on medium-to-high dose inhaled corticosteroids.
Cromolyn and Nedocromil				
Cromolyn	MDI 1 mg/puff Nebulizer 20 mg/ampule	2–4 puffs tid-qid 1 ampule tid-qid	1–2 puffs tid-qid 1 ampule tid-qid	• One dose prior to exercise or allergen exposure provides effective prophylaxis for 1–2 hours.
Nedocromil	MDI 1.75 mg/puff	2–4 puffs bid-qid	1–2 puffs bid-qid	• See cromolyn above.
Leukotriene Modifiers				
Montelukast	4 mg or 5 mg chewable tablet 10 mg tablet	10 mg qhs	4 mg qhs (2–5 years of age) 5 mg qhs (6–14 years of age) 10 mg qhs (>14 years of age)	• Montelukast exhibits a flat dose-response curve. Doses >10 mg will not produce a greater response in adults.
Zafirlukast	10 or 20 mg tablet	40 mg daily (20 mg tablet bid)	20 mg daily (7–11 years of age) (10 mg tablet bid)	• For zafilukast, administration with meals decreases bio-availability; take at least 1 hour before or 2 hours after meals.
Zileuton	300 or 600 mg tablet	2,400 mg daily (give tablets qid)		• For zileuton, monitor hepatic enzymes (ALT).
Methylxanthines				
Theophylline	Liquids, sustained-release tablets, and capsules	Starting dose 10 mg/kg/day up to 300 mg max; usual max 800 mg/day	Starting dose 10 mg/kg/day; usual max: <1 year of age: 0.2 (age in weeks) + 5 = mg/kg/day >1 year of age: 16 mg/kg/day	• Adjust dosage to achieve serum concentration of 5–15 mcg/mL at steady-state (at least 48 hours on same dosage). • Due to wide interpatient variability in theophylline metabolic clearance, routine serum theophylline level monitoring is important.

(Continues)

Table 24-10 Usual Dosages for Asthma Medications (*Continued*)

MEDICATION	DOSAGE FORM	ADULT DOSE	CHILD DOSE*	COMMENTS
Short-Acting Inhaled Beta-2 Agonists				
	MDI			
Albuterol	90 mcg/puff, 200 puffs	2 puffs 5 minutes prior to exercise 2 puffs tid-qid PRN	1–2 puffs 5 minutes prior to exercise 2 puffs tid-qid PRN	• An increasing use or lack of expected effect indicates diminished control of asthma. • Not generally recommended for long-term treatment. Regular use on a daily basis indicates the need for additional long-term-control therapy. • Differences in potency exist, but all products are essentially comparable on a per puff basis. • May double usual dose for mild exacerbations. • Nonselective agents (i.e., epinephrine, isoproterenol, metaproterenol) are not recommended due to their potential for excessive cardiac stimulation, especially in high doses.
Albuterol HFA	90 mcg/puff, 200 puffs			
Pirbuterol	200 mcg/puff, 400 puffs			
	DPI			
Albuterol rotahaler	200 mcg/capsule	1–2 capsules q 4–6 hours as needed and prior to exercise	1 capsule q 4–6 hours as needed and prior to exercise	
	Nebulizer solution			
Albuterol	5 mg/mL (0.5%) 2.5 mg/3 mL 1.25 mg/3 mL 0.63 mg/3 mL	1.25–5 mg in 3 mL of saline q 4–8 hours	0.05 mg/kg (min 1.25 mg, max 2.5 mg) in 3 mL of saline q 4–6 hours	• May mix with cromolyn or ipratropium nebulizer solutions. May double dose for severe exacerbations.
	Nebulizer solution			
Bitolterol	2 mg/mL (0.2%)	0.5–3.5 mg (0.25–1 mL) in 2–3 mL of saline q 4–8 hours	Not established	• May not mix with other nebulizer solutions.
	Nebulizer solution			
Levalbuterol (R-albuterol)	0.31 mg/3 mL 0.63 mg/3 mL 1.25 mg/3 mL	0.63 mg–2.5 mg q 4–8 hours	0.025 mg/kg (min. 0.63 mg. max. 1.25 mg) q 4–8 hours	• 0.63 mg of levalbuterol is equivalent in efficacy and side effects to 1.25 mg of racemic albuterol. The product is a sterile-filled preservative-free unit dose vial.

(Continues)

Table 24-10 Usual Dosages for Asthma Medications (*Continued*)

MEDICATION	DOSAGE FORM	ADULT DOSE	CHILD DOSE*	COMMENTS
Anticholinergics				
	MDI			
Ipratropium	18 mcg/puff, 200 puffs	2–3 puffs q 6 hours	1–2 puffs q 6 hours	• Evidence is lacking for anticholinergics producing added benefit to beta-2 agonists in long-term-control asthma therapy.
	Nebulizer solution	0.25 mg q 6 hours	0.25–0.5 mg q 6 hours	
	0.25 mg/mL (0.025%)			
	MDI			
Ipratropium with albuterol	18 mcg/puff of ipratropium bromide and 90 mcg/puff of albuterol. 200 puffs/ canister	2–3 puffs q 6 hours	1–2 puffs q 8 hours	
	Nebulizer solution			
	0.5 mg/3 mL ipratropium bromide and 2.5 mg/ 3 mL albuterol	3 mL q 4–6 hours	1.5–3 mL q 8 hours	• Contains EDTA to prevent discoloration of the solution. This additive does not induce bronchospasm.
Systemic Corticosteroids				
			(Applies to all three corticosteroids)	
Methylprednisolone	2, 4, 6, 8, 16, 32 mg tablets	Short course "burst": 40–60 mg/day as single or 2 divided doses for 3–10 days	Short course "burst" 1–2 mg/kg/day, maximum 60 mg/ day, for 3–10 days	• Short courses or "bursts" are effective for establishing control when initiating therapy or during a period of gradual deterioration.
Prednisolone	5 mg tablets, 5 mg/5 mL, 15 mg/5 mL			• The burst should be continued until patient achieves 80% PEF personal best or symptoms resolve. This usually requires 3–10 days but may require longer. There is no evidence that tapering the dose following improvement prevents relapse.
Prednisone	1, 2.5, 5, 10, 20, 50 mg tablets; 5 mg/mL, 5 mg/5 mL			
	Repository injection			
Methylprednisolone acetate	40 mg/mL 80 mg/mL	240 mg IM once	7.5 mg/kg IM once	• May be used in place of a short burst of oral steroids in patients who are vomiting or if adherence is a problem.

*Children ≤12 years of age

Source: National Asthma Education and Prevention Program. (2003). *Expert panel report: Guidelines for the diagnosis and management of asthma: Update on selected topics 2002.* Bethesda, MD: National Heart, Lung, and Blood Institute; National Institutes of Health; U.S. Department of Health and Human Services. NIH Publication No. 02-5074, pp. 117–118, 120–121. Retrieved September 8, 2005, from http://www.nhlbi.nih.gov.

Table 24-11 Estimated Comparative Daily Dosages for Inhaled Corticosteroids in Children

DRUG	LOW DAILY DOSE		MEDIUM DAILY DOSE		HIGH DAILY DOSE	
	CHILD 0-4	CHILD 5-11	CHILD 0-4	CHILD 5-11	CHILD 0-4	CHILD 5-11
Beclomethasone HFA 40 or 80 mcg/puff	NA	80–160 mcg	NA	>160–320 mcg	NA	>320 mcg
Budesonide DPI 90, 180, or 200 mcg/inhalation	NA	180–400 mcg	NA	>400–800 mcg	NA	>800 mcg
Budesonide Inhaled Inhalation suspension for nebulization (child dose)	0.25–0.5 mg	0.5 mg	>0.5–1.0 mg	1.0 mg	>1.0 mg	2.0 mg
Flunisolide 250 mcg/puff	NA	500–750 mcg	NA	1,000–1,250 mcg	NA	>1,250 mcg
Flunisolide HFA 80 mcg/puff	NA	160 mcg	NA	320 mcg	NA	≥640 mcg
Fluticasone **HFA/MDI:** 44, 110, or 220 mcg/puff **DPI:** 50, 100, or 250 mcg/inhalation	176 mcg NA	88–176 mcg 100–200 mcg	>176–352 mcg NA	>176–352 mcg >200–400 mcg	>352 mcg NA	>352 mcg >400 mcg
Mometasone DPI 200 mcg/inhalation	NA	NA	NA	NA	NA	NA
Triamcinolone acetonide 75 mcg/puff	NA	300–600 mcg	NA	>600–900 mcg	NA	>900 mcg

Key: HFA, hydrofluoroalkane; NA, not approved and no data available for this age group.

Notes:

- **The most important determinant of appropriate dosing is the clinician's judgment of the patient's response to therapy.** The clinician must monitor the patient's response on several clinical parameters and adjust the dose accordingly. The stepwise approach to therapy emphasizes that once control of asthma is achieved, the dose of medication should be carefully titrated to the minimum dose required to maintain control, thus reducing the potential for adverse effect.
- Some doses may be outside package labeling, especially in the high-dose range. Budesonide nebulizer suspension is the only ICS with FDA approval labeling for children <4 years of age.
- Metered-dose inhaler (MDI) dosages are expressed as the actuator dose (the amount of the drug leaving the actuator and delivered to the patient), which is the labeling required in the United States. This is different from the dosage expressed as the valve dose (the amount of drug leaving the valve, not all of which is available to the patient), which is used in many European countries and in some scientific literature. Dry powder inhaler (DPI) doses are expressed as the amount of the drug in the inhaler following activation.
- For children <4 years of age: The safety and efficacy of ICSs in children <1 year has not been established. Children <4 years of age generally require delivery of ICS (budesonide and fluticasone HFA) through a face mask that should fit snugly over nose and mouth and avoid nebulizing the eyes. Wash face after each treatment to prevent local corticosteroid side effects. For budesonide, the dose may be administered 1–3 times daily. Budesonide suspension is compatible with albuterol, ipratropium, and levalbuterol solutions in the same nebulizer. Use only jet nebulizers, as ultrasonic nebulizers are ineffective for suspensions.
- For fluticasone HFA, the dose should be divided 2 times daily; the low dose for children <4 years is higher than for children 5–11 years of age due to lower dose delivered with face mask and data on efficacy in young children.
- Comparative dosages are based on published comparative clinical trials (Adams et al., 2005; Barnes et al., 1998; Kelly, 1998; Lasserson et al., 2005; Pedersen and O'Byrne, 1997). The rationale for some key comparisons is summarized as follows:
  - The high dose is the dose that appears likely to be the threshold beyond which significant hypothalamic-pituitary-adrenal (HPA) axis suppression is produced, and, by extrapolation, the risk is increased for other clinically significant systemic effects if used for prolonged periods of time (Martin et al., 2002; Szefler et al., 2002).
  - The low- to medium-doses reflect findings from dose-ranging studies in which incremental efficacy within the low- to medium dose ranges was established without increased systemic effect as measured by overnight cortisol excretion. The studies demonstrated a relatively flat dose-response curve for efficacy at the medium-dose range; that is, increasing the dose of high-dose range did not significantly increase efficacy but did increase systemic effect (Adams et al., 2001; Martin et al., 2002; Szefler et al., 2002).
  - The doses for budesonide and fluticasone MDI or DPI are based on recently available comparative data. These new data show that fluticasone requires one-half the microgram dose of budesonide DPI to achieve comparable efficacy (Adams et al., 2005; Barnes et al., 1998; Nielsen and Dahl, 2000).
  - The dose of budesonide/formoterol in children is based on product information and current literature (Pohunek et al., 2006; Tal et al., 2002; Zimmerman et al., 2004).
  - The dose for fluticasone HFA in children <5 years of age is based on clinical studies demonstrating efficacy at this dose of 176 mcg/day (Bisgaard et al., 2004; Guilbert et al., 2006).

Source: National Asthma Education and Prevention Program. (2007). Expert panel report 3: Guidelines for the diagnosis and management of asthma. U.S. Department of Health and Human Services. National Institutes of Health. National Heart Lung and Blood Institute. NIH Publication Number 08-5846. Retrieved September 8, 2005, from http://www.nhlbi.nih.gov.

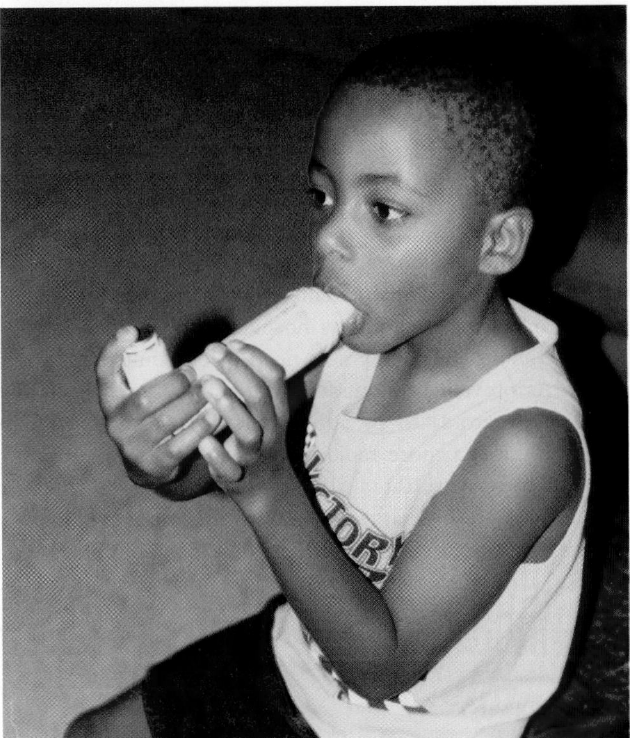

FIGURE 24-10 Child Using an MDI with Spacer and Mouthpiece. DELMAR CENGAGE LEARNING.

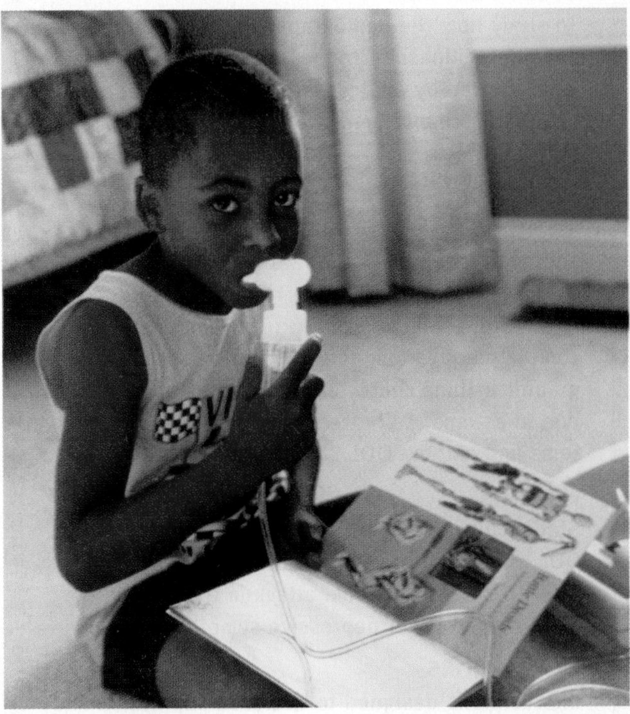

FIGURE 24-11 Administration of a Short-Acting Beta-2 Agonist Via Nebulizer. DELMAR CENGAGE LEARNING.

Characteristics associated with an increased risk for a severe asthma attack are repeated emergency room or hospital admissions, marked morning and evening fluctuations in lung functioning, and a prior life-threatening asthma attack.

NURSING TIP

Proper MDI Technique with Spacer

FOR INFANT USING MASK AND SPACER:

1. Remove the cap from the canister.
2. Attach MDI canister to spacer and shake well.
3. Cover the child's mouth and nose with the mask, making sure there is a good seal.
4. Activate the canister by pressing the top of the canister.
5. Allow child to take 6–10 breaths while holding mask in tight seal on the face. Make sure the valve moves with each breath.
6. Wait 60 seconds and repeat if second inhalation is prescribed.

FOR OLDER CHILD USING MOUTHPIECE AND SPACER:

1. Attach MDI canister to mouthpiece.
2. Shake to increase pressure in canister.
3. Expire to functional residual capacity (if coughing occurs, exhale less vigorously).
4. Place mouthpiece in mouth and make a seal with lips.
5. Activate the canister.
6. Inspire slowly to total lung capacity.
7. Hold breath for 5–10 seconds, and then breathe normally. For infants, and children unable to hold their breath, a mask should be used and remain in place until they have taken 5–6 breaths.
8. Wait 60 seconds.
9. Repeat steps 2–7.

A thorough respiratory assessment is clearly indicated for children with asthma symptoms. Assessment of activity tolerance, cardiovascular functioning, and fluid balance are also important. Additionally, the nurse needs to assess the child's and family's understanding related to asthma and its treatment. Ongoing management, early recognition of symptoms, and the initiation of emergency intervention for acute attacks are skills the child and family need in order to successfully manage the disease. Clarification of information and teaching directed to resolving deficient knowledge are critical for the safety of the child.

Nursing Diagnosis

1. *Risk for suffocation* related to airway obstruction.
2. *Ineffective airway clearance* related to allergic and inflammatory processes.
3. *Interrupted family processes* related to child with chronic illness.

Outcome Identification

1. The child will be free from life-threatening asthma exacerbations.
2. The child will have clear lung sounds, normal respiratory effort, and be free from cough.

NURSING TIP

Directions for Use of PEF Meters

- Make sure the sliding marker on the monitoring device is at the bottom of the scale.
- Sit up straight or stand.
- Take a deep breath and seal lips around mouthpiece.
- Blow out as hard and fast as possible into the device.
- Repeat these steps two more times. Record the highest of the three readings.
- Readings should be taken in the morning, evening, and other times as directed.

3. The family will demonstrate positive adaptation in meeting the child's needs.

Planning and Implementation While nurses are in a position to provide acute and emergency asthma-related care, most children with asthma are managed at home. Family education related to self-management of asthma is a primary focus of nursing care. The family may need help in identifying possible triggers and exploring feasible ways of limiting the affected child's exposure to these. They also need to ensure the child has appropriate follow-up care and that they have quick access into the health care system in case the child has an asthma attack. The nurse should collaborate with social services and other agencies when families need help with resources to meet their child's health needs. In addition, the school nurse is an excellent resource for children with asthma and their parents and, for school-age children, their school nurse should be made aware of the child's diagnosis of asthma.

Language or cultural barriers that prohibit the child from getting appropriate and timely health care need to be addressed. Different cultural practices that do not create potential health problems should be supported and integrated with necessary conventional treatments. Interpreters need to be utilized to ensure the family has the information they need to meet the child's health needs. If possible, reading materials in the family's native language should be made available to literate families. Additionally, it is important that the family acquire the language needed to access emergency care in the event of an attack.

Evaluation The effectiveness of the nursing care plan is based on the client's achievement of outcomes. If the education the family receives is effective, the child's asthma should be managed successfully. Certainly, the child should be free from life-threatening attacks. Effective management also means the child will be free from the classic manifestations of wheezing, shortness of breath, and cough. Support, education, and referrals for needed services are ways the nurse can help the family make the adaptations necessary to meet the child's needs.

Family Teaching

Family education is focused on prevention of exacerbations, avoiding triggers if possible, early recognition of exacerbations, treatments, proper administration of medications, and the use of PEF monitoring devices and metered-dose inhalers. The importance of education in the management of asthma has been discussed. Caregivers need a thorough understanding of asthma, including learning to identify the child's triggers, and maintenance of optimal health to prevent asthma attacks requiring hospitalization.

The child and family also need to be competent using MDIs. As previously discussed, MDIs allow for bronchodilators and steroids to be administered via inhalation. This route produces a more rapid onset than oral administration and has fewer associated side effects. Sometimes children with asthma are discharged home with nebulizer treatments, another form of aerosolized medication administration.

RESEARCH Highlight

Adolescents with Asthma: Predictors of Quality of Life

STUDY PURPOSE

To study how the demographic, personal, interpersonal, and illness factors associated with asthma as self-reported by adolescents from the United States (USA) and Iceland predict quality of life (QOL). Asthma affects 12% of American children and an estimated 9% in Iceland.

METHODS

This cross-sectional exploratory study included adolescents with asthma (n = 15 from the USA; n = 15 from Iceland), aged 13–17 years. Participants completed questionnaires measuring sociodemographic asthma characteristics, degree of limitations due to asthma, self-rated health, depressive symptoms and asthma QOL.

FINDINGS

Statistically significant predictors of higher asthma QOL were a better rating of overall health, not having had a severe asthma attack in the last six months, and lower depressive symptoms.

IMPLICATIONS

Interventions designed to decrease depression and prevent asthma exacerbations may improve QOL for adolescents for asthma.

REFERENCE

Burkhart, P. V., Svavarsdottir, E. K., Rayens, M. K., Oakley, M. G., & Orlygsdottir, B. (2009). Adolescents with asthma: Predictors of quality of life. *Journal of Advanced Nursing*, 65(4), 860–866.

Reflections from Families

My son, Antonio, is 6 years old. He has had asthma since he was a baby. When he was 6 months old, he had to be hospitalized because he had such a hard time breathing. He was very sick for several days. I was so worried, so scared that he would die. Since then, whenever he gets a cold, I wonder if he has just a cold or the beginnings of a full-blown attack. When you have a child with asthma, you worry a lot. You also miss a lot of sleep. Antonio has problems breathing at night sometimes. I am also afraid to travel with him. Even though we take all his medicines and equipment with us on trips, we are still away from his doctor and from the hospital. And he always seems to get sick when we travel. Will the worrying ever end?

Nebulizers may be used for younger children and developmentally delayed children, who cannot reliably take deep breaths. When a family is utilizing a nebulizer, education about the nebulizer needs to be included in the family education.

Exercise is another focus of family education. Most children with asthma can participate in physical exercise and athletic activities as long as their asthma is under control. The ability to participate in specific sport activities is based on individual responses to the activity. Premedication with a short-term beta-2 agonist may be used prophylactically, approximately 20–30 minutes prior to physical exercise to minimize exacerbation of symptoms. Asthma triggers are child-specific. Recognizing these specific triggers is an important step in minimizing exposure. The child should avoid his or her triggers as much as possible. The nurse is positioned to help the child and family adjust to necessary environmental and lifestyle changes dictated by the child's health needs. The reinforcement of asthma education should be ongoing. Warning signs should be reviewed regularly. The family is counseled to notify the child's health care provider if symptoms such as wheezing, frequent coughing, shortness of breath, tightness in the chest, and drop in peak expiratory flow rates are present.

LESS COMMON RESPIRATORY ALTERATIONS

Less common pediatric respiratory alterations include cystic fibrosis, respiratory distress syndrome, and tuberculosis. Nurses must have a thorough understanding of these alterations in order to effectively care for affected children and their families.

CYSTIC FIBROSIS

Cystic Fibrosis (CF) is an autosomal, recessive, genetic disease primarily affecting the respiratory and gastrointestinal tracts. It is the most common profoundly life-shortening genetic illness in the Caucasian population, but can be found in all ethnicities. CF is caused by genetic abnormalities in the seventh chromosome which result in impaired function of the CFTR protein, a critical protein in the functioning of multiple organs in the body. While one specific genetic mutation, DF508 affects a wide majority of individuals with CF, well over a thousand different mutations have been identified worldwide. Additionally there is wide variation in disease severity thought to be due to the specific genetic mutations in any given individual, in concert with other individual modifying genetic influences, as well as external factors, both environmental and treatment-related. While CF is a chronic progressive illness that requires daily treatment and care, with advances in understanding and treatment, the majority of affected individuals now live well into adulthood, and nearly half of affected individuals in the United States are now adults.

Incidence and Etiology

CF affects over 30,000 individuals in the United States. On the basis of data from U.S. newborn screening programs, less than 90% of diagnoses are in non-Hispanic whites with a birth prevalence of 1 in 2,500–3,500 births. CF occurs in 1 in 4,000–10,000 births among Hispanics, and 1 in 15,000–20,000 births among non-Hispanic blacks (Grosse et al., 2004). The median survival for individuals with CF was 37.4 year in 2007 with an age range of 0–70 years.

Approximately 45% of individuals in the United States living with CF are over the age of 18.

Diagnosis

Over half of patients are diagnosed in the first 6 months of age, and close to 75% by age 2 (CF Foundation, 2009). However a recent recommendation from the Centers for Disease Control and Prevention (2004) now mandates newborn screening for CF. Implementation of this has varied state to state but will soon be part of the newborn screening process in every state in the United States. Additionally the American College of Geneticists and the American College of Obstetricians and Gynecologists recommend carrier screening for all couples considering pregnancy or who are pregnant, regardless of family history for CF. It is important to note that newborn screening for CF is *not* diagnostic; further evaluation with a sweat chloride test or confirmatory CF genetics is necessary to make the diagnosis. In the absence of newborn screening, diagnosis continues to be made based on history, physical examination, laboratory findings, chest films, and DNA analysis, with the sweat test remaining as the gold standard for diagnosis.

CRITICAL THINKING

Cystic Fibrosis and Sterility

Andrew, an 18-year-old with cystic fibrosis, asks about what he heard in a CF chat room that all men with CF are sterile. How are you prepared to this question? Who are the best resources to help Andrew sort out rumors from factual information?

NURSING ALERT

Signs of a Pneumothorax

A pneumothorax is suspected in a patient with CF who experiences an acute onset of chest or back pain, increased work of breathing, dyspnea, pallor, or cyanosis.

Pathophysiology

Cystic fibrosis results from a defective protein causing exocrine gland dysfunction that leads to abnormal levels of sodium and chloride, an increased viscosity of mucus secretions, and increased susceptibility to pulmonary colonization of bacteria. The epithelium of body tissues exhibits marked impermeability to chloride and an excessive reabsorption of sodium. These ion alterations lead to dehydration of airway secretions, causing impaired expectoration and airway obstruction in the lungs. In addition to causing airway obstruction, the stasis of thick, sticky pulmonary secretions increases the risk for pathogen invasion and bacterial colonization.

Thick mucus as a result of CFTR dysfunction leads to obstructions in other body system structures as well. Gastrointestinal manifestations include impairment of pancreatic, intestinal, and liver function. The sweat glands and the reproductive glands are also affected; almost all males with CF are sterile due to absence or impairment of the vas deferens, while females have reduced fertility. The impact in the sweat gland gives rise to abnormally high chloride secretion; individuals with CF are at risk for easily provoked dehydration.

Clinical Manifestations

Lung disease accounts for most illness and mortality in CF. Inflammation exists even in the airways of young asymptomatic infants. This inflammation leads to mucus secretions and debris from the influx of inflammatory cells creating the ideal environment for bacterial growth. The most common organisms to invade the CF airway are *Hemophilus influenzae, Staphylococcus Aureus, Methicillin*-resistant *Staphylococcus Aureus (MRSA),* and *Pseudomonas Aeruginosa.* Bacterial infections cause the release of toxins and other products that generate more inflammation in the airway creating a cycle of inflammation, infection, and impaired airway clearance. Chronic infection and airway obstruction lead to bronchial epithelium destruction and bronchiectasis (a lung condition characterized by irreversible dilation and destruction of the bronchial walls). Atelectasis, hemoptysis, or pneumothorax can be complications of this process. In the most severe stages of lung disease pulmonary vasculature changes can result in pulmonary hypertension and cor pulmonale. Digital clubbing occurs as a result of chronic lung disease. Pulmonary exacerbations (an acute decline in respiratory status), as a result of respiratory infection, occur sporadically in individuals with CF and are a hallmark of the disease. Manifestations of a pulmonary exacerbation include increased cough, new or increased sputum production, weight loss, malaise, fever, and a drop in lung function (as measured by pulmonary function testing).

Clinical manifestations in the gastrointestinal tract are variable and can range from mild constipation, normal liver function, and intermittent pancreatitis to severe loss of pancreatic function, malabsorption, CF-related diabetes, and end stage liver disease. The majority of children with CF have pancreatic insufficiency as a result of obstruction of the pancreatic ducts and consequent autoingestion of the pancreas. Untreated pancreatic insufficiency causes malabsorption of fat and protein from the diet with subsequent malnutrition steatorrhea, fat-soluble vitamin deficiencies

BOX 24-4
REASONS TO SUSPECT A DIAGNOSIS OF CF

meconium ileus
failure to thrive
bulky, foul-smelling, oily or greasy stools
hypoproteinemia
deficiency of fat soluble vitamins (A, D, E, K)
easily provoked hyponatremic dehydration
rectal prolapse
nasal polyps
pansinusitis
recurrent pneumonia or bronchitis
respiratory infection with *Pseudomonas aeruginosa*

(A, D, E, and K), and failure to thrive despite adequate intake. Slow transit of stool through the intestinal tract due to abnormalities in the intestinal lumen can also cause chronic constipation and intestinal obstruction (particularly in children receiving adequate pancreatic enzyme supplementation to correct steatorrhea). Meconium ileus at birth is the presenting symptom of CF in about 20% of patients. Glucose intolerance and insulin deficiency leading to CF-related diabetes can develop in adolescents and young adults with CF, causing a sub-acute decline in nutritional status and pulmonary status. Close to 10% of individuals with CF will have some degree of liver disease.

Treatment

Daily lifelong airway clearance, attention to infection prevention, reducing the frequency of exacerbations as well as early aggressive treatment of pulmonary exacerbations when they occur, are the mainstay of therapy aimed at slowing decline and preserving lung function. Additionally, supporting normal growth and nutrition over the lifespan is associated with improved pulmonary outcomes in all ages.

CF is marked by intermittent pulmonary exacerbations in lung disease as a result of new or increased bacterial growth in the lungs. Specific therapies aimed at reducing pulmonary exacerbations and maintaining lung function includes inhaled recombinant human deoxyribonuclease (DNase), inhaled hypertonic saline, and high-dose ibuprofen (Flume et al., 2007). Additionally daily airway clearance therapy is recommended to promote removal of mucous from the airways. This can be done through a variety of methods: chest physiotherapy, mechanical oscillation with a chest vest, handheld oscillation devices, or autogenic drainage (Flume et al., 2009). A mechanical chest vest is often the choice for young children. This vest provides high-frequency oscillation, which loosens airway secretions and facilitates their removal.

Aggressive treatment of pulmonary exacerbations, when they do occur, is associated with improved outcomes and helps to slow the progression of lung disease (Johnson, Butler, Konstan, Morgan, & Wohl 2003). Antibiotics, both oral and inhaled, in conjunction with an increase in airway clearance therapies, are used to treat mild exacerbations at home. Failure to improve with these therapies, or more severe exacerbations, result in hospitalization for intravenous antibiotics, extensive airway clearance, and other supportive measures (oxygen, nutritional supplementation) as needed. The choice of antibiotics is based on airway cultures (oropharyngeal, expectorated sputum, or bronchoscopic washings). Less common complications requiring additional treatment include pneumothorax and hemoptysis. Both complications are associated with more advanced lung disease, requiring more complex intervention. Lung transplantation is an end stage treatment that offers promise to children and young adults facing death because of respiratory insufficiency.

The treatment for pancreatic insufficiency and nutritional deficits in CF can be challenging. The goal for all children with CF is to grow normally and maintain a BMI above 50% for optimal health (Stallings, Stark, Robinson, Feranchak, & Quinton, 2008). In pancreatic insufficient patients, pancreatic enzyme supplementation is required with almost all foods to properly digest nutrients. Even with good pancreatic enzyme supplementation, the absorption of food is not completely normalized and patients require a calorie-dense diet high in fat, protein, and carbohydrates to reach nutritional goals. Caloric needs can be as high as four times the recommended calories for children without CF. This often creates a need for oral supplements or enteral feedings. Both infants and children should have fat-soluble vitamin supplementation as well as added salt in their diet, particularly during warm weather. This can be accomplished with the addition of table salt to infant formula, and liberal salt intake in the diet of children.

Infants with a meconium ileus may be treated medically with laxatives or enemas but surgical intervention may be required. Laxatives are typically used to manage intestinal obstructions in older infants and children and may be needed on a chronic basis to manage constipation and prevent recurrent obstruction. Liver transplantation is an option for those with end-stage liver disease.

Nursing Management

Cystic fibrosis, like other chronic illnesses, has enormous physical, financial, social, and emotional consequences for the child and family. Extensive treatment regimens, aggressive therapies required during exacerbations, interruptions in life routines, and the uncertainty around the variable course and prognosis of a life-shortening disease are sources of stress on the family. Assisting the family to develop strategies for successful adaptation to the demands of the disease is an integral component of the nursing care for CF. Care

KIDS WANT TO KNOW

Does CF affect my ability to have a family?

Michelle is a 15-year-old with CF. She is being seen in the pediatric pulmonary clinic for a routine check-up. She confides to Lori, the pediatric pulmonary nurse specialist, that she's worried about something. "My friends have started their periods and I haven't. I'm feeling left out and wondering if I am going to be able to have children when I get older." Lori tells Michelle that while puberty can be delayed in children with CF, she sees signs that Michelle's sexual development is on target. Lori explains that the development of breast tissue and pubic hair are mid-puberty indicators. Since Michelle has developed these signs, Lori believes she will begin her menstrual periods soon. Lori also explains to Michelle that almost all men with CF are infertile; most women with CF can have children if their health allows for the demands of pregnancy. Therefore, Michelle needs to recognize that if she engages in unprotected intercourse she runs the risk of acquiring a sexually transmitted disease or having an unwanted pregnancy. Additionally, before Michelle and a future partner plan a pregnancy, they need to understand the increased demands pregnancy can have on a woman with CF, as well as the challenges of caring for a child while managing a chronic illness. For this reason, they should explore associated health risks and family planning options with Michelle's CF care provider. Having addressed Michelle's immediate concerns, the two turned to a discussion surrounding dating, relationships, and intimacy.

Reflections from Families

I remember the first time I thought that something was wrong with Charmaine. After her bath, Charmaine and I played peek-a-boo for a while and then I gave her a big, fat, loud kiss on her cheek. She tasted salty, like a potato chip! That scared me—I called the clinic and they told me to come right in. I had never heard of CF before—now it's our entire life.

also includes collaborating with home health providers, coordinating input from a multidisciplinary team, implementing social and community service referrals, and providing ongoing family education.

During hospitalizations, nursing care for the child with CF includes respiratory, cardiovascular, nutritional, and developmental assessments. Other nursing interventions include managing the child's IV or long-term venous access device, administering IV antibiotics and other medications, providing nutritional support, and reinforcing teaching about the child's disease and medical regimen. Ensuring that adequate nutrition is provided during times of exacerbation is also an essential nursing intervention. Pancreatic enzymes must be taken before meals and snacks. Most children with CF are taught to swallow their enzymes whole at a young age; however capsules may be opened in applesauce and taken this way if needed. Favorite foods are incorporated into the child's diet and nutritional supplements between meals are encouraged. Collaboration with a nutritionist is recommended if the child's growth is impaired or less then acceptable. Nursing management may also include administering tube feedings to children who use enteral feedings to maintain their nutritional status.

Facilitating family development of coping strategies to address anxiety and stress related to the CF diagnosis and its management is another important nursing intervention. Families also need to understand the child's treatment plan and be competent with related care. Anticipatory guidance should include information related to general parenting and child developmental needs and address issues related to chronic illness, feelings of guilt, sibling reactions, and anticipatory grieving.

Family Teaching

The educational needs of families who have children with CF evolve as the children grow and develop and health status changes. Teaching is based on these needs. Clearly, families need to understand the disease, its management, and measures to prevent exacerbations. The focus of CF care is rooted in maintaining good nutrition, adherence to preventive therapies and interventions to minimize disease progression and complications. Infection prevention is one of these interventions. Good hand washing is one of the most important ways to decrease the incidence of infections. Peers or older adults with CF may be excellent sources of support, but this interaction should be limited to indirect contact via Internet or telephone. Families also need to be educated about the importance of routine follow-up care and monitoring for disease progression or complications (Figure 24-12). Recognizing the signs or symptoms of disease changes is important for early and aggressive interventions. Follow-up visits not only serve to address the medical needs of the child, they also provide an excellent opportunity for reviewing previously taught information, clarifying family understanding, and presenting new information.

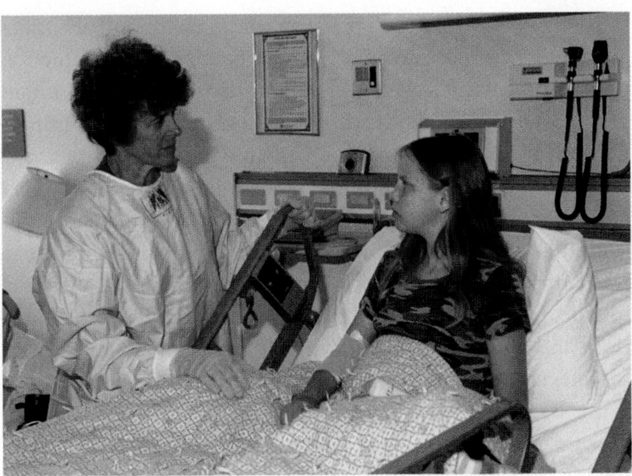

FIGURE 24-12 **Client education of cystic fibrosis should include the need for adequate nutrition, rest, and ongoing follow-up care.** DELMAR CENGAGE LEARNING.

RESPIRATORY DISTRESS SYNDROME

Premature infants born at less than 36 weeks' gestation may develop respiratory distress syndrome (RDS). This occurs because the lungs of premature infants are underdeveloped and lack enough surfactant to keep the alveoli open. At this age, there is also innate structural immaturity of the lungs (Pickerd & Kotecha, 2008). Without being able to get enough oxygen into their bodies, these premature infants develop dyspnea, hypoxia, hypercapnia, and cyanosis and require immediate oxygen administration and, possibly, ventilator use (Dudell & Stoll, 2004).

INCIDENCE AND ETIOLOGY

RDS is the most common condition found and managed in neonatal intensive care units (Jeenakeri & Drayton, 2009). The more premature the newborn, the more likely that RDS will occur. For example, about 60–80% of 28-week gestation infants develop RDS while only 15–30% of those born at 32–36 weeks do so. Infants born beyond 37 weeks' gestation have only about a 5% chance of developing RDS (Dudell & Stoll, 2004). RDS is also more common in male infants and children of mothers who have diabetes (Pickerd & Kotecha, 2008).

PATHOPHYSIOLOGY

Infants with RDS have poor lung compliance. As a result, they generally require mechanical ventilation and supplemental oxygen. The result is trauma to pulmonary structures, which leads to interstitial edema and epithelial destruction. The inflammatory response and accumulation of cellular debris from tissue necrosis causes airway obstruction. Hyperinflation, atelectasis, and tissue fibrosis result. The process may also damage pulmonary vasculature. The overall effect of the disease process is a ventilation-perfusion ratio imbalance that leads to **hypercapnia** and hypoxemia.

CLINICAL MANIFESTATIONS

Infants with RDS have varying degrees of respiratory distress depending on the severity of their illness. Signs and symptoms can appear within minutes of birth and can progressively worsen. Characteristic manifestations include signs and symptoms associated with pulmonary edema and cor pulmonale. Crackles and wheezing are commonly audible with auscultation. Other common signs of RDS are increased work of breathing with retractions, shallow respirations and tachypnea of at least 60 breaths per minute (Dudell & Stoll, 2004). Fluid retention can occur as a result of the infant's heart failure. Although oxygen administration is needed initially to keep these infants ventilated, too much oxygen can cause problems, which should always be kept in mind. Oxygen toxicity from the long-term RDS treatment leads to bronchopulmonary dysplasia (Dudell & Stoll, 2004).

Bronchopulmonary dysplasia (BPD) is a chronic lung disease that primarily affects extremely low birthweight premature infants with respiratory distress syndrome (RDS). Respiratory distress syndrome occurs as a result of premature infants' pulmonary system immaturity and surfactant insufficiency. Without medical intervention, premature infants require treatments to ensure adequate ventilation. Mechanical ventilation, the primary treatment modality, causes trauma to the infant's lungs. The combined effects of mechanical ventilation and a fragile pulmonary system predispose premature infants to BPD.

DIAGNOSIS

The diagnosis of RDS is based on the infant's history, physical examination, laboratory results, and chest X-rays. The diagnosis is suspected when the infant is born prematurely and is exhibiting the clinical symptoms noted above. Chest radiography in infants with RDS can vary, but typically show alveolar hyperinflation, atelectasis, and **fibrosis**. Lab results usually reveal hypoxemia, hypercapnia, and signs of metabolic acidosis. The diagnosis of RDS is made only after other illnesses, such as pneumonia, sepsis, and patent ductus arteriosus, have been ruled out (Dudell & Stoll, 2004).

TREATMENT

Prevention is the primary focus of medical management of RDS, if prevention is possible. Prenatal steroids promote the maturation of fetal lungs. Giving steroids to a mother before delivery, if the baby is going to be born between 24–34 weeks' gestation, has been shown to decrease the risk of mortality and morbidity associated with RDS. The administration of exogenous surfactant lowers alveolar surface tension, allowing the alveoli to open more easily with inspiration and preventing collapse on expiration. The result is more effective ventilation. Pharmacologic agents used to treat RDS include diuretics, steroids, and bronchodilators. Diuretics are used to help manage the infant's pulmonary and systemic edema. Steroids are used to reduce the inflammatory response associated with the disease and its treatment. Mechanical ventilation may be necessary for weeks to months, especially in infants with severe RDS and complications such as persistent apnea, hypoxemia, and hypercapnia. Mechanical ventilation is normally instituted after other modes of oxygen delivery alone or continuous positive airway pressure (CPAP) has failed. A tracheostomy is indicated for infants requiring long-term ventilation. Many infants with RDS are discharged to home still requiring oxygen therapy (Dudell & Stoll, 2004).

For infants who are extremely ill that cannot be ventilated efficiently via mechanical ventilation, an intervention called ECMO may be needed. ECMO stands for extracorporeal membrane oxygenation and is a way to oxygenate a patient's blood outside of their body. It is reserved for very sick babies who have heart or lung problems so significant that they are not able to oxygenate on their own. Some of the common diagnoses requiring ECMO are congenital diaphragmatic hernia, pneumonia, and severe pulmonary hypertension. There are major risks that come along with ECMO, including bleeding, blood clots, and infections. Children placed on ECMO tend to be at risk for death without its use.

Nursing Management and Family Teaching

Nursing management for infants with RDS includes addressing physical needs and providing family support and education. Family-centered, developmentally supportive care is also an important aspect of nursing management of this respiratory alteration. Physical care includes conducting ongoing physical assessment and providing respiratory, nutritional, and developmental support. Respiratory support generally includes managing the infant's artificial airway, ensuring appropriate settings and functioning of the ventilator, monitoring the child's oxygenation and laboratory data, and performing endotracheal suctioning on an as-needed basis. Premature infants, particularly those in respiratory distress, tend to become further compromised with frequent handling. Noninvasive monitoring and coordination of care are measures that help promote the infant's rest, conserve energy, and ease the work of breathing.

A significant challenge for nursing is ensuring that infants with RDS have sufficient nutritional intake. These infants tire easily and their increased work of breathing impairs the coordination of sucking, swallowing, and breathing during feedings. Further, infants with RDS have increased nutritional requirements because of the elevated metabolic rate associated with prematurity. These patients are also at increased risk for developing gastroesophageal reflux, which further interferes with their nutritional intake. Nasogastric feedings are indicated until infants with RDS are stable and can tolerate breastfeeding or bottle feeding. Breast milk is preferred over formula because it is more easily digested and has immunologic benefits. Additionally, small, more frequent feedings are generally better tolerated than large volume feedings.

Infants with a history of RDS have an increased risk for developing respiratory infections and usually continue to have chronic respiratory problems into childhood. Families are taught to recognize early signs of respiratory infection or compromise and to seek medical care for their infant should these signs develop. They are also taught the importance of immunizations as a primary prevention measure. In addition to routine immunizations, infants with a history of RDS frequently receive respiratory syncytial virus immune globulin to lower their risk for developing an RSV infection. The combined effects of this hospitalization, inappropriate environmental stimulation, inadequate nutrition, and respiratory insufficiency place these infants at risk for developmental delays. Developmental considerations must be incorporated into the infants' care in order to maximize their long-term outcomes. This includes minimizing noxious stimuli associated with neonatal nurseries and providing stimuli appropriate for their developmental needs. Caregivers are encouraged to communicate and have physical contact with their infants. They are also encouraged to participate in their infants' care.

Infants with RDS are discharged to their families as soon as they are stable, meet weight requirements, and the family demonstrates its ability to care for the infant. Home care is clearly preferred for infants because of caregiver-infant attachment, and developmental, health, and cost-containment benefits. In addition to general anticipatory guidance, family education for infants with RDS includes teaching related to medications, oxygen therapy, cardiopulmonary monitoring and resuscitation, and follow-up care.

TUBERCULOSIS

Tuberculosis (TB) is an infection caused by the rod-shaped bacterium, *Mycobacterium tuberculosis* (NIAID, 2007). The incidence of TB is increasing worldwide in both affluent countries and poverty-stricken countries (Aberle et al., 2007). The disease can cause very severe symptoms if left untreated. It can manifest both in the pulmonary system and in other body systems, as well (AAP Red Book, 2006).

Incidence and Etiology

Almost one-third of the population of the world is infected with tuberculosis (almost 2 billion people). In 2005, there were about 9 million new cases of tuberculosis (TB) diagnosed (Patel & DeSantis, 2008). TB cases are seen more prevalently in urban and lower socioeconomic areas and in nonwhite racial and ethnic groups. Some of the highest incidence of latent TB infection is seen in international adoptees, immigrants, homeless people, and travelers to countries where TB is more common (AAP Red Book, 2006).

Pathophysiology

The transmission of TB occurs through droplets from the respiratory tract of individuals with active pulmonary infections. The bacilli enter the respiratory tract on droplets of air. Once in the lung, the pathogen reproduces and spreads through the body via the lymph and circulatory systems. Granulomas are formed in the lungs as an inflammatory response to the initial pathogen invasion. These granulomas serve to contain and consume areas of infection. They are eventually replaced by scar tissue as the body heals itself. Pockets of infection in the primary or metastatic sites, however, may survive the immune response and lie dormant until something precipitates its reactivation. The disease causes destruction of the lung parenchyma and pulmonary vasculature, which impairs ventilation and pulmonary blood flow.

There is a difference between latent TB disease and active TB disease. In latent TB disease, the bacteria can enter a persons' lungs but not cause them to become sick. It can lie dormant for a lengthy period of time and not cause symptoms or be transferred to others. However, at any time, the latent disease can progress to active TB disease. For someone to develop active TB the bacteria have to enter the person's body and cause TB infection and then the immune system of the affected person must not be able to stop the TB from spreading (NIAID, 2007).

Clinical Manifestations

During the initial period of infection in children and adolescents, they are asymptomatic and cannot pass the organism to others. The TB infection will progress to TB disease if the body's defenses are unable to fight the disease. When TB disease does occur, symptoms usually are noted 1–6 months after infection. Individuals who do not receive preventive pharmacologic therapy are at risk of developing the disease later in life.

As the TB infection progresses to TB disease in children, some of the most notable symptoms are fever, weight loss or poor weight gain, failure to thrive, cough, and night sweats. Symptoms associated with metastatic infections are specific to the area of involvement. Complications of the disease include TB meningitis, lymphadenopathy and inflammation of the joints and skin (AAP Red Book, 2006).

Diagnosis

The diagnosis of TB is based on the combined findings from physical examinations, X-rays, and positive Mantoux skin tests or the isolation of the *Mycobacterium tuberculosis* organism in body fluids. Isolating *Mycobacterium tuberculosis* from gastric aspirates, sputum, pleural fluid, CSF, urine or other body fluids would establish the diagnosis of TB. The TB skin test is most effective at diagnosing those who have latent TB infection with no symptoms. Prior to performing the skin test in children, a risk assessment should be reviewed with the family. Only if the child is at risk, should they get the skin test. Using the skin test as a screening measure for school, camps, or daycares for children at low-risk should be discouraged. This testing can yield large numbers of false-positive results. The skin test is unreliable in children under 3 months of age. If possible, the risk assessment should be performed annually for children over 2 years old (AAP Red Book, 2006).

Treatment

The treatment for TB depends on whether or not the patient is diagnosed with latent TB infection (LTBI) or TB disease. The goal is to use antituberculosis medications to kill *Mycobacterium tuberculosis* in order to stop the LTBI from progressing to TB disease and to prevent as many complications as possible. The main medications used for TB are ethambutol, isoniazid, pyrazinamide, and rifampin. These drugs should be used in combination in order to prevent new strains of drug-resistant TB from developing (AAP Red Book, 2006).

For infants, children, and adolescents with LTBI (positive skin test, but no signs or symptoms of TB disease and have never taken medications for TB before), the therapy includes isoniazid daily for nine months. For infants, children and adolescents with drug-susceptible pulmonary TB disease, directly observed therapy is highly recommended. For active TB disease, a six-month regimen of multiple medications is recommended. The first two months consist of isoniazid, pyrazinamide, and rifampin. This is followed by four months of isoniazid and rifampin (AAP Red Book, 2006).

Nursing Management and Family Teaching

The nursing management for TB is centered on family and community education. This education should include information related to the prevention and treatment of the disease. Prevention measures include teaching the public about infection control measures and promoting routine Mantoux skin testing. Health teaching also needs to include information about drug therapy used for prophylaxis or treatment regimens. Children generally become infected through contact with adults with active pulmonary disease. Therefore, the most effective way to minimize children's risk for becoming infected is to identify and treat adult contacts.

Migrant and minority families may benefit from additional education and support regarding TB prevention and treatment. Their care needs to be culturally appropriate. Nursing care also should address environmental, structural, and language barriers that may exist. These barriers are thought to play a primary role in disproportionate rates of TB in these populations.

ADDITIONAL RESPIRATORY ALTERATIONS

Additional respiratory alterations include foreign body aspiration, and smoke inhalation injury. Although their epidemiologic impact is limited, a discussion of these conditions is warranted because of their serious, life-threatening potential.

FOREIGN BODY ASPIRATION

Foreign body aspiration in infants and young children is a common and life threatening condition. It occurs most commonly in children under 3 years of age (Altkorn et al., 2008). The cough reflex generally protects the airway from foreign body obstruction. When objects do become lodged in the airway, they can cause partial or complete airway obstruction. Partial airway obstruction leads to atelectasis and air trapping beyond the point of obstruction with subsequent respiratory distress. The majority of foreign body aspiration is into the right main bronchus although less commonly the left main bronchus or trachea can be affected (Heyer et al., 2006; Yadav, Singh, Aggarwal, & Goeal, 2007). Complete airway obstruction in the trachea results in hypoxia and death.

Clinical Manifestations

Children with foreign body aspiration can have symptoms for hours to months prior to an actual diagnosis. Symptoms of foreign body aspiration are variable and can include cough, wheezing, fever, elevation in WBC count, or abnormalities on chest radiograph, and these symptoms can easily be contributed to an upper respiratory infection, asthma or even pneumonia. The most reliable signs of foreign body aspiration are a witnessed choking episode, hyperinflation of one area of the lung, and unilateral wheezing or crackles (Heyer et al., 2006; Righini et al., 2007). Children with complete obstructions are unable to cough, speak, or make vocalization. Cyanosis, loss of consciousness, and death will result if the obstruction is not relieved.

Treatment

Suspected foreign body aspiration is a medical emergency. If the child is conscious, pink, and able to cough, observation and further evaluation is indicated. If the child is not able to cough or make vocalizations, loses consciousness, or turns cyanotic, the Heimlich maneuver should be implemented. Even if a child suspected of having a foreign body aspiration appears stable, shifting of the foreign body could cause further blockage and respiratory compromise and in this situation a child should remain under close medical observation. Ongoing evaluation and surgical retrieval with bronchoscopy should be performed as soon as medically available.

Education is an essential component in the prevention of foreign body aspiration. Infants and young children learn about their environment through oral exploration. They also have fewer teeth, which affects their ability to safely manage foods such as raw fruits and vegetables. Their limited motor and cognitive skills also play a role in their increased risk for foreign body aspiration. Caregivers need to understand these developmental factors and make necessary adjustments in their environments to protect children from harm. Additionally, all caregivers should be encouraged to learn basic first-aid intervention, included management of the obstructed airway.

> **NURSING ALERT**
>
> **Common Causes of Choking in Infants and Young Children**
>
> The most common items that cause foreign body aspiration in infants and young children are small, round, hard, or crunchy foods such as nuts, berries, seeds, corn, or beans (Gregori et al., 2008). The most common item is the peanut. The food associated most with fatal outcomes is the hot dog (Altkorn et al., 2008).

SMOKE INHALATION INJURY

Smoke inhalation injury can be divided into three basic categories: thermal injury, chemical injury throughout the respiratory tract, and systemic toxicity. Patients that suffer from thermal, chemical, or systemic toxicity injuries have high incidence of morbidity and mortality. Even one episode of smoke inhalation can carry long-term pulmonary effects. Often along with the inhalation injury, there are cutaneous burns which can contribute to the poor prognosis in this patient population (Woodson, 2009).

Clinical Manifestations

Immediate manifestations of smoke inhalation are related to inflammatory response from the thermal and chemical injury. Varying degrees of respiratory distress are related to the degree of injury. Pulmonary edema, airway obstruction, decreased airway compliance, and multisystem effects from systemic toxicity are not uncommon manifestations seen with smoke inhalation (Woodson, 2009).

Treatment

The treatment for smoke inhalation depends on the degree of injury. Ongoing assessment and monitoring, oxygen therapy, and supportive care are commonly indicated. Aggressive clearing of mucous and secretions is often necessary, along with antibiotics to prevent infection and ventilatory support as needed (Fidkowski, Fuzaylov, Sheridan, & Cote, 2008).

PREVENTION OF RESPIRATORY ALTERATIONS

Various health promotion strategies can be implemented to reduce the pediatric population's risk for developing respiratory alterations. These strategies include controlling environmental hazards such as secondhand smoke, air pollution, and allergens; minimizing the risk of infection through immunizations and infection control practices; genetic counseling; prenatal care; and anticipatory guidance. Nurses, as child and family advocates, need to educate families about these health promotion strategies. Caregivers are better equipped to create healthy environments for their children when they have the requisite knowledge to create such an environment.

One of the major concerns in relation to respiratory illness related to environmental exposure is secondhand smoke. Secondhand smoke, or passive smoking, has been demonstrated to increase the numbers of respiratory infections in infants and children. Specifically, an increased incidence of pneumonia, otitis media, bronchitis, asthma, allergies, pharyngitis, and colds are connected with passive smoking. Children with asthma who live in homes where there are smokers are twice as likely to be admitted to an emergency room with a respiratory emergency. These children also have a slower recovery from their illness. It is important when obtaining a history on a patient to ask if anyone who interacts regularly with the child smokes at any time, whether it is in the child's presence or not. Smoke on clothing and in automobiles can easily be a trigger, as well.

Even taking a child out to get "fresh air" can, in certain instances, put them at risk for a respiratory episode. Pollution in the air resulting from automotive and industrial emissions can cause or exacerbate certain respiratory conditions. Allergens in the air, such as pollen and mold, can also trigger alterations. At-risk children, such as those with chronic lung disorders, should avoid being outdoors when pollution and allergen indexes are high. Cold weather can also be a trigger for some children with asthma and allergens during spring and fall can be a trigger for children with asthma or hay fever.

Ensuring that children are properly immunized will help decrease their risk for developing a respiratory alteration. Several pediatric respiratory conditions, such as pneumonia, pertussis, and diphtheria, can be either prevented or minimized with the appropriate immunizations. These immunizations are discussed in Chapter 15. Additional immunizations may be used to prevent respiratory alterations in high-risk children such as those with immune, cardiac, or lung disorders. Regular hand washing is a primary strategy for minimizing the spread of pathogens. It is easy and extremely effective. Other common infection control methods include teaching children to cover their mouth and nose when sneezing and to avoid sharing eating utensils, drinks, and towels.

Genetic counseling is indicated when a child is born with an inherited respiratory disorder or when parents are known carriers. For example, a couple who has a child with cystic fibrosis needs to understand that there is a 25% probability that each additional child they have will have the disorder. This information is critical for parents as they make decisions about future children. Prenatal care is a critical health promotion strategy that optimizes health outcomes for children. Comprehensive prenatal care is associated with a decreased incidence of prematurity. Reducing prematurity is important because it is linked to several health alterations including respiratory distress syndrome, bronchopulmonary dysplasia, apnea, and respiratory infections.

Anticipatory guidance about the care and safety of infants and children in the home is another important

IN THE REAL WORLD

I was assigned to care for Khalil, age 3, the day after his tonsillectomy. He had been admitted to the hospital because he was refusing oral fluids. When I performed my initial assessment I noted that he was congested, mouth breathing, and crying. His father stated he could not get his son to eat or drink. He was also quite concerned because he was not able to calm his son. I noted that Khalil had received no pain medication since surgery. His father, who was an ear, nose, and throat (ENT) physician, indicated that his son had been refusing his pain medication because it burned his throat. Clearly, Khalil needed to get his pain under control. I collaborated with Khalil's father and physicians to get an order for IV morphine. Once Khalil's pain was controlled he stopped crying, started drinking, and was able to take his oral pain medication. Within 4 hours he was discharged from the hospital. I was surprised that Khalil's dad had not solved the problem situation beforehand. I was even more surprised that the nursing staff had not gotten the child's pain under control.

This experience, and later personal experiences, taught me that we, as health care providers, sometimes make assumptions about the understanding and coping of health professionals that are on the receiving end of health care. Khalil's father was not his son's health care provider. He was a father. And like other fathers, his focus was on meeting the needs of his son, juggling family and job responsibilities, and dealing with the overwhelming fatigue of being up all night and worrying about his child. The nursing staff and the father's ENT colleagues, yielding to the father's expertise, had stepped away from the situation and were unaware of the need for an intervention. Instead, what we needed to remember was that Khalil's father was not an expert in providing postoperative care to his son. This was a new experience. As health care providers, it is our responsibility to collaborate with families to ensure that interventions are employed that optimize the health outcomes for children. In addition to planning and providing care for children, we also have a responsibility to support and educate the families.

strategy for preventing respiratory alterations. The AAP released a position statement in 2005, recommending that babies be put to sleep in the supine position, an initiative dubbed "Back to Sleep," to help prevent Sudden Infant Death Syndrome (SIDS). The incidence of otitis media can be diminished through breastfeeding, not propping bottles, and keeping the infant away from those who smoke. Breastfeeding provides immune complexes that can protect infants from respiratory infections. Further, caregivers can help protect their children from asthma exacerbations and allergic rhinitis by controlling the amount of allergens in the home. The establishment of a fire evacuation plan in the home, and ensuring that children understand the plan, can lower a child's risk for burns and smoke inhalation injuries. Water safety education can help prevent drowning or near-drowning incidents. Finally, keeping small toys and other items away from infants and young children minimizes choking and the risk of foreign body aspirations.

KEY CONCEPTS

- The primary function of the respiratory tract is to facilitate gas exchange.
- Several anatomic and physiological variations increase infants' and young children's risk for developing a respiratory system dysfunction. These variations include smaller airways, fewer alveoli, increased chest compliance, immature immune systems, and increased oxygen demands.
- Viral respiratory infections are treated with supportive care. Antibiotics are not indicated for these infections unless a secondary bacterial infection has developed.
- A serious complication following a tonsillectomy is hemorrhage. Frequent swallowing is the earliest manifestation of bleeding during the postoperative period.
- Otitis media is the most common infectious disease of childhood and is often a complication of an upper respiratory tract infection.
- Croup is characterized by hoarseness, a "barky" or croupy cough, inspiratory stridor, and varying degrees of respiratory distress.
- Acute epiglottitis is a life-threatening bacterial infection that can lead to complete airway obstruction. Respiratory distress, dysphagia, drooling, fever, agitation, and lethargy are classic manifestations of this condition.
- Bronchiolitis is an acute infection of the bronchioles. The respiratory syncytial virus is the most common etiologic agent. Symptoms include labored respirations, wheezing, prolonged expiratory phase, and intermittent cyanosis.
- Pneumonia is the result of the accumulation of secretions, cellular debris, and other exudate resulting from airway infection and inflammation.
- Asthma is the leading cause of chronic illness in children. Nursing management is focused on educating the family and child regarding preventive medications, symptoms, triggers, treatments, and the importance of follow-up care.
- Cystic fibrosis is an autosomal recessive disorder that primarily affects the lungs and digestive tracts. The disorder is managed with aggressive therapies to prevent lung function decline and to sustain normal nutrition. Most individuals with this disease live well into adulthood.
- Respiratory distress syndrome (RDS) is a respiratory dysfunction in premature infants. It occurs because the lungs of premature infants are underdeveloped and lack enough surfactant to keep the alveoli open.
- Tuberculosis is significant in terms of global morbidity and mortality. Prevention is a prime focus of care.
- Health promotion strategies that can reduce the pediatric population's risk for developing respiratory alterations include controlling environmental pollutants, routine immunizations, prenatal care, genetic counseling, infection control practices, and anticipatory guidance related to care and safety in the home.

REVIEW ACTIVITIES

1. Describe the anatomic differences in a child's respiratory tract from those in the adult's tract that make the child more susceptible to respiratory tract infections.
2. Develop a family teaching plan for care of a child during the pre- and post-tonsillectomy periods.
3. Develop a care plan for a child with croup.
4. Describe the clinical manifestations of nasopharyngitis.
5. Differentiate between OME and AOM.
6. Develop a family teaching plan for the care of a child with AOM.

7. Discuss the clinical manifestations of pneumonia in a child.
8. Explain the treatment approaches for the different categories of asthma.
9. Describe some of the latest advances in therapy for children with cystic fibrosis.
10. Identify five ways to minimize a child's risk for developing a respiratory alteration.

STUDY QUESTIONS

1. Why is it that infants and children are at more risk for complications due to respiratory infections than adults?
   a. Infants and children are still "learning how to breathe" and have uncoordinated, inefficient breathing until a later age.
   b. Infants and young children have smaller respiratory passageways and are more vulnerable to obstruction.
   c. Infants and children have more rigid chest walls, making them less pliable and more resistant to change.
   d. Infants and children are more vulnerable and more frequently exposed to other children with germs.
2. What are the most common causes of acute otitis media infections in children?
   a. Viral
   b. Mycobacterium tuberculosis and Group A beta-hemolytic streptococci
   c. Strep pneumoniae, *haemophilus influenzae*, moraxella catarrhalis
   d. Foreign body in the ear
3. Which of the risk factors below, combined, would put a child at most risk for acquiring RSV?
   a. A full-term infant with history of wheezing in the past, born in March
   b. A 3-year-old little girl who does not yet attend daycare or school and lives in a home where both parents smoke
   c. A 10-year-old boy who had been pneumonia when he was 2 years old and admitted into the hospital at that time
   d. An infant who is now 4 months old who was born at 30 weeks' gestation as one of twins in the month of September
4. What are the major ways in which pneumonia is diagnosed?
   a. History, physical findings, and sputum culture
   b. Complete blood count and chest X-ray
   c. Blood culture and sputum culture
   d. Pulmonary function tests and spirometry
5. What are the major symptoms in allergic rhinitis?
   a. Wheezing, cough, and itchy eyes
   b. Not sleeping well, congestion, and cough
   c. Congestion, sneezing, and itchy eyes and nose
   d. Temperature and sore throat
6. For a child with moderate persistent asthma, which elevated therapies would you recommend him or her to be on?
   a. Herbal supplements, a multivitamin, and acupuncture
   b. An inhaled corticosteroid, a long-acting bronchodilator, and a short-acting beta agonist to use with exacerbations
   c. A daily oral steroid and a leukotriene modifier
   d. An antibiotic
7. What symptoms in a child might lead a provider towards testing for cystic fibrosis?
   a. Chronic cough and wheeze, improves with short-acting beta agonist
   b. Congestion, itchy eyes, sneezing
   c. Recurrent otitis infections and chronic nasal discharge
   d. Recurrent respiratory infections, poor weight gain, and mucous-like stools
8. What needs to occur for someone to develop active TB disease?
   a. They need to drink out of the same glass as someone who has latent or active TB, and they need to have a genetic predisposition for developing TB.
   b. They need to have been exposed to TB so Mycobacterium tuberculosis has entered their body, and they need to have a compromised immune system which cannot fight off the TB bacteria.
   c. They need to be exposed to the blood or mucous of someone who has latent or active TB.
   d. They need to have a relative or close friend with active TB.
9. Which of the following children would most likely be diagnosed with sinusitis?
   a. An 11-year-old with cold symptoms for twelve days, complaining of headache, facial pain and postnasal drip
   b. A 3-year-old with fever of 100°F and runny nose for 4 days
   c. A 10-month-old with audible wheezing, congestion, and cough
   d. A 9-year-old who says that there have been numerous children absent from her class and has sore throat, abdominal pain, and low-grade fever

10. What are the most important preventive measures when it comes to respiratory illnesses in children?
    a. Taking your child to the pediatrician as soon as he or she presents with any respiratory symptoms at all, and giving antibiotics as soon as possible.
    b. Attempting to raise the child in a mild, warm environment, with less exposure to winter weather and extreme changes in temperature.
    c. Controlling inhalation of second-hand smoke and exposure to pollutants, good hand-washing techniques, immunizations, and good parental teaching.
    d. Making sure the child lives in a home with hardwood floors and no pets.

REFERENCES

Aberle, N., Bublic, J., Feric, M., Bukvic, B., Simic, A., Trtica, B. et al. (2007). Increasing rate of childhood tuberculosis in a region of east Croatia. *Pediatrics International, 49*, 183–189.

Altkorn, R., Chen, X., Milkovich, S., Stool, D., Rider, G., Bailey, C. M., Haas, A. et al. (2008). Fatal and non-fatal food injuries among children (aged 0–14 years). *International Journal of Pediatric Otorhinolaryngology, 72*(7), 1041–1046.

American Academy of Pediatrics Red Book Online. (2006). Antimicrobial agents and related therapy; principles of appropriate use for upper respiratory tract infections. Retrieved March 24, 2009, from http://aapredbook.aappublications.org.

American Lung Association. (2009). Trends in asthma morbidity and mortality. American Lung Association Epidemiology and Statistics Unit, Research and Program Services Division. Available at http://www.lungusa.org/.

Barson, W. (2009). Epidemiology, pathogenesis, and etiology of pneumonia in children. www.UpToDate version 17.1.

Bjornson, C. L., & Johnson, D. W. (2008). Croup. *Lancet, 371*(9609), 329–339.

Bolt, P., Barnett, P., Babl, F. E., & Sharwood, L. N. (2008). Topical lignocaine for pain relief in acute otitis media: Results of a double blind placebo controlled randomized trial. *Archives of Disease in Childhood, 93*, 40–44.

Brashers, V. (2004). Alterations of pulmonary function. In S. Huether & K. McCance (Eds.). *Understanding pathophysiology* (3rd ed.). St. Louis: Mosby.

Brook, I., & Gober, A. E. (2008). Concurrent influenza A and group A beta-hemolytic streptococcal pharyngotonsillitis. *Annals of Otology, Rhinology & Laryngology, 117*(4), 310–312.

Burkhart, P. V., Svavarsdottir, E. K., Rayens, M. K., Oakley, M. G., & Orlygsdottir, B. (2009). Adolescents with asthma: Predictors of quality of life. *Journal of Advanced Nursing, 65*(4), 860–866.

Carr, W. W. (2008). Pediatric allergic rhinitis: A current focus and future state of the art. *Allergy and Asthma Proceedings, 29*(1), 14–23.

Carter, N. (2006). Delivery of 100%, 40% and below by humidity did not differ for change in croup scores in children with moderate croup. *Evidence Based Nursing, 9*(4), 105.

Centers for Disease Control and Prevention. (2007). Infant deaths associated with cough and cold medications—two states, 2005. *Morbidity and Mortality Weekly Report, 56*(1), 1–4.

Chao, J. H., Kunkow, S., Reyes, L.B., Licten, S., & Crain, E. F. (2008). Comparison of two approaches to observation therapy for acute otitis media in the emergency department. *Pediatrics, 121*(5), e1352–e1356.

Checchia, P. (2008). Identification and management of severe respiratory syncytial virus. *American Journal of Health-System Pharmacists, 65*(8), S7–S12.

Cherry, J. D. (2008). Clinical Practice: Croup. *New England Journal of Medicine, 358*(4), 384–391.

Chetty, K., & Thomson, A. H. (2007). Management of community-acquired pneumonia in children. *Paediatric Drugs, 9*(6), 410–411.

Cystic Fibrosis Foundation. (2009). Treatment of Pulmonary Exacerbation of Cystic Fibrosis, Clinical Practice Guidelines. Retrieved March 24, 2009, from http://www.cff.org.

De Sutter, A., Lemiengre, M., Van Maele, G., van Driel, M., De Meyere, M., Christians, T., et al. (2006). Predicting prognosis of effect of antibiotic treatment in rhinosinusitis. *Annals of Family Medicine, 4*(6), 486–493.

Dudell, G. G., & Stoll, B. J. (2004). Respiratory tract disorders—respiratory distress syndrome (hyaline membrane disease). *Nelson textbook of pediatrics* (18th ed.). Philadelphia: Saunders, pp. 731–742.

Fanta, C. (2009). Asthma. *New England Journal of Medicine, 360*(10), 1002–1014.

Fidkowski, C. W., Fuzaylov, G., Sheridan, R. L., & Cote, C. J. (2008). Inhalation burn injury in children. *Paediatric Anaesthesia*, December 2008: 1–8.

Fifoot, A. A., & Ting, J. (2007). Comparison between single dose oral prednisolone and oral dexamethaosone in the treatment of croup: A randomized double-blind clinical trial. *Emergency Medicine Australia, 19*, 15–18.

Flume, P., O'Sullivan, B., Robinson, K., Goss, C., Mogayzel, P., Willey-Courand, D. B., et al. (2007). Cystic fibrosis pulmonary guidelines: Chronic medications for maintenance of lung health. *American Journal of Respiratory and Critical Care Medicine, 176*, 957–969.

Flume, P. A., Robinson, K. A., O'Sullivan, B. P., Finder, J. D., Vender, R. L., Willey-Courand, D. B., et al. (2009). Clinical practice guidelines for Pulmonary Therapies Committee. Cystic fibrosis pulmonary guidelines: Airway clearance therapies. *Respiratory Care, 54*(4), 522–537.

Foxlee, R., Johansson, A., Wejalk, J., Dawkins, J., Dooley, L., & Del Mar, C. (2006). Topical analgesia for acute otitis media. *Cochrane Database of Systematic Reviews*, 3: CD005657.

Gregori, D., Salerni, L., Scarinzi, C., Morra, B., Berchialla, P., Corradetti, R. et al. (2008). Foreign bodies in the upper airways causing complications and requiring hospitalization in children 0–14 years; results from ESFBI study. *European Archives of Otolaryngology, 265*(8), 971–978.

Griffen, G. H., Flynn, C., Bailey, R. E., & Schultz, J. K. (2006). Antihistamines and/or decongestants for otitis media with effusion in children. *Cochrane Database of Systematic Reviews, 4*: CD003423.

Grosse, S. D., Boyle, C. A., Botkin, J. R., Comeau, A. M., Kharrazi, M., Rosenfeld, M., & Wilfond, B. S. (2004) Newborn screening for CF: Evaluation of benefits and risk and recommendations for state newborn screening programs. *Morbidity and Mortality Weekly Review, 53*, 1–36.

Hale, K. A., & Issacs, D. (2006). Antibiotics in childhood pneumonia. *Paediatric Respiratory Reviews, 7*(2), 145–151.

Harrison, C. J. (2004). Pediatric practice: The new guideline for managing otitis media. *Patient Care for the Nurse Practitioner.* Retrieved February 7, 2006, from http://www.patientcarenp.com/pcnp/article/articleDetail.jsp/id5119431.

Heyer, C. M., Bollmeier, M. E., Rossler, L., Nuesslein, T. G., Stephan, V., Bauer, T. T., et al. (2006). Evaluation of clinical radiologic and laboratory prebronchoscopy findings in children with suspected foreign body aspiration. *Journal of Pediatric Surgery, 41*(11), 1882–1888.

Huabin, L. I., Quan, S., Zuo, K., Hongyan, J., Cheng, L., Shi, J., et al. (2009). Nasal saline irrigation facilitates control of allergic rhinitis by topical steroid in children. *Journal of Otorhinolaryngology, 71*(1).

Jeenakeri, R., & Drayton, M. (2009). Management of respiratory distress syndrome. *Peadiatrics and Child Health, 19*(4), 158–164.

Johnson, C., Butler, S., Konstan, M., Morgan, W., & Wohl, M. E. (2003). Factors influencing outcomes in cystic fibrosis. *Chest, 123,* 20–27.

Kaari, J. (2006). The role of intranasal steroids in the management of pediatric allergic rhinitis. *Clinical Pediatrics, 45*(8), 697–704.

Koopman, L., Hoes, A. W., Glasziou, P. P., Appelman, C. L., Burke, P., McCormick, D. P., et al. (2008). Antibiotic therapy to prevent the development of asymptomatic middle ear effusion in children with acute otitis media: A meta-analysis of individual patient data. *Archives of Otolaryngology, 134*(2), 128–132.

Kurugol, Z., Bayram, N., & Atik, T. (2007). Effect on zinc sulfate on common cold in children: Randomized, double blind study. *Pediatrics International, 49,* 842–847.

Lieberthal, A. S., Ganiats, T. G., Cox, E. O., Culpepper, L., Mahoney, M., Miller, D., et al. (2004). American Academy of Pediatrics and American Academy of Family Physicians: Clinical Practice Guideline for the diagnosis and management of acute otitis media. *Pediatrics, 113*(5), 1451–1465.

McWilliams, D. B., Jacobson, R. M., Van Houten, H. K., Naessens, J. M., Ytterberg, K. L., & Berman, S. (2008). A program of anticipatory guidance for the prevention of emergency department visits for ear pain. *Archives of Pediatric and Adolescent Medicine, 162*(2), 151–156.

Meltzer, E. O. (2006). Allergic rhinitis: Managing the pediatric spectrum. *Allergy and Asthma Proceedings, 27*(1), 2–8.

Milgrom, H., & Leung, D. Y. M. (2004). Allergic rhinitis. In R. E. Behrman, R. M. Kliegman, & H. B. Jenson, *Nelson Textbook of Pediatrics* (17th ed.). Philadelphia: Saunders, pp. 759–760.

Moore, M., & Little, P. (2007). Humidified air for treating croup: A systematic review and meta analysis. *Family Practice, 24*(4), 295–301.

National Asthma Education and Prevention Program. (2003). Expert panel report: Guidelines for the diagnosis and management of asthma: Update on selected topics 2002. Bethesda, MD: National Heart, Lung, and Blood Institute; National Institutes of Health; U.S. Department of Health and Human Services. NIH Publication No. 02-5074, pp. 117–118, 120–121. Retrieved September 8, 2005, from http://www.nhlbi.nih.gov.

National Asthma Education and Prevention Program. (2007). Expert panel report 3: Guidelines for the diagnosis and management of asthma. US Department of Health and Human Services; National Institutes of Health; National Heart Lung and Blood Institute. NIH Publication Number 08-5846. Retrieved June 24, 2010, from http://www.nhlbi.nih.gov/guidelines/asthma/asthsumm.pdf.

National Heart, Lung, and Blood Institute, a part of the National Institutes of Health and the U.S. Department of Health and Human Services. Retrieved December 9, 2010, from http://www.nhlbi.nih.gov/guidelines/asthma.

National Institute of Allergy and Infectious Diseases. (2007). Available at http://www3.niaid.nih.gov.

National Institute of Allergy and Infectious Diseases. (2008). Available at http://www3.niaid.nih.gov.

Nayak A., & Langdon, R. B. (2007). Monteleukast in the treatment of allergic rhinitis: An evidenced based review. *Drugs, 67*(6), 887–901.

Ostapchuk, M., Roberts, D. M., & Haddy, R. (2004). Community acquired pneumonia in infants and children. *American Academy of Family Physicians, 70,* 899–908.

Patel, S., & DeSantis, E. R. (2008). Treatment of congenital tuberculosis. *American Journal of Health-System Pharmacists, 65,* 2027–2031.

Pickerd, N., & Kotecha, S. (2008). Pathophysiology of respiratory distress syndrome. *Paediatrics and Child Health, 19*(4), 153–157.

Righini, C. A., More, N., Karkas, A., Reyt, E., Ferretti, K., Pin, I. et al. (2007). What is the diagnostic value of flexible rigid bronchoscopy in the initial investigation of children with suspected foreign body aspiration? *International Journal of Pediatric Otorhinolaryngology, 71*(9), 1383–1390.

Robinson, R. (2008). Impact of respiratory syncytial virus in the United States. *American Journal of Health-System Pharmacists, 65*(8), S3–S6.

Roder, E., Berger, M. Y., deGroot, H., & Van Wijk, R. G. (2008). Immunotherapy in children and adolescents with allergic rhinoconjunctivitis: A systematic review. *Pediatric Allergy and Immunology, 19*(3), 197–207.

Rosenfeld, R. M., Culpepper, L., Doyle, K. J., Grundfast, K. M., Hoberman, A., & Kenna, M. A. et al. (2004). American Academy of Pediatrics Clinical Practice Guideline for otitis media with effusion. *Pediatrics, 113*(5), 1412–1429.

Rote, N., Huether, S., & McCance, K. (2004). Hypersensitivities, infection, and immunodeficiencies. In S. Huether & K. McCance (Eds.), *Understanding Pathophysiology* (3rd ed.). St. Louis: Mosby.

Scadding, G. (2008). Optimal management of nasal congestion caused by allergic rhinitis in children: Safety and efficacy of medical treatments. *Paediatric Drugs, 10*(3), 151–162.

Scottish Intercollegiate Guidelines Network (SIGN). (2006). Bronchiolitis in Children: A National Clinical Guideline. Retrieved on June 26, 2010, from http://www.sign.ac.uk/pdf/sign91pdf.

Smyth, R. L., & Openshaw, P. J. M. (2006). Bronchiolitis. *Lancet, 368,* 312–322.

Spiro, D. M., & Arnold, D. H. (2008). The concept and practice of a wait and see approach to acute otitis media. *Current Opinion in Pediatrics, 20*(1), 72–78.

Stallings, V., Stark, L., Robinson, K., Feranchak, A., & Quinton, H. (2008). Clinical practice guidelines on growth and nutrition subcommittee; ad hoc working group. Evidence-based practice recommendations for nutrition-related management of children and adults with cystic fibrosis and pancreatic insufficiency: Results of a systematic review. *Journal of the American Dietician Association, 108,* 832–839.

Sung, V., Massie, J., Hochmann, M. A., Carlin, J. B., Jamsen, K., & Robertson, C. F. (2008). Estimating inspired oxygen concentration delivered by nasal prongs in children with bronchiolitis. *Journal of Paediatrics and Child Health, 44,* 14–18.

Traynor, K. (2007). FDA investigating nonprescription cough and cold products. *American Journal of Health-System Pharmacists, 64,* 802–803.

Turkoski, B. B. (2007). Medicating young or very young patients—part II. *Orthopaedic Nursing, 26*(3), 194–201.

van Driel, M., De Sutter, A., Deveugele, M., Peersman, W., Butler, C. C., Meyere, M. D. et al. (2006). Are sore throat patients who hope for antibiotics actually asking for pain relief? *Annals of Family Medicine, 4*(6), 494–498.

Vilagoftis, H., Kouranos, V. D., Betsi, G. I., & Falagas, M. E. (2008). Probiotics for the treatment of allergic rhinitis and asthma: A systematic review of randomized controlled trials. *Annals of Allergy, Asthma, and Immunology, 101*(6), 570–579.

West, J. B. (2004). *Respiratory physiology: The essentials* (7th ed.). Philadelphia: Lippincott Williams & Wilkins.

Woodson, L. C. (2009). Diagnosis and grading of inhalation injury. *Journal of Burn Care & Research, 30*(1), 143–145.

Wright, C. M., Williams, G., & Ludeman, L. (2007). Comparison of two rapid tests for detecting Group A Streptococcal Pharyngitis in the pediatric population at Wright-Patterson Air Force Base. *Military Medicine, 172,* 644–646.

Yadav, S. P., Singh, J., Aggarwal, N., & Goeal, A. (2007). Airway foreign bodies in children: experience of 132 cases. *Singapore Medical Journal, 48*(9), 850–853.

SUGGESTED READINGS

Arruda, L. K., Sole, D., Baena-Cagnani, C. E., & Naspitz, C. K. (2005). Risk factors for asthma and atopy. *Current Opinion in Allergy and Clinical Immunology, 5,* 153–159.

Asthma. (2004). *The Nurse Practitioner, 30*(4), 49–50.

Bulechek, G., Butcher, H., & Dochterman, J. (2008). *Nursing Interventions Classification (NIC)* (5th ed). St. Louis, MO: Mosby.

Kimball, C. T. (Ed.). (2004). *Childhood diseases and disorders sourcebook.* Detroit, MI: Omnigraphics.

Laumbach, R. J., & Kipen, H. M. (2005). Bioaerosols and sick building syndrome: Particles, inflammation, and allergy. *Current Opinion in Allergy and Clinical Immunology, 5,* 135–139.

Moorhead, S., Johnson, M., Maas, M., & Swanson, E. (2008). *Nursing Outcomes Classification (NOC)* (4th ed). St. Louis, MO: Mosby.

Ngoc, L. P., Gold, D. R., Tzianabos, A. O., Weiss, S. T., & Celedon, J. C. (2005). Cytokines, allergy, and asthma. *Current Opinion in Allergy and Clinical Immunology, 5,* 161–166.

Reznick, M., Ozuah, P. O., Franco, K., Cohen, R., & Motlow, F. (2002). Use of complementary therapy by adolescents with asthma. *Archives of Pediatrics and Adolescent Medicine, 156*(10), 1042–1044.

RESOURCES

Refer to the online student StudyWARE for Potts & Mandleco at http://www.CengageBrain.com for additional content and study aids.

Organization: **Allergy and Asthma Network** (Mothers of Asthmatics, Inc.)
Description: Allergy & Asthma Network Mothers of Asthmatics (AANMA) is the leading nonprofit family health organization dedicated to eliminating suffering and death due to asthma, allergies, and related conditions. The website is a wealth of information regarding publications, advocacy, and related health topics.
Website/Resource: http://www.aanma.org

Organization: **American Academy of Allergy, Asthma & Immunology**
Description: The American Academy of Allergy, Asthma & Immunology (AAAAI) is the largest professional medical organization in the United States devoted to the allergy/immunology specialty. The AAAAI represents asthma specialists, clinical immunologists, allied health professionals and others with a special interest in the research and treatment of allergic disease. The website offers links to information for patients/consumers, professionals, and members.
Website/Resource: http://www.aaaai.org

Organization: **American Lung Association**
Description: The American Lung Association is the leading organization working to save lives by improving lung health and preventing lung disease through education, advocacy, and research. The website offers readers a wealth of information regarding lung diseases, current and future cures, smoking cessation, and air pollution concerns.
Website/Resource: http://www.lungusa.org

Organization: **Asthma & Allergy Foundation of America (AAFA)**
Description: The Asthma and Allergy Foundation of America (AAFA) is the leading patient organization for people with asthma and allergies, and the oldest asthma and allergy patient group in the world. AAFA provides practical information, community based services and support to people through a network of regional chapters, educational support groups and other local partners around the United States. AAFA develops health education, organizes state and national advocacy efforts, and funds research to find better treatments and cures. The mission of AAFA's website is to provide online access to reliable, validated asthma and allergy information and tools to families, patients, parents, health care providers, policymakers, and others.
Website/Resource: http://www.aafa.org

Organization: **Centers for Disease Control and Prevention**
Description: The Centers for Disease Control and Prevention (CDC) serves as the national focus for developing and applying disease prevention and control, environmental health, and health promotion and health education activities designed to improve the health of the people of the United States. The CDC website offers readers information regarding current disease conditions, emergency preparedness and response, life stages and populations, healthy living, workplace environment and health, traveler's health, and much more.
Website/Resource: http://www.cdc.gov

Organization: **Cystic Fibrosis Foundation**
Description: The mission of the Cystic Fibrosis Foundation, a nonprofit donor-supported organization, is to assure the development of the means to cure and control cystic fibrosis and to improve the quality of life for those with the disease. The website offers users

access to general cystic fibrosis information and information regarding available treatments.

Website/Resource: http://www.cff.org

Organization: **Mayo Clinic Web Site**

Description: Mayohealth.org is an information database in which more than 3,300 physicians, scientists, and researchers from Mayo Clinic share their expertise to empower good health around the world. The website offers users access to a wealth of information regarding diseases/conditions, symptoms, drugs/supplements, tests/procedures, healthy lifestyle, and first aid.

Website/Resource: http://www.mayohealth.org

Organization: **NIH/National Heart, Lung, and Blood Institute Information Center**

Description: The National Heart, Lung, and Blood Institute (NHLBI) provides global leadership for a research, training, and education program to promote the prevention and treatment of heart, lung, and blood diseases and enhance the health of all individuals so that they can live longer and more fulfilling lives. The website provides information regarding networks, research, clinical trials, careers/training, and education campaigns.

Website/Resource: http://www.nhlbi.nih.gov

Organization: **National Asthma Education & Prevention Program**

Description: The National Asthma Education and Prevention Program (NAEPP) was initiated in March 1989 to address the growing problem of asthma in the United States. The NAEPP is administered and coordinated by the National Heart, Lung, and Blood Institute (NHLBI). The NAEPP works with intermediaries including major medical associations, voluntary health organizations, and community programs to educate patients, health professionals, and the public. The ultimate goal of the NAEPP is to enhance the quality of life for patients with asthma and decrease asthma-related morbidity and mortality. The website offers users information regarding program descriptions and committee rosters.

Website/Resource: http://www.nhlbi.nih.gov

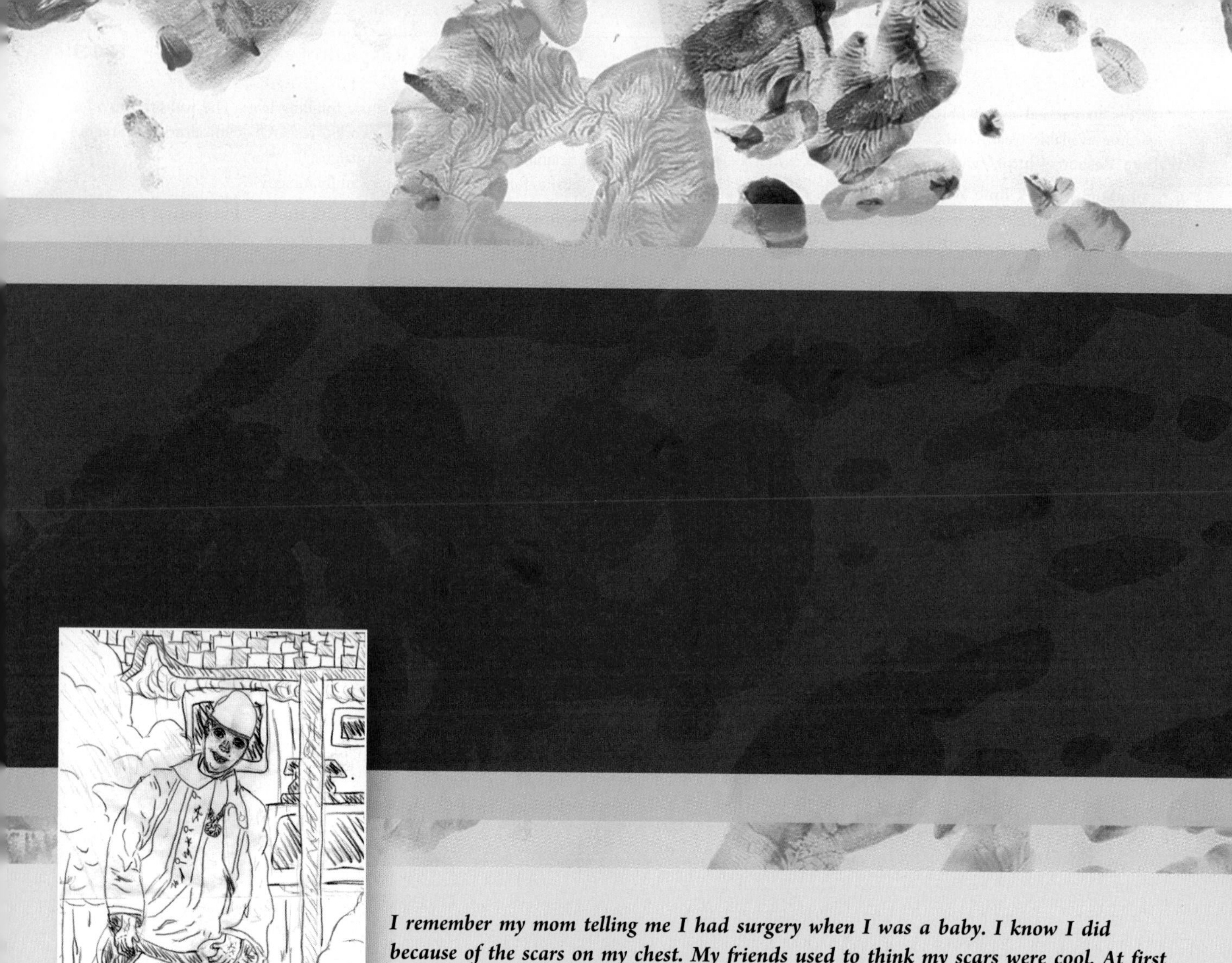

I remember my mom telling me I had surgery when I was a baby. I know I did because of the scars on my chest. My friends used to think my scars were cool. At first I felt like everyone else, until middle school. Then it got to be hard to play sports or even to do PE. I couldn't keep up with my friends. Now I try to do things but I have to take my time. I go to the cardiologist twice a year for a check up. She says that I am doing well.... what does THAT mean? All I want is to be like everyone else in my class.

From the Mother's Perspective:

A child is a precious gift that should not be taken for granted. When a child is diagnosed with heart disease, this becomes a parent's nightmare. They become numb to reality, living in a world of disbelief and fear. Parents don't want statistics and evasive answers for their many questions; they want support, education ... the truth. Parents and family members need to understand the quality of life their child will have based on the decisions they will make. There will always be the doubts, fears, and questions.

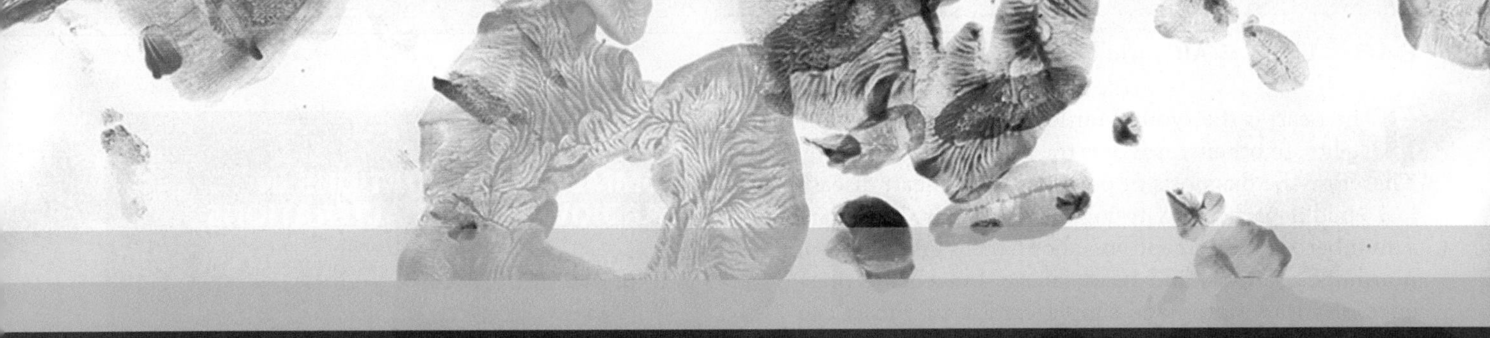

CHAPTER 25

Cardiovascular Alterations

JANET CRAIG, RN, MS, PNP
BONNIE CLAY, RN, MS, CCRN, PNP

COMPETENCIES

Upon completion of this chapter, the reader will be able to:

- Explain the differences in anatomy and physiology of the child's cardiovascular system as compared to the adult's.
- Perform an assessment of the child with heart disease.
- Describe the clinical symptoms of congestive heart failure and identify appropriate interventions.
- Identify two congenital heart lesions that increase pulmonary blood flow.
- Identify two congenital heart lesions that decrease pulmonary blood flow, resulting in cyanosis.
- Develop a plan of care for the child who has undergone open heart surgery.
- Describe the disorder and treatment for acute rheumatic fever, Kawasaki disease, and infectious endocarditis.
- Identify the three forms of shock.
- Identify interventions to support the psychosocial well-being of the child with heart disease and caregivers.
- Successfully complete the games and activities in the online student StudyWARE.

The heart is the symbol for love, emotion, and mortality. In other words, it is the essence of well-being. Therefore the diagnosis of possible or real heart disease in a child is particularly trying for the family. There are a number of misperceptions about the significance of murmurs, cyanosis, and heart failure. Indeed the presence of an asymptomatic simple cardiac diagnosis can evoke fears and concerns that are very real to the family. Many times family concerns over a simple cardiac condition exceed those raised by a more life-threatening condition in another body part.

The estimated prevalence of congenital heart disease is 4–50 per 1,000 live births, and 40% of these children will be diagnosed in the first year of life. However this may underestimate the true prevalence since many simple defects may not be identified until well into adulthood (Pierpont et al., 2007). This number does not include those children who develop acquired heart disease. Over the last 50 years significant advances have been made in the diagnosis, treatment, and evaluation of the child with heart disease. As a result of these advances the vast majority will survive into adulthood. Nevertheless, concerns about treatment plans, possibility of death, lifestyle changes, and finances remain for the child and family.

Pathophysiology in pediatric heart disease is widely variable and challenging to even the most experienced clinician. Care of the child with heart disease requires a multidisciplinary approach. A sound knowledge of normal and abnormal physiology is critically important to the understanding of pathology, therapeutic interventions, and responses to treatments.

Caring for children with heart disease can also be rewarding. Innovations and technological advances continue to improve outcomes. However, a number of life issues remain for the family and child. The nurse is in a pivotal position to support innovative technologies, assess response to intervention, provide education, and facilitate growth and development. Often the nurse serves as the liaison between the family and health care team. A sound understanding of anatomy, physiology, and pathophysiology provides the basis for nursing intervention. Exciting opportunities await those who are interested in participating in this specialty. Opportunities are available for nursing research in a number of areas, including physiological responses, psychosocial effects, and development of children with heart disease.

As more of these children survive into adulthood a whole new subspecialty has emerged—the adult with congenital heart disease. These clients require knowledgeable, skillful nurses who understand congenital heart disease as well as the normal life issues that young adults face. Concerns regarding pregnancy, work, insurance, parenting, and healthy lifestyles become paramount. Life is a continuum; therefore, we can no longer afford to segregate pediatric cardiac issues from adult health issues. Nurses are the key to improved outcomes in *all* clients with congenital and acquired heart disease.

This chapter will review normal cardiovascular anatomy and physiology, congestive heart failure, congenital and acquired heart disease, and shock. Nursing concerns specific to this population will be addressed providing a sound basis for future practice and stimulating further investigation into the nursing care of the child with heart disease. Box 25-1 provides a list of common terms and abbreviations used in the discussion of cardiovascular alterations.

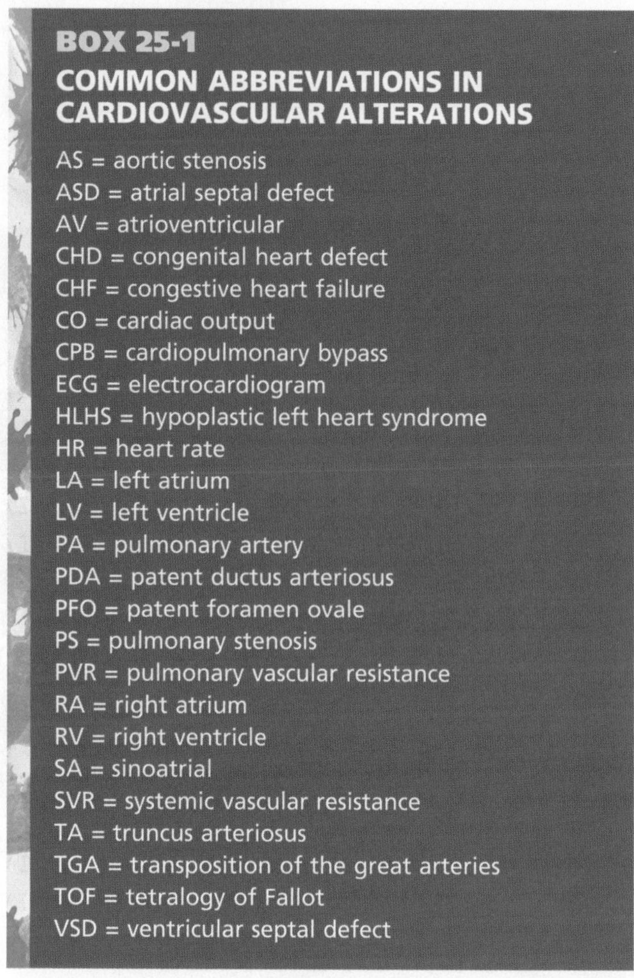
BOX 25-1
COMMON ABBREVIATIONS IN CARDIOVASCULAR ALTERATIONS

AS = aortic stenosis
ASD = atrial septal defect
AV = atrioventricular
CHD = congenital heart defect
CHF = congestive heart failure
CO = cardiac output
CPB = cardiopulmonary bypass
ECG = electrocardiogram
HLHS = hypoplastic left heart syndrome
HR = heart rate
LA = left atrium
LV = left ventricle
PA = pulmonary artery
PDA = patent ductus arteriosus
PFO = patent foramen ovale
PS = pulmonary stenosis
PVR = pulmonary vascular resistance
RA = right atrium
RV = right ventricle
SA = sinoatrial
SVR = systemic vascular resistance
TA = truncus arteriosus
TGA = transposition of the great arteries
TOF = tetralogy of Fallot
VSD = ventricular septal defect

ANATOMY AND PHYSIOLOGY

NORMAL CARDIAC ANATOMY

The cardiovascular system is the first system to function in the developing fetus. The heart begins as a tube by the third week of gestation. This tube loops to the right and begins to fold into itself (Figure 25-1). Incomplete partitioning of the atria leaves a small opening called the foramen ovale (normal in utero connection in the atrial septum), which normally closes after birth. In addition the ductus arteriosus (a blood vessel connecting the aorta with the pulmonary artery) serves to divert blood from the fetal lungs to the fetal aorta as the lungs do not participate in gas exchange in utero. This structure usually closes after birth. Final formation of the ventricular septum occurs by the seventh week of gestation (Figure 25-2) (VanPraagh, 2006). Cardiac

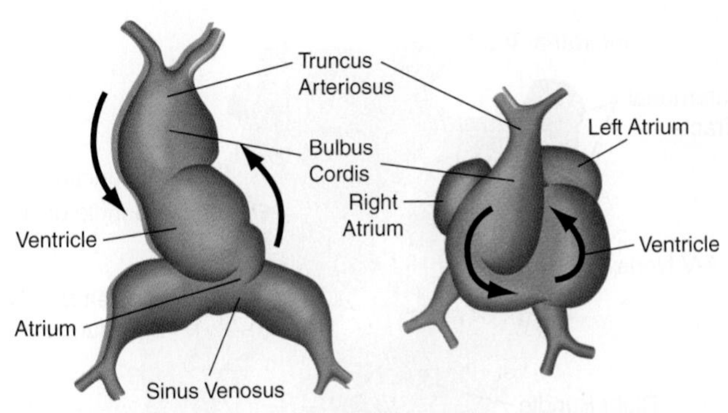

FIGURE 25-1 Normal Folding of the Heart Tube that Occurs Between 23 and 28 Days of Gestation. DELMAR CENGAGE LEARNING.

development is nearly complete by 8 weeks of gestation. Cardiac abnormalities account for about 25% of all congenital malformations. Most malformations are multifactorial secondary to genetic defects, abnormal fetal hemodynamics, and environmental factors. Many defects occur before the pregnant woman knows she has conceived (Jenkins et al., 2007; Pierpont et al., 2007).

The fully developed heart is a four-chambered structure that lies between the lungs in the mediastinum. Heart size corresponds with the size of the child's fist; this correlation continues into adulthood. Normal position is distinguished by the ventricular apex, which is directed downward and toward the left (Figure 25-3). The atria are thin-walled low-pressure chambers that serve as reservoirs for the ventricles. The ventricles are the cardiac pumps. The right ventricle is a low pressure chamber that drives blood to the low resistance pulmonary circulation (lungs) via the pulmonary artery. The left ventricle is a high pressure chamber that drives blood to the high resistance systemic circulation (body) via the aorta. There are four cardiac valves: the tricuspid, mitral, pulmonary, and aortic, which allow for unidirectional blood flow during the cardiac cycle. The great vessels of the heart are the pulmonary artery and aorta. After birth the pulmonary artery is the only artery in the body that carries deoxygenated blood; all other arterial

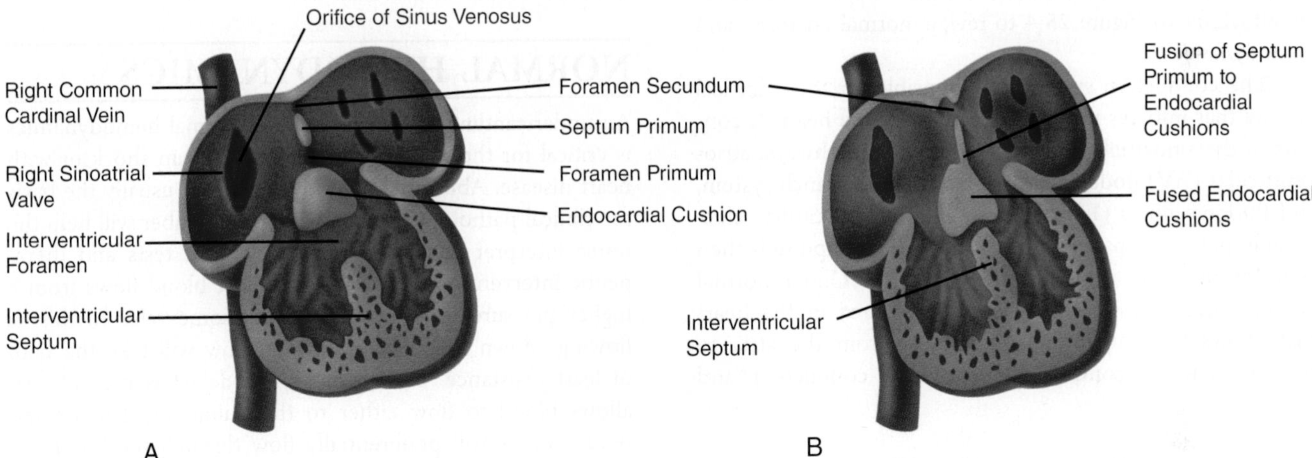

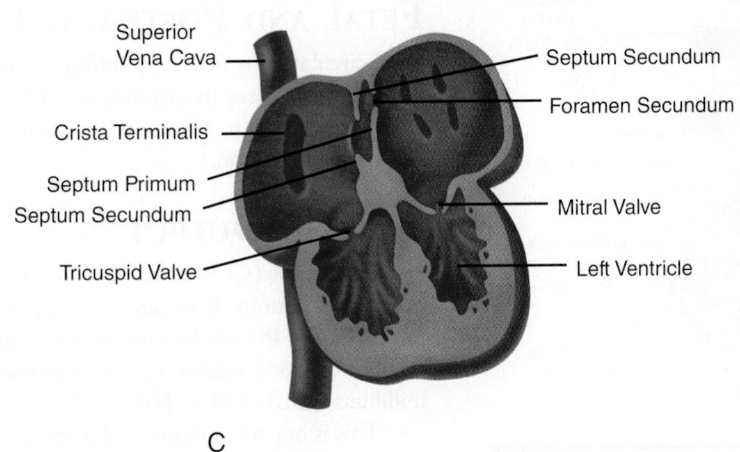

FIGURE 25-2 Sequential Development of the Heart Tube (A, B, C). Final development occurs by 7 weeks' gestation. DELMAR CENGAGE LEARNING.

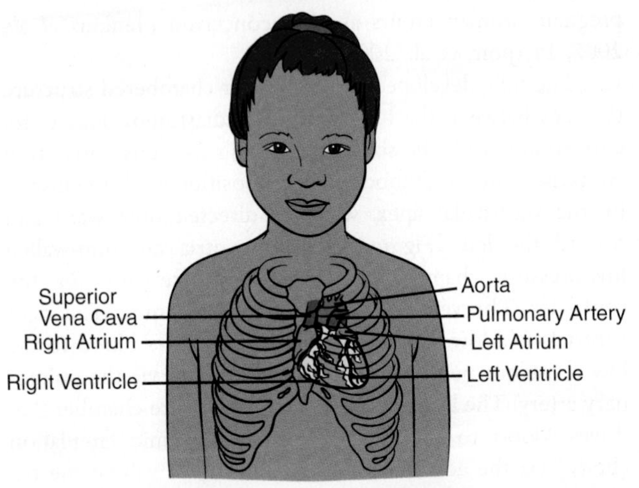

FIGURE 25-3 Normal Placement of the Heart in the Chest. DELMAR CENGAGE LEARNING.

beds, including the aorta, carry oxygenated blood. Under normal conditions in children (outside of the newborn) the pulmonary vascular bed is a low pressure, low resistance circuit. Refer to Figure 25-4 to review normal anatomy and hemodynamics.

The conduction system is responsible for the electrical activity that initiates mechanical activity of the heart. It consists of the sinoatrial (SA) node, internodal pathways, atrioventricular (AV) node, bundle of His, bundle branch system, and Purkinje fibers (Figure 25-5). The normal cardiac electrical impulse originates in the SA node. The impulse is then sent through the atrium to the AV node. Under normal circumstances the AV node is the only area in the heart that allows transmission of an impulse from the atria to the ventricle. It controls the speed of conduction and

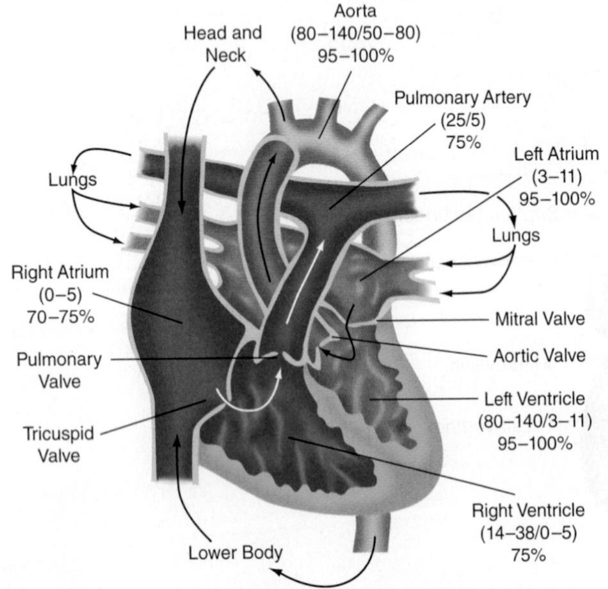

FIGURE 25-4 Normal Anatomy of the Heart and Blood Flow. Percentages are intracardiac oxygen saturations. Normal pressures are in parentheses. DELMAR CENGAGE LEARNING.

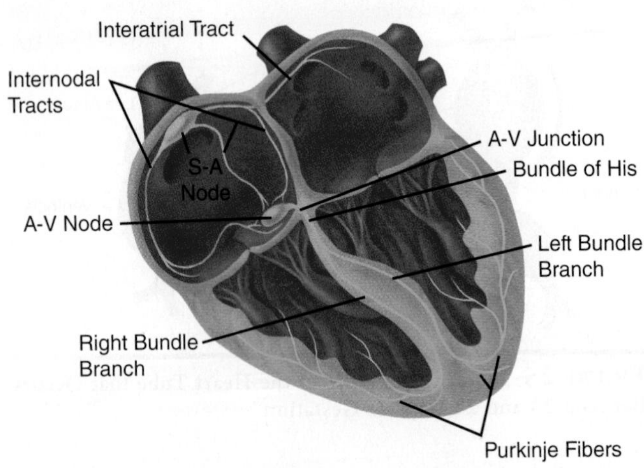

FIGURE 25-5 Normal Conduction System. DELMAR CENGAGE LEARNING.

number of impulses allowed to enter the ventricle. The Purkinje fibers infiltrate and transmit the electrical impulses into the ventricle. This well-orchestrated process results in a uniform cardiac contraction.

NORMAL HEMODYNAMICS

An understanding of transitional and normal hemodynamics is critical for the nurse caring for the child in shock or with heart disease. Abnormal hemodynamics are usually the basis for clinical pathology. Key caveats to remember will help the nurse interpret and understand diagnostic tests and therapeutic interventions. First and foremost blood flows from a higher pressure to a lower pressure; some refer to this as flowing "down hill." Second, blood flow will take the path of least resistance. For example, if a defect is present that allows blood to flow either to the pulmonary bed or systemic bed, it will preferentially flow through the low resistance pulmonary bed. With increasing expertise the nurse will be able to apply these simple concepts to more complex defects in clinical practice.

FETAL AND POSTNATAL CIRCULATION

Fetal circulation is distinctly different from postnatal circulation. In some cases persistence of fetal circulation can occur after birth. Refer to Chapter 7 for a discussion of fetal and postnatal circulation.

CARDIAC OUTPUT

Cardiac output (CO) is the volume of blood ejected by the heart in 1 minute. It is calculated by multiplying the heart rate (HR) by the stroke volume (SV). Stroke volume is the amount of blood ejected by the ventricles per contraction in milliliters (mL): $CO = HR \times SV$.

This is one measurement of blood flow. Normal CO in an infant is 200 mL/kg/min; in adolescents it is 100 mL/kg/min.

The determinants of stroke volume are preload, afterload, and contractility. Preload is the amount of blood in the ventricle at the end of diastole and just prior to systole. It is the volume of blood returning to the heart. Preload is responsible for the stretching of the cardiac muscle and is primarily influenced by intravascular volume and the compliance of the ventricle.

Afterload is the resistance that the ventricle must overcome when ejecting blood. Clinically this value is used during cardiac catheterization to measure the degree of ventricular work. Afterload is influenced by the size of the ventricular outflow tract and accompanying semilunar valve, resistance of the associated vascular bed, and blood viscosity (hematocrit). Right ventricular afterload is subject to pulmonary vascular resistance, which is normally low after about 8 weeks of life. In utero the pulmonary vascular resistance is very high to divert blood away from the fetal lung. In general it takes up to 8 weeks after birth for this resistance to fall to normal levels that are maintained into adulthood. Left ventricular afterload is subject to systemic vascular resistance, which is high relative to the pulmonary bed.

Contractility is the intrinsic ability of the myocardial fiber to shorten and produce a forceful contraction. It is influenced by preload, oxygen supply, circulating catecholamines (epinephrine and norepinephrine), maturity of the **myocardium** (the cardiac muscle; middle layer of the heart), and serum calcium. It should be noted that the newborn and infant myocardium is immature with fewer contractile fibers and limited intracellular calcium stores (Freed, 2006).

Heart rate is also important in determining cardiac output. Rates that are too fast result in decreased diastolic filling because the resting phase of the heart is shortened. Rates that are too slow will result in low cardiac output because there are fewer beats per minute in which to eject blood. Abnormal rhythms can also interfere with cardiac output.

ASSESSMENT OF THE CHILD WITH A CARDIOVASCULAR ALTERATION

HISTORY

A concise thorough history is crucial to the assessment, diagnosis, and evaluation of the response to therapeutic intervention. Many caregivers have obvious concerns about the implications of cardiac symptomatology. An important outcome of history taking is the opportunity to assess caregiver and child interaction and coping skills. The chief complaint should be elicited, particularly in children who are being evaluated for the first time. Presenting symptoms such as when a murmur was first heard can help with the establishment of a possible diagnosis.

When evaluating an infant, a prenatal and postnatal history must be obtained. Pertinent data include maternal infections (rubella, HIV), lifestyle, prenatal drug and alcohol exposure, complications of pregnancy, gestational age at birth, and birth complications. Eating is the exercise of the neonate; therefore, feeding behaviors should be evaluated. Does the infant exhibit excessive diaphoresis, shortness of breath, fatigue, or cyanosis (a bluish tinge to the skin and mucous membranes) with feeding? The nurse should specifically determine where cyanosis is observed. Peripheral cyanosis of the extremities is usually caused by vasomotor instability typically seen in the young infant. Cyanosis of the lips (not perioral, which is the skin around the lips) and tongue is worrisome, and the presence of **hypercyanotic spells** (extreme cyanosis that results in a deep blue or purple color of the entire body) requires further investigation. Often infants with heart disease will be irritable, inconsolable, have poor weight gain, excessive diaphoresis, and poor feeding (Geggel & Fyler, 2006).

When evaluating the older child, height and weight should be documented and compared with previous trends to evaluate for growth retardation. Exercise tolerance relative to developmental norms and their peers is evaluated. Care must be taken to obtain the caregiver's as well as the child's perceptions on exercise tolerance, as these can be quite divergent. Unnecessary restrictions may have been placed on the child by the caregiver caused by anxiety about real or presumed heart disease. The presence of color changes, shortness of breath, dizziness, **syncope** (fainting), frequent respiratory infections, or **palpitations** (sensation of abnormal heart beats) should be investigated and documented.

When interviewing an adolescent, the primary historian should be the child, using the caregivers to corroborate information. Ability to keep up with peers while undertaking normal activities (climbing the stairs, physical education, dancing, walking in the mall) is assessed. Various limitations include shortness of breath, dizziness, fatigue, syncope, or chest pain. In addition the nurse should query the family about any genetic syndrome the child may have. It is often helpful to know if the child has been formally evaluated by a geneticist, since a number of syndromes are associated with congenital heart disease.

Obtaining a family history is very important as a number of cardiac conditions are familial; incidence is increased when a first degree relative (parent or sibling) has congenital heart disease. A number of cardiac defects are associated with various conditions and syndromes. For a list of these see Table 25-1.

PHYSICAL EXAMINATION

The following section outlines specific findings that are salient to the cardiac examination.

INSPECTION

Physical abnormalities such as **dysmorphic** (abnormal or unusual) facial features, edema, chest wall deformities, and skin color (pallor, cyanosis, or jaundice) should be assessed. Cyanosis is best evaluated under bright natural light. Changes in skin color may be difficult to discern in children

TABLE 25-1 Conditions Associated with Congenital Heart Disease

SYNDROME	ANOMALY
DiGeorge syndrome	Interrupted aortic arch, tetralogy of Fallot (TOF), truncus arteriosus
Williams syndrome	Pulmonary stenosis, aortic stenosis
Trisomy 21 (Down)	Primum ASD, VSD, atrioventricular septal defect
Turner's syndrome	Pulmonary stenosis, coarctation of aorta
Trisomy 18	VSD, PDA
Apert syndrome	VSD
Glycogen storage disease	Cardiomyopathy
Duchenne's and Becker's muscular dystrophy	Cardiomyopathy
Noonan's syndrome	Pulmonary stenosis
Long QT	Arrhythmias
Marfan syndrome	Aortic valve regurgitation, aortic aneurysms, mitral valve prolapse
Fetal alcohol syndrome	VSD, ASD, TOF
Lithium ingestion (maternal)	Ebstein's anomaly, ASD
Amphetamines	VSD, PDA, ASD, TGA
Maternal lupus	Congenital heart block
Maternal diabetes	Cardiomyopathy, VSD, TGA
Thyroid dysfunction	Supraventricular tachycardia, cardiomyopathy

with deeply pigmented skin, so particular attention should be paid to the color of the lips, tongue, and nail beds.

The fingers should be evaluated for the presence of clubbing. This is a soft-tissue deformity that is the result of chronic cyanosis with the subsequent development of the loss of the normal angle between the nail and the nail bed. The finger tips eventually become wider and rounder (Figure 25-6) (Geggel & Fyler, 2006).

AUSCULTATION FOR MURMURS

Refer to Chapter 14 for an in-depth review of cardiac auscultation. Murmurs are noises that occur from turbulent blood flow which can be abnormal or "innocent." Murmurs are described by their location, timing, frequency, and intensity. When auscultating the chest four traditional areas are utilized (Figure 25-7). Landmarks on the chest such as left lower sternal border, left axilla, right upper sternal border, and so forth are used to denote location. Systolic murmurs are heard between the first and second heart sounds. Holosystolic murmurs are heard throughout systole, incorporating the second heart sound into the murmur. Diastolic murmurs are heard after S2 but before S1. Continuous murmurs are heard throughout the entire cardiac cycle. There is a standardized way to grade murmurs that is universally accepted (Box 25-2). Systolic murmurs that are loud (grade III or greater) are generally considered abnormal and require further evaluation by a cardiologist. Holosystolic, diastolic,

Normal Angle

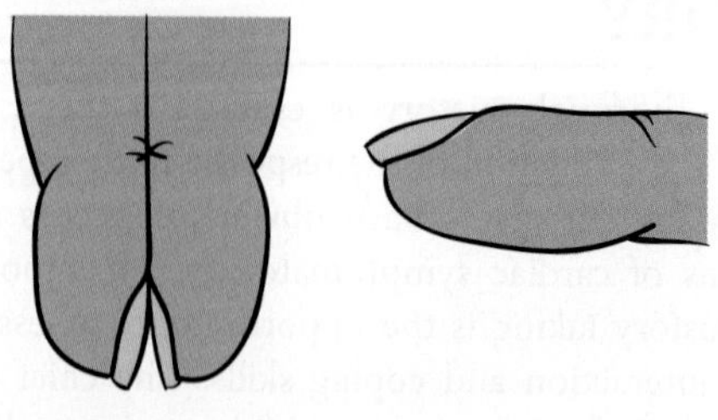

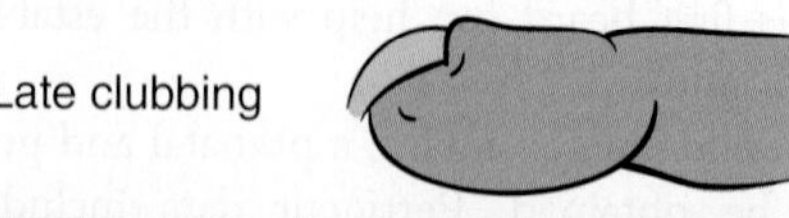

FIGURE 25-6 Changes in the Nailbed that Result in Clubbing. DELMAR CENGAGE LEARNING.

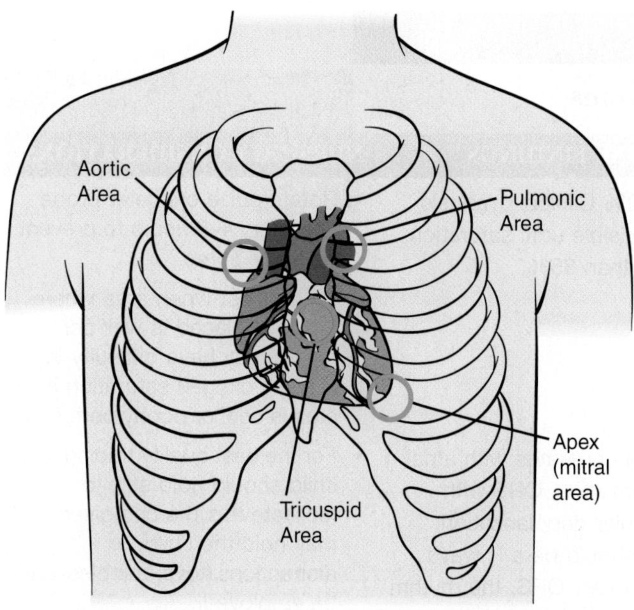

FIGURE 25-7 **Normal Areas of Cardiac Auscultation.** DELMAR CENGAGE LEARNING.

and most continuous murmurs are abnormal. Pathologic murmurs associated with congenital defects are discussed with each specific defect in the congenital heart disease section.

It must be clarified that not all murmurs are pathologic. Many murmurs are denoted as innocent, indicating there is no structural or functional heart disease. Nonetheless the presence of a murmur often invokes caregivers' fears regarding their child's health and well-being. The quality of an innocent murmur is quite characteristic (soft, short, systolic, and vibratory in quality). Therefore experienced clinicians are able to determine if a murmur is innocent without obtaining special tests. Children who are found to have innocent murmurs require no intervention or specific follow-up since these murmurs often disappear with age. Activity restrictions are not necessary, and the child should be treated normally. It should be noted that the intensity of an innocent murmur will increase with fever, illness, or stress. This should be communicated to the family as a normal phenomenon and it does not indicate the sudden occurrence of heart disease. Careful education is critically important since many families will continue to presume their child has heart disease, even though it has been determined that the murmur is innocent.

BOX 25-2
CLASSIFYING MURMURS BY GRADE

Grade 1—Barely audible, may require listening to several cardiac cycles to appreciate

Grade 2—Soft murmur that is readily heard

Grade 3—Moderately loud murmur without a thrill

Grade 4—Moderately loud murmur with a thrill

Grade 5—Loud murmur heard with the edge of the stethoscope touching the chest

Grade 6—Loud murmur that can be heard without the stethoscope touching the chest

Palpation for Hepatomegaly

Refer to Chapter 14 for more in-depth review regarding palpation of the chest and extremities. The abdomen is palpated for **hepatomegaly** (liver enlargement). In normal infants the liver edge may be as far as 1–2 centimeters below the right costal margin. In older children and adolescents the liver edge may be at the right costal margin or nonpalpable. Hepatomegaly can be associated with congestive heart failure.

Blood Pressure Measurement

Blood pressure (BP) measurement is a common maneuver for all nurses to perform. However, in children this can be fraught with error if not executed correctly. Most important is selecting the appropriately sized cuff in order to obtain a correct measurement. Refer to Chapter 14 for information about BP cuff size and normal values for BP according to age, sex, and height. There are a number of different cuff sizes available. Simultaneous arm and leg blood pressures are obtained to rule out coarctation of the aorta (the right arm and either leg are used). Normally lower extremity BP is equal to or greater than the arm BP. A right arm BP greater than a leg BP can indicate coarctation of the aorta.

Serial BP measurements must be taken on repeat visits before a child is determined to be hypertensive. Anxiety around a clinic visit, particularly with a new health care provider, can elevate BP. Repeat visits will help the child to accommodate to the environment, allowing the accurate reflection of the true BP. Body size, age, and sex are the most important determinants of BP in children (Urbina et al., 2008). **Pulsus paradoxus** is an excessive variation in systolic pressure with respiration. Normally the systolic BP drops no more than 10 mm Hg with inspiration (in the spontaneously breathing child). A drop of more than 10 mm Hg is pathologic and is characteristic of those conditions that interfere with cardiac filling, that is, cardiac **tamponade** (accumulation of fluid around heart that restricts filling of heart), **pericardial effusion** (collection of fluid in pericardial sac that can lead to tamponade), and **pericarditis** (inflammation of the pericardium).

DIAGNOSTIC TESTS

A number of diagnostic studies can be utilized in the diagnosis and evaluation of the child with heart disease. These include laboratory tests, pulse oximetry, electrocardiogram (ECG), holter monitor, event monitoring, chest radiograph (CXR), echo cardiogram (ECHO), magnetic resonance imaging (MRI), and cardiac catheterization. Not all tests are used for every child. The selection of appropriate tests is based on diagnosis and symptoms. Table 25-2 offers a listing

Table 25-2 Diagnostic Tests for Cardiac Alterations

NAME OF TEST	PURPOSE AND DESCRIPTION	NORMAL FINDINGS	NURSING CONSIDERATIONS
Pulse oximetry (SpO_2)	Evaluates degree of oxygen saturation in the blood using a small infrared light probe that is placed on a finger, toe, earlobe, or bridge of the nose.	95–100% Clinical cyanosis is not visible until saturation is less than 85%.	• Rotate pulse oximeter probe site every 4–6 hours to prevent pressure sores. • Works best when area where probe is placed is well perfused; may have difficulty in reading oxygen saturation if area is cool or poorly perfused.
Electrocardiogram (ECG)	Detects electrical events, normal and abnormal cardiac rhythms in the heart. Waveforms are produced via the use of 12 or 15 electrodes that are placed on the chest and extremities (Figure 25-8). These waveforms can be used to assess cardiac rhythm.	P wave correlates with atrial depolarization, QRS with ventricular depolarization. There should be a P wave before every QRS, the rhythm should be regular, and rate normal for child's age.	• For the best quality tracing, the child should hold still; to facilitate this the caregivers may hold the child, or distractions (toys, bubbles) can be employed. • If lotion or powder is on the skin, it should be cleansed gently with alcohol prior to placement of the electrodes. Otherwise, vigorous cleansing or shaving is not indicated in children.
Holter monitor	Continuous 24-hour ECG recorder that utilizes five chest leads and a recording device to produce a two-channel recording. This is used if symptoms or arrhythmia occur daily. A diary is kept by the caregiver or child while the holter is worn.	Normals should be similar to ECG.	• As the monitor should stay on for 24 hours the skin must be prepped with alcohol or other solvent to remove oils. The electrode adhesive is strong so adhesive remover is recommended for removal. If the skin is inflamed following removal a 1% steroid cream may be applied. • The caregiver or child should be instructed to write in the diary symptoms, activities, and sleep times so that appropriate correlation of rhythm can be made with diary entries.
Event recorder	Small pager-sized recorder that is client activated to record heart rhythm during symptoms. This is used when symptoms do not occur daily. It is generally worn for a month. Once the recorder is activated it stores the ECG; this can be transmitted via telephone at a later time.	Normal would be the same as ECG.	• Event recorder does not need to be worn during sleep (unless the symptoms occur during sleep and awaken the child). It should not be worn while bathing or swimming. • If inflammation occurs from the electrodes then the placement may be rotated slightly and 1% steroid cream applied.
Chest radiograph (CXR)	Chest X-ray that is used to determine cardiac size, contour, and alterations in pulmonary vascularity.	Heart size should be no greater than 50% of widest intercostal diameter of chest. Pulmonary arteries should not appear large, lung fields should be clear.	• Best quality CXR is ensured if child is still and X-ray is obtained during inspiration. (The heart size is falsely increased during expiration.) Diversional activities, or caregiver assistance, may be required.

(Continues)

Table 25-2 Diagnostic Tests for Cardiac Alterations (*Continued*)

NAME OF TEST	PURPOSE AND DESCRIPTION	NORMAL FINDINGS	NURSING CONSIDERATIONS
			• Lead shields are placed over the child's gonads and are worn by any assistive personnel or family member.
Echocardiogram (ECHO)	Two-dimensional, three dimensional and Doppler evaluation of cardiac anatomy, size, and function. Utilizes sound waves (ultrasound) emitted by a transducer that is placed on the chest in different positions.	Cardiac structures should be normal without evidence of valve leakage or septal defects. Heart thickness is normal for body surface area.	• Client cooperation is imperative. Children less than 2 years may require sedation to hold still. Pulse oximetry and heart rate should be monitored during sedation. For client comfort the ultrasound gel should be warmed. See Figure 25-9.
	Transesophageal echo uses a transducer that is placed in the esophagus to visualize posterior cardiac structures or to evaluate for intracardiac thrombi.	Function is evaluated by determining shortening fraction (normal 28–44%) and ejection fraction (normal >55%).	
Cardiac catheterization (card cath)	An invasive procedure performed under fluoroscopy that allows determination of cardiac anatomy, function, cardiac pressures, and oxygen saturations. Catheters are inserted into the heart via a large vein or artery. A contrast agent (dye) is sometimes injected to aid in the recording of blood flow and help evaluate the coronary arteries.	For normal intracardiac oxygen saturations and pressures, see Figure 25-4.	• Sedation or anesthesia is necessary to prevent client movement. For pre- and post-catheterization nursing care see section under cardiac catheterization. See Figure 25-10.
	Electrophysiology (EP) studies and catheter ablation are performed to diagnose and treat some arrhythmias. Intracardiac electrodes are inserted into the heart as in a cardiac cath. Some systems are capable of creating an electroanatomic 3D reconstruction. The focus of the abnormal rhythm can then be identified and obliterated with a special warm or cool tip catheter.		
Magnetic resonance imaging (MRI)	Uses large magnet that stimulates atomic nuclei in body to emit energy in form of radio waves that are then transformed into a picture of the structure(s) being evaluated. Assists in defining cardiac anatomy that cannot be well evaluated by ECHO.	Anatomic structures should be normal.	• Client cooperation is imperative; sedation is employed with young children, toddlers, and infants. • MRI is avoided if permanent pacemaker, metal implants, or implantable defibrillator is in place.

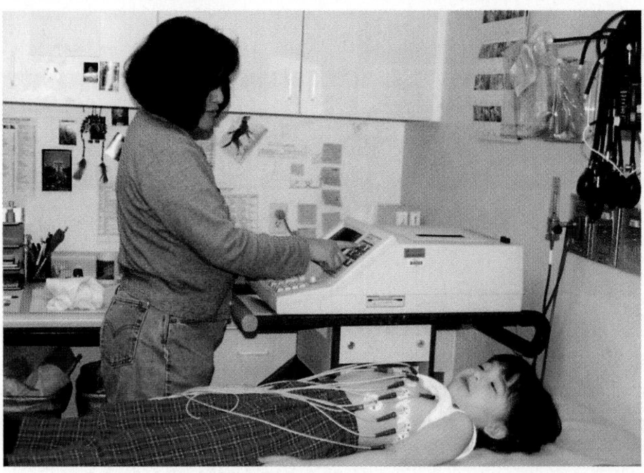

FIGURE 25-8 A Child with Heart Disease Getting a 12-lead ECG. DELMAR CENGAGE LEARNING.

of the most common diagnostic tests used in diagnosing cardiovascular alterations in infants and children. Figure 25-8 shows a child getting an ECG.

Nursing Considerations for the Child Undergoing Cardiac Catheterization

This is a procedure that is generally performed on an outpatient basis. Children who have undergone therapeutic cardiac cath or small infants may require overnight hospitalization. Even though routine, this procedure can be very stressful for the child and family and is not completely risk free.

Prior to the procedure a complete nursing history must be obtained. Pretesting can include an ECG, ECHO, CBC, and platelet count. The child should be NPO for 4 to 6 hours prior to the procedure, depending on hospital policy. Assessment includes accurate height and weight as these measurements are used to determine catheter size and calculate body surface area. Obtaining a history of allergies is critically important. Many contrast materials contain iodine; therefore, allergies to iodine, contrast dyes, or shellfish must be brought to the attention of the cardiologist. Any history of fever or previous illness, as well as signs and symptoms of infection, must be assessed. The presence of illness or infection may require postponement of the procedure. Baseline assessment of pedal pulses and pulse oximetry are documented so that post procedural findings can be compared to baseline.

Preprocedural preparation is important for the child and family. Child life specialists, puppet therapy, or therapeutic play can all facilitate the alleviation of anxiety. The sights and sounds of the cath lab should be explained to the child, utilizing age-appropriate language. Often a tour of the lab is helpful. Specific aspects of the procedure should be explained such as the placement of the IV and the ECG electrodes, washing of the groin with betadine (brown soap), use of the numbing medicine (lidocaine) to put the skin to

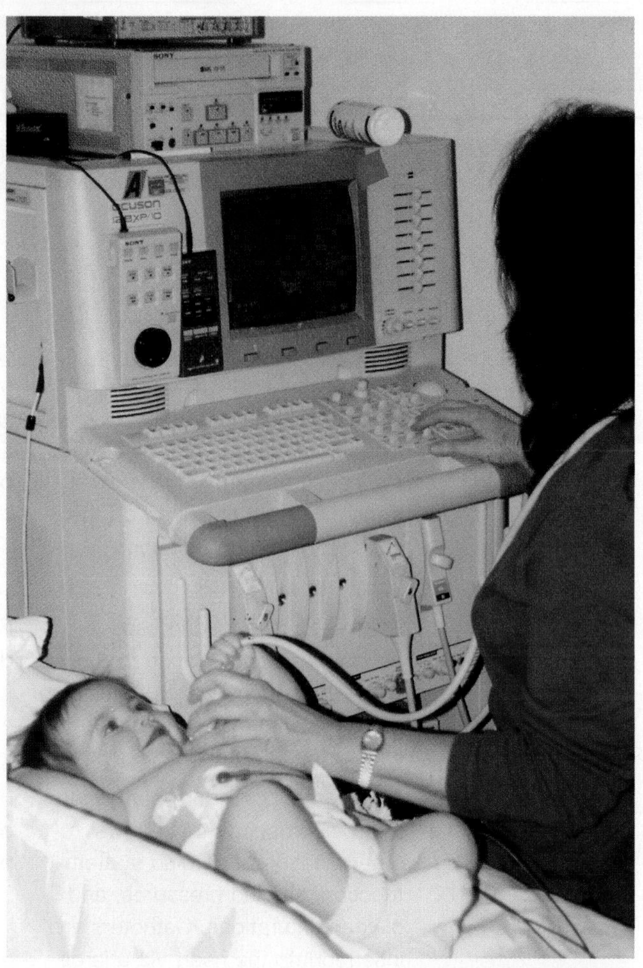

FIGURE 25-9 A Baby Getting an Echocardiogram. DELMAR CENGAGE LEARNING.

sleep, humming of the fluoroscopy when turned on, how injection of the contrast will create a warm flushed feeling, and how the sedative will make the child feel. The family and child must be assured that sedatives will be given appropriately as needed. The type of sedative used varies among practitioners and institutions.

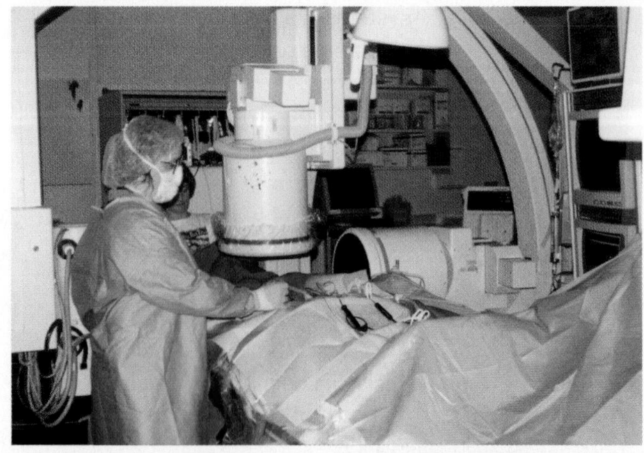

FIGURE 25-10 A Child Undergoing Cardiac Catheterization. DELMAR CENGAGE LEARNING.

Following the procedure the child is monitored for a number of hours prior to discharge, often with a cardiac monitor and pulse oximeter. It is critically important that the nurse monitor the following:

1. Temperature and color of the extremity distal to the catheter insertion site.
2. Pulse of the extremity distal to the catheter insertion site.
3. Check vital signs frequently, for example, every 15 minutes for the first hour and hourly thereafter. Particular attention should be paid to HR and BP. The nurse must monitor trends and assess for the development of hypotension, tachycardia, and bradycardia.
4. Intake and output, as contrast material can promote brisk diuresis.
5. Bleeding at the insertion site; observe for evidence of hematoma. The nurse must inspect the dressing with each vital sign check, and if bleeding is noted, apply direct pressure and notify practitioner.
6. Oxygen saturation. This must be compared to the child's baseline.

The child should be kept in bed with the affected extremity straight for 4 to 8 hours, depending on hospital policy. Younger children can be held by their caregiver to ensure better compliance. Diet is advanced as tolerated. The pressure dressing can be removed in 24 hours. An effort should be made to keep the dressing dry in infants and toddlers who still wear diapers. Discharge teaching includes family education on site care, observing the site for signs of inflammation and infection, monitoring for fever, restriction from strenuous activities for a few days, avoiding tub baths for 48–72 hours (showers are fine), and the use of acetaminophen or ibuprofen for pain.

NURSING ALERT

Children with Latex Allergies

Some catheters used in the catheterization laboratory have latex balloons. Therefore, it is very important that the nurse determine if the child has a latex allergy prior to the cath as use of the balloon can precipitate a life-threatening reaction. If the child has a possible latex allergy then they can be premedicated with steroids, Benadryl, and Tylenol. Or the intervention is deferred and the child is referred for alternative interventions or evaluation.

NURSING TIP

Avoid Sandbags to Prevent Bleeding after Cardiac Catheterization

Sandbags should never be used to prevent or treat bleeding from the catheter site. Use of a sandbag can severely compromise distal circulation and increase the child's agitation.

CONGESTIVE HEART FAILURE

Congestive heart failure (CHF) is the inability of the cardiovascular system to provide adequate cardiac output to meet the metabolic demands of the body. To understand the pathophysiological and clinical manifestations of CHF the nurse must have a working knowledge of normal determinants of cardiac output, as well as an understanding of the normal compensatory mechanisms. Refer to the previous section on cardiac output for review of the normal determinants. A discussion of the compensatory mechanisms is located in the pathophysiology segment in this section.

INCIDENCE AND ETIOLOGY

The absolute incidence of CHF in infants and children is unknown because of the wide range of causes. Congenital heart defects are the most common causes of CHF in infants. Structural defects can impose either a volume load or pressure load on the heart. Defects with left to right shunts (ventricular septal defect) impose a volume load. Left-sided obstructive defects (hypoplastic left heart syndrome, aortic stenosis, coarctation of the aorta) impose a pressure load as there is obstruction to forward flow of blood. Excessive volume or pressure can contribute to pulmonary edema. Most infants with significant defects will develop symptoms within weeks to months following birth (Penny & Mynard, 2006).

The most common cause of CHF in infants is congenital heart disease. Acquired heart disease is the most common cause in older children or adolescents. These include **cardiomyopathy** (disease of the heart muscle resulting in poor pump function), **endocarditis** (infection of the inner lining of the heart), rheumatic fever (refer to section on rheumatic fever), and **myocarditis** (inflammation of the heart muscle). These diseases result in impaired myocardial contractility with a subsequent fall in cardiac output. This phenomenon causes volume overload and resultant pulmonary and systemic venous congestion.

Tachyarrhythmias (abnormally fast heart rates) or **bradyarrhythmias** (abnormally slow heart rates) can also be responsible for CHF. Acute onset, very fast heart rates that are abnormal (supraventricular tachycardia, junctional ectopic tachycardia) will produce heart failure if not identified in a timely manner. Chronic incessant tachyarrhythmias (atrial flutter, atrial ectopic tachycardia) can produce CHF if the arrhythmia is present for a significant portion of the day. Very slow heart rates (complete heart block) can also be an etiology for heart failure. CHF secondary to arrhythmias will resolve once the rhythm returns to normal.

PATHOPHYSIOLOGY

The previously discussed etiologies are responsible for the hemodynamic changes and symptoms of CHF. Figure 25-11 illustrates the physiological mechanisms of CHF. Inadequate emptying of the heart caused by volume overload or poor contractility results in cardiac failure. This will generate an increase in venous volume with a subsequent increase in venous congestion. Systemic venous congestion results in liver engorgement (hepatomegaly). Pulmonary venous congestion results in pulmonary edema. Large left to right shunts result in an increased amount of blood circulating through the lungs, also contributing to pulmonary congestion.

Reduced ejection of the blood from obstruction or diminished contractility results in a pressure load. As the pressure in the heart increases from inadequate emptying of the heart, pulmonary and venous congestion results. The normal physiological responses to low cardiac output are increased sympathetic activity and activation of the renin-angiotensin aldosterone system. These compensatory responses can provide cardiovascular support for a limited period of time, but can be detrimental to the failing heart.

Epinephrine increases heart rate and cardiac output. Norepinephrine release results in vasoconstriction and elevation of BP. Both of these processes result in increased cardiac work. This is initially helpful; however, the increase in heart rate and cardiac work will eventually contribute to worsening failure.

Activation of the renin-angiotensin aldosterone system is in response to low renal perfusion. This mechanism produces an increase in aldosterone and angiotension release. Aldosterone is responsible for reabsorption of sodium and water, which causes an increase in blood volume. Initially, this is successful in improving cardiac output, but over time it contributes to volume overload. As end diastolic volume increases so does myocardial stretch. Initially this increase in stretch improves contraction; however, as stretch progresses cardiac dilation occurs. Over time an abnormal pressure load causes the heart muscle to **hypertrophy** (become abnormally thick). A dilated or hypertrophied ventricle is a poor pump as these mechanisms interfere with normal myocardial fiber shortening.

Other mechanisms to maintain cardiovascular function include tachycardia and redistribution of blood flow. Since cardiac output is a function of heart rate multiplied by the stroke volume, the body will normally increase heart rate to support cardiac output. Perfusion to major organs (heart and brain) is initially preserved. Vasoconstriction of the vessels in the skin and gut will redirect blood flow to other areas of the body. If perfusion is significantly compromised,

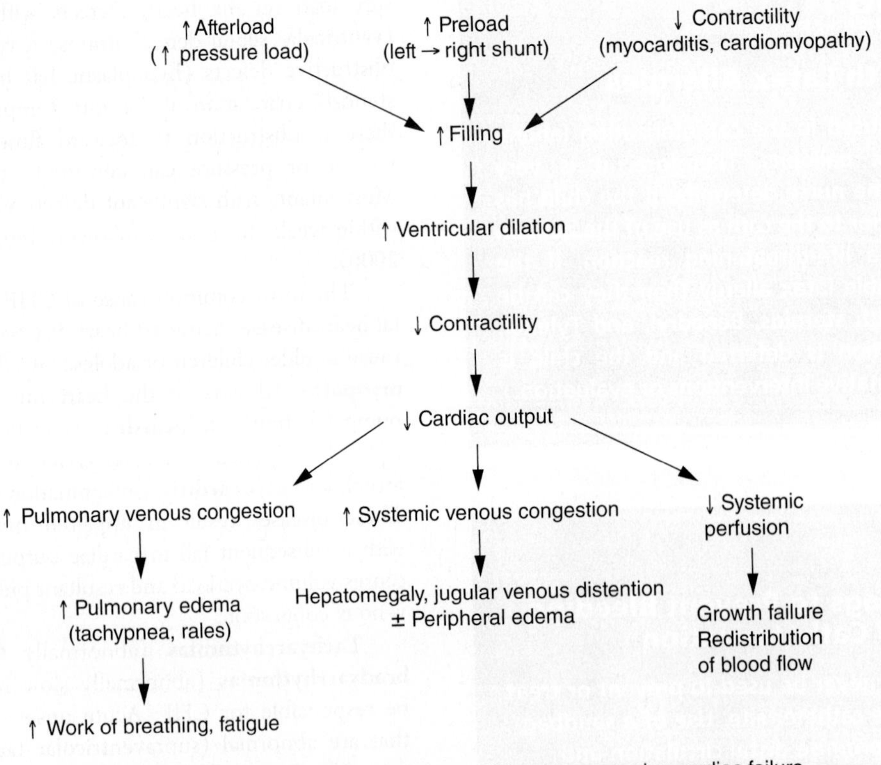

FIGURE 25-11 Physiological Mechanisms of Congestive Heart Failure. DELMAR CENGAGE LEARNING.

CRITICAL THINKING

Relationship of Metabolic Acidosis to Pathophysiology in CHF

- What is metabolic acidosis and why does it occur?
- Why does metabolic acidosis occur with CHF?
- What laboratory blood test is used to evaluate acid-base balance?

metabolic acidosis will result from inadequate delivery of oxygen to the cells.

CLINICAL MANIFESTATIONS

Clinical manifestations occur when mechanisms of compensatory response are exceeded and cardiac output begins to fall. These symptoms can vary depending on the underlying etiology and age of the child. Box 25-3 lists clinical manifestations of CHF according to age.

Tachypnea is commonly seen in children with CHF. The respiratory rate can be ≥60 in infants and toddlers, and ≥40 in children over 2 years. There may be retractions, nasal flaring, or rapid shallow respirations and restlessness in neonates and infants. Older children may demonstrate dyspnea with exertion or orthopnea. Crackles and rhonchi can also be present. These symptoms commonly indicate that there is pulmonary congestion. As pulmonary congestion progresses there is a subsequent leaking of fluid into the alveoli and interstitium of the lung leading to pulmonary edema. Oxygen saturation may fall if the increase in lung fluid interferes with the diffusion of oxygen into the blood.

Systemic venous congestion indicates right ventricular failure. Signs of this include hepatomegaly, jugular venous distention, peripheral edema, and changes in urine output and body weight. Hepatomegaly is observed in children more frequently than jugular venous distention, which is usually seen in the child older than 10–12 years of age. Liver congestion reflects an increase in central venous pressure and blood volume. Jugular venous distention generally cannot be observed in infants because of their short necks. In the older child distention of the neck veins is evaluated when the child is sitting. Peripheral edema is a rare finding in infants, but when present, it is usually localized to the periorbital area. The older child will exhibit edema of the hands and feet in addition to periorbital edema. Ascites indicates severely compromised cardiac function.

The cardiac symptoms of CHF include tachycardia, gallop rhythms, diaphoresis, and decreased peripheral pulses. A gallop rhythm (S3) or extra heart beat is often heard in severe CHF. Excessive diaphoresis is caused by sympathetic stimulation. Diaphoresis is frequently noted during feeding in infants with heart failure. Cool, mottled extremities and weak, thready pulses indicate poor perfusion. The blood pressure is usually maintained; therefore, hypotension is a late and ominous sign.

Growth failure and poor weight gain are very common in infants and children with CHF. Respiratory difficulties make feeding exhausting for infants, demonstrated by dyspnea and fatigue during feedings. Older children have exercise intolerance and excessive fatigue.

BOX 25-3
CLINICAL MANIFESTATIONS OF CHF

Newborns or Infants

- Tachycardia
- Tachypnea
- Gallop rhythm
- Retractions
- Diminished pulses
- Wheezing
- Diaphoresis
- Rales or rhonchi
- Cool, mottled extremities
- Hepatomegaly
- Pallor
- Low urine output
- Edema
- Failure to thrive or poor weight gain
- Restlessness

Children or Adolescents

- Jugular venous distention
- Tachycardia
- Wheezing
- Gallop rhythm
- Rales or rhonchi
- Diminished pulses
- Dyspnea
- Pallor
- Orthopnea
- Edema
- Hepatomegaly
- Low urine output
- Ascites
- Exercise intolerance
- Poor weight gain

DIAGNOSIS

A number of noninvasive tests provide supportive data for the diagnosis of CHF. Chest X-rays can demonstrate cardiac enlargement, although in some instances heart size can be normal. CXR can also be used to determine if there is pulmonary over circulation or edema. The best diagnostic tool is echocardiography, which can be used to determine if congenital defects or cardiomyopathy are present. It can also assess for heart size, cardiac function, hypertrophy, and dilation.

TREATMENT

Therapies are directed at reducing volume overload, improving contractility, reducing afterload, and decreasing cardiac work. In infants who have heart failure secondary to congenital defects, surgical correction is the primary treatment (Warnes et al., 2008).

NURSING ALERT

Serum Potassium Levels and Digoxin Administration

Prior to the initiation of digoxin, serum potassium must be checked and levels should be normal. Hypokalemia in combination with digoxin can result in ventricular arrhythmias and can enhance digoxin toxicity. Signs and symptoms of toxicity include nausea, vomiting, bradycardia, heart block, and premature ventricular contractions. Use with caution in renal failure.

Diuretic therapy is the primary intervention used for volume overload. Furosemide (Lasix) is the primary diuretic used in children. These agents can decrease pulmonary and venous congestion, improving symptoms. Fluid restriction should be avoided in the infant as the primary source of calories is in formula or breast milk.

Medications directed at improving contractility are referred to as positive **inotropes**. There are three classes of agents primarily used: cardiac glycosides, sympathomimetics, and phosphodiesterase inhibitors. These agents work through a number of different mechanisms of action (Table 25-3).

Digoxin is a cardiac glycoside and is the most commonly used oral inotrope in infants and children. Benefits of digoxin are improved myocardial contractility, a reduction in heart rate, and a reduction of cardiac work. Dosing depends on body size and age of the child (Table 25-4). Children receiving digoxin should have their heart rate and rhythm monitored with periodic ECGs because it can cause heart block and bradycardia. Other side effects include nausea and vomiting. If any of these are noted, a digoxin level should be obtained 8–12 hours after the last dose. Therapeutic levels are 0.8–2 ng/mL. It should be noted that serum digoxin levels in infants do not correlate well with clinical effect; however they are still helpful in assessing for toxicity. Digoxin should be withheld if levels are elevated above the therapeutic range or if the heart rate is lower than normal for age. Digoxin is frequently used in combination with diuretics. Because of the development of hypokalemia that is associated with diuretics, periodic serum potassium levels should be evaluated.

FAMILY TEACHING

Administering Digoxin

- Avoid giving the medication with meals. Give it 1 hour before or 2 hours after feedings.
- Give the medication at regular intervals.
- Measure the amount of digoxin exactly using a syringe, not the dropper provided with the medication.
- Check the child's apical pulse for 1 full minute before giving digoxin. As a general rule, the drug is not given if the pulse is below 90–110 beats per minute in infants and young children.
- Maintain adequate amounts of potassium in the child's diet to decrease the risk of hypokalemia.
- A fall in serum potassium level enhances the effects of digoxin, increasing the risk of toxicity.
- Do not double up on the next dose if a dose is missed. If a dose is missed and more than 4 hours have elapsed, caregivers should hold the dose and give the next dose at the regular time. If less than 4 hours have elapsed, give the missed dose.
- Notify the health care practitioner for any of the following symptoms: decrease in appetite, nausea, vomiting, abdominal pain, diarrhea, or visual changes occur.
- Do not give a repeat dose if the child vomits after being administered digoxin.

Sympathomimetics and phosphodiesterase inhibitors are generally used for acute heart failure in those children who do not respond to other medications. These agents are given intravenously by continuous infusion. Dopamine, dobutamine, and epinephrine are sympathomimetics that work via their stimulation of the sympathetic nervous system. They increase blood pressure, heart rate, and cardiac output. Amrinone (Inocor) and milrinone (Primacor) are phosphodiesterase inhibitors that improve cardiac contraction and promote vascular dilation. These drugs increase cardiac output without an increase in heart rate. They can also decrease cardiac work through afterload reduction.

Vasodilators augment cardiac output through a reduction in vascular resistance. If resistance is decreased, then cardiac output can increase. There are a number of oral and intravenous agents. Oral agents are used in those children with mild to moderate heart failure. Intravenous agents are used in the acutely ill child in severe failure.

Angiotensin-converting enzyme (ACE) inhibitors and angiotensin II receptor blockers are used for afterload reduction. ACE inhibitors suppress the conversion of angiotensin I to angiotensin II, thus augmenting vasodilation. The end result is vasodilation with a fall in vascular resistance. The most commonly used ACE inhibitors are captopril (Capoten) and enalapril (Vasotec). Angiotensin II receptor blockers inhibit the action of angiotensin II, therefore modulating cardiac neurohormonal activity with a favorable effect on the heart (Stayer, 2006). Intravenous afterload reducing agents are the nitrates and phosphodiesterase inhibitors. The nitrates consist of sodium nitroprusside and nitroglycerine. These medications produce vasodilation and a decrease in afterload. Data suggests that use of a recombinant brain-type natriuretic factor (BNP) in critically ill children improves cardiac output, perfusion, and urine output. Nesiritide (Natrecor) is a recombinant BNP given as a continuous infusion to treat severe decompensated CHF (Marshall, Berkenbosch, Russo, & Tobias, 2004; Taketomo, Hodding, & Kraus, 2008).

TABLE 25-3 Commonly Used Medications for the Treatment of CHF

MEDICATION	DOSAGE	ACTIONS	SIDE EFFECTS	NURSING CONSIDERATIONS
Inotropes				
Cardiac Glycosides				
Digoxin	See Table 25-4	↑ Ventricular contraction ↓ HR, ↓ cardiac work	Bradycardia, heart block Nausea, vomiting	Monitor potassium levels, should be normal before giving digoxin. Hold digoxin if PR interval is greater than 0.2 on ECG or if HR is less than normal for age. Check HR prior to administration.
Sympathomimetics				
*Dopamine	1–20 mg/kg/min	↑ CO ↑ Renal blood flow ↑ BP ± ↑ HR ± ↑ SVR (high dose)	Tachycardia, arrhythmias Tissue necrosis if IV infiltrates Hypertension	Monitor HR and BP for arrhythmias or hypertension; decrease infusion for either. If infiltration occurs, administer subcutaneous phenolamine.
*Dobutamine	2–20 mg/kg/min	↑ CO ↑ BP ± ↓ SVR	Arrhythmias Tachycardia	Monitor HR and BP for arrhythmias or hypertension; decrease infusion for either. Do not mix with sodium bicarbonate.
*Epinephrine	0.05–0.3 mg/kg/min	↑ CO ↑ BP ↓ Renal blood flow ↑ SVR (high dose)	Tachycardia Hypertension ↓ Urine output Vasoconstriction	Monitor HR and BP for hypertension or arrhythmias; decrease infusion for either. Do not mix with sodium bicarbonate.
Phosphodiesterase Inhibitors				
*Milrinone	50 mg/kg/load then 0.5–0.75 mg/kg/min	↑ CO ↓ Afterload ↓ Cardiac work ↓ Filling pressures	Hypotension Arrhythmias Thrombocytopenia Hepatic or GI dysfunction	If hypotension occurs, administer volume, monitor for arrhythmias. Thrombocytopenia resolves when infusion is discontinued. Monitor liver function tests, discontinue infusion if values are elevated.
*Amrinone	0.75–5 mg/kg load then 5–10 mg/kg/min	Same as milrinone	Same as milrinone except greater risk of thrombocytopenia	Same as milrinone.
Diuretics				
Furosemide (Lasix)	1–2 mg/kg q 6, 8, 12 or 24 hours Oral or IV	Loop diuretic Renal loss of H_2O, sodium, and potassium	Hypovolemia Hypokalemia Hyponatremia Metabolic alkalosis	Monitor I&O and electrolytes; may require electrolyte replacement if values are low. Excessive diuresis can produce hypotension—monitor BP if urine output excessive.
Bumetanide (Bumex)	Oral 0.015–0.1 mg/kg/dose every 6–24 hours, maximum dose 10 mg/day	Loop diuretic Same as furosemide	Same as furosemide	Same as furosemide.

(Continues)

TABLE 25-3 Commonly Used Medications for the Treatment of CHF (*Continued*)

MEDICATION	DOSAGE	ACTIONS	SIDE EFFECTS	NURSING CONSIDERATIONS
Spironolactone (Aldactone) Diuril	1–3 mg/kg/day oral divided BID Oral 10–20 mg/kg/day in 1 or 2 divided doses; IV 4 mg/kg/day in 1 or 2 divided doses	Potassium sparing diuretic Thiazide diuretic	Hypovolemia Hyperkalemia Contraindicated in renal failure Hypovolemia, electrolyte imbalances, nausea, vomiting. Use with caution in patients with renal or hepatic disease.	Same as furosemide; however, aldactone can cause hyperkalemia; if this occurs, discontinue. Monitor fluid balance, electrolytes, uric acid and bicarbonate.
Vasodilators				
ACE Inhibitors				
Captopril (Capoten)	Start with 0.05–0.5 mg/kg/dose TID; titrate up to max 6 mg/kg/day in 1–4 divided doses, oral	↓ SVR & PVR ↑ Sodium excretion	Hypotension Rash, GI upset	Monitor BP during initiation of drug—if hypotension occurs, hold next dose. Avoid concurrent administration of potassium.
Enalopril (Vasotec)	Start with 0.1 mg/kg/day divided BID; titrate up to max 0.5 mg/kg/day, oral	Similar to captopril	Similar to captopril	Same as captopril.
Nitrates				
*Nitroprusside (Nitropress)	0.5–10 mg/kg/min	Direct arterial and venous dilation ↓ SVR ↓ Afterload ↑ CO	Hypotension Thrombocytopenia Nitroprusside is metabolized to thiocyanate and cyanide—monitor for cyanide toxicity (i.e., metabolic acidosis) Tachypnea Tachycardia	Monitor BP continuously, stop infusion for significant hypotension (may need to administer fluids). If using high dose or long-term therapy, monitor cyanide and thiocyanate levels; discontinue if elevated. Monitor serum pH; if metabolic acidosis occurs, discontinue drug.
*Nitroglycerine	0.25–3 mg/kg/min	Direct arterial dilation ↓ SVR ↓ Afterload ↑ CO	Hypotension Headache	Monitor BP continuously; decrease or discontinue for hypotension (may need to administer fluids).
Angiotensin II Receptor Blockers				
Losartan (Cozaar)	25–50 mg/day (pediatric dosing not determined)	Vasodilation, ↓ SVR	Hypotension, dizziness, palpitations, cough	Monitor BP, particularly with initiation and escalation of therapy. Treat hypovolemia prior to starting losartan.
Beta Blockers				
Carvedilol (Coreg)	Initial dose 0.025 mg/kg/dose BID for 2 weeks; titrate up to 0.4mg/kg/dose BID	Beta-adrenergic blocker with non-selective alpha blocking properties	Hypotension, bradycardia, depression, malaise, syncope	Monitor BP with initial dose and each dosing increase. Monitor HR and liver function.

* These medications are given via continuous infusion in the PICU. Dose is titrated to therapeutic effect.
Key: CO cardiac output, SVR systemic vascular resistance, PVR pulmonary vascular resistance, GI gastrointestinal, BP blood pressure, daily, BID twice daily, TID three times daily, mcg microgram, mg milligram,

TABLE 25-4 Digoxin Therapy in Infants and Children

AGE	DIGITALIZATION DOSE*	MAINTENANCE DOSE
Neonate	20–35 mcg/kg PO 20–30 mcg/kg IV	5–8 mcg/kg/day divided BID
1 mo–2 yrs	30–40 mcg/kg PO 25–40 mcg/kg IV	8–12 mcg/kg/day divided BID
2 yrs–10 yrs	20–40 mcg/kg PO 15–35 mcg/kg IV	5–9 mcg/kg/day daily or divided BID
10 yrs to adults	1–1.5 mg PO 0.5–1 mg IV	0.125–0.500 mg/day

*This is total digitalization dose. Total dose is divided into three divided doses. 50% of total dose is given initially, then 8 hours later 25% of dose is given and 8 hours later final 25% of dose is given. It should be noted that not all patients are given digitalization dose, particularly when digoxin is started as an outpatient therapy. Decrease dose in patients with renal disease. Avoid IM administration.

Data from Taketomo, C., Hodding, J., & Kraus, D. (2008). *Pediatric dosage handbook* (15th ed.). Hudson, OH: Lexi Company, Inc.

Beta blocker use in heart failure is currently utilized in severely symptomatic children with chronic congestive heart failure. Although the exact mechanism of action is still being delineated, it has been shown to reverse or prevent cardiac dysfunction that is secondary to sympathetic activation. Carvedilol is a third generation beta blocker that can help improve symptoms and ventricular systolic performance in children (Shaddy, 2006). Due to its side effects profile patients must be monitored closely while the drug is being initiated and up titrated. Side effects include hypotension, depression, dizziness, and headaches. It is contraindicated in asthma, severe bradycardia, heart block, and diabetes (due to masking of the manifestation of hypoglycemia).

Nutritional support is critically important in the infant or child in CHF. Because of increased work of breathing, tachypnea, and fatigue these fragile children may not be able to consume enough calories to meet their increased metabolic needs. Caloric density in formula can be increased by adding less water to the concentrate or powder, therefore increasing the calories per ounce. Breast milk fortifier or powdered formula can be added to expressed breast milk to increase caloric density. Increasing caloric density should be accomplished slowly over a number of days, as a sudden increase will increase the osmotic load in the gut, producing diarrhea. A maximum of 27–30 calories per ounce is sufficient for most infants. If the infant is a slow feeder, or is incapable of consuming an appropriate amount of formula to promote growth, then gavage feedings are implemented. A nasogastric (NG) or nasojejunal (NJ) tube can be placed to provide feedings, either bolus or continuous. It should be noted that bolus feedings should never be given in an NJ tube since the jejunum does not have the capacity to hold large volumes (as does the stomach). Continuous feedings can be given all day or only at night. Volume and calories consumed over a 24-hour period should be sufficient to promote normal growth and development (Schwalbe-Terilli et al., 2009) (Table 25-5).

Older children are offered high-calorie foods, milkshakes, or supplemental nutritional products. Fluid restriction is not necessary because of concomitant use of diuretics. Rarely NG or gastrostomy tube feedings are implemented in the older child. Tube feedings should be given at night to encourage normal eating habits during the day.

Many children with CHF will have low arterial oxygen saturations. The etiology for this may be congenital defects or pulmonary edema. Oxygen therapy is withheld until determination is made of the child's structural defect. Oxygen stimulates closure of the ductus arteriosus and also dilates the pulmonary vascular bed. In the presence of structural defects that depend on a patent ductus arteriosus to support life until surgical correction, oxygen therapy could be lethal. In some patients with large L→R shunts oxygen therapy can increase pulmonary blood flow, worsening congestive failure. Oxygen administration is carefully implemented only after a thorough evaluation of the patient's cardiac anatomy is completed.

TABLE 25-5 Normal Caloric Requirements to Support Growth

AGE	CALORIES/KG/24 HOURS
Neonates	100–150
1–2 years	90–100
2–6 years	80–90
7–9 years	70–80
>10 years	50–60
Adolescents or adults	50

RESEARCH Highlight

Enteral Feeding and Caloric Intake in Neonates After Cardiac Surgery

STUDY PURPOSE

Adequate nutrition is essential to wound healing and growth. This study was to determine if neonates who have undergone congenital heart surgery obtain optimal calories from enteral feedings while in the cardiothoracic intensive care unit (CTICU).

METHODS

Retrospective chart review of all full-term neonates admitted to a CTICU at a major tertiary care pediatric facility were reviewed between November 2003 and August 2004. Exclusion criteria included those infants who did not require cardiopulmonary bypass and those who were enterally fed for less than two days prior to discharge from the CTICU. Assessed data included diagnosis, institution of enteral feeding, discontinuation of parental nutrition, total caloric intake, weight, method of feeding (oral vs. tube feeding), and reasons for discontinuation of feedings.

FINDINGS

100 infants were evaluated; median age at time of surgery was 4 days. Median length of stay in the CTICU was 13 days after surgery. Enteral feedings were started on post-operative day 3 (median). 18.9% were fed orally exclusively, 40.6% were fed via NG tube exclusively and 37.6% were fed both NG and PO. Median caloric intake was 93 cal/kg/day. 100 cal/kg/day was achieved in 48.4% and 120 cal/kg/day was achieved in 19.7%.

IMPLICATIONS

Caloric intake by enteral feedings alone was suboptimal for most neonates after cardiac surgery. Authors suggest that new strategies to maximize caloric intake be investigated. Further study is needed to evaluate feeding behaviors and feeding interventions in neonates with congenital heart disease.

REFERENCE

Schwalbe-Terilli, C. R., Hartman, D. H., Nagle, M. L., Gallagher, P. R., Ittenbach, R. F., Burnham, N. B., Gaynor, J. W., & Ravishankar, C. (2009). Enteral feeding and caloric intake in neonates after cardiac surgery. *American Journal of Critical Care*, 18, 52–57.

Maneuvers to decrease cardiac work are used along with pharmacologic agents to help improve outcomes. Measures to limit energy expenditure are important nursing interventions. Bed rest is only recommended in children with severe CHF. Client care should be clustered to allow for periods of quiet. Occasionally the extremely fussy infant or small child may benefit from small, carefully monitored doses of sedatives.

Children with severe CHF that is refractory to medical treatment and who do not have the option for surgical repair may be offered heart transplantation. In this setting heart transplantation offers the only hope of survival. Once the decision is made to move forward with transplantation then a full evaluation is undertaken by the heart transplant team. See the section on heart transplantation for more detail.

NURSING MANAGEMENT

Assessment

Negative sequela of decreased cardiac output is assessed. Physical examination includes the determination of heart rate, blood pressure, peripheral perfusion, urine output, and level of consciousness. If pharmacologic treatment has been implemented, response to therapy must be assessed. Respiratory function and oxygen saturation are evaluated and compared to the baseline assessment to monitor for trends or changes. Height, weight, and developmental milestones are determined to assess the impact CHF has had on growth and development. Nutritional assessment can be made in collaboration with a dietician.

Family supports, caregiver role, and interaction with the child are assessed. Coping skills must be determined, particularly in the family with a child who has been newly diagnosed with heart failure. Response to family teaching is evaluated to determine deficient knowledge. Reinforcement of teaching is frequently required, particularly during periods of stress.

Nursing Diagnosis

1. *Decreased cardiac output* related to decreased contractility, increased preload, increased afterload as evidenced by edema, shortness of breath, decreased urine output, hepatomegaly.
2. *Excess fluid volume* related to increased preload and decreased contractility secondary to CHF as evidenced by peripheral edema, hepatomegaly, and pulmonary edema.
3. *Imbalanced nutrition: Less than body requirements* related to poor caloric intake and increased metabolic demands as evidenced by poor weight gain, weight loss, and poor caloric intake.

Outcome Identification

- The child will have optimal cardiac output as evidenced by normal blood pressure, and normal urine output along with absence of difficult or labored breathing and edema.
- The child will be alert and interactive indicating normal cerebral perfusion.
- The child will not exhibit signs or symptoms of venous congestion such as hepatomegaly or edema.
- The child will exhibit normal electrolyte levels.
- The child will ingest the appropriate number of calories for his age (see Table 25-5).
- The child will exhibit normal growth.

Planning and Implementation

Nurses should monitor vital signs, tissue perfusion, and evaluate and monitor trends and changes. Monitor heart rate and rhythm, document ECG, and treat rhythm abnormalities as indicated as many arrhythmias will adversely affect cardiac output. Administer medications as appropriate and monitor for clinical efficacy and side effects (see Table 25-3). If vasodilators are initiated or dose is adjusted, monitor blood pressure 30 minutes to 1 hour after dose as hypotension may occur.

Nurses should assess fluid status: mucous membranes are moist, pulses are strong, anterior fontanel is not sunken, and hepatomegaly is absent or does not worsen. Daily weight and I&O are assessed. Specific gravity of urine is to be checked daily. Excessive weight gain or new onset edema can mean fluid retention. Urine output is at least 1 cc/kg/hour, indicating normal renal perfusion and volume status. Diuretics are administered as ordered and electrolytes monitored if diuretic dose is increased. Potassium replacement is indicated if diuretic induced hypokalemia is present.

Nurses should document height and weight on growth chart and evaluate for changes (particularly weight loss). Weigh daily to weekly depending on acuity of child. Calorie counts help to determine if adequate calories are being consumed. Consultation with a dietician can assist in providing appropriate diet and calories. Gavage feedings are administered if necessary, and caloric density of formula is increased to maximize caloric intake if necessary.

Evaluation

Vital signs are within normal limits for age without evidence of hepatomegaly or jugular venous distention. The CXR is clear without evidence of cardiomegaly or pulmonary venous congestion. No arrhythmias are evident. Peripheral perfusion is normal; urine output is normal at 1 cc/kg/hour. The blood pressure is normal without evidence of hypotension. The medications are well tolerated without side effects. Intake and output is equal. Urine output and specific gravity are normal. Serum electrolytes are maintained within normal limits. Normal caloric intake and weight gain are supported, and feedings are tolerated without diarrhea or emesis. The family understands the rationale for dietary plan and is comfortable with NG or NJ feedings.

FAMILY TEACHING

The family is taught the signs and symptoms of worsening heart failure so that notification of the cardiologist can be made in a timely manner. They are taught how to

Reflections from Families

We waited three years to have our first baby. When she was born I thought she was the most beautiful thing I had ever seen. Then I noticed a large birthmark on her hand and thought that was no big deal and could be removed. My little girl was still perfect as far as I was concerned. Upon further examination the doctors told me she had what they called an imperforate anus and would need major surgery to correct it. I couldn't believe this was happening but I was encouraged because the doctors told me she would have a normal life after a couple of surgeries. My wife and I agreed that we could handle this. While she was being prepared for surgery they told us she had a heart murmur and needed more tests. What we heard next was very hard to handle. Our baby had two holes in the wall between the chambers of her heart and a serious narrowing of her aorta, the biggest artery in the body. She would need open heart surgery as a tiny baby and there was a chance she wouldn't live at all. Imagine how I felt being worried about her silly birthmark. I was sad, angry, worried, and hopeful that things would be okay all at the same time. As a religious man I questioned why this was happening to our precious little girl.

Our special girl has survived her open heart surgery and is doing okay. Our next step will be to have her imperforate anus surgery. My wife and I are grateful that she is doing as well as she is and have learned to love her even more and appreciate our time with her. We know the trips to the hospital are not over but we've learned to accept life's troubles with a new attitude.

administer all medications. The nurse must also review all medication side effects with the caregivers. Reinforcement of teaching will most likely be required, particularly upon discharge from the hospital. Questions are encouraged to clarify misconceptions.

Prior to discharge from the hospital all family members involved in the care of the child should learn CPR. Many hospitals have programs designed specifically for caregivers that are simple and straightforward. Emergency phone numbers should be provided as well. Clinic appointments are made prior to discharge from the hospital.

For many children the definitive treatment for CHF will be surgery, so outcome is somewhat less uncertain. However, CHF can also mean end stage disease and an uncertain future. Support systems must be in place in the scenario of end stage disease. If the future holds a possible heart transplant, then early contact with the transplant team is critical.

Family teaching should include:

- Allow frequent short periods of time for feedings.
- Pay attention to infant cues during a feeding—back arching or averting of eyes means child wants to disengage and take a break. If feeding disengagement cues are demonstrated, allow infant to take a break.
- For tube feedings allow infant to nipple as much as possible, then gavage the rest. If the infant is tube fed at night, do not awaken to try to nipple feed.
- Concentrate formula as prescribed. Teach family how to do this and have them give a return demonstration.
- If feeding the infant becomes a full-time job, get family or friends to help.
- Use home nursing to help with feeding tube placement and problem-solve tube feeding issues.
- Call health care provider if questions arise. Have family develop rapport with one health care provider who is familiar with them and their infant.

CONGENITAL HEART DEFECTS

Congenital heart defects (CHD) occur in approximately 4–50 per 1,000 live births (Pierpont et al., 2007). There are a minimum of 35 types of recognized defects ranging from mild, easily corrected defects such as a patent ductus arteriosus to more serious and complex anomalies such as hypoplastic left heart syndrome. Heart defects are one of the most common birth defects and the leading cause of birth defect related deaths.

It should be pointed out that although these defects will be discussed separately, it is not uncommon for the infant to present with a combination of defects. It should also be noted that many of these defects can be diagnosed with prenatal echocardiogram. The following section will be divided into defects that result in *increased pulmonary flow, decreased pulmonary blood flow,* and those with *left-sided obstruction.* In the modern era the vast majority of complex defects are repaired or palliated in the first year of life. It is believed by many surgeons and cardiologist's that when complete repair is possible in the neonatal period, there are advantages to providing normal cardiac function, normal respiratory function, and brain maturation. Many complex defects require staged repairs, that is, more than one surgery is ultimately required for final correction. Even in this scenario completion of staged repairs generally occurs by age 2 to 4 years. Repair of defects that impose little or no hemodynamic alteration may be deferred until age 2 or 3 years. Mild isolated defects may never require surgery.

> **NURSING TIP**
>
> **Blood Flow, Pressure, and Resistance**
>
> Remembering that blood will always flow from an area of high pressure to an area of lower pressure and will take the path of least resistance will help the reader understand the hemodynamic effect of all congenital heart defects.

Because the heart is the size of the child's fist, intracardiac or open heart surgery can be complex. To support the child during this type of surgery, cardiopulmonary bypass (CPB) is implemented. It must be clarified that CPB is not a *treatment* but a form of life support used during open heart surgery only. Although technological advances have improved CPB, there remain a number of sequelae that have an impact on the child's condition following surgery.

CPB, which is used for the repair of many congenital defects, is a mechanical pump and artificial oxygenator that provides, for a short period, substitution for the heart and lungs. The general principles of CPB include the removal of unoxygenated blood via a venous cannula and the delivery of oxygenated blood back to the patient via an aortic cannula. The work of the heart and lungs is therefore performed by the bypass pump, allowing the surgeon to work on the heart in a bloodless field.

DEFECTS WITH INCREASED PULMONARY BLOOD FLOW

Defects that increase pulmonary blood flow are caused by a shunting of the blood from the left side of the heart to the right side through an abnormal connection (left to right shunt). The blood flows from the left to the right side because the pressures are greater on the left side of the heart. The increased amount of blood in the right side leads to increased pulmonary blood flow. Infants with these defects exhibit the clinical manifestations of CHF. Atrial septal defects, ventricular septal defects, patent ductus arteriosus, atrioventricular septal defects, and truncus arteriosus are all in this category.

Atrial Septal Defect

An atrial septal defect (ASD) is an abnormal connection between the right and left atria and is illustrated in Figure 25-12. This is an acyanotic defect and can be missed by the practitioner until school age.

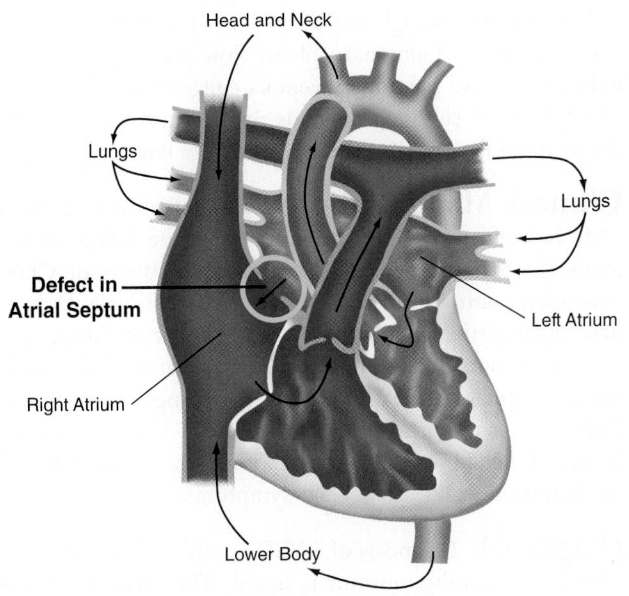

FIGURE 25-12 Atrial Septal Defect. DELMAR CENGAGE LEARNING.

Incidence ASDs account for approximately 6–10% of all congenital heart disease and are usually present in combination with other more severe heart defects (Backer & Mavroudis, 2003).

Pathophysiology Because of the normal increased pressure on the left side of the heart, blood flows from the left to the right across the ASD. This leads to increased volume on the right side of the heart, with a subsequent increase in right atrial and ventricular size, as well as an increase in pulmonary artery (PA) size.

Clinical Manifestations The infant or child with an ASD is generally asymptomatic. There is often a soft systolic murmur and more classically a widely split S2, unaffected by respiratory pattern.

Diagnosis Diagnosis is often made after a murmur is detected during a routine health care examination. Chest X-rays will usually demonstrate increased heart size. An echocardiogram demonstrates the location and size of the defect. Cardiac catheterization is not routinely indicated for diagnosis of an isolated ASD.

Treatment Preoperative intervention is only indicated in the infant or child with a large ASD that results in CHF. Diuretics are given to control the symptoms of CHF until repair is performed. Surgical repair is generally performed in the preschool age period because there is a possibility of spontaneous closure in the first 2 years of life, and the child is usually asymptomatic. Traditionally, surgery has been performed via a median sternotomy (vertical incision along the sternum). For closure of an isolated ASD, a limited lower partial sternotomy is the choice for minimally invasive surgery. This type of incision is much smaller than a normal sternotomy and therefore more cosmetic for the child (Jonas, 2004a). The defect is repaired via stitch closure or patch closure through an incision made in the right atrium, often a prepared piece of the child's pericardium is used to close the defect.

Recently, the treatment of choice for certain ASDs has been closure via nonsurgical device placement, performed in the cardiac catheterization lab. The device is placed via a catheter in a large femoral vessel, threaded up into the heart and across the ASD, occluding the opening. The ASD must be of a

EYE ON...

Interventional Procedures for Congenital Heart Disease

A number of technological innovations are in use or evolving that will allow those with congenital heart disease to avoid surgery. Treatment options include interventional procedures performed in the cardiac catheterization laboratory. These include, but are not limited to, balloon valvuloplasty, stent placement, placement of coils, and occluding devices.

Balloon valvuloplasty can be used for balloon dilation of stenotic pulmonary, aortic, and mitral valves. A catheter with a balloon tip is passed percutaneously into the femoral artery or vein and then advanced to cross the appropriate valve. The balloon is then expanded to dilate the valve subsequently relieving the stenosis. As technology and skill improve, clinical indications are continuing to expand. Balloon dilation of recurrent coarctation of the aorta can also be used in lieu of surgical correction.

Stents can be placed in narrowed vessels such as the aorta or pulmonary arteries. Again a special catheter (with the stent loaded on the tip of the catheter) is placed percutaneously in the femoral vein or artery. Once the catheter tip is in the area of narrowing the stent is deployed, resulting in widening of the narrowed area. This procedure often obviates the need for surgery to correct either peripheral pulmonary stenosis or recurrent coarctation of the aorta.

Coils can be placed in abnormal vessels or a patent ductus arteriosus to occlude the vessel without surgery. Occluding devices are used for nonsurgical treatment of most atrial septal defects and are becoming more popular for the closure of some ventricular septal defects. These occluding devices are small, round mesh containing devices that are loaded into the tip of a special catheter. Once the catheter is placed across the septal defect the device is deployed and attaches to the rim of tissue around the defect, thereby effectively closing the hole. With both coil and occluding devices native tissue will eventually cover the device.

Interventional cardiac catheterization represents a rapidly growing frontier in health care. As skill and knowledge increase clinical indications will continue to expand.

certain size, and the device, when in place, must not obstruct flow across any valve. The major advantage of this procedure is the avoidance of open heart surgery and generally a decrease in hospital stay.

The main complications of an ASD repair are atrial arrhythmias or heart block secondary to edema around or surgical interruption of the conduction system. This can occur with either surgical closure or device closure. This is often temporary and normal conduction returns with time. For children with a repaired ASD long-term survival is comparable to normal individuals when matched for age and sex. A small percentage can develop atrial arrhythmias following surgery so periodic follow-up is warranted. Natural history and resultant sequela of *unrepaired* ASD may not become apparent until the third or fourth decade of life. The result of many years of increased pulmonary blood flow often leads to severe pulmonary hypertension.

VENTRICULAR SEPTAL DEFECT

A ventricular septal defect (VSD) is an abnormal connection between the right and left ventricles (Figure 25-13). The defect can be located in various positions along the septum.

Incidence VSDs are among the most common congenital heart defects. Isolated VSDs and those VSDs associated with other congenital anomalies account for approximately 50% of infants with congenital heart disease (Mavroudis, Backer, & Jacobs, 2003).

Pathophysiology Because of normally increased pressures on the left side of the heart, blood flow through a VSD is *left to right*. The blood that flows through the VSD will recirculate through the pulmonary artery to the lungs. The increase in pulmonary blood flow leads to left heart enlargement and pulmonary venous congestion. The degree of left to right shunting depends on two major factors: *the size of the defect* and the child's *pulmonary resistance*.

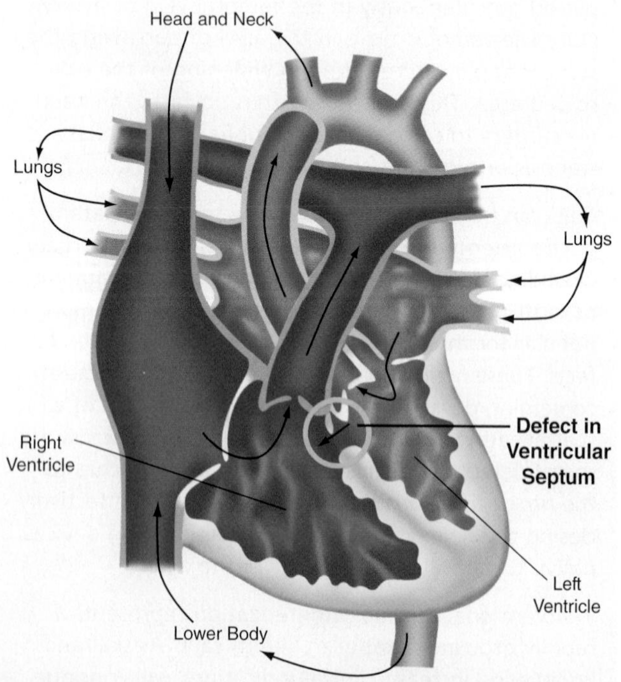

FIGURE 25-13 **Ventricular Septal Defect.** DELMAR CENGAGE LEARNING.

Clinical Manifestations The infant with a small VSD is likely to be asymptomatic while the infant with a moderate to large defect will demonstrate signs of CHF. The infant with a moderate to large VSD is usually tachypneic, diaphoretic, fatigues easily, and is underweight for age; cyanosis is not usually present. Feeding history will usually reveal an infant that tires before a feeding is completed. VSDs are also seen in older children. If a VSD is detected in an older child for the first time, it is because the defect is small and the child has had no symptoms.

Diagnosis Diagnosis of a VSD is often suspected when a loud holosystolic murmur is heard. The intensity of the murmur can reflect the size of the defect. The X-ray of a child with a small VSD can be normal while the X-ray of a child with a moderate to large defect will often show cardiomegaly with an increase in pulmonary blood flow. Echocardiogram is indicated to determine the size and location of the defect. Cardiac catheterization is rarely indicated.

Treatment The infant with a small VSD who does not demonstrate signs of congestive heart failure usually requires no treatment, as 75–80% of these defects will close spontaneously (Miyake et al., 2004). Many children with small hemodynamically insignificant VSDs never require surgery. These children are asymptomatic without cardiac enlargement. It is felt that the risks of surgery outweigh the benefits. Large defects are unlikely to close; therefore, the infant is treated medically for the first few months of life and watched closely for appropriate weight gain and for any signs of complicating respiratory infections. Digoxin, ACE inhibitors, and diuretics are given to relieve symptoms of CHF. High-calorie formula may be utilized to promote growth. Nasal gastric feedings are used in infants who are excessively tachypneic or who tire with feedings. If symptoms persist despite these therapies then surgical closure is indicated (Jonas, 2004e).

Surgical repair is indicated between 3 and 12 months of age. This is necessary to prevent the development of

NURSING TIP

Pulmonary Vascular Resistance (PVR)

Pulmonary vascular resistance falls in the first few weeks of life. This can dramatically change intracardiac blood flow patterns. Therefore, a newborn with a VSD may not demonstrate symptoms until after PVR falls.

pulmonary vascular disease in children who have large L→R shunts. Surgery is indicated earlier in the small infant who is failing to thrive. The defect is closed with a stitch or with synthetic material while on CPB. Postoperative complications include atrial arrhythmias, complete heart block, ventricular arrhythmias, and residual shunt or leaking at the site of the VSD patch. Increasing experience is also being gained closing VSDs in the catheterization lab with nonsurgical devices. However, due to the varied location of many VSDs and their association with other forms of congenital heart disease, not all defects are amenable to device closure

Children with small unrepaired VSDs exhibit life span and health similar to the unaffected population. For children with large VSDs repaired in the first two years of life, the long-term outlook for normal health is excellent. Surgical mortality is less than 5% when performed in the first year of life. Those who have surgery after 2 years of age may have residual problems with arrhythmias, depressed myocardial function, and pulmonary hypertension. When and if this will occur is difficult to predict.

Patent Ductus Arteriosus

The ductus arteriosus is a direct connection between the main pulmonary artery and the aorta (Figure 25-14). In the fetus the ductus arteriosus is necessary for survival. In the preterm infant it is a common finding simply based on developmental immaturity. In the term newborn the ductus begins to close within 12 hours and should be completely closed by 2–3 weeks. A PDA results from failure of normal transition from fetal to postnatal circulation (Jonas, 2004c).

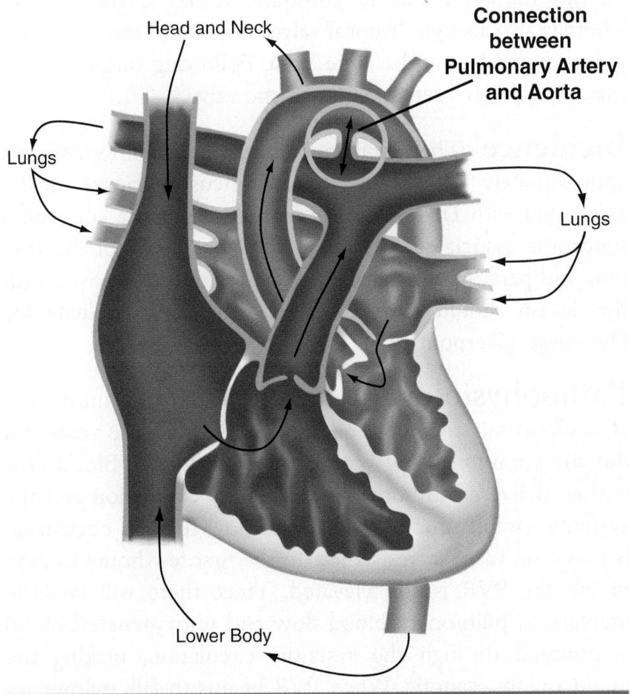

Figure 25-14 Patent Ductus Arteriosus. DELMAR CENGAGE LEARNING.

Incidence The incidence of PDA in a nonpremature infant is approximately 5–10% of all CHD. The incidence in the premature infant is dramatically higher at 45% in infants who weigh less than 1,750 grams and up to 80% in infants weighing less than 1,000 grams.

Pathophysiology The hemodynamic effect of a PDA is similar to other defects with left to right shunts. Blood from the high pressure aorta flows directly into the low pressure pulmonary artery and pulmonary circulation. The degree of shunting depends on the size of the PDA as well as the pulmonary vascular resistance. This increase in pulmonary blood flow can contribute to CHF.

Clinical Manifestations The degree of symptoms experienced by the infant will depend on the size of the shunt. The infant with a small PDA will generally be asymptomatic. The infant with a large PDA will have signs of CHF.

Diagnosis The murmur of a PDA is often continuous and is best heard just below the left clavicle. A chest X-ray is usually normal and diagnosis is generally made with an echocardiogram. Cardiac catheterization is not necessary for the diagnosis of a PDA.

Treatment In the premature infant, closure of the PDA is attempted medically with the infusion of indomethacin, which inhibits the synthesis of prostaglandin. Prostaglandins are a group of fatty acid substances present in many tissues and are responsible for a number of cellular interactions. They are responsible for maintaining patency of the ductus arteriosus. More recently intravenous or oral ibuprofen has been used to medically close the PDA. It is believed to be as effective as Indomethacin with fewer side effects, in particular there are fewer renal abnormalities (Ohlsson, Walia, & Shah, 2008). Closure is indicated in the full-term symptomatic (CHF) infant with a PDA. Indomethacin and ibuprofen are not effective in full-term infants. Older asymptomatic children undergo elective closure before 5 years of age. Technique for nonsurgical closure involves the use of coils to occlude the PDA. This is performed in the cardiac catheterization lab. For those PDAs deemed too large for coil occlusion, surgical ligation, or tying off, is indicated. This is performed via left thoracotomy incision without the use of CPB. Rare postoperative complications include injury to the recurrent laryngeal nerve causing hoarseness, or injury to the left phrenic nerve resulting in paralysis of the left hemidiaphragm.

Normal survival and quality of life are excellent for the infant and child with a repaired, isolated PDA. Because mortality approaches zero, it is therefore recommended that all PDAs without pulmonary vascular disease be closed. Unrepaired PDAs produce large left to right shunts with left atrial dilation, left ventricular volume overload, and pulmonary hypertension, leading to the development of pulmonary vascular disease (Hillman, Mavroudis, & Backer, 2003). The presence of severe pulmonary vascular disease precludes PDA closure.

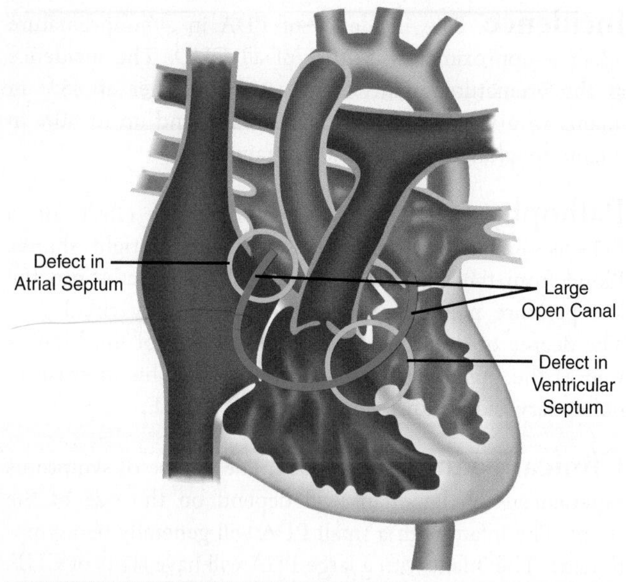

FIGURE 25-15 Atrioventricular Canal Defect. DELMAR CENGAGE LEARNING.

ATRIOVENTRICULAR SEPTAL DEFECT

Atrioventricular defect or atrioventricular canal (AVC) is associated with a septal defect in the atrium and ventricle, as well as involvement of the AV valves. In this defect, when the heart is developing, the atrial and ventricular septums are not fully completed and never meet (Figure 25-15). This, in turn, causes the tricuspid and mitral valves to develop inappropriately. The severity of the defect depends on the amount of the septum that is involved as well as the degree of AV valve involvement.

Incidence AVC accounts for about 4–10% of all congenital heart defects (AHA, 2007). It should also be noted that approximately 40% of children with Trisomy 21 (Down syndrome) have some form of congenital heart defect and almost half of these have AVC (Setty, Shaun, & Shen, 2006).

Pathophysiology Because of the fact that there is free communication between all chambers of the heart, blood flow patterns are dependent on the resistance to the pulmonary and systemic circulations. In the infant whose PVR is decreasing with age, blood flow will be left to right causing increased blood flow to the lungs. Increased pulmonary blood flow will result in increased pulmonary venous return to the left side of the heart with left atrial and ventricular enlargement.

Clinical Manifestations The infant with an AVC demonstrates signs and symptoms of CHF. The murmur can be quite variable, depending on the size of the septal defects. It is usually a long systolic or holosystolic murmur. Virtually all infants are symptomatic by their first birthday.

Diagnosis On chest X-rays the heart and main pulmonary artery are enlarged. An echocardiogram will demonstrate the degree of septal involvement and the commitment of the common AV valve to the left or right ventricle. In certain cases cardiac catheterization may be indicated.

Treatment The infant with AVC is treated for CHF prior to surgical repair. Many centers around the country perform surgical correction within the first few months of life, but surgery should be completed by 1 year of age to prevent the development of irreversible pulmonary vascular disease (Jonas, 2004b). The goal of the repair is to close the atrial and ventricular septal defects and then construct new mitral and tricuspid valves from the common AV valve. This surgery is performed while the infant is on CPB. Potential postoperative complications include heart block, arrhythmias, bleeding from the multiple intracardiac suture lines, or pulmonary hypertension. Another potential postoperative problem includes poor cardiac output secondary to poorly functioning or incompetent AV valves. A postoperative echocardiogram will demonstrate the degree of incompetency of the valves and any residual ASD or VSD.

Surgical mortality rate for AVC repair is less than 4% (Jonas, 2004b). Regurgitation through the affected AV valve (mitral or tricuspid) is not uncommon with AVC. Long-term outcomes are quite variable and are dependent upon the degree of AV valve incompetence. Natural history for the *unrepaired* AVC is quite poor, with most children dying by 15 years of age.

TRUNCUS ARTERIOSUS

The primary anatomical features of a truncus arteriosus result from failure of the embryologic trunk to divide into the pulmonary arteries and the aorta. Therefore, a single arterial trunk arises from the heart giving rise to the pulmonary arteries, the aorta, and the coronary arteries (Figure 25-16). There is also a single "truncal valve" in place of the aortic and pulmonary valves and a large VSD. Following surgical repair this truncal valve serves as the aortic valve.

Incidence The incidence of truncus arteriosus is approximately 1.4% of all CHD. Truncus arteriosus can be associated with **DiGeorge syndrome**, which is a congenital syndrome associated with hypoplasia or aplasia of the thymus and parathyroid gland. Any child who is diagnosed with this lesion should have a genetic workup to evaluate for DiGeorge (Pierpont et al., 2007).

Pathophysiology Both oxygenated and unoxygenated blood mix together and are ejected from the ventricles out the common trunk (common great vessel). Blood flow is then delivered to both the pulmonary circulation and the systemic circulation. The degree of flow to each circulation is based on vascular resistance. In the first few hours to days of life the PVR is still elevated. Thus, there will be little increase in pulmonary blood flow and unoxygenated blood is pumped through the systemic circulation, making the infant mildly cyanotic. When PVR begins to fall, pulmonary

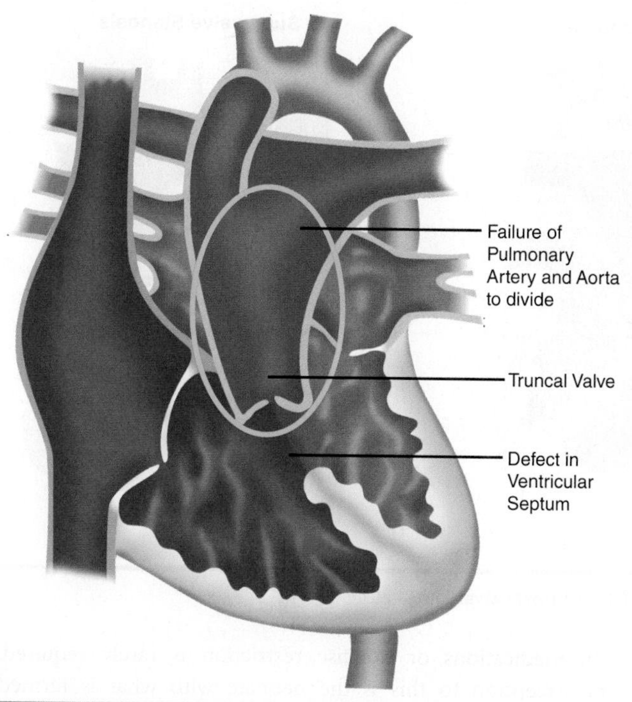

FIGURE 25-16 **Truncus Arteriosus.** DELMAR CENGAGE LEARNING.

flow increases, making the shunt left to right. The infant will no longer be cyanotic but may develop CHF.

Clinical Manifestations The newborn infant, as previously described, may be mildly cyanotic despite supplemental oxygen. As PVR falls the newborn will develop signs and symptoms of CHF. Auscultation will reveal a loud continuous murmur along with a loud click associated with the closing of the truncal valve. Symptoms almost always develop in the first month of life.

Diagnosis A chest X-ray demonstrates moderate cardiomegaly. Echo-cardiogram is diagnostic for truncus arteriosus, but cardiac catheterization is still indicated to determine any questionable anatomic variations and hemodynamics.

Treatment The infant is treated for symptoms of CHF. Surgical repair is performed within the first 1–2 weeks of life (Jonas, 2004d). The repair is performed as follows: The PAs are removed from the common trunk and the defect left in the trunk wall is sutured closed. The VSD is closed and a valved homograft conduit is placed connecting the RV to the PAs. A homograft conduit is a chemically treated human aorta or pulmonary artery, obtained from a cadaver that is placed like a tube to conduct blood from the right ventricle to the pulmonary artery. The conduit will require replacement as the child grows. Research is ongoing to determine the best material that will provide the most longevity and efficiency.

Postoperative circulation is as follows. Systemic venous return enters the RA to the RV and flows through the conduit to the pulmonary artery and to the lungs. Pulmonary venous return enters the LA to the LV and flows out through the truncal valve to the aorta. There is no longer mixing of oxygenated and unoxygenated blood so oxygen saturations should be normal. Postoperative complications include arrhythmias, low cardiac output, and truncal valve regurgitation. Without treatment the prognosis is poor: 1) mortality is approximately 80% during the first year of life with about half of these infants dying during the neonatal period (St. Louis, 2006); 2) those who survive infancy will often die in the first years of life secondary to complications of pulmonary vascular disease.

DEFECTS WITH DECREASED PULMONARY BLOOD FLOW

In these defects the amount of blood flow to the pulmonary system is decreased, resulting in shunting of unoxygenated blood from the right side of the heart to the left. There is a mixing of oxygenated and unoxygenated blood in the systemic circulation. Infants with such a defect are hypoxic and cyanotic. An increase in the hematocrit (polycythemia) is frequently observed in these infants with chronic cyanosis. **Erythrocytosis** is an adaptive mechanism in which red cell production is increased in an attempt to compensate for decreased oxygen delivery, leading to an increase in hematocrit.

A hematocrit of 65–75% can lead to increased blood viscosity. Increases in viscosity will also increase afterload and ventricular work. The risk of cerebral strokes also increases if hematocrit rises above 65%. These individuals can also develop bleeding disorders caused by a decrease in circulating clotting factors and platelets. Fortunately, most children now undergo early surgical intervention, preventing or minimizing erythrocytosis. Defects with decreased pulmonary blood flow include pulmonary stenosis, tetralogy of Fallot, transposition of the great arteries, and tricuspid atresia. Of note, transposition of the great vessels can cause an increase in pulmonary blood flow but is listed here because of the hallmark cyanosis that is associated with it.

PULMONARY STENOSIS

Pulmonary stenosis (PS) refers to narrowing of the pulmonary valve and obstruction to blood flow from the right ventricle to the lungs. The obstruction can be at the valve (valvar, Figure 25-17A), just before the pulmonary valve itself (subvalvar, Figure 25-17B), above the valve (supravalvar, Figure 25-17C), or in varying places along the pulmonary artery. This discussion will focus on infants with valvar pulmonary stenosis. Valvar pulmonary stenosis results from abnormal fusion of the leaflets of the pulmonary valve. A smaller number of patients will have thickened valves known as dysplastic valves.

Incidence The incidence of pulmonary stenosis is approximately 8%–10% of all CHD (Mitchell & Clarke, 2003).

Pathophysiology Secondary to the obstruction of blood flow from the RV to the PA, there is a significant

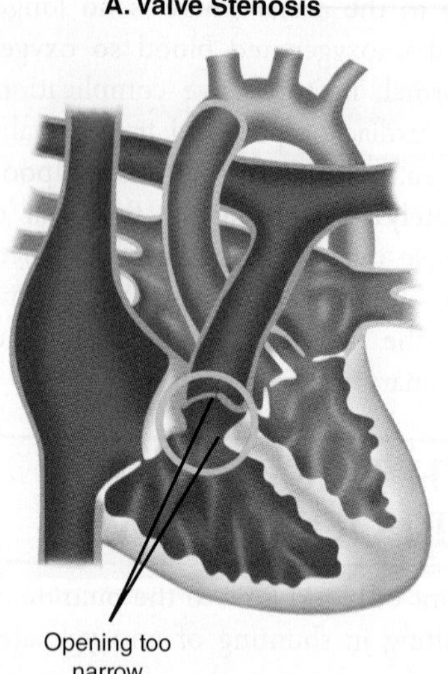

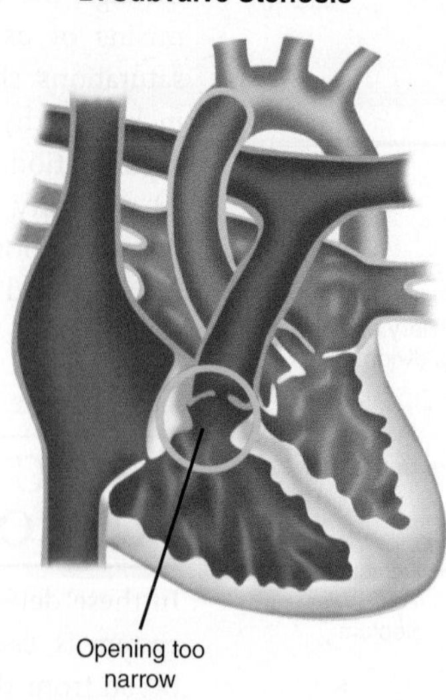

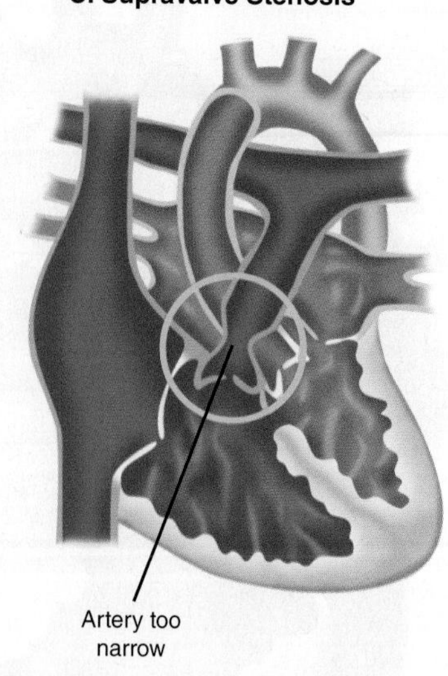

FIGURE 25-17 Pulmonary Stenosis: (A) Valvar, (B) Subvalvar, and (C) Supravalvar. DELMAR CENGAGE LEARNING.

increase in the right ventricular pressure. This may eventually lead to RV failure. There is also a decreased amount of blood flow that is able to get to the lungs. At rest, the body can compensate for this decrease in pulmonary blood flow so there are no symptoms. However, with increase in exertion, such as crying or feeding in the infant, or exercises in the child, exertion compensation is no longer effective, and the individual may develop exercise intolerance or, occasionally, cyanosis. The amount of exercise that promotes intolerance and cyanosis is dependent on the individual infant or child and could be something as simple as walking up a flight of stairs.

The degree of PS is determined by the RV systolic pressure at rest. If the pressure is low, then the defect is considered mild. If the RV and LV pressures are equal, the defect is classified as moderate. The infant with an RV pressure greater than LV is considered to have severe pulmonary stenosis.

Clinical Manifestations The infant with mild to moderate PS is asymptomatic, and generally a murmur is discovered on routine examination. Growth is generally normal for infants and children with PS, and symptoms are usually present only in those with severe PS. The symptoms of severe PS include dyspnea upon exertion and fatigue. Cyanosis is common with *severe* PS but is not usually seen with the milder forms.

Diagnosis The diagnosis can often be made on clinical examination alone. Supportive diagnostic tests are usually obtained to confirm the diagnosis. The chest X-ray of the child with mild to moderate PS is generally normal, while the child with severe PS may have cardiomegaly. Echocardiogram will demonstrate the size and function of the RV and the anatomy of the pulmonary valve. Cardiac catheterization is not necessary for diagnosis of PS.

Treatment Treatment for PS is recommended for those with moderate to severe forms. Preoperative management with medications or exercise restriction is rarely required. The exception to this is the neonate with what is termed *critical PS.* These infants are critically ill and require the infusion of prostaglandins to maintain patency to the ductus arteriosus. This provides adequate blood flow to the lungs until catheterization or surgical intervention.

In most children with valvar PS a balloon **valvuloplasty** can be performed. This is done in the cardiac catheterization laboratory. A valvuloplasty involves using a balloon-tipped catheter to dilate a cardiac valve (the pulmonary). If a valvuloplasty cannot be performed, a surgical **valvotomy** (an incision into a cardiac valve to correct a defect) is the treatment of choice. Short-term complications of valvuloplasty include ventricular arrhythmias *during* the procedure; over the long term, the child may develop pulmonary valve insufficiency. This is often mild and requires no intervention.

Infants with mild PS are unlikely to have progression of their obstruction and are therefore not treated. However, it is recommended that they be monitored with several echocardiograms during their childhood. Because of the safety and effectiveness of balloon valvuloplasty, this treatment is recommended for those with moderate to severe PS as the obstruction may worsen over time.

TETRALOGY OF FALLOT

Tetralogy of Fallot (TOF) is made up of four components: (1) VSD, (2) pulmonary stenosis, (3) right ventricular hypertrophy, and (4) an overriding aorta (Figure 25-18). The degree of PS is the most important component of TOF, as its severity will determine clinical presentation, timing of surgery, and preoperative management. The right ventricle is hypertrophied because of resistance to pumping its blood through the pulmonary artery, which is stenosed or narrowed. The placement of the aorta, overriding the VSD, is of little clinical importance but is part of the anatomic features of this defect.

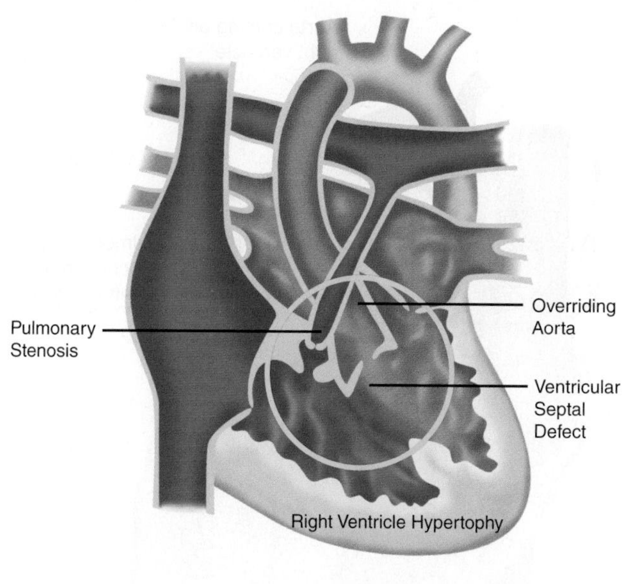

FIGURE 25-18 Tetralogy of Fallot. DELMAR CENGAGE LEARNING.

Incidence TOF is the most common cyanotic heart defect accounting for approximately 9–14% of all CHD (AHA, 2007).

Pathophysiology The large VSD associated with this defect leads to equal pressures in the R and L ventricles. The amount of pulmonary blood flow and, therefore, the amount of cyanosis, will depend on the degree of pulmonary stenosis. Even with mild PS there is usually enough obstruction to pulmonary flow that these infants have some decrease in pulmonary blood flow. In some individuals there is such minimal obstruction that they are not cyanotic; thus, the term *pink tet* is often used to describe them.

Clinical Manifestations Clinical symptoms vary greatly depending on the degree of PS. The infant or child may be profoundly cyanotic, or may display no signs of cyanosis and be growing normally. A characteristic systolic murmur results from the right ventricular outflow tract obstruction and is generally moderate in severity. One of the most common conditions associated with TOF is hypercyanotic episodes. These episodes are also known as "tet spells" and are usually initiated by some type of activity such as crying, feeding, or defecating. There are several theories as to the cause of hypercyanotic spells but in general the following occurs. There is likely a decrease in pulmonary blood flow caused by spasm of the infundibular muscle (the area below the valve) within the right ventricular outflow tract. This leads to an increase in R→L shunt, worsening cyanosis and development of **hyperpnea**, deep, rapid respirations. In the normal individual this increase in respiratory rate leads to an increase in venous return to the heart (systemic venous return). In the infant with TOF, increased systemic venous return of a large amount of unoxygenated blood leads to a decrease in arterial saturation (caused by R→L shunt) with continuation of profound cyanosis. If left untreated, the infant or child may become unconscious or die.

Diagnosis The chest X-ray of the child with TOF is often within normal limits although sometimes the classic boot-shaped heart (caused by hypertrophy of the right ventricle) is observed. Echocardiogram will demonstrate the clinical features of TOF and is the best diagnostic tool.

Treatment Management of the infant and child with TOF is definitive surgical correction, but preoperative medical management is important as well. A hypercyanotic spell can be frightening to watch and difficult to manage. Caregivers should be taught simple measures to alleviate these symptoms. The simplest treatment for a hypercyanotic spell is to place the infant in the knee-chest position (Figure 25-19). This measure will decrease systemic venous return of unoxygenated blood as well as increase systemic vascular resistance in the hope of decreasing R→L shunt, allowing more blood flow to the lungs. In the hospital, acutely ill infants are also treated with morphine sulfate to relieve symptoms of agitation and break the cycle of hyperpnea. Other interventions include volume resuscitation to decrease blood viscosity, supplemental oxygen and, if necessary, medications such

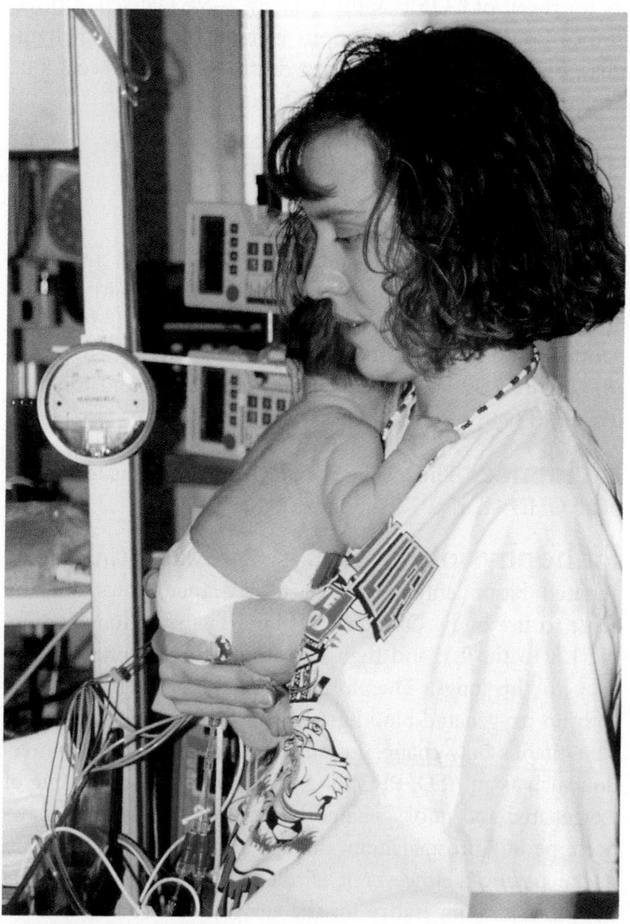

FIGURE 25-19 An Infant with Tetralogy of Fallot in Knee-Chest Position. DELMAR CENGAGE LEARNING.

as phenylephrine (administered intravenously) to increase systemic vascular resistance. An increase in the number and severity of spells should lead to surgical palliation or complete repair.

For the infant with multiple hypercyanotic spells, a palliative modified Blalock-Taussing (BT) shunt may be performed to assure pulmonary blood flow until complete surgical repair is performed. A **palliative** procedure relieves or reduces the symptoms of a cardiac defect but does not correct the defect. The shunt provides a fixed amount of blood flow to the pulmonary bed and cannot grow with the child. Complete repair for the child with TOF is usually performed between 3 and 12 months of age, but varies by institution. The goals of the repair are to widen the right ventricular outflow tract and to close the VSD. If a modified BT shunt is present, it is taken down or occluded at the time of the definitive repair.

Postoperative complications include low cardiac output and arrhythmias. Long-term complications include residual VSD (leaking at the patch of the VSD) and pulmonary regurgitation across the patch. TOF accounts for the largest number of adults with congenital heart disease. Approximately 11% of patients who have not had any surgical repair will live past 20 years of age, but this decreases to 3% by age 40. Death is secondary to ventricular failure. Surgical mortality for repair of TOF is approximately 2–5% (Hirsch & Bove, 2003). Long-term complications include ventricular arrhythmias, cardiac failure, and sudden death. As surgical technique evolves, long-term outcomes continue to improve.

Transposition of the Great Arteries

Transposition of the great arteries (TGA) is a defect in which the great vessels (aorta and the pulmonary artery) are transposed or reversed. The aorta comes off the right ventricle and the pulmonary artery comes off the left ventricle (Figure 25-20). There is almost always a patent foramen ovale (PFO) present.

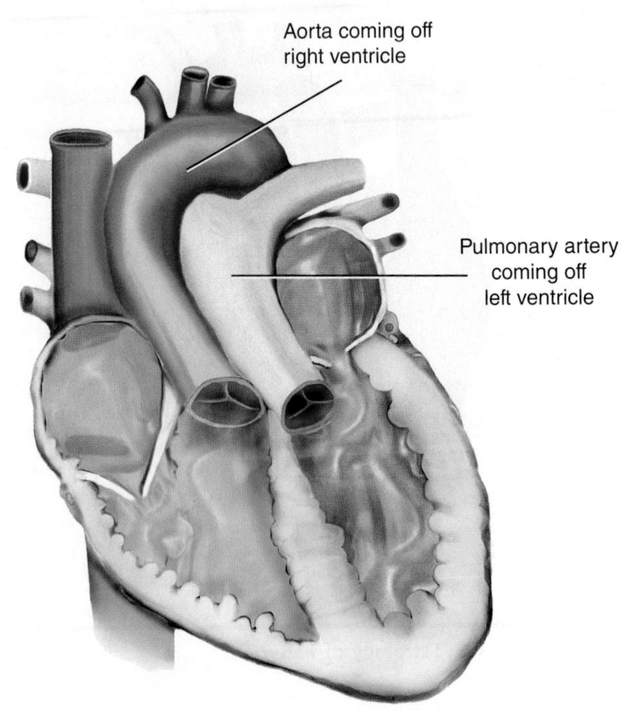

Figure 25-20 Transposition of the Great Arteries. DELMAR CENGAGE LEARNING.

Incidence
The incidence of TGA is approximately 7–8% of all CHD (Karl & Kirshbom, 2006).

Pathophysiology
In the infant with TGA, unoxygenated blood enters the RA to RV then flows out the aorta to the body. Oxygenated blood from the lungs enters the LA to the LV and then flows out the pulmonary artery back to the lungs. Therefore, there is a parallel circulation with no oxygenated blood getting to the systemic circulation. The infant's only chance for survival is an intra-atrial connection such as an ASD, PFO, or a PDA that will allow mixing of oxygenated and unoxygenated blood. In the immediate newborn period prostaglandin therapy is initiated to maintain ductal patency. However it is adequate mixing at the atrial level that it is imperative for the survival of these infants.

Clinical Manifestations
Cyanosis within the first few hours of birth is the most important clinical finding in the infant with TGA. These neonates otherwise appear quite healthy and are generally of normal size and weight. Clinicians should be suspicious of TGA in an otherwise healthy newborn with acute cyanosis that is not responsive to oxygen.

Diagnosis
Diagnosis is made on clinical presentation and echocardiogram. Chest X-rays may be within normal limits or show a mildly enlarged right heart. Echocardiogram will confirm the diagnosis of TGA but cardiac catheterization is sometimes used to confirm the relationships of the ventricles to the great vessels, to delineate the coronary artery anatomy, and to document other associated defects.

Treatment
Once diagnosis is made, stabilization of the infant is essential. Often these neonates are placed on

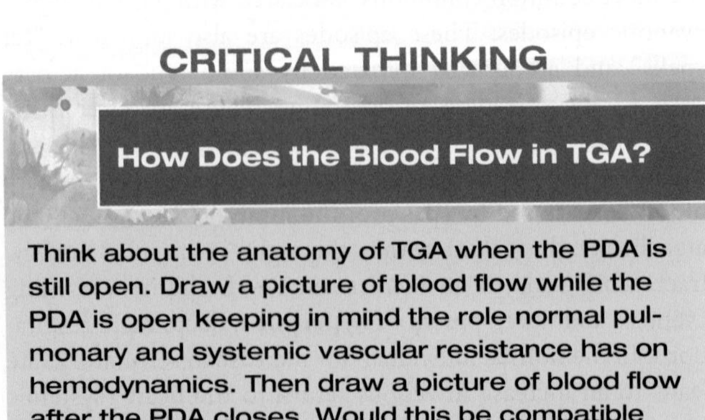

Think about the anatomy of TGA when the PDA is still open. Draw a picture of blood flow while the PDA is open keeping in mind the role normal pulmonary and systemic vascular resistance has on hemodynamics. Then draw a picture of blood flow after the PDA closes. Would this be compatible with life? Why?

mechanical ventilation; some will need pharmacologic support for poor cardiac output and correction of metabolic acidosis. Prostaglandin (PGE1) is initiated to promote oxygenated blood flow from the pulmonary artery to the aorta via **retrograde** (backward) blood flow through a PDA.

In many centers a balloon **atrial septostomy** is performed. During this procedure a balloon-tipped catheter is threaded via a femoral vein into the RA. It is then passed through the PFO to the left atrium. Once in position the balloon is inflated and then rapidly pulled back across the atrial septum resulting in a tear in the septum creating an ASD. This will ensure enough intra-atrial mixing to provide adequate oxygenation until the child can be surgically repaired. At some institutions PGE1 is discontinued and the child is allowed to orally feed until the time of surgery. However, other cardiac centers prefer to continue prostaglandins to maintain the work of the left ventricle.

The arterial switch procedure is the treatment of choice for the neonate with TGA. This procedure is performed via median sternotomy with the infant on CPB. The aorta is resected from the aortic trunk and similarly the pulmonary artery is resected from the pulmonary trunk. These great vessels are then switched, resulting in anatomic correction. One of the more difficult tasks during this procedure is the removal and reimplantation of the coronary arteries from the old aortic trunk onto the newly created aorta (previous pulmonary trunk). Timing of this procedure is important and is normally done within the first week or two of life. This helps to ensure that the left ventricle will remain strong as it will become the systemic ventricle.

Postoperative complications may include poor cardiac output related to decreased ventricular function, bleeding, arrhythmias, and a risk of coronary artery occlusion or kinking, leading to sudden death. Long-term complications include supravalvar pulmonary stenosis that in some individuals requires re-operation. With increasing experience with the arterial switch procedure, operative mortality is now similar to such lesions as VSD closure and Tetralogy of Fallot (Karl & Kirshbom, 2006).

Tricuspid Atresia

Tricuspid atresia is characterized by absence of or complete closure of the tricuspid valve and therefore no connection between the RA and the RV (Figure 25-21). Other associated defects include ASD, VSD, and varying degrees of RV hypoplasia. Hypoplasia refers to incomplete or underdevelopment of an organ, in this case the RV.

Incidence The incidence of tricuspid atresia is approximately 1–3% of all CHD.

Pathophysiology In infants with tricuspid atresia there is complete mixing of systemic and pulmonary venous return at the atrial level. Blood flow is as follows: Systemic venous return enters the RA but cannot pass to the RV through the tricuspid valve and must flow through an intra-atrial connection to the LA. Blood then flows to the LV and if there is a VSD, some blood flows through the VSD to the PA. The remainder of the blood in the left ventricle will flow out the aorta. If there is no associated VSD, then blood flow to the lungs must be through a PDA. This defect is termed a *ductal dependent lesion* as the infant would not survive without the PDA.

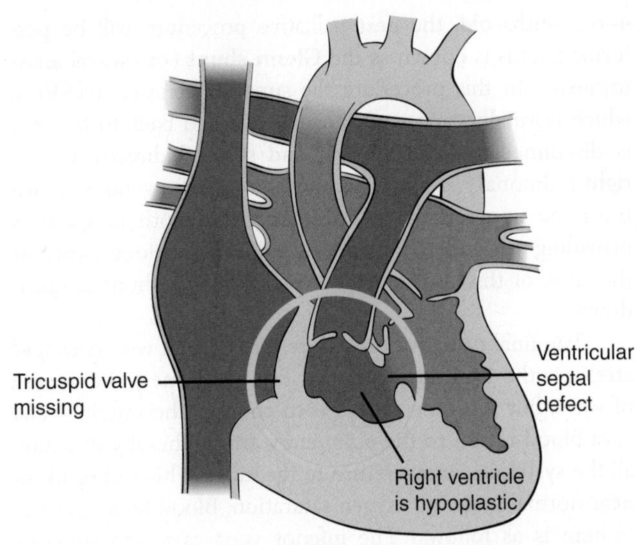

FIGURE 25-21 **Tricuspid Atresia.** DELMAR CENGAGE LEARNING.

Clinical Manifestations The infant with tricuspid atresia is generally cyanotic within the first day of life. Cyanosis is secondary to a R→L shunt at the atrial level. Severe hypoxic spells can occur and are related to closure of the VSD or closure of the PDA.

Diagnosis CXR in these infants usually demonstrates enlargement of the RA, LA, and LV with decreased pulmonary markings suggestive of decreased pulmonary blood flow. Diagnosis is made with echocardiogram. Often cardiac catheterization is indicated to determine the size of the RV. Unfortunately, in many infants with tricuspid atresia the right ventricle is so small that it will never function normally, so a univentricular repair is indicated. This will be described in the following section.

Treatment Definitive treatment for the infant with tricuspid atresia is surgical. In the preoperative period the neonate with no VSD (and therefore no pulmonary blood flow) is treated with PGE1 to keep the ductus arteriosis open or patent until surgery can be performed. Surgical repair for the infant with a small or no VSD and a hypoplastic RV is considered palliative, as complete correction is not possible. This is true with any defect that will require the child to live his or her life with only one functioning ventricle, known as a univentricular repair.

The first stage of the repair is the placement of a modified BT shunt as previously described. Over the next several months as the infant begins to grow, the amount of pulmonary blood flow will decrease secondary to the fixed diameter of the BT shunt. When the infant is approximately

4–6 months old, the next palliative procedure will be performed. This is known as the **Glenn shunt** (or bicaval anastomosis). In this procedure the superior vena cava (SVC), which normally carries unoxygenated blood back to the RA, is disconnected from the RA and sutured directly to the right pulmonary artery. This allows for all the venous return from the upper body to flow directly to both lungs, thus providing the infant with more pulmonary blood flow. At the time of this procedure the modified BT shunt is taken down.

The final palliative procedure for children with tricuspid atresia is the **Fontan** procedure. It is performed in a variety of ways, but the general goal is to connect the inferior vena cava blood return to the pulmonary artery, thereby directing all the systemic venous return to the lungs. This will result in near normal systemic oxygen saturation. Blood flow after the Fontan is as follows: The inferior vena cava and superior vena cava flow blood directly to the pulmonary artery. Pulmonary venous return flows to the LA then to the LV and out the aorta. There are in effect two separate circulations. The Fontan is generally performed when the child is about 2 years of age.

The natural history of the unrepaired infant with tricuspid atresia without a VSD is poor with few infants surviving past 6 months. Survival and better quality of life are improving for the infant who has undergone the three palliative phases associated with this defect. Long-term complications include arrhythmias, protein losing enteropathy, need for pacemakers, stroke, and exercise intolerance. Ventricular failure may occur later in life and the need for heart transplantation is a possibility for some of these infants. The goal of newer surgical techniques and medications is to provide longer and better quality of life.

DEFECTS THAT OBSTRUCT LEFT VENTRICULAR OUTFLOW

These defects increase afterload to the left ventricle in varying degrees. Therefore, systemic cardiac output can be limited in some individuals. Defects in this category that will be discussed are coarctation of the aorta, aortic stenosis, and hypoplastic left heart syndrome.

Coarctation of the Aorta

Coarctation of the aorta is a stenosis or narrowing located most commonly within the thoracic aorta. The area of stenosis as well as the degrees of obstruction may vary. The most common position of the coarctation is opposite the insertion of the PDA (Figure 25-22).

Incidence The incidence of coarctation is approximately 8 to 11% of all CHD (AHA, 2007).

Pathophysiology Coarctation causes narrowing of the aorta and therefore increases resistance to blood flow out the left ventricle. Because all the systemic blood flow must go past the stenotic area of the aorta, an increase in left ventricular pressure and work occurs with resulting LV hypertrophy.

Clinical Manifestations The symptomatic infant with severe coarctation is likely to present in CHF once the PDA has closed. This is secondary to the inability of the LV to eject its contents with a subsequent backup of blood from the left side of the heart to the lungs. A decrease in systemic cardiac output will lead to shock, acidosis, and death unless medical intervention is initiated.

The older child with coarctation is generally asymptomatic, and the diagnosis is made when the child is sent for evaluation of a murmur or hypertension. The classic clinical finding in the child with coarctation is upper extremity hypertension and a noticeable difference in blood pressure between the arms and legs. There are also diminished pulses in the lower extremities. The simple tasks of palpating four extremity pulses and taking four extremity blood pressures should be part of all routine pediatric examinations.

Diagnosis Diagnosis of coarctation is made on clinical examination and echocardiogram. Chest X-rays of the infant may be normal or there may be cardiomegaly. Cardiac catheterization is not indicated for diagnosis. MRI is indicated if there is a need to define associated defects or **collateral** circulation. The severity of coarctation is determined by the arm or leg pressure gradient. Upper extremity blood pressure should be measured in the right arm, as this will always be the proximal pressure. A lower extremity blood pressure will always be the distal pressure. Measurements less than 20 mm Hg are associated with mild coarctation.

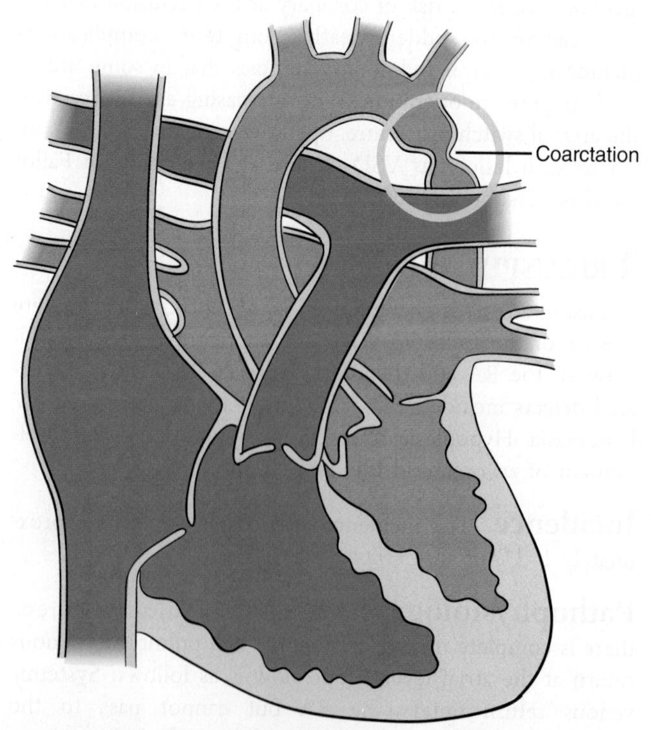

Figure 25-22 Coarctation of the Aorta. DELMAR CENGAGE LEARNING.

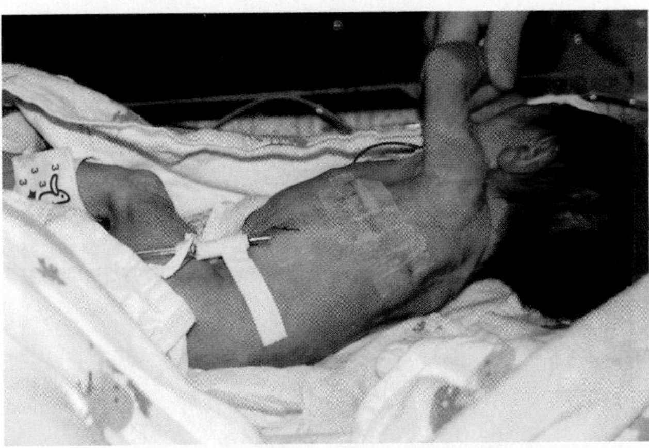

FIGURE 25-23 **Thoracotomy Incision with a Chest Tube in an Infant After Repair of Coarctation.** DELMAR CENGAGE LEARNING.

Treatment Definitive treatment for the child with coarctation is relief of the obstruction by either surgical or balloon dilation. The most common surgical repair for the infant with coarctation of the aorta is dissection of the stenotic area and end-to-end anastomosis (or bringing together) of the two segments of the aorta (Figure 25-23). Surgical timing for the infant with coarctation depends on his or her hemodynamic stability. The older child should have an elective repair after 3 to 5 years of age. There appears to be a decreased risk of recoarctation when the repair is performed at this age.

Balloon angioplasty can be used to dilate the stenotic area. During this procedure a catheter with a balloon at the tip is passed via the femoral artery to the area of coarctation. The balloon is then inflated and the area of stenosis dilated reducing the obstruction. Angioplasty is most often used for correction of recurrent coarctation.

Medications are used in the postoperative period to control the residual hypertension that is often present in children with coarctation of the aorta. It is essential to control postoperative hypertension to prevent bleeding from the multiple sutures at the area of repair in the high pressure aorta. Long-term complications after repair include recoarctation (particularly when the original procedure was performed during infancy) and residual hypertension. The latter complications appear to be more significant when the repair is performed in patients over 6 years of age.

AORTIC STENOSIS

Aortic stenosis (AS) is a narrowing of the aortic valve that causes obstruction to the left ventricular outflow and decreases the amount of blood that can be ejected from the LV. Similar to pulmonary stenosis, there are three types of AS: subvalvar, valvar, or supravalvar (Figure 25-24).

Incidence The incidence of AS is approximately 3–6% of individuals with CHD with a 4:1 ratio of males to females.

Pathophysiology The primary hemodynamic impacts of this lesion are an increase in afterload, increased ventricular work, and left ventricular hypertrophy.

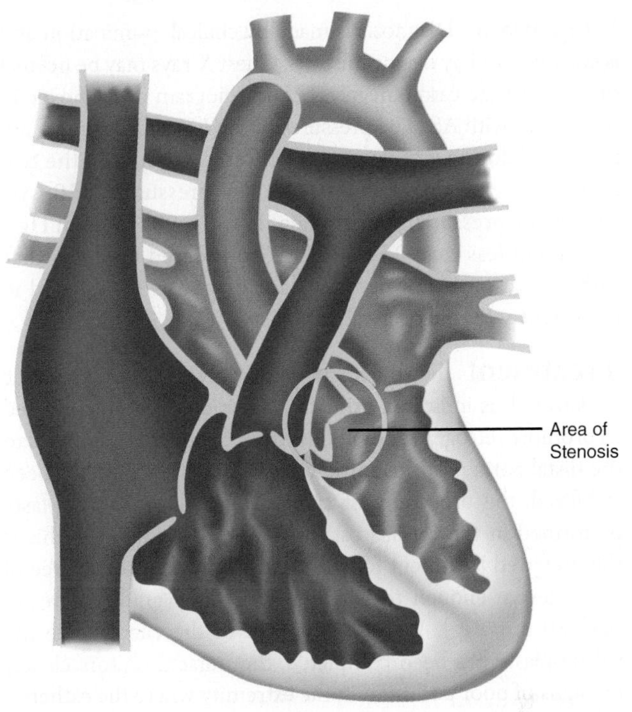

FIGURE 25-24 **Aortic Stenosis.** DELMAR CENGAGE LEARNING.

Clinical Manifestations Most infants with AS grow normally, and the diagnosis is often not made until the older child is referred for evaluation of a murmur. The exception to this is the infant with critical aortic stenosis. Critical AS is a very serious form of AS diagnosed in the newborn. These infants present critically ill and in shock. Critical AS in an infant is a medical emergency, and death will occur without intervention.

Symptoms of AS in the older child are subtle with exertional fatigue, dyspnea, and angina. Severe AS may present with syncope. Syncope in these clients may be related to the inability of the LV to increase cardiac output during exercise, thus limiting blood flow to the brain.

NURSING TIP

How to Determine Arm or Leg Gradients

To determine pressure gradient across a coarctation: Take right arm and leg BP; it is very important to use the appropriate size cuff. Subtract the *leg systolic* pressure from the *arm systolic* pressure; this will equal the gradient. Example: Right arm 150/70, right leg 100/68 gradient is 150 – 100 = 50 mm Hg.

Diagnosis Diagnosis is made by clinical examination and is corroborated by diagnostic tests. Chest X-rays may be normal or demonstrate cardiomegaly. Echocardiogram is diagnostic in the patient with AS. The pressures of the LV and the aorta are measured during systole and the difference between the two is the gradient. (Example: Systolic LV pressure is 150, systolic aortic pressure is 90; gradient is 150 – 90 = 60 mm Hg.) A gradient less than 25 mm Hg is considered mild. Cardiac catheterization is not necessary for diagnosis but is used in treatment with balloon valvuloplasty.

Treatment For the infant with critical AS, hemodynamic stabilization is indicated prior to correction. PGE1 is initiated to promote retrograde blood flow from the ductus arteriosus to the distal aorta past the aortic valve. Once the infant has been stabilized, the procedure of choice is a balloon valvuloplasty performed in the cardiac catheterization lab. Likewise, this is the preferred treatment for the older child when the degree of AS is severe enough to warrant correction (gradient greater than 50 mm Hg). Whatever the age of the client, once the valvuloplasty has been completed, the nurse monitors closely for signs of poor perfusion in the extremity where the catheterization was performed (see Nursing Care for the Child Undergoing Cardiac Catheterization). The main complication of valvuloplasty is aortic regurgitation. If this becomes severe, the aortic valve may need to be surgically repaired or replaced.

Valve replacement can be performed with an artificial valve or with a pulmonary autograft (Ross procedure). Children who are recipients of mechanical artificial valves that replace the aortic valve have traditionally been on anticoagulation medications such as warfarin (Coumadin) to prevent clot formation in the valve. This is a lifetime requirement. Experience is being gained with newer porcine valves that can be used to replace the aortic valve and may not require long term anticoagulation (Lemaire et al., 2009). An alternative to an artificial valve is to use the infant or child's own pulmonary valve and move it to the aortic position. A pulmonary conduit then replaces the relocated pulmonary valve. The advantage of the Ross procedure is that anticoagulation is not required. The disadvantage is that the pulmonary conduit will require replacement during the child's lifetime. Postoperative complications of any type of aortic valve surgery include arrhythmias, heart block, and bleeding.

Natural history of unrepaired AS varies depending on the severity of the stenosis. In general, gradients of less than 25 mm Hg are followed medically and do not require intervention. If gradients are between 25 and 50 mm Hg, the child is followed for potential progression. Unrepaired children with a gradient of greater than 50 mm Hg are at risk for **arrhythmias** (abnormal heart rhythm) and sudden death. Based on this, and with the safety of balloon valvuloplasty, those with moderate to severe AS should be corrected.

Hypoplastic Left Heart Syndrome (HLHS)

HLHS encompasses a variety of deformities characterized by lack of development of the left ventricle secondary to mitral valve atresia or aortic atresia. The left ventricle is essentially small, hypoplastic, and not capable of any cardiac function (Figure 25-25).

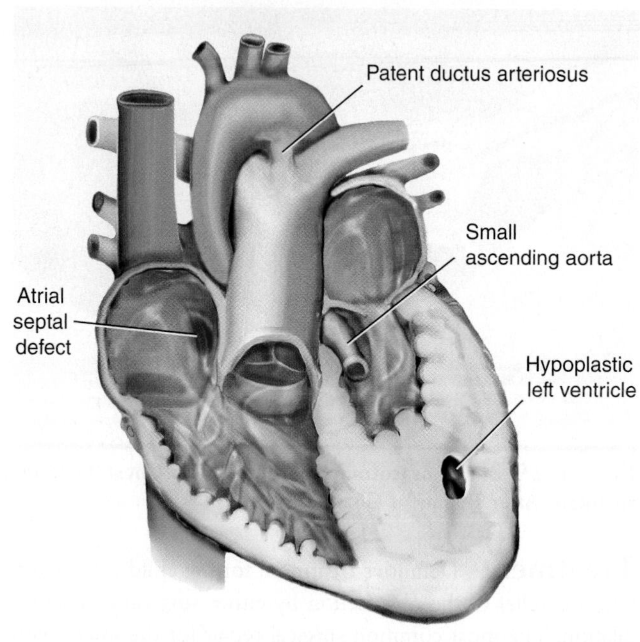

Figure 25-25 Hypoplastic Left Heart Syndrome (HLHS).
DELMAR CENGAGE LEARNING.

Incidence The incidence of HLHS is approximately 4% to 8% of CHD (AHA, 2007). HLHS is the leading cause of cardiac death in the infant less than 1 month old.

Pathophysiology Blood flow with HLHS is as follows: Systemic venous return enters the RA and flows to the RV, out the PA to the lungs, and then returns to the LA. Secondary to atresia of the mitral valve and resulting hypoplasia of the LV, blood cannot pass into the LV and must cross the patent foramen ovale into the RA via a left to right shunt. The only way blood can enter the aorta is through retrograde flow across the PDA.

Clinical Manifestations The infant with HLHS is generally cyanotic within hours of birth; one-third will present in cardiovascular collapse. The infant will present with hypotension, tachycardia, cyanosis, and tachypnea.

Diagnosis Diagnosis is made by clinical presentation and echocardiogram. A chest X-ray of the infant with HLHS is generally not diagnostic but may show increased right heart size. Echocardiogram will demonstrate the structural defects and is diagnostic.

Treatment In the recent past HLHS was an inoperable cardiac defect, and the infant was offered only comfort measures until death occurred. These infants died because the PDA closed, resulting in no systemic blood flow. Presently there are three treatment options that are presented to the family: no intervention, cardiac transplantation, or some form of palliative surgery. These should be presented with no bias on the part of the health care provider and in no

CASE STUDY / CARE PLAN

FIVE-YEAR-OLD CHILD WITH TRISOMY 21 AND SEVERE MITRAL REGURGITATION AFTER AVCD REPAIR AS AN INFANT

Marcela is a 5-year-old Hispanic female with a clinical history significant for atrioventricular canal defect, repaired at 6 months of age, and Trisomy 21. She did very well after her initial surgery but over the last few months her mother has noted that she cannot keep up with her siblings and is taking 3–4 hour naps every day. Her physical examination demonstrates typical Down Syndrome facies, a well-healed surgical incision, cardiomegaly on chest X-ray, and a harsh systolic and diastolic murmur consistent with significant valve regurgitation. Echocardiogram confirms severe left AV valve regurgitation. After extensive discussion with the parents through a Spanish interpreter, the decision is made to attempt surgical repair versus replacement of her valve. An important part of this discussion is the fact that if the valve cannot be repaired it will need to be replaced with a mechanical valve that will require life-long anticoagulation. Assuring that the parents understand this is an essential part of the preoperative workup.

Marcela is taken to the operating room and undergoes successful repair of her left AV valve, then returns to the Pediatric Intensive care unit where she is cared for for two days before her transfer to the surgical unit.

NURSING CARE PLAN

ASSESSMENT

Accurate and frequent ongoing assessment of the cardiovascular system in the postoperative child is an essential part of care. Nurses should monitor for signs of decreased cardiac output such as tachycardia, poor perfusion, mottling of the skin, decreased or absent distal pulses, and poor urine output. Listen to the child's heart sounds to note changes in heart tones or murmurs. After a reoperation on a valve, sutures may come apart and a new murmur may herald signs that the valve is not working as it should. An Echocardiogram is frequently indicated in the postoperative period to evaluate the repair if concerns arise and before discharge to home. Assess the rhythm strip for arrhythmias.

Nurses should auscultate breath sounds bilaterally. Listen to the quality of the breath sounds; listen for rales or coarse rhonchi. Observe the child's color and work of breathing either spontaneously or while on mechanical ventilation. Monitor for tachypnea, retractions, and nasal flaring. Monitor oxygen saturations, keeping in mind the child's anatomy. It is essential that the nurse understand the surgical repair and the expected norm for each defect. When the child has awakened from anesthesia, the nurse assesses the neurologic function by noting equal movement of all extremities, absence of any signs of seizures, and pupillary function. Pain in the nonverbal child is expressed by an increase in heart rate and blood pressure and by grimacing and crying. In a child with a syndrome, such as Down syndrome, it is important to obtain information from the caregivers as to how the child expresses fear and pain. Older children can convey their degree of pain by verbalization or through the use of one of the multiple pain scores and charts available to nurses. Refer to Chapter 18 for more information about pain assessment.

Many cardiac repairs involve multiple suture lines in and around a very small heart. These sutures combined with the destruction of platelets secondary to cardiopulmonary bypass can lead to excessive bleeding in the postoperative period. The child is monitored for signs of bleeding from surgical incisions and intravenous insertion sites.

NURSING DIAGNOSIS 1

Ineffective breathing pattern related to pulmonary edema, pleural effusions, poor respiratory effort, atelectasis, or phrenic nerve damage, as indicated by prolonged intubation, tachypnea, and increased work of breathing.

(Continues)

CASE STUDY / CARE PLAN (Continued)

EXPECTED OUTCOMES

1. Child will have adequate respiratory function as evidenced by respiratory rate normal for age and comfortable respiratory pattern.
2. Child will have no increased work of breathing.

NOC: Respiratory Status: Gas Exchange

NIC: Respiratory Monitoring

INTERVENTIONS/*RATIONALES*

1. Frequently reassess breath sounds. *Unequal aeration may signal pleural effusion, pneumothorax, or damage to the phrenic nerve.*
2. Provide analgesia and sedation. *A child who is in pain related to a sternal or thoracotomy incision is unlikely to take deep breaths.*
3. Obtain chest X-ray as ordered. *To evaluate for presence of pneumothorax or pleural effusion.*
4. Administer scheduled diuretics. *To prevent interstitial fluid from accumulating in the lungs.*
5. Provide good pulmonary toilet (i.e., deep breathing, coughing, head of bed elevated, early ambulation) to prevent atelectasis. *Will assist in establishing good respiratory function.*
6. Provide supplemental oxygen as needed. *To maintain oxygen saturations in desired range. Often children with Down syndrome have elevated pulmonary pressures and require supplemental oxygen to help decrease the pulmonary pressure. Many of these children are discharged on oxygen even though their measured oxygen saturations are greater than 90%.*
7. Obtain arterial blood gases as ordered. *To evaluate for CO_2 retention and hypoxia.*

EVALUATION

Supplemental oxygen is weaned over the expected time period. Oxygen saturations are within normal limits for child's physiology. There is no increased work of breathing, and arterial blood gases are within normal limits.

NURSING DIAGNOSIS 2

Decreased cardiac output related to decreased stroke volume as a result of mechanical, structural, or electrophysiological problems as demonstrated by poor perfusion, hypotension, arrhythmias, decreased urine output, or increased chest tube output.

EXPECTED OUTCOMES

1. The child will have warm, well-perfused extremities, strong peripheral pulses, and blood pressure within normal range to minimize stress on the mitral valve.
2. The child's cardiac rhythm will be normal.
3. The child's urine output will be at least 1 cc/kg/hour.
4. Child's chest tube output will gradually decrease over 24–48 hours.

NOC: Tissue Perfusion: Cardiac

NIC: Cardiac Care: Acute

INTERVENTIONS/*RATIONALES*

1. Administer volume resuscitation for hypovolemia. *Prevent hypotension.*
2. Monitor ongoing losses through chest tubes and dressings. *Normal chest tube output is approximately 2–3 cc/kg/hr over the first few hours and should then slowly taper off.*
3. Monitor for an abrupt cessation in chest tube output, tachycardia, narrow pulse pressure, or acute deterioration in cardiac output. *May indicate cardiac tamponade.*

(Continues)

CASE STUDY / CARE PLAN (Continued)

4. Add pharmacologic support if the child shows signs of decreased cardiac output. *Maintain normal perfusion.*
5. Record rhythm strip upon arrival and anytime there is a change in rhythm. *Document any arrhythmia.*
6. Use temporary external pacemaker as needed. *Temporary external pacing will be initiated for bradycardia, complete heart block, or any abnormal rhythm that results in poor cardiac output.*
7. Monitor calcium, magnesium, and potassium levels and infuse ordered replacements for low levels. *Maintaining normal electrolytes will help prevent arrhythmias and support cardiac output.*

EVALUATION

Extremities are warm and well-perfused. Urine output is within normal limits. Heart rate and rhythm are normal and cardiac tamponade is avoided.

NURSING DIAGNOSIS 3

Acute pain related to operative site as evidenced by crying, verbalization of pain, tachycardia, diaphoresis, hypertension.

EXPECTED OUTCOME

The child's pain will be adequately controlled.

NOC: Pain Control

NIC: Pain Management

INTERVENTIONS/*RATIONALES*

1. Perform neurologic checks upon arrival and frequently until fully awake. *Evaluate baseline and observe for trend in neurologic function.*
2. Administer ordered analgesics. *To prevent postoperative pain. Opiates can cause respiratory depression and are used with caution in the extubated child.*
3. Administer sedatives as ordered while on mechanical ventilation. *To alleviate anxiety and provide amnesia. These medications can cause respiratory depression and are generally not administered once the child is extubated.*
4. Provide nonpharmacologic pain relief measures. These can include soft music, audio tapes from home, a favorite toy or blanket, and relaxation exercises. *To augment pharmacologic intervention.*

EVALUATION

The child demonstrates adequate anxiety and pain control. There are no abnormal neurologic sequelae.

NURSING DIAGNOSIS 4

Ineffective family coping related to illness and hospitalization, as demonstrated by prolonged, disabling feelings of guilt or sadness and lack of involvement in child's care.

EXPECTED OUTCOMES

1. Caregivers will have their questions answered and will be kept aware of their child's progress and complications. This will be done with the use of Spanish translators, providing daily updates and written instructions.
2. The family will be prepared for their child's postoperative course and will be better able to handle the stress.
3. Family will be actively involved in the plan of care for their child.

NOC: Coping

NIC: Coping Enhancement

(Continues)

CASE STUDY / CARE PLAN (Continued)

INTERVENTIONS/*RATIONALES*

1. Encourage participation in preoperative tour or teaching session. *Decrease anxiety and help answer questions and allay fears. Provide handouts in Spanish.*
2. Allow caregivers to visit as soon as possible after surgery. *Support family unit. Caregivers provide support for the child and decrease his anxiety.*
3. Explain all lines and tubes. *Educate caregivers to prevent deficient knowledge.*
4. Encourage caregivers to participate in child's care when possible. These times include diaper changes, bathing, and feeding. *Support caregiver role and family unit.*
5. Encourage home routines when possible. *Normalize routine for child. Allow for food the child is familiar with, once a regular diet is re-established.*
6. Involve child life team to assist with relaxation prior to painful procedures. *Provide strategies for mastery of difficult situations.*
7. Involve social workers or clergy if family continues to have problems coping with the child's illness. *Support family to help with crisis intervention.*
8. Encourage caregivers to ask questions and *listen* to their concerns. No one knows a child as well as the caregivers. *Educate caregivers and provide support.*

EVALUATION

Caregiver role is maintained, and the caregiver–child interaction is normal. Stress of hospitalization will be minimized and family unit will be maintained.

particular order of preference. The first is to allow the infant to die without surgical intervention, although this remains controversial. The second option is cardiac transplantation. The final choice is a three-stage palliative procedure. This can be accomplished in two different pathways. The first pathway includes the modified Norwood procedure with a modified BT shunt or Sano modification, the Glenn shunt and then the modified Fontan. The latter two procedures were discussed in the section on tricuspid atresia and are performed in a similar fashion in infants with HLHS. The other pathway is a newer procedure typically referred to as a "hybrid" procedure and will be discussed below.

If the caregivers decide to pursue surgical transplant or palliation, medical management in the preoperative stage is extremely important in the attempt to keep the infant alive. For infants having either heart transplantation or the modified Norwood procedure, it is mandatory to maintain patency of the ductus arteriosus. Therefore, all of these infants are started on PGE1. Preoperative support of these critically ill infants is often difficult, with little margin for error. Survival depends on the appropriate balance between systemic and pulmonary blood flow. This balance is a function of an adequately sized PDA and the pulmonary or systemic vascular resistances. These infants are sometimes treated with subambient oxygen (delivered at less than 21%) or inhaled carbon dioxide in an attempt to mildly vasoconstrict the pulmonary bed and prevent excessive pulmonary blood flow. The infant should have an oxygen saturation of approximately 75%. Alkalosis should also be avoided because this can result in too much pulmonary blood flow.

The following discussion will focus on staged repair. The initial stage of palliation is the Norwood procedure and is performed within the first week of life. The goals of this procedure are to provide systemic blood flow independent of the PDA, to provide consistent pulmonary blood flow, and to eliminate any obstruction to pulmonary venous return by eliminating the atrial septum. During the procedure the main pulmonary artery is transected and attached to the ascending aorta, creating a new aorta. A modified BT shunt is then performed to supply pulmonary blood flow, and an atrial septectomy, or complete removal of the atrial septum, is performed (Figure 25-26). A more recent advancement in the first stage palliation is the Sano procedure, which includes the use of a small conduit from the right ventricle to the pulmonary artery in place of the modified BT shunt (Figure 25-27). The main goals of this modification are to avoid the major complications of pulmonary over circulation and hemodynamic instability seen in the early postoperative period.

For some infants too ill to undergo the stress of the Norwood procedure, the hybrid approach may be an alternative. This procedure coordinates the cardiac catheterization lab with the operating room to perform the following: two small bands or ties are placed around the right and left branch pulmonary arteries to decrease the amount of blood flow to the lungs. At the same time a stent is placed

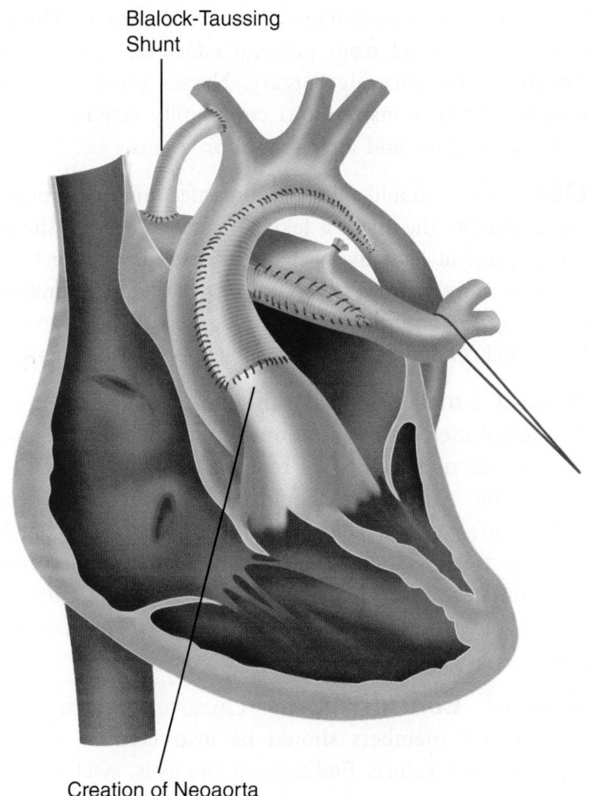

FIGURE 25-26 Norwood Procedure with Modified Blalock-Taussing (BT) shunt. DELMAR CENGAGE LEARNING.

across the ductus arteriosis to keep it open without the use of prostaglandin E. A stent may also be placed across the PFO to allow for mixing at the atrial level (Figure 25-28). This is all performed without the use of CPB. For these infants the second surgery at about 4–6 months involves

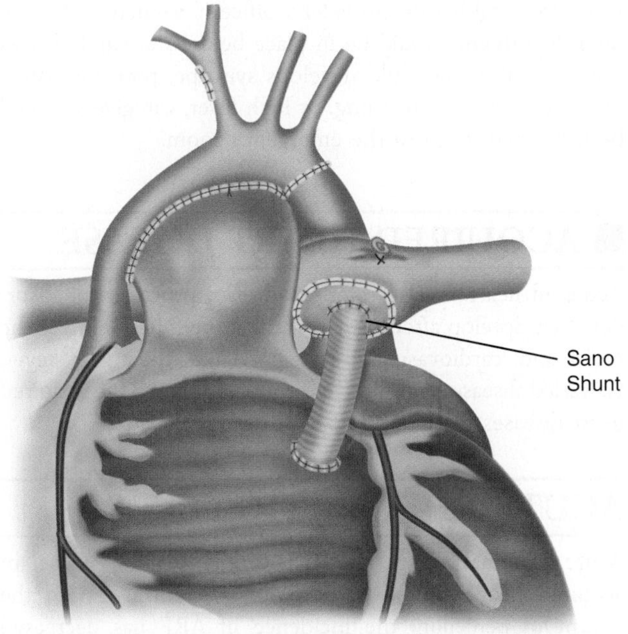

FIGURE 25-27 Norwood Procedure with Sano Shunt. DELMAR CENGAGE LEARNING.

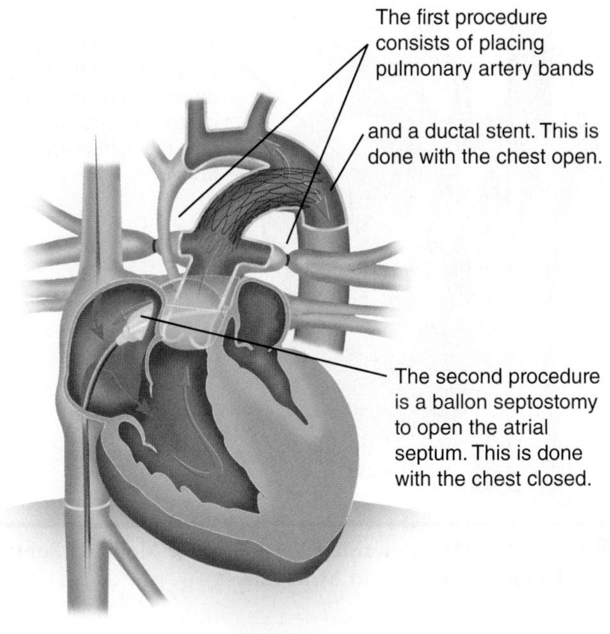

FIGURE 25-28 Hybrid Approach to Hypoplastic left heart syndrome. DELMAR CENGAGE LEARNING.

the arch reconstruction of the Norwood with the Glenn and becomes the most difficult of the three palliative procedures. For some of these infants the hybrid procedure permits longer waiting time on the transplant list (Akinturk et al., 2007). The decision to proceed with transplantation, the staged Norwood procedure, or the hybrid is made by the cardiac team based on the infant's individual status, the wish of the parents, and the preferences and experiences of the institution.

The other palliative procedures for HLHS are the Glenn (Figure 25-29) and the modified Fontan (Figure 25-30), as previously discussed in the section on tricuspid atresia. The Glenn is generally performed at 4–6 months of age and the Fontan at approximately 2–3 years of age.

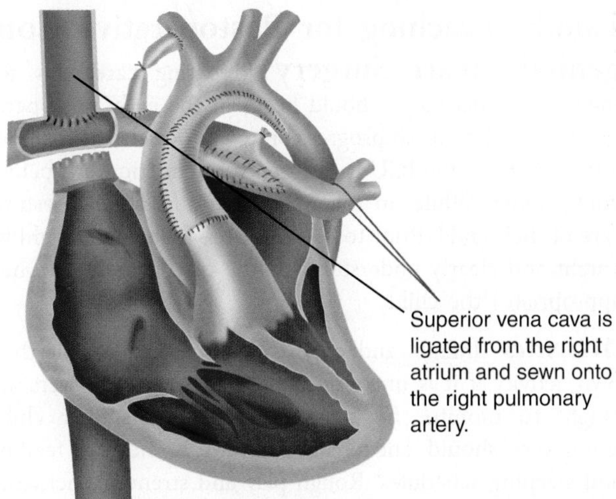

FIGURE 25-29 Bidirectional Glenn for Hypoplastic Left Heart Syndrome. DELMAR CENGAGE LEARNING.

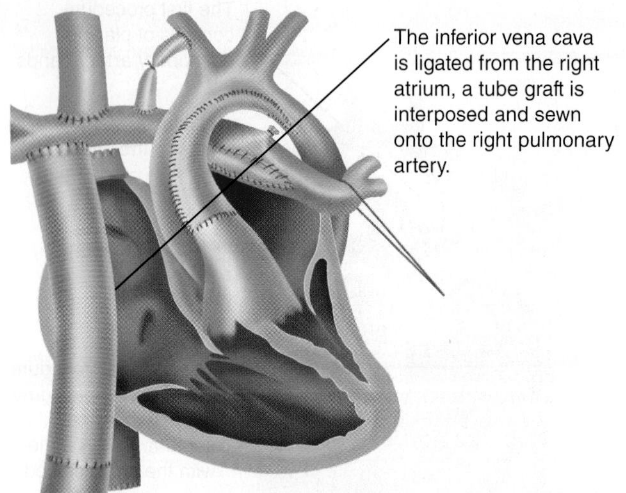

FIGURE 25-30 Extracardiac Version of the Modified Fontan for Hypoplastic Left Heart Syndrome. DELMAR CENGAGE LEARNING.

Despite astute medical and nursing care these infants or children can deteriorate rapidly with maneuvers as simple as suctioning the endotracheal tube. Sudden death is sometimes seen in the immediate postoperative period and remains a potential complication when the individual has been discharged. Other complications include arrhythmias, bleeding, and poor cardiac output.

Survival data for the infant who has undergone the modified Norwood procedure are evolving. Five-year survival for all three palliative procedures was 61% but is improving steadily. Long-term survival data for the infant with HLHS who has undergone palliative repair remain to be seen. One of the most important factors that will influence long-term survival is that the right ventricle will be the systemic ventricle for life. The right ventricle is not designed to be the "high pressure" pump for a lifetime, so it may fail. These children may present for transplantation in the future.

Family Teaching for Postoperative Congenital Heart Surgery Preparing caregivers for their child's discharge should begin in the early postoperative period. The usual progression toward discharge includes a transfer from the ICU to the general pediatric ward before going home. While on the ward caregivers should resume care of their child. Prior to discharge the following should be taught and clearly understood by the caregivers and (when appropriate) the child.

Activities Infants and children will generally limit their own activity if it is uncomfortable for them. Caregivers are taught to monitor for tiring and fatigue in their child. Caregivers should encourage a return to normal feeding and sleeping schedules. Rough play and strenuous activities are avoided until six weeks following discharge. Children may return to school within approximately two weeks, but home tutoring is encouraged prior to this time. The child should be excused from physical education classes during the six weeks following surgery. Nurses should encourage involvement in nonstrenuous community activities such as scouting, church, and after-school programs.

Diet Infants should return to breastfeeding or formula. To assess whether the infant is taking in adequate fluids, she or he should have at least five wet diapers per day. Since formula contains more calories than cereal or baby food, families are encouraged to limit these foods and give additional formula or breast milk. Older children are encouraged to eat a regular diet.

Wound Care Generally the sutures used to close either the sternal incision or the thoracotomy incision are absorbable and do not need to be removed. Children may sit in a shallow tub. Caregivers should cleanse around the wound and pat the area dry. The wound should not be soaked for the first week. Showers and normal baths can resume in approximately two weeks. Caregivers are instructed to inspect the wound looking for signs of redness, swelling, drainage, or tenderness.

General Considerations Caregivers, teachers, and other family members should be instructed to watch for signs of heart failure. Puffiness of the eyes, swelling of the feet, shortness of breath, poor feeding, and excessive irritability all warrant further investigation by the medical team.

Medications Many children are discharged on medication to promote cardiac function. Frequently these medications are similar to those the child was taking before surgery. Refer to Table 25-3 for a listing of cardiac medications and their side effects. Schools should be notified of any medications (and possible side effects) the child is on.

Finally, before discharge the family must demonstrate an understanding of these instructions and know how to reach the health care provider's office if needed. A follow-up appointment should be in place before the family leaves the hospital. If the child develops syncope, poor perfusion, increased work of breathing, or high fever, caregivers should be instructed to go to the emergency room.

ACQUIRED HEART DISEASE

Acquired heart disease refers to disease processes or disorders that develop after birth and affect the functioning of the heart and cardiovascular system. Acute rheumatic fever, Kawasaki disease, and infective endocarditis are the acquired heart diseases discussed in this section.

ACUTE RHEUMATIC FEVER

Acute rheumatic fever (ARF) is the leading cause of acquired heart disease in developing countries. With the advent of penicillin, the incidence of ARF has decreased substantially in the United States.

Incidence and Etiology

An estimated 12 million individuals are affected by rheumatic fever: as many as 150 cases/100,000 in developing countries versus <1/100,000 in countries such as the United States. In the United States, rheumatic fever is most frequently observed in the age group most susceptible to group A streptococcal infections, children ages 5–15. Only 5% of pediatric ARF cases are less than 5 years of age (Miyake, Gauvreau, Tani, Sundel, & Newburger, 2007; Tani, Veasy, Minich, & Shaddy, 2003). ARF follows an untreated or partially treated group A streptococcal **pharyngitis** (sore throat) (AAP, 2006). Although group A streptococci can produce infection in any number of bodily tissues, rheumatic fever will only follow a throat infection. It has never been identified subsequent to a group A streptococci skin infection (impetigo). With the advent of antibiotic therapy the mortality has been reduced substantially.

Pathophysiology

The exact pathogenesis of ARF is unknown. It is generally felt to be an autoimmune response to untreated group A streptococcal pharyngitis in genetically predisposed individuals. The three organ systems primarily affected by this autoimmune response are the heart, central nervous system, and the joints (Gerber et al., 2009).

The entire heart can be affected during the acute inflammatory phase of illness. Pericarditis, myocarditis, and **valvulitis** (inflammation of the heart valves) can occur. The most significant cardiac pathophysiological phenomenon is valvulitis. The most frequently affected valve is the mitral valve. Valvulitis is responsible for mitral valve deformity that results in mitral regurgitation. The aortic valve can also be affected and develop insufficiency; however, isolated aortic insufficiency without mitral regurgitation is uncommon in ARF. Myocarditis and pericarditis are never encountered in rheumatic fever without valvar involvement. Therefore, myocarditis or pericarditis in isolation should not be considered rheumatic in origin. Joint involvement consists of **polyarthritis**. Unfortunately, polyarthritis can also mimic many childhood illnesses such as juvenile rheumatoid arthritis. The involved joints are usually the larger ones, such as the knees, ankles, hips, and shoulders. Presentation of arthritis is quite variable. The pain can be mild or so severe the child is unable to bear weight. The arthritis of ARF does not result in permanent disability.

Central nervous system manifestations often present late, sometimes years after the initial illness. Inflammatory changes in the neurons result in **chorea** (classically known as Sydenham's chorea). Chorea is characterized by involuntary, purposeless movements of the extremities and the trunk. Because this is a late manifestation of rheumatic fever there may be no antecedent evidence of recent group A streptococcal pharyngitis (Rogness, 2008).

Chronic changes in the heart are responsible for the long-term sequela of ARF. Valvar regurgitation can progress to stenosis. In many situations evidence of a previous episode of rheumatic fever is not uncovered until an adult develops valvar stenosis, requiring replacement with an artificial valve.

Clinical Manifestations

The clinical presentation of rheumatic fever can be quite varied. The American Heart Association (Gerber et al., 2009) has established clinical criteria for ARF and has categorized these into major and minor manifestations. These criteria are the Jones Criteria, in honor of T. Duchett Jones who first set forth diagnostic standards for rheumatic fever in 1944.

The criteria have been recently reviewed by the AHA and are found in Box 25-4 (Gerber et al., 2009). To make the diagnosis of ARF the presence of two major manifestations or of one major and two minor manifestations must be present. In addition, there must be supportive evidence of an antecedent group A streptococcal infection. Generally the child presents with a nondescript febrile illness and antecedent group A streptococcal throat infection. Unfortunately, some children have no history of febrile illness or pharyngitis.

The manifestations of valvulitis are the most significant clinical features. In the presence of mitral regurgitation a new systolic murmur is appreciated. If aortic insufficiency is present there will be a diastolic murmur. Sometimes the murmur is soft. Occasionally there can be "silent" mitral regurgitation with no appreciable murmur, although it will be identified on echocardiogram (Lanna, Tonelli, Barros, Goulart, & Mota, 2003).

BOX 25-4
CRITERIA FOR THE DIAGNOSIS OF INITIAL ATTACK OF ARF

Major Manifestations

- Carditis
- Polyarthritis
- Chorea
- Erythema marginatum
- Subcutaneous nodules

Minor Manifestations

- Arthralgia
- Fever
- Elevated acute phase reactants
  - Erythrocyte sedimentation rate (ESR)
  - C-reactive protein (CRP)
- Prolonged PR interval on ECG

Supporting Evidence of Previous Group A Streptococcal Infection

- Positive throat culture (not rapid streptococcal test)
- Elevated or rising streptococcal antibody titer

Polyarthritis is the most frequent benign major manifestation. The arthritis is migratory, meaning the joint pain moves from one joint to another. There is tenderness, pain, swelling, heat, and limitation of movement in the affected joints. An isolated severely swollen red joint that is not migratory in nature must be considered septic until proven otherwise, as this is not characteristic of ARF.

Erythema marginatum is a distinctive, fine, pink rash noted on the trunk and extremities, never on the face. It becomes more pronounced with heat, such as when the child first comes out of a hot bath. This is always seen with **carditis** (inflammation of the heart) or polyarthritis. Subcutaneous nodules are firm painless nodules over the extensor surfaces of the elbows, knees, and wrists. The skin over the nodules is not inflamed. These are rare and are never seen in isolation; they always accompany carditis. Arthralgia and fever are frequently present but are nonspecific for rheumatic fever.

Diagnosis

Those who have had a previous episode of ARF are at higher risk for a recurrent episode. The diagnosis is made on the presence of the clinical manifestations, supported by laboratory data. There is a high probability of rheumatic fever if evidence exists of antecedent group A streptococcal throat infection, and either two major manifestations of ARF or one major and two minor manifestations.

Laboratory findings support the presence of an inflammatory process and document an antecedent group A streptococcal infection. Elevation of sedimentation rate and C-reactive protein are nonspecific blood tests used to document an inflammatory process. A throat culture can document the organism responsible for pharyngitis; unfortunately, many children will have recovered by the time rheumatic fever is suspected, and thus a throat culture may be negative. In addition, a number of asymptomatic children can be carriers of group A streptococci; hence, a positive culture would result.

Fortunately there are blood tests that are sensitive and reliable in establishing a previous streptococcal infection. These are antibody determinations that can be elevated for weeks following the initial infection. Antistreptolysin O-titer (ASO) and anti-DNAs B are obtained together. In combination these two tests will increase the confirmation of rheumatic fever to 92%.

ECG can demonstrate PR interval prolongation with first-degree heart block, although this is nonspecific and not always observed. Echocardiogram is the most sensitive tool for the diagnosis of valvar disease. The echocardiographic findings of mitral regurgitation in rheumatic fever are quite characteristic, so a firm diagnosis can be made. An ECHO should be obtained in any child suspected of having rheumatic fever because mitral regurgitation and aortic insufficiency may be "silent."

Treatment

The treatment of ARF during the acute phase is directed at eradicating the organism and implementing anti-inflammatory agents. Oral penicillin is used for the initial treatment. Aspirin is the primary anti-inflammatory agent used for the treatment of ARF. Aspirin in high doses is begun at 100 mg/kg/day for two days, and then decreased to 70 mg/kg/day until the sedimentation rate returns to normal. Polyarthritis responds very quickly to high-dose aspirin. Once acute phase reactants (sedimentation rate) are normal aspirin can be discontinued. If aspirin side effects are noted, then the dose can be decreased slightly. Some clinicians use naproxen (Aleve) in the treatment of ARF; however the primary anti-inflammatory agent in this scenario remains aspirin. Concurrent administration of antacids helps with the stomach pain associated with high-dose aspirin.

Initially the child should be placed on bed rest until inflammation has resolved; this can be done as an outpatient. In the presence of new mitral or aortic regurgitation, activities should be restricted for a number of weeks to months. Compliance in this area can be quite difficult, particularly when the child begins to feel better. Frequent follow-up with a pediatric cardiologist is essential. Repeat ECHOs are obtained to evaluate for resolution of valvar involvement. Unfortunately, in many cases the valves do not completely return to normal.

Secondary prophylaxis is essential in all cases of rheumatic carditis. This consists of oral penicillin 250 mg BID, or monthly intramuscular injections of penicillin. Secondary prophylaxis is carried out for at least 5 years or well into adulthood (Box 25-5). This is critically important as a recurrence of rheumatic fever can induce severe cardiac damage. Those children with residual valvar disease must also follow endocarditis prophylaxis (see section on endocarditis). However, because these children are on chronic penicillin therapy a different antibiotic agent must be used. Compliance with secondary prophylaxis is very difficult. Many clients either forget to take their medication or feel it is unnecessary since they are not "sick." Although traumatic for young children, intramuscular injections allow for more individual freedom resulting in better compliance.

Over the last few decades death rates from rheumatic fever in the United States have dropped significantly. This is

BOX 25-5
DURATION OF SECONDARY RHEUMATIC FEVER PROPHYLAXIS

Rheumatic fever with carditis and residual persistent valvular disease	10 years or until 40 years of age (whichever is longer), sometimes lifelong prophylaxis
Rheumatic fever with carditis but no residual heart disease (no valvular disease)	10 years or until 21 years of age (whichever is longer)
Rheumatic fever without carditis	5 years or until 21 years of age (whichever is longer)

due to timely identification and antibiotic therapy. However, because the incidence has been declining some children are missed because of lack of experience on the part of the health care provider. Although mortality has dropped, morbidity remains a risk for many. This is in the form of chronic valvar disease and progressive mitral stenosis. Many individuals will require either aortic valve or mitral valve replacement for treatment of rheumatic heart disease in adulthood.

Nursing Management

Unless the child is in severe heart failure the management of acute rheumatic fever is handled as an outpatient. The treatment of congestive heart failure has been discussed previously. Timely identification and diagnosis of rheumatic fever is essential to the prevention of adverse sequelae. Community and family education are critical to the prevention and recurrence of ARF. The community must be made aware that strep throat infections must be treated in a timely manner, and the full course of antibiotics completed (to prevent undertreatment).

Family Teaching

Education is the most important nursing intervention with this disease. The family is educated on the importance of antibiotic therapy, both in the acute phase and for secondary prophylaxis. If the child is on aspirin, the family must be made aware of the side effects. Compliance with activity restrictions is important; the nurse can offer suggestions for diversional activities or home schooling can be instituted. The length and type of restriction varies between clients and is determined by clinical condition. For any child who has had an episode of ARF, the family must be vigilant in looking for the signs and symptoms of group A streptococcal throat infection in order to facilitate timely treatment. Even those children on chronic penicillin therapy can have a recurrent streptococcal infection. Adolescents must be made accountable for their own treatment. This is a high-risk group for noncompliance with secondary prophylaxis. Ongoing education with frequent reinforcement is of prime importance. The importance of follow-up must also be stressed.

KAWASAKI DISEASE

Kawasaki disease (KD) was first described by Tomisaku Kawasaki in 1967 in Japan. Since that time KD has been widely recognized throughout the world, and is currently the leading cause of acquired heart disease in the United States. Early diagnosis and treatment is imperative to prevent the coronary vascular disease associated with KD (Minich et al., 2007).

Incidence and Etiology

Peak incidence occurs in children 2 years of age and younger; the majority of cases occur in children less than 5 years old. Boys are affected more commonly than girls, and prevalence is increased in those children of Asian descent. Incidence rates in Japan approximate 145 cases/100,000 children, in the United States incidence approximates 45 cases/100,000 in children less than 5 years (Burns et al., 2005).

To date, a specific etiology is unknown. Most clinicians believe that the etiology is microbial because of the clinical presentation, response to treatment, and epidemiology. Nonetheless, viral and bacterial cultures do not reveal consistent findings.

Epidemiologic evidence suggesting an infectious etiology is as follows. It is uncommon for KD to manifest in infants less than 3 months of age, inferring protection from acquired immunity from the mother. KD in children over 12 years of age is almost unheard of, suggesting the possibility of natural immunity through subclinical infection. Epidemics occur in the winter and spring. Past epidemiologic studies have identified community-wide outbreaks of KD at regular 3–5 year intervals, although this trend may be subsiding. To date, the most attractive hypothesis for the etiology of KD is one of a widespread infectious agent that is responsible for disease in susceptible (possibly genetically predisposed) individuals (Burns et al., 2005).

Pathophysiology

KD is a multisystem **vasculitis** (inflammation of the blood vessels) with a proclivity to affect the coronary arteries. The pathogenesis is felt to be an antibody-mediated vascular injury, in which the vascular endothelium plays a major role. Infiltration of the vessel wall with inflammatory cells is responsible for the early manifestations and symptoms found in KD (Baker & Newburger, 2008).

During the first 10 days of illness there is infiltration and hypertrophy of the vascular vessel. At this stage aneurysms do not form, although **ectasia** (larger than normal for age) of the coronary arteries can be seen on ECHO. The vascular changes that occur lay the groundwork for possible aneurysm formation in the future. During this stage of illness there is **pancarditis** (inflammation of entire heart) and pericardial inflammation often with effusion. Some clients can develop congestive heart failure.

From day 10 to day 40 of the illness there is a decrease in the inflammatory process. Because of earlier pathophysiological processes, vessels have undergone destructive changes. It is during this period that coronary artery aneurysm can develop. Coronary artery abnormalities and aneurysms are more pronounced at the origins of the coronaries, proximal segments, and distal branching segments. Other arteries such as the iliac, femoral, axillary, and renal can be involved, although this is rare.

After 40 days there is progressive fibrosis and healing of coronary artery abnormalities. Aneurysms and dilation usually regress in 1 to 2 years. Individuals with aneurysms can develop progressive stenosis and calcification of the affected coronary arteries (Baker & Newburger, 2008). Death caused by myocardial ischemia can occur.

Clinical Manifestations

The onset of illness is abrupt and begins with the first day of fever. There is no prodrome and the majority of children are healthy prior to illness. The first symptom is a high (38°–41°C; 100.4°–105.8°F) remittent fever lasting more than five days. Within two to five days other signs of KD manifest. These include conjunctival injection (redness of conjunctiva), **erythematous** (diffuse redness) rash, oral changes, unilateral cervical swollen lymph nodes (**lymphadenopathy**), and changes in the feet and hands.

Eye involvement consists of nonexudative conjunctival injection with photophobia, which occurs within the first five days of illness. The rash is **polymorphous** erythematous without vesicles, and appears within five days of fever. There is extensive involvement of the trunk and limbs, and perineal desquamation (peeling of skin) may occur in 10% of individuals. Changes in the oral mucosa consist of erythema and cracking of the lips, strawberry tongue, and diffuse erythema of oropharyngeal mucosa.

The most characteristic findings of this disease are changes of the hands and feet. The hands and feet become tensely edematous and very erythematous. By the tenth day of illness desquamation begins. This starts just under the finger and toenails and progresses to involve the palms and soles, with skin peeling in sheets.

Cervical lymphadenopathy, although a widely recognized clinical finding, remains the least consistent manifestation, occurring in only 50% of clients. (Previously described symptoms occur in 90% of clients.) When present the enlarged lymph node is nontender and nonfluctuant. It can occur on the first day of fever.

Associated findings of KD include marked irritability, arthralgia, arthritis, aseptic meningitis, sterile pyuria (white cells in the urine), and diarrhea. Hepatic dysfunction with elevated liver function tests is observed in up to 40% of clients, although it is transitory and requires no intervention. White cell count and sedimentation rate are elevated secondary to the overwhelming inflammatory response. Platelet counts are significantly elevated: 450,000/mm3 by day 10 of illness to 650,000–2,000,000/mm3 by day 20 of illness.

Cardiac manifestations are the most serious, contributing to morbidity and mortality. Sixty percent of clients will develop tachycardia and gallop rhythm. Up to 20% can develop congestive heart failure. Coronary artery lesions are seen in 25% of those *not treated* with intravenous gamma globulin (IVIG). This has dropped to 5% with the advent of gamma globulin therapy. Coronary artery ectasia is transient and usually disappears during the acute phase of illness. Coronary artery aneurysms generally develop after day 10 of illness; prognosis differs according to size. Small aneurysms are $<$ 4 mm, medium 4–8 mm, and giant $>$ 8 mm. Small and medium aneurysms regress after one year, albeit medium aneurysms may develop local stenosis in the future. Giant aneurysms have a tendency to develop stenosis and calcification, even though regression occurs within one to two years. Those children at the highest risk for the development of giant aneurysms include males, infants less than 1 year, and those not treated before the tenth day of illness or who are refractory to treatment (Minich et al., 2007).

BOX 25-6
PRINCIPAL DIAGNOSTIC CLINICAL CRITERIA FOR KAWASAKI DISEASE

- Remittent fever of 38° to 41°C (101° to 104°F), lasting longer than five days
- Conjunctival injection
- Oral changes: strawberry tongue, erythema of lips and oropharynx, cracked lips
- Polymorphous erythematous rash
- Changes in hands and feet: tense edema, diffuse erythema, desquamation
- Unilateral cervical lymphadenopathy

Diagnosis

Kawasaki disease is a clinical diagnosis augmented by laboratory findings. Other entities that may have a similar presentation must be excluded. The diagnosis is made in children with a high fever who meet four or five of the clinical diagnostic criteria (Box 25-6). Infants may not meet diagnostic criteria and manifestations may be subtle. "Atypical" KD may be diagnosed if coronary artery aneurysms are noted on ECHO in the absence of criteria. ECHO is the primary tool for the initial evaluation and follow-up of children with coronary artery lesions. Unfortunately, it cannot evaluate for the presence of stenosis in aneurysms that have regressed.

Differential diagnoses include bacterial infection, measles, toxic shock syndrome, and scarlet fever. Laboratory data and cultures are helpful in supporting the diagnosis. Unfortunately, there is no specific laboratory test to diagnose KD.

Treatment

Intravenous immune globulin (IVIG) and aspirin therapy provide the mainstay in the therapeutic intervention for KD. These interventions are the most beneficial if administered during the first 10 days of illness, as they have demonstrated significant improvement in outcome. The child who has been ill for longer than 10 days, or has become afebrile, may have less benefit from IVIG. However, IVIG can still be administered if KD is suspected.

IVIG should be administered 2 gm/kg over 10–12 hours intravenously. IVIG usually results in rapid resolution of CHF, defervescence of fever, and normalization of sedimentation rate. IVIG markedly reduces the incidence of coronary artery aneurysms. Some children will not initially respond to IVIG, so a repeat dose of 1 gm/kg may be

NURSING TIP

Administration of Aspirin

Give aspirin with meals or an antacid to prevent GI upset. If flu or chickenpox is suspected in the child on aspirin it should be discontinued or changed to dipyridamole (Persantine).

administered. Methylprednisolone has been used in select clients who were refractory to multiple doses of IVIG in combination with aspirin (Burns et al., 2005).

Initial aspirin therapy consists of 100 mg/kg/day in four divided doses until fever subsides; the dosage is then changed to 3–5 mg/kg/day as one dose for 6–8 weeks. If small or medium coronary artery aneurysms are present, aspirin is continued until they resolve; long-term therapy is indicated in those with giant aneurysms. If the child is exposed to varicella or influenza, the aspirin should be temporarily discontinued and dipyridamole substituted, to minimize the risk of Reye's syndrome.

Anticoagulation with warfarin is recommended in children with giant aneurysms to prevent coronary artery thrombosis and occlusion. Those with acute coronary artery occlusion may be treated with thrombolytics such as tissue plasminogen activator or streptokinase. Novel interventions such as percutaneous transluminal coronary angioplasty, coronary artery bypass and graft, and heart transplant have been used on select patients with severe ischemic coronary artery disease (Burns et al., 2005).

Most patients do quite well if diagnosed and treated in a timely manner. The occurrence of aneurysms, most notably giant aneurysms, has decreased markedly with the use of IVIG. Currently the mortality rate is less than 1%. Long-term issues remain unsolved. The coronary arteries in patients with a history of aneurysms demonstrate abnormalities in dilation and flow. Giant aneurysms can become stenotic and calcified, contributing to ischemic heart disease years after the initial illness (Baker & Newburger, 2008). Children who have suffered from KD may be at high risk for the development of coronary artery disease as adults. Longitudinal studies are ongoing to evaluate long-term sequelae in Kawasaki disease.

Nursing Management

It is recommended that children with KD be admitted to the hospital during the acute phase (days 1–10) of illness. During this period close observation and assessment of cardiac status are important. Vital signs, intake and output, and daily weights are recorded. The child should be frequently assessed for signs and symptoms of CHF (see section on CHF) such as tachycardia, gallop rhythm, poor perfusion, and decreased urine output.

Guidelines for the administration of IVIG should be the same as blood product administration. Vital signs and perfusion are assessed and documented frequently according to hospital policy. Adverse reactions include hypotension, tachycardia, chills, nausea, and hypersensitivity reaction (rare). Most side effects can be minimized by slowing the rate of infusion, or with the concurrent administration of benadryl. The infusion should be discontinued and the physician notified immediately in the case of hypersensitivity.

Most nursing care is supportive, focusing on symptomatic relief. These young children are usually miserable and very irritable. The child should be cared for in a quiet, soothing environment to minimize the extreme discomfort of fever, edema, and joint pain. Timely administration of aspirin and analgesics is critically important. Lip balm, skin lotions, cool cloths, and tepid baths may provide temporary alleviation of symptoms. The parent or primary caregiver should be allowed to stay throughout the hospitalization, and the family should be involved in the development of the plan of care. Because of oral lesions soft foods and fluids should be offered frequently. Adequate fluid intake, intake and output, and calorie counts should be monitored closely. As the child improves, child life therapists, occupational therapists, and physical therapists can be utilized as appropriate.

Family Teaching

Discharge planning includes family education for aspirin administration, warfarin administration if warranted, and

NURSING ALERT

Administration of Warfarin (Coumadin)

Warfarin has a multitude of drug and food interactions. Antibiotics, vitamin K, birth control pills, and soy-based formulas can all affect International Normalization Ration (INR), the blood test used to determine the degree of anticoagulation present. Family education is imperative; monitoring of INR should be adjusted accordingly.

NURSING ALERT

Administration of Intravenous Immune Globulin (IVIG)

IVIG is a blood product. The nurse should be familiar with hospital guidelines prior to administration. Frequent monitoring of vital signs should occur during the first hour or two of administration. If an adverse reaction is noted (rash, fever, shaking, chills) discontinue infusion immediately and notify practitioner.

follow-up with pediatric cardiology. Clinic appointments are best made prior to discharge from the hospital. In addition, families should be given a phone number for the cardiology clinic in case they have questions following discharge.

INFECTIVE ENDOCARDITIS

Infective endocarditis (IE) is an infection with subsequent inflammation of the heart valves and lining of the heart. Although it is relatively uncommon it can be life-threatening. Considerable morbidity and mortality continue to result from this disease process, in spite of advances in diagnosis and treatment.

Incidence and Etiology

Absolute incidence of IE is difficult to determine. In pediatrics many children who develop endocarditis have underlying structural heart disease. Those at the highest risk are children with complex cyanotic heart disease, prosthetic cardiac valves, and a previous history of endocarditis. The second most common group of clients to develop endocarditis are critically ill infants and children with normal hearts who have multiple invasive lines and tubes. School-age children and adolescents who are IV drug abusers are also at high risk for the development of IE. Although uncommon, previously healthy children with normal hearts can develop IE as well.

IE is caused by an initial **bacteremia** (bacteria in the blood) that can occur spontaneously, following an invasive procedure (dental work, GI/GU surgery, instrumentation) or be secondary to a focal infection (abscess or urinary tract infection) (Wilson et al., 2007). The most common organisms are group A streptococci, *Staphylococcus aureus*, enterococci, and *Candida*. However, any number of infectious agents have been reported to cause endocarditis (AAP, 2006).

Pathophysiology

Infectious organisms enter the blood and can lodge on areas of the heart that are irregular or where there is turbulent blood flow (abnormal valves, VSD). See Box 25-7 for procedures commonly associated with bacteremia and subsequent endocarditis.

The invading organism will lodge and grow on the **endocardium** (serous inner membrane of the heart) forming **vegetations**, or abnormal growths, contributing to inflammation. Fibrin deposits and platelet thrombi form on the vegetations. Vegetations can break off and embolize to other parts of the body. Adjacent tissues and valves may be invaded, contributing to progressive cardiac damage.

BOX 25-7
PROCEDURES ASSOCIATED WITH INFECTIVE ENDOCARDITIS

- Only dental work that involves manipulation of gingival tissue or the periapical (tissues around the root of teeth) region of teeth or perforation of the mucosa
- Tonsillectomy or adenoidectomy

Clinical Manifestations

Early symptoms can be quite mild; sometimes the only symptom is prolonged fever. On the other end of the spectrum the child can experience an acute onset of very high fever and exhaustion. However, most symptoms are nonspecific consisting of low-grade fever, fatigue, headache, nausea, vomiting, and cyclic afternoon chills. A new or changing murmur may be noted on auscultation, particularly in a child with known structural heart disease. Tachycardia can be seen, and, infrequently, arrhythmias or heart failure.

There are some fairly classic skin lesions seen with IE. However, these usually appear late in the illness and are seldom seen if the child is treated in a timely manner. The lesions include Osler nodes and Janeway lesions. Osler nodes are tender pea-sized nodules on the pads of the fingers and toes. Janeway lesions are small areas of hemorrhage on the soles and palms.

Diagnosis

The diagnosis of IE is based on a high index of suspicion in concert with clinical and laboratory findings. The most important diagnostic tools are blood cultures and ECHO. Blood cultures are obtained immediately prior to the administration of antibiotics. Careful antiseptic preparation of the phlebotomy site will help prevent contamination of the cultures with normal skin flora. Serial cultures may need to be obtained for definitive diagnosis. ECHO can identify the presence, location, and size of vegetations. ECHO is also helpful in predicting whether a vegetation is at risk for embolization.

Treatment

Prevention is the best treatment of IE. The American Heart Association has set forth guidelines for antibiotic prophylaxis of children with congenital heart disease (Wilson et al., 2007). Cardiac conditions at the highest risk for IE include unrepaired complex cyanotic lesions and prosthetic valves (Box 25-8). Prophylaxis is recommended prior to those procedures associated with endocarditis. Amoxicillin is the primary drug used for prophylaxis; for those children with penicillin allergies clindamycin is used. For dosage recommendations see Box 25-9.

In those individuals who have documented endocarditis, antibiotic treatment should be instituted immediately (after appropriate blood cultures have been obtained). The most frequently used antibiotic is penicillin; however antibiotic therapy is determined by the causative organism and its sensitivity to antibiotic therapy. The course is 4–6 weeks of intravenous drug therapy. Amphotericin B is administered to treat fungal endocarditis.

BOX 25-8

CARDIAC CONDITIONS ASSOCIATED WITH INFECTIVE ENDOCARDITIS

Prophylaxis Recommended

- Prosthetic cardiac valves
- Previous history of infective endocarditis
- Unrepaired cyanotic heart disease (TGA, TOF, TA, HLHS)
- Surgically constructed arterial to pulmonary shunts (BT shunt)
- Completely repaired CHD with prosthetic material or device, whether placed by surgery of catheter intervention, during the first six months after the procedure
- Repaired CHD with residual defects at the site or adjacent to the site of a prosthetic patch or device

Prophylaxis Not Recommended (Risk is no greater than general population)

- Acyanotic defects
- Repaired CHD without residual shunt six months after surgery
- Mitral valve prolapse without regurgitation
- Innocent murmurs
- Previous history of rheumatic fever with or without heart involvement
- Isolated cardiac pacemakers or defibrillators without structural heart disease

Adapted from Wilson et al. (2007). Prevention of infective endocarditis: Guideline from the American Heart Association, *Circulation*, http://circ.ahajournals.org, DOI: 10.1161/CIRCULATIONAHA.106.183095.

Rarely, surgical intervention is undertaken to replace severely abnormal leaking valves. The ideal is to provide antibiotic administration for as long as possible prior to surgery. Active infection (persistent positive blood cultures) is a contraindication for surgery.

If preprocedural antibiotic prophylaxis is instituted appropriately, the incidence of endocarditis will remain low. Unfortunately, IE is difficult to treat, and mortality can be as high as 20%. Morbidity in the form of persistent valvar disease can be as high as 50%. Clearly the best intervention is prevention.

Nursing Management

It is imperative that the nurse caring for the child with suspected IE obtain blood cultures and institute antibiotic therapy in a timely manner. Early treatment is critically important to improving outcomes. Because of the need for long-term intravenous therapy a percutaneous peripherally inserted catheter (PICC line) should be inserted early in the hospitalization. These are small (2.0–4.0 French) silastic catheters that can be left in place long-term (weeks to months), have low risk for infection, and allow for client mobility. It is very important that antibiotic doses are *not missed*. Therefore, if intravenous access is interrupted, a new line is inserted immediately. Bed rest is implemented early in the illness. Quiet diversional activities (video games, board games, books) are offered at age-appropriate levels. If CHF is present, it is treated appropriately (see section on CHF).

BOX 25-9

PROPHYLACTIC REGIMENS FOR DENTAL PROCEDURES

Amoxicillin	50 mg/kg up to the adult dose of 2 grams taken orally 1 hour prior to procedure
Ampicillin	50 mg/kg up to adult dose of 2 grams IV 30 minutes prior to procedure
Clindamycin	20 mg/kg up to adult dose of 600 mg orally 1 hour prior to procedure, or 20 mg/kg up to adult dose of 600 mg IV 30 minutes prior to procedure

If the preprocedure dose is missed it can be given within 2 hours after the procedure to infer some protection. Pediatric dose should not exceed adult dose. Cephalosporins (cephalexin, cefadroxil, cefaxolin) can be used in select patients who are allergic to penicillin. The above is also recommended for those children undergoing procedures of the respiratory tract that involve incision or biopsy of the mucosa.

Adapted from Wilson et al. (2007). Prevention of infective endocarditis: Guideline from the American Heart Association, *Circulation*, http://circ.ahajournals.org, DOI: 10.1161/CIRCULATIONAHA.106.183095.

Family Teaching

Family education regarding the need for endocarditis prophylaxis is done when the initial diagnosis of congenital heart disease is made. Follow-up reinforcement is mandatory. It has been demonstrated that many children and adults with congenital heart disease have inadequate knowledge of endocarditis prophylaxis. The AHA has developed wallet-sized cards for individual use that should be given to every child requiring prophylaxis.

The family and child should be educated regarding the treatment plan, including the need for prolonged hospitalization and intravenous antibiotic therapy. Reinforcement of AHA recommendations for prophylaxis should be made prior to discharge in children with congenital defects.

In addition, the importance of good dental hygiene must be emphasized at each encounter. Evidence supports the prevention and eradication of dental disease in helping to decrease the incidence of bacteremia following routine and invasive dental procedures.

HYPERTENSION

Hypertension is defined as systolic or diastolic blood pressure equal to or greater than the 95th percentile for age, sex, and height on at least three separate occasions. High-normal or borderline BP elevation is defined as systolic or diastolic BP between the 90th and 95th percentile for age, sex, and height. Normal BP is defined as systolic and diastolic BP below the 90th percentile for age, sex, and height (Urbina et al., 2008). Although clinical hypertension occurs less frequently in children than adults, evidence is accumulating that the roots of essential hypertension extend back to childhood. Children and adolescents whose BPs are in the upper percentiles are more likely to become young adults who have elevated BP, which is associated with an increased risk of cardiovascular disease morbidity and mortality.

INCIDENCE AND ETIOLOGY (PATHOPHYSIOLOGY)

The incidence (and prevalence) of hypertension in childhood is low, only about 1%. African Americans and Asians have higher BP levels than whites.

When no known underlying disease is present, hypertension is referred to as primary or essential. When the cause of the elevated BP can be explained by an associated disease, hypertension is referred to as secondary. In infants and young children below 6 years of age, secondary hypertension is more common than primary hypertension. The main causes are renal diseases, followed by cardiovascular (coarctation of the aorta), endocrine, and some neurologic disorders. After age 6 years, primary hypertension is the more common type.

Many factors play a role in the development of primary hypertension. These include heredity, obesity, stress, smoking, physical activity, and salt intake. Most children and adolescents with BP measurements exceeding the 95th percentile are overweight and have family histories of hypertension.

CULTURAL CONSIDERATION

Hypertension in Children

African-American children have a higher incidence of primary hypertension than Caucasians. It develops at a younger age, is frequently more severe, and may result in early death.

CLINICAL MANIFESTATIONS

Most children and adolescents with primary hypertension are asymptomatic until the BP elevation is detected, usually during a routine examination or during physical evaluation prior to athletic participation. These individuals tend to have mild elevation in BP and are somewhat overweight. Children with secondary hypertension will usually not have symptoms unless BP has been sustained or is rising rapidly. However, with substantial elevation, headache, dizziness, changes in vision, and seizures may occur. Infants and young children cannot communicate symptoms such as a headache so observation of their behavior may provide clues. However, their behavior may not be considered abnormal until complications of hypertension are present. In retrospect, many caregivers report that their child had become increasingly irritable before the hypertension was detected.

DIAGNOSIS

Elevated BP must be confirmed on repeated visits before characterizing an individual as having hypertension. In general, the younger the individual, the higher the level of BP, the presence of symptoms, and the less family history of hypertension, the more likely it is that the child has secondary hypertension. The diagnostic evaluation for children whose history or physical examination suggests a specific cause of hypertension should be guided by the suspected problem, initially focusing on the renal system. Physical examination should determine the presence of flank masses. Screening tests should include CBC, serum electrolytes, urinalysis, blood urea nitrogen (BUN), serum creatinine, and uric acid. Renal ultrasonography may be useful to evaluate structural renal abnormalities. Diminished femoral pulses suggest the presence of coarctation of the aorta, and measurement of BP in the legs should be performed to determine if it is substantially lower than in the arms. Imaging studies such as echocardiography should be obtained on these children.

Children suspected of having primary hypertension require few diagnostic tests other than a urinalysis and blood profiles to examine serum creatinine. A lipid profile may provide useful information as many overweight children and adolescents with hypertension have elevated triglycerides and low high-density lipoprotein (HDL) cholesterol and high low-density lipoprotein (LDL) cholesterol.

TREATMENT

Both nonpharmacologic and pharmacologic approaches to treatment are useful in managing children and adolescents with hypertension. Nonpharmacologic therapy includes weight reduction, dietary intervention, and exercise. This approach should be used not only with individuals with hypertension but also in children with high-normal BPs (90th to 95th percentile BP distribution) and those with severe hypertension to complement drug therapy. If the

RESEARCH Highlight

Cholesterol-Lowering Diet in Children with Elevated Low-Density Lipoprotein Cholesterol (LDL-C)

STUDY PURPOSE

To test the long-term efficacy and safety of a cholesterol-lowering dietary intervention in children. Diets reduced in fat and cholesterol are recommended for children over 2 years of age, yet long-term safety and efficacy are unknown.

METHODS

For 7.4 years, 666 children 8 to 10 years of age with elevated low-density lipoprotein cholesterol (LDL-C) were randomized to a dietary intervention or usual care group. The dietary behavioral intervention promoted adherence to a diet with 28% of energy from total fat, 8% from saturated fat, up to 9% from polyunsaturated fat, and 75 mg/1,000 calories of cholesterol per day. Those assigned to the usual care group were given educational publications on heart-healthy eating available to the public and were examined annually for study-wide measurements.

FINDINGS

Reductions in dietary total fat, saturated fat, and cholesterol were greater in the intervention than in the usual care group. A salient finding is the safety of an intervention to promote a fat-reduced diet in actively growing children with elevated LDL-C, when they are instructed properly and instructions are followed at regular intervals.

IMPLICATIONS

Dietary fat modification can be achieved and safely sustained in actively growing children with elevated LDL-C. Improvements in these levels can be made without adverse effects on children's growth and maturational development.

REFERENCE

Obarzanek, E., Kimm, S., Barton, B., Van Horn, L., Kwiterovich, P., & Simons-Morton, D. et al. (2001). Long-term safety and efficacy of a cholesterol-lowering diet in children with elevated low-density lipoprotein cholesterol: Seven-year results of the dietary intervention study in children (DISC). *Pediatrics*, 107(2), 256–264.

child is obese, efforts should be directed at reducing obesity by lowering excessive calorie intake and increasing physical exercise. Dietary intervention includes ingestion of a low-fat, high-fiber diet with an increase in fresh fruits and vegetables, and elimination of foods high in sodium and added salt. Increased physical exercise, especially aerobic exercise, and sports participation help with weight reduction and stress management.

Because of the lack of data on drug therapy outcomes in children, guidelines for treatment are conservative. Children with mild hypertension should include lifestyle changes such as weight reduction and physical activity. For those with secondary hypertension treatment should focus on the underlying cause. Drug therapy is considered for children with significant elevation of BP that has not responded to lifestyle changes. When drugs are used, the goals are to reduce BP to below the 95th percentile. The oral antihypertensive drugs used most often in children include diuretics, beta blockers such as propranolol (Inderal), angiotensin-converting enzyme inhibitors such as captopril (Capoten) and enalapril (Vasotec), and calcium channel blockers such as nifedipine (Adalat).

NURSING MANAGEMENT AND FAMILY TEACHING

The nurse focuses on teaching the child and family and supporting them in adhering to the treatment plan. Education about lifestyle habits and changes such as diet, exercise, weight control, and attitudes about smoking should include the entire family. When all members participate in any of the treatment strategies, lifestyle changes tend to be more consistent and long-lasting and the child's compliance is likely to be greater. An exercise program should include physical activities the child likes. School-age children and adolescents may prefer team sports rather than solitary activities such as running, swimming, and bicycling. Praise and encouragement for even minor changes are important for motivation to continue to follow the prescribed program. Blood pressure measurements should be performed as part of all routine physical examinations on all children older than 3 years of age. Baseline and serial measurement need to be documented in the child's record.

HEART TRANSPLANTATION

Heart transplantation is the process by which a failing heart is removed from a recipient and replaced with a functional heart from a brain dead donor. While heart transplantation offers a chance for reasonable quality of life for the recipient it must be remembered that this procedure is not a cure, but a palliation and with it come a host of potential and real complications. Heart transplantation is a lifelong commitment for the child and family.

INDICATIONS

Heart transplantation is indicated in children with heart failure who have a significant decrease in their quality of life related to their heart failure. These children have failed medical management and are unlikely to survive without a new heart. Unfortunately, not all clients are deemed physically or emotionally capable of withstanding the lifelong issues associated with transplantation.

There are two major groups in whom heart transplant is indicated. The first group includes individuals with dilated cardiomyopathy, and the second group includes those children with complex congenital heart disease. HLHS is the leading indication for heart transplantation in the infant population. Dilated cardiomyopathy is the most common cause in children over the age of 1 year (Boucek & Chrisant, 2004). Dilated cardiomyopathy can be caused by a number of etiologies (ischemia, familial conditions, or viral infections) that result in a thin-walled poorly contractile ventricle. Contraindications to transplantation include malignancy, serious systemic infection, or a systemic disease such as diabetes. Psychosocial instability within the family may preclude heart transplantation because of an inability to follow the lifelong treatment plan.

TRANSPLANT LISTING

Once the extensive pretransplant workup has been completed, the child is listed with the United Network for Organ Sharing (UNOS). This is a national organization that oversees transplant activity. Children are listed by their blood type and weight and are prioritized according to their severity of illness.

The waiting period can be a very stressful time for both the child and the family. Relocation may be necessary so the family will be in closer proximity to the transplant center. This can result in major disruption for the whole family. The waiting period may be quite extensive and the possibility exists that the child may die before a donor organ becomes available. According to a recent study of a cohort of more than 3,000 children awaiting heart transplantation, 17% died before a heart became available (Almond et al., 2009). In the last several years the option of a Ventricular Assist Device (VAD) has given new hope for the family of a child awaiting a heart donor. Several temporary devices exist that allow for support of the failing heart. These devices can provide support for the left, right, or both ventricles. The procedure involves placement of cannula or tubes directly into the failing ventricle with a pump outside the child's body providing cardiac support. Although this does provide some hope for the families, placement of a VAD carries significant risks of bleeding and infection and may not maintain the child until a donor heart is available. One of the major predictors of mortality on the waiting list is the degree of invasive procedures required to keep the child alive. These procedures include VAD support (Almond et al., 2009). In one recent study 9 children were bridged to transplant with the use of a biventricular assist device. At 19-month follow-up there was 100% survival post transplantation (Gandhi et al., 2008).

SURGICAL PROCESS

When a child has been declared brain dead, he or she is considered a potential organ donor. If the donor family agrees to organ donation the local transplant organization is notified. A member of the organization will evaluate the donor to determine if he or she is suitable for organ donation. Donor organs are removed in the operating room by the procurement team. Once the donor heart has been removed the maximum time before reimplantation into the

REFLECTIVE THINKING

A Teenager Awaits a New Heart

My name is Eric and I am 17 years old. Four years ago I had to have radiation, chemotherapy, and my left leg amputated below my knee because I had a bone cancer called osteosarcoma. It was a scary nightmare and I never knew if I was going to get better. By the time I was 16, I was much better. My family really helped me. I was back at school and my friends didn't care that I had a prosthesis for a leg.

Then when I was in school I started feeling really tired and I just couldn't get my work done. I didn't want to tell anyone, I was so afraid the cancer was back, but my doctor said no. Then I went to another doctor who took a chest X-ray and my heart was much bigger than it was supposed to be. Then I started with new doctors who did all kinds of testing and then told me that one of the medications I needed for my bone cancer, Adriamycin, caused my heart to fail and I had what is called cardiomyopathy. After all I've been through, now they tell me I need a new heart.

At first I was really mad. Why should I have to go through all this? It's not fair. I feel like I can't plan for anything with my friends. They are all talking about college and future careers. Me, I just wait for the phone to ring or for one of my parent's pagers to go off saying they might have an available heart. It's really weird that someone else will have to die before I can get a new heart. What will it feel like to have someone else's heart in my body? What will all these medications do to me? They tell me I have to take them for the rest of my life. My parents are pretty stressed worrying about me, but I think as a family we do pretty well together. Part of me hopes that this happens soon so I can get it over with and part of me still hopes that my own heart gets better.

Some issues for the nurse to think about:

1. What other hurdles do you think these children face?
2. How would you talk with them if you were taking care of them before surgery?
3. How do you feel about organ donation yourself?
4. Could you be nonjudgmental if your beliefs differed from this patient?
5. Do you have religious or personal beliefs for or against transplantation?

recipient should be less than 6–8 hours to prevent cardiac dysfunction. The recipient's heart is explanted and the donor heart is implanted into the recipient.

POSTTRANSPLANT ISSUES

Postoperative complications include decreased cardiac function, rejection, arrhythmias, and infection. Cardiac function is supported by medications to improve cardiac output (refer to Table 25-3). The new heart is perceived by the recipient's immune system as foreign, stimulating the immune system, which results in rejection. Therefore, the use of antirejection medications is the mainstay of therapy for the heart transplant recipient. Despite the initiation of antirejection medications such as cyclosporin and FK503 (Prograf) in the immediate postoperative period, rejection does occur and is the leading cause of death during the first 6–12 months posttransplant. Acute rejection is seen in the first few days while chronic rejection is seen after months and years. Signs and symptoms of rejection are unfortunately subtle and often nonspecific. Clients can have fever, tachycardia, arrhythmias, hypotension, shortness of breath, and irritability. Because of the nonspecific nature of the signs of rejection, routine heart biopsies are scheduled to monitor for rejection.

All clients receiving immunosuppressive medications are at increased risk for infection. Strict handwashing is essential before contact with these children. Prophylactic medications are given to prevent infections from organisms such as CMV, *Pneumocystis carinii*, and *Candida* infections. Acyclovir, trimethoprim or sulfamethoxazole (Septra), and nystatin are used, respectively, to prevent the previously listed infections. Fevers are treated aggressively.

Long-term complications include the development of coronary artery disease requiring re-transplantation, poor growth and development secondary to steroids, and lymphoproliferative disease (LPD). LPD is a form of cancer that can occur in any type of solid organ transplant. Mortality for heart transplantation is 15–20% in the first 30 days. Recent results from the transplant registry indicate that recipients who were less than 1 year of age at the time of transplant and who survive the first year have an approximately 95% chance to survive to 4 years of age (Boucek & Chrisant, 2004). In a study of patients with either HLHS, cardiomyopathy, or complex congenital heart disease the 15-year survival is approximately 55% (Dionigi, Razzouk, Hasaniya, Chinnock, & Bailry, 2008). Outcomes for those awaiting heart transplant is suboptimal. Approximately 25% of patients listed for a heart transplant will die waiting for a donor to become available.

Heart transplantation is a viable palliation for the failing heart that may provide the recipient with years of quality life. The major roadblock to transplantation at this time is the lack of available organs to meet the needs of the listed recipients. As members of the health profession we must examine our own feelings regarding transplantation and let our families and loved ones know how we feel. Many nurses will find themselves taking care of both potential organ donors and children who need organs at some time during their careers. In dealing with families who are faced with the question of whether or not to donate their child's organs we must be nonjudgmental and supportive. Education regarding the process of transplantation for both medical and nonmedical people must continue if we are to decrease the number of individuals that will die before an organ becomes available.

FAMILY TEACHING

It cannot be emphasized enough that transplantation is a lifetime commitment. The child must remain on antirejection medications for his or her entire life. Lifetime follow-up is necessary to identify noncompliance and complications in a timely manner. Immunizations should be administered as scheduled, but no live viruses are to be given. Large crowds should be avoided for the first several months after transplant; children are permitted back in school approximately six months after successful transplant. Children who are still at home should always be encouraged to participate in school assignments and home education. Community resources that can be utilized include home schooling and home nursing visits to minimize exposure to infection. Many communities have heart transplant support groups that are helpful to both the child and caregivers.

Once the child returns to school, the teachers should be apprised of the treatment regimen and any precautions. The medications are taken frequently throughout the day so assistance from the school is imperative. If any child in the class comes down with varicella, the family of the transplant client should be notified immediately. During periods of seasonal illness it may be beneficial for the child to be home schooled to prevent infection secondary to immunosuppression.

CARDIAC ARRHYTHMIAS

A number of children with acquired or congenital heart disease can develop cardiac arrhythmias. Many cardiac rhythm abnormalities in children are not life-threatening; however, some require close monitoring and treatment. It must be remembered that several important differences exist between children and adults, although they may have the same rhythm abnormality. Although an in-depth review of ECG interpretation is beyond the scope of this text, a brief review is warranted.

The P wave correlates with atrial depolarization and the QRS with ventricular depolarization. The PR interval is the time it takes an electrical impulse to travel from the normal pacemaker of the heart (SA node) to the AV node. The QT interval represents ventricular repolarization. Every normal beat should have a P wave before every QRS and the rhythm should be regular. Heart rates are faster in infants and children. PR interval and QRS duration are generally shorter and increase with age as the heart rate slows.

Many arrhythmias are caused by the conduction system changes that occur as a consequence of heart surgery and may not be appreciated until adolescence. Early postoperative arrhythmias may be transient, resolving in the first few weeks after surgery. The following is a discussion of the more significant arrhythmias found in infants and children.

SUPRAVENTRICULAR TACHYCARDIA

Supraventricular tachycardia (SVT) is the most common arrhythmia seen in infants and children. It usually occurs in the presence of a structurally normal heart; however, it can occur in individuals with congenital heart disease. Many of these patients present prenatally or during the first year of life (Gilljam, Jaeggi, & Gow, 2008; Massin, Benatar, & Rondia, 2008). Half of all infants who develop this in the first few months of life will outgrow it by 1 year of age. The other most common period for the occurrence of SVT is during adolescence. SVT is characterized as a narrow QRS tachycardia that is abrupt in onset and termination (Figure 25-31). Heart rates in infants can be as high as 300 beats per minute, older children are >220 beats per minute. Although this arrhythmia is not life-threatening it can cause significant symptoms (Massin et al., 2008; Vos, Pulles-Heintzberger, & Delhaas, 2003).

Presentation is quite variable. Some children will have infrequent episodes that terminate spontaneously. Others can have incessant tachycardia that is difficult to treat. Symptoms in infants are nonspecific, so frequently this diagnosis is initially missed. Symptoms include poor feeding, irritability, fussiness, and pallor. If SVT persists then cardiac failure will ensue. Once the tachycardia is terminated cardiac function returns to normal.

Older children can often identify the sudden onset of SVT. Therefore, intervention is much more timely. SVT can produce chest pain and dizziness, and syncope rarely occurs. SVT is sudden in onset and termination. It is often not associated with any specific activity and can occur at rest or with exercise.

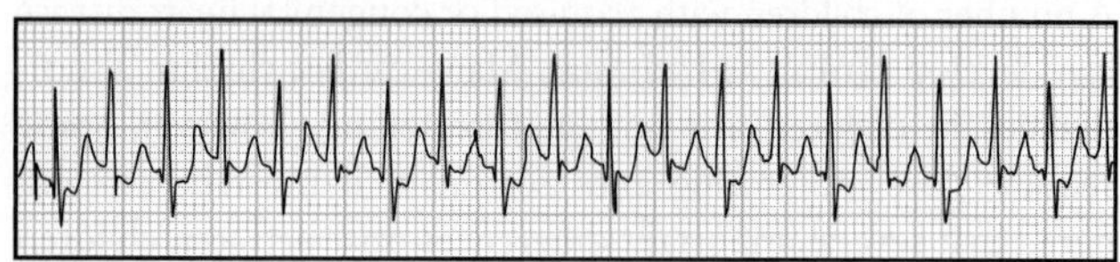

FIGURE 25-31 Supraventricular Tachycardia in a 12-Year-Old Boy. Heart rate is 240. DELMAR CENGAGE LEARNING.

Diagnosis is made by ECG while the patient is in SVT. The decision to treat SVT is determined by client choice (in that SVT episodes are frequent and interfere with lifestyle), syncope associated with SVT, or presence of structural heart disease (Vos et al., 2003).

Initial maneuvers to treat SVT are simple in the stable child. Vagal maneuvers are quite successful in terminating tachycardia if implemented shortly after onset. These include valsalva maneuver (holding their breath and then bearing down), headstand for a few minutes, or placing their face in a tub of ice water for as long as tolerated. Application of an ice bag to the face of an infant is often successful in tachycardia termination. Care must be taken to avoid prolonged application of the ice bag to prevent fat necrosis from profound vasoconstriction. If vagal maneuvers are not successful in tachycardia termination, or if the tachycardia does not terminate spontaneously, then the child should be taken to the nearest emergency room for treatment. The first-line intervention for hard-to-treat SVT is intravenous adenosine. This medication blocks conduction at the AV node for 10–15 seconds, thus terminating the rhythm. Although transient, there can be a short period of asystole following administration (Figure 25-32). This can make the child lightheaded without loss of consciousness. Other side effects include tightness in the chest and difficulty breathing. All symptoms are very transient. The child should be warned ahead of time of the effects of adenosine to prevent undue anxiety.

Infrequently a child will develop re-onset of SVT after termination with adenosine, or the child may have frequent episodes that interfere with lifestyle. In these situations, chronic therapy can be implemented. Medications used to treat SVT include beta blockers (propranolol, atenolol), sotalol procainamide, or amiodarone. All have different mechanisms of action and different side effects. The nurse should become familiar with all options when administering these medications.

Acute management for unstable children who do not respond to adenosine includes overdrive pacing or **synchronized cardioversion**. For overdrive pacing, esophageal pacing is utilized. A special pacing electrode is passed down the esophagus to the level of the heart. Short bursts of rapid pacing, faster than the tachycardia rate, are applied. This

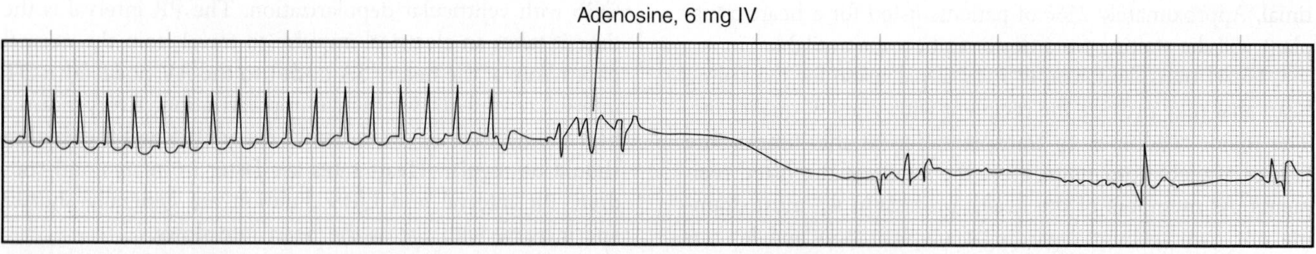

FIGURE 25-32 Cardioversion of SVT to Normal Sinus Rhythm with IV Adenosine; Note Long Pause of Heart Block. DELMAR CENGAGE LEARNING.

maneuver can break the tachycardia and is the most effective treatment in younger children.

Synchronized cardioversion uses the defibrillator to produce an electrical shock to convert the arrhythmia to sinus rhythm. Prior to cardioversion the child must be NPO for 4–6 hours and *must be well sedated,* as this is *very* painful. Following the procedure the nurse should document the subsequent rhythm with an ECG. Overall outcomes are very good with SVT. Many infants will have no recurrence of SVT after the first year of life. A number of older children learn to terminate their tachycardia without pharmacologic intervention by vagal maneuvers as previously discussed.

For select children, definitive treatment is radiofrequency catheter ablation performed in the cath lab (see Table 25-2). This is generally very successful, and many will have no subsequent episodes of SVT.

NURSING ALERT

How to Safely Perform Cardioversion

The nurse must be familiar with the defibrillator prior to use. The child is placed on the defibrillator ECG; a consistent upright R wave must be present on the ECG. The "synch" button must be on, and the nurse must assess for the synch mark on the R wave. Usual output for synchronized cardioversion is 1/2–1 joule/kg. Multifunction pads are recommended rather than the paddles, as these allow for pacing in cases of asystole. Prior to discharge make sure no one is touching the child or the bed, and shout "clear" prior to discharge.

COMPLETE HEART BLOCK (CHB)

Complete heart block can be either acquired or congenital. CHB is diagnosed on ECG. There is no conduction through the AV node so there is complete atrial and ventricular dissociation, and the atrial rate is much faster than the ventricular rate (Figure 25-33).

Acquired heart block can be secondary to myocarditis, endocarditis, or cardiac surgery. Congenital heart block is diagnosed in utero on fetal echocardiogram or in the immediate neonatal period. The most common reason for congenital heart block is maternal systemic lupus erythematosus. Other maternal connective tissue diseases can cause heart block as well.

The treatment for heart block is a permanent pacemaker. The need for a pacemaker in congenital heart block is determined by the child's resting heart rate, presence of symptoms, CHF, or ventricular arrhythmias. Heart rates lower than 55 when awake are associated with increased risk for death. Children with syncope, dizziness, PVCs, or VT also require a pacemaker. Without a permanent pacemaker the mortality rate is estimated to be 5%. Long-term sequelae include CHF and mitral regurgitation. Once a pacemaker is implanted, and sinus rhythm is restored, outcome is excellent. The pacemaker system consists of leads attached to the heart and a generator. The generator contains the battery and the microcircuitry needed to pace the heart. The generator is changed when the battery voltage is low.

VENTRICULAR TACHYCARDIA

Ventricular tachycardia (VT) is a wide complex tachycardia (ventricular rates greater than 200 bpm) that is generated from the ventricles and can result in diminished cardiac output and may deteriorate to a pulseless rhythm or ventricular fibrillation. Although it is relatively uncommon in the general pediatric population it is more prevalent in children with underlying heart disease. Particularly since many of these children are now surviving into adolescence and adulthood in the current era of early identification and treatment of pediatric heart disease.

On ECG the QRS complex is wide and the P waves may not be identifiable or the ventricular rate (as determined by the number or R waves) will be greater than the atrial rate (as determined by the number of P waves) (Figure 25-34). Children at the greatest risk for developing VT are those with ventricular scarring secondary to surgery, abnormal hemodynamics despite surgery, and those with long QT syndrome. Long QT syndrome is a genetic

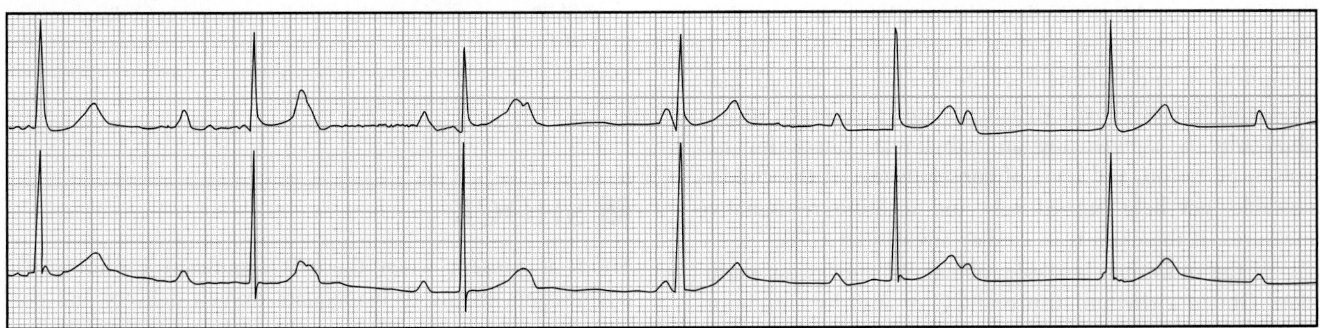

FIGURE 25-33 **Complete Heart Block in a 14-Year-Old Girl. Atrial rate is 65. There is complete atrial and ventricular dissociation; ventricular rate is 39.** DELMAR CENGAGE LEARNING.

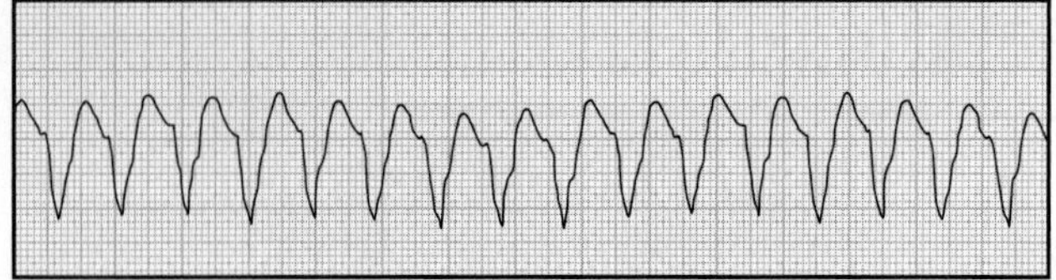

FIGURE 25-34 Ventricular Tachycardia. DELMAR CENGAGE LEARNING.

arrhythmia syndrome that is due to mutations in the genes responsible for the electrical behavior of the heart (Roos-Hesselink & Karamermer, 2008; Wilde, 2008).

Treatment is determined by the frequency of VT, how rapid the ventricular rate is, associated heart disease, the presence of symptoms (syncope) or sudden death. Antiarrhythmics are often employed to suppress the focus of the arrhythmia and/or to slow the ventricular rate. Often correction of any underlying hemodynamic abnormalities will help prevent future episodes. Implantable cardiac defibrillators (ICDs) are used in patients who have experienced sustained VT or have survived an episode of sudden death (Walsh, 2008). Some centers implant ICDs in children who are at risk for the development of VT or ventricular fibrillation as a secondary prevention.

The ICD system consists of one or two leads placed either inside or on the outside (epicardial leads) of the ventricle and/or atria. One lead is the shock (defibrillating) lead. The leads are connected to the ICD device that is similar to a pacemaker, only slightly larger. The device is then programmed to detect specific rhythms and heart rates. If the detected rhythm or rate is in the appropriate zone then the device will discharge a small amount of energy in an attempt to terminate the rhythm. Rate, rhythms, and discharge energy are all programmable. If the client is conscious they will feel the discharge (shock). This is quite uncomfortable and is frightening, particularly if the discharge was inappropriate. All shocks should be reported to the primary cardiologist by the patient.

NURSING MANAGEMENT

The care of the child with arrhythmias can be challenging for the nurse. Most rhythm abnormalities are not life-threatening. The nurse should become familiar with the identification and treatment of life-threatening arrhythmias. First and foremost hemodynamic status is assessed in any child who is experiencing an arrhythmia. Check for BP, pulses, perfusion, and level of consciousness. If the child is unstable, get help immediately and institute resuscitative measures. If the child is in cardiac arrest, start CPR.

If the individual is stable, obtain BP and assess perfusion. Obtain a rhythm strip or ECG of any rhythm abnormality to document in the chart. An ECG will help to finalize the diagnosis. Treatment depends on the underlying etiology and type of rhythm abnormality.

EVIDENCE-BASED PRACTICE

Implantable Defibrillator Therapy in Patients with Congenital Heart Diseaes

CLINICAL PROBLEM

Implantable cardiac defibrillators (ICDs) have been shown to improve outcomes in pediatric patients with malignant ventricular arrhythmias. Technological advances have downsized leads and ICDs so they are now suitable for children. What are the implications of ICD placement in infants and children?

BEST CLINICAL PRACTICE

- In those patients with known malignant ventricular arrhythmias or those who have survived a sudden death event an ICD can treat and terminate lethal cardiac rhythms (secondary prevention).
- As primary prevention use of ICDs is less clear.
- Appropriate shocks are more common in secondary prevention patients.
- Most inappropriate shocks are due to lead failure not device failure.
- Strategies to minimize inappropriate shocks include: optimizing device programming and optimizing medical therapies.

IMPLICATIONS FOR NURSING

- Patient education regarding compliance with medical therapy is critical. Patients must continue to take all prescribed medications after ICD implant.
- Patients should report all shocks so the health care provider can check the device to insure that the shocks were appropriate.
- Identified inappropriate shocks should be further investigated with possible reprogramming of the ICD.

Reference: Berul, C. I., Van Hare, G. F., Kertesz, N. J., Dubin, A. M., Cecchin, F., Collins, K. K., Cannon B. C., Alexander, M. E., Triedman, J. K., Walsh, E. P., & Friedman, R. A. (2008). Results of a multicenter retrospective implantable cardioverter-defibrillator registry of pediatric and congenital heart disease patients. *Journal of American College of Cardiology, 51*(17), 1685–1691. Walsh, E. P. (2008). Practical aspects of implantable defibrillator therapy in patients with congenital heart disease, *PACE, 31*, S38–S40).

SHOCK

Shock is present when there is significant cardiovascular dysfunction leading to inadequate oxygen delivery and perfusion of vital organs. This results in anaerobic metabolism and production of lactic acid. If left untreated, the final pathway will be cell destruction, multi-organ system failure, and

KIDS WANT TO KNOW

Life with a Pacemaker

1. *What can I do after I get my pacemaker?*
   - The only restrictions are no contact sports (tackle football, ice hockey, and karate).
   - Other competitive and recreational sports are safe.
   - No scuba diving deeper than 100 feet.
2. *What equipment is dangerous for a pacemaker?*
   - Microwave ovens are safe.
   - Cell phones should be used on the side opposite where the generator has been implanted.
   - No arc welding, as this interferes with pacemaker function.
   - Some antitheft devices and metal detectors can temporarily affect pacemaker function; avoid these if possible or pass through detectors quickly.
   - Avoid being around large electric generators (power plants).
3. *Can the pacemaker ever be turned off by accident?*
   - No. Although some of the equipment mentioned above can temporarily affect function or set the pacemaker to the default settings, it will never be turned off. If you feel like your pacemaker is not working right or your heart rate is too slow, leave the area immediately. This should rectify the problem. If you still feel bad, call your health care provider immediately.
4. *How long does the battery in the generator last?*
   - 2–10 years, depending on how much you use the pacemaker.
5. *How do you change the battery?*
   - The battery is not changed like you would a flashlight; it is sealed into the generator so the whole generator must be changed when the battery gets low.
6. *How can you tell when the battery is low?*
   - At your clinic visits your health care provider will check the pacemaker and find out how much voltage is left.

death. Because of the morbidity and mortality of untreated or inadequately treated shock in the pediatric population it is essential that clinicians caring for these children learn to recognize the early signs and symptoms of impending shock. Early and aggressive management is likely to improve outcome and survival.

Generally shock can be divided into three major classifications: *hypovolemic, maldistributive,* and *cardiogenic.* Hypovolemic shock is secondary to intravascular volume loss. Maldistributive shock is a **maldistribution** of blood flow secondary to vasomotor instability or capillary leak. Cardiogenic shock is caused by cardiac pump dysfunction. When providing therapy for shock of any form all caretakers must remember to follow the principles of basic life support and the ABCs of resuscitation. These include airway, breathing, and circulation. Only then should one proceed to more specific treatment of the child in shock.

INCIDENCE AND ETIOLOGY

Hypovolemic shock is by far the most common form of shock in the pediatric population. In developing nations, hypovolemic shock continues to claim millions of lives secondary to illnesses leading to severe diarrhea. In the United States, this trend has decreased in the last 30 years because of many factors, including early recognition and aggressive fluid management in sick children. Recently the cholera outbreak in Zimbabwe has reached epidemic proportions. Thousands of people have succumbed to the severe vomiting, diarrhea, and dehydration that lead to hypovolemic shock and death. The etiology of hypovolemic shock varies. Box 25-10 lists the common causes.

BOX 25-10
COMMON CAUSES OF HYPOVOLEMIC SHOCK

Fluid and Electrolyte Losses
- Vomiting
- Diarrhea
- Excessive use of diuretics
- Heat stroke
- Inadequate water

Hemorrhage
- Trauma
- Surgical blood loss
- Fractures

Plasma Losses
- Burns
- Sepsis
- Intestinal obstruction

Endocrine
- Diabetes mellitus
- Diabetes insipidus

In the general pediatric population, the most common cause of fluid and electrolyte loss is gastroenteritis. This is associated with vomiting, diarrhea, and inadequate oral intake with concomitant ongoing losses. Dehydration with hypovolemic shock is the leading cause of death in children worldwide (AHA, 2006). Traumatic injury and hemorrhage is another cause of hypovolemic shock in children. The incidence of liver or spleen lacerations is significant in trauma clients. Large amounts of blood can also be lost from long bone fractures and deep lacerations. Intracranial hemorrhages from subdural hematomas in the neonate and newborn, such as those associated with shaken baby syndrome can also cause significant blood loss. Plasma losses from extensive burns can quickly lead to shock as intravascular fluid leaks into the damaged tissues. Sepsis will also lead to extensive plasma loss or "capillary leak" of fluid into the extravascular space.

The most common cause of maldistributive shock is sepsis, generally caused by systemic infection from a variety of bacteria, viruses, or fungi. The incidence of sepsis in the hospitalized child is much higher than the general population. These children are at increased risk from nosocomial infection from indwelling catheters and intravascular lines. This is particularly true for the immunocompromised or critically ill child. Anaphylactic shock is another form of maldistributive shock and is caused by the exposure of an allergic individual to a specific antigen. As this individual is exposed to an antigen (food, medication, and insect bite) the antigen–antibody response causes massive vasomotor tone abnormalities and widespread vasodilation.

Major causes of cardiogenic shock include preexisting congenital heart disease, cardiomyopathy, myocarditis, arrhythmias, drug toxicity, and hemolytic uremic syndrome. Cardiogenic shock is seen less frequently in children than other forms of shock.

PATHOPHYSIOLOGY

Although specific etiologies can vary, there are a number of common pathophysiological phenomena found in all children suffering from shock. A decrease in intravascular volume leads to a decrease in venous return to the heart with a subsequent fall in preload. This will lead to inadequate cardiac output. The normal compensatory mechanism is to increase heart rate. Therefore an early sign of shock is tachycardia. Antidiuretic hormone is released by the hypothalamus to facilitate the reabsorption of free water by the kidney in a compensatory attempt to increase intravascular volume.

If infection or inflammation is present, then subsequent release of toxins produces a decrease in sympathetic tone with resulting vasodilation and a decrease in systemic vascular resistance (SVR). Endothelial damage also occurs leading to the leaking of fluid from the intravascular to the interstitial space. This is known as capillary leak syndrome and can be a source of significant fluid loss internally. The initial response to vasodilation and decreased SVR is an increase in cardiac output to support blood pressure. Excessive vasodilation leads to a relative hypovolemia and hypotension.

In maldistributive shock the child may develop disseminated intravascular coagulopathy (DIC) secondary to the inflammatory process. DIC is an abnormal response of the clotting system leading to prolonged and inappropriate clotting. This is often seen as petechiae, small purplish hemorrhagic spots on the skin, and bleeding from IV sites and puncture wounds.

Ventricular pump dysfunction is frequently seen and is caused by a number of etiologies (structural heart disease, myocarditis, ischemia, or inflammatory mediators of septic shock). Contractility is depressed so cardiac output falls. This phenomena triggers sympathetic activation and the renin-angiotensin-aldosterone system previously discussed in the section on congestive heart failure.

If cardiac output remains low, oxygen delivery to the tissues will decrease. This will result in conversion of metabolism from aerobic to anaerobic with ensuing metabolic acidosis. The lungs will attempt to compensate for metabolic acidosis by increasing the respiratory rate to exhale CO_2, so respiratory alkalosis may develop as well. If left untreated, metabolic acidosis will depress myocardial function. Therefore cardiac output decreases further, and compensatory mechanisms fail resulting in cardiovascular collapse and death.

CLINICAL MANIFESTATIONS

Cardiovascular signs are often the most prominent. Poor perfusion will manifest as cool extremities, diminished or absent distal pulses (radial, dorsalis pedis), a capillary filling time (CPT) of greater than 3 seconds, and mottling of the skin. Blood flow shunted away from the skin will cause extensive mottling of the extremities and eventually the trunk. However, in distributive shock skin will be warm and flushed because of intense vasodilation. Tachycardia and tachypnea are common in the child with early shock. Blood pressure should be measured; however, because of compensatory mechanisms, blood pressure can be normal until the child deteriorates. Hypotension is a late and often sudden sign of cardiovascular compensation. Even mild hypotension must be vigorously treated (AHA, 2006).

NURSING ALERT

Severe Hypotension

One of the hallmarks of septic shock is *severe hypotension* in the face of increased cardiac output. Frequently it is the diastolic blood pressure that is most affected secondary to vasodilation. Therefore, a low diastolic pressure and wide pulse pressure is seen.

From a respiratory standpoint the child initially will be mildly tachypneic with a minimal need for supplemental oxygen. As acidosis worsens, work of breathing will increase. Increased work of breathing is manifested by increased respiratory rate, retractions, and nasal flaring. Neurologically, the child in early shock may be irritable and hard to console. In the face of shock, compensatory mechanisms will attempt to deliver oxygen to the brain; therefore, the development of lethargy is an ominous sign. Clients with anaphylactic shock often present with severe hypotension immediately after exposure to an antigen. Often the child will develop urticaria (hives), have swollen lips, and develop respiratory difficulties secondary to airway swelling.

DIAGNOSIS

The diagnosis is based on clinical findings, history of preceding illness, and results of diagnostic tests. Laboratory studies, including complete blood count, electrolytes, blood gases, and blood cultures, are commonly obtained. A chest X-ray is obtained to evaluate heart size. In a child with hypovolemia the heart silhouette will be quite small and narrow. If the heart is larger than normal (cardiomegaly), the concern of cardiogenic shock must be ascertained. Echocardiograms can evaluate cardiac size and function.

TREATMENT

Early recognition and therapy can make the difference in the survival of the child with shock. Clients should be treated with supplemental oxygen via nasal cannula or oxygen mask. If the child's respiratory status has deteriorated to the point that he or she is unable to support him- or herself, endotracheal intubation and mechanical ventilation must be initiated.

Once the airway is established, management is directed toward volume replacement, particularly in hypovolemic and septic shock. Intravenous lines are placed in any number of locations in the infant and child. For rapid fluid resuscitation a large bore, short catheter is preferable to small scalp or extremity IV. If perfusion is very poor, a femoral or subclavian line may be required as peripheral veins may be difficult to visualize and palpate in the child with shock. In the severely ill child intraosseous (IO) access may be necessary to save the child's life. In this case a special needle is placed in the anterior surface of the tibia 1–3 cm below the tibial tuberosity (Figure 25-35). Other locations for placement of intraosseous needles include the distal femur, the medial malleolus, and the distal tibia (AHA, 2006). Fluid and medications may be administered through an IO line. Fluid replacement begins with a minimum of 20 cc/kg of crystalloid fluid such as lactated Ringer's or normal saline (AHA, 2006). Dextrose-containing fluids are *initially avoided* as a rapid increase in the glucose level may lead to an osmotic diuresis, further complicating the hypovolemic state. If the child is a trauma victim and blood loss is documented it must be replaced. This is usually in the form of whole blood or packed red blood cells. Normal saline or lactated Ringer's is given until blood is available. Until proper typing and cross matching can be performed O-negative blood (universal donor) should be given. Therapy for the hypovolemic client continues with ongoing and frequent reassessment of initial clinical signs. Fluid boluses are repeated if perfusion does not improve. It is not unusual for the child in hypovolemic shock to require up to 100 cc/kg of fluid to improve cardiac output and perfusion. The clinician must also be vigilant in assessing any ongoing losses (e.g., bleeding, vomiting, diarrhea, chest tube drainage) that have not been controlled.

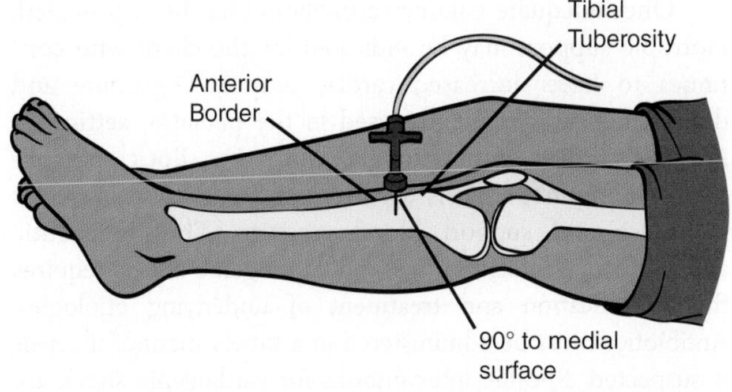

FIGURE 25-35 Placement of Intraosseous Needle. DELMAR CENGAGE LEARNING.

CRITICAL THINKING

The Three Types of Shock

Compare the pathophysiology and clinical manifestations of all three types of shock. Identify similarities for all three and identify appropriate interventions. Then identify specific interventions that are unique to each type of shock.

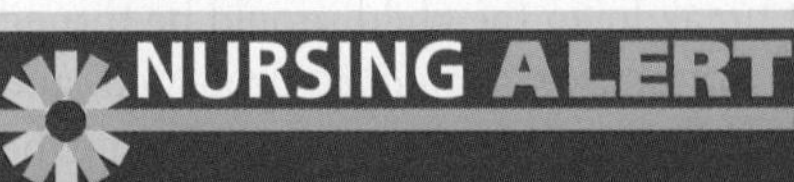

NURSING ALERT

Blood Pressure in Shock

A fall in blood pressure is a very late sign of shock. Do not be falsely reassured by a child who appears ill but has a normal BP.

NURSING ALERT

Volume Replacement in Shock

A frequent error in the management of shock in pediatric clients is insufficient volume replacement.

Once adequate volume resuscitation has been provided, inotropic support may be indicated for the client who continues to have decreased cardiac output. Dopamine and dobutamine are frequently used in the pediatric setting to improve cardiac output. In maldistributive shock epinephrine or norepinephrine is used to increase systemic vascular resistance and support blood pressure. The therapeutic approach for maldistributive and cardiogenic shock requires the identification and treatment of underlying etiologies. Antibiotics must be administered in a timely manner if sepsis is suspected. Specific interventions for cardiogenic shock are driven by the pathophysiology of the underlying etiology.

Anaphylaxis is a true life-threatening emergency and must be recognized immediately. Once an airway is secured, or if the child is adequately breathing spontaneously, treatment is aimed at increasing blood pressure by systemic vasoconstriction. The use of epinephrine either subcutaneously or intravenously is the treatment of choice. Airway management and hemodynamic support are the mainstays of treatment until airway swelling has subsided and the cardiovascular system has returned to normal.

Children with hypovolemic shock who are appropriately resuscitated have an excellent chance to return to their previous state of health. The child in sepsis-induced maldistributive shock unfortunately continues to have a high rate of morbidity and mortality. Research in this area continues. Ongoing research is investigating specific pathophysiological responses to sepsis to better delineate therapeutic intervention. Studies have also been done to look at specific indicators to predict survival in the pediatric population. Such parameters as heart rate, arterial blood pressure, serum lactate levels, and degree of acidosis have been studied as potential indicators. Outreach education is also important to teach emergency and clinic staffs the early signs of impending shock and the deleterious effects of failing to recognize these signs with adequate treatment. Survival for the child in cardiogenic shock will depend on accuracy of diagnosis, the underlying etiology, and the ability to provide surgical or medical support. Refer to the sections on acquired and congenital heart disease for specific outcomes for these conditions.

NURSING MANAGEMENT

Assessment

Ongoing and frequent assessment of the child in shock is essential. The nurses assess pulses, perfusion, CFT, color and temperature of skin, vital signs, urine output, level of consciousness, and respiratory effort. Frequent reassessment after intervention is critical to evaluate for therapeutic response.

Nursing Diagnosis

1. *Decreased cardiac output* related to decreased cardiac function or inadequate intravascular volume as evidenced by hypotension, tachycardia, poor urine output, lethargy, or poor perfusion.
2. *Ineffective peripheral tissue perfusion* related to vasodilation and coagulopathy as evidenced by altered neurologic status, decreased urine output, and metabolic acidosis.

Outcome Identification

- The child will show restoration of normal volume status, heart rate, urine output, blood pressure, and level of consciousness within 24–48 hours.
- The child suffering from sepsis-induced maldistributive shock will exhibit restoration of normal vascular tone.
- The child's blood cultures will be negative for sepsis.
- The child's coagulation studies will be normal without evidence of bleeding disorders.

Planning and Implementation

Vital signs, perfusion, and pulses are assessed on presentation and followed for changes. These parameters are also monitored to evaluate clinical response to therapeutic intervention. IV access is maintained for the administration of fluids and medications. Many of these children require continuous infusions of inotropes to maintain heart rate and blood pressure. The nurse should ensure accurate delivery of these medications and monitor for efficacy. The nurse should record accurate intake and output and any ongoing losses such as vomiting, diarrhea, or chest tube or surgical drain output.

Nurses should monitor for any changes in respiratory status that may indicate the child is becoming fatigued. Interventions such as oxygen administration and endotracheal intubation may be necessary to support respiratory function during the acute illness.

Neurologic status should be closely monitored as changes in level of orientation may indicate poor cerebral perfusion. Any child with decreased level of consciousness requires airway protection with either an artificial airway or endotracheal intubation. Airway suction is implemented if there is a poor cough, as this will facilitate clearance of secretions.

Many of these children (particularly those suffering from septic shock) will have positive blood cultures and coagulation disorders. Blood cultures are obtained for the identification of infectious organisms and should be obtained prior to the initiation of antibiotics. As determined by blood culture and sensitivities, appropriate antibiotics will be administered as ordered. If coagulopathy is present, interventions such as fresh frozen plasma, cryoprecipitate, and vitamin K are administered as ordered. Careful inspection of the skin to monitor for worsening petechia and skin breakdown is imperative. To prevent breakdown the child should be turned every two hours, heels and elbows should be protected, and mobility encouraged as soon as tolerated. Fever should be treated with antipyretics or tepid sponge baths.

Evaluation

The child will be hemodynamically stable with good respiratory function and appropriate level of consciousness. Ongoing losses will be accounted for and adequately replaced. Cardiac output and BP will be normal. There will be no evidence of bleeding from intravascular lines or orifices. All lab work will be normal. Fever will diminish to normal and white blood cell count will be normal.

FAMILY TEACHING

To prevent hypovolemic shock caregivers should be taught the signs of dehydration as well as potential causes. Infants are at high risk for dehydration and hypovolemic shock if diarrhea or vomiting becomes protracted. All caretakers should be taught good handwashing techniques and proper mixing of formulas. It is not uncommon for an infant to become severely dehydrated because not enough water was mixed with powdered formula. Caregivers should also be instructed on appropriate diets for infants and children with gastroenteritis.

For the child with anaphylactic shock the caregivers are educated to avoid the triggering antigen. Caregivers and the child (when old enough) should be instructed in the use of an EpiPen. These are precalculated doses of epinephrine that the child should have with her at all times in the case of accidental exposure to a known allergen. They are administered subcutaneously or intramuscularly in the event of exposure. Medical alert bracelets should also be worn by all of these clients.

It is every nurse's responsibility to be aware of medication and food allergies that a child may be exposed to while in the hospital setting. Nurses should always check the child's charts and ID bracelets prior to the administration of any medication. This is especially true in pediatrics where the individual is often too young to know his or her own allergies. For the child with a newly diagnosed heart disease, whether acquired or congenital, child and family education will center on the specific disease or defect. Interventions generally involve a combination of medications and nutritional support.

PSYCHOSOCIAL ISSUES FOR CHILDREN WITH HEART DISEASE

A number of issues become apparent when a child is born with, or develops, heart disease. At birth the parents must grapple with the fact that their newborn is not perfect. If the newborn is in distress it is quickly taken away from the parents in the delivery suite, interrupting the normal bonding that occurs in the immediate post partum period. If the child remains ill and on life support, the parents are not afforded the opportunity to hold or nourish their newborn. Parents frequently feel grief at their loss of an anticipated healthy infant. Inability to form an attachment to the infant and marital stress can result.

As the child grows, the family must deal with the dilemma of life adjustments. After the family adjusts to the initial shock of having something wrong with their infant, they must be able to incorporate the child into the family and society. Health care providers advise parents to treat their child "normally," as if there were no existing heart disease. Unfortunately, health care providers do not always offer tools to the family on how to do this. Some families are able to look past their child's condition, while others continue to impose unnecessary restrictions. As the child grows, physical limitations become more apparent, and the child may withdraw from peer interactions. Support groups can be helpful in this situation. Many congenital heart programs have an ongoing cardiac support group facilitated by social workers who can offer therapeutic strategies. Nurses working with these children must be able to listen, and apply reflective feedback and support for both the child and family. Creative solutions for such necessary treatments as oxygen, medication administration, and exercise restrictions can be implemented in concert with school nurses or community agencies. Cyanotic children, particularly adolescents, benefit from fashion consultants who can select colors for makeup and clothing that will minimize the appearance of cyanosis.

Caregivers of newly diagnosed children and adolescents with heart disease must decide to whom they disclose medical information. How information regarding heart disease is transmitted to family and friends is an early issue for caregivers. Extended family can pressure the family to not disclose information to the child. When the child enters school this issue reemerges. Should the family tell teachers about the child's condition? On the surface the answer would be yes, as a logical means to keep the school informed and treat emergencies. However, this frequently backfires because teachers and principals can form incorrect judgments about the child's capabilities. As teenagers are struggling to develop their own identity, peer acceptance is very important. Many teenagers prefer not to tell friends and peers of their condition. Some will avoid group activities, dances, dating, or swimming. Surgical scars or exercise intolerance can become a source of embarrassment.

As adolescents gain independence, they must be able to assume their own care. Many caregivers struggle with this issue and do not allow normal self-determination to develop. Therefore, the chronically ill adolescent may never achieve true mastery of life skills. Caregivers must be encouraged to allow their teenagers to care for themselves. Teenagers should become responsible for taking their own medicines, limiting their own activities, and paying attention to their bodies' cues. The primary historian during follow-up clinic visits must be the adolescent. Teenagers must never be excused to allow private discussion with the caregivers, as this will hinder the development of a trusting relationship.

Family lifestyles and activities change. Because of the extra attention received by the child with heart disease sibling rivalry and jealousy are common. Older siblings can feel displaced and resentful. These feelings can carry on throughout childhood and adolescence. Previously enjoyed athletic activities such as hiking, skiing, or camping are no longer pursued. Divorce is a possible consequence in some families.

Coping with uncertainty is difficult for caregivers and child (Arafa, Zaher, El-Dowaty, & Moneeb, 2008). There is always the uncertainty of another operation, worsening symptoms, or an untimely death. Support systems must be identified. Social workers, therapists, church leaders, community services, and support groups can all be accessed to provide support. Each family must be assessed individually to make the appropriate fit. Financial stresses are almost inevitable. Early referral to financial counselors can be made on a proactive basis to prevent financial catastrophes.

Family issues are multifaceted. Some families have the personal resources to effectively deal with the stresses and uncertainties of a child with heart disease. Others can decompensate over minor issues. Every child and family is assessed individually to determine suitable intervention. A multidisciplinary team is best suited to meet the needs of these families. Health care providers, nurses, social workers, and therapists work together to develop an individualized plan of care. Community and national organizations such as the American Heart Association can be tapped to provide ancillary support.

Physical activity is necessary for psychological as well as physical well-being. Today's society places much well-deserved significance on the positive effects of regular exercise. Technological and surgical advances have improved the physical status of children with heart disease. Consequently more and more of these children will be participating in both recreational and competitive athletics. However, families and health care providers continue to place restrictions on children with heart disease, regardless of the severity of disease.

Exercise can be divided into two types: static (isometric) or dynamic. Static exercise generates a large intramuscular tension with little muscular movement. High static activities include weight lifting, rock climbing, and gymnastics. This form of exercise primarily increases blood pressure and afterload. Dynamic exercise is aerobic in that muscle length and movement change rhythmically. Dynamic activities include running, soccer, basketball, and swimming. This form of exercise increases oxygen consumption, heart rate, and cardiac output. It also decreases systemic vascular resistance (afterload).

The child is evaluated on an individual basis as to which form of exercise is appropriate and safe. The potential risks as well as the benefits must be considered. Recreational activities versus competitive athletics must be evaluated separately for each patient. The nurse must remember that many forms of competitive athletics incorporate both static and dynamic levels of training (e.g., football employs weight training and running as part of training).

Most congenital defects are minor, therefore imposing no limitation on physical performance. Children with more complex defects will often limit their own level of activities, especially when they are young. However, many adolescents wish to participate with peers in a variety of physical activities. Simple defects such as repaired ASD, VSD, or PDA impose little or no limitation. Children with obstructive lesions such as severe AS or coarctation of the aorta should not participate in static exercise or those competitive sports requiring weight lifting for training. The increase in afterload imposed by this form of exercise in combination with their obstructive lesion will significantly impede cardiac output and increase ventricular work. Over the long run this will affect myocardial function (Maron et al., 2004).

Cyanotic children will have severe exercise limitations because of decreased cardiovascular function as well as pulmonary abnormalities. This is also true for children with single ventricle physiology following a Fontan procedure. These children should be allowed to participate in recreational activities to the best of their abilities, but competitive athletics are discouraged. Of note, altitude is generally not well tolerated by these children so caution must be used when planning activities in the mountains.

Children with cardiac arrhythmias are evaluated with an exercise test to ensure that abnormal heart rhythms are suppressed with exercise. If rhythm abnormalities persist or worsen with exercise, then the child is restricted from vigorous competitive sports. An inability to increase heart rate (chronotropic incompetence) with exercise will also impose physical limitations. Many times these children will benefit from a permanent pacemaker (Villian, 2008).

A small group of individuals is at high risk for sudden death with exercise so these children are restricted from physical education classes, competitive sports, and strenuous activities. These include hypertrophic cardiomyopathy, long QT syndrome, pulmonary hypertension, syncope with exercise, and exercise-induced ventricular tachycardia. Contact sports are prohibited for those on warfarin therapy and those with artificial conduits placed under the sternum. Nonstrenuous recreational activities with friends, family, community, or church groups are generally safe.

As longevity of children with heart disease improves, so must quality of life. Exercise is important to a sense of well-being. Unfortunately there are few objective data to make judgments about exercise in this population; most recommendations are based on collective experience. Nonetheless, physical activity should be encouraged to the best of the child's abilities. Emphasis should be on the enjoyable and fun aspects of regular exercise, and not on competitive rewards.

Congenital heart disease can affect normal growth and development in infants and children. The impact of early parental stress, multiple hospitalizations, cyanosis, child temperament, parent–child relationships, and health status all play a role in development. It is also well-known that children with chronic illnesses are at high risk for the development of behavioral problems.

Early maternal interaction and bonding are critical to the development of the infant. This includes the mother's ability to read her infant's cues and respond appropriately. Frequently postnatal growth is compromised by cardiac disease. Social interactions around feedings can be hampered by respiratory difficulties, infant fatigue, and poor stamina. These infants are frequently irritable and difficult to console. Mothers of infants with heart disease report high levels of stress, frustration, and inadequacy. If these difficulties become prolonged, then the infant will have low levels of engagement and will demonstrate more aversion behaviors (arching the back, lack of eye contact). If the mother is sensitive to these cues, she will allow the infant time to rest and regroup cognitive processes. Unfortunately, many mothers respond to these behaviors by over-stimulating their infant in an attempt to regain their attention. Unfortunately this will only serve to aggravate the infant further. Sensitive and responsive interaction must be developed. The nurse is in a crucial position to assist caregivers by giving them the tools they need to provide a solid foundation for infant attachment. Educating caregivers about common aversion behaviors is helpful. Continuous support will help strengthen maternal sensitivity to her infant's cues. This can be started early in the neonatal period with positive feedback and encouragement.

A number of physiological phenomena also unfavorably affect development. Poor nutritional intake and weight gain adversely affect brain growth and psychosocial development. Chronic cyanosis has been long recognized to adversely affect cognitive function and intelligence. Other neurologic complications of cyanosis include risk for stroke, cerebral abscess, and abnormal cerebral metabolism. Chronic illness with associated hospitalizations will slow achievement of developmental milestones, or in some cases, cause regression.

Other significant factors in developmental dysfunction in this population are the intraoperative events that can cause damage to the central nervous system. Cardiopulmonary bypass is associated with micro thrombi and inflammatory response that can affect the whole body, including the brain. Hypothermia is intended to decrease the metabolic rate of the body, therefore protecting it from adverse sequela of ischemia. The organ most sensitive to ischemic injury is the brain. If cooling occurs too slowly, there is an associated delay in subsequent developmental achievements.

As the child approaches preschool and school age, behavior problems may become apparent. A sense of well-being, physical health and activity, child-parent relationships, and family environment all contribute to a child's psychosocial development. Children with congenital heart disease also have adjustment problems, possibly caused by low self-esteem. Caregiver stress can contribute to family dysfunction and inadequate coping, but is not always related to the severity of illness. Frequently less severe illness is associated with high stress. This may be caused by perceived uncertainty of medical outcome and lack of control. If caregivers make extensive accommodations for perceived illness and overestimate severity, then the risk for future behavior problems is very high. All these issues can manifest as behavioral problems in the child or adolescent.

Developmental issues for the adolescent are compounded by peer pressures. Frequently these young people have struggled with motor and language delays, learning disabilities, insecurities, exercise intolerance, and social withdrawal. It is not uncommon for teenagers with heart disease to act out and test limits during this period. Experimentation with alcohol, drugs, and alternative lifestyles is not uncommon. Frequently peer support groups with other teens who have similar illnesses are very helpful during this time. Caregivers have more difficulty allowing their teen increasing freedom if there are concerns about chronic illness. They should be counseled to allow their teenager more autonomy and freedom, as long as health care interventions (medications) are not ignored. Teenagers should be expected to begin assuming their own health care.

Issues continue into adulthood. Professional achievement, job ability, and livelihood become significant issues for the young adult. Many adults with congenital heart disease can go on to be productive members of society. Others, because of physical limitations, may only be able to work part time or not at all. Job counseling, occupational therapy, and financial planning are beneficial and should be offered. Health insurance may be denied because of preexisting conditions. Ongoing medical expenses can be quite high so referral must be made to social service agencies when needed. Frank and open discussions about contraception and pregnancy should first occur during adolescence. Many women with heart disease can have children without complications; unfortunately for many others pregnancy can be life-threatening. This must be discussed prior to conception so the woman is well informed about potential complications and choices (Warnes et al., 2008).

Pediatric heart disease imposes physiological, psychological, and social concerns. Some can be quite small and insignificant, others seemingly insurmountable. As with other life problems, perceived severity of these concerns influences coping and outcomes. Nurses are in a pivotal position to assist families with all these issues. Continuity of care allows for timely problem identification, intervention, and follow-up.

IN THE REAL WORLD

As a student nurse, nothing can prepare you for when you see your first patient coming back from having a cardiac procedure. My first patient scared and overwhelmed me. The infant came to the pediatric intensive care unit following an intensive cardiac procedure. The infant had four chest tubes, numerous IV pumps, and an external pacemaker. This poor infant was so sick and had so many things happening to him at once. No matter how much theory we are taught as students the complexity of these patients is terrifying. The heart is not the only organ that potentially is affected and luckily I had a great nurse mentor me on what this child was going through. She sat and explained everything to me and the more she talked the less frightened I was. From this experience I decided I really enjoyed learning about cardiac patients and I look forward to taking care of them.

KEY CONCEPTS

- Normally, the three fetal shunts (ductus venosus, foramen ovale, and ductus arteriosus) close at birth or shortly thereafter. The cardiac output of an infant is normally 200 mL/kg/min. Cardiac output per minute decreases during childhood and by the age of 15 years; it is the same level as an adult, 100 mL/kg/min.
- Normal determinants of cardiac output are heart rate and stroke volume. The determinants of stroke volume are preload, afterload, and contractility.
- Assessment of the child with a cardiovascular alteration should include health history and a physical examination.
- The physical exam of a child with a cardiovascular alteration should include an inspection of facial features, edema, chest wall deformities, skin color, presence of finger clubbing, auscultation for murmurs, palpation for hepatomegaly, and blood pressure along with other routine exam procedures.
- Congestive heart failure can be caused by volume overload, pressure overload, or poor contractility. Many different cardiac lesions can produce CHF for one or more of these reasons.
- Clinical manifestations of CHF are numerous and can include gallop rhythm, diaphoresis, jugular venous distention, tachycardia, and poor weight gain.
- The primary treatments of CHF are diuretics, inotropes, and afterload reducing agents. Infants with structural heart defects responsible for CHF should have surgical repair.
- Nutritional support and maneuvers to decrease metabolic demands of CHF clients are important nursing interventions to promote growth and development.
- Congenital defects that produce L→R shunt result in excessive pulmonary blood flow (ASD, VSD, PDA, AV canal).
- Congenital defects with R→L shunt result in decreased pulmonary blood flow and are associated with cyanosis (tetralogy of Fallot, tricuspid atresia).
- Acquired rheumatic fever follows an untreated or partially treated group A streptococcal pharyngitis.
- Kawasaki disease is the number one reason for acquired heart disease in pediatrics in the United States.
- Children with structural heart defects require prophylaxis against endocarditis before surgical or dental procedures.
- Heart transplantation is not a cure; it is trading one chronic disease for another.
- There are three major classifications of shock: hypovolemic, maldistributive, and cardiogenic.
- If an abnormal heart rhythm is noted, check the client's blood pressure and perfusion to ensure stability. Document with an ECG.
- Psychosocial issues surrounding children with heart disease and their families include grief and loss, dilemma of normality, and marital and family stress.

REVIEW ACTIVITIES

1. What are the determinants of cardiac output? Define preload, afterload, and contractility.
2. Draw a diagram of fetal circulation and identify those structures that close after birth.
3. What diagnostic tests would be ordered in a child you suspect of having congenital heart disease?
4. What are the clinical manifestations of congestive heart failure? What are the corresponding treatments?
5. Draw the blood flow for a VSD.
6. Draw the blood flow for transposition of the great arteries.
7. Why is it necessary to keep the ductus arteriosus open in children with severely decreased pulmonary blood flow? How is it kept open?
8. Write a nursing care plan for an infant with coarctation of the aorta.
9. What are the criteria for the diagnosis of rheumatic fever?
10. Describe the treatment for Kawasaki disease; include nursing interventions.
11. What are the three types of shock? Compare physiology and treatment of the three types of shock.
12. What are some of the psychosocial concerns for the family with a child who has heart disease?

STUDY QUESTIONS

1. A 6-month-old female presents to the ED after 24 hours of vomiting and diarrhea. Her HR is 180, she is cool and mottled and barely cries when she is examined. Based on her history, a diagnosis of hypovolemic shock is suspected. Which of the following fluids should be given to her for *initial* resuscitation?
   a. Whole blood
   b. 5% dextrose solution and water (D5W)
   c. Normal saline solution
   d. 5% albumin
2. Which of the following congenital defects puts an infant at risk for developing congestive heart failure while awaiting surgical repair?
   a. Atrioventricular canal defect
   b. Tetralogy of Fallot
   c. Pulmonary valve stenosis
   d. Atrial septal defect
3. Which of the following clinical signs should NOT necessarily be considered reassuring in a patient admitted with hypovolemic shock?
   a. Warm extremities
   b. Normal urine output
   c. Normal blood pressure
   d. Awake and alert infant
4. Adenosine is an antiarrhythmic agent used to treat which of the following arrhythmias?
   a. Bradycardia
   b. Normal sinus rhythm
   c. Supraventricular tachycardia
   d. Complete heart block
5. Which of the following congenital defects requires that the ductus arteriosus remains open for pulmonary blood flow so that the infant can survive until surgical intervention?
   a. AVCD
   b. Tricuspid atresia with no VSD
   c. Ventricular septal defect
   d. Atrial septal defect
6. Which clinical findings are often associated with a hypercyanotic spell (Tet spell) in an infant with tetralogy of Fallot?
   a. Tachycardia, normal oxygen saturations
   b. Severe cyanosis, pallor, tachypnea
   c. Normal respirations with cyanosis
   d. Apnea and tachycardia
7. The best treatment for hypertension in the obese child with no underlying heart or renal disease is:
   a. ACE inhibitors
   b. Weight loss
   c. Fluid restriction
   d. Digoxin
8. You are caring for a 4-month-old infant who has a large ventricular septal defect and a known left-to-right shunt. Which of the following clinical pictures best fits the description of an infant with a left-to-right shunt?
   a. Small heart on chest x-ray, adequate weight gain, good feeder
   b. Cardiomegaly on chest x-ray, diastolic murmur, good feeder
   c. Bradycardia, no murmur, good stamina
   d. Cardiomegaly, poor weight gain, poor feeder
9. Pacemakers are indicated for:
   a. Complete heart block
   b. SVT
   c. Ventricular fibrillation
   d. Normal sinus rhythm
10. Acute rheumatic fever primarily affects which two heart valves?
   a. Mitral and tricuspid
   b. Pulmonary and aortic
   c. Mitral and aortic
   d. Tricuspid and pulmonary

REFERENCES

Almond, C., Thiagarajan, R., Piercey, G., Gauvreau, K., Blume, E., Bastardi, H., Flynn-Thompson, F., & Singh T. (2009). Waiting list mortality among children listed for heart transplantation in the United States. *Circulation, 119*, 717–727.

Akinturk, A., Michel-Benke, I., Valeske, K., Mueller, M., Thul, J., Bauer, J., Hagel, K., & Schranz, D., (2007). Hybrid transcathete—Surgical palliation basis for univentricular or biventricular repair: The Giessen Experience. *Pediatric Cardiology, 28*, 79–87.

American Academy of Pediatrics, Committee on Infectious Diseases. (2006). *2006 Red Book: Report of the Committee on Infectious Diseases* (26th ed.). Elk Grove, IL: Author.

American Heart Association. (2006). *Pediatric advanced life support manual*. Dallas, TX: Author.

American Heart Association. (2007). Congenital cardiovascular defects: statistics. Retrieved July 28, 2010, from http://www.americanheart.org/presenter.jhtml?identifier=4576.

Arafa, M. A., Zaher, S. R., El-Dowaty, A. A., & Moneeb, D. E. (2008). Quality of life among parents of children with heart disease. *Health and Quality of Life Outcomes, 6*, 91–97.

Backer, C., & Mavroudis, C. (2003). Atrial septal defect, partial anomalous pulmonary venous connection and scimitar syndrome. In C. Mavroudis & C. Backer (Eds.). *Pediatric cardiac surgery*. Philadelphia: Mosby.

Baker, A. L., & Newburger, J. W. (2008). Kawasaki disease. *Circulation, 118*, e110–e112.

Berul, C. I., Van Hare, G. F., Kertesz, N. J., Dubin, A. M., Cecchin, F., Collins, K. K., Cannon, B. C., Alexander, M. E., Triedman, J. K., Walsh, E. P., & Friedman, R. A. (2008). Results of a multicenter retrospective implantable cardioverter-defibrillator registry of pediatric and congenital heart disease patients. *Journal of the American College of Cardiology, 51*, 1685–1691.

Boucek, R. J. Jr., & Chrisant, M. R. (2004). Cardiac transplantation for hypoplastic left heart syndrome. *Cardiology in the Young, 14* (Supp. 1), 83–87.

Burns, J. C., Taubert K., Rowley, A. H., Newburger J. W., Gewitz M., Takahashi M., & McCrindle, B. W. (2005) Summary of the 8th International Kawasaki Disease Symposium: Presentation of Selected Abstracts. Retrieved July 28, 2010, from http://www.americanheart.org/presenter.jhtml?identifier=3043252.

Dionigi, B., Razzouk, A. J., Hasaniya, N. W., Chinnock, R. E., & Bailey, L. L. (2008). Late outcomes of pediatric heart transplantation are independent of pre-transplant diagnosis and prior cardiac surgical intervention. *Journal of Heart and Lung Transplantation, 27*(10), 1090–1095.

Freed, M. D. (2006). Fetal and transitional circulation. In J. F., Keane, J. E. Lock, & D. C. Fyler (Eds.). *Nada's pediatric cardiology*, Philadelphia: Saunders Elsevier.

Gandhi, S., Huddleston, C., Balzer, D., Epstein, D., Boschert, T., & Canter, C. (2008). Biventricular assist devices as a bridge to heart transplantation in small children. *Circulation, 118*, S89–S93.

Geggel, R. L., & Fyler, D. C. (2006). History, growth, nutrition, physical examination and routine laboratory tests. In J. F., Keane, J. E. Lock, & D. C. Fyler (Eds.). *Nada's pediatric cardiology*, Philadelphia: Saunders Elsevier.

Gerber, M., Baltimore, R., Eaton, C., Gewitz, M., Rowley, A., Shulman, S. & Taubert, K. (2009). Prevention of rheumatic fever and diagnosis and treatment of acute streptococcal pharyngitis: A scientific statement from the American Heart Association Rheumatic Fever, Endocarditis, and Kawasaki Disease Committee of the Council on Cardiovascular Disease in the Young, the Interdisciplinary Council on Functional Genomics and Translational Biology, and the Interdisciplinary Council on Quality of Care and Outcomes Research: Endorsed by the American Academy of Pediatrics. *Circulation, 119*. 1541–1551.

Gilljam, T., Jaeggi, E., & Gow, R. M. (2008). Neonatal supraventricular tachycardia: Outcomes over a 27-year period at a single institution. *ACTA Paediatrica, 97*, 1035–1039.

Hillman, N., Mavroudis, C., & Backer, C. (2003). Patent ductus arteriosus. In C. Mavroudis & C. Backer (Eds.). *Pediatric cardiac surgery*. Philadelphia: Mosby.

Hirsch, J. C., & Bove, E. (2003). Tetralogy of Fallot. In C. Mavroudis and C. Backer (Eds.). *Pediatric cardiac surgery*. Philadelphia: Mosby.

Jenkins, K. J., Correa, A., Feinstein, J. A., Botto, L., Britt, A. E., Daniels, S. R., Elixson, M., Warnes, C. A., & Well, C. L. (2007). Noninherited risk factors and congenital cardiovascular defects: Current knowledge: A scientific statement from the American Heart Association Council on Cardiovascular Disease in the Young: Endorsed by the American Academy of Pediatrics. *Circulation, 115*, 2995–3014.

Jonas, R. (2004a). Specific advantages of primary repair for the patient. In R. Jonas (Ed.). *Comprehensive surgical management of congenital heart disease*. New York: Oxford University Press.

Jonas, R. (2004b). Complete atrioventricular canal defect. In R. Jonas (Ed.), *Comprehensive surgical management of congenital heart disease*. New York: Oxford University Press.

Jonas, R. (2004c). Patent ductus arteriosus, aortopulmonary window, sinus of valsalva fistula, aortoventricular tunnel. In R. Jonas (Ed.). *Comprehensive surgical management of congenital heart disease*. New York: Oxford University Press.

Jonas, R. (2004d). Truncus arteriosus. In R. Jonas (Ed.). *Comprehensive surgical management of congenital heart disease*. New York: Oxford University Press.

Jonas, R. (2004e). Ventricular septal defect. In R. Jonas (Ed.). *Comprehensive surgical management of congenital heart disease*. New York: Oxford University Press.

Karl, T. R., & Kirshbom P. (2006). Transposition of the great arteries and the arterial switch procedure. In D. Nichols (Ed.), *Critical heart disease in infants and children*. Philadelphia: Mosby.

Lanna, C. C. D., Tonelli, E., Barros, M. V. L., Goulart, E. M. A., & Mota, C. C. C. (2003). Subclinical rheumatic valvitis: A long-term follow-up. *Cardiology in the Young, 13*, 431–438.

Lemaire S. A., Green, S. Y., Sharma, K., Cheung, C. K., Sameri, A., Tsai, P. I., Adams, G., & Coselli, J. S. (2009). Aortic root replacement with stentless porcine xenografts: Early and late outcomes in 132 patients. *Annals of Thoracic Surgery, 87*, 503–513.

Maron, B. J., Chaitman, B. R., Ackerman, M. J., de Luna, A. B., Corrado, D., Crosson, J. E., Deal, B. J., Driscoll, D. J., Estes, N. A. M., Araujo, C. G. S., Liang, D. H., Mitten, M. J., Myergurg, R. J., Pelliccia, A., Thompson, P. D., Towbin, J. A., & VanCamp, S. P. (2004). Recommendations for physical activity and recreational sports participation for young patients with genetic cardiovascular diseases. *Circulation, 109*, 2807–2816.

Marshall, J., Berkenbosch, J. W., Russo, P., & Tobias, J. D. (2004). Preliminary experience with nesiritide in the pediatric population. *Journal of Intensive Care Medicine, 19*(3), 164–170.

Massin, M. M., Benatar, A., & Rondia, G. (2008). Epidemiology and outcome of tachyarrhythmias in tertiary pediatric cardiac centers. *Cardiology, 111*, 191–196.

Mavroudis, C., Backer, C., & Jacobs, J. (2003). Ventricular septal defect. In C. Mavroudis & C. Backer (Eds.). *Pediatric cardiac surgery*. Philadelphia: Mosby.

Minich, L. L., Sleeper, L. Y., Atz, A. M., McCrindle, B. W., Lu, M., Colan, S. D., Printz, B. F., Klein, G. L., Sundel, R. P., Takahasi, M., Li, J. S., Vetter, V. L., & Newburger, J. W. (2007). Delayed diagnosis of Kawasaki Disease: What are the risk factors? *Pediatrics, 120*, e1434–e1440.

Mitchell, M., & Clarke, D. (2003). Isolated right ventricular outflow tract obstruction. In C. Mavroudis & C. Backer (Eds.). *Pediatric cardiac surgery*. Philadelphia: Mosby.

Miyake, C. Y., Gauvreau, K., Tani, L. Y., Sundel, R. P., & Newburger, J. W. (2007). Characteristics of children discharged from hospitals in the United States in 2000 with the diagnosis of acute rheumatic fever. *Pediatrics, 120*, 503–508.

Miyake, T., Shinohara, T., Nakamura, Y., Fukuda, T., Tasato, H., Toyohara, K., & Tanihara, Y. (2004). Spontaneous closure of ventricular septal defects followed up from 3 months of age. *Pediatrics International, 46*(2), 135–140.

Obarzanek, E., Kimm, S., Barton, B., Van Horn, L., Kwiterovich, P., & Simons-Morton, D., et al. (2001). Long-term safety and efficacy of a cholesterol-lowering diet in children with elevated low-density lipoprotein cholesterol: Seven-year results of the dietary intervention study in children (DISC). *Pediatrics, 107*(2), 256–264.

Ohlsson, A., Walia, R., & Shah, S. (2008). Ibuprofen for the treatment of patent ductus arteriosus in preterm and/or low birth weight infants. *Cochrane Database Systemic Review (1)*: CD003481.

Penny, D. J., & Mynard, J. P. (2006). The pressure-volume relationship in heart failure. In A. C. Chang & J. A. Towbin, (Eds.), *Heart failure in children and young adults.* Philadelphia: Saunders Elsevier.

Pierpont, M. E., Basson, C. T., Benson, W., Gelb, B. D., Giglia, T. M., Goldmuntz, E., McGee, G., Sable, C. A., Srivastava, D., & Webb, C. (2007). Genetic basis for congenital heart defects: Current knowledge: A scientific statement for the American Heart Association Congenital Cardiac Defects Committee, Council on Cardiovascular Disease in the Young: Endorsed by the American Academy of Pediatrics. *Circulation, 115,* 3015–3038.

Rogness, C. (2008). Can't stop dancing: Could it be St. Vitus dance? *Journal of the American Academy of Nurse Practitioners, 20,* 353–358.

Roos-Hesselink, J. W., & Karamermer, Y. (2008). Significance of postoperative arrhythmias in congenital heart disease. *PACE, 31,* S2–S6.

Schwalbe-Terilli, C. R., Hartman, D. H., Nagle, M. L., Gallagher, P. R., Ittenbach, R. F., Burnham, N. B., Gaynor, J. W., & Ravishankar, C. (2009). Enteral feeding and caloric intake in neonates after cardiac surgery. *American Journal of Critical Care, 18,* 52–57.

Setty, S., Shaun, P., & Shen, I. (2006). Atrioventricular septal defects. In D. Nichols (Ed.). *Critical heart disease in infants and children.* Philadelphia: Mosby.

Shaddy, R. E. (2006). β-adrenergic receptor blockade. In A. C. Chang & J. A. Towbin (Eds.). *Heart failure in children and young adults.* Philadelphia: Saunders Elsevier.

Stayer, S. A. (2006). Use of vasodilators in heart failure. In A. C. Chang, & J. A. Towbin (Eds.), *Heart failure in children and young adults.* Philadelphia: Saunders Elsevier.

St. Louis, J. D. (2006). Persistent truncus arteriosus. In D. Nichols (Ed.), *Critical heart disease in infants and children.* Mosby, Philadelphia.

Taketomo, C., Hodding, J., & Kraus, D. (2008). *Pediatric dosage handbook.* Hudson, OH: Lexi Company, Inc.

Tani, L. Y., Veasy, G., Minich, L. L., & Shaddy, R. E. (2003). Rheumatic fever in children younger than 5 years: Is the presentation different? *Pediatrics, 112,* 1065–1068.

Urbina, E., Alpert, B., Flynn, J., Hayman, L., Harshfield, G. A., Jacobson, M., Mahoney, L., McCrindle, B., Mietus-Snyder, M., Steinberger, J., & Daniels, S. (2008). Ambulatory blood pressure monitoring in children and adolescents: Recommendations for standard assessment: A scientific statement from the American Heart Association Atherosclerosis, Hypertension, and Obesity in Youth Committee of the Council of Cardiovascular Disease in the Young and the Council for High Blood Pressure Research. *Hypertension, 52,* 433–451.

VanPraagh, R. (2006). Embryology. In J. F. Keane, J. E. Lock, & D. C. Fyler (Eds.). *Nada's pediatric cardiology,* Philadelphia: Saunders Elsevier.

Villian, E. (2008). Indications for pacing in patients with congenital heart disease. *PACE, 31,* S17–S20.

Vos, P., Pulles-Heintzberger, C. F., & Delhaas, T. (2003). Supraventricular tachycardia: An incidental diagnosis in infants difficult to prove in children. *Acta Paediatrica, 92*(9), 1058–1061.

Walsh, E. P. (2008). Practical aspects of implantable defibrillator therapy in patients with congenital heart disease. *PACE, 31,* S38–S40.

Warnes, C. A., Williams, R. G., Bashore, T. M., Child, J. S., Connolly, H. M., Dearani, J. A., del Nido, P., Fasules, J. W., Graham, T. P., Hijazi, Z. M., Hunt, S. A., King, M. E., Landzberg, M. J., Miner, P. D., Radford, M. J., Walsh, E., & Webb, G. D. (2008). ACC/AHA 2008 Guidelines for the management of adults with congenital heart disease: A report for the American College of Cardiology/American Heart Association task force on practice guidelines. *Circulation, 118,* e714–e833.

Wilde, A. M. (2008). Channelopathies in children and adults. *PACE, 31,* S41–S45.

Wilson, W., Taubert, K. A., Gewitz, M., Lockhart, P. B., Baddour, L. M., Levison, M., Bolger, A., Cabell, C. H., Takahashi, M., Baltimore, R. S., Newburger, J. W., Strom, B. L., Tani, L. Y., Gerber, M., Bonow, R. O., Pallasch, T., Shulman, S. T., Rowley, A. H., Burns, J. C., Ferrieri, P., Gardner, T., Goff, D., & Durack, D. T. (2007). Prevention of infective endocarditis. Guidelines from the American Heart Association. *Circulation.* http://circ.ahajournals.org/cgi/content/full/116/15/1736.

SUGGESTED READINGS

Ascuitto, R., Ross-Ascuitto, N., Wiesman, J., & DeLeon, S. (2007). Bidirectional Glenn Shunt as an adjunct to surgical repair of congenital heart disease associated with pulmonary outflow obstruction: Relevance of the fluid pressure drop-flow relationship. *Pediatric Cardiology, 29,* 910–917.

Baranchuk, A., Shaw, C., Alanazi, H., Campbell, D., Bally, K., Redfearn, D. P., Simpson, C. S., & Abdollah, H. (2009) Electrocardiography pitfalls and artifacts: The 10 commandments. *Critical Care Nurse, 29,* 67–73.

Gerber, M. S. (2008). *My heart vs. the real world: Children with heart disease, in photographs & interviews.* Cold Spring Harbor, NY: Cold Spring Harbor Laboratories Press.

Karpawich, P. (2008). Technical aspects of pacing in adult and pediatric congenital heart disease. *PACE, 31,* S28–S31.

Keane, J. F., Lock, J. E., & Fyler, D. C. (Eds.). (2006). *Nada's pediatric cardiology,* Philadelphia: Saunders Elsevier.

Saul, J. P. (2008). Role of catheter ablation in postoperative arrhythmias. *PACE 31,* S7–S12.

RESOURCES

Refer to the online student StudyWARE for Potts & Mandleco at http://www.CengageBrain.com for additional content and study aids.

Organization: **American Association of Critical Care Nurses**
Description: The American Association of Critical Care Nurses (AACN) is the largest specialty nursing organization in the world, representing the interests of more than 500,000 nurses who are charged with the responsibility of caring for acutely and critically ill patients. The association is dedicated to providing our members with the knowledge and resources necessary to provide optimal care to critically ill patients. The website offers users information regarding certification, membership and guidelines for clinical practice.
Website/Resource: http://www.aacn.org

Organization: **American Heart Association National Center**
Description: The American Heart Association is a national voluntary health agency whose mission is: "Building healthier lives, free of cardiovascular diseases and stroke." The association's impact goal is to reduce coronary heart disease, stroke and risk by 25 percent by 2010. The website offers users a wealth of information regarding heart attack/stroke warning signs and healthy lifestyle standards.
Website/Resource: http://www.americanheart.org

Organization: **California Heart Connection**
Description: California Heart Connection (CHD) resources is committed to helping those with congenital heart defects reach their potential by providing important resources and questions to ask physicians. CHD created a set of FREE materials for physicians to distribute to patients. All materials can be customized to include physician contact information and personalized for each patient.
Website/Resource: http://www.CHDResources.org

Organization: **Children's Heart Institute**
Description: The Children's Heart Institute's website helps parents understand in plain language the heart problems of their child. The website accomplishes this by providing information about cardiac testing, medications, and general patient education.
Website/Resource: http://www.childrenheartinstitute.org

Organization: **Congenital Heart Information Network**
Description: Congenital Heart Information Network (CHIN) is a national organization that provides reliable information, support services, financial assistance, and resources to families of children with congenital heart defects and acquired heart disease, adults with congenital heart defects, and the professionals who work with them. CHIN's website offers users countless links to helpful resources and community information.
Website/Resource: http://www.tchin.org

Organization: **Congenital Heart Surgeons' Society**
Description: Congenital Heart Surgeons' Society (CHSS) is a not-for-profit charitable corporation. The CHSS' purpose is to associate persons interested in, and carry on activities related to, the science and practice of congenital heart surgery and sponsor clinical studies. CHSS's website offers users access to information regarding funding, annual meetings, and membership.
Website/Resource: http://www.chss.org

Organization: **Heart Rhythm Society**
Description: The Heart Rhythm Society is the international leader in science, education and advocacy for cardiac arrhythmia professionals and patients, and the primary information resource on heart rhythm disorders. Its mission is to improve the care of patients by promoting research, education and optimal health care policies and standards. The website offers users access to information regarding professional education, health policy, and specialist referrals.
Website/Resource: http://www.hrsonline.org

Organization: **Little Heart, Inc.**
Description: **Little Hearts, Inc.** is a national organization providing support, education, resources, networking, and hope to families affected by congenital heart defects. Membership consists of families nationwide who have or are expecting a child with a congenital heart defect. The website offers information about donors, programs, and services.
Website/Resource: http://www.littlehearts.org

Organization: **National Down Syndrome Congress**
Description: It is the purpose of the National Down Syndrome Congress to create a national climate in which all people will recognize and embrace the value and dignity of people with Down syndrome. The website offers users access to affiliates, self-advocates, and informational resources.
Website/Resource: http://www.ndsccenter.org

Organization: **NIH/National Heart Lung and Blood Institute Information Center**
Description: The National Heart Lung and Blood Institute (NHLBI) provides global leadership for a research, training, and education program to promote the prevention and treatment of heart, lung, and blood diseases and enhance the health of all individuals so that they can live longer and more fulfilling lives. The website provides information regarding networks, research, clinical trials, careers/training, and education campaigns.
Website/Resource: http://www.nhlbi.nih.gov

Patient Education Materials

Organization: **American Heart Association National Center**
Description: The American Heart Association is a national voluntary health agency whose mission is: "Building healthier lives, free of cardiovascular diseases and stroke." The association's impact goal is to reduce coronary heart disease, stroke, and risk by 25 percent by 2010. The website offers users a wealth of information regarding heart attack/stroke warning signs and healthy lifestyle standards.
Website/Resource: http://www.americanheart.org

Organization: **California Heart Connection**
Description: California Heart Connection (CHD) resources is committed to helping those with congenital heart defects reach their potential by providing important resources and questions to ask physicians. CHD created a set of FREE materials for physicians to distribute to patients. All materials can be customized to include physician contact information and personalized for each patient.
Website/Resource: http://www.CHDResources.org

Organization: **Children's Heart Institute**
Description: The Children's Heart Institute's website helps parents understand in plain language the heart problems of their child. The website accomplishes this by providing information about cardiac testing, medications, and general patient education.
Website/Resource: http://www.childrenheartinstitute.org

Organization: **Sudden Arrhythmia Death Syndromes Foundation**
Description: The mission of the Sudden Arrhythmia Death Syndromes (SADS) Foundation is to save the lives and support the

families of children and young adults who are genetically predisposed to sudden death due to heart rhythm abnormalities. The website provides users with information regarding living with SADS, medical profession education, and awareness.
Website/Resource: http://www.sads.org

Organization: **United Network for Organ Sharing**
Description: The United Network for Organ Sharing (UNOS) is a non-profit, scientific and educational organization that administers the nation's only Organ Procurement and Transplantation Network (OPTN), established by the U.S. Congress in 1984. Through the OPTN, the UNOS collects and manages data about every transplant event occurring in the United States, facilitates the organ matching and placement process using UNOS-developed data technology and the UNOS Organ Center, and brings together medical professionals, transplant recipients, and donor families to develop organ transplantation policy. The UNOS website offers information regarding organ transplant recipients, donors, and patients still on the waiting list.
Website/Resource: http://www.unos.org

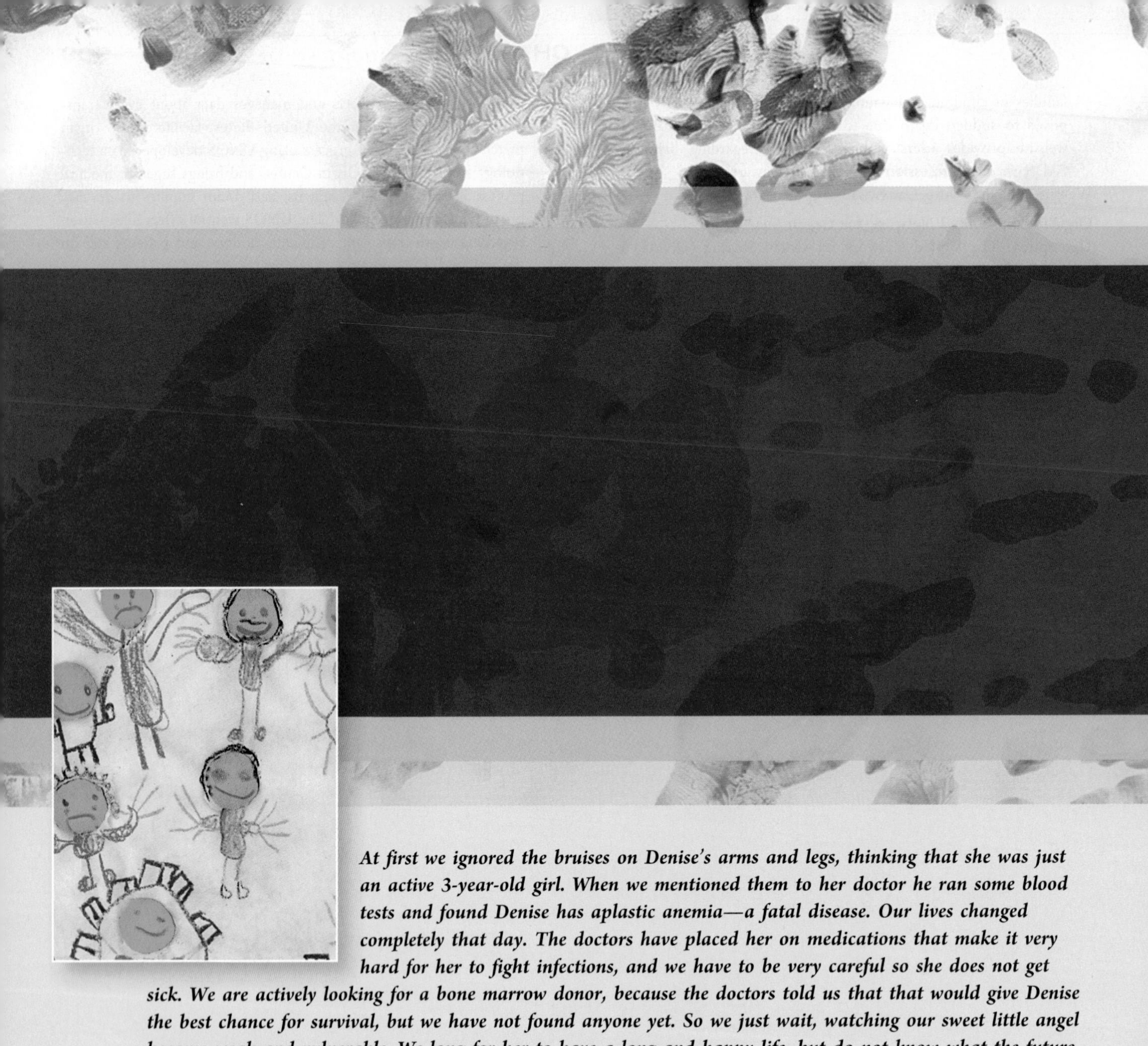

At first we ignored the bruises on Denise's arms and legs, thinking that she was just an active 3-year-old girl. When we mentioned them to her doctor he ran some blood tests and found Denise has aplastic anemia—a fatal disease. Our lives changed completely that day. The doctors have placed her on medications that make it very hard for her to fight infections, and we have to be very careful so she does not get sick. We are actively looking for a bone marrow donor, because the doctors told us that that would give Denise the best chance for survival, but we have not found anyone yet. So we just wait, watching our sweet little angel become weak and vulnerable. We long for her to have a long and happy life, but do not know what the future holds.

CHAPTER 26

Hematological Alterations

KAREN M. LUNDBERG, RN, MS, CNE
CHRISTINA LINTON, FNP, PhD

COMPETENCIES

Upon completion of this chapter, the reader will be able to:

- Discuss the anatomy and physiology of the hematological system.
- Identify differences between child and adult hematological systems.
- Explain and identify different types of anemia and discuss the etiology, treatment, and nursing care for these types.
- Identify several types of coagulation disorders and discuss the etiology, treatment, and nursing care for these disorders.
- Successfully complete the games and activities in the online student StudyWARE.

In a healthy child, the hematological system enables the body to transport oxygen, fight infection, and minimize hemorrhage. These functions, which are essential for survival, are a direct result of the functions of the cellular components of the blood. Alterations involving these cellular components can cause illnesses such as iron-deficiency anemia, sickle cell anemia, beta-thalassemia major, aplastic anemia, hemophilia, von Willebrand's disease, immune thrombocytopenic purpura, and disseminated intravascular coagulation. The etiology of each alteration is discussed in this chapter, along with the treatment and nursing care for children with these disorders.

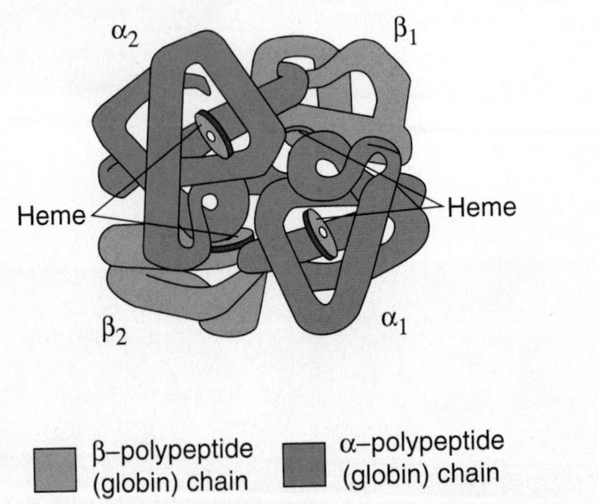

FIGURE 26-1 The Structure of Normal Hemoglobin. DELMAR CENGAGE LEARNING.

ANATOMY AND PHYSIOLOGY

Human blood has two major components: the plasma, which consists primarily of water with a small percentage of solutes, and the formed elements, which consist of cells and proteins. The **cellular elements** of the blood are the erythrocytes or red blood cells, the leukocytes or white blood cells, and the thrombocytes or platelets. During fetal development blood cells are produced in the liver and the spleen. After birth, new blood cells are synthesized from stem cells in the bone marrow through the processes of hematopoiesis. Red blood cell volume varies with age. A unique circumstance exists in newborns immediately following birth. At this time there is a period of inactive erythropoiesis during which the iron obtained from catabolized red blood cells is stored as hemosiderin in the bone marrow and the liver tissue. These stores are greatest at 4 to 8 weeks of age and function to protect the infant from anemia because the stores can be used in lieu of dietary iron intake. Premature infants use up these stores within 6 to 12 weeks, whereas the iron stores of full-term infants last up to 20 weeks. Each component of the blood has a specific purpose and together enables the blood to carry out the following functions: (1) transporting substances needed for cellular metabolism in the tissues; (2) regulating acid-base balance; and (3) protecting against infection and injury (Rote & McCance, 2010a).

RED BLOOD CELLS

The primary function of **red blood cells** (RBCs) is to supply the tissues of the body with oxygen, made possible by the shape, size, and structure of these cells. They are the most abundant cells in the blood, although the number of RBCs varies with age (see Appendix E for normal RBC values in children). The RBCs remain in circulation for approximately 120 days and are removed from circulation, mainly by the spleen. Because RBCs are not capable of replication, the bone marrow releases new, immature erythrocytes called reticulocytes to replace the RBCs removed from circulation. The characteristic biconcave shape of RBCs allows for a maximal amount of surface area while maintaining a small volume. This feature, in addition to their small size and ability to squeeze through small spaces, allows them to reach all the tissue sites in the body (Rote & McCance, 2010a).

The ability of the RBCs to supply oxygen to the tissues is further facilitated by the oxygen-carrying protein **hemoglobin** (Hb), the most abundant protein within a RBC, numbering nearly 300 molecules per cell. There are several types of Hb, the two most common being adult hemoglobin (Hb A) and fetal hemoglobin (Hb F). Hb F is the primary Hb found in newborns. This form of Hb is gradually replaced with Hb A as the child ages. Normal Hb molecules are made up of four globin components, composed of polypeptide chains, and four heme sections, composed of iron and a substance called protoporphyrin (Figure 26-1). With its unique structure, hemoglobin enables RBCs to transport 100 times more oxygen than could be transported dissolved in plasma alone (Rote & McCance, 2010a).

WHITE BLOOD CELLS

The primary function of **white blood cells** (WBCs) is to defend against invading microorganisms and remove debris. These functions are carried out primarily in the injured tissues themselves, but the circulatory system provides a method of transportation that delivers the WBCs to the site of the injury. When invasion by a foreign organism or substance occurs, the body first responds with the inflammatory response, followed by the immune response. The inflammatory response is rapid and nonspecific, whereas the immune response is slower and requires previous sensitization to the foreign organism or substance. This prior sensitization allows the body to recognize and remember the foreign organism, resulting in a more specific response. Members of a subcategory of WBCs called the lymphocytes are responsible for the immune response, whereas the inflammatory response involves other WBCs, namely, the monocytes, macrophages, neutrophils, eosinophils, and basophils. Table 26-1 outlines the functions of these cells in

TABLE 26-1 Functions of the White Blood Cells

LEUKOCYTE	FUNCTION	OTHER IMPORTANT CHARACTERISTICS
Lymphocytes	Immune response	• Majority are located in lymphoid tissue • B cells are responsible for humoral immunity • T cells are responsible for cell-mediated immunity
Monocytes and macrophages	Phagocytosis	• Monocytes are immature macrophages in the bloodstream • Macrophages reside in lymphoid tissue • Both make up the mononuclear phagocyte system (along with cells in the marrow), which destroys unwanted materials in the blood and organs
Eosinophils	Phagocytosis	• Prevalent in parasitic infections and allergic reactions • Associated with Hodgkin's disease • Involved in the recovery phase of infection
Neutrophils	Phagocytosis	• Prevalent in early phases of inflammation • Also called polymorphonuclear neutrophils (PMNs) • Immature cells are called bands or stabs • Mature cells are called segmented neutrophils
	Unknown	• Associated with allergic reactions and mechanical irritation

Adapted from Rote, N. R., & McCance, K. L. (2010a). Structure and function of the hematologic system. In K. L. McCance & S. E. Huether (eds.), *Pathophysiology: The biologic basis for disease in adults and children* (6th ed.). St. Louis, MO: Mosby, pp. 952–988.

more detail (Rote & McCance, 2010a). The proportions of each WBC type within the blood vary with age, as does the total number of WBCs (see Appendix E for normal WBC values in children). The complete blood count (CBC) with differential is the primary method of assessing WBC prevalence and function, and therefore is helpful in determining the presence of infection.

PLATELETS

The **platelets** are disk-shaped cytoplasmic fragments and are not considered cells. As such, they do not have a nucleus or DNA strands and cannot reproduce. Instead, they live for approximately 10 days and are then removed from circulation, primarily by the spleen. Their primary function is to facilitate blood coagulation in order to control bleeding. This is accomplished when platelets adhere to the injured vessel wall, release biochemical mediators, and form platelet plugs, which soon turn into clots (Rote & McCance, 2010a).

ANEMIA

Anemia is not a disease, but rather a term used to describe a decrease in the oxygen-carrying capacity of the blood caused by underlying disease or injury. Anemia is the most common blood disorder in children (Kline, 2010). In a study monitoring the nutritional status of low-income children in federally funded maternal and child health programs, the prevalence of anemia in the United States was over 13% for children under 5 years of age (Polhamus, Dalenius, Borland, Smith, & Grummer-Strawn, 2007). This alteration is manifested by a decrease in the hemoglobin concentration of the blood to less than 11.0 g/dl or a hematocrit (HCT) less than 33%. Anemias can be classified either by morphology or etiology. The morphology system uses the terms *microcytic, normocytic,* and *macrocytic* to describe the size of RBCs and the terms *hypochromic, normochromic,* and *hyperchromic* to describe the color and Hb content of the cells. Within this classification system, abnormally sized RBCs indicate alterations in RBC formation and abnormally colored RBCs indicate alterations in the hemoglobin content of the cells. The etiology system of classification is based on the idea that anemia develops because production of RBCs (**erythropoiesis**) is decreased, destruction of RBCs (**hemolysis**) is increased, or blood is lost (Tcheng, 2008a). This system of classification according to etiology lends itself better to a discussion of the causes of anemia, and is the system used in this chapter. The types of anemia discussed in this chapter are listed according to this classification system in Box 26-1. Information regarding the morphology of specific anemias is presented in the laboratory findings section for each type of anemia.

KIDS WANT TO KNOW

What are blood cells?

Many children are curious about their bodies, especially if there is something that is different about them. When caring for a child with a hematological disorder, questions about blood cells can be answered in the following manner:

- Cells are very small parts of our bodies, so small we cannot see them one at a time. We can only see them when they are all piled together. They are in every part of our bodies, even the blood.
- The cells in our blood are either red or white or a special kind of cell called a platelet.
- Just like us, cells need air in order to live. This is why we need red blood cells. They pick up the air from the lungs and take it to the other cells in the body. If these cells are not working right, we might get tired or dizzy.
- The white blood cells are like watchdogs. They look for anything they have not seen before and if they find something, they fight it so it cannot hurt the body. If we do not have enough cells, they may not be able to fight hard enough to stop something that could make us sick.
- The platelets are special cells that help stop bleeding. When we get hurt and start to bleed, these cells become sticky and form a big clump that blocks the hole where the blood is getting out. This is why we get a scab. If we do not have enough of these cells, it is hard for our bodies to stop the bleeding.

BOX 26-1
ANEMIAS CLASSIFIED ACCORDING TO ETIOLOGY

- Decreased production of RBCs
  - Iron-deficiency anemia
  - Aplastic anemia
- Increased destruction of RBCs
  - Sickle cell anemia
  - Thalassemia
- Blood loss
- Iron deficiency anemia

Adapted from Tcheng, W. Y. (2008a). Anemia. In C. D. Berkowitz (ed.), *Pediatrics: A primary care approach* (3rd ed.). Elk Grove Village, IL: American Academy of Pediatrics, pp. 411–418.

EVIDENCE-BASED PRACTICE

Prevention of Iron Deficiency in Early Infancy

CLINICAL PROBLEM

Iron deficiency is estimated to be the most common nutritional deficiency worldwide and is particularly persistent among infants and children. The high prevalence of anemia in 6- to 9- month-old children raises the concern that birth iron stores in some infants are inadequate to sustain growth and development through the first 6 months of life. Maternal iron status, infant birth weight, and gestational age as well as the timing of umbilical cord clamping at birth all contribute to the establishment of adequate total body iron at birth. Postnatally, feeding practices and growth rate are factors that will affect how quickly birth iron is depleted during the first 6 months of life.

BEST CLINICAL PRACTICE

- Primary prevention approaches for iron-deficiency anemia include dietary and medicinal iron interventions.
- Delayed cord clamping has a beneficial effect on infant iron status.
- Treating maternal anemia during pregnancy may be another important approach to use in treating iron deficiency in high-risk infants and toddlers.

IMPLICATIONS FOR NURSING

- Educate parents about the importance of providing a diet high in iron for infants and toddlers (iron-fortified cereals, meats).
- Educate parents of toddlers that widespread consumption of cow's milk may inhibit iron absorption.
- Educate parents on the importance of following the primary care provider's recommendations regarding medicinal iron prescriptions.
- Educate high-risk women of child-bearing age on the importance of taking prenatal vitamins with iron prior to becoming pregnant.
- Educate health care providers of the benefits of 2–3 minute delayed cord clamping to allow for redistribution of blood between the placenta and newborn.

Reference: Chaparro, C. M. (2008). Setting the stage for child health and development; Prevention of iron deficiency in early infancy, *American Society for Nutrition, 138,* 2529–2533.

IRON-DEFICIENCY ANEMIA

Iron-deficiency anemia is the most common hematologic disorder of infancy and childhood.

INCIDENCE AND ETIOLOGY

In the United States, prevalence of iron-deficiency anemia has remained low and unchanged since the 1980s. Specifically, iron-deficiency anemia affects < 2% of U.S. children ages 1 to 5 years. These low prevalence rates are likely the result of concerted efforts to prevent iron-deficiency anemia through iron fortification of infant formulas and the establishment of the Special Supplemental Nutrition Program for Women, Infants, and Children in the early 1970s (Cusick et al., 2008). However, several recent studies (Brotanek, Gosz, Weitzman, & Flores, 2007; Cusick, Mei, & Cogswell, 2007) have identified disparities between the average rate and the rate of iron-deficiency anemia in the same age group from poor or minority households at 15%. The incidence of iron-deficiency anemia is not innately related to race, but children with low socioeconomic status, those who are between the ages of 6 months and 2 years, and adolescent girls are particularly at risk. Young children are at risk due to their high need of iron for normal growth and development (Kline, 2010). Iron-deficiency anemia occurs predominantly in adolescence because adolescence is a period of rapid growth and is often associated with poor food choices. Pregnant adolescents are particularly at risk for iron-deficiency anemia because of the increased demand for iron imposed by the developing fetus (Dunn, 2008; Kline, 2010; Rote & McCance, 2010b).

Inadequate intake of dietary iron is the most common cause of iron-deficiency anemia in the first few years of life and during adolescence in the United States. In school-age children, however, the most common cause is blood loss. In developing countries, the most common cause of iron-deficiency anemia is hookworms. Less common causes include inadequate iron stores at birth, impaired iron absorption, and excessive demands for growth (Kline, 2010; Rote & McCance, 2010b). No matter the cause of the iron deficiency, the result is the same. The body eventually does not have enough iron to synthesize the hemoglobin necessary to carry oxygen to the tissues and, as a result, anemia develops.

Pathophysiology

In children of all ages, dietary iron is absorbed in the small intestine and either passed into the bloodstream or stored in the intestinal epithelial cells as **ferritin**. The iron in the intestinal cells is often lost when the epithelial cells slough off into the intestinal lumen, but can be used for hemoglobin synthesis if necessary. The iron in the bloodstream binds to the iron-transport molecule **transferrin** and is then delivered to the RBCs in the bone marrow where it combines with the other components of hemoglobin. If the iron is not used for hemoglobin formation, it is stored as ferritin or **hemosiderin** and later excreted if it remains unused. Normally, approximately 67% of the body's iron is bound to heme and 30% of the iron is stored as ferritin or hemosiderin. Iron for hemoglobin formation can also be obtained from RBCs that have been removed from the bloodstream and catabolized. Like dietary iron, this iron is either stored as ferritin or hemosiderin or released into the bloodstream where it can bind to transferrin and travel to the bone marrow to participate in hemoglobin formation (Kline, 2010; Rote & McCance, 2010a).

When a child or adolescent does not ingest enough dietary iron, the normal process of obtaining iron for hemoglobin synthesis is impaired because there is not enough iron absorbed by the small intestine. When blood loss occurs there are fewer RBCs to be catabolized by the body and consequently the iron contained in these cells cannot be recycled by the body for future use. One of the most common forms of blood loss in children with iron-deficiency anemia is chronic intestinal blood loss caused by a heat-labile protein in cow's milk. This protein causes an inflammatory reaction in the gastrointestinal system, which damages the mucosa and results in diffuse hemorrhage (Kline, 2010).

As mentioned earlier, because premature infants use up their iron stores within 6–12 weeks from birth, they are at greater risk for iron-deficiency anemia (Kline, 2010).

Clinical Manifestations

The signs and symptoms of iron-deficiency anemia are directly related to the severity of the tissue hypoxia and the effectiveness of the compensatory mechanisms employed by the body. Iron-deficiency anemia, like other types of anemia, can be classified as mild (Hb of 11 g/dl), moderate (Hb of 3–7 g/dl), or severe (Hb < 3 g/dl) (Kline, 2010; Tcheng, 2008a). With mild anemia, caregivers commonly do not notice the gradual increase in lethargy and lassitude in their young child or adolescent. Once the child becomes moderately anemic, he or she presents with general irritability, weakness, and lack of interest in play. At this point, the compensatory mechanisms of the body (Box 26-2) are still able to make up for much of the decreased oxygen-carrying

BOX 26-2
COMPENSATORY MECHANISMS FOR ANEMIA

- Interstitial fluids enter bloodstream (if the anemia is caused by blood loss)
- Vasodilatation occurs
- Heart rate increases
- Rate and depth of respiration increase
- Hemoglobin releases oxygen to tissues more readily
- Erythropoiesis increases
- Peripheral vasoconstriction occurs (with severe anemia)
- Renin-angiotensin system retains salt and water

Adapted from Rote, N. S., & McCance, K. L. (2010a and 2010b). Structure and function of the hematologic system, and Alterations of erythrocyte function. In K. L. McCance & S. E. Huether (eds.), *Pathophysiology: The biologic basis for disease in adults and children* (6th ed.). St. Louis, MO: Mosby, pp. 952–1013.

capacity of the blood. Eventually, the compensatory mechanisms cannot keep up with the anemia and manifestations such as pallor, anorexia, and systolic murmurs begin to appear (Kline, 2010). Additional signs and symptoms common to all types of anemia, according to severity, are listed in Box 26-3. The distinction between these categories is not rigid and there may be an overlap of symptoms between categories.

In addition to the common manifestations of anemia, there are several specific signs and symptoms for iron-deficiency anemia. These include hair that falls out, nails that are brittle and spoon shaped, and spleen enlargement. Long-standing iron-deficiency anemia can also cause decreased physical growth, developmental delays, and widening of cranial sutures. Children with iron-deficiency anemia can be underweight, normal weight, or overweight (Kline, 2010; Tcheng, 2008a). The signs and symptoms of iron-deficiency anemia generally resolve with adequate treatment, although some studies suggest developmental delays may persist (see Research Highlight).

BOX 26-3

SIGNS AND SYMPTOMS OF ANEMIA ACCORDING TO SEVERITY

Mild Anemia

- Generally asymptomatic
- May experience symptoms of moderate anemia during exertion

Moderate Anemia

Effects of compensatory mechanisms:

- Shortness of breath
- Rapid, pounding heart beat
- Dizziness, fainting, lethargy, irritability

Severe Anemia

Effects of compensatory mechanisms:

- Cardiac murmurs
- Congestive heart failure

Effects of tissue hypoxia:

- Pale skin, mucous membranes, lips, nail beds, and conjunctiva
- Impaired healing and loss of skin elasticity
- Thinning and early graying of the hair
- Abdominal pain, nausea, vomiting, and anorexia
- Low-grade fever

Other:

- Yellowish skin color (if the anemia is from increased RBC destruction)

Rote, N. S., & McCance, K. L. (2010b). Alterations of erythrocyte function. In K. L. McCance & S. E. Huether (Eds.). *Pathophysiology: The biologic basis for disease in adults and children* (6th ed.). St. Louis, MO: Mosby, pp. 989–1013.

DIAGNOSIS

For all ages, a diagnosis of iron-deficiency anemia is made on the basis of history, clinical presentation, and laboratory data. The assessment should include questions about family history, recent blood loss, and dietary history. The child's clinical presentation should be evaluated according to the signs and symptoms listed in Box 26-3. Initial laboratory tests for a child suspected of having iron-deficiency anemia are listed in Table 26-2.

TREATMENT

Treatment of iron-deficiency anemia takes two directions: correction of the underlying problem responsible for the iron-deficiency and replacement of depleted iron stores. If the cause of the iron-deficiency is blood loss, the bleeding must be stopped before treatment will be effective. Once the bleeding has stopped, or if the cause is purely nutritional, an adequate teaching plan for the caregiver and child needs to be implemented. For infants, breast milk should be encouraged as the exclusive source of nutrition because the bioavailability of iron in human milk is greater than the iron found in iron-fortified formulas. Once a child is started on solid foods at 4–6 months of life, he or she should be given iron-fortified cereal (Hui & Grover, 2008). For a school-age child with iron-deficiency anemia, cow's milk restriction may be implemented to increase the child's hunger for other iron-rich foods and also to prevent blood loss in those children who have an inflammatory reaction to cow's milk proteins (Kline, 2010). Both school-age children and adolescents should be encouraged to increase their intake of foods high in iron (Box 26-4) and vitamin C, which increase the body's absorption of iron. Pregnant adolescents need to be especially aware of their iron intake. Iron supplementation is recommended both to prevent and treat iron-deficiency anemia in this population (Wardlaw & Hampl, 2006).

In addition to dietary supplementation, iron supplementation is given either orally or parenterally. However, parenteral iron is reserved for use in clients with iron malabsorption, chronic blood loss, or inability to tolerate oral iron. This is because oral iron corrects iron-deficiency just as rapidly and completely as parenteral iron, with potentially less severe side effects. The recommended form of oral iron supplementation is ferrous iron because it is the most efficiently absorbed. The common side effects of oral iron supplementation are listed in Box 26-5. If children cannot tolerate these side effects, they can often be overcome by either switching to a different type of oral iron, lowering the daily dose of iron, or by taking the tablets immediately after

TABLE 26-2 Common Laboratory Tests and Findings for Anemia

LABORATORY TEST	NO ANEMIA PRESENT	IRON-DEFICIENCY ANEMIA	SICKLE CELL ANEMIA	COOLEY'S ANEMIA	APLASTIC ANEMIA
Hemoglobin—measures the total amount of Hb in the peripheral blood	9–16 g/dl (see Appendix E)	Decreased	Decreased	Decreased	Decreased
Hematocrit—measures the percentage of RBCs in the total blood volume	28–49% (see Appendix E)	Decreased	Decreased	Decreased	Decreased
Reticulocyte count—measures immature RBCs in order to measure RBC production	Infant: 0.5–3.1% Child & Adolescent: 0.5–2%	Normal	Increased	Normal	Decreased
Mean corpuscular volume (MCV)—measures average RBC volume and size	86–98 μ^3	Decreased	Normal	Decreased	Normal
Mean corpuscular hemoglobin (MCH)—measures the average weight of Hb within a RBC	28–33 pg	Decreased	Normal	Decreased	Normal
Mean corpuscular hemoglobin concentration (MCHC)—measures the average concentration of Hb in one RBC	32–36 g/dl	Decreased	Normal	Decreased	Normal
Hemoglobin electrophoresis—enables detection of abnormal forms of Hb	Predominantly Hb A with decreasing amounts of Hb F as the child ages	Normal	Predominantly Hb S	Abnormally high Hb F	Normal
Peripheral smear—reveals variations in RBC size, color, and shape	Normocytic, normochromic	Microcytic Hypochromic	Normocytic Normochromic Sickle shaped cells	Microcytic Hypochromic	Normocytic Normochromic
Serum iron—measures the iron levels in the blood	50–150 mg/dl	Decreased	Normal	Increased	Increased
Serum ferritin—measures available iron stores	6 mo–15 yrs: 7–140 mg/mL Male adolescents: 12–300 mg/mL Female adolescents: 10–150 mg/mL	Decreased	Normal	Increased	Normal
Total iron binding capacity (TIBC) measures tansferrin	250–450 mcg/dl	Increased	Decreased	Normal	Normal

Adapted from Wilson, D. D. (2008). *McGraw-Hill's manual of laboratory & diagnostic tests.* New York: McGraw-Hill.; Kee, J. L. (2009). *Prentice Hall handbook of laboratory and diagnostic tests with nursing implications* (6th ed.). Upper Saddle River, NJ: Pearson Prentice Hall; Linker, C. A. (2009). Blood Disorders. In S. J. McPhee, M. A. Papadakis & L. M. Tierney (Eds.). *Current medical diagnosis & treatment. 2009*. Retrieved January 21, 2009, from http://www.accessmedicine.com/content.aspx?aID=5476.

or with meals (Masters, 2007). The recommended dosage for oral iron supplementation is based on the weight of the child. In order to ensure iron stores are replenished, treatment is continued for at least two months after RBC indexes have returned to normal. If hemoglobin levels do not increase after one month of oral therapy, the oral supplementation should be stopped and the child evaluated for other causes of anemia (Tcheng, 2008a).

BOX 26-4
GOOD DIETARY SOURCES OF IRON

Meat: Lean beef, veal, pork, lamb, poultry, liver

Seafood: Clams, shrimp, oysters

Vegetables: Spinach, okra, sweet potatoes, winter squash, white potatoes

Legumes: Dried peas, dried beans, legumes

Grains: Whole grain breads and fortified cereals, brown rice, enriched pasta, tofu, soybeans

Fruits: Tomato and prune juice, prunes, raisins, figs

Miscellaneous: Molasses, egg yolk, nutritional yeast

Adapted from Centers for Disease Control and Prevention. (2007, May 22). Iron Deficiency. Retrieved August 13, 2010, from http://www.cdc.gov/nutrition/everyone/basics/vitamins/iron.html.

BOX 26-5
COMMON SIDE EFFECTS OF IRON SUPPLEMENTATION

ORAL IRON	PARENTERAL IRON
Nausea	Local pain
Epigastric discomfort	Tissue staining
Abdominal cramps	Headache
Constipation	Lightheadedness
Diarrhea	Fever
Black stools	Arthralgias
	Nausea and vomiting
	Back pain
	Flushing
	Urticaria
	Bronchospasm
	Anaphylaxis (rare)
	Death (rare)

Adapted from Masters, S. B. (2007). Drugs used in anemias: Hematopoietic growth factors. In B. G. Katzung (ed.), *Basic and clinical pharmacology* (10th ed.). New York: McGraw-Hill, pp. 527–541, 549–563.

Nursing Management

Assessment The assessment of a child with iron-deficiency anemia consists mainly of observing for the signs and symptoms listed in Box 26-3. A good client history will also provide valuable information, and should include a detailed dietary history along with a history of bowel movements.

Nursing Diagnosis Appropriate nursing diagnoses for a child with iron-deficiency anemia include:

1. *Ineffective tissue perfusion* related to anemia.
2. *Imbalanced nutrition: less than body requirements* related to inadequate iron intake.
3. *Deficient caregiver knowledge* related to age-appropriate iron intake.
4. *Activity intolerance* related to decreased oxygen delivery to the tissues.

Outcome Identification The desired outcomes for these nursing diagnoses include:

1. The child will maintain an adequate Hb level for his/her age.
2. The child will consume at least the minimum recommended daily allowance (RDA) of iron each day.
3. The caregiver will be able to describe the appropriate feeding guidelines for the child's age.
4. The child will be able to engage in age-appropriate play without signs or symptoms of excessive exertion.

Planning and Implementation In order to achieve these outcomes, the primary focus of nursing intervention is caregiver education. This education should include a discussion of iron-deficiency anemia, age-appropriate dietary guidelines, and information regarding the administration of oral iron supplements. This education, which is included in the family teaching section, will help caregivers overcome their lack of knowledge in relation to iron intake, and increase their child's iron intake, tissue perfusion, and activity tolerance.

Evaluation Follow-up with the family should focus on evaluating the desired outcomes and reviewing education concepts as needed. The caregiver and child should be asked about how and when the child has been taking iron supplements. Laboratory work will also be helpful in determining the success of the interventions. A dietary history should be obtained to determine if the child has consumed at least the minimum RDA of iron each day. The nurse should ask the caregiver to explain the appropriate feeding guidelines for his or her child's age and observe the child's actions for any signs or symptoms of excessive exertion.

Family Teaching

The nurse should explain adequate iron is necessary for the blood to be able to transport oxygen to the tissues. If a child does not eat enough iron, the body will use up all the extra iron it has stored. Once the stores of iron have been used, the child will have symptoms, such as weakness, irritability, pale skin, decreased appetite, and a fast heart beat. Eating more iron and taking iron supplements will help replenish the body's stores of iron and allow adequate oxygen to be transported to the tissues.

The nurse should also reinforce age-appropriate dietary guidelines. These include:

Under 12 months of age:

- Encourage exclusive breastfeeding of infants for 4–6 months after birth.
- When exclusive breastfeeding is stopped, encourage intake of approximately 1 mg/kg per day of iron, preferably from supplementary foods (see Box 26-4).

RESEARCH Highlight

Delay in Cognitive Development Related to Early Iron Deficiency in Infants

STUDY PURPOSE

To determine whether iron-deficiency anemia in infancy presents a risk factor for deficits in early attention and memory development.

METHODS

Brain electrical activity data was obtained at 9 and/or 12 months from 15 infants with iron-deficiency anemia and 19 who were iron sufficient during a test of the infant's ability to discriminate their mother's face from a stranger's face.

FINDINGS

After controlling for background factors, iron-sufficient infants at 9 months showed a greater attentional response to the mother and a greater memory for the stranger. The iron-deficient children did not show a similar response until 12-months of age thus suggesting a delay in cognitive development.

IMPLICATIONS

This study suggests that iron-deficiency anemia adversely affects infants' development of attention and memory relating to familiar and unfamiliar stimuli. This delay in cognitive development may reflect alterations of the central nervous system related to early iron deficiency. Additional studies are needed to understand the degree early iron deficiency has on cognitive development and subsequent development in children.

REFERENCE

Burden, M. J., Westerlund, A. J., Armony-Sivan, R., Nelson, C. A., Jacobson, S. W., Lozoff, B., Angelille, M., & Jacobson, J. L. (2007). An event-related potential study of attention and recognition memory in infants with iron-deficiency anemia. *Pediatrics, 120*, e336–e345.

- For infants who are not breastfed or who are partially breastfed, recommend only iron-fortified infant formula as a substitute for breast milk.
- For breastfed infants who receive less than 1 mg/kg per day of iron from supplementary foods by age 6 months, suggest 1 mg/kg per day of iron drops.
- For breastfed infants who were preterm or had a low birth weight, recommend 2–4 mg/kg per day of iron drops (to a maximum of 15 mg/day) starting at one month after birth and continuing until twelve months after birth.

NURSING ALERT

Iron Supplements

Although oral iron supplementation is generally perceived as a safe treatment alternative, an overdose can be lethal for children. Initial signs and symptoms of overdose include vomiting, abdominal pain, and bloody diarrhea. These manifestations are typically followed by shock, lethargy, and dyspnea. Often the child will appear to improve before the onset of severe metabolic acidosis, coma, and death. Urgent treatment is essential and includes flushing out unabsorbed pills, administration of Desferal (see Beta-Thalassemia section), and supportive therapy (Masters, 2007).

- Encourage the use of only breast milk or iron-fortified infant formula for any milk-based part of the diet (e.g., in infant cereal).
- Discourage the use of low-iron milks (e.g., cow's milk, goat's milk, and soy milk).
- At age 4–6 months two or more servings per day of iron-fortified infant cereal can meet an infant's requirement for iron.
- By approximately age 6 months, encourage one feeding per day of foods rich in vitamin C (e.g., fruits, vegetables, or juice) to improve iron absorption, preferably with meals.
- Suggest introducing plain, pureed meats after age 6 months or when the infant is developmentally ready to consume such food.

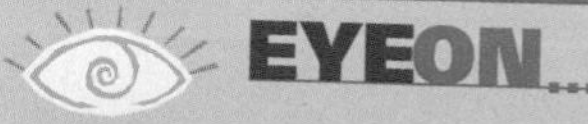

Alternative Approaches to Iron Supplementation

In at-risk populations, routine iron supplementation is a method of preventing iron-deficiency anemia. In addition to the iron-fortified foods and oral iron supplements used in the United States, alternative methods of iron supplementation are surfacing in other countries, with promising results.

In India, researchers investigated the use of inexpensive iron-fortified candies to improve the iron status of over 400 children ages 3 to 6. The children ate three iron-fortified candies a week and after twelve weeks researchers concluded that the candies were successful in raising hemoglobin levels and decreasing the anemia prevalence in the children (Anand et al., 2006).

School-age children, preschool children and adolescents:

- Suggest children ages 1–5 years consume no more than 24 oz of cow's milk, goat's milk, or soy milk each day.
- Encourage consumption of iron-rich foods (see Box 26-4).
- Recommend cooking acidic foods in iron cookware.
- Increase dietary intake of foods rich in vitamin C (e.g., fruits, vegetables, or juice) to improve iron absorption, preferably with meals.

The nurse should provide the following information about oral iron supplements:

- Give exactly the prescribed amount. More is not better and can actually harm the child.
- Keep the iron locked in a safe place to prevent accidental overdoses.
- The side effects listed in Box 26-5 are common and can be avoided by taking the tablets immediately after or with meals.
- If the child is getting enough iron, stools should be a tarry green color.
- Constipation will often persist and may require the use of stool softeners or laxatives.
- Liquid iron supplements may stain teeth. If the child is old enough, give the iron solution with a straw. Otherwise, give with a dropper or syringe in the back part of the mouth.
- Avoid giving the child fluoride, antacids, tetracycline, coffee, tea, dairy products, eggs, or whole-grain breads within one hour before or two hours after the oral iron supplement because these substances interfere with iron absorption.

Much of the teaching provided to caregivers for home management of iron-deficiency anemia applies in the school setting as well. If the child eats foods prepared by the school, these foods should provide adequate iron intake and include vitamin C if possible. If the iron supplements need to be given at school, instructions should also be provided concerning their proper administration and storage.

Refer the family to the Iron Disorders Institute; the National Heart, Lung and Blood Institute Information Center; or the Children's Cancer & Blood Foundation (see the Resources section at the end of this chapter).

CRITICAL THINKING

What Is the Diagnosis?

While working in the community you encounter 10-month-old Adrienne, who is irritable and appears weak for her age. Her mother states she seems more tired than usual and does not play as much as she used to. She has tried giving Adrienne a bottle of milk like she usually does when she appears unhappy, but that does not seem to pacify her. You ask more about dietary habits and find that when Adrienne's mother stopped breastfeeding, she started her on a cow's-milk bottle. She usually uses this bottle to calm her and when it is time for meals. Adrienne typically does not eat very much. What do you think Adrienne's diagnosis is and what nursing interventions would be appropriate?

SICKLE CELL ANEMIA

Sickle cell anemia (SCA) is one of three disorders that fall under the classification of sickle cell disease. Each disorder in this class is characterized by the presence of **hemoglobin S** (Hb S), also known as sickle hemoglobin. The other types of Hb inherited from the parents of a child with sickle cell disease determine which sickle cell disorder the child will manifest. In addition to SCA, the other two types of sickle cell disease are sickle cell-hemoglobin C disease and sickle cell-thalassemia disease. Of these disorders, SCA is the most severe, although every type of sickle cell disease is a lifelong disorder with no known cure (Kline, 2010).

INCIDENCE AND ETIOLOGY

Like the other sickle cell disorders, SCA is an autosomal recessive disorder that can be transmitted to the offspring of those with the disease, as well as to the offspring of carriers. In order for either of these possibilities to occur, both parents must carry at least one of the recessive genes (Figure 26-2). If both parents do not have the gene, the child will either be a carrier for sickle cell disease or will not have the sickle cell gene. Carriers of sickle cell disease are said to have the sickle cell trait (SCT), although they generally have no symptoms (DeBaun & Vichinsky, 2007).

Sickle cell disease has been traced back thousands of years to the inhabitants of countries that were plagued by malaria, particularly in certain parts of Africa. However, researchers have found children in these areas who had the sickle cell trait were able to survive the malaria epidemics more often than those who did not. Thus, the gene for sickle

CULTURAL CONSIDERATION

Sickle Cell Anemia

Sickle cell anemia occurs most frequently in African Americans, with an estimated 2,000 babies born with sickle cell disease each year in the United States. It also occurs in persons from South or Central America, Caribbean islands, Mediterranean countries, India, and Saudi Arabia (Brawley et al., 2008).

(A) When both parents carry the disease gene, there is a 25% chance each child conceived will not have the disease or carry the disease. There is a 50% chance each child conceived will carry the gene, and a 25% chance each child conceived will have the disease.

	B	b
B	BB 25% Normal	Bb 25% Carrier
b	Bb 25% Carrier	bb 25% Disease

(B) When one parent has the disease and the other is a carrier for the disease, there is a 50% chance each child conceived will carry the disease and a 50% chance each child conceived will have the disease.

	b	b
B	Bb 25% Carrier	Bb 25% Carrier
b	bb 25% Disease	bb 25% Disease

Legend
b = Recessive disease gene
B = Dominant normal gene
bb = Disease state
Bb or bB = Carrier state
BB = Normal state

FIGURE 26-2 Autosomal Recessive Inheritance. DELMAR CENGAGE LEARNING.

cell disease was passed on to the children of these survivors. At present, however, possessing the sickle cell gene may be a serious threat to those not likely to be exposed to malaria (Heeney & Dover, 2009; Kline, 2010).

Sickle cell anemia affects millions of people throughout the world. However, because of the benefits of the sickle cell trait in regard to malaria exposure, SCA is particularly common among individuals whose ancestors originated in Africa. In the United States, SCA occurs among African Americans at a rate of 1/396 births and among Hispanics at a rate of 1/36,000 births (DeBaun & Vichinsky, 2007). The sickle cell trait is even more common with 1/14 black Americans possessing the asymptomatic carrier genotype (Platt, 2008).

PATHOPHYSIOLOGY

In children who have the recessive sickle cell gene one amino acid replaces another, resulting in the production of sickle hemoglobin (Hb S). This abnormal form of hemoglobin contains a semisolid gel that aggregates within the RBC, causing it to stretch into an elongated crescent or sickle shape (Figure 26-3). When compared to normal RBCs, sickled cells are stiffer and less able to change shape. As a result, they are often unable to pass through the microcirculation, causing vaso-occlusion, pain, and organ infarction. They can also cause infarction of the splenic vessels and blood pooling in the spleen because the cells are destroyed or sequestered there. This phenomenon results in an anemia of increased RBC destruction. The body tries to compensate by increasing RBC production. This anemic condition is worsened by the fact that sickled RBCs die after only about 10 to 20 days, resulting in an abnormally low number of RBCs in circulation (Heeney & Dover, 2009; Kline, 2010, McMahon, 2006).

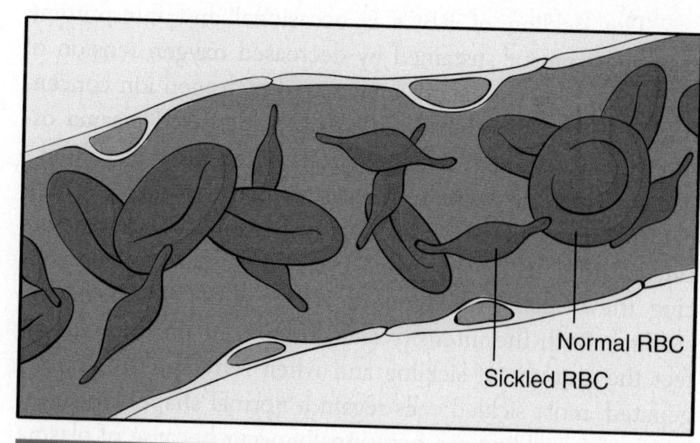

FIGURE 26-3 Regular and Sickled RBCs. DELMAR CENGAGE LEARNING.

EVIDENCE-BASED PRACTICE

Parents' Perspectives on Pain Management in Pediatric Sickle Cell Disease

CLINICAL PROBLEM

Children with sickle cell disease commonly have unpredictable and recurrent severe pain also called vaso occlusive crises. Typically children with sickle cell disease experience pain episodes on an average of 5–7 times per year and require hospitalization 1–2 times each year for pain. These painful episodes have both physical and emotional implications that impact the child experiencing the pain and the family helping the child cope. Most of these painful episodes are managed at home. Parent's perceptions on care and the relationships between coping, family function, and health care utilization can offer nurses insight when planning effective nursing interventions.

BEST CLINICAL PRACTICE

Parents' expressed the need for increased support, education, and sensitivity to parents and patients and for improved staff training and medication dispensing options. They also highlighted the need for more activities that allow children with sickle cell disease to interact.

IMPLICATIONS FOR NURSING

- Educate health care workers and community groups about the special needs of children and families coping with sickle cell disease. Information should include input from parents and patients.
- Explore drug dispensing policies that offer options and include patient and parental input.
- Nurses should provide patient support group information to families that include opportunities for children with sickle cell disease to interact with each other.

Reference: Mitchell, M. J., Lemanek, K., Palermo, T. M., Crosby, L. E., Nichols, A., & Powers, S. W. (2007). Parent perspectives on pain management, coping, and family function in pediatric sickle cell disease. *Clinical Pediatrics*, *46*(4), 311–319.

The sickling of RBCs is occasional and intermittent, resulting from or sustained by decreased oxygen tension of the blood (i.e., hypoxemia), increased hydrogen ion concentration in the blood (decreased pH), increased plasma osmolality (increased concentration of solutes in blood), decreased plasma volume (increased viscosity), and low temperature (associated with vasoconstriction). These factors can create a self-perpetuating cycle because as sickled cells clog the vessels, hypoxemia develops and perpetuates the sickling. Both the intensity and duration of the stimulus affect the amount of sickling and when rehydrated or reoxygenated, most sickled cells regain a normal shape. However, irreversible sickling can occasionally occur because of plasma membrane damage (Kline, 2010).

Sickle cell anemia has the highest prevalence of Hb S, with approximately 75–95% of the Hb within a RBC being Hb S. The severity of sickling is directly correlated with the percentage of Hb S, thus making SCA the most severe type of sickle cell disease. On the other end of the spectrum, children who have the sickle cell trait rarely experience RBC sickling because Hb F (fetal hemoglobin) and Hb A (adult hemoglobin) do not participate in sickling. These children may experience anemia, however, because of the prevalence of Hb F. Hb F does not live as long as Hb A and therefore causes these children to have lower Hb concentrations (Kline, 2010). Figure 26-4 illustrates the effect on the body.

Clinical Manifestations

The clinical manifestations of SCA can vary widely in severity and frequency. During the first 6 months of life most newborns are asymptomatic because Hb F does not sickle. As Hb S replaces Hb F, however, sickling increases and symptoms begin to develop. The anemia of SCA is manifested by the same signs and symptoms of other anemias, including pallor, fatigue, shortness of breath, irritability, and jaundice (see Box 26-3 for additional signs and symptoms). Children with SCA also experience delayed growth and delayed onset of puberty. However, the principal symptom experienced by children with this disorder is pain. This pain can occur unpredictably in any body organ or joint and is typically associated with the occurrence of vaso-occlusive crises. These crises are the most common type of sickle cell crisis, although sequestration crisis and aplastic crisis can also occur (Heeney & Dover, 2009; Kline, 2010).

The term **vaso-occlusive crisis** refers to the aggregation of sickled cells within a vessel, causing obstruction. If the process is not reversed, infarction of the distal tissues will ensue. This type of crisis causes extreme pain and can last from a few hours to several weeks (Kline, 2010; U.S. Department of Health and Human Services [DHHS], 2004). The most common sites of vaso-occlusive crises are listed in Table 26-3 along with the common manifestations associated with each type of obstruction. Of particular importance in the pediatric population is the vaso-occlusive manifestation of **hand-foot syndrome** (tender, warm, and swollen hands, feet, or both) because it is typically the first manifestation of SCA in infants. The pain associated with this syndrome is severe, causing children to cry and refuse to bear weight (Heeney & Dover, 2009). Another commonly occurring manifestation in children is a cerebral vascular accident (CVA). Approximately 11% and 20% of children with sickle cell disease experience either overt or silent strokes respectively, before their 18th birthday. These CVAs typically occur without warning, but may be preceded by severe headaches or deterioration in school performance (DeBaun & Vichinsky, 2007).

The term **sequestration crisis** refers to the excessive pooling of blood in the liver and spleen. As more and more of the child's blood leaves circulation, the decreased

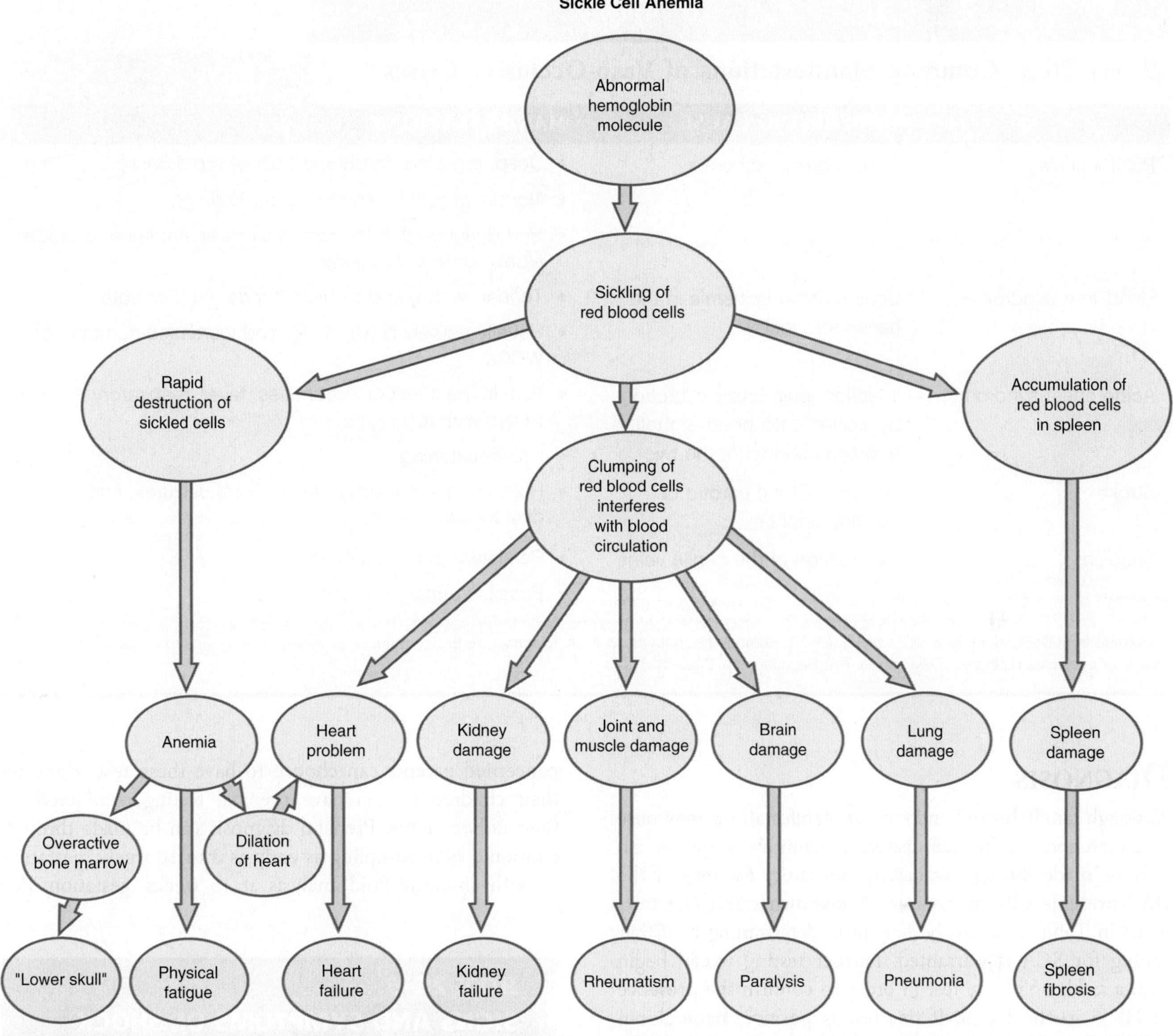

FIGURE 26-4 The Consequences of Sickled RBCs. DELMAR CENGAGE LEARNING.

blood volume results in shock (see Box 26-6 for the signs and symptoms of shock). This type of crisis can cause fatal cardiovascular collapse, because the spleen is capable of holding as much as one-fifth of the body's blood volume. This type of crisis is most commonly seen in children ages 3 months to 5 years of age. Sequestration crisis is associated with a mortality rate of up to 50%. Removal of the spleen is the treatment for recurrent sequestration crises in children over 5 years of age (Kline, 2010).

Aplastic crisis occurs when there is a decrease in erythropoiesis, despite the shortened life span of sickled RBCs and the body's need for increased RBC production. Frequently this type of crisis is precipitated by an infection with human parovirus B19. The infection is self-limited, but highly contagious and warrants isolation from persons vulnerable to infection. Aplastic crisis results in severe anemia, manifested by the signs and symptoms listed in Box 26-3 (Kline, 2010; Krishnamurti, Landord, & Munoz, 2007).

Many children with SCA will eventually experience organ damage as a direct result of sickled RBCs reducing blood flow to the organ. Nearly every organ system of the body is affected. In addition to the common sites of vaso-occlusive crisis, sickle cells can reduce blood flow to the eyes, gastrointestinal tract, and the kidneys, and result in blindness, abdominal pain, and **enuresis** (urinary incontinence). Sickled cells can also cause damage to the spleen and reduce its ability to destroy bacteria in the blood, leaving the child immunocompromised and susceptible to serious infections, usually caused by common pathogens. For this reason, the single most common cause of death in children with SCA is streptococcus pneumoniae infection (DeBaun & Vichinsky, 2007; Linker, 2009; U.S. DHHS, 2004).

Table 26-3 Common Manifestations of Vaso-Occlusive Crises

	UNDERLYING CAUSE	MANIFESTATIONS
Painful crisis	Bone marrow ischemia	• Deep, gnawing, throbbing pain of rapid onset • Normal physical and laboratory findings • Usually located in the lumbosacral spine, knee, shoulder, elbow, or femur regions
Hand-foot syndrome	Bone marrow ischemia in the hands and feet	• Tender, warm, and swollen hands, feet, or both • Usually acutely ill with fever and increased numbers of WBCs
Acute chest syndrome	Infection, pulmonary infarction by sickled cells or fat emboli, or a combination of the two	• Pain in the chest or extremities, fever, respiratory distress or hypoxemia • Life-threatening
Stroke	Infarction of the carotid or cerebral arteries	• Hemiparesis, speech defects, focal seizures, and gait dysfunction
Priapism	Obstruction of the penile veins	• Persistent penile erection • Possible urinary retention

Adapted from DeBaun, M. R. & Vichinsky, E. (2007). Hemoglobinopathies. In R. M. Kliegman, R. E. Behrman, H. B. Jenson & B. F. Stanton (Eds.). *Nelson textbook of pediatrics* (18th ed.). Philadelphia, PA: Saunders, pp. 2023–2031.

Diagnosis

Although family history and clinical manifestations may raise suspicion about sickle cell disease, a definitive diagnosis can only be made through evaluating laboratory findings. If the child presents with an anemia of unknown cause, the tests listed in Table 26-2 can be helpful in determining if further testing for SCA is warranted. Further testing would begin with a sickle solubility test in order to confirm the presence of Hb S in the blood. If this test is positive, hemoglobin electrophoresis would then be conducted to determine the amount of Hb S in the blood. The results of this test can then be used to differentiate SCA from other types of sickle cell disease. These two tests would also be appropriate in evaluating children who present with the clinical manifestations of SCA. If there is a family history of sickle cell disease, concerned parents can choose to have these tests done on their children or can have prenatal testing conducted on their unborn fetus. Prenatal diagnosis can be made through chorionic villus sampling as early as 8 to 10 weeks' gestation or with amniotic fluid analysis at 15 weeks' gestation. For

NURSING ALERT

Children with SCA and SCT

Children with sickle cell anemia, and on rare occasions children who have the sickle cell trait, can experience vaso-occlusive episodes and severe hypoxia caused by shock, vigorous exercising at high altitudes, flying at high altitudes in unpressurized aircraft, or undergoing anesthesia (Kline, 2010).

BOX 26-6 SIGNS AND SYMPTOMS OF SHOCK

Early Signs

- Tachycardia
- Delayed capillary refill
- Cool, clammy, pale, or mottled skin
- Decreased urine output

Late Signs

- Altered mental status
- Weak, thready, or absent pulses
- Hypotension
- Tachycardia or bradycardia
- Delayed capillary refill
- Severely mottled or cyanotic skin
- Decreased or absent urine output

Adapted from Young, K. D. (2008). Shock. In C. D. Berkowitz (ed.), *Pediatrics: A primary care approach* (3rd ed.). Elk Grove Village, IL: American Academy of Pediatrics, pp. 265–270.

those families without a known family history of sickle cell disease, the routine testing of newborns conducted in over 44 states is able to detect both sickle cell disease and sickle cell trait (Kline, 2010; U.S. DHHS, 2004).

Treatment

The primary treatment for children with sickle cell disease is prevention of RBC sickling in order to prevent anemia and sickle cell crises. This entails avoiding stimuli such as fever, infection, acidosis, dehydration, constricting clothing, and exposure to cold. Adherence to the recommended childhood immunization schedule, including the hepatitis B and pneumococcal vaccines, is essential for children with this disease because of their increased risk for infection. For this reason, children with SCA are also maintained on prophylactic oral penicillin until age 5. Blood transfusions are also an effective treatment, though this intervention must be weighed against risks such as iron overload (see Beta-Thalassemia major section) (DeBaun & Vichinsky, 2007; Heeney & Dover, 2009; U.S. DHHS, 2004).

If a vaso-occlusive crisis does occur, pain can usually be managed with acetaminophen or ibuprofen if mild or if the child is under 6 years of age. For more severe pain, the use of narcotics such as morphine is appropriate. IV fluids may be necessary to achieve optimal hydration and reverse RBC sickling. A sequestration crisis requires the transfusion of red blood cells to treat the rapid decrease in circulating blood volume. If sequestration crises occur frequently, a splenectomy may be performed to alleviate the danger of cardiovascular collapse. Most aplastic crises are short, mild, and do not require therapy (Heeney & Dover, 2009; McMahon, 2006). Hydroxyurea, a myelosuppressive agent, is a new drug that reduces the frequency of painful episodes related to sickle cell disease in adults but has not been approved yet for use in children (Strouse et al., 2008).

Fortunately, sickle cell trait is not associated with decreased life expectancy. However, sepsis and meningitis develop in as many as 10% of SCA children under the age of 5, with a mortality rate of 25%. Many children who survive past age 5 only live into their twenties (Kline, 2010). However, overall survival rates have been improving steadily following the institution of comprehensive care, immunizations, antibiotics, hydroxyurea, and more rapid treatment of disease complications.

Nursing Management

Assessment

In addition to observing for the signs and symptoms of anemia listed in Box 26-3, nurses should also assess for pain related to vaso-occlusive crises or shock related to sequestration crisis.

Nursing Diagnosis

Potential nursing diagnoses for the child with sickle cell anemia include:

1. *Acute pain* related to vaso-occlusive crisis.
2. *Ineffective tissue perfusion* related to impaired arterial blood flow.
3. *High-risk for infection* related to splenic malfunction and chronic immunocompromised state.
4. *Ineffective coping of child and family* related to chronic and potentially life-threatening disease.

Outcome Identification

The desired outcomes for these diagnoses include:

1. The child will report pain relief is adequate.
2. The child will not demonstrate the manifestations of anemia.
3. The child will be afebrile.
4. Caregivers will be aware of resources available to help them cope with difficulties inherent in having a child with SCA.

Planning and Implementation

Pain management is most commonly needed when a child experiences a vaso-occlusive crisis. In this instance, analgesics should be given around the clock, rather than on an as-needed basis. Children experiencing sickle cell crisis are often undermedicated, resulting in "clock watching" and requests for additional doses occurring sooner than prescribed. Many misinformed health care professionals interpret this behavior as a sign of drug addiction, whereas the actual problem is inadequate pain control. Other nursing interventions include

REFLECTIVE THINKING

Family Planning for a Person with Sickle Cell Disease

1. **If you and your partner were carriers of the sickle cell gene, would you make a decision to attempt a pregnancy and hope for a child born without the disease?**
2. **If you decided to conceive, would you use prenatal testing to determine if the child you were carrying was positive for the disease or the trait? Why or why not?**
3. **If the fetus was positive for the disease, what would you do? Would you terminate the pregnancy? Would you carry to term? Would it make a difference if the fetus had the trait rather than having the disease? Why or why not?**
4. **What if you and your partner decided not to conceive but accidentally became pregnant? Would you go through prenatal testing, carry the fetus to term, and hope for a healthy outcome, or abort the pregnancy without determining the sickle cell status of the fetus? Why or why not?**
5. **What are options two people who are both carriers for the disease might have in terms of having children?**

(1) applying heat to the painful area (cold is contraindicated because it promotes sickling); (2) allowing the child to determine the amount of activity he or she can tolerate; (3) providing passive range of motion exercises to prevent venous stasis; (4) administering intravenous fluids to maintain hydration status; (5) frequent hand washing; and (6) proper aseptic techniques. If blood transfusions are administered, hospital protocol should be followed (see Beta-Thalassemia section). As the nurse interacts with the child and caregivers, he or she should take the time to talk with them about their emotions related to their child's situation. The nurse should also refer the caregivers to social workers or community resources for the clients and their families.

Evaluation Once nursing interventions have been implemented, the desired outcomes can be evaluated by assessing the child for pain, anemia, and fever. Assessment should also include thorough observation and discussion to determine if the child and caregiver are aware of the resources available to help them. Nurses should also evaluate the families need for support while caring for a child with a potentially fatal and chronic disease.

Family Teaching

Caring for a child with sickle cell anemia at home requires a clear understanding of the situations that precipitate sickling, including dehydration, infection, and exposure to cold. The child and caregivers should be taught to avoid any known sources of infection and maintain adequate nutrition and hand washing. They should also be taught to seek medical help if they notice fever, pallor, pain, or enlargement in the area of the spleen.

The child's teachers should be made aware of the child's condition, the situations that the child needs to avoid, and indications of a need for medical help. If the child participates in any school sports it is essential to maintain adequate hydration. There are numerous agencies that provide information and support for both caregivers and children with SCA, including the Sickle Cell Disease Association of America; the Center for Sickle Cell Disease; the Sickle Cell Association of Ontario; and the Information Center for Sickle Cell and Thalassemic Disorders (see the Resources section at the end of this chapter).

BETA-THALASSEMIA MAJOR

The **thalassemias** are a group of inherited autosomal recessive disorders, characterized by an impaired rate of hemoglobin chain synthesis (see Figure 26-2). These lifelong disorders are classified as alpha- or beta-, according to which globin chain of hemoglobin synthesis is impaired, and as major or minor, depending on how many genes are defective. That is, thalassemia major refers to the inheritance of recessive genes from both parents and thalassemia minor refers to the inheritance of recessive genes from only one parent. Of all thalassemias, the beta-thalassemias are more common and present the most significant health concerns for children (Kline, 2010).

Incidence and Etiology

The beta-thalassemias are common among children of Mediterranean descent, such as Italians, Greeks, and some Arabs and Sephardic Jews. In the United States, an estimated 2,000 individuals have beta-thalassemia (DeBaun & Vichinsky, 2007). The alpha-thalassemias are common among Chinese, Vietnamese, Cambodians, and Laotians. Both alpha-thalassemias and beta-thalassemias are common among black Americans. Children with thalassemia minor, also referred to as having the thalassemia trait, carry the gene for thalassemia without manifesting significant health problems. In these children, the lack of alpha- or beta-globin is generally not great enough to cause altered hemoglobin function, other than causing mild anemia. In contrast, **beta-thalassemia major** (also called Cooley's anemia) is associated with a life-threatening form of anemia that requires regular blood transfusions and ongoing medical care. Death from cardiac failure usually occurs between ages 20 and 30 (Cooley's Anemia Foundation [CAF], 2009; Kline, 2010; Linker, 2009).

Pathophysiology

Each normal Hb A contains four globin components, or polypeptide chains. Two of these globins are alpha polypeptide chains and two are beta polypeptide chains. These four chains combine with four heme complexes, the oxygen-carrying component, to form one Hb molecule (see Figure 26-1). In beta-thalassemia the synthesis of beta-globin chains is impaired, resulting in RBCs that contain less hemoglobin. In addition, these RBCs contain free alpha chains that are unstable and precipitate, causing many of the RBCs in the marrow to be destroyed; thus, an anemia of decreased RBC production results. The RBCs that do mature and enter the bloodstream are destroyed prematurely in the spleen, resulting in a concomitant anemia of increased RBC destruction (Kline, 2010; Rote & McCance, 2010a).

The severe anemia associated with beta-thalassemia major causes the kidneys to release **erythropoietin**, a hormone that stimulates the bone marrow to produce more RBCs. The resulting increase in hematopoiesis is ineffective, however, because of the increased rate of RBC destruction that is characteristic of the disorder. As a result of this process, the bone marrow eventually becomes hyperplastic. This **hyperplasia** (abnormal proliferation) of the bone marrow cells causes the bones themselves to enlarge in order to accommodate the increased bone marrow volume (Linker, 2009; Rote & McCance, 2010a).

Clinical Manifestations

Beta-thalassemia major typically manifests itself during the second six months of life when Hb F is replaced by Hb A. As they grow older, children with this disorder not only develop the signs and symptoms of severe anemia (Box 26-3),

TABLE 26-4 Clinical Manifestations of Beta-Thalassemia Major

MANIFESTATIONS	UNDERLYING CAUSE
Facies of beta-thalassemia major:	Expansion of bones to accommodate hyperplastic marrow
Prominent and protruding forehead	
Maxillary prominence	
Wide-set eyes	
Flattened nose	
Pathologic fractures	Expansion of bones to accommodate hyperplastic marrow
Decreased bone mineralization	Expansion of bones to accommodate hyperplastic marrow
Malocclusion	Maxillary overgrowth
Splenic enlargement	Extramedullary hematopoiesis and increased hemolysis
Jaundice	Increased RBC hemolysis
Bronze coloring of the skin	Iron accumulation in the skin

Adapted from Kline, N. E. (2010). Alterations of hematologic function in children. In K. L. McCance & S. E. Huether (Eds.). *Pathophysiology: The biologic basis for disease in adults and children* (6th ed.). St. Louis, MO: Mosby, pp. 1062–1090; Linker, C. A. (2009). Blood disorders. In S. J. McPhee, M. A. Papadakis & L. M. Tierney (Eds.). Current medical diagnosis & treatment: 2009. Retrieved January 21, 2009, from http://www.accessmedicine.com/content.aspx?aID=5476.

but also exhibit numerous other manifestations associated with beta-thalassemia major (Table 26-4 and Figure 26-5). All these factors contribute to the impaired growth and development manifested by these children. If children with this disorder are not treated, they will die by the age of 5 to 6 years. This clinical course can be modified with transfusion therapy, which can increase life span by 1 to 2 decades. However, as will be discussed in the treatment section, severe symptoms of iron overload can develop (Kline, 2010; Linker, 2009).

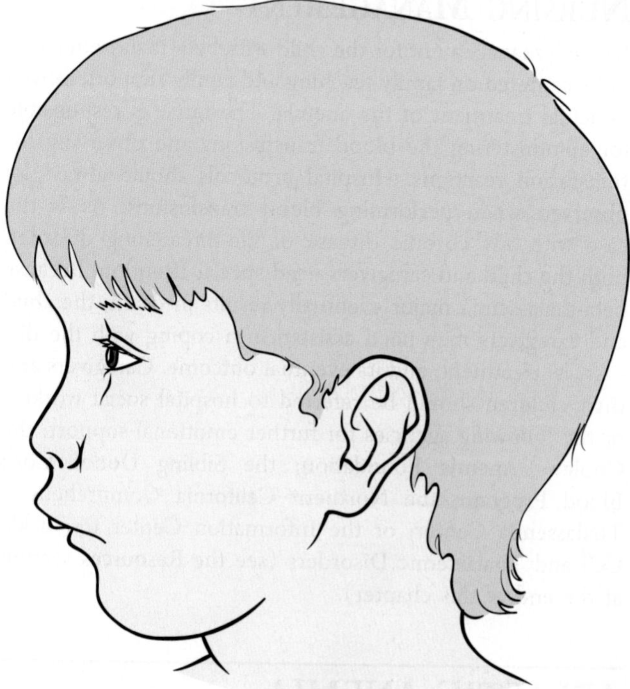

FIGURE 26-5 Facies of a Child with Beta-Thalassemia. DELMAR CENGAGE LEARNING.

DIAGNOSIS

The diagnosis of thalassemia is based on family disease history, clinical presentation, and laboratory findings. Thalassemia can be detected through specific newborn screening tests, which are collected according to state law. Prenatal diagnosis is also possible. The laboratory tests for children or adolescents suspected of having thalassemia are listed in Table 26-2, along with findings typically associated with beta-thalassemia major. One of the most striking laboratory findings is the extremely low hematocrit, which can fall to less than 10% of normal if not treated with transfusions. Thalassemia minor, however, often presents with an anemia so mild, it is mistaken for iron-deficiency anemia (Kline, 2010; Linker, 2009).

TREATMENT

Unlike thalassemia minor, which does not require any specific treatment, beta-thalassemia major requires medical intervention to support and prolong life. There is no cure for thalassemia, so the goal of treatment is to normalize the Hb and HCT of the child, thus alleviating the symptoms of severe anemia. This is accomplished via a regular schedule of transfusions, with many children requiring transfusions every 2 to 3 weeks. Along with these transfusions, a splenectomy is often performed because eliminating the site of hemolysis can decrease the child's need for frequent transfusions (CAF, 2009; Kline, 2010).

Repeated transfusions eventually result in a buildup of excess iron in the body, causing iron overload or **hemosiderosis.** In hemosiderosis, the excess iron is stored as hemosiderin in the cells of many organs and tissues, particularly in the liver and heart. Iron is toxic to the tissues and organs and eventually causes organ failure and death. This condition is exacerbated by the increased rate of hemolysis is present if the spleen has not been removed (CAF, 2009; Linker, 2009; McCance & Grey, 2010).

In order to reduce hemosiderosis, a chelating agent is given to reduce the amount of stored iron. A **chelating agent** is a drug used to either prevent or reverse the toxic effects of a heavy metal or to accelerate the elimination of the metal from the body. For many years the only iron-chelating agent available in the United States was Desferal (Deferoxamine) which has to be administered subcutaneously over 8–12 hours 5–7 days per week through a painful and difficult process (Box 26-7). An oral iron chelating drug, Exjade (Deferasirox), was approved in 2005 for use in the United States. This medication appears to be safe and effective in children over the age of 2 (Children's Hospital & Research Center Oakland [CHRCO], 2008; VanOrden & Hagemann, 2006). Exjade (deferasirox) is a tablet to be dissolved in water or juice and drunk orally, once per day. Adverse effects are relatively mild and transient and are most likely to include nausea, abdominal pain, diarrhea, and skin rash (VanOrden & Hagemann, 2006). In an attempt to eliminate the need for lifelong blood transfusions, both bone marrow transplants and cord blood transplants have been used in children with beta-thalassemia major. The goal of both interventions is to introduce healthy stem cells into the marrow so normal red blood cells and hemoglobin production will occur. Bone marrow transplantation is a difficult option because the bone marrow donor must be a genetic match, usually a family member (refer to Chapter 29). However, those children who find a suitable donor and who have not yet experienced iron overload or chronic organ toxicity experience long-term survival in more than 80% of cases. Cord blood transplants are similar to bone marrow transplants, except the stem cells are taken from the placenta or umbilical cord of a suitable donor. These donors do not have to be as close genetically; there appears to be a lower probability of rejection in this type of treatment (CHRCO, 2008; Linker, 2009).

BOX 26-7
POTENTIAL SIDE EFFECTS OF DESFERAL

- Hypotension with rapid IV infusion
- Orange-red colored urine
- Flushing
- Blotchy erythema
- Intestinal irritation
- Urticaria
- Pulmonary complications with infusion >24 hrs
- Neurotoxicity after long-term therapy

Adapted from Kosnett, J. J. (2001). Heavy metal intoxication & chelators. In B. G. Katzung (Ed.), *Basic and clinical pharmacology* (8th ed., pp. 999–1010). New York: McGraw-Hill.

Reflections from Families

When Anna was diagnosed with beta-thalassemia major, I was devastated. My husband and I had no idea that we carried the gene for this disease, but that is the only way she could have gotten it. I hate to think it is my fault that Anna is so sick, but it is. She needs blood transfusions every three weeks now, but even those harm her body. I do not know how much longer she will live, but I am trying to cherish every moment I have with her.

Nursing Management

Nursing management for the child with beta-thalassemia major is centered on family teaching and family support, as well as actual treatment of the anemia. The nurse is responsible for administering the blood transfusions and observing for transfusion reactions. Hospital protocols should always be observed when performing blood transfusions. As is the case with any chronic disease or life-threatening disorder, both the child and caregivers need special attention. Because beta-thalassemia major eventually results in death, the child and caregivers may need assistance in coping with the disease, its treatment, and its eventual outcome. Caregivers and their children should be referred to hospital social workers or the following agencies for further emotional support: the Cooley's Anemia Foundation; the Sibling Donor Cord Blood Program; the Northern California Comprehensive Thalassemia Center; or the Information Center for Sickle Cell and Thalassemic Disorders (see the Resources section at the end of this chapter).

APLASTIC ANEMIA

Aplastic anemia is a condition wherein injury to or abnormal expression of the stem cells in the bone marrow results in the production of inadequate numbers of erythrocytes, leukocytes, and platelets.

Incidence and Etiology

Aplastic anemia can be categorized as either hereditary or acquired. The hereditary form of aplastic anemia, **Fanconi's anemia** (FA), is a rare autosomal recessive disorder that develops early in life and is accompanied by multiple congenital abnormalities (see Figure 26-2). FA should be suspected in all children and adolescents with aplastic anemia, especially if they have any birth defects. Acquired aplastic anemia can be either idiopathic or due to secondary causes. Idiopathic aplastic anemia is rare in children and adolescents, and for this reason, secondary causes should always be investigated in these age groups (Rote & McCance, 2010b).

The most common cause of aplastic anemia is autoimmune suppression of blood cell production. The toxins and pharmacological agents implicated in the development of this disorder are listed in Box 26-8. They each cause direct stem cell injury, but using appropriate dosages and monitoring blood levels when using these agents are generally effective in preventing aplastic anemia. In rare instances, aplastic anemia has resulted from abnormal responses to appropriate doses of these substances. In addition to toxins and pharmacological agents, factors such as radiation, chemotherapy, and infections are also known to play a role in the development of this condition. Of the implicated infections, viral infections are the most common. The severity of the infection does not predict the severity of the resulting anemia (Linker, 2009; Rote & McCance, 2010b).

The incidence of aplastic anemia in the world is relatively rare, with two per million in the West and about two or three times higher rates in Asia (Young, Calado, & Scheinberg, 2006). The onset of acquired aplastic anemia is dependent on exposure to the causal factor. The onset of FA is quite variable, with some infants demonstrating symptoms at birth and other individuals going into their fifth decade of life before a diagnosis is made. The median age of diagnosis of FA is 8–9 years of age (Freedman, 2007). Following onset, the progression of aplastic anemia may be gradual or rapid, with the severity defined by laboratory values. Without treatment, children with at least three of the four criteria for severe aplastic anemia have a median survival rate of three months (Box 26-9). Only 20% of children with this disorder will survive for one year (Linker, 2009).

Pathophysiology

In the fetus, hematopoiesis occurs in the liver and the spleen. After birth, however, hematopoiesis normally occurs only in the bone marrow. Within the marrow, the stem cells, from which all blood cells originate, proliferate and differentiate into the cellular components of the blood. If these stem cells are abnormal, as is the case with aplastic anemia, the body experiences **pancytopenia**, a condition in which all three types of blood cells are either decreased or absent. The life span of each type of blood cell affects the rate of reduction experienced by that cellular line. Thus, RBCs are the last to demonstrate a reduction in number because of their relatively long life span (Rote & McCance, 2010b).

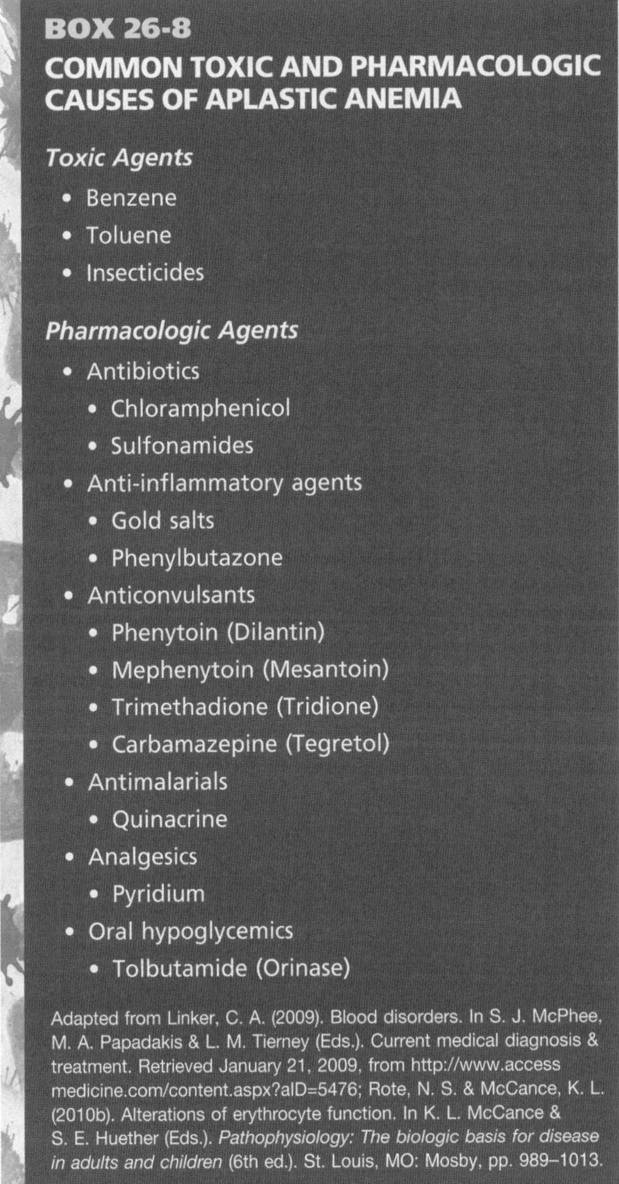

BOX 26-8
COMMON TOXIC AND PHARMACOLOGIC CAUSES OF APLASTIC ANEMIA

Toxic Agents

- Benzene
- Toluene
- Insecticides

Pharmacologic Agents

- Antibiotics
  - Chloramphenicol
  - Sulfonamides
- Anti-inflammatory agents
  - Gold salts
  - Phenylbutazone
- Anticonvulsants
  - Phenytoin (Dilantin)
  - Mephenytoin (Mesantoin)
  - Trimethadione (Tridione)
  - Carbamazepine (Tegretol)
- Antimalarials
  - Quinacrine
- Analgesics
  - Pyridium
- Oral hypoglycemics
  - Tolbutamide (Orinase)

Adapted from Linker, C. A. (2009). Blood disorders. In S. J. McPhee, M. A. Papadakis & L. M. Tierney (Eds.). Current medical diagnosis & treatment. Retrieved January 21, 2009, from http://www.accessmedicine.com/content.aspx?aID=5476; Rote, N. S. & McCance, K. L. (2010b). Alterations of erythrocyte function. In K. L. McCance & S. E. Huether (Eds.). *Pathophysiology: The biologic basis for disease in adults and children* (6th ed.). St. Louis, MO: Mosby, pp. 989–1013.

Clinical Manifestations

Although the age of onset varies, the clinical manifestations of both FA and acquired aplastic anemia are similar in all age groups and directly related to the decrease in each of the three cell types. Typically, the first sign noted is increased bruising caused by the decreased number of platelets. After this, the child becomes more vulnerable to infection because of the decreased number of WBCs. Once the RBCs have decreased in number, the signs and symptoms of anemia begin to manifest themselves. These typically begin with pallor, weakness, and difficulty breathing, and proceed as shown in Box 26-3. Children with aplastic anemia will also experience impaired growth and development and may even develop acute myelogenous leukemia (Linker, 2009; Rote & McCance, 2010b).

Diagnosis

History and clinical manifestations are helpful in the diagnosis of aplastic anemia, but laboratory tests are essential. A CBC with differential will show pancytopenia, although not all cell lines will be reduced early in the development of the disorder. Other initial laboratory tests and their results are listed in Table 26-2. The definitive diagnosis must be based on a bone marrow biopsy, which will typically show hypocellular marrow, although all of the cells that are seen will appear normal. To differentiate FA from acquired aplastic anemia, bone marrow chromosome studies must be done (Linker, 2009).

Treatment

If the aplastic anemia is acquired, the first line of treatment is to alleviate the underlying disorder or prevent further exposure to the causal agent. Once this has been accomplished, or if FA is present, the effects of pancytopenia may need to be treated. If any symptoms of bleeding are present or the platelet count is less than 10,000 cells/mL, platelet transfusions are used to increase the number of platelets in circulation. If the symptoms of anemia interfere with normal functioning, packed RBCs should be administered to increase the Hb level. If a fever develops in a child with decreased numbers of WBCs, an intensive work-up should be initiated in conjunction with administering broad-spectrum antibiotics (Teo & Dror, 2006).

For children with acquired aplastic anemia, remission can generally be achieved with either a bone marrow transplant or immunosuppressive therapy. If a suitable donor can be found, bone marrow transplantation is a very effective treatment for aplastic anemia. In previously untransfused children and young adults with an HLA-matched sibling, the durable complete response rate exceeds 80% (Linker, 2009). Slightly less effective is the use of antithymocyte globulin combined with cyclosporine to suppress the immune system. Together these drugs selectively attack the immune response and can alter the course of aplastic anemia if the aplastic anemia is caused by an autoimmune process. If effective, this treatment increases blood counts within three months. However, in as many as 25% of children will relapse after discontinuation of immunosuppressant therapy and will need to continue cyclosporine for several years (Hord, 2007). While cyclosporine has been shown to promote remission in clients, it has the potential for many toxic side effects (Box 26-10). Most cyclosporine side effects are manageable with dose reduction (Young, Calado, & Scheinberg, 2006).

The only potential cure for FA is a bone marrow transplant. Unfortunately, the chemotherapy or irradiation associated with the procedure may accelerate the development of cancer. For this reason, this method of treatment must be considered with caution. The other common treatment option for children with FA is androgen therapy. The most commonly given androgen is oxymetholone. The recommended dosage is 2–5 mg/kg each day and may cause obstructive liver disease, hepatitis, or liver tumors. Most clients respond to the treatment and relapse if the treatment is discontinued. Often the child develops resistance to the androgen being administered and must change to another androgen. On average, this treatment approach can prolong the life of a child with FA for a few years. Corticosteroids are often given in conjunction with the androgens in order to decrease bleeding and counteract the accelerated growth stimulation of the androgens (Dror, 2006).

BOX 26-9
CRITERIA FOR SEVERE APLASTIC ANEMIA

Severe Aplastic Anemia

- Neutrophils < 500 mcg
- Platelets < 20,000 mcg
- Reticulocytes < 1%
- Bone Marrow Cellularity < 20%

Adapted from Linker, C. A. (2009). Blood disorders. In S. J. McPhee, M. A. Papadakis & L. M. Tierney (eds.), *Current medical diagnosis & treatment: 2009*. Retrieved January 21, 2009, from http://www.accessmedicine.com/content.aspx?aID=5476.

Nursing Management

The nursing management for a child with aplastic anemia begins with assessment of the child for potential health care needs. This assessment should include observation for any of the signs and symptoms of anemia listed in Box 26-3 in addition to observation for excessive bruising. A baseline temperature should be recorded and the child monitored for any fever or signs and symptoms of infection. The nurse is also responsible for implementing and teaching precautions for preventing infection including proper hand washing, aseptic technique, and adequate fluid intake. Hospital care of a child with aplastic anemia may include the administration of platelets or other blood products (see Beta-Thalassemia section), or bone marrow transplantation (see Chapter 29). Because this is a life-threatening illness, the emotional needs of both the child and the family should also be assessed. The child or other family members may need education about aplastic anemia, reassurance, or just

BOX 26-10
COMMON SIDE EFFECTS OF CYCLOSPORINE

- Hypertension
- Excessive body hair
- Gingival hypertrophy
- Hyperkalemia
- Nephrotoxicity

Adapted from Furst, D. E., & Ulrich, R. W. (2007). Nonsteroidal anti-inflammatory drugs, disease-modifying antirheumatic drugs, nonopiod analgesics, and drugs used in gout. In B. G. Katzung (ed.), *Basic and clinical pharmacology* (10th ed.). New York: McGraw-Hill, pp. 573–598.

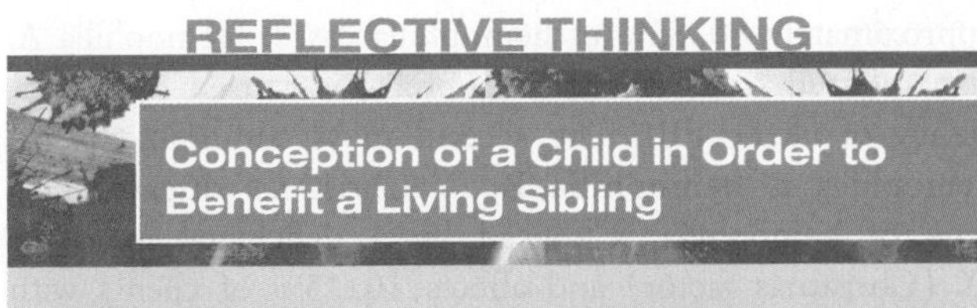

Conception of a Child in Order to Benefit a Living Sibling

Occasionally in the news we read about a family with a living child who needs a bone marrow transplant or another type of transplant. If a suitable donor cannot be found for the child, the family may choose to conceive another child in hopes of supplying the living child with a suitable donor for the transplant. What are your feelings about this?

a listening ear. Some of these needs can also be met by community agencies such as the Fanconi Anemia Research Fund or the Aplastic Anemia & MDS International Foundation (see the Resources section at the end of this chapter).

Family Teaching

If bone marrow transplantation occurs, caregivers can be a tremendous resource and support to their child if they understand each pre-procedure treatment and its rationale. The child will need to be hospitalized for approximately 1 month prior to the actual transplant to provide adequate time to pharmacologically suppress the child's immune system. The rationale is to ensure all diseased cells are destroyed, and any immunity that could adversely affect the donor marrow is also eliminated. To achieve immune depletion, the child will receive very large doses of cyclophosphamide. If the child has already received a number of blood transfusions, total body irradiation will be performed. This severe immunosuppression carries with it a number of risks including infection, stomatitis, diarrhea, and skin breakdown. However, a successful transplant will result in the child's own bone marrow beginning to produce normal cells.

Because the most common type of transplant is allogenic, with a relative serving as the donor, caregivers also need to be educated about the procedures involved in being a donor. The donor, often a sibling, is placed under general anesthesia, and several bone marrow aspirates are taken, usually from the hip area. The donor is then recovered as a typical postoperative client. The bone marrow aspirates are washed and irradiated, then transfused to the recipient in a manner similar to a blood transfusion.

DISORDERS OF COAGULATION

Coagulation is the main mechanism of **hemostasis** (control of bleeding) and is vital in maintaining blood volume, pressure, and flow through injured vessels. The three integral components in this effort are the platelets, the clotting factors, and the vasculature. When a blood vessel is injured, it undergoes endothelial sloughing in order to expose the subendothelial tissue. The platelets are then attracted to this tissue and adhere to the vessel wall. Following adhesion, platelets release biochemical mediators such as serotonin and histamine to direct platelet activity and promote temporary vasoconstriction. The vasoconstriction minimizes blood loss and is followed by vasodilation so WBCs can be transported to the site of injury. The platelets then aggregate into plugs, which are stabilized by blood clot formation. Blood clots are made up of fibrin strands that form around the plug and trap other blood cells. **Fibrin** is a protein that is formed through a series of reactions called the coagulation cascade. The coagulation cascade involves numerous blood clotting factors and can be initiated by either damage to body tissues or vessel walls (Figure 26-6). Although fibrin is created only

	Intrinsic Pathway Activated by damage to blood vessels	**Extrinsic pathway** Activated by damage to body tissues
Phase 1:	Sequence of enzymatic reactions involves factors listed below in the order listed: 1) Factor XII 2) Factor XI 3) Factor IX 4) Factor VIII 5) Factor X	Sequence of enzymatic reactions involves factors listed below in the order listed: 1) Factor VII 2) Factor X

The last step of phase 1 for each pathway leads to phase 2 and the Common Pathway

	Common Pathway
Phase 2:	Prothrombin activator complex facilitates Prothrombin → Thrombin
Phase 3:	Thrombin facilitates Fibrinogen → Fibrin

Figure 26-6 The Coagulation Cascade. Adapted from Kline, N. E. (2010). Alterations of hematologic function in children. In K. L. McCance & S. E. Huether (Eds.). *Pathophysiology: The biologic basis for disease in adults and children* (6th ed.). St. Louis, MO: Mosby, pp. 989–1013; McCance, K. L. (2010). Structure and function of the hematologic system. In K. L. McCance & S. E. Huether (Eds.). *Pathophysiology: The biologic basis for disease in adults and children* (6th ed.). St. Louis, MO: Mosby, pp. 952–988.

when an injury occurs, all clotting factors, in addition to prothrombin and fibrinogen, circulate continually in the blood of healthy individuals (Rote & McCance, 2010a).

Conditions that alter the delicate balance of platelets, clotting factors, and vasculature can have effects ranging from bruising to life-threatening illness. Within this portion of the chapter the etiology and treatment of the following coagulation disorders are discussed: hemophilia, von Willebrand's disease, immune thrombocytopenic purpura, and disseminated intravascular coagulation. Both hemophilia and von Willebrand's disease involve a decrease in specific factors necessary for coagulation. Immune thrombocytopenic purpura is characterized by a decreased number of platelets. In disseminated intravascular coagulation, the normal mechanisms that regulate coagulation are ineffective.

HEMOPHILIA

The **hemophilias** are a group of bleeding disorders in which one factor in the first phase of coagulation is deficient.

Incidence and Etiology

The most common type of hemophilia, **hemophilia A**, occurs in approximately 1 in 5,000 males and accounts for approximately 80–85% of hemophilia cases. Hemophilia A, also referred to as classic hemophilia, is caused by a deficiency of factor VIII. The second most common type of hemophilia is **hemophilia B**, or Christmas disease. This type of hemophilia is caused by a deficiency in factor IX (Christmas factor) and affects 10–15% of clients with hemophilia. The least common type of hemophilia is **hemophilia C**, a factor XI deficiency (Kline, 2010; Scott & Montgomery, 2007). Each type of hemophilia impairs the body's ability to control bleeding and can result in fatal hemorrhage. With proper monitoring and the use of prophylactic treatment, however, children with hemophilia can lead relatively normal lives.

Both hemophilia A and hemophilia B are X-linked recessive disorders (Figure 26-7). Because the female genotype consists of two X chromosomes, a female would need two recessive genes for disease expression to occur. Males, however, only have one X chromosome and, therefore, the possession of just one recessive hemophilia gene results in disease expression. Hence, a female can only have the disorder when both the mother and the father have the recessive gene. A male, however, only needs to have a mother who carries the gene in order for the disease to be expressed in his phenotype. For this reason, hemophilia is much more commonly expressed in males. One exception is

(A) When the mother is a carrier for the disease, there is a 50% chance each child conceived will not have nor carry the disease. There is a 25% chance each child conceived will carry the disease and a 25% chance each child conceived will have the disease.

	Y	X
X	XY 25% Normal (Male)	XX 25% Normal (Female)
x	xY 25% Disease (Male)	Xx 25% Carrier (Female)

(B) When the father has the disease, there is a 50% chance each child conceived will not have the disease or carry the disease and a 50% chance each child conceived will carry the disease.

	Y	x
X	XY 25% Normal (Male)	Xx 25% Carrier (Female)
X	XY 25% Normal (Male)	Xx 25% Carrier (Female)

Legend
x = Recessive disease gene
X or Y = Dominant normal gene
xx or xY = Disease state
Xx = Carrier state
YX or XX = Normal state

Figure 26-7 X-Linked Recessive Inheritance. DELMAR CENGAGE LEARNING.

hemophilia C, an autosomal recessive disorder that occurs equally in males and females (Kline, 2010).

Pathophysiology

Although there are several different types of gene deletions and mutations that can cause hemophilia, the genetic alteration appears to be the same among members of a given family and, therefore, the severity of symptoms among family members is typically very similar. In each child with hemophilia, regardless of the cause, there is either a missing or a deficient clotting factor. This factor, whether it is VIII, IX, or XI, is an integral part of the coagulation cascade and, as such, enables the body to create adequate fibrin for clot formation to repair damaged blood vessels (see Figure 26-6). Hence, a decreased amount, or the complete absence of any factor, impairs or completely prevents the body from forming clots (Kline, 2010).

Clinical Manifestations

The clinical manifestations of hemophilia A and hemophilia B vary, depending on the concentration of clotting factor VIII or IX in the blood. The three levels of severity, along with their associated frequency of bleeding episodes, are listed in Table 26-5. Generally, hemophilia C is less severe than either hemophilia A or hemophilia B, and presents with only mild bleeding (Kline, 2010).

During the first year of life spontaneous bleeding in hemophiliacs is rare, although injections or firm holding of the infant can result in **hematomas**, pockets of blood under the skin caused by excessive bleeding following trauma. As the child learns to walk he may bruise easily and bleed into his joints, a condition called **hemarthrosis**. By 3–4 years of age, episodes of persistent bleeding from minor lacerations occur in 90% of children with this disorder. Hemarthrosis continues to be a problem, causing pain and limited movement in the elbows, knees, and ankles. Hemarthrosis also predisposes the child to degenerative joint changes later in life. Other complications of hemophilia include minor occurrences of **hematuria** (blood in the urine) and **epistaxis** (nose bleed), as well as major events such as intracranial hemorrhage and bleeding into the neck or abdomen (Kline, 2010).

Diagnosis

After a client history or physical examination reveals evidence of excessive bleeding, several laboratory tests can be used to determine the presence of hemophilia. These diagnostic tests and the results typically associated with hemophilia are listed in Table 26-6. Often the type of hemophilia present is determined by using the thromboplastin generation test, which can precisely identify deficiencies of factors VIII and IX. A positive family history of hemophilia can also lead to testing asymptomatic children in order to determine carrier status (Kline, 2010).

Treatment

The treatment of hemophilia A consists mainly of replacing the missing coagulation factor through infusion of recombinant factor VIII concentrates. The advent of recombinant factor concentrates replaced the previously used plasma-derived products in 1989. The new recombinant factor concentrates are similar in their treatment effect without the danger of transmitting diseases such as HIV or hepatitis to the recipient. The amount of recombinant factor concentrate given varies with the severity of the hemophilia, must be calculated for each child's situation, and is routinely given when excessive bleeding or hemarthrosis occurs. For many children, prophylactic treatment is administered three or four times a week. This preventive approach, which is started after the child manifests hemarthrosis, is generally effective in preventing spontaneous bleeding. As the child ages, caregivers can be taught to administer the factor concentrates at home. This is more convenient for the child and caregiver and allows for immediate administration following an injury (Kline, 2010; Scott & Montgomery, 2007).

For many pediatric clients with mild hemophilia A, desmopressin acetate (Stimate) has proven to be an effective treatment for spontaneous bleeding and is also effective in preventing excessive bleeding when administered prior to dental or surgical procedures. Responses to desmopressin

Table 26-5 Classifying the Severity of Hemophilia A and Hemophilia B

	CONCENTRATION OF CLOTTING FACTOR VIII OR IX IN THE BLOOD	OCCURRENCE OF EXCESSIVE BLEEDING
Mild	5–35% of normal	Only after severe trauma or surgery
Moderate	1–5% of normal	Only after trauma
Severe	Less than 1% of normal	Spontaneously

Adapted from Kline, N. E. (2010). Alterations of hematologic function in children. In K. L. McCance & S. E. Huether (Eds.). *Pathophysiology: The biologic basis for disease in adults and children* (6th ed.). St. Louis, MO: Mosby, pp. 1062–1090.

TABLE 26-6 Common Laboratory Tests and Findings for Coagulation Disorders

LABORATORY TEST	NO DISORDER PRESENT	HEMOPHILIA	VON WILLEBRAND'S DISEASE	ITP	DIC
Platelet count—measures the number of platelets in the blood	See Appendix E	Normal	Normal	Decreased	Decreased
Standard bleeding time (Ivy Method)—evaluates the vascular and platelet factors	1–9 minutes	Normal	Prolonged	Prolonged	Prolonged
Prothrombin time (PT or INR)—evaluates the extrinsic system and common pathway of coagulation	11.0–12.5 sec	Normal	Normal	Normal	Prolonged
Partial thromboplastin time (PTT)—evaluates the intrinsic system and common pathway of coagulation	60–90 sec	Prolonged	Prolonged	Normal	Prolonged

Adapted from Wilson, D. D. (2008). *McGraw-Hill's manual of laboratory & diagnostic tests.* New York: McGraw-Hill.; Kee, J. L. (2009). *Prentice Hall handbook of laboratory and diagnostic tests with nursing implications* (6th ed.). Upper Saddle River, NJ: Pearson Prentice Hall.

vary considerably and a therapeutic trial is necessary to determine the adequacy of the treatment for a specific child. The recommended dosage for bleeding disorders is one intranasal spray (1.5 mg) for young children under 50 kg and increases to one spray in each nostril for adolescents over 50 kg. IV doses of 0.3 mcg/kg can also be given. Potential side effects are mild and include headache, flushing, low sodium levels, and slight alterations in heart rate or blood pressure. Low sodium levels are a rare complication, but can cause seizures. Consequently, fluid intake should be monitored (Scott & Montgomery, 2007; Zehnder, 2007).

Because of the propensity of children with hemophilia to experience mucosal bleeding, antifibrinolytic agents such as aminocaproic acid (Amicar) or tranexamic acid (Cyklokapron) may be used following dental extractions. These medications inhibit the breakdown of fibrin and thereby delay the degradation of blood clots. The agents are administered for 7–10 days following the procedure and are generally effective in preventing recurrent bleeding from the site. Potential side effects include thrombosis, hypotension, muscle wasting, abdominal discomfort, diarrhea, and nasal stuffiness (Casella, Takemoto, & Pelidis, 2006; Zehnder, 2007).

The treatment of hemophilia B is similar to that of hemophilia A, except factor IX concentrates are given instead of factor VIII concentrates. The factor concentrates currently in use for hemophilia B are plasma-derived, but treated to reduce the likelihood of disease transmission. Desmopressin is not an effective treatment for clients with hemophilia B and subsequently should not be used (Scott & Montgomery, 2007). Aggressive treatment of hemophilia C is rarely necessary because of the mild nature of the disease. Instead, these clients should be given supportive therapy and education about how to control minor bleeding episodes.

NURSING ALERT

Child with Hemophilia

If a child with hemophilia is showing signs and symptoms of neurological impairment such as irritability, altered level of consciousness, or vomiting, the child may have an intracranial bleed and should be taken to the hospital immediately. If head trauma occurs, a child with hemophilia should be treated as if he or she were experiencing an intracranial bleed, even if the child does not manifest these signs or symptoms.

VON WILLEBRAND'S DISEASE

Von Willebrand's disease is the most common congenital disorder of homeostasis. It is a genetic disorder in which **von Willebrand's factor** (vWF), a protein that facilitates adhesion between platelets and injured vessels, is either deficient or defective.

INCIDENCE AND ETIOLOGY

This deficiency of normal vWF results in a mild bleeding disorder that is rarely as severe as hemophilia. It is estimated 1% of the population may have this disorder, but many are undiagnosed because of the mildness of their symptoms. Therefore, the prognosis for von Willebrand's disease is excellent (Casella, Takemoto, & Pelidis, 2006; Linker, 2009; Scott & Montgomery, 2007).

CASE STUDY / CARE PLAN

CHILD WITH HEMOPHILIA TYPE A

Spencer is an 18-month-old diagnosed with hemophilia type A during the neonatal period. He was circumcised shortly after birth and noted to have prolonged bleeding from the site. He has moderate hemophilia and has received frequent factor infusions because of falls and subsequent hemarthrosis. His caregivers now want to learn how to better manage and cope with his illness.

NURSING CARE PLAN

ASSESSMENT

The main focus of nursing assessment in this instance is to determine the history of the child's illness and the current knowledge level of his caregivers. The history should focus on: (1) any factors that precipitated the child's bleeding episodes; (2) the frequency of the bleeding episodes; and (3) how bleeding episodes have been managed in the past. Finally, the child and caregiver need to be given the opportunity to express any emotional concerns that they may have in relation to the child's illness. While having this discussion, the nurse should observe for any behaviors that indicate the child's and caregivers' level of coping.

NURSING DIAGNOSIS 1

Ineffective tissue perfusion related to bleeding episodes.

EXPECTED OUTCOMES

1. Caregivers will be able to prevent bleeding episodes.
2. Caregivers will be able to manage mild bleeding episodes.
3. Caregivers will be able to manage an episode of hemarthrosis.

NOC: Circulation Status; Pain Control

NIC: Hemodynamic Regulation; Pain Management

INTERVENTIONS/*RATIONALES*

1. Educate caregivers about the following strategies to prevent bleeding episodes:
   - Make the home and play environment as safe and clutter-free as possible. *Minimizes accidental injuries and falls during time when the child is learning to ambulate.*
   - Provide close supervision during the toddler years. *Prevents the child from engaging in dangerous activities.*
   - Pad the crib and playpen. *Allows for safer play and prevention of injury from accidental falls.*
   - Use protective equipment while the child learns to walk and when playing. *Prevents injuries to the joints and the head.*
   - As the child gets older, encourage participation in low contact sports such as swimming or tennis. *Prevents injuries to the joints and the head.*
   - Use soft-bristled toothbrushes, water picks, and so forth. *Prevents oral mucosal bleeding.*
   - Help the child maintain a healthy weight. *Prevents undue stress and strain on joints.*
2. Educate caregivers about the following interventions for a mild bleeding episode:
   - In preparation for bleeding episodes, contact the Medic Alert Foundation (see Resources section at the end of this chapter) and obtain a medic alert bracelet. *Ensures proper care and treatment of child in the event of a bleeding episode.*
   - Apply pressure to any bleed for 10 to 15 minutes. *Promotes clot formation.*
   - Immobilize and elevate the extremity where the bleed is occurring. *Decreases blood flow to the area of bleeding.*
   - Apply ice or cold to bleeding area. *Promotes vasoconstriction.*

(Continues)

CASE STUDY / CARE PLAN (Continued)

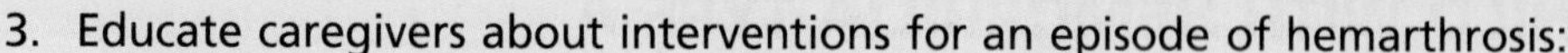

3. Educate caregivers about interventions for an episode of hemarthrosis:
   - Elevate and immobilize the affected extremity. *Decreases the amount of bleeding into the joint space.*
   - Provide pain relief for joint pain. *Allows for more feasible range of motion exercises without pain.*
   - Avoid taking aspirin. *Prevents the blood-thinning effects of aspirin from exacerbating the bleeding.*
   - Institute active range of motion exercises after 48 hours. *Prevents joint contractures.*

EVALUATION

After the nursing interventions have been completed, a follow-up visit with the family is necessary to assess the success of the interventions and the need for additional education. During this follow-up visit, the nurse should again elicit a history from the family and compare it to the baseline information collected before the interventions were started. If the desired outcomes have been met, this history will demonstrate the number of bleeding episodes has decreased and the family was able to manage any mild bleeding episodes or hemarthrosis that had occurred.

NURSING DIAGNOSIS 2

Interrupted family processes related to having a child with an inherited, potentially fatal disease.

EXPECTED OUTCOMES

1. The family members will be able to express an understanding of the disease process.
2. The family members will be able to cope effectively with the child's illness.

NOC: Knowledge: Disease Process; Family Coping
NIC: Teaching: Disease Process; Family Support

INTERVENTIONS/*RATIONALES*

1. Assess caregivers' knowledge of the disease process. *Aids in delivering appropriate teaching content.*
2. Teach family members appropriate content related to the disease process. *Facilitates understanding and acceptance of the diagnosis of hemophilia.*
3. Listen to and be aware of caregivers' feelings related to the disease, remembering that if they are Spencer's biological parents they may have feelings of guilt related to the transmission of the disease to him. *Provides the caregivers with an opportunity to express and work through their emotions.*
4. Refer caregivers to social workers or community agencies that can provide additional education and emotional support (see the Resources section at the end of this chapter). *Ensures proper support and resources are known to the family.*

EVALUATION

During the follow-up visit with the family, the nurse can determine if the desired outcomes have been reached by asking caregivers to explain the disease process. The nurse should also observe the caregivers for effective coping skills and the presence of guilt. A discussion of the caregivers' emotions regarding the child's illness may also be appropriate in order to assess their current level of coping and the need for further interventions.

As shown in Table 26-7, there are three major variants, with type I accounting for approximately 80% of cases. Both type I and type II are transmitted via autosomal dominant inheritance and affect males and females equally. With this method of genetic inheritance there can be no carriers (Figure 26-8). Type III von Willebrand's disease is a rare autosomal recessive disorder.

PATHOPHYSIOLOGY

When a person without von Willebrand's disease sustains injury to the wall of a blood vessel, the concentration of vWF in the area of the injury increases. This is important because vWF binds to the platelets and is essential in adhering them to the damaged vessel wall, one of the first steps of

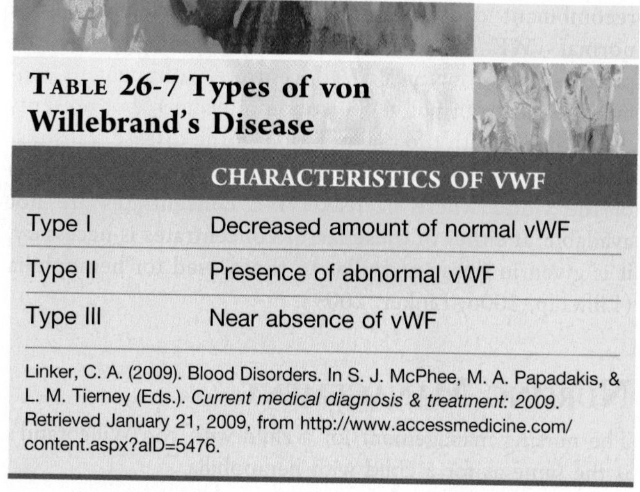

Table 26-7 Types of von Willebrand's Disease

	CHARACTERISTICS OF VWF
Type I	Decreased amount of normal vWF
Type II	Presence of abnormal vWF
Type III	Near absence of vWF

Linker, C. A. (2009). Blood Disorders. In S. J. McPhee, M. A. Papadakis, & L. M. Tierney (Eds.). *Current medical diagnosis & treatment: 2009*. Retrieved January 21, 2009, from http://www.accessmedicine.com/content.aspx?aID=5476.

clot formation. Hence, when vWF is not present in sufficient quantities or is dysfunctional, as in von Willebrand's disease, the body is unable to adequately form clots and control bleeding. In addition to its role in facilitating platelet adhesion, vWF also carries and protects factor VIII. For this reason, children with von Willebrand's disease may also experience secondary factor VIII deficiencies (Casella, Takemoto, & Pelidis, 2006).

Clinical Manifestations

Children with von Willebrand's disease, unlike those with hemophilia, usually do not experience spontaneous hemarthrosis. Rather, the most common types of bleeding are mucosal such as epistaxis, **ecchymoses** (bruises), and gingival bleeding. In females, abnormally long and heavy menstrual periods, referred to as **menorrhagia**, can also occur. Other possible bleeding manifestations include gastrointestinal bleeding and excessive bleeding following surgery or dental extractions. These manifestations commonly vary in severity over time, and are generally aggravated by the intake of aspirin and lessened by pregnancy or estrogen administration (Casella, Takemoto, & Pelidis, 2006; Linker, 2009).

Diagnosis

Because the manifestations of von Willebrand's disease are typically mild in nature, many families dismiss their increased

(A) When both parents are heterozygous for the disease, there is a 25% chance each child conceived will not have the disease and a 75% chance each child conceived will have the disease.

	B	b
B	BB 25% Disease	Bb 25% Disease
b	Bb 25% Disease	bb 25% Normal

(B) When one parent is heterozygous for the disease, there is a 50% chance each child conceived will not have the disease, and a 50% chance each child conceived will have the disease.

	b	b
B	Bb 25% Disease	Bb 25% Disease
b	bb 25% Normal	bb 25% Normal

Legend
b = Recessive normal gene
B = Dominant disease gene
bb = Normal state
Bb or bB = Heterozygous disease state
BB = Homozygous disease state

Figure 26-8 Autosomal Dominant Inheritance. DELMAR CENGAGE LEARNING.

incidence of epistaxis or ecchymoses as normal and do not seek medical attention. For this reason, many children with von Willebrand's disease remain undiagnosed until they bleed excessively following a surgical or dental procedure. In addition to the clinical manifestation characteristic of the disease, a family history is helpful in making the diagnosis. Because most cases of von Willebrand's disease are transmitted via autosomal dominant inheritance, there will almost always be a family history of excessive bleeding. Once a suspicion of von Willebrand's disease has been raised, laboratory tests can then be conducted to make a definitive diagnosis. The laboratory tests commonly used to assess bleeding disorders, along with the results typical for von Willebrand's disease, are listed in Table 26-6. In addition to these tests, immunoassays for vWF can further differentiate von Willebrand's disease from other bleeding disorders and determine which type of the disease is present (Casella, Takemoto, & Pelidis, 2006: Linker, 2009).

Treatment

The first line of treatment for type I, or mild type II, von Willebrand's disease is desmopressin. Desmopressin is believed to promote the release of stored vWF and should be given in the same dosages as for hemophilia A (refer to the Hemophilia section for dosages and side effects). In order to prevent depletion of the vWF stores, Desmopressin doses should not be given more often than 24 hours apart. Desmopressin should be avoided in type III von Willebrand's because of potentially adverse effects. As with hemophilia, antifibrinolytic agents such as Amicar or Cyklokapron may be used to control the bleeding associated with dental extractions (refer to the Hemophilia section) (Casella, Takemoto, & Pelidis, 2006; Linker, 2009). For clients who do not respond to desmopressin or who experience adverse reactions, plasma-derived vWF containing factor VIII concentrates or licensed vWF concentrates are used. Some (not all) of the newer, disease-free recombinant concentrates now have sufficient levels of normal vWF to be therapeutic. Cryoprecipitate is the plasma-derived factor VIII concentrate is thought to contain the most normal vWF protein molecules, but presents the recipient with the risk of blood-borne disease transmission. For this reason, cryoprecipitate is used only in areas of the world where licensed vWF concentrates are not available. If either of these factor concentrates is necessary, it is given in dosages similar to those used for hemophilia (Lillicrap, 2006; Linker, 2009).

NURSING TIP

Care of a Child Experiencing a Nosebleed

Blood coming from a child's nose can be a frightening experience for a caregiver and for the child. The most important thing to remember is to remain calm. Have the child sit up and lean forward. The child should not lean his or her head back because he or she could aspirate blood if the bleeding is profuse. The child should pinch his or her nose between two fingers and hold it with pressure for 10 minutes. This should stop the bleeding, but if it does not, the caregiver can apply ice to the bridge of the nose.

Nursing Management

The nursing management for a child with von Willebrand's is the same as for a child with hemophilia.

IMMUNE THROMBOCYTOPENIC PURPURA (ITP)

As the name suggests, the thrombocytopenic purpuras are a group of acquired diseases characterized by thrombocytopenia and purpura. **Thrombocytopenia** is a decrease in the platelet count below 150,000 mm^3 (see Appendix E for normal values in children) and **purpuras** are areas of blood underneath the skin or mucous membranes.

Incidence and Etiology

The thrombocytopenic purpuras are classified as either intrinsic or immune, depending on the cause of the symptoms. In children the most common form is **immune thrombocytopenic purpura** (ITP). This disease was formerly called idiopathic thrombocytopenic purpura, but has since been found to be an autoimmune disorder. Consequently, the name was changed to reflect this discovery. ITP can occur at any age, but the peak incidence in children is between 2 and 4 years of age. The ITP of children differs from the ITP

Table 26-8 Different Presentations of ITP in Children and Adults

CHILDREN	ADULTS
Generally preceded by viral infection	Rarely preceded by a viral infection
Usually self-limiting	Usually chronic (>6 months)
Affects males and females equally	Females affected 2–3 times more often than males

Adapted from Rote, N. S., & McCance, K. L. (2010c). Alterations of leukocyte, lymphoid, and hemostatic function. In K. L. McCance & S. E. Huether (Eds.). *Pathophysiology: The biologic basis for disease in adults and children* (6th ed.). St. Louis, MO: Mosby, pp. 1014–1061.

BOX 26-11
VIRUSES ASSOCIATED WITH ITP

- Cytomegalovirus (CMV)
- Epstein-Barr virus (EBV)
- Human immunodeficiency virus (HIV)
- Parovirus
- Viral respiratory infection

Adapted from Kline, N. E. (2010). Alterations of hematologic function in children. In K. L. McCance & S. E. Huether (Eds.). *Pathophysiology: The biologic basis for disease in adults and children* (6th ed.). St. Louis, MO: Mosby, pp. 1062–1090.

of adults in several ways (Table 26-8). Because of these differences, the prognosis for children is excellent, even without therapy. Approximately 75% of children recover completely in three months. Within six months of onset, 80–90% of affected children have regained normal platelet counts (Kline, 2010; Rote & McCance, 2010c; Tcheng, 2008b).

Pathophysiology

One of the essential components of maintaining hemostasis is the process whereby the platelets adhere to injured vessel walls, release biochemical mediators, and form plugs. Through these actions, platelets block the many minute ruptures occurring daily in the microcirculation. When there are inadequate numbers of platelets, these ruptures are not repaired, resulting in purpura under the skin and throughout the tissues. In ITP the inadequate supply of platelets results from an autoimmune process, which in approximately 70% of ITP cases is triggered by a viral infection (Box 26-11). Once the autoimmune process has been triggered, antiplatelet antibodies bind to the platelets, causing them to become sequestered and destroyed prematurely in the spleen. This increased rate of platelet destruction exceeds the bone marrow's ability to create new platelets, resulting in a decreased platelet count. No other blood cell types are affected by this process (Kline, 2010; Rote & McCance, 2010c).

Clinical Manifestations

The most common presentation of ITP is one of acute onset. With this presentation, ecchymoses and a general petechial rash (small purpuras) will often occur 1–4 weeks following the viral infection. The child's presenting complaint is often spontaneous bleeding of the skin or hemorrhagic blisters of the mucous membranes. Asymmetrical bleeding is typical, especially on the legs and trunk. Bleeding in gastrointestinal or urinary tracts may occur. Nose bleeding may also be present and difficult to control. These are the only manifestations of ITP, and the child otherwise appears healthy. The spontaneous hemorrhage of the acute stage lasts for 1 to 2 weeks and is associated with a platelet count below 20,000 mm^3. In some children the onset is more gradual with clinical manifestations of moderate bleeding and a few petechiae (small purpuras). The most severe complication is intracranial hemorrhage, which occurs in only 1% of patients (Kline, 2010; Tcheng, 2008b).

Diagnosis

The diagnosis is based on history, clinical presentation, and laboratory tests. The child's history should be examined for other causes of thrombocytopenia such as aspirin or heparin use. The child's clinical presentation will also demonstrate the signs and symptoms discussed previously. Enlargement of the liver, spleen, or lymph nodes suggests other causes of thrombocytopenia such as leukemia or HIV infection. The common laboratory tests and findings for a child with ITP are listed in Table 26-6. Other than the platelet count, all CBC values should be normal. A peripheral blood smear will reveal very few platelets, with normal amounts of all other cell types. The platelets seen on the smear will be large and more immature. A bone marrow aspiration will appear normal, although there may be increased numbers of megakaryocytes, the precursor cells of platelets (Kline, 2010; Tcheng, 2008b).

Treatment

Because ITP in children is generally a self-limiting condition with excellent prognosis, treatment is largely supportive. Children and their caregivers should receive information on how to prevent injury or trauma and control bleeding episodes (see Nursing Management section). If severe symptoms are present, the severity and duration of the initial acute phase may be lessened by administering medications that suppress the immune system. These medications, listed in Box 26-12, decrease the autoimmune process and thereby

BOX 26-12
IMMUNOSUPPRESSIVE MEDICATIONS USED IN ITP

- Prednisone
- Vincristine (Oncovin)
- Cyclophosphamide (Cytoxan)
- Mercaptopurine (Purinethol)
- Azathioprine (Imuran)
- Gamma globulin
- Danazol (Danocrine)
- Cyclosporine (Sandimmune)

Adapted from Lake, D. F., Briggs, A. D., & Akporiaye, E. T. (2007). Immunopharmacology. In B. G. Katzung (Ed.). *Basic and clinical pharmacology* (10th ed.). New York: McGraw-Hill, pp. 908–933; Linker, C. A. (2009). Blood disorders. In S. J. McPhee, M. A. Papadakis & L. M. Tierney (Eds.). *Current medical diagnosis & treatment: 2009.* Retrieved January 21, 2009, from http://www.accessmedicine.com/content.aspx?aID=5476.

Reflections from Families

Last winter it seemed like my daughter Rose Ann was always getting sick. Every few weeks she had something new and I was starting to get used to it. About 2 weeks after one of her illnesses, I noticed she had several blood blisters. I was immediately worried and thought Rose Ann might have something very serious—like cancer. I took her to the doctor and was relieved to find out she had a disease called ITP. It was difficult to see her suffer until the disease resolved on its own three months later, but it was much better than a diagnosis of something potentially terminal.

decrease the destruction of platelets. Of these medications, prednisone is the drug of choice, followed by intravenous immunoglobulin. The other medications are used only when these two safer alternatives are ineffective. Splenectomy is reserved for children with chronic ITP who do not respond to less invasive interventions. Because of the short life span of platelets, transfusion of fresh blood or platelets is ineffective unless life-threatening hemorrhage is present (Kline, 2010; Lake, Briggs, & Akporiaye, 2007; Rote & McCance, 2010c).

Nursing Management

Nursing management for the child with ITP centers mainly on educating the child and caregivers about preventing injury and managing bleeding episodes. The amount of activity restriction placed on the child depends on illness severity, but the child should be given the opportunity to help decide what the restrictions will be. This will help the child understand and comply. The use of safety equipment should be emphasized to prevent trauma and bleeding. Aspirin should not be taken since it may aggravate the bleeding. If an external bleeding episode occurs, the area should be elevated while pressure is applied for at least ten minutes. Application of ice to the area will further reduce the amount of bleeding. The child and caregivers should also be taught to recognize the signs and symptoms of internal bleeding: pallor, altered level of consciousness, and increased pulse. If any manifestations occur, the child should be seen by a physician. Children with ITP and their families can also be referred to the National Organization for Rare Disorders; the NIH/National Heart, Lung and Blood Institute Information Center; and the Genetic Alliance for additional information and support (see Resources section at the end of this chapter).

DISSEMINATED INTRAVASCULAR COAGULATION (DIC)

Disseminated intravascular coagulation (DIC) is a coagulation disorder in which the stimulus for coagulation overwhelms the control mechanisms that normally confine coagulation to the area of bleeding. This sequence of events can lead to either an acute and potentially life-threatening process of ischemia and hemorrhage, or a chronic and low-grade condition of mild hemorrhage and microcirculatory thrombosis.

Incidence and Etiology

A variety of precipitating factors can over stimulate the coagulation mechanism and cause DIC. Of these factors, which are listed in Box 26-13, infection and sepsis are the most common. Any time a child or adolescent is very ill with one of these conditions, he or she is at risk for DIC (Rote & McCance, 2010; Scott & Montgomery, 2007).

Pathophysiology

When one of the precipitating factors listed in Box 26-13 abnormally stimulates the first stage of the coagulation process, thrombin is generated in greater amounts than can be neutralized by the body. This excess thrombin leads to excessive conversion of fibrinogen to fibrin, leading to excessive clot formation (see Figure 26-6). As this process continues, blood clots can eventually obstruct the blood vessels, causing ischemia, infarction, and necrosis. This necrotic tissue damage then activates the coagulation cascade and stimulates the formation of more clots. As more and more clots are formed, the components of the clotting process are consumed at an accelerated pace. The depletion of platelets and coagulation factors leads to thrombocytopenia and hemorrhage. The presence of numerous clots also triggers the release of factors to dissolve the clots. The by-products of this process are potent anticoagulants that exacerbate the hemorrhage. This process continues until the initial precipitating factor is removed or the child is treated with the appropriate therapeutic interventions (Rote & McCance, 2010c; Scott & Montgomery, 2007).

Clinical Manifestations

Depending on the intensity of the precipitating stimulus and the intensity of the damage incurred by the endothelium and

BOX 26-13

CAUSES OF DISSEMINATED INTRAVASCULAR COAGULATION

Sepsis

- Especially gram-negative bacteria

Any widespread infection

- Bacterial
- Fungal
- Protozoal
- Viral

Severe tissue injury

- Especially burns and head injury

Obstetric complications

- Abruptio placentae
- Amniotic fluid embolus
- Septic abortion
- Retained fetus

Cancer

- Acute promyelocytic leukemia
- Mucinous adenocarcinomas

Major hemolytic transfusion reactions

- Anaphylaxis

Hypotension or hypoxia

- Shock
- Cardiopulmonary arrest

Snake bites

- Snake venom

Organ injury

- Pancreatitis
- Liver disease

Adapted by Rote, N. S., & McCance, K. L. (2010c). Alterations of leukocyte, lymphoid, and hemostatic function. In K. L. McCance & S. E. Huether (Eds.). *Pathophysiology: The biologic basis for disease in adults and children* (6th ed.). St. Louis, MO: Mosby, pp. 1014–1061; Scott, J.P. & Montgomery, R.R. (2007). Hemorrhagic and thrombotic diseases. In R. M. Kliegman, R. E. Behrman, H. B. Jenson & B. F. Stanton (Eds.). *Nelson textbook of pediatrics* (18th ed.). Philadelphia, PA: Saunders, pp. 2060–2066.

BOX 26-14

CLINICAL MANIFESTATIONS OF ORGAN DAMAGE IN DIC

- Altered level of consciousness
- Behavioral changes
- Mental activity changes
- Confusion
- Seizure activity
- Oliguria
- Hematuria
- Hypoxia
- Hypotension
- Coughing up blood
- Chest pain
- Tachycardia

Adapted from Rote, N. S., & McCance, K. L. (2010c). Alterations of leukocyte, lymphoid, and hemostatic function. In K. L. McCance & S. E. Huether (Eds.). *Pathophysiology: The biologic basis for disease in adults and children* (6th ed.). St. Louis, MO: Mosby, pp. 1014–1061.

tissues, the clinical presentation of DIC can be either acute or chronic. The acute form is associated with massive hemorrhage and thrombosis. This is manifested by oozing from venipuncture sites, arterial lines, or surgical sites. Bleeding may also occur in the nose, gums, and sclera or conjunctiva of the eyes. Typically the bleeding will be apparent in at least three unrelated sites and will be accompanied by purpura, petechiae, and hematomas. Bleeding can also occur in closed compartments of the body but will often be less obvious. The damage resulting from thrombosis may be localized to one organ or generalized to many organs. The organ systems most commonly damaged are the cardiovascular, pulmonary, central nervous, renal, and hepatic systems. The resulting alterations in organ function cause a variety of clinical manifestations (Box 26-14). If not treated, children with acute DIC can also develop end organ failure. Children with chronic DIC do not present with these overt manifestations of hemorrhage and thrombosis because the pathological mechanisms are partially compensated for by the body. Instead these children experience mild hemorrhage and thrombosis confined to the microcirculation. As a result, these children may present with confusion, jaundice, hypoxia, and **oliguria** (a decreased ability to form and excrete urine) (Rote & McCance, 2010c; Scott & Montgomery, 2007).

Diagnosis

A diagnosis of DIC is based on the clinical manifestations already discussed, in addition to several laboratory findings. The preliminary tests used to distinguish between various bleeding disorders are listed in Table 26-6, along with the findings typically associated with DIC. Because no one test exists to definitively diagnose DIC, a combination of several laboratory findings needs to be used. Additional tests may include serum fibrinogen levels, which will be decreased, and measures of fibrin degradation products (D-dimer), which will be increased (Rote & McCance, 2010c; Scott & Montgomery, 2007).

Treatment

The first step in treating acute DIC is identification and correction of the underlying cause. The next step, replacement therapy, provides the client with adequate amounts of platelets, fibrinogen, and possibly coagulation factors. The platelets are replaced via platelet transfusion. Cryoprecipitate administration is effective in increasing fibrinogen levels (see von Willebrand's disease for a discussion of cryoprecipitate). The liver generally is able to restore coagulation factors, but fresh-frozen plasma can be used for replacement if necessary. The use of heparin in the treatment of DIC is controversial, but if given, it should be administered in conjunction with the replacement of these coagulation components (Rote & McCance, 2010c; Scott & Montgomery, 2007).

Nursing Management

The nursing management for a child with DIC takes place in an intensive care setting and involves assessment, the administration of blood products, and supportive care. Because of the potential for severe hemorrhage, the nurse must frequently assess for overt bleeding, manifestations of internal bleeding such as pallor and tachycardia, and signs and symptoms of shock (see Box 26-6). The administration of blood products should be done in accordance with hospital policy (see Beta-Thalassemia section). The supportive role of the nurse focuses on the anxiety and fear likely to be present in both the child and caregivers. Some nursing interventions that can help calm the child and their caregivers are to: (1) explain all procedures to the family; (2) allow the child to make choices about care when possible; (3) encourage open conversation about the situation; and (4) offer to listen to and address the family's questions and concerns.

IN THE REAL WORLD

When I entered nursing school, I never imagined that there were so many children in the prosperous country of America whose health care needs were not being met. Before I started working with poor families in the clinics, I thought that those individuals with inadequate nutrition either chose not to or did not know any better. Now I know that even with education many families cannot provide the nutrition necessary to keep their children healthy. I have also learned a great deal about the difficulties faced by children trying to find suitable bone marrow donors. It seems amazing that with our advanced system of medical care we are unable to match potential donors and recipients more efficiently, but that is a reality that many potential recipients must face.

KEY CONCEPTS

- Human blood has two major components: plasma and formed elements.
- The formed elements of the blood include red blood cells, white blood cells, and platelets.
- During fetal development blood cells are produced in the liver and spleen. After birth new blood cells are synthesized from stem cells in the bone marrow.
- red blood cells, white blood cells, and platelet counts vary with age.
- Iron-deficiency anemia, the most common pediatric hematological disorder, occurs when there is not enough iron available for adequate hemoglobin production and can usually be treated with age-appropriate dietary modification and oral iron supplementation.
- Sickle cell anemia, a genetic disorder, is characterized by red blood cells that undergo sickling and cause an anemia of increased red blood cell destruction.
- Beta-thalassemia major, a genetic disorder resulting in altered hemoglobin formation, causes a life-threatening anemia requiring regular blood transfusions to sustain life.
- Aplastic anemia can be either an inherited or an acquired disorder characterized by altered stem cells in the bone marrow. The resulting pancytopenia may need treatment with platelet

transfusions, red blood cell transfusions, or broad spectrum antibiotics.

- Hemophilia A is an inherited coagulation disorder in which there is a deficiency of coagulation factor VIII. The episodes of excessive bleeding that result from this deficiency are treated with either recombinant factor VIII concentrates or desmopressin.
- Von Willebrand's disease is the most common pediatric coagulation disorder. This genetic disorder is characterized by a deficiency of von Willebrand's factor, which causes a mild anemia that is often undiagnosed. If necessary, desmopressin or licensed vWF concentrates can be used for treatment.
- Immune thrombocytopenic purpura is an autoimmune disease wherein the platelets are destroyed prematurely. The associated bleeding is usually mild enough to only require supportive treatment, and spontaneous resolution generally occurs in affected children within a few months of onset.
- Disseminated intravascular coagulation occurs when a stimulus for coagulation overwhelms the control mechanisms that normally confine coagulation to the area of bleeding, resulting in a potentially life-threatening combination of hypercoagulation and hemorrhage. Treatment may include platelet transfusion, cryoprecipitate administration, and the use of fresh-frozen plasma.

REVIEW ACTIVITIES

1. Which of the anemias are inherited disorders?
2. Describe the signs and symptoms associated with mild anemia, moderate anemia, and severe anemia.
3. Discuss the most common cause of iron-deficiency anemia in young children and adolescents, in school-age children, and in children living in third-world countries.
4. What are ten points discussed when educating a child or caregiver about iron supplementation and dietary modification for iron-deficiency anemia?
5. Describe the type of hemoglobin characteristic of sickle cell disease. What change does it cause in the red blood cells?
6. Describe five situations that could cause red blood cells to sickle in a child with sickle cell anemia. Which syndrome is usually the first manifestation of sickle cell disease in an infant?
7. What treatment is necessary to sustain the life of a child with beta-thalassemia disease?
8. What condition develops after repeated blood transfusions? How is it treated?
9. Which cells are affected by aplastic anemia?
10. What condition may occur in the joints of a child with hemophilia?
11. What should a child or caregiver do to stop a bleeding episode in a child with hemophilia or von Willebrand's disease?
12. Describe the most common coagulation disorder in children. How severe is this condition?
13. What cells are destroyed in immune thrombocytopenic purpura? What manifestations result?
14. How is immune thrombocytopenic purpura treated?
15. Describe the two paradoxical conditions present in disseminated intravascular coagulation.

STUDY QUESTIONS

1. A man and woman both test positive for the sickle cell trait. The couple asks the nurse how many of their children with have sickle cell disease. The nurse understands that when both parents carry the sickle cell trait gene:
   a. Out of four children, only one will have the sickle cell disease.
   b. Only male children will be affected.
   c. All of their children will carry the sickle cell trait.
   d. Each pregnancy will have a 25% chance of having the disease.
2. A 6-year-old child has been admitted to the emergency department with the diagnosis of vaso-occlusive crisis. What should the nurse anticipate as a priority medical intervention?

a. IV pain medications and IV fluids
b. CBC and IV fluids
c. IV antibiotics and oxygen
d. Transfuse platelets

3. The nurse identifies which group as being most at risk for developing iron-deficiency anemia?
a. School-aged children enrolled in an after-school program
b. Breast-fed infants under the age of 6 months
c. Children ages 6 months to 2 years of age
d. 3- to 5-year-old children in daycare five days a week

4. An important nursing intervention for the prevention of infection in a child with sickle disease includes which of the following?
a. Encouraging compliance of regular exchange transfusions
b. Administering hepatitis b and pneumococcal vaccines
c. Explaining the importance of frequent urination
d. Preparing the child for IV replacement therapy

5. A mother of a 3-month-old infant newly diagnosed with sickle cell anemia asks the nurse why her baby does not have any symptoms. The nurse understands that most newborns are asymptomatic because:
a. Newborns have sufficient maternal stores of iron.
b. Newborns have a higher percentage of HbF.
c. Newborns' blood is relatively high in water content.
d. Newborns have immature liver function.

6. The nurse is caring for a 5-year-old hemophiliac complaining of knee pain. The nurse understands that hemarthrosis predisposes the child to long-term joint dysfunction. What is an important nursing intervention?
a. Starting active range of motion exercises
b. Administering aspirin for pain relief
c. Appling heat to the affected joint
d. Immobilizing and elevating the extremity

7. A child is admitted with immune thrombocytopenic purpura (ITP). What will the nurse anticipate the history to include?
a. Petechial rash following a viral infection
b. Frequent urinary tract infections
c. Recent transfusion of platelets
d. Recent aspirin use

8. The nurse is caring for a child with septicemia in the intensive care unit and notices blood oozing from around the arterial line. The nurse would suspect which of the following?
a. Hand-foot syndrome
b. Aplastic anemia
c. Hemosiderosis
d. Disseminated intravascular coagulation

9. The nurse is performing a well-baby checkup on a 12-month-old infant. What finding would be of most concern?
a. Cannot walk yet
b. Has increased bruising
c. Eating less variety of foods
d. Straining during bowel movements

10. Which of the following foods are a good dietary sources of iron? Check all that apply.
a. Meat
b. Red potatoes
c. Whole grains
d. Green beans
e. Canned peaches
f. Raisins
g. Seafood

REFERENCES

Anand, K., Lakshmy, R., Janakarajan, V. N., Ritvik, A., Misra, P., Pandey, R. M., Kapoor, S. K., Sankar, R., & Bulusu, S. (2006). Effect of consumption of micronutrient fortified candies on the iron and vitamin A status of children aged 3–6 years in rural Haryana. *Indian Pediatrics, 44*, 823–829.

Brawley, O. W., Cornelius, L. J., Edwards, L. R., Northingtion Gamble, V., Green, B. L., Intuisi, C., & Schori, M. (2008). National institutes of health consensus development conference statement: Hydroxyurea treatment for sickle cell disease. *Annuals of Internal Medicine, 148*, 932–938.

Brotanek, J. M., Gosz, J., Weitzman, M., & Flores, G. (2007). Iron-deficiency in early childhood in the United States: Risk factors and racial/ethnic disparities. *Pediatrics, 120*, 568–575.

Burden, M. J., Westerlund, A. J., Armony-Sivan, R., Nelson, C. A., Jacobson, S. W., Lozoff, B., Angelille, M., & Jacobson, J. L. (2007). An event-related potential study of attention and recognition memory in infants with iron-deficiency anemia. *Pediatrics, 120*, e336–e345.

Casella, J. F., Takemoto, C. M., & Pelidis, M. A. (2006). Disorders of coagulation factors. In J. A. McMillan, R. D. Feigin, C. D. DeAngelis, & M. D. Jones, Jr., (Eds.). *Oski's pediatrics* (4th ed.). Philadelphia: Lippincott Williams & Wilkins, pp. 1737–1748.

Centers for Disease Control and Prevention (2007). *Iron Deficiency*. Retrieved August 13, 2010, from http://www.cdc.gov/nutrition/everyone/basics/vitamins/iron.html.

Chaparro, C. M. (2008). Setting the stage for child health and development: Prevention of iron-deficiency in early infancy. *American Society for Nutrition, 138*, 2529–2533.

Children's Hospital & Research Center Oakland. (2008). Standards of care guidelines for thalassemia. Retrieved January 24, 2010, from http://www.thalassemia.com/documents/thalhandbook2008.final.pdf.

Cooley's Anemia Foundation. (2009). What is thalassemia? Retrieved January 23, 2009, from http://www.thalassemia.org/sections.php?option=com.content&view=article&id=19<emid=27#5.

Cusick, S. E., Mei, Z., & Cogswell, M. E. (2007). Continuing anemia prevention strategies are needed throughout early childhood in low-income preschool children. *The Journal of Pediatrics, 150*, 422–428.

Cusick, S. E., Mei, Z., Freedman, D. S., Looker, A. C., Ogden, C. L., Gunter, E., & Cogswell, M. E. (2008). Unexplained decline in the prevalence of anemia among U.S. children and women between 1988–1994 and 1999–2002. *American Journal of Clinical Nutrition, 88*, 1611–1617.

DeBaun, M. R., & Vichinsky, E. (2007). Hemoglobinopathies. In R. M. Kliegman, R. E. Behrman, H. B. Jenson, & B. F. Stanton (Eds.). *Nelson textbook of pediatrics* (18th ed.). Philadelphia, PA: Saunders, pp. 2023–2031.

Dror, Y. (2006). Inherited bone marrow failure syndromes. In R. J. Arceci, I. M. Hann, & O. P. Smith (Eds.). *Pediatric hematology* (3rd ed.). Malden, MA: Blackwell, pp. 30–63.

Dunn, A. M. (2008). Nutrition. In C. E. Burns, A. D. Dunn, M. A. Brady, N. B. Starr, & C. G. Blosser (Eds.). *Pediatric primary care* (4th ed.). St. Louis, MO: Saunders Elsevier, pp. 191–234.

Freedman, M. H. (2007). The pancytopenias. In R. M. Kliegman, R. E. Behrman, H. B. Jenson, & B. F. Stanton (Eds.). *Nelson textbook of pediatrics* (18th ed.). Philadelphia, PA: Saunders, pp. 2047–2053.

Furst, D. E., & Ulrich, R. W. (2007). Nonsteroidal anti-inflammatory drugs, disease-modifying antirheumatic drugs, nonopiod analgesics, and drugs used in gout. In B. G. Katzung (Ed.). *Basic and clinical pharmacology* (10th ed.). New York: McGraw-Hill, pp. 573–598.

Heeney, M., & Dover, G. J. (2009). Sickle cell disease. In S. H. Orkin, D. G. Nathan, D. Ginsburg, A. T. Look, D. E. Fisher, & S. E. Lux (Eds.). *Nathan and Oski's hematology of infancy and childhood* (7th ed.). Philadelphia, PA: Saunders Elsevier, pp. 949–1014.

Hord, J. D. (2007). The acquired pancytopenias. In R. M. Kliegman, R. E. Behrman, H. B. Jenson, & B. F. Stanton (Eds.). *Nelson textbook of pediatrics* (18th ed.). Philadelphia, PA: Saunders, pp. 2053–2060.

Hui, W. T., & Grover, G. (2008). Nutritional needs. In C. D. Berkowitz (Ed.). *Pediatrics: A primary care approach* (3rd ed.). Elk Grove Village, IL: American Academy of Pediatrics, pp. 63–69.

Kee, J. L. (2009). *Prentice Hall handbook of laboratory and diagnostic tests with nursing implications* (6th ed.). Upper Saddle River, NJ: Pearson Prentice Hall.

Kline, N. E. (2010). Alterations of hematologic function in children. In K. L. McCance & S. E. Huether (Eds.). *Pathophysiology: The biologic basis for disease in adults and children* (6th ed.). St. Louis, MO: Mosby, pp. 989–1013.

Kosnett, J. J. (2001). Heavy metal intoxication & chelators. In B. G. Katzung (Ed.). Basic and clinical pharmacology (8th ed.). New York: McGraw-Hill, pp. 999–1010.

Krishnamurti, L., Landord, L., & Munoz, R. (2007). Life-threatening parvovirus B19 and herpes simplex virus associated acute myocardial dysfunction in a child with homozygous sickle disease. *Pediatric Blood & Cancer, 49*, 1019–1021.

Lake, D. F., Briggs, A. D., & Akporiaye, E. T. (2007). Immunopharmacology. In B. G. Katzung (Ed.). *Basic and clinical pharmacology* (10th ed.). New York: McGraw-Hill, pp. 908–933.

Lillicrap, D. (2006). von Willebrand disease. In R. J. Arceci, I. M. Hann, & O. P. Smith (Eds.). *Pediatric hematology* (3rd ed.). Malden, MA: Blackwell, pp. 598–607.

Linker, C. A. (2009). Blood Disorders. In S. J. McPhee, M. A. Papadakis, & L. M. Tierney (Eds.). *Current medical diagnosis & treatment: 2009*. Retrieved January 21, 2009, from http://www.accessmedicine.com/content.aspx?aID=5476.

Masters, S. B. (2007). Drugs used in anemias: Hematopoietic growth factors. In B. G. Katzung (Ed.). *Basic and clinical pharmacology* (10th ed.). New York: McGraw-Hill, pp. 527–541.

McCance, K. L. (2010). Structure and function of the hematologic system. In K. L. McCance & S. E. Huether (Eds.). *Pathophysiology: The biologic basis for disease in adults and children* (6th ed.). St. Louis, MO: Mosby, pp. 952–988.

McCance, K. L., & Grey, T. C. (2010). Altered cellular and tissue biology. In K. L. McCance & S. E. Huether (Eds.). *Pathophysiology: The biologic basis for disease in adults and children* (6th ed.). St. Louis, MO: Mosby, pp. 46–95.

McMahon, C. (2006). Sickle cell disease. In R. J. Arceci, I. M. Hann, & O. P. Smith (Eds.). *Pediatric hematology* (3rd ed.). Malden, MA: Blackwell, pp. 213–230.

Mitchell, M. J., Lemanek, K., Palermo, T. M., Crosby, L. E., Nichols, A., & Powers, S. W. (2007). Parent perspectives on main management, coping, and family function in pediatric sickle cell disease. *Clinical Pediatrics, 46*(4), 311–319.

Platt, O. S. (2008). Hydroxyurea for the treatment of sickle cell anemia. *The New England Journal of Medicine, 358*, 1362–1369.

Polhamus, B., Dalenius, K., Borland, E., Smith, B., & Grummer-Strawn, L. (2007). *Pediatric nutrition surveillance 2006 report.* Atlanta: U.S. Department of Health and Human Services, Centers for Disease Control and Prevention.

Rote, N. S., & McCance, K. L. (2010a). Structure and function of the hematologic system. In K. L. McCance & S. E. Huether (Eds.). *Pathophysiology: The biologic basis for disease in adults and children* (6th ed.). St. Louis, MO: Mosby, pp. 952–988.

Rote, N. S., & McCance, K. L. (2010b). Alterations of erythrocyte function. In K. L. McCance, & S. E. Huether (Eds.). *Pathophysiology: The biologic basis for disease in adults and children* (6th ed.). St. Louis, MO: Mosby, pp. 989–1013.

Rote, N. S., & McCance, K. L. (2010c). Alterations of leukocyte, lymphoid, and hemostatic function. In K. L. McCance & S. E. Huether (Eds.). *Pathophysiology: The biologic basis for disease in adults and children* (6th ed.). St. Louis, MO: Mosby, pp. 1014–1061.

Scott, J. P., & Montgomery, R. R. (2007). Hemorrhagic and thrombotic diseases. In R. M. Kliegman, R. E. Behrman, H. B. Jenson, & B. F. Stanton (Eds.). *Nelson textbook of pediatrics* (18th ed.). Philadelphia, PA: Saunders, pp. 2060–2066.

Strouse, J. J., Lanzkron, S., Beach, M. C., Haywood, C., Park, H., Witkop, C., & Segal, J. B. (2008). Hydroxyurea for sickle cell disease: A systematic review for efficacy and toxicity in children. *Pediatrics, 122*, 1332–1342.

Tcheng, W. Y. (2008a). Anemia. In C. D. Berkowitz (Ed.). *Pediatrics: A primary care approach* (3rd ed.). Elk Grove Village, IL: American Academy of Pediatrics, pp. 411–418.

Tcheng, W. Y. (2008b). Bleeding Disorders. In C. D. Berkowitz (Ed.). *Pediatrics: A primary care approach* (3rd ed.). Elk Grove Village, IL: American Academy of Pediatrics, pp. 419–426.

Teo, A., & Dror, Y. (2006). Acquired aplastic anemia. In R. J. Arceci, I. M. Hann, & O. P. Smith (Eds.). *Pediatric hematology* (3rd ed.). Malden, MA: Blackwell, pp. 64–76.

U.S. Department of Health and Human Services. (2004). *The management of sickle cell disease* (NIH Publication No. 02-2117). Bethesda, MD: National Institutes of Health.

VanOrden, H. E., & Hagemann, T. M. (2006). Deferasirox: An oral agent for chronic iron overload. *The Annals of Pharmacotherapy, 40,* 1110–1117.

Wardlaw, G. M., & Hampl, J. (2006). *Perspectives in nutrition* (7th ed.). Boston: McGraw-Hill.

Wilson, D. D. (2008). *McGraw-Hill's manual of laboratory & diagnostic tests.* New York: McGraw-Hill.

Young, K. D. (2008). Shock. In C. D. Berkowitz (Ed.), *Pediatrics: A primary care approach* (3rd ed.). Elk Grove Village, IL: American Academy of Pediatrics, pp. 265–270.

Young, N. S., Calado, R. T., & Scheinberg, P. (2006). Current concepts in the pathophysiology and treatment of aplastic anemia. *Blood, 108,* 2509–2519.

Zehnder, J. L. (2007). Drugs used in disorders of coagulation. In B. G. Katzung (Ed.). *Basic and clinical pharmacology* (10th ed.). New York: McGraw-Hill, pp. 542–559.

SUGGESTED READINGS

Beard, J. L. (2008). Why iron-deficiency is important in infant development, *The Journal of Nutrition, 138,* 2534–2540.

Blanchette, V., & Bolton-Maggs, P. (2008). Childhood immune thrombocytopenic purpura: Diagnosis and management. *Pediatric Clinics of North America, 55,* 393–420.

Chang, T. T. (2008). Transfusion therapy in critically ill children. *Pediatrics and Neonatology, 49,* 5–12.

Frempong, T., & Pearson, H.A. (2007). Newborn screening coupled with comprehensive follow-up reduced early mortality of sickle cell disease in Connecticut. *Connecticut Medicine, 71,* 9–12.

Hankins, J., Hinds, P., Day, S., Carroll, Y., Li, C-S., Garvie, P., & Wang, W. (2006). Therapy preference and decision making among patients with severe sickle cell anemia and their families. *Pediatric Blood & Cancer, 48,* 705–710.

Hoots, W. K., & Nugent, D. J. (2006). Evidence for the benefits of prophylaxis in the management of hemophilia A. *Thrombosis and Haemostasis, 96,* 433–440.

Iannotti, L. L., Tielsch, J. M., Black, M. M., & Black, R. E. (2006). Iron supplementation in early childhood; Health benefits and risks. *American Journal of Clinical Nutrition, 84,* 1261–1275.

Karras, N. A., & Hemenway, C. S. (2007). Hurricane Katrina's impact on pediatric and adult patients with sickle cell disease. *Journal of Health Care for the Poor & Underserved, 18,* 382–393.

King, A. A., DeBaun, M. R., & White, D. A. (2008). Need for cognitive rehabilitation for children with sickle cell disease and strokes. *Expert Review of Neurotherapeutics, 8,* 291–296.

Kosnett, J. J. (2001). Heavy metal intoxication & chelators. In B. G. Katzung (Ed.). *Basic and clinical pharmacology* (8th ed., pp. 999–1010). New York: McGraw-Hill.

Kullip, S., Bennett, J. M., & Chambers, M. D. (2007). Iron-deficiency anemia. *American Family Physician, 75,* 671–678.

Lozoff, B. (2007). Iron-deficiency and child development. *Food and Nutrition Bulletin, 28,* S560–S571.

Lozoff, B., Beard, J., Connor, J., Felt, B., Georgieff, M., & Schallert, T. (2006). Long-lasting neural and behavioral effects of iron-deficiency in infancy. *Nutrition Review, 64,* S34–S91.

Lutter, C. K. (2008). Iron-deficiency in young children in low-income countries and new approaches for its prevention. *American Society for Nutrition, 138,* 2523–2528.

Maguire, J. L., deVeber, G., & Parkin, P. C. (2007). Association between iron-deficiency anemia and stroke in young children. *Pediatrics, 120,* 1053–1057.

McClain, B. C. (2007). Pediatric palliative care: A novel approach to children with sickle cell disease. *Pediatrics, 119,* 612–614.

Morris, P. J. (2008). Physical activity recommendations for children and adolescents with chronic disease. *Current Sports Medicine Reports, 7,* 353–358.

Robertson, J., Lillicrap, D., & James, P. D. (2008). Von willebrand disease. *Pediatric Clinics of North America, 55,* 377–392.

Schatz, J., & Roberts, C. W. (2006). Neurobehavioral impact of sickle cell disease in early childhood. *Journal of the International Neuropsychological Society, 13,* 933–943.

Sherry, D. D. (2008). Avoiding the impact of musculoskeletal pain on quality of life in children with hemophilia. *Orthopaedic Nursing, 27,* 103–108.

Sutcliffe, T., Kambalia, A., Westergard, S., Jacobson, S., Peer, M., & Parkin, P. (2006). Iron depletion is associated with daytime bottle-feeding in the second and third years of life. *Archives of Pediatric & Adolescent Medicine, 106,* 1114–1120.

Valentino, L. A., & Oza, O. M. (2006). Blood safety and the choice of anti-hemophilic factor concentrate. *Pediatric Blood & Cancer, 47,* 245–254.

Will, A. M. (2006). Disorders of iron metabolism: Iron deficiency, iron overload and the sideroblastic anemias. In R. J. Arceci, I. M. Hann, & O. P. Smith (Eds.). *Pediatric hematology* (3rd ed.). Malden, MA: Blackwell, pp. 79–104.

RESOURCES

Refer to the online student StudyWARE for Potts & Mandleco at http://www.CengageBrain.com for additional content and study aids.

Organization: **American Association of Blood Banks**
Description: Offers information regarding blood and cellular therapies, blood donation, and blood programs/services.
Website/Resource: http://www.aabb.org

Organization: **American Sickle Cell Anemia Association**
Description: Offers information regarding Sickle Cell Anemia Association programs/services, FAQs, and donations.
Website/Resource: http://www.ascaa.org

Organization: **Aplastic Anemia & MDS International Foundation, Inc.**

Description: Provides readers with information regarding clinical trials, news, calendar, and diseases/drugs related to aplastic anemia, myelodysplastic syndromes, paroxysmal nocturnal hemoglobinuria, and related bone marrow failure diseases.

Website/Resource: http://www.aamds.org

Organization: **Canadian Hemophilia Society**

Description: Strives to improve health/quality of life/find a cure for people with inherited bleeding disorders; website provides information regarding research/treatment centers/educational materials.

Website/Resource: http://www.hemophilia.ca

Organization: **Center for Sickle Cell Disease**

Description: Committed to goals including medical care, research, testing, education, counseling and community outreach; provides information regarding patient services/research/education/faculty/staff.

Website/Resource: http://www.sicklecell.howard.edu

Organization: **Children's Cancer and Blood Foundation**

Description: Supports clinical care of children living with cancers/blood disorders, fosters research, sponsors fellowship training; provides information about medical conditions/news/support.

Website/Resource: http://www.childrenscbf.org

Organization: **Cooley's Anemia Foundation**

Description: Offers information regarding clinical trials, research, fundraising, and local chapters for people afflicted with various forms of thalassemia.

Website/Resource: http://www.thalassemia.org

Organization: **Fanconi Anemia Research Fund, Inc.**

Description: Provides information regarding research, family services, publications, and fundraising about Fanconi anemia.

Website/Resource: http://www.fanconi.org

Organization: **Genetic Alliance**

Description: Offers information regarding membership services, training, programs, policy advocacy, research, publications, and events related to genetics.

Website/Resource: http://www.geneticalliance.org

Organization: **Information Center for Sickle Cell and Thalassemic Disorders**

Description: Offers links to information on hemoglobin disorders, particularly sickle cell disease and thalassemia, as well as disorders of iron metabolism.

Website/Resource: http://sickle.bwh.harvard.edu

Organization: **Iron Disorders Institute, Inc.**

Description: Provides links for health care providers and patients to access information regarding iron disorders.

Website/Resource: http://www.irondisorders.org

Organization: **March of Dimes**

Description: Provides information regarding March of Dimes professionals/researchers, and pregnancy/newborn conditions.

Website/Resource: http://www.marchofdimes.com

Organization: **Medic Alert Foundation**

Description: Medic Alert (a 24-hour emergency response service that relays vital medical information to emergency responders); provides health information, access to online ID, and membership instruction.

Website/Resource: http://www.medicalert.org

Organization: **NIH/National Heart, Lung and Blood Institute Information Center (NHLBI)**

Description: Provides information regarding networks, research, clinical trials, careers/training, and education campaigns related to heart, lung, and blood conditions.

Website/Resource: http://www.nhlbi.nih.gov

Organization: **National Hemophilia Foundation**

Description: Provides information regarding coagulation disorders, blood product safety, advocacy, and educational conferences.

Website/Resource: http://www.hemophilia.org

Organization: **National Organization for Rare Disorders (NORD)**

Description: Offers access to information regarding research, programs/services, and news/current issues about rare disorders.

Website/Resource: http://www.rarediseases.org

Organization: **Northern California Comprehensive Thalassemia Center**

Description: Provides information regarding treating thalassemia, living with thalassemia, cultural and genetic significance, research, and support.

Website/Resource: http://www.thalassemia.com

Organization: **Sibling Donor Cord Blood Program**

Description: Provides basic information regarding cord blood donation; helps families who want to save umbilical cord blood for their children when there is a specific medical indication for banking.

Website/Resource: http://www.childrenshospitaloakland.org

Organization: **Sickle Cell Association of Ontario (SCAO)**

Description: Provides information regarding SCAO programs/services, news/events, and donations.

Website/Resource: http://www.sicklecellontario.com

Organization: **Sickle Cell Disease Association of America (SCOA)**

Description: Provides information regarding SCOA membership, educational opportunities, research, and news/events.

Website/Resource: http://www.sicklecelldisease.org

Organization: **Sickle Cell Information Center**

Description: Provides sickle cell patient and professional education, news, research updates, and worldwide sickle cell resources.

Website/Resource: http://www.scinfo.org

Organization: **Thalassemia Foundation of Canada**

Description: Provides information addressing program fundraisers, events, and research related to thalassemia

Website/Resource: http://www.thalassemia.ca

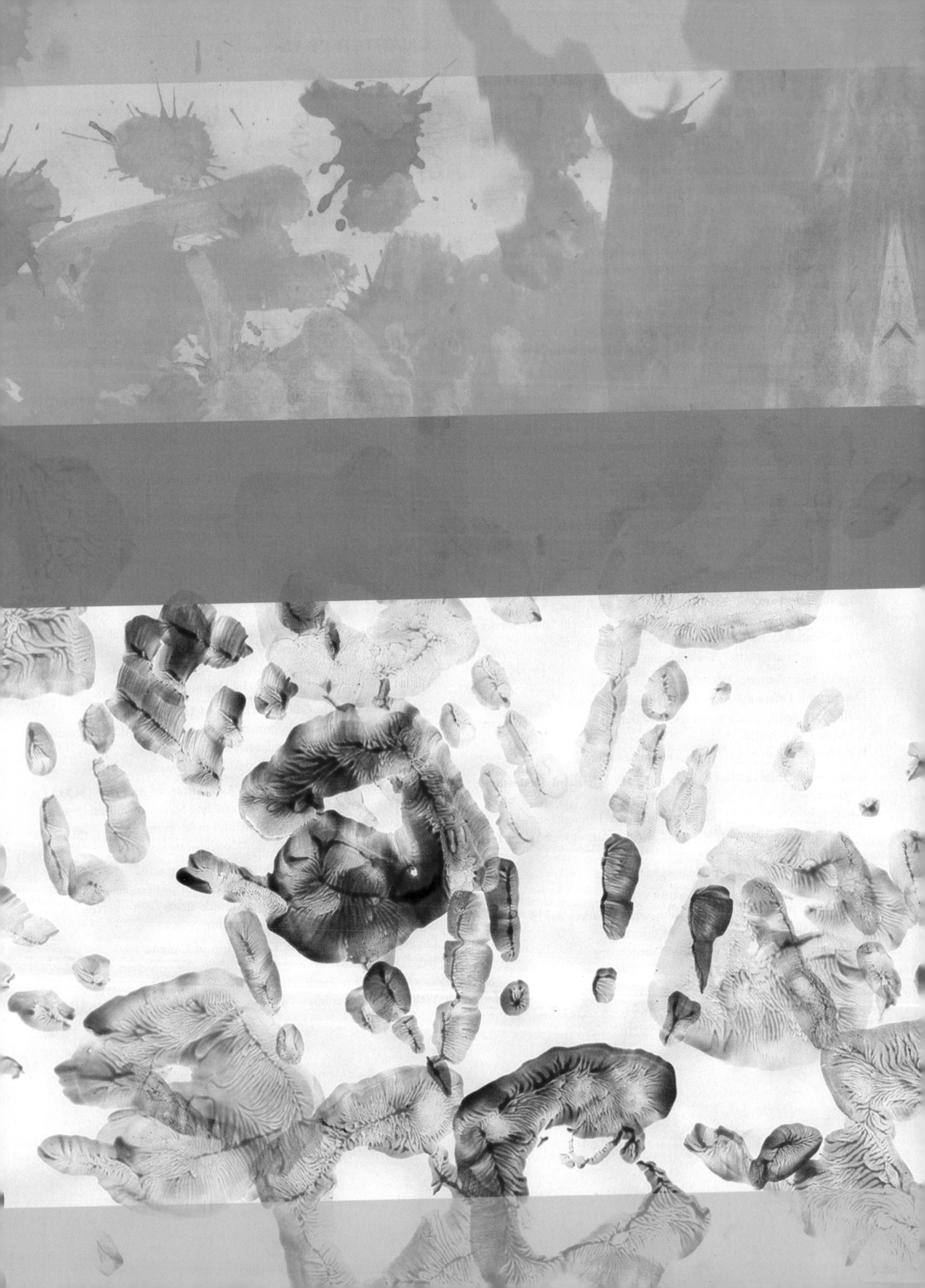

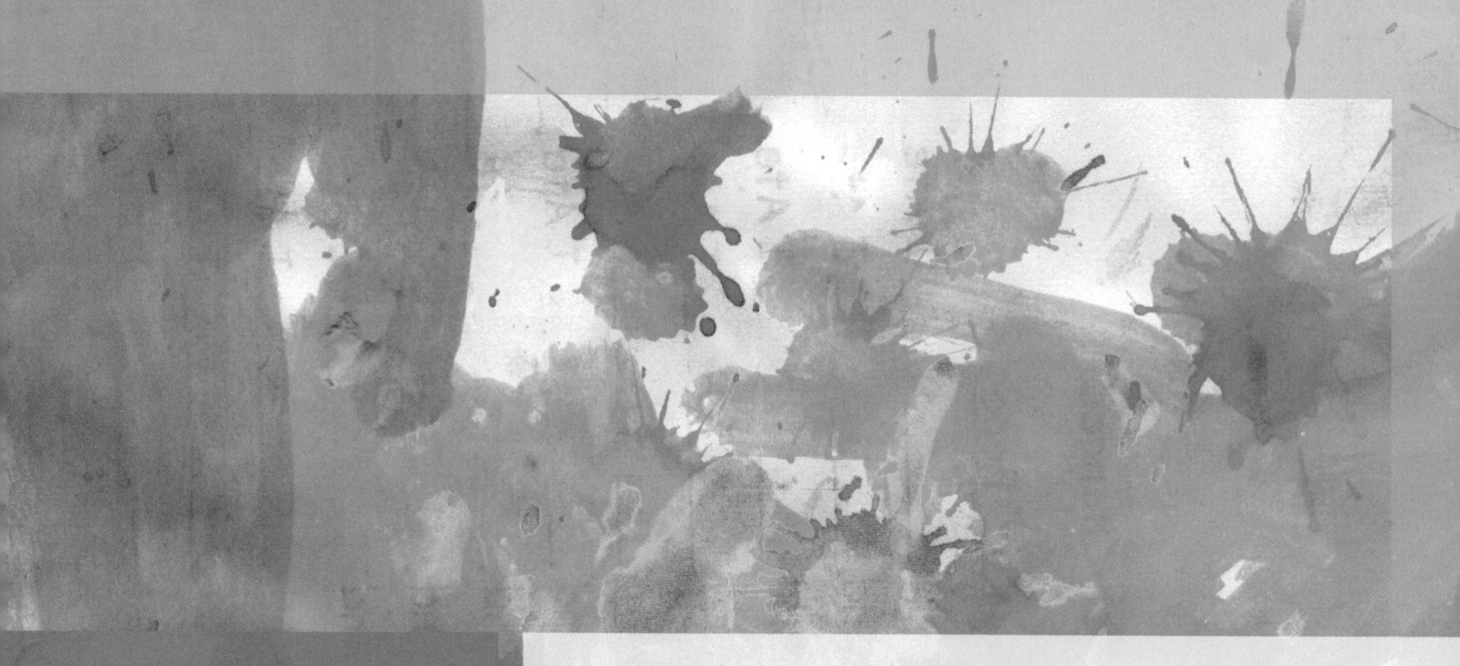

UNIT 6 Alterations in Protective Mechanisms

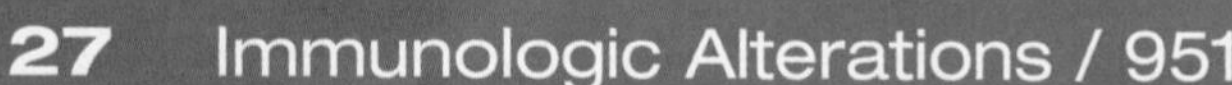

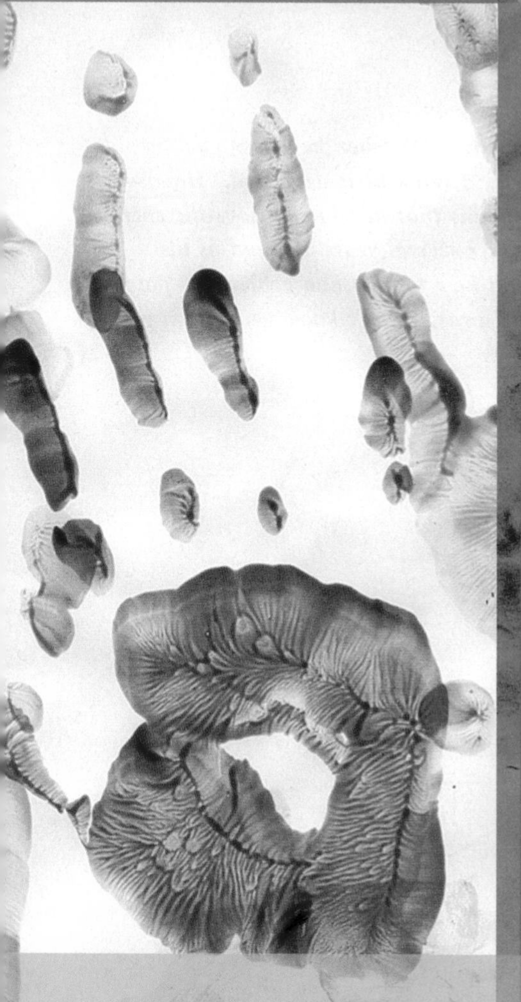

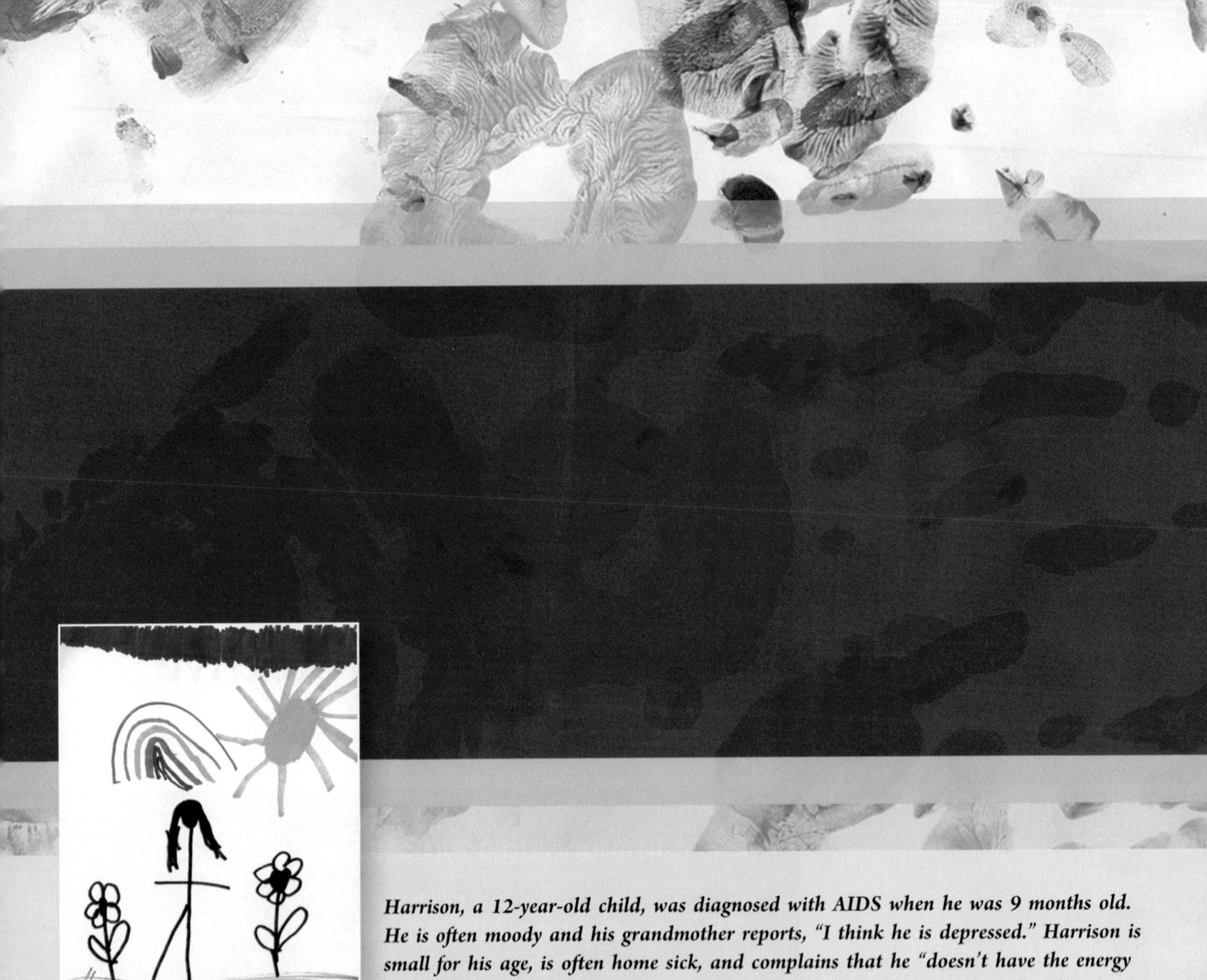

Harrison, a 12-year-old child, was diagnosed with AIDS when he was 9 months old. He is often moody and his grandmother reports, "I think he is depressed." Harrison is small for his age, is often home sick, and complains that he "doesn't have the energy to play with his friends." Harrison lost his mother several years ago and as his grandmother and caregiver, I am anxious about how to help him achieve his potential. I feel overwhelmed and worry that Harrison "will wither up and fly away, I don't know what I am going to do."

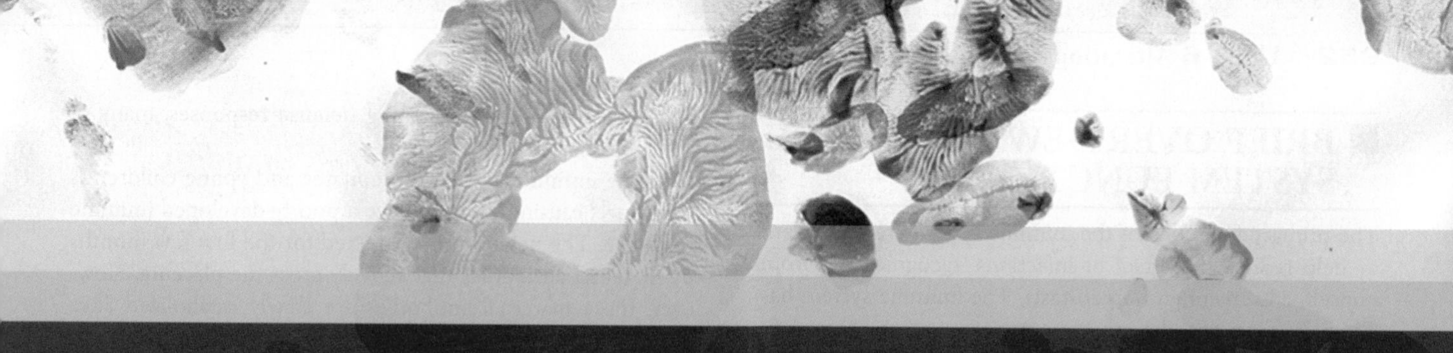

CHAPTER 27
Immunologic Alterations

Debra Ann Mills, RN, MS

COMPETENCIES

Upon completion of this chapter, the reader will be able to:

- Discuss the normal functions of the immune system.
- Discuss the etiology, clinical manifestations, and medical treatment for the common immune system alterations: juvenile idiopathic arthritis (JIA), systemic lupus erythematosus (SLE), human immunodeficiency virus (HIV), and allergic reaction to drugs.
- Use knowledge of immune system alterations when delivering care to children who have juvenile idiopathic arthritis (JIA), systemic lupus erythematosus (SLE), human immunodeficiency virus (HIV), or allergic reaction to drugs.
- Discuss the educational, resource, and support needs of families who have children with immune system alterations.
- Successfully complete the games and activities in the online student StudyWARE.

BRIEF OVERVIEW OF IMMUNE SYSTEM FUNCTION

The primary functions of the immune system are to prevent or help reduce the effect of infections, recognize self from nonself, and maintain homeostasis. The immune system has two basic divisions: the innate immune system and the adaptive immune system. The **innate immune system** acts as the first line of defense against infections and includes biochemical and physical barriers. The **adaptive immune system** produces a specific reaction to each infectious agent, remembers that agent, and can prevent a later infection by the same agent. Even though the two systems interact considerably, they are discussed here separately.

The **immune system** includes the spleen, lymph nodes, and lymphoid tissue, along with cellular elements such as the leukocytes (white blood cells), phagocytes, and natural killer cells. It also includes the skin, mucus produced by the body, cilia, sebaceous gland secretions, stomach acid, normal intestinal flora, and sperm in the semen. Biochemicals such as cytokines, complement factors, and interferon also play crucial roles.

A number of disorders and conditions can cause profound changes in how the body's immune system functions. These changes may lead to alterations in a family's and child's lifestyle as well as present life-threatening challenges. This chapter will present a brief overview of the immune system as well as describe examples of the most common immune system alterations. These common diseases are primarily immune based, but demonstrate multisystem involvement. Clinically significant immune system alterations are (1) autoimmunity, such as juvenile idiopathic arthritis and systemic lupus erythematosus; (2) immunodeficiency, such as human immunodeficiency virus (HIV) disease; and (3) hypersensitivity reactions, such as drug sensitivities. Illnesses primarily associated with other systems, although with immune system implications (asthma, transplants), are described elsewhere (refer to Chapters 24 and 29 for more information about these topics).

Although immune system alterations occur less commonly in children than other types of alterations, the effects are often disabling or terminal. In addition, the immune system interacts with other body systems so symptoms may not appear to be immune related but rather primarily musculoskeletal, such as in juvenile idiopathic arthritis (JIA), or integumentary, such as with systemic lupus erythematosus (SLE). HIV, another immune system disease, can affect all organ systems. However, much of how the immune system functions and dysfunctions is still poorly understood, so therapies described may not be clearly related to a known pathologic entity (Lupus Foundation of America, 2008).

ANATOMY AND PHYSIOLOGY

The basic role of the immune system is to recognize "self" from "nonself" and to initiate a protective process to eliminate the "foreign danger," or antigen. This protective process is complex and has overlapping defense responses, many of which are not mature.

The immune system of neonates and young children is immature, causing them to have a poorly developed immune response. The newborn is protected for the first few months by maternal antibodies that actively cross the placenta. However, these maternal antibodies are slowly catabolized after birth and are completely gone by about 10 months of age. The newborn begins to produce IgG at birth and is usually fully protected by 6 months of age. Different immunoglobins are present but in smaller and differing amounts. Manufacturing of these immunoglobins begins by 2 weeks of age and normal values are achieved by about 7 years of age. Because of this immaturity, infants and young children are susceptible to infectious organisms that can cause illness and its associated morbidity. Lymphoid tissue reaches adult size by 6 weeks of age, becomes larger in the prepubertal ages, and then goes back to normal by puberty. The spleen becomes full-size at adulthood. (Yogev & Chadwick, 2007). Immunizations in early childhood can help prevent many viral and bacterial infections, thus decreasing morbidity and mortality caused by major infectious illnesses. The risks of being infected by invading organisms are lower when the immune system is fully functioning. However, autoimmune disorders may appear at later ages if the body incorrectly begins to recognize its own proteins as foreign.

The term **immunity** refers to all the processes used by the body to protect against foreign material from environmental sources, including microorganisms or their toxins, foods, chemicals, pollen, dander, or drugs. It is important to remember all facets of the immune system work together

> **NURSING ALERT**
>
> **The Importance of Preventing Infection and Maintaining Immunizations for Immunologically Compromised Children**
>
> Nurses play a pivotal role in teaching families to prevent infection and to promptly identify infections so that appropriate treatment takes place quickly. This is especially important for the infant or child whose immune defenses are compromised, e.g., a child with idiopathic juvenile rheumatoid arthritis. The nurse should also keep in mind that the Centers for Disease Control and Prevention (CDC) continues to focus on the importance that immunizations play in keeping the world's population healthy. Keep two factors in mind when providing education regarding immunizations. One is the health status of the infant/child who will be receiving the immunization and two is the type of immunization to be given (Mink, 2008).

to provide the immune response; alterations in one area may stimulate changes in other areas. These changes may be beneficial, that is, compensate for a damaged function, or be harmful to a person if the response is dramatic or causes more symptoms.

Innate or **natural immunity** functions against most threats to the body in a broad sense, and consists of physical barriers (skin, mucous membranes, and cough reflex); chemical barriers (pH of the stomach, fatty acids and proteolytic enzymes of the small intestine); and fever. This immunity also includes nonspecific immune cells such as phagocytes and lymphocytes which release lysing chemicals, and **inflammation** where increased vasodilation brings an increased blood supply and is responsible for chemical messengers.

Acquired immunity is a specific immunity, triggered when a person has had prior contact with a foreign agent. Upon initial contact with the foreign agent, the **humoral system** consisting of primarily **B lymphocytes** (formed in the bone marrow and producer of **immunoglobulins**, including IgG, IgM, IgA, IgE, and IgD) or the **cell-mediated system** is activated. Each of the five immunoglobulins has different functional properties, thereby increasing the complexity of immune response. Their essential role is to "tag" or identify an **antigen** or pathogen for destruction by other immune cells. Refer to Table 27-1 for specific information about the immunoglobulins.

Cell-mediated immunity has an antigen-specific arm consisting of the **T lymphocytes** or cells, developed in the thymus gland (hence "T" cells), and accounting for 70–80% of all lymphocytes. There are many subclasses of T lymphocytes identified to date; each performs different functions. The four main subclass types include the **helper T cells**, which cooperate with B lymphocytes to induce antibody production and activate cytotoxic T cells; **cytotoxic** or **killer T lymphocytes**, which attack infected or pathogenic cells; **suppressor cells** whose release of **cytokines** slows the immune response; and **memory cells**, distinctive for their memory and specificity in immune responses. T lymphocytes are the immune system's main defense against viruses, and direct and regulate the immunologic response by secreting lymphokines which in turn affect other T cells and attract and activate mononuclear cells, particularly macrophages. Both the humoral and cell-mediated systems specifically recognize antigens and interact with each other and

TABLE 27-1 Immunoglobulins

IG TYPE AND %	WHERE FOUND	ACTION	WHEN APPEARS
IgG 70–80%	All body fluids	• Longest and strongest response. • Neutralizes bacterial toxins. • Activates phagocytosis. • Thought to influence B cell differentiation.	• Crosses placenta. • Disappears by 6–8 months. • Reaches adult levels by 7–8 years.
IgA 10–15%	Secretions of gastrointestinal, respiratory, and genitourinary tract, including breast milk	• Prevents infections.	• Not present at birth.
IgM 5–10%	Intravascular spaces	• Agglutinates antigen. • Lyses cell walls. • First immunoglobulin produced in response to bacterial and viral infections. • Responsible for transfusion reactions in the ABO blood typing system.	• Low at birth. • Adult levels reached at 1 year. • Produced 48–72 hours after an antigen enters the body. • Presence in cord or infant blood suggests an infection in utero or during the newborn period.
IgD 0.2%	Plasma	• May be receptor that binds antigen to lympocyte surfaces. • May influence B cell differentiation.	• Not present at birth. • Adult values achieved at 6–7 years.
IgE 0.004%	Internal or external body fluid	• Binds to mast cells on tissue surfaces. • Associated with allergy and parasitic infections.	• Seen in hypersensitivity reactions.

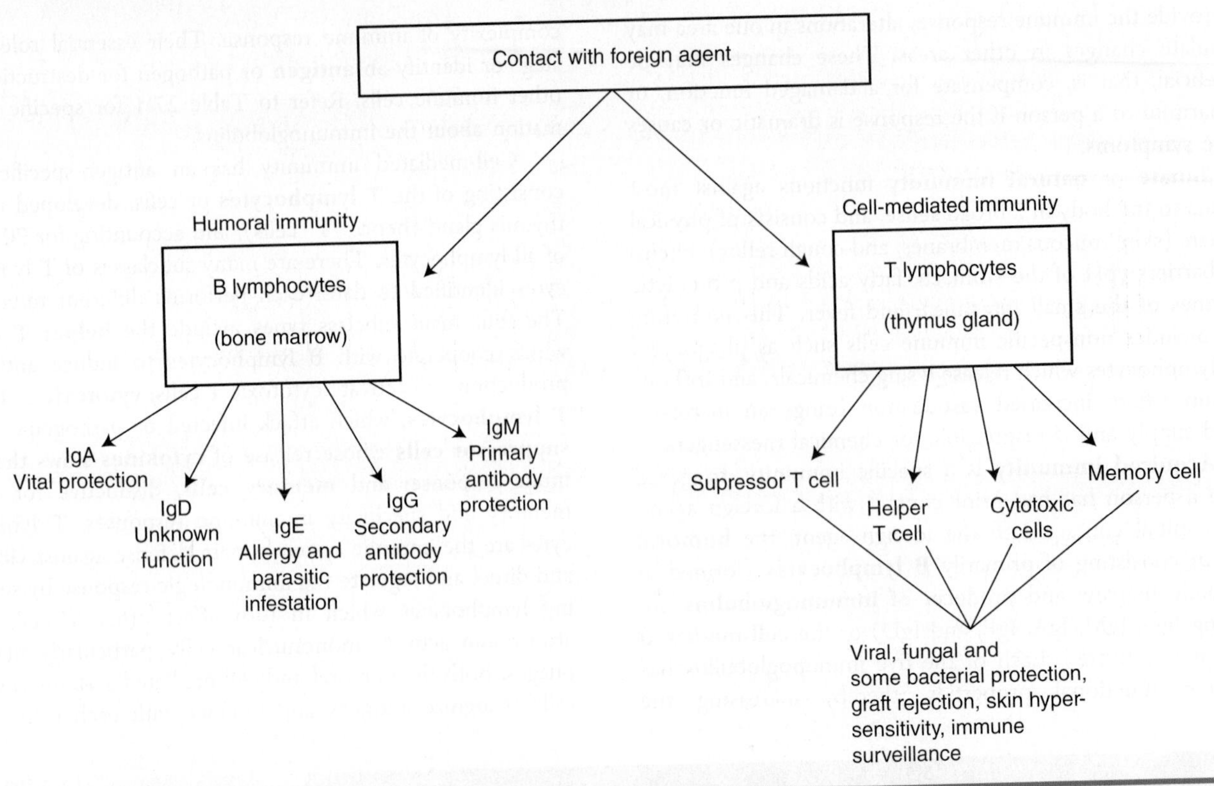

FIGURE 27-1 Acquired Immunity. DELMAR CENGAGE LEARNING.

with components of the innate system to inactivate the immune challenge (Buckley, 2007). Figure 27-1 illustrates acquired immunity.

The chemical mediators that communicate throughout the immune process are called **interleukins**, and include the lymphokines, produced by lymphocytes, and the **monokines**, produced by monocytes and macrophages. **Interferons** are also important messengers, but are host-specific rather than antigen-specific as infected cells secrete them, inhibit replication of many viruses, and have antitumor effects. The final major component of the immune response is **complement**, a group of about 25 serum proteins activated by the onset of the immune response on a pathogen surface, which amplifies the immune response and "complements" antibody activity by facilitating phagocytosis by macrophages or attacking the pathogen's cell membranes (Rote & Huether, 2010a; Yogev & Chadwick, 2007). **Passive immunity** refers to the passing or administration of preformed antibodies to someone, such as the transfer of maternal antibodies to an infant through breast milk. Human or animal antibodies are also sometimes administered to prevent/minimize the effects of an infectious disease in people with congenital or acquired B lymphocyte defects, when a person is susceptible to a disease, when there is a high risk of complications from a disease, or when there is no time for active immunization. Antibodies may also help suppress the effect of some toxins when a disease is already present (American Academy of Pediatrics, 2006).

An important factor in acquired immunity is determining what is self and what is nonself. For various reasons, the identification of "self" is sometimes made as nonself and an immune response mounted, called **autoimmunity**, which causes illnesses that are difficult to treat.

Immune responses are also sometimes directed against substances foreign to the body but not necessarily harmful, such as pollen, animal fur or dander, and food proteins. Here, the immune response is initiated as these innocuous substances sensitize a person, so on re-exposure to the same substance, the person has a hypersensitive or allergic reaction that can be severely pathologic or cause death if the dose of the **allergen** (foreign antigen) is high or the antibody response is excessive.

Humoral or cell-mediated immunity may also be involved in hypersensitivity. **Immediate hypersensitivity** results in release of chemical mediators such as histamine, or damage to tissue by lysosomal enzymes, and has a short duration between exposure and reaction. **Delayed hypersensitivity** is a cellular reaction involving T cells and macrophages and has a longer duration between exposure and reaction.

RHEUMATOLOGICAL AUTOIMMUNE INFLAMMATORY DISEASES

Common rheumatological autoimmune inflammatory diseases include juvenile idiopathic arthritis (JIA), a new name for juvenile rheumatoid arthritis (JRA), and systemic lupus erythematosus (SLE). See Box 27-1.

BOX 27-1
TERMINOLOGY

Autoimmunity

The inability of the body to distinguish "self" from other, leads to an immune response aimed at parts of one's own body.

Inflammation

Increased blood flow and permeability of blood vessels; results in increased fluid production and attraction of lymphocytes and leukocytes to the area, caused by the release of inflammatory substances called cytokines.

JUVENILE IDIOPATHIC ARTHRITIS

Juvenile idiopathic arthritis (JIA), previously classified as juvenile rheumatoid arthritis (JRA), is a heterogeneous group of autoimmune chronic inflammatory diseases affecting joints and connective tissues in children. JIA represents the most common rheumatic condition of childhood and may present as one of three major disease courses: systemic onset; pauciarticular (pauci), involving five or fewer joints; or polyarticular, simultaneous involvement of four or more joints.

Incidence and Etiology

Juvenile Idiopathic Arthritis (JIA) is the most common pediatric rheumatological disease, and one of the more common chronic diseases affecting children. It is thought that 18 out of 100,000 children are diagnosed with JIA each year (Bernatsky et al., 2007). The Arthritis Foundation estimates that approximately 71,000 children under the age of 18 have JIA in the United States. Globally the incidence is 0.8 to 22 per 100,000 children. Females experience JIA more frequently than males, and it is more common in Caucasians than minority children in the United States. However, Native-American children are most frequently affected than African-American and Asian children. A child is generally diagnosed with JIA after experiencing more than 6 weeks of persistent arthritis with an onset of symptoms at less than 16 years of age (Edgerton, 2008; Hashkes & Laxer, 2005; Miller & Cassidy, 2007).

Although rarely life-threatening, the outcome for most children with JIA is impossible to predict. Recent research indicates many children with JIA continue to have active disease 10 years after onset and do not achieve long-term remission. Approximately 70% of children with JIA may experience permanent remission and function optimally. It is important to diagnose JIA as early as possible to prevent joint damage, growth retardation, long-term disabilities, and poor quality of life. Treatment combines anti-inflammatory and immune modulatory medications, physical and occupational therapy, nutritional support, psychosocial and emotional support, client and family education, and occasional surgery. Future considerations for health care evaluation should include annual cardiovascular risk assessments because of issues with chronic inflammation. It is important to also recognize that clients with JIA may require eventual joint replacement as the arthritis progresses into adulthood (Edgerton, 2008; Hashkes & Laxer, 2005; Lovell et al., 2008). Children at most risk for these impairments (1) have a later age of onset, (2) exhibit prominent systemic manifestations, and (3) develop early symptomatic involvement of the small joints (hands, feet) or progressive hip disease (Edgerton, 2008). Two peak ages of onset have been identified: between 2 and 4 years of age (more commonly in girls) and between 10 and 12 years of age (most often in boys) (Miller & Cassidy, 2007). Overall, girls are affected twice as often as boys. Additionally, there are variations within the subgroups. (See Table 27-2.) The cause of JIA is unknown, but is generally linked to interactions of genetic, environmental, and immunologic factors (Petty & Cassidy, 2005). The current theory is an immunogenetic susceptibility in an individual along with an external trigger, probably viral or bacterial, are both necessary to start the inflammatory process in genetically targeted body cells. Chronic inflammation of the synovium with joint effusion eventually erodes, destroys, and causes fibrosis of the articular cartilage. In systemic arthritis other organs, such as the heart and skin, may also be affected. In susceptible individuals chronic and acute uveitis (inflammation of the iris and cillary body) can cause damage to the eye and possible permanent vision loss (Miller & Cassidy, 2007).

Pathophysiology

Current research suggests T cell activation triggers development of antigen-antibody complexes, which cause release of inflammatory substances called cytokines in targeted organs such as joints and skin. This causes inflammation of the synovial membranes and other tissues leading to joint effusion and swelling. Chronic inflammation eventually evolves into erosion of articular cartilage and other symptoms of inflammatory diseases (Miller & Cassidy, 2007).

Clinical Manifestations

The most common symptoms of JIA are persistent joint swelling, pain, and stiffness ("jelling") that is typically worse in the morning. The child may also exhibit limited mobility or range of motion in the limb of the affected joint. Swelling is secondary to joint effusion, edema, and thickening of the synovium. Surrounding muscle spasms and joint inflammation are the main causes of impaired mobility early in the disease process. Children may also experience a high fever and a light skin rash. These may appear and disappear very quickly. There are periods when the symptoms are better or

TABLE 27-2 Comparison of Juvenile Idiopathic Arthritis by Onset Criteria

	SYSTEMIC	RF–POLY	RF+POLY	YOUNG PAUCI	OLDER PAUCI
INCIDENCE	30%	25%		45%	
Female-male ratio	F=M	F>M	F>M	F>M	F<M
Rheumatoid factor	Neg	Pos	Neg	Neg	Neg
Antinuclear antibody	Neg	Neg	Neg	Pos	Neg
Median age of onset	5 yr	3 yr	12 yr	2 yr	10 yr
Most common joints	Any	Any—usually symmetric		Knee most common	Lower extremities
Other common clinical manifestation	Fever, fatigue, malaise, rash	Rheumtatic Nodules		Iritis	
Other labs	↑ ESR Moderate anemia ↑ WBC ↑ Platelet	↑ ESR Mild anemia	↑ ESR Moderate anemia	↑ ESR	↑ ESR +HLA-B27
Course or prognosis	Systemic symptoms remit; progress to poly arthritis	Usually burns out	Persistent, chronic joint destruction; poor functional outcome	Bony overgrowth; Good prognosis	May progress to ankylosis

ESR = Erythrocyte sedimentation rate (normal: neonatal to puberty: 3 to 13 mm/hr)
WBC = White blood count (normal: 4,500–10,000 white blood cells per microliter)
HLA = Human leukocyte antigen (normal: identification of specific leukocyte antigens, HLA-A, HLA-B, HLA-C and HLA-D).

disappear (remission) and when they are worse (flare-ups). Each child is unique in the frequencies of remission and flare-ups. Some children have many flare-ups, with symptoms never going away. Others may have one or two flare-ups and never have symptoms again. JIA classification reflects disease onset, not progression of the disease (see Box 27-2 and Table 27-2 for specifics) (Edgerton, 2008).

DIAGNOSIS

Diagnosis is made primarily on the basis of history and assessment findings. The American College of Rheumatology (1999) determined diagnostic criteria for JIA that include onset before 16 years of age; arthritis (objectively observed) of at least 6 weeks' duration; a defined subtype (by onset characteristics); and exclusion of other conditions such as other rheumatic diseases, infectious arthritis, inflammatory bowel disease, and nonrheumatic conditions of bones and joints. Objectively observed arthritis is defined as joint swelling or effusion, *or* two of the following: warmth, pain on motion, or limited range of motion. Diagnosis also considers the child's age, gender, race, ethnicity, history of presenting symptoms, and serology results (Edgerton, 2008).

The diagnosis and categorization of the disease is based on history, physical examination, the American College of Rheumatology onset criteria, and laboratory and radiographic testing for both inclusion and exclusion criteria. Systemic symptoms such as fevers, rash, and lymphadenopathy may complicate the diagnosis, as they can precede joint involvement by months or years and may suggest other diseases that must first be ruled out.

The clinical manifestations of the varied forms of juvenile arthritis are also often the presenting symptoms of many childhood diseases, both rheumatological and non-rheumatological. For instance, fever and lymphadenopathy may indicate an infection or certain malignancies (leukemia, lymphoma). Arthralgia and arthritis can also be symptoms of systemic lupus erythematosus, juvenile dermatomyositis, and inflammatory bowel disease, as well as malignancies, trauma, and infections of the bone. Other conditions that have to be ruled out are benign arthralgia of childhood (growing pains), rheumatic fever, and school phobia.

BOX 27-2
SYMPTOMS OF JIA

Systemic Onset

- Fevers—High, daily or more than once a day as high as 40.56°C (105°F), returning back to baseline between spikes
- Rash—Salmon-pink, migratory, macular or papular, most common in late afternoon or early evening
- Arthralgia or myalgia
- Arthritis; usually multiple joints are involved
- Fatigue or malaise
- Lymphadanopathy—Usually cervical, epitrochlear, axillary, or inguinal
- Hepatosplenomegaly
- Can also present with signs of carditis—chest pain, tachycardia

Polyarticular Onset

- Arthritis in many joints (five or more)—any joint can be affected, but most particularly the joints of the knees, wrists, ankles, and proximal interphalangeal joints of the fingers. Often neck and temporomandibular (TMJ) joints are affected
- Fever—occasionally, low grade

Pauciarticular Onset

- Arthritis in a few joints (four or fewer)—often, though not exclusively, joints of the knees and ankles; some children may present with single joint involvement
- Some children, especially girls who are antinuclear antibody positive, have iritis, or inflammation of the eyes

There are no specific laboratory tests for JIA. Even though test results reflecting inflammation are completed and used to help diagnose and monitor rheumatological diseases, they are nonspecific and can reflect other conditions causing inflammation. These tests and results include elevated erythrocyte sedimentation rate (ESR), elevated c-reactive protein (CRP), elevated white blood count, decreased hemoglobin, and increased platelet count. Antinuclear antibody (ANA) and rheumatoid factor (RF) are positive in a proportion of children with arthritis (see Table 27-2). A positive ANA is not itself diagnostic as there are positive results in about 5% of the nonarthritic population, and it is very closely associated with systemic lupus erythematosus. Positive RF test results occur in approximately 10% of children, and is associated with a poor prognosis, rheumatoid nodules, and eventual decrease in functional ability. Some feel this may be early onset of adult rheumatoid arthritis (Miller & Cassidy, 2007).

X-rays can demonstrate characteristic changes such as soft-tissue swelling and joint effusion. With continued disease activity, bony erosions and narrowing of the joint spaces are seen. Subluxations and malalignment may also be visible. Late changes include increased bone destruction and fusion. Bone scans can rule out malignancies and MRI can help evaluate both joints and soft tissues.

TREATMENT

Treatment is best undertaken by a multidisciplinary team, including the child and family, nurse, physician, occupational and physical therapists, and social worker. Overall goals include decreasing inflammation, maintaining joint function, and preventing psychosocial complications. Treatment includes medications, physical-occupational therapies, nutrition, and education.

A variety of medications are the mainstay of treatment for arthritis in children (Edgerton, 2008), and the goal is to minimize inflammation, control pain, preserve joint function, and promote normal growth and development. Refer to Table 27-3 for specific information about medications prescribed. Currently, combinations of disease-modifying antirheumatic drugs (DMARDs), nonsteroidal anti-inflammatory drugs (NSAIDs), and tumor necrosis factor inhibiting agents have become standard therapy. Not only do they decrease inflammation by decreasing production of the inflammatory substance prostaglandin, but they help to reduce pain and are also antipyretic. NSAIDs approved for use in children include ibuprofen, naproxen, indomethacin, tolmetin, and salicylates. NSAIDs commonly cause stomach pain or bleeding and medications may be needed to prevent or minimize symptoms of ulceration (Miller & Cassidy, 2007). Aspirin may also be prescribed but it has been linked to Reye's syndrome in children exposed to the flu virus and should not be administered if a child develops flu symptoms. A newer

TABLE 27-3 Common Medications Used to Control Inflammation

MEDICATION	ACTION	COMMON SIDE EFFECTS	NURSING IMPLICATION
NSAIDs	Interferes with production of prostaglandins	Stomach upset, ulcers	Give with food or milk. Monitor for GI bleeding, blood in stool, anemia.
Aspirin	Interferes with production of prostaglandins	Stomach upset, ulcers, Reye's syndrome	Give with food. D/C if develops flu symptoms.
Sulfasalazine	Antibiotic, anti-inflammatory	Allergic reaction (sulfa)	Begin slowly at low doses, gradually increase.
Hydroxychloroquine	Antimalarial	Retinopathy	Eye exams q 6 months–1 yr.
Methotrexate	Folic acid antagonist	Nausea, ↑ liver enzymes	Folic acid supplement may ↓ side effects, monitor liver enzymes.
Corticosteroids	Anti-inflammatory	Round face, ↑ BP, weight gain, ↓ bone density	↓ Na, ↑ fat diet. Monitor bone density, encourage calcium in diet, do not abruptly D/C.
Cytotoxics	Interferes with cell production	Hair loss, possible fertility problems; risk of infection	Discuss side effects before starting, protect from infection.

type of NSAID is the COX-2 inhibitor such as Celebrex, which causes fewer gastrointestinal side effects.

Slow-acting antirheumatic drugs (SAARDs), such as sulfasalazine, may also be used in combination with NSAIDs and other medications to control inflammation. Methotrexate is the most common DMARD used to treat children with persistent joint disease. It is important for the nurse working with the child and family to alert them to possible side effects of gastrointestinal disturbance associated with taking methotrexate. Families should also be educated about discontinuing the methotrexate during viral illnesses, or if the child has varicella, as it suppresses the immune system (Albers et al., 2009; Edgerton, 2008). Although the majority of children can be treated adequately using these medications in conjunction with other measures such as physiotherapy, occupational therapy, and psychosocial support, there is continued research into new therapies including biological therapies and stem cell transplantation for severe JIA. Etanercept, a biologic agent, is approved for the use in children and is typically begun when NSAIDS and methotrexate has been unsuccessful in reducing inflammation. Parents should be educated about withholding Etanercept in the presence of an infection and to report to their health care provider any unusual symptoms their child has. At issue, though, are cost and accessibility, as newer and more expensive medications are developed. This is particularly true for children and families that lack health care provider resources and may be facing economic disparity (Haines, 2007; McCann & Woo, 2007; Wulffraat, et al., 2008).

Parents with infants or children with juvenile idiopathic rheumatoid arthritis who are receiving aspirin therapy need to be educated regarding their child's risk for developing Reye's syndrome. Aspirin should not be administered if flu symptoms develop. Nurses should also educate parents about the resources available to ensure their infant or child will be immunized with influenza vaccine in the fall of each year. This is particularly important for families experiencing financial challenges that need a resource referral. Corticosteroids such as prednisone, or increasingly intravenous "pulses" of high dose solumedrol, are often used to help control systemic onset and polyarticular disease, especially

NURSING TIP

Including School Based Management of Children with Chronic Illnesses

Approximately 275,000 children are affected by arthritis nationwide. These children may miss a few days of school or may require frequent home or hospital care requiring tutoring to help keep up with schoolwork and assignments. Other concerns can include the social impact of required medications and their side effects, altered growth and development, altered socialization with peers, and psychological fears of "being different." School-based case management is one strategy that may improve academic and social success. Potential outcomes include improved quality of life and increased independence as knowledge and skills improve in self-management of the disease.

Reflections from Families

My name is Jonah. I am 16 years old and live with my mother and brother on the reservation. When I was 12 I loved to run and play basketball. I don't know if I'll ever be able to do that again. The doctor told me I have arthritis. All I know is that I can hardly move in the mornings and my knees and hips hurt so bad that I don't know if I can take any more. I took something to help, and it made my face puffy and I gained 15 pounds. All my friends leave me behind. My mother worries that I'm getting fat and lazy. She says if I don't want to go to school I need to get a job. She just doesn't understand how I feel, how much I hurt. Next week I'm going to see Woman Who Walks. She is our Medicine Woman. I think I'll get better after she blesses me. Someday maybe I'll be able to run and play ball again.

during the acute phase, to bring relief until the slower-acting medications have time to take effect. Common side effects are weight gain, round face, increased blood pressure, cataracts, decreased bone density, "buffalo hump," increased body hair, acne, and striae of skin from weight gain.

As integral members of the team, physical and occupational therapists evaluate the status of affected joints for range of motion, alignment, and strength. Heat and cold application may be recommended to help lessen pain. A therapeutic home exercise program will also be useful for maintaining or increasing range of motion and improving strength/endurance. Splinting may be needed to protect a joint, decrease pain, or help with alignment.

Physical activity options for a child with arthritis are swimming, walking, and biking, and should continue unless a joint is acutely inflamed. High impact and contact sports should be avoided. Although activity is important, rest periods may be necessary.

It is important for children with arthritis to eat well-balanced meals and maintain a healthy body weight. Increased weight gain puts additional stress on tender joints and makes movement more difficult. Calcium intake should be 3–4 servings daily to maintain strong bones, and if necessary, calcium supplements with vitamin D may be recommended. Low-fat and low-sodium intake is important, especially if the child is on corticosteroids. Additionally there is evidence that folate supplementation can help to reduce the oral and gastrointestinal side effects of methotrexate (Ortiz et al., 2000).

The nurse should not forget to consider the child/adolescent's school experience since pain and fatigue may cause school absences and prevent participation in many types of school activities. The nurse also needs to provide support and encouragement when parents and children have questions about what to do when this happens and how to access

EVIDENCE-BASED PRACTICE

Promoting Health and Well-Being, The Role of Adequate Nutrition in the Life of a Child with Juvenile Idiopathic Arthritis

CLINICAL PROBLEM

Studies have shown that bone density is decreased in children with juvenile idiopathic arthritis (JIA) even when not receiving glucocorticoid medications. Data shows that approximately 40% of children with JIA develop osteopenia and that diminished bone mass may persist into adulthood. Children with osteopnia may also be at higher risk for fractures.

BEST CLINICAL PRACTICE

- General health can be promoted with a well balanced diet.
- Children with JIA may suffer from decreased mobility, pain, and emotional crisis that can decrease metabolic needs.
- Children with JIA who are overweight or obese may have additional muscle and bone strain which can further interfere with activity, impair physical mobility, increase pain, and affect body image.

IMPLICATIONS FOR NURSING

- It is important to recognize the impact of nutrition on the child with JIA and the interrelationship adequate intake of calories as well as calcium and vitamin D has on overall health.
- Nurses will need to consult with dietary professionals to ensure appropriate nutritional planning is included in the child's plan of care.
- Nurses will need to assess for and recognize the implications of JIA on emotional well-being and consider providing psychosocial support for the child/family.
- Nurses will need to be aware of cultural diet restrictions and/or common ethnic foods consumed by the child and family. Supplements may be necessary.

Reference: Lovell, D. J. et al. (2006). A randomized controlled trial of calcium supplementation to increase bone mineral density in children with juvenile rheumatoid arthritis. *Arthritis and Rheumatism, 54*, 2235–2242.

RESEARCH Highlight

Differences in Disease Outcomes between Medicaid and Privately Insured Children: Possible Health Disparities in Juvenile Ideopathic Arthritis

STUDY PURPOSE

To identify the relationship and implications of health care insurance states and disease outcomes in children with juvenile idiopathic arthritis

METHODS

Children with JIA from a tertiary pediatric rheumatology clinic were assessed using a variety of tools including the Childhood Health Assessment Questionnaire, Pediatric Quality of Life Inventory (PedsQL) Generic Core scale, and the PedsQL Rheumatology Module. The number of active joints, number of joints with limited range of motion, well-being, and pain were also evaluated. Children were placed into two groups: those who were covered by private health care resources and those who covered by Medicaid or other similar state programs for low income families. Disease outcomes were compared between these two groups.

FINDINGS

Forty (14%) of 195 children with JIA were covered by Medicaid. These children were more often of nonwhite race and had a polyarticular or systemic disease course more frequently compared to the other children in the study. Children with Medicaid status were shown to have significantly higher disability and lower mean PedsQL Generic Scale scores even after correcting for differences in disease duration, race, onset of JIA, and disease course. Health resource utilization was similar between groups.

IMPLICATIONS

Nurses need to be alert to the role disparity plays when planning and providing care to children with chronic illnesses such as JIA. Despite similarities in accessing health care resources and the degree of joint involvement, children impacted by disparity (Medicaid status) may have significantly lower health-related quality of life and greater disability. The nursing plan of care needs to carefully assess for needs and seek out appropriate resources, provide adequate child and family teaching, and communicate with essential members of the interdisciplinary team such as the dietician, physical therapist, occupational therapist, and school nurse to facilitate the plan of care.

REFERENCE

Brunner, H. I. et al. (2006). Differences in disease outcomes between Medicaid and privately insured children: Possible health disparities in juvenile rheumatoid arthritis. *Arthritis and Rheumatism*, 55, 378–384.

resources in the community that can facilitate normal social and physical development. This may include a referral to the Arthritis Foundation and the American Juvenile Arthritis Foundation.

Family Teaching

Education for caregivers and other family members should include information about the disease and medications, diagnostic tests and their significance, physical activity, sleep, and nutrition. Because arthritis is a disease affecting the entire family, time should be spent describing the adjustment process, and addressing parental, sibling, and child issues. The nurse's role is to coordinate and facilitate family contact with appropriate caregivers.

SYSTEMIC LUPUS ERYTHEMATOSUS

Systemic lupus erythematosus, commonly called SLE or lupus, is one of the most common, complex, and serious chronic autoimmune disorders. The inflammatory process of SLE affects multiple systems. Presently, there is no cure for SLE and specific therapies should be targeted to the symptoms, severity of the disease, and the child's response. SLE can be effectively treated with a multidisciplinary approach that includes medication therapies, nutritional therapies, and physical activities.

Incidence and Etiology

Although SLE can develop at any age, onset in childhood usually occurs at about 12 years (Edgerton, 2008). Similar to other autoimmune diseases, females are impacted ten times

NURSING TIP

Corticosteroid Treatment for Juvenile Idiopathic Arthritis (JIA) and Systemic Lupus Erythematosus (SLE)

Children with JIA and SLE may need corticosteroids, effective anti-inflammatory and immunosuppressive agents, as part of their therapeutic management. Common side effects include increased appetite and weight gain. Children and their families should be educated about these as well as provided support regarding changes in physical appearance, appropriate exercise choices, and diet. Nurses should also take every opportunity to help children/adolescents adjust to changes in appearance/limitations and emphasize their positives. Because of the immunosuppressive effect, it is also important to teach the child and family about good hand washing and to avoid others who are ill because of immunosuppression. Parents should also be encouraged to keep immunizations up to date.

CASE STUDY / CARE PLAN

CHILD WITH JUVENILE IDEOPATHIC ARTHRITIS

Madison is a 7-year-old who was diagnosed with JIA when she was 4 years old. She currently complains of joint stiffness and swelling and is beginning to lose mobility in the affected joints (hands, feet, knees). She "doesn't feel well" and complains of nausea. She has a 9-year-old brother, Henry, who doesn't know much about JIA.

NURSING CARE PLAN

ASSESSMENT

Swelling, inflammation, and stiffness are noted on the joints of the fingers and knees. She limps and complains of moderate pain when asked to walk across the examination room. Her temperature is 37.8°C (100°F), pulse 85, and respirations 24, BP 90/68.

NURSING DIAGNOSES 1

Chronic pain and fatigue related to swollen/inflamed joints, restricted movement.

EXPECTED OUTCOME

Madison's pain and fatigue will be decreased and her mobility will be increased.

NOC: Energy Conservation; Mobility; Pain Control

NIC: Analgesic Administration; Calming Technique; Environment Comfort; Exercise Therapy: Joint Mobility; Presence

INTERVENTIONS/*RATIONALES*

1. Administer medications in an accurate and timely manner. *Will minimize pain.*
2. Use heat/cold and positioning to relieve and support affected joint. *Will relieve pain.*
3. Encourage participation in activities that maximize the child's capability allowing normal involvement in family, school, and other social activities. *To facilitate growth and development and minimize fatigue.*
4. Encourage participation in occupational/physical therapy and home exercise programs. *Will minimize deformity.*
5. Maintain adequate body alignment. *Will minimize deformity.*

EVALUATION

Madison will exhibit increased mobility and less fatigue as activities and medications are adjusted to appropriate levels.

NURSING DIAGNOSIS 2

Deficient knowledge related to etiology, pathophysiology, and treatment of JIA.

EXPECTED OUTCOME

Madison and her family will verbalize understanding of JIA and the treatment regime.

NOC: Knowledge: Disease Process, Illness Care, Treatment Regime

NIC: Learning Facilitation; Medical Management; Teaching Disease Process

INTERVENTIONS/*RATIONALES*

1. Provide information regarding JIA, and prescribed medications. *With improved knowledge they will be better able to manage JIA.*
2. Provide information regarding limitations on activity and occupational/physical therapy exercises that can be done at home. *Improves knowledge, empowers client.*

EVALUATION

Madison and her family will learn about JIA as well as the treatment and management plan.

more often than males; SLE is eight times more common in African-American females than males. Genetic links also exist with an increased incidence in twins (Rote, 2010).

The exact etiology of SLE, a chronic, complex disease with unpredictable multisystem impact and complications, is unknown. However, there is general agreement that it is an autoimmune process requiring a genetic susceptibility and an interaction with an environmental, viral or bacterial, or hormonal trigger (Klein-Gitelman & Miller, 2007; Rote, 2010).

Pathophysiology

The process is one of autoimmunity. It is thought that immune complexes recognize normal body tissues as foreign, bind, then deposit these proteins in the vascular system of targeted organs (skin, kidneys, joints, heart, lungs, bone marrow, brain) causing inflammation and damage. Because so many organs can be affected, symptoms may be different (Rote, 2010).

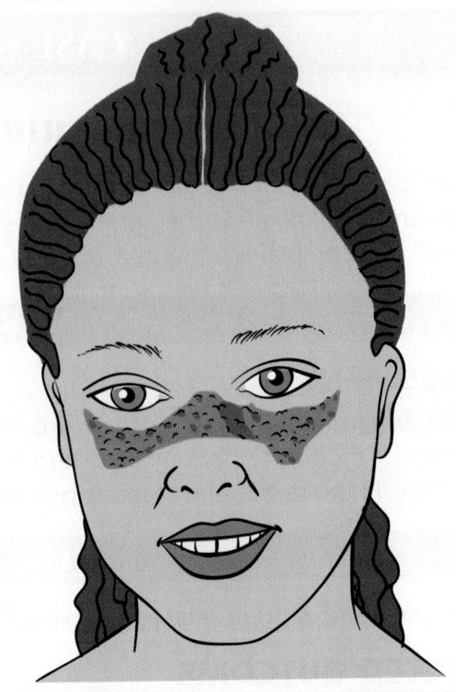

Figure 27-2 Butterfly Rash Often Seen in SLE. DELMAR CENGAGE LEARNING.

Clinical Manifestations

Individuals with SLE may exhibit a range of symptoms, from mild to severe that may come and leave over a period of time. Symptoms include fever, fatigue, weight loss, lymphadenopathy, and hepatosplenomegaly. A predominant manifestation is a malar or butterfly rash on the face resulting from mucocutaneous involvement. Clinical manifestations depend on which organs are targeted by the immune complexes, are chronic, and are characterized by remissions and exacerbations. Refer to Box 27-3 for criteria used to diagnose SLE and see Figure 27-2.

Diagnosis

Diagnosing SLE can be difficult and is based on history, physical exam, laboratory test results, and the presence of four of the eleven criteria listed in Box 27-3 (Edgerton, 2008; Klein-Gitelman & Miller, 2007; Rote, 2010). The disease is diagnosed when positive antinuclear antibodies and other blood tests reveal anemia, an elevated BUN, an

BOX 27-3
DIAGNOSTIC CRITERIA FOR SYSTEMIC LUPUS ERYTHEMATOSUS

- Malar (butterfly) rash: Erythematosus, flat or raised over the cheeks
- Discoid rash: Erythematosus raised patches with scaling
- Photosensitivity
- Oral or nasal ulcers
- Nonerosive arthritis: Two or more peripheral joints with tenderness, swelling, or effusion
- Serositis, pleuritis, or pericarditis
- Persistent proteinuria progressing to hypertension, nephrotic syndrome, renal insufficiency, and end stage renal disease requiring transplantation
- Seizures or psychosis without other cause
- Hemolytic anemia, leucopenia, lymphopenia, or thrombocytopenia
- Positive systemic lupus erythematosus (LE) cell preparation
- ANA: Positive antinuclear antibody (ANA)

Note: Four out of the eleven criteria are required when classifying the disease as systemic lupus erythematosus.

Adapted from American College of Rheumatology Ad Hoc Committee of Systemic Lupus Erythematosus Guidelines. (1999). Guidelines for referral and management of systemic lupus erythematosus in adults. *Arthritis and Rheumatism*, *42*(9), 1785–1796; Edgerton, 2008.

EVIDENCE-BASED PRACTICE

The Connection between Quality of Life and SLE Activity and Damage in Children Over Time

CLINICAL PROBLEM

SLE in children often is associated with significant morbidity because the treatment effects psychological, physical, and functional well being. Quality of life is an important outcome measure for evaluating the response to treatment. Children with higher disease activity have a lower quality of life.

BEST CLINICAL PRACTICE

- When caring for children with SLE it is important to assess their disease activity and indicators of their quality of life since they are different concepts and may be related.
- Parents may or may not be aware of how the SLE has affected their child's quality of life.

IMPLICATIONS FOR NURSING

- Gather data from children who have SLE and their parents related to the child's quality of life.
- Provide opportunities to improve a child's quality of life by assessing the child's disease activity and then planning with the child activities he or she is interested in and can participate in so his or her quality of life is improved.

Reference: Brunner, H., Higgins, G., Wiers, K., Lapidus, S., Olson, J., Onel, K., Punaro, M., Ying, J., & Klein-Gitelman, M. (2009). Health-related quality of life and its relationship to patient disease course in childhood-onset systemic lupus erythematosus. *Journal of Rheumatology, 36*(7), 1536–1545; Moorthy, L. N., Peterson, M. G., Hassett, A. L., Baratelli, M., Chalom, E. C., Hashkes, P. J., Hong, S., Reiff, A., & Lehman, T. J. (2009). Relationship between health-related quality of life and SLE activity and damage in children over time. *Lupus, 18*, 622–629.

elevated erythrocyte sedimentation rate (ESR), and a positive lupus erythematosus (LE) cell reaction (indication of inflammation) (Gotlieb & Itowite, 2006). However, it can take many months for doctors to correctly interpret the significance of the symptoms, medical history data, physical examination findings, and laboratory results.

TREATMENT

Many choices are available in the management and treatment of SLE. Children and their families must work closely with members of the health care team and take an active role in managing the disease and in promoting health and well-being. The treatment plan is usually based on the child's age, sex, health, symptoms, and lifestyle. Treatment is targeted at preventing exacerbations, treating them when they do occur, and minimizing organ damage and complications. Initial treatment is often targeted to treat musculoskeletal symptoms, such as arthritis, with NSAIDS combined with an antimalarial drug. If symptoms persist or worsen steroids or methotrexate may ordered. Other medications may be used to treat neuropsychiatric symptoms. These include immunosuppressive medications, antidepressants, and antiepileptics. Additional treatment strategies are included as other body system symptoms develop (Edgerton, 2008). Nurses need to educate children and families about medications and to report any new symptoms or responses to the physician promptly. Refer to Table 27-3 for medications also used in SLE.

CULTURAL CONSIDERATION

Treatments for SLE

Because of frequent health care visits, the cost of medications, the risk of serious drug side effects, and the chronic nature of the disease, many families may seek other methods for treating the disease. This may be particularly true for families without insurance, families of ethnic diversity, or families who prefer alternative/complementary healing. These alternative approaches may include special diets, nutritional supplements, ointments, massage therapy, acupuncture, and homeopathy. The nurse needs to be aware that, although these alternative methods may not be harmful, current research does not suggest these methods will suppress or affect the disease process or prevent organ damage. However, complementary methods may help reduce anxiety and assist the child and family cope with SLE.

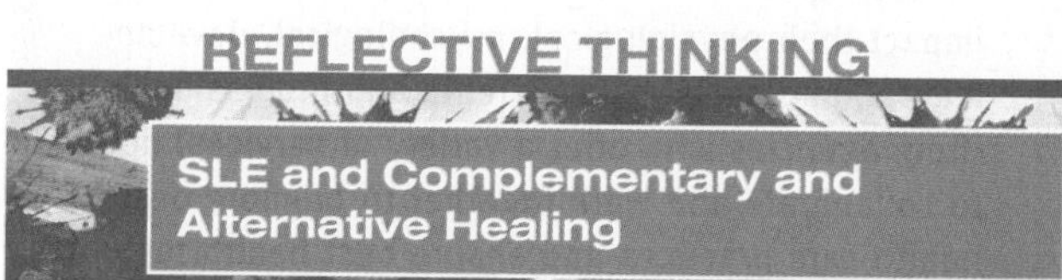

Complementary and alternative healing methods are increasingly being selected by families for treating and managing SLE, particularly for stress relief and pain management. How do you feel about the use of these unproven methods? How can you support families' selection of these methods? What should your education include if your family chooses to use a complementary or alternative strategy such as aromatherapy or acupuncture?

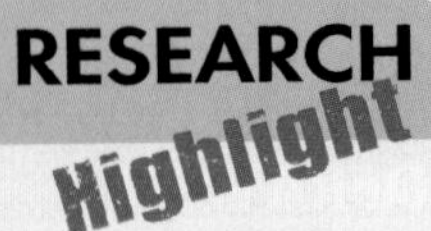

Exploring Best Practices for Working with Families Raising Children with Complex Health Problems. What Works Well and What Needs to Improve?

STUDY PURPOSE

This study explored examples of best multiagency practices for working with families raising children with complex health needs. The objective was to determine what worked well, why it worked well, and what best collaborative practices could be accomplished in the future.

METHODS

The study used interviews, and workshops to develop a set of ten guidelines that reflected best practices perspectives from all participants.

FINDINGS

Ten "best practice" statements were used to serve as a guide of what works well in providing multidisciplinary services and considered the following issues: communication, accessing and providing information, decision making regarding plan of care, accessibility, collaboration, respect, and a shared mission and vision. The study pointed out the value of this guidance to help parents and children get the support they need from a variety of resources, including receiving support from other parents of children with complex health care needs.

IMPLICATIONS

Children with JIA, SLE, and other chronic illnesses have complex health care needs. Their diseases impact their physiological, psychological, developmental, and social care. Parents and professionals (from agencies who offer a variety of services) need to collaborate and work together to promote best health care practices and ensure best health for children experiencing complex chronic health care issues.

REFERENCE

Carter, B., Cummings, J., & Cooper, L. (2007). An exploration of best practice in multi-agency working and the experience of families with children with complex health needs. What works well and what needs to improve practice for the future? *Journal of Clinical Nursing*, *16*, 527–539.

Nursing Management

SLE is a chronic illness; nursing care needs to include support, recognition and treatment of infection, education about the importance of adequate fluid and electrolyte balance, nutrition, activity and rest, as well as developmental considerations. Anti-inflammatory medications are a significant part of the treatment plan. Therefore, it is necessary for the child and family to understand the importance of complying with timeliness, dosing, and side effects. In addition, families need to know exposure to the sun can trigger a "flare-up" so it should be avoided or limited (Burns, Dunn, Brady, Strarr & Blosser, 2009).

Teenagers need to know they are more susceptible to STDs because of immunosuppressive medications. Pregnancy can stress the body and increase disease activity, and cytotoxic medications increase the risk of birth defects. However, if pregnancy is planned for and closely monitored, it is more likely to be successful. Adolescents must also think of vocational issues, including interests and professions likely to include good health insurance benefits and allow for the possibility of absence in the event of serious disease flare-ups.

It is also helpful for families to know the course of the disease may become frustrating and discouraging at times because of its lifelong nature, remissions, exacerbations, and body image issues from medications. They also need to be able to identify resources to help them through the difficult times. Participation in age-appropriate activities should be encouraged.

HUMAN IMMUNODEFICIENTY VIRUS (HIV)

Human immunodeficiency virus (HIV), and the subsequent development of acquired immunodeficiency syndrome (AIDS), is the most serious life-threatening immune system disease. HIV has affected a broad social and geographical community worldwide. However, with the advancement of antiretroviral therapies children are living longer. The World Health Organization now considers HIV/AIDS as a chronic illness that can be managed through strict adherence to the plan of care and adequate nutritional, psychosocial, and developmental support (WHO, 2005).

INCIDENCE AND ETIOLOGY

HIV is the virus responsible for a range of symptoms, conditions, and **opportunistic infections**. **HIV infection** is a multisystem disease known primarily for its effects on the immune system. **HIV disease** is an illness continuum, from asymptomatic to death, with an acquired immunodeficiency syndrome (AIDS) diagnosis usually occurring in the latter part of the continuum. **AIDS** is a term used when the immune system has become compromised enough to allow one of the many diagnoses or conditions known to be associated with advanced HIV disease to occur (AAP, 2006). These diagnoses or conditions are caused by either the direct or indirect effects of the virus on the immune system, or because of HIV's affinity for other cells of the body with CD4 receptors, including the lining of the intestines causing diarrhea, or neurological cells leading to cerebral atrophy.

Since AIDS was first diagnosed it is estimated that 8,460 children have been infected perinatally, and approximately 1000 to 2000 infants were born with HIV during the 1990s, primarily as a result of infected mothers (CDC, 2006a). McKenna and Hu (2007) estimate that about 96 to 186 infants were infected with HIV in 2004. Statistics provided by 33 states from 2005 indicate that 142 children under the age of 13 years were diagnosed with HIV/AIDS (CDC, 2007a).

The diagnosis of HIV in children is often a difficult task. Two definitions of the infection are utilized, one for prenatal exposure up to 15 months of age, and one for older children (Mink, 2008). Although infants and children are infected through various sources, it is believed that 90% of pediatric AIDS cases in the United States are through perinatal transmission (CDC, 2007b; 2007c). However, in 2006 the Centers for Disease Control (CDC) announced a new initiative to help further reduce the incidence of HIV infections in children. The "Revised Recommendations for HIV Testing of Adults, Adolescents, and Pregnant Women in Health-Care Settings" calls for routine "opt out" HIV screening for all pregnant women with repeat HIV screening for high-risk pregnant women during the third trimester. Prenatal HIV efforts have made significant improvements in decreasing the numbers of prenatally exposed infants infected with HIV. In addition to prenatal testing, antiretroviral therapy administered during pregnancy, labor, delivery, and to the newborn has reduced perinatal transmission to 2% or less (CDC, 2006b).

Infants born to positive mothers have serological tests to detect the virus within 48 hours of birth with tests repeated at 1 to 2 months and again at 3 and 6 months. Children less than 13 years of age are considered infected based on whether or not their symptoms meet the CDC criteria for AIDS, if their blood or tissue is HIV positive, or if they have HIV antibodies. When it is determined that the child is infected he/she is placed into a staging classification. The CDC revised the classification for HIV infection in children in 1994. (See Box 27-4.)

BOX 27-4

REVISED PEDIATRIC CLASSIFICATION SYSTEM (AIDS): CLINICAL CATEGORIES

Category N: Not Symptomatic

No signs or symptoms the result of HIV infection, or only one condition listed in category A.

Category A: Mildly Symptomatic

Two or more of the conditions listed below but none of the conditions listed in categories B and C.

- Lymphadenopathy (0.5 cm at more than two sites; bilateral at one site)
- Hepatomegaly
- Splenomegaly
- Dermatitis
- Parotitis
- Recurrent or persistent upper respiratory infection, sinusitis, or otitis media

Category B: Moderately Symptomatic

Symptomatic conditions other than those listed for category A or C that are attributed to HIV infection. Examples of conditions in clinical category B include but are not limited to:

- Anemia (<8 gm/dl), neutropenia (<1,000/mm^3), or thrombocytopenia (<100,000 mm^3) persisting ≥30 days
- Bacterial meningitis, pneumonia, or sepsis (single episode)
- Candidiasis, oropharyngeal (thrush) persisting >2 months in children >6 months
- Cardiomyopathy
- Cytomegalovirus infection with onset <1 month age
- Diarrhea, recurrent or chronic
- Hepatitis
- Herpes Simplex Virus stomatitis, recurrent (>2 episodes within 1 yr)
- Herpes Simplex Virus bronchitis, pneumonitis, or esophagitis <1 month age

(Continues)

BOX 27-4
REVISED PEDIATRIC CLASSIFICATION SYSTEM (AIDS): CLINICAL CATEGORIES (CONTINUED)

- Herpes zoster (shingles) involving at least 2 distinct episodes or >1 dermatome
- Leiomyosarcoma
- Lymphoid interstitial pneumonia or pulmonary lymphoid hyperplasia complex
- Nephropathy
- Nocardiosis
- Persistent fever lasting >1 month
- Toxoplasmosis, onset <1 month age
- Varicella, disseminated (complicated chickenpox)

Category C: Severely Symptomatic

Any condition listed in the 1987 surveillance case definition for AIDS, with the exception of LIP, which is a category B condition.

- Serious bacterial infections, multiple or concurrent (≥2 within 2-yr period) of the following types: septicemia, pneumonia, meningitis, bone or joint infection, or abscess of an internal organ or body cavity (excluding otitis media, superficial skin or mucosal abscesses, and indwelling catheter-related infections)
- Candidiasis, esophageal, or pulmonary (bronchi, trachea, or lungs)
- Sisseminated Coccidioidomycosis
- Extrapulmonary Cryptococcosis
- Cryptosporidiosis or isosporiasis with diarrhea persisting >1 month
- Cytomegalovirus disease with onset of symptoms at age >1 month at site other than liver, spleen, or lymph nodes
- Encephalopathy (at least one of the following progressive findings present for at least 2 months in the absence of a concurrent illness other than HIV infection that could explain findings): (1) failure to attain or loss of developmental milestones or loss of intellectual ability, verified by standard developmental scale or neuropsychological tests; (2) impaired brain growth or acquired microcephaly demonstrated by head circumference measurements or brain atrophy demonstrated by CT or MRI (serial imaging is required for children <2 years age); (3) acquired symmetric motor deficit manifested by two of the following: paresis, pathologic reflexes, ataxia, or gait disturbance
- Herpes Simplex Virus infection causing a mucocutaneous ulcer persisting for >1 month or bronchitis, pneumonitis, or esophagitis for any duration affecting a child >1 month age
- Histoplasmosis, disseminated at a site other than or in addition to lungs or cervical or hilar lymph nodes
- Kaposi's sarcoma
- Lymphoma, primary, in brain
- Lymphoma, small, noncleaved cell (Burkitt's), or immunoblastic or large cell lymphoma of B cell or unknown immunologic origin

Centers for Disease Control and Prevention. (1994). Revised classification system for human immunodeficiency virus infection in children less than 13 years of age. *Morbidity and Mortality Weekly Report, 43* (RR-12), 1–10; Working Group on Antiretroviral Therapy and Medical Management of Infants, Children and Adolescents with HIV Infection. (1998). Antiretroviral therapy and medical management of pediatric HIV infection. *Pediatrics, 102*, 1005–1062S.

For many infants and children, an AIDS diagnosis often follows the progression of nonspecific findings. HIV affects all systems of the body, eventually destroying the immune system's ability to respond to infections. The initial clinical manifestations often progress slowly but many times will advance rapidly to an acute life-threatening course. The central nervous system is particularly vulnerable to the virus. HIV infection often presents as HIV encephalopathy (may be present in acute presentations) or occurs as the disease progresses, causing cognitive and functional motor skill delay or deterioration. Lymphoid interstitial pneumonitis is a common disease associated with AIDS in children, while Pneumocystis jiroveci pneumonia (formerly known as Pneumocystis carinii), Haemophilus influenza, Streptococcus, Haemaophilus influenza, Salmonella, and malinganceis occur as the disease progresses (Kline, 2006; Michaels & Green, 2007; Mink, 2008; Plowfield, 2007; Rote & Huether, 2010b). Adolescents' AIDS-defining illnesses are the same as adults. Adolescents diagnosed with AIDS are primarily males and ethnic minorities, infected via sexual contact or

Table 27-4 Revised Pediatric Classification System (AIDS): Immunologic Categories Based on Age-Specific CD4+ Lymphocyte Count and Percentage

	AGE OF CHILD		
IMMUNE CATEGORY	<12 MO	1–5 YR	6–12 YR
1: No suppression	≥1500	≥1000	≥500
2: Moderate suppression	750–1499	500–900	200–499
3: Severe suppression	<750	<500	<200

Centers for Disease Control and Prevention. (1994). Revised classification system for human immunodeficiency virus infection in children less than 13 years of age. *Morbidity and Mortality Weekly Report, 43* (RR-12), 1–10; Working Group on Antiretroviral Therapy and Medical Management of Infants, Children and Adolescents with HIV Infection. (1998). Antiretroviral therapy and medical management of pediatric HIV infection. *Pediatrics, 102*, 1005–1062S.

injected drug use (Sifuentes, 2008). The Joint United Nations Programme on HIV/AIDS (2007) reported that globally 2.5 million children younger than 15 years were living with AIDS.

Another useful tool for monitoring and reporting HIV infection in children is the Immunologic and Clinical Categories of the revised Pediatric Classification System (CDC, 1994), which consider age as a variable, as infants' CD4+ T lymphocyte counts and percentage values are much higher than those of adults. Adult values are reached by the age of 6. (Refer to Table 27-4.)

Over 84% of perinatally infected children are African American and Hispanic, demonstrating this disease disproportionately affects children and families of color. The rate continues to be disproportionately higher among African-American adults and adolescents. In 2007 the rate among the African-American population was 48% (CDC, 2007a; 2008).

The pediatric nurse plays an important role in recognizing high-risk factors for HIV or informational alerts from the child's care provider. These alerts, such as suspected maternal diagnosis, high-risk environmental conditions, failure to thrive presentation, or a history of recurrent bacterial infections, necessitate appropriate follow-up and discussion with the health care provider. There have been significant reductions in morbidity and mortality in recent years because of the availability of HAART (**highly active antiretroviral therapy**), early diagnosis, and supportive treatment. The importance of early diagnosis and therapeutic intervention cannot be understated as the advances made in caring for children with HIV have been dramatic in the last decade, changing the grim statistics and offering greater quality and quantity of lives.

Children acquire HIV infection through perinatal transmission, during delivery, unprotected sexual behaviors, or injection drug use. The risk of perinatal infection may be higher if the mother acquires HIV infection during the first trimester of pregnancy, has a high viral load, or delivers a premature infant. Contact with the mother's vaginal secretions during delivery is thought to be the highest risk for perinatal transmission, supported in part by the reduction in transmission with elective cesarean sections (CDC, 2007b). The presence of maternal sexually transmitted diseases (STDs) and chorioamnionitis may increase the risk of transmission, as does the prolonged rupture of membranes prior to delivery.

Postnatally, infants may become infected through breast milk (CDC, 2007b). For this reason, mothers with HIV in developed countries are advised to bottle-feed formula to their infants.

It is important to note only a very small percentage of infants born to infected mothers will be infected themselves. The incidence of perinatal HIV transmission is currently declining in the United States due to women taking highly active antiretroviral therapy (HAART) during pregnancy and delivery, and neonates receiving one or two antiretroviral drugs, such as zidovudine and epivir, for six weeks after birth. The transmission rate with these regimens has decreased to less than 2% in many urban HIV care centers, compared to a transmission rate of approximately 23% in infants whose mothers do not take antiretroviral therapy (Perinatal HIV Guidelines, 2001).

REFLECTIVE THINKING

HIV Disease and the Challenge of Life with a Chronic Communicable Disease

Advances in the medical care and treatment of HIV infection have led to a longer life expectancy for children with HIV. This leads to safety, developmental, psychological, financial, and social challenges. Consider the importance of communication and listening skills in developing a trusting relationship with children and families faced with the fear and anxiety that accompany the diagnosis of HIV. How would you facilitate return to day care or school knowing the community may be ignorant about the transmission of the virus and most schools lack health services support? What would you plan for if you were the school nurse working with children with HIV/AIDS?

NURSING ALERT

HIV/AIDS and Lack of Access to Health Care

Many children with HIV/AIDS have poor access to health care. Many of these children are economically and socially disadvantaged, and often culturally diverse. It is essential for the pediatric nurse to have the knowledge and skills necessary to assist these families cope and access appropriate resources in the community. It may be helpful to create an information guide or passport listing some of the available resources and services. There are now CDC-funded programs designed to provide community-based free clinics.

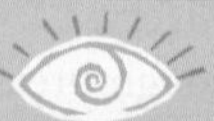

EYE ON...

The Global Pandemic

The care of people with AIDS changes rapidly due to the huge worldwide impact of the pandemic and the amount of research conducted internationally. HIV care in the United States and Europe differs dramatically from developing countries, most notably in Africa. New knowledge and therapies are rapidly integrated into care in the United States, creating vast discrepancies in care and international debates over medication patents and availability and who should receive the medications.

Older adolescents may have acquired HIV through contaminated blood or blood products prior to 1985, when testing was first licensed for the HIV antibody in donated blood. Beginning in 1984, coagulation factors were heat treated to inactivate the virus, which also significantly decreased the number of pediatric infections. Therefore, older adolescents with hemophilia, other bleeding disorders, or idiopathic thrombocytopenia may have acquired HIV during treatment for their disease.

Children and adolescents are also at risk for HIV infection through sexual contact with an infected person. Even though the number of children who acquire HIV through abuse is relatively low, it should always be considered when evaluating a child with a history of abuse. In addition, drug use among children and adolescents continues to be prevalent in some areas of the country and should be assessed as it also is a risk factor for HIV transmission because of the potential for sharing needles with an infected person, exchanging sex in return for drugs, and consensual sex with a drug-using person infected with HIV. Use of drugs, including alcohol, is known to inhibit thought, impair gross and fine motor ability, and, as a consequence, decrease the likelihood safer sex including using condoms will be practiced.

PATHOPHYSIOLOGY

HIV belongs to the family of lentiviruses, which are retroviruses and known to cause an illness trajectory with long periods of clinical latency and asymptomatic infection, weak humoral response, and persistent viremia (Yogev & Chadwick, 2007). There are two known types of HIV: HIV-1, which is worldwide, and HIV-2, which exists primarily in West Africa. Both types cause primary immunodeficiency in humans. HIV-1 is highly mutant and has a number of different subtypes based on their nucleotide sequences. Most HIV testing carried out in the United States is for HIV-1 subtypes, although worldwide there are different subtypes, which affect the sensitivity and specificity of antibody tests, and different DNA and RNA assays, necessitating the need for using a combination of tests and the further development of broader tests (Yogev & Chadwick, 2007).

HIV is composed of inner and outer envelopes of two glycoproteins, gp120 and gp41 (gp160 together), and a viral core. The outer glycoproteins bind HIV-1 to CD4+ lymphocytes. The viral core capsule, consisting of the core proteins p24, p7, and p9, has two single strands of viral RNA and essential viral enzymes for replication. The structure of HIV and the replication of viral components are directed by at least nine different genes with specific functions (Rote & Huether, 2010b; Yogev & Chadwick, 2007).

HIV-1 penetrates into the host cell, uncoats its viral core, releases two single strands of viral RNA into the host cytoplasm, and makes a DNA copy from the RNA using reverse transcriptase. The other viral enzymes separate the RNA and DNA and join two DNA strands together, which move into the host nucleus's DNA forming the HIV-1 provirus, which remains quiet until CD4+ cell activation causes it to replicate (Yogev & Chadwick, 2007). When activated, the CD4+ cell transcribes the proviral DNA into messenger RNA, which moves out of the nucleus facilitating the production of viral polyproteins precursors to the HIV envelope and core (Yogev & Chadwick, 2007).

An initial infection with HIV is marked by high levels of plasma HIV and a decrease in CD4+ lymphocytes, which fluctuate as the immune response attempts to contain the infection. These values stabilize after about six months of infection and the levels depend on a client's strength of immune response, the number of infected cells, and the virulence of the HIV strain. Clients with higher plasma levels after stabilization are at higher risk of disease progression (Yogev & Chadwick, 2007).

HIV infection affects the immune system directly and indirectly. Directly, the virus infects cells that possess the CD4+ marker or receptor which then kills the CD4+ cell. The CD4+ mononuclear cells (lymphocytes, macrophages, and monocytes) also travel to many tissue sites, infecting

NURSING ALERT

Infections Prior to a Diagnosis of HIV

Chronic otitis media, thrush, and *Pneumocystis carinii* (PCP) are infections common in HIV-infected infants even before they are diagnosed with HIV.

other organs, and adding to its multisystem effects and variety of clinical signs and symptoms (Burns et al., 2009; Yogev & Chadwick, 2007). Indirect effects result from the immune response, which depletes the CD4+ cells, resulting in dysfunction and cellular death (Yogev & Chadwick, 2007). However, if viral glycoprotein binds to CD4+ receptors the immune system may not respond to infectious challenges (**anergy**). On the other hand, superantigens can cause CD4+ cells to become more susceptible to infections by binding to them and causing massive stimulation and destruction (Yogev & Chadwick, 2007).

CLINICAL MANIFESTATIONS

Clinical manifestations range from being completely asymptomatic with normal CD4+ counts to having associated symptoms of the presenting opportunistic infection or condition that meet the criteria for an AIDS diagnosis. The symptoms are variable depending on the mode of transmission and the age a child becomes infected. In general, the younger a child is at the time of acquisition, the more severe the symptoms, the more quickly the disease progresses, and the poorer the prognosis. However, there have been tremendous gains in understanding HIV and in developing new effective therapies that slow disease progression, thus delaying the appearance of symptoms.

The severity of each clinical manifestation varies by organ system and often is the result of several factors, including viral replication in the affected tissue, an opportunistic infection of the organ, concurrent autoimmune or immunodeficiency processes in the organ, or the side effects of medication therapies for treatment of HIV or prophylaxis. Infants who acquire HIV perinatally are at greatest risk of poor health outcomes and premature death, because they may experience failure to thrive, developmental delays, generalized lymphadenopathy, hepatomegaly, splenomegaly, *Pneumocystis jiroveci* pneumonia, bacterial pneumonia, anemia, thrombocytopenia, recurrent candidiasis, nephropathy, cardiomyopathy, and cancers (Yogev & Chadwick, 2007).

Older children may exhibit recurrent bacterial infections, generalized lymphadenopathy, hepatomegaly, splenomegaly, lymphoid interstitial pneumonitis, poor school performance, fatigue, and so forth. Laboratory data may show decreased T cells, elevated or decreased B cells, or anemia. If other organ systems are involved, lab tests pertaining to those systems may be altered. For example, in nephropathy, an elevated BUN and creatinine may be evident (Burns et al., 2009; Yogev & Chadwick, 2007).

Adolescents present with symptoms similar to adults, although many will be asymptomatic for many years. Many adults diagnosed with HIV are thought to have become infected during adolescence, demonstrating the initial benign course of HIV disease. Some people who become infected have an initial illness resembling the flu, then appear to recover fully without symptoms of any illness.

DIAGNOSIS

A careful history is important in determining whether testing for HIV is indicated, although testing should be offered to anyone who (1) is sexually active, (2) has drug-using sexual partners, (3) has a suspicious or documented history of sexual abuse, (4) is pregnant, (5) is an infant whose mother used drugs, (6) uses drugs, or (7) has symptoms suggestive of HIV infection.

The timing of transmission of HIV from mother to child is particularly important in the correct diagnosis of infants. The standard ELISA (enzyme linked immunosorbent assay) HIV antibody test can be used for anyone older than 15–18 months of age. It cannot be used for younger infants because of the persistence of maternal antibodies (IgG) until this age, so the test would actually only be indirectly testing the mother. The antibody will be positive (i.e., antibodies are detected) from 3 weeks to 6 months after

TABLE 27-5 Diagnosis of HIV Infection in Infants, Children, and Adolescents

AGE FOR TEST	NAME OF TEST	SENSITIVITY	COMMENTS
Birth, 1, 3–6 months	HIV DNA PCR	38% @ 48 hrs age, 93% age 14 days	Most common test
	HIV plasma RNA assay	May or may not be more sensitive	More expensive
	HIV cultures	Same as DNA PCR	More complex, expensive, results in 2 weeks
>18 months	HIV IgG EIA "antibody test"	99%	Most commonly known test
Any	P24 antigen	Less sensitive	Very specific

initial infection. A positive result on the ELISA is confirmed by the Western Blot test, which identifies specific proteins and glycoproteins found in antibodies specific to HIV (Table 27-5) (Alvarez & Rathore, 2007).

Infants from birth to 18 months of age should be tested by using a viral diagnostic assay. The HIV DNA polymerase chain reaction (PCR) is the preferred test to confirm HIV infection in infants. Plasma HIV RNA assay or HIV whole cell viral culture can also be used to confirm HIV status in infants. A positive test indicates probable infection and should be confirmed on a second specimen as soon as possible. Testing for HIV by a PCR test should be done at birth or before the infant is 48 hours of age, at 14 days, at 1–2 months, and at 3–6 months of age (Alvarez & Rathore, 2007; United States Department of Health and Human Services [USDHHS], 2008a; Working Group on ART, 1998) to determine actual infection status in an infant known to have a mother with HIV, and at any time up to 18 months of age in an infant having other indications for testing. Many treatment decisions are made based on lymphocyte subsets (primarily CD4+ T lymphocytes and percentage) in conjunction with the DNA viral load level, particularly in determining when to initiate medications and when to change them.

TREATMENT

The management of HIV is complex and requires a coordinated multidisciplinary team approach for the many physiological, psychosocial, and spiritual issues involved. It is a unique infectious illness because multiple family members may be infected and the course of illness is unpredictable. Advances in medical care and treatment of the disease are evolving HIV infection into a chronic illness, with an eventual outcome of death. Multidisciplinary team members usually include physicians, nurses, social workers, dieticians, physical therapists, occupational therapists, pharmacists, and case managers. It is helpful to offer other support services, particularly in this overwhelmingly low socioeconomic group of affected clients, transportation assistance, child care, and interpreter services.

The goals of management are to slow the progression of disease and improve the quality of life of infected persons. Prophylactic treatment begins with highly active antiretroviral therapy (HAART). Antiretroviral (AVR) medications should begin early, no later than 6 weeks of age for the infant with the infection or born to an infected mother. This is done primarily through a combination of several antiretroviral drugs (AVRs). The medication regime consists of at least three medications from a minimum of two different categories. Fourteen from these categories have been approved to be used in treating children (Alvarez & Rathore, 2007; USDHHS (2008a). (See Table 27-6 for the medications that are used in treating AIDS). Other essential measures in managing HIV/AIDS is preventing, detecting, and providing early treatment of opportunistic infections, as well as supporting and promoting growth and development.

Guidelines for initiating HAART and when to change drug regimens are updated frequently by collaborations between a number of clinicians, researchers, and health policy groups. Initial medication drug regimens usually include three from at least two of the following categories: nonnucleoside reverse transcriptase inhibitors (NNRTIs), nucleoside reverse transcriptase inhibitor (NRTIs), protease inhibitors (PsI), and fusion inhibitors (Alvarez & Rathore, 2007; USDHHS 2008a;

TABLE 27-6 Antiretroviral Agents for HIV

FAMILY	MODE OF ACTION	NAME
Nonnucleosides Reverse Transcriptase Iinhibitors (NNRTIs)	Bind directly to viral reverse transcriptase and prevent conversion of RNA to DNA	Nevirapine Efavirenz
Nucleoside/ Nucleotide Reverse Transcriptase Inhibitors (NNRTIs)	Inhibits action of viral reverse transcriptase in the conversion of RNA to DNA	Abacavir Zidovudine (AVD) Didanosine Lamivudine Stavudine Emtricitabine
Protease Inhibitors	Prevents protease function in assemblage and growth of HIVs	Nelfinavir Ritonavir Atazanvir Fosamprenavir Lopinovir/Ritonavir
Fusion Inhibitors	Blocks viral entry	Enfuvirtide

Information taken from Alvarez & Rathore, 2007; USDHHS, 2008a; Blosser, Brady, & Muller, 2009. Infectious diseases and immunizations. In C. Burns, A. Dunn, M. Brady, N. Strarr & C. Blosser (Eds.). *Pediatric primary care* (4th ed.). St. Louis, MO: Saunders Elsevier, pp. 477–552.

USDHHS, 2008b). Children being treated with antiretroviral drugs will have a complete blood count and blood chemistry, prior to beginning treatment, six weeks into treatment, and every three to four months during treatment. It is highly recommended that CD4+ cell counts and HIV RNA levels also be drawn to evaluate effectiveness of the treatment and to monitor compliance. It is very important that nurses provide education to caregivers regarding the side effects that are associated with Antiretroviral Drugs (ARVs) and what actions to take if any of these occur. Research continues to be conducted to find other treatments and strategies to help strengthen the immune system.

The prevention of opportunistic infections includes the use of sulfamethoxazole or trimethoprim as prophylaxis against *Pneumocystis carinii* pneumonia (for CD4+ cells <200), which is still the primary cause of death for both children and adults, and possibly prophylaxis for *Mycobacterium avium-intracellulare* and cytomegalovirus retinitis, which are of more concern with very low CD4+ cells (<50). In addition, azithromycin may be prescribed as a prophylactic agent against *Mycobacterium Avium-intracellulare,* and Nystatin may be used to help prevent *Candida* (Mink, 2008). However, these, and other opportunistic infections (OI), are becoming less frequent with the use of HAART.

Much of the remaining ongoing medical management is related to early detection of HIV clinical manifestations and opportunistic infections. Early intervention can then be initiated, often making the effects of the illness through appropriate treatment and referrals more tolerable. It is also important to incorporate well-child care with the usual anticipatory guidance topics, which are often overlooked in many chronic illnesses. Important considerations in immunizations include following the recommended schedule with the exceptions of using only the inactivated formulation for polio (IPV), receiving an annual influenza vaccine, considering varicella only for children with milder disease and excluding those with severe suppression from measles vaccine (Yogev & Chadwick, 2007).

EVIDENCE-BASED PRACTICE

The Art of Nursing: Supporting Self-Concept and Emotional Status of Children with HIV/AIDS

CLINICAL PROBLEM

The Joint United Nations Program on HIV/AIDS reported that by the end of 2007 there were 2.5 million children under the age of 15 years of age living with HIV/AIDS. With the availability of antiretroviral therapies these children are living longer and with issues of chronic illness, managing multiple medications frequently during the day, nutritional issues, diarrhea, skin conditions, etc. Children with other chronic conditions deal with developmental changes, social, emotional, functional, and behavioral challenges, and suffer from depression, low self-esteem, and anxiety. These effects can adversely impact overall quality of life.

BEST CLINICAL PRACTICE

Nurses concerned about the well being of children with HIV/AIDS need to provide holistic nursing care, including therapeutic interventions, communication, and nurturing behaviors. Children with adequate social support tend to thrive and cope with their disease more effectively.

IMPLICATIONS FOR NURSING

Nurses need to:

- Be cued to use tools and to assess self-concept and emotional indicators of children with HIV/AIDS or other chronic illnesses.
- Consider all aspects of life when providing care to children with HIV/AIDS, not only managing disease implications, but recognizing spiritual, developmental, social, familial, and economic factors.
- Assess a child's self-concept and emotional indicators as a factor in developing a holistic plan of care.
- Use alternative strategies to evaluate self-concept, such as art therapy, if children are housed in orphanages or group homes since they also need more positive reinforcement and caring responses.
- Be alert to how much and what kinds of social, emotional, physical, developmental, spiritual, and economic support children and families may need to promote coping skills and managing the impact of HIV/AIDS upon the child and family's lives.

Reference: Waweru, S. M., Reynolds, A., & Buckner, E. B. (2008). Perceptions of children with HIV/AIDS from the USA and Kenya: Self-concept and emotional indicators. *Pediatric Nursing, 34,* 117–124.

NURSING MANAGEMENT

ASSESSMENT

The assessment of children with HIV can be extensive. Family processes must always be considered, particularly around issues of diagnosis, disclosure, grieving, caregiver strain, involvement of extended family, fears/hopes/hopelessness, spiritual beliefs, support systems, loneliness/social isolation, altered parenting, and coping.

NURSING DIAGNOSIS

1. *Deficient knowledge* related to managing acute episode and chronic illness.
2. *Imbalanced nutrition* related to taking in less than daily requirements.
3. *Altered growth and development* related to effects of chronic disease.
4. *Impaired care at home* due to insufficient finances, unfamiliarity with community resources, and/or inadequate support systems.

CASE STUDY / CARE PLAN

A CHILD LIVING WITH HIV

Penelope is an 18-month-old child with HIV. She lives with her mother Anna, her sister Catherine, and her mother's boyfriend. Anna was diagnosed with AIDS four months prior to Penelope's birth. They live in government housing and rely on Medicaid and the state for medical assistance, housing, and food. Anna brings Penelope to the emergency department because she has been "feeling hot," is fussier than usual, and has had "liquid poop." Anna is "tired of dealing with it all."

NURSING CARE PLAN

ASSESSMENT

Temperature 38.9°C (102°F), heart rate 98, BP 110/70, and respirations 48. Breath sounds congested bilaterally, oxygen saturation 89%, increased work of breathing. Penelope is listless and whimpers. She hasn't wanted to eat for the last 3 days. Diaper change × 4 in 20 minutes, stool is green and watery. She has lost 4 pounds since her last ED visit 4 weeks ago. Anna is hovering and very anxious appearing. She is teary and looks exhausted.

NURSING DIAGNOSIS 1

Impaired gas exchange related to inadequate immune system and pulmonary disease (*Pneumocystis jiroveci* [PJP]).

EXPECTED OUTCOME

Oxygen saturations >94% on room air, respiratory rate 12 – 20 tissue oxygenation 70%, and child is able to engage in physical activity.

NOC: Respiratory Status: Gas Exchange

NIC: Oxygen Therapy, Calming Technique

INTERVENTIONS/*RATIONALES*

1. Maintain patient airway. *Facilitates tissue oxygenation.*
2. Position for maximum ventilatory efficiency. *Facilitates tissue oxygenation.*
3. Monitor vital signs, pulse oximetry readings. *To detect or prevent hypoxemia.*
4. Administer supplemental oxygen (as ordered). *To prevent hypoxemia.*

EVALUATION

Child has effective gaseous exchange based on assessment and tissue oxygen level.

NURSING DIAGNOSIS 2

Imbalanced nutrition: Less than body requirements related to diarrheal losses, loss of appetite, metabolic needs, and recurrent infections.

EXPECTED OUTCOME

Penelope's nutrition improves and she gains at least 1 pound a week.

NOC: Nutritional Status: Nutrient Intake, Energy

NIC: Diarrheal Management, Energy Management, Nutritional Monitoring and Management

INTERVENTIONS/*RATIONALES*

1. Provide high-calorie,high-protein meals. *To meet body's requirements for metabolism, healing, and growth.*
2. Provide small frequent feedings. *Requires less energy; meets body's requirements for metabolism, healing, and growth.*

(Continues)

CASE STUDY / CARE PLAN (Continued)

3. Supplement intake with protein shakes. *To maximize quality of intake.*
4. Monitor weight daily. *To assess need for alternative nutritional interventions if growth is not progressing or if weight decreases*

EVALUATION

Penelope gains 1 pound a week.

NURSING DIAGNOSIS 3

Interrupted family processes related to having a life-threatening disease

EXPECTED OUTCOME

Anna verbalizes understanding of plan of care, accepts support and encouragement, asks for assistance in planning for care after discharge, and accepts support from social services.

NOC: Caregiver Emotional Health

NIC: Caregiver Support

INTERVENTIONS/*RATIONALES*

1. Recognize concern and need for information and support. *To provide what is needed.*
2. Encourage participation in care planning meetings. *To facilitate parent involvement in care.*
3. Assess understanding of plan of care. *To provide what is needed.*
4. Reinforce or increase understanding of therapies and treatment. *To facilitate parent involvement in care.*
5. Acknowledge feelings of anxiety and fear. *To lessen feelings of anxiety.*
6. Support and provide comfort. *To lessen feelings of anxiety.*
7. Identify available resources (e.g., social services, clergy). *To facilitate parent involvement in care.*
8. Identify and support coping abilities. *To facilitate parent involvement in care.*

EVALUATION

Anna able to verbalize plan of care.

Outcome Identification

1. Family will understand disease, how transmission occurs, and how to manage acute episode and chronic illness.
2. Child's nutritional status will be maintained/improved to optimal state.
3. Child's immunizations will be up-to-date.
4. Child will not develop secondary or opportunistic infections.
5. Child's development will be minimally affected by disease state.
6. Family care at home will be adequate and community resources/supports will be utilized.

Planning and Implementation

1. Teach family about signs and symptoms of acute illness, how to manage symptoms, and when to call health care provider.
2. Teach family principles of adequate nutrition; suggest foods high in protein and calories, use of dietary supplements if needed, small frequent meals and snacks.
3. Suggest appropriate activities to facilitate development. Teach family developmental milestones. Provide appropriate community resources. Provide encouragement.
4. Listen to family's concerns related to caring for the child;

Evaluation

1. Family verbalizes understanding of how to manage acute episode and chronic illness.
2. Child's nutritional status is improved from baseline.
3. Child's development follows expected patterns.
4. Family care at home is supportive. Community resources are used.

Family Teaching

The waiting period to determine the infection status of the young infant at about 4 months of age is one of uncertainty, anxiety, and distress for caregivers. Encourage the family to

EVIDENCE-BASED PRACTICE

Increasing Adherence to Therapy in HIV-Infected Adolescents

CLINICAL PROBLEM

Adherence to highly active antiretroviral medication regimens is a problem in the adolescent population. Mental health barriers, high/low self-efficacy and outcome expectancy, and the presence of specific structural barriers are related to non adherence, which is associated with poorer outcomes of increased morbidity and premature death.

BEST CLINICAL PRACTICE

- Indicators for non adherence of antiretroviral medication regimen include mood disorders, one's sense of being able to adhere to the medications prescribed, one's impression of the impact of taking antiretroviral therapy, and several barriers including a place to sleep, the presence or absence of medical insurance, transportation to get needed medications, transportation to the clinic for appointments, getting the medication prescriptions filled, problems related to one's school or employment, and problems related to family or child care, if they had children.

IMPLICATIONS FOR NURSING

Since most youth with adherence issues are struggling with more than one issue that is a barrier, it is important to thoroughly assess adolescents who are HIV positive in order to assist them overcome barriers that influence their adherence to prescribed therapy.

- Provide developmentally appropriate nursing care to adolescents.
- Intervention programs should identify a clear purpose, identify essential knowledge concepts, emphasize self-examination, present life skills, and emphasize family and peers.

Reference: Rudy, B. J., Murphy, D. A., Harris, D. R., Muenz, L., Ellen, J., for The Adolescent Trials Network for HIV/AIDS Interventions. (2009). Patient-related risks for nonadherence to antiretroviral therapy among HIV-infected youth in the United States: A study of prevalence and interactions. *AIDS Patient Care and Standards, 23*(3), 185–194. DOI: 10.1089=apc.2008.0162

RESEARCH Highlight

Does Disclosing that a Child has HIV Affect Quality of Life?

STUDY PURPOSE

To discover how disclosing that a child has HIV impacts the child's quality of life and how old the child is when the disclosure occurs.

METHODS

This longitudinal study asked primary caregivers of HIV-infected youths to complete an age-specific quality-of-life instrument before and after disclosure that the child had HIV that examined symptom distress, psychological status, physical functioning, general health perception, social/role functioning, and health care utilization. In addition, the age when disclosure occurred was obtained.

FINDINGS

The median age of the children at disclosure was 11 years of age (range: 9–12 years). There was no significant difference in the quality of life indicators before and immediately after disclosure even though the scores dropped, except for general health perception. In addition, the study discovered over time, disclosure is occurring at younger ages, perhaps suggesting there is less fear and stigma surrounding the diagnosis.

IMPLICATIONS

Since disclosing that a child has HIV does not decrease the child's quality of life, caregivers should not worry that such disclosure will affect the child's quality of life. Disclosure should also be encouraged at a younger age.

REFERENCE

Butler, A., Williams, P., Howland, L., Storm, D., Hutton, N., Seage, G., for the Pediatric AIDS Clinical Trials Group 219C Study Team (2009). Impact of disclosure of HIV infection on health-related quality of life among children and adolescents with HIV infection. *Pediatrics, 123*(3), 935–943.

talk to health care providers. However, if the diagnosis is positive, referral to support groups is warranted. Even though most children generally are healthy for a number of years, they will be closely monitored. For example, infants and children will be evaluated at the usual well-child intervals, and often at three-month intervals when older. Children's growth and development will be closely monitored for early signs of growth failure and developmental delays. Caregivers should be encouraged to consult with their health care provider if they notice anything that seems delayed. Transmission of HIV should be discussed and clarified, as misconceptions continue to abound. Encourage living as "normal a life" as possible with the restrictions imposed by the illness. Families and individuals can be assisted through social support systems, peer networks, community resources, ongoing formal education, and spiritual beliefs. It is important to establish strong trusting relationships with health care providers in a multidisciplinary team, as the relationships are likely to be long term. Infants and children need to be integrated into all aspects of their respective communities and cultures to maximize their full developmental potentials.

Children with HIV/AIDS should attend school. Schools have a legal obligation to provide for a child's education and to provide medications when indicated during school hours.

There is a continuing concern about transmitting HIV through biting, although there has not been a single documented case of this occurring in the United States. HIV-positive children are at greater risk of contracting illnesses at school, such as varicella (chickenpox) or influenza. Common childhood illnesses can be treated or minimized; it is important to notify the child's health care provider if exposures occur.

ALLERGIC REACTIONS TO MEDICATIONS

Medication allergies are adverse reactions to medications or their metabolites caused by immunologic responses. Children with these allergies can have reactions after ingestion, injection, or application of medication to the skin (e.g. ointments, creams). The reactions demonstrate either systemic hypersensitivity or organ-specific patterns. They usually recur on re-exposure to the same medication, but may also occur with prolonged administration (Redjal, 2008). Sensitivity and reactions occur from an individual's intolerance to a particular medication or its concentration.

INCIDENCE AND ETIOLOGY

Allergic and immunologic medication reactions account for 6–10% of adverse reactions in hospitalized clients. The risk of such an allergic reaction is 1–3%. Some people may be allergic to all medications in the same or similar class based on antigen properties. Common allergens are a phenolophalein, sulfonamides, NSAIDS, tetracyclines, barbiturates, and oral contraceptives.

Medication allergies are less common and less severe in infants. However, some children may have a genetic predisposition to develop medication allergies, and if one parent has an allergy, his/her children may have a 40% chance of developing an allergy. The rate goes up when both parents have allergies (Rote, 2010).

PATHOPHYSIOLOGY

Medication reactions have an immunological basis and are usually IgE mediated. This is a matter of concern because of the risk for anaphylaxis. Histamine is the most potent mediator of IgE mediated hypersensitivity causing bronchial constriction and increased blood flow to the affected area. Reactions may also be caused by nonspecific histamine release, when the medications cause the release of mediators from mast cells which cannot be distinguished clinically from IgE-mediated responses. Hypersensitivity responses result from sensitization against an antigen that causes an immune response, and can occur immediately or are delayed. The timing of the reaction and clinical manifestations are linked to exposure. Anaphylaxis is the most rapid and severe form of immediate hypersensitivity, occurring within minutes of re-exposure to the antigen, and can be either cutaneous or systemic (Rote, 2010).

CLINICAL MANIFESTATIONS

Reactions can be classified into cutaneous or multiple organ system manifestations. Cutaneous reactions are the most common, while multiple organ system involvement is the more life-threatening and dramatic presentation. Cutaneous reactions include urticaria (**angioedema**), pruritis, erythematosus, maculopapular exanthems, and allergic contact dermatitis. **Urticaria**, the wheel-like lesions, can move from one body part to another and appear after beginning the medication. Urticaria resolves fairly rapidly after the medication is discontinued; however, occasionally, chronic urticaria lasting six weeks or more may persist despite medication stoppage.

Maculopapular rashes are the most common form of cutaneous reactions. They are symmetric, often confluent erythematous lesions, which typically spare the palms and soles, and are more common in people with concurrent viral infections. The eruptions usually appear within one week of starting the medication, may subside even with use of the medication, may not recur with repeated exposure, or may occasionally progress to an exfoliative dermatitis.

Contact dermatitis is an example of delayed-type hypersensitivity and occurs with medications applied directly to the skin. It is usually pruritic, erythematous, vesicular, or maculopapular. Contact dermatitis usually takes 5–7 days to develop, and can occur within 24 hours after re-exposure.

Multiple organ system manifestations include anaphylaxis, nonspecific histamine release, erythema multiforme or Stevens-Johnson syndrome, toxic epidermal necrolysis (TEN), hypersensitivity syndromes, and medication fever). **Anaphylaxis** is an acute, life-threatening reaction with diffuse erythema, urticaria, angioedema, pruritis, bronchospasm, laryngeal edema, hyperperistalsis, hypotension, or cardiac dysrhythmias Anaphylaxis, sometimes known as anaphylactic shock, occurs rapidly, within 5 to 30 minutes after exposure. Physiologic responses include: vasodilatation, pooling of blood in the extremities, inadequate blood flow which leads to poor tissue perfusion and impaired cellular metabolism. Nonspecific histamine release

NURSING ALERT

Medication Allergies

Nurses are key in educating parents about possible medication reactions. When obtaining a health history it is important to obtain information about past medications taken, if the child experienced any difficulties taking the medication (e.g., rash, fever), and to verify any known allergies, which should be clearly documented and highlighted in the child's health history. Nurses should be careful and always follow appropriate policies and procedures when administering medication. It is also helpful to have the child wear an alert bracelet which identifies any allergy the child might have, especially if there is sensitivity to medications.

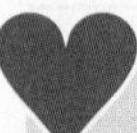

FAMILY**TEACHING**

Anaphylaxis

- Know the offending medication or allergen such as latex, insect stings, drugs, or foods.
- Teach child or caregiver to use and carry an EpiPen.
- Remind family that prevention is critical.

reactions, although having a different etiology, have the same systemic manifestations as anaphylaxis (Rote, 2010; Sheikh, Shehata, Brown, & Simons, 2009).

Erythema multiforme, a syndrome characterized by inflammation of the skin and mucous membranes, may be caused by medications in 10–20% of all cases, and is an erythematous, maculopapular, vesicular, urticarial rash that may include target lesions. It is relatively rare, occurring 1–2 cases per million people per year (Levi et al., 2009) but can be life threatening. The most severe form is **Stevens-Johnson syndrome (SJS)**, which may exhibit widespread blisters, ulcerations, and erosions of the mucosa and involve conjunctival lesions. A rash follows 1–2 days later (Figure 27-3). The lesions, bullae, and erosions spread and may cover up to 10% of the body surface area. The skin may become so fragile that full thickness epidermis peels off in sheets with only light touch. Lungs and gastroiintestinal slouging of the mucous membrane may occur as well as corneal abrasions potentially causing scarring or even blindness. **Toxic epidermal necrolysis** is an acute illness of fever, epidermal loss of more than 30% of the body surface area, and visceral involvement with an associated 30–40% mortality rate (Nicol & Huether, 2010).

Hypersensitivity syndromes, such as with anticonvulsant therapy, usually occur within 1 to 3 weeks after initiating therapy, but can occur within three months or later. Manifestations include fever, erythematous papules, tender and generalized lymphadenopathy, hepatitis, nephritis, and leukocytosis. Periorbital edema, myalgias, or arthralgias may also occur. The fever associated with a reaction to a medication is manifested by an elevated temperature, rash, eosinophilia, leukocytosis, and elevated sedimentation rate, can occur with any medication, and almost always resolves within 72 hours of discontinuing the medication.

DIAGNOSIS

The diagnosis of allergic medication reactions is usually made by a history of initiation and use, onset and presentation of clinical manifestations, and improvement of symptoms after discontinuing the medication. Administration of the offending medication again is occasionally used to confirm the diagnosis, although this can cause a serious reaction. Diagnostic skin testing is available for some medications, which can limit the systemic symptoms. Certain laboratory tests can be ordered, such as white cell count and sedimentation rate.

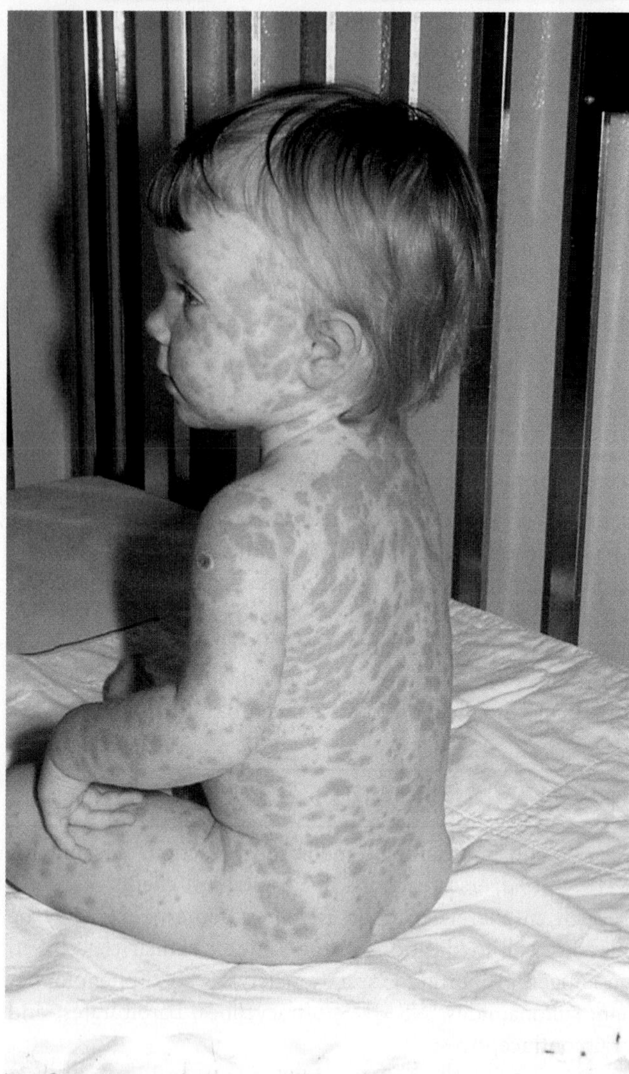

FIGURE 27-3 Photo of a toddler with erythema multiforme major, an allergic rash, associated with Stevens-Johnson Syndrome. PHOTOGRAPHY BY ALLEN W. MATHIES, MD, & JOHN LEEDOM, MD, CALIFORNIA EMERGENCY PREPARED OFFICE, IMMUNIZATION BRANCH. PHOTO OBTAINED HTTP://WWW.WRONGDIAGNOSIS.COM/PHIL/HTML/ALLERGIES/4652.HTML

TREATMENT

Treatment varies based on the pathophysiology and severity of the reaction. Avoidance of contact with the offending medication is the first intervention. Anaphylaxis and histamine release reactions are an emergency and should be treated with Epinephrine, which inhibits further mediator release, reduces vascular permeability, and improves vasomotor tone. Oxygen should be administered if indicated, along with measurement of blood oxygen levels. An intravenous infusion of normal saline may be indicated for hypotension. Breathing may need to be supported through intubation or tracheostomy for laryngeal spasm or edema. Antihistamines may attenuate the reaction, although they are limited in usefulness during the acute onset of symptoms. Corticosteroids may decrease the possible late-phase reactions occasionally occurring 6 to 12 hours after the onset of anaphylaxis.

CRITICAL THINKING

Stevens-Johnson Syndrome

Twelve-year-old Ron was admitted to the unit with an erythematous papular rash covering his arms, legs, abdomen, the soles of his feet, and the palms of his hands. His mother Helen said that he had a sore throat, headache, fever, and "just didn't feel well" a day or two before he broke out with his rash. He also had been on penicillin for 5 days because of a throat infection. He was diagnosed with Stevens-Johnson Syndrome. What nursing care would be appropriate?

IN THE REAL WORLD

I was diagnosed with JIA as an early teen, around the time when I started my period. My joints really hurt and were so swollen. I was really miserable. I remember the nurses who took care of me. They were so kind and patient. I am sure I was not an easy child to care for, and at the time, thought I would never be able to lead a normal life. But, I was one of the lucky ones. I have no problems today and no residual effects from that disease. Perhaps those early experiences were why I decided to become a nurse. I hope the children I care for feel the same way about me that I did about those nurses who cared for me so long ago.

Treatment is primarily supportive for erythema multiforme and toxic epidermal necrolysis, although corticosteroids are recommended in the former to prevent visceral involvement and shorten the duration of symptoms. Corticosteroids are also indicated in hypersensitivity syndromes. Benadryl relieves symptoms of most milder cutaneous reactions, and other symptoms of histamine release such as pruritis, erythema, and swelling. Refer to the nursing alert box.

NURSING MANAGEMENT

General nursing care for a child with a medication reaction involves being sure there is an effective airway if the child is having an acute reaction; providing comfort measures related to pruritis, pain, and itching; providing oral hygiene and skin care; teaching the child and family about the treatments ordered and experienced; administering and watching for the side effects of any medications ordered; teaching the child and caregivers about medications that should be avoided; providing opportunities for the child to rest; providing age-appropriate activities; and encouraging the child to wear a medic alert bracelet with the name of the medication the child is allergic to listed on the back.

FAMILY TEACHING

Encourage caregivers and children to know the name of the offending medication(s) to avoid exposure or being prescribed that medication in the future. Although it cannot be known for certain the medication will cause the same reaction, it is more likely than not to cause a similar reaction.

Some medications may be required for lifesaving treatment in the future; drug sensitization may be needed, such as for penicillin, when there is a history of reactions to a particular class of medications.

KEY CONCEPTS

- The function of the immune system is to prevent or eliminate infections, recognize self from nonself, and maintain homeostasis.
- Immune system alterations are almost always chronic illnesses that are managed rather than cured, using a multidisciplinary team approach.
- Immune system dysfunction demonstrates a wide variety of clinical manifestations
- Juvenile idiopathic arthritis (JIA), an autoimmune disorder involving joints and occasionally the eyes or heart, causes pain and affects mobility and activities of daily living and has multiple psychosocial consequences.
- Systemic lupus erythematosus (SLE), a lifelong autoimmune disorder characterized by multiple system involvement, requires a delicate balance between symptoms of the disease, side effects of medication and treatment, and psychosocial aspects of both.
- HIV or AIDS is an infectious disease known for affecting primarily the immune system, but demonstrates multiple clinical manifestations directly related to its multi-organ system involvement and requires many of the same considerations as other chronic diseases
- Children with HIV/AIDS are living longer and experience chronic health issues; most children will be impacted by HIV encephalopathy which adversely impacts growth and development.
- Highly active antiretroviral therapy (HAART) involves using a combination of several antiretroviral drugs; at least three medications from a minimum of two categories are used.
- Medication reactions may vary from a mild rash to a serious systemic reaction.
- Nursing care of children with immune system alterations involves knowing about the etiology, treatment, medications, management, and educational needs.

REVIEW ACTIVITIES

1. Describe the three subgroups of juvenile idiopathic arthritis (JIA).
2. Discuss nursing management goals of JIA.
3. Describe the pathophysiology of systemic lupus erythematosus (SLE).
4. Discuss issues related to pregnancy for a teen age female with SLE.
5. Discuss the clinical criteria used to make treatment decisions for children with HIV/AIDS.
6. Discuss the major nursing management goals and care for children with HIV/AIDS.
7. Discuss the nursing diagnoses for the child with HIV/AIDS and appropriate nursing care.
8. Describe the multiple organ system patterns involved in allergic drug reactions and the appropriate nursing care required.

STUDY QUESTIONS

1. Juvenile rheumatoid arthritis (JIA), a chronic autoimmune inflammatory disease, is characterized by:
   a. Abnormal joint function and appearance.
   b. Decreased mobility and pain.
   c. Severe pain and abnormal joint appearance.
   d. Swelling and abnormal joint function.
2. Melissa, a 13-year-old adolescent, who has missed the last seven days of school, is being seen for reassessment of her juvenile rheumatoid arthritis. The nurse should most likely consider which of the following nursing diagnoses based on this information?
   a. Risk for disturbed body image related to physical appearance
   b. Pain related to joint inflammation
   c. Anxiety related to stress of chronic illness and altered daily life
   d. Activity intolerance related to chronic pain
3. A client with JIA is placed on Etanercept, a biologic response modifier. Your nursing management should include:
   a. Teaching the client to monitor for side effects of abdominal pain, bleeding, and gastrointestinal complaints.
   b. Teaching the client how to administer the medication subcutaneously.
   c. Scheduling a follow-up appointment to monitor liver function.
   d. Teaching the client and her family about the importance of avoiding NSAIDS.
4. A client requests information on reducing joint inflammation. Which should the nurse not recommend?
   a. Applying ice packs to help reduce joint swelling and inflammation
   b. Using braces and splints to help promote proper alignment
   c. Applying warm moist compresses to the involved joints in the morning
   d. Using anti-inflammatory agents
5. A child diagnosed with systemic lupus erythematosus (SLE) may require special dietary considerations. The nurse needs to educate the parents on reasons for the dietary changes. Which statement is correct?
   a. Altered renal function may occur secondary to the diagnosis of SLE.
   b. The need for increased protein and complex carbohydrates is associated with immunosuppressants.
   c. An increasing magnesium intake will prevent loss of bone density secondary to the chronic joint inflammation.
   d. A supplement can help fight infection and prevent bleeding.
6. The nurse is providing education to a mother whose infant has human immunodeficiency virus (HIV infection). Which of the following statements indicates that the parent understands infection control precautions?
   a. "I will need to use gloves whenever I hold my baby."
   b. "I will need to monitor my baby's rectal temperature every day."
   c. "When I change my baby's diaper I will need to wear gloves."
   d. "I need to wash my hands after feeding my baby."
7. The nurse is caring for a 6 year old who has HIV/AIDs. Which of the following nursing diagnoses is most appropriate based on complications of HIV/AIDS?
   a. Risk for altered body image related to skin irritation
   b. Pain related to hepatosplenomegaly
   c. Altered nutrition related to chronic diarrhea and lack of appetite
   d. Risk for noncompliance related to taking 12 medications each day
8. An 8-year-old refugee from Somalia is brought to the local emergency department by a social worker. Since arriving in the United States the child has been ill with fever, upper respiratory symptoms, diarrhea, and sores in his mouth. The social worker explains that the child does not want to eat, has lost weight, and only wants to

sleep. Based on the clinical categories for children with HIV infection under the age of 13 you would anticipate that the child will be classified as:
   a. Category N.
   b. Category A.
   c. Category B.
   d. Category C.

9. The nurse is teaching an 8-year-old child with asthma and multiple allergies about emergency care for symptoms of anaphylaxis. Instruction should include which of the following?
   a. Carry and use oxygen at the first signs of distress.
   b. Carry and take the prescribed amount of a bronchodilator at the first signs of distress.
   c. Carry and use an EpiPen at the first signs of distress.
   d. Carry and use an Albuterol inhaler at the first signs of distress.

10. A 2-year-old is admitted to your unit with a diagnosis of Stevens-Johnson-Syndrome (SJS). Based on your understanding of SJS, which of the following nursing diagnoses should the nurse recognize as a high priority?
   a. Altered skin integrity related to an allergic skin allergy
   b. Risk for altered fluid and electrolyte balance related to chronic diarrhea
   c. Altered skin integrity related to erythema multiforme major
   d. Risk for altered nutrition related to medication therapy

REFERENCES

Albers, H. M., Wessels, J. A., van der Straaten, R. J., Brinkman, D. M., Suijlekom-Smit, L. W., Kamphuis, S. S. et al. (2009). Time to treatment as an important factor for the response to methotrexate in juvenile rheumatoid arthritis. *Arthritis Rheumatism, 61*, 46–51.

Alvarez, A. M., & Rathore, M. H. (2007). Hot topics in pediatric HIV/AIDS. *Pediatric Annals, 36*, 423–432.

American Academy of Pediatrics. (2006). *Red book: Report of the Committee on Infectious Diseases* (27th ed.). Elk Grove Village, IL: Author.

American College of Rheumatology Ad Hoc Committee of Systemic Lupus Erythematosus Guidelines. (1999). Guidelines for referral and management of systemic lupus erythematosus in adults. *Arthritis and Rheumatism, 42*(9), 1785–1796.

Bernatsky, S., Suffy, C., Malleson, P., Feldman, D. E., St. Pierre, Y., & Clarke, A. E. (2007). Economic impact of juvenile idiopathic arthritis. *Arthritis and Rheumatism, 57*, 44–48.

Blosser, C., Brady, M., & Muller, W. (2009). Infectious diseases and immunizations. In C. Burns, A. Dunn, M. Brady, N. Strarr, & C. Blosser, (Eds.). *Pediatric primary care* (4th ed.). St. Louis, MO: Saunders Elsevier, pp. 477–552.

Brunner, H. I., et al. (2006). Differences in disease outcomes between Medicaid and privately insured children: Possible health disparities in juvenile rheumatoid arthritis. *Arthritis and Rheumatism, 55*, 378–384.

Brunner, H., Higgins, G., Wiers, K., Lapidus, S., Olson, J., Onel, K., Punaro, M., Ying, J., & Klein-Gitelman, M. (2009). Health-related quality of life and its relationship to patient disease course in childhood-onset systemic lupus erythematosus. *Journal of Rheumatology, 36*(7), 1536–1545.

Buckley, R. H. (2007). The T-, B-, and NK-cell systems. In R. M. Klingman, R E. Behrman, H. B. Jenson & B. F. Stanton, *Nelson textbook of pediatrics* (18th ed.). Philadelphia: Saunders Elsevier, pp. 873–879.

Burns, C., Dunn, A., Brady, M., Strarr, N., & Blosser, C. (2009). *Pediatric primary care* (4th ed.). St. Louis. MO: Saunders Elsevier.

Butler, A., Williams, P., Howland, L., Storm, D., Hutton, N., Seage, G., for the Pediatric AIDS Clinical Trials Group 219C Study Team (2009). Impact of disclosure of HIV infection on health-related quality of life among children and adolescents with HIV infection. *Pediatrics, 123*(3), 935–943.

Carter, B., Cummings, J., & Cooper, J. (2007). An exploration of best practice in multi-agency working and the experiences of families and children with complex health needs. What works and what needs to be done to improve practice for the future? *Journal Clinical Nursing, 16*, 527–539.

Centers for Disease Control and Prevention (CDC). (1994). Revised classification system for human immunodeficiency virus infection in children less than 13 years of age. *Morbidity and Mortality Weekly Report, 43* (RR-12), 1–10.

Centers for Disease Control and Prevention (CDC). (2006a). *CDC recommends routine, voluntary HIV screening in health care settings.* Retrieved on May 1, 2009, from http://www.cdc.gov/od/oc/media/[ressre;/r060921.htm.

Centers for Disease Control and Prevention (CDC). (2006b). Revised recommendations for HIV testing of adults, adolescents, and pregnant women in health-care settings. *Morbidity and Mortality Weekly Report, 55* (No. RR–14), 1–24.

Centers for Disease Control and Prevention (CDC). (2007a). Cases of HIV infection and AIDS in the United States and dependent areas. *2005 HIV/AIDS Surveillance Report, 17.* Retrieved on May 1, 2009, from http://www.cdc,gov/hiv/topics/surveillance/resources/reports/2005/report/default.htm.

Centers for Disease Control and Prevention (CDC). (2007b). *Mother to child (perinatal) HIV transmission and prevention.* Retrieved on January 23, 2010, from http://www.cdc.gov/hiv/topics/perinatal/resources/factsheets/pdf/perinatal.pdf.

Centers for Disease Control and Prevention (CDC). (2007c). *HIV and its transmission.* Retrieved on May 1, 2000, from http://www.cdc.gov/hiv/resources/factsheets/PDF/transmission.pdf.

Centers for Disease Control and Prevention (CDC). (2008). *HIV/AIDS among African Americans.* Retrieved on May 20, 2009, from http://www.cdc.gov/hiv/topics/aa/resources/factsheets/pdf/aa.pdf.

Edgerton, E. A. (2008). Juvenile idiopathic arthritis/collagen vascular disease. In C. Berkowitz, (Ed.). *Pediatrics: A primary care approach* (3rd ed.). Elk Grove Village IL: American Academy of Pediatrics, pp. 801–808.

Gotlieb, B. S., & Ilowite, N. T. (2006). Systemic lupus erythematosus in children and adolescents. *Pediatrics, 27*, 323–328.

Haines, K. A. (2007). Juvenile idiopathic arthritis: Therapies in the 21st century. *Bulletin of NYU Hospital Joint Disease, 65*, 205–211.

Hashkes, P. J., & Laxer, R. M. (2005). Medical treatment of juvenile idiopathic arthritis. *Journal of the American Medical Association, 294*, 1671–1684.

Joint United Nations Programme on HIV/AIDS (UNAIDS). (2007). Report on global AIDS epidemic, AIDS, epidemic update, 2007. Retrieved on May 31, 2009, from http://www.Unaids.org/en/Knowledge Centre/HIVData/EpiUpdate/EpUpdArchive/2007default.asp.

Klein-Gitelman, M., & Miller, M. (2007). Systemic lupus erythematosus. In R. M. Kliegman, R. E. Behrman, H. B. Jenson, & B. F. Stanton, *Nelson textbook of pediatrics* (18th ed.). Philadelphia, PA: Saunders Elsevier, pp. 1015–1019.

Kline, M. W. (2006). Perspectives on the pediatric HIV/AIDS pandemic: Catalyzing access of children to care and treatment. *Pediatrics, 117,* 1388–1393.

Levi, N. et al. (2009). Medications as risk factors of Stevens-Johnson Syndrome and toxic epidermal necrolysis in children. *Pediatrics, 123,* e297–e304.

Lovell, D. J., Glass, D. et al. (2006). A randomized controlled trial of calcium supplementation to increase bone mineral density in children with juvenile rheumatoid arthritis. *Arthritis and Rheumatism, 54,* 2235–2242.

Lovell, D. J., Reiff, A. et al. (2008). Safety and efficacy of up to eight years of continuous Etanercept therapy in patients with juvenile rheumatoid arthritis. *Arthritis and Rheumatism, 58,* 1496–1504.

Lupus Foundation of America. (2008). "About Lupus." Retrieved on January 23, 2010, from http://www.lupus.org/webmodules/webarticlesnet/templates/new_aboutintroduction.aspx?articleid=311&zoneid=9.

McCance, K. L., & Huether, S. E. (2010). *Pathophysiology: The biologic basis for disease in adults and children* (6th ed.). St. Louis, MO: Mosby.

McCann, L. J., & Woo, P. (2007). Biologic therapies in juvenile idiopathic arthritis: Why and for whom? *Acta Rheumatology Port., 32,* 15–26.

McKenna, M. T. & Hu, X. (2007). Recent trends in the incidence and morbidity associated with perinatal human immunodeficiency virus infection in the United States. *American Journal of Obstetrics and Gynecology,* 197, S10–S16.

Michaels, M. G., & Green, M. (2007). Infections in immunocompromised persons. In R. M. Kliegman, R. E. Behrman, H. B. Jenson, & B. F. Stanton, (Eds.). *Nelson textbook of pediatrics* (18th ed.). Philadelphia, PA: Saunders Elsevier, pp. 1100–1107.

Miller, M., & Cassidy, J. (2007). Juvenile rheumatoid arthritis. In R. M. Kliegman, R. E. Behrman, H. B. Jenson, & B. F. Stanton, (Eds.). *Nelson textbook of pediatrics* (18th ed.). Philadelphia, PA: Saunders Elsevier, pp. 1001–1010.

Mink, C. M. (2008). Pediatric HIV. In C. Berkowitz, (Ed.). *Pediatrics: A primary care approach* (3rd ed.). Elk Grove Village, IL: American Academy of Pediatrics, pp. 115–120.

Moorthy, L. N., Peterson, M. G., Hassett, A. L., Baratelli, M., Chalom, E. C., Hashkes, P. J., Hong, S., Reiff, A., & Lehman, T. J. (2009). Relationship between health-related quality of life and SLE activity and damage in children over time. *Lupus, 18,* pp. 622–629.

Nicol, N. H., & Huether, S. E. (2010). Structure, function, and disorders of the integument. In McCance, K. L., & Huether, S. E., *Pathophysiology: The biologic basis for disease in adults and children,* (6th ed.). St. Louis, MO: Elsevier Mosby, pp. 1644–1679.

Ortiz, Z., Shea, B., Suarez, A. M., Moher, D., Well, G., & Tugwell, P. (2000). Folic acid and follinic acid for reducing side effects in patients receiving methotrexate for rheumatoid arthritis. *Cochrane Database Systematic Review, 2,* CD000951.

Perinatal HIV Guidelines Working Group Members. (2001). Public Health Service Task Force recommendations for use of antiretroviral drugs in pregnant HIV-1-infected women for maternal health and interventions to reduce perinatal HIV-1 transmission in the United States, 1–54.

Petty, R. E., & Cassidy, J. T. (2005). Polyarthritis. In J. T. Cassidy, R. E. Petty, R. M. Laxer, & C. B. Lindsley, (Eds.). *Textbook of pediatric rheumatology* (5th ed.). Philadelphia: Saunders Elsevier, pp. 261–278.

Plowfield, L. A. (2007). HIV disease in children 25 years later. *Pediatric Nursing, 33,* 273–278.

Redjal, N. (2008). Allergic disease. In C. Berkowitz, (Ed.). *Pediatrics: A primary care approach* (3rd ed.). Elk Grove Village, IL: American Academy of Pediatrics, pp. 387–302.

Rote, N. (2010). Alterations in immunity and inflammation. In K. L. McCance & S. E. Huether (Eds.), *Pathophysiology: The biologic basis for disease in adults and children.* 256–292.

Rote, N., & Huether, S. (2010a). Innate immunity: Inflammation. In K. L. McCance & S. E. Huether (Eds.), *Pathophysiology: The biologic basis for disease in adults and children* (6th ed.). St. Louis, MO: Mosby. 183–216.

Rote, N., & Huether, S. (2010b). Infection. In K. L. McCance & S. E. Huether (Eds.), *Pathophysiology: The biologic basis for disease in adults and children.* 293–335.

Rudy, B. J., Murphy, D. A., Harris, D. R., Muenz, L., Ellen, J., for the Adolescent Trials Network for HIV/AIDS Interventions. (2009). Patient-related risks for nonadherence to antiretroviral therapy among HIV-infected youth in the United States: A study of prevalence and interactions. *AIDS Patient Care and Standards, 23*(3), 185–194.

Sheikh, A., Shehata, Y. A., Brown, S. G. A., & Simons, F. E. R. (2009). Adrenaline for the treatment of anaphylaxis: Cochrane systematic review. *Allergy, 64,* 204–212.

Sifuentes, M. (2008). Sexually transmitted infections. In C. Berkowitz, (Ed.). (2008). *Pediatrics: A primary care approach,* 3rd edition. Elk Grove Village, IL: American Academy of Pediatrics, pp. 503–512.

United States Department of Health and Human Services. (2008a). *Guidelines for the use of antiretroviral agents in pediatric HIV infection.* Retrieved on January 23, 2010, from http://aidsinfo.nih.gov/contentfiles/PediatricGuidelines.pdf.

United States Department of Health and Human Services. (2008b). *Pediatric antiretroviral drug information.* Retrieved on January 23, 2010, from http://www.aidsinfo.nih.gov/ContentFiles/PediatricGL_SupI.pdf.

Waweru, S. M., Reynolds, A., & Buckner, E. B. (2008). Perceptions of children with HIV/AIDS from the USA and Kenya: Self-concept and emotional indicators. *Pediatric Nursing, 34,* 117–124.

Working Group on Antiretroviral Therapy and Medical Management of Infants, Children and Adolescents with HIV Infection. (1998). Antiretroviral therapy and medical management of pediatric HIV infection. *Pediatrics, 102,* 1005–1062S.

World Health Organization. (2005). Chronic disease. Retrieved on May 15, 2009, from http://www.who.int/topics/chronic_disease/en/.

Wulffraat, N. M., van Rooijen, E. M., Tewarie, R., Brinkman, D., Prakken, B., & Kuis, W. (2008). Current perspectives of autologous stem cell transplantation for severe juvenile rheumatoid arthritis. *Autoimmunity, 41,* 632–638.

Yogev, R., & Chadwick, E. (2007), Acquired immunodeficiency syndrome (Human Immunodeficiency Virus). In R. M. Kliegman, R. E. Behrman, H. B. Jenson, & B. F. Stanton, (Eds.). *Nelson textbook of pediatrics* (18th ed.). Philadelphia, PA: Saunders Elsevier, pp. 1427–1442.

SUGGESTED READINGS

Benner, P. (2004). Relational ethics of comfort, touch, and solace—endangered arts? *American Journal of Critical Care, 13,* 346–349.

Bonilla, F. A., & Geha, R. S. (2006). Update on primary immunodeficiency diseases. *Journal of Allergy and Clinical Immunology, 117,* S435–S440.

Borchers, A. T., Selmi, C., Cheema, G., Keen, C. L., Shoenfeld, Y., & Gershwin, M. E. (2006). Juvenile rheumatoid arthritis. *Autoimmunity Review, 5,* 279–289.

Burgos-Vargos, R. (2009). A case of childhood-onset ankylosing spondylitis: Diagnosis and treatment. *National Clinical Practice of Rheumatology, 5,* 52–57.

Cibulka, N. J. (2006). Mother-to-child transmission of HIV in the United States. *American Journal of Nursing, 106,* 56–63.

Food Allergy and Anaphylaxis Network. (2006). *School guidelines for managing students with food allergies.* Retrieved May 31, 2009, from http://www.foodallergy.org/school/guidelines.html.

Greenswald, J. L., Burstein, G. R., Pincus, J., & Branson, B. (2006). A rapid review of rapid HIV antibody tests. *Current Infectious Disease Report, 8,* 125–131.

Hamra, M., Ross, M. W., Karuri, K., Orrs, M., & D'Agostino, A. (2005). The relationship between expressed HIV/AIDS-related stigma and beliefs and knowledge about care and support of people living with AIDS in families caring for HIV-infected children in Kenya. *AIDS, 17,* 911–922.

Keehner, E. M., Guttu, M., Warren, M. B., & Swanson, M. (2008). School nurse case management for children with chronic illness: Health, academic, and quality of life outcomes. *Journal of School Nursing, 24,* 205–214.

Len, C. A., Terreri, M. T., Puccini, R. F., Wechsler, R., Silva, E. K., Oliveira, L. M. et al., (2000). Folic acid and folinic acid for reducing side effects in patients receiving methotrexate for rheumatoid arthritis. *Cochrane Database Systematic Review, 2,* CD000951.

Lewis, J. (2006). New CDC guidelines for HIV testing will change health care. *Infectious Disease News.*

Malattia, C., Damasio, M. B., Magnaguagno, F., Pistorio, A., Valle, M., Martinoli, C. et al. (2008). Magnetic resonance imaging, ultrasonography, and conventional radiography in the assessment of bone erosions in juvenile rheumatoid arthritis. *Arthritis and Rheumatism, 59,* 1764–1772.

Marinescu, L. M., & Ilowite, N. T. (2007). Update on pediatric rheumatology: Growth spurt in the knowledge base. *Consultant for Pediatricians,* 397–404.

McElhone, K., Abbott, J., & Teh, L-S. (2006). A review of health related quality of life in systemic lupus erythematosus. *Lupus, 15,* 633–643.

Moorthy, L. N., Harrison, M. J., Peterson, M., & Onel, K. B. (2005). Relationship of quality of life and physical function measures with disease activity in children with systemic lupus erythematosus. *Lupus, 14,* 280–287.

Naar-King, S., Templin, T., Wright, K., Frey, M., Parsons, J. T., & Lam, P. (2006). Psychosocial factors and medication adherence in HIV-positive youth. *AIDS Patient Care and STDs, 20,* 44–47.

Palmer, K., & Burks, W. (2006). Current developments in peanut allergy. *Current Opinion in Allergy and Clinical Immunology, 6,* 202–206.

Pedroso, G. C., & Hilario, M. O. (2006). Development of a tool for early referral of children and adolescents with signs and symptoms suggestive of chronic arthropathy to pediatric rheumatology centers. *Arthritis and Rheumatology, 55,* 373–377.

Perinatal HIV Guidelines Working Group Members. (2001). Public Health Service Task Force recommendations for use of antiretroviral drugs in pregnant HIV-1-infected women for maternal health and interventions to reduce perinatal HIV-1 transmission in the United States, 1–54.

Pongmarutani, T., Alpert, P. T., & Miller, S. K. (2006). Pediatric systemic lupus erythematosus: Management issues in primary practice. *Journal of the American Academy of Nurse Practitioners, 18,* 258–267.

Saarinen, J., Lehtonen, K., Maikia, E., & Lahdenne, P. (2008). Lower extremity isometric strength in children with juvenile idiopathic arthritis. *Clinical Exp Rheumatology, 26,* 947–953.

Sanzo, M. (2008). The child with arthritis in the school setting. *Journal of School Nursing, 24,* 190–196.

Sheffer, A. L., Feldweg, A., & Castells, M. (2006). Anaphylaxis. In S. T. Holgate, M. K. Church, & L. M. Lichtenstein, (Eds.). *Allergy* (3rd ed.). Philadelphia: Saunders Elsevier, pp. 167–178.

Thurgate, C., & Warner, H. (2005). Living with disability: Part 1. *Paediatric Nursing, 17,* 37–44.

Thurgate, C. (2006). Living with disability: Part 3. Communication and care. *Paediatric Nursing, 18,* 40–44.

Tork, H., Lohrmann, C., & Dassen, T. (2007). Care dependency among school-aged children: Literature review. *Nursing Health Science, 9,* 142–149.

Ward, T. M. Brandt, P., Archbold, K., Lentz, M., Ringold, S., Wallace, C. A., & Landis, C. A. (2008). Polysomnograpy and self-reported sleep, pain, fatigue, and activity in children with active and inactive juvenile rheumatoid arthritis. *Journal of Pediatric Psychology, 33,* 232–241.

Williams, P. L., Storm, D., Montepiedra, G., Nichols, S., Kammerer, B., Sirois, P. A., et al. (2006). Predictors of adherence to antiretroviral medications in children and adolescents with HIV infections. *Pediatrics, 118,* e1745–e1757.

RESOURCES

Refer to the online student StudyWARE for Potts & Mandleco at http://www.CengageBrain.com for additional content and study aids.

Organization: **Association of Rheumatology Health Professionals**
Description: Offers information to students, members/professionals, patients/public, and the press concerning rheumatologic issues.
Website/Resource: http://www.rheumatology.org

Organization: **HIV/AIDS Treatment Information Service**
Description: Hivatis.org is a website that offers links to helpful resources regarding HIV symptoms, drugs, and awareness.
Website/Resource: http://www.hivatis.org

Organization: **Information About HIV Clinical Trials for Children and Adults**
Description: Offers links to helpful resources regarding HIV testing, transmission, infection, statistics, treatment, and research.
Website/Resource: http://www.actis.org

Organization: **Lupus Foundation of America, Inc.**
Description: Offers users information regarding helpful resources, research, and membership communities for people with lupus.
Website/Resource: http://www.lupus.org

Organization: **National AIDS Clearinghouse**
Description: Offers countless sources of information including data about HIV prevention, CDC guidelines, and education/outreach.
Website/Resource: http://www.cdcnpin.org

Organization: **National Association of People with AIDS (NAPWA)**
Description: Provides information regarding NAPWA programs, media, advocacy, resources, and membership.
Website/Resource: http://www.napwa.org

Organization: **The Arthritis Foundation**
Description: The largest private, not-for-profit contributor to arthritis research in the world, website provides information regarding advocacy, research, news/events, and helpful resources.
Website/Resource: http://www.arthritis.org

Organization: **The Elizabeth Glaser Pediatric AIDS Foundation**
Description: Offers information regarding publications, careers, grants/awards, and program accomplishments related to Pediatric AIDS.
Website/Resource: http://www.pedaids.org

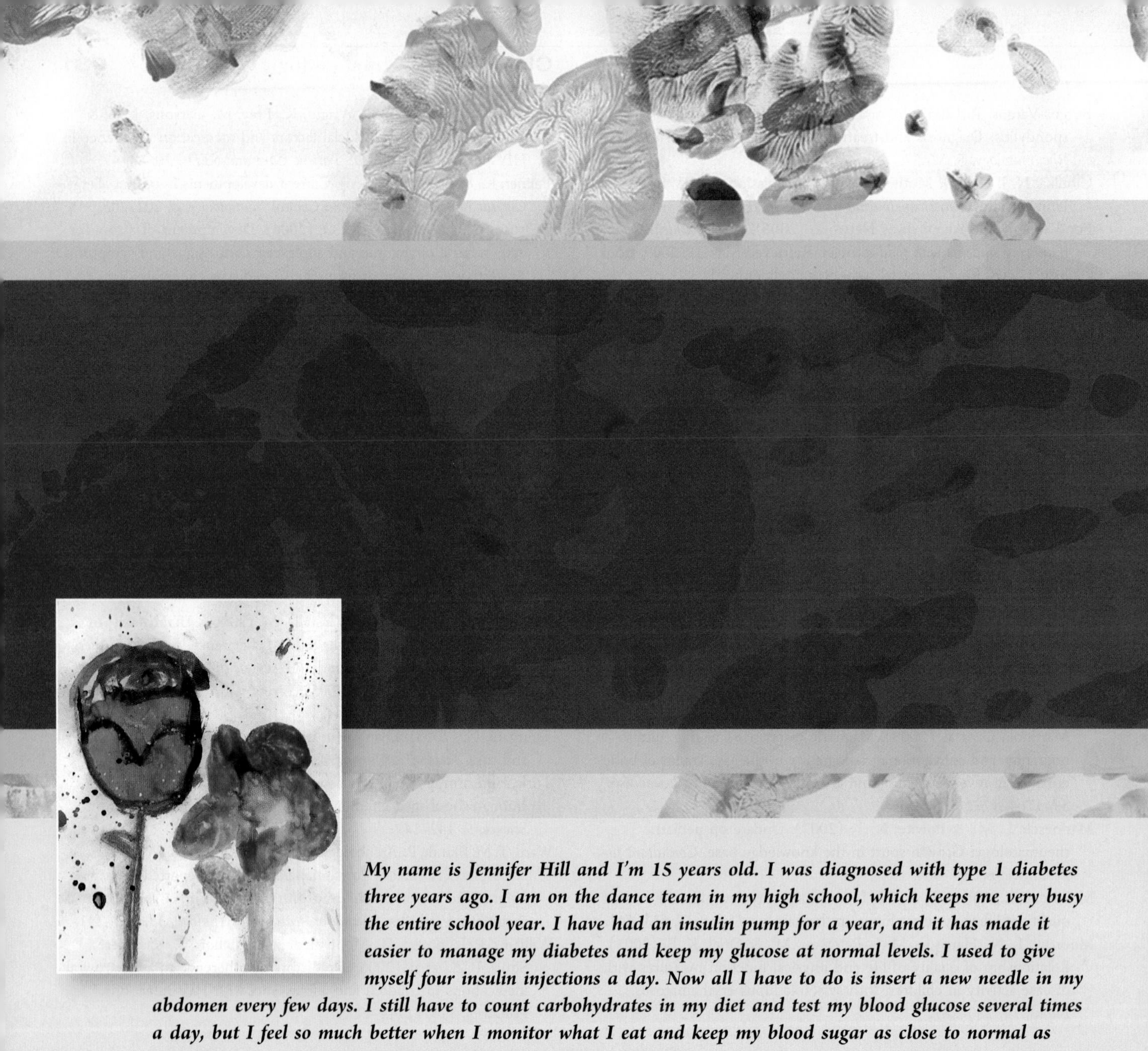

My name is Jennifer Hill and I'm 15 years old. I was diagnosed with type 1 diabetes three years ago. I am on the dance team in my high school, which keeps me very busy the entire school year. I have had an insulin pump for a year, and it has made it easier to manage my diabetes and keep my glucose at normal levels. I used to give myself four insulin injections a day. Now all I have to do is insert a new needle in my abdomen every few days. I still have to count carbohydrates in my diet and test my blood glucose several times a day, but I feel so much better when I monitor what I eat and keep my blood sugar as close to normal as possible.

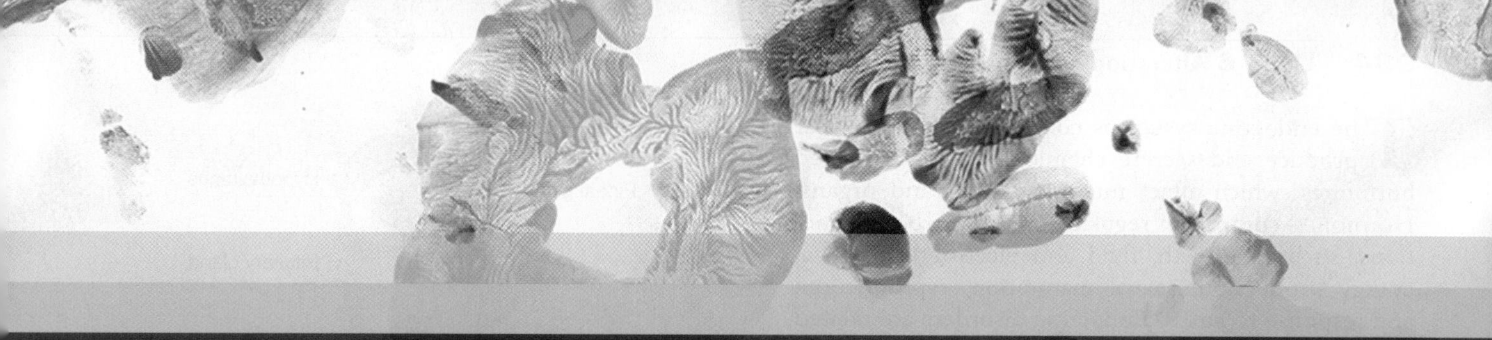

CHAPTER 28

Endocrine Alterations

Shirley Goodman, RN, BSN, CDE

COMPETENCIES

Upon completion of this chapter, the reader will be able to:

- Describe the endocrine glands, their hormones, and functions.
- Explain the principle of negative feedback.
- Describe the etiology, clinical manifestations, treatment, and nursing management of common endocrine alterations.
- Discuss the management goals for the child with type 1 and type 2 diabetes mellitus.
- Develop a teaching plan for a child with newly diagnosed type 1 diabetes.
- Compare the causes, clinical manifestations, and treatment of hypoglycemia and hyperglycemia.
- Successfully complete the games and activities in the online student StudyWARE.

The endocrine system is composed of glands that produce and secrete chemical substances called hormones, which affect multiple tissues and organs. Hormones control or regulate important body functions, such as growth, fluid and electrolyte balance, energy production, sexual maturation, reproduction, and response to stress. Endocrine disorders are related to either a deficiency (hypofunction) or an excess (hyperfunction) of a specific hormone. In children, most endocrine disorders are caused by insufficient production of hormones. Additionally, disorders can be classified based on the origin of the defect that results in a malfunction. Primary disorders occur when the target gland itself is not functioning normally. Secondary disorders are ones in which the origin of the disorder is in the pituitary, resulting in inadequate stimulation of the target gland. A tertiary disorder is one in which the hypothalamus is the cause of the problem. Early identification of endocrine disorders is imperative because they can cause significant problems, some of which are life-threatening. The onset of these disorders is insidious, and most do not become clinically apparent for a long time.

This chapter will include an overview of the anatomy and physiology of the endocrine system. Common childhood endocrine disorders will be discussed, including lifelong management of the diseases. Understanding the mechanisms of action of the endocrine system is essential for interpreting the various laboratory values and is helpful when providing education to a family about an endocrine abnormality.

ANATOMY AND PHYSIOLOGY

The endocrine system consists of glands that affect numerous body functions through the production of hormones. These glands include the pituitary, thyroid, parathyroids, adrenals, pancreas, ovaries, and testes (Figure 28-1). A **hormone** is a chemical substance produced by an endocrine gland, which is secreted into the bloodstream and affects other tissues or organs (target tissues or organs). Table 28-1 lists the endocrine glands and the major hormones they produce. The endocrine system is incompletely developed at birth. It is less mature than any other body system. Hormonal control of many body functions is lacking until 12 to 18 months of age.

The endocrine system has a close relationship with the nervous system, and the integration of both is necessary to maintain homeostasis. The central nervous system (CNS) receives and reacts to stimuli and transmits a message to the hypothalamus. The hypothalamus responds to the stimuli and produces either releasing or inhibiting hormones, which are transported to the pituitary gland. Box 28-1 lists the hormones produced by the hypothalamus. The anterior pituitary in response secretes **tropic hormones**, which cause the target tissue or organ to produce its hormones.

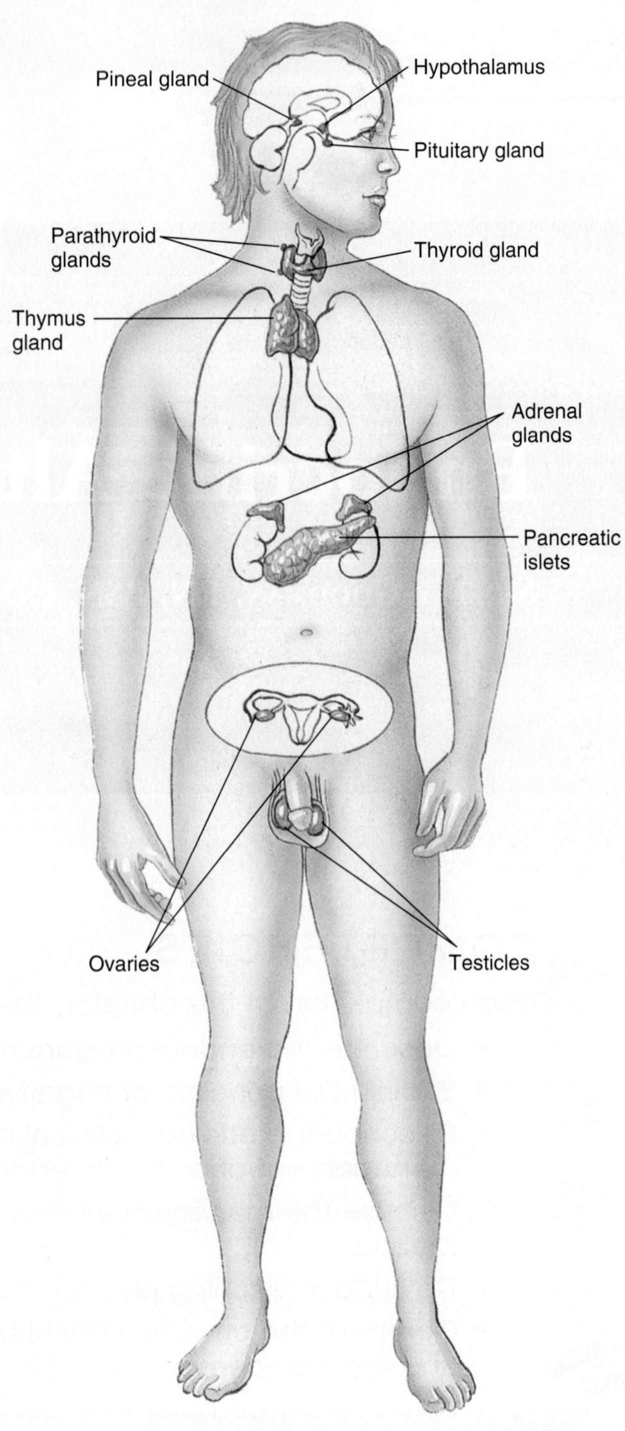

FIGURE 28-1 The Endocrine System. DELMAR CENGAGE LEARNING.

An example of this process is seen in the stress response of the body. A stimulus (psychological stress) is received by the CNS, a message is conveyed to the hypothalamus, and corticotropin-releasing hormone (CRH) is produced. CRH stimulates the anterior pituitary to release adrenocorticotropic hormone (ACTH). The adrenal glands in turn secrete glucocorticoids (cortisol) and mineralocorticoids (aldosterone).

TABLE 28-1 Endocrine Glands and Hormones

GLAND	HORMONES
Anterior pituitary	Thyroid-stimulating hormone (TSH)
	Growth hormone (GH)
	Adrenocorticotropic hormone (ACTH)
	Luteinizing hormone (LH)
	Follicle-stimulating hormone (FSH)
	Prolactin (PL)
	Melanocyte-stimulating hormone (MSH)
Posterior pituitary	Vasopressin [antidiuretic hormone (ADH)]
	Oxytocin
Thyroid	Triiodothyronine (T_3)
	Thyroxine (T_4)
	Calcitonin
Parathyroids	Parathyroid hormone (PTH)
Adrenal cortex	Glucocorticoids (cortisol)
	Mineralocorticoids (aldosterone)
	Androgens
Adrenal medulla	Epinephrine
	Norepinephrine
Ovaries	Estrogen
	Progesterone
Testes	Testosterone
Pancreas	Insulin
	Glucagon
	Somatostatin

BOX 28-1

HORMONES PRODUCED BY THE HYPOTHALAMUS

- Corticotropin-releasing hormone (CRH)
- Gonadotropin-releasing hormone (Gn-RH)
- Growth hormone-releasing hormone (GH-RH)
- Growth hormone-inhibiting hormone (somatostatin) (GN-IH)
- Melanocyte-inhibiting hormone (MIH)
- Prolactin-inhibiting hormone (PIH)
- Thyrotropin-releasing hormone (TRH)

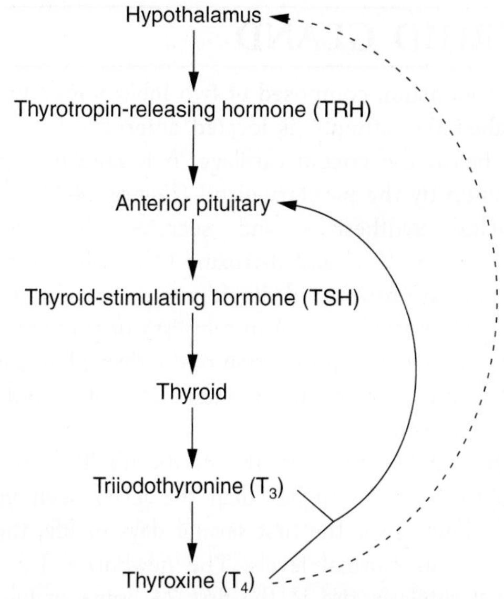

FIGURE 28-2 Negative Feedback System of the Hypothalomic–Pituitary–Thyroid Gland Axis. The hypothalamus secretes TRH, stimulating the anterior pituitary to release TSH. TSH stimulates the thyroid gland to release its hormones T_3 and T_4. The levels of T_3 and T_4 directly stimulate the anterior pituitary production of TSH and indirectly affect the hypothalamus production of TRH. DELMAR CENGAGE LEARNING.

The production and secretion of hormones is controlled by a negative feedback system. The example in Figure 28-2 illustrates the hypothalamic–pituitary–thyroid gland axis. The hypothalamus secretes a hormone, thyrotropin-releasing hormone (TRH), which stimulates the anterior pituitary. The anterior pituitary then secretes thyroid-stimulating hormone (TSH), which in turn acts on the thyroid gland (target organ) to increase the production of the thyroid hormones, triiodothyronine (T_3) and thyroxine (T_4). Feedback occurs when an increased secretion of T_3 and T_4 leads directly to a decrease in the secretion of the stimulating pituitary hormone (TSH) and indirectly to a decrease in the hypothalamic production of TRH.

PITUITARY GLAND

Located in the sella turcica (at the base of the brain), the pituitary gland is commonly referred to as the master gland of the body. It is divided into the anterior and posterior lobes. The anterior lobe is larger, occupying 80% of the gland. It produces growth hormone (GH), luteinizing hormone (LH), follicle-stimulating hormone (FSH), ACTH, TSH, and prolactin hormone (PL). The posterior gland produces oxytocin and stores the hormone arginine vasopressin or antidiuretic hormone (ADH), which is produced in the hypothalamus. By the fourth month of gestation the pituitary gland is formed, and measurable amounts of hormones can be detected.

THYROID GLAND

The thyroid gland, composed of two lobes joined by a thin band called the isthmus, is located anteriorly in the neck, directly below the cricoid cartilage. It is regulated in feedback fashion by the pituitary gland (Figure 28-2). The thyroid gland synthesizes and secretes the hormones triiodothyronine (T_3) and thyroxine (T_4), which are essential for normal growth and development, maturation of the central nervous system, and metabolism of proteins, carbohydrates, and fat. The production of the thyroid hormones is dependent on sufficient dietary intake of protein and iodine in food and water.

Immediately after birth the newborn's TSH rises rapidly, up to 10 times higher than the levels seen in older children. Then, over the first several days of life, the TSH declines to the normal levels. The newborn's T_3 and T_4 levels will similarly rise in the first 24 hours of life in response to the stimulation by the TSH. The newborn's initial thyroid function tests cannot be interpreted using the normal standards of childhood or adults.

PARATHYROID GLANDS

The parathyroid glands, usually four in number, are located on the posterior surface of the thyroid gland and secrete parathyroid hormone (PTH). PTH regulates calcium and phosphorus as a result of its effect on three target organs: bone, kidney, and the gastrointestinal tract. PTH secretion influences the bone mobilization of calcium, thus increasing serum calcium. In the kidneys, PTH decreases urinary excretion of calcium and increases excretion of phosphate. In the intestines, PTH causes increased absorption of calcium. Lastly, PTH influences vitamin D metabolism. PTH is secreted in response to a decrease in systemic calcium levels. Conversely, a rise in serum calcium causes decreased secretion of PTH.

ADRENAL GLAND

The adrenal glands are located on top of each kidney and are divided into two parts, the cortex and the medulla. Each operates independently of the other. The primary function of the cortex is to synthesize and secrete glucocorticoids, mineralocorticoids, and sex steroids. The adrenal medulla secretes catecholamines, epinephrine, and norepinephrine. Cortisol, the most potent glucocorticoid produced by the adrenal cortex, is regulated directly by the anterior pituitary hormone ACTH and indirectly by the hypothalamic corticotropin-releasing hormone. Cortisol provides feedback to the hypothalamic–pituitary–adrenal system, which regulates glucocorticoid synthesis. In a classic example of the feedback system, when serum levels of cortisol are low, the hypothalamus secretes CRH, which stimulates the anterior pituitary to secrete ACTH. ACTH then stimulates the adrenal cortex's conversion of cortisol from its substrate cholesterol. Stress and the sleep–wake cycle affect the secretion of CRH and ACTH, thereby influencing the secretion of cortisol. Aldosterone is the most important mineralocorticoid, causing sodium retention and potassium excretion. Its secretion is regulated by the renin–angiotensin system. The synthesis of the sex steroids, androgens and estrogens, produced by the adrenal cortex is mediated by events of puberty.

PANCREAS

The pancreas is located behind the stomach and is both an exocrine (duct-type) and endocrine (ductless) organ. Between 4 and 8 weeks of fetal development the differentiation of cells of the exocrine and endocrine portion of the pancreas occurs. The exocrine function is to secrete enzymes that are essential for digestion. The endocrine function is the secretion of the hormones from the islets of Langerhans. The islets, clusters of endocrine cells within the pancreas, produce glucagon by its alpha cells, insulin by the beta cells, and somatostatin by the delta cells. Glucagon increases blood glucose levels by stimulating the liver to convert its stored glycogen into glucose (**glycogenolysis**). Insulin, an anabolic hormone produced by the fetus by 20 weeks' gestation, promotes synthesis and storage in carbohydrate metabolism and prevents the breakdown of fat and protein. In carbohydrate metabolism, nutrients are consumed and digested. Carbohydrate is broken down into glucose through digestion and enters the peripheral system. The changes in glucose stimulate the beta cells to secrete additional insulin. Insulin promotes the transportation of glucose into muscle and fat cells. Somatostatin inhibits the release of insulin and glucagon from the islets of Langerhans.

DISORDERS OF THE ANTERIOR PITUITARY

The anterior pituitary gland regulates growth, sexual development, and metabolic activity. Common disorders of childhood that are discussed are growth hormone deficiency and precocious puberty.

GROWTH HORMONE DEFICIENCY

Growth hormone deficiency (GHD) is characterized primarily by poor growth and short stature caused by failure of the pituitary to produce sufficient GH. Growth hormone plays a primary role in postnatal growth. It is released in a pulsatile (pulsating) fashion throughout the day; however, most is secreted primarily after the onset of sleep.

INCIDENCE AND ETIOLOGY

Growth hormone deficiency occurs in 0.05–0.25 per 1,000 live births. The frequency of occurrence is equal in both sexes. Boys are evaluated for GHD more often and earlier than girls because historically, the social pressures placed on the short male are of greater magnitude than those placed on "petite" females (Grimberg, Kutikov, & Cucchiara, 2005). GHD may result from injury, destruction of the anterior pituitary gland by a brain tumor, infection, or irradiation, but in 75% of the children diagnosed with GHD no cause for the dysfunction is found (idiopathic).

Pathophysiology

The hypothalamus secretes growth hormone-releasing hormone (GH-RH), which stimulates the production of GH by the pituitary. GH stimulates growth and has metabolic actions. In GHD the pituitary is unable to respond and produce GH, which has an impact on growth and can result in short stature.

Clinical Manifestations

A child with GHD presents with short stature and a deteriorating (<4–5 cm/yr) or absent **rate of growth** (a calculation of the amount of growth in a defined period of time, usually a year). Children with GHD tend to have a higher weight to height ratio and a delayed **bone age**, a determination of skeletal maturation by X-ray of the hand, wrist, or knee. Additional clinical manifestations include:

- increased fat in the trunk area
- childlike face with a large, prominent forehead
- high-pitched voice
- hypoglycemia
- micropenis and small testes in males
- delayed sexual maturation
- delayed dentition

Diagnosis

The growth concern is typically identified by the family or primary care provider in an outpatient setting. A clinician who carefully and consistently plots the growth of the child on a standardized growth chart will note the deteriorating rate of growth. The diagnostic work-up includes a review of the previous growth records, determination of growth rate, radiographic bone studies (the bone age), MRI, and baseline blood testing. Further pituitary function testing may be done to evaluate peak growth hormone production. This testing consists of provocative tests in which a growth hormone stimulant such as glucagon, clonidine, insulin, arginine, or L-dopa is given to stimulate the pituitary to release a burst of growth hormone. Because up to 20% of non-GHD children will randomly not respond to a single provocative growth hormone test, two or more tests with peak growth hormone levels below 7–10 ng/l can be used to assist in establishing the diagnosis.

Treatment

The goal of treatment is to promote normal growth rates by the administration of growth hormone. It is administered as a subcutaneous injection, typically given 6–7 days each week at a dosage of 0.15–0.35 mg/kg/wk in divided doses for children and up to 0.7 mg/kg/wk in divided doses in an adolescent. Response to the therapy is more pronounced in the younger child as compared to an adolescent, in the more obese child compared to the thinner individual, and in the more severely growth hormone-deficient child compared to one with partial growth hormone deficiency. Growth hormone deficiency may or may not persist into adulthood. After the child has obtained adult height, with closure of the epiphyseal growth plates, growth hormone is discontinued for several months. Rescreening is then done for adult GHD.

There are potential complications to growth hormone therapy. Growth hormone is now produced through recombinant DNA technology by several different drug companies. It is essentially free from contaminants. At physiological replacement doses, side effects can include slipped femoral epiphysis, pseudotumor cerebri, edema, and sodium retention. Several studies raised a concern that GH treatment would increase the risk for leukemia and cancer. In an

NURSING TIP

Measuring the Child

- Under age two years and in children with motor problems who cannot stand independently, it is customary to do length measurements in the supine position, ideally using a measuring board developed for supine measurements.
- The growth charts from birth to 36 months are based on supine measurements. The 2- to 18-year-old growth charts are based on standing heights.
- A supine measurement requires two individuals. One person holds the child's head against the headboard of the measuring board. The child's face and pelvis are in a horizontal plane, the hips and knees are gently extended. A movable footboard is placed against the soles of the feet in a 90-degree angle.
- Standing measurements should be done on a stadiometer (a standing measuring board). The child should stand barefoot on a level surface (no inclines or carpeting). The child's back and heels are in the same vertical plane as the measuring instrument. The arms should be relaxed. The child's face should be placed with the outer canthus of the eye and the outer external auditory meatus horizontal. A gentle upward traction is exerted on the child's mastoid process.
- Height is measured to the nearest full millimeter.
- Measurement should be plotted accurately on a standardized growth chart.

analysis of over 19,000 children on GH, when the child had no additional risk factors, GH was not associated with any increased occurrence of leukemia or CNS tumors. Recently there has been an association made between high growth factors and breast and colorectal cancer. Current GH therapy includes regular monitoring of insulin-like growth factors with GH dosages titrated to avoid high levels of these growth factors.

Nursing Management

Assessment For any child, growth monitoring is a basic and essential part of health monitoring. It is even more important for the child with GHD to be measured accurately. In a study of 55 pediatric and primary care practices in the United States, caring for a total of 4,000 children, correct measurement techniques were demonstrated on 30% of the observed measurements. Proper equipment was used in only 58% of standing measurements, and in 18% of recumbently measured children. The measurements differed on average 1.2 cm in the same child between the office professional staff (mostly nurses) and the study staff, with a range up to 12.1 cm (Lipman et al., 2004). The child should be evaluated and measured no less than every 6 months. Growth charts should be maintained properly, rates of growth calculated, and drug dosage recalculated as the child gains weight and with lab evidence of need to increase dose (low insulin-like growth factors) to ensure that the appropriate dose of growth hormone is being prescribed.

Nursing Diagnosis

1. *Delayed growth and development* related to inadequate growth hormone secretion.
2. *Disturbed body image* related to short stature.
3. *Deficient knowledge (caregiver)* related to treatment.

Outcome Identification

1. The child will demonstrate an improvement in growth rate, yielding a minimum of 4–5 cm/yr of linear growth.
2. The child will express positive feelings about his or her body image.
3. Caregiver and child will verbalize a realistic understanding of the likely response to GH replacement therapy.
4. The caregiver will demonstrate correct medication preparation and injection technique.
5. The caregiver will be able to verbalize the side effects of GH replacement therapy.

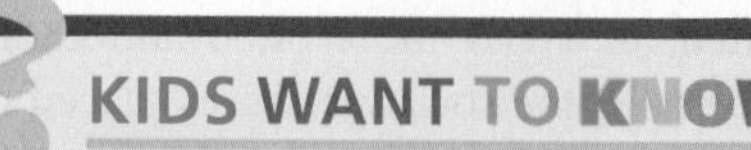

What do growth hormone shots feel like?

An 8-year-old boy with short stature is to start daily, subcutaneous growth hormone for a new diagnosis of growth hormone deficiency. He asks "How much do the shots hurt?" "Will I have to give them to myself?" and "How soon will I be really taller?" Be honest in your reply that the injections may pinch but are given with the smallest needles into the fat areas of the body. Reassure him that when he is ready and interested, he can also learn to do the injections, but until that time, the adults in his life will be responsible for them. Reassure him that the growth hormone is expected to help him grow and he will be monitored to see how well his body responds.

Planning and Implementation The nurse fills the role of coordinator, teacher, and provider of support to the child and the caregivers. Nursing care initially focuses on providing the child (if appropriate) and caregivers with information about normal development, normal growth rates, bone age, and growth potential. Many caregivers and children are unaware of normal growth patterns and genetic expectations for a child's growth. The nurse should explore with the child and the caregivers their expectations of treatment, which at times are unrealistic. Counseling referrals should be considered. Many children with short stature and GHD are emotionally immature. Because these children look much younger than they are, caregivers, teachers, peers, and relatives tend to have expectations similar to those for a younger child. The nurse and other health care providers need to pay particular attention to how they talk to the child with short stature. The health care team should speak to the child in an age-appropriate manner. Discreetly provide step stools to aid the child's ability to independently get onto the exam table.

Caregivers need to be prepared for the financial implications of growth hormone therapy, which costs between \$35–\$55 per milligram for the growth hormone. Over a year, the cost is approximately \$20,000–\$30,000 per year to treat the average 30 kg GHD child. Many third-party payers, with the appropriate documentation of the diagnosis, will cover the cost of the treatment once the child's deductible has been met. Should the third-party payer deny coverage, or in situations where the family's financial obligation for the drug exceeds their ability to pay, the numerous pharmaceutical companies that market GH have indigent drug programs that assist qualified families.

Evaluation The child shows an increase in height and acceptance of his or her body image. The child and caregivers accept the eventual height increase. Caregivers are able to correctly prepare and administer injections. They also know to observe for expected side effects.

Family Teaching

Growth hormone can come as a powder that must be mixed with its packaged diluent or already in solution. Several of the growth hormone preparations come in the form of an injection pen. The nurse needs to teach caregivers how to properly prepare the medication for injection and how to give the correct dose. The potential side effects of growth hormone replacement therapy need to be communicated. The caregiver should alert the health care provider of the child's complaints of headaches, rapid weight gain, or painful hip joints. Because the treatment can continue for many years, the nurse needs to prepare the child and family about this issue before therapy begins. They need guidance in setting realistic goals and expectations. During adolescence, the child should dress in clothing that reflects his or her age, not size. Counseling referrals for the child and family should be considered if appropriate.

PRECOCIOUS PUBERTY

Precocious puberty is defined in Caucasian girls as breast development before the age of 7–8 years and before 6–7 years old in African Americans. In boys less than 9 years of age, the onset of testicular enlargement (>2.5 cm or 4 mL if using an orchidometer) is precocious puberty.

Incidence and Etiology

The incidence of precocious puberty is approximately 0.1–0.5 per 1,000 children and is 4–10 times more common in girls (Muir, 2006). Precocious puberty is more common in African Americans than in Caucasians. The cause is most frequently idiopathic in girls. In contrast, in boys, the cause is most likely related to abnormalities in the central nervous systems such as lesions.

Pathophysiology

The normal fetus and infant's hypothalamic–pituitary–gonadal axis is activated, with the hypothalamus secreting GnRH in a pulsatile fashion. GnRH, in turn, stimulates the pituitary to produce LH and FSH, which are measurable for months after birth. By the age of 4 years and throughout childhood, the level of the gonadotropins is minimal. Negative feedback of sex steroids on the hypothalamus and pituitary is evident, although the exact mechanism for this inhibition of the axis is not yet understood. Puberty begins when the secretion of GnRH increases, and gonadotropins are again released.

True or central precocious puberty can be distinguished from precocious pseudopuberty. True precocious puberty results from premature activation of the hypothalamic–pituitary–gonadal axis, with GnRH, LH, FSH, and estrogen or testosterone produced (Figure 28-3). Precocious pseudopuberty occurs when there is evidence of secondary sexual characteristics (breast or sexual hair growth) but no activation of the axis (i.e., normal levels of GnRH, LH, and FSH).

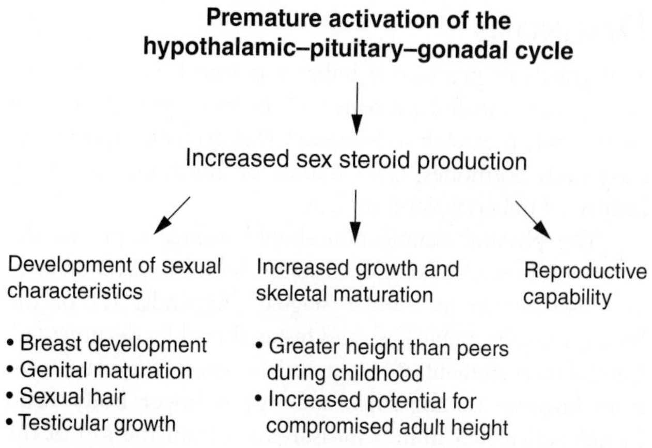

Premature activation of the hypothalamic–pituitary–gonadal cycle

↓

Increased sex steroid production

↙ ↓ ↘

Development of sexual characteristics
- Breast development
- Genital maturation
- Sexual hair
- Testicular growth

Increased growth and skeletal maturation
- Greater height than peers during childhood
- Increased potential for compromised adult height

Reproductive capability

Figure 28-3 True Precocious Puberty. DELMAR CENGAGE LEARNING.

Clinical Manifestations

The child with precocious puberty will have an accelerated growth rate, an advanced bone age, evidence of secondary sexual characteristics, acne, an adult body odor, and sometimes behavioral changes. Psychosocial development is typically age-appropriate, and not a reflection of the physical maturation. Inappropriate sexual behavior is not commonly observed in children with precocious puberty; however, emotional lability, aggressive behavior, and mood swings may occur. A child with untreated central precocious puberty is potentially fertile.

NURSING TIP

Hormone Containing Products

When taking the history of a child with the complaint of precocious puberty, ask about the use of skin lotions or hair products. Some over-the-counter beauty products contain estrogen. A child could absorb enough estrogen from one of these products to have measurable levels of estrogen and physical changes reflecting exposure to estrogen. If you are unfamiliar with a product, ask the family to bring the product with them. You may then need to contact the manufacturer to determine if there is estrogen in the product. If birth control pills are available in the house, verify that the child has not had access to them, possibly ingesting the pills to be "just like mommy." This exposure to exogenous hormones could promote the development of secondary sexual characteristics. There are reports of children absorbing testosterone from topical testosterone products used by the male caretakers in their lives. Children who have absorbed testosterone from skin contact will have evidence of hair growth but not testicular enlargement or breast development.

Diagnosis

A diagnosis of precocious puberty is based on a complete history, which includes a review of the linear growth chart to identify when growth acceleration was evident, exposure to exogenous hormones, CNS trauma or infection, and family history of pubertal development.

The physical examination should include a precise description of the child's pubertal status. Sexual maturation staging, also known as Tanner staging (Appendix D) of the breast, genitalia, pubic hair, and testes should be documented. Careful measurement of height, weight, **span** (a measurement from fingertip to fingertip), and **upper/lower body ratio** (a ratio calculated from a measurement from the top of the head to the top of the synthesis pubis and from the synthesis pubis to the bottom of the feet) also need to be documented. Radiological exams should be ordered and the child's bone age calculated. In girls, a pelvic ultrasound to identify size of the uterus and ovaries may be helpful. Given the high incidence of CNS lesions with boys, a CT, MRI, or skull film is usually warranted, and commonly performed in girls also.

The child will need screening lab tests for LH, FSH, estradiol, or testosterone. Because LH, FSH and estradiol is secreted in puberty in a pulsitile fashion, and levels of these hormones are most elevated at night, first morning labs are done to most accurately capture the peak of these levels. Provocative testing to evaluate the child's response to stimulation may be necessary to confirm the diagnosis of central precocious puberty, should the screening labs not be in the pubertal range. This stimulation test is done by administering a GnRH agonist to the child and drawing serial blood levels of LH, FSH, and estrogen or testosterone. A child whose hypothalamic–pituitary–gonadal axis has been activated will exhibit a pubertal or adult level of these hormones in response to the administration of GnRH.

Treatment

Treatment initially focuses on the underlying cause of sexual precocity. In cases of a CNS tumor, surgery, radiation, or chemotherapy is indicated. Precocious puberty itself is treated with GnRH analogs. When the GnRH analog is initially given, it will stimulate gonadotropin release. When given on a long-term basis, it will suppress gonadotropin release. GnRH analog is available as a depot injection given every 3–4 weeks, subcutaneous injection given daily, an intranasal compound given 2–3 times each day, or a histrelin implant.

Treatment results in a decrease in growth rate, usually to an age-appropriate level. Secondary sexual development stabilizes or regresses. In girls, breasts may decrease in size and pubic hair fails to progress. The ovaries and uterus also decrease in size. In boys, there is a decrease in the size of the testes and in the frequency of erections and variable regression of pubic hair. Effectiveness of the treatment is gauged through accurate growth records and intermittent serum gonadotropin and sex steroid measurements. When therapy is discontinued, puberty resumes promptly.

NURSING TIP

Histrelin Implant

Histrelin implant is a new treatment for the continuous, slow release of GnRH agonist histrelin. A small 50 mg histrelin implant (a thin, flexible tube) is inserted subcutaneously in the inner, upper arm while the child is under anesthesia (local, twilight, or general). The implant of histrelin achieves and maintains suppression of LH and the sex steroids (estrogen and testosterone) in children with central precocious puberty for one year. The most common side effect, different from other GnRH agonists, is a skin reaction where the implant was placed.

CRITICAL THINKING

Precocious Puberty

Draw a diagram of the activated hypothalamic–pituitary–gonadal axis, including the various hormones excreted by each endocrine gland that would be consistent with puberty. Can this be differentiated from the axis seen in the child with precocious pseudopuberty? At what age is puberty precocious?

The child's family will need to be prepared for the financial aspect of treatment. The GnRH analog depot cost averages $700–$1,000 per injection. The Histrelin implant is $10,000–$14,000 for the implant, not including physician and institute fee for insertion. Third-party payers, with appropriate documentation, will frequently cover the cost of the therapy after the child's deductible has been met. For children who choose the monthly injectable drug, in order to get fully covered by the third-party payer, some will need to have the injectable GnRH analog administered in a health care provider's office. Others may need to obtain the drug through a specific home care company, and some children will not be eligible for coverage for either the injectable or implantable medication. In these situations, the pharmaceutical companies often have indigent drug programs to assist with the financial impact of treatment.

Disorders of the Posterior Pituitary

Disorders of the posterior pituitary are related to a deficiency or excess of vasopressin or antidiuretic hormone (ADH). Diabetes insipidus (DI) is one of these disorders.

DIABETES INSIPIDUS

Diabetes insipidus or neurogenic DI is a disorder of water regulation. The function of antidiuretic hormone (ADH) is to concentrate urine by stimulating reabsorption of water in the renal collecting tubules. A deficiency of ADH results in excretion of large amounts of dilute urine.

INCIDENCE AND ETIOLOGY

DI is most often seen in children as a complication following head trauma or cranial surgery to remove tumors of the hypothalamic–pituitary region. DI that develops after surgery may be transient or permanent. Other causes include vascular anomalies (cerebral aneurysms), infection (encephalitis or meningitis), and a genetic defect in the synthesis of ADH.

PATHOPHYSIOLOGY

The posterior lobe of the pituitary gland secretes arginine vasopressin (also known as ADH), which is produced in the hypothalamus and stored in the pituitary gland. ADH acts at the level of the renal collecting ducts, increasing their permeability to water, in order to limit water loss. A deficiency in ADH secretion results in massive loss of water and retention of sodium in the serum.

CLINICAL MANIFESTATIONS

In infants, failure to thrive, a history of fevers, vomiting, constipation, dehydration, and poor growth are the initial clinical manifestations. In the older child, polyuria (excretion of an abnormally large amount of urine) and **polydipsia** (excessive thirst) are the most common first symptoms (over 50% of children have these initial reported symptoms). Children experience nocturnal enuresis, which interrupts their sleep, and increased thirst. Urine output can range from a few liters to 18 liters a day. Urine specific gravity is 1.005 or less, urine osmolarity is $<$200 mmol/L, and serum sodium concentration and plasma osmolarity are elevated. In an infant, urine output is $>$100 mL/kg/24 hours.

DIAGNOSIS

An initial screen, rather than a full work-up, is valuable in a child who presents with a history that suggests DI. An outpatient screening includes obtaining a first morning urine sample for osmolarity, specific gravity, and sodium after attempting an overnight fast. Caution should be exercised in instructing the caregivers to do an overnight fast, in that the child with DI can become hypernatremic if fluids are discontinued. A child with hypernatremia is at risk for seizure. If the history of the child strongly suggests that the child has DI, an overnight fast should not be conducted. The child who does have an outpatient screening should be evaluated for hydration status, which includes a weight before the fast has been terminated. Serum osmolarity, sodium, and creatinine levels are also checked.

Further investigation is pursued should the urine be dilute ($<$1.005, osmolarity $<$200 mmol/L), especially if the serum is hypertonic and hypernatremic. A water deprivation test is commonly performed at this point. The object of the water deprivation test is to measure the vasopressin release from the pituitary in response to depriving the child of water. The test requires several hours to complete with close monitoring (I&O, weight, vital signs, hydration assessment, and urine and blood samples), most frequently by the nurse.

TREATMENT

As long as a child has a normal thirst drive and free access to water, treating DI is not necessary to maintain life. Treatment, however, greatly improves the quality of life because of the inconvenience of polyuria and polydipsia. The usual

> **NURSING TIP**
>
> **Symptoms of DI**
>
> A common symptom of DI is the child who is much more satisfied with water in copious amounts than other liquids. The child will awaken at night to drink. Young children who have been denied fluids have been known to drink from a toilet or a puddle on the ground.

> **NURSING TIP**
>
> **Use of Rhinal Tube to Administer Desmopressin Acetate (DDAVP)**
>
> While the use of a rhinal tube to deliver medication is rare, in the infant with DI, whose dose of DDAVP is quite small, this may be the best choice. Some older children may continue to use the rhinal tube. Below are tips for using a rhinal tube to administer the DDAVP intranasally:
>
> 1. Have the child blow the nose before administering (if age appropriate).
> 2. Have the child lay on a side (same side where the medication was administered) for several minutes after the medication is given. Observe for evidence that DDAVP has trickled out of the nares.
> 3. If age appropriate, ask the child if he or she swallowed the medication, which would indicate that it "overshot" the nasal choana, and will, therefore, not be absorbed.

treatment is daily replacement of the hormone ADH (vasopressin). The drug of choice is desmopressin acetate (DDAVP), a long-acting vasopressin analog, which is given intranasally or orally. DDAVP is also available in a parenteral form. The mechanism for delivery is based on the dosage, ease of administration, and ability of the child and family to reach the treatment goals. Common goals of therapy include antidiuresis, uninterrupted sleep, and increased ability to participate in school and other programs. In order to avoid possible water intoxication and hyponatremia, a brief period of time each day when the DDAVP begins to wear off and unrestrained urination can occur is planned as part of the therapy.

Nursing Management

Children with a damaged thirst center provide a special challenge to both the health care providers and families. Fluid intake regimens will need to be devised, and families will need to carefully monitor the child's fluid status by measuring intake, urine output, and daily weights. A journal or log is essential for these caregivers. Infants present special treatment concerns. They excrete more dilute urine, consume large volumes of free water, and secrete lower amounts of vasopressin than older children. Treatment typically calls for more frequent feeds or, if breastfed, supplements of water. DDAVP dosing is controversial in this age group.

A child who is NPO (i.e., pre- or post-surgery) with DI will require careful titration of the medication and fluid volumes and concentration. Frequent electrolytes, I&Os, and reassessment of the fluid management plan are necessary. Medical identification jewelry should be encouraged.

DISORDERS OF THE THYROID GLAND

The disorders of the thyroid gland are some of the most common endocrine abnormalities of childhood and include congenital hypothyroidism, acquired hypothyroidism, and hyperthyroidism.

CONGENITAL HYPOTHYROIDISM

Congenital hypothyroidism (CH), a disorder present at birth, is a reduced rate of metabolism caused by a low concentration of circulating thyroid hormones (T_3 and T_4). The early detection and treatment of hypothyroidism can prevent **cretinism** (severe mental retardation). In North America and most of Europe and Japan, mass screening of newborns for CH is routine and identifies the majority of those affected. Since TSH surges in the first 24–48 hours of life, screening of newborns occurs in most instances after 48 hours to minimize false positives.

Incidence and Etiology

Congenital hypothyroidism affects 1 in 3,000–4,000 newborns. Female infants are affected 2:1 in comparison to male infants. Incidence is higher in Hispanic populations and lower in African Americans. Infants with Down Syndrome also have a higher incidence of CH (AAP, 2006). CH may develop from a variety of conditions. The majority of cases are caused by a defect in the embryonic development of the thyroid gland in which it is absent, partially present, or ectopic (in the wrong position). Other causes include an inborn error of thyroid hormone synthesis (**dyshormonogenesis**), which is inherited as an autosomal, recessive trait, and pituitary dysfunctions.

Pathophysiology

CH is caused by an absent, underdeveloped, or ectopic placement of the thyroid gland or an error of thyroid hormone synthesis. The thyroid gland is unable to produce T_3 and T_4 in response to increasingly elevated levels of TSH secreted by the pituitary gland.

Clinical Manifestations

The majority of affected infants are asymptomatic at birth. The most common neonatal clinical signs are a large posterior fontanel, an umbilical hernia, constipation, and prolonged jaundice. Other clinical manifestations may include the following:

- Pallor
- Hypothermia
- Enlarged tongue
- Hypotonia, hypoactivity
- Feeding difficulties
- Delayed mental responsiveness or dull expression
- Cool, dry, scaly skin
- Swollen eyelids

Diagnosis

Mandatory newborn screening identifies the majority of newborns with CH and allows early treatment, thereby reducing the incidence of mental retardation. Different states and countries may use a different method of screening for congenital hypothyroidism. When the initial test is positive, the newborn should have a second confirming laboratory test performed. Persistent elevation in TSH, irrespective of thyroxine level, indicates CH in the newborn. A thyroid scan to evaluate for absence or ectopic placement of the gland may be performed. It is the practice of some pediatric endocrinologists to have radiological films of the infant's knee to evaluate for growth retardation, a reflection of the severity of the hypothyroidism in utero.

Treatment

Thyroid hormone is vital to the growing, developing central nervous system. A delay in treatment is associated with lower mean intelligence quotients (IQ). Thyroid replacement with sodium L-thyroxine (Synthroid) is initiated as soon as possible with a recommended starting dose of 10–15 mcg/kg/day (AAP, 2006). Given in physiological doses, the medication does not have side effects. There are no contraindications for this therapy or any alternate options for therapy. Thyroid function tests should be closely monitored to ensure proper dosing, initially as often as every 2 weeks. The goal of therapy is to quickly normalize thyroid function. In the newborn, the goal is to maintain the level of T_4 in the upper half of the normal range and TSH in the normal range. Lifelong thyroid replacement is necessary to maintain normal metabolism in most cases of CH.

Nursing Management

The child's growth should be accurately measured and plotted on a standardized growth chart at regular intervals, often corresponding with visits during which lab values are obtained. Lab tests are performed initially every 2–4 weeks until thyroid function is within the target range on a stabilized dose of medication. Tests will be performed every 3–4 months for the first several years of life, with the interval lengthening as the child grows older, to every 6–12 months in adolescence.

Initially, the urgency to begin treatment must be communicated to the caregivers. Most newborns with CH are asymptomatic, and the initial notification by the health care provider is unexpected. Caregivers will need reassurance that the occurrence of CH is random and not a reflection of the mother's actions during pregnancy. Developmental screening may be recommended as the child gets older.

Family Teaching

L-thyroxine is an oral medication and is available only as a pill. While compounding pharmacies may be able to make a liquid preparation, the stability of these preparations are unknown. L-thyroxine should never be given in a compounded liquid form. Caregivers will need to be instructed in the preparation and administration of the pill, which must be crushed for infants and young children. The preferred method involves crushing the pill, mixing the powder with a drop of formula or breast milk, placing the paste on the infant's tongue, and then feeding the infant. Teach the caregivers about the need to continue thyroid hormone replacement for the child's life. They also need to be prepared for the importance of frequent blood tests for ongoing evaluation of thyroid function. If appropriate, the nurse must help them identify a lab that is convenient for them to use. The nurse should provide information about soy-containing formulas to avoid.

Reflections from Families

When I received a phone call from the nurse at my son's pediatrician's office a few days after he was born to tell me his newborn blood tests indicated a problem, I was shocked. He looked so healthy, right from the time he was born. His APGAR was perfect. I didn't even know that they had done blood tests before I took him home from the hospital. (I'd wished someone had told me about this while I was pregnant.) When I was told that his thyroid gland didn't seem to be working, I was sure I did something to cause it. While the nurse assured me that this was unrelated to anything I had done during pregnancy, it frightened me when she insisted that I bring him in immediately to confirm the diagnosis and start treatment. I had a million questions. Would he be slow? Would he look different? At our appointment, I was relieved that this could be managed but I worry about how I will give him his medicines so that he's getting the right amount.

NURSING TIP

Absorption of L-thyroxine

L-thyroxine's absorption is affected by formulas that are soy based; therefore, caregivers should avoid using these. Soy formulas include Alsoy (Nestle), Gerber Soy, Isomil (Mead Johnson), Nursoy (Wyeth-Ayerst), ProSobee (Mead Johnson), and Soyalac (Loma Linda). Iron also impacts absorption. Therefore, iron should not be given concurrently with L-thyroxine. To maximize L-thyroxine absorption, the family should administer the medication in the same fashion each time.

ACQUIRED HYPOTHYROIDISM

Acquired hypothyroidism, recognized after the age of 2 years, is a condition in which there are inadequate thyroid hormones.

Incidence and Etiology

Acquired hypothyroidism is categorized as primary, secondary, or tertiary. Primary is the most common form and is usually caused by autoimmune chronic lymphocytic thyroiditis, called Hashimoto's thyroiditis. This condition occurs during childhood and adolescence and more frequently in girls. It occurs in greater frequency with other autoimmune-mediated diseases like type 1 diabetes or chromosal abnormalities such as Down syndrome. Secondary and tertiary hypothyroidism are associated with pituitary or hypothalamic dysfunction.

Pathophysiology

Acquired hypothyroidism is commonly caused by an autoimmune disorder. Antibodies are developed against the thyroid gland. The gland becomes inflamed, infiltrated by the antibodies, and is progressively destroyed. Serum T_4 levels decrease and concurrently TSH levels increase.

Clinical Manifestations

The child may present with complaints of fatigue, weakness, constipation, and dry skin. Some children will present with a **goiter**, an enlargement of the thyroid gland. The course of acquired hypothyroidism may be silent, with a subtle shift in the child's growth parameters (i.e., a decrease in the linear rate of growth, change in the linear growth percentiles evident on a standardized growth chart, and weight increase). There is often a delay in puberty and teeth eruption. Box 28-2 lists the clinical manifestations of acquired hypothyroidism.

Diagnosis

The diagnostic evaluation for primary acquired hypothyroidism is relatively simple, requiring serum thyroid function studies (TSH, T_4, free T_4). Confirmation of autoimmune thyroiditis is made with serum thyroid antibodies.

Treatment

Treatment involves replacing thyroid hormone with L-thyroxine, with the dosage based on the weight of the child and the severity of the hypothyroidism. While in the newborn, the prevailing advice is a rapid restoration to a **euthyroid** (normal) state; in the child or adolescent with severe or chronic hypothyroidism the advice is different. The child or adolescent with hypothyroidism is more likely to experience side effects if the restoration phase is too rapid, which mimics symptoms of hyperthyroidism and can include aggressive behavior and deterioration in school performance. Increased intracranial pressure has also been demonstrated in the child or adolescent with severe hypothyroidism with rapid restoration. Therefore, the initiating dose in these cases is small and titrated upwards based on symptoms and thyroid lab tests, usually every few weeks until a euthyroid state is reached.

HYPERTHYROIDISM

Hyperthyroidism or hyperfunction of the thyroid gland is characterized by excessive levels of circulating thyroid hormones.

Incidence and Etiology

Hyperthyroidism is uncommon in children and adolescents. Exact pediatric incidence rates are not available. However, it rarely occurs before age 10, with the predominance of cases diagnosed between ages 11 and 15 years. The most common cause of hyperthyroidism in children is Graves' disease, which is five times more common in girls than in boys. There is a common genetic marker in individuals with this disease, and approximately 60% have a family history of autoimmune thyroid problems. In identical twins, the concordance rate is less than 50%, thereby suggesting that factors other than genetics play a role in the development of Graves' disease.

BOX 28-2
CLINICAL MANIFESTATIONS OF ACQUIRED HYPOTHYROIDISM

- Decreased rate of growth
- Weight gain
- Constipation
- Dry skin
- Thinning or coarse hair
- Fatigue
- Cold intolerance
- Edema of face, eyes, and hands
- Delayed deep tendon reflexes
- Delayed puberty and tooth eruption

NURSING TIP
Consistency of Medication

Many third party payers will cover generics at a higher rate than name brand drugs. L-thyroxine is no exception. With respect to L-thyroxine, each manufacturer's preparation may result in different levels of T_4. It is essential in the first three years of life that the child's thyroid hormone level remain stable. If a child is using a generic product, that product manufacturer could change several times. For stability in thyroid function, it is best for the child to remain on one drug preparation. If this is not possible, the child's thyroid function should be reassessed with every change in drug manufacturer.

CASE STUDY / CARE PLAN

A CHILD WITH ACQUIRED HYPOTHYROIDISM

A 10-year-old female is seen in the office during a routine visit. In her review of symptoms, both child and parent mention that she has been mildly fatigued. In reviewing her growth chart, her weight continues on its usual percentile, but her height has dropped just below her previous height percentiles. On physical exam, her vital signs are within normal range (consistent with previous measurements). Her skin is drier than had been noted on previous exams. Her thyroid gland is palpable, and mildly enlarged. Lab work reveals positive thyroid antibodies, a TSH of 54.3 units (normal range 0.5–5.0 units) and a Free T_4 of 0.87 ng/dL (normal range 0.9–1.4 ng/dL). A diagnosis of acquired autoimmune hypothyroidism is made, and thyroid hormone replacement therapy is initiated.

NURSING CARE PLAN

ASSESSMENT

The most common cause of hypothyroidism outside the neonatal period is autoimmune in nature. Autoimmune destruction of the thyroid gland results in impairment of the cells for secretion of thyroid hormone. As thyroid hormone levels decrease, the feedback loop to the pituitary gland results in an increase in TSH, in an effort to increase thyroid hormone secretion by the impaired gland. The gland enlarges with this increased stimulation, resulting in a goiter. To achieve a diagnosis of hypothyroidism, only the TSH needs to be elevated. Thyroid antibodies confirm the autoimmune cause of the disease. Initially, thyroid replacement dosing is small, with incremental changes in the dose (based on thyroid function labs) over several weeks to achieve normal thyroid levels.

NURSING DIAGNOSIS 1

Altered growth and development: Decelerating growth, related to altered metabolic processes and inadequate thyroid hormone levels.

EXPECTED OUTCOMES

1. Child will achieve appropriate development for age.
2. Child will achieve normal rate of growth for age.

NOC: Growth, Child Development

NIC: Teaching, Counseling

INTERVENTIONS/*RATIONALES*

1. Obtain accurate, serial height and weight measurements, and plot on standardized growth charts. *Assessment for growth and impact of therapy on growth.*
2. Reassure caregivers that the child has the best chance of normal development when the hormone replacement therapy is given as prescribed. *Reinforces need for the medication to be given every day to have optimal effect.*
3. Reinforce the importance of follow-up visits. *To assess growth rate, developmental progress, response to therapy, and to regulate drug doses as the child grows.*

EVALUATION

During therapy the child's rate of growth should improve as thyroid function returns to normal. Child is likely to experience "catch up growth," an increase in the rate of growth to reestablish growth along the same percentile the child grew along prior to the thyroid impairment.

(Continues)

CASE STUDY / CARE PLAN (Continued)

NURSING DIAGNOSIS 2

Deficient knowledge related to lack of information about the disorder.

EXPECTED OUTCOMES

1. Caregivers will verbalize an understanding of the cause and treatment for hypothyroidism.
2. Caregivers will explain the method for medication administration and list its action and side effects.

NOC: Knowledge: Disease Process, Treatment Procedure

NIC: Teaching: Disease Process, Procedure

INTERVENTIONS/*RATIONALES*

1. Assess caregivers' knowledge of disorder and replacement therapy. *Provides information needed to develop plan of instruction to ensure compliance with medical regimen.*
2. Provide information about normal thyroid function and impact of thyroid dysfunction. *Providing this information helps caregivers understand the child's delayed growth and development.*
3. Teach caregivers about medication administration including:
   (a) administering daily for life;
   (b) giving at least one hour prior to a meal;
   (c) chewing, crushing, or mixing the medication with food. *Provides information to enhance medication compliance and empowers caregivers to adhere to medical plan.*
4. Discuss plan for monitoring thyroid function. Lab evaluation of thyroid function is done every few weeks until dose is titrated for normal thyroid levels. Once a dose of medication is stabilized, thyroid function labs are done every 4–6 months while a child continues to grow. Once adult height is achieved, labs are done every 6–12 months. *Providing information regarding routine of lab work prepares the child and caregiver for the lifelong need to evaluate dosing.*
5. Teach caregivers signs indicating overdose, such as rapid pulse, dyspnea, irritability, insomnia, fever, sweating, and weight loss. *Indicates an excess of thyroid hormone and need for an adjustment in dosage.*

EVALUATION

Caregiver and child (if appropriate) are able to verbalize about the disorder and correct method of medication administration, impact of thyroid dysfunction, plan for monitoring thyroid function, and signs of overdose. Caregivers are consistent in administering medication. This consistency in medication delivery results in normal thyroid hormone levels, normal growth and development, and a cessation of the symptoms associated with hypothyroidism.

NURSING DIAGNOSIS 3

Activity intolerance related to fatigue and decreased endurance.

EXPECTED OUTCOME

Child will return to her usual level of activity and endurance.

NOC: Disease process

NIC: Disease process, teaching

INTERVENTIONS/*RATIONALES*

1. Fatigue and decreased endurance are symptoms of underactive thyroid function. Provide education about signs and symptoms of hypothyroidism. *Providing information helps child and caregiver better understand the physical nature of the current complaints of fatigue.*

(Continues)

CASE STUDY / CARE PLAN (Continued)

2. Reinforce benefits of medication compliance. Normal thyroid function, even when established by medication, will eliminate symptoms that were caused by hypothyroidism. Should symptoms return in the future, thyroid function should be reassessed to determine if that is a cause of the complaint. *Reassure caregivers and child that medication will eventually relieve the symptoms of fatigue and decreased endurance. If it does not, the symptoms could indicate too low a dose that needs to be adjusted.*

EVALUATION

The child overcomes the activity intolerance, no longer complains of fatigue, and returns to her usual level of endurance.

Pathophysiology

Graves' disease occurs when antibodies are formed against antigens in the thyroid gland, orbital tissue, and dermis. The antibodies that are directed against the thyroid gland mimic the action of TSH, thereby causing the gland to inappropriately produce thyroid hormone. A goiter is usually present in the child with Graves' disease.

Clinical Manifestations

Initially, the symptoms may be mild and easily overlooked by the child's family (Box 28-3) and include ophthalmic changes (Box 28-4). Growth patterns may include increased growth velocity, rapidly advancing bone age, and decreasing weight.

Diagnosis

The diagnosis of hyperthyroidism is confirmed with serum thyroid tests. The active circulating thyroid hormones will be markedly elevated. TSH levels will be suppressed because increased levels of T_3 and T_4 inhibit the anterior pituitary from producing TSH.

BOX 28-3
CLINICAL MANIFESTATIONS OF HYPERTHYROIDISM

- Increased rate of growth
- Weight loss despite excellent appetite
- Warm, moist skin
- Tachycardia
- Ophthalmic changes
- Heat intolerance
- Emotional lability
- Insomnia
- Fine tremors

BOX 28-4
OPHTHALMIC CHANGES WITH HYPERTHYROIDISM

- Exophthalmos (bulging of the eyeballs)
- Proptosis (downward displacement of the eyeball)
- Lid lag
- Lid retraction
- Staring expression
- Periorbital edema
- Diplopia

Treatment

Treating Graves' disease is difficult because of the chronic nature of the disorder and because the treatment options all have disadvantages. Current treatment options include antithyroid medication, radioactive iodine therapy, and subtotal thyroidectomy. Spontaneous remissions of Graves' disease do occur and may last for years. Others will have a disease course that is persistent. Antithyroid drug therapy has been used the longest and includes the use of propylthiouracil (PTU) or methimazole (MTZ; Tapazole), which block the synthesis of T_3 and T_4. It may be 4–8 weeks before the child becomes euthyroid on this therapy. Adjunct therapy of beta-adrenergic blockers such as propranolol (Inderal) may be considered in the individual with marked symptoms. These drugs relieve tachycardia, restlessness, and tremors. The major problems with drug therapy are the risk of toxic effects and the duration of the therapy, which may last for years. Approximately 11–22% of children treated with antithyroid medication will have side effects from the medication. (Glase & Slyne, 2008). The side effects of antithyroid medication can be serious, and if suspected, therapy must be promptly discontinued (Table 28-2). Alternative drugs should be initiated when appropriate.

Table 28-2 Side Effects of Antithyroid Medication

MILD EFFECTS	SEVERE (POSSIBLY FATAL)
Skin rash	Agranulocytosis (manifested by sore throat, high fever)
Mild leukopenia	Lupus-like syndrome
Loss of taste	Hepatitis
Arthralgia	Hepatic failure
Loss or abnormal pigmentation of hair	Glomerulonephritis

The second treatment option for hyperthyroidism is radioactive iodine therapy (RAI). Used for years with adults, this therapy is becoming more acceptable for children over the age of 15 years as an alternative to long-term drug therapy. Oral radioactive iodine is administered, with tissue damage and destruction of the thyroid gland occurring in approximately 6–18 weeks. Hypothyroidism is one of the most frequent complications of this treatment, and L-thyroxine therapy is initiated if this occurs. While RAI is effective, its long-range potential for cancer and gonadal damage has not been established in pediatric populations.

The third option, subtotal thyroidectomy, is used when adequate caregiver cooperation with drug therapy is not possible, or when treatment has failed to result in permanent remission. Approximately 25% of children will go into remission after two years (Glase & Slyne, 2008). Surgery is performed after the child has been brought to a euthyroid state, which is accomplished with antithyroid medication. Hypothyroidism frequently occurs as a complication following thyroidectomy. Hypoparathyroidism and laryngeal nerve damage are also a risk. A surgeon, skilled and experienced with pediatric thyroidectomy, is essential to optimize a successful surgical outcome.

NURSING ALERT

Academic Performance of Children with Hyperthyroidism

Children who are in school may have a change in behavior with increased difficulty staying on task, inability to sit still, and decreased academic performance. Some of these children may have been referred for evaluation of learning disabilities or attention-deficit hyperactivity disorder (ADHD).

Nursing Management

The majority of children with hyperthyroidism are diagnosed and treated in an ambulatory environment. A history of the child's behavior including the pattern of sleep, school performance (past and current), and distractibility need to be obtained. Nursing intervention should focus on providing information about the disorder. In the acute phase, teaching centers on providing information to the caregiver about the treatment options. If radioactive therapy or thyroidectomy is the treatment of choice, the caregivers need to be prepared with information about the procedure, goals of treatment, and complications. If surgical intervention is chosen, nurses should explore with the child and caregivers their perceptions and fears of having an incision in the neck.

Family Teaching

When working with a child with hyperthyroidism that is being treated with medication, it is important to teach the family the medication regimen, the side effects of the drugs, and the need to continue with the medication despite resolution of symptoms of hyperthyroidism. The nurse must familiarize the family with the routine of blood tests and help them to identify a lab facility that is convenient for them to use.

Nurses should teach caregivers about the symptoms of hypothyroidism and provide guidelines for contacting the health care provider (e.g., presence of symptoms of drug reaction, tachycardia, fatigue). The child with heat intolerance caused by increased basal metabolic rate may be more comfortable in lightweight clothing, using fans or air conditioning if available, and taking frequent baths or showers. Until symptoms disappear with drug therapy, children need a low-stress, low-pressure environment. Emotional lability may be evidenced by sudden episodes of crying and irritability or elation. Caregivers need to be taught that these emotions are uncontrollable and can be minimized by encouraging the child to discuss these feelings.

If the child attends school, instruct the family on activity restrictions if medically appropriate. Nurses should discuss with school personnel restrictions for physical education and when these will be reevaluated. Nurses should provide the school with information regarding the symptoms of hyperthyroidism that may have an impact on the child's ability to focus during class, and thereby affect the child's school performance. If appropriate, nurses may request that the school nurse monitor the child's pulse and blood pressure changes in response to the medication or symptoms of hyperthyroidism. Once recovery is evident, the caregivers may consider tutoring to assist the child who may have fallen behind in school work. It is important to refer caregivers to community resources for any local support groups or educational opportunities.

DISORDERS OF THE ADRENAL GLAND

The adrenal glands are composed of the inner cortex and the outer medulla. The cortex produces hormones called steroids: glucocorticoids and mineralocorticoids. The main glucocorticoid, cortisol, has an effect on the metabolism of glucose, proteins, and fats; stress reactions; and inhibition of inflammation. Aldosterone is the most important mineralocorticoid. It is responsible for maintaining extracellular fluid volume and blood pressure by conservation of sodium, chloride, and water, and excretion of potassium by the kidneys. The adrenal medulla secretes the catecholamines epinephrine and norepinephrine. These hormones are produced by the sympathetic nervous system (SNS); therefore, when the adrenal supply is decreased or absent, it is not life-threatening.

CONGENITAL ADRENAL HYPERPLASIA

Congenital adrenal hyperplasia (CAH) is a group of inherited disorders in which a genetic defect results in the deficiency of an enzyme essential for synthesis of cortisol and, at times, aldosterone.

Incidence and Etiology

The incidence of CAH is 0.06 to 0.08 in 1,000 live births. There are several forms of CAH, the most common of which is 21-hydroxylase (21-OH) deficiency, occurring in about 95% of all cases.

Pathophysiology

In a child with CAH, cortisol synthesis is blocked by the lack of the enzyme 21-OH. This reduction of cortisol leads to increased ACTH production by the anterior pituitary. Prolonged over secretion of ACTH causes enlargement or hyperplasia of the adrenal glands and excess production of androgens.

Clinical Manifestations

The enzyme deficiency of 21-OH exposes the fetus to excessive production of androgens. In the male fetus, this causes no physical changes; however, in the female, excessive androgens will **virilize** (to develop sexual characteristics of a male) the external genitalia, resulting in an enlarged clitoris (possibly to the extent of resembling the male phallus), fusion of the labial folds, and a rugated appearance to the labia. This is known as ambiguous genitalia or **pseudohermaphrodism**. The ovaries, fallopian tubes, and uterus are normal.

Approximately 75% of cases of 21-OH deficiency have salt wasting from a defect in the ability to synthesize aldosterone. If not diagnosed at birth, the neonate with 21-OH deficiency and salt wasting will develop a life-threatening hyponatremia, hyperkalemia, and hypovolemia by day 10–14 of life. This is known as adrenal crisis.

Children with atypical 21-OH deficiency will present later (often in the toddler or preschool years) with premature **adrenarche** (pubic hair development), accelerated growth velocity, advanced bone age, acne, and **hirsutism** (excessive body hair in a masculine distribution pattern).

Diagnosis

Prenatal diagnosis and treatment of CAH is possible with the objective of preventing prenatal virilization in affected female infants and early recognition of the potential for salt wasting in newborn infants. This is performed most commonly in families with a previously affected child with CAH with a defined genetic defect. Forty two states currently test for 21-OH deficiency in their newborn screening programs (AAP, 2006). The major objectives of this screening are to identify infants at risk for the development of life-threatening adrenal crisis and to prevent the incorrect male sex assignment of affected female infants with ambiguous genitalia. Health care practitioners are notified of abnormal screens, similar to that for congenital hypothyroidism. Confirmation of the diagnosis through repeat blood testing, electrolyte levels (to screen for abnormalities associated with salt wasting), and physical examination are done immediately.

REFLECTIVE THINKING

The Newborn with Ambiguous Genitalia

Gender identification is most commonly based on the appearance of the external genitals. Think about one of the very first questions asked when a child is born. "Is it a boy or a girl?" Think about the answer: "The sex of the child cannot be determined yet." When the newborn presents with ambiguous genitalia, this is the response in the delivery room. Sometimes the ambiguity of the genitalia is missed and a sex assignment is made at birth. The caregivers announce the gender of the baby to their friends and families, yet the gender is not consistent with the child's genetic makeup or gonads.

For the child with 21-OH deficiency, gender misidentification is problematic only for the females. Most of these girls who have mildly virilized external genitalia are rapidly identified as ambiguous. However, some go home with a male sex assignment and are thought of as a male by caregivers, relatives, and friends. These children and caregivers present a special challenge.

What is your own personal view of what makes a girl a girl or a boy a boy?

In the child who presents with clinical symptoms suggestive of CAH, hormonal testing is pursued. While the most common type of CAH is 21-OH deficiency, there are other enzyme deficiencies that cause CAH, and each type has its own unique hormonal profile. Several different adrenal steroids and their precursors should be measured to seek the most appropriate diagnosis. Bone age films should also be obtained to evaluate future growth potential and to monitor response to therapy.

TREATMENT

The goal of treatment is suppression of adrenal secretion of androgens and prevention of progressive virilization and includes lifelong replacement of the steroids the adrenal gland is unable to produce. The vast majority of individuals with 21-OH deficiency will take both the glucocorticoid hydrocortisone and the mineralocorticoid fludrocortisone (Florinef). At physiological replacement doses, there are no side effects related to these drugs, but at doses that are elevated, hypertension, growth impairment, and acne can occur. Regular and ongoing follow-up are essential for titrating doses of the medication and for monitoring treatment goals of normal growth and development.

The genetic female infant with CAH is often born with varying degrees of ambiguous genitalia. The parents, together with the clinical and surgical team, should make the decision for surgical intervention after discussing all pertinent factors and available options. They should consider the child's fertility potential, capacity for normal sexual function, endocrine function of the gonads, testosterone imprinting, and timing of surgery. All females with virilizing CAH are potentially fertile. Goals of surgery are to have good adult sexual and reproductive function, to have unobstructed urinary opening without incontinence or infections, and to make the genital appearance compatible with gender (although this goal is less compelling than the first two goals). Recommended timing for surgery is after stability on medical treatment for the CAH and between ages 2–6 months.

There is a growing movement in the United States, driven by individuals whose gender was previously described as ambiguous, to delay decision of cosmetic correction of the genitalia until the child is of an age to participate in the decision making. Surgical intervention most often results in a loss of the nerve endings in the clitoris, which has an impact on sexuality and sexual experiences later. It can also have an impact on the appearance of the genitalia. The decision to surgically intervene immediately versus delaying the decision is a complex one. The decision to raise a child with an ambiguous gender in today's society raises numerous concerns and problems. Yet many of the individuals who have experienced surgical intervention of the genitalia are adamant that the decision is too complex to be decided solely by the caregivers and health care provider of a newborn or young child.

NURSING TIP

Cortisol Replacement

In the event of an illness, stress, or surgery that would normally cause an increase in the production of cortisol, changes in the dose of medication will need to be made. Caregivers need to be taught when to increase the cortisol dose and by how much for common illnesses. They should be instructed that any surgical procedure will require increases in the child's medication and should be discussed with their health care provider well in advance of any planned procedure, and as soon as possible for any emergency procedure. The most common cause of adrenal insufficiency is a result of glucocorticoid omission in a patient on chronic glucocorticoid therapy (Shulman, Palmert, & Kemp, 2007). Adrenal insufficiency is a life threatening emergency.

NURSING MANAGEMENT AND FAMILY TEACHING

Nursing management with the newborn in adrenal crisis is focused on interventions necessary to maintain homeostasis through administration of fluids and cortisone, and monitoring electrolytes and vital signs. Nurses need to also provide a safe environment for the caregivers to ask questions and explore their feelings. They need to address the newborn with ambiguous genitalia as "your baby" or "your child," not as he, she, or it. The genitals should be described as sex organs, not as a penis or clitoris. Nurses should describe to the caregivers that the penis and clitoris develop from the same fetal tissue. Most infants in the United States have been assigned a sex at birth; delaying a sex assignment is stressful for the family and often the health care team. Depending on the severity of the virilization of the genitalia in the female and the sex assignment decision made by the caregivers and health care provider, corrective surgery may be immediately considered. If the genitals remain in an ambiguous state, nurses should discuss with the caregivers how they feel about handling diaper changes in public or by other family members. If a birth certificate was issued at birth, nurses should discuss how to best change the sex identification and possibly the child's name if there is a sex reassignment. It is important to discuss with the caregivers how to best handle notifying those people whom they have already contacted about the baby and gender identification.

Medication administration and the lifelong nature of treatment need to be taught to the caregivers. Intramuscular injection technique will need to be taught. Cortisone is necessary to sustain life, and at times when the oral medication cannot be taken, intramuscular injections are given.

Nursing management for the child diagnosed later focuses on coordinating the testing for establishing the diagnosis. Most caregivers will have little understanding of adrenal function and will benefit from education. If the child who is diagnosed later has been assigned a sex that is not consistent with the child's gonads or chromosomes, the issues and focus of management will quickly include this new dilemma. The full ramifications of reassigning the sex of the child versus raising the child with the sex as assigned at birth will need to be considered.

DISORDERS OF THE PANCREAS

The most common disorder of the pancreas is diabetes mellitus (DM), in which the islets of Langerhans fail to produce adequate insulin.

DIABETES MELLITUS

Diabetes mellitus is a group of diseases in which carbohydrate and lipid metabolism are impaired. Diabetes mellitus, as a whole, is one of the leading causes of health problems and death in the United States. Traditionally DM had been classified according to the type of treatment needed. The old categories were: (1) type I, or insulin-dependent diabetes mellitus (IDDM), or juvenile type; and (2) type II or non-insulin dependent diabetes (NIDDM). In 1997 these terms were eliminated because treatment can vary (some with NIDDM require insulin). The new terms are type 1 and type 2 (not type I and type II). Type 1 DM is the second most common chronic disease of childhood in the United States and much of Europe. In the past, type 2 DM occurred most commonly in adults over age 40 and accounted for 90% of the diagnosed cases in the United States.

INCIDENCE AND ETIOLOGY

Diabetes mellitus is an umbrella diagnosis, under which several diseases that result in an alteration in insulin-mediated glucose metabolism are grouped. Type 1 diabetes results from insulin-producing pancreatic beta-cell destruction and usually results in absolute insulin deficiency. Type 1 DM has two forms: (1) immune-mediated, which results from an autoimmune destruction of the beta cells and (2) idiopathic, which refers to rare forms of the disease with no known cause. Several environmental factors, such as viruses or chemicals in the environment, have been implicated in the process of developing type 1 diabetes. In a genetically susceptible individual exposed to environmental factors, the immune system begins a T lymphocyte-mediated process that damages and destroys the beta cells of the pancreas (Figure 28-4). Islet cell antibodies (ICA), insulin autoantibodies (IAA), glutamic acid decarboxylase (GAD), and other antibodies specific to the beta cell can be measured in the serum of individuals who are in the process of developing type 1 diabetes for years before the clinical appearance. By the time symptoms are evident and diagnosis is commonly made, approximately 90% of the beta cells have been destroyed.

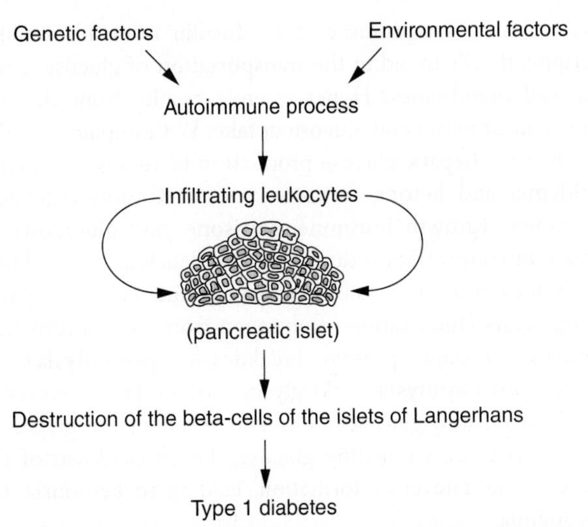

FIGURE 28-4 Development of Type 1 Diabetes. DELMAR CENGAGE LEARNING.

Type 1 diabetes is the most common form of diabetes found in young people. In the United States, the prevalence of type 1 DM among all children ages 19 and younger is 1.82 per 1000 (SEARCH for Diabetes in Youth Study Group, 2006). There is an equal distribution between males and females. Caucasians experience a higher incidence of type 1 DM than any other ethnic group. There is a small peak in diagnosis at age 2, again at ages 4–6, with the major peak in diagnosis from age 10–14 years.

In the past, type 2 DM occurred in those who were older than 45, were overweight and sedentary, and had a family history of diabetes. Changes in food consumption and exercise patterns have increased the incidence of type 2 DM in children and adolescents in the United States, especially among children of ethnic minority populations (Cowell, 2008). Characteristics common in children diagnosed with type 2 diabetes are obesity, family history of type 2 diabetes, and being of a non-European ancestry (Americans of African, Hispanic, Asian, or American Indian descent). The problem of obesity is so prevalent that even in the type 1 diabetes population, 16% of children at diagnosis met the criteria for obesity (Jones, 2008). Additionally, as many as 90% of children diagnosed with type 2 diabetes have acanthosis, a skin finding characterized by velvety, hyperpigmented patches that are most prominent in areas with creases like the armpit or back of the neck.

PATHOPHYSIOLOGY

In type 1 diabetes the autoimmune destruction, mediated by the T lymphocyte, of the beta cells results in inadequate insulin secretion and eventually insulin deficiency. When beta-cell insulin production is less than 10–20% of normal, overt clinical symptoms emerge. Insulin is unable to alter peripheral cells to aid in the transportation of glucose across the cell membranes. Hyperglycemia results from this impairment of peripheral glucose uptake. With impaired insulin production, hepatic glucose production increases, and hyperlipidemia and ketone formation occur. Counterregulatory hormones (growth hormone, cortisone, and glucagon) increase in concentration during insulin-deficient states. These hormones promote insulin resistance and enhance **glyconeogenesis** (the fixation of glycogen from noncarbohydrate sources) through protein breakdown (**proteolysis**), fat breakdown (**lipolysis**), and glycogenolysis (the conversion of glycogen into glucose). The end result of the glyconeogenesis is more circulating glucose. The breakdown of fats increases ketone body formation, leading to ketonuria and ketonemia.

When the blood glucose exceeds 150–180 mg/dL, the renal threshold for glucose is exceeded and it is filtered out of the serum and into the urine. When glucose is excreted in the urine, an osmotic shift begins. Additional water is excreted, and polyuria, the first of the classic symptoms of diabetes, is evident. The osmotic shift and increasing fluid loss from the glucosuria stimulate the thirst center and polydipsia, the second of the classic symptoms, develops. **Polyphagia** (excessive hunger) occurs as less glucose is used for energy production and storage and the hunger center is stimulated. As the hyperglycemia becomes even more pronounced and persistent, fluid loss becomes severe, and oral consumption will not replenish the loss. Dehydration occurs, and weight loss ensues, caused by fluid loss from the osmotic diuresis and inadequate storage of nutrients. Electrolyte disturbances result from the osmotic diuresis and cell death.

Ketones are acid bodies that are initially buffered by stores of bicarbonate. The kidney eventually loses its ability to buffer the ketone bodies, and bicarbonate stores are depleted, worsening the metabolic acidosis. Respiratory compensation of the metabolic acidosis begins with the clinical symptoms of increased respiratory rate, **Kussmaul respirations** (deep, slow, labored breathing), flushed cheeks, and an acetone odor to the breath, resembling nail polish remover or rotten apples.

Type 2 diabetes is a complex metabolic disorder. Its etiology is a result of social, behavioral, and environmental factors. It is a genetic disease, with identical twin studies showing a concordance of diagnosis at nearly 100%, but the genetics of this form of diabetes has not yet been defined. Glucose homeostasis is dependent on both insulin secretion and insulin action. In children with type 2 diabetes, it appears that the initial abnormality is impaired glucose action followed by beta-cell failure. The target cells in the body resist insulin-stimulated glucose uptake, resulting in hyperinsulinism or insulin resistance, hallmark characteristics of type 2 diabetes. Eventually, beta cells fail to hypersecrete insulin, resulting in insulin insufficiency, marked hyperglycemia, and clinical diabetes.

NURSING TIP

History Taking in the Evaluation of New Onset Type 1 Diabetes

When taking a history on a child with symptoms of diabetes, explore for new onset nocturia or newly developed bed-wetting. Ask caregivers of infants and toddlers about a recent increase in frequency of diaper changes, which would indicate polyuria, a symptom of diabetes.

Clinical Manifestations

The individual with type 1 diabetes presents most commonly with a history of polyuria, polydipsia, polyphagia, weight loss, and dehydration. In some individuals, abdominal pain and vomiting will be present, leading to a misdiagnosis of appendicitis or gastroenteritis. In the early diagnosis of type 1 diabetes, there may be a virtual lack of symptoms. Children and adolescents are sometimes diagnosed early through a routine urinalysis done in the course of a yearly physical examination by their primary care provider. Typically, the child with type 2 diabetes is overweight at diagnosis, with a body mass index over the 95th percentile for age. Some will have a history of polyuria that was mild in nature, others may report significant polyuria, and others will report none. Fatigue and frequent infections may be present; sometimes but not always, the child would have ketosis. Table 28-3 presents the characteristics of type 1 vs. type 2 diabetes.

Diagnosis

The individual with type 1 diabetes can present in a variety of ways, from the most critical to the most stable. In the vast majority of children, the diagnosis is immediately apparent. They present with a history of polyuria, polydipsia, and polyphagia (the classic triad of symptoms of diabetes) and glucose in excess of 200 mg/dL. Most will also have experienced weight loss and fatigue. Some will present in diabetic ketoacidosis (DKA). Oral glucose tolerance testing (OGTT) and fasting serum glucose determination, the historical hallmark used in diagnosing type 2 diabetes, are not commonly needed in children because of their unequivocal presentation. The fasting plasma glucose is the preferred test to diagnose diabetes in children. The use of the A1c for diagnosis is not recommended. Diagnosis of the child with type 2 diabetes with symptoms is preferably established with a fasting glucose level greater than or equal to 126 or a random glucose level greater than or equal to 200. If an oral glucose tolerance test is performed, the two hour plasma glucose needs to be 200 or greater, using a glucose load of 1.75 gm/kg to a max dose of 75 grams of anhydrous glucose dissolved in water. If the child is asymptomatic, then the abnormality of glucose should be evident on two different days (ADA, 2008a).

Table 28-3 Characteristics of Type 1 and Type 2 Diabetes

DISTINGUISHING CHARACTERISTICS	TYPE 1 DIABETES	TYPE 2 DIABETES
Clinical features (onset)	Young	Prepubertal
Duration of symptoms	Days to weeks	Months
Acute Presentation	Yes	No
DKA at presentation	Sometimes (30–40%)	Rare (5–25%)
Family History	Infrequent	Frequent
Lab Values		
Immune markers	Frequent	Infrequent
C-peptides	Low to normal	Normal to high

Treatment

Treatment of type 1 and type 2 diabetes in pediatrics ideally involves a team consisting of the child, caregivers, health care practitioner, nurse, nutritionist, and mental health professional. Each discipline brings to the management a unique and helpful perspective. The general goals for therapy for type 1 diabetes include achieving normal growth and development, optimal glucose control, minimal complications, and a positive adjustment to the disease. It requires daily injections of insulin, blood glucose monitoring, following a meal plan, exercise, self-management skills, and decision making. The goal of treatment of type 2 diabetes is normalization of blood glucose levels and hemoglobin A1c, achievement of normal growth and development, development of minimal complications, and a positive adjustment to the disease and its management. Other metabolic parameters include normalization of any hypertension or hyperlipidemia. The initial treatment plan (diet, oral medication, or insulin) for type 2 diabetes will vary dependent on clinical presentation. Children presenting with metabolic compromise, such as DKA, will require insulin therapy, at least initially. Insulin regimens used in the treatment of type 1 diabetes are the same regimens used for the treatment of type 2 diabetes.

Children who present with type 2 diabetes without metabolic decompensation may be treated with oral agents. Glucophage has an indication for use in adolescents and is the typical first oral agent used. Glucophage is an antihyperglycemic agent that works by both improving insulin sensitivity by increasing peripheral uptake and utilization of glucose and by decreasing hepatic glucose production. It does not increase insulin production and therefore does not cause hypoglycemia. Its common side effects are gastrointestinal in nature and are often avoided by starting at a low dose and taking the medication with the meal. It has a less common but a serious side effect of lactic acidosis. Clients should be instructed to discontinue the medication when they are vomiting, have an illness, and prior to surgery. Table 28-4 lists the acute, intermediate, and chronic complications of diabetes.

NURSING TIP

Characteristics of Kussmaul Respirations

Kussmaul respirations sound like a train. They are deep and laborious. The respiratory system is attempting to eliminate excess carbon dioxide to compensate for the metabolic acidosis.

Table 28-4 Complications of Diabetes

ACUTE	INTERMEDIATE	CHRONIC
Ketoacidosis	Lipohypertrophy	Retinopathy
Hypoglycemia	Lipoatrophy	Nephropathy
Weight loss	Growth failure	Neuropathy
	Pubertal delay	Cardiopathy
	Menstrual disturbances	
	Impaired cognitive function	
	Hyperlipidemia	
	Emotional disturbances	
	Cataracts	

Reflections from Families

When my child was first diagnosed with diabetes, I was so frightened. My father had also had diabetes diagnosed when he was a young boy. I can remember when I was a child that he would act so different when his blood sugar was low. (As a teenager, I found his behavior during those events so embarrassing.) When I was in my later teenage years, he started to have real problems with his vision and we learned that he might lose his eyesight. But nothing prepared me for his developing kidney failure and death when I was in my twenties. He was only 48 years old and had diabetes for 35 years when he died from diabetes complications.

Diabetes management is so different today than when my father was diagnosed. He never knew what his blood sugar was (he could only test his urine) and he could never adjust his insulin doses to keep himself in control. He never really knew when he was younger what kind of control he was in. When my child was diagnosed, the nurses and physicians took so much time helping me to understand that my child and I could manage the diabetes by monitoring blood sugar levels, how food affects blood sugar, and how to adapt the dose of insulin my child receives. I feel more in control, more empowered to manage the diabetes, because of the tools I have and the knowledge of the health care professionals on the diabetes team. I still worry, but my fear of the future and my child's health is not stopping me from envisioning a healthy future for my child.

Insulin Management Insulin replacement is the cornerstone of management. Daily insulin is administered by subcutaneous injections or a portable insulin pump. The frequency of injection is based on the goals of management for the child. Multiple daily injections (3–7 injections) has become commonplace in the management of type 1 diabetes. The use of insulin pumps in children and teens with diabetes is rapidly growing. Types of insulin preparations are categorized by their actions as short, intermediate, or long-acting (Table 28-5). The most common insulin used

Table 28-5 Insulin Types and Action

NAME	TYPE	ONSET	PEAK	DURATION
Lispro (Humalog)	Rapid-acting	5–15 min	30–90 min	5 hours
Aspart (Novolog)	Rapid-acting	5–15 min	30–90 min	5 hours
Apidra	Rapid-acting	5–15 min	30–90 min	5 hours
Regular	Short-acting	20–60 min	2–3 hours	5–8 hours
NPH	Intermediate-acting	2–4 hours	4–10 hours	10–16 hours
Detemir (Levemir)	Long-acting	1–2 hours	minimal	22–24 hours
Glargine (Lantus)	Long-acting	1–2 hours	None	20–24 hours
Premixed 70/30	70% NPH with 30% regular or Novolog	20 min–4 hours	4–10 hours	10–16 hours
Premixed 75/25	75% NPH with 25% Humalog	5 min–4 hours	4–10 hours	10–16 hours

EVIDENCE-BASED PRACTICE

Use of Insulin Analogs in Type 1 Diabetes

CLINICAL PROBLEM

Does the use of insulin analogs result in improvement in glucose control in the management of type 1 diabetes?

BEST CLINICAL PRACTICE

- Insulin analogs were introduced to the U.S. market in 1990s, with the rapid-acting Lispro, followed by Aspart, and then Glulisine. In 2000, basal analog Glargine became available, followed several years later by Detemir.
- Insulin analogs are designed to be more physiologic in their action (pharmacokinetics and pharmacodynamics), resulting in a reduced risk of hypoglycemia.
- Insulin analogs are more predictable in absorption and action than human insulin preparations (regular insulin, NPH, lente series); therefore, there is less variability in their action.
- From the largest clinical study linking glucose control to complications, intensive diabetes management (usually accomplished with multiple daily injections or insulin pump therapy) resulted in exceptional glucose control but at the expense of increased frequency of hypoglycemia (62 episodes per 100 patient-years of therapy). This study was done prior to the introduction of insulin analogs.
- Insulin analogs are associated with a reduction in hypoglycemia without loss of glucose control.
- Insulin analogs should be used as the insulin preparation for glucose management of diabetes.

IMPLICATIONS FOR NURSING

- Rapid-acting insulin analogs are absorbed and have peak impact within 100 minutes of administration. Unless the patient is experiencing hyperglycemia, these insulin preparations should be given 15 minutes before the start of a meal.
- Basal insulin analogs only provide insulin for basal requirements. Whenever food is consumed or if glucose becomes elevated, a rapid-acting insulin is given. Caregivers and children need to be instructed on dose determination of rapid-acting insulin, usually based on carbohydrate intake, premeal glucose concentration, and anticipated activity.
- Basal analogs and rapid-acting analogs cannot be mixed together into one injection.
- Hypoglycemia continues to be a risk; therefore, glucose monitoring should be continued. The patient should have access to treatment for hypoglycemia at all times.
- Regimens of basal analog with premeal rapid-acting analog is a multiple daily injection regimen, usually requiring four or more injections each day.

Reference: American Diabetes Association. (2008a). Standards of medical care in diabetes. *Diabetes Care* (31), S12–S54.

in the United States is synthetic human, produced through DNA recombinant technology. Dosage of insulin is based on the needs of the child or adolescent. Common dosage for a child with type 1 diabetes more than 1 year post-diagnosis is 0.75–1.0 units/kg/day. The insulin dose in the adolescent with type 1 tends to exceed 1.0 units/kg/day, sometimes reaching 1.6–1.7 units/kg/day. Different types of insulin can be mixed together. It is common for insulin regimens to incorporate mixed insulins. Regular, Aspart, and Lispro insulin are stable when mixed with NPH.

No insulin is compatible when mixed in the same syringe with Glargine or Detemir. Insulin regimens can be described as either physiologic or nonphysiologic. The traditional routine of using rapid- or short-acting insulin (e.g., Humalog or Novolog) with NPH using a 2–3 injection per day routine is nonphysiologic. In this regimen, the insulin actions do not mimic normal beta-cell secretion of basal and prandial (or meal bolus) insulin secretion. Timing of meals and snacks is essential to prevent hypoglycemia while insulin is in its peak effect, and for avoiding snacks and meals when insulin is in low concentration to prevent hyperglycemia. Insulin regimens that utilize a long-acting insulin like Glargine or Detemir or using an insulin pump are more physiologic, with a better approximation of normal beta-cell insulin secretion. With the physiologic regimens, Glargine, Detemir, or the insulin pump provides a steady rate of insulin at a low dose throughout the day, in an attempt to replicate the basal insulin production of the beta cell. Prior to meals, rapid-acting insulin is given to provide peaking insulin to coincide with glucose increases because of eating.

Blood Glucose Monitoring Home blood glucose monitoring (HBGM) became available in the late 1970s to early 1980s. Prior to its introduction, daily glucose monitoring was often done through urine testing. Urine glucose monitoring did not supply quantitative data that could aid in making decisions about insulin doses or success of treatment. The introduction of HBGM facilitated the introduction of insulin regimens geared toward tighter glucose control, the use of supplemental insulin to correct or prevent hyperglycemia, and the ability of clients and caregivers to become skilled at self-management. HBGM is done by lancing the fingertip or other appropriate area (several meters today can test small samples of blood obtained from a forearm, thigh, or side of the hand) with a small lancet to obtain a blood sample. The blood sample is placed on a testing strip in a glucose meter. The glucose level is measured by the meter. Home blood glucose meters are commercially available and are frequently covered by third-party insurers; however, the test strips can be one of the more costly items, ranging up to $1.00 per testing strip. Frequency of blood glucose testing is based on the goals of the individual's management.

National standards for medical monitoring are listed in Box 28-5. This monitoring reflects the ongoing needs of the individual with type 1 diabetes, and the assessment of

EYE ON...

Insulin Pumps and Continuous Glucose Monitoring—A Growing Trend

Insulin pumps have been available commercially since the 1980s. Current pumps are the size of a cell phone, weigh 2.7–3.2 ounces, and contain a reservoir that holds up to 300 units of insulin. The pump delivers insulin through a tiny catheter that is placed every 2–3 days into subcutaneous fat. The pump is programmed to deliver insulin continuously in small amounts throughout the day and night. With each meal or snack, the pump is programmed to deliver an immediate bolus of insulin based on the dose of insulin necessary for the carbohydrate consumed and the individual's blood glucose level. Pumps (called "smart pumps") can be programmed with dosing guidelines and can recommend doses of insulin to patients when given information about blood glucose levels and carbohydrates to be consumed. Some pumps are programmed with carbohydrate data bases for easy access to information on carbohydrate contents of specific foods. Some pumps operate in a wireless fashion, downloading glucose information from a meter to the pump wirelessly or programming a bolus through a remote operator. Pump therapy has demonstrated a reduction in severe hypoglycemia in pediatric populations and an increase in client satisfaction (Weissberg-Benchell, Antisdel-Lomaglio, & Seshardi, 2003).

Continuous glucose monitoring (CGMS) is new technology. A small sensor is placed subcutaneously into the interstitial fluid. Interstitial glucose is measured and wireless transmitted to a receiver. While not actual blood glucose, and not accurate enough to obtain FDA approval to replace glucose monitoring, interstitial glucose is a close approximation of blood glucose levels. These systems can be set up to alert patients to a declining glucose that is likely to result in hypoglycemia, or a rising glucose trend. This information can lead to improvement in glycemia, with a reduction in hypoglycemic excursions (Wolpert, 2008). Some of these systems are reporting to insulin pumps as a receiver. Insulin pumps are not using the information to alter insulin dosing, but, as technology improves the accuracy of the readings, may be able to in the future.

the various body systems that are affected by the disease. The individual is monitored for immediate, intermediate, and long-term complications.

As with type 1 diabetes, children with type 2 diabetes monitor their blood glucose levels. The frequency of monitoring is dependent on therapy they are using and whether they are meeting their metabolic goals.

NURSING TIP

Monitoring for Long-term Glucose Control: The Hemoglobin A1c

The hemoglobin A1c (HgbA1c), or glycosolated hemoglobin, measurement reflects the average blood glucose control of the individual over the previous 8–12 weeks. It measures the amount of glucose that attaches to protein in the red blood cells. The greater the amount of glucose in the blood overall, the higher the HgbA1c will be. A1c goals for type 1 by age are 0–6 years, 7.5–8.5%; 6–12 years, <8.0%; and 13–19 years, <7.5% (ADA, 2008a). The national standards recommend that this be measured semiannually to quarterly for individuals with type 1 diabetes. It is an invaluable tool for the assessment of overall glucose control, and is an outcome measurement used to describe comparable risk for the development of the long-term (or chronic) complications.

Nutrition Modifications (2004) to new nutritional recommendations established in 2002 for diabetes were released by the American Diabetes Association in conjunction with the American Dietetics Association (ADA, 2008b). Now known as medical nutrition management (MNT), the recommendations include evidence-based nutritional and meal planning principles. MNT should reflect the management goals of the individual. In children, the meal plan should be updated at least annually and should reflect their growing needs. The meal plan is no longer a plan that excludes foods. The previous philosophy (pre-1994) was that foods that were simple sugars, for example candy or pie, were automatically forbidden. The change in philosophy is that while some foods are better nutritional choices than others, no food is automatically excluded. The dietary pattern will include carbohydrates from fruits, vegetables, whole grains, legumes, and low-fat milk. Sucrose containing foods can be incorporated by substituting for other carbohydrate containing foods or covering with glucose lowering medication. Saturated fat is limited to <7% of total calories, with a dietary cholesterol <200 mg/day. Protein should not exceed 15–20% of calories (0.8 grams protein/kg/day) (ADA, 2008b).

Perhaps even more essential in children with type 2 diabetes is MNT. Meal planning, with the goal that meets all the metabolic needs of the child and provides adequate calories and nutrients for ongoing growth and development, yet promoting weight loss or stabilization, can be a challenge for many families, especially those that struggle with adult members who have been unsuccessful with weight management themselves. Set realistic, specific goals that can be met. Build on the success of small goals to begin reaching the child's target metabolic levels of normalized blood glucose and A1c levels, weight reduction or stabilization, and the absence of complications.

BOX 28-5

MEDICAL MONITORING RECOMMENDATIONS FOR TYPE 1 DIABETES (ADA, 2008A)

- Semiannual or quarterly exams
- Height measurement (until maturity)
- Weight
- Blood pressure (quarterly)
- Sexual maturation staging (periodically in the peripubertal client)
- Foot exam with quarterly exam
- Comprehensive eye exam for all clients over age 10 after 3–5 years of diagnosis with diabetes
- Medical history: include frequency or severity of hypoglycemia HBGM results, regimen adjustments made by client, lifestyle changes, symptoms of complications, medications, psychosocial issues
- Annual physical exam (any abnormality noted is reevaluated at next visit)
- Laboratory evaluation
- Hemoglobin A1c: 2–4 times per year (preferably 4 times)
- Fasting lipid panel soon after diagnosis, (after glycemic control is improved) if family history of hypercholesterolemia or cardiovascular event before age 55, or if family history unknown in children under 10 years of age. If child is 10 years or older, run fasting lipid panel irrespective of family history. Repeat annually if abnormal, otherwise every 5 years.
- Urine screening for microalbumin. Annual after 5 years of diagnosis, and older than 10 years.
- Celiac Disease—Children who are symptomatic should be screened with tissue transglutaminase or antiendomysial antibodies with documentation of normal serum IgA levels.
- Thyroid screen – Screen at diagnosis with thyroid peroxidase and thyroglobulin antibodies. TSH should be measured after metabolic control is established after diagnosis, and if symptomatic in the future.
- Review of management plan—each encounter.

Exercise Exercise plays an important role in diabetes management as it potentiates the hypoglycemic effect of insulin. Regular activity and exercise may assist in blood glucose control. For some individuals, higher levels of activity may permit a larger meal plan or lower doses of insulin. Exercise and activity are rarely restricted, but preparation for increased activity (i.e., insulin dose changes, changes in food) may be necessary to maintain blood glucose control. Exercise and activity are also basic components of therapy for type 2 diabetes. Exercise improves insulin sensitivity, thereby addressing one of the fundamental problems of type 2 diabetes, as well as assisting with weight control.

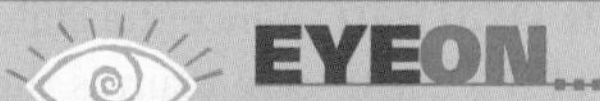

Micronutrients and Antioxidants

Many clients with diabetes are beginning to incorporate vitamins, antioxidants, and herbal supplements into their daily management. There is theoretical evidence that supplements with antioxidants may have benefits, but there is little if any confirmation of these reported benefits. Some of the reported benefits of micronutrients like chromium and magnesium are evident in deficient individuals and include a reduction of insulin resistance, a causative factor of type 2 diabetes. Research into the benefits of antioxidants and other micronutrients continues. There continues to be no clear evidence as to the benefits of vitamin or mineral supplementation, antioxidants, or chromium in people with diabetes (ADA, 2008b).

Nursing Management

Assessment Diabetes management is fluid and should reflect the growing and changing needs of the client. The success of the management is based on achieving the established goals for the client. The nurse is vigilant for evidence of complications, problems with management, and opportunities to provide education that will expand the child and caregiver's understanding and skills for diabetes management.

Nursing Diagnosis The following nursing diagnoses are pertinent to the child with type 1 diabetes:

1. *Risk for injury* related to insulin insufficiency and deficiency.
2. *Risk for injury* related to hypoglycemia or hyperglycemia.
3. *Disturbed body image* related to developing a chronic disease.
4. *Deficient knowledge* related to management of both types of diabetes.
5. *Interrupted family processes* related to management of a chronic illness.

Outcome Identification

1. Child will have adequate insulin levels, with normalized glucose levels.
2. Child will exhibit no evidence of hypoglycemia or hyperglycemia.
3. Child will have a positive body image.
4. Child and caregiver will be capable of managing diabetes in the home environment with the support and guidance of the other team members.
5. Family members will show evidence of healthy family processes.

Planning and Implementation

Once the child is medically stable, the priority of the health care team is the education of the child and caregivers. Initial education has traditionally occurred over several inpatient hospital days, but there is a growing movement to develop ambulatory educational programs for the newly diagnosed child and family. Education does not only occur at diagnosis, but is an ongoing process. Every meeting with a family or child with diabetes is an opportunity to provide ongoing education or assessment of knowledge. Excellent information is available to the family on the American Diabetes Association website at http://www.diabetes.org.

Survival Education The initial goal is to provide survival education, which encompasses the management skills and decision-making processes necessary for the caregiver or child to be safe at home. Once basic management skills are understood and the caregiver and child are proficient, the goals of education shift. Self-management becomes the overall goal at this time, and the role of the health care team is to empower the family and child to accomplish this goal.

The following concepts and skills are considered survival level:

1. Essential nature of insulin therapy
2. Identifying prescribed insulin
3. Preparing an accurate injection
4. Giving an injection with proper technique
5. Blood glucose monitoring and documentation
6. Urine testing for ketones
7. Understanding how to obtain supplies and equipment
8. Hypoglycemia and hyperglycemia, their causes, signs and symptoms, treatments
9. Understanding whom to call and when
10. Identifying the daily routine (timing of injection, when to do blood testing, when to eat)
11. Wearing medical identification
12. Meal planning

Most families and children will want to understand the "why and how come" of type 1 diabetes. To best understand the reason for the management regimen, they will need information on the function and action of insulin, carbohydrate metabolism, and the relationship the blood glucose level has to food intake, insulin level, and exercise. Caregivers tend to have many questions. Providing answers will increase their confidence and sense of security.

Education should be given to the caregiver and also in a developmentally appropriate manner to the child. Box 28-6 identifies diabetes management skills and the common age the skill is introduced to children. The nurse and family need to clarify at the beginning of the education who the primary caregiver will be initially. With the growing trend for short inpatient stays or ambulatory education programs, there may be insufficient time to prepare several individuals and offer them direct experience with diabetes care. Helping the primary caregiver identify who else in the family can assist with the diabetes care and incorporating that individual in the primary education sessions is an important nursing responsibility.

BOX 28-6

DEVELOPMENTAL TARGET AGES FOR TECHNICAL SKILL TRAINING

- Urine testing—4 to 6 years
- Blood testing—4 to 8 years
- Insulin injections—8 to 10 years
- Nutrition decision skills—10 to 14 years
- Management decision skills—12 to 18 years

Insulin Preparation and Injection Insulin preparation and injection require one-on-one time with the caregiver and child. Learning to give an injection is a task many caregivers and children approach with fear and anxiety. Both demonstration and return demonstration should be provided. Nurses should emphasize accuracy and consistency of the preparation technique. Refer to the accompanying "Nursing Tip" for specifics on the insulin injection.

Nurses should provide information about site selection and rotation. The sites for injections are the abdomen (which has the most consistent absorption rate), arms, legs, and buttocks (Figure 28-5). The absorption of insulin is fastest in the abdomen, followed by the arms. Leg and buttock insulin injections are absorbed the slowest. Injection sites may have evidence of **lipoatrophy** (indentation or atrophy of subcutaneous fat) or **lipohypertrophy** (lumpiness or hypertrophy of subcutaneous fat). Lipoatrophy is currently uncommon with the purified insulin preparations available and is treated by injecting insulin into the edges of the area of atrophy. Lipohypertrophy occurs commonly and is caused by trauma to the injection sites from repeatedly giving injections into the same area. Lipohypertrophy results in a cosmetically unsightly area that has decreased sensation and absorption. It resolves only by avoiding the area for injections.

Blood Glucose and Urine-Ketone Monitoring The technique of blood glucose monitoring will need to be taught to caregivers and the child (if appropriate). Specific instruction should concentrate on the technique of performing the blood-letting procedure and applying an adequate sample to the testing area of the meter to be used in the home. The instructor needs to be familiar with the glucose meter being used, aware of the volume of blood necessary for the performance of the test, how the blood sample is applied to the strip, and how the meter itself operates. Nurses should instruct and reinforce the practice of writing the results in a log, even with meters that have memories, and emphasize that the blood glucose monitoring, and its ongoing evaluation, play a major role in the success of the

NURSING TIP

Insulin injection

1. Encourage the caregiver or child (if child is doing self-injection) to receive a practice saline injection. This will help them to have knowledge about the comfort of the injection and will often allay their fear of performing the procedure. This practice session also allows caregivers an opportunity to role model cooperation for the child on receiving an injection.
2. Provide practice materials for the caregiver and child to use outside the educational sessions.
3. Initially when the caregiver is preparing the first injection, the child's anxiety may make the caregiver anxious and interfere with the ability to prepare it successfully. Should this occur, offer to have the caregiver prepare the injection in an area away from the child.
4. Most insulin bottles in use can be stored at room temperature or in the refrigerator for up to 30 days or to the expiration date on the bottle, whichever comes first. Unopened bottles are stored refrigerated up to the expiration date on the bottle. Insulin that is stored at temperatures that exceed 85°F (29.44°C) or below 50°F (10°C) should be discarded. Room temperature injections are considered more comfortable.
5. Recommend and provide insulin syringes that are the smallest volume for the dose. For example, use a 30 unit (3/10 mL) insulin syringe for insulin doses that are less than 30 units. This strategy will help to ensure more accuracy with prepared doses. Syringes are also available with 1/2 unit marking for clients who use 1/2 unit insulin doses.
6. Insulin pens are also available. Containing small containers of insulin, these pens (the size of a magic marker) can be dialed to deliver a single dose of insulin. A needle is attached to the end of the pen, the dose dialed, needle inserted into the subcutaneous fat, and the insulin injected. Insulin pens come in Lispro, Aspart, Apdidra, NPH, Regular, Detemir, and Glargine insulin, along with premixed insulin (70/30 or 75/25 insulin). Expiration of pens is variable; check drug insert for specifics.

regimen by identifying problem areas and successful strategies for management (Figure 28-6).

The technique and rationale for urine testing should be taught to the family. Given that most children and caregivers will be doing blood glucose testing, urine is monitored for ketones. Ketones are tested when there is a question about insulin deficiency. Common recommendations are

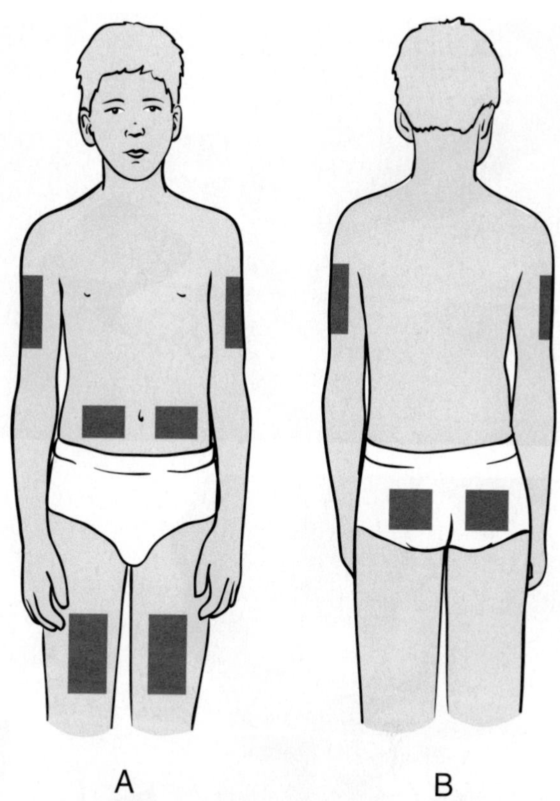

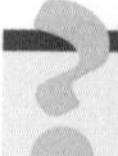

FIGURE 28-5 Insulin injections need to be rotated among the sites illustrated. (A) Front (B) Back. DELMAR CENGAGE LEARNING.

KIDS WANT TO KNOW

Do I really have to check my blood sugars so often?

The 10-year-old child you are caring for has been diagnosed with type 1 diabetes and is preparing to be discharged home. In preparing for her discharge, she asks "Do I really have to check my blood sugars so often? Can't I just test them in the morning and then test my urine the rest of the day? Every time I test, it hurts so much!"

A child of 10 has not developed an abstract cognitive thought process and may not understand the relationship between the blood glucose testing and the ongoing evaluation of the success of diabetes management. Additionally, blood glucose testing does require a small lancing of the skin, which can be uncomfortable. Review with her the techniques for doing less painful blood testing, using the sides of her upper fingers, not the tips or the pads, or using a meter that allows for less painful testing sites like the forearm. Reassure her that over the next several weeks, the discomfort will ease a bit as her fingers become slightly callused.

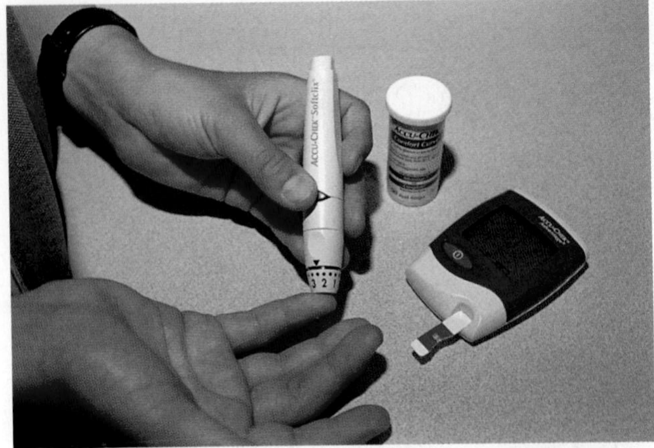

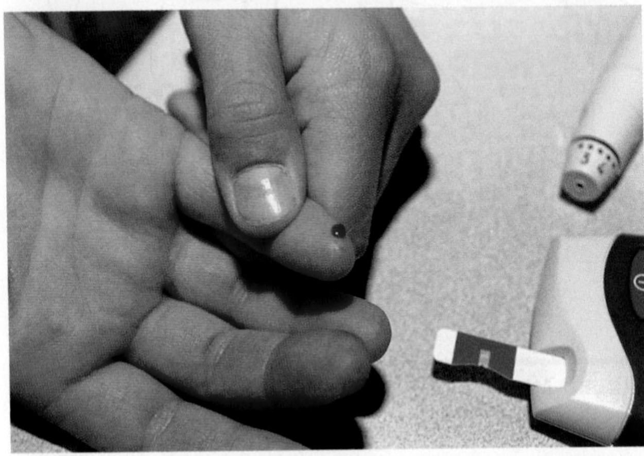

FIGURE 28-6 **This school-age child is able to perform his own blood glucose monitoring.** DELMAR CENGAGE LEARNING.

that the urine is tested for ketones when a client is ill, has a glucose over 250 mg/dL, or is experiencing unexplained weight loss. Return demonstration should be done. Results should be documented. There is one commercial home product that will measure serum ketones. Families who want more precise information about ketone status or whose child is uncooperative with urine collection may prefer this system.

Hypoglycemia Hypoglycemia, or low blood glucose or an insulin reaction, is also a survival topic. Hypoglycemia is a short-term complication of diabetes and occurs when the blood glucose level falls below 60 mg/dL. It is caused by more insulin being available than is necessary and may result from an insulin dose that is too large, insufficient food consumption, or increased activity. The most common symptoms of mild to moderate hypoglycemia include drowsiness, lightheadedness, irritability, tremors, sweating, and confusion. Severe hypoglycemia, which is rare, may lead to unconsciousness and convulsions and, if not treated promptly, can be life-threatening. Causes, symptoms, and treatment of hypoglycemia should be taught, reviewed, and assessed for retention of knowledge. Mild episodes will typically respond to 10–15 grams of carbohydrate (e.g., 3–4 glucose tablets, 4 ounces of juice or soda, 6 ounces of milk, 6–7 lifesaver-type candies) within 10–15 minutes. Moderate episodes should also resolve with treatment of 10–15 grams of carbohydrate, but the individual will likely require assistance. Severe

RESEARCH Highlight

Insulin Pump Therapy in Young Children

STUDY PURPOSE

To assess the effects of insulin pump therapy in young children on diabetes management, control, and family quality of life.

METHODS

Subjects (26 total) were children between the ages of 1–6 years who had had diabetes for > 6 months. Subjects were randomly assigned to a current treatment module of NPH insulin with a rapid-acting insulin analog given two to three times per day or to a continuous subcutaneous insulin pump (CSII) for six months. At the end of six months, the group on current therapy was offered the opportunity to change to CSII. Hemoglobin A1c (HbA1c), mean blood glucose, frequency of hypoglycemia, parental adjustment, and diabetes-related quality of life were recorded.

FINDINGS

Eleven subjects from each group completed the study. The results of the study found no change in mean HbA1c or mean blood glucose from baseline to the end of six months in either group. There was no difference in reports of severe hypoglycemia, hospitalization, or ketoacidosis between the two groups. There was a difference in the report of mild-moderate hypoglycemia, with the CSII group reporting more fasting and predinner hypoglycemia than the conventional group. The diabetes-related quality of life improved in the fathers of the children in the CSII group in comparison to the injection group. In mothers, psychological distress increased in the conventional group from baseline. All subjects chose to remain with CSII at the conclusion of the study.

IMPLICATIONS

CSII can be an effective and safe management tool for young children. This study identified no deterioration in control, improvement in quality of life, and a reduction in psychological distress as experienced by parents. Health care professionals should be open to the options of treatment for diabetes, identifying with the families and child the most appropriate method and treatment modality to help them reach metabolic and psychological goals. Age, while a factor, is not an exclusion for CSII. This study was limited in both the number of participants and the length of data collection.

REFERENCE

Fox, L., Buckloh, L. M., Smith, S. D., Wysocki, T., & Mauras, N. (2005). A randomized controlled trial of insulin pump therapy in young children with type 1 diabetes. *Diabetes Care, 28,* 1277–1281.

episodes will require IV glucose or IM glucagon. As IV glucose is an unrealistic intervention by a caregiver, glucagon preparation (which requires reconstitution) and administration will need to be taught. Caregivers should be instructed on treatment options, glucagon preparation, and injection technique. Caregivers and children should be instructed to always carry a source of oral carbohydrate for hypoglycemia.

Whom to Call and When Caregivers will need to understand who to call and how to reach the health care team for questions, advice, problem solving, and emergency situations. The plan of care should include guidelines for routine phone calls and for what constitutes a more urgent call. Telephone, email, and fax numbers, including emergency instructions, should be provided. Medical identification jewelry should be worn by the child.

Medical Nutrition Treatment: Meal Planning
Typically the instruction for meal planning is provided by a nutritionist. The extent of meal planning at diagnosis is based on the ability of the caregivers and child to understand the plan. For some families, the concept of three meals and two snacks at routine, regular times of the day is revolutionary. For other families, counting grams of carbohydrate is quickly and easily understood and the meal plan is sophisticated. From a baseline, survival standpoint, the minimal understanding needed to be demonstrated by the caregivers are the concepts that food intake will increase blood glucose levels and that consistent times for eating are essential.

Family Teaching: Beyond the Survival Stage As mentioned previously, the education provided to prepare a family to care for a child with type 1 diabetes at the time of diagnosis is just the beginning of the educational process. Ongoing and advanced education begins as the caregivers and child gain experience with the diabetes care. For some families, this occurs quickly, and some of these topics are addressed at the time of the initial education. Topics that are addressed after the initial diagnosis phase include:

1. Hyperglycemia, its causes, symptoms, treatment options
2. Exercise and activity
3. Sick day care
4. Community resources
5. Adjustment and adaptation process
6. Complications of diabetes
7. Hygiene
8. Meal planning
9. Areas of research
10. Anticipatory planning
11. Insulin dose adjustment and use of supplemental insulin

This level of education begins to require the skills of an individual who has experience with diabetes management, such as a nurse certified as a diabetic educator. The educational process is ongoing and neverending. The goals of education are to empower the child and caregivers, to provide them with support and knowledge to make management decisions and plans, and to evaluate their success.

NURSING TIP

Blood Glucose Testing

1. The pads and tips of the finger contain many nerve endings and few capillaries. For a less painful finger puncture, use the sides of the fingertips or a meter that allows testing from an alternative site.
2. Warm the fingers by rubbing the hands together or milking the finger to aid in obtaining a blood drop. Cleaning the area with soap and warm water will help draw the blood to the surface and cleans the area at the same time. Using soap and water eliminates the need to cleanse the area with alcohol.
3. Once finger punctures are done repeatedly, small calluses form. As long as an adequate sample can be obtained from a finger puncture, using these areas with calluses is less painful and should be encouraged.
4. Finger puncture devices (lancet devices) come in many styles. Some allow the client to adjust the depth of penetration, which can be helpful for obtaining blood samples in young children.
5. Several glucose monitors and devices are becoming available that allow for a client to lance the forearms or thighs for drops of blood to do glucose monitoring, increasing a client's options of sites for testing.

Hyperglycemia Hyperglycemia or high blood glucose occurs when the body gets too little insulin, too much food, or too little exercise. It may also be caused by stress, an illness, or surgery. The most common symptoms are thirst, polyuria, fatigue, and blurred vision. Hyperglycemia can lead to diabetic ketoacidosis if untreated over a period of several days. Table 28-6 compares hypoglycemia and hyperglycemia.

Diabetic Ketoacidosis Diabetic ketoacidosis (DKA), a common and potentially life-threatening acute complication of type 1 diabetes, is characterized by a severe insulin deficit, hyperglycemia, acidosis, and ketosis. While 30–40% of all newly diagnosed individuals with type 1 diabetes will present in DKA, it is also the primary reason for rehospitalization or emergency care of the previously diagnosed. DKA is also the leading cause of death in children with this type of diabetes. The basic cause of DKA is absolute or relative insulin deficiency. In the known individual with type 1 diabetes, DKA may be precipitated by an illness, particularly an infection, but up to 75% of cases are caused by insulin omission or treatment error.

There usually will be a history of classic signs and symptoms of polyuria, polydipsia, and weight loss. Once the child is sufficiently acidotic and ketotic, the breath will have a fruity or acetone odor. Many will have nausea, vomiting, and abdominal pain. The individual's state of consciousness varies

CASE STUDY / CARE PLAN

THE CHILD WITH TYPE 1 DIABETES MELLITUS

Brian is a 12-year-old African-American boy diagnosed 2 months ago with type 1 diabetes. He was started on an insulin regimen of glargine (Lantus) once a day in the evening and lispro (Humalog) at meals to cover his carbohydrates at a dose of 1 unit for every 15 grams of carbohydrate he is eating. His correction dose is 1 unit of Humalog for every 60 mg/dL he wants to reduce his glucose, to a goal of 120. He was instructed to monitor his blood glucose levels prior to meals and to follow a carbohydrate-counting meal plan, usually eating three meals and one to two snacks.

Brian has been noticing that some of his blood glucose levels are below his target and that he has had repeated episodes of symptoms of hypoglycemia over the last 2 weeks. He often treats his low symptoms without testing, especially when he is in school. He wasn't sure if it is better to have lower glucose levels than higher ones, nor is he sure that he's actually low as often as he is having symptoms. He wasn't really worried until he started having several episodes with significant, more severe symptoms of hypoglycemia. He is now so afraid of having a severe low glucose level at school that he is eating extra food between classes.

NURSING CARE PLAN

ASSESSMENT

At time of diagnosis with type 1 diabetes, approximately 90% of the beta cells in the pancreas have been damaged and destroyed. As blood glucose levels rise, glucose toxicity at the cellular level results and can cause the remaining functioning beta cells to not respond to glucose by making insulin. After diagnosis and the initiation of insulin treatment, as glucose levels decline, those beta cells not yet destroyed begin to be able to make insulin. This period is called the honeymoon or remission stage of diabetes. During the honeymoon, insulin needs can decrease because of beta cells' production of endogenous insulin. Doses of insulin that achieved the glucose target shortly after diagnosis may be higher than necessary to achieve the same glucose target during the honeymoon phase. While this honeymoon phase can last anywhere from a few weeks to a few years, typically it is gone by the first anniversary of diagnosis. The honeymoon phase may explain why Brian's glucose levels are suddenly lower than they were shortly after diagnosis. Brian's management plan is not achieving its goals, and he has not made appropriate changes to the plan to achieve his goals more successfully.

NURSING DIAGNOSIS 1

Risk for injury related to hypoglycemia.

EXPECTED OUTCOMES

1. Child will not experience an injury related to a hypoglycemic event.
2. Child and caregivers will identify safety plan to avoid injury.

NOC: Risk Detection
NIC: Surveillance

INTERVENTIONS/*RATIONALES*

1. Child will have access to blood glucose monitoring supplies at all times. *Ability to monitor glucose levels and the easy accessibility to testing equipment will encourage the child and caregivers to test glucose frequently. Symptoms of hypoglycemia, such as headaches and hunger, can be caused by events other than hypoglycemia, and should not be treated in the same manner.*
2. Child will wear medical identification. *Should an injury or accident occur and the child is unable to communicate, the presence of medical identification jewelry will provide diagnosis information for emergency personnel.*

(Continues)

CASE STUDY / CARE PLAN (Continued)

3. Child will have access to immediate treatment for hypoglycemia. *Delays in treating mild hypoglycemia can result in moderate to severe hypoglycemia.*
4. Adults who have supervision or care responsibilities for the child, and peers who spend time with the child, will be educated in the signs, symptoms, and treatment of hypoglycemia. *Providing education to the adults who care for the child and the people the child spends time with will increase the chances that hypoglycemia will be recognized earlier, and that the child will be supported in obtaining treatment for the hypoglycemic episode. This includes developing a safety plan at school, and notifying sports coaches and club directors of the risk of hypoglycemia, its symptoms, and its treatment.*
5. Adjust the diabetes management plan to decrease risk of hypoglycemia. *Developing prevention strategies to decrease the risk of hypoglycemia and its actual event eliminates the risk of injury.*

EVALUATION

Safety plan will be in place at school and for the other organizations that the child attends. Child will carry treatment for hypoglycemia with him at all times, and have access to treatment supplies at home, school, and work. Child and caregiver express confidence with the plan.

NURSING DIAGNOSIS 2

Deficient knowledge related to lack of information about the disease and management.

EXPECTED OUTCOMES

1. Child and caregivers verbalize understanding of type 1 diabetes and a plan for avoiding hypoglycemia.
2. Child and caregivers express confidence with knowledge and plan for avoiding hypoglycemia.
3. Child and caregivers will demonstrate correct blood glucose monitoring, insulin administration, and dietary management.

NOC: Knowledge: Disease Process and Management
NIC: Teaching: Disease Process and Management

INTERVENTIONS/*RATIONALES*

1. Assess child's or caregivers' current knowledge related to the relationship between insulin, activity, and carbohydrate intake. *Assessing understanding of the child and family identifies knowledge deficits and will assist in determining the scope and extent of required teaching.*
2. Assess child's or caregivers' understanding of insulin action. *Assessing understanding identifies knowledge deficits which may be playing a role in the occurrence of hypoglycemia.*
3. Provide information and education related to self-management. *Self-management and plan adjustment of diabetes is an educational topic that is approached from the basic education provided at diagnosis to the education provided after basic understanding is evident. Self-management is the cornerstone for all individuals with diabetes and an essential component to the successful achievement of health-related outcomes. Knowledge and understanding grow with time and experience. Now that the child and caregiver have had time to understand the information provided at the initial education, they can build and learn more complex skills and knowledge.*
4. Adjust insulin as appropriate based on pattern assessment to avoid hypoglycemia. *Adjusting dose based on the assessment of hypoglycemia caused by inappropriate insulin doses will reduce its occurrence. Hypoglycemia is an acute complication of diabetes. Episodes of hypoglycemia can result in mild to severe symptoms. The more severe the symptoms, the more at risk the child is for injury. Dose adjustment can be done by the practitioner as a demonstration of how to adjust the insulin or can be a joint effort between child or caregiver and practitioner.*

(Continues)

CASE STUDY / CARE PLAN (Continued)

EVALUATION

1. Child and caregivers express confidence that they can identify causes of current problems and can identify possible solutions to management problems.
2. Child has a reduction in frequency and severity of hypoglycemia.

NURSING DIAGNOSIS 3

Impaired adjustment related to the chronic health care needs of a child with type 1 diabetes.

EXPECTED OUTCOMES

1. Child and family will explore and recognize their coping skills and their emotional challenges with management responsibilities.
2. They will recognize areas that challenge them in caring for diabetes and problem-solve solutions.

NOC: Family Coping
NIC: Coping Enhancement

INTERVENTIONS/*RATIONALES*

1. Discuss with child and family the areas of diabetes management that they find most difficult. *Having the family identify where they are struggling will allow the team to develop a plan of care and treatment goals directed at the individual challenges and needs of diabetes management.*
2. Include mental health professionals in diabetes education. *Diabetes is a chronic, complex disease that requires constant intervention. The rate of mental health disorders is higher in this population than the population as a whole. A mental health professional will be able to identify children and caregivers at higher risk for coping and adjustment disorders. Additionally, the inclusion of mental health care professionals as part of the health care team from the beginning acknowledges the emotional component of diabetes care and successful management.*
3. Develop with child and family treatment goals and a management plan. *Treatment goals and strategies need to be patient centered and involve the child in the decision-making process.*
4. Suggest community agencies for the child and caregivers such as summer camps, support groups, and so on. *Community agencies offer an alternative to relying solely on family coping skills.*

EVALUATION

Child and caregivers will gain understanding of their personal response to the stress of diagnosis and care responsibilities. Child and caregiver will gain understanding of how their response impacts their caregiving and their management goals and will develop effective coping and care strategies.

from alertness to coma, and the degree of compromise does not always correlate with the degree of acidosis or hyperglycemia. Kussmaul respirations and dehydration are also seen. The diagnosis of DKA, while at times readily apparent, is based on clinical presentation and laboratory data. Confirmation of the diagnosis is based on the following criteria: blood glucose over 200 mg/dL, ketonuria or ketonemia, an arterial pH < 7.30 or serum bicarbonate < 15 mEq/L.

Treatment of DKA focuses on the problems of fluid deficit, electrolyte imbalances, alteration in acid-base balance, and insulin deficiency. It is a process that does not follow a specific protocol, but requires ongoing assessment and readjustment of the plan. The ultimate goal of therapy is to restore normal hemodynamic status and acid-base balance, and to slowly reduce and stabilize the blood glucose level.

Fluids are most often the first priority. Hypovolemic shock may be imminent. Fluids should be isotonic in concentration, and the volume should be geared toward replenishing the deficit over 24–48 hours. Rehydration is a slow process, and is limited to a volume of 4 liters/m^2/day, a rate suggested as a maximum rate that will not increase the individual's risk of complications to the therapy.

The goal of electrolyte replacement is to correct the imbalance and is most often integrated with the fluid replacement guidelines. In DKA, potassium is depleted. The hydrogen ions circulating in acidosis will replace intracellular potassium and the serum potassium level will

TABLE 28-6 Symptoms of Hypoglycemia and Hyperglycemia

HYPOGLYCEMIA	HYPERGLYCEMIA
Shakiness	Polyuria
Dizziness	Polydipsia
Pallor	Flushed face
Headaches	Dry skin
Disturbed vision	Blurred vision
Hunger	Hunger
Fatigue	Weakness
Tachycardia	Weaker, slower pulse rate
Disorientation	Fruity odor to breath
Confusion	Rapid respiratory rate
Seizure	Confusion
Coma	Coma

NURSING TIP

Insulin Infusion

Insulin will adhere to plastic and glass tubing. When preparing an insulin infusion, some hospital pharmacies will add albumin to decrease this tendency. Flushing the tubing with the insulin infusion to saturate the binding sites is also recommended in many hospitals.

be falsely elevated. However, the total body potassium is depleted. Correction of potassium is initiated once there is evidence of a renal output. Other electrolytes are potentially diminished (sodium, phosphorus, magnesium, calcium), and replacement may be necessary. Correction of acid-base imbalance, by the infusion of bicarbonate, is initiated in the most severe cases of DKA, where the acid-base imbalance is not improving. Bicarbonate infusion does not cross the blood–brain barrier and can accentuate the cerebral acidosis.

Fluid, electrolyte replacement, and bicarbonate will not, in and of themselves, halt the process of DKA. Insulin is the essential intervention for the correction of DKA. Insulin is necessary to stop glucosuria and is essential to facilitate the transportation of glucose across the cell membrane to halt cellular death and loss of potassium. Acid-base imbalance will correct as insulin stabilizes counter-regulatory hormone production and halts ketosis.

Except in mild cases of DKA, insulin is given by infusion (using Regular insulin). Insulin cannot be absorbed from subcutaneous or intramuscular injection sites in the dehydrated or acidotic individual. The rate of the infusion is titrated to achieve the established goal for the rate of glucose decline. A decrease of 100–150 mg/dL/hour is the maximum acceptable glucose drop in DKA in order to minimize the risks of therapy. When the blood glucose reaches approximately 200–300 mg/dL, stabilization of the glucose may be warranted with dextrose added to the fluid regimen.

The most serious risk associated with the treatment of DKA in pediatrics is cerebral edema, which occurs in 0.2 to 1% of cases. Risk factors for cerebral edema include newly diagnosed, age (<5 years), high initial BUN, hyperventilation and a presenting arterial pH <7.00 (Koul, 2009). Cerebral edema accounts for between 57–87% of all DKA deaths (Hoorn et al., 2007). It occurs in the first 4–12 hours of treatment, more commonly in infants and young children and in cases of new-onset type 1 diabetes. Symptoms (signs of increased intracranial pressure) include sudden complaint of a headache, confusion, difficulty in arousing the child, widening pulse pressure, tachycardia, or bradycardia. Immediate assessment and intervention are essential.

NURSING TIP

Check for Adherence to Diabetes Regimen

In the known client with diabetes, evaluate for adherence to the diabetes regimen. Evaluate the child's fingers for the small marks indicating blood glucose monitoring. Assess the injection sites for bruising (a benign indication of receiving injection) or hypertrophy, a lumpy appearance to the sites (indicating tissue damage caused by repeatedly giving injections to a specific area). Ask the child or caregivers how much insulin the child takes, how long it takes to empty a bottle of insulin, and compare the answers to determine if the child is receiving the prescribed dose of insulin. If you are uncertain about the accuracy of the questions, calling the pharmacy to inquire how often the prescriptions are filled for insulin may provide insight into how much insulin a child is using. If the child states he is taking about 40 units of insulin a day, but only getting a bottle of insulin every 6 weeks, there is a discrepancy. At 40 units a day, a child would use approximately 1200 units in 30 days. With a bottle of insulin holding 1000 units of insulin, the information of dose is not consistent with supply.

The child in DKA is often managed in the ICU. Nursing plays a vital role in the management of DKA. Time is essential, and the assessment should be done quickly. Nurses should assess fluid status by determining recent changes in weight, skin turgor, blood pressure, pulse rate, and neurological function with a fundi exam and level of consciousness. Acidosis is assessed with complaints of back pain or abdominal pain, presence of Kussmaul respirations, flushed cheeks, and the odor of acetone on the breath of the child. Electrolytes, blood gas, serum or urine ketones, and glucose should be obtained.

It is the nurse at the bedside who has been monitoring the child, whose concern is first heightened when the child just doesn't seem to be responding in the same way as he or she was earlier, and intervenes appropriately. This nurse needs to be skilled in assessment and understand the goals of therapy in the stabilization and treatment of DKA. Careful, accurate records must be maintained documenting the course of care and the child's response. These records should document the child's vital signs, fluids administered, laboratory results (electrolytes, glucose, ketones, and pH), insulin infused or administered, intake and output, level of consciousness, and weight. The successful clinical course of DKA resolves in 24–48 hours, and the child is advanced to subcutaneous insulin and oral nutrition.

The ultimate, ideal goal of therapy is to develop a diabetes management plan that is user-friendly and provides the most normal glucose levels on average. Diabetes is the leading cause of blindness, kidney failure, and amputations in the United States. Children with diabetes face these health risks as they age into adulthood. Among people with an age at diagnosis <30 years, type 1 diabetes reduces life expectancy by at least 15 years. The research that has been done on the relationship between glucose control and the development of long-term complications clearly defines that near normal glucose control provides the greatest protection against the development of long-term complications (Diabetes Control and Complications Trial Research Group, 1993).

NURSING TIP

School Nursing and Type 1 Diabetes

Because type 1 diabetes is the second most common chronic disease of childhood, the school nurse is likely to have responsibility for a child with type 1 diabetes at some time. Monitoring, adherence to the meal plan, medication administration, education of school personnel, and communication with the caregivers will be part of the school nurse's plan of care. The school nurse can play a vital role in the health management of the child with type 1 diabetes by helping to facilitate the management regimen that may conflict with the typical school routine.

REFLECTIVE THINKING

Injections and School Policy

School policy forbids students from carrying any medication. Sally, a high school junior who has had type 1 diabetes for 6 years, has found Lispro insulin given pre-lunch is the best way to control her afternoon glucose. Her lunch period is 20 minutes in length. It takes her 4 minutes to reach the nurse's office; another 5 minutes on average to test her blood glucose and do her insulin injection, and 3 minutes to get to the cafeteria. This leaves her 8 minutes on average to consume her lunch and get on to her next class. Sally, whose nurse educator and physician have provided permission, would like to administer her insulin in the restroom outside the cafeteria. How would you, as the school nurse, approach Sally's dilemma? How would you, as her diabetes nurse educator, approach her dilemma?

ADDITIONAL ENDOCRINE DISORDERS

The following disorders are rare in children; therefore, they are discussed only briefly.

HYPOPARATHYROIDISM

Hypoparathyroidism is characterized by a deficiency in the secretion of parathyroid hormone (PTH), whose main function is maintenance of serum calcium. The impaired secretion of PTH affects calcium and phosphorus metabolism. This very rare disorder can be congenital or acquired. A frequent cause of congenital hypoparathyroidism is aplasia or hypoplasia of the parathyroid glands. The acquired type is primarily caused by inadvertent removal of the glands during a thyroidectomy. A deficit of PTH results in hypocalcemia and hyperphosphatemia.

CLINICAL MANIFESTATIONS

The neonate may present with jittery movements, convulsions, apnea, lethargy, poor eating, and vomiting. Symptoms outside the neonatal period include tetany, stridor, **Chvostek's sign** (elicited by tapping the facial nerve, which produces a facial muscle spasm), **Trousseau's sign** (a carpopedal spasm that results from oxygen deficiency), complaints of tingling of the hands or around the mouth, diarrhea, seizures, papilledema, and skin and dental enamel changes. The skeleton is the storage area for calcium and phosphorus, and abnormalities of these substances will have an impact on bone formation. In the growing child, severe disease may result in permanent bone deformities and limited growth.

Treatment

Acute treatment, in cases of seizures or tetany, includes giving intravenous calcium in the form of calcium gluconate. The infusion should be given slowly except in the direst of emergencies. Rapid infusion can lead to cardiac dysrhythmias. Calcium given IV is caustic, and extravasation will cause severe tissue burns. The nonacute treatment of transient hypocalcemia involves oral calcium gluconate. Chronic hypocalcemia is treated with an active metabolite of vitamin D, calcitriol. Calcium gluconate orally is usually added as an adjunct to therapy, as it may help to bind phosphorus in the gut.

ADDISON'S DISEASE

Damage or destruction of the adrenal glands caused by tuberculosis, fungal infections, autoimmune disease, and HIV result in decreased production of adrenal steroids, cortisol, and aldosterone. The disease can also result from dysfunction of the hypothalamus or pituitary gland or from discontinuation of high levels of glucocorticoids for treatment of other diseases. The decrease in production of cortisol has an impact on the metabolism of glucose, fat, and protein. Aldosterone plays a primary role in sodium and potassium excretion; therefore, a deficit of this hormone has an impact on blood pressure and electrolytes.

Clinical Manifestations

The presentation of Addison's may be as an acute or chronic problem. The acute phase is life-threatening, with symptoms of severe hypotension, shock, electrolyte imbalances, dehydration, weakness, cardiovascular changes, fever, mental status changes, and hypoglycemia. An acute crisis can occur with febrile illnesses, infection, or stress.

Treatment

Treatment for Addison's involves replacing the deficient or absent hormones. In acute Addison's, IV hydrocortisone is given at regular intervals, and IV hydration is given to correct the dehydration and prevent hypovolemia. Electrolyte replacement will also be pursued in the acute phase. Chronic, nonacute treatment involves oral hydrocortisone and florinef. The dose of hydrocortisone will need to be increased with illness, stress, or surgery to meet the physiological needs of the body. If oral medication cannot be used or tolerated, intramuscular or intravenous cortisone should be used. The child and caregivers should be counseled on the essential need for lifelong treatment, with the information that untreated Addison's disease can be life-threatening. A medical identification should be worn by the individual with Addison's irrespective of age.

CUSHING'S SYNDROME

Cushing's syndrome is a cluster of signs and symptoms caused by hypercortisolism or excessive circulating free cortisol. The most common cause of hypercortisolism in children is caused by the prolonged or excessive corticosteroid therapy. Other possible etiologies are an adrenal tumor or a pituitary tumor that produces excessive ACTH. This disorder is rare in childhood and adolescence.

Clinical Manifestations

The most obvious sign of Cushing's syndrome is rapid weight gain, particularly in the abdomen, the face (moon-shaped), and the cervical fat pad (buffalo hump). Linear growth is decreased or stops because the excessive cortisol suppresses the release of the growth hormone. The child may complain of muscle weakness and fatigue. The skin may be thin and fragile, with an increased tendency to bruise. Reddish purple striae appear in the abdomen, as might acne and increased hair growth in inappropriate locations (hirsutism). Other symptoms include poor wound healing, increased susceptibility to infections, and decreased inflammatory response.

Treatment

Treatment is based on the cause. Adrenal or pituitary tumors should be surgically removed if possible. When the cause is steroid therapy, the effects may be lessened if the medication is given early in the morning or on an alternate day schedule. Morning administration mimics the normal diurnal pattern of cortisol secretion. Alternate day administration allows the anterior pituitary to maintain a more normal hypothalamic–pituitary–adrenal control mechanism.

SYNDROME OF INAPPROPRIATE ANTIDIURETIC HORMONE

Syndrome of inappropriate antidiuretic hormone (SIADH) occurs when ADH (vasopressin) is secreted in the presence of low serum osmolality. Normally a decrease in serum osmolality inhibits ADH production and secretion. In children with SIADH the feedback mechanism that regulates ADH does not function properly, and ADH continues to be released. This leads to water retention, dilutional hyponatremia (decrease in serum sodium level due to dilution), and extracellular fluid volume expansion. SIADH is caused by various conditions such as CNS infection (meningitis), head trauma, brain tumors, intracranial surgery, and certain medications (analgesics, barbiturates, chemotherapy).

Clinical Manifestations

Clinical manifestations related to water retention include decreased urine output and weight gain. Gastrointestinal symptoms such as anorexia, nausea, and vomiting develop. As the sodium level continues to decrease, neurological manifestations appear, including lethargy, behavioral changes, headaches, changes in level of consciousness, seizures, and finally coma.

Treatment

Treatment consists of fluid restriction to correct the hyponatremia, raising the serum sodium level with intravenous sodium chloride, and increasing the serum osmolality. The underlying disorder is also treated.

IN THE REAL WORLD

As a student, I became overwhelmed with the hormonal feedback loops my biology teacher diligently taught me. I remember thinking to myself, "Thank goodness I only need to learn this for the exam. I'll never need to understand this in real life." Then, I started working with children with hormonal problems. When I started to see the impact of the various hormones on the children in my practice and had to explain this to caregivers and children, I began to understand the process. Teaching them by illustrating the feedback system of the hormones produced by the various endocrine organs helped me conceptualize the information. My teaching, for the families, children, and my colleagues, became more comprehensive and accurate, helping them be fully prepared for the management of each endocrine abnormality.

KEY CONCEPTS

- The endocrine system is composed of glands that produce chemical substances called hormones in response to stimulation from the nervous system.
- Hormones have an intrinsic role in reproduction, growth and development, maintenance of the internal environment, and energy production, utilization, and storage.
- Feedback loops are characteristic of the endocrine system.
- The pituitary gland is the master gland, producing hormones that stimulate the other glands of the endocrine system.
- Growth hormone deficiency (GHD) is characterized primarily by poor growth and short stature caused by failure of the anterior pituitary to produce sufficient GH.
- Precocious puberty is a result of early or premature activation of the hypothalamic–pituitary–gonadal cycle, which causes the child to develop secondary sex characteristics earlier than expected.
- Diabetes insipidus is an endocrine disorder of water regulation caused by a deficiency of antidiuretic hormone. Common symptoms are polyuria, polydipsia, and dehydration.
- Thyroid dysfunction is the most common endocrine abnormality in pediatrics.
- Early diagnosis and treatment of congenital hypothyroidism is important to prevent severe mental retardation.
- Symptoms of hyperthyroidism include nervousness, weight loss, increased growth rate, ophthalmic abnormalities, emotional lability, and heat intolerance.
- Congenital adrenal hyperplasia results from a genetic defect, which causes a breakdown in steroid synthesis and an overproduction of androgens. The goal of treatment is suppression of adrenal secretion of androgens, prevention of progressive virilization, and includes lifelong replacement of glucocorticoids and mineralocorticoids.
- Type 1 diabetes is an autoimmune form of diabetes that has its peak onset in childhood and is the second most common chronic disease of children.
- Type 1 diabetes results from damage and destruction of the beta cells of the pancreas, resulting in insulin insufficiency and deficiency. Insulin treatment is essential to preserve the life of the affected individual.
- Type 2 diabetes is a new epidemic among children and adolescents that results from insulin resistance. Children most commonly affected are obese, and the majority have family members with the same type of diabetes.
- Diabetic ketoacidosis is a medical emergency, and in pediatric cases of diabetes is the most common cause of death.

REVIEW ACTIVITIES

1. Describe a feedback loop system characteristic of an endocrine system.
2. Discuss the relationship between the clinical manifestations and pathophysiology of diabetes insipidus.
3. Describe the impact of neonatal screening on congenital hypothyroidism.
4. Differentiate the symptoms of hypothyroidism and hyperthyroidism.
5. List the clinical manifestations of type 1 diabetes.
6. Identify the clinical manifestations of diabetic ketoacidosis (DKA).
7. What is the most serious complication of the treatment of DKA?
8. Describe the difference in time action of Lispro, Regular, NPH, and Glargine/Detemir insulin.
9. Differentiate the symptoms of hypoglycemia and hyperglycemia.
10. Differentiate the diagnosis of type 1 diabetes from type 2 diabetes.

STUDY QUESTIONS

1. Which of the following is an example of a negative feedback system?
   a. Hypothalamus secretes ACTH, stimulating the anterior pituitary to secrete TRH, which stimulates the thyroid gland to make TSH. The TSH then directly influences the anterior pituitary gland's production of TRH.
   b. Hypothalamus secretes TSH which stimulates the thyroid gland to secrete Thyroxine (T_4). The T_4 levels indirectly stimulate the hypothalamus' production of TSH.
   c. Anterior pituitary gland secretes triiodothyronine (T_3) which stimulates the hypothalamus to secrete TRH, which stimulates the thyroid gland to make T_4. The T_4 then indirectly influences the anterior pituitary gland's production of T_3.
   d. Hypothalamus secretes TRH which stimulates the anterior pituitary to secrete TSH. TSH stimulates the thyroid gland to produce Triiodothyronine (T_3) and Thyroxine (T_4). T_3 and T_4 directly stimulate the pituitary's secretion of TSH.
2. Common clinical characteristics of growth hormone deficiency in a school-age child are:
   a. Short stature, rate of growth 6–7 cm/year, normal bone age, truncal obesity, history hypoglycemia, delayed dentition.
   b. Short stature, rate of growth 5–6 cm/year, delayed bone age, history of hyperglycemia, delayed dentition, delayed sexual maturation
   c. Short stature, rate of growth <4–5 cm/year, delayed bone age, history of hypoglycemia, delayed dentition, high pitched voice.
   d. Short stature, growth velocity <3 cm/90 days, advanced bone age, history of delayed dentition, family history of GHD.
3. When measuring and recording the linear growth of a less than cooperative 2 year, 2 month old boy:
   a. Use a supine measuring board. Ask the parent to hold the child's shoulders in a vertical plane to the board and place a movable foot board against the feet. Record the height on the 2–18 year old growth chart.
   b. Use a supine measuring board. Have a second, trained person hold the child's head against the head board with the child's face and hips in a horizontal plane. Place the movable foot board against the soles of the feet in a 90 degree angle. Record the height on a 0–36 month growth chart.
   c. Ask the parent to help keep the child cooperative with standing height. Have the child stand barefoot on a standing measuring board. With the child's back and heels against the standing board obtain the measurement. Record the height on the 0–36 month growth chart.
   d. Lay child on exam table. With one person holding the child's head in a horizontal plane, the second person will take a tape measure from the crown of the head to the sole of the heel. Record the measurement on the 0–36 month growth chart.
4. In teaching a family about medication for treatment of congenital hypothyroidism (CH) in a newborn, instructions should include which one of the following?
   a. Generic l-thyroxine is a viable option for all children with CH.
   b. L-thyroxine comes in tablet form. Since the medication should not be taken with food, the tablet can be crushed and added to a small bottle of water. Give one hour before a feed or two hours after.
   c. Compound pharmacies can prepare a liquid l-thyroxine for infants. Once a child is able to chew, the pill form can be used.
   d. L-thyroxine tablet should be crushed and made into a paste with a small drop of formula or

breast milk. Stroke the paste on the infant's tongue and feed the child in a normal fashion.

5. One treatment option for hyperthyroidism is subtotal thyroidectomy. This option is:
   a. Typically considered once medication therapy has not resulted in a permanent remission.
   b. Typically considered after medication therapy has stabilized hyperthyroidism.
   c. Typically considered as a treatment of last resort, when all else fails.
   d. Is not an option in pediatrics. Its complications are severe and too risky for children.
6. What are the clinical manifestations in a female of viralizing, salt wasting congenital adrenal hyperplasia (CAH)?
   a. Hypotonia, elevated androgens, normal genitalia, hirsutism
   b. Hypertonia, hypernatremia, hyperkalemia, ambiguous genitalia
   c. Hirsutism, acne, advanced bone age, adrenarche, normal genitalia
   d. Hypotonia, hyponatremia, hyperkalemia, ambiguous genitalia
7. When planning the education for the parents of a child with type 1 diabetes mellitus (DM), which of the following should the nurse include?
   a. Restrict the activity of the child.
   b. Rotate the insulin injection sites.
   c. Avoid letting the child perform the home testing of blood sugar.
   d. Encourage a high-carbohydrate diet.
8. The nurse is admitting a child suspected of having acquired hypothyroidism. Which of the following assessments should the nurse evaluate as confirming the diagnosis?
   a. Goiter
   b. Exophthalmos
   c. Proptosis
   d. Hirsutism
9. The parents of a child with newly diagnosed type 2 diabetes mellitus want to know more about the condition. The nurse should include which of the following?
   a. Activity is not important with type 2 diabetes.
   b. Daily insulin injections are required.
   c. Type 2 diabetes does not require intervention.
   d. Type 2 diabetes is increasing in frequency in children.
10. The nurse identifies which of the following adolescents with type 1 diabetes mellitus as being at greatest risk for complications? An adolescent:
   a. With frequent *Candida albicans* urinary infections
   b. Who has an eating disorder
   c. Who has a fever and sore throat
   d. Who is sexually active and taking birth control

REFERENCES

American Academy of Pediatrics. (2006). Introduction to the newborn screening fact sheet. *Pediatrics, 118*(3), 1304–1312.

American Diabetes Association. (2008a). Standards of medical care in diabetes. *Diabetes Care, 31*(1), S12–S54.

American Diabetes Association. (2008b). Nutrition recommendations and interventions for diabetes. *Diabetes Care, 31*(1), S61–S78.

Cowell, K. (2008) Focus on diagnosis: Type 2 diabetes mellitus. *Pediatric Review, 29*, E289–E292.

Diabetes Control and Complications Trial Research Group. (1993). The effect of intensive treatment of diabetes on the development and progression of long-term complications in insulin dependent diabetes mellitus. *The New England Journal of Medicine, 329*, 977–986.

Fox, L., Buckloh, L. M., Smith, S. D., Wysocki, T., & Mauras, N. (2005). A randomized controlled trial of insulin pump therapy in young children with type 1 diabetes. *Diabetes Care, 28*, 1277–1281.

Glase, N., & Slyne, D. (2008). Predicting the likelihood of remission in children with Graves disease: A prospective multicenter study. *Pediatrics, 121*, e481–e488.

Grimberg, A., Kutikov, J. K., & Cucchiara, A. J. (2005). Sex differences in patients referred for evaluation of poor growth. *Journal of Pediatrics, 146*(2), 212–216.

Hoorn, E., Carlotti, A., Costa, L. A., MacMahon, B., Bohn, G., Zietse, R. et al. (2007). Preventing a drop in effective plasma osmolality to minimize the likelihood of cerebral edema during treatment of children with diabetic ketoacidosis. *Journal of Pediatrics, 150*, 467–473.

Jones, K. (2008). Role of obesity in complicating and confusing the diagnosis and treatment of diabetes in children. *Pediatrics, 121*, 361–368.

Koul, P. (2009). Diabetic ketoacidosis: A current appraisal of pathology and management. *Clinical Pediatrics, 48*(2), 135–144.

Lipman, T., Hench, K., Benyi, T., Delauen, J., Gilluly, K., Johnson, L. et al. (2004). A multicenter randomized controlled trial of an intervention to improve the accuracy of linear growth measurement. *Archives of Diseases in Childhood, 89*(4), 342–346.

Muir, A. (2006) Precocious puberty. *Pediatrics in Review, 27*, 373–381.

SEARCH for Diabetes in Youth Study Group. (2006). Burden of diabetes mellitus among U.S. youth. *Pediatrics, 11*(4), 1510–1518.

Shulman, D., Palmert, M., & Kemp, S. (2007) Adrenal insufficiency–Still a case of morbidity and death in childhood. *Pediatrics Online.* DOI:10.1542/peds.20061612.

Weissberg-Benchell, J., Antisdel-Lomaglio, A., & Seshadri, R. (2003). Insulin pump therapy. A meta-analysis. *Diabetes Care, 26*(4), 1079–1087.

Wolpert, H. (2008). The nuts and bolts of achieving end points with real-time continuous glucose monitoring. *Diabetes Care, 31*, S146–S149.

SUGGESTED READINGS

American Diabetes Association. (2008). Diabetes care in the school and day care setting: Position statement. *Diabetes Care, 31*(1), S79–S86.

American Diabetes Association. (2008). Diagnosis and classification of diabetes mellitus: Position statement. *Diabetes Care, 31*(1), S55–S60.

RESOURCES

Refer to the online student StudyWARE for Potts & Mandleco at http://www.CengageBrain.com for additional content and study aids.

Organization: **American Association of Diabetes Educators**
Description: The American Association of Diabetes Educators (AADE) is an association of health care professionals dedicated to integrating successful self-management as a key outcome in the care of people with diabetes and related conditions. The website offers users access to information regarding diabetes education and professional resources.
Website/Resource: http://www.aadenet.org

Organization: **American Diabetes Association**
Description: The mission of the American Diabetes Association (ADA) is to prevent and cure diabetes and to improve the lives of all people affected by diabetes. ADA's website provides users with information regarding living with diabetes, community events, and food and fitness plans.
Website/Resource: http://www.diabetes.org

Organization: **American Dietetic Association**
Description: The American Dietetic Association (ADA) is a science-based food and nutrition information source. As the world's largest organization of food and nutrition professionals, ADA is committed to improving the nation's health and advancing the profession of dietetics through research, education, and advocacy. The website offers links to nutrition information for the public, for students, for the media, and for health professionals.
Website/Resource: http://www.eatright.org

Organization: **Children with Diabetes**
Description: The mission of Children with Diabetes, Inc. is to promote understanding of the care and treatment of diabetes, especially in children; to increase awareness of the need for unrestricted diabetes care for children at school and daycare; to support families living with diabetes; and to promote understanding of research into a cure. The website connects individuals with diabetes, offers diabetes information, and provides information regarding forums and conferences.
Website/Resource: http://www.childrenwithdiabetes.com

Organization: **Congenital Adrenal Hyperplasia Education and Support Network**
Description: The Congenital Adrenal Hyperplasia Education and Support Network is an organization dedicated to increasing awareness of congenital adrenal hyperplasia. The website is a wealth of information concerning congenital adrenal hyperplasia including medical sites, frequently asked questions, and message boards.
Website/Resource: http://www.congenitaladrenalhyperplasia.org

Organization: **Human Growth Foundation**
Description: The Human Growth Foundation is a voluntary, non-profit organization whose mission is to help children and adults with disorders of growth and growth hormone through research, education, support, and advocacy. The foundation is dedicated to helping medical science to better understand the process of growth. The website offers access to recent publications, programs, and resources.
Website/Resource: http://www.hgfound.org

Organization: **Juvenile Diabetes Research Foundation**
Description: The Juvenile Diabetes Research Foundation (DRF) is the worldwide leader for research to cure type 1 diabetes. DRF sets the global agenda for diabetes research, and is the largest charitable funder and advocate of diabetes science worldwide. The DRF's website provides users with information concerning research, publications, and advocacy.
Website/Resource: http://www.jdf.org

Organization: **MAGIC (Major Aspects of Growth in Children) Foundation**
Description: Major Aspects of Growth In Children (MAGIC) is made up of 25,000+ families whose children (and affected adults) have growth hormone deficiency or other medical conditions which affect their growth. The website offers users access to educational conventions and foundation information.
Website/Resource: http://www.magicfoundation.org

Organization: **National Diabetes Information Clearinghouse**
Description: The National Diabetes Information Clearinghouse is a service of the National Institute of Diabetes and Digestive and Kidney Diseases (NIDDK). The website offers advanced information regarding diabetes awareness, treatments, complications, statistics, and much more.
Website/Resource: http://diabetes.niddk.nih.gov

Organization: **National Graves' Disease Foundation**
Description: The Graves' Disease Foundation is committed to reaching out to those affected by Graves' and other thyroid related diseases. Programs provide patients and caregivers counseling, support, and referrals to medical professionals. The website provides general information about Graves' disease and access to recent publications.
Website/Resource: http://www.ngdf.org

Organization: **Pediatric Endocrinology Nursing Society**
Description: PENS is a voluntary non-profit specialty nursing organization committed to the advancement of the art and science of pediatric endocrine nursing. The website offers users information regarding online scholarships, committees, conventions, journals, and helpful links.
Website/Resource: http://www.pens.org

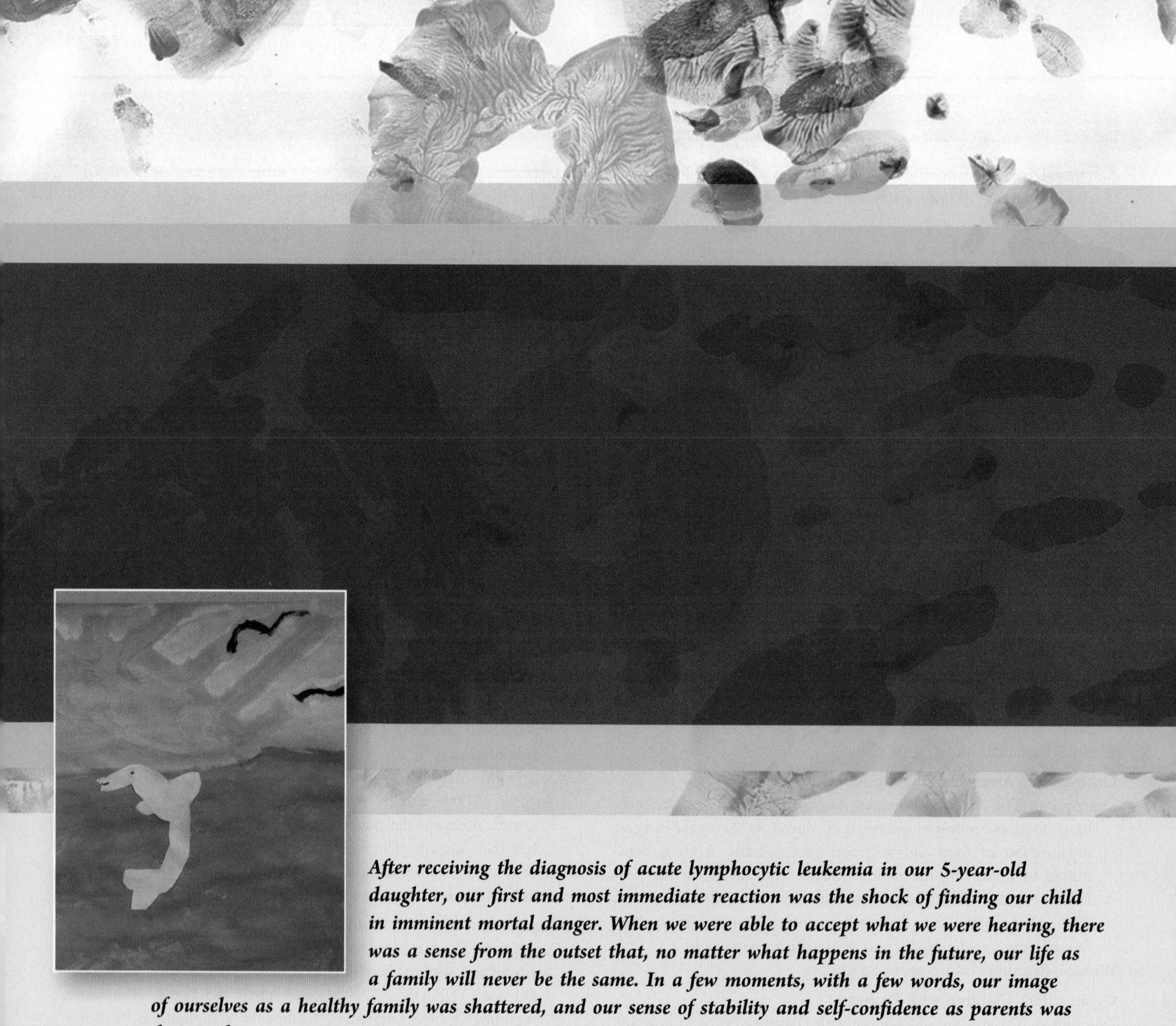

After receiving the diagnosis of acute lymphocytic leukemia in our 5-year-old daughter, our first and most immediate reaction was the shock of finding our child in imminent mortal danger. When we were able to accept what we were hearing, there was a sense from the outset that, no matter what happens in the future, our life as a family will never be the same. In a few moments, with a few words, our image of ourselves as a healthy family was shattered, and our sense of stability and self-confidence as parents was destroyed.

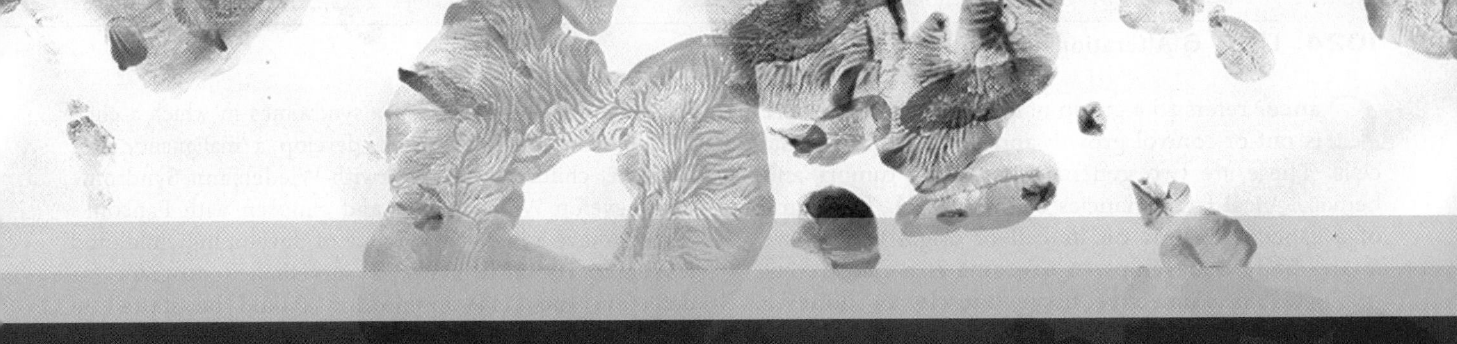

CHAPTER 29

Cellular Alterations

MARY NARVAEZ YEANEY, MSN, CPNP; MARY H. CHANDLER, MSN; and KATHLEEN A. SCARBALIS, PA-C

COMPETENCIES

Upon completion of this chapter, the reader will be able to:

- Describe the clinical manifestations, treatment, and nursing management of common malignancies in children.
- Identify the different treatment modalities used to treat cancer in children.
- Explain how the different treatment modalities affect malignant cells.
- Discuss the nursing management of common side effects of treatment modalities.
- Identify the emotional and educational needs of families who have children with cancer.
- Discuss the importance of clinical trials and research in pediatric oncology.
- Discuss the long-term, late effects of childhood cancer therapy.
- Successfully complete the games and activities in the online student StudyWARE.

Cancer refers to a group of diseases in which there is out-of-control growth and spread of abnormal cells. There are two general types: solid tumors and hematological (malignancies of the blood). The name of a cancer depends on its cell of origin and where in the body it develops. A **sarcoma** is a cancer that originates in connective tissue, muscle, or bone; a **carcinoma** originates from epithelial tissue that consists of cells from glands, hollow organs, and the outer layer of skin that lines the blood vessels.

The most common childhood malignancy is leukemia, followed by tumors of the central nervous system, lymphoma, neuroblastoma, soft tissue sarcomas, Wilms' tumor, and bone tumors (see Figure 29-1). This chapter discusses these malignancies and their treatment modalities as well as the nursing management of a child with cancer. The late effects of therapy in children who are long-term cancer survivors are also addressed.

ANATOMY AND PHYSIOLOGY

Childhood cancer differs from adult cancer. Common childhood malignancies usually arise from primitive embryonic tissue or are sarcomas. Adult malignancies are of epithelial origin and are carcinomas (Ruccione, 2007). In adult malignancies there is a strong relationship between environmental factors and the development of cancer. Children have not lived long enough for exposure to carcinogens to cause a malignancy. Routine screening, which leads to early detection, is a key to survival in many adult cancers. Screening evaluations for childhood cancer have generally not proved advantageous and the diagnosis of cancer in children is usually made when symptoms warrant a diagnostic work-up. Exceptions to this are the rare syndromes in which a child has an increased potential to develop a malignancy. For example, children with Beckwith-Wiedemann Syndrome may develop Wilms' tumor and children with Fanconi's Anemia have a higher incidence of developing childhood leukemia. In these cases, a surveillance program for detection and close monitoring should be started in early childhood (Ruccione, 2007; Drigan & Androkites, 2007).

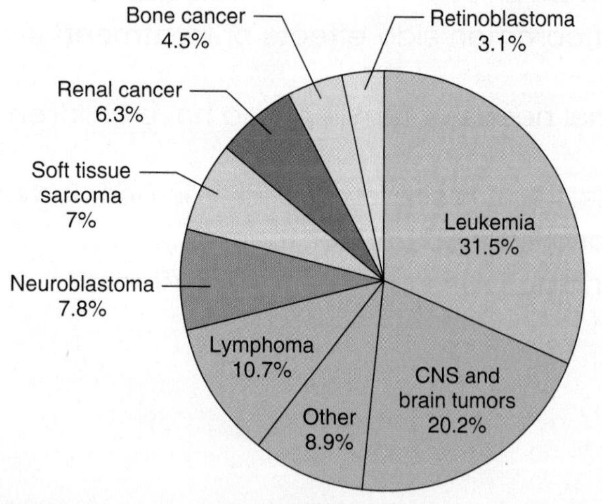

FIGURE 29-1 Incidence of Childhood Cancer in the United States. ADAPTED FROM RIES, L. A. G., SMITH, M. A., GURNEY, J. G., LINET, M., TAMRA, T., YOUNG, J. L., BUNIN, G. R. (EDS.). *CANCER INCIDENCE AND SURVIVAL AMONG CHILDREN AND ADOLESCENTS: UNITED STATES SEER PROGRAM 1975–1995.* BETHESDA, MD: NATIONAL CANCER INSTITUTE, SEER PROGRAM, 1999.

Many children's cancers are metastatic at the time of diagnosis whereas adult's tumors are often localized. Fortunately the prognosis in children with cancer is much better, with a 70–90% survival rate, compared to less than 60% in adults. This may be due to the fact that children have a much better response rate to treatment and tolerate higher doses of chemotherapy with less toxicity than adults (Ruccione, 2007).

Childhood cancer has become a curable disease, with greater than 80% of children diagnosed with cancer surviving (O'Leary, Krailo, Anderson, & Reaman, 2008). Organized multidisciplinary approaches to providing care for these children, as well as greatly improved supportive care measures, have been essential to this success. The Children's Oncology Group (COG) is a national collaborative study group composed of pediatric oncology professionals. Cooperative study groups have provided an organized, coordinated approach to cancer treatment with the use of **clinical trials**, which are protocols or guidelines used to treat specific diseases (Table 29-1). Following these guidelines and submitting treatment results to the study group provides the necessary data to improve therapy, decrease morbidity, and increase the survival of children with cancer. In the United States, 90–95% of all children under age 15 years with a newly diagnosed malignancy are seen at a COG institution. Of these, 50–60% will be registered on a clinical trial if one is available. It is clinical research of this type that has been responsible for the dramatic improvement in the survival rates of children with cancer. Cure rates have improved from less than 10%, when the cooperative groups started 50 years ago, to nearly 80% at present (O'Leary et al., 2008).

REFLECTIVE THINKING

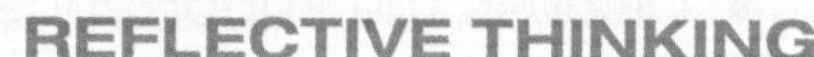

Clinical Trials: How Would a Parent Respond?

Newly diagnosed children are eligible for front-line treatment in **clinical trials** where there is a comparison of the existing standard treatment to a new therapeutic approach. The decision to receive either approach is by random selection. What would it be like to be the caregiver of a child, newly diagnosed with cancer, and be asked to sign consent to participate in a clinical trial?

TABLE 29-1 Clinical Trials

Clinical trials are research studies designed to test the value of a medical treatment. All clinical trials have protocol guidelines that provide information and describe how the study is to be conducted under controlled conditions. An informed consent is obtained after explaining to the parent the reasons to conduct the study including all the benefits and risks.

Phase I	Purpose is to determine the maximum tolerated dose of an investigational drug or combination of drugs. Usually offered to patients with good organ function who have advanced disease that is resistant to standard therapy. Patients are monitored very closely for drug toxicity.
Phase II	Purpose is to determine the efficacy of a new drug in the treatment of a specific disease or group of diseases. The tumor response rate is measured. Clients are carefully monitored for side effects and toxicity.
Phase III	Purpose is to compare the efficacy of at least two different treatments. Generally, the comparison is the current standard therapy with an experimental arm.
Phase IV	Purpose is to determine further toxicity or side effects and safety after the drug has been approved by the Food and Drug Administration and is commercially available.

All clinical trials researchers have to abide by the Food and Drug Administration's strict guidelines. All clinical trials must be approved by an Institutional Review Board (IRB) to ensure that all of the rights and the welfare of clients are observed and protected.

TREATMENT MODALITIES

The goal of cancer therapy is to rid the body of all malignant cells, thereby curing the cancer. Therapy may include surgery, chemotherapy, radiation therapy, **hematopoietic stem cell transplantation** (HSCT), and biological response modifiers (BRM). A combination of these modalities is frequently used (Table 29-2).

The type of cancer and the extent of metastasis, known as **stage**, determine the appropriate treatment. In general, staging ranges from stage I (1), which is localized disease in just one area or organ, to stage IV (4), with disseminated metastatic disease. Stage V applies to the case of bilateral kidney or eye tumors in children. Staging is used to establish a prognosis and treatment plan. There are several disease-specific staging classifications for pediatric tumors. Tumor

TABLE 29-2 Cancer Treatment Modalities

MODALITY	GOAL	FUNCTION
Surgery	Remove all existing cancer cells; biopsy excise tumor, decrease tumor burden, provide palliative procedures	Remove existing cancer, provide tissue for identification, provide comfort when cure is not possible such as debulking a tumor causing pain or obstruction and; insertion of Venous Access Device (VAD)
Chemotherapy	Kill all malignant cells and microscopic metastasis	Provide systemic treatment for cancer
Radiation therapy	Kill malignant cells and provide comfort	Eradicate all local tumor cells and provide local control of malignancy for comfort and palliation when cure is not possible
Hematopoietic stem cell transplantation	Replace bone marrow that has been destroyed by disease or treatment	Provide new hematopoietic system with all its components
Biological response modifiers	Destroy cancer cells, or stimulate specific processes of hematopoiesis	Stimulate immune system to destroy cancer cells or accelerate hematopoiesis

TABLE 29-3 Staging of Pediatric Tumors

STAGING SYSTEMS USED FOR PEDIATRIC SOLID TUMORS	
SPECIFIC TUMOR	STAGING SYSTEM
Hodgkin's Lymphoma	Ann Arbor Classification
Non-Hodgkin's Lymphoma	St. Jude Children's Research Hospital Murray Classification
Rhabdomyosarcoma	Intergroup Rhabdomyosarcoma (IRS)
Wilms' Tumor	National Wilms' Tumor Study V
Neuroblastoma	International Neuroblastoma Staging System (INSS)
Retinoblastoma	Reese-Ellsworth Classification

biology and location are used for appropriate staging (see Table 29-3).

Staging studies are done according to the client's diagnosis. In leukemia a bone marrow aspirate and biopsy are done to diagnose and determine the type of leukemia. Staging of solid tumors again depends on the specific cancer and its known areas to metastasize. Common studies are: computerized tomography (CT scan), bone scans, magnetic resonance imaging (MRI), and positron emission tomography (PET). An MIBG scan is specific to neuroblastoma. Each tumor staging system specifies the necessary imaging studies and biology studies needed to accurately stage a specific tumor. The pediatric oncologist can then decide the client's treatment and eligibility for a clinical trial (Table 29-1).

SURGERY

The goal of surgery in cancer therapy is to remove all visible and microscopic malignant cells when possible. Surgery is used to obtain a biopsy (a sample of the tumor), which is examined microscopically for diagnosis. Surgery also aids in tumor staging by noting the presence and extent of metastatic disease. Later, a "second look" surgical procedure may be performed to assess the response to therapy. Reconstructive surgery corrects defects caused by previous therapy or the tumor itself. Palliative care is given to relieve pain and improve quality of life when cancer treatment is no longer effective. It may include a surgical procedure such as the excision of an abdominal tumor that is causing severe pain and obstruction. Surgery is also used for the insertion of venous access devices.

CHEMOTHERAPY

Chemotherapy is the most frequently used treatment modality in pediatric oncology and is unique because it is effective for systemic cancers that cannot be managed by surgery or radiation therapy. Dramatic advances in the successful use of multi-agent chemotherapy have increased the rate of survival of many children with cancer. Chemotherapy drugs are classified into six major categories according to their chemical structure. These categories are alkylating agents, antimetabolites, antitumor antibiotics, plant alkaloids, enzymes, and miscellaneous agents. Unfortunately, these drugs do not exclusively affect malignant cells, but also affect normal cells that reproduce rapidly, such as the intestinal mucosa, blood cells, and hair follicles. Chemotherapy drugs are given in cycles to allow normal cells to recover. The child's disease and treatment regimen determine which drugs are used. The route and method of administration of a particular agent is influenced by the drug's pharmacology, side effects, classification, the child's disease, and the treatment regimen. Routes of administration include intravenous (IV), oral (PO), intramuscular (IM), subcutaneous (SC), intrathecal (IT), and intra-arterial (IA). Table 29-4 lists common chemotherapeutic agents and biologic response modifiers, their route of administration, side effects, and nursing actions for the administration of these drugs.

SIDE EFFECTS OF CHEMOTHERAPY

The hematopoietic, gastrointestinal, hepatic, renal, integumentary, and reproductive systems are most commonly affected by side effects of chemotherapy.

Hematopoietic Effects The hematopoietic side effects include myelosuppression (transient decrease in blood cell production), anemia, thrombocytopenia, neutropenia (a decrease in the number of circulating neutrophils), and immunosuppression (a condition in which the patient's immune system is functioning at a lower than normal level). The lowest point in the child's blood counts or myelosuppression is called a nadir and occurs approximately 10 to 14 days after the administration of most chemotherapy agents. If a child becomes anemic while undergoing chemotherapy, red blood cell transfusions may be given. The caregivers and child should be told when to expect anemia and taught to recognize pallor, fatigue, and headache. Thrombocytopenia is a decrease in the number of circulating platelets. When thrombocytopenic, the child is at risk of bleeding. A platelet count of 50,000/mm^3 is associated with only a slight risk of bleeding, while a platelet count of less than 20,000 poses a higher risk of spontaneous bleeding. Common sites of bleeding include the skin, oral mucosa, conjunctiva, and nose. Intracranial and visceral bleeding, although uncommon, can be life-threatening. When IM injections or venipunctures are necessary in the thrombocytopenic child, the sites require the application of direct pressure for 10 minutes to prevent bleeding. Rectal temperatures or suppositories are avoided to prevent bleeding or infection in this area. Caregivers are taught to look for signs of thrombocytopenia (easy bruising, petechiae, and purpura) and instructed when to notify the health care provider. If the

Table 29-4 Chemotherapeutic Agents

DRUG	ROUTE	SIDE EFFECTS	NURSING ACTIONS
CLASSIFICATION: ENZYMES			
Asparaginase (L-asparaginase, Elspar) ***Erwinia*** **Asparaginase** **PEG-Asparaginase** (Oncaspar)	• IM • IV	• Allergic reactions, from mild urticaria to anaphylaxis (have emergency medications with doses available) • Coagulation abnormalities • Hepatotoxicity • Pancreatitis • Hyperglycemia	• Have emergency equipment available for allergic reaction • Make sure platelet count is acceptable before giving IM injection • Check urine for glucose prior to giving • When volume requires that the dose be divided, two injections may be given simultaneously by two nurses • Observe client for 30–60 minutes after injection for allergic reaction
ANTIMETABOLITES			
Cladrabine (Leustatin, CDA)	• IV	• Myelosuppression • Injection site reaction, rash • Nausea • Headache • Fatigue • Neurotoxic • Fever	• Monitor child for infection and side effects
Cytarabine (Ara-C, Cytosine arabinoside, Cytosar-U)	• IV • SQ • IT • IM	• Myelosuppression • Nausea, vomiting, diarrhea • Hepatotoxicity • Fever and malaise • Alopecia, rash • Conjunctivitis • Stomatitis • Neurotoxicity	• Premedicate with antiemetics • High dose: close monitoring for neurotoxicity and chemical conjunctivitis requiring steroid eye drops
Fludarabine (Fludara)	• IV	• Myelosuppression • Nausea, vomiting, diarrhea • Stomatitis • CNS toxicity • Interstitial pulmonary infiltrate	• Monitor pulmonary function tests regularly
5 Fluorouracil (5-FU)	• IV • PO	• Myelosuppression • Nausea, vomiting (mild) • Mucositis (severe) • Hyperpigmentation of nails • Dermatitis	• Give on empty stomach • Parenteral solution is given PO. Do not mix in acidic fruit juices
Gemcitabine (Gemzar)	• IV	• Radiation recall • Myelosuppression • Peripheral edema • Nausea, vomiting	• Observe for signs of infection • Monitor client weight • Teach client and parents of flu-like symptoms

(Continues)

TABLE 29-4 Chemotherapeutic Agents (*Continued*)

DRUG	ROUTE	SIDE EFFECTS	NURSING ACTIONS
Gemcitabine (continued)	• IV	• Skin changes • Proteinuria • Flu-like illness	• Provide antiemetics • Dip urine for proteinuria on follow-up
Hydroxyurea (Hydrea, HU)	• PO	• Myelosuppression • Nausea, vomiting	• Give on empty stomach • Do not mix in acidic or carbonated drinks
Mercaptopurine (6-MP, purinethol)	• PO	• Myelosuppression (mild) • Nausea, vomiting (mild) • Anorexia • Hepatotoxicity • Stomatitis	• Take on empty stomach • Watch for mouth sores
Methotrexate (MTX)	• PO • IM • IV • IT	• Myelosuppression • Nausea, vomiting, stomatitis • Alopecia • Hepatotoxicity • Neurotoxicity • Photosensitivity • Rash	• Give oral dose on empty stomach • Use sunscreen • Avoid vitamins containing folic acid (methotrexate is a folate antagonist) • When given in high doses Leucovorin rescue must be given on time • Watch for mouth sores
Thioguanine (6-TG, 6 thioguanine)	• PO	• Myelosuppression • Nausea, vomiting (mild) • Anorexia, stomatitis • Hepatotoxicity	• Give on empty stomach • Watch for mouth sores
ANTITUMOR ANTIBIOTICS			
Bleomycin Sulfate (Blenoxane, Bleo)	• IV • SQ • IM	• Anaphylaxis (rare) • Pulmonary toxicity • Myelosuppression • Nausea, vomiting, anorexia • Hepatotoxicity	• Have emergency meds available for allergic reaction • Always give test dose and observe for one hour before starting medication • Monitor with pulmonary function tests regularly • Monitor with pulse oximetry
Dactinomycin (Actinomycin D, Act-D, Cosmegen)	• IV	• Vesicant • Myelosuppression • Nausea and vomiting • Radiation recall • Alopecia • Stomatitis	• Vesicant-avoid extravasation • Protect drug from light
Daunorubicin *Also classified as Anthacycline* (Daunomycin, Cerubidine)	• IV	• Vesicant • Myelosuppression • Cardiotoxicity, arrhythmias—acute, cardiomyopathy—delayed	• Vesicant-avoid extravasation • Inform client and parent that child's urine will be discolored pink for several voids after drug is given

(Continues)

Table 29-4 Chemotherapeutic Agents (*Continued*)

DRUG	ROUTE	SIDE EFFECTS	NURSING ACTIONS
Doxorubicin *Also classified as an Anthracycline* (Adriamycin, Adria, DOX)	• IV	• Nausea, vomiting, stomatitis • Radiation recall • Alopecia, rash, • Hyperpigmentation of nails	• Monitor for mouth sores • Monitor cardiac function for toxicity
Idarubicin (Idamycin, IDA) *Also classified as Anthracycline*	• IV	• See daunorubicin	• See daunorubicin • Does not discolor urine
Mitoxantrone (Novantrone) *Also classified as topoisomerase II inhibitor*	• IV dark blue color solution	• Vesicant • Cardiac arrhythmias • Nausea, vomiting • Radiation recall • Myelosuppression • Alopecia • Anaphylaxis	• See daunomycin • Discolors urine a blue-green color
ALKALATING AGENTS			
Busulfan (Myleran)	• PO	• Myelosuppression • Nausea, vomiting, diarrhea • Seizures • Sterility • Skin changes—"bronzing"	• May have prophylactic anticonvulsants ordered when given in high doses as for BMT cytoreduction
Carboplatin (Paraplatin, CBDCA) *Also classified as Heavy metal*	• IV	• Myelosuppression • Nausea, vomiting, diarrhea • Renal and liver toxicity • Ototoxicity • Alopecia • Neuropathy	• Monitor kidney function; children unable to collect urine for 24 hours may need GFR • Monitor hearing with audiograms; small children may need BAER evaluation under anesthesia • Deliver in glass bottles and polyethylene lined tubing sets for stability • Strict monitoring of I&O. Child may need diuretic to assist urinary output
Cisplatin (Platinol, platinum, CDDP) *Also classified as Heavy metal*	• IV	• Myelosuppression • Nausea, vomiting (severe) • Nephrotoxicity with electrolyte wasting (Mg, Ca) • Ototoxicity • Peripheral neuropathies • Allergic reactions (rare)	• See Carboplatin • No restriction on IV tubing or bags • Antiemetics prior to delivery
Cyclophosphamide (Cytoxan, CTX, CPM)	• IV • PO	• Myelosuppression • Nausea, vomiting, anorexia, • and diarrhea	• Monitor strict I&O • Maintain adequate hydration and urine output • Monitor urine for blood

(Continues)

Table 29-4 Chemotherapeutic Agents (*Continued*)

DRUG	ROUTE	SIDE EFFECTS	NURSING ACTIONS
Cyclophosphamide (continued)	• IV • PO	• Hepatotoxicity • Hemorrhagic or nonhemorrhagic cystitis • Alopecia • Sterility • Syndrome of inappropriate antidiuretic hormone (SIADH) • Cardiac toxicity (rare) • May cause second neoplasm	• Give during the day so child can void frequently to prevent accumulation of toxic end products in bladder • Make sure child empties bladder before bed; if CTX given later in day, awaken child to void several times at night • Causes delayed nausea and vomiting; give antiemetics around the clock for 24 hours • Give Mesna on time to prevent hemorrhagic cystitis
Ifosfamide (IFEX)	• IV	• Myelosuppression • Nausea, vomiting, diarrhea • Neurotoxicity (encephalopathy peripheral neuropathy) • Hepatotoxicity • Hemorrhagic cystitis • Renal tubular damage • Alopecia • Sterility potential • May cause second neoplasm	• See cyclophosphamide
Mechlorethamine (nitrogen mustard, Mustargen, NH2)	• IV	• Vesicant • Myelosuppression • Nausea, vomiting (severe) • Sterility potential • Pain and phlebitis at IV site • May cause second neoplasm	• Avoid extravasation • May cause discoloration of vein • Deliver within one hour of reconstitution
Procarbazine (Matulane)	• PO	• Myelosuppression • Nausea, vomiting, stomatitis • Alopecia, pruritus, rash • CNS toxicity • Sterility potential • May cause second neoplasm	• Avoid cheese, wine, bananas, yogurt that are rich in tyramine; avoid phenytoin, MOA inhibitors, phenothiazines, tricyclic antidepressants, and barbiturates to prevent hypotension and or CNS depression. Give client list of drugs and foods to avoid. • Give on empty stomach
Temozolamide (Temodar)	• PO	• Myelosuppression • Fatigue • Nausea, vomiting, diarrhea • Hepatotxicity • Headache • Rash	• Do not take with food • Instruct parents on safe handling-use gloves • Have client take pill as a whole if possible • Instruct parents to give antiemetics prior to giving drug and suggest giving at bedtime to decrease nausea and vomiting.

(Continues)

Table 29-4 Chemotherapeutic Agents (*Continued*)

DRUG	ROUTE	SIDE EFFECTS	NURSING ACTIONS
CLASSIFICATION: PLANT ALKALOID			
Etoposide (VP-16, VePesid) *Also Classified as: Epipodophyllotoxin*	• IV • PO	• Myelosuppression • Hypotension • Nausea, vomiting • Alopecia • Rash • Radiation sensitivity • Allergic reaction • Peripheral neuropathy • May cause second malignancy	• Monitor BP during infusion • Administer over 60 minutes to avoid severe hypotension
Paclitaxol (Taxol)	• IV	• Alopecia • Diarrhea • Myelosuppression • Arthralgia, myalgia • Peripheral neuropathy • Anaphylaxis	• Avoid extravasation-irritant • Premedicate with antihistamine, antiemetics and steroid • Use filter for delivery
Teniposide (VM-26) *Also classified as Epipodophylloto-xin*	• IV	• Hypotension • Nausea, vomiting, mucositis • Alopecia • Hypersensitivity reactions • May cause secondary leukemia	• Avoid extravasation-irritant
Thiotepa (TESPA)	• IV • PO • IT • IM • Intra-tumor	• Nausea, vomiting • Anorexia • Myeolsuppression • Infertility • At higher doses for BMT: esophga-gitis, mucositis • Increased liver enzymes and bilirubin • Pain at injection site • Headache, inappropriate behavior, confusion, somnolence	• Deliver with filter • Monitor renal function • Instruct parents that Thiotepa sweats out of the skin and can cause irritation to the point of skin breakdown. Sheets have to be changed, washed at least twice a day
Topotecan (Hycamtin) *Also classified as: Topoisomerase inhibitor*	• IV • IT	• Myelosuppression • Alopecia • Nausea, vomiting • Diarrhea • Mucositis • Flu-like symptoms • Abnormal liver enzymes • asthenia	• Provide antiemetics • Instruct caregiver on management of flu-like symptoms

(Continues)

TABLE 29-4 Chemotherapeutic Agents (*Continued*)

DRUG	ROUTE	SIDE EFFECTS	NURSING ACTIONS
Vinblastine (Velban, VLB)	• IV	• Vesicant • Peripheral neuropathy • Alopecia • Constipation • SIADH (rare)	• Avoid extravasation-vesicant
Vincristine (Oncovin, VCR)	• IV	• Vesicant • Peripheral neuropathy • Alopecia • Constipation • SIADH (rare) • Seizure (rare)	• Avoid extravasation-vesicant • Check for foot drop before giving • Provide stool softeners prophylactically and laxatives as needed • Dose is limited to 2mgs maximum
MISCELLANEOUS			
Alemtuzumab (Campath) *Classification: BRM* **Alemtuzumab** (Campath) *Classification: Immunological agent and monoclonal antibody*	• IV	• Allergic reaction • Severe immune suppression • Diarrhea • Hypotension, cardiac dysrhythmias • Rash	• Have emergency drugs available for allergic reaction • Do not give as IV bolus or IV push; give over two-hour infusion • Alert parents of prolonged immunosuppression and to call immediately if fever develops
Arsenic (Trisenox) *Classification: Antineoplastic Agent*	• IV	• Edema • Pruritus, rash • Lightheadedness, headache, insomnia, dizziness • Abdominal pain, nausea, vomiting, diarrhea • Abnormal EKG–QT prolongation	• Monitor EKG; watch for QT wave abnormalities • Slow infusion if child becomes lightheaded
CCNU (Lomustine, CeeNU)	• PO	• Myelosuppression • Nausea and vomiting • Anorexia • Abnormal liver enzymes • Pulmonary toxicity	• Give on an empty stomach • Monitor pulmonary function tests
Corticosteroids *(Prednisone, Dexamethasone, hydrocortisone, methylprednisolone, solucortef)*	• PO • IV • IT	• Hyperphagia, weight gain • Immunosuppression • Acne, hirsutism, striae • Cushingoid features • Osteoporosis, delayed growth • Hypertension • Mood swings • Hyperglycemia • Gastritis, peptic ulcer	• Instruct parents to avoid salty and high sugar intake • Watch for hyperglycemia • Inform parents of mood swings • Give with antacids to prevent GI upset • Mask taste in food—very bitter

(Continues)

TABLE 29-4 Chemotherapeutic Agents (*Continued*)

DRUG	ROUTE	SIDE EFFECTS	NURSING ACTIONS
Epogen (Epo) *Classification: BRM, Erythropoietic, hematopoietic*	• SC	• Injection site reaction • Constipation • Fever • Allergic reaction • Kidney failure	• When preparing, do not shake vial • Monitor hemoglobin • Monitor kidney function • Monitor BP • Instruct parents in SQ administration technique
Gemtuzimab (Mylotarg) *Classification: BRM, monoclonal antibody*	• IV	• Myelosuppression-thrombocytopenia, neutropenia and anemia • Allergic reaction within 24 hrs of infusion can include anaphylaxis • Liver toxicity • Vomiting • Headache	• Given as IV infusion, do not give IVP or as bolus.
Imatinib (Gleevec) *Classification: Tyrosine Kinase Inhibitor*	• PO	• Nausea, vomiting, diarrhea • Fluid retention • Muscle pain • Hepatotoxicity	• Do not crush tablets, but can be stirred in apple juice or water until disintegrated and given immediately • Take with meal or large amount of water
Irinotecan (Camptosar) *Classification: Topoisomerase I inhibitor*	• IV	• Diarrhea, nausea, vomiting • Myelosuppression • Alopecia • Abdominal pain	• Monitor stool output; charting number, frequency and consistency of stools. Instruct parents to chart stooling at home • Instruct parents on when to call for increased stooling and when to give antidiarrheal medication to prevent dehydration • Monitor electrolytes
Isotretinoin (Cis-Retinoic Acid) *Classification: Antineoplastic Agent, Retinoid*	• PO	• Cheilitis, dry skin, retinoid dermatitis • Itching, sweating • Xerostomia • Nausea and vomiting • Dry eyes, eyesight changes • Arthralgia and back pain	• Do not use in combination with Vitamin A supplements • Pregnancy precautions—drug is known to cause deformities in a fetus • Instruct patient to avoid grape juice • Instruct patient to avoid exposure to the sun; use sunscreen
Nelarabine (Arranon) *Classification: Antineoplastic Agent*	• IV	• Edema • Constipation, diarrhea, nausea, vomiting • Myelosuppression • Dizziness, headache, somnolence • Cough, dyspnea • Cerebral hemorrhage, coma, seizures • Pleural effusions	• Do not dilute medication further after prepared by pharmacy • Monitor client for tumor lysis syndrome • First course given in the in-patient setting to observe closely for neurological side effects

(*Continues*)

Table 29-4 Chemotherapeutic Agents (*Continued*)

DRUG	ROUTE	SIDE EFFECTS	NURSING ACTIONS
Neupogen (gcsf) *Classification: BRM, Colony stimulating factor*	• SC	• Bone pain • Nausea and vomiting • Anaphylaxis	• First dose given in clinic setting to monitor for allergic reaction • Monitor CBC with differential.
Tarceva (Erlotinib) *Classification: Antineoplastic agent, Tyrosine Kinase Inhibitor)*	• PO	• Rash • Diarrhea • Headache • Fatigue • Gastrointestinal hemorrhage, deep vein thrombosis, CVA • Myocardial infarction, pleural effusion	• Monitor closely for rash • Monitor closely for bleeding • Monitor renal function • Instruct parent to avoid grapefruit and grapefruit juice • Administer on empty stomach
Thalidomide (Thalomid) *Classification: Leprostatic*	• PO	• Birth defects • Rash • Hypocalcemia • Constipation • Nausea • Confusion, somnolence, tremor • Leucopenia, thrombotic disorder • Peripheral neuropathy • Edema	• Healthcare personnel must be registered providers in order to prescribe the drug
Rituximab *Classification: BRM Antineoplastic agent and monoclonal antibody*	• IV	• Allergic reaction • Pruritus • Nausea and vomiting • Aesthenia, dizziness, headache • Fever • Myelosuppression • Bowel obstruction • Cardiac dysrhythmias	• First infusion to be given in-patient for close observation for hypersensitivity reactions which may occur at any time but especially with initial infusion • Never give as an IV bolus or IV push
Avastin *Classification: BRM Immunological agent and monoclonal antibody*	• IV	• Hypertension • Alopecia • Abdominal pain, constipation, diarrhea, stomatitis • Asthenia, dizziness, headache • Proteinuria • Dyspnea • Thromboembolism, • Gastrointestinal hemorrhage, hemorrhagic cerebral infarction	• Instruct client to report any signs of bleeding, headache, hemoptysis or abdominal pain • Have client call for any skin changes

NURSING TIP

How to Calculate an ANC (absolute neutrophil count) to Determine the Severity of Neutropenia

Formula: $\frac{(\%\ \text{Segs} + \%\ \text{Bands})}{100} \times \text{WBC}$

Example: The child's CBC shows the following:

Total WBC = 2000
2% Segs
8% Bands

Calculation: $\frac{(2+8)}{100 \times 2000} = \frac{10 \times 2000}{100} = 200$

This child has an ANC of 200 and is severely neutropenic

platelet count is very low or if there is active bleeding, a platelet transfusion may be ordered. Children should be inspected daily for signs of bleeding. Those with low platelet counts need to be protected from trauma. Prevention measures include instructing the child and caregiver to avoid playing or engaging in any contact sports or activity that has a risk of physical injury such as roller skating or riding a bicycle. Menstruating girls who have prolonged or heavy periods may require oral contraceptives to control the vaginal bleeding.

Neutrophils are cells that perform phagocytosis and destroy bacteria. When the neutrophil level is low the child has neutropenia and is at risk for serious life-threatening infections. To determine the severity of neutropenia a calculation is made to determine the absolute neutrophil count (ANC) (see Nursing Tip). A child with an ANC of $500/\text{mm}^3$ or less is at risk for serious life-threatening bacterial infections, which are usually caused by normal body flora. Infection in the

NURSING ALERT

Aspirin, Aspirin-Containing Products, and NSAIDs (Nonsteroidal Anti-Inflammatory Drugs)

These products are not to be given to a child receiving chemotherapy because they interfere with normal platelet function. While on chemotherapy, a child is at increased risk of developing thrombocytopenia so the function of the circulating platelets should not be further compromised. Nurses are responsible to educate caregivers of this restriction.

NURSING TIP

Neutropenic Children May Not Show Signs of Infection

Children who are neutropenic will not mount an immune response to infection. They may not show signs of inflammation such as redness or the production of pus because they lack the neutrophils to do so. Some will complain of pain and swelling in the area. These symptoms are to be considered indicative of infection and should be treated promptly. Fever may be the only sign of infection.

neutropenic child can quickly progress to septic shock and death. Handwashing is the cornerstone of infection prevention and control in and out of the hospital. When a child is neutropenic, any signs of infection must be treated emergently. The goal is to have antibiotics given within 30 minutes. (See research highlight on page 1049.) All children with fever and neutropenia should have a sepsis work-up that includes peripheral and venous access device (VAD) blood cultures, a chest X-ray, and urine and wound cultures. If the fever does not subside with IV antibiotics and if the causative organism has not been isolated, it may be necessary to start an antifungal agent. This protects the child, as fungal organisms are slow to grow and isolate in culture medium. Invasive procedures should be avoided when possible. These include rectal temperatures, use of suppositories, and use of urinary catheters. Infectious organisms can be introduced through the mucosal lining of these areas.

The child's immune system is suppressed (immunosuppression) and not able to respond or mount a response because of lack of lymphocytes. Management of the immunosuppressed child includes prevention and prompt treatment of infections. Also, exposure to viral diseases such as varicella (chickenpox) and measles is to be avoided if possible. Many children on chemotherapy regimens receive *Pneumocystis carinii pneumonia* (PCP) prophylaxis, with Trimethoprim-sulfamethoxazole. Children allergic to sulfa will get intravenous or inhaled Pentamidine.

Gastrointestinal Effects

Gastrointestinal (GI) side effects are common. **Mucositis**, also called stomatitis, is an inflammation of the oral mucosa that ranges from mild redness to severe painful ulceration. The entire gastrointestinal tract can be affected. Mucositis is one of the most difficult and painful side effects of cancer therapy, and usually presents several days after the administration of chemotherapy. The primary management is pain control and good oral care, which includes using a cleansing solution such as warm water or chlorhexidine to clean and rinse the oral cavity of food particles and debris several times a day, particularly after meals. Gentle cleansing with oral sponges or ultra-soft toothbrushes may be necessary to minimize pain

NURSING ALERT

Varicella (Chickenpox)

Caregivers should be taught that varicella can be an overwhelming infection in the immunosuppressed child, and exposure is to be avoided if at all possible. If the child is exposed, caregivers need to notify the health care provider and seek prompt treatment with VZoster IG if available or Intravenous Immune Globulin (IVIG) within 72 hours of exposure as a preventive measure (American Academy of Pediatrics, 2006b). Children who present with an active case of varicella are hospitalized and receive antiviral therapy in respiratory isolation. It is recommended that healthy siblings of an immunosuppressed child who have not had varicella receive the vaccine. If the vaccinated sibling develops a rash, the individual should avoid contact with the child with cancer until the rash is no longer present. The goal is to prevent widespread dissemination of the virus to the lungs, liver, or central nervous system.

and to prevent further trauma to the oral mucosa. Painful mouth lesions may cause a decrease in oral intake and lead to dehydration, poor nutrition, and weight loss.

Other GI side effects are nausea and vomiting, which may range from mild nausea to severe vomiting. Some children experience anticipatory vomiting, which occurs when the child associates a certain situation with chemotherapy and vomiting, such as riding to the hospital or entering the outpatient clinic. Prolonged nausea, vomiting, and anorexia can lead to significant weight loss and weakness, which can further compromise the child's immune status. The administration of antiemetics and nonpharmacologic interventions can help to control the nausea and vomiting. Maintaining adequate hydration and monitoring fluids and electrolytes is necessary in children with severe nausea and vomiting.

NURSING ALERT

Immunosuppression and Vaccines

Immune responses of immunocompromised children to inactive vaccines (diphtheria, tetanus, and pertussis (DTaP), hepatitis A and B, inactive polio vaccine (IPV), hemophilus influenza B (HIB), pneumococcal conjugate, and influenza may vary and be inadequate. Measles, mumps, rubella (MMR), varicella, and flu mist are live vaccines and should not be given to immunosuppressed children, since they are at risk of developing the disease. MMR, varicella, rotavirus, and inactive flu vaccines are recommended for household contacts. Once immunosuppressive therapy is discontinued an immune response to vaccines occurs between three months to a year. Inactive flu vaccine is recommended for children six months of age and older, including immune compromised children, before each flu season (American Academy of Pediatrics, 2006a). Many institutions recommend inactive flu vaccine in immunocompromised children.

Hepatic Effects Liver toxicity seen with different chemotherapeutic agents ranges from the elevation of hepatic enzymes to liver fibrosis caused by long-term use of these drugs. Periodic monitoring of hepatic function allows for the adjustment of liver toxic chemotherapeutic agents to prevent severe long-term liver damage. A liver function evaluation is performed routinely by examining liver transaminases and bilirubin levels prior to chemotherapy administration. The nurse, prior to administering the chemotherapy, must check the results and notify the health care provider of any abnormal findings. High transaminases and bilirubin may require a dose reduction adjustment or postponement of the chemotherapeutic agent.

Renal Effects Various chemotherapeutic agents, especially high dose methotrexate and cisplatin, can cause significant renal toxicity. Renal toxicity will be manifest as an increase in blood urea nitrogen (BUN) and serum creatinine and decrease in urine creatinine clearance. Factors that compound renal toxicity include the use of certain antibiotics, antifungal agents, and radiation to the kidney area. Children receiving cytoxan and ifosfamide are at risk for **hemorrhagic cystitis** (abnormal bleeding of the bladder), which may occur during the administration of the agent or months after. To prevent stasis of the end products of these drugs in the bladder, the child must be well hydrated and encouraged to void every two hours while, and after, the drug is given. Mesna, a bladder protectant, is given before, during, and after administration of these drugs. Continued periodic urine examination for blood is recommended because it may occur months after the drug is given. Kidney function is also determined by the client's ability to handle body fluids; therefore, monitoring intake and output is essential. A discrepancy in intake and output must be reported as this may be the first indication of renal toxicity.

NURSING TIP

Nausea and Vomiting

Giving chemotherapy at bedtime may alleviate nausea and vomiting in children. It may allow them to sleep through the emetic effects. Playing soft music, such as lullabies, or recording a caregiver singing soft songs is soothing and distracting and may alleviate symptoms of nausea and vomiting.

NURSING ALERT

Nothing by Rectum

Giving rectal medications, taking a rectal temperature, or performing a rectal examination can lead to breaks in the rectal mucosa, allowing bacteria into the bloodstream, which may lead to sepsis, a rectal abscess, or bleeding. Children undergoing chemotherapy have fragile intestinal mucosa and are not to receive anything per rectum.

Integumentary Effects **Alopecia** or hair loss is often the side effect most associated with cancer treatment, but not all children undergoing chemotherapy will lose their hair (Figures 29-2, 29-3, 29-4). When it does occur it can be devastating to the child and family. Hair loss from chemotherapy is not permanent, and regrowth often starts while the child is still receiving treatment. Children less than five years of age are not as concerned with hair loss as an adolescent whose body image and peer acceptance are of utmost importance. If the child requests a wig, arrangements for the purchase should be done prior to the alopecia. Many young children are bothered by wigs and prefer to use scarves and hats or to wear nothing at all. All children experiencing alopecia should protect their heads from sunburn or cold weather.

Some chemotherapy drugs are **vesicants** or skin irritants and cause discomfort with the sensation of burning, redness, and inflammation if they **extravasate** or leak out of the vein during administration. Vesicants cause a skin reaction that may range from a slight hyperpigmentation at the area of extravasation to a severe burn leading to loss of function and mobility of the extremity where the drug was given. To prevent extravasation, the nurse should assure venous patency prior to the administration of a chemotherapeutic agent. A free-flowing intravenous access with a blood return should be present. Venous blood return

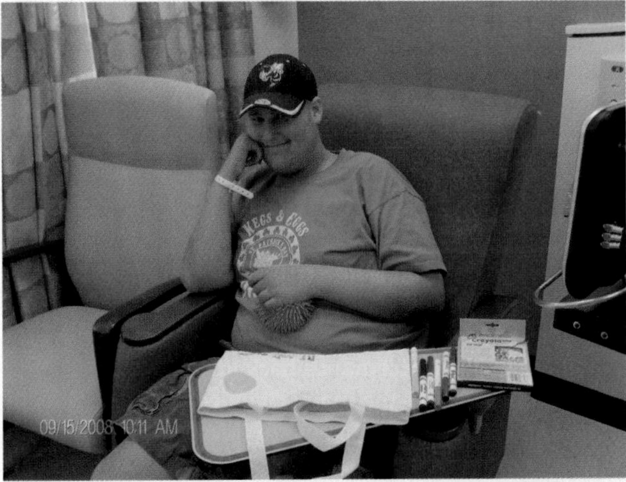

FIGURE 29-2 Alopecia is a common side effect of chemotherapy and a threat to body image especially in the older child. Many adolescents prefer to wear a wig, hat, or scarf. DELMAR CENGAGE LEARNING.

RESEARCH Highlight

Blood Sampling from Central Venous Access Devices

STUDY PURPOSE

To determine whether a push-pull method for obtaining blood samples from a central venous access device (CVAD) will produce laboratory results comparable to blood samples obtained using a standard method.

METHODS

The sample group consisted of pediatric oncology inpatients with CVADs who required CBC and chemistries. A 10 cc syringe was connected to the CVAD. 5 cc of blood was withdrawn and then reinfused. This process was repeated two more times. Using a second syringe, a 5 cc "waste" specimen was withdrawn and transferred to lab tubes as the research specimen. A third 5 cc blood sample was aspirated and placed into lab tubes for the ordered lab tests. Both the "research" sample obtained with the push-pull method and the standard draw specimen were tested for CBC and Chemistry.

FINDINGS

Of the 18 serum chemistries and 3 CBC values studied, results from blood samples obtained using the push-pull method showed no significant differences from the samples obtained using the discard method. Additionally the push-pull method did not result in increased hemolysis or hemodilution.

IMPLICATIONS

Based on the findings, discarding blood does not seem to be necessary when drawing some labs from CVADs. In the pediatric oncology population, frequent blood sampling is the norm. Central Venous Access devices (CVAD) are often used for this purpose. The widely used discard method may contribute to anemia and the need for transfusions in children with cancer. Pediatric oncology nurses should be familiar with the blood draw policy in their institutions and promote further research to confirm best practice in the clinical setting.

REFERENCE

Adlard, K. (2008). Examining the push-pull method of blood sampling from central venous access devices. *Journal of Pediatric Oncology Nursing*, *25*(4), 200–207.

is checked during the infusion, and if there is a loss of blood return, the infusion is stopped immediately, and any residual medication is aspirated to reduce the extent of extravasation. Vesicants are not to be administered over joints, bony prominences, in the anticubital fossa, or above tendons, as extravasation damage in these areas can affect limb function.

Reproductive Effects The reproductive system is also adversely affected by chemotherapy. Most children have normal pubertal development, but fertility may still be affected. Prepubertal girls may have delayed pubertal development, and girls who have already started menstruating may develop **oligomenorrhea** (abnormally light or reduction in menstruation), amenorrhea, excessive bleeding, or menopausal symptoms. The effect of cancer treatment on male fertility is more severe than on female fertility. Sterility may result from the use of alkylating agents, which have a dramatic effect on spermatogenesis. A decrease in spermatogenesis may be reversible in months or years after completion of chemotherapy, but sterility is frequently permanent. The increased risk of infection during neutropenic episodes poses additional potential problems. Condoms should be used to reduce the risk of infection and also to prevent pregnancy. Oral contraceptive pills are sometimes ordered to control excessive menstrual bleeding. The adolescent female should be instructed to use sanitary pads instead of tampons to reduce the risk of trauma and infection. Sexually mature males can be offered the option of sperm banking if they are well enough prior to initiating chemotherapy. This is to be done as expeditiously as possible in order to not delay cancer treatment. At the present time egg banking for adolescent girls is not routinely recommended. If puberty is delayed, it may be managed with hormonal therapy in both males and females.

Complementary and Alternative Therapies

The use of Complementary and Alternative Medicine (CAM) is not uncommon in pediatric oncology when parents want to help alleviate their child's side effects from

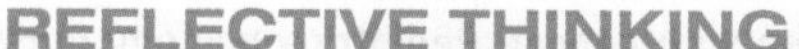

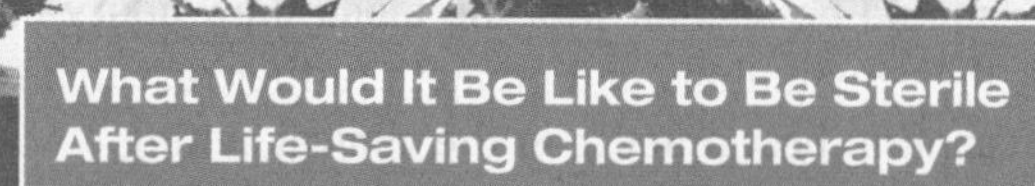

What Would It Be Like to Be Sterile After Life-Saving Chemotherapy?

In a Long Term Cancer Survivor Clinic, a young man who survived Ewing's Sarcoma as a child (before sperm banking was available) has found out that he is now sterile. His sperm count showed no viable sperm. His parents came to the clinic with him and he looked at them after being informed of this news, and in anger asked "How could you do this to me?"

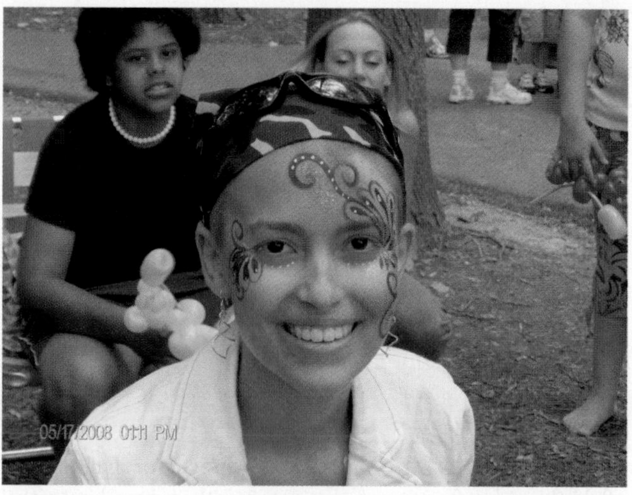

FIGURE 29-3 Children with alopecia must protect their heads from cold weather and sunburn. DELMAR CENGAGE LEARNING.

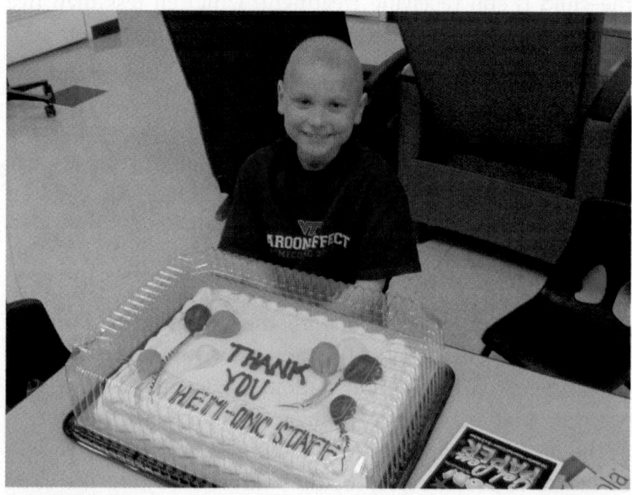

FIGURE 29-4 Alopecia is less of a threat to body image in younger children. DELMAR CENGAGE LEARNING.

NURSING TIP

Coping with Alopecia

Role-play with the child as to what to say when someone asks, "What happened to your hair?" Children returning to school have many anxieties regarding their acceptance back into their peer group because of the many changes in their appearance. This activity helps to develop coping strategies to deal with alopecia. A school visit from the oncology team nurse to speak with the child's teacher and classmates can help the transition back to school.

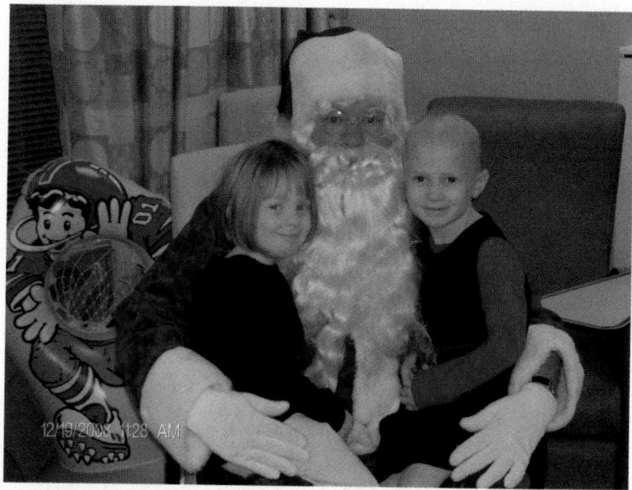

FIGURE 29-5 It's important to include siblings in the care of the child with cancer. DELMAR CENGAGE LEARNING.

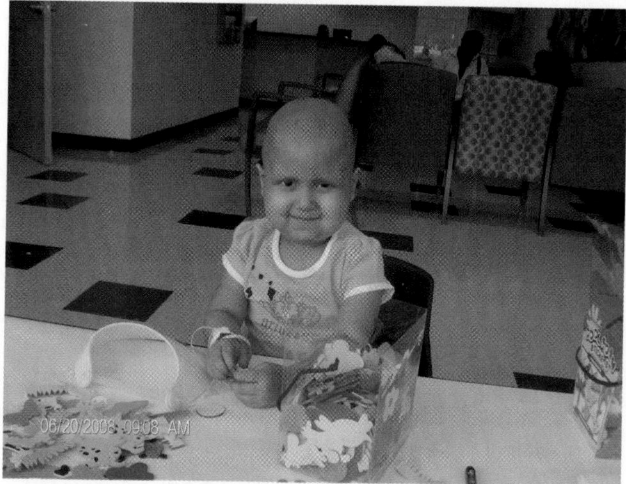

FIGURE 29-6 Supportive care, such as art or play therapy, will help children endure long treatment days. DELMAR CENGAGE LEARNING.

treatment that may range from stress and pain to nausea and vomiting. Several of the most common CAM therapies used by children with cancer are: prayer, massage, vitamins, supplements, relaxation, and imagery. The most important factor in a child's use of CAM is whether or not the child's parents used CAM. (Post-White, Fitzgerald, Hageness, & Sencer, 2009). Other complementary therapies are art therapy, music therapy, and play therapy (Figures 29-5, 29-6).

VENOUS ACCESS DEVICES

The most frequent route of delivery of antineoplastic drugs is IV, which is also one of the most difficult in children. Venipuncture is painful and disturbing for children who may not have a full understanding of the importance of cancer therapy. Hundreds of venipunctures may be needed during the course of cancer treatment. For therapeutic as well as psychological reasons, most children will have a **venous access device** (VAD), which is a catheter that is usually inserted into the superior vena cava. It is utilized for chemotherapeutic drug delivery, blood sampling and blood product administration, intravenous fluids, medications, and total parenteral nutrition (TPN). The most common devices used with children are external catheters (i.e., Broviac, Hickman, Groshong) and implanted ports (i.e., Port-A-Cath, Infusaport). An external catheter requires exit site care and frequent flushing with a heparinized saline solution to maintain patency. Implanted ports are accessed with a special nonboring needle and require monthly flushing when not used more frequently. There are no restrictions on activities, such as swimming, for a child with a port. Complications of VADs include increased risk of infection, occlusion with fibrin sheath formation, and dislodgment. Fibrin sheath formation requires the use of a fibrinolytic agent to restore patency. A dislodged device must be surgically repaired or replaced. Figures 29-7 and 29-8 illustrate an external catheter and an implanted port, respectively.

> **NURSING ALERT**
>
> **Use of Complementary and Alternative Medicine (CAM)**
>
> It is very important to ask parents if they are using CAM to help alleviate their child's side effects of cancer therapy. Many vitamin supplements contain folic acid that should not be given to children receiving methotrexate, a folic acid antagonist.

> **KIDS WANT TO KNOW**
>
> **Will I Lose My Hair, and If So, When Will It Grow Back?**
>
> A 12-year-old girl recently diagnosed with osteogenic sarcoma is admitted for her first course of chemotherapy. She says to you, "I know I need this chemotherapy to fight the tumor in my leg, but I really think it's awful that my hair is going to fall out. Will it fall out as soon as I get the chemotherapy?" This girl's worry about her appearance is a real concern. You should explain that her hair will probably start to fall out in 10 days to 2 weeks. The hair will come out over several days and it can be messy. Some clients cut the hair short to prevent this. When the chemotherapy is complete, the hair will grow back. You should advise the girl of the options available (wig, hat, scarf, nothing). Emphasis should be on personal choice. Speaking with another girl of the same age who has also lost her hair may be helpful.

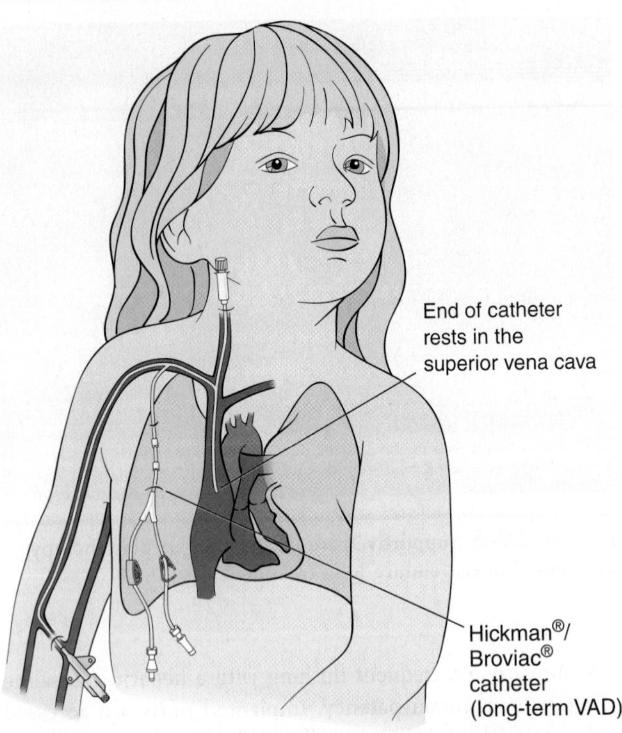

FIGURE 29-7A **External catheters allow chemotherapy, IV medications, and TPN to be administered without piercing the child's skin with a needle.** DELMAR CENGAGE LEARNING.

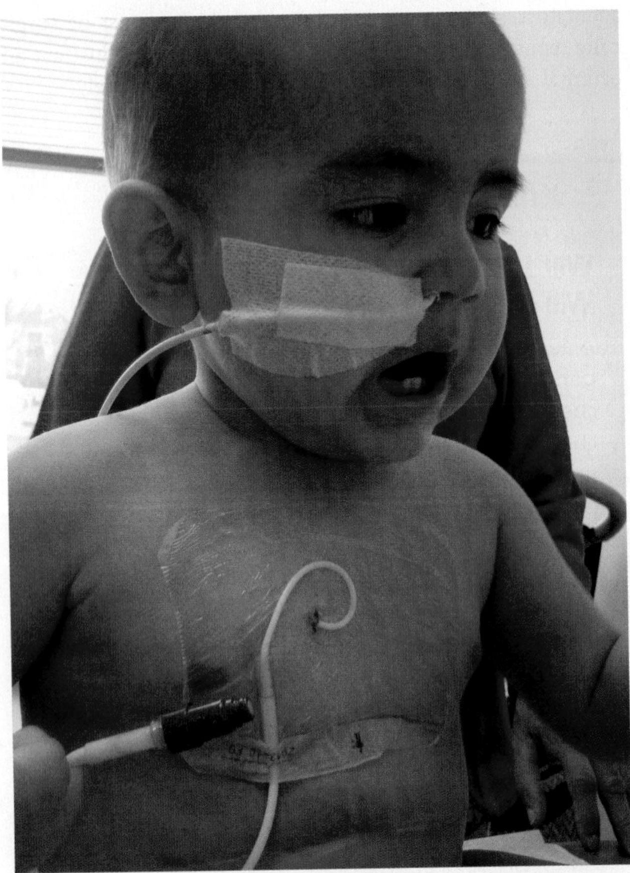

FIGURE 29-7B **A Child with a Broviac Catheter.** DELMAR CENGAGE LEARNING.

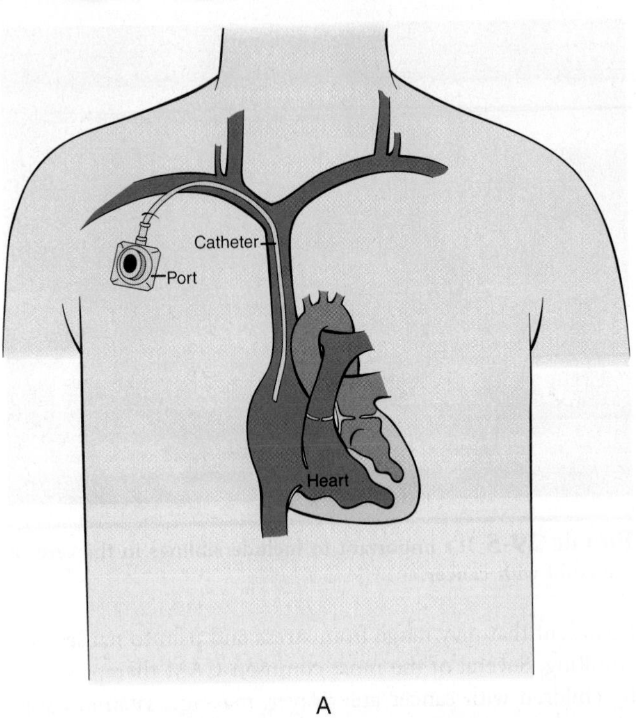

FIGURE 29-8A **An implanted port is surgically inserted under the skin, and the catheter tip is frequently placed in the superior vena cava for long term chemotherapy administration.** DELMAR CENGAGE LEARNING.

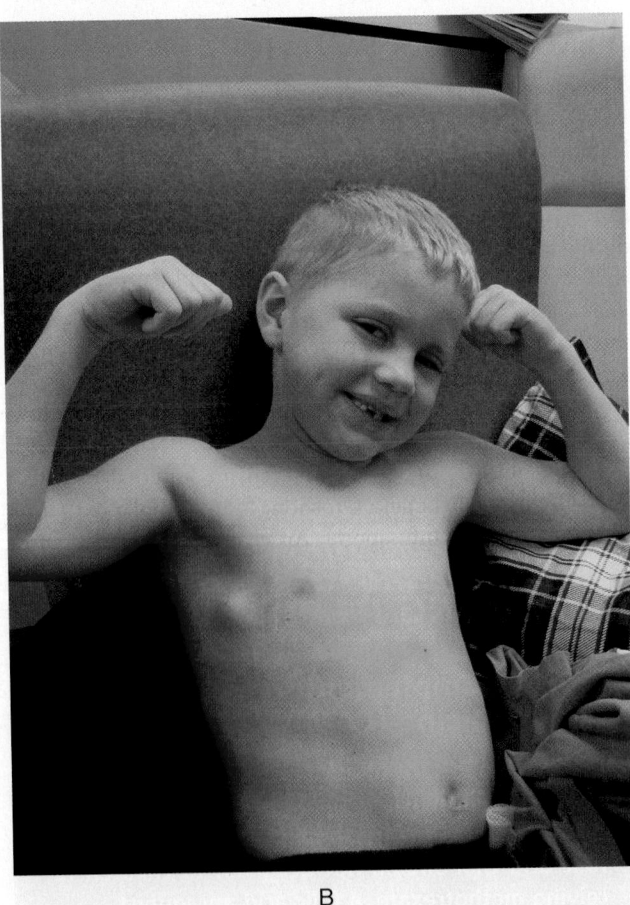

FIGURE 29-8B **A Child with an Implanted Port.** DELMAR CENGAGE LEARNING.

KIDS WANT TO KNOW

How Will the Other Students React to My VAD?

A 17-year-old high school student is undergoing chemotherapy and has an external venous access device. While the adolescent appreciates the device and the ease it provides for blood drawing, as well as administration of medications and blood products, she is very concerned about returning to school with the device. "What if someone notices it? What if someone bumps into me? What if someone pulls it?" Unlike hair loss, a central venous access device is for the most part unnoticeable. It still is a constant reminder of the diagnosis, and a feature that makes the adolescent stand out as different from his or her peers. It is important to stress that a central venous device is unnoticeable when covered by clothing and would not be pulled by an unknowing person. Trauma to the device is unlikely, because of its location on the upper chest wall. Stress the importance of continuing school and maintaining friendships. Meeting another adolescent who has had a VAD will also help.

Teaching the family to care for a VAD begins before it is surgically placed. Implanted devices require no home care once the initial incision from placement is healed. External catheters require more care. Daily assessment for signs of infection at the exit site, such as drainage, redness, or pain, is needed. To maintain patency, the catheter is flushed daily with a heparinized solution. Sterile dressing changes of the catheter site and change of catheter injection caps need to be done on a schedule. The caregiver must be instructed to notify the health care provider if the child has a fever or signs of infection. The inability to flush the catheter with ease may be caused by a catheter malposition, anatomical obstruction, or the formation of a fibrin sheath. The caregiver must be instructed not to force flush the catheter at any time and to call should any problems with flushing exist. Direct pressure at the insertion site is applied if an external catheter is accidentally pulled out. Consistency of catheter care methods between the hospital and home is essential to avoid confusion and anxiety in the child and caregiver.

NURSING ALERT

Safe Handling of Chemotherapy

Many chemotherapeutic agents have been found to be carcinogenic, mutagenic, and teratogenic in animals, although further research is needed to determine the implications to human exposure. Nurses can be exposed to these agents through inhalation, absorption, or ingestion, while mixing, administering, or handling the agents or the body excreta of the client. To prevent absorption of cytotoxic agents through the skin, chemotherapy is given with the protection of nonporous gloves. A gown is used during administration to prevent self-contamination should a spill occur. Precautions must be taken for 48 hours after single-agent chemotherapy and 5 days after multi-agent chemotherapy. The Occupational Safety and Health Administration (OSHA) has developed guidelines to protect workers. Guidelines include the use of an airflow hood while mixing chemotherapy and the use of protective gowns, gloves, masks, and eyeshields when handling the agents. Gowns are not needed for patient contact only but are needed along with gloves when disposing of patient waste and body secretions. All equipment and linen contaminated with chemotherapy waste must be disposed of in labeled, sealed containers. The nurse is responsible to follow the guidelines found in the policy and procedure manual of his or her institution, and must also teach caregivers safe handling procedures and disposal (Figure 29-9).

RADIATION THERAPY

Radiation therapy is used to deliver a therapeutic dose of ionizing radiation to a tumor with minimal effects to the healthy surrounding tissue. It is the primary treatment for several pediatric malignancies such as lymphomas, solid tumors, and brain tumors. Radiation therapy can also be given for pain control as a part of palliative care in terminally ill clients in which it is used to enhance the quality of remaining life.

Radiation therapy is delivered by several methods:

1. External Beam—a two dimensional beam of radiation is aimed at a specific tumor site or tumor volume.
2. Brachytherapy—the implantation of radioactive "seeds" or "pellets" placed directly into a body cavity, skin surface, or tissue. It provides localized radiation therapy. May be used with external beam radiation for a tumor radiation boost. In pediatric oncology it is used in children with retinoblastoma and central nervous system tumors.
3. Three-dimensional conformal radiation therapy (3D-CRT)—uses CT imaging to map out the specific location of a tumor in three dimensions. The radiation beams are then delivered to the tumor from several different locations, sparing local nonaffected tissue.
4. Intensity modulated radiation therapy (IMRT)—external radiation therapy using photons. As with

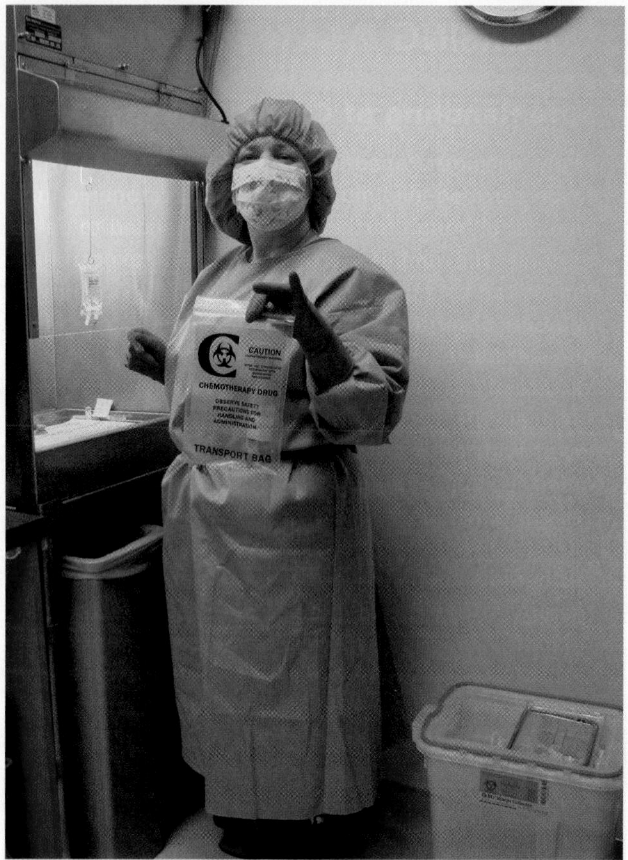

FIGURE 29-9 OSHA Approved Personal Protective Equipment (PPE) and Hazardous Waste Container. DELMAR CENGAGE LEARNING.

3D-CRT the tumor is mapped with CT imaging and radiation therapy is delivered in several directions, along with photon beams, to increase the intensity of the radiation.

5. Intraoperative radiation therapy—delivered directly to an exposed tumor or tumor bed preserving nonaffected tissue.
6. Proton beam radiation—high-energy external radiation therapy that uses streams of protons that are small, positively charged particles.

Radiation is given daily in divided doses until the total prescribed dose is delivered. This method spares damage to normal tissues, allowing them to repair between doses. Hyperfractionation is the delivery of radiation in smaller doses, divided two or three times a day, to give a higher total dose and to further reduce the effects to the surrounding tissue. Total body irradiation (TBI) is external beam radiation delivered to the whole body in preparation for hematopoietic stem cell transplantation.

At each radiation treatment the child must remain immobile on a hard flat surface. This may be uncomfortable for the 10–15 minutes it takes for the preparation, positioning, and delivery of the treatment. The actual treatment only lasts minutes. Depending upon the developmental level of the child, sedation or anesthesia may be necessary to complete the treatments. Immobilization devices such as plastic casts and molds are often necessary for children, so that accurate delivery of the treatment can be accomplished.

Nursing care of the child undergoing radiation therapy involves teaching about the process and its effects on the child. Children and caregivers need to know that radiation therapy is not painful, yet it may be frightening to the child and caregiver. Preradiation teaching and role-playing decrease the child's anxiety and promote more cooperation. Caregivers need to know the daily time schedule and any sedation or anesthesia protocol, if used.

FAMILY TEACHING

Chemotherapy

- Teach the child and family the chemotherapeutic regimen. Include the drug's side effects and reasons to notify the medical team, such as signs of an infection.
- Using the child's protocol roadmap as a guide, write a calendar of daily medications, clinic visits, admissions, lab tests, radiographic studies, and procedures. Update the calendar as needed.
- Familiarize the family with routine CBC results. Teach caregivers to calculate the ANC and to understand the consequences of being neutropenic.
- Teach the caregivers how to care for the child's VAD. Provide written instruction. Set up a visit from a home care nurse to reinforce home care of the VAD and reassure caregivers.
- Provide telephone numbers to call for questions or concerns.
- Provide the school with information regarding the return to school of the child who is receiving chemotherapy. Offer a school visit to facilitate the re-entry.
- Provide instructions in writing to the school nurse and teacher regarding infection precautions, exposure to communicable diseases, and bleeding precautions.
- Give caregivers information regarding support groups such as the Leukemia and Lymphoma Society.

SIDE EFFECTS OF RADIATION THERAPY

Children who are receiving radiation to large bones, such as the pelvis, cranium, and spine, may show signs of anemia, thrombocytopenia, and neutropenia caused by the effects of ionizing radiation on the blood producing bone marrow. Ionizing radiation suppresses the bone marrow and causes a drop in all blood cell lines. Care of the child with these hematopoietic effects is addressed in the chemotherapy section of this chapter.

Radiation therapy delivered to the head and neck area will cause an alteration of the oral mucosa. The epithelial cells of the mouth are very sensitive to ionizing radiation, leading to mucositis after the start of therapy. **Xerostomia**, or dryness of the mouth, occurs from a decreased or arrested production of salivary secretions. Pain, teeth sensitivity, and difficulty speaking may accompany this dryness. Mouth care is essential to promote comfort, prevent infection, and provide lubrication to the mucosa. Nurses should offer relief by encouraging fluids, sucking hard candy, or chewing sugarless gum to stimulate saliva production. Continued use of fluorinated water and toothpaste can help prevent caries caused from a decrease in saliva production. Esophagitis is caused by radiation to the chest and upper back area. A burning pain behind the sternum is a common complaint. Regurgitation and indigestion may accompany this side effect. Milk and milk products frequently can relieve this discomfort, but medication is sometimes necessary. Radiation to the abdomen, pelvis, or lower back may cause nausea, vomiting, and diarrhea, which may be alleviated by the use of antiemetics and antidiarrheal agents. Weight should be monitored frequently, and a loss greater than 10% is an indication for parenteral nutrition to maintain the child's nutritional needs until the effects of radiation subside.

Skin in the radiated field may exhibit changes such as dryness, erythema, or pruritus. More serious reactions with skin breakdown and desquamation may warrant a delay in treatments. Good nutrition and hydration are important to maintain skin integrity, healing, and recovery. Skin care is to be given daily with a mild soap with care not to wash off any skin markings made by the radiation oncologist, which identify the treatment field. Friction, tight clothing, hot water, tape, and strong soaps should be avoided because they can contribute to skin breakdown. The use of creams, lotions, or deodorants should be discussed with the radiation oncologist. All children are to avoid sun exposure in the treatment area because radiated skin may burn more easily. Moist desquamated skin requires a culture of the wound, and further skin care may be ordered by the radiologist.

Radiation recall is a phenomenon that occurs as an inflammatory skin reaction in a previously irradiated area when a client is receiving certain chemotherapy agents such as Actinomycin-D, adriamycin, and carboplatin. This recall phenomenon can occur from months to years following the conclusion of radiation therapy (Ayoola & Lee, 2006). The skin reaction can range from mild erythema to a severe sunburn effect.

Radiation to the scalp produces alopecia that may be permanent. The child and caregivers should be made aware of this and encouraged to obtain appropriate head coverings. A warm head covering is important during the colder months to prevent heat loss, and coverings are also necessary to prevent sunburn.

Radiation pneumonitis is an acute reaction, caused by the swelling and sloughing of the endothelial cells of the small vessels of the lung, which allows fluid to accumulate in the interstitial tissues. Signs and symptoms include tachypnea, orthopnea, a dry cough, and respiratory difficulty. Radiation pneumonitis can be a serious condition that may lead to a hospital admission and at times mechanical ventilation. Caregivers need to seek medical attention if their child shows any signs of respiratory difficulty.

Whole-brain radiation can cause acute, subacute, and delayed toxicity. Acute toxicity occurs during or shortly after radiation and is caused by inflammation, edema, and increased intracranial pressure. Headache, nausea, and vomiting are common signs and symptoms of acute toxicity. Subacute toxicity is seen five to seven weeks after radiation and resolves within one to three weeks. This is called **somnolence syndrome**. Children will experience drowsiness and may sleep up to 20 hours a day. Nausea and malaise frequently accompany this sleepiness, and fever, dysphasia,

FAMILY TEACHING

Radiation Therapy

- Families have an appointment with the radiation oncologist prior to starting therapy.
- Provide the caregiver with a daily schedule of appointments and sedation or anesthesia instructions. Written literature about radiation therapy is helpful and provides the caregiver the opportunity to review the details of treatment at his or her own pace and to ask questions at a later time.
- Teach the child and family about acute side effects and their management. Instruct parents if radiation recall is a concern.
- Provide specific instructions about the amount of fluid intake that is adequate.
- Provide instructions about when and how to contact the medical team if side effects or concerns occur.
- Plan a school visit or phone call to facilitate the child's school reentry. A school visit will assure school staff and classmates that the child is not radioactive and no radiation precautions are necessary for children who have undergone external beam radiation therapy.
- Help to schedule the radiation treatment later in the day, so the child can continue to go to school in the morning.
- Provide written guidance for teachers and the school nurse, so they know when to contact the child's caregiver should an acute side effect occur.
- Refer the family and child to appropriate support groups such as the Childhood Brain Tumor Foundation.

ataxia, and transient **papilledema**, an inflammation of the optic disk, may also occur.

Caregivers and the child may view the nausea, vomiting, and headache of acute neurological toxicity as a tumor recurrence or progression, and must be reassured that it is a side effect of the radiation treatment. Steroids may be prescribed to reduce the swelling and pressure on the brain and thereby alleviate the symptoms. The child and caregivers must also be prepared for somnolence syndrome because the symptoms can be very worrisome. The family often fears that there has been a recurrence. Repeated reassurance that somnolence syndrome will resolve is helpful, but occasionally imaging studies are performed to assure the child and family that there has not been a relapse.

Radiation to the bones, soft tissue, and blood vessel areas of a growing child will affect growth in the treated area. Effects of radiation include impaired growth of bone and soft tissue resulting in an asymmetry as the child grows. Children who are most susceptible are those less than six years of age or undergoing pubertal growth spurts. These bones are also susceptible to fractures and recurrent tumors later in life. Teaching to protect the affected bones from trauma must be repeated, even when the child's therapy has been completed.

Families always have an appointment with the Radiation Oncologist prior to starting therapy. At this time, the radiation oncologist reviews the importance of radiation therapy, why and how it will be delivered, and the side effects to expect. Long-term side effects are also discussed. Parents then sign consent for treatment.

HEMATOPOIETIC STEM CELL TRANSPLANTATION

Hematopoietic stem cell transplantation (HSCT), previously known as bone marrow transplantation, is the replacement of a person's hematopoietic stem cells after his or her own bone marrow has been destroyed by disease or by the treatment of a malignant disease. Stem cells are the precursors of red and white blood cells and platelets. Stem cells can be obtained from a variety of sources, such as bone marrow or umbilical cord blood. In cancer therapy the use of hematopoietic stem cell transplantation has become increasingly accepted as treatment for leukemia, lymphoma, and certain solid tumors. See Table 29-5, which describes different types of hematopoietic stem cell transplant.

For all types of HSCT (except autologous) donor stem cells must be found. A suitable donor is one whose tissue type closely matches the client's. Genetic markers on the surface of white blood cells, called human lymphocyte antigens (HLA), define a person's tissue type. These antigens are proteins that play a critical role in protecting the body against invading organisms such as bacteria, viruses, and other foreign matter. These HLA markers are inherited, so siblings are more likely to be compatible donors. If a donor must be located in the general population, the chances of finding an HLA match vary widely, depending upon the child's ethnicity. Several unrelated donor registries in the United States have listings of the HLA tissue types of people who are willing to donate stem cells, such as the National Marrow Donor Program. Most potential donors are Caucasian. Only about 30% of clients who need a bone marrow transplant have a matched sibling donor, meaning that 70% of patients have to consider alternative donors (Bollard, Krance, & Hesop, 2007).

Obtaining donors for minorities has been a challenge for bone marrow registries. Some problems identified within the African-American community are lack of knowledge regarding the importance of marrow donation, information on the process of donation, and cost of donating (Glasgow, Smith, & Bello, 2008). The National Marrow Donor Program has reached out to potential minority donors with programs such as African Americans Uniting for Life, Asian/Pacific Islander Donors Can Save Lives, and Hispanics Giving Hope.

TABLE 29-5 Types of Hematopoietic Stem Cell Transplant

TYPE	DESCRIPTION
Autologous	The client receives his own stem cells, which is possible if the disease afflicting the bone marrow is in remission, or if the condition does not involve the bone marrow (e.g., Hodgkin's disease lymphoma and brain tumor). Stem cells are extracted from the client prior to transplant and may be "purged" to remove lingering malignant cells.
Allogeneic	The client receives stem cells from a donor. The new stem cells must match the genetic makeup of the client's own marrow as perfectly as possible.
Syngeneic	The donor is an identical twin, whose marrow genetically matches the client.
Umbilical cord blood	Hematopoietic stem cells collected from the placenta, after birth, are used as the source of cells for marrow regeneration. These cells must match the genetic makeup of the client as perfectly as possible.

Hematopoietic stem cell transplantation consists of three phases: (1) pretransplant, (2) transplant, and (3) posttransplant. The pretransplant phase involves thorough evaluation and testing of the child to assure he or she is physically capable of undergoing transplant. The donor must also undergo several tests to assure that the individual is healthy to undergo anesthesia and free of infectious diseases such as hepatitis or HIV.

During the transplant phase, the **cytoreduction** or conditioning regimen is initiated. Lethal doses of chemotherapy, often combined with radiation, are used to eradicate all malignant cells and to suppress the child's immune system to prevent rejection of the transplanted stem cells. Cytoreduction therapy induces a profound and prolonged decrease in the production of blood cells. The toxicity associated with cytoreduction, such as immunosuppression, may appear soon after transplant and last for many months to years. After the conditioning regimen is delivered, the hematopoietic stem cell infusion is given by IV, similar to the transfusion of a blood product.

During the posttransplant phase, all children have a period of prolonged **pancytopenia** (a marked decrease in the number of RBCs, WBCs, and platelets) immediately after the conditioning, lasting at least three weeks. This period includes the greatest risk of infection, bleeding, and anemia. Clients who receive an allogeneic or cord blood HSCT are also at risk for **graft versus host disease** (GVHD). This immune response is the result of disparities in the HLA match between donor and recipient. The donor white cells perceive the child's body as foreign material to be attacked and destroyed. Graft versus host disease is usually restricted to certain organs such as the skin, gastrointestinal tract, liver, and other organs. The symptoms of GVHD can be minimal to life-threatening and include skin rash beginning on the hands and feet, spreading to other parts of the body; diarrhea; jaundice; and infection. These symptoms are managed with symptomatic support, immunosuppressive drugs, and steroids.

Nurses are responsible for the family orientation, education, and coordination of the pretransplant evaluation. Caregivers and older children may be acutely aware that the only chance of long-term survival may rest on finding a suitable donor for transplantation. Providing emotional support to a family who is waiting for a donor before the child relapses or becomes too ill to undergo HSCT is crucial. During the hospitalization for the transplant phase the nurse is responsible for monitoring the side effects of therapy and maintaining isolation precautions to provide infection control. When the child becomes pancytopenic (marked reduction of white blood cells, red blood cells and platelets), he or she will be dependent upon transfusion support of both red cells and platelets. Mucositis and other side effects of the cytoreduction may make it impossible for the child to eat. Accurate monitoring of intake, output, and the child's weight are necessary. Total parenteral nutrition (TPN) is used in many cases to provide all essential nutrients by the IV route. Careful assessment for signs of infection, vigilant handwashing, and isolation technique is of the utmost importance. Family teaching about infection control should be emphasized daily. At the first sign of infection, cultures are obtained and then IV antibiotics are started. This supportive care posttransplant is a major component that affects the survival of children undergoing HSCT.

EYE ON...

Ethnic Minorities and HSCT Donors

Not all clients who may benefit from an HSCT transplant have a suitable donor. According to the National Cancer Institute (www.cancer.gov), close relatives, especially siblings, are likely to offer a match (25–35%). The chances of obtaining an unrelated donor match are closer to 50% in general. However, children from minority (racial or ethnic) backgrounds have more difficulty finding suitable donors because minority groups are not as well represented in the donor registries. Nursing efforts must continue to concentrate on recruiting minority donors.

Careful nursing assessment of the child's skin, GI tract, and liver function is essential to diagnose and treat GVHD. The earliest sign of GVHD is often a skin rash, first appearing on the hands and feet. It may spread to other parts of the body and include redness and blistering. Graft versus host disease of the gastrointestinal tract presents with diarrhea stools, abdominal pain and cramping, malaise, anorexia, nausea, and vomiting. All stools are monitored for quantity, consistency, and the presence of blood and mucus. The diarrhea may be copious and the need to monitor fluids and electrolytes is essential. Jaundice may indicate that GVHD has affected the liver. The child with elevated liver transaminases and bilirubin must be evaluated for GVHD. Obtaining a biopsy of the affected tissue or organ confirms the diagnosis.

Immunosuppressive drugs increase the risk of infection. Precautions must be taken and taught to the child and family to limit the exposure to harmful bacteria, viruses, and fungi. Each institution has its own infection control measures which may include special air-filtering of the client's room; frequent handwashing; use of masks, gloves, and gowns by anyone coming in contact with the child; the elimination of fresh fruits and vegetables from the child's diet; and not permitting flowers in the room, which can harbor bacteria.

Discharge planning starts when the child's condition stabilizes. With home care nursing services now able to provide parenteral nutrition, antibiotics, and other intravenous medications, children are able to return home sooner than they used to. Hospitalizations that used to last months or years are now typically six weeks or so in duration. Understandably, given the acutely life-threatening condition from which the child is emerging, all families have concerns regarding returning home. Nursing support to prepare the family for this transition is essential.

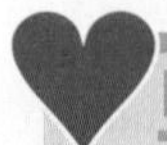

FAMILY TEACHING

Going Home from Stem Cell Transplant

- Obtain all medications prior to discharge. Each medication should be reviewed and a written time schedule given for the administration of each drug.
- Provide caregivers with a follow-up appointment schedule prior to discharge.
- Instruct the child and caregivers of the studies such as blood tests and bone marrow aspirates that will be needed to monitor the child's recovery status.
- Teach caregivers and the child the signs and symptoms of GVHD, and instruct them to report these immediately to the health care provider.
- Reinforce the need to contact the health care provider immediately for fever, signs of infection, or exposure to varicella.
- Refer the child for homebound schooling if available through the local school district.
- Notify school personnel that the child may not be allowed to return for several months posttransplant. The return to school may be facilitated by a visit from the stem cell transplant team nurse to answer questions from the other students, school nurse, or staff.
- Encourage families to ask for help from friends, church groups, and local social service agencies.

BIOLOGIC RESPONSE MODIFIERS

Biologic response modifier (BRM) therapy is also known as biotherapy or immunotherapy. BRM is a relatively new and rapidly expanding modality of cancer treatment (Vizcarra & Belcher, 2006). BRMs are naturally occurring or synthetic agents used to alter biologic responses. They can be used both to stimulate the body's immune system to destroy cancerous cells and to enhance the body's ability to replace normal cells damaged by cancer treatment. Examples of BRMs include colony stimulating factors (CSFs), interleukins, interferons, and monoclonal antibodies.

CSFs are responsible for stimulating and regulating the physiological process of hematopoiesis, which can be accelerated to accommodate the body's needs. They are used to accelerate hematopoietic recovery after chemotherapy, which leads to the reduction of treatment-related hospital admission days and permits the use of aggressive dose-intensive chemotherapy. Epoetin is a CSF that stimulates red cell production. Granulocyte-macrophage colony stimulating factor (GM-CSF) and granulocyte-colony stimulating factor (G-CSF) are examples of CSFs that increase the number of white cells. These factors are used to counteract the myelosuppressive effects of radiation and chemotherapy. Side effects of CSFs include low-grade fever, myalgia, headache, and bone pain (McCune, 2008).

Interleukins and interferons are produced by immune system cells. Interleukins help regulate the intensity and duration of immune responses. They do not directly kill cancer cells, but act as messengers to immune cells, such as lymphocytes, that can destroy cancer cells. Interferons are capable of inhibiting viral replication, modulating immune responses, and altering cellular proliferation. Research is ongoing to determine the best way these agents can aid cancer treatment in children. Side effects of interleukin and interferon therapy include flu-like symptoms among others (McCune, 2008).

Monoclonal antibodies are produced in the laboratory to target specific antigens. This class of drugs is rapidly expanding, with many studies currently in progress, as researchers identify more tumor-related antigens (Vizcarra & Belcher, 2006). Monoclonals have several mechanisms of action. For example, some work by marking cancer cells for immune system destruction while others act to interfere with growth of cancer cells. They are also used in cancer therapy for the delivery of immunotoxins, early cancer detection, and the delivery of radioactive isotopes. The delivery of immunotoxins is achieved by attaching a toxin to the monoclonal antibody, which penetrates the malignant cell and delivers the lethal toxin. Monoclonal antibodies used to detect specific tumors can be "tagged" with radioactive isotopes. This approach can be used for both diagnostic scans and the delivery of therapeutic radiation doses. Because monoclonal antibodies are target-specific, toxicities are generally mild as compared to standard chemotherapy

FAMILY TEACHING

Biologic Response Modifiers

- Instruct the caregivers in subcutaneous injection technique.
- Teach the family about the medication, including the schedule, dose, and side effects. Recommend measures to alleviate symptoms of side effects such as antipyretics for fever.
- Teach the family the importance of frequent monitoring of blood counts.
- Instruct caregivers in precautions required with monoclonal antibodies combined with chemotherapy or radioisotopes.
- Provide written information about the BRM to the caregiver to share with the school.

REFLECTIVE THINKING

The Side Effects of Cancer Therapy

Caregivers of children newly diagnosed with cancer suddenly find themselves in a medical environment inundated with information. By the time the diagnosis is made, many caregivers are emotionally distraught and physically exhausted. At this time of emotional stress, they are told of the potentially lifesaving treatments, which have a high risk of creating new lifelong side effects. The treatment in some cases may seem as horrible as the cancer, but not treating will ensure the death of the child. The health care team must take the time to teach the caregivers about the disease and the proposed treatment so that a truly informed consent can be granted. How can you support caregivers who find themselves in this situation?

(Smith, 2006). Side effects include fever, arthralgia, pruritus, and, in some cases, anaphylaxis (McCune, 2008).

Nurses who care for children receiving BRM therapy must be familiar with the biology of the disease being treated and the function and side effects of the specific BRM in order to safely treat the patient. Each BRM has specific potential side effects ranging from mild fatigue to severe anaphylaxis. Caregivers must be taught about the agent and learn potential side effects. Colony-stimulating factors (CSFs) and interferons are given subcutaneously and usually in the home; therefore, caregivers will need to learn how to administer the agent. Children who receive BRMs, especially CSF, will need frequent monitoring of their CBC to make decisions regarding the continuation of the drug. Caregivers should be instructed to give acetaminophen prior to giving interferon to prevent the fever associated with this agent. It is important that caregivers assess for fever associated with infection prior to the administration of acetaminophen. Caregivers of children receiving monoclonal antibodies combined with chemotherapy or radioisotopes must be taught appropriate body fluid precautions.

LEUKEMIA

Leukemia is a broad term describing a group of malignant diseases in which normal bone marrow elements are replaced by abnormal immature lymphocytes, known as blast cells. It is the most common childhood malignancy in those under 15 years of age. In children, two forms of leukemia are generally recognized: acute lymphocytic leukemia (ALL) and acute myelogenous leukemia (AML).

ACUTE LYMPHOCYTIC LEUKEMIA

Incidence and Etiology

Acute lymphocytic leukemia (ALL) is the most common cancer diagnosed in children. There are approximately 2,400 new cases diagnosed in the United States each year (Westlake & Bertolone, 2007). A variety of agents have been implicated that might increase the risk of developing leukemia, including viruses, irradiation, exposure to certain toxic chemicals or drugs such as benzene, and a genetic predisposition. The etiology of most cases of ALL is unknown.

Pathophysiology

Acute lymphocytic leukemia develops when a single lymphoid cell undergoes malignant transformation and proliferates uncontrollably. In the bone marrow of an individual with ALL the invasion of these malignant **lymphoblasts**, or immature white cells, causes a "crowding out" of normal red blood cells, platelets, and white blood cells, resulting in pancytopenia and immunosuppression.

Clinical Manifestations

The most common presenting signs of ALL are fever, bone pain, pallor, and bruising. Most children diagnosed with ALL have been symptomatic for only one or two weeks. The clinical manifestations arise from the affected organs.

Diagnosis

A bone marrow aspirate (BMA) is required to make the diagnosis of ALL, and a finding of more than 25% of abnormal lymphoblasts in the bone marrow confirms the diagnosis. Other samples of the bone marrow are sent for further testing, which can show chromosomal changes and better identify the biological markers of the leukemia. The child's white blood count and age at diagnosis are the most important prognostic signs in ALL. The best prognosis is a WBC less than 5,000/mm^3 and an age of 2–9 years, and the worst prognosis is an initial WBC of 50,000/mm^3 or more and an age younger than two years and older than 10 years. A lumbar puncture is done to assess for the presence of leukemia cells in the cerebral spinal fluid. If leukemia cells are present, central nervous system (CNS) involvement is verified. A chest X-ray is obtained to detect a mediastinal mass. Laboratory findings will show liver or kidney involvement. Optimal treatment depends on identifying the origin of the leukemia, such as B cell precursor, mature B cell precursor, or T cell. Knowing the origin, chromosomal abnormalities and biological markers of the leukemic blast cells is significant in determining the treatment and the prognosis of the child.

Treatment

ALL is treated with systemic chemotherapy and includes three phases: induction, consolidation, and maintenance. The goal in the **induction phase** is to reduce the tumor burden to an undetectable level, a state known as remission. In remission there is no evidence of leukemia on physical exam, bone marrow evaluation, peripheral blood counts, in the CSF, or any other **extramedullary** (outside the bone marrow) site. Ninety-five percent of children with ALL achieve remission during induction, which usually lasts four weeks. Once remission is achieved most children will relapse within a few months if treatment is stopped, indicating the existence of undetectable blasts and the necessity of continuation of therapy. Remission induction is achieved by treating the child with the chemotherapeutic agents, vincristine (Oncovin), L-asparaginase (Elspar), and prednisone. Children who have a poorer prognosis will have an **anthracycline** drug (chemotherapeutic agents known to affect the heart by damaging cardiac myocytes), such as doxorubicin (Adriamycin), added to this phase (Table 29-4). Once the child is stable, this phase of treatment is administered in the outpatient clinic. Presenting symptoms, such as anemia, infection, or bleeding are treated at the time of diagnosis. Once chemotherapy begins, the release of purines from the destroyed leukemic lymphoblasts causes an elevation of uric acid, which can lead to acute renal failure. This is called **tumor lysis syndrome**. This complication is prevented with IV hydration containing sodium bicarbonate to alkalinize the urine to a pH of 7 or 8. Allopurinol (Zyloprim) is also given to aid in the excretion of uric acid through the kidneys, preventing renal obstruction and failure. Tumor lysis syndrome occurs more frequently and severely with children who have a greater tumor burden, such as those with a high WBC of 50,000 or greater or extensive lymphadenopathy.

Leukemia cells can cross the blood-brain barrier and most drugs that are effective treatment do not. Children with ALL receive CNS prophylaxis with chemotherapy instilled **intrathecally** (IT), into the cerebral spinal fluid space during a lumbar puncture. Children who present with CNS disease at diagnosis will also receive radiation therapy to the brain and spinal cord to eradicate malignant leukemic cells. Some clinical trials treat children with radiation to the brain if they present with WBC of 50,000/mm^3 or greater, to reduce their risk of CNS disease. Radiation to the testes is reserved for males with testicular involvement of ALL.

The next phase of treatment is called **consolidation** or intensification and aims at eradicating any residual leukemic cells, and starts promptly once remission is attained. Chemotherapy is frequently given in high doses, often requiring hospitalization during this phase of treatment. The administration of IT medications is frequent and radiation therapy to the brain may be given for CNS prophylaxis or treatment during this phase. Children who have extramedullary disease, such as testicular involvement, will receive radiation to those sites at this time. This phase of therapy is intense and lasts several months.

Reflections from Families

My child and the entire family had been counting the admissions, spinal taps, and weeks of chemotherapy left until the treatment was complete. As the "big day" grew near, though, we were all surprised to find ourselves anxious. Although the treatment was stressful, we all felt some comfort that the chemotherapy was keeping the cancer away. What will happen when the chemotherapy ends?

The **maintenance** phase follows consolidation and maintains control of the leukemia with most chemotherapeutic agents administered by the oral, IV, or IM routes. During this phase, occasional intravenous injections of vincristine and lumbar punctures with IT chemotherapy may be given. Most centers continue therapy for two-and-a-half to three years after diagnosis. Children who maintain a complete continuous remission during this time electively discontinue treatment. Today, remission can be induced in 95% of children. With current treatment regimens, event-free survival rates for childhood acute lymphocytic leukemia approach or exceed 80% (Vrooman & Silverman, 2009).

The completion of chemotherapy is a goal that many caregivers and children look forward to with a hope to return to a "normal life" again. It is also met with high anxiety and fear that if no further therapy is given, the child will relapse. The family needs to be assured that there is no significant advantage to

NURSING TIP

Medication Swallowing

Prednisone, a frequently used medication in leukemia therapy, tastes very bitter and many children have difficulty taking it. Prednisone may be given crushed in ice cream, mixed in chocolate syrup, crushed and placed in blank capsules, mixed in applesauce, or placed in a fruit roll-up. It should be given with milk or an antacid to prevent heartburn. Enteric-coated or time-released tablets and capsules should never be crushed before giving.

Antibiotics in 30 Minutes or Less for Febrile Neutropenic Patients: A Quality Control Measure in a New Hospital

STUDY PURPOSE

To identify what prompt antibiotic administration means. Medical literature reports that prompt empiric antibiotic therapy to prevent death caused by virulent organisms is the standard of care; however, the literature fails to identify what prompt antibiotic delivery means.

METHODS

Nurses, as part of an education series at the opening of a new center, were informed of the goal of antibiotics delivery within 30 minutes to all febrile neutropenic patients. Standardized orders were developed. Two months after admitting patients, an antibiotic tracking log was placed on the units to monitor patient's arrival, temperature spike, and delivery of medications to the floor and patient. Causes for delays of antibiotic delivery were monitored.

FINDINGS	ACTIONS
Not all patient rooms were set up for a potentially septic patient, with the presence of manual resuscitation and suction equipment at the bedside, causing the nurse to gather these before initiating antibiotics.	Required verification of equipment for patient to be admitted to room.
A delay was noted when patient information was not entered in the computer system until the patient arrived on the unit causing a delay in getting the antibiotics from pharmacy.	Admission process altered to accept the admission of patient information into computer before patient's arrival to hospital. Physician calls bed control to inform of patient's pending admission and provides verbal and written orders to the admitting nurse. Pharmacy will then prepare antibiotics and may potentially have them on the floor before patient's arrival. The clinical pharmacist provided orientation to pharmacy staff on the importance of prompt delivery of antibiotic. Pharmacy developed their own tracking system of arrival of orders and delivery to floor time. After several months, the pharmacy also provided the unit with standard doses of antibiotics for the units automatic medication station to cover the initial STAT dose.
Ordering practitioners were forgetting to use the readily available antibiotics in the automatic medication systems.	Staff nurses were asked to remind practitioners of the availability of antibiotics on the unit.
Nurses reported being unfamiliar with how to override the medication doses in the automatic medication stations.	Signs were posted in the medication rooms listing the steps needed to give STAT antibiotics. Incident reports were issued on any case where the goal of 30-minute door-to-administration-of-antibiotics was unmet.
Disruption in paging system.	Back-up with cell phones provided.

IMPLICATIONS

After 20 months of monitoring the delivery of antibiotics to febrile neutropenic patients within 30 minutes of arrival to hospital, no patients were transferred to the intensive care unit due to septic shock. No deaths were reported due to bacteremia. Monitoring is ongoing. With the collaboration and willingness to change previous practices, physicians, nursing, pharmacy, and hospital bed control of a new hospital all contributed and achieved the goal of antibiotic delivery within 30 minutes of arrival to hospital. Months of monitoring and implementing changes to achieve this goal were promptly addressed and instituted.

REFERENCE

Corey, A., & Snyder, S. (2008). Antibiotics in 30 minutes or less for febrile neutropenic patients: A quality control measure in a new hospital. *Journal of Pediatric Oncology Nursing*, *25*(4), 208–212.

continuing therapy beyond this period. All phases of therapy depend upon guidelines set by each child's specific clinical trial.

Unfortunately, regardless of all the success in the treatment of ALL, a number of children will relapse and those who relapse while on therapy or within six months of completing treatment have a very poor prognosis. Hematopoietic stem cell transplant is a treatment option for children with ALL who attain a second remission after relapse and who have a compatible bone marrow donor.

ACUTE MYELOGENOUS LEUKEMIA

Acute myelogenous leukemia (AML) is the second most common type of leukemia in children. Children with AML have a poorer prognosis than those with ALL. Greater than 30% of leukemia deaths are attributed to AML (Golub & Arceci, 2007).

Incidence and Etiology

AML represents about 15% of all children diagnosed with leukemia, with approximately 1,000 children diagnosed each year in the United States. It is more common in the Hispanic population and has a higher incidence in African Americans when compared to Caucasians (McCarthy, 2008). The frequency of AML remains stable throughout childhood but there is a slight increase during adolescence (Golub & Arceci, 2007).

The etiology is not known, but certain predisposing factors have been associated with AML. Risk factors such as exposure to radiation and chemotherapy for the treatment of a previous cancer, exposure to benzene, genetic predisposition in children with Down syndrome, and Fanconi's anemia have been identified (Golub & Arceci, 2007).

Pathophysiology

As in ALL, the malignant myeloid blasts crowd out the normal WBC, platelets, and red blood cells, causing neutropenia and immunosuppression, thrombocytopenia, and anemia.

Clinical Manifestations

Children with AML may present with seemingly benign symptoms resembling the flu (i.e., fever, fatigue, malaise, anorexia) or may be severe and life-threatening (i.e., bleeding and severe hemorrhage). Bleeding at the time of diagnosis is usually associated with thrombocytopenia but may also be caused by disseminated intravascular coagulation (DIC). A particular subtype of AML, specifically acute promyelocytic leukemia, is associated with DIC. Children with AML may present with gingival hypertrophy caused by infiltration of the gums with malignant myeloid cells. **Chloromas** are localized collections of malignant cells. When this occurs in the skin or subcutaneous tissue, it presents as a nodular protuberance in the skin. There is a higher incidence of CNS disease at diagnosis with AML than with ALL, but the clinical manifestations are the same. In AML the CNS symptoms may also be caused by a chloroma in the brain. An epidural chloroma may manifest by difficulty walking or incontinence of urine and stool caused by spinal cord compression. Enlargement of the liver and spleen is often seen at initial presentation; significant lymphadenopathy occurs less often.

Diagnosis

A bone marrow aspirate, showing 25% malignant myeloid blasts, confirms the diagnosis of AML.

Treatment

Once a diagnosis is made, treatment begins promptly, attending to the presenting symptoms such as anemia, bleeding from thrombocytopenia or DIC, infection, and metabolic abnormalities such as hyperuricemia. The treatment of hyperuricemia, anemia, thrombocytopenia, and neutropenia are addressed in the ALL section of this chapter. DIC is best treated with the aggressive management of the underlying disease process. Many children will require platelet transfusions as well as the replacement of coagulation factors such as cryoprecipitate, and fresh frozen plasma to control bleeding. Red cell transfusions may be necessary to replace blood loss and maintain tissue perfusion.

Treatment of AML is with systemic chemotherapy. The phases of AML treatment are remission induction and continuation therapy. Chemotherapy drugs such as cytarabine (Ara-C) and an anthracycline agent such as daunorubicin (Daunomycin) are used in the induction phase. After remission is achieved many clinical trials call for a continuation with intense high dose chemotherapeutic agents such as cytarabine, cyclophosphamide (Cytoxan), anthracyclines, and etoposide (VePesid). Treatment of the CNS is with cytarabine or methotrexate (MTX) given intrathecally. Radiation to the head may be part of CNS therapy and prophylaxis. Hematopoietic stem cell transplantation has been used for the treatment of AML once remission is achieved and a suitable donor is available. Therapy for AML is very intense, and is usually given as an inpatient. Children who receive this intense chemotherapy often are hospitalized for lengthy periods of time because of pancytopenia and fever.

Children in first remission, with identical HLA matched siblings, will be referred for hematopoietic stem cell transplantation since this approach is superior to continuation chemotherapy with the exclusion of children with Down syndrome (Landier, 2007).

Nursing Management

Nursing management is similar to that of ALL. Children with AML are at high risk for bleeding related to DIC. Assessment for signs of bleeding such as a change in vital signs, including a decrease in blood pressure or increase in heart rate, is important. Physical assessment of the mucous membranes and skin includes looking for petechiae or bruising. Bleeding may be seen at needle puncture sites even hours after the puncture. Trends in laboratory findings that suggest DIC include a prolongation of the prothrombin time, a decrease in platelet count, and a decrease in fibrinogen levels.

BRAIN TUMORS

Brain tumors are the most common solid tumor of childhood, and are second only to leukemia among childhood malignancies. Brain tumors are the third leading cause of death in children under 16 years, and prognosis varies depending upon the age of the child at diagnosis, pathology, and location of the tumor. Histology, or cell structure, and location determine the classification of brain tumors.

INCIDENCE AND ETIOLOGY

Approximately 3,750 children younger than 20 years old are diagnosed annually with central nervous system (CNS) tumors in the United States with a slightly greater risk for boys than girls. While the cause of most pediatric brain tumors remains unknown, this is the most common solid tumor in children. A strong link exists between hereditary and environmental factors and the occurrence of certain brain tumors. Certain hereditary diseases such as neurofibromatosis and tuberous sclerosis are associated with certain rare brain tumors. Environmental factors, such as industrial and chemical toxins and ionizing radiation, have been related to an increase in pediatric brain tumors, although epidemiologic evidence is lacking. Children who received cranial irradiation for the treatment of previous malignancies have an increased risk of brain tumors (American Brain Tumor Association, 2007).

PATHOPHYSIOLOGY

Brain tumors are classified according to their histology and location. Sixty percent of pediatric brain tumors arise from **glial cells**, which are the supporting cell structures of the brain. These include astrocytoma, brain stem gliomas, and ependymomas. Brain tumors arising from neurons or their precursors include primitive neuroectodermal tumors (PNET) and medulloblastoma.

The location of the tumor makes a further classification and includes infratentorial, supratentorial, and midline tumors. About 60% of all pediatric brain tumors are **infratentorial** (in the posterior third of the brain, primarily in the cerebellum and brain stem and below the tentorium). The **tentorium** is the dura mater located between the cerebrum and cerebellum supporting the occipital lobes. These include the following types of tumors: medulloblastoma, cerebellar astrocytoma, brain stem glioma, and ependymoma. **Supratentorial** tumors occur in the anterior two-thirds of the brain above the tentorium, primarily in the cerebrum. These include cerebral astrocytomas. Other brain tumors occur in the midline (third and fourth ventricles, optic chiasm, and brain stem) and include optic nerve gliomas, craniopharyngiomas, and pineal region tumors. Astrocytomas are the most common type of CNS tumors in children (50%), followed by medulloblastomas (20%), brain stem gliomas (10–15%), ependymomas (10%), and others (5%) (Ryan-Murray & Petriccione, 2007).

CLINICAL MANIFESTATIONS

Initial symptoms of childhood brain tumors are often vague and mimic common childhood illnesses. They include irritability, vomiting, and anorexia. Increased intracranial pressure is frequently seen in the infratentorial tumors of the posterior fossa, caused by the tumor itself or indirectly by an obstruction of the flow of cerebrospinal fluid. Symptoms include headache and vomiting, which may be worse in the morning. The vomiting may temporarily relieve the headache. Younger children may present with irritability and an increase in head circumference. Infants with increased intracranial pressure may have a raised or tense anterior fontanel, which may not close as expected between 8 and 18 months. Loss or delay of developmental milestones is a frequent finding in infants and toddlers with brain tumors. A young child who no longer does an activity he or she has mastered, such as walking or sitting up, needs a careful evaluation. Diplopia or double vision may be present but is difficult to diagnose in a young child. The young child with diplopia may tilt the head or use a hand to cover one eye. Ataxia, unsteady uncoordinated movement, nystagmus, rhythmic oscillation of the eyes and impaired upward gaze can also be signs of increased intracranial pressure (Watral, 2008).

Brain stem tumors are associated with cranial nerve abnormalities, hemiparesis, a weakness of one side of the body, and a spastic gait. A complete neurological examination will show a positive Babinski's sign. The symptoms associated with increased intracranial pressure caused by tumor growth will not appear until late in the course of the disease with brain stem tumors. Children with supratentorial tumors commonly present with a hemiparesis, **hemisensory** loss, a decrease or loss of function of a sense organ on one side of the body, seizures, visual field changes, and cognitive problems. Midline tumors are associated with visual field and acuity changes, personality changes, and endocrine system problems such as precocious puberty. Isolated spinal cord tumors are rare and comprise a small percentage of CNS tumors. Presenting symptoms may include leg weakness or difficulty walking, change in bowel or bladder habits, and back pain that could extend toward the extremities. Again, developmental milestones may be delayed. The presenting symptoms of a child with a brain

TABLE 29-6 Common Pediatric Brain Tumors: Symptoms and Treatment

TUMOR TYPE	TUMOR & INCIDENCE	SYMPTOMS	TREATMENT
Infratentorial or posterior fossa	Medulloblastoma 20%	Increased ICP, headache, morning vomiting, ataxia, lethargy, irritability, loss of appetite, increased head size	Maximal surgical resection and cranial or spinal radiation* and chemotherapy
	Ependymoma 3–6%	Neck pain, increased ICP, increased head size, irritability, sleepiness, vomiting, morning headache	Maximal surgical resection and radiation* or chemotherapy
	Brain stem glioma 10–20%	Eye movement abnormalities, diplopia, headache, nausea, vomiting, Cranial nerve deficits, increased ICP, hemiparesis	Radiation chemotherapy if there is tumor progression after radiation; surgery only if the tumor appears contained or outside of the brain stem.
Supratentorial	Low-grade astrocytoma 15–25%	Seizures, visual changes, endocrinopathies, incidental finding: hemiparesis	>90% surgical removal and observation <90% surgical removal, observation or radiation* or chemotherapy
	High-grade astrocytoma 9%	Seizures, increased ICP, mental status change, hemiparesis, seizure	Maximal surgical removal and radiation or chemotherapy
Midline	Optic-nerve chiasmal gliomas 5%	Seizures, endocrinopathies, increased ICP, visual changes	Observation, chemotherapy, radiation or surgical debulking
	Craniopharyngiomas 6–9%	Seizures, visual changes, increased ICP, endocrinopathies—short stature, delayed puberty	<95% surgical removal, observation >95% surgical removal, reoperation, or radiation*
	Pineal region 2%	Increased ICP, no upward gaze, diplopia, nausea, vomiting, Headache	Low-grade: surgery alone, radiation High-grade: surgery, radiation,* and chemotherapy

** Delay radiation therapy in children younger than five years of age.*

References: Adapted from American Brain Tumor Association. (2007) *A primer of brain tumors, a patient's reference manual* (8th ed.). Des Plaines, IL: Author. Source: Blaney, S. M., Kun, L. E., Hunter, J., Rorke-Adams, L. B., Lau, C., Strother, D., & Pollack, I. F. (2006). Tumors of the Central Nervous System. In P. A. Pizzo & D. G. Poplack (Eds.). *Principles and practice of pediatric oncology* (5th ed.). Philadelphia, PA: Lippincott, Williams & Wilkins, pp. 786–851.

tumor can lead the health care providers to suspect specific locations of the tumor. See Table 29-6 for the common presenting symptoms and treatment of specific pediatric brain tumors.

DIAGNOSIS

Any child who displays signs of increased intracranial pressure or other neurological symptoms such as ataxia, visual disturbances, or hemiparesis needs to be referred for a complete physical and neurological examination. The diagnostic work-up of a child with neurological symptoms includes magnetic resonance imaging (MRI), which has replaced computerized tomography (CT) as the most common first diagnostic test obtained. Both tests have advantages and disadvantages.

MRI creates an image of the brain in three different planes, which allows for exact localization of the tumor. MRI best defines neuroanatomy and tumor margins. This complete picture of the tumor can be helpful to the neurosurgeon in planning the surgical approach and to the oncologist in evaluating growth of the tumor over time. MRI of the spine is the diagnostic method most used to evaluate spread of the tumor to the spinal cord.

There are disadvantages of MRI, which relate to the lengthy time that the child must remain motionless inside a dark noisy tube to obtain the scan. It takes about one hour and can be frightening to a young child. Sedation or anesthesia may be needed to obtain the scan. It is difficult to safely monitor a seriously ill child during this test especially when sedation or anesthesia is required.

CT scan is still a useful diagnostic tool for the evaluation of a child with a brain tumor. It is easier and less expensive to perform than MRI. CT scan is a quick test, taking five to ten minutes and is less affected by body motion than MRI. Many children can tolerate a CT without sedation. It is most useful when there is a sudden change in neurological status that needs evaluation.

Other studies are used in limited situations. Angiography contributes to preoperative evaluation of the vascularity of the tumor, which is helpful to the neurosurgeon in planning how to approach the tumor surgically. Magnetic resonance angiography (MRA) has replaced angiography in many situations because it is noninvasive and can often provide the same information. The positron-emission tomography (PET) scan and the thallium single photon emission computed tomography (SPECT) scan both provide information about residual abnormalities after treatment. They help to distinguish between recurrent tumor cells versus cells killed by radiation versus scar tissue. With advances in computer technology, more and more specific diagnostic tests will be made available. A biopsy is performed in all but brain stem tumors, where the risk of surgical complication is too great and the knowledge gained will add little to treatment decisions. A biopsy may be done as a separate surgical procedure or as part of the surgery to remove the tumor.

TREATMENT

Pediatric brain tumors are treated on an individual basis and may include surgery, radiation therapy, or chemotherapy, or a combination of all these modalities. The actual plan of treatment depends upon the location and pathology of the tumor and the age of the child (Figure 29-10). Radiation or chemotherapy are often major components of the plan. Surgery is used to remove as much of the tumor as possible while preserving normal brain function. Prognosis is improved when all or most of the tumor can be surgically removed. In the postoperative period, intravenous steroids such as dexamethasone (Decadron) are used to prevent edema within the brain and are tapered gradually. Anticonvulsants are indicated for children with supratentorial lesions where seizures are possible.

The goal of radiation therapy is to destroy tumor cells while sparing normal brain tissue. Because of the damage that radiation causes to the developing brain, such as intellectual and growth impairment, it is avoided in children who are less than three years old, if possible. When radiation therapy is used to treat brain tumors, the dose is usually high, and the toxicity can be severe.

Continued care will be required for many CNS tumor children. A multidisciplinary approach provides the best continuity for the child, family, and the medical team. Ophthalmology, audiology, physical therapy, occupational therapy, and speech may need to be part of the team with routine oncology, surgery, and radiation follow-up.

> **NURSING TIP**
>
> **Sedation for Neurodiagnostic Testing**
>
> Adequate sedation is necessary in obtaining the needed neurodiagnostic information to confirm the diagnosis of a brain tumor. Sedation protocols vary from institution to institution, but sleep deprivation can enhance the effects of sedation. Advising caregivers to put the child to sleep an hour or two later the night before a procedure and then waking her or him a few hours earlier will enhance the effects of the medication. All children who are sedated must be monitored carefully with pulse oximetry and telemetry to prevent complications of over-sedation.

In the last decade, chemotherapy has emerged as standard care in the treatment of certain pediatric brain tumors. The drugs most commonly used in brain tumor treatment include the nitrosoureas (carmustine [BCNU] and lomustine [CNU]), cisplatin, vincristine, etoposide, carboplatin, ifosfamide, avastin, and topotecan (Table 29-4 Chemotherapeutic Agents). These agents are given in intense doses and are sometimes included in a regime with autologous hematopoietic stem cell transplant to rescue the child from the toxic effects of the drugs. Chemotherapy is

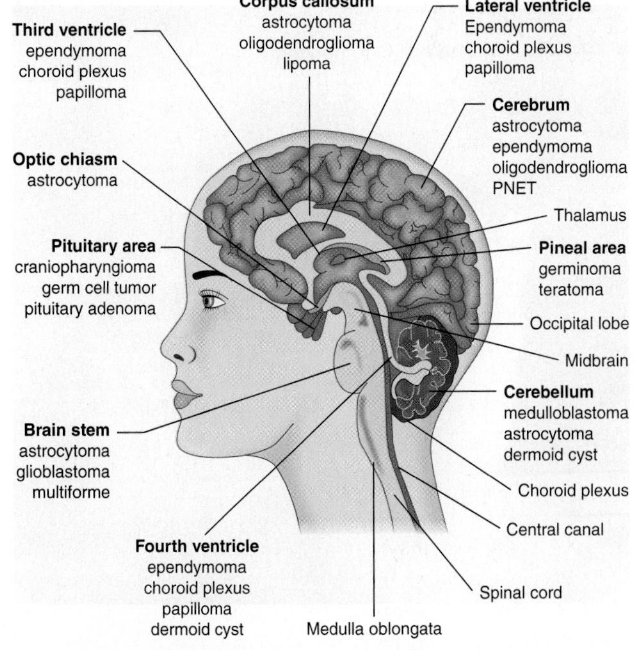

FIGURE 29-10 Common Childhood Brain Tumors and Their Location. SOURCE: CHILDHOOD BRAIN TUMOR FOUNDATION. (2009). JEANNE YOUNG, ARTIST. RETRIEVED MARCH 30, 2009, FROM WWW.CHILDHOODBRAINTUMOR.ORG (USED WITH PERMISSION).

often used in children younger than three years of age to delay or eliminate the necessity of radiation therapy.

NURSING MANAGEMENT

The focus of the physical assessment of the child with a brain tumor is dictated by the clinical manifestations. A thorough neurological assessment is performed before surgery and includes vital signs; pupil size, equality, and response to light; level of consciousness; and strength and equality of grip. Head circumference measurement and assessment of the anterior fontanel in infants is necessary to evaluate increasing intracranial pressure. Seizure precautions are instituted both preoperatively and postoperatively. The nurse assesses the child for developmental and behavioral alterations. Behavior changes, school performance, and social interactions should be ascertained.

Caregivers, whose child has been diagnosed with a brain tumor, as with other tumors, are faced with the real concern of having their child die. They must also face the possibility that their child, who was healthy and active only a short time ago, may now have severe physical, intellectual, and growth impairments. During the prediagnosis period, nursing care includes providing support and coordination of the many diagnostic procedures, which can help reduce some of the stress experienced by the child and caregiver. Using role-play to teach the child about the tests can sometimes reduce the need for sedation during scans.

Once a tumor is identified, surgery is planned. Caregivers often do not have adequate time to comprehend all that is being asked of them. Being available, answering questions, providing written information, and providing emotional support are important nursing responsibilities. Preparing the child and caregivers for the postoperative stay in the intensive care unit is crucial. Postoperative care of the child who has had a craniotomy usually includes several days in an intensive care unit. Because of the surgical trauma to the brain, there is a chance of developing edema and increased intracranial pressure; therefore, frequent neurological assessment and monitoring of vital signs is essential. Careful monitoring of fluid and electrolyte balance is another important aspect of nursing care. The need to identify and prevent increased intracranial pressure is paramount. Usually the child has an MRI within a few days postoperatively to determine the extent of any residual tumor. Steroids are given intravenously at first but later changed to the oral route, and then the dosage is slowly tapered. Caregivers and the child must be made aware of the side effects of this medication, including mood swings, increased appetite, and changes in body shape and weight. Assurance that the moon face and weight gain from steroids is temporary and will disappear once the medication is withdrawn is helpful (Figure 29-11). The combination of chemotherapy and radiation can result in heightened toxicity. For example, cisplatin with radiation increases the risk of ototoxicity, resulting in severe hearing loss. After the immediate postoperative period, the child is often evaluated with audiologic, neuropsychological, and repeated scans to determine the response to therapy and side effects.

Caregivers may become overwhelmed with the physical, emotional, and financial demands that the diagnosis of a

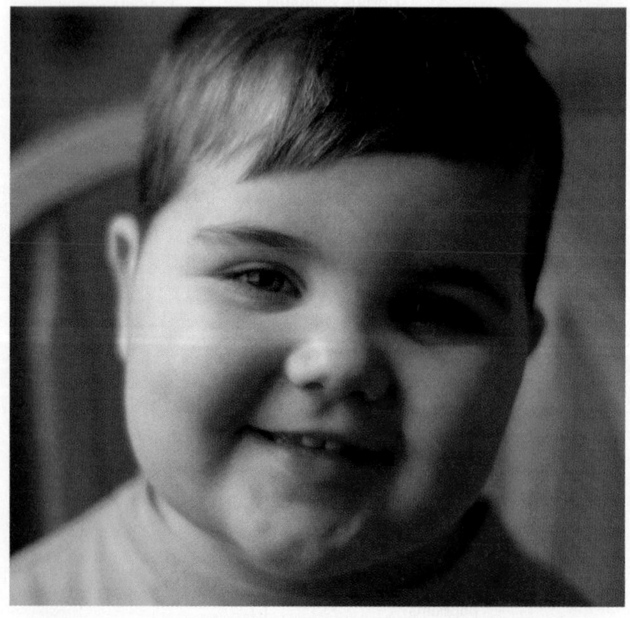

A

FIGURE 29-11A The child received corticosteroids as a chemotherapeutic agent. Notice the "moon face" and prominent cheeks. DELMAR CENGAGE LEARNING.

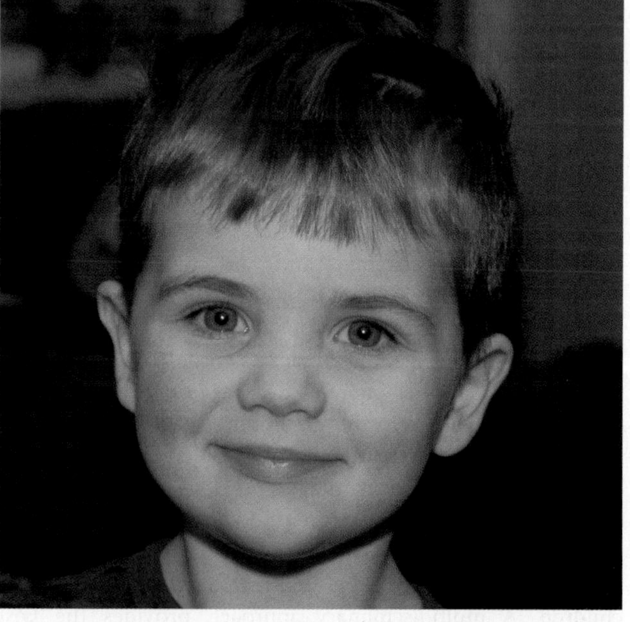

B

FIGURE 29-11B Resolution of the steroid "moon face" will take several weeks after the medication is discontinued. DELMAR CENGAGE LEARNING.

NURSING ALERT

Safety Precautions for Children with Ataxia

Children with ataxia have difficulty walking and are at risk of falling and injury. Some children need pediatric walkers or the assistance of an adult to walk. They should be referred to physical therapy for neuromuscular retraining and muscle strengthening. Safety issues to be addressed prior to going home include gates for stairways and doors and placing pads on sharp furniture corners.

brain tumor in their child brings. Nurses can be instrumental in helping them cope by introducing them to other members of the multidisciplinary team and families who have managed a similar difficult situation. It is also important for nurses to help families identify other sources of support, such as the extended family, friends, religious organizations, and childhood cancer support groups.

LYMPHOMAS

Lymphoma is a malignancy that arises from the lymphoid system. Lymphatic tissue is present throughout the body and is responsible for recognizing and destroying foreign invaders. Lymphatic tissue is responsible for developing competent lymphocytes to perform this task. Lymphomas are a malignant transformation of these cells. There are two types of lymphomas seen in children: Hodgkin's disease (HD) and non-Hodgkin's lymphoma (NHL). Malignant lymphomas are the third most common type of childhood cancer.

HODGKIN'S DISEASE

Hodgkin's disease (HD) usually originates in a cervical lymph node. It spreads to other lymph node regions. If left untreated, it spreads to the organs.

Incidence and Etiology

Hodgkin's disease (HD) has a unique bimodal age distribution that differs based on geography, ethnicity, and socioeconomic status. In industrialized countries the early peak incidence occurs in the middle to late twenties with the second peak after the age of 50. In developing countries the early peak occurs before adolescence. There is a slight overall male predominance. HD is rarely diagnosed before the age of five years. The etiology is unknown; however, the role of an infectious agent has been implicated. Indirect associations between Epstein-Barr virus (EBV) and HD have been reported, but the DNA of EBV has not been isolated in tumor tissue (Androkities, 2008).

Pathophysiology

HD originates in the lymphatic system and is differentiated from other lymphomatous diseases by its histology. The malignant cell is more differentiated than with NHL, and the pattern of infiltration is more specific. HD is classified by histology into four types: nodular sclerosing, mixed cellularity, lymphocyte predominant, and lymphocyte depleted.

Clinical Manifestations

The onset of HD is commonly not acute in nature, and the child may have had symptoms for a prolonged time prior to seeking medical attention. The disease is usually localized at the time of diagnosis. The usual presentation is painless enlarged lymph nodes. The most common sites of presentation are the cervical and supraclavicular areas. Other symptoms may include malaise, anorexia, night sweats, and fever. Most children have localized disease at the time of diagnosis, but HD can metastasize to the spleen, bone marrow, and lungs (Figure 29-12). It is necessary to obtain a staging evaluation to determine the extent of disease and to plan treatment.

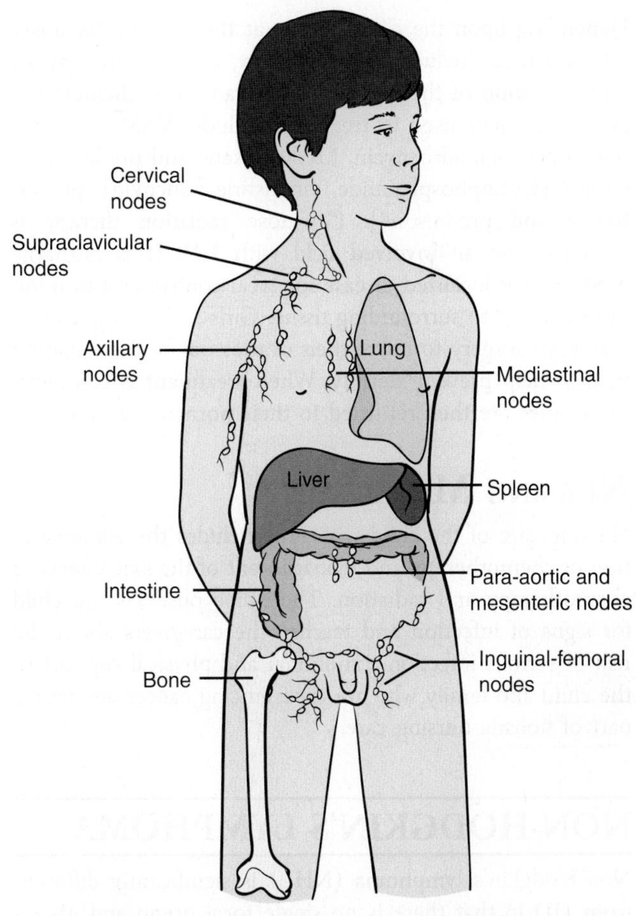

Figure 29-12 Lymph Nodes Affected by Hodgkin's Disease.

Diagnosis

Diagnosis of HD is made by biopsy of an affected node and histologic classification by the pathologist. Staging of the disease helps determine the prognosis and is determined by the extent of lymph node involvement. A staging evaluation includes chest X-ray and CT of the chest, abdomen, and pelvis to assess for distant lymph node involvement. Stages range from I to IV, with I having the best prognosis and IV the worst. A gallium scan may be used to assess for metastatic disease. Bone marrow aspirates and biopsies are performed to assess for marrow involvement. Laboratory tests will include a CBC and liver function tests. Abnormalities noted in these tests suggest marrow or liver disease, respectively. The child's erythrocyte sedimentation rate (ESR), ferritin, and copper levels may be elevated at the time of diagnosis.

For those children who will undergo chemotherapy or radiation therapy, pulmonary function tests and a cardiac evaluation are needed as a baseline evaluation of these organs. Bleomycin (Bleo) and doxorubicin (Adriamycin) are two commonly used drugs in HD that may affect these organs. Baseline thyroid studies are helpful, especially if the treatment plan will include radiation to the neck area.

Treatment

Depending upon the clinical stage at the time of diagnosis, HD treatment includes chemotherapy, radiation therapy, or a combination of these modalities. Traditional chemotherapeutic regimens used to treat HD include: VAMP (vincristine [oncovin], adriamycin, Methotrexate, and prednisone); COPP (Cyclophosphaimide, vincristine [oncovin], procarbazine and prednisone). Low-dose radiation therapy is used to treat an involved field with HD. It is primarily used to treat localized disease for local control and to minimize damage to surrounding tissue. Girls and young women may have surgery to move their ovaries out of the radiation field to help prevent sterility. When treatment is complete, the ovaries are then returned to their normal position.

Nursing Management

Nursing care of the child with HD includes the administration of chemotherapy and management of the side effects of chemotherapy and radiation. The nurse observes the child for signs of infection and teaches the caregivers about the risk of serious infection. Emotional and physical support to the child and family who are experiencing cancer are always part of holistic nursing care.

NON-HODGKIN'S LYMPHOMA

Non-Hodgkin's lymphoma (NHL) is significantly different from HD in that there is no single focal origin and, therefore, the malignant cells are rarely localized. Also, NHL has a rapid onset and presents with widespread involvement.

Incidence and Etiology

NHL is more common than HD in children less than 10 years old. There are approximately 750–800 new cases each year in the United States. Boys are affected more than girls; and like HD it is uncommon under the age of five years (Androkities, 2008). The cause of NHL is unknown although viral, genetic, immunologic, and environmental factors have been implicated. Children with congenital and acquired immune deficiencies, including children post-organ transplant, have a higher risk of developing NHL. Children with AIDS often present with primary lymphoma of the CNS.

Pathophysiology

Because NHL is a malignancy of the lymph system, which is widely spread throughout the body, this disease is often generalized at diagnosis. Non-Hodgkin's lymphomas of childhood are distinct from the lymphomas of adults. Childhood NHL is extremely aggressive in its ability to proliferate and is divided into four high-grade types: (1) Burkitt's lymphoma; (2) lymphoblastic lymphoma; (3) large B cell lymphoma; and (4) anaplastic large cell lymphoma.

Clinical Manifestations

The presenting complaint of a child with NHL is usually pain or swelling with acute onset and progression. Children with lymphoblastic NHL commonly present with a mediastinal mass, pleural effusion, and lymphadenopathy, and have a tendency for spread to the bone marrow and CNS. Burkitt's NHL manifests with an abdominal mass, which can mimic appendicitis, and can also spread to the CNS and bone marrow.

Because of the rapidity with which this tumor can proliferate, most children have advanced disease at diagnosis even though they may have had symptoms for only a short period of time. Most have stage III and IV disease when diagnosed. Children with advanced disease may present with CNS symptoms, including headaches, nausea, and vomiting. Petechiae, bruising, bleeding, and bone pain are present if the bone marrow is involved. Those with a large mediastinal mass may present with respiratory distress.

Diagnosis

The diagnosis of NHL is made from a biopsy. The cells or tissue may be obtained from the bone marrow, pleural effusion, ascites, or an affected node or mass. The diagnostic studies and staging of NHL must be done expeditiously to avoid delay in treatment.

Staging evaluation includes a bone marrow aspirate and biopsy, and lumbar puncture to assess for marrow and CNS involvement, respectively. Radiologic studies include CT of the affected area, the chest, abdomen, and pelvis. Nuclear studies including bone and PET scans are done to identify any other sites of disease. Laboratory evaluations include a

NURSING ALERT

Mediastinal Mass Can Cause Obstruction

A child with NHL and a large mediastinal mass may present with respiratory distress caused by compression of the trachea by the malignant lymphoma. The distress will be more pronounced when the child is lying down. A mediastinal mass can also cause superior vena cava syndrome (SVC), which is obstruction of the superior vena cava resulting in edema of the face, neck, and upper trunk. Both respiratory distress and SVC syndrome are oncologic emergencies.

CBC, liver and kidney function tests, electrolytes, calcium, phosphorus, magnesium, lactate dehydrogenase (LDH), uric acid, and urinalysis.

Treatment

Aggressive multi-agent chemotherapy is started as soon as possible once the diagnosis is made and the staging of the tumor is complete. Like the child with leukemia, these children are at risk for tumor lysis syndrome, and all precautions to prevent renal injury are followed. Children who have stage I and II disease receive a shorter and less aggressive course of treatment than those with stages III and IV. Intrathecal chemotherapy is given for CNS prophylaxis, and cranial radiation is used with children who have disease in their CNS. In the past, radiation therapy was commonly used in treatment, but studies have demonstrated that with intensive chemotherapy there is no benefit to adding irradiation. Children with NHL now have survival rates that approach or exceed 90% (Wayne, Reaman, & Helman, 2008). Hematopoietic stem cell transplant may be recommended as a treatment option for those children who relapse.

Nursing Management

The nursing management of the child with NHL is similar to the care of the child with leukemia. In NHL there is a high incidence of tumor lysis syndrome, and these children are often admitted to an intensive care unit for initiation of treatment. Because of the intense chemotherapy these children receive, side effects are common, and nursing care involves managing these.

NEUROBLASTOMA

Neuroblastoma is a tumor originating from neural crest cells, which are embryologic precursors of the sympathetic nervous system. These cells are present in tissue found in the brain, adrenal medulla, pelvis, mediastinum, and sympathetic ganglia. A neuroblastoma may occur at any of these sites.

INCIDENCE AND ETIOLOGY

Neuroblastoma is the most common extracranial solid tumor in children. It accounts for 8–10% of childhood cancers (Brodeur & Maris, 2006). Because neuroblastoma is an embryonal tumor, it is usually seen in early childhood with 40% of cases diagnosed in children less than one year of age. Over 95% are identified in children less than 10 years of age (Park, Eggert, & Caron, 2008). The true incidence of neuroblastoma is unknown because this tumor can spontaneously regress (Tonini & Pistoia, 2006). This phenomenon occurs more commonly in neonates and infants and results in cases being undetected and uncounted.

The etiology of neuroblastoma remains unknown. Studies have failed to link this tumor with sex, race, or geographical location. Environmental factors have been implicated but none have been confirmed (Park et al., 2008). There are rare cases of neuroblastoma occurring in more than one child in a family. Children with a familial occurrence tend to be diagnosed at an early age and have multiple primary sites.

PATHOPHYSIOLOGY

Neuroblastoma is a solid mass which usually contains areas of necrosis, calcification, and hemorrhage. Within the same tumor the histology may be highly variable with areas of more mature cells called ganglioneuroblastoma or even benign cells called ganglioneuroma in addition to the malignant neuroblastoma cells. Several genetic and biologic features of this tumor have been identified, including the gene that is capable of causing cells to transform to neuroblastoma. This **oncogene** is called *MYCN*. An increase in the number of copies, or amplification of *MYCN*, is related to rapid tumor progression and a poorer prognosis (Brodeur & Maris, 2006).

CLINICAL MANIFESTATIONS

Children with neuroblastoma can present with a wide variety of symptoms, depending upon the location of the tumor and the extent of the disease. The most common primary site is in the abdomen with involvement of the adrenal gland or the paraspinal ganglia. Less common primary sites include the paraspinal areas in the thorax, neck, or pelvis. Metastasis at diagnosis is present about 50% of the time, most often in children over four years (Tonini & Pistoia, 2006). The most common metastatic sites include bone marrow, bones, and liver (Park et al., 2008).

The tumor is most often detected by palpation of an abdominal mass that can be firm and irregular in shape and frequently crosses the midline. The child may complain of abdominal pain or fullness. Large abdominal or pelvic tumors can cause edema to the lower extremities, as a result of vascular compression. Masses of the thorax can be seen on chest X-ray, and if large enough, can cause respiratory symptoms or superior vena cava syndrome. When the tumor presents in any paraspinal area, it can grow into the spinal foramen and cause spinal cord compression. When neuroblastoma presents behind the orbit, it causes ecchymosis of the eyelid and proptosis. Metastatic disease often results in systemic symptoms such as fatigue and low grade fever. Bone marrow involvement usually presents with pain and refusal to bear weight or limping.

DIAGNOSIS

Although signs and symptoms, blood and urine tests, and imaging studies may indicate that a neuroblastoma is present, a conclusive diagnosis can be made only when neuroblastoma cells in tissue samples are seen under a microscope. When neuroblastoma is suspected, a complete history and physical examination is done. Laboratory tests include a CBC, liver and kidney function tests, and a chemistry profile. Neuroblastoma often causes an elevation in the catecholamine metabolites vanillymandelic acid (VMA) and homovanillic acid (HVA), which can be measured in the urine. With treatment leading to remission, these metabolites become undetectable in the urine and are important markers of a recurrence. Other neuroblastoma tumor markers include elevated LDH and ferritin levels.

Bone marrow aspiration and biopsy from bilateral iliac crest sites can often confirm the diagnosis of neuroblastoma and are necessary to determine bone marrow involvement. Chest X-ray may reveal thoracic or paravertebral primary tumor and abdominal ultrasound can show the extent of any mass. In order to determine if the tumor is surgically resectable, a CT or MRI scan is done, which more accurately defines the location of the mass and identifies whether the tumor is impinging upon other organs.

A metastatic work-up is conducted to determine the stage of the disease. Along with bone marrow testing, a bone scan and skeletal survey are done to determine if bony metastases are present. A nuclear medicine imaging study called an MIBG scan is also used. The radioactive agent ^{131}I-MIBG is highly specific to neuroendocrine tissue and localizes in a variety of tumors, including neuroblastoma. After this isotope is injected, the scan can screen the body for both primary and metastatic sites. A PET scan is done to identify metastatic disease that is not sensitive to MIBG. Brain imaging is done if neurologic symptoms are present.

The International Neuroblastoma Staging System (INSS) is used throughout the world to standardize the definition of diagnosis. Staging is based upon the extent of dissemination of the tumor. The prognosis for a child with neuroblastoma is determined by several variables: stage, age of the individual at diagnosis, *MYCN* amplification and other genetic factors, and various biologic features of the tumor. Children diagnosed with neuroblastoma are placed into risk categories, low, intermediate or high. Based on these factors treatment varies with risk stratification. Children in the low risk group, for example, those with stage 1 or 2 neuroblastoma and single *MYCN* amplification have an excellent prognosis with surgical resection alone. In contrast, standard therapy for children in the high risk group, while very intensive, results in only a 30–40% survival rate (Park et al., 2008). There is a "special" group of infants less than 12 months of age who present with a localized primary tumor and dissemination limited to the liver, skin, or bone marrow in which the malignant neuroblastoma will often spontaneously mature and disappear without treatment. These children are said to have stage 4S and are generally low risk (Brodeur & Maris, 2006).

> **NURSING ALERT**
>
> **Safety in Handling Radioactive Fluids**
>
> Because ^{131}I-MIBG contains the radioisotope, iodine^{131}, precautions should be taken by health care personnel and family members. The patient's thyroid gland must be protected from this iodine isotope. A solution of saturated potassium iodine (SSKI) is given 24 to 48 hours before and 3 days after the injection. Gloves should be worn when handling the child's body fluids for at least 48 hours after the isotope injection. As always, good hand washing technique is needed. Caregivers should be instructed to not allow the child to sleep with them or siblings for at least 48 hours while the isotope is being excreted. The half-life of iodine^{131} is 8 days.

TREATMENT

The treatment plan is determined by risk category and other prognostic markers of the disease. Treatment can include surgery, chemotherapy, radiation therapy, biotherapy, and hematopoietic stem cell transplantation. Surgery can be both diagnostic and therapeutic. An initial surgery is performed to establish a diagnosis by biopsy, stage the extent of the disease, and completely resect or partially reduce the tumor. Complete surgical resection is often the only therapy needed for the child who presents with stage 1 or 2 disease. Second-look surgery is used to evaluate the response of treatment and to excise any residual tumor. The majority of children with neuroblastoma with advanced disease at diagnosis are in a high-risk category. Aggressive multi-agent chemotherapy is the predominant modality of treatment for these children. Chemotherapy agents used include cyclophosphamide, adriamycin, vincristine, cisplatin, and etoposide (D'Andrea, 2008). Initial response rates are high, greater than 85%, but the disease frequently recurs. The consolidation phase of treatment consists of myeloablative chemotherapy with hematopoietic stem cell rescue. Neuroblastoma is radiosensitive, but radiation therapy is not curative when used alone. Radiation is used for local tumor control in conjunction with chemotherapy and is important in palliation of pain in end stage patients. Biologic response modifiers, including 13-cis-Retinoic acid (isotretinoin) and monoclonal antibodies are a more recent addition to the treatment of high risk neuroblastoma. Several novel approaches to the challenge of progressive disease are currently in clinical study (Brodeur & Maris, 2006).

NURSING MANAGEMENT AND FAMILY TEACHING

Nursing assessment is similar to the assessment of children with other tumors such as leukemia or lymphomas. Emphasis is on the expeditious completion of the metastatic work-up. The initial care focuses on alleviating the child's discomfort associated with the presenting symptoms and supporting the child and family through the diagnostic work-up. The nurse will need to assist with the coordination of tests and procedures, and teach the family the importance of these in determining the extent of tumor involvement.

Subsequent nursing interventions will vary based on the treatment plan as prescribed by stage and risk category. Frequently the child and caregivers must be prepared for major surgery in a relatively short time period following the discovery of a malignant mass. Feelings of fear and uncertainty may occur in all family members, and they need support. High risk neuroblastoma causes even greater fear and anxiety for caregivers because of the poor prognosis of advanced stage disease. The therapy for these patients is intense, and the child spends long periods of time in the hospital. Chemotherapy or radiation therapy will begin quickly once the child is stable postoperatively. Caregivers will need to be educated about the side effects of these treatments. Radiological scans to evaluate the efficacy of treatment are frequently performed, requiring the family to attend many outpatient appointments. If the disease progresses, nursing care will focus on pain control and other palliative measures as well as support and counseling for family members.

CRITICAL THINKING

Identification of Infection in the Neutropenic Child

You are caring for a 4-year-old boy who has an ANC of 300. He was admitted the previous evening with a fever of 102.3°F (39.1°C). He is receiving intravenous antibiotics. While you are bathing him, he complains of pain in the perianal area. You do not note any redness or inflammation in the area. You suspect the source of infection is a rectal abscess. What would you do?

WILMS' TUMOR

Wilms' tumor, also called nephroblastoma, is a tumor that arises in the kidney. It is a renal embryoma, meaning that the tumor is derived from undifferentiated primitive cells.

INCIDENCE AND ETIOLOGY

Wilms' tumor is the most common primary malignant kidney tumor of childhood. It represents 6% of childhood cancer, and the total incidence in the United States is estimated at 500 cases per year. The tumor usually presents between two and three years of age. There is a slightly higher incidence rate of Wilms' tumor in the African-American population than in the white population and an even lower rate for Asians. Girls present more often than boys and unilateral disease is more common than bilateral (Dome et al., 2006). The cause of Wilms' tumor is unknown in most cases. Rare cases are associated with certain congenital anomalies such as **aniridia** (a congenital absence of the iris), **hemihypertrophy** (a relative increase in size of one-half of the body as compared to the other), Beckwith-Weidemann Syndrome, and urinary defects. Therefore, children who have these anomalies need close surveillance, including frequent abdominal examination and ultrasound as part of their primary care. Genetics plays an important role in clinical research of Wilms' tumor. Several genes specific to Wilms' have been identified; two of these are WT1 and WT2. There is predictive value for tumor risk after gene characterization (Dome et al., 2006).

PATHOPHYSIOLOGY

Wilms' tumor grows rapidly and may be very large at the time of diagnosis. A fragile thin capsule that may be easily torn or broken usually encloses the tumor, which may be present in one or both kidneys. There are two categories to describe the histology of a Wilms' tumor, favorable and unfavorable. Favorable histology tumors are more responsive to therapy and, as the name implies, have a favorable prognosis; whereas, children having the unfavorable histology tumors have a poorer prognosis. Histology type and the stage of tumor at diagnosis determine prognosis and treatment decisions. Wilms' tumor may metastasize to the lungs, liver, brain, bones, or to the unaffected kidney.

CLINICAL MANIFESTATIONS

An abdominal mass is the most common presentation of Wilms' tumor. A large flank mass is usually found in a healthy child by a family member. The mass presents on one side and seldom crosses the midline, as does neuroblastoma. Some children experience pain, microscopic or gross hematuria, hypertension, and general malaise.

DIAGNOSIS

Any child with an abdominal mass needs a timely and thorough diagnostic work-up. Abdominal ultrasound is often the first test ordered and can detect a solid intrarenal mass. Rapidly growing tumors migrate toward the point of least resistance, and it is not unusual to find Wilms' tumor infiltrating the renal veins or inferior vena cava. Ultrasound will also evaluate the unaffected kidney and abdominal lymph nodes for any signs of disease. An abdominal CT scan or MRI will give a clearer preoperative view of the abdomen. Because the lungs are the most common site of distant metastatic disease, a CT scan of the chest is ordered. Laboratory studies including a CBC, urinalysis, blood chemistries, and liver function tests are performed. The diagnosis is confirmed at surgery when the mass is removed, usually with the entire kidney, and biopsied.

TREATMENT

The usual treatment for unilateral Wilms' tumor is surgical resection of the affected kidney (nephrectomy) followed by chemotherapy and, at times, radiation. The treatment used depends upon the extent of disease and histology of the mass.

Preoperatively, it is important to monitor the child's blood pressure. Hypertensive children are at risk of hypotension during a nephrectomy when the renal vessels are tied off. A tumor that is completely enclosed within one kidney will be resected, and the child will receive a short course of chemotherapy postsurgery. With bilateral kidney disease (Stage V) presurgical chemotherapy is given with the goal of decreasing tumor burden and preserving normal kidney function. Chemotherapeutic agents used are dactinomycin (Actinomycin D) and vincristine. Children with more extensive disease will have additional chemotherapeutic agents added to their regimens and possibly radiation therapy.

Wilms' tumor is highly radiosensitive, and in the past all children received radiation. Today radiation therapy is used only in those who have metastatic disease, residual tumor after surgical resection, and recurrent tumors. When radiation is necessary, it can cause defects in the spine including a decrease in linear growth or scoliosis. Children who present with or develop bilateral kidney disease pose a special problem. Usually the most affected kidney is removed, and an excisional biopsy of the tumor in the other kidney is performed. The remaining kidney is then irradiated and followed closely for signs of recurrent disease. These children usually have "second look" surgery to determine the effectiveness of therapy.

The prognosis for children with Wilms' tumor continues to improve. The overall five-year survival rate is 92% (Duffy-Lind, 2008). The long-term survivor must continue to have active surveillance of the remaining kidney and follow-up for late effects. Irradiation to the trunk can cause scoliosis, and pulmonary radiation can cause fibrosis of lung tissue. Survivors of Wilms' tumor are at higher risk for a second neoplasm, especially those children who received radiation.

NURSING MANAGEMENT

Caregivers have little time to prepare for the major surgery involved with a nephrectomy and the diagnosis of cancer. The nurse should remain available to answer questions and describe what they can expect. Chemotherapy is started soon after surgery, usually before the child is discharged postoperatively. Pain control is necessary after the nephrectomy and is given around the clock in the first 24 hours postoperatively, with a weaning of analgesia over the following few days. By discharge most children are no longer receiving pain medication. Postoperatively the nurse also needs to make certain that the child's oral fluid intake is

NURSING ALERT

Manipulation of the Abdomen in a Child with Wilms' Tumor

A precaution is to limit manipulation of the abdomen or liver in these children that might cause spread of malignant cells should the encapsulated mass rupture. A sign placed on the child's crib or bed that warns all health care providers to avoid palpation of the abdomen, and instructions to caregivers to use caution when handling and bathing their child, can prevent trauma to the tumor.

NURSING TIP

Avoid Trauma to Remaining Kidney

A child who has one kidney must avoid trauma and injury to that kidney. The caregiver and the child must learn that contact sports, such as football and basketball, pose a special risk. Activities that do not have great potential for injury should be encouraged such as swimming, golf, bike riding, and hiking.

CASE STUDY / CARE PLAN

A CHILD WITH WILMS' TUMOR

Shannon is a 6-year-old girl who was referred to a pediatric oncologist after her pediatrician palpated an abdominal mass. Shannon had been complaining of abdominal pain for several weeks and her parents reported that they had been using acetaminophen for pain. They noticed that Shannon would bend over when walking and reported that her energy level was decreased as was her appetite. Shannon had no recent fever. Shannon's medical history has been unremarkable up until now. Her immunizations are up to date and she has no allergies. She lives with her parents and three sisters and attends kindergarten.

On exam, Shannon's abdomen was protuberant and firm, with a palpable mass on her right side, extending to midline from her ribs to her pelvis. An ultrasound revealed a large renal mass, confirmed by biopsy to be a nonmetastatic Wilms' tumor. Shannon's diagnosis and treatment plan, which would include surgical resection, chemotherapy and radiation therapy, were discussed with the family. She was admitted for a biopsy and VAD placement. Because of concerns that the tumor was expanding rapidly, it was determined that chemotherapy would be started prior to surgical resection. After several weeks of chemotherapy, a right nephrectomy was performed. Additional chemotherapy and radiation were planned as outpatient treatment postdischarge.

NURSING CARE PLAN

ASSESSMENT

Nursing assessment of a newly diagnosed oncology patient includes a thorough physical evaluation. A baseline evaluation is needed to determine the level of improvement or deterioration of the child's physical status over the course of treatment. Physical assessments should be done at least daily in the hospital setting and at each outpatient visit. The family's cultural, spiritual, and social background must be assessed to be able to provide individualized holistic care. Emotional support is given differently to a family with strong extended member ties than to a family with a limited social support network. Cultural differences may result in disease perceptions that vary tremendously from Western scientific reasoning; therefore, the nurse must take time to talk with family members about the meaning of the illness. Many families find comfort in the support of their spiritual leaders while others would prefer the support of a team member such as the social worker. An assessment of the support systems of families should be obtained. Nursing assessment of the child's developmental level and emotional maturity will determine the appropriate approach to use during the many painful procedures involved in diagnosis and treatment. The child and caregiver's cognitive abilities and preferred learning style should be assessed prior to the initiation of teaching. This includes the educational and reading level of the caregiver, his or her stress level, and the child's developmental level. Once this assessment is made, appropriate written and verbal instructions can be given.

NURSING DIAGNOSIS 1

Acute pain related to disease process, and treatment (nephrectomy and chemotherapy).

EXPECTED OUTCOME

1. Shannon states or exhibits an increased level of comfort.

NOC: Comfort Status: Physical; Pain Level

NIC: Pain Management; Analgesic Administration

INTERVENTIONS/*RATIONALES*

1. Use a developmentally appropriate pain assessment scale to determine pain level. *A pain scale provides objective data that can be used for both assessment and evaluation.*

(Continues)

CASE STUDY / CARE PLAN (Continued)

2. Assess painful areas for location, severity, and signs of infection. *Pain is an indicator of infection in a neutropenic patient who may not be able to mount an immune response.*
3. Provide Shannon with pain medication on a preventive schedule (around the clock). *Pain is easier to prevent than to treat. Postoperative pain continues for one to two days after surgery.*
4. Reassess for relief from medication given. *To determine need for changes in drug, dosage, and frequency.*
5. Implement and teach nonpharmacological pain reduction methods, including position of comfort and distraction techniques. *Positioning can help decrease strain on the incisional site. Age-appropriate toys and activities help the child focus on something other than pain.*

EVALUATION

Shannon will report or exhibit an increased level of comfort and be able to participate in age-appropriate activity.

NURSING DIAGNOSIS 2

Excess fluid volume related to potential renal insufficiency as a result of diseased kidney (preop) and nephrectomy (post-op).

EXPECTED OUTCOME

1. Shannon will exhibit adequate renal functioning

NOC: Kidney Function

NIC: Fluid/Electrolyte Management

INTERVENTIONS/*RATIONALES*

1. Maintain IV hydration to induce urine output of 1 cc/kg/hour or greater both pre- and post-operatively. *Urine output of less than 1 cc/kg/hour can be the first sign of impending renal compromise. Close monitoring of the child's intake and output allows early detection of renal problems.*
2. Monitor blood urea nitrogen (BUN), creatinine, electrolytes, and minerals (potassium, calcium, phosphorus, and uric acid) pre- and post-operatively. *Normal levels confirm that the healthy kidney is functioning adequately.*
3. Monitor blood pressure at least every two to four hours. *High blood pressure can result from a damaged kidney. Intraoperatively, hypotension may occur when renal vessels are tied off. Hypertension may occur postoperatively as the remaining kidney equilibrates.*
4. Instruct parents on the importance of protecting the remaining kidney through the avoidance of contact sports and other potential trauma. *To prevent injury to the only remaining kidney contact sports or any other activity that has a high risk potential should be avoided.*

EVALUATION

Shannon will have normal blood pressure and adequate urine output both pre- and post-operatively. BUN, creatinine, electrolytes and mineral levels will remain within acceptable limits.

NURSING DIAGNOSIS 3

Risk for infection related to neutropenia from chemotherapy treatment.

EXPECTED OUTCOMES

1. Shannon will remain free of infection.
2. Shannon and her caregivers will demonstrate infection prevention actions.

NOC: Risk Control

NIC: Infection Control; Infection Protection

(*Continues*)

CASE STUDY / CARE PLAN (Continued)

INTERVENTIONS/*RATIONALES*

1. Assess child for any signs of infection. Pay close attention to incision site, oral ulcerations, needle punctures, lesions or breaks in skin for localized signs of infection (pain, erythema, indurations). *Skin is the first line of defense against infection.*
2. Monitor vital signs frequently for signs of infection. Report temperatures above 101°F (38.3°C). *The child with neutropenia has no immune defense against infection and sepsis can develop quickly. Because of the risk of overwhelming infection, prompt interventions must be instituted when the child develops fever. Increased temperature, pulse, and respirations may indicate an infection.*
3. Administer antibiotics as ordered; monitor for expected and toxic effects. *Antibiotic therapy is started in the child with fever and neutropenia.*
4. Use meticulous handwashing techniques at all times and teach Shannon and family about the importance of good handwashing. The *most important intervention in preventing infections is strict handwashing. Educating Shannon and her family allows them to observe and question all persons coming in contact with her about washing their hands.*
5. Use aseptic technique for all invasive procedures. *To minimize exposure to infective organisms.*

EVALUATION

Shannon and her caregivers, and anyone entering the room, will carry out measures to prevent infection. Shannon's vital signs will remain stable and within normal limits. She will be free of infection. If an infection develops, Shannon will be promptly and effectively treated.

NURSING DIAGNOSIS 4

Imbalanced nutrition: Less than body requirements related to surgical NPO status, post-op discomfort, and chemotherapy-related loss of appetite, nausea/vomiting, and mucositis.

EXPECTED OUTCOMES

1. Shannon will ingest a sufficient number of calories to maintain and support normal growth.
2. Shannon will maintain baseline weight during hospitalization.

NOC: Nutritional Status

NIC: Nutrition Management; Nutritional Monitoring

INTERVENTIONS/*RATIONALES*

1. Assess bowel function pre- and postoperatively and introduce foods slowly after bowel sounds return post-operatively. *A large mass may cause pain and diminished appetite. Bowel sounds are indicative of normal intestinal peristalsis.*
2. Encourage high-protein and high-calorie foods. *This will maximize nutritional quality of intake.*
3. Offer small amounts of food frequently throughout the day. *Small portions are usually better tolerated by children with chemotherapy-induced nausea.*
4. Encourage caregivers to bring child's favorite foods from home. *Children are more likely to eat foods they like.*
5. Make breakfast as high in caloric intake as possible. *Children often lose their appetite as the day progresses.*
6. Administer antiemetics as ordered. *Antiemetics decrease anticipatory or actual nausea related to chemotherapy.*
7. Provide mouth analgesics as ordered before food and fluid intake if the child develops mucositis. *Mucositis is painful. Analgesics will improve comfort and increase interest in eating.*
8. Avoid making food an issue for power or control and emphasize this to caregivers. *A child may resist eating even when he or she has an increase in appetite.*

(Continues)

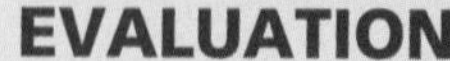

CASE STUDY / CARE PLAN (Continued)

EVALUATION

Shannon will experience no more than 5% weight loss and will show normal growth for age.

NURSING DIAGNOSIS 5

Deficient knowledge related to diagnosis, treatment, and long-term plan of care.

EXPECTED OUTCOMES

1. Shannon will have a basic understanding of her treatment plan and what to expect with chemotherapy and after her surgery
2. Shannon's caregivers will have adequate understanding of the diagnosis, initial treatment, and long-term plan for Wilms' tumor and will have the necessary knowledge and resources needed to participate in Shannon's plan of care

NOC: Knowledge: Disease Process, Treatment Regimen, Cancer Management

NIC: Teaching: Disease Process, Chemotherapy Management, Venous Access Device Maintenance

INTERVENTIONS/*RATIONALES*

1. Assess the educational level and cognitive ability of Shannon and her caregivers. *To be effective, teaching plans for both the child and caregivers must be educationally and developmentally appropriate.*
2. Upon admission, assess caregivers' understanding of diagnosis and initial treatment plan, provide the child's parents with information about the initial chemotherapy and surgical intervention and be available to answer questions. *Treatment, including surgical resection, of Wilms' tumor occurs shortly after diagnosis giving caregivers little time to prepare.*
3. Use simple terms and concrete examples, such as demonstration dolls, when teaching Shannon about her diagnosis, treatment, and upcoming surgery. *Teaching should be developmentally appropriate.*
4. Provide more detailed information about the long-term treatment plan and chemotherapy after the acute phase of treatment. *The shock and fear of a cancer diagnosis combined with the immediate treatment considerations and decisions make processing large amounts of information difficult for caregivers.*
5. Provide parents with pamphlets and other sources of information (websites) about Wilms' tumor and treatment. *Individuals differ in their preferred style of learning and education is enhanced when multiple teaching strategies are employed.*
6. Continually assess/reassess caregiver understanding of the long term treatment plan, post hospitalization follow-up plan, administration of chemotherapy and side effects to watch for, concerns related to the nephrectomy, and care of a venous access device. *Treatment for Wilms' tumor will continue for several months after the initial surgery and chemotherapy. Family members will need to have a good understanding of their role in the plan of care to ensure optimal outcome.*

EVALUATION

Shannon's caregivers will verbalize understanding of important concepts related to disease and treatment plan and will demonstrate the ability to care for Shannon appropriately.

adequate and that any nausea, vomiting, or constipation from the chemotherapy is under control before discharge. Wound care and activity restrictions should be reviewed. The surgical wound site is usually a large abdominal incision and signs of increased pain, redness, or drainage should be reported. When radiation is necessary, caregivers will be told of the potential side effects of altered growth and increased risk of second malignancies. Because these are late effects of treatment, continued education regarding the need for long-term follow-up is necessary.

CRITICAL THINKING

Oncological Emergencies

Can you recognize these oncological emergencies?

1. Neutropenic child, temperature 104°F (40.0°C), low blood pressure, pale and diaphoretic with shaking chills.
2. Child newly diagnosed with ALL, WBC 89,000 with significant hepatosplenomegaly, increased uric acid level, increased serum potassium, and poor urine output.
3. Toddler with stage 4 neuroblastoma who recently stopped walking or pulling to a stand. Decreased tone in lower extremities and loss of bowel control.
4. Five-year-old with large mediastinal mass who refuses to lie down; has edematous eyelids, and fullness in upper chest and neck.

BONE TUMORS

Malignant bone tumors account for approximately 5% of all childhood cancers. The two most common bone tumors are osteogenic sarcoma and Ewing's sarcoma.

OSTEOGENIC SARCOMA

Osteogenic sarcoma, also called osteosarcoma, is a tumor of bone that usually occurs in the growth metaphysis or the end of the long bones. Trauma is frequently associated with the diagnosis of osteosarcoma. Rather than being a cause of the tumor, trauma is the event that brings the malignancy to the attention of the child, the family, and the health care team.

Incidence and Etiology

Osteogenic sarcoma is the most common bone cancer in children, with approximately 400 new cases diagnosed each year in the United States. There is a peak incidence in the second decade of life when adolescents are gaining rapid vertical height. Girls are diagnosed earlier because of their earlier growth spurt but overall males are affected more often due to their larger bone volume. The cause of most osteosarcoma tumors is unknown. Children with the hereditary form of retinoblastoma, an eye tumor, have an increased risk of developing osteogenic sarcoma (Holloway, 2008).

Pathophysiology

The bones are composed of different cell types that include osteoblasts and osteoclasts. Osteosarcomas derive from primitive bone-forming cells similar to the osteoblasts that make bone matrix. These malignant cells do not function normally and have the potential to spread to other areas of the body such as the lungs and other bones. Osteogenic sarcoma occurs most frequently in the rapidly growing bones of the distal femur, proximal tibia, and proximal humerus. Children with tumors arising in sites such as the skull or vertebrae have a poorer prognosis because these bones are not surgically resectable.

Clinical Manifestations

Pain at the site of the tumor is almost always present and frequently is associated with a swelling or palpable mass. The pain increases with activity and weight bearing and may cause the child to limp. Signs and symptoms of the tumor may have a short duration but a history with average duration of pain of three months is not uncommon. Osteosarcoma tumors that have destroyed normal bone place the child at risk for fracture. Occasionally the fractured bone is the first clinical manifestation of the tumor.

Diagnosis

A child with a suspected tumor of the bone requires a complete evaluation, including history, physical examination, and X-rays of the primary site and chest. Often characteristic patterns seen on the X-rays suggest the histology of the bone tumor, but a more complete evaluation and biopsy are necessary. Metastatic evaluation is necessary, as approximately 15–20% of children have metastasis at diagnosis, most often pulmonary in nature (Holloway, 2008). The lung is the most common site of metastasis, but distant bone lesions can also be seen. Other organ involvement is rare. The presence of metastasis at diagnosis is an important prognostic indicator and helps to determine the specifics of therapy. Metastatic evaluation includes CT scan of the chest and a radionuclide bone scan to identify bone lesions. MRI of the primary lesion is performed to assess the extent of the bone and soft-tissue tumor and its relationship to blood vessels, nerves, and other bones prior to definitive surgery. Whole-body PET scan performed prior to initiation of treatment provides a very sensitive means of monitoring tumor changes throughout the course of therapy. Laboratory evaluation includes a CBC, blood chemistries, serum alkaline phosphatase, and lactic dehydrogenase (LDH). A biopsy is required to confirm the diagnosis of osteogenic sarcoma.

Treatment

Osteosarcoma is treated with surgical resection of the affected bone and multiagent chemotherapy to eradicate any microscopic disease that could lead to metastasis. Many clinical trials use several courses of preoperative chemotherapy to reduce tumor size and permit a less radical surgical procedure. A complete radiographic evaluation is repeated prior to surgery.

Amputation was the surgical treatment used almost exclusively in the past, but now many children can be offered a limb-sparing procedure. Limb-sparing surgery uses a cadaver bone or an endoprosthetic device, such as a total hip joint or knee, to replace the section of bone with tumor that must be excised. Both amputation and limb-sparing surgery seek to excise the tumor completely and preserve the adjacent nerves and vessels. Limb-sparing surgery should be a consideration, over amputation, only if there is no compromise to the child's ultimate prognosis. Contraindications to limb-sparing surgery include displaced pathologic fractures at the tumor site, and skeletal immaturity, which would create problems with leg length discrepancies. A grafted cadaver bone will not grow, so a child who still has significant growth to achieve will have an unacceptable leg length discrepancy with limb-sparing surgery of the leg.

Endoprosthetic devices can have mechanical malfunctions or become infected; this may require additional surgery. The family must be educated about the advantages and disadvantages of all possible surgical procedures so they can make informed decisions. Issues of body image and the amount of function to be expected through rehabilitation must be discussed. The client, who is usually an adolescent, must be made an active participant in the discussion and decision-making process.

Aggressive chemotherapy is restarted after a few weeks of postoperative recovery. The overall five year survival rate for children with osteosarcoma who respond well to chemotherapy is 65–70%. Patients receive chemotherapy with surgery since there are presumed microscopic metastases. Surgery-only patients have an 80% relapse rates (Holloway, 2008). Complete surgical resection of all overt metastatic disease is necessary for long-term survival. Children who develop metastatic lesions after treatment has begun have a poorer long-term prognosis. Osteosarcoma is radiation resistant and this modality is rarely used in primary treatment. Occasionally, radiation is used for pain palliation in clients whose disease is unresponsive to chemotherapy.

Nursing Management

Adolescents and their families need ongoing explanations about the disease, treatment, equipment, and expected outcomes. Explanations before a procedure or treatment is initiated help keep the adolescent informed and take into consideration the need for autonomy. Introducing the adolescent to another adolescent who has undergone the same procedures and therapy may help alleviate some stress and provide another support system.

Pain from bone lesions of osteosarcoma in many cases requires analgesics prior to surgery. Postoperative pain medication needs to be given around the clock the first 24 hours. Clients who undergo amputation may experience **phantom limb pain**, which is pain perceived to be coming from the amputated limb. After limb-sparing surgery the client is at risk for altered tissue perfusion and nerve damage in the affected limb. Checking nail beds for capillary refill and assessing sensation of the limb distal to the surgery site every 15–30 minutes is important to assess nerve damage. Infection risks are great in individuals who undergo extensive and lengthy orthopedic surgery such as in a limb-sparing procedure. This risk is compounded when immunosuppressive chemotherapy is instituted after surgery. Wound care must be meticulous, and signs of infection such as redness, drainage at the site, or fever should be reported.

Adolescents who have either limb-sparing surgery or amputation will have major alterations in their body image. Aside from the surgery, they will also face body changes related to chemotherapy such as alopecia. Normal activities with friends may be curtailed and previous activities such as sports or dance may have to be given up completely. The nurse can support these adolescents by listening to their concerns, encouraging them to dress in their own clothes while in the hospital, and suggesting peer support groups.

EWING'S SARCOMA

Ewing's sarcoma is a highly malignant bone tumor with a histiologic appearance and presentation that is different from osteosarcoma. Ewing's sarcoma can present in any bone of the skeleton but is often seen in the bones of the pelvis, tibia, fibula, humerus, and femur.

Incidence and Etiology

Ewing's sarcoma represents about one-third of all childhood malignant bone tumors with approximately 200 children and adolescents diagnosed every year in the United States. Ewing's sarcoma is a disease of older children and young adults. It is rare in children less than five years old or in older adults. African-American children in the United States rarely develop Ewing's sarcoma, but the protective etiology has yet to be found (D'Amore, 2008).

Pathophysiology

Ewing's sarcoma is a highly malignant tumor that arises from primitive undifferentiated cells. Bone is the most likely location for these abnormal small round blue cells. Extraosseous Ewing's sarcoma can occur in soft tissue. This is very rare and difficult to treat.

Clinical Manifestations

As with osteosarcoma, pain and swelling at the site of the tumor are the usual presenting symptoms of Ewing's sarcoma. Pain may be caused by tumor under the periosteum or the tissue covering the bone, or by a fracture of the weakened bone. Unlike osteosarcoma, children with Ewing's sarcoma may present with systemic signs and symptoms, including weight loss, fever, and an increased sedimentation rate (Betcher, Simon, & McHard, 2007).

Diagnosis

The diagnosis of Ewing's sarcoma is made by biopsy of the bone lesion. Ten to thirty percent of newly diagnosed clients have metastatic disease, with the lung, other bones, or the bone marrow as the most common sites. A complete staging evaluation must be done prior to beginning treatment, including CT scan of the lungs, MRI of the primary site, a radionuclide bone scan, and a PET scan to assist in detecting metastases. As with other pediatric malignancies the stage of the disease at the time of diagnosis is an important prognostic factor in Ewing's sarcoma. Widespread metastatic disease to other bones and the bone marrow has a poor prognosis. Location of the primary tumor is also a significant factor with pelvic and sacral lesions having a worse prognosis because these tumors are not resectable.

Treatment

The primary lesion of Ewing's sarcoma is treated with surgical resection of the bone when possible, and radiation therapy. If the bone is expendable, such as a rib or fibula, then the entire bone is removed. Control of the primary lesion can be achieved in this fashion. Multiagent, intense chemotherapy is used to prevent and control metastatic disease. Most current protocols use chemotherapy prior to definitive surgery and the amount of tumor decreased prior to resection is a prognostic factor, with more tumor decrease associated with a better prognosis.

When complete removal of the primary lesion cannot be achieved surgically, then radiation therapy is added to the treatment. With increases in the survival rate of Ewing's sarcoma, secondary malignancies in the radiation field have become an issue. Long-term follow-up must be stressed as an essential part of these clients' care. The addition of the chemotherapy agents ifosfamide and etoposide to a standard regimen of vincristine, doxorubicin, and cyclophosphamide, in addition to local tumor control with surgery or radiation therapy has significantly improved outcome for patients with nonmetastatic Ewing's sarcoma (Bernstein et al., 2006). Nursing management is similar to the management of osteogenic sarcoma.

SOFT-TISSUE SARCOMA

A sarcoma is a malignant tumor that arises from mesenchymal cells. Mesenchymal cells normally mature into skeletal muscle, smooth muscle, fat, fibrous tissue, bone, and cartilage. Rhabdomyosarcoma arises from tissue resembling striated muscle and contains primitive muscle cells. There are several types of rhabdomyosarcoma seen in children. Embryonal is the most favorable histology and has the best prognosis. Alveolar, solid alveolar, and undifferentiated are the other subtypes, all with unfavorable histology. Some rhabdomyosarcoma cells are too primitive to classify and are referred to as undifferentiated sarcoma. The treatment of rhabdomyosarcoma and soft-tissue sarcoma is similar (Triche, Hicks, & Sorensen, 2006).

INCIDENCE AND ETIOLOGY

In the United States 850–900 children and adolescents are diagnosed with malignant soft-tissue sarcomas each year, of which approximately 350 are rhabdomyosarcomas (Okcu et al., 2006). There is no known definitive cause of soft-tissue sarcoma.

PATHOPHYSIOLOGY

Rhabdomyosarcoma cells resemble rhabdomyoblasts, which in the human embryo will eventually form voluntary and skeletal muscle tissue. The embryonal type of rhabdomyosarcoma usually affects infants and young children in the area of the genitourinary tract and the head and neck area. The alveolar type usually occurs in the large muscles of the trunk, arms, and legs, affecting older children and teenagers. Most often sarcomas metastasize via the blood and lymphatic systems to the lung, bone, and bone marrow.

CLINICAL MANIFESTATIONS

As with other solid tumors, the presentation of soft-tissue sarcoma depends upon the location, with the most common symptom being a hard nontender mass. Orbital involvement may present with **ptosis**, a drooping of the eyelid, and **proptosis**, a protrusion of the eyeball. These signs may also be associated with eye movement abnormalities. Tumors in the orbit are usually detected early because of the visible physical changes. Nasopharyngeal tumors may present with nasal obstruction, chronic sinusitis, epistaxis, or pain. Tumors that arise in the paranasal sinuses or middle ear result in signs and symptoms of chronic otitis media and sinusitis. Rhabdomyosarcoma in these areas may invade through foramina and cause intracranial spread, which results in cranial nerve palsies and signs of increased intracranial pressure. Intracranial disease reduces overall survival. Tumors in the extremities are similar to traumatic hematomas, which are raised and easily palpable. The tumor is fixed to the underlying muscle and can involve the skin. When rhabdomyosarcoma arises in the retroperitoneal area, it is usually asymptomatic until the disease is widespread and the mass is very large. A tumor in this location can cause bowel and urinary obstruction. Genitourinary involvement may cause urinary obstruction, hematuria, vaginal discharge, or a mass. Pain, swelling, and limping may be seen in bone involvement. Metastatic spread of rhabdomyosarcoma is seen in about 18% of children at the time of diagnosis. Most children with bone marrow involvement have their primary tumor in an extremity or in the trunk and usually have widespread metastatic disease to other organs.

DIAGNOSIS

The diagnosis of rhabdomyosarcoma and soft-tissue sarcoma is confirmed after tumor biopsy or resection. It is imperative that the surgeon obtain sufficient tissue sample to meet the needs of the required studies. The biopsy sample is submitted for specialized tests to determine cytogenetic abnormalities. There are specific gene variations associated with certain soft tissue sarcomas. These evaluations are included in the staging of the disease. The diagnostic evaluation includes a history and physical examination. Radiographic studies include CT and MRI of the primary tumor site and CT scan of the lungs to assess for metastases. A radionuclide bone scan and skeletal survey look for metastatic disease of bone. PET scan has a high sensitivity for lymph node metastases (Volker et al., 2007). Bone marrow aspirates and biopsies are usually performed at multiple sites, and lumbar puncture is performed to examine the CSF for the presence of malignant cells. Laboratory evaluation includes a CBC, urinalysis, blood chemistries, and liver function studies.

As with other malignancies, the treatment and prognosis of rhabdomyosarcoma depends upon the stage and histology of the disease.

TREATMENT

The primary treatment of rhabdomyosarcoma and soft-tissue sarcoma is wide surgical resection, whenever feasible. Only about one in six tumors can be completely removed because of the location or metastatic dissemination. When complete excision is done, the child will still receive adjuvant therapy to treat microscopic spread. Second-look surgery is often done to try to excise the remaining tumor completely and to evaluate the response to treatment.

Radiation therapy is used to control tumor growth by eradication of gross or microscopic disease. It usually follows surgery to treat residual disease and at times may be given preoperatively to decrease tumor size in inoperable masses or to spare radical surgical excision, as in the orbit. Radiation given to young children will cause decrease in growth in the radiated field. If the field includes a part of the face, the child may develop a noticeable asymmetry with aging.

Chemotherapy is recommended in all children with rhabdomyosarcoma and soft-tissue sarcoma. The use of chemotherapy has increased the survival rate in these children whether they have metastatic disease at diagnosis or not. The regimens for advanced stage disease are severely myelosuppressive.

NURSING MANAGEMENT AND FAMILY TEACHING

Nursing management of the child with rhabdomyosarcoma emphasizes emotional support and education of the client and family. Therapy is multimodal and intense in nature. As with other malignancies, teaching about prevention and early recognition of side effects of treatment or recurrence cannot be overemphasized. Children who receive this intense therapy are at risk for late effects.

RETINOBLASTOMA

Retinoblastoma is a rare form of cancer in children and exceptionally uncommon in adults. It is a tumor of the eye that develops when immature retinal cells, called retinoblasts, become malignant and grow out of control. In the United States approximately 200 children are diagnosed with retinoblastoma each year (Baniewicz, 2008). This tumor is usually found in infants and very young children; most are diagnosed before age four years. About 40% of cases of retinoblastoma are hereditary, with 60% nonhereditary. The retinoblastoma cells can spread along the optic nerve to reach the brain, or through the covering layers of the globe into the eye socket. Once tissues outside the globe are affected, the cancer may then spread to lymph nodes, bones, bone marrow, or other organs. Most retinoblastoma tumors are discovered before they spread outside the globe of the eye. Overall prognosis is excellent, as 96% of children with retinoblastoma survive more than five years (Baniewicz, 2008).

CLINICAL MANIFESTATIONS

Usually retinoblastoma is detected by the caregiver, who notices a whitish glow in the pupil. Leukocoria or **cat's eye reflex** is seen, instead of the typical red reflex that appears in photographs. This is the most common manifestation. Other signs include strabismus and red painful eyes and blindness (late manifestations).

DIAGNOSIS

Children with suspected retinoblastoma are referred to an ophthalmologist to confirm the diagnosis. Retinoblastoma is diagnosed with a thorough eye examination under anesthesia. Ultrasound, CT, or MRI are the most often ordered imaging studies when verifying this tumor. Bone marrow aspirate and lumbar puncture also provide information on metastatic disease spread for staging prior to treatment.

TREATMENT

Treatment of retinoblastoma depends upon whether the tumor is unilateral or bilateral, quality of vision, and whether the tumor extends beyond the globe. Surgery, radiation therapy, laser therapy, cryotherapy (using very cold probes to freeze and kill the tumor), and chemotherapy are all used to treat this tumor. When the tumor is found in only one eye and vision has been destroyed, the usual treatment is **enucleation**, or surgical removal of the eye. If bilateral disease is present, and there is still some useful vision, then

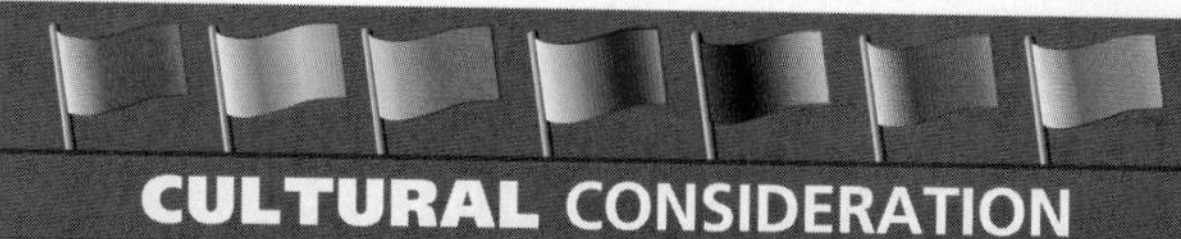

CULTURAL CONSIDERATION

How Would You Support an International Family Whose Disease Perception Varies from Western Scientific Reasoning?

An international family who came to the United States for treatment of bilateral retinoblastoma refuses to consent for bilateral enucleation which would probably cure their child. They refuse because in their country a blind child has no support or hope for an education—in other words, "no future." They prefer to take her home, care for her as best they can, and allow her to die.

other forms of treatment are used. Recent clinical trials using local tumor control with laser therapy combined with chemotherapy have shown much promise in preserving vision and curing the disease. When retinoblastoma spreads locally beyond the globe or metastasizes to distant sites, systemic therapy is used. This may include chemotherapy, radiation therapy, and hematopoietic stem cell transplantation. Once retinoblastoma metastasizes, chemotherapy may control the disease, but usually is not curative.

NURSING MANAGEMENT AND FAMILY TEACHING

Nursing management is important for the child. Family teaching for retinoblastoma includes several therapeutic approaches; ophthalmic surgery, chemotherapy, and radiation therapy. The multidisciplinary approach also includes genetic counseling and services for the visually impaired.

LATE EFFECTS OF CANCER THERAPY

The number of childhood cancer survivors has increased dramatically over the past few decades as pediatric cancer approaches a nearly 80% overall cure rate (O'Leary et al., 2008). The upturn in survival can be attributed to more effective therapies, organized treatment protocols, and advances in supportive care for children with cancer. One of these includes the development of pediatric oncology nursing as a specialty.

The definition of a long-term childhood cancer survivor is one who has been free of cancer for five years and off all cancer therapy for two years. With the increase in numbers of survivors, new family and child support options have developed and many pediatric oncology centers now have clinics where the special needs of long-term survivors are addressed. Survivors often have complex psychosocial and physical problems. Some may not show up for many years after treatment (Oeffinger et al., 2006). Late effects are complications from cancer and its treatment, which persist or become apparent after treatment is completed. Nearly two out of three childhood cancer survivors experience at least one late effect (Bhatia, Blatt, & Meadows, 2006). The degree to which an individual experiences late effects is related to the type of cancer, the type and intensity of treatment, the child's age at diagnosis, and the physiologic and developmental status of the individual at the time of diagnosis and treatment (Nathan, 2009). Survivors of bone tumors, CNS tumors, Hodgkin's disease, and those whose treatment plans included chest, abdominal, or pelvic irradiation are most at risk for severe long-term health conditions (Oeffinger et al., 2006). Late effects of childhood cancer therapy have been identified in all major organs.

Children who have received radiation therapy to the brain may show growth retardation and cognitive impairments. These effects are dose- and age-related, with children less than five years of age at the time of radiation being the most affected. As a result, cranial irradiation has been replaced by intrathecal chemotherapy in the treatment of most ALL patients. Cognitive impairment may be manifest as a significant decrease in the child's general intelligence or as problems with visual spatial skills, attention span, short-term memory, verbal fluency, and the rapidity with which information can be processed.

The endocrine system can be affected by damage to end organs such as the ovaries and testes or by damage to endocrine pathways. Radiation to the head or neck can damage the hypothalamus resulting in growth issues. The thyroid gland is very sensitive to radiation therapy. Children who have received radiation to the head and neck area may develop primary hypothyroidism. Impaired ovarian function in women or testicular dysfunction in men is seen in clients who have received alkylating chemotherapeutic agents such as cyclophosphamide. These findings are related to the age of the child and dose of the alkylating agents. Gonadal irradiation, including total body irradiation, affects the function of reproductive organs. Treatment can produce sterility and decrease hormone production, leading to an absence or delay in pubertal development. As childhood cancer survival rates increase, fertility preservation becomes an increasingly important topic (Zakak, 2009).

Radiation that includes the ear canal may lead to chronic radiation otitis. The chemotherapeutic agent, cisplatin, is known to cause hearing loss. When radiation therapy is also given, the severity of the hearing loss is increased. Radiation to the head and neck may also produce abnormalities in the teeth, including incomplete calcification, tooth and root agenesis, and arrested tooth development. Chronic changes to the oral mucosa may be seen postradiation, including xerostomia, loss of mucosal pliability, and chronic oral ulcers. Skin changes postradiation may include permanent hyperpigmentation, atrophy, and hair loss of the affected area.

EVIDENCE-BASED PRACTICE

What Is the Role of the Professional Nurse in Addressing Fertility Issues Related to Childhood Cancer Treatment?

CLINICAL PROBLEM

How can health care providers improve quality of life issues related to fertility in pediatric cancer survivors?

BEST CLINICAL PRACTICE

- Studies report that while fertility issues are viewed as important by pediatric cancer survivors, infertility often comes as a surprise
- Surveys of pediatric hematologist/oncologists have found that fertility preservation is often not discussed with childhood and adolescent cancer patients
- Fertility preservation options for both males and females are currently available with several others in the experimental stages
- Patients and families report finding open discussion about fertility options to be beneficial

IMPLICATIONS FOR NURSING

- Nurses should familiarize themselves with fertility issues and fertility options available to pediatric cancer patients
- As patient educators and advocates, nurses are in a position to provide fertility information and make sure that fertility issues are addressed with all pediatric oncology patients
- Nurses should work cooperatively with all disciplines to develop fertility screening tools and educational resources that are developmentally appropriate and easy to understand

Reference: Zakak, N. (2009). Fertility issues of childhood cancer survivors: The role of the pediatric nurse practitioner in fertility preservation. *Journal of Pediatric Oncology Nursing, 26*(1), 48–59.

NURSING TIP

Camps for Children with Life-Threatening Illnesses

Around the country there are summer camps designed especially for children with life-threatening illnesses, cancer included. These camps offer these children a respite where they can get to know others that may struggle with the same emotions as they do and just be a kid. These camps offer activities that foster self confidence. The activities (like swinging from a rope over a net) can be done with special equipment or with an adult so that all children can have the experience if they feel up to it.

Doctors, nurses, and other health care professionals often donate a week or two of their time to work at these camps. Thus the campers always have medical care available to them to address their particular needs.

Impaired lung and thoracic development and chronic pulmonary compromise can occur after radiation or chemotherapy. Pulmonary compromise is manifest as acute pneumonitis and pulmonary fibrosis. Bleomycin is the chemotherapeutic agent most commonly associated with pulmonary complications. Dyspnea, dry cough, and low exercise tolerance are all signs of pulmonary fibrosis.

The heart may experience long-term effects from chemotherapy or radiation, which can be life-threatening. These treatments may cause irreversible damage to the heart. Anthracyclines are chemotherapeutic agents known to affect the heart by damaging cardiac myocytes. Chronic effects manifest as cardiomyopathy, pericarditis, or both. Cardiac toxicity from radiation alone may result in pericardial effusions or constrictive pericarditis. Decreased bone marrow function and immunosuppression may be long-term sequelae of cancer therapy and contribute to the increased risk of second malignancies. Bone marrow transplantation also places the child at great risk for hematopoietic late effects.

Musculoskeletal defects involving the bones, soft tissues, and teeth have been reported most frequently in children with solid tumors. Survivors of bone tumors may experience disfigurement and functional limitations related to limb amputation or limb salvage surgeries. Other musculoskeletal late effects include scoliosis, atrophy, and osteoporosis. These effects are usually the result of radiation therapy to the area. Higher doses of radiation delivered to the younger child results in more pronounced late effects to the treated area. Corticosteroids have been implicated in the development of avascular necrosis.

Children and adolescents cured of cancer have an increased risk of developing a second malignant neoplasm, defined as a tumor whose histologic type is different from the primary malignancy. The risk of developing a second malignancy is up to six times greater in survivors compared to the risk of first cancers in the population at large. The most common second malignancies are AML, breast, bone, and thyroid cancers. Those most at risk include survivors of Hodgkin's disease, hereditary retinoblastoma, and children who received high doses of radiation or alkylating agents (Bhatia et al., 2006).

Childhood cancer survivors also experience psychosocial issues that can impact their quality of life. Survivors must deal with feelings of loss, fear, and uncertainty and may be at risk for depression (Sharp, Kinahan, Didwania, & Stolley, 2007). Treatment can impact education and occupational achievement due to cognitive impairments. Survivors may have difficulty obtaining health and life insurance and many have inadequate long-term follow-up care.

Long-term surveillance and the recognition of the potential for the development of these late effects allow the nurse to provide anticipatory guidance, supportive care, and interventions for symptom management. Long-term evaluations specific to the child's cancer therapy need to be done at least annually (or more frequently as necessary). A long-term follow-up visit provides the opportunity to encourage clients to follow the recommendations for risk reduction and early detection. Long term follow-up care has become a specialty of its own, with comprehensive programs that monitor and manage late effects, provide education, address psychosocial issues, encourage wellness activities, and assist with financial issues specific to cancer survivors (Children's Oncology Group, 2007). Those in the pediatric oncology field look forward to the day when late effects of therapy can be prevented; in the meantime helping clients and their families anticipate and cope with late effects remains a critical element in the care of survivors of childhood cancer.

IN THE REAL WORLD

As a pediatric oncology nurse I am often asked, "Isn't it depressing to be around kids who are so sick and die? How can you go and work there everyday?" I respond that this is the most rewarding job I can ever imagine. Yes, there are sad days; when a child relapses or dies, the entire staff feels the family's pain, but oncology nursing is not depressing. Most children will have their cancer go into remission, and many will be cured. New advances in science improve the survival rates every year. Few other areas of nursing allow the nurse to get to know their clients and families so well. Pediatric oncology nursing is working on the cutting-edge of new scientific discoveries. I can counsel the caregiver and child, provide information, and offer comfort measures, whether it is pain medication or even rocking a child while reading him a book. The families whom I provide care to suffer great hardships, and I have the privilege to get to know them and be able to ease some of their burden.

CHALLENGES OF THE PEDIATRIC ONCOLOGY NURSE

Pediatric oncology nursing involves cutting edge technology and knowledge. It is easy to see only the disease and the technology. Both can be very dehumanizing and demeaning. A constant challenge for the oncology nurse is to focus beyond the technology and focus on the child and family. The oncology nurse must connect with them in such a way that their dignity, uniqueness, and strengths are enhanced and preserved (Foley & Fergusson, 2007).

KEY CONCEPTS

- Cancer is the leading cause of death from disease in children 1–14 years of age. Only accidents claim more lives.
- The primary treatment modalities for childhood cancer may include surgery, chemotherapy, radiation therapy, hematopoietic stem cell transplantation (HSCT), and biologic response modifiers (BRMs).
- Colony stimulating factors are now widely used with children on chemotherapy to decrease the time the child is neutropenic and at risk for infection. Nurses are responsible for teaching the caregivers the administration of these agents in the home. Frequent monitoring of the CBC is needed to know when these agents can be stopped.
- The hematopoietic, gastrointestinal, hepatic, renal, integumentary, and reproductive systems are most commonly affected by side effects of chemotherapy. The nurse caring for the child undergoing chemotherapy is responsible for side effect management.
- Infection is the leading cause of death in the immunosuppressed child. Good hand washing and infection control measures are essential for the nurse to practice and teach the child and caregiver.
- Children with venous access devices are at increased risk of infection. Caregivers need to be taught the proper care of the devices and signs of infection.

- Hematopoietic stem cell transplant is a treatment modality for leukemia, lymphomas, and certain solid tumors.
- The most common childhood malignancies are leukemia, brain tumors, and lymphomas.
- Children with leukemia commonly present with anemia, thrombocytopenia, and neutropenia, manifested as bleeding and fever. Pain is also a presenting symptom caused by bone destruction from leukemic infiltrates.
- Acute renal compromise can result from tumor lysis syndrome in children with leukemia and lymphoma. Nursing management includes IV hydration, alkalization of the child's urine with sodium bicarbonate, and the administration of allopurinol, prior to starting chemotherapy.
- Children with brain tumors may present with subtle neurological findings or signs of increased intracranial pressure.
- Children with neuroblastoma commonly present with advanced disease. Nursing care includes management of the presenting symptoms such as pain and, once chemotherapy has started, management of the side effects of therapy.
- Wilms' tumor is a malignancy of childhood that arises from the kidney. This tumor usually presents as an abdominal mass. Treatment is with surgery, chemotherapy, and sometimes radiation therapy.
- Limb-sparing surgery is commonly used for osteogenic sarcoma (bone tumors). Children with this type of cancer need to be prepared preoperatively both physically and emotionally. These individuals and their caregivers are to be informed of issues of body image and the expected amount of limb function prior to the procedure.
- Rhabdomyosarcoma and soft-tissue sarcoma are the most common sarcomas of childhood. These children usually present with a hard, nontender mass. Sarcomas are primarily treated with wide surgical excision, radiation therapy, and chemotherapy.
- Long-term effects of cancer therapy involve all major organs. Nurses in the outpatient settings need to assess for these specific side effects and provide prompt management and support. Cancer survivors are followed for life for late effects of therapy.

REVIEW ACTIVITIES

1. List and describe the three most common childhood malignancies.
2. Describe how chemotherapy and radiation therapy are used in treating cancer.
3. List at least four common side effects of chemotherapy and describe how the nurse should manage these.
4. What are the client and family teaching needs of a child receiving a venous access device?
5. Describe the nursing interventions to prevent tumor lysis syndrome in a child who has recently been diagnosed with lymphoma.
6. Identify the nursing interventions for a child presenting with fever and neutropenia.
7. What is the single most important means of preventing infection?
8. How would you treat a child presenting with mucositis?
9. What should be included in a discharge care plan for the child recently diagnosed with a brain tumor?
10. Describe why screening for late effects of cancer therapy is important for cancer survivors.

STUDY QUESTIONS

1. To alleviate nausea and vomiting caused by chemotherapy the administration of antiemetics is started:
   a. One hour before the administration of chemotherapy and continued for 24 hours after the completion of chemotherapy.

b. After nausea and vomiting has occurred and for 24 hours after the completion of chemotherapy.
c. 30 minutes before chemotherapy and for 8 hours after the completion of chemotherapy.
d. 30 minutes before chemotherapy and for 24 hours after the resolution of nausea and vomiting.

2. A 4-year-old with ALL has just completed a course of chemotherapy. She was noted to have an ANC of 300 yesterday in clinic. She presents to the ER today with fever. Your first assessment reveals: T 102.5 axillary, HR 120, RR 23, BP 98/70. The child is talkative, her color is pink, she has good capillary refill, and her O2 saturation is 100%. She does not have a VAD and she has been stuck two times for her CBC. No cultures were obtained because of the difficult stick. What are your next steps?
   a. Recognize fever and neutropenia as a medical emergency. Get an experienced phlebotomist and start antibiotics within 30 minutes. Obtain blood cultures, urine culture, and chest X-ray as soon as possible.
   b. Get an experienced phlebotomist. Get blood cultures, urine cultures, and a chest X-ray, then start antibiotics.
   c. Because the child is not neutropenic, you can give antibiotics IM and send the child home.
   d. Recognize fever and neutropenia as a medical emergency and have the child transferred to the ICU, where the ICU staff will place an IV draw blood, get urine cultures and a chest X-ray, and start IV antibiotics.
3. A 16-year-old with rhabdomyosarcoma of the sinuses completed a course of chemotherapy last week consisting of vincristine, cytoxan, and adriamycin. Today he presents to clinic with a headache, pallor, and fatigue on exertion. His CBC revealed a WBC of 3.0, Hgb 7 gms, platelet count 50,000, ANC 700. His other measurements include: T 98.1°F HR 122 RR 26 BP 116/74. What is the probable cause of his symptoms?
   a. Side effects of chemotherapy resulting in anemia
   b. Side effects of chemotherapy resulting in thrombocytopenia
   c. Side effects of chemotherapy resulting in neutropenia
   d. Side effect of chemotherapy resulting in immunosuppression
4. An 8-year-old with a brain tumor comes to clinic today for Cyclophosphamide. In addition to double-checking the client's chemotherapy doses with the orders, maintaining good hydration, and using gloves for the administration of the drug, what other precaution will you take before administration of this drug?
   a. Monitor the client's stool frequency.
   b. Monitor the client's urine for glucose.
   c. Monitor the client's urine for hematuria.
   d. Monitor the client's blood pressure for hypotension.
5. Chemotherapy waste is disposed of in a:
   a. Trash receptacle.
   b. Receptacle with lid and plastic bag.
   c. Red plastic bag receptacle for hazardous waste.
   d. Chemo-approved hazardous waste receptacle.
6. Children and adolescents who have completed cancer therapy are carefully followed for late effects of therapy for what period of time?
   a. 6 months after therapy
   b. For life
   c. 5 years after therapy
   d. 1 year after therapy
7. A 10-year-old boy with AML will soon be discharged from the hematopoietic stem cell transplantation (HSCT) unit. It has been twelve weeks since his transplant. His ANC is 1100. He is anxious to get back to school. You inform him and his family that:
   a. Since he is no longer neutropenic he can go home, restart his immunizations, and go to school. Immunosuppression is not an issue.
   b. He is still neutropenic and immunocompromised so he cannot return to school for six months.
   c. He is no longer neutropenic so he can go home. However he is still immunocompromised and will have to wait six months for immune recovery before he can go back to school.
   d. Since he is no longer neutropenic he can go home. His immunosuppression may continue for up to a year posttransplant. He will have to wait until he remains nonneutropenic for several months to return to school.
8. Nurses administering chemotherapy should use what personal protective equipment:
   a. Use of nonporous gloves only
   b. Nonporous gloves and a gown
   c. A gown, mask, nonporous gloves, and eye shields
   d. Only standard precautions are required
9. Chemotherapy most commonly affects which of the following normal cells?
   a. Skin, oral mucosa, GI tract, liver and kidneys
   b. Skin, GI tract, bone marrow, and liver
   c. Hair follicles, GI tract, and bone marrow
   d. Hair follicles, bone marrow, gonads, and kidneys

10. The nurse is assigned to a child who has a platelet count of 15,000 per cubic millimeter. The nurse realizes that which of the following is true?
    a. A blood thinner such as Coumadin needs to be considered by the physician.
    b. There is serious danger of infection even from normal skin bacteria.
    c. This is a normal platelet count, and no precautions need to be taken.
    d. The child has a high risk of spontaneous bleeding which can be life threatening.

REFERENCES

Adlard, K. (2008). Examining the push-pull method of blood sampling from central venous access devices. *Journal of Pediatric Oncology Nursing, 25*(4), 200–207.

American Academy of Pediatrics. (2006a). Immunocompromised children. In L. K. Pickering (Ed.). *Red book: 2006 report of the committee on infectious diseases* (27th ed.). Elk Grove Village, IL: American Academy of Pediatrics, pp. 71–80.

American Academy of Pediatrics. (2006b). Varicella zoster infections. In L. K. Pickering (Ed.). *Red book: 2006 report of the committee on infectious diseases* (27th ed.). Elk Grove Village, IL: American Academy of Pediatrics, pp. 711–717.

American Brain Tumor Association. (2007). *A primer of brain tumors: A patient's reference manual* (8th ed.). Des Plaines, IL: Author.

Androkities, A. (2008). Non-Hodgkin's Lymphoma. In N. Kline (Ed.), *Essentials of pediatric hematology/oncology nursing: A core curriculum* (3rd ed.). Glenview, IL: Association of Pediatric Hematology/Oncology Nurses, pp. 20–25.

Ayoola, A., & Lee, L. Y. (2006). Radiation recall dermatitis with cefotetan: A case study. *The Oncologist, 11*, 1118–1120.

Baniewicz, D. (2008). Retinoblastoma. In N. Kline (Ed.). *Essentials of pediatric hematology/oncology nursing: A core curriculum* (3rd ed.). Glenview, IL: Association of Pediatric Hematology/Oncology Nurses, 52–54.

Bernstein, M., Kovar, H., Paulussen, M., Randall, R. L., Schuck, A., Teot, L. A., & Juergens, H. (2006). Ewing sarcoma family of tumors: Ewing sarcoma of bone and soft tissue and the peripheral primitive neuroectodermal tumors. In P. A. Pizzo & D. G. Poplack (Eds.), *Principles and practice of pediatric oncology* (5th ed.). Philadelphia, PA: Lippincott, Williams & Wilkins, pp. 1002–1032.

Betcher, D. L., Simon, P. J., & McHard, K. M. (2007). Bone Tumors. In N. Kline (Ed.), *Essentials of pediatric hematology/oncology nursing: A core curriculum* (3rd ed.). Glenview, IL: Association of Pediatric Hematology/Oncology Nurses, pp. 575–587.

Bhatia, S., Blatt, J., & Meadows, A. T. (2006). Late effects of childhood cancer and its treatment. In P. A. Pizzo & D. G. Poplack (Eds.), *Principles and practice of pediatric oncology* (5th ed.). Philadelphia, PA: Lippincott, Williams & Wilkins, pp. 1490–1514.

Blaney, S. M., Kun, L. E., Hunter, J., Rorke-Adams, L. B., Lau, C., Strother, D., & Pollack, I. F. (2006). Tumors of the central nervous system. In P. A. Pizzo & D. G. Poplack (Eds.). *Principles and practice of pediatric oncology* (5th ed.). Philadelphia, PA: Lippincott, Williams & Wilkins, pp. 786–851.

Bollard, C., Krance, R. A., & Hesop, H. E. (2007). Hematopoietic stem cell transplantation in pediatric oncology. In P. A. Pizzo & D. G. Poplack (Eds.). *Principles and practice of pediatric oncology* (5th ed.). Philadelphia, PA: Lippincott, Williams & Wilkins, pp. 476–500.

Brodeur, G. M., & Maris, J. M. (2006). Neuroblastoma. In P. A. Pizzo & D. G. Poplack (Eds.). *Principles and practice of pediatric oncology* (5th ed.). Philadelphia, PA: Lippincott, Williams & Wilkins, pp. 933–970.

Children's Oncology Group. (2007). *Long term follow up program resource guide.* Retrieved March 30, 2009, from http://survivorshipguidelines.org/pdf/LTFUResourceGuide.pdf.

Corey, A., & Snyder, S. (2008). Antibiotics in 30 minutes or less for febrile neutropenic patients: A quality control measure in a new hospital. *Journal of Pediatric Oncology Nursing, 25*(4), 208–212.

D'Amore, R. (2008). Ewing's sarcoma of bone and soft tissue and peripheral primitive neuroectodermal tumors. In N. Kline (Ed.), *Essentials of pediatric hematology/oncology nursing: A core curriculum* (3rd ed.). Glenview, IL: Association of Pediatric Hematology/Oncology Nurses, pp. 40–43.

D'Andrea, L. (2008). Neuroblastoma. In N. Kline (Ed.). *Essentials of pediatric hematology/oncology nursing: A core curriculum* (3rd ed.). Glenview, IL: Association of Pediatric Hematology/Oncology Nurses, pp. 32–36.

Dome, J. S., Cotton, C. A., Perlman, E. J., Breslow, N. E., Kalapurakal, J. A., Ritchey, M. L., Grundy, P. E., Malogolowkin, M., Beckwith, J. B., Shamberger, R. C., Haase, G. M., Coppes, M. J., Coccia, P., Kletzel, M., Weetman, R. M., Donaldson, M., Macklis, R. M., & Green, D. M. (2006). Treatment of anaplastic histology Wilms' tumor: Results from the fifth national Wilms' tumor study. *Journal of Clinical Oncology, 24*(15), 2352–2358.

Drigan, R., & Androkites, A. L., (2007). Wilms, tumor. In C. R. Baggott, K. P. Kelly, D. Fochtman, & G. V. Foley (Eds.). *Nursing care of children and adolescents with cancer* (3rd ed.). Philadelphia: W. B. Saunders, pp. 568–574.

Duffy-Lind, E. Care After Cure: Improving the Quality of Life of Children Cancer Survivors, March, 2008, University of Massachusetts Memorial Medical Center, Worcester, MA.

Foley, G., & Fergusson, J. (2007). History, issues and trends. In C. R. Baggott, K. P. Kelly, D. Fochtman, & G. V. Foley (Eds.). *Nursing care of children and adolescents with cancer* (3rd ed.). Philadelphia: W. B. Saunders, pp. 2–21.

Glasgow, M., Smith, E., & Bello, G. (2008). Bone marrow donation: Factors influencing intentions in African Americans. *Oncology Nursing Forum Online, 34*(2), 369–377.

Golub, T. D., & Arceci, R. J. (2007). Acute myelogenous leukemia. In P. A. Pizzo & D. G. Poplack (Eds.), *Principles and practice of pediatric oncology* (5th ed.). Philadelphia, PA: Lippincott, Williams & Wilkins, pp. 591–644.

Holloway, J. A. (2008). Osteosarcoma. In N. Kline (Ed.). *Essentials of pediatric hematology/oncology nursing: A core curriculum* (3rd ed.). Glenview, IL: Association of Pediatric Hematology/Oncology Nurses, pp. 36–40.

Landier, W. (2007). Myeloid diseases. In C. R. Baggott, K. P. Kelly, D. Fochtman, & G. V. Foley (Eds.). *Nursing care of children and adolescents with cancer* (3rd ed.). Philadelphia: W. B. Saunders, pp. 491–502.

McCarthy, K. (2008). Leukemia. In N. Kline (Ed.). *Essentials of pediatric hematology/oncology nursing: A core curriculum* (3rd ed.). Glenview, IL: Association of Pediatric Hematology/Oncology Nurses, pp. 15–20.

McCune, R. (2008). Biologic response modifiers. In N. Kline (Ed.). *Essentials of pediatric hematology/oncology nursing: A core curriculum* (3rd ed.). Glenview, IL: Association of Pediatric Hematology/Oncology Nurses, pp. 108–112.

Nathan, P. (2009). *Late effects of childhood cancer: Current research & the impact on health.* Teleconference, 1-20-09. Sponsored by: The National Children's Cancer Society.

O'Leary, M., Krailo, M., Anderson, J., & Reaman, G. (2008). Progress in childhood cancer: 50 years of research collaboration, a report from the Children's Oncology Group. *Seminars in Oncology, 35*(5), 484–493.

Oeffinger, K., Mertens, A., Sklar, C., Kawashima, T., Hudson, M., Meadows, A., Freidman, D., Marin, N., Hobbie, W., Kada-Lottick, N., Schwartz, C., Leisenring, W., & Robinson, L. (2006). Chronic health conditions in adult survivors of childhood cancer. *New England Journal of Medicine, 355*(15), 1572–1582.

Okcu, M. F., Hicks, J., Merchant, T. E., Andrassy, R. J., Pappo, A. S., & Horowitz, M. E. (2006). Nonrhabdomyosarcomatous soft tissue sarcomas. In P. A. Pizzo & D. G. Poplack (Eds.). *Principles and practice of pediatric oncology* (5th ed.). Philadelphia, PA: Lippincott, Williams & Wilkins, pp. 1033–1073.

Park, J., Eggert, A., & Caron, H. (2008). Neuroblastoma: Biology, prognosis, and treatment. *Pediatric Clinics of North America, 55*, 97–120.

Post-White, J., Fitzgerald, M., Hageness, S., & Sencer, S. F. (2009). Complementary and alternative medicine use in children with cancer and general and specialty pediatrics. *Journal of Pediatric Oncology Nursing, 26*(1), 7–15.

Ries, L. A. G., Smith, M. A., Gurney, J. G., Linet, M., Tamra, T., Young, J. L., Bunin, G. R. (Eds.). (1999). Cancer incidence and survival among children and adolescents: United States SEER Program 1975–1995. Bethesda, Md: National Cancer Institute, SEER Program.

Ruccione, K. (2007). Biological basis of cancer in children and adolescents. In C. R. Baggott, K. P. Kelly, D. Fochtman, & G. V. Foley (Eds.), *Nursing care of children and adolescents with cancer* (3rd ed.). Philadelphia: W. B. Saunders, pp. 24–63.

Ryan-Murray, J., & Petriccione, M. (2007). Central nervous system tumors. In C. R. Baggott, K. P. Kelly, D. Fochtman, & G. V. Foley (Eds.), *Nursing care of children and adolescents with cancer* (3rd ed.). Philadelphia: W. B. Saunders, pp. 503–523.

Sharp, L., Kinahan, K., Didwania, A., & Stolley, M. (2007). Quality of life in adult survivors of childhood cancer. *Journal of Pediatric Oncology Nursing, 24*(4), 220–226.

Smith, M. (2006). Evolving molecularly targeted therapies and biotherapeutics. In P. A. Pizzo & D. G. Poplack (Eds.). *Principles and practice of pediatric oncology* (5th ed.). Philadelphia, PA: Lippincott, Williams & Wilkins, pp. 366–404.

Tonini, G. P., & Pistoia, V. (2006). Molecularly guided therapy of neuroblastoma: A review of different approaches. *Current Pharmaceutical Design, 12*(18), 2303–2317.

Triche, T. J., Hicks, J., & Sorensen, P. H. B. (2006). Diagnostic pathology of pediatric malignancies. In P. A. Pizzo & D. G. Poplack (Eds.), *Principles and practice of pediatric oncology* (5th ed.). Philadelphia, PA: Lippincott, Williams & Wilkins, pp. 185–231.

Vizcarra, C., & Belcher, D. (2006). Management of the patient receiving parental biologic therapy. *Journal of Infusion Nursing, 29*(2), 63–71.

Volker, T., Denecke, T., Steffen, I., Misch, D., Schonberger, S., Plotkin, M., Ruf, J., Furth, C., Stover, B., Hautzel, H., Henze, G., & Amthauer, H. (2007). Positron emission tomography for staging of pediatric sarcoma patients: Results of a prospective multicenter trial. *Journal of Clinical Oncology, 25*(34), 5435–5441.

Vrooman, L. M., & Silverman, L. B. (2009). Childhood acute lymphoblastic leukemia: Update on prognostic factors. *Current Opinions in Pediatrics, 21*, 1–8.

Watral, M. (2008). Central-nervous-system tumors. In N. Kline (Ed.), *Essentials of pediatric hematology/oncology nursing: A core curriculum* (3rd ed.). Glenview, IL: Association of Pediatric Hematology/Oncology Nurses, pp. 28–32.

Wayne, A., Reaman, G., & Helman, L. (2008). Editorial. *Journal of the National Cancer Institute, 100*(18), 1271–1273.

Westlake, S. K., & Bertolone, K. L. (2007). Acute lymphoblastic leukemia. In C. R. Baggott, K. P. Kelly, D. Fochtman, & G. V. Foley (Eds.), *Nursing care of children and adolescents with cancer* (3rd ed.). Philadelphia: W. B. Saunders, pp. 466–490.

Zakak, N. (2009). Fertility issues of childhood cancer survivors: The role of the pediatric nurse practitioner in fertility preservation. *Journal of Pediatric Oncology Nursing, 26*(1), 48–58.

SUGGESTED READINGS

Echevarría, M. E., Fangusaro, J., & Goldman, S. (2008). Pediatric central nervous system germ cell tumors: A review. *Oncologist, 13*(6), 690–699.

Esper, P., Gale, D., & Muehlbauer, P. (2007). What kind of rash is it? Deciphering the dermatologic toxicities of biologic and targeted therapies. *Clinical Journal of Oncology Nursing, 11*(5), 659–666.

Meeske, K., & Nelson, M. B. (2008). The role of the long term follow-up clinic in discovering new emerging late effects in adult survivors of childhood cancer. *Journal of Pediatric Oncology Nursing, 25*(4), 213–219.

Shankar, A., Fiumara, F., & Pinkerton, R. (2008). Role of FDG PET in the management of childhood lymphomas-case proven or is the jury still out? *European Journal of Cancer, 44*(2008), 663–673.

RESOURCES

Refer to the online student StudyWARE for Potts & Mandleco at http://www.CengageBrain.com for additional content and study aids.

Organization: **American Brain Tumor Association**
Description: The American Brain Tumor Association exists to eliminate brain tumors through research and to meet the needs of brain tumor patients and their families. The website provides users with information regarding tumor treatment, research progress, and advocacy.
Website/Resource: http://www.abta.org

Organization: **American Cancer Society**
Description: The American Cancer Society is the nationwide, community-based, voluntary health organization dedicated to eliminating cancer as a major health problem by preventing cancer, saving lives, and diminishing suffering from cancer, through research, education, advocacy, and service. The website provides users with a wealth of information including access to health care, clinical trials, and much more.
Website/Resource: http://www.cancer.org

Organization: **Association of Pediatric Hematology/Oncology Nurses**
Description: The Association of Pediatric Hematology/Oncology Nurses (APHON) is the professional organization for pediatric hematology/oncology nurses and other pediatric hematology/oncology healthcare professionals. APHON provides the leadership and expertise to pediatric hematology/oncology nurses by defining and promoting the highest standards of practice and care to the pediatric, adolescent, and young adult communities. The website provides users with information regarding education, practice, products, and publications.
Website/Resource: http://www.aphon.org

Organization: **Candlelighters Childhood Cancer Foundation**
Description: The mission of Candlelighters Childhood Cancer Foundation is to provide information and awareness for children and adolescents with cancer and their families, to advocate for their needs, and to support research so every child survives and leads a long and healthy life. The website offers information regarding awareness, advocacy, research, and affiliates.
Website/Resource: http://www.candlelighters.org

Organization: **Childhood Brain Tumor Foundation**
Description: The Childhood Brain Tumor Foundation (CBTF) mission is to raise funds for scientific research; heighten public awareness of this most devastating disease; and improve prognosis and quality of life for those that are affected. CBTF's website provides a wealth of information regarding brain tumor types, diagnostics, therapies, and late effects of treatments.
Website/Resource: http://www.childhoodbraintumor.org

Organization: **Children's Oncology Group**
Description: This site offers long-term follow-up guidelines for survivors of childhood, adolescent, and young adult cancers. The purpose of these guidelines is to provide recommendations for screening and management of late effects that may potentially arise as a result of therapeutic exposures used during treatment for pediatric malignancies. They are intended to increase awareness of potential late effects and to standardize and enhance follow-up care provided to survivors.
Website/Resource: http://survivorshipguidelines.org/

Organization: **CureSearch: National Childhood Cancer Foundation Children's Oncology Group**
Description: CureSearch represents the combined efforts of the National Childhood Cancer Foundation and the Children's Oncology Group. The website helps parents and families of children with cancer find educational and support resources.
Website/Resource: http://www.childrensoncologygroup.org

Organization: **The Leukemia & Lymphoma Society, Inc.**
Description: The Leukemia & Lymphoma Society (LLS) is the world's largest voluntary health organization dedicated to funding blood cancer research, education, and patient services. LLS's mission: Cure leukemia, lymphoma, Hodgkin's disease and myeloma, and improve the quality of life of patients and their families. The website is a wealth of information about patient services, disease facts, advocacy, and science/professionals.
Website/Resource: http://www.leukemia-lymphoma.org

Organization: **National Cancer Institute**
Description: The National Cancer Institute coordinates the National Cancer Program, which conducts and supports research, training, health information dissemination, and other programs with respect to the cause, diagnosis, prevention, and treatment of cancer, rehabilitation from cancer, and the continuing care of cancer patients and the families of cancer patients. The website offers information regarding clinical trials, cancer topics, and cancer statistics.
Website/Resource: http://www.cancer.gov

Organization: **National Marrow Donor Program**
Description: The National Marrow Donor Program (NMDP) is a nonprofit organization dedicated to creating an opportunity for all patients to receive the bone marrow or umbilical cord blood transplant they need, when they need it. The website provides access to a donor registry as well as special links for physicians and families.
Website/Resource: http://www.marrow.org

Organization: **Oncology Nursing Society**

Description: The Oncology Nursing Society (ONS) is a professional organization of over 37,000 registered nurses and other healthcare providers dedicated to excellence in patient care, education, research, and administration in oncology nursing. It's also the largest professional oncology association in the world. The website provides information regarding education, clinical practice resources, publications, and membership services.

Website/Resource: http://www.ons.org

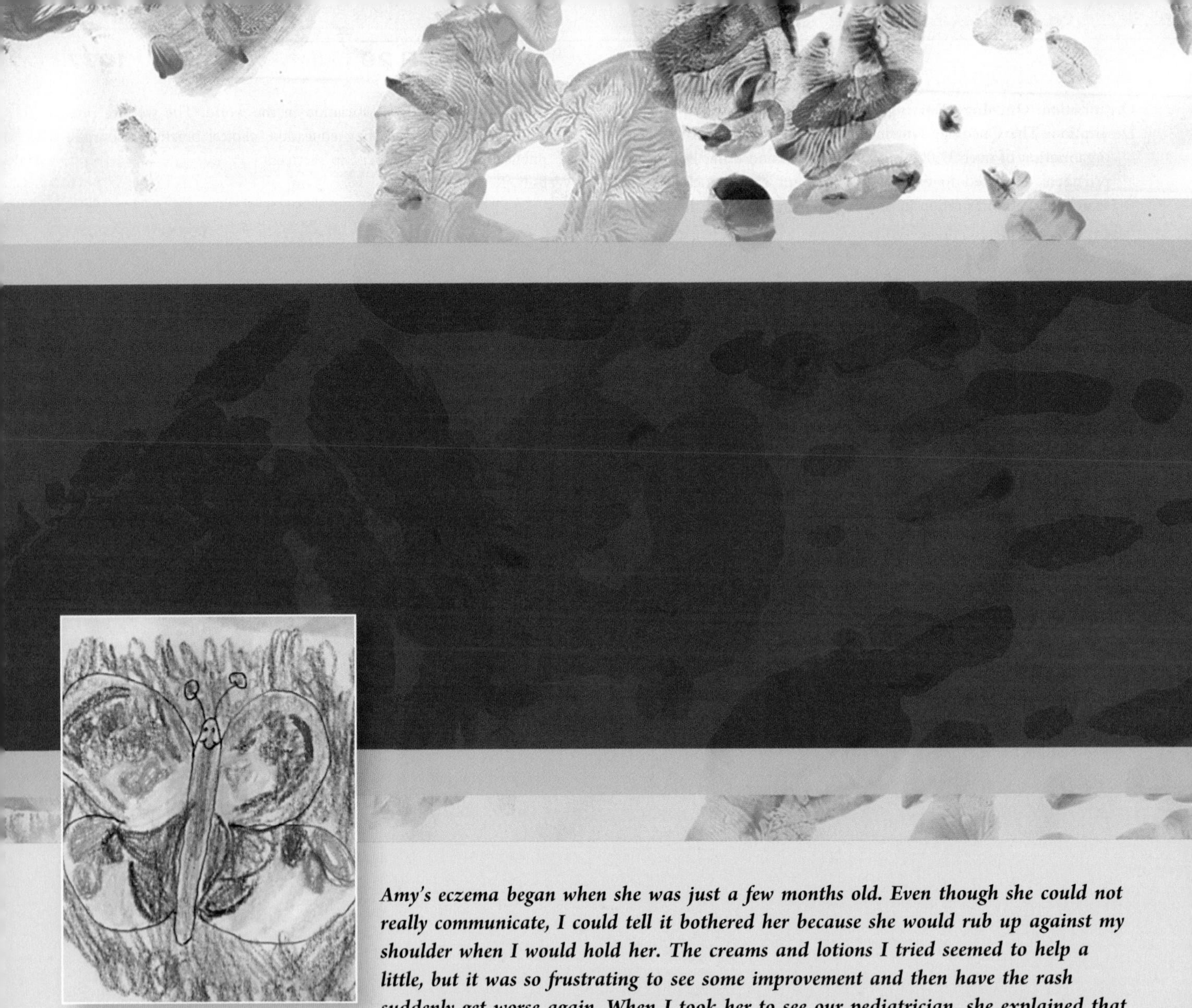

Amy's eczema began when she was just a few months old. Even though she could not really communicate, I could tell it bothered her because she would rub up against my shoulder when I would hold her. The creams and lotions I tried seemed to help a little, but it was so frustrating to see some improvement and then have the rash suddenly get worse again. When I took her to see our pediatrician, she explained that eczema is a chronic condition that involves both treatment for flares and preventive steps to reduce flares. She gave me some prescription ointment that helps Amy when her rash is really bad and her nurse gave me some good tips about what I can do everyday to help Amy's skin not get bad as often. It has been an adjustment to bathe her more often and put moisturizers on every day, but I am so glad that there are things I can do that make my daughter more comfortable. Amy is 5 years old now. Sometimes she complains about me putting cream on her, but she can go several months without a flare now. I am so happy to see her enjoying the life of a typical kindergartener without itching all the time or being embarrassed about her skin.

CHAPTER 30

Integumentary Alterations

CHRISTINA P. LINTON, PhD, FNP-BC

COMPETENCIES

Upon completion of this chapter, the reader will be able to:

- Discuss the anatomy and physiology of the skin, including developmental changes and racial differences.
- Discuss the etiology, pathophysiology, clinical manifestations, and management of common pediatric integumentary disorders.
- Discuss the appropriate nursing management and family teaching for children with various integumentary disorders.
- Prepare a family-centered plan of care for a child with a skin condition.
- Evaluate evidence-based practice related to the care of children with integumentary disorders.
- Successfully complete the games and activities in the online student StudyWARE.

The pediatric integumentary system plays a vital role in the child's health and well-being. From a physiological standpoint, it serves as a protective barrier against infectious organisms, external agents, and mechanical trauma. From a psychosocial perspective, the appearance of the skin can influence the child's self-image and others' perceptions of the child. Alterations of the pediatric integumentary system can occur from many different causes including infectious and noninfectious sources. Although integumentary disorders are rarely life-threatening, they can have a major impact on the child's comfort and social functioning. This chapter begins with an overview of the anatomy and physiology of the child's integument. A discussion of several pediatric integumentary disorders is then presented: bacterial infections, fungal infections, viral infections, infestations, dermatitis, acne, bites and stings, and sunburn.

BOX 30-1
FUNCTIONS OF THE SKIN

Provides a barrier to physical agents
Protects against mechanical injury
Prevents loss of body fluids
Helps regulate body temperature
Acts as a sensory organ
Reduces penetration of ultraviolet radiation
Plays a role in vitamin D production
Performs immune surveillance functions
Contributes to physical appearance

Adapted from: Gawkrodger, D. J. (2008). *Dermatology: An illustrated colour text* (4th ed.). Philadelphia, PA: Elsevier.

ANATOMY AND PHYSIOLOGY

The skin and its appendages (nails, hair, and certain glands) comprise one of the largest organs of the body, making up about 16% of the body's weight (Gawkrodger, 2008). As shown in Box 30-1, the integumentary system performs many functions. There are three distinct layers of the skin: the epidermis, the dermis, and the subcutaneous tissue. Figure 30-1 illustrates the structures of epidermal and dermal layers of the skin. The outer layer of the skin, the **epidermis**, acts as a physical and biological barrier to the environment and aids in maintaining internal homeostasis (Lawton, 2006a). This skin layer does not contain any blood vessels and is therefore dependent on the underlying dermis for nutrient delivery and waste disposal. The epidermis is primarily composed of keratinocytes which differentiate and move up through the layers of the epidermis until they reach the outermost layer, the **stratum corneum**, and are shed (desquamation). The stratum corneum consists of flattened dead keratinocytes and a mixture of lipids and proteins, which forms the skin's barrier against water loss and penetration by allergens and irritants. The cells in this layer normally have a high water content that keeps the stratum corneum pliable and prevents the formation of fissures and cracks.

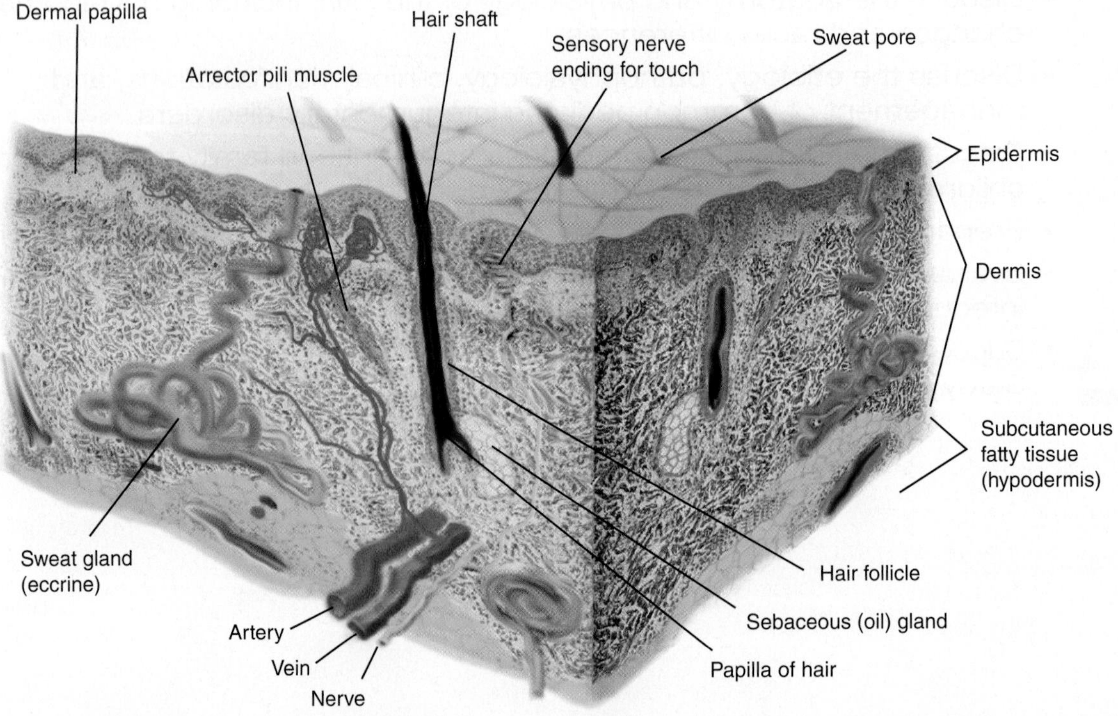

FIGURE 30-1 Structures of the Skin. DELMAR CENGAGE LEARNING.

NURSING ALERT

Sun Exposure and Vitamin D Synthesis

Many children and caregivers may feel that sun exposure is healthy because it is a source of vitamin D. However, it takes less than five minutes of unprotected sun exposure and about 20 minutes of exposure using an SPF 15 sunscreen to maximize vitamin D synthesis. Furthermore, vitamin D can also be obtained through dietary supplementation without exposing one's skin to the harmful effects of ultraviolet radiation.

In addition to keratinocytes, the epidermis contains **melanocytes**, which produce the pigment **melanin**. Melanin absorbs ultraviolet radiation, and thus, provides important protection from these potentially harmful rays (Lawton, 2006a). The absorption of ultraviolet radiation by the skin also promotes the synthesis of vitamin D. Current research supports that maximal vitamin D photosynthesis occurs after less than five minutes of unprotected sun exposure and about 20 minutes of exposure using an SPF 15 sunscreen. After this period of time, exposure to ultraviolet radiation produces only deleterious effects.

The middle layer of the skin, the **dermis**, has several functions: to sustain and support the epidermis, to protect and cushion the deeper structures, and to play a role in wound healing (Lawton, 2006b). This skin layer consists largely of fibroblasts, which synthesize collagen, the main component of the dermis. In addition, the dermis contains mast cells, which are involved in immune and inflammatory responses; blood vessels, which promote thermoregulation and supply nutrients; and lymphatic structures, which scavenge foreign material. Sensory nerve endings are also found in both the epidermis and dermis to facilitate detection of pain, irritation, and temperature. Below the dermis, the subcutaneous layer consists largely of fat. It provides the main support for the skin, insulates the body from cold, and provides shock absorption (Lawton, 2006a).

NURSING ALERT

Topical Medications and Infants

Topical medications should be used with caution in young infants because they have an increased rate of absorption, which may lead to toxicity.

The skin appendages all lie within the dermis and connect with the surface of the skin. Hair is a keratin structure that is found on all areas of the body except the palms, soles, and lips. Hair is important for temperature regulation, protection from UV radiation, and physical appearance. **Terminal hair** is found on the scalp, eyebrows, eyelashes, beard, axillae, and pubic areas. **Vellus hair** is the finer hair that covers the rest of the body. Fine **lanugo hairs** are present in utero and shed before or at birth. The nails consist of hardened, densely packed keratin. They protect the fingers and toes, facilitate grasping, and enhance the tactile sensitivity of the fingers (Lawton, 2006c).

The **sebaceous glands** are located along the hair follicles and secrete sebum, which lubricates the skin and hair. In addition, there are two types of sweat glands, both of which aid in the body's thermoregulation. The **eccrine glands** are found over the entire body, but are most prevalent on the forehead, axillae, palms, and soles. These glands have a duct that leads to the surface of the skin. In contrast, the **apocrine glands** have ducts that open into hair follicles. These glands are less numerous and are localized to the axillae, nipples, perineum, and scalp. The apocrine glands become active during puberty and produce a viscous material that causes body odor when it interacts with surface bacteria (Lawton, 2006c).

Table 30-1 presents several of the important differences between the integument of infants when compared to that

TABLE 30-1 Infant Skin Characteristics

SKIN CHARACTERISTICS	IMPLICATIONS
Thinner epidermis, blood vessels closer to the surface, less subcutaneous fat	Loses heat more readily through the skin's surface Allows substances to be absorbed through the skin more easily Microorganisms can gain entry more easily
Epidermis is loosely bound to the dermis and the skin contains more water	Friction can more easily result in blister formation or skin breakdown
Less skin pigmentation, regardless of race	Increased risk from ultraviolet radiation

Adapted from: Kyle, T., & Kyle, T. (2007). *Essentials of pediatric nursing*. Philadelphia, PA: Lippincott Williams & Wilkins.

of older children and adults (Kyle & Kyle, 2007). Infants are born with thin skin and limited subcutaneous fat, which limits thermoregulation and enhances infants' susceptibility to topical substances and microorganisms. In addition, the epidermis is loosely bound to the dermis and the infant's skin has a higher water content, thus making infants more susceptible to damage caused by friction. The presence of reduced pigment in neonates' skin also makes them more prone to the harmful effects of ultraviolet radiation. Over time, children's skin toughens and becomes less hydrated and thus less susceptible to microorganism invasion.

At birth, the infant's sebaceous glands function immaturely (Kyle & Kyle, 2007; Lawton, 2006c). During puberty, the sebaceous glands become very active and sebum production is increased. The infant's eccrine glands are somewhat functional and will produce sweat as a response to emotional stimuli and heat. Maturation of these glands during the middle childhood years allows for more effective thermoregulation. The apocrine glands remain small and nonfunctional until puberty.

As shown in Table 30-2, there are several notable differences in the integumentary system among various racial groups. The differing skin pigments of each racial group are due to the relative prevalence of four substances: hemoglobin and oxyhemoglobin (pinkish color), melanin (brown and black shades), and caretinoids (yellow-orange coloration) (Rawlings, 2006). It is also of interest to note that among some racial groups, the epidermis does not provide the same degree of protection from irritants. The clinical presentation of some dermatologic conditions also varies among children of different races. For instance, skin pigmentation can mask the appearance of erythema. Therefore, eruptions that appear red or brown in light-skinned children may appear black, grey, or purple in darker-skinned children (Gawkrodger, 2008). Darker-skinned individuals are also more prone to develop hyperpigmented or hypopigmented lesions, particularly after trauma or inflammatory eruptions. When compared to lighter-skinned children, darker-skinned children are also more prone to develop follicular responses, skin thickening, and blistering reactions (Kyle & Kyle, 2007).

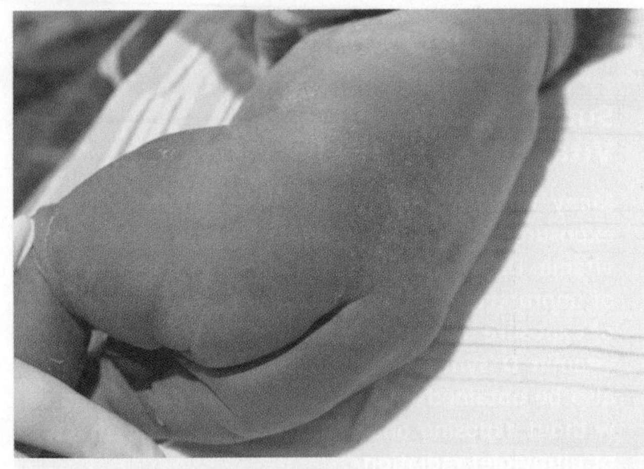

FIGURE 30-2 Mongolian Spots. DELMAR CENGAGE LEARNING.

TABLE 30-2 Skin Variations by Race

RACE	SKIN COLOR	MOLES AND CANCER	HAIR COLOR	HAIR TEXTURE	BODY HAIR	POTENTIAL FOR IRRITATION	OTHER SKIN ISSUES
White	Lightest skin color pink to white	Highest propensity	Red, black, blonde, brown	Wavy, straight, helical	More likely to have more	Moderate	Less pigmentation; increased risk from ultraviolet radiation
Black	Darkest skin color	Lowest propensity	Black	Short, spiraled, drier & more brittle	More likely to have less	Minimal	Larger pores, increased number of sweat glands, greater sebum production, more skin surface microbial flora
Asian	Medium skin color	Moderate risk for moles and cancer	Black	Straight, largest hair diameter	Almost none	Highest	None

Adapted from: Gawkrodger, D. J. (2008). *Dermatology: An illustrated colour text* (4th ed.). Philadelphia, PA: Elsevier; Rawlings, A. V. (2006). Ethnic skin types: Are there differences in skin structure and function? *International Journal of Cosmetic Science*; *28*(2), 79–93.

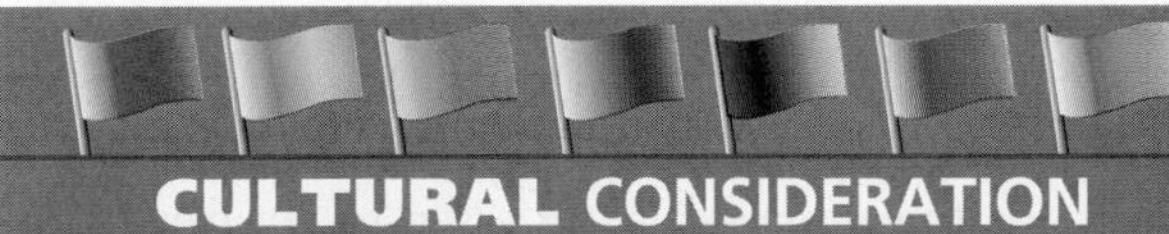

CULTURAL CONSIDERATION

Mongolian Spots

Mongolian spots are areas of slate-brown to blueish-black pigmentation over the lumbosacral area of infants and young children (Figure 30-2). They occur in 100% of Asians, 70% of blacks, and 10% of whites (Gawkrodger, 2008). These normal variations in skin color fade as the child gets older, generally with complete resolution by 6 years of age. The presence of Mongolian spots should be documented to prevent future misdiagnosis as a bruise with protecting children from abuse in mind.

BACTERIAL INFECTIONS

Most pediatric bacterial infections are caused by *Staphylococcus aureus* (*S. aureus*) and/or *Streptococcus pyogenes* (*S. pyogenes*). The clinical manifestations of a particular infection depend on several factors, including the type of bacteria involved, as well as the location and depth of the infection. Impetigo is a superficial bacterial infection that commonly affects children. Cellulitis is a deeper infection that is not as common, but can lead to serious complications.

IMPETIGO

Impetigo is a highly contagious, superficial bacterial skin infection. Two major disease forms exist: (1) nonbullous impetigo, which is characterized by crusted lesions; and (2) bullous impetigo, which is characterized by fragile blisters.

NURSING TIP

Assessing Cutaneous Eruptions in Dark-skinned Children

Skin eruptions can have a different clinical appearance among children with varying skin color. When inspecting darker skin look for black, grey, or purple discoloration as a sign of inflammation. Using palpation can also help nurses make a more accurate assessment of various cutaneous eruptions. It is also important to be aware that as lesions heal, it is common for dark-skinned children to develop hyperpigmentation or hypopigmentation.

Incidence and Etiology

Impetigo is one of the most frequently observed skin infections in children and typically affects children under the age of 5 years (Bernard, 2008; Johnston & Mansouri, 2007). Although either form of impetigo can occur at any age, bullous impetigo is most common in newborns and infants, while nonbullous impetigo is most common in young children (Hirschmann, 2007). Regarding relative incidence, nonbullous impetigo is more common than bullous impetigo.

In many cases, impetigo is preceded by minor trauma to the skin such as a scratch, laceration or insect bite which disrupts the skin barrier and allows the introduction of bacteria (Hirschmann, 2007; Johnston & Mansouri, 2007). In nonbullous impetigo, *S. aureus* is the most common causative agent. *S. pyogenes* may also be present or, less commonly, can be the single causative agent. Nonbullous impetigo only results from certain strains of *S. aureus.*

Impetigo is considered a highly contagious infection (Johnston & Mansouri, 2007). The responsible bacteria are typically spread from individual to individual by direct skin contact. Once an individual is infected, **autoinoculation** may occur. Autoinoculation is the transfer of infection from one site to another on the same individual, usually due to scratching. Individuals colonized with *S. aureus or S. pyogenes* are at risk for recurrent infections, as are children with atopic dermatitis (Johnston & Mansouri, 2007). In addition, the incidence of nonbullous impetigo has been reported to be more prevalent during the summer months and in hot, humid climates (Bernard, 2008; Hirschmann, 2007).

Pathophysiology

Both *S. aureus* and group A beta-hemolytic streptococci (usually *S. pyogenes*) can cause nonbullous impetigo, though the most common causative bacterium is *S. aureus* (Hirschmann, 2007; Johnston & Mansouri, 2007). However, only certain strains of *S. aureus* produce the exfoliative toxins that result in the development of bullous impetigo. Regardless of the type of bacteria responsible, bullous and nonbullous impetigo infections involve only the epidermis. Because the lesions are so superficial, they are fragile and rupture easily, leading to local expansion (Hirschmann, 2007; Johnston & Mansouri, 2007).

Clinical Manifestations

The lesions of nonbullous impetigo begin as small red **macules** (small flat lesions) or **papules** (small raised lesions) that quickly progress into small, thin-roofed **vesicles** (small blisters) and then pustules. The resulting lesions rupture easily and spill their serous contents, which results in a characteristic honey-colored or dark brown crust (Hirschmann, 2007; Johnston & Mansouri, 2007) (Figure 30-3). The crusted plaques may enlarge to be up to two centimeters in diameter. If left untreated, lesions generally resolve spontaneously within two weeks without scarring (Hirschmann, 2007; Johnston & Mansouri, 2007).

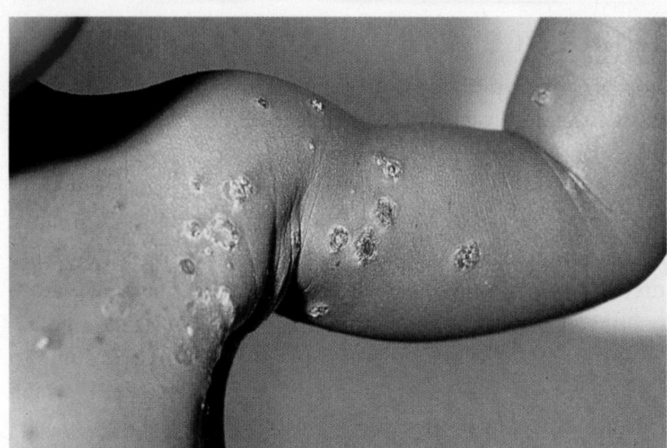

FIGURE 30-3 **Impetigo.** COURTESY OF ROBERT A. SILVERMAN, M.D., CLINICAL ASSOCIATE PROFESSOR, DEPARTMENT OF PEDIATRICS, GEORGETOWN UNIVERSITY.

The lesions of bullous impetigo begin as superficial vesicles that rapidly enlarge to form fragile **bullae** (large blisters) without surrounding erythema (Hirschmann, 2007). The fluid may be clear or turbid. The bullae rupture easily and may then have the appearance of shiny, erythematous erosions or honey-colored crusting. Individual lesions may also coalesce to form one or more larger lesions.

The lesions of bullous impetigo tend to favor the extremities, while nonbullous impetigo eruptions commonly affect the legs, buttocks, and face; in particular, around the mouth and nose (Hirschmann, 2007; Johnston & Mansouri, 2007). Widespread involvement is possible and lesions may be present on any surface of the skin. Such involvement typically occurs in the presence of an underlying skin disorder such as atopic dermatitis.

Diagnosis

The diagnosis of impetigo is based on the child's history and clinical presentation. The patient history should inquire about prior injuries or rashes in the affected areas. In addition, the child and caregivers should be asked about any history of similar infections. Such information can aid in the diagnosis and may indicate nasal carriage of the causative organism (Johnston & Mansouri, 2007). Upon physical examination, the presence of honey-colored crusts is considered the hallmark characteristic of impetigo (Hirschmann, 2007; Johnston & Mansouri, 2007). In addition, the child should be assessed for signs of underlying skin diseases such as atopic dermatitis, herpes simplex, scabies, or tinea capitis that may have become secondarily infected (Johnston & Mansouri, 2007). If needed, a bacterial culture of the exudate can assist in confirming the diagnosis (Johnston & Mansouri, 2007).

Treatment

Although impetigo is a self-limiting condition, treatment is generally initiated to reduce complications, prevent spread, and provide faster relief (Johnston & Mansouri, 2007). For localized infections, treatment typically consists of topical antibiotic therapy. In such instances, mupirocin ointment (Bactroban or Centany) has proven to be as effective as oral antibiotic therapy (Bernard, 2008; Hirschmann, 2007; Johnston & Mansouri, 2007). The recommended dosing for mupirocin is three times daily for seven to ten days. Alternatively, retapamulin (Altabax) is the first agent in a new class of topical antibiotics that has shown promising efficacy against mupirocin resistant strains of *S. aureus* (Bernard, 2008). Topical treatment is generally easy to apply and lacks systemic side effects. However, potential disadvantages include difficulty treating numerous lesions, failure to eradicate nasal carriage, and concerns about emerging mupirocin resistance (Bernard, 2008; Hirschmann, 2007).

If lesions are widespread or do not respond to topical therapy, the administration of oral, systemic antibiotics is indicated. A seven-day course of penicillinase-resistant penicillin such as dicloxacillin or a cephalosporin such as cephalexin is likely to be effective (Bernard, 2008; Hirschmann, 2007). However, health care providers need to be aware of the local antibiotic resistance patterns as well as the increasing prevalence of community-acquired methicillin-resistant *S. aureus* (CA-MRSA). Presently CA-MRSA is rarely associated with impetigo (Hirschmann, 2007).

Nursing Management

Assessment

Nurses should ask the child and caregivers about any known exposure to someone with similar lesions, any history of similar eruptions, and any observed injuries or rashes that first occurred in the affected areas. During the physical assessment, nurses should note the presence of vesicles, bullae and/or crusting as well as the location of the eruption. As with any infection, nurses should observe for presence of elevated temperature, respiratory rate, and heart rate and ask about the child's comfort. The child should also be assessed for any underlying skin disorders such as atopic dermatitis.

Nursing Diagnosis

Nursing diagnoses for the child with impetigo include:

1. *Infection* related to presence of infective organisms.
2. *Impaired skin integrity* related to presence of lesions.
3. *Risk for infection (secondary)* related to scratching or picking.
4. *Deficient knowledge* related to treatment and measures to prevent the spread of infection.

Outcome Identification

1. Child's lesions will heal and the infection will resolve.
2. Child's infection will not spread beyond the primary site of infection.
3. Child will not manifest signs of a secondary infection.
4. Child and caregivers will verbalize understanding of the treatment regimen and implement strategies to prevent spread of infection.

Planning and Implementation

The nursing management of children with impetigo focuses on resolution of the infection and family teaching. When providing nursing care, gloves should be worn and careful hand washing before and after contact with the child is essential. Both the child and caregivers should be educated about the treatment regimen and on methods to prevent spread of the infection to other areas or to other individuals. Included in this education should be information about not picking or scratching at the primary lesions.

Evaluation The child and caregivers are able to convey proper understanding of and demonstrate adherence to the antibiotic treatment regimen. They will also be able to implement strategies to prevent spread of the infection to others and minimize picking and scratching, resulting in the affected area remaining free from signs of secondary infection. These measures should also result in containment of the primary lesions to the initial site of infection. Implementation of these steps, in addition to the antibiotic therapy, should lead to resolution of the infection.

Family Teaching

Strict adherence in taking the prescribed topical or oral antibiotics as directed is essential. This necessitates that the nurse carefully explain the medication usage instructions and answer any questions about the treatment. In addition, the nurse must emphasize the need to take the full course of antibiotic medication, even if the infection appears to be gone. The child and caregivers also need to understand the contagious nature of impetigo and be instructed in proper hygiene principles, including the need to use good hand washing with antibacterial soap. Towels, clothing, and other personal items should not be shared. Older children may be able to understand instructions about not scratching or picking at the lesions, but younger children will likely need other interventions such as keeping the child's nails cut short, placing mittens over the child's hands, closely supervising the child, and utilizing distraction techniques. If the affected child participates in sports that involve direct skin contact, the lesions should be covered or the child should be excluded from participation. Finally, instructions for seeking medical attention should be provided if the infection is not resolving.

CELLULITIS

Cellulitis is an acute, spreading inflammation of the skin and subcutaneous tissue that is characterized by a painful area of warm, swollen erythema. This localized bacterial infection generally responds well to treatment, although serious sequelae can result if treatment is delayed or inadequate.

Incidence and Etiology

Cellulitis is not an infection that is prevalent among pediatric patients, although facial cellulitis has been reported to be more commonly observed in children less than 3 years old (Micali, Dhawan, & Nasca, 2009). Those children who are affected have been reported to be at higher risk for serious complications such as gangrene, metastatic abscess, and grave sepsis (James, Berger, & Elston, 2006). For this reason, prompt recognition and treatment of cellulitis in children is critical.

Cellulitis usually results from a discernable wound such as a fissure, laceration, insect bite, or puncture wound (James et al., 2006; Micali et al., 2009). It is also common for the skin breakdown of tinea pedis to allow the entry of bacteria and result in cellulitis of the leg. *S. pyogenes* and *S. aureus* are the most common organisms isolated from cellulitis infections (Gabillot-Carre & Roujeau, 2007; Hirschmann, 2007; James et al., 2006; Micali et al., 2009). Unlike in adults, *S. aureus* is the most common pathogen involved in pediatric cellulitis (Hirschmann, 2007; Micali et al., 2009). This organism is also more likely to cause cellulitis that occurs around an open wound or an abscess. An emerging problem in pediatric bacterial infections is the involvement of community-acquired methicillin-resistant *S. aureus* (CA-MRSA). Presently, CA-MRSA is reported to cause about half of the cases of cellulitis with purulent exudates (Bernard, 2008; Gabillot-Carre & Roujeau, 2007) (Box 30-2).

Pathophysiology

Among pediatric patients, *S. aureus* is the most common bacterial organism responsible for the development of cellulitis (Micali et al., 2009). In order for this pathogen to cause the clinical manifestations of cellulitis, it must gain entry into the dermis. This bacterial invasion is facilitated by impairment of the skin barrier, often due to trauma or a pre-existing rash

BOX 30-2

ANTIBIOTIC RESISTANCE IN PEDIATRIC INFECTIONS

Community acquired methicillin-resistant *S. aureus* (CA-MRSA) infections have been increasing, especially in children. Children at risk include athletes and young children who attend daycare. Fortunately, CA-MRSA infections are less drug-resistant than hospital acquired strains and life-threatening infections are not common. CA-MRSA usually presents as skin and soft-tissue infections, especially abscesses. Incision and drainage of the abscess is considered essential as this is often sufficient treatment and resolution of the lesion may not be achieved without this intervention even if an appropriate antibiotic is prescribed. Bacterial cultures should be collected to guide therapy. If an antibiotic is needed, oral clindamycin or trimethoprim/sulfamethoxazole (Bactrim, Septra) are good choices for pediatric patients (Elston, 2007a; Swanson, 2006).

(Hirschmann, 2007; James et al., 2006; Micali et al., 2009). Once introduced into the dermis, the invading bacteria multiply and trigger an immune response. The resulting infection extends into the dermis and subcutaneous fat, but does not involve the fascia or muscles (James et al., 2006; Micali et al., 2009).

Clinical Manifestations

The classic symptoms of cellulitis are those of an acute infectious process: erythema, swelling, warmth, and pain (Hirschmann, 2007; Micali et al., 2009). The erythema rapidly intensifies and spreads (Figure 30-4). The affected area also becomes infiltrated and progressive infection may cause the central portion to become nodular and surmounted by a vesicle that ruptures and discharges purulent material (James et al., 2006). **Lymphangitis**, red streaks leading from the affected area to adjacent lymph nodes, and/or lymphadenopathy may be observed (James et al., 2006; Micali et al., 2009). The affected child may also complain of systemic symptoms such as fever, chills, and malaise.

Diagnosis

Cellulitis is typically diagnosed based on history and clinical presentation. The history should inquire about any initial injury or rash in the area, the progression of the infection, and the presence of any systemic symptoms. The physical exam should assess for characteristic manifestations as well as any lymph node involvement. Diagnostic procedures such as tissue aspirates, skin biopsies, and blood cultures often yield negative results and are not recommended for routine diagnosis (Gabillot-Carre & Roujeau, 2007; Micali et al., 2009). If purulent drainage is present, however, bacterial culture and sensitivities should be collected to evaluate for resistant bacterial strains and guide antibiotic therapy (Bernard, 2008; Gabillot-Carre & Roujeau, 2007).

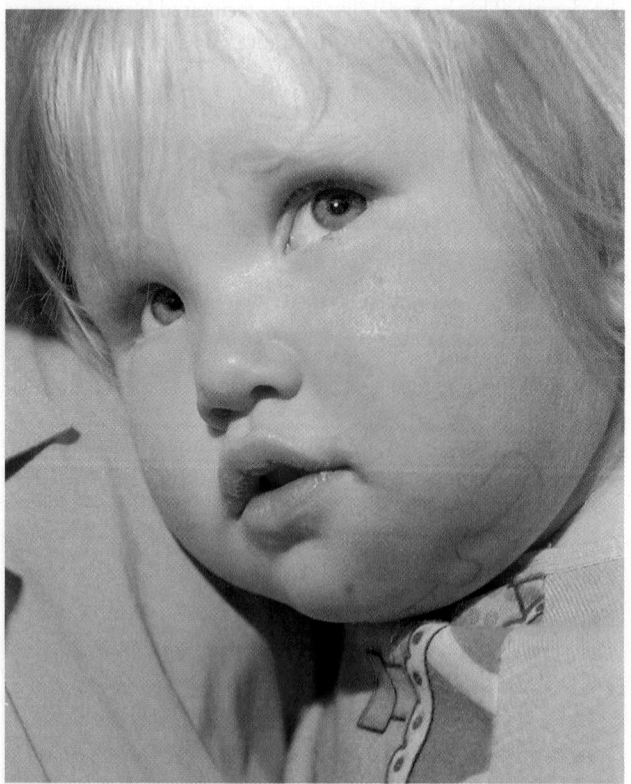

Figure 30-4 Cellulitis of the Face. DELMAR CENGAGE LEARNING.

Treatment

Prompt administration of systemic antibiotics is essential for treating cellulitis. Penicillinase-resistant penicillins (dicloxacillin), cephalosporins (cephalexin), or clindamycin are generally appropriate agents for treatment (Bernard, 2008; Gabillot-Carre & Roujeau, 2007; Micali et al., 2009). If CA-MRSA is suspected, clindamycin or trimethoprim/sulfamethoxazole (Bactrim, Septra) are appropriate choices (Elston, 2007a; Swanson, 2006). In most cases, appropriate oral antibiotic therapy is sufficient to lead to full resolution. In severe cases, hospitalization and administration of IV antibiotics may be necessary to minimize complications and obtain resolution (Gabillot-Carre & Roujeau, 2007; Micali et al., 2009).

Nursing Management

Priorities for nursing management include eradication of the infection, promotion of the child's comfort, preventing spread of the infection, and minimizing complications. The assessment should include questioning the child or caregivers about a history of trauma or rash in the affected area. The nurse also should ask about the development of symptoms related to the cellulitis such as fever, chills, or malaise. Planning and implementation should include precautions such as wearing gloves and practicing proper hand washing. Nurses should monitor the affected child for signs and symptoms of worsening infection. Family education should also be provided about the treatment regimen, comfort measures, and preventing the spread of infection.

Family Teaching

The child and caregivers should be educated about the importance of taking the prescribed antibiotics as directed, even if the infection appears to be gone. The child and caregivers also need to understand that if there is drainage or an open wound, then precautions are necessary to prevent the spread of infection, including the need to use good hand washing and to avoid contact with the wound whenever possible. To promote comfort, the affected area should be immobilize and elevated. Caregivers may also be instructed to use acetaminophen or ibuprofen to relieve pain and reduce fever. Close observation for early signs of potentially serious systemic infections is required and instructions should be provided for seeking medical attention if the infection is not resolving.

FUNGAL INFECTIONS

Fungal infections can be caused by yeasts or dermatophytes. The *Candida* species of yeast are responsible for the development of the cutaneous infection candidiasis. Candidiasis can occur at any age, but is most common among infants. **Dermatophytes** are a group of fungi that invade keratinized tissues (Crawford & Hollis, 2007; Sarabi & Khachemoune, 2007; Theos, 2007). There are three genera of dermatophytes: *Trichophyton, Microsporum,* and *Epidermophyton* and approximately 40 species (Sarabi & Khachemoune, 2007). Depending on the type of dermatophyte involved, the epidermis and its structures, the hair and nails, are infected. Tinea capitis (head ringworm) is the most common fungal infection in children, followed by tinea corporis (body ringworm), tinea pedis (athlete's foot), and tinea unguium (nail fungus) (Theos, 2007).

CANDIDIASIS

Candidiasis most commonly presents during infancy in the oral cavity or diaper area, though other anatomic locations and age groups may be affected. Most infections are minor and respond well to topical treatment, though candidiasis may be a sign of a more serious underlying problem, such as immunocompromise.

Incidence and Etiology

The peak prevalence of candidiasis occurs within the first year of life (Kalyoussef, Tolan, & Greenberg, 2008). During this time, candidal infections commonly present as oral candidiasis (thrush) or candidal diaper dermatitis. The incidence of thrush in healthy newborns is approximately 2–5%, (Kalyoussef et al., 2008). The exact incidence of candidal diaper dermatitis is difficult to estimate, but this form of candidiasis is considered to be more common than the oral variant.

The most common pathogen responsible for the development of candidiasis is *Candida albicans (C. albicans). C. albicans* is part of the body's normal flora, but under certain circumstances this organism can invade the epidermis and cause clinical infection (James et al., 2006; Rudy, 2007). Factors that place children at risk for developing candidal infections include antibiotic therapy, immunocompromise, corticosteroid use (inhaled, topical, or oral), prematurity, and irritation or maceration of the skin (James et al., 2006; Kalyoussef et al., 2008; Rudy, 2007). Newborns may also acquire candidal infections from the vaginal tract of their mother during birth (James et al., 2006).

Pathophysiology

C. albicans, the most common cause of candidiasis, is part of the normal flora of the skin and mucous membranes (James et al., 2006; Kalyoussef et al., 2008; Rudy, 2007). *C. albicans* is considered an **opportunistic organism**, meaning it acts as a pathogen when the resistance of the host is impaired and conditions favor its growth (James et al., 2006). Several factors may prompt *C. albicans* to overgrow (James et al., 2006; Rudy, 2007). Often the use of systemic antibiotics can reduce the competing normal flora and thus lead to a proliferation of *C. albicans.* Similarly, conditions that are associated with an impaired immune response, such as immunocompromise or corticosteroid use, reduce a child's ability to suppress the growth of candidal organisms. *C. albicans* growth can also be promoted by high pH conditions, such as those found in the diaper area as well as by the presence of warmth and moisture. In addition to *C. albicans* proliferation, the clinical manifestations of candidiasis result from the invasion of the overgrown yeast into the epidermis. Such invasion is facilitated by impairment of the skin barrier by warmth, moisture, maceration, and/or contact with irritating substances.

Clinical Manifestations

Thrush is characterized by the development of adherent, white plaques with an erythematous base on the buccal mucosa, lips, tongue, and/or palate (James et al., 2006; Kalyoussef et al., 2008; Rudy, 2007). The lesions gradually become confluent and may cover the entire oral cavity (Figure 30-5). The affected infant may experience discomfort and present with a history of fussiness or poor feeding.

Candidiasis in the diaper area is characterized by intensely erythematous plaques that are often macerated and display scalloped borders (James et al., 2006; Kalyoussef et al., 2008). Unlike noncandidal diaper dermatitis, these plaques originate in the skin folds. Satellite papules and pustules are also commonly observed surrounding the plaques. Itching, burning, or soreness may be associated with this eruption.

In adolescents, candidiasis also may present as **intertrigo**, a pruritic, erythematous skin eruption occurring in intertriginous areas (James et al., 2006; Kalyoussef et al., 2008). Intertriginous areas are those anatomic regions where opposing skin surfaces rub together, often creating a warm, moist environment. In adolescents with intertrigo, commonly involved areas include the groin, gluteal cleft, axillae, and

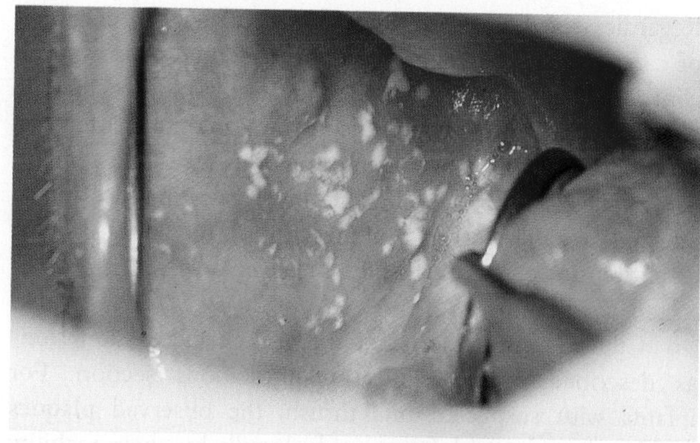

FIGURE 30-5 Oral Candidiasis (Thrush). COURTESY OF DR. JOSEPH KONZELMAN, SCHOOL OF DENTISTRY, MEDICAL COLLEGE OF GEORGIA.

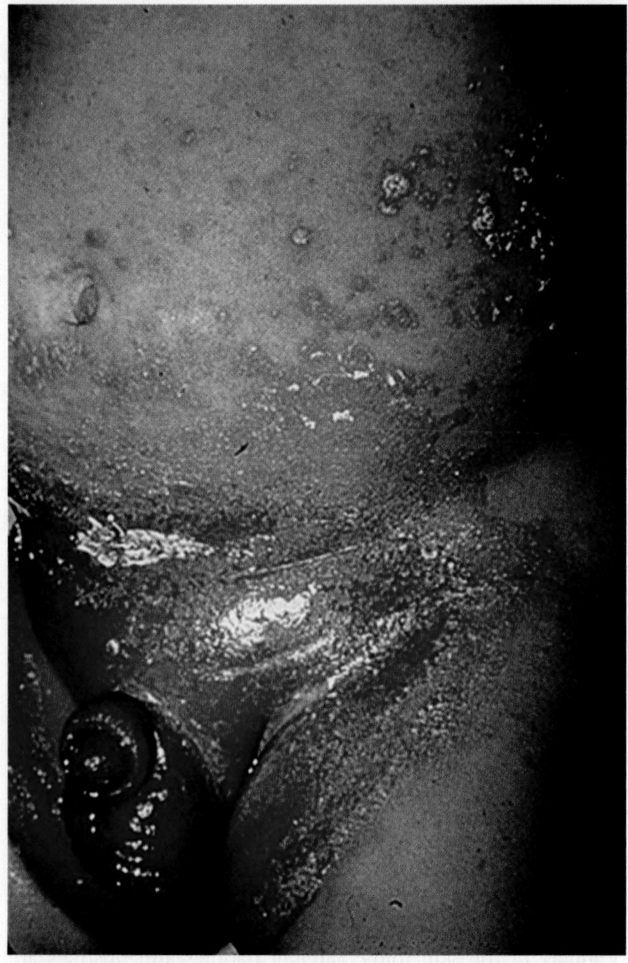

FIGURE 30-6 **Candidiasis-Intertrigo.** COURTESY OF THE CENTERS FOR DISEASE CONTROL AND PREVENTION.

abdominal folds. The presentation of intertrigo is similar to that of candidal diaper dermatitis with areas of well-defined beefy erythema and satellite lesions (Figure 30-6).

DIAGNOSIS

Regardless of the anatomic location involved, the diagnosis of candidiasis is based primarily on the child's history and clinical presentation. For infants, the history should include feeding habits and the presence of any maternal infection. For children with diaper or intertriginous area involvement, caregivers should be asked about any preexisting rash in the affected area. The use of any prescription medications, such as antibiotics or steroids, should also be assessed for all affected children.

Clinical examination should reveal characteristic lesions as described in the clinical manifestations section. For infants with suspected oral thrush, the observed plaques can be distinguished from residual milk by their inability to be scraped off easily (Kalyoussef et al., 2008). Microscopic potassium hydroxide (KOH) examination of scrapings from oral or cutaneous lesions can help to confirm the diagnosis (James et al., 2006; Kalyoussef et al., 2008). Observation of budding yeast spores or pseudohyphae are indicative of a positive result. Other alternative tests include gram stains or PAS stains. If it is necessary to identify the strain of *Candida* involved, yeast cultures can provide this information.

TREATMENT

The treatment of choice for thrush is oral nystatin suspension, which is administered topically to the affected mucous membranes four times a day. Treatment should continue for 48 hours following symptom resolution (James et al., 2006; Kalyoussef et al., 2008). Gentian violet is considered an effective second-line treatment. The recommended dosing is three times a day, but caution is advised as this topical option stains skin and clothing. If the mother of a breastfeeding infant is infected with cutaneous candidiasis, it is recommended that she undergo simultaneous treatment. If the affected infant is bottle-feeding, adequate cleaning of the bottles will help to prevent re-infection (Kalyoussef et al., 2008).

Candidal diaper dermatitis and intertrigo are most often managed successfully with nystatin cream (Kalyoussef et al., 2008). As with the treatment of thrush, topical therapy for cutaneous candidiasis should be continued for 48 hours after the resolution of visible lesions. Alternative topical treatments include clotrimazole cream and miconazole cream. For refractory cases, the use of oral antifungal agents such as fluconazole (Diflucan), itraconazole (Sporanox), and ketoconazole may be indicated (Kalyoussef et al., 2008). Measures to prevent irritant diaper dermatitis will help reduce a child's risk of developing future candidiasis of the diaper area. For adolescents with intertrigo, preventive measures should focus on keeping intertriginous areas cool and dry (Kalyoussef et al., 2008).

NURSING MANAGEMENT

Nursing care priorities for the infant or child with candidiasis include resolution of the infection, promotion of the child's comfort, and preventing the spread of infection. The nursing history should include prior antibiotic or steroid, prior rashes in the affected area, and the presence of any discomfort. If the affected child is an infant with thrush, feeding habits should be discussed, as should the mother's use of prescription medications or the presence of any rashes. Physical examination should note the characteristics and location of the lesions. Planning and implementation should include precautions such as wearing gloves and practicing proper hand washing. Family education should also be provided about the treatment regimen, comfort measures, and preventing the spread of infection.

FAMILY TEACHING

Family teaching should address proper use of the prescribed antifungal preparation. If nystatin suspension or

NURSING ALERT

Inhaled Corticosteroids and Oral Candidiasis

Children with asthma who use inhaled corticosteroids are at increased risk for the development of oral candidiasis. To prevent thrush, these children should be taught to rinse the mouth after using the meter dose enhaler (includes the use of spacers).

cream is utilized, the mechanism of action requires direct contact with the affected area, and thus, it should be administered in a manner that will allow for optimum contact with the lesions. The nurse should also explain that treatment should be continued for 48 hours following the resolution of visible lesions. In order to prevent the spread of infection, family teaching should also address proper hand washing and the importance of minimizing direct contact with the affected areas when possible. If applicable, caregivers should be instructed on the proper cleaning of breast pumps, bottles, and pacifiers. To prevent recurrence of candidiasis in intertriginous or diaper areas, the skin in these locations should be kept cool, dry, and separated from irritating substances.

TINEA CAPITIS

Tinea capitis is a fungal infection of the scalp and hair shaft that is associated with scaling, pruritus, and hair loss. Treatment involves a relatively long course of oral antifungal medication as well as precautions to prevent the spread of infection.

Incidence and Etiology

Tinea capitis is the most common fungal infection in children under the age of 12 (Sarabi & Khachemoune, 2007; Theos, 2007). While tinea capitis can occur at any age, most cases are found in preadolescent children, particularly between the ages of 3–7 years old (Ali, Graham, & Forgie, 2007; Gonzalez, Seaton, Bergus, Jacobson, & Martinez-Monzon, 2007; Muirhead, 2007; Trovato, Schwartz, & Janniger, 2006). In the United States, the overall incidence of tinea capitis has been estimated to be approximately 4%. However, incidence rates have been reported to be over 12% among African-American children (Ali et al., 2007; Trovato et al., 2006). Current research evidence discredits the hypothesis that this increase in incidence is due to hair products, hairstyling, frequency of washing, or other hair care practices (Trovato et al., 2006).

Trichophyton tonsurans (*T. tonsurans*) is the causative organism responsible for most cases of tinea capitis in the United States (Ali et al., 2007; Muirhead, 2007; Trovato et al., 2006). Transmission of the responsible dermatophyte may result from contact with infected humans, animals, or **fomites** (Gonzalez et al., 2007; Trovato et al., 2006). Fomites are inanimate objects that may harbor and transmit a disease agent. In tinea capitis, possible fomites include combs, bedding, couches, and toys. Even infected individuals who do not have signs of clinical infection can play a role in the spread of tinea capitis (Ali et al., 2007; Gonzalez et al., 2007; Trovato et al., 2006). Because of its contagious nature, tinea capitis infections are more common among those who live in crowded living conditions and disadvantaged communities.

Pathophysiology

Although *T. tonsurans* is the dermatophyte most commonly responsible for tinea capitis infections in the United States, fungi from any of the three main genera of fungi may be responsible: *Trichophyton, Microsporum,* or *Epidermophyton* (Ali et al., 2007; Sarabi & Khachemoune, 2007; Trovato et al., 2006). Regardless of the specific dermatophyte involved, the infection involves both the scalp and the hair shaft (Ali et al., 2007; Gonzalez et al., 2007). Disruption of the hair shaft is-hyphae and accomplished differently by different dermatophytes. In some instances, the hair shaft becomes covered with spores; while in other instances, the hair shaft becomes filled with hyphae and spores (Sarabi & Khachemoune, 2007; Trovato et al., 2006). Exaggerated cell-mediated responses to the dermatophyte can result in severe inflammation and manifestations such as kerion and permanent hair loss (Ali et al., 2007; Gonzalez et al., 2007; Sarabi & Khachemoune, 2007).

Clinical Manifestations

The clinical presentation of tinea capitis is very diverse. The most typical features of tinea capitis are single, or multiple, patches of **alopecia** (hair loss) that may be accompanied by inflammation, scaling, pustules, and pruritus (Ali et al., 2007; Gonzalez et al., 2007; Trovato et al., 2006) (Figure 30-7). In some children, the presentation may be subtle with dandruff-like scale, minimal pruritus, and very slight hair loss. In more severe cases, inflammatory kerion may be produced. Kerion are boggy, tender, and pustular scalp nodules that are often mistaken for abscesses (Ali et al., 2007; Sarabi & Khachemoune, 2007; Trovato et al., 2006). Children with kerion may also develop scarring and permanent hair loss.

The most commonly affected areas of the scalp are the crown, occipital region, and parietal region (Trovato et al., 2006). The eyelashes and eyebrows may also be affected. It is typical for the areas of hair loss to be well defined and irregularly shaped, with both long and short broken hairs present. Careful inspection may also reveal black dots at the site of the broken hairs (Ali et al., 2007; Gonzalez et al., 2007; Trovato et al., 2006). Particularly in children with pustules or kerion, cervical lymphadenopathy may also be present (Ali et al., 2007; Muirhead, 2007; Sarabi & Khachemoune, 2007; Trovato et al., 2006).

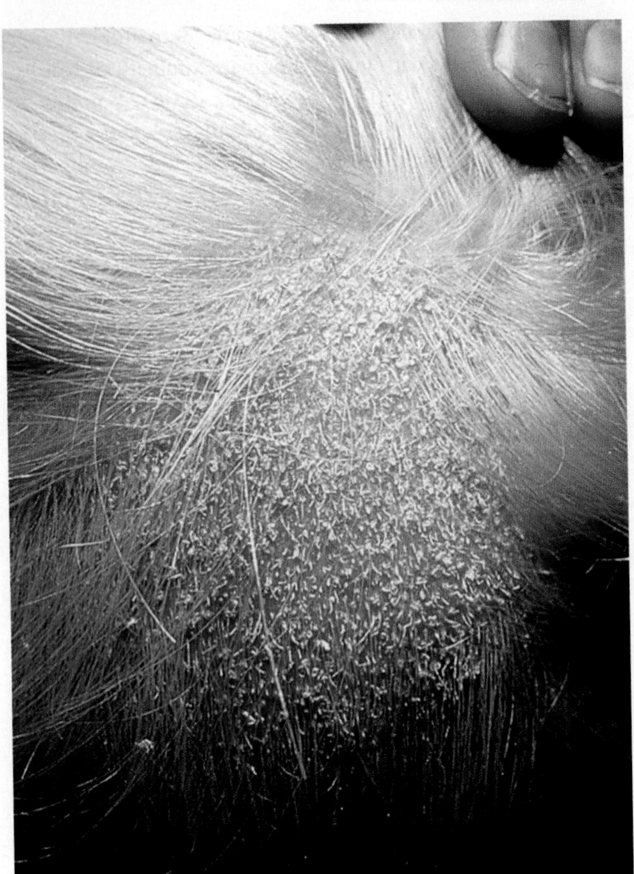

FIGURE 30-7 **Tinea Capitis.** COURTESY OF ROBERT A. SILVERMAN, M.D., CLINICAL ASSOCIATE PROFESSOR, DEPARTMENT OF PEDIATRICS, GEORGETOWN UNIVERSITY.

Diagnosis

Although the diagnosis of tinea capitis may be suspected based on clinical presentation, it is essential to confirm the diagnosis via laboratory testing because treatment may be lengthy and associated with undesirable side effects (Ali et al., 2007; Gonzalez et al., 2007; Muirhead, 2007; Trovato, 2007). Common sources of laboratory confirmation are microscopic potassium hydroxide (KOH) examination and fungal cultures. KOH preparations are advantageous because they can produce immediate results, but fungal cultures are more sensitive and can provide antifungal sensitivities (Ali et al., 2007; Gonzalez et al., 2007).

Samples for KOH preparations or fungal cultures can be obtained in several ways: plucking hair, scraping skin and hair with a scalpel or microscope slide, brushing hair, or using adhesive tape (Ali et al., 2007). To make the collection process less traumatic for children, two additional collection methods have proven efficacious: rubbing the scalp with a sterile toothbrush or using a sterile, moist cotton swab that is rubbed over the scalp and then applied to the transport media (Ali et al., 2007; Trovato, 2007). In some instances, a skin biopsy with fungal stains may be necessary to confirm the diagnosis (Trovato, 2007). The use of Wood's lamp is not routinely recommended because although it may detect strains of *Microsporum*, the most common dermatophyte implicated in tinea capitis, *T. tonsurans*, does not fluoresce under Wood's lamp (Gonzalez et al., 2007; Sarabi & Khachemoune, 2007).

Treatment

Systemic therapy is indicated for the treatment of tinea capitis because topical preparations cannot effectively penetrate the hair shaft (Ali et al., 2007; Gonzalez et al., 2007). In addition to treating the affected child, it is recommended that even asymptomatic family members be screened, as one study found that up to 50% of affected children has at least one family member who was culture-positive (Ali et al., 2007; Trovato et al., 2006). All affected household members should then be treated simultaneously.

Griseofulvin remains the standard treatment for tinea capitis, as well as the only systemic antifungal medication approved for this indication (Ali et al., 2007; Muirhead, 2007; Sethi & Antaya, 2006). Treatment typically lasts for a minimum of 6–8 weeks and possibly extends as long as 16 weeks. It is recommended that treatment be continued for 1–2 weeks after the resolution of symptoms (Ali et al., 2007; Trovato et al., 2006). Alternatively, the off-label use of terbinafine (Lamisil), itraconazole (Sporanox), or fluconazole (Diflucan) may offer similar efficacy for *Trichophyton* infections with a shorter duration of treatment (Gonzalez et al., 2007; Muirhead, 2007; Sethi & Antaya, 2006). For infections due to *Microsporum*, however, it appears that griseofulvin remains more effective.

Adjunctive therapy with topical agents, such as shampoos containing 1% or 2.5% selenium sulfide or 2% ketoconazole, is potentially advantageous as the use of these agents reduces surface fungal colony counts and may help reduce fungal transmission (Ali et al., 2007; Muirhead, 2007; Sarabi & Khachemoune, 2007; Trovato et al., 2006). The shampoo should be applied for 5–10 minutes at least 3 times a week. Some experts advise that asymptomatic family members should use 1% selenium sulfide or 2% ketoconazole shampoo for several weeks to prevent infection and carrier states (Ali et al., 2007; Sarabi & Khachemoune, 2007).

In addition to pharmacologic therapy, clinical management must also include precautions to prevent the spread of infection. The home environment should be evaluated for objects that have come into contact with the infected child's hair. Floors should be mopped with a strong disinfectant, all washable objects should be laundered, and all non-washable items should be vacuumed (Trovato et al., 2006). To prevent transmission via fomites, the affected child should not share items such as brushes, combs, or hats with others until treatment is complete (Ali et al., 2007; Sarabi & Khachemoune, 2007). It is also recommended that close physical contact of the head with the infected child be avoided.

Nursing Management

Assessment The nursing assessment should include inquiry regarding any known exposure to others with similar lesions as well as the presence of lesions in other household members. The child should also be asked about the presence and extent of pruritus. The physical assessment should note the extent of hair loss and scaling as well as the presence of pustules, kerion, or lymphadenopathy. Family members should also be screened to detect any asymptomatic carriers.

Nursing Diagnosis Nursing diagnoses for the child with tinea capitis include:

1. *Infection* related to presence of infective organisms.
2. *Risk for infection (secondary)* related to scratching or picking.
3. *Deficient knowledge* related to treatment and measures to prevent the spread of infection.

Outcome Identification

1. Child's lesions will heal and the infection will resolve.
2. Child will not manifest signs of a secondary infection.
3. Child and caregivers will verbalize understanding of the treatment regimen and implement strategies to prevent spread of infection.

Planning and Implementation The planning and implementation of nursing care for children with tinea capitis focus on resolution of the infection, prevention of secondary infection, and family teaching. When providing nursing care, gloves should be worn at all times and careful hand washing should be conducted before and after contact with the child. Both the child and caregivers should be educated about the treatment regimen and on methods to prevent spread of the infection to other individuals. This education should also include information about not picking or scratching at the primary lesions.

Evaluation The child and caregivers are able to convey proper understanding and demonstrate adherence to the antifungal treatment regimen. They will also be able to implement strategies to prevent spread of the infection to others and prevent picking and scratching, resulting in the affected area remaining free from excoriations and signs of secondary infection. Implementation of these steps, in addition to the antifungal therapy, should lead to resolution of the infection.

Family Teaching

Family teaching must include the importance of taking the prescribed antifungal treatment as directed. Because of the long-term nature of tinea capitis treatment, poor adherence is more likely and could result in incomplete clearance or recurrence of the infection. Furthermore, nurses should explain to caregivers the importance of continuing the treatment for 1–2 weeks after the resolution of symptoms. The child and caregivers also need to understand the contagious nature of tinea capitis and be instructed in proper hygiene principles, including the need to use good hand washing. Older children should be instructed to not scratch or pick at their scalp. For younger children, caregivers should be instructed to keep the child's nails cut short and place mittens over the child's hands if necessary. The child and caregivers should also be educated about cleaning the home environment, avoiding contact with the affected area, and not sharing items such as brushes, combs, or hats with others until the treatment is complete.

TINEA CORPORIS

Tinea corporis, or "ringworm," is a superficial fungal infection that can occur on most areas of the body. The infection usually occurs due to contact with another infected individual and is most common among preadolescent children. The resulting clinical lesions are typically ring-shaped and generally respond well to topical treatments.

Incidence and Etiology

Tinea corporis is the term used to refer to superficial fungal infections that occur anywhere on the body, except the scalp, groin, palms and soles (Lott, Zember, & Lesher, 2008; Pleacher & Dexter, 2007; Theos, 2007). This dermatophyte infection can occur at any age, though prevalence rates are highest among preadolescents (Lott et al., 2008).

The dermatophyte most commonly associated with tinea corporis in the United States is *Trichophyton rubrum (T. rubrum)*, followed by *Trichophyton tonsurans (T. tonsurans)* and then *Microsporum canis (M. canis)* (James et al., 2006; Lott et al., 2008; Theos, 2007). Acquisition of these dermatophytes occurs most commonly from contact with infected humans; though infection can also result from contact with infected animals, fomites (such as towels or wrestling mats) or, less frequently, directly from the soil (Lott et al., 2008; Pleacher & Dexter, 2007; Theos, 2007). Tinea corporis infections can also occur due to the spread of dermatophytes from other anatomic locations on the same individual, such as tinea pedis (Lott et al., 2008). Risk factors for developing tinea corporis infections include

> **KIDS WANT TO KNOW**
>
> **What kind of worm causes ringworm?**
>
> It is a common misperception that ringworm infections are caused by worms. It is important to reassure children, and if necessary their caregivers, that the affected child does not have any worms or parasites. In addition, nurses should explain that fungi are commonly found in the environment, like bacteria, and do not indicate poor hygiene.

immunosuppression, participation in sports involving skin contact, and travel to hot, humid climates (Lott et al., 2008; Theos, 2007).

Pathophysiology

After being transferred onto the skin, dermatophytes release keratinases that allow them to invade the stratum corneum (Lott et al., 2008; Pleacher & Dexter, 2007). After an incubation period of 1–3 weeks, the dermatophytes then invade the epidermis peripherally (Lott et al., 2008). The body responds to this invasion by increasing proliferation of the basal cell layer, which results in epidermal thickening and the formation of scale on the border of the lesion (Pleacher & Dexter, 2007). The lesion eventually takes on a ring-shaped appearance because as the infection spreads peripherally, the originally infected skin is shed, leaving an area of new, healthy skin in the center of the lesion (Lott et al., 2008).

Clinical Manifestations

The classic presentation of tinea corporis is one or more **annular** (ring-shaped) lesions with an erythematous, scaly border and central clearing (Pleacher & Dexter, 2007; Rudy, 2007; Theos, 2007) (Figure 30-8). The appearance of the lesion has led to the infection being commonly known as "ringworm," despite the fact that worms do not cause this eruption. Alternatively, there may be a lack of central clearing or concentric circles/polycyclic lesions (James et al., 2006; Theos, 2007). In some cases the advancing border may also manifest pustules, vesicles, crusts, verrucous lesions, or follicular involvement (Lott et al., 2008; Rudy, 2007; Theos, 2007). Although tinea corporis is most commonly observed on exposed areas, it can involve any part of the skin surface, except the scalp, groin, palms and soles (Lott et al., 2008; Pleacher & Dexter, 2007; Theos, 2007). Pruritus or a burning sensation may be associated with tinea corporis eruptions (Lott et al., 2008; Pleacher & Dexter, 2007; Theos, 2007).

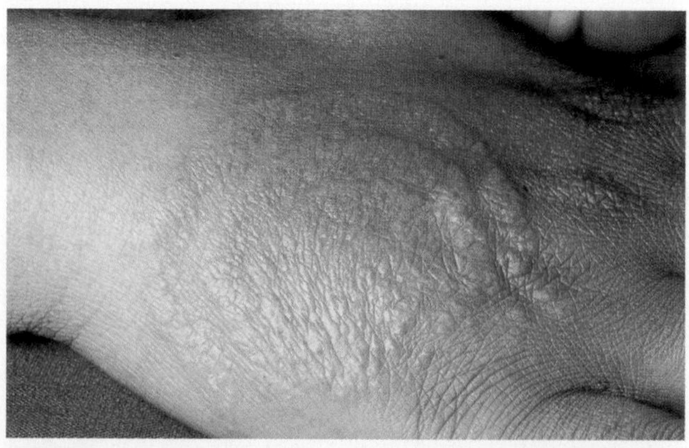

Figure 30-8 Tinea Corporis. COURTESY OF ROBERT A. SILVERMAN, M.D., CLINICAL ASSOCIATE PROFESSOR, DEPARTMENT OF PEDIATRICS, GEORGETOWN UNIVERSITY.

Diagnosis

Clinical presentation alone is often suggestive of tinea corporis, but the use of diagnostic testing is recommended because many other skin conditions may resemble dermatophyte infection (James et al., 2006; Lott et al., 2008; Theos, 2007). The two most commonly utilized tests to confirm the diagnosis of tinea corporis are microscopic potassium hydroxide (KOH) examination and fungal culture. For either of these two tests, scale should be scraped from the border of the lesion (Lott et al., 2008; Rudy, 2007; Theos, 2007). A positive KOH preparation will reveal the presence of septate hyphae, but cannot identify the specific species of dermatophyte involved, as can be accomplished with a fungal culture. As previously mentioned, KOH preparations allow for rapid assessment, but fungal cultures are more sensitive (Ali et al., 2007; Gonzalez et al., 2007; Lott et al., 2008).

Treatment

Most cases of tinea corporis respond well to topical agents (Lott et al., 2008; Rudy, 2007; Theos, 2007). Over-the-counter options include ketoconazole, miconazole, clotrimazole, tolnaftate, and terbinafine. Prescription agents such as econazole, oxiconazole, naftifine, butenafine, and ciclopirox olamine are also effective. Most topical treatments are applied once or twice daily until clinical resolution occurs, which typically takes two to four weeks (James et al., 2006; Lott et al., 2008; Pleacher & Dexter, 2007; Theos, 2007). Combination antifungal/corticosteroid preparations are not recommended, as they have been shown to cause persistent and recurrent infections and often result in longer treatment durations (James et al., 2006; Theos, 2007).

Systemic antifungal treatment may be necessary if the lesions are widespread, the child is immunocompromised, or topical treatments have failed (James et al., 2006; Lott et al., 2008; Pleacher & Dexter, 2007; Theos, 2007). Griseofulvin is considered the systemic drug of choice for children with tinea corporis (Theos, 2007). This oral agent is approved for use in children over 2 years of age and should be administered for two to four weeks. Other off-label treatment options include itraconazole, terbinafine, and fluconazole (James et al., 2006; Lott et al., 2008; Pleacher & Dexter, 2007; Theos, 2007).

Nursing Management

The nursing management of a child with tinea corporis focuses on eradication of the infection, preventing spread of the infection, and family teaching. The nursing history should include inquiry regarding any known exposure to others with similar lesions, any fungal infections on other anatomic areas, and the presence of lesions in other household members. The child should also be asked about the presence and extent of pruritus. The physical assessment should note the characteristics of the lesions as well as their distribution. Planning and implementation should include precautions such as wearing gloves and practicing proper hand washing. Family education should also be provided about the treatment regimen and preventing the spread of infection.

Family Teaching

Family teaching must include the importance of using the prescribed antifungal treatment as directed. The child and caregivers should specifically be advised that poor adherence, particularly stopping the medications too soon, could result in incomplete clearance or recurrence of the infection. Furthermore, if fungal infections are present on different anatomic locations, such as tinea pedis, these infections should be adequately treated in order to reduce the risk of recurrent tinea corporis infections. The child and caregivers also need to understand the contagious nature of tinea corporis and should be instructed to use good hand washing and avoid contact with the lesions whenever possible. In addition, fomites such as towels should not be shared until the eruption is resolved. When tinea corporis is present in an athlete who engages in direct skin contact with others, fomites such as wrestling mats should be cleaned. Furthermore, athletes should be disqualified from practice and competition until treated with topical agents for at least 72 hours (Pleacher & Dexter, 2007). Lesions should be covered before contact sports are resumed.

TINEA PEDIS

Tinea pedis, or "athlete's foot," is a fungal infection that affects the soles of the feet and/or interdigital spaces. The infection is generally not serious and responds well to topical treatments. However, it is important to take measures to prevent recurrence of the infection.

Incidence and Etiology

Tinea pedis is the most common dermatophyte infection in the world (James et al., 2006; Robbins & Elewski, 2008). Tinea pedis aoccurs almost exclusively in postpubertal adolescents and affects males more often than females (Robbins & Elewski, 2008; Rudy, 2007). Tinea pedis is rare among preadolescent children, with incidence rates estimated to be only 1.3% to 2.3% (Theos, 2007).

The organism most commonly responsible for tinea pedis infections is *Trichophyton rubrum* (*T. rubrum*), followed by *Trichophyton mentagrophyte* (*T. mentagrophytes*) and *Epidermophyton floccosum* (*E. floccosum*) (James et al., 2006; Robbins & Elewski, 2008; Theos, 2007). Often these dermatophytes are transmitted during the use of communal changing rooms or shared bathing facilities (Crawford & Hollis, 2007; Robbins & Elewski, 2008). Other pediatric risk factors for tinea pedis include hyperhidrosis (excessive perspiration), sports participation, and a household member with tinea pedis or tinea unguium (Pleacher & Dexter, 2007; Robbins & Elewski, 2008; Theos, 2007). Tinea pedis is also more common in hot, humid climates and in individuals who wear occlusive footwear. Some individuals may also have a genetic predisposition for the development of tinea pedis (James et al., 2006; Robbins & Elewski, 2008).

Pathophysiology

After being transferred onto the skin, dermatophytes release keratinases that allow them to invade the epidermis (Crawford & Hollis, 2007; Robbins & Elewski, 2008). The presence of maceration and impaired skin barrier function can further facilitate dermatophyte invasion. Depending on the specific dermatophyte involved, the cell walls of the organism may contain elements that inhibit the body's immune function and reduce the rate of skin sloughing, thus prolonging the infectious process (Robbins & Elewski, 2008). The body's response to the dermatophyte invasion and thus the clinical presentation of the infection is determined by the type of infecting dermatophyte and the host's immune system.

Clinical Manifestations

Tinea pedis has three main clinical presentations. The interdigital form consists of scaling, erythema, maceration, and possibly fissures, occurring between the toes (Pleacher & Dexter, 2007; Theos, 2007) (Figure 30-9). This form of tinea pedis occurs most often between the fourth and fifth toes and is the most commonly observed form of tines pedis (Robbins & Elewski, 2008). Among children, tinea pedis can

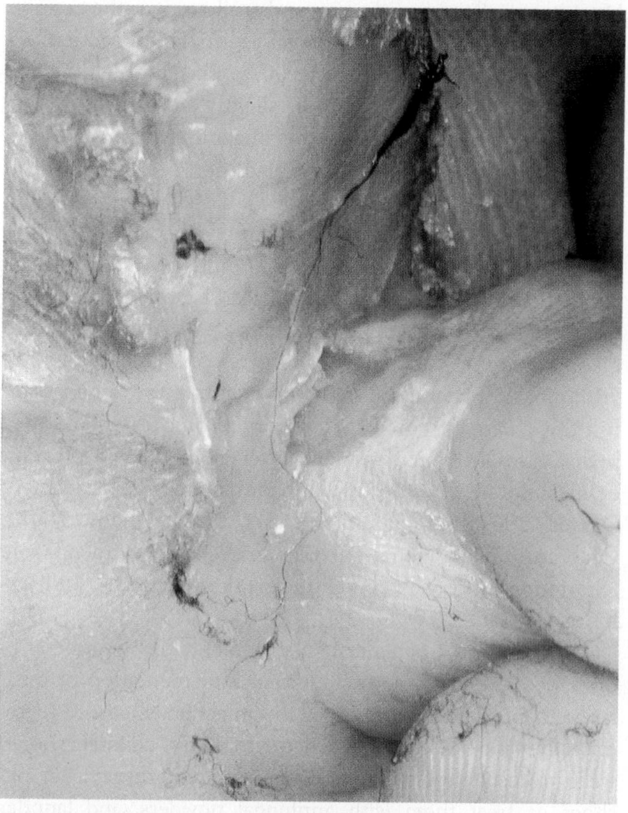

FIGURE 30-9 Tinea Pedis. COURTESY OF ROBERT A. SILVERMAN, M.D., CLINICAL ASSOCIATE PROFESSOR, DEPARTMENT OF PEDIATRICS, GEORGETOWN UNIVERSITY.

also present with vesicular or bullous lesions on the instep of the foot (James et al., 2006; Theos, 2007). The vesicles can contain clear or purulent fluid and are followed by scaling with erythema (Robbins & Elewski, 2008). The moccasin-type presentation, which consists of a dry, hyperkeratotic scale covering the sole and lateral surface of the foot, is more common in adults than children (Crawford & Hollis, 2007; James et al., 2006; Pleacher & Dexter, 2007; Theos, 2007). With all three presentations, involvement may be unilateral or bilateral, and the affected child may complain of pain or pruritus (Crawford & Hollis, 2007; James et al., 2006; Theos, 2007). Toenail involvement may also be present (James et al., 2006; Robbins & Elewski, 2008; Theos, 2007).

DIAGNOSIS

As with other dermatophyte infections, the diagnosis of tinea pedis may be suspected based on clinical presentation, but the use of the diagnostic testing such as microscopic potassium hydroxide (KOH) examination and fungal culture are recommended (Pleacher & Dexter, 2007; Theos, 2007). Specimens for laboratory examination generally consist of skin scrapings taken from areas of prominent scaling, but if vesicles are present the specimen should be collected from the roof of the blister (James et al., 2006; Robbins & Elewski, 2008).

TREATMENT

Most cases of tinea pedis respond well to over-the-counter and prescription topical antifungal agents (Pleacher & Dexter, 2007; Rudy, 2007; Theos, 2007). Presently, terbinafine and naftifine are considered to be slightly more effective than other topical agents such as clotrimazole, econazole, butenafine, tolnaftate, and ciclopiroxolamine (Crawford & Hollis, 2007; Robbins & Elewski, 2008). Topical agents should be applied once or twice daily for four to six weeks (Pleacher & Dexter, 2007). Patients should be instructed to apply the medication for the entire recommended duration, even if symptoms resolve sooner, because premature discontinuation can lead to recurrence of the infection (Robbins & Elewski, 2008). Oral agents may be necessary for the treatment of extensive or chronic cases of tinea pedis, cases in which toenail involvement is also present, or in children who are immunocompromised (Pleacher & Dexter, 2007; Robbins & Elewski, 2008; Theos, 2007). Oral antifungal agents include griseofulvin, itraconazole (Sporanox), fluconazole (Diflucan), ketoconazole, and terbinafine (Lamisil).

In addition to medical management, the treatment of tinea pedis should also include the implementation of measures to prevent recurrence of the infection. In order to reduce the risk of exposure to dermatophytes, children should wear protective footwear in communal areas, throw away old shoes or treat them with antifungal powders, and launder clothing that has contacted the infected area (Robbins & Elewski, 2008; Theos, 2007). Furthermore, if household contacts have tinea pedis or tinea unguium it is recommended that they undergo treatment as well (Theos, 2007). Recommended measures to reduce hyperhidrosis and maceration include drying one's feet thoroughly after bathing, changing socks frequently, alternating shoes, avoiding occlusive footwear, and using medicated powders in socks and shoes (James et al., 2006; Robbins & Elewski, 2008; Theos, 2007).

NURSING MANAGEMENT

The nursing management for a child with tinea pedis focuses on eradication of the infection, preventing recurrence of the infection, and family teaching. The nursing history should ask the child and caregivers about any known exposure to someone with similar lesions, any fungal infections in other household members, and assess for high risk behaviors such as sports participation or use of communal changing rooms. The physical assessment should note the characteristics of the lesions, their distribution, and the presence of pruritus. Planning and implementation should include precautions such as wearing gloves and practicing proper hand washing. Family education should also be provided about the treatment regimen and preventing recurrence of infection.

FAMILY TEACHING

Family teaching must include the importance of using the prescribed antifungal treatment as directed. The child and caregivers should specifically be advised that poor adherence, particularly stopping the medications too soon, could result in incomplete clearance or recurrence of the infection. If household contacts are found to have tinea pedis or tinea unguium infections, it should be recommended that they be adequately treated as well.

The child and caregivers also need to understand the contagious nature of tinea pedis and should be instructed to use good hand washing and avoid contact with the lesions whenever possible. In addition, instructions should be provided regarding the importance of wearing protective footwear in communal areas, throwing away old shoes or treating them with antifungal powders, and laundering clothing that has contacted the infected area. Nurses should also recommend drying the child's feet thoroughly after bathing, changing socks frequently, alternating shoes, avoiding occlusive footwear, and using medicated powders in socks and shoes.

TINEA UNGUIUM

Tinea unguium is a dermatophyte infection of the toenails and/or fingernails that is uncommon in children. However, its presence can cause psychological distress and predispose children to recurrent cutaneous fungal infections in other anatomic locations (Blumberg , Kantor, & Ratz, 2007; Crawford & Hollis, 2007). Treatment often requires relatively long courses of oral antifungal medications and is associated with a high recurrence rate.

Incidence and Etiology

The term tinea unguium refers to dermatophyte infections of the nail. Often the term **onychomycosis** is used to refer to fungal infections of the nail, as this term also includes nail infections due to nondermatophyte molds and yeasts (James et al., 2006; Sethi & Antaya, 2006). However, the majority (90%) of onychomycosis infections are caused by dermatophytes (Blumberg et al., 2007; James et al., 2006). Within the pediatric population, tinea unguium is estimated to affect only 0.3–2.6% of children (Blumberg et al., 2007; Theos, 2007).

Trichophyton rubrum (*T. rubrum*) is the dermatophyte most commonly associated with tinea unguium in children, followed by *Trichophyton mentagrophytes* (*T. mentagrophytes*) (Blumberg et al., 2007; James et al., 2006; Sethi & Antaya, 2006; Theos, 2007). Risk factors for the development of tinea unguium in children include personal history of tinea pedis, family history of tinea pedis or tinea unguium, immunosuppression, and Down syndrome (Blumberg et al., 2007; Theos, 2007). Additional factors that are associated with tinea unguium infection include warm climates, the use of occlusive foot wear, participation in athletic activities, and the use of communal changing rooms or shared bathing facilities (Blumberg et al., 2007; Crawford & Hollis, 2007).

Pathophysiology

The exact pathophysiology of tinea unguium varies depending on the dermatophyte involved and the site of initial nail penetration (Blumberg et al., 2007). Most commonly, the dermatophyte originates on the plantar skin lateral to the nail and then invades the underside of the nail (Blumberg et al., 2007; James et al., 2006). The dermatophyte then triggers an inflammatory response that results in thickening of the nail plate, the formation of subungual debris, and separation of the nail from the nail bed. Gradually, the infection worsens and spreads proximally. Alternatively, the responsible dermatophyte may affect the surface of the nail, the cuticle, or the proximal nail fold. In some cases, the causative organism affects the entire nail unit and may cause permanent scarring of the nail matrix (Blumberg et al., 2007).

Clinical Manifestations

The classic presentation of pediatric tinea unguium is distal and lateral **onycholysis** (separation of the nail plate from the nail bed), **subungual hyperkeratosis** (accumulation of keratin debris under the nail), yellowish nail discoloration, and thickening of the nail (Blumberg et al., 2007; James et al., 2006; Crawford & Hollis, 2007; Theos, 2007). These features may affect a portion of the nail or the entire nail plate (Blumberg et al., 2007; Crawford & Hollis, 2007). One, several or all of a child's nails can be affected, with infection occurring more frequently in toenails than fingernails (Blumberg et al., 2007; Crawford & Hollis, 2007; Theos, 2007).

Although the early stages of tinea unguium do not usually cause physical discomfort, the affected child and his/her caregivers may express cosmetic concerns (James et al., 2006; Blumberg et al., 2007). The psychosocial and emotional effects associated with the clinical appearance of tinea unguium can have a significant impact on quality of life (Blumberg et al., 2007). Specifically, adolescents affected by onychomycosis have been found to experience loss of self-esteem and lack of social interaction. When children are affected, it is reasonable to assume that caregivers may also experience emotional concerns on behalf of their child.

Diagnosis

A diagnosis of tinea unguium is suspected when characteristic nail changes are present, but confirmation of the diagnosis via laboratory testing is essential prior to starting long-term oral antifungal treatment (Blumberg et al., 2007; Sethi & Antaya, 2006; Theos, 2007). When microscopic potassium hydroxide (KOH) examination or fungal cultures are utilized, the specimen should be collected from the subungual debris closest to the proximal nail fold (James et al., 2006; Theos, 2007). Another alternative is to clip the affected nail, along with the subungual debris, and submit the specimen for histologic evaluation with fungal staining. This method may be more effective than KOH preparations and fungal cultures for diagnosing tinea unguium, with sensitivity rates ranging from 41–93% (Blumberg et al., 2007; James et al., 2006; Theos, 2007).

Treatment

The treatment of tinea pedis focuses on achieving a **mycologic cure** (defined as no dermatophytes detected with laboratory testing) and a **clinical cure** (defined as resolution of clinical signs and symptoms). When successful, the treatment of tinea unguium results in a mycologic cure before a clinical cure is observed because it can take up to a year for the affected nail to grow out (Blumberg et al., 2007). However, no antifungal treatment is 100% effective for treating tine unguium and in many patients clinical cure is achieved without a complete mycologic cure.

Topical antifungal treatments have proven to be effective in some patients, but due to poor nail plate penetration these medications generally require daily application for at least one year (Blumberg et al., 2007; James et al., 2006; Crawford & Hollis, 2007). When compared to adults, the thinner nail plate in children may enhance the penetration and, therefore, the efficacy of topical antifungals in pediatric tinea unguium (Theos, 2007). Therefore, the use of topical antifungal agents may be considered as first-line therapy if mild disease is present on the distal nail plate (Blumberg et al., 2007; Theos, 2007). Topical antifungal agents may also be used as adjuncts to oral antifungal therapy or as prophylaxis to prevent recurrence.

Systemic antifungal treatment is indicated for most cases of tinea unguium (Blumberg et al., 2007, James et al., 2006; Theos, 2007). Griseofulvin is generally considered the oral antifungal treatment of choice for children; however, when used for tinea unguium it has been associated with long treatment duration, poor response rates, and high recurrence rates (Blumberg et al., 2007; Sethi & Antaya, 2006). Therefore, the use of newer oral antifungal agents such as fluconazole, itraconazole, and terbinafine should be considered. All three of these systemic antifungals have been reported to be efficacious for tinea unguium when used over a period of several months, though results with terbinafine appear to be superior (Blumberg et al., 2007; James et al., 2006; Sethi & Antaya, 2006; Theos, 2007). The use of **pulse dosing**, in which the treatment alternates between periods of medication administration and drug-free intervals, has been proposed to help minimize side effects associated with long-term antifungal therapy (James et al., 2006; Sethi & Antaya, 2006).

Even with successful treatment, the recurrence rate for tinea unguium is high (Blumberg et al., 2007; Sethi & Antaya, 2006; Theos, 2007). It is therefore recommended that preventive precautions be taken such as wearing protective footwear and cotton socks, using antifungal or absorbent powders applied daily, and frequently clipping the nails (Blumberg et al., 2007; Theos, 2007). In addition, old shoes can harbor dermatophytes and should be discarded or treated with antifungal powders. If tinea pedis or tinea unguium infections are present in family members, appropriate treatment should be initiated to prevent the spread of infection to others.

Nursing Management

The nursing management for a child with tinea unguium focuses on eradication of the infection, preventing recurrence of the infection, and family teaching. The nursing history should ask the child and caregivers about the presence of any fungal infections in other household members and assess for high risk behaviors such as sports participation or use of communal changing rooms. The physical assessment should note the characteristics and severity of the affected nails, including both fingernail and toenails. Planning and implementation should include precautions such as wearing gloves and practicing proper hand washing. Family education should also be provided about the treatment regimen and preventing recurrence of infection.

Family Teaching

Family teaching must include the importance of using the prescribed antifungal treatment as directed. Because of the long-term nature of tinea unguium treatment, poor adherence is more likely and could result in incomplete clearance or recurrence of the infection. If household contacts are found to have tinea pedis or tinea unguium infections, it should be recommended that they be adequately treated as well. The child and caregivers also need to understand the contagious nature of tinea unguium and should be instructed to use good hand washing. In addition, instructions should be provided regarding the importance of wearing protective footwear, using cotton socks, throwing away old shoes or treating them with antifungal powders, frequently clipping the nails, and using antifungal or absorbent powders daily.

VIRAL INFECTIONS

There are several viral infections that commonly cause cutaneous eruptions in children. The human papilloma virus is responsible for the formation of **verrucae** (warts) in children of all ages. Molluscum contagiosum are the manifestation of a poxvirus infection, which is particularly common among young children. Another common pediatric viral infection involves the herpes simplex virus, which can cause eruptions such as herpes labialis (cold sores) in infected children and adolescents.

VERRUCAE

Verrucae, also known as warts, are benign epidermal tumors caused by the human papilloma virus (HPV). Although individuals of any age may get warts, the highest incidence generally occurs during childhood and adolescence. The availability of multiple treatment options allows for individualization based on the characteristics of the wart and the affected child.

Incidence and Etiology

Reported wart prevalence estimates among children and young adults range from just under 5% to over 20% (Gibbs & Harvey, 2009; James et al., 2006; Wenner et al., 2007). Warts may occur at any age, but it is generally agreed that warts are uncommon in infancy, increasingly common in childhood, peak in the teenage years, and sharply decline thereafter (Gibbs & Harvey, 2009; James et al., 2006).

Warts develop as a result of infection with HPV, which is spread through direct contact. To date over 80 types of HPV have been identified, with different HPV types favoring particular anatomical sites (Gibbs & Harvey, 2009; Gawkrodger, 2008; James et al., 2006). Children with compromised cell-mediated immunity are at increased risk for developing verrucae (James et al., 2006; Gawkrodger, 2008).

Pathophysiology

HPV infection occurs in the epidermal cells, which form the outer layer of skin or lining of body cavities (Gibbs & Harvey, 2009). Viral transmission may occur through direct skin contact with an infected individual (direct inoculation) or via autoinoculation (Gawkrodger, 2008; James et al., 2006). Once the HPV is introduced, viral replication leads to keratinocyte proliferation, resulting in the clinical manifestation of a verrucous papule or plaque (Gibbs & Harvey, 2009; Rudy 2007). Over a period of a few weeks to months, the wart typically grows larger and may spread to form new lesions (James et al., 2006). In some cases, HPV infection remains dormant within the epithelial cells without visible disease

(Gibbs & Harvey, 2009; James et al., 2006). There are currently conflicting reports regarding how often and how quickly warts resolve spontaneously (Boschert, 2008; Gibbs & Harvey, 2009; James et al., 2006). Estimates range from several months to several years. Some of this variation is likely due to differences in individual host immunity as well as HPV type and the site of infection (Gibbs & Harvey, 2009).

Clinical Manifestations

The exact presentation of verrucae varies with the type of HPV involved and the anatomic area affected. Verrucae are classified according to their clinical presentation. Frequently occurring types include verrucae vulgaris (common warts), verrucae plantaris (plantar warts), and verrucae plana (flat warts) (Gawkrodger, 2008; James et al., 2006).

As their name implies, verrucae vulgaris are the most frequently occurring warts. These warts appear predominantly on the hands, though they may be present anywhere on the skin (Gawkrodger, 2008; James et al., 2006). When observed on the proximal or lateral nail folds, these warts are referred to as **periungual** warts. Individuals may have a single lesion or multiple warts, with sizes ranging from pinpoint to over 1 cm (James et al., 2006). Verrucae vulgaris typically present as elevated, flesh-colored papules with a rough grayish surface (Figure 30-10). Small black spots may also be apparent due to the presence of dilated, thrombosed capillaries (James et al., 2006). Verrucae vulgaris generally are not painful unless secondary lesions such as fissures develop.

Verrucae plantaris (plantar warts) develop on the soles of the feet and are more commonly observed in adolescents and young adults (Gawkrodger, 2008). Plantar warts are most often located on weight-bearing areas such as the ball of the foot or the mid-metatarsal area (James et al., 2006). The clinical appearance of these lesions is similar to that of verruca vulgaris, though verrucae plantaris are typically flatter because pressure causes them to grow into the dermis. Frequently there are several lesions, which may grow together to form a single plaque called a mosaic wart (Gawkrodger, 2008; James et al., 2006). Plantar warts commonly present with small black spots representing dilated, thrombosed capillaries and may be associated with pain or discomfort.

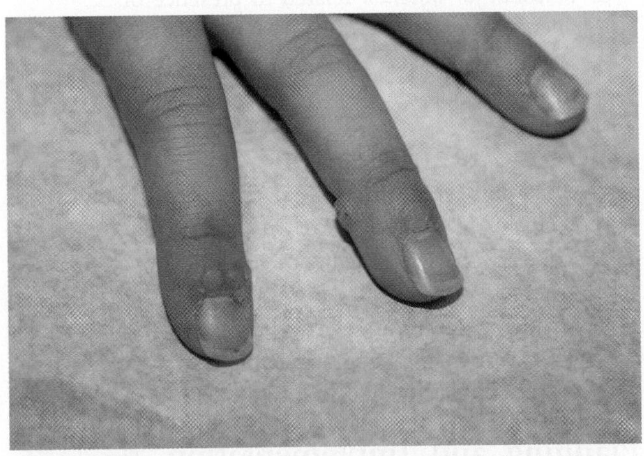

Figure 30-10 Verrucae Vulgaris. DELMAR CENGAGE LEARNING.

Verrucae plana (flat warts) are most commonly observed on the face and dorsal surface of the hands (Gawkrodger, 2008; James et al., 2006). Lesions typically present as multiple flat-topped papules that are slightly erythematous or brown and measure 2–4 mm in diameter. Of all clinical HPV infections, this form of verruca has the highest rate of spontaneous remission (James et al., 2006).

Diagnosis

Verrucae are typically diagnosed based on clinical presentation. If differential diagnosis is difficult, gentle paring or abrasion of the lesion will reveal small black dots (dilated, thrombosed capillaries). The presence of these capillaries can help distinguish verrucae from molluscum contagiosum or callus formation, in which black dots will not be observed (Gawkrodger, 2008; James et al., 2006). Observing a child's fingerprints or footprints can also be beneficial, as prints are undisturbed in calluses, but are interrupted by verrucae (Gawkrodger, 2008; James et al., 2006).

Treatment

No single wart treatment is recommended for all situations. Rather, treatment selection should be based on the unique circumstances of each child. Among factors to be considered are the size, number, location, and duration of the warts as well as response to any prior treatments. One should also consider the child's age, child and caregiver treatment preferences, as well as the degree to which the warts are problematic. Many children and caregivers want warts removed because of cosmetic concerns or social stigma. The removal of certain warts may also be indicated because they are a source of pain or inhibit function because of their size and/or location.

Regardless of the therapeutic approach utilized, warts can be frustrating to treat because of resistance to treatment or recurrence (James et al., 2006). Warts are even more difficult to treat in immunocompromised children. Because verrucae are generally harmless and often spontaneously resolve within months or years, no treatment can be considered as a treatment option. However, because of conflicting reports regarding how often and how quickly warts resolve spontaneously, there are currently differing opinions about how frequently watchful waiting should be advised (Boschert, 2008; Gibbs & Harvey, 2009; James et al., 2006).

Currently available wart treatments are intended to destroy the affected epidermal cells and/or stimulate an immune response to the HPV. A common first-line treatment is the use of topical agents containing salicylic acid. Over-the-counter and prescription preparations are available in the form of solutions, gels, pads, patches, or plasters containing salicylic acid in concentrations of 17–40% (Boschert, 2008). These treatments are readily available, relatively inexpensive, and can be applied at home with minimal pain. However, these treatments require diligent, daily application and it can take weeks or months before complete resolution is achieved.

Consequently, many caregivers find this option too laborious to be practical, particularly if numerous warts are present. The efficacy of this relatively simple treatment is supported by several studies, with an average cure rate of 73% (Boschert, 2008; Gibbs & Harvey, 2009).

Cryotherapy, often referred to as "freezing", can be used as a first-line or second-line treatment or as an adjunct to topical treatment (Boschert, 2008; Gibbs & Harvey, 2009; James et al., 2006). Typically, liquid nitrogen is applied to the lesion by a health care provider with a cotton swab or spray device. Within hours or days of application, a blister forms, followed by scabbing and sloughing of the lesion. Treatments are repeated every 2–4 weeks until resolution of the wart is achieved Reported cure rates for this therapy range from 50–80% (Boschert, 2008). Over-the-counter versions are also available, but they produce less than half the chill of liquid nitrogen and are therefore less efficacious. The potential advantages of cryotherapy with liquid nitrogen include simplicity, acceptable cure rates, and in some cases resolution after just one treatment. However, liquid nitrogen treatments are also painful, potentially expensive, and may result in scarring. As with other wart therapies, repeat treatments may be needed and there is a risk for recurrence.

Cantharidin, a topical medication made from the purified secretions of a blister beetle (*Cantharis vesicatoria*), is often used off-label for the treatment of warts (Boschert, 2008; James et al., 2006). This agent should only be applied by medical providers. The application is generally painless and is followed by blistering and desquamation that begins within a few hours. Treatment can be repeated in two weeks if necessary and is associated with a low risk of scarring.

REFLECTIVE THINKING

Alternative Wart Treatments

Caregivers may ask about alternative wart treatments such as duct tape, rubbing the wart with a sliced potato, or paying the child to borrow his/her wart. There are many "old wives tales" about warts because the placebo cure rate for warts is relatively high (0–73%). For instance, a randomized controlled trial comparing duct tape and moleskin for wart treatment found that although moleskin was intended to be the control group, 21–22% of patients in each group had their warts resolve. These findings demonstrate that duct tape may not be a highly efficacious treatment, but both treatments did provide benefit for some patients (Wenner et al., 2007; Gibbs & Harvey 2009). Based on this information, what should nurses tell patients when they ask about alternative treatments? Is it ethical to encourage treatments that may not be supported by clinical trials? Will it do any harm to have patients try easy, inexpensive treatments at home first?

Aldara (5% imiquimod cream) is a topical immunomodulatory treatment used off-label for the treatment of pediatric warts (Boschert, 2008; James et al., 2006). Therapy generally involves daily application for several months and may induce immunity to warts. The treatment is typically painless, though the cream can be expensive and erythema has been reported in about 30% of cases (Boschert, 2008). One study found clearance rates of only 27%, though the efficacy of imiquimod is likely higher when used on flat warts (James et al., 2006).

Other treatment modalities that are generally reserved for more severe cases include surgical interventions and immunotherapy (Boschert, 2008; Gibbs & Harvey, 2009; James et al., 2006). The use of curettage with cautery or surgical resection has been reported to be effective, but may result in scarring. As with other therapies, recurrence is a potential outcome, even if complete destruction of the wart is achieved (James et al., 2006). Squaric acid dibutyl ester and dinitrochlorobenzene are topical forms of immunotherapy that can induce immunity to HPV. Application is painless, but can result in contact dermatitis (Boschert, 2008; James et al., 2006). Intralesional candida antigen is another immunotherapy option, though it may be too painful for young children. Cure rates for topical and intralesional immunotherapy have been reported to range from 60–80% (James et al., 2006). Other treatment alternatives include topical 5-fluorouracil, bleomycin injections, oral cimetidine, and laser treatment (Boschert, 2008; Gibbs & Harvey, 2009; James et al., 2006).

Nursing Management

Assessment Nurses should ask the child and caregiver about the location and duration of the lesions as well as the use of any previous treatments. It is also important to assess for any pain or limited function associated with the warts. The physical assessment should focus on the character, size, number, and location of the lesions.

Nursing Diagnosis Nursing diagnoses appropriate for the child with verrucae include:

1. *Body image disturbance* related to lesions.
2. *Potential for infection* related to presence of microorganisms.
3. *Deficient knowledge* related to course of infection and treatment options.

Outcome Identification

1. Child and caregivers will utilize positive coping mechanisms to manage impact on body image.
2. Child's warts will remain contained to the original site of infection.
3. Child and caregivers will verbalize understanding of the treatment regimen and implement strategies to prevent spread of infection.

Planning and Implementation The nursing care of children with verrucae should emphasize promotion of the child's self-image and family teaching about the typical course of HPV infections, preventing the spread of infection, and specifics about their chosen wart treatment. When interacting with the affected child, nurses should reassure the child that warts are common and not serious. Self-image can further be promoted by complimenting the child's other desirable qualities such as their hair, clothes, or polite manner. When possible, the correct use of topical preparations should be demonstrated. If treatments such as cryotherapy or surgical excision are to be used, the nurse should help with the physical and emotional preparation of the child and caregivers.

Evaluation The child will display signs of satisfaction with their body image and maintain their usual activities and relationships. The child and caregivers should be able to convey proper understanding of and demonstrate adherence to the chosen treatment regimen. The primary lesions should remain contained to the initial sites of infection and eventually resolve.

Family Teaching

Appropriate teaching for the child and caregivers is an essential aspect of nursing care for patients with warts. Education should address the typical course of HPV infections, measures to prevent the spread of infection, and specifics about the chosen wart treatment. The child and/or caregivers should be made aware that warts are a viral infection that can be spread by direct inoculation or autoinoculation. Because of the infectious nature of warts, instructions should be provided about proper hand washing and the importance of not scratching or picking at the warts. In younger children, keeping the warts covered may be necessary to prevent picking or scratching. Family teaching should also include information about the often chronic nature of warts as well as the possibility of spontaneous resolution. Regarding wart treatment, the child and caregivers should be taught how the selected therapy is intended to treat the warts, what the child may expect during the treatment, and specific instructions on how to apply the treatment and/or how to care for the area following treatment. Nurses should also provide information about the expected duration of treatment, any risk for scarring, and the likelihood of recurrence.

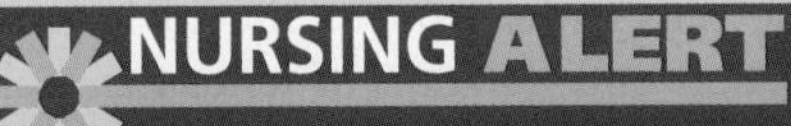

Impact of Immune Function on Verrucae and Molluscum Contagiosum

Widespread warts or molluscum may be present in children who have an underlying compromised immune system. Examples include children with HIV infection or those receiving chemotherapy.

MOLLUSCUM CONTAGIOSUM

Molluscum contagiosum is a common childhood condition in which single or multiple benign papular lesions erupt. Because of the contagious nature of the responsible poxvirus, treatment must focus on resolving the primary lesions as well as initiating precautions to prevent autoinoculation and spread of the infection to others.

Incidence and Etiology

It is estimated that slightly less than 5% of children in the United States are affected by molluscum contagiosum, with the majority of cases occurring in children who are 2–5 years of age (Dohil et al., 2006; Mansouri & Johnston, 2007). Molluscum are quite contagious, with transmission of the responsible poxvirus occurring most commonly by direct skin contact (Dohil et al., 2006; James et al., 2006; Mansouri & Johnston, 2007; McNamara, 2008a; Nelson & Morrell, 2007). Viral transmission can also occur via autoinoculation (due to scratching or occlusion in intertriginous areas), via fomites (such as bath towels) or warm water (such as a pool or bath). Adolescents who participate in sports that involve significant skin contact area are at risk for developing molluscum (Dohil et al., 2006; James et al., 2006; McNamara, 2008a; Nelson & Morrell, 2007). Molluscums have also been reported to be more common and to spread more extensively in patients with atopic dermatitis (Dohil et al., 2006; Nelson & Morrell, 2007).

Pathophysiology

Following exposure to the poxvirus, there is an incubation period of two to eight weeks before lesions begin to appear (McNamara, 2008a). New lesions occur over a period of many months, though individual lesions last for only two to four months (James et al., 2006; Mansouri & Johnston, 2007). The cell-mediated immune system appears to play an important role in the resolution of molluscum, which can take up to two years for one or multiple lesions (Dohil et al., 2006; McNamara, 2008a). For this reason, immunocompromised children are at risk for a greater number of lesions, longer duration of lesions and greater resistance to therapy (Nelson & Morrell, 2007).

Clinical Manifestations

The lesions of molluscum contagiosum are discrete, single or multiple, flesh-colored papules or nodules. Each lesion is generally 1–6mm in size with a characteristic dome-shaped appearance and a central dimple (Dohil et al., 2006; James et al., 2006; Mansouri & Johnston, 2007; McNamara, 2008a) (Figure 30-11). Healthy individuals typically develop 11–20 lesions on average, though immunocompromised patients may have hundreds of lesions. Although any cutaneous (and rarely mucosal surface) may be affected, molluscum are typically observed in clusters that favor the trunk, axillae, antecubital and popliteal fossae, and crural folds

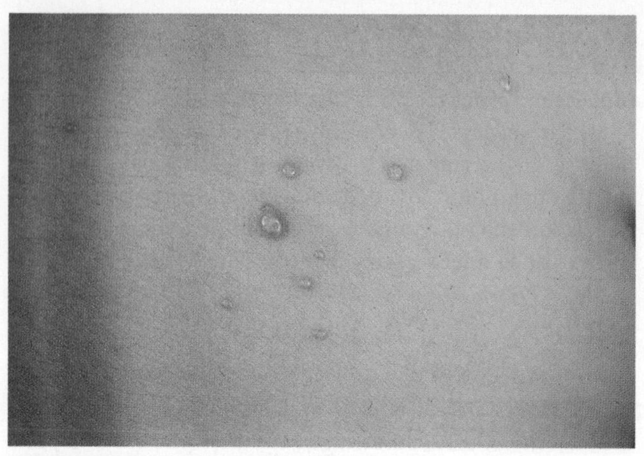

FIGURE 30-11 Molluscum Contagiosum. COURTESY OF ROBERT A. SILVERMAN, M.D., CLINICAL ASSOCIATE PROFESSOR, DEPARTMENT OF PEDIATRICS, GEORGETOWN UNIVERSITY.

(Dohil et al., 2006; Mansouri & Johnston, 2007). Lesions are generally asymptomatic, though itching or tenderness may occur, particularly if secondary infection is present (Mansouri & Johnston, 2007). Irritation and crusting may also indicate the onset of spontaneous lesion resolution (James et al., 2006). Treated and untreated lesions may resolve leaving small, pit-like depressions that will disappear with time (Nelson & Morrell, 2007).

DIAGNOSIS

The diagnosis of molluscum contagiosum is based on history and clinical observation. The history should include any known exposure to individuals with similar lesions, the location and character of the lesions, and the use of any previous treatments. Identification of typical lesions is generally sufficient to diagnose molluscum. In some instances inflammation, scabbing, or secondary infection may mask the primary lesion and obscure the diagnosis. If necessary, biopsy can be performed to confirm the diagnosis (Nelson & Morrell, 2007).

TREATMENT

The treatment of molluscum contagiosum should be tailored to the child's age as well as the number and location of lesions. The psychological impact of the lesions on the child as well as his/her caregivers should also be considered. The presence of other siblings in the household may also indicate the need for treatment in order to prevent spread of the lesions to other family members. Because many cases of molluscum resolve spontaneously, reassurance and observation may be an appropriate therapeutic approach, though caregivers should be educated that resolution can take months to years (Hanna et al., 2006; James et al., 2006; Nelson & Morrell, 2007).

Curettage is a common treatment for molluscum which involves nicking each lesion and removing the viral core (McNamara, 2008a). Prior to the procedure, each lesion is covered with a topical anesthetic cream, such as eutectic mixture of local anesthetics (EMLA) or topical lidocaine (Nelson & Morrell, 2007). Curettage can be very effective and typically yields immediate results. In one study, over 80% of children treated with curettage required only one office visit to achieve complete resolution of their molluscum (Hanna et al., 2006). Disadvantages of curettage include potential for pain and scar formation (Nelson & Morrell, 2007). Furthermore, some providers feel that this option is too time consuming and is impractical for young children who may be scared by the procedure and have difficulty holding still (Hanna et al., 2006; McNamara, 2008a).

Another common treatment for molluscum in pediatric patients is Cantharidin, a topical medication made of purified secretions from a blister beetle (Hanna et al., 2006; McNamara, 2008a; Nelson & Morrell, 2007). Application of this topical agent to individual lesions is generally painless and followed by blistering and desquamation that begins within a few hours. On average, reapplication is required every 2–4 weeks for a total of 2–3 visits to obtain complete clearance (Nelson & Morrell, 2007). Clearance rates have been reported to be as high as 90%, with an average of 2.1 visits (James et al., 2006; McNamara, 2008a). In addition, treatment of 7–10 lesions has been reported to incite immune clearance of additional nontreated lesions in some patients (Nelson & Morrell, 2007).

Aldara (5% imiquimod cream) is a topical immunomodulatory treatment intended to foster immune recognition of the poxvirus (Nelson & Morrell, 2007). Application by caregivers is painless, though the resulting inflammation may be uncomfortable. Evidence from large clinical trials is lacking, but efficacy has been reported, particularly on areas of thinner skin (Hanna et al., 2006; Nelson & Morrell, 2007). If successful, resolution may take weeks to months. It should also be considered that this prescription medication can be expensive and its use in molluscum is off-label. Other treatment alternatives include cryotherapy with liquid nitrogen, topical tretinoin, and trichloroacetic acid (James et al., 2006; McNamara, 2008a).

NURSING MANAGEMENT

The nursing management for children with molluscum should focus on promoting the child's self-image and educating the child and caregivers about molluscum infections, preventing the spread of infection, and specifics about their chosen treatment. The nursing assessment should include queries about the location and duration of lesions as well as the psychological impact of the lesions on the child and caregivers. It is also important to ascertain if other young children live in the household and if they have similar lesions. When interacting with the affected child, nurses should reassure the child and caregivers that molluscum are common, not serious, and usually resolve without scarring. Self-image can further be promoted by complimenting the child's other desirable qualities such as their hair, clothes, or polite manner. If topical treatments are to be used at home, the correct application should be demonstrated when possible. If curettage is going to be performed, the nurse should help with the physical and emotional preparation of the child and caregivers.

Family Teaching

The family teaching for children with molluscum should address the typical course of molluscum infections, measures to prevent the spread of infection, and specifics about the chosen treatment. The child and/or caregivers should be made aware that molluscum contagiosum is a viral infection that can be spread by direct inoculation or autoinoculation. Because of the infectious nature of this condition, instructions should be provided about proper hand washing and the importance of not scratching or picking at the lesions. In addition, precautions should be taken to prevent the spread of infection to other children in the household. The affected child should not take baths with other children or share possible fomites, like towels, until the lesions are resolved. If the affected child participates in sports that involve direct skin contact, the lesions should be covered or the child should be excluded from participation. Family teaching should also include information about the possibility of spontaneous resolution. Regarding treatment, the child and caregivers should be taught how the selected therapy is intended to treat the lesions, what the child may expect during the treatment, and how many treatments will likely be needed. Nurses should also provide specific information about how to apply the treatment at home and/or how to care for the area following in-office treatment.

Reflections from Families

When Jacob was 6 years old, he got a little bump on his neck that I though was a pimple. I kept an eye on it, but it did not go away. Then, several weeks later a whole bunch of them popped up around the first one. They didn't seem to bother him, but I worried about what they could be and how to get rid of them. I checked the rest of his body and found a few more bumps under one of his arms. Some were red and scabbed and I was concerned that they might be infected. When I took him to our pediatrician, she explained that they were molluscum contagiosum and gave us a cream to use at night. It took several weeks, but finally they went away. During the treatment I was nervous that the bumps might leave scars on my handsome little boy, but now Jacob is as cute as ever, without any sign of where those awful bumps used to be.

HERPES SIMPLEX VIRUS

Of the eight identified herpes viruses that may cause infections in humans, herpes simplex virus type I (HSV-1) is the most commonly encountered strain in children (Alter, 2007). Infection with HSV-1 most commonly results in oral lesions, such as cold sores. There is no cure for herpes simplex infections. Rather, after the resolution of an eruption, the virus remains dormant in the host until it may be reactivated by physical, emotional, or environmental triggers.

Incidence and Etiology

Primary infection with HSV-1 occurs most commonly in children, with more than 40% of infections occurring by the age of 15 (Drugge & Allen, 2008; Xu et al., 2007). Within the United States, the prevalence of HSV-1 is strongly influenced by race and socioeconomic status. It has been reported that among 5-year-old children, nearly twice as many black children (35%) test positive for HSV-1 when compared with white children (18%) (Alter, 2007; Fatahzadeh & Schwartz, 2007). Among children 6 to 13 years old, 48% of blacks and 42% of Mexican Americans tested positive for HSV-1, while only 25% of white children were positive (Xu et al., 2007). Regarding socioeconomic status, more than twice as many 6- to 13-year-old children of lower socioeconomic status (52%) test positive for HSV-1 when compared to those of improved socioeconomic status (24%) (Xu et al., 2007). By late adolescence, 70–80% of lower socioeconomic status children are positive, while only 40–60% of improved socioeconomic status children are positive (Fatahzadeh & Schwartz, 2007).

Primary infection with HSV-1 occurs as a consequence of direct contact with the virus via skin contact or bodily fluids, such as saliva, respiratory secretions, or vesicle fluid from active lesions (Drugge & Allen, 2008; Fatahzadeh & Schwartz, 2007). HSV-1 can also remain viable on the skin, clothing, and plastics for brief periods of time. Transmission may occur during a primary infection, recurrent infection, or during viral shedding in the absence of clinical manifestations. Infants are protected from HSV-1 infection through maternal immunity for the first six months of life (Fatahzadeh & Schwartz, 2007).

Once an individual has been infected with HSV-1, internal and external triggers can reactivate the virus and lead to the development of clinical lesions (Drugge & Allen, 2008; Fatahzadeh & Schwartz, 2007). Only 15–40% of individuals who are infected with HSV-1 will have recurrent infections (Drugge & Allen, 2008; Fatahzadeh & Schwartz, 2007).

Potential internal triggers include emotional stress, physical stress, fatigue, fever, illness, immunosuppression, use of corticosteroids, and local tissue trauma (Alter, 2007; Drugge & Allen, 2008; Fatahzadeh & Schwartz, 2007). Exposure to heat, cold, sunlight, and wind can also trigger recurrent HSV-1 infections.

Pathophysiology

After initial HSV-1 exposure, the virus invades the epithelial cells, replicates at the site of exposure (Figure 30-12), and leads to the development of clinical lesions (Alter, 2007; Fatahzadeh & Schwartz, 2007). The time between when the HSV-1 first enters the body and when symptoms first appear ranges from two to fourteen days in children (Alter, 2007; Drugge & Allen, 2008). After the primary infection, the virus travels down the peripheral sensory neuron to the dorsal root ganglia where it remains dormant for life, or until a trigger stimulates reactivation of the virus (Alter, 2007; Drugge & Allen, 2008; Fatahzadeh & Schwartz, 2007). If the virus becomes reactivated, it travels along the sensory neurons to the innervated mucocutaneous sites, undergoes replication, and leads to the formation of clinical lesions in the vicinity of the initial anatomic site of exposure (Fatahzadeh & Schwartz, 2007). Reactivation may also lead to viral shedding in the absence of clinical symptoms.

Clinical Manifestations

In children, the majority of herpes simplex infections are oral lesions caused by HSV-1 (Drugge & Allen, 2008; Fatahzadeh & Schwartz, 2007). In instances where herpes simplex virus type 2 (HSV-2) causes oral lesions, the outbreaks are usually clinically indistinguishable. The term primary infection refers to the first time an individual is infected with the herpes simplex virus. A majority of primary infections are asymptomatic (Fatahzadeh & Schwartz, 2007; Xu et al., 2007). However, for children who do develop clinical manifestations, primary infections are generally more severe than recurrent infections and may be associated with symptoms such as lymphadenopathy, headache, fever, or malaise (Alter, 2007; Drugge & Allen, 2008; Fatahzadeh & Schwartz, 2007; James et al., 2006). Primary infections often present as primary herpetic gingivostomatitis, which is most common among children between 6 months and 5 years old (Alter, 2007; Fatahzadeh & Schwartz, 2007; Xu et al., 2007).

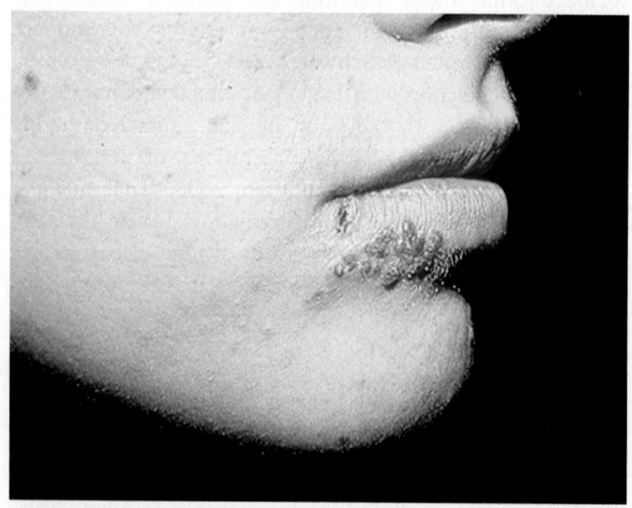

Figure 30-12 Herpes Simplex Type 1. COURTESY OF ROBERT A. SILVERMAN, M.D., CLINICAL ASSOCIATE PROFESSOR, DEPARTMENT OF PEDIATRICS, GEORGETOWN UNIVERSITY.

Primary herpetic gingivostomatitis is typically preceded by a prodrome characterized by localized pain, tingling, burning, tenderness, or parasthesia (Drugge & Allen, 2008; Fatahzadeh & Schwartz, 2007). One or two days later, vesicles and superficial ulcerations appear inside and around the mouth, potentially covering the hard and soft palate, gingiva, buccal mucosa, lips, tongue, and floor of the mouth. Recovery generally occurs within 10–14 days, though viral shedding continues for several weeks (Alter, 2007; Fatahzadeh & Schwartz, 2007).

Herpes simplex labialis, also known as fever blisters or cold sores, are the most common form of recurrent herpes simplex infection (Alter, 2007; Drugge & Allen, 2008; Fatahzadeh & Schwartz, 2007; James et al., 2006). Recurrent lesions tend to be fewer in number, less painful, and heal more rapidly. The most common site for recurrence is the outer edge of the lips. A prodrome sensation of localized tingling, burning, or pain may be present for nearly 6 hours before the appearance of clinical lesions. Multiple vesicles then appear on an erythematous base and rupture to form erosions that rapidly crust over. Lesions heal within 2 weeks and viral shedding continues for 3–5 days after resolution of the lesions.

In addition to the clinical lesions of oral herpes simplex infections, affected children may exhibit difficulty eating or swallowing, increased drooling, listlessness, irritability, or dehydration (Alter, 2007; Drugge & Allen, 2008; James et al., 2006). Oral herpes simplex outbreaks have also been associated with distress, anxiety, and embarrassment due to the visible nature of the lesions (Drugge & Allen, 2008). Among affected children, lower self-esteem can occur due to teasing by other children. Caregivers may also be fearful about the affected child transmitting the infection to other household members.

Diagnosis

Herpes simplex infections can often be diagnosed based on the child's history and clinical appearance. The history should assess for any prodrome sensations as well as any known exposure to herpes simplex, including the presence of infection in household members. However, viral cultures remain the "gold standard" for confirming the diagnosis of herpes simplex infection (Alter, 2007; Drugge & Allen, 2008). Viral culture samples are obtained by swabbing the most recent lesion, preferably collecting some vesicular fluid. Viral cultures are highly sensitive and are able to distinguish between HSV-1 and HSV-2. Serologic testing is generally not recommended because positive results only indicate a history of infection and cannot determine if the herpes virus caused the current clinical lesions (Alter, 2007; James et al., 2006).

TREATMENT

Treatment priorities for HSV-1 infection are to relieve associated discomfort, limit the duration and severity of lesions, prevent complications, and decrease the duration of viral shedding (Drugge & Allen, 2008). Two prescription topical antiviral medications are available to help accomplish these goals: acyclovir (Zovirax), which is approved for children over 1 year old, and penciclovir (Denavir), which is approved for children over 13 years old. Docosanol (Abreva) is available over-the-counter and is approved for use in children over 12 years old. Each of these medications are applied every 2–3 hours for several days, preferably with application starting in the prodrome phase (Alter, 2007; Drugge & Allen, 2008). To further help relieve discomfort, several over-the-counter anesthetic creams and ointments are available that contain benzocaine, lidocaine, tetracaine, benzoyl alcohol, camphor, and phenol (Drugge & Allen, 2008). Acetaminophen and ibuprofen can also be used for pain management if needed (Alter, 2007; Drugge & Allen, 2008).

For more severe infections, the use of oral antiviral medications may be necessary. Acyclovir (Zovirax) and valacyclovir (Valtrex) are indicated for use in children over 1 year of age and famciclovir (Famvir) is indicated for use in children 13 years old and older (Alter, 2007; Drugge & Allen, 2008). Because herpes simplex replicates quickly, these medications are most effective when initiated early in the infection. Oral antiviral medications can also be used for prophylaxis if trauma or other known triggers are anticipated (James et al., 2006). Herpes simplex is more common among immunocomprised children. If severe herpes simplex eruptions are associated with significant dehydration, the affected child may require hospitalization for pain control and administration of IV fluids (Alter, 2007).

NURSING MANAGEMENT

Nursing management priorities for the child with an oral herpes simplex eruption should include resolving the eruption, preventing spread of the virus, promoting the child's comfort, preventing complications, and providing family teaching. The nursing history should assess the presence of any prodrome sensations, any known contact with infected individuals, and the severity of discomfort, if present. In order to prevent complications, nurses should also evaluate for systemic symptoms and poor feeding. The physical assessment should note the appearance, severity, and location of clinical lesions. The presence of fever and lymphadenopathy should also be noted, if present. The planning and implementation of nursing care should include precautions such as wearing gloves and practicing proper hand washing. If the child is hospitalized, nurses should monitor the child's fluid intake and observe for signs and symptoms of worsening infection. Family education should also be provided about the treatment regimen, comfort measures, preventing the spread of infection, and the potential for recurrent infections.

FAMILY TEACHING

An important aspect of family teaching for children with herpes simplex infections is conveying to the child and caregivers that the herpes virus will remain latent and can cause recurrent infections in response to physical, emotional, or environmental triggers. Nurses should encourage the identification and avoidance of the child's most common triggers. The child and caregivers should also be educated about the prodrome phase that typically occurs before the appearance of the eruption. Identification of these sensations can help identify future outbreaks quickly.

The child and caregivers should also be warned about the contagious nature of herpes simplex infections. Nurses should encourage families to use proper hand washing and avoid contact with the lesions whenever possible. While the outbreak is present, the affected child should refrain from sharing objects that touch the lesions, such as cups and utensils (Drugge & Allen, 2008). If the affected child participates in sports that involve direct skin contact, he/she should be excluded from participation until the outbreak resolves (Drugge & Allen, 2008; Pleacher & Dexter, 2007).

If antiviral medications are recommended, the child and caregivers should be educated about the use of the topical or oral medication chosen. For children with recurrent infections, it is recommended that a supply of medication be kept on hand so that treatment can be initiated as soon as possible (Drugge & Allen, 2008). Education should also be provided about comfort measures such as over-the-counter topical anesthetics and oral analgesics. To reduce the discomfort of oral lesions, it is also recommended that the child avoid acidic or salty foods (Drugge & Allen, 2008). Caregivers should also be instructed about the importance of monitoring hydration and encouraging fluid intake.

INFESTATIONS

Pediculosis capitis and scabies are caused by ectoparasites that live on the skin surface and rely on their human host for survival. Both infestations generally respond well to topical medications, though these highly contagious disorders may become epidemic if left untreated.

PEDICULOSIS CAPITIS

Pediculosis capitis (head lice) is a skin disorder in which the scalp of the affected individual is infested by lice. Head lice most frequently affect school-age children and can cause pruritus as well as embarrassment and social stigma.

INCIDENCE AND ETIOLOGY

Pediculosis capitis is most common among young children, affecting 6 to 12 million children age 3 to 12 years old in the United States each year (Sciscione & Krause-Parello, 2008; Wyndham, 2008). The ratio of infestation among girls vs. boys is 2:1, though hair length has not proven to be a factor affecting infestation rates (Sciscione & Krause-Parello, 2008). All socioeconomic groups are affected, though incidence is more common among those who live in poor economic conditions (Silva, Alencar, & Madeira, 2008). In the United States, African-American children have fewer reported infestations (Sciscione & Krause-Parello, 2008). This is believed to be because of racial differences in hair shaft shape and possibly due to the use of oil or grease hair preparations. Lice also seem to prefer red or brown hair over blonde or black hair.

Head lice are spread primarily via direct head-to-head contact, most often among family members (Lebwohl, Clark, & Levitt, 2007; Sciscione & Krause-Parello, 2008). Fomites such as hats, combs, bedding, and clothing have also been implicated in lice transmission, though this method of spread is considered much less common (Lebwohl et al., 2007; Sciscione & Krause-Parello, 2008; Wyndham, 2008). Lice do not fly, jump, swim, or crawl long distances. Home cleanliness is not a factor in lice transmission (Sciscione & Krause-Parello, 2008).

Pathophysiology

Pediculus humanus capitis, the head louse, is an ectoparasite that can only survive by feeding on blood drawn from the scalp of human hosts (Sciscione & Krause-Parello, 2008). Lice feed every 4–6 hours and will die within 1–2 days without a host (Lebwohl et al., 2007; Sciscione & Krause-Parello, 2008). Lice range in size from 2.1–3.3mm (about the size of a sesame seed) and reside mainly on the scalp and neck hair of their hosts (Sciscione & Krause-Parello, 2008; Wyndham, 2008). The female louse lays 5–10 eggs per day that are attached firmly to the proximal end of the hair shaft, usually within 6mm of the scalp. Nymphs emerge from the egg casings (nits) within 7 days, leaving the nits attached to the hair shaft. Nymphs grow from the size of a pinhead into mature adults in about 7 days. Lice live for approximately 30 days after they hatch. At any given time, the average infected host has approximately 20 active, live lice. As lice feed, the saliva may trigger an immune response that results in pruritus (Sciscione & Krause-Parello, 2008). Sensitivity to their saliva may take 4–6 weeks to develop. The fecal matter excreted by the lice may also contribute to scalp irritation.

> **NURSING TIP**
>
> **Racial Variations in Pediculosis Capitis**
>
> Racial factors appear to influence the development of pediculosis capitis. African-American children have fewer reported cases of head lice, presumably because of differences in the shape of their hair shafts when compared to children of other ethnicities. Lice also seem to prefer red or brown hair over blonde or black hair. Despite these differences in incidence, all children should be considered at risk for developing pediculosis capitis regardless of race or ethnicity.

Clinical Manifestations

Most children with pediculosis capitis are asymptomatic (Lebwohl et al., 2007; Sciscione & Krause-Parello, 2008). When symptoms do develop, the most common presenting complaint is persistent itching, most commonly on the occipital and postauricular scalp (Sciscione & Krause-Parello, 2008; Silva et al., 2008). Some affected children may report a sensation of crawling on their scalp.

Live adult lice may be apparent, but nits are much more easily identifiable. Nits are smooth, teardrop-shaped masses that are firmly attached to the hair shaft (Figure 30-13). Nits measure 0.5–0.8 mm and range in color from silvery-white to dark brown. Nits that are viable are generally found within 6 mm of the scalp. Scalp inspection may also reveal bite marks on the scalp or louse feces, which resemble small black specks. The only known physical complication of head lice is secondary bacterial infection, which may cause localized lymph node enlargement (Sciscione & Krause-Parello, 2008; Wyndham, 2008).

In addition to the physical manifestations of pediculosis capitis, there are also several psychosocial sequelae that commonly affect both caregivers and the affected child. Children

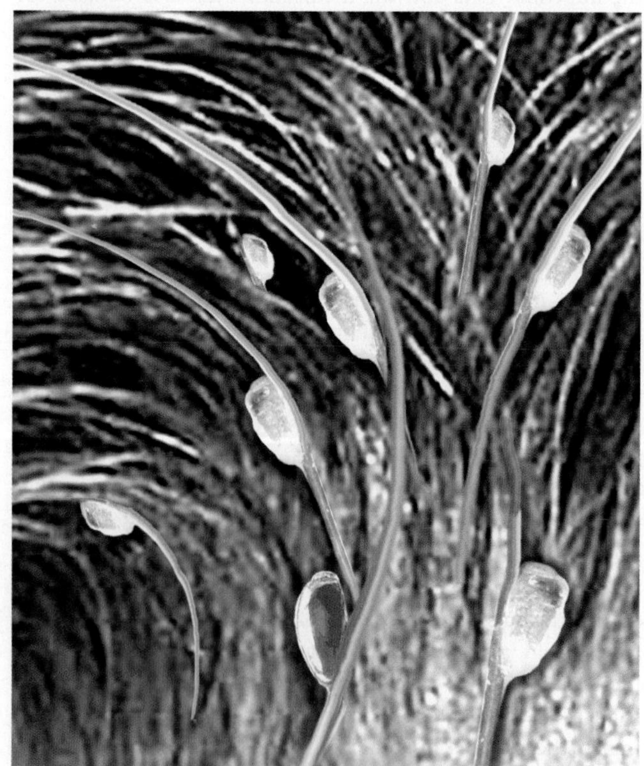

Figure 30-13 Louse Eggs (Nits) Attached to the Hair Shaft.

with head lice often experience embarrassment, low-self-esteem, and are teased by peers (Lebwohl et al., 2007; Sciscione & Krause-Parello, 2008). Caregivers can likewise experience social stigma and embarrassment regarding their child's condition (Silva et al., 2008). In most situations, the onus of resolving head lice rests on the caregiver and this may be perceived as overwhelming. In addition, the presence of pruritus can cause the affected child to develop poor sleep patterns (Lebwohl et al., 2007; Silva et al., 2008). Among younger children who are not be able to express the source of their discomfort, behavior changes such as restlessness, inattention, or irritability may be observed (Sciscione & Krause-Parello, 2008).

Diagnosis

The "gold standard" for diagnosing pediculosis capitis is identification of a live louse on the scalp (Sciscione & Krause-Parello, 2008). However, such identification can be difficult because lice are generally few in number and move very quickly. Visual identification of nits can indicate head lice, but the presence of nits should be evaluated carefully because misdiagnosis frequently results from failure to distinguish viable nits from other material such as dandruff, hairspray, or old dried nits. For this reason, screeners should be educated about the characteristic appearance of live nits. Gently shaking the hair can also help distinguish nits from dandruff, as dandruff will become dislodged and nits will not (Wyndham, 2008). Furthermore, nits found only at distances greater than 6 mm from the scalp most likely indicate a previous infestation and do not indicate the need for treatment (Sciscione & Krause-Parello, 2008). Another factor resulting in misdiagnosis is the fact that many infestations are missed by visual inspection. In such instances, wetting the hair and using a nit comb can make the identification of characteristic findings easier (Lebwohl et al., 2007; Wyndham, 2008).

Treatment

Current recommendations advise that pediculosis capitis treatment should be administered only to children in whom viable eggs, living nymphs, or adult lice have been observed (Centers for Disease Control and Prevention [CDC], 2008a; Sciscione & Krause-Parello, 2008). In addition, all other household members and close contacts should be carefully checked for signs of active infection. If a current infestation is detected, affected contacts should be treated simultaneously with the affected child.

There are several pharmacologic and nonpharmacologic treatments available to treat head lice. The most commonly used pharmacologic treatments are available over-the-counter, such as 1% permethrin lotion (Nix) and pyrethrin combined with piperonyl butoxide (A-200 or Rid) (CDC, 2008a; Chayavichitsilp & Barrio, 2007; Lebwohl et al., 2007). Permethrin has been recommended as a preferred first-line treatment for head lice (Lebwohl et al., 2007). Both over-the-counter products are considered safe and effective, though permethrin is not approved for use in children less than 2 years old (CDC, 2008a; Lebwohl et al., 2007). Because these products are only **pediculocidal** (kills live lice), but not **ovicidal** (kills unhatched eggs), a second

Reflections from Families

I was horrified when the school nurse called and told me that my 7-year-old daughter had head lice. I had not seen her scratching her scalp and didn't notice anything when I helped her do her hair. It was so embarrassing to have someone else find those little bugs on her! I keep our home very clean, and I wash her hair several times a week. I wondered what the other parents would think of me when they found out! What about the other kids? Were they going to make fun of my daughter? How could this have happened?

I was really nervous about choosing the right treatment at the drug store. Once I got home, I read the instructions carefully to make sure I did the treatment right. The hardest part, though, was combing out her long red hair. It was very tedious, but we decided to make a game of it and play "going to the beauty parlor." Then we went through the house and cleaned all of the bedding, hairbrushes, hats, and hair clips and ribbons. Fortunately, no one else in our family got lice. This experience definitely made me more sympathetic to other families who have a child with head lice. It can happen to anyone.

NURSING ALERT

Use of Hair Products Before and After Topical Lice Treatment

Do not use a cream rinse or any type of conditioner before using topical lice medications. Do not re-wash the hair for one to two days following treatment.

treatment is recommended in nine to ten days to kill any newly hatched lice before they can produce new eggs (CDC, 2008a). Unlike pyrethrins, permethrin may continue to kill newly hatched lice for several days after treatment. Depending on the patient's geographic location, lice may be resistant to either of these treatments (CDC, 2008a; Chayavichitsilp & Barrio, 2007; Lebwohl et al., 2007).

Prescription topical treatments available in the United States for the treatment of head lice include 5% permethrin, 0.5% malathion (Ovide) and 1% lindane. Permethrin 5% is considered a second-line option when 1% permethrin is not effective. The higher concentration may overcome failure due to poor treatment adherence, but the treatment will not be effective if resistance is an issue (Chayavichitsilp & Barrio, 2007). Malathion is a safe and effective pediculocide that is also partially ovicidal. A second treatment is recommended if live lice are present after seven to nine days. Malathion is flammable and is not recommended for use in children under age 6 (CDC, 2008a). Resistance to malathion has not yet been reported in the United States, but is common in Britain, where malathion has been available longer (Lebwohl et al., 2007; Ross, 2008). Because of toxicity concerns, lindane is not recommended for use in infants or children (CDC, 2008a).

Oral ivermectin may also prove to be a useful agent in the treatment of pediculosis capitis (Chayavichitsilp & Barrio, 2007; Lebwohl et al., 2007). Thus far, ivermectin has demonstrated pediculocidal activity without any resistance observed, though ivermectin does not appear to be ovicidal. Because of potential neurotoxicity concerns, the use of ivermectin is not recommended in children who weigh less than 15kg. The oral antibiotic trimethoprim/sulfamethoxazole (Bactrim, Septra) has also been reported to have pediculocidal effects, presumably by ridding lice of symbiotic bacteria in their gut (Chayavichitsilp & Barrio, 2007; Lebwohl et al., 2007). However, the efficacy of this treatment is currently controversial.

Several nonpharmacologic treatment options are also available, though there is little research to support which, if any, of these options are effective enough to be used as monotherapy. At present, these options are considered adjunct treatments. Perhaps the most common of these treatments is nit combing (removal of nits with a fine-tooth comb). Although this method is questionably effective as monotherapy, performing nit combing immediately after use of a topical pediculocide is thought to reduce the risk of self-reinfestation. Presently, it is recommended that nit combing be performed initially following treatment and every two to three days for two to three weeks after treatment is initiated (CDC, 2008a).

Although pediculocide resistance has been increasing, more common causes of treatment failure are poor compliance or reinfestation (Chayavichitsilp & Barrio, 2007). Poor treatment compliance has been attributed to the amount of time and effort that is required for caregivers to correctly apply pediculocides and/or comb lice out of hair as well as children's reluctance to undergo the often lengthy and bothersome treatment process. In order to prevent reinfestation, treatment of the environment is recommended. All potentially contaminated clothing, linens, and stuffed animals used by the child two days prior to treatment should be washed in hot water, placed in a hot dryer for 5–15 minutes, or dry cleaned (CDC, 2008a; Chayavichitsilp & Barrio, 2007; Lebwohl et al., 2007). Items that cannot be washed should be placed in a sealed plastic bag for two weeks. Contaminated combs and brushes should be immersed in boiling water for 5–10 minutes. Floors and furniture should be vacuumed thoroughly. Use of pediculocide sprays on inanimate objects is not recommended as this can result in toxicity (CDC,

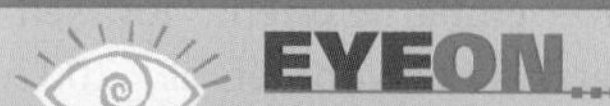

Nonpharmacologic Treatments for Pediculosis Capitis

Presently, there is little research to support which, if any, of these treatment options are effective enough to be used as monotherapy.

- Nit combing is theoretically highly efficacious when performed rigorously for several minutes over many days, but real-life success rates have been quite variable.
- Head shaving has not been formally tested, but is anecdotally effective.
- Hot air devices have shown promising ovicidal effects, but fail to consistently kill live lice.
- Occlusive agents such as petroleum jelly, olive oil, and butter have thus far failed to produce successful enough suffocation to be considered pediculocidal.
- Cetaphil Gentle Skin Cleanser, when applied to the scalp, dried with a hair dryer for 30 minutes, and then left in place for one day, has shown promising results (96% success rate), but valid clinical trials have yet to be conducted.

Adapted from: Chayavichitsilp, P., & Barrio, V. (2007). Choosing the best treatment to eradicate lice infestations. *Practical Dermatology*, *4*(11), 43–47; Lebwohl, M., Clark, L., & Levitt, J. (2007). Therapy for head lice based on life cycle, resistance, and safety considerations. *Pediatrics*, *119*(5), 965–974.

2008a; Chayavichitsilp & Barrio, 2007; Lebwohl et al., 2007). As previously mentioned, it is also critical to carefully check all other household members and close contacts for signs of active infection and initiate treatment if indicated.

Nursing Management

Assessment When taking the client history for a child suspected of having head lice, it is important to ask about any known contact with another individual who is suspected of having head lice. Caregivers should also be asked if they have observed any live lice or nits. Nurses should also assess for pruritus, sleep disturbance, or irritability in the affected child. The physical exam should assess for the presence of live lice, viable nits, signs of secondary infection, or lymph node enlargement. The assessment should also ascertain the psychological effects of having head lice on the child and/or caregivers. Finally, all other symptomatic or asymptomatic household members and close contacts should be screened so that if infestations are detected, all affected individuals can be treated simultaneously.

Nursing Diagnosis Nursing diagnoses for the child with pediculosis capitis include:

1. *Infection* related to presence of infective organisms.
2. *Body image disturbance* related to the presence of lice.
3. *Risk for infection (secondary)* related to scratching or picking.
4. *Deficient knowledge* related to treatment and measures to prevent the spread of infection.

Outcome Identification

1. Child's infestation will resolve.
2. Child and caregivers will utilize positive coping mechanisms to manage impact on body image.
3. Child will not manifest signs of a secondary infection.
4. Caregivers will verbalize understanding of the treatment regimen and implement strategies to prevent spread of infection.

Planning and Implementation The nursing management of children with pediculosis capitis focuses on resolution of the infestation, promotion of the child's self-image, and family teaching. When providing nursing care, thorough hand washing before and after contact with the child is essential. When interacting with the affected child, nurses should reassure the child that head lice are common, not serious, and are not an indication of poor hygiene. Self-image can further be promoted by complimenting the child's other desirable qualities such as their smile, clothes, or polite manner. Both the child and caregivers should be educated about the treatment regimen and methods to prevent the spread of the infestation to other individuals. Included in this education should be information about not picking or scratching the scalp. When possible, the correct use of topical preparations should be demonstrated. If nursing care is provided in the school setting, nurses are responsible for coordinating care with the caregivers, informing and educating teachers, and ensuring that treated children not be excluded from school (Sciscione & Krause-Parello, 2008).

Evaluation The child will display signs of satisfaction with their body image and maintain their usual activities and relationships. The child and caregivers will also be able to convey proper understanding of and demonstrate adherence to the treatment regimen. They will also be able to implement strategies to prevent spread of the infestation to others and prevent picking and scratching, resulting in the affected area remaining free from excoriations and signs of secondary infection. Implementation of these steps should lead to resolution of the infestation.

Family Teaching

It is essential that caregivers strictly comply with the pediculocide treatment. This necessitates that the nurse carefully explain the medication usage instructions and answer any questions about the treatment. Regardless of whether a prescription or over-the-counter topical product is used, caregivers should be instructed that the hair should first be washed with regular shampoo. The child should not use a cream rinse or any type of conditioner before using the medication. The pediculocide should be applied and left on the hair according to label instructions. It is recommended that nit combing be performed initially following treatment and every two to three days for two to three weeks after treatment is initiated. The caregiver should work with small sections of hair at a time, working from the scalp outward. Hair should be recombed every two to three days until no nits are found. The child's hair should not be washed for one to two days following treatment (CDC, 2008a).

In order to prevent secondary infection, older children should be instructed not to scratch or pick at their scalp. If younger children experience pruritus, caregivers should be instructed to keep the child's nails cut short and place mittens over the child's hands if necessary. The child and caregivers also need to be made aware that head lice can be spread by direct head to head contact or, less commonly, by fomites. To prevent the spread of infection, direct head contact should be avoided and children should be instructed to not share items such as brushes, combs, backpacks, jackets, scarves, or hats with others until the treatment is complete. To prevent reinfestation, all potentially contaminated items should be washed, placed in a hot dryer for fifteen minutes, dry cleaned, sealed in a plastic bag for two weeks, or immersed in boiling water for five to ten minutes. Floors and furniture should be vacuumed thoroughly. Use of pediculocide sprays on inanimate objects is not recommended as this can result in toxicity (CDC, 2008a; Chayavichitsilp & Barrio, 2007; Lebwohl et al., 2007).

SCABIES

Scabies is a papular rash caused by the *Sarcoptes scabiei* mite. Although the condition is generally not serious, the associated pruritus is often intense and can result in depression or sleep disturbance.

Incidence and Etiology

Scabies infestations are a significant public health problem, with an estimated global prevalence of 300 million cases (Strong & Johnstone, 2007). The burden of disease is greatest among individuals living in areas of poor sanitation, overcrowding, and social disruption (Dupuy et al., 2007; Heukelbach & Feldmeier, 2006; Jacobson & Abel, 2007; Leone, 2007; Strong & Johnstone, 2007). Sporadic cases occur in industrialized countries, while epidemics occur in institutions such as hospitals and long-term care facilities (Dupuy et al., 2007; Heukelbach & Feldmeier, 2006; Leone, 2007). In contrast, scabies is endemic in many underdeveloped countries (Dupuy et al., 2007; Leone, 2007).

Within the United States, the prevalence of scabies is less than 1%, with higher incidence observed among children and sexually active adults (Jacobson & Abel, 2007). Scabies mites are transmitted primarily by direct skin contact. Mites have also been found to survive for two to three days on fomites, though fomite transmission is considered rare (Heukelbach & Feldmeier, 2006; Leone, 2007).

Pathophysiology

The *Sarcoptes scabiei* mite is an obligate human parasite that completes its entire 30–60 day life cycle on human hosts (Jacobson & Abel, 2007; Leone, 2007). Once scabies mites infest a new host, symptoms do not develop for three to six weeks. After this time period, the host develops an immune response to the mites and their excrement, resulting in a pruritic rash. Reinfestation is associated with a brisk immune response and the onset of symptoms within 24–72 hours (Mansouri & Johnston, 2007; Heukelbach & Feldmeier, 2006; Leone, 2007; Strong & Johnstone, 2007).

While on their human host, male scabies mites explore the skin for an unfertilized female. Once impregnated, female mites burrow into the stratum corneum of the epidermis to lay their eggs (Heukelbach & Feldmeier, 2006; Leone, 2007). The eggs hatch after two to four days, and the larvae mature on the skin surface over the course of 10–14 days. On average, approximately 10–15 mites live on an infected host. The presence of saliva, eggs, and fecal material stimulates a host hypersensitivity reaction, leading to pruritus that is often intense (Heukelbach & Feldmeier, 2006; Strong & Johnstone, 2007).

Clinical Manifestations

Once sensitization occurs, the affected child will develop a rash consisting initially of small erythematous papules. However, these primary lesions often progress into vesicles, excoriations, crusts, eczematous lesions, or secondary infections (Heukelbach & Feldmeier, 2006; Leone, 2007). These changes are more common in infants and young children because of scratching (Mansouri & Johnston, 2007).

The most characteristic lesion of scabies is the burrow (Heukelbach & Feldmeier, 2006; Leone, 2007; Mansouri & Johnston, 2007). When apparent, these subcutaneous tunnels look like a thin, short wavy line that is slightly elevated. Burrows can be up to 1 cm long, though they are rarely visible unless a local host reaction occurs around the tunnel. Occasionally a female mite can be observed as a black dot at the end of the burrow. However, female mites are only 0.3–0.5 mm long and are, consequently, at the limit of visibility (Heukelbach & Feldmeier, 2006).

The extent of lesions may range from a few erythematous papules to hundreds of excoriated lesions. Skin lesions most commonly involve the interdigital spaces and flexor surfaces of the wrist, axillae, waist, groin, feet, and ankles (Heukelbach & Feldmeier, 2006; Leone, 2007; Mansouri & Johnston, 2007; Strong & Johnstone, 2007) (Figure 30-14). Among infants and children the face, neck, palms, and soles are commonly involved, though these areas are rarely involved in other age groups.

Although some patients are asymptomatic, most affected individuals experience intense pruritus that typically worsens at night and can inhibit sleep (Heukelbach & Feldmeier, 2006; Leone, 2007; Mansouri & Johnston, 2007). This persistent itch can result in emotional manifestations such as depression and reduced ability to carry out usual tasks (Strong & Johnstone, 2007).

Diagnosis

Several factors may contribute to the diagnosis of scabies. The patient history should include details about the child's living situation, any known contact with scabies, and the presence of symptoms in other household members. The presence and severity of pruritus should also be assessed. Careful clinical observation is also required to assess for the presence of burrows and typical scabies lesions in a classic distribution (Page, Eiff, & Judkins, 2007). The progression of the initial erythematous papules to secondary excoriations or infected lesions can obscure the diagnosis, though primary and secondary lesions can be present

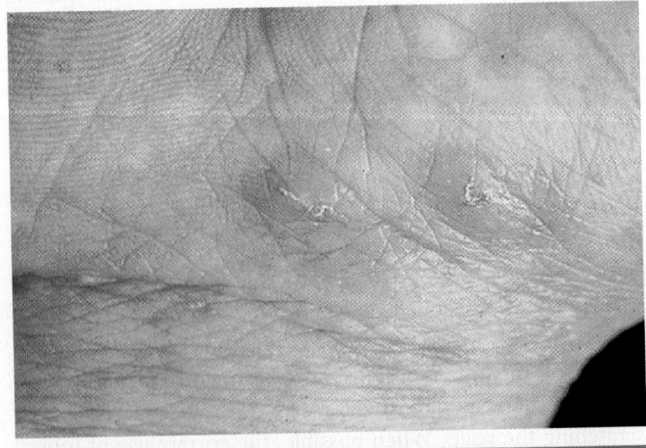

Figure 30-14 Scabies. COURTESY OF ROBERT A. SILVERMAN, M.D., CLINICAL ASSOCIATE PROFESSOR, DEPARTMENT OF PEDIATRICS, GEORGETOWN UNIVERSITY.

simultaneously (Heukelbach & Feldmeier, 2006; Mansouri & Johnston, 2007). Because female mites are at the limit of visibility, using a dermatoscope for magnification can be useful to identify their presence (Dupuy et al., 2007; Heukelbach & Feldmeier, 2006).

In some cases, a careful history and complete physical exam are sufficient to diagnose scabies (Leone, 2007; Page et al., 2007). If additional evidence is needed to help distinguish the diagnosis, a microscopic examination of skin scrapings can be useful. Mineral oil is placed on a scalpel blade, which is then used to scrape several skin lesions. Microscopic observation of mites, eggs, or feces can provide a definitive diagnosis (Dupuy et al., 2007; Heukelbach & Feldmeier, 2006; Leone, 2007; Page et al., 2007; Strong & Johnstone, 2007). However, the accuracy of this technique varies greatly and false negative findings are often obtained (Heukelbach & Feldmeier, 2006; Page et al., 2007).

Treatment

Permethrin 5% cream (Elimite) is considered the first-line treatment for scabies (Heukelbach & Feldmeier, 2006; Jacobson & Abel, 2007; Strong & Johnstone, 2007). Clearance rates of up to 98% have been reported after a single application (Chosidow, 2006). If needed, a second application may be used one week after the initial application (Mansouri & Johnston, 2007). Permethrin has a low risk for toxicity and has proven safe for use in infants as young as 1 month of age (Heukelbach & Feldmeier, 2006; Jacobson & Abel, 2007). Topical lindane is no longer recommended for the treatment of scabies because of toxicity concerns and increasing resistance (Heukelbach & Feldmeier, 2006; Leone, 2007).

Another treatment alternative is the off-label use of oral ivermectin. Clearance rates have been reported to range from 70–88% following a single dose (Chosidow, 2006; Leone, 2007). Administration of a second dose after one to two weeks has been associated with 95–100% treatment success (Jacobson & Abel, 2007; Leone, 2007). Use in children as young as 6 months old has not been associated with serious adverse events (Chosidow, 2006; Jacobson & Abel, 2007). Ivermectin is not recommended for use in children less than 15kg (Jacobson & Abel, 2007; Mansouri & Johnston, 2007). The use of ivermectin may be especially useful for children who have failed topical treatment, are immunosuppressed, have diffuse eczematous dermatitis, or are unable to comply with topical treatment (Chosidow, 2006; Jacobson & Abel, 2007).

Because of the long incubation period associated with scabies, it is generally recommended that all household members and close physical contacts be treated prophylactically (Heukelbach & Feldmeier, 2006; Jacobson & Abel, 2007; Page et al., 2007; Strong & Johnstone, 2007). This recommendation is based on the premise that since an initial scabies infestation may take several weeks to become symptomatic, household members may be infected without realizing it. However, no controlled trials address whether empiric treatment of asymptomatic family members or close personal contact decreases the spread of scabies (Page et al., 2007). Although fomite transfer is less common, the household environment should also be treated. Clothing, bedding, and linens used by the affected child should be washed in warm or hot water and dried in a hot dryer. Items that cannot be washed should be isolated from use for 3–7 days (Heukelbach & Feldmeier, 2006; Jacobson & Abel, 2007; Leone, 2007).

Even with successful treatment, pruritus and skin manifestations may persist for several weeks (Jacobson & Abel, 2007; Leone, 2007; Mansouri & Johnston, 2007; Strong & Johnstone, 2007). Persistence of symptoms beyond this point may indicate resistance, poor treatment compliance, or reinfection. Dermatitis may also result from the use of topical mediations and mimic scabies persistence.

Nursing Management

Priorities for nursing management include successful eradication of the infestation, preventing secondary infection, preventing spread of the infestation to others, and providing family teaching. The nursing assessment should inquire about any known contact with scabies, the presence and severity of pruritus, sleep disturbances, and the emotional impact on the child and caregivers. Nurses should also assess the child for the typical clinical manifestations of scabies. Until a definitive diagnosis is made the nurse should assume that the child might be contagious. Thorough hand washing should be implemented before and after client contact, and gloves should be worn during examination and care. When interacting with the child and caregivers, nurses should reassure the family that scabies infestations are common, are not an indication of poor hygiene, and usually respond well to treatment. Family education should also be provided about the treatment regimen and preventing secondary infection and spread of infestation to others. If the affected child attends school or day care, nurses should advise the family to notify them of the child's condition so that peers and teachers may be monitored for signs and symptoms of infestation.

Family Teaching

When educating the family of a child with scabies, nurses should recommend that all members of the household be treated because asymptomatic individuals may have an infestation that has not manifested clinical signs yet. Caregivers must be instructed to follow the directions for the chosen scabicide treatment carefully. If topical treatment is being used, it should be applied to whole body from neck down and washed off after 8–14 hours (Jacobson & Abel, 2007; Leone, 2007). In children less than 2 years of age, the medication should be applied to the whole body including face, neck, ears, and scalp (Mansouri & Johnston, 2007). In young children it may be necessary to cover the feet and hands with mittens or socks to prevent the child from sucking off the medication. Caregivers should also be instructed that treated individuals put clean clothes on after applying the treatment.

In order to prevent secondary infection, older children should be instructed to not scratch or pick at their skin. If younger children experience pruritus, caregivers should be instructed to keep the child's nails cut short and place mittens over the child's hands if necessary. The child and caregivers also need to be made aware that the rash and itching may persist for a few weeks following successful treatment. To prevent spread of the infestation, direct skin contact should be avoided until treatment is complete and proper hand washing should be utilized. To prevent reinfestation, all clothing and linens should be washed in warm or hot water and dried in a hot dryer. Items that cannot be washed should be isolated from use for three to seven days (Heukelbach & Feldmeier, 2006; Jacobson & Abel, 2007; Leone, 2007).

DERMATITIS

Dermatitis is a term that literally means "inflammation of the skin." There are several types of dermatitis that commonly affect children: atopic dermatitis, contact dermatitis, diaper dermatitis, and seborrheic dermatitis. Although the exact cause and appearance of these rashes differs, many of the management strategies are similar for these four diagnoses.

ATOPIC DERMATITIS

Atopic dermatitis, commonly referred to as eczema, is a chronic, pruritic, inflammatory skin condition that is most commonly observed among young children. Affected children typically experience disease remissions and flares and therefore require long-term management. Because of its chronic nature, atopic dermatitis can have significant impact on the quality of life of the affected child and his/her caregivers.

INCIDENCE AND ETIOLOGY

Atopic dermatitis is the most common pediatric skin condition in developed countries (Buys, 2007). Furthermore, the overall incidence of atopic dermatitis in the United States and other industrialized countries has been steadily increasing over the past 30 years (Buys, 2007; Fleischer, 2008; Peterson & Chan, 2006). Currently, the prevalence of atopic dermatitis among children in the United States is estimated to be between 7–30% (Bieber, 2008; Buys, 2007; Fleischer, 2008; Krakowski, Eichenfield & Dohil, 2008; Peterson & Chan, 2006).

Although it can occur at any time of life, atopic dermatitis most commonly affects infants and young children. In the United States, 45% of cases appear by 6 months of age, 60–65% by the age of 1 year old, and 85–90% of cases present by 5 years of age (Bieber, 2008; Fleischer, 2008; Krakowski et al., 2008; Peterson & Chan, 2006; Sidbury & Poorsattar, 2006). When children reach school age, they typically stop having significant flares (Kiken & Silverberg, 2006a). Approximately 40–70% of children "outgrow" atopic dermatitis and achieve complete clearing by adolescence (Buys, 2007; Kiken & Silverberg, 2006a; Peterson & Chan, 2006). Persistent cases are associated with early disease onset, increased disease severity, concomitant asthma or hayfever, and a family history of atopic dermatitis (Buys, 2007; Kiken & Silverberg, 2006a; Peterson & Chan, 2006).

There are multiple factors that appear to play a role in the etiology of atopic dermatitis. One such factor is genetic predisposition. It has been found that 70% of atopic dermatitis patients have a positive family history for the condition (Kiken & Silverberg, 2006a). Atopic dermatitis is also associated with a personal or family history of other forms of atopy such as asthma, hay fever, allergic rhinitis, and food or environmental allergies (Bieber, 2008; Kiken & Silverberg, 2006a; Peterson & Chan, 2006). Furthermore, children with atopic dermatitis are at increased risk to develop these related conditions.

The incidence of atopic dermatitis is slightly higher in females, though incidence has not been found to vary with ethnicity (Kiken & Silverberg, 2006a; Peterson & Chan, 2006). Other factors associated with an increased incidence of atopic dermatitis include smaller family size, higher socioeconomic status, caregivers with higher education, increased use of antibiotics, and residing in urban locations (Kiken & Silverberg, 2006a; Peterson & Chan, 2006). Although it has been debated, experts presently use the "hygiene hypothesis" to explain these findings. Within this hypothesis, a lack of exposure to infectious agents early in life predisposes children to the development of atopic dermatitis (Bieber, 2008; Kiken & Silverberg, 2006a).

In addition to the numerous factors that appear to be involved in the development of atopic dermatitis in children, there are several specific triggers that have been shown to exacerbate atopic dermatitis (Box 30-3) (Kiken & Silverberg, 2006a; Peterson & Chan, 2006). For many patients, environmental triggers include animal dander, dust mites, molds, and pollens. Commonly identified topical irritants are fragrances, soaps or detergents, household solvents, and hot water. Food allergens such as peanuts, fish, wheat, eggs, milk, and soy have been identified as triggers for 20–40% of children with atopic dermatitis. Emotional stress, summer sweating, and winter reductions in humidity have also been linked to disease flares.

PATHOPHYSIOLOGY

The pathophysiology of atopic dermatitis involves a complex interplay of skin barrier defects, dysregulation of the immune system, and susceptibility to infectious organisms (Bieber, 2008; Buys, 2007; Fleischer, 2008; Kiken & Silverberg, 2006a; Krakowski et al., 2008). Because of the multifactorial etiology of atopic dermatitis, the pathophysiology of this disorder is complex and not yet fully understood. Impaired skin barrier function, one of the main physiologic mechanisms involved in atopic dermatitis development, is thought to be due in part to mutations of the filaggrin (an epidermal barrier protein) gene, as well as decreased production of ceramides (the major lipid in the stratum corneum). The resulting transepidermal water loss can lead to dry skin, cracks, and microfissures that allow entry of infectious

BOX 30-3

FACTORS ASSOCIATED WITH EXACERBATIONS OF ATOPIC DERMATITIS

Environmental

- Dust mites
- Animal dander
- Molds
- Pollens

Irritants

- Fragrances
- Soaps or detergents
- Household solvents
- Hot water

Food allergies

- Peanuts
- Fish
- Wheat
- Eggs
- Milk
- Soy

Climate

- Reduced humidity in winter
- Sweating in summer

Emotional stressors

Adapted from: Kiken, D. A., & Silverberg, N. B. (2006a). Atopic dermatitis in children, Part 1: Epidemiology, clinical features, and complications. *Cutis, 78*, 241–247; Peterson, J. D., & Chan, L. S. (2006). A comprehensive management guide for atopic dermatitis. *Dermatologic Nursing, 18*(6), 531–542.

agents and greater exposure to irritants (Bieber, 2008; Fleischer, 2008; Kiken & Silverberg, 2006a; Krakowski et al., 2008; Peterson & Chan, 2006).

Dysregulation of the immune system is another important mechanism in atopic dermatitis patients. In about 60–80% of affected children, atopic dermatitis is currently thought to be an immunoglobulin E (IgE) mediated disorder (Bieber, 2008; Kiken & Silverberg, 2006a; Peterson & Chan, 2006). In these individuals, food and/or environmental allergens bind to IgE on the surface of Langerhan's cells, resulting in the activation of type 2 T-helper lymphocytes which then release a combination of **cytokines** (Buys, 2007; Kiken & Silverberg, 2006a; Krakowski et al., 2008). Cytokines are substances secreted by cells that facilitate cell-to cell communication. Cytokine production is also stimulated by the mechanical injury that results from scratching. The proinflammatory cytokines associated with atopic dermatitis induce an inflammatory response that leads to eczematous skin eruptions and pruritus. It appears that among atopic dermatitis patients, unique patterns of cytokine production are associated with the acute and chronic phases of skin inflammation (Krakowski et al., 2008).

Another major factor in the development of atopic dermatitis is colonization of the skin by *S. aureus*, which occurs in more than 90% of affected individuals (Bieber, 2008; Kiken & Silverberg, 2006a; Krakowski et al., 2008; Peterson & Chan, 2006). Factors contributing to these high colonization rates include defects in the skin barrier and the fact that scratching increases the binding of *S. aureus* to the skin. *S. aureus* enterotoxins then further stimulate the inflammatory process and exacerbate the eczema (Bieber, 2008; Kiken & Silverberg, 2006a).

Clinical Manifestations

The hallmark clinical manifestations of atopic dermatitis are **xerosis** (dry skin) and pruritus (Peterson & Chan, 2006). Xerosis is a direct result of impaired skin barrier function and is found on both affected and unaffected skin (Fleischer, 2008). Pruritus, resulting from the release of proinflammatory cytokines, is frequently worse at night (Bieber, 2008; Kiken & Silverberg, 2006a; Peterson & Chan, 2006). Although the appearance of lesions varies with age, the classic presentation of atopic dermatitis is erythematous, excoriated plaques with serous discharge (Kiken & Silverberg, 2006a). Another classic feature of atopic dermatitis is the progression through disease remissions and flares (Kiken & Silverberg, 2006a).

The distribution and appearance of skin lesions can be categorized into one of three age-dependent phases (Kiken & Silverberg, 2006a; Peterson & Chan, 2006). The infantile stage is characterized by pruritic, erythematous papules, patches and vesicles on the cheeks and **extensor surfaces** of the extremities. The extensor surfaces are the skin surfaces that do not come into direct contact when the extremity is flexed. There may be additional involvement of the scalp, forehead, chin and trunk, though the diaper area is typically not involved. Lesions may also have a weeping and exudative appearance.

The childhood phase begins around 2 years of age and lasts until puberty. During this time frame, the distribution of lesions favors the **flexural surfaces** (Figure 30-15). The flexural surfaces are the skin surfaces that come into direct contact when the extremity is flexed. The antecubital and popliteal fossae are the two most commonly affected areas. Other common areas of involvement include the wrists, ankles, hands, feet, and neck as well as the periorbital and perioral skin. During this phase, chronic rubbing and scratching cause the lesions to become less weeping and exudative and more excoriated and lichenified. **Lichenification** manifests with visible thickening of the skin and accentuated skin markings, usually due to scratching. Children who do not experience remission of their atopic dermatitis by puberty will begin to manifest the disease characteristics of the adult phase. During this phase, the flexural folds are still affected, with lesions also potentially affecting the face, hands, wrists, feet, upper arms, and back. Lesions commonly manifest as

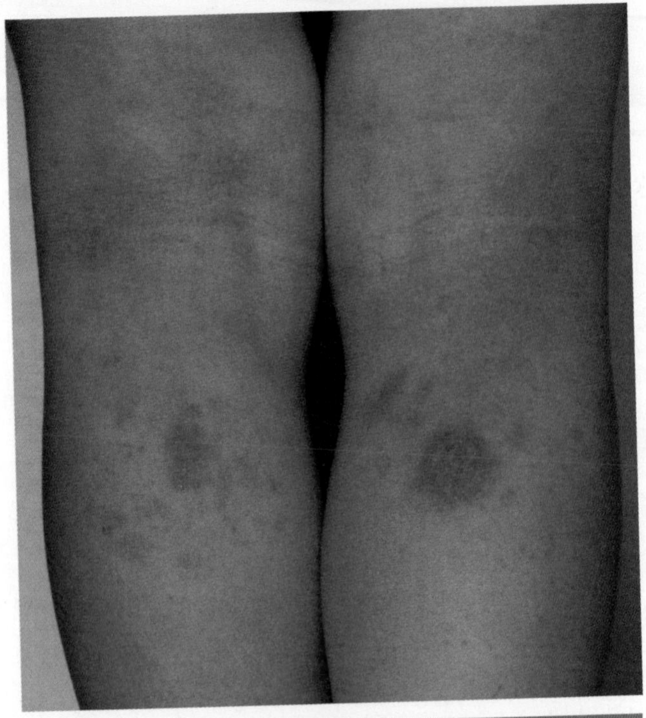

FIGURE 30-15 Atopic Dermatitis. DELMAR CENGAGE LEARNING.

scaling, erythematous papules, and plaques or large lichenified plaques.

Because of the high rates of *S. aureus* colonization among children with atopic dermatitis, there is an increased risk of secondary bacterial infection. Secondary infections due to *S. aureus* commonly manifest with superficial pustules or weeping honey-colored crusts (Krakowski et al., 2008; Peterson & Chan, 2006). Impaired skin barrier function may also lead to other secondary infections such as streptococcal infections, herpes simplex, dermatophytes, yeast, warts, and molluscum contagiosum (Fleischer, 2008; Krakowski et al., 2008; Peterson & Chan, 2006; Sidbury & Poorsattar, 2006).

In addition to the physical manifestations of atopic dermatitis, there are several social, emotional, and behavioral manifestations that are commonly observed in children with eczema. As a result of pruritus, chronic sleep disorders are very common, affecting both children and caregivers (Buys, 2007; Fleischer, 2008; Jancin, 2007; Kiken & Silverberg, 2006a; Krakowski et al., 2008). In older children, sleep disturbance can lead to irritability, diminished school performance, or behavioral problems (Buys, 2007; Fleischer, 2008; Krakowski et al., 2008). Affected children may also show signs of stress, anxiety, low self-esteem, and isolation from activities that involve skin exposure (Buys, 2007; Fleischer, 2008; Krakowski et al., 2008).

In addition to disturbing the establishment of normal sleep patterns, severe eczema during infancy may compromise maternal-infant bonding (Jancin, 2007). Children and caregivers may also experience frustration due to the chronic, relapsing nature atopic dermatitis and the inconvenience of frequently applying topical products. The financial burden of eczema can also be substantial due to the expense of doctor's visits, medications, home care, diminished work productivity, and lost wages (Fleischer, 2008).

DIAGNOSIS

The diagnosis of atopic dermatitis is often challenging because of the multifactorial etiology and the wide variety of clinical presentations (Fleischer, 2008). Furthermore, no objective laboratory criteria exist for the diagnosis of atopic dermatitis. Rather, diagnosis is made based on the child's history and clinical manifestations. A family history of atopic conditions should be collected, as should a history of the current outbreak including the location, duration, and appearance of the rash. Also helpful in diagnosing eczema is information about remissions or flares as well as any response to previous over-the-counter or prescription medications.

Hanifin and Rajka (1980) proposed a set of diagnostic criteria based on major and minor characteristic features of atopic dermatitis, which continues to be used in clinical practice (Fleischer, 2008; Peterson & Chan, 2006). These guidelines propose that a diagnosis of atopic dermatitis can be established if three major and three minor criteria are present. The major criteria for diagnosis are: (1) pruritus; (2) chronic relapsing dermatitis; (3) typical distribution and morphology of lesions; and (4) a personal or family history of **atopy** (asthma, allergic rhinitis, or atopic dermatitis). Among the minor diagnostic criteria are xerosis, early age of onset, tendency toward cutaneous infections, tendency toward nonspecific hand or foot dermatitis, food intolerances, and a clinical course influenced by environmental or emotional factors.

Allergy testing may be beneficial in children with a suspected, specific allergic trigger or who experience refractory dermatitis (Fleischer, 2008; Sidbury & Poorsattar, 2006). Commonly utilized tests include serum RadioAllergoSorbent Testing (RAST) or pick testing (Peterson & Chan, 2006; Sidbury & Poorsattar, 2006). Negative results can be valuable to rule out suspected allergens, but positive results are often poorly correlated with clinical improvement (Fleischer, 2008; Peterson & Chan, 2006; Sidbury & Poorsattar, 2006).

TREATMENT

Presently, no cure for atopic dermatitis exists. Rather, treatment focuses on adequately treating flares as well as taking proactive steps to reduce the severity and frequency of flares (Bieber, 2008; Fleischer, 2008; Krakowski et al., 2008). More specifically, a combination of various management strategies are utilized to achieve the treatment goals of repairing and maintaining the stratum corneum, reducing inflammation, treating any secondary infections, stopping the itch-scratch cycle, and avoiding triggers/irritants (Fleischer, 2008; Kiken & Silverberg, 2006b; Krakowski et al., 2008; Peterson & Chan, 2006). Treatment recommendations should be tailored to the individual child's age, the location and severity of the eczema, and the frequency of disease flares. Caregiver and child preferences should also be considered,

BOX 30-4

VEHICLES USED IN TOPICAL MEDICATIONS

Topical prescription and over-the-counter medications are available in a variety of vehicles. Each vehicle has its own potential advantages and disadvantages. Product selection should be individualized for each child's situation.

PROPERTIES	*LOTIONS*	*CREAMS*	*OINTMENTS*
Water content	Highest	Medium	Least
Consistency	Light, most subject to evaporation	Medium, less subject to evaporation	Heavy, greasy, least subject to evaporation
Other irritants	Fragrances; preservatives	Fragrances, preservatives	Most hypoallergenic
Skin Hydration	Least hydrating	Medium hydrating	Most hydrating
Steroidal delivery	Least capable	Medium capability	Most capable
Sting from application	Most likely to sting	More likely to sting	Least likely to sting

Adapted from: Buys, L. M. (2007). Treatment options for atopic dermatitis. *American Family Physician, 75*(4), 523–528; Gawkrodger, D. J. (2008). *Dermatology: An illustrated colour text* (4th ed.). Philadelphia, PA: Elsevier; Kiken, D. A., & Silverberg, N. B. (2006b). Atopic dermatitis in children, Part 2: Treatment options. *Cutis, 78*, 401–406.

as should the child's response to previous over-the-counter and prescription treatments.

Because of the defects in the skin barrier that are associated with atopic dermatitis, it is essential to repair and maintain the stratum corneum by promoting adequate hydration of the skin. Previously, bathing had been thought to increase water loss and promote drying of the skin. However, current practice recommends short, daily baths in lukewarm water followed by patting the skin dry and immediate application of an emollient (Buys, 2007; Fleischer, 2008; Kiken & Silverberg, 2006b; Krakowski et al., 2008; Peterson & Chan, 2006; Sidbury & Poorsattar, 2006). Emollients are topical products containing varying amounts of lipid and water that are used to reestablish the surface lipid barrier and enhance rehydration of the epidermis (Gawkrodger, 2008). In addition, emollients provide a mechanical barrier that reduces the exacerbating effects of irritants (Fleischer, 2008). Emollients are available in various formulations, such as ointments, creams, and lotions (See Box 30-4). Thicker emollients, such as ointments, should be used in the winter and thinner emollients, such as creams or lotions, should be used in the summer (Kiken & Silverberg, 2006b; Sidbury & Poorsattar, 2006). It is particularly important to liberally apply moisturizing emollients at least once to twice daily, as this at-home intervention has been shown to reduce the need for topical steroids (Buys, 2007; Kiken & Silverberg, 2006b; Peterson 2006).

Topical corticosteroids are the mainstay of therapy for atopic dermatitis (Buys, 2007; Kiken & Silverberg, 2006b; Peterson & Chan, 2006; Sidbury & Poorsattar, 2006). This class of medications reduces inflammation and pruritus and has been reported to reduce the density of *S. aureus.* Topical corticosteroids are available in several vehicles and potency (Box 30-4). Ointments are more potent, hydrating, hypoallergenic, and result in less stinging following application (Buys, 2007; Kiken & Silverberg, 2006b; Peterson & Chan,

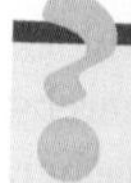

KIDS WANT TO KNOW

Will these steroids make me stronger?

I have a steroid cream that I use to help the eczema on my arms and legs go away. If I rub it over my muscles will they make me stronger?

It is important for kids to understand that topical and oral corticosteroids are not the same as anabolic steroids. They will not increase muscle strength or athletic performance. Athletes can safely use these medications and will not have problems if they are screened for steroid use.

2006). However, children and caregivers may not like using greasy topical products, especially during the day.

Potential side effects associated with the use of topical steroids include atrophy (skin thinning), striae (stretch marks), telangiectasia (dilated capillaries), skin lightening, and hypothalamic-pituitary-adrenal (HPA) axis suppression (Buys, 2007; Fleischer, 2008; Kiken & Silverberg, 2006b; Peterson & Chan, 2006). The likelihood of developing these side effects is increased with the use of more potent steroids, longer treatment duration, use in thin-skinned or occluded areas, or with widespread application (Kiken & Silverberg, 2006b; Peterson & Chan, 2006). Consequently, it is generally reasonable to begin with over-the-counter 1% hydrocortisone and move to more potent steroids if needed, particularly in infants (Kiken & Silverberg, 2006b; Sidbury & Poorsattar, 2006). For more advanced disease, it is often prudent to utilize stronger products which will likely result in rapid improvement and thus allow for less medication use (Peterson &

Chan, 2006; Sidbury & Poorsattar, 2006). It is currently recommended that active flares be treated with topical steroids once to twice daily for the shortest duration necessary and then be tapered and replaced with emollients for maintenance (Buys, 2007; Fleischer, 2008; Krakowski et al., 2008; Sidbury & Poorsattar, 2006; Peterson & Chan, 2006).

Oral corticosteroids (Prednisolone, Prednisone) are generally not recommended for the treatment of pediatric atopic dermatitis because the potential risks are thought to outweigh the benefits (Kiken & Silverberg, 2006b; Peterson & Chan, 2006; Sidbury & Poorsattar, 2006). Furthermore, oral corticosteroids, while they have been associated with transient improvement, may demonstrate rebound flares (Buys, 2007; Peterson & Chan, 2006; Sidbury & Poorsattar, 2006). In severe cases, use should be limited to the smallest necessary dose. With continued application, possible side effects from oral steroids include growth retardation, striae, weight gain, osteoporosis, and mood changes (Kiken & Silverberg, 2006b).

Also available for the reduction of inflammation in atopic dermatitis patients are topical calcineurin inhibitors (TCIs). These medications, pimecrolimus (Elidel) and tacrolimus (Protopic), are immune modulators that block early T-cell activation and the release of cytokines, thereby inhibiting the inflammatory process (Buys, 2007; Fleischer, 2008; Krakowski et al., 2008). Both medications have proven to be beneficial in treating atopic dermatitis without the side effects associated with topical steroid use, though they work more slowly than topical steroids and commonly cause stinging or burning when placed on open skin (Fleischer, 2008; Kiken & Silverberg, 2006b; Krakowski et al., 2008; Peterson & Chan, 2006; Sidbury & Poorsattar, 2006). TCIs also have a black box warning stating that cancers have been reported. The warning advises localized use, short-term or intermittent long-term use, avoidance in children younger than 2 years old, and use as a second-line agent (Kiken & Silverberg, 2006b; Krakowski et al., 2008; Peterson & Chan, 2006; Sidbury & Poorsattar, 2006). Experts have questioned the likelihood of cancer being caused by TCIs, but generally agree that providers should follow the usage instructions advised by the black box warning.

Children with atopic dermatitis are at increased risk for secondary bacterial infections because of the high rates of *S. aureus* colonization among this population. If there are signs of an active bacterial infection or signs of heavy *S. aureus* colonization, topical antibiotics (such as mupirocin) or oral antibiotics (such as cephalexin) are recommended (Buys, 2007; Kiken & Silverberg, 2006b; Peterson & Chan, 2006; Sidbury & Poorsattar, 2006). Treatment with oral antibiotics for common *S. aureus* colonization is generally not advised because of concerns about antibiotic resistance. The use of antibacterial soaps has been associated with decreased *S. aureus* colonization and greater clinical improvement (Kiken & Silverberg, 2006b). Diluted bleach baths (half a cup of bleach in a full tub of water) have also been found to decrease the occurrence of local skin infections in patients with heavy *S. aureus* colonization (Krakowski et al., 2008). If signs of other infections are present, such as herpes simplex or molluscum contagiosum, appropriate treatment should be initiated.

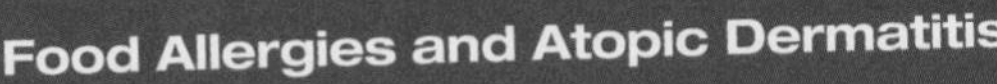

CRITICAL THINKING

Food Allergies and Atopic Dermatitis

Many caregivers want to do everything possible to help minimize their child's eczema flares and will ask about whether their child should undergo allergy testing. Current research suggests that food allergens are triggers for 20–40% of children with atopic dermatitis (Kiken & Silverberg, 2006a; Peterson & Chan, 2006). In addition, children with atopic dermatitis are at higher risk for developing other atopic conditions, including allergies. For this reason, many eczema patients have positive food allergy tests, but do not experience clinical improvement when these foods are avoided (Fleischer, 2008; Peterson & Chan, 2006; Sidbury & Poorsattar, 2006). Based on this evidence, how should nurses answer caregivers who inquire about the role of food allergies in atopic dermatitis? When should allergy testing be recommended? If caregivers are already excluding foods from the child's diet based on suspicion, does current medical knowledge indicate that nurses should recommend resuming consumption of these foods?

Managing the pruritus and scratching associated with atopic dermatitis is a critical component of eczema treatment. The itch-scratch cycle begins when the release of inflammatory cytokines promotes pruritus and is perpetuated when the child's scratching results in tissue injury and promotes ongoing cytokine release/pruritus (Leung, Bogunmiewicz, Howell, Nomura, & Hamid, 2004). Because the pruritus of atopic dermatitis is due to proinflammatory cytokines and not due to histamine, antihistamines have not proven to be beneficial in reducing itching (Bieber, 2008; Kiken & Silverberg, 2006b; Sidbury & Poorsattar, 2006). However, sedating antihistamines, such as diphenhydramine (Benadryl) and hydroxyzine (Vistaril, Atarax), can be useful to promote sleep and interrupt the itch-scratch cycle when severe (Kiken & Silverberg, 2006b; Krakowski et al., 2008; Sidbury & Poorsattar, 2006).

In patients with severe eczema or excessive scratching, wet wrap therapy may be considered. Wet wrap dressings provide a barrier to scratching, enhance the penetration of topical medications, promote increased hydration, and help to relieve pruritus (Krakowski et al., 2008). However, wet wraps can cause maceration and secondary infection if overused or used incorrectly. Consequently, this treatment should only be conducted under the supervision of a health care provider. To apply wet wraps, the topical agent is applied to the skin, followed by bandages or cotton-blend pajamas dampened in warm water, and then dry bandages or pajamas are worn over the wet layer. These dressings are best tolerated at night because of their cumbersome nature.

Another important goal of atopic dermatitis treatment is the avoidance of triggers and irritants (see Box 30-3). Methods to reduce exposure to irritants such as fragrances, soaps, and detergents are incorporated into the skin care recommendations listed in Box 30-5. When advising caregivers about selecting fragrance-free products, it is important to explain that products labeled as "unscented" and "scent-free" often contain masking fragrances and are not the same as those that are labeled "fragrance-free." As previously mentioned, daily bathing with a mild temperature and soap, followed by liberal application of an emollient, is recommended (Fleischer, 2008; Kiken & Silverberg, 2006b; Krakowski et al., 2008; Sidbury & Poorsattar, 2006). Children's clothing should be loose fitting and can be made from either natural or synthetic fibers, as neither have been found to aggravate eczema (Kiken & Silverberg, 2006b). Particularly among infants, the chronic wetting and drying that occurs from drool, food, and saturated bibs can exacerbate eczema (Kiken & Silverberg, 2006b; Peterson & Chan, 2006). To prevent these items from irritating the skin, it is recommended that caregivers apply a thick emollient or barrier cream to potentially affected areas prior to and immediately following mealtime. In the summer, children should be dressed in light clothing and isolated from extreme heat when possible (Kiken & Silverberg, 2006b; Peterson & Chan, 2006). The use of humidifiers in the winter can help to reduce winter dryness (Kiken & Silverberg, 2006b). If emotional stressors are identified as significant, children may require psychological consultation to address these concerns (Peterson & Chan, 2006). Based on current research, the evidence regarding the benefits of minimizing exposure to animal dander and dust mites is inconclusive (Fleischer, 2008; Krakowski et al., 2008; Sidbury & Poorsattar, 2006).

BOX 30-5
SKIN CARE RECOMMENDATIONS FOR CHILDREN WITH ATOPIC DERMATITIS

Bathing

- Avoid washcloths and sponges
- Pat dry after bathing
- Mild, fragrance-free soaps or soap-free cleansers
- No bubble baths
- Liberally apply emollients immediately after bathing
- Use lukewarm water (not hot water)

Clothing

- Avoid clothing made from rough or abrasive fabrics
- Wear natural materials
- Avoid tight-fitting clothing
- Use only fragrance-free detergents
- Avoid fabric softeners

Feeding

- Avoid chronic wetting and drying from drool, food, saturated bibs
- Apply thick emollient or barrier cream prior to and immediately following mealtime

Adapted from: Kiken, D. A., & Silverberg, N. B. (2006a). Atopic dermatitis in children, Part 1: Epidemiology, clinical features, and complications. *Cutis*, *78*, 241–247; Peterson, J. D., & Chan, L. S. (2006). A comprehensive management guide for atopic dermatitis. *Dermatologic Nursing*, *18*(6), 531–542.

NURSING ALERT
Selecting Fragrance-Free Products

Products that are labeled as "unscented" and "scent-free" often contain masking fragrances. These products are not the same as those that are labeled "fragrance-free."

The role of avoiding potential food triggers is also controversial. Although food allergens have been found to act as disease triggers for 20–40% of children with atopic dermatitis, current immunologic evidence supports the conclusion that food allergies are a contributor to atopic dermatitis, but not the cause (Kiken & Silverberg, 2006a; Peterson & Chan, 2006). Furthermore, studies on dietary restriction, including those based on positive allergy test results, have thus far demonstrated inconsistent benefits and poor correlation with clinical improvement (Fleischer, 2008; Peterson & Chan, 2006; Sidbury & Poorsattar, 2006). Consequently, the practice of broad food restrictions is not recommended because clinical improvement may not result and such diets can lead to malnutrition (Fleischer, 2008; Krakowski et al., 2008; Peterson & Chan, 2006; Sidbury & Poorsattar, 2006). If foods are to be excluded, dietary recommendations should be made on an individual basis after the affected child has been allergy tested and the caregivers have engaged in detailed discussions with their health care provider about their child's specific situation.

Nursing Management

Assessment The nursing assessment should begin with a detailed client history including the location, duration, and appearance of the rash. If pruritus is reported, the nurse should assess the severity as well as any associated sleep disturbances. The emotional impact of the rash on the child and caregivers should also be noted. The nurse should inquire about any remissions or flares as well as any response to previously used over-the-counter or prescription medications. A family history of atopic conditions should also be collected. The nursing assessment should note the type of lesions present, as well as their distribution and severity. Any indications of secondary infection should also be noted.

Nursing Diagnosis

1. *Impaired skin integrity* related to the presence of lesions.
2. *Pain* related to pruritus.
3. *Disturbed sleep pattern* related to pruritus.
4. *Risk for infection (secondary)* related to scratching of lesions.
5. *Interrupted family processes* related to having a child with a chronic skin condition.

Expected Outcomes

1. Child's lesions will resolve.
2. Child will exhibit decreased pruritus.
3. Child will sleep undisturbed.
4. Child will not manifest signs of a secondary infection.
5. Caregiver will demonstrate positive coping skills.

Planning and Implementation

Because of the chronic nature of atopic dermatitis, the nursing management for this condition focuses a great deal on family teaching and the emotional well-being of both the affected child and the caregivers. The main goals of nursing management for children with eczema are to resolve flares, reduce the frequency and severity of flares, prevent secondary infection, reduce pruritus, promote sleep, and foster positive coping skills. The majority of these goals are achieved through family teaching. When providing care to the child, nurses should practice careful hand washing before and after contact with the child to prevent secondary infection. Nurses can also promote positive coping skills by modeling these behaviors when interacting with the affected child and caregivers.

Evaluation

Caregivers will exhibit positive coping skills as evident by conveying an understanding of the rationale for acute and chronic eczema treatment. They will express a sense of competence in their ability to provide eczema care, and openly share their thoughts and emotions about the child's condition and care. The child and caregivers will be able to implement strategies to minimize pruritus and scratching, resulting in the affected area remaining free from excoriations and signs of secondary infection. The affected child will also be able to sleep through the night with minimal waking and return to normal sleep patterns including naps. Implementation of these steps, in addition to following the treatment regimen, should lead to resolution of the eruption.

Family Teaching

One of the most important aspects of family teaching for children with eczema and their caregivers is education regarding the chronic nature of atopic dermatitis. It is important that caregivers understand that flares are expected and that they

RESEARCH

The Use of Alternative Medicine in Pediatric Patients with Atopic Dermatitis

STUDY PURPOSE

To investigate the prevalence of alternative medicine use among children with atopic dermatitis. In addition, the researchers evaluate the type, duration and success of the reported alternative medicine treatments. Parents were also asked about the rationale for choosing to treat their child with alternative medicine.

METHODS

The study sample consisted of 80 pediatric patients and their parents. Participants were recruited from a university dermatology clinic. The pediatric subjects ranged in age from 2 months to 17 years old, with an average age of 3.9 years. Data was collected via self-report questionnaires.

FINDINGS

Nearly half of the sample (43%) reported that they had used alternative medicine. Herbal remedies (41%) and homeopathy (23.5%) were used most often, with majority of treatments being used for one month or longer. Reasons for selecting alternative medicine included recommendation from others (47%), fear of steroid side effects (26%), and dissatisfaction with conventional treatment (18%). Most treatments resulted in no improvement (58%) and when improvement was reported, reduction of itch was the most commonly observed benefit.

IMPLICATIONS

Because the use of alternative medicines among pediatric patients with atopic dermatitis is fairly common, it is important for nurses to ask caregivers about the use of these treatments. In addition, the prevalence of dissatisfaction with conventional treatments and fear of steroid use among the caregivers in this sample indicates the need for nurses to clearly explain conventional treatments, including rationale, intended benefit, expected duration, and likelihood of potential side effects. Finally, although alternative treatments did not often lead to resolution of the dermatitis, pruritus was improved in some cases. This finding suggests that alternative treatments may be helpful adjuncts to conventional treatment. However, there is clearly a need for additional research to determine which alternative treatments are efficacious and safe.

REFERENCE

Hughes, R., Ward, D., Tobin, A. M., Keegan, K., & Kirby, B. (2007). The use of alternative medicine in pediatric patients with atopic dermatitis. *Pediatric Dermatology*, 24(2), 118–120.

do not necessarily represent inadequate treatment or poor adherence to the maintenance plan. This knowledge can help caregivers to better cope with the frustrating cycle of atopic dermatitis. Throughout the teaching process, the child and caregivers should be encouraged to share their thoughts and emotions about the diagnosis and the treatment. Encouragement should also be provided as they demonstrate an understanding of the disease process and its treatment. When educating families about eczema treatment, it is critical that nurses not only explain how to use the recommended treatment to resolve the current flare, but also provide education about maintenance strategies that will help to reduce the frequency and severity of flares. If caregivers are fearful of using topical steroids, it may be necessary to provide reassurance that side effects are rare when these medications are used properly. Regarding the prevention of secondary infection, the child and caregivers should be instructed about proper hand washing. Older children may be able to understand instructions about not scratching or picking at the lesions, but younger children will likely need other interventions such as keeping the child's nails cut short, placing mittens over the child's hands, closely supervising the child, and utilizing distraction techniques. To reduce pruritus and promote sleep, families should also be taught about trigger avoidance, proper skin care guidelines, and the importance of emollients.

CONTACT DERMATITIS

Contact dermatitis can occur as a result of direct skin contact with either an irritant or an allergen. Irritant contact dermatitis is a local, nonimmunologic reaction whereas allergic contact dermatitis is an immune-mediated hypersensitivity response. The treatment for both types of contact dermatitis focuses on resolving the eruption and taking steps to avoid the irritant or allergen in the future.

INCIDENCE AND ETIOLOGY

The two major forms of contact dermatitis are irritant contact dermatitis and allergic contact dermatitis. Irritant contact dermatitis is more common and accounts for approximately 80% of all cases of contact dermatitis (Nijhawan, Matiz & Jacob, 2009). Irritant contact dermatitis is a nonimmunologic skin reaction that occurs following exposure to any substance that is irritating to the skin. The severity of the resulting dermatitis depends on the status of the skin barrier, the type of irritant, and the duration of contact (James et al., 2006). Common irritants for children include saliva, urine, feces, certain foods, harsh detergents, soaps, wipes, and bubble baths (Nijhawan et al., 2009).

Allergic contact dermatitis is an immune-mediated hypersensitivity reaction that occurs in response to allergen exposure. It is estimated that allergic contact dermatitis represents approximately 20% of all pediatric cases of dermatitis, though this estimate is thought to be low because the role of contact allergens is often overlooked among pediatric patients (Militello, Jacob, & Crawford, 2006; Nijhawan et al., 2009). Allergic contact dermatitis occurs less frequently during the first few months of life and its prevalence increases with age (Allen, 2006; Militello et al., 2006). As with irritant contact dermatitis, the penetration of allergens is facilitated by skin barrier impairment (Militello et al., 2006). In addition the frequency, type and duration of allergen exposure also contributes to a child's susceptibility to developing this type of hypersensitivity reaction (Nijhawan et al., 2009). There is substantial individual variation in sensitization thresholds, though females appear to be at higher risk for developing allergic contact dermatitis (Militello et al., 2006; Nijhawan et al., 2009).

The most common contact allergen in the United States is urushiol, which is the substance found in poison ivy, poison oak, and poison sumac (Allen, 2006) (Box 30-6). The next most common contact allergen among children is nickel, with sensitization rates reported to range from 10–24% (Militello et al., 2006). Nickel can be found in a variety of items including jewelry, jean snaps, buckles, orthodontics, eye glasses, and school chairs (Militello et al., 2006; Nijhawan et al., 2009). Other common pediatric contact allergens include neomycin and bacitracin (topical antibiotics), potassium dichromate and carba mix (found in athletic equipment), and fragrances (commonly used in lotions, soaps, deodorants, cosmetics, perfumes, and colognes) (Militello et al., 2006; Nijhawan et al., 2009).

BOX 30-6
URUSHIOL

Urushiol is the active allergen in plants belonging to the *Toxicodendron* genus, which include poison ivy, poison oak, and poison sumac. It is a very potent resin that may cause an intense rash, blisters, and pruritus. Approximately 50% of people are highly or moderately sensitive to urushiol, and another 30–40% will only react if they come in contact with a large quantity of the plant oil. Urushiol is widely distributed through the leaves, stems, and roots of *Toxicodendron* plants, including dead plants. Direct contact with the plant is the primary source of sensitization. If this occurs, the exposed areas should be washed immediately (within ten minutes) with soap and water. Urushiol can also be carried on clothing, pets, tools, and toys for weeks unless washed off with soap and water. Urushiol can even become airborne when these plants are burned. However, the serum released from the resulting vesicular lesions is not antigenic and does not spread the allergic contact reaction.

Adapted from: Allen, P. L. (2006). Leaves of three, let them be: If it were only that easy! *Dermatology Nursing*, *18*(3), 236–242.

Pathophysiology

Irritant contact dermatitis occurs as a consequence of an irritating substance coming in contact with the skin. The irritant involved triggers an inflammatory process that results in the typical clinical manifestations of irritant contact dermatitis. No previous exposure to the irritant is necessary. The condition of the skin barrier and the concentration of the irritant are the only two factors that affect the severity of the resulting dermatitis (James et al., 2006).

In contrast, allergic contact dermatitis is a delayed T-cell mediated hypersensitivity reaction (type IV) that involves two phases: first, a **sensitization phase**, and second, an **elicitation phase** (Allen, 2006; Militello et al., 2006; Nijhawan et al., 2009). During the sensitization phase, an allergen penetrates the epidermis, attaches to Langerhans' cells, and is transported to the lymph nodes where it is presented to naïve T-lymphocytes. The T-lymphocytes then develop recognition of the antigen and are released into the bloodstream to circulate throughout the body. When a sensitized individual again comes in contact with the antigen, the elicitation phase begins. During this phase, the sensitized T-lymphocytes proliferate and release inflammatory mediators that lead to the clinical manifestations of dermatitis. The dermatitis most often occurs within 24 to 48 hours following reexposure to the allergen (Allen, 2006; Militello et al., 2006). Many contact allergens are weak and require repeated exposures to establish an immune response, but stronger allergens, like urushiol, typically require only two exposures to establish sensitization in susceptible children (Allen, 2006).

Clinical Manifestations

Irritant contact dermatitis typically manifests as a large erythematous patch in a discrete geometric pattern that matches the distribution of the irritating substance (Nijhawan et al., 2009). Pruritus is commonly present. The pattern may be a pruritic eczematous dermatitis with linear configurations. Edema, vesicles, papules, and lichenification may also be present (Militello et al., 2006; Nijhawan et al., 2009) (Figure 30-16). If allergic contact dermatitis is not treated and exposure is discontinued, symptoms generally resolve over a period of two to four weeks (Allen, 2006; Militello et al., 2006). However, if exposure to the allergen continues, the resulting dermatitis can last indefinitely (Militello et al., 2006). Commonly the areas of greatest allergen exposure will manifest the most severe dermatitis, but it is also possible for clinical lesions to erupt distant to the site of exposure (Militello et al., 2006; Nijhawan et al., 2009).

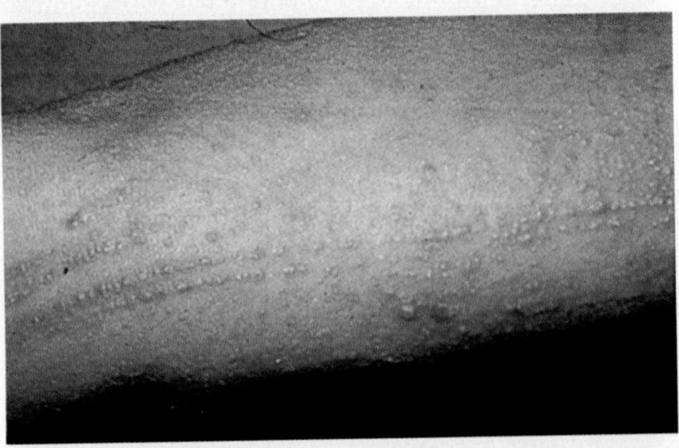

Figure 30-16 **Allergic Contact Dermatitis from Poison Oak.**
COURTESY OF THE CENTERS FOR DISEASE CONTROL AND PREVENTION.

Diagnosis

The diagnosis of both irritant and allergic contact dermatitis should be suspected in children whose dermatitis becomes progressively severe or does not respond as expected to standard therapy (Militello et al., 2006; Nijhawan et al., 2009). Suspicion of contact dermatitis may also be raised by the appearance and distribution of the rash. For example, repeated lip licking or drooling can cause an irritant dermatitis that is localized around the mouth of young children. Conversely, an edematous dermatitis on the earlobes is suggestive of nickel allergy associated with wearing earrings. If a linear distribution of vesicles is observed on the extremities, a urushiol-induced allergic contact dermatitis may be suspected (Allen, 2006).

Distinguishing between irritant and allergic contact dermatitis is often challenging because the clinical presentations of both diagnoses are similar (Nield & Kamat, 2007). Often a thorough exposure history can help refine the diagnosis. This history should include questions about hygiene products, clothing, footwear, jewelry, cosmetics, topical medications, and time spent outdoors. These questions should address products used on the affected child as well as those used on other household members.

For suspected allergic contact dermatitis, the diagnostic gold standard is epicutaneous patch testing (Militello et al., 2006; Nijhawan et al., 2009). Patch testing involves the placement of specific antigens on the skin for 48 hours and then monitoring for evidence of a localized reaction. However, when performing patch testing, it is important to remember that not all positive results will be clinically relevant (Militello et al., 2006; Nijhawan et al., 2009).

Treatment

Recognition and avoidance of the offending irritant or contact allergen is the cornerstone of treatment for contact dermatitis (Militello et al., 2006; Nijhawan et al., 2009). This component of treatment should include educating children and caregivers about potential sources of the offending substance, methods to avoid exposure, and suggestions about alternative products that do not contain the substance. For cases of irritant contact dermatitis, this education may also include advising caregivers to routinely apply emollients to the commonly exposed areas to provide barrier protection (Nijhawan et al., 2009). If a child has been exposed to urushiol, the affected area should be thoroughly washed immediately (within ten minutes) with soap and water. Clothing should be removed and washed. Tools, toys, or other contaminated objects should be washed thoroughly with soap and water to remove any residual resin (Allen, 2006).

The treatment of contact dermatitis is similar to that of atopic dermatitis. Topical corticosteroids and/or topical calcineurin inhibitors can be used to reduce inflammation and pruritus. In severe cases, oral corticosteroids may be necessary (Allen, 2006; Militello et al., 2006; Nijhawan et al., 2009). Evening doses of antihistamines, such as diphenhydramine or hydroxyzine, may also help control the associated pruritus and promote sleep. Wet compresses, tepid baths, oatmeal baths, and over-the-counter topical products containing menthol, camphor, or phenol can help to soothe the skin and relieve pruritus (Allen, 2006). Topical antihistamines or benzocaine are not recommended as they can cause allergic contact dermatitis and may have systemic absorption.

Nursing Management

The nursing management for children with contact dermatitis focuses on resolving the eruption, alleviating pruritus, and educating the child and caregivers about avoiding the irritant or contact allergen in the future. The nursing history should focus on exposure to common environmental irritants and allergens. The presence and severity of pruritus should also be determined. The physical assessment should note the characteristics, location, and severity of the clinical lesions. The planning and implementation of nursing care focuses primarily on family teaching. If patch tests are to be applied, the nurse may be responsible for explaining the testing procedure to the child and caregivers and applying the patches.

Family Teaching

The family teaching for children with contact dermatitis should address specifics about the chosen treatment, recommendations to reduce pruritus, and measures to avoid exposure to the irritant or contact allergen in the future. The child and caregivers should be educated about how to use the prescribed medications, including the expected duration of treatment. Caregivers should also be made aware of nonprescription options to help relieve pruritus, such as wet compresses, tepid baths, oatmeal baths, and over-the-counter topical products containing menthol, camphor, or phenol. One of the most important aspects of family teaching for children with contact dermatitis is advice about potential sources of the irritant or contact allergen, methods to avoid exposure, and suggestions about alternative products that do not contain the substance. In some cases, it can also be helpful to advise routine application of emollients to the commonly exposed areas to provide barrier protection. When exposure to poison ivy, poison oak, or poison sumac is possible, long pants, shirts with long sleeves, and shoes with socks should be worn to avoid exposure.

DIAPER DERMATITIS

Diaper dermatitis or "diaper rash" is an irritant contact dermatitis that occurs in the diaper area. Although medication use may be indicated in some cases, the primary management approach focuses on hygienic measures.

Incidence and Etiology

Diaper dermatitis is the most common dermatologic problem in infancy and accounts for approximately 16% of pediatric skin complaints (Fleischer, 2008; Nield & Kamat, 2007; Nijhawan et al., 2009). Any child wearing diapers is at risk for the development of diaper dermatitis; however, peak incidence occurs between 9 and 12 months of age (Fleischer, 2008; Nijhawan et al., 2009).

Common diaper dermatitis is an irritant contact dermatitis that results from moisture, warmth, urine, feces, and friction (Fleischer, 2008; Humphrey, Bergman, & Au, 2006; Nield & Kamat, 2007). Consequently, cloth diapers are associated with increased incidence of diaper dermatitis when compared to super-absorbent disposable diapers (Fleischer, 2008; Humphrey et al., 2006; Nield & Kamat, 2007). Other risk factors for developing diaper dermatitis include infrequent diaper changes and inappropriate diaper area hygiene.

Pathophysiology

The development of diaper dermatitis involves the interaction of several factors that contribute to skin breakdown and irritation. The increased wetness and warmth in the diaper area results in maceration of the stratum corneum and leads to impaired barrier function (Fleischer, 2008; Humphrey et al., 2006). As a result of impaired barrier function, the skin is more vulnerable to penetration by irritants and frictional damage (Fleischer, 2008; Humphrey et al., 2006). In addition, the degradation of urine by bacterial ureases in the stool results in an increased pH in the diaper environment. Fecal enzymes are then activated by the increased pH, leading to further irritation and disruption of epidermal barrier function (Humphrey et al., 2006). The warm, humid, and high pH diaper environment also places the infant at increased risk for overgrowth of microorganisms such as *C. albicans* and, less commonly, *S. aureus* (Humphrey et al., 2006).

Clinical Manifestations

Diaper dermatitis most commonly presents as erythema and mild scaling, though shiny plaques, erosions, papules, vesicles, and maceration may also develop (Fleischer, 2008; Humphrey et al., 2006). Because the rash affects skin that is in direct contact with the diaper, the most commonly involved areas are the convex skin surfaces of the buttocks, genitalia, lower abdomen, and upper thighs (Fleischer, 2008; Humphrey et al., 2006; Nield & Kamat, 2007). The skin folds commonly are spared. If the diaper dermatitis is secondarily infected with *C. albicans*, there will likely be an intense erythema that affects the skin creases and perianal skin, along with scattered papules and pustules (Humphrey et al., 2006; Nield & Kamat, 2007). If erosions and honey-colored crusts are apparent, *S. aureus* infection should be suspected (Humphrey et al., 2006).

Diagnosis

The diagnosis of diaper dermatitis is made based on the child's history and the clinical presentation (Nield & Kamat,

2007). The history should focus on the child's diaper-changing routine, including frequency of diaper changes and any topical products used. Physical examination should evaluate for the classic clinical manifestations of diaper dermatitis, including involvement of the expected areas. If secondary infection is suspected, bacterial cultures or a KOH preparation may be beneficial.

Treatment

First-line treatment for diaper dermatitis involves the implementation of hygienic measures (Fleischer, 2008; Humphrey et al., 2006; Nield & Kamat, 2007). Frequent diaper changes are essential for treating and preventing diaper dermatitis. Between changes, air and light is beneficial. Leave the diaper off when possible for ten to fifteen minutes. Diapers should be changed at least every two to four hours, preferably as soon as they are wet or soiled. Super-absorbent disposable diapers should be used instead of cloth diapers. Harsh soaps or detergents should be avoided, as should the use of baby wipes that contain alcohol or fragrances. Children with diaper dermatitis should be bathed frequently with a mild soap or cleanser. In addition, the use of barrier creams, such as zinc oxide, helps to protect the skin from moisture and friction, particularly in patients with recurrent diaper dermatitis. When using zinc oxide, reapply between changes until the next bath time. For infants with moderate to severe inflammation, low-dose topical steroids, such as 1% hydrocortisone, may be beneficial (Fleischer, 2008; Humphrey et al., 2006; Nield & Kamat, 2007). The use of topical steroids should be limited to once or twice daily application and they should not be used for more than two weeks. If secondary infection due to *C. albicans* or *S. aureus* is present, treatment with a topical antifungal or antibacterial agent is warranted (Fleischer, 2008; Humphrey et al., 2006; Nield & Kamat, 2007).

Nursing Management

The nursing management for children with contact dermatitis focuses on resolving the eruption and providing education about how to prevent recurrence in the future. The nursing assessment should begin with a thorough history, including the type of diaper used, frequency of diaper changes, and the use of any baby care products. The character and duration of the rash should also be assessed, as should the use of any previous treatments. When examining the child, the nurse should note the distribution of the rash, the type of lesions present, and any signs of secondary infection. The planning and implementation of nursing care focuses primarily on family teaching. In addition, nurses should take precautions such as wearing gloves and practicing proper handwashing when touching the affected area to prevent secondary infection.

> **NURSING TIP**
>
> **Baby Wipes and Diaper Dermatitis**
>
> Baby wipes containing fragrances or alcohol may exacerbate the rash and cause pain or stinging. In some cases they can even cause allergic contact dermatitis. An alternative is to use mild soap (or a nonsoap cleanser), warm water, and a cotton cloth.

> **CRITICAL THINKING**
>
> **Diaper Dermatitis**
>
> What instructions about diaper changing would you give to the caregivers of an infant with diaper dermatitis?

Family Teaching

The family teaching for caregivers of a child with diaper dermatitis focuses on implementing measures to resolve the eruption and prevent recurrence. This education should begin with an explanation of the factors that contribute to the development of diaper dermatitis. Caregivers should be instructed about the importance of frequent diaper changes, the use of super-absorbent disposable diapers if possible, and avoidance of harsh soaps and baby wipes that contain alcohol or fragrances. Nurses should also recommend frequent baths with a mild soap or cleanser and the use of barrier creams. If prescription medications are indicated, caregivers should be instructed on their use, including a demonstration of topical medication application if possible.

SEBORRHEIC DERMATITIS

Among children, seborrheic dermatitis most commonly presents as a self-limiting inflammatory condition on the scalp of infants (cradle cap). A more chronic form of seborrheic dermatitis may also be observed during adolescence as mild scalp flaking (dandruff) or more severe flaking, erythema, and pruritus. The exact etiology of seborrheic dermatitis is unclear, but the condition typically responds well to topical treatments.

Incidence and Etiology

During infancy, seborrheic dermatitis is also known as "cradle cap." It most commonly presents within the first 3 months of life, and resolves spontaneously by 6 to 12 months of age (Elish & Silverberg, 2006; Fleischer, 2008; Sheffield & Wright, 2007). Cradle cap is estimate to affect approximately 42% of infants (Fleischer, 2008; Schwartz, Janusz, & Janniger, 2006). The incidence of seborrheic dermatitis then drops sharply until adolescence, with only about 6% of children age 2–10 years old being affected (Fleischer, 2008). After puberty, the prevalence of seborrheic dermatitis again rises and becomes more common in boys (Dawson, 2006; Schwartz et al., 2006). Mild adolescent seborrheic dermatitis is often referred to as "dandruff." For many adolescents, regardless of severity, seborrheic dermatitis is often chronic and recurrent (Elish & Silverberg, 2006; Fleischer, 2008; Grimalt, 2007).

The etiology of seborrheic dermatitis is not yet clearly understood. In children of all ages, seborrheic dermatitis has been linked to an overgrowth of the *Malassezia* species of yeast, which is normally found on the scalp (Dawson, 2006; Fleischer, 2008; Grimalt, 2007; Sheffield & Wright, 2007). In addition, personal susceptibility and sebaceous gland activity also appear to play a significant role. Other factors that have been implicated in the development of seborrheic dermatitis include nutritional deficiencies, altered essential fatty acid patterns, and neurogenic factors (Fleischer, 2008; Schwartz et al., 2006).

Pathophysiology

Although an overgrowth of *Malassezia* yeast has been observed in conjunction with the development of seborrheic dermatitis, the causative mechanism is not clearly understood (Fleischer, 2008; Grimalt, 2007; Sheffield & Wright, 2007). Currently, it is thought that increased sebum production by the sebaceous glands due to hormonal influences plays a role in *Malassezia* yeast overgrowth. During infancy, transplacental maternal hormones have been implicated; while the increased levels of circulating androgens that occur during puberty are suspected to trigger the development of adolescent seborrheic dermatitis (Dawson, 2006; Fleischer, 2008). In either age group, it appears that once sebum is produced, the yeast digests the sebaceous triglycerides in the sebum, creating fatty acid byproducts (Dawson, 2006; Sheffield & Wright, 2007). In susceptible individuals, these byproducts then disrupt skin barrier function and induce a hyperproliferative response. In adolescents, an inflammatory response is also stimulated which results in the development of erythema and pruritus (Grimalt, 2007).

Clinical Manifestations

Cradle cap commonly manifests as thick, greasy patches of white, off-white, or yellow scaling on the vertex of the scalp (Elish & Silverberg, 2006; Fleischer, 2008; Sheffield & Wright, 2007) (Figure 30-17). Cradle cap is generally nonpruritic (Fleischer, 2008; Sheffield & Wright, 2007). In adolescents, mild cases of dandruff may present with dry scalp and loosely adherent white or gray flakes (Grimalt, 2007). More severe cases of seborrheic dermatitis often manifest yellowish, oily flakes. Adolescents also typically experience erythema and pruritus. The distribution of lesions among adolescent patients may be localized or distributed diffusely across the scalp surface.

Although the scalp is the most commonly affected area, both infants and adolescents can develop seborrheic dermatitis anywhere that sebaceous glands are plentiful (Elish & Silverberg, 2006; Fleischer, 2008). Specifically, lesions may

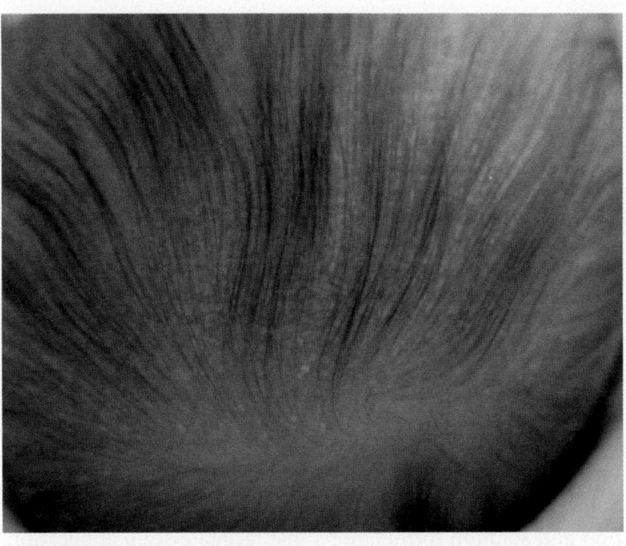

Figure 30-17 Seborrheic Dermatitis (Cradle Cap). DELMAR CENGAGE LEARNING.

also involve the eyebrows, eyelids, forehead, nasolabial folds, ears, and even intertriginous areas. During infancy, generalized lesions may indicate immunodeficiency (Fleischer, 2008). However, most cases (72%) of pediatric seborrheic dermatitis are classified as minimal or mild (Schwartz et al., 2006).

In addition to the clinical manifestations of seborrheic dermatitis, psychosocial manifestations may also affect the child and/or caregivers. Infant seborrheic dermatitis is not typically bothersome for the infant, but caregivers may be overly concerned about the appearance of the lesions (Sheffield & Wright, 2007). Similar concerns may be present in adolescents with seborrheic dermatitis.

Diagnosis

In children of any age, the diagnosis of seborrheic dermatitis is made based on history and physical examination (Fleischer, 2008). The history should include physical factors such as duration, recurrences, and the presence of pruritus. The psychosocial impact of the condition on the child and/or affected caregivers should also be assessed as this may impact treatment choices. The physical examination should confirm the presence of characteristic lesions in the expected anatomic locations. In difficult cases, biopsy can be used to confirm the diagnosis (Schwartz et al., 2006).

Treatment

Mild cases of cradle cap often respond to daily shampooing with a mild, nonmedicated shampoo or a baby shampoo (Elish & Silverberg, 2006; Fleischer, 2008; Sheffield & Wright, 2007). Another alternative is the application of mineral oil, olive oil, or white petrolatum to the scalp and left overnight. The scales can then be gently removed with an infant hairbrush or fingertips. When prescription treatments are needed, once daily use of ketoconazole shampoo or cream are safe and effective options (Elish & Silverberg,

2006; Sheffield & Wright, 2007). Low-potency topical corticosteroids, such as 1% hydrocortisone, are also beneficial, particularly if signs of inflammation are present (Elish & Silverberg, 2006; Fleischer, 2008; Sheffield & Wright, 2007). However, there are concerns about the potential for systemic absorption of even mild steroids in infants.

As with infant seborrheic dermatitis, affected adolescents can benefit from frequent cleansing to help remove excess oil from the skin and the application of emollients help to relieve dryness (Fleischer, 2008). In addition, the treatment of adolescent seborrheic dermatitis often involves the use of anti-inflammatory agents, keratolytics, and/or antifungal medications. Anti-inflammatory agents, such as topical corticosteroids and topical calcineurin inhibitors, can help relieve erythema and pruritus (Fleischer, 2008; Schwartz et al., 2006). Topical steroids are available in shampoo and solution formulations that facilitate scalp application. These medications can be used as adjuncts to other treatments or as a first-line treatment (Schwartz et al., 2006).

Also recommended as first-line agents are topical antifungal medications (Fleischer, 2008). Antifungal shampoos such as zinc pyrithione, selenium sulfide, ketoconazole, and ciclopirox have been shown to improve flaking and restore the condition of the skin (Elish & Silverberg, 2006; Grimalt, 2007). The use of keratolytic agents such as salicylic acid shampoo, tar shampoo, and zinc pyrithione shampoo two to three times per week can also be helpful for removing flakes (Grimalt, 2007; Schwartz et al., 2006). Because of the often chronic nature of adolescent seborrheic dermatitis, treatment for this population may require long-term use of therapeutic agents (Elish & Silverberg, 2006; Grimalt, 2007).

Nursing Management

Priorities for nursing management include resolution of the condition and providing family education regarding the nature of seborrheic dermatitis and the treatment regimen. The nursing history should inquire about the characteristics of the lesions, duration of the condition, and any accompanying symptoms. The presence of any psychosocial concerns should also be assessed. Upon examination, the nurse should note the appearance, location, and distribution of the lesions. When interacting with the caregivers of an infant with cradle cap, the nurse should offer reassurance that the condition is self-limiting and not serious. Similarly, during interactions with adolescents, nurses should convey that seborrheic dermatitis is not serious and not an indication of poor hygiene.

Family Teaching

One of the key components of family teaching for the child with seborrheic dermatitis is providing information about the nature of the condition. In addition to providing reassurance that the condition is not serious, nurses should advise caregivers of affected infants that the condition is self-limiting. For affected adolescents, it is important that the child and caregivers understand the typically chronic nature of the condition and that continued, intermittent medication use may be necessary to maintain clearance. The child and caregivers should also be educated about the specific treatments they will be using, including the manner of application, amount to be used, recommended duration of contact, and expected length of treatment.

ACNE

Acne is a chronic cutaneous disorder that affects most adolescents. In addition to the presence of acne lesions, acne is commonly associated with scarring, emotional distress, and poor adherence to treatment. For these reasons, successful acne management must address not only physiological factors but also emotional well-being and compliance.

Incidence and Etiology

The most common form of acne, acne vulgaris, is estimated to affect 85–95% of adolescents (Amin, Riddle, Aires, & Schweiger, 2007; Collier et al., 2008; James et al., 2006). The onset of acne typically occurs during early adolescence, and it is generally expected to spontaneously regress during the late teenage or early adult years. However, acne often persists well into adulthood or initially presents in adulthood. Acne is more commonly observed among males before the age of 16, but after adolescence acne prevalence is higher in females (Collier et al., 2008).

The exact etiology of acne is complex and not completely understood. Acne is known to be associated with the increased androgen and sebum production that normally occurs during puberty (James et al., 2006; Roebuck, 2006; Zaenglein & Thiboutot, 2006). Genetic influences have also been observed. In addition, factors such as occlusive skin care products, friction, and emotional stress can exacerbate acne (James et al., 2006; Magin Adams, Heading, Pond, & Smith, 2006). Dietary factors have also been investigated as potential contributors to acne development, though the evidence collected thus far has been inconclusive (Magin, Adams, Heading, Pond, & Smith, 2006; Webster, 2008; Webster, 2009).

Pathophysiology

Acne is a chronic cutaneous disorder involving the **pilosebaceous unit**, which consists of a hair follicle (pore), a hair shaft, and a sebaceous gland (James et al., 2006, Roebuck, 2006, Zaenglein & Thiboutot, 2006). Pilosebaceous units are most abundant on the face, chest, and upper back. Consequently, these are the body areas most commonly affected by acne.

There are four primary factors involved in the development of acne lesions (Amin et al., 2007; James et al., 2006; Roebuck, 2006; Webster 2009; Zaenglein & Thiboutot, 2006). One such factor is excessive sebum production. Beginning around 7 to 8 years of age, and continuing throughout puberty, circulating androgens act on the sebaceous glands and stimulate increased sebum production. Sebum is a complex lipid mixture that helps to maintain normal hydration of the skin. Another factor involved in acne development is abnormal epithelial keratinization within the pilosebaceous units. In individuals with acne, the epithelial cells (keratinocytes) lining the hair follicle shed more frequently and become more cohesive. The exact trigger for this process has not been determined. This alteration leads to the accumulation of sebum and keratinized material within the pilosebaceous unit. The consequence of this obstruction is the development of a microcomedo, the precursor to all acne lesions.

A third factor in acne development is the proliferation of *Propionibacterium acnes* (*P. acnes*). *P. acnes* is a gram-positive anaerobic bacterium, which often colonizes the pilosebaceous follicle and uses sebum as a nutrient for growth. *P. acnes* is believed to contribute to the development of acne by hydrolyzing sebum into free fatty acids and stimulating chemotaxis which then triggers the inflammatory response. The presence of inflammation is the fourth factor in the development of acne.

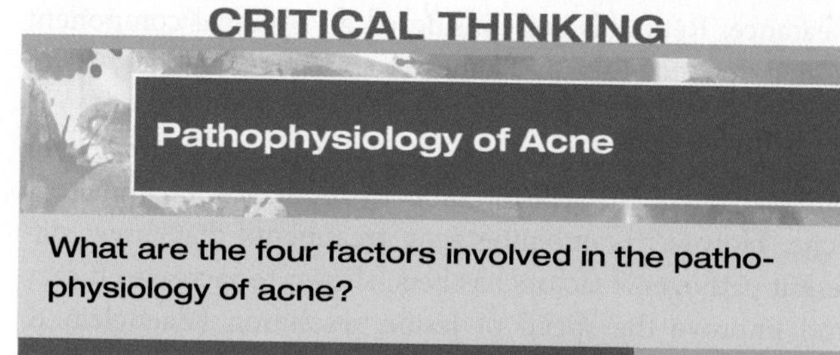

What are the four factors involved in the pathophysiology of acne?

Clinical Manifestations

Acne lesions can be classified as either: (1) noninflammatory lesions, characterized by **comedones** or (2) inflammatory lesions, which are characterized by papules, pustules, and nodules. Many individuals with acne have more than one type of lesion present. There are two types of comedones (Roebuck, 2006; Zaenglein & Thiboutot, 2006). Closed comedones, commonly referred to as whiteheads, are small (1 to 3 mm), slightly elevated papules with microscopic openings that are whitish or flesh colored. Open comedones, commonly referred to as blackheads, are slightly larger, flat or raised lesions with dilated openings. The characteristic black color of these lesions is not dirt, but occurs as a consequence of oxidation.

Inflamed acne lesions are characterized by the proliferation of *P. acnes* (Roebuck, 2006; Zaenglein & Thiboutot, 2006). Papules are erythematous, elevated lesions that range from 2 to 5 mm in diameter. Pustules are papules that contain visible purulent material. Nodules exceed 5 mm in diameter, are often tender, and are seated more deeply in the dermis than papules and pustules. The term cyst is no longer recommended to describe these lesions. The extension of inflammation into the surrounding dermis results from rupture of the follicular wall due to the effects of *P. acnes* (Roebuck, 2006; Zaenglein & Thiboutot, 2006).

As acne lesions resolve, they often leave a short lived, reddish-purple scar in light-skinned patients. In dark-skinned patients, a hyperpigmented macule may result from acne lesions. The most common types of permanent acne scarring are pitted scars, depressed scars, and keloids (James et al., 2006). In addition to the presence of acne lesions, psychological effects such as anxiety, low self-esteem, or depression may also be apparent (Amin et al., 2007; Jancin, 2007; Roebuck, 2006; Webster, 2009). Caregivers may also show an unhealthy preoccupation with their child's face, which can lead to negative emotional sequelae for the acne patient (Roebuck, 2006). Furthermore, it is important to remember that there is large individual variation in the emotional impact of acne lesions or scars, and the degree of impact is not necessarily correlated with the severity of acne lesions (Collier et al., 2008).

Diagnosis

The diagnosis of acne is made based on the history and physical examination (Roebuck, 2006). No biopsy or laboratory testing is routinely recommended. The history should address acne duration and severity, as well as factors associated with acne flares. Adolescents with acne should also be asked to describe their facial care routine, including current and previous prescription and over-the-counter products, their effectiveness, and any irritation or side effects. The adolescent's face, chest, and back should be examined to determine the type of acne lesions present, as well as their distribution and severity. The presence of comedones is diagnostic for acne. If typical comedones are not present, alternate diagnoses should be considered. The effect that the disease has on the adolescent, as well as the presence of scarring, should also be assessed. Each of these factors are important in determining the appropriate course of treatment.

Treatment

The main objectives of acne treatment are to target pathogenic factors, improve physical appearance, decrease discomfort, reduce scar formation, and minimize adverse psychological outcomes. Treatment should be individualized to the adolescent based on the type, location, duration, and severity of lesions. The adolescent's personal preferences regarding treatment, response to prior treatments, and the psychological impact of the acne should also be taken into consideration.

Both topical and oral medications are available for the treatment of acne. The most commonly used topical medications include benzoyl peroxide, retinoids, and topical antibiotics. Commonly used oral agents include antibiotics, hormonal agents, and isotretinoin (Accutane). No single treatment formula works for all adolescents and it may take time to find the best combination of treatments for a particular adolescent. Regardless of the medications selected, it may take six to eight weeks to observe significant improvement and two to three months to reach maximal improvement (James et al., 2006; Webster, 2009). Medications should be continued until complete resolution is achieved and then the focus of treatment shifts to maintaining acne clearance. Retinoids are considered an essential component of maintenance therapy (James et al., 2006; Roebuck, 2006; Strauss et al., 2007; Zaenglein & Thiboutot, 2006).

Topical medications may be used as monotherapy for purely comedonal acne or mild to moderate inflammatory acne. However, combining acne treatments that target different pathogenic factors has been shown to increase efficacy and improve the speed of lesion resolution (Zaenglein & Thiboutot, 2006). Retinoids (adapalene, tretinoin, and tazarotene) are considered the mainstay of topical treatment because they inhibit microcomedo formation by normalizing keratinocyte desquamation, thereby reducing obstruction of the pilosebaceous unit (James et al., 2006; Roebuck, 2006; Strauss et al., 2007; Webster, 2009; Zaenglein & Thiboutot, 2006). Retinoids have also been shown to have direct anti-inflammatory properties as well as to enhance the penetration of other topical treatments. Therefore, retinoids are indicated for use in both comedonal and inflammatory acne. When first initiated, retinoids may cause mild burning/irritation for the first few weeks that gradually improves.

Benzoyl peroxide is a useful bactericidal agent with the ability to reduce *P. acnes* colonization and minimize inflammation. In addition, this agent has been found to prevent the development of antibiotic resistant strains of *P. acnes* (James et al., 2006; Roebuck, 2006; Strauss et al., 2007). Benzoyl peroxide is available in several over-the-counter and prescription formulations. However, use is somewhat limited by the fact that benzoyl peroxide may cause skin irritation and can bleach clothing, bedding, carpet, and hair.

Topical antibiotics, such as clindamycin and erythromycin, are also commonly used treatments for inflammatory acne. However, because of the development of antibiotic resistance to these agents, they are no longer recommended as monotherapy (James et al., 2006; Zaenglein & Thiboutot, 2006). Rather, it is advised that topical antibiotics be combined with benzoyl peroxide because of increased efficacy and reduced development of antibiotic resistant strains of *P. acnes*. Separate products may be used or combination formulations are available that integrate a topical antibiotic and benzoyl peroxide into the same vehicle. Other less frequently used prescription topical acne treatments include azelaic acid, dapsone, sodium sulfacetamide, and sulfur (James et al., 2006; Strauss et al., 2007; Webster, 2009). Salicylic acid is also available over-the-counter and is considered moderately effective.

Oral antibiotics are recommended for use in adolescents with moderate to severe inflammatory acne and treatment resistant forms of inflammatory acne (Strauss et al., 2007; Zaenglein & Thiboutot, 2006). These agents reduce the colonization of *P. acnes* and also have intrinsic anti-inflammatory properties (Amin et al., 2007; Roebuck, 2006; Zaenglein & Thiboutot, 2006; Webster, 2009). Current evidence supports the use of tetracycline, doxycycline, minocycline, erythromycin, trimethoprim-sulfamethoxazole, and azithromycin (Amin et al., 2007; Strauss et al., 2007). Antibiotic resistance has occurred with all of these antibiotics, but is most common with erythromycin. Ideally, oral antibiotics should be taken for three to six months and then tapered/discontinued as soon as possible to decrease the incidence of antibiotic resistance (James et al., 2006; Roebuck, 2006; Webster, 2009).

NURSING ALERT

Antibiotic-Resistant Bacteria

Antibiotic-resistant strains of *P. acnes* have been emerging. Increased use of topical antibiotics has been credited for this change. The development of antibiotic resistance can be minimized by limiting the initiation of antibiotics, avoiding long-term antibiotic use, and refraining from using topical antibiotics as monotherapy. Utilizing benzoyl peroxide in combination with topical antibiotics is also recommended because this treatment combination has been shown to inhibit the development of antibiotic resistance.

Treatment with isotretinoin is limited to individuals with severe nodular acne, individuals with acne that has not responded to standard therapies, and individuals with significant physical or psychological scarring (James et al., 2006; Strauss et al., 2007). Isotretinoin is the most effective acne treatment available, with nearly all patients experiencing complete acne resolution after a five- or six-month course of treatment and 80% never relapsing (Roebuck 2006; Webster, 2009). Common side effects include dry skin and mucous membranes, joint and muscle aches, mild hypertriglyceridemia, and headaches (James et al., 2006; Strauss 2007; Webster, 2009). Mood disorders, depression, and suicide have been reported in individuals treated with isotretinoin, though a causal relationship has not been established (James et al., 2006; Strauss et al., 2007; Webster, 2009). In addition, mood improvement has often been associated with the acne improvement that results from isotretinoin treatment. Because isotretinoin is highly teratogenic, it can only be prescribed by providers registered with iPLEDGE, the federal risk management program for isotretinoin. Patients are also required to register with the program and female patients must adhere to strict contraceptive requirements (Strauss et al., 2007).

The two most commonly used hormonal agents are oral contraceptives and spironolactone, which are both utilized for their antiandrogenic properties (James et al., 2006; Roebuck, 2006; Strauss et al., 2007; Webster, 2009). These treatments have been shown to be effective, though they are indicated for use in female patients only. Several adjunct therapies are also available to treat adolescents with acne. These include comedone extraction, steroid injections, chemical peels, and light/laser treatments. Often referral to a dermatologist is required for treatment. Manual comedone extraction may be indicated for treatment resistant lesions or when rapid improvement in appearance is desired, though the process may result in increased scarring (Strauss et al., 2007; Webster, 2009). Intralesional steroid injections are effective for the treatment of individual acne nodules (James et al., 2006; Straus et al., 2007; Webster, 2009). There is currently limited evidence to support the efficacy of chemical peels (Strauss et al., 2007). Finally, light and laser therapies are used by some providers, though additional research is needed to determine the efficacy of these interventions as compared to other treatments as well as to develop standardized treatment protocols (James et al., 2006; Webster, 2009).

When selecting acne treatments, it is important to consider that acne treatment failure is often attributed to poor compliance (James et al., 2006; Webster, 2009). Prescribers can enhance treatment adherence by selecting medications that are well tolerated, tailored to the adolescent's needs, affordable, and conveniently dosed. Adequate patient education is also essential as this intervention has been shown to increase compliance and overall treatment success (James et al., 2006; Roebuck, 2006; Zaenglein & Thiboutot, 2006). Client education should include an explanation of the pathogenic factors involved in acne development as well as a discussion about common myths regarding acne formation, such as dirt or certain foods as causual factors (Magin et al., 2006). Education should also explain why specific treatments were chosen, expected response to the medication, and potential side effects and their management. Adolescents with acne also need to be made aware of the

NURSING TIP

Assessing Acne Treatment Adherence

When assessing adherence to acne treatments, it can be helpful to ask how many bottles of pills the adolescent has used. A typical bottle of antibiotics for acne is a one-month supply. Nurses can also ask how much is left in the tube of topical medication. A typical 45-gram tube should last two to three months if used daily for the entire face.

KIDS WANT TO KNOW

Is eating chocolate making my acne worse?

My mom keeps telling me that my acne will not get better unless I stop eating so much chocolate and soda. Do I really have to choose between having acne and eating the foods I love?

Several studies have investigated the potential influence of diet on acne. The results of this research do not provide clear evidence that eating foods like chocolate, pizza, and soda affect acne development (Strauss et al., 2007; Webster 2008; Webster 2009). Investigations focusing on the relationship between milk consumption and acne have likewise produced conflicting and inconclusive results. However, when counseling adolescents that scientific studies do not show a correlation between eating certain foods and acne, it is important to emphasize the importance of maintaining a healthy, balanced diet. Furthermore, if consumption of a particular food item seems to aggravate an individual's acne, then discontinuation of that item may be warranted.

EVIDENCE-BASED PRACTICE

Treatment for Acne

CLINICAL PROBLEM

What are the most effective treatments for various forms of acne and how should treatments be administered to obtain the best results with minimal complications?

BEST CLINICAL PRACTICE

- Topical therapy is a standard of care in acne treatment.
- A topical retinoid should be the foundation of treatment for most individuals with acne because retinoids target the microcomedo, the precursor to all acne lesions.
- Because of their effect on the microcomedo, topical retinoids also are recommended as an important facet of maintenance therapy.
- Topical antimicrobial agents are effective acne treatments, but when used alone they are associated with the development of bacterial resistance.
- Combining a topical retinoid with an antimicrobial agent results in significantly faster and greater clearing as opposed to antimicrobial therapy alone.
- Oral antibiotics are a standard of care in moderate to severe acne, as well as in treatment-resistant forms of inflammatory acne.

IMPLICATIONS FOR NURSING

- The availability of numerous acne treatments allows for individualization of the treatment regimen based on the characteristics of the adolescent's acne.
- Adolescents with acne should be taught about the pathophysiology of acne and how various acne treatments target these factors.
- Nurses need to educate adolescents and caregivers about antibiotic resistance as well as methods to decrease the emergence of resistant *S. aureus* strains.

References: Strauss, J. S., Krowchuk, D. P., Leyden, J. J., Lucky, A. W., Shalita, A. R., Siegfried, E. C., et al. (2007). Guidelines of care for acne vulgaris management. *Journal of the American Academy of Dermatology, 56*, 651–63; Zaenglein, A. L., & Thiboutot, D. M. (2006). Expert committee recommendations for acne management. *Pediatrics, 118*, 1188–1199.

CASE STUDY / CARE PLAN

AN ADOLESCENT WITH ACNE

Rebecca is a 14-year-old who started getting acne about one year ago. At first she only got little bumps and blackheads on her nose, cheeks, and forehead. Recently she has started noticing deep, tender zits along her jaw line. She has tried over-the-counter products, but is frustrated because they make her skin dry and flaky. They help a little, but every time she stops the acne gets bad again. Rebecca is concerned because she thinks it may be her make-up that is making the acne worse, but she is embarrassed to go to school without make-up on.

NURSING CARE PLAN

ASSESSMENT

The main focus of the nursing assessment for adolescents with acne is obtaining a detailed client history. The history should address acne duration and severity, as well as factors associated with acne flares. The adolescent should be asked to describe their facial care routine, including current or previous use of prescription and over-the-counter products, their effectiveness, and any irritation or side effects. The emotional impact of the acne on the adolescent and her caregivers should also be assessed, as should any treatment preferences.

In addition, a physical assessment should be conducted which focuses on the adolescent's face, chest, and back. The nurse should note the type of acne lesions present, as well as their distribution and severity. In particular, it is important to identify the presence of comedones, as these lesions are diagnostic for acne. The presence and severity of any scarring should also be noted.

NURSING DIAGNOSIS 1

Impaired skin integrity related to the presence of acne lesions and the use of potentially irritating topical products.

EXPECTED OUTCOMES

1. Adolescent will exhibit signs of acne clearing.
2. Adolescent will exhibit decreased irritation while using topical products.

NOC: Tissue Integrity: Skin

NIC: Skin Care: Topical Treatments

INTERVENTIONS/*RATIONALES*

1. Educate the adolescent about properly using common prescription and over-the-counter acne treatments. Provide specific instructions for the use of recommended topical and oral medications. *Adolescents are often not very experienced in managing medication use and require specific instructions to encourage proper use.*
2. Warn patient about potential side effects and what to do if they arise. *Having prior knowledge of what to do if side effects occur can help prevent complications and help patients manage nuisance side effects without unnecessarily stopping the medication.*
3. Explain that benefit from treatment may take six to eight weeks to become apparent. *Misunderstanding about the length of time required to see improvement can cause the adolescent to give up on the treatment prematurely.*
4. Advise the adolescent that the medications should be continued until complete resolution is achieved and then the focus of treatment will shift to maintaining acne clearance. *Knowledge about the need for maintenance treatment can help prevent premature medication cessation.*

(Continues)

CASE STUDY / CARE PLAN (Continued)

5. Explain that consistent daily application of topical medications is necessary to see the full benefit of the medication. *Adolescents may be more likely to use the medication regularly if they understand that this will help them see more acne improvement.*
6. Topical medications should be applied to the entire affected area and not just individual lesions. *It is important for adolescents to understand that acne treatments can have preventive benefits and should not be used to just treat existing lesions.*
7. Explain that a pea-sized amount of topical medication should be sufficient to cover the entire face. *Use of too much medication can cause unnecessary irritation and using too little medication may not produce sufficient improvement.*
8. No single treatment formula works for all adolescents and it may take time to find the best combination of treatments for a particular adolescent. *This information can help reduce frustration if the first acne treatments do not lead to complete acne resolution.*
9. If caregivers are present, they should be encouraged to support the adolescent in using the medications appropriately. *Having a support system at home can help improve acne treatment adherence and lead to greater improvement.*
10. Advise adolescents to wash their face twice a day with a mild skin cleanser and lukewarm water. *Vigorous washing and harsh cleansers can disrupt the skin barrier, increase inflammation, and decrease tolerance of other topical treatments.*
11. Teach adolescents to use their hands to wash their face and to avoid aggressive scrubbing. *Aggressive washing does not improve acne clearance and the resulting friction can actually worsen inflammation.*
12. Warn adolescents that it is normal to experience mild burning/irritation with some topical acne products for the first few weeks that gradually improves. *It can be reassuring for adolescents who experience irritation to know that this is normal and will get better as they keep using the product.*
13. If needed, adolescents can be advised to apply the product less frequently or shorten the duration of contact by washing the product off after a period of time. *These measures can help minimize irritation while still allowing for use of the product.*
14. If necessary, adolescents can be instructed to apply an oil-free/noncomedogenic moisturizer before or after the topical medication is applied. *Using these products can help minimize irritation without clogging pores and making the acne worse.*

EVALUATION

The adolescent will experience healing of her acne as evident by decreased inflammation and the presence of fewer acne lesions. The adolescent's skin should also manifest minimal signs of irritation, including reduced dryness and sensitivity.

NURSING DIAGNOSIS 2

Disturbed body image related to perception of appearance.

EXPECTED OUTCOME

Adolescent will maintain a positive self-image as evident by expressions of positive self-perceptions and engagement in usual activities and relationships.

NOC: Body Image

NIC: Body Image Enhancement

INTERVENTIONS/*RATIONALES*

Implement the following strategies to promote positive body image perceptions:

1. Allow the adolescent to verbalize her feelings about her appearance. *Providing an opportunity for adolescents to discuss their emotions regarding their acne can help identify areas of need and is often an intervention on its own.*

(Continues)

CASE STUDY / CARE PLAN (Continued)

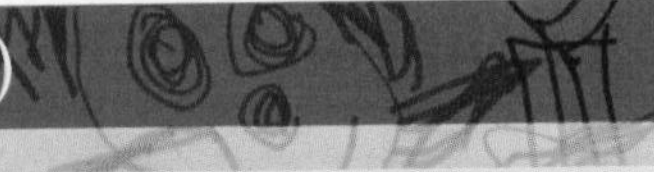

2. Provide realistic reassurance about future clearance of the acne lesions. *While it is counterproductive to provide unrealistic expectations of clearing, it can be helpful for adolescents to know that with time their acne will improve.*
3. Compliment the adolescent's other desirable qualities such as their hair, clothes, or personality. *Providing positive feedback about desirable traits can help enhance the adolescent's self-image.*
4. Give the adolescent positive feedback when improvement is noticed, even when complete clearing has not yet been achieved. *Adolescents can become discouraged when their acne is not totally clear, but complimenting partial clearing can help adolescents to view their appearance with a more positive perspective.*
5. Encourage the adolescent to continue age-appropriate activities with family and friends. *Interactions with others are an important part of socialization and development for adolescents.*
6. Encourage caregivers to provide a safe emotional environment for their adolescent and to focus on providing positive statements about the adolescent. *It can be detrimental to the adolescent's self-image if her caregiver focuses primarily on how the acne negatively impacts her appearance.*
7. If psychological conditions such as anxiety or depression are apparent, referral to a psychologist or psychiatrist may be warranted. *In some cases, professional help is needed to prevent the adolescent from progressing to more serious psychological problems.*
8. Psychological referral should be considered if caregivers show an unhealthy preoccupation with their adolescent's acne. *If the acne is a source of conflict between the adolescent and her caregiver or if the caregiver continually provides negative feedback to the adolescent, psychological assistance can help promote an environment that fosters the adolescent to develop a positive self-image.*

EVALUATION

The adolescent will be able to express her emotions regarding her condition. She will express a positive self-image through her body language, verbalization, and interactions with others. She will also participate in age-appropriate activities.

NURSING DIAGNOSIS 3

Deficient knowledge related to the causes of acne.

EXPECTED OUTCOME

The adolescent will be able to express an understanding of the causes of acne.

NOC: Knowledge: Disease Process

NIC: Teaching: Disease Process

INTERVENTIONS/RATIONALES

1. Assess what the adolescent and her caregivers already know about the formation of acne and identify potential areas for improving knowledge. *Providing information better enables the adolescent and her caregivers to take control of the condition.*
2. Explain the pathophysiology of acne. Describe the role of increased sebum production, abnormal epithelial keratinization, proliferation of *P. acnes*, and inflammation in the formation of acne. *Explaining the role of these internal factors can help adolescents understand why multiple products are often necessary to target all of the factors involved in ane development.*
3. Adolescents should be made aware of the typically chronic nature of acne. *This knowledge can promote medication adherence and reduce frustration if the treatment is stopped and acne lesions recur.*
4. Explain that as acne lesions resolve, they often leave a short-lived reddish-purple scar. *Because the presence of these lesions can lead adolescents to believe that their acne is not improving, it can be helpful to reassure them that these spots are not active acne lesions or permanent scars.*

(Continues)

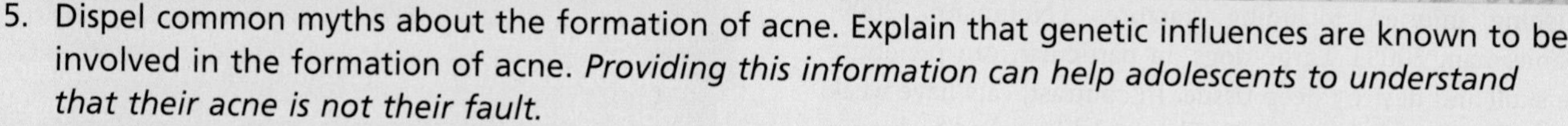

CASE STUDY / CARE PLAN (Continued)

5. Dispel common myths about the formation of acne. Explain that genetic influences are known to be involved in the formation of acne. *Providing this information can help adolescents to understand that their acne is not their fault.*
6. Explain that the use of occlusive skin care products can produce or worsen acne. *If adolescents are using oil free/noncomedogenic cleansers, moisturizers, or make-up they can be reassured that these products will not make their acne worse.*
7. Explain that the black color of open comedones is not dirt, but occurs as a consequence of oxidation. *Conveying this information can help dispel feelings of uncleanliness and frustration that washing does not improve the appearance of these lesions.*
8. Explain that friction can exacerbate acne, so aggressive washing should be avoided. *This information can be helpful to adolescents who feel that their acne will get better if they wash harder.*
9. Explain that studies do not provide clear evidence that eating foods like chocolate, pizza, and soda affect acne development. *This information can help reassure adolescents that they do not need to feel guilty that their diet is causing their acne or restrict their diet unnecessarily.*

EVALUATION

The adolescent and her caregivers will be able to explain the causes of acne and express realistic expectations about acne clearance. They will also be able to identify lifestyle factors that she can change to improve her acne, as well as factors that do not need to be changed.

typically chronic nature of acne, the delayed onset of acne improvement once treatment is initiated, and the need to utilize measures to maintain clearance of the acne lesions once the initial treatment has been successful.

Because of the often irritating nature of topical acne products, skin care education that focuses on reducing irritation is also essential (James et al., 2006; Roebuck, 2006; Webster, 2009). Vigorous washing and harsh cleansers can disrupt the skin barrier, increase inflammation, and decrease tolerance of other topical treatments. Instead, adolescents should gently wash their face twice a day with a mild skin cleanser and lukewarm water. If irritation occurs with topical medications, adolescents can apply the product less frequently or shorten the duration of contact by washing the product off after a period of time. As their skin adjusts to the medication, they can then gradually increase the frequency/duration of application until the medication is being used as recommended. If necessary, adolescents can also use an oil-free/non-comedogenic moisturizer before or after the topical medication is applied.

BITES AND STINGS

Although most bites and stings sustained by children are minor, life-threatening consequences can result. Animal bites can inflict extensive damage and introduce polymicrobial infection, particularily among young children. Likewise, arthropod bites and stings can transfer serious diseases or cause potentially fatal allergic reactions. Consequently, educating children and their caregivers about the prevention of injuries from animals and arthropods is of critical importance.

ANIMAL BITES

Children are more likely than adults to sustain animal bites, usually from dogs. Although the majority of injuries from animal bites are minor, potentially serious complications and even death may result.

INCIDENCE AND ETIOLOGY

Of the more than 5 million Americans bitten by animals each year, children aged 5–14 are the most common victims (Spanierman, 2008). In addition, most of the fatalities resulting from dog bites occur among young children. Dog bites account for 80–90% of all domestic animal bites in the United States and cat bites account for 5–15% (Neumann, 2009). Other commonly involved animals include rodents, ferrets, and rabbits.

Dog breeds that are associated with serious bite injuries include pit bulls, German shepherds, rottweilers, wolf mixes, Saint Bernards, and Akitas (Spanierman, 2008). Pit bulls are responsible for nearly 75% of all dog bite fatalities (Spanierman, 2008). However, any dog can attack. Male, unneutered dogs tend to be more aggressive (Schalamon et al., 2006). Children are most likely to be bitten by a dog that is known to them (Schalamon et al., 2006). Although the majority of dog bites involving children do not involve the family pet, children who have a dog in the home are more likely to be bitten (CDC, 2008b; Schalamon et al., 2006). Dog bites are also more likely in the summer and when a dog is provoked (Schalamon et al., 2006). Boys tend to be bitten by dogs more frequently than are girls, though girls tend to be bitten more frequently by cats (Spanierman, 2008).

Pathophysiology

Dogs have strong jaws and wide, dull teeth which can cause crushing injuries, including fractures (Neumann, 2009; Spanierman, 2008). Large dogs, in particular, can penetrate the skull and destroy deep tissue. In contrast, cats have weak bite strength and sharp teeth. Thus, cat bites tend to have a puncture quality that can inoculate bacteria deep into the tissues. In addition to the truma that animal bites can inflict, the transfer of infection from the oral flora of the animal to the bite victim is common. Infection occurs in about 15–20% of dog bite cases and can involve *Staphylococcus, Streptococcus, Capnocytophaga canimorsus, Klebsiella, Bacillus subtilis, Pseudomonas* and *Enterobacteriaceae.* The rate of infection associated with cat bites ranges from 30–50% and commonly involves *Staphylococcus, Streptococcus,* and *Pasteurella multocida.*

Clinical Manifestations

The most common types of injuries resulting from animal bites include puncture wounds, lacerations, crushing damage, or **avulsion** (major tearing of tissue) (Neumann, 2009). Injuries to the face, head, and neck occur more frequently in younger children (Schalamon et al., 2006).

Infection is a common complication resulting from animal bites. Infection rates are significantly greater following cat bites than dog bites, and puncture wounds are more likely to become contaminated than lacerations (Spanierman, 2008). Bites on the hand are more likely to develop infection and facial wounds are less likely to become infected (Neumann, 2009). Cat bites may appear minor, but introduce bacteria into the joint space (Spanierman, 2008).

Potentially serious complications from animal bites include cellulitis, septic arthritis, osteomyelitis, and meningitis (Spanierman, 2008). Permanent deformity, scarring, and limb loss are also possible. Rabies is an uncommon, but potentially fatal consequence of animal bites (Box 30-7). In addition, there are often psychosociological sequelae that burden the quality of life of the affected child and his/her caregivers (Schalamon et al., 2006). For instance, children may have nightmares and a lasting fear of dogs. It can also be traumatic if an animal familiar to the family requires euthanization.

BOX 30-7
RABIES

Rabies is a preventable, fatal viral infection. The majority of cases involve wild animals, such as bats, raccoons, skunks, and foxes. Less than 10% of cases involve domesticated animals such as dogs, cats, and cattle. However, any mammal is believed to be susceptible to the disease. The rabies virus is transmitted when the saliva of an infected animal is introduced into bite wounds, open cuts, or onto mucous membranes. The average incubation period for rabies is four to six weeks, after which flu-like symptoms progress to cerebral dysfunction, hallucinations, and abnormal behavior. Once these signs appear, the disease is almost always fatal.

If suspected transfer of the rabies virus occurs, rabies prophylaxis should be initiated immediately, and the case should be reported to the local health department as soon as possible. The wound should be washed immediately with soap and water and both the human rabies vaccine and human rabies immune globulin should be administered. In addition, a stray or unwanted animal that has bitten a child and is suspected of being rabid should be captured and euthanized. Other animals should be confined and observed for ten days. In order to prevent rabies, it is recommended that all dogs, cats, and ferrets should be vaccinated and given a booster dose one year later. The animal can be considered immunized 28 days after the initial vaccination and immediately after the booster dose.

Adapted from: Centers for Disease Control and Prevention. (2007). Compendium of animal rabies prevention and control, 2007. *Morbidity & Mortality Weekly Report, 56*(22), 1–8; Serota, J. A. (2006). A bite in the night. *Journal of Pediatric Health Care, 20*(6), 407, 431–432.

Diagnosis

A thorough history and physical examination are necessary to assess the severity of animal bites. The initial history should address the type of animal, whether the bite was provoked or unprovoked, and the duration of time that has elapsed since the injury (Neumann, 2009; Spanierman, 2008). The health and behavior of the involved animal and its immunization status should also be assessed as should the tetanus immunization status of the child. The physical examination should determine the type of injury, the size and depth of the wound, the presence of foreign material in the wound, and the integrity of underlying structures (Neumann, 2009). When applicable, the exam should also assess the range of motion, nerve function, and the vascular supply at the site and distal to the site of injury.

X-rays should be obtained when there is a risk of fracture, such as in the case of children with deep tissue injuries or bites to the head (Spanierman, 2008). Radiology can also be helpful for detecting the presence of foreign bodies. Because of the risk for infection associated with animal bites, cultures of the wound site should also be considered, particularly if the wound is more than eight hours old or if signs of localized infection are present (Neumann, 2009).

Treatment

After the appropriate cultures have been obtained, the wound should be thoroughly irrigated with copious amounts of sterile saline under high pressure (Neumann, 2009; Spanierman, 2008). Local anesthesia may be necessary to accomplish adequate cleansing of the wound. If less than eight hours have passed since the injury and the wound does not appear to be infected, it may be sutured (Neumann, 2009; Spanierman, 2008). Facial wounds also typically undergo surgical closure because they rarely become infected and their cosmetic outcome is important. However, improved outcomes are noted if certain wounds are left open: bites to the hand, bites more than 24 hours old, deep wounds or puncture wounds, entensive injuries, and infected wounds. Surgical care may also involve debridement and wound excision (Spanierman, 2008).

In addition to the need for antibiotic usage for children with signs of infection, the use of prophylactic antibiotics should also be considered. It has been suggested that antibiotics be given to children who have puncture wounds or evidence of crushing wounds to the face, hands, feet or genitals; or have medical conditions such as diabetes or splenectomy (Neumann, 2009). Infections should be assumed to be polymicrobial (Spanierman, 2008). The commonly recommended first-line antibiotic is amoxicillin-clavulanate (Augmentin). Other alternatives include ceftriaxone (Rocephin), trimethoprim/sulfamethoxazole (Bactrim, Septra) plus clindamycin, or doxycycline (Neumann, 2009; Spanierman, 2008). Appropriate tetanus prophylaxis should also be administered to children who have not been immunized previously, whose immunization status is unknown, or who have not had a tetanus booster within the past five years. An assessment of the biting animal's rabies status, in conjunction with the local health department, should guide decisions about initiating rabies prophylaxis.

Although most cases of animal bites have a good-to-excellent prognosis, there are several instances that indicate the need for in-patient care: airway compromise, hemodynamic instability, penetrating skull injuries, or severe soft tissue injuries (Spanierman, 2008).

BOX 30-8
PREVENTING DOG BITES IN CHILDREN

The following safety principles should be taught to children and reviewed regularly:

- Do not play aggressive games with dogs.
- Do not hug or kiss a dog.
- Do not approach an unfamiliar dog.
- Do not run past or from a dog. Do not scream.
- Remain motionless when approached by an unfamiliar dog (e.g., "be still like a tree").
- Do not play with a dog unless supervised by an adult.
- Immediately report stray dogs or dogs displaying unusual behavior to an adult.
- Avoid direct eye contact with a dog.
- Do not disturb a dog that is sleeping, eating, or caring for puppies.
- Do not stop two fighting dogs.
- Do not pet a dog without allowing it to see and sniff you first.
- If knocked over by a dog, roll into a ball, keep your face down, cover your ears, and lie still (e.g., "be still like a log").

Adapted from: Centers for Disease Control and Prevention. (2008b). *Dog bite prevention.* Retrieved March 20, 2009, from http://www.cdc.gov/HomeandRecreationalSafety/Dog-Bites/biteprevention.html; Schalamon, J., Ainoedhofer, H., Singer, G., Petnehazy, T., Mayr, J., Kiss, K., et al. (2006). Analysis of dog bites in children who are younger than 17 years. *Pediatrics, 117*(3), e374–e379.

Nursing Management

The nursing management for a child who has sustained an animal bite varies greatly with the severity of the injuries. The initial nursing assessment should include a detailed history focused on determining the type of animal involved, the rabies status of the animal, the tetanus immunization status of the child, and the duration of time that has elapsed since the injury. The physical examination should focus on determining the severity of the injuries, including the type, size, and depth of the wound, as well as the integrity of the underlying structures (Neumann, 2009). If the child is hospitalized for extensive injuries, monitoring of breathing and circulation are of critical importance. If the child is cared for in an out-patient setting, family education regarding the treatment regimen and preventing future attacks is paramount. Nurses may also be involved with public education regarding animal bite and rabies prevention.

Family Teaching

When care for the bitten child will be completed at home, family teaching should include instructions about the use of any prescribed medications, proper wound care techniques, and signs and symptoms of infection. After all bite injuries, education regarding strategies for preventing future bite injuries should also be given. Children must be taught a healthy respect for animals, including those that are familiar to them. General dog bite prevention strategies for children are presented in Box 30-8. Education of the caregiver should include factors to consider when selecting a family pet, measures to socialize animals to interact with humans, and the importance of carefully supervising children around animals (CDC, 2008b). Spaying/neutering should also be recommended as this tends to decrease aggressive behavior.

ARTHROPOD BITES AND STINGS

Arthropods that inflict bites or stings on humans include mosquitoes, fleas, bedbugs, ticks, spiders, ants, bees, and wasps. Most bites and stings produce only local skin reactions. However, in some cases serious or even fatal sequelae may result.

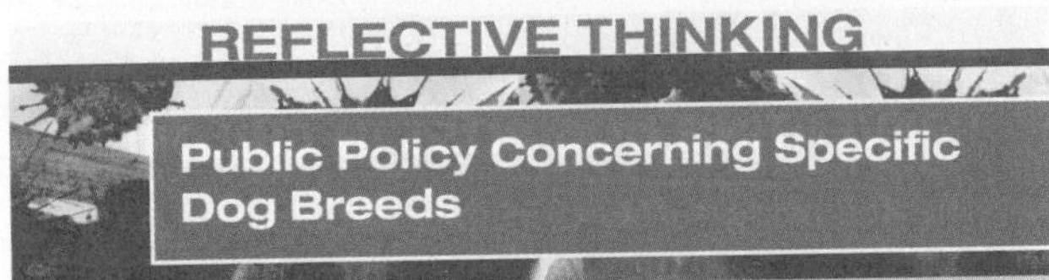

Public Policy Concerning Specific Dog Breeds

Because certain dog breeds, such as pit bulls, are more frequently involved in dog-bite-related fatalities, many individuals support legislation to regulate these breeds. Do you think that this is an appropriate approach to reducing injury by these dogs? What legal responsibility should owners of these dogs be required to assume for their animals' actions?

Incidence and Etiology

It is difficult to estimate the incidence of arthropod bites because the resulting injury is usually minor and does not require medical attention. However, even common insects such as mosquitoes and fleas can serve as disease vectors for serious illnesses. For instance, mosquitoes are known to spread conditions such as West Nile fever, Dengue fever, and viral encephalitis. Similarly, fleas can carry plague, endemic typhus, and cat scratch disease. Unlike mosquitoes, fleas are wingless but they are capable of jumping long distances. Gender and race do not appear to play a role in determining one's susceptibility to insect bites. Rather, factors that are associated with an increased incidence of insect bites include body heat, body odor, the use of fragrances, and carbon dioxide secretion (Elston, 2007b; James et al., 2006).

At one time, bedbugs were nearly eradicated in the United States. However, there has been a recent resurgence of bedbug infestations, presumably because of international travel (Hernandez & Cohen, 2006). Bedbugs can survive in many geographic regions and are able to live for up to 1 year without a blood meal. Commonly, bedbugs infest birds' nests and bats' roosts and then wander into houses after seasonal migration causes the birds and bats to leave (Elston, 2007b; James et al., 2006). Once indoors, bedbugs often hide in cracks or crevices and descend to feed while their victim sleeps.

Ticks often are found in backyards and recreational areas adjacent to wooded areas. Once transferred to their human host, ticks attach to their victims and feed on superficial blood vessels for seven to twelve days. They then become engorged and fall off. Ticks are vectors for diseases such as Lyme disease and Rocky Mountain spotted fever. Typically, a sustained tick attachment of more than 24 hours is required for effective disease transmission (Elston, 2007b; James et al., 2006).

Spiders are commonly found in shoes, trash, woodpiles, attics, and garages. Though several spiders may bite children, very few are dangerous. The reaction a child experiences from a spider bite depends on the type of spider, age and size of the patient, and amount of venom injected (Elston, 2007b). One spider that can inflict significant harm is the brown recluse. Brown recluse spiders, common throughout North America, are small brown spiders with a large leg span and a dark brown "violin case" pattern on their cephalothorax (Elston, 2007b; James et al., 2006). The bite of this spider typically causes localized tissue necrosis and may cause disseminated intravascular coagulation (DIC). Another dangerous spider common in North America is the black widow. Black widows are large shiny black spiders with long legs and a red hourglass on the abdomen (Elston, 2007b; James et al., 2006). They are not aggressive arthropods and only bite when they are disturbed. A single bite quickly leads to the development of acute abdominal pain and systemic symptoms. Children appear to be more susceptible to the effects of black widow spider bites (Elston, 2007b).

The Hymenoptera order of arthropods includes bees (honeybees and bumblebees), vespids (hornets, wasps, and yellow jackets), and ants (Lewis & Smith, 2007; Vankawala & Park, 2008). The most aggressive species of ant, fire ants, fiercely guard their territory and attack in large numbers. Ants sting approximately 9.3 million people each year, while the other Hymenoptera cause about 1 million stings annually (Vankawala & Park, 2008). In those who are stung, 17–56% experience large local reactions and 1–2% experience a generalized reaction. An estimated 0.5–3.0% of the general population is considered allergic to Hymenoptera venom and together wasp and bee stings cause 30–120 deaths each year in the United States (Lewis & Smith, 2007; Vankawala & Park, 2008).

The frequency of Hymenoptera stings is not age dependent, though males are more commonly stung. Factors that place children at risk for Hymenoptera stings include proximity to the colony, noisy or vigorous activity, wearing bright or dark colors, and perfumes. In addition, if a stinging insect is smashed or stings a child it releases pheromones that attract other insects and induce them to sting (Lewis & Smith, 2007; Vankawala & Park, 2008). Stings are also more common in the spring and summer months and in the Southern states (Lewis & Smith, 2007).

Pathophysiology

The actual arthropod bite or sting typically inflicts minimal injury. However, the antigens that are introduced trigger the body's immune response and can result in a variety of clinical manifestations (Elston, 2007b; Hernandez & Cohen, 2006). Immunoglobulin E (IgE) mediated hypersensitivity responses result in the formation of immediate hive-like skin lesions. Delayed hypersensitivity (type IV cell-mediated immunity) responses can cause pruritic papules, nodules, and vesicles within 48 hours. In the case of Hymenoptera stings, the components of the venom are potent activators of the immune system and anaphylaxis may result (Vankawala & Park, 2008).

Less commonly, clinical lesions occur as a direct result of the toxins that are introduced. For instance, the toxin contained in brown recluse spider venom initiates a neutrophillic reaction that causes tissue necrosis (Elston, 2007b;

James et al., 2006). In some cases, the resulting damage to the endothelial cells of the blood vessels results in the development of DIC. The venom of brown recluse spiders also contains substances that dissolve the dermal ground substance and thereby promote local spread of the toxin. In addition, toxic reactions from Hymenoptera stings can be fatal if the amount of venom introduced is sufficient (about 30 vespid stings or 200 honeybee stings) (Vankawala & Park, 2008).

Clinical Manifestations

Insect bites typically present as erythematous papules that are clustered in the area where the bites occurred (Elston, 2007b). The lesions are pruritic, so excoriations are common. Vesicular, bullous, and urticarial reactions may also occur (Elston, 2007b; Hernandez & Cohen, 2006). A single urticarial lesion manifests as a smooth, erythematous lesion that is slightly edematous and may have central clearing. The term **urticaria** (hives) refers to a generalized eruption of these lesions, such as the generalized reactions that can occur from insect stings. Mosquitoes are a common cause of urticarial papules. However, more severe local reactions can occur, particularly in young children (James et al., 2006). Fleabites typically manifest as clustered lesions on the legs or waist. Bedbug bites are most commonly observed on the head and neck and usually appear as a linear arrangement of three bites in a row.

Tick bites are usually painless and may not be noticed for hours or days. As long as the tick is attached, the child may experience allergic reactions, fever, chills, headache, vomiting, and abdominal pain. Removal of the tick usually leads to symptom resolution in 12–36 hours. Tick bites may be followed by small, severely pruritic fibrous nodules or pruritic, circular localized erythemas, either of which may continue for months (James et al., 2006).

Brown recluse spiders usually cause a severe localized reaction. Within the first eight hours, a painful area of edema occurs with the development of a central bulla surrounded by zones of erythema and ischemia. In about a week the central portion becomes dark, demarcated, and gangrenous. Rarely, systemic toxicity may develop and result in DIC. If a black widow spider bite is sustained, the victim typically experiences severe pain within minutes that spreads throughout the extremities and trunk. Within a few hours there may be chills, vomiting, violent cramps, delirium or partial paralysis, spasms, and abdominal rigidity. These symptoms may be mistaken for appendicitis or food poisoning (Elston, 2007b; James et al., 2006).

The clinical manifestations of Hymenoptera stings can be classified as local reactions, urticaria without systemic symptoms, and generalized reactions. Most children who are stung will experience only local reactions which consist of pain, pruritus, erythema, and edema at the site of the sting (Lewis & Smith, 2007; Vankawala & Park, 2008). Vasodilation may produce a sensation of warmth in the affected area. Although the pain is immediate, the symptoms usually resolve within a few hours in children who are not allergic.

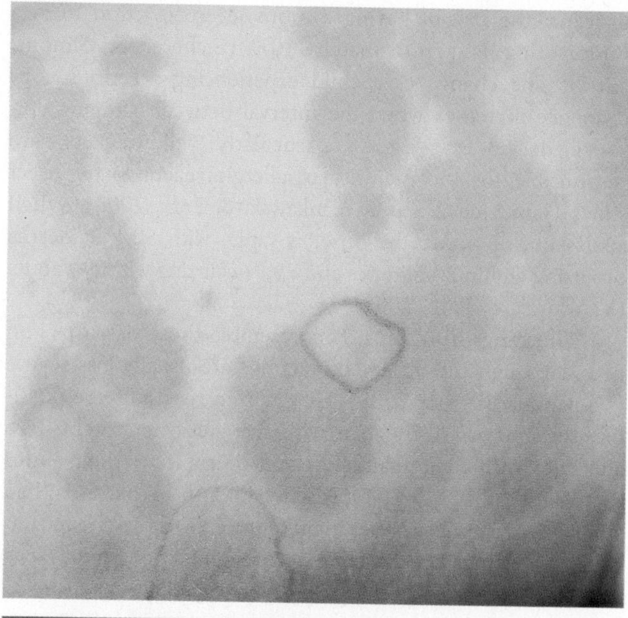

FIGURE 30-18 Urticaria. COURTESY OF ROBERT A. SILVERMAN, M.D., CLINICAL ASSOCIATE PROFESSOR, DEPARTMENT OF PEDIATRICS, GEORGETOWN UNIVERSITY.

Large local reactions may occur up to 48 hours after the sting, with edema extending up to 10 cm from the originally affected area. In some cases, the location of the sting may compromise distal sensation or circulation. Nausea or vomiting may also occur in the absence of a generalized reaction. Large, local reactions do not put children at increased risk for developing generalized reactions. However, local reactions can cause airway occlusion due to local swelling. Symptoms of large local reactions may persist for seven to ten days. In some children, urticaria may be present with or without the classic symptoms of a local reaction or systemic symptoms (Figure 30-18).

In allergic children, generalized anaphylactic reactions usually develop within ten to twenty minutes of the sting (Lewis & Smith, 2007). Mild generalized reactions are similar to large local reactions, but occur in areas that are not contiguous with the sting site. Moderate generalized reactions present with typical allergy symptoms such as sneezing, itchy watery eyes, generalized pruritus, and/or cough. In addition, lightheadedness, headaches, fever, muscle spasms, gastrointestinal tract distress, and difficulty breathing may occur. Severe generalized reactions may also include the following symptoms: urticaria or confluent red rash; vomiting; hypotension; edema of the airway, tongue, or uvula; shortness of breath and wheezing; weakness or syncope; anxiety and confusion; or chest pain (Lewis & Smith, 2007; Vankawala & Park, 2008). Anaphylactic shock can lead to cardiovascular collapse, respiratory arrest, and death. Toxic reactions from large amounts of Hymenoptera venom can mimic the clinical manifestations of anaphylaxis.

Although fatal allergic reactions can occur as the first generalized reaction, it is more common for individuals to experience a milder generalized reaction first (Vankawala & Park, 2008). For children who have experienced generalized urticaria, the risk of having a more severe reaction from a future sting is approximately 10% (Sicherer & Simons, 2007). The chance of a child experiencing a serious consequence increases when the interval between stinging episodes decreases. Vespids, particularly yellowjackets, are responsible for the majority of allergic reactions to insect stings (James et al., 2006; Vankawala & Park, 2008). When fatal sequelae occur, the onset is rapid, with 50% of deaths occurring within 30 minutes and 75% occurring within 4 hours (Vankawala & Park, 2008).

The stings from most ants resemble those of wasps and bees, although the observed reactions are usually less severe (Vankawala & Park, 2008). Generalized reactions are possible, though less likely than with flying Hymenoptera. Fire ants bite with their mandibles and then swivel their abdomen and inflict stings repeatedly in an arc pattern. The stings form sterile vesicles that rupture to form crusted lesions. Ant stings on the conjunctiva or mucous membranes can cause dramatic swelling in sensitive patients.

DIAGNOSIS

The diagnosis of arthropod bites and stings is usually based on the child's history and clinical presentation. In some cases, multiple minor bites may present a diagnostic challenge because they can resemble other dermatologic conditions, such as dermatitis (Hernandez & Cohen, 2006). In these instances, a thorough history should be conducted to assess the duration, location, and symptoms associated with the condition as well as any remissions or flares. The presence of an eruption in other family members and the activities of the child prior to the eruption should also be assessed. When possible, accurate identification of the arthropod is valuable as this information can guide decisions about prophylactic treatment (Elston, 2007b). In some cases, serologic testing may be needed to assess for exposure to arthropod-borne diseases. When a child presents with a stinger or attached tick present, the diagnosis is simplified.

If a child presents with symptoms of systemic reaction, the diagnostic focus is on determining the severity of the reaction. Both the physical exam and history should focus on assessing for the presence of anaphylactic signs and symptoms. Assessing the child's respiratory and circulatory status is of critical importance. Following resolution of the allergic event, diagnostic confirmation/reconfirmation of the triggering allergen by an allergist is recommended (Sicherer & Simons, 2007). Radio Allergo Sorbent Testing (RAST) is a commonly used method to confirm sensitivity to Hymenoptera (Elston, 2007b). Because cross-reactivity between vespid and bee venoms is uncommon, the majority of children who are allergic to honeybee venom are not allergic to yellow jacket venom and vice versa (Lewis & Smith, 2007).

TREATMENT

Supportive care measures are sufficient to manage the majority of arthropod bites and stings. If the stinger is present, it should be promptly removed (Box 30-9). Over-the-counter anesthetics, such as pramoxine, and antipruritics, such as camphor and menthol, can provide symptomatic relief (Elston, 2007b). Topical or intralesional steroids of varying strengths can also be used, with the more potent formulations providing superior relief. For minor, local Hymenoptera sting reactions a mild analgesic, such as acetaminophen, can be helpful, as are cool compresses and elevation of the extremity (Lewis & Smith, 2007; Vankawala & Park, 2008). For larger local reactions, an oral antihistamine such as diphenhydramine (Benadryl) or oral corticosteroid (Prednisone) may be utilized.

If the child presents with an attached tick, extraction is best accomplished by using forceps to grasp the tick near the head and then pull or twist the tick gently from the skin (Elston, 2007b). Care should be taken to avoid squeezing or breaking the tick. Although no standard guidelines exist, antibiotic prophylaxis may be administered to prevent illness such as Lyme disease and Rocky Mountain spotted fever. If a brown recluse spider bite has been sustained, treatment consists of rest, ice, and elevation. Additional treatment options include conservative surgical debridement, antibiotics if infection develops, dapsone, and systemic or intralesional steroids (Elston, 2007b; James et al., 2006). Children with

BOX 30-9
STINGER REMOVAL

All flying Hymenoptera inject their venom from a gland or sac through a long tapered structure on the posterior portion of their body called an ovipositor. When honeybees sting the ovipositor and venom sac remain embedded in the flesh of the victim and the honeybee dies after a single sting. The musculature between the venom glands will continue to pump venom through the stinger for up to one minute. In contrast, the ovipositors of bumble bees, wasps, hornets, and yellow jackets do not detach, so a single insect can sting multiple times.

If the stinger remains in the skin, prompt removal is essential to minimize the amount of venom introduced. It is commonly agreed that the method of stinger removal is not as important as the speed of removal. One commonly used technique is to pluck out the stinger with fingers or tweezers. This is a fast method that may forcibly instill more venom. Alternatively, a credit card or similar object can be used to scrape the stinger out of the skin without squeezing it. However, this method may be more time consuming because of the need to search for a card and there is a chance that the tip of the stinger will break off and remain in the skin.

Adapted from: Lewis, F. S., & Smith, L. J. (2007). What's eating you? Bees, part 1: Characteristics, reactions, and management. *Cutis, 79*, 439–444; Vankawala, H. H., & Park, R. (2008). *Bee and hymenoptera stings*. Retrieved March 20, 2009, from http://emedicine.medscape.com/article/768764-print.

minor appearing wounds should be monitored for several days because of the potential for tissue necrosis to lead to systemic toxin absorption and DIC (Elston, 2007b). The sequelae of black widow bites may be treated with narcotics, intravenous calcium gluconate, benzodiazepines, or antivenin (Elston, 2007b; James et al., 2006).

In the event of an anaphylactic reaction, emergency measures are required. Epinephrine is the primary medical therapy for these children (Sicherer & Simons, 2007). Epinephrine is a direct acting sympathomimetic agent that results in increased vasoconstriction, reduced mucosal edema, bronchodilation, and down regulation of inflammatory mediators such as histamine. Delayed administration of epinephrine in anaphylaxis is associated with poor outcomes, including death. The desired route of administration is intramuscular injection in the lateral thigh. Potential side effects include pallor, tremor, anxiety, palpitations, headache, and nausea.

Individuals with a history of an anaphylactic reaction should have an emergency epinephrine kit (EpiPen) available for self-administration in the event of a sting (Lewis & Smith, 2007; Sicherer & Simons, 2007). The child and caregivers should be instructed to err on the side of immediately injecting the medication rather than waiting too long. The injection may be given through clothing, though care should be taken to avoid obstructions such as seams or items in the pockets. If accidental injection into a digit occurs, medical care should be sought immediately because vasoconstriction and necrosis can result. The child and caregivers should also be instructed to routinely check the expiration date of the kit and to store it away from extreme temperatures and direct sunlight. Children with a documented history of anaphylaxis may also be referred to an allergist for desensitization by means of venom immunotherapy (Elston, 2007b; James et al., 2006; Vankawala & Park, 2008).

In addition to pharmacologic treatment, the occurrence of arthropod bites and stings indicates the need to implement preventive measures to reduce the incidence of future arthropod injuries. Measures to protect against Hymenoptera stings are listed in Box 30-10. The incidence of spider bites can be reduced by educating children and caregivers to exercise caution in areas where spiders are commonly found, such as garbage bins, woodpiles, attics, and garages. In regions that have prominent spider populations, it is also prudent to shake out one's shoes before putting them on (Elston, 2007b).

BOX 30-10

PREVENTING INSECT STINGS IN CHILDREN

- Avoid using perfumed products.
- Avoid wearing dark or bright colored clothing.
- Avoid known hive or nest locations.
- Avoid blooming flowers or overripe fallen fruit.
- Do not use noisy equipment close to hives.
- Avoid drinking or eating sweets outside during the summer months.
- Do not walk barefoot outside in grassy areas during summer months.
- Drive with car windows up and air-conditioning on.
- Have a qualified expert destroy nests near houses and other structures.
- If a nest is encountered, retreat slowly and do not panic.
- If attacked, cover head, nose, and mouth with arms or clothing and move away quickly.
- Do not flail arms when confronted with bees or wasps because smashing one can incite others to sting.

Adapted from: Lewis, F. S., & Smith, L. J. (2007). What's eating you? Bees, part 1: Characteristics, reactions, and management. *Cutis, 79*, 439–444; Vankawala, H. H., & Park, R. (2008). *Bee and hymenoptera stings*. Retrieved March 20, 2009, from http://emedicine.medscape.com/article/768764-print.

Mosquito populations can be reduced by draining stagnant water and spraying preferred breeding grounds (James et al., 2006). Additional measures to avoid bites from these insects include wearing protective clothing and limiting time outdoors during dawn and dusk, when mosquitoes are most likely to bite (Katz, Miller, & Herbert, 2008). Tick populations can be reduced by clearing leaf debris from wooded areas (Elston, 2007b; James et al., 2006). In addition, protective clothing, frequent tick checks, and prompt tick removal are important steps for preventing the transmission of tick-borne illnesses (James et al., 2006; Katz et al., 2008).

In households with pets, precautions should be taken to reduce fleas such as flea collars, flea medication, frequent bathing of the pet, and frequent washing of personal bedding in hot water (Hernandez & Cohen, 2006). Measures to reduce bedbug bites include washing bedding and mattress pads every two to four weeks as well as applying double-sided tape to the legs of the bed. In addition, elimination efforts may require the destruction of nearby bird nests and bat roosts (James et al., 2006). For both fleas and bedbugs, families can also consider professional pesticide treatments (Hernandez & Cohen, 2006; James et al., 2006).

NURSING TIP

Maintenance of Epinephrine Kits

Epinephrine kits should be stored away from extreme temperatures and direct sunlight to prevent degradation. The child and caregivers should also be instructed to check the expiration date of the kit routinely. Kits need to be promptly replaced before the expiration date has passed.

Although they do not protect against stinging insects, insect repellants can be effective in reducing bites from mosquitoes, flies, and ticks (Elston, 2007b; Katz et al., 2008). Insect repellents containing N, N-diethyl-3-methylbenzamide (DEET) have historically been the most broad-spectrum and efficacious products available. Concentrations are available from 5–100%. However, there have been rare reports of toxicity and even fatalities, most of which were associated with overuse or incorrect use of the product. Because of the dose-dependent nature of DEET toxicity, it is recommended that DEET concentrations should not exceed 30% in children (Elston, 2007b; James et al., 2006; Katz et al., 2008). Care should also be taken to avoid contact with the mouth and eyes, including avoiding application to the hands of children who may touch their mouth or eyes. Toxicity risk can also be reduced by limiting the amount of insect repellent applied. For this reason, combination products containing both DEET and sunscreen should be avoided because sunscreens need to be reapplied frequently. Additional precautions for using DEET products in children are listed in Box 30-11. Other alternative insect repellants approved by the Environmental Protection Agency for cutaneous application include picardin (for children 2 years old or older), oil of citronella (only lasts 20–30 minutes), and oil of lemon eucalyptus (for children 3 years old and older, does not repel ticks) (James et al., 2006; Katz et al., 2008; McNamara, 2008b). Picardin is commonly recommended as an acceptable DEET alternative, though the efficacy when compared to DEET has been debated.

BOX 30-11

DEET INSECT REPELLENT USE IN CHILDREN

- Apply product to skin sparingly; best to spray outside surfaces of shoes, socks, pants
- Avoid using under clothing or near open wounds
- Avoid combination sunscreen/insect repellent products
- Do not apply product to the child's hands or fingers
- Do not apply product directly to the child's face
- Do not leave product on overnight
- Do not use product on infants younger than 2 months
- Do not apply product more than once a day

Adapted from: Katz, T. M., Miller, J. H., & Herbert, A. A. (2008). Insect repellents: Historical perspectives and new developments. *Journal of the American Academy of Dermatology*, *58*(5), 865–871; McNamara, D. (2008b). Answering parents' questions about DEET, "natural" repellents. *Skin & Allergy News*, *39*(4), 36.

Nursing Management

The nursing management for a child who has sustained an arthropod bite or sting varies greatly with the severity of the injuries. For minor reactions, the initial nursing assessment should include a detailed history and exam focused on determining the type of arthropod involved as well as the duration, location, and symptoms associated with the bite or sting reaction. If a stinger or attached tick presents prompt removal is indicated. If the child presents with symptoms of a systemic reaction, assessing the child's respiratory and circulatory status are of critical importance. Severe allergic reactions also indicate the need for prompt administration of epinephrine. If the child is cared for in an out-patient setting, nursing care should include family education regarding supportive care measures and precautions to prevent future bites or stings. After allergic reactions have resolved, nurses may also be involved in developing an emergency plan and coordinating the child's care with his/her school, daycare, or summer camp.

Family Teaching

Priorities for family teaching include strategies to avoid insect bites and stings and appropriate management if they occur. Children and caregivers should be advised of common areas where biting and stinging insects are likely to be found as well as measures to reduce arthropod populations. In addition, proper insect repellent use should be explained (Box 30-11). Particularly in children who are allergic to Hymenoptera, preventive measures specific to avoiding insect stings should also be reviewed (see Box 30-10). Children with allergies to Hymenoptera venom should also be instructed to wear medical identification bracelets or tags indicating their allergy and to call 911 immediately after any arthropod sting. If an emergency epinephrine kit is provided, caregivers and older children should be educated about when and how to administer the medication, as well as proper storage of the medication. If a minor bite or sting occurs in a child who is not allergic, recommendations for supportive care include prompt stinger removal (if applicable), application of cool compresses, elevation of the extremity, and administration of over-the-counter analgesics or anesthetics.

SUNBURN

Sun exposure is a major health concern for individuals of all ages. Skin cancer is the most common form of cancer in the United States and sun exposure has been deemed responsible for 65–90% of all skin cancers (Boe & Tillotson, 2006; Cokkinides et al., 2006; Lim & Wang, 2007). However, despite current awareness of the dangers of sun exposure, a significant proportion of children and adolescents still do not receive adequate sun protection and sustain sunburns (Cokkinides et al., 2006; Guenther, Barankin, & Powell, 2007; James et al., 2006).

INCIDENCE AND ETIOLOGY

It has been estimated that 80% of an individual's lifetime sun exposure occurs before 18 years of age (Boe & Tillotson, 2006). This is largely because children spend significantly more time outdoors than do adults. Furthermore, children are at increased risk for sunburn because a significant amount of their sun exposure occurs during peak hours of the day (10am–4pm) and during the summer. Experts agree that among children and adolescents, the incidence of sunburn generally increases with age (Cokkinides et al., 2006; Guenther et al., 2007). Specifically, one survey found that during the summer, 13% of children reported having had a sunburn in the previous week (Guenther et al., 2007). Another survey of adolescents found self-reported sunburn incidence rates to be 69% (Cokkinides et al., 2006).

Sunburns occur more frequently in children with skin type I or II, though any skin type can sunburn with prolonged exposure (Guenther et al., 2007). A list of skin types and associated characteristics is presented in Table 30-3. Children who freckle easily and have blue or green eye color also sunburn more easily (Guenther et al., 2007). A number of medications including tetracyclines, fluoroquinolones, and ibuprofen can cause increased photosensitivity (Boe & Tillotson, 2006; Guenther et al., 2007; Lim & Wang, 2007). Certain diseases, such as systemic lupus erythematosus, can also increase a child's sensitivity to sunlight (Guenther et al., 2007).

Table 30-3 Fitzpatrick Skin Types

SKIN TYPE	SKIN COLOR	SUN HISTORY
I	White	Always burns, never tans
II	White	Usually burns, tans minimally
III	White	Sometimes burns, tans gradually to light brown
IV	White	Burns minimally, always tans to moderate brown
V	Brown	Rarely burns, tans darkly
VI	Black	Never burns, tans darkly black

Adapted from: American Academy of Dermatology. (2009). *Facts about sunscreens*. Retrieved March 20, 2009, from http://www.aad.org/media/background/factsheets/fact_sunscreen.htm; Fitzpatrick, T. B. (1988). The validity and practicality of sun-reactive skin types I through IV. *Archives of Dermatology, 124*, 869–871; James, W. D., Berger, T. G., & Elston, D. M. (2006). *Andrew's diseases of the skin: Clinical dermatology* (10th ed.). Philadelphia, PA: Elsevier.

Table 30-4 UV Index

INDEX	LEVEL OF RISK	EXPOSURE REQUIRED TO SUNBURN*
0–2	Minimal	1 hour
3–4	Low	20 minutes
5–6	Moderate	< 15 minutes
7–9	High	< 10 minutes
10 or more	Extreme	< 5 minutes

*Estimated duration of exposure required to cause a sunburn in a fair-kinned person.
Adapted from: Guenther, L., Barankin, B., & Powell, J. (2007). *Sunburn*. Retrieved March 20, 2009, from http://emedicine.medscape.com/article/911358-print

Exposure to ultraviolet B radiation, which is responsible for most sunburn, is greatest between the hours of 10 a.m. and 4 p.m. (Boe & Tillotson, 2006; James et al., 2006). Increases in ultraviolet exposure also occur at higher altitudes and at locations closer to the equator (Guenther et al., 2007; James et al., 2006; Lim & Wang, 2007). Up to 80% of ultraviolet rays are reflected by snow, sand, water, and concrete, creating an increased potential for sunburn (AAD, 2009; Guenther et al., 2007; Lim & Wang, 2007). In addition, approximately 80% of the sun's rays can penetrate clouds (AAD, 2009; Lim & Wang, 2007). Because of the variability of ultraviolet radiation exposure based on weather, the Environmental Protection Agency developed the UV index to help inform the public about the risk of sunburn on any given day (Guenther et al., 2007) (Table 30-4).

PATHOPHYSIOLOGY

Sunburn is a manifestation of skin damage that occurs as a consequence of exposure to ultraviolet radiation from the sun or tanning beds. The two types of ultraviolet rays responsible for damage to the skin are ultraviolet A (UVA) and ultraviolet B (UVB). Ultraviolet B rays make up only a small percentage of UV radiation exposure (0.5–5%); however, UVB is the primary cause of sunburn (AAD, 2009; Boe & Tillotson, 2006; Guenther et al., 2007). UVB rays are absorbed primarily in the epidermis, while UVA rays are able to penetrate the dermis (AAD, 2009; Guenther et al., 2007). UVA rays potentiate the effects of UVB radiation and are also responsible for photoaging and immunosuppression as well as sunburns that result from drug-induced photosensitivity or tanning bed use (AAD, 2009; Boe & Tillotson, 2006; Guenther et al., 2007; James et al., 2006). Exposure to both forms of ultraviolet radiation can lead to skin cancer (AAD, 2009).

NURSING ALERT

Medications and Sunburn

Be certain to identify all over-the-counter and prescription medications the child is taking when obtaining a client history. Certain medications can increase the child's sensitivity to sunlight and result in sunburn.

Following exposure to ultraviolet light, the epidermal keratinocytes absorb the radiation, causing damage to their DNA (Guenther et al., 2007). This damage leads to the release of inflammatory mediators and cytokines. These molecules affect the blood vessels resulting in erythema, edema, and burning/stinging sensations (Lim & Wang, 2007). Also in response to the DNA damage, the body produces melanin which increases the pigmentation of the skin (AAD, 2009; Guenther et al., 2007; James et al., 2006). The resulting tan appearance begins two to three days after exposure, and lasts ten to fourteen days.

CLINICAL MANIFESTATIONS

The erythema of a typical UVB induced sunburn appears two to six hours following exposure (Guenther et al., 2007; James et al., 2006). The erythema reaches a peak in 12–36 hours and can persist for several days. When a UVA induced sunburn occurs, the erythema is immediate, peaks at eight hours, and persists for 24–48 hours (Guenther et al., 2007). Mild sunburns are characterized by erythema and warmth. Moderate to severe sunburns may manifest edema, vesicle formation, pain, and/or pruritus. Scaling or peeling follows a few days after the sun exposure. Severe sunburn may be associated with systemic symptoms such as tachycardia, nausea, abdominal cramping, weakness, malaise, fever, chills, and/or headache (Guenther et al., 2007; James et al., 2006).

DIAGNOSIS

The diagnosis of sunburn is based on history and the clinical presentation. The history should assess for recent ultraviolet radiation exposure, including the type, duration, and anatomic location of exposure. The physical exam should assess for indicators of sunburn severity including the extent of erythema and edema, the observance of vesicles and bullae, and the presence of systemic symptoms (AAD, 2009; Guenther et al., 2007; James et al., 2006).

TREATMENT

Because sunburns are self-limiting, they are most often managed with supportive measures such as cool compresses or baths, moisturizers, pramoxine lotion, and low potency topical corticosteroids (AAD, 2009; Guenther et al., 2007; James et al., 2006). Oral analgesics such as acetaminophen, aspirin, or ibuprofen are beneficial in relieving the associated pain (AAD, 2009; James et al., 2006). Topical anesthetic preparations pose the risk of contact dermatitis and should be avoided (AAD, 2009). If necessary, higher potency topical corticosteroids are beneficial in diminishing the inflammation and pain (James, et al., 2006). If blisters are present, they should be left intact to protect against secondary infection (AAD, 2009; Guenther et al., 2007). Severe sunburns may require admission to a burn unit for fluid replacement, pain control, and prophylaxis against infection (Guenther et al., 2007).

Experts agree that because of the potentially serious sequelae associated with ultraviolet radiation exposure, sunburn is better prevented than treated (AAD, 2009; Boe & Tillotson, 2007; Guenther et al., 2007; James et al., 2006). Box 30-12 lists the most commonly recommended precautions for protecting one's skin from ultraviolet radiation. When selecting protective clothing, features that provide more protection include synthetic fabrics, dark color, tight weave, loose fit, and dry fabrics (Boe & Tillotson, 2006; Guenther et al., 2007; James et al., 2006). Guidelines for proper sunscreen application are listed in Box 30-13.

It is currently recommended that everyone over 6 months of age use sunscreen daily to protect from sunburn, photoaging, and skin cancer (AAD, 2009; Lim & Wang, 2007). The risks and benefits of sunscreen use in children under 6 months of age are unknown. Some experts recommend against using sunscreen in young infants because of concerns about how much systemic absorption occurs, while others advise that sunscreen can be applied to infants under 6 months of age on limited areas (James et al., 2006; Lim & Wang, 2007; Meurer & Jamieson, 2006). Whenever possible, it is best to keep young infants covered with protective clothing and out of direct sunlight.

BOX 30-12
ULTRAVIOLET PROTECTION MEASURES

- Use a broad spectrum sunscreen with SPF 15 or higher
- Wear protective clothing such as long-sleeved shirt, pants, wide-brimmed hat, and sunglasses
- Seek the shade
- Avoid prolonged sun exposure when the UV index is high
- Avoid prolonged exposure between 10 am and 4 pm
- Avoid tanning beds

Adapted from: American Academy of Dermatology. (2009). *Facts about sunscreens*. Retrieved March 20, 2009, from http://www.aad.org/media/background/factsheets/fact_sunscreen.htm; Guenther, L., Barankin, B., & Powell, J. (2007). *Sunburn*. Retrieved March 20, 2009, from http://emedicine.medscape.com/article/911358-print.

BOX 30-13
PROPER SUNSCREEN APPLICATION

- Use a broad spectrum product with SPF 15 or higher
- Apply product to dry skin 15–60 minutes before exposure
- Use a generous amount and coat the skin liberally
- Reapply every two hours
- Reapply sooner if swimming, perspiring heavily, or toweling dry
- If swimming, use a waterproof product as this provides more protection than water-resistant or sweat-resistant products
- Check the expiration date of the sunscreen prior to use

Adapted from: American Academy of Dermatology. (2009). *Facts about sunscreens*. Retrieved March 20, 2009, from http://www.aad.org/media/background/factsheets/fact_sunscreen.htm; Guenther, L., Barankin, B., & Powell, J. (2007). *Sunburn*. Retrieved March 20, 2009, from http://emedicine.medscape.com/article/911358-print.

Both chemical and physical sunscreens are available. Chemical sunscreens absorb ultraviolet radiation whereas physical sunscreens block ultraviolet radiation (James et al., 2006). Physical sunscreens, such as titanium dioxide and zinc oxide, provide better sun protection but are thicker and more opaque (Guenther et al., 2007). Many high SPF sunscreens contain both chemical and physical sunscreens. The UVA and UVB protection offered by various sunscreens is described in Box 30-14. Among children and adolescents, sunscreen is the most commonly used method of sun protection (Boe & Tillotson, 2006; Cokkinides et al., 2006). Unfortunately, sunscreen provides inadequate protection for many children because it is not applied properly and is not used in conjunction with other ultraviolet protection behaviors.

NURSING MANAGEMENT

Assessment

Nurses should discuss with the child and caregivers the type and duration of ultraviolet radiation exposure as well as the use of any sun protection measures. Nurses should also ask about any over-the-counter or prescription medications that the child is taking that may increase his or her susceptibility to sunburn. Upon exam, the nurse should note the extent of the sunburn as well as the presence of edema or vesicles. The nursing assessment should also determine the presence of associated complications such as pain, nausea, fever, tachycardia, or headache.

Nursing Diagnosis

Nursing diagnoses appropriate for the child with sunburn include:

1. *Impaired skin integrity* related to epidermal injury secondary to the sunburn.
2. *Acute pain* related to inflammation secondary to injury from the sunburn.
3. *Risk for further injury from additional sun exposure.*
4. *Deficient knowledge* related to inadequate understanding of factors that increase the risk for sunburn and actions to decrease such risk.

Outcome Identification

1. Child will experience healing of the injured skin.
2. Child will experience relief from pain.
3. Child and caregivers will utilize appropriate sun protection measures to avoid sunburn in the future.
4. Child and caregivers will convey understanding of the factors that increase the risk of sun-related skin damage and actions to decrease that risk.

BOX 30-14
UVA AND UVB SUNSCREEN PROTECTION

The sun protection factor (SPF) is a measure of the sunscreen's ability to block UVB. There is currently no rating system for UVA protection. Instead the term "broad spectrum" is used to refer to products that protect against UVB and UVA radiation.

SPF is calculated by comparing the amount of time needed to produce a sunburn on unprotected vs. protected skin. For example, if a child could usually remain in the sun for 10 minutes without burning, he or she would be protected for 150 minutes when using a product with an SPF of 15. However, the SPF of a product is calculated in a laboratory setting under ideal conditions. In actual practice, most people only apply 20–60% the recommended amount of sunscreen and are consequently inadequately protected.

It is estimated that an SPF 15 sunscreen blocks 93% of the UVB rays and an SPF 30 sunscreen blocks 97% of the UVB rays. No sunscreen provides 100% protection. Therefore, sunscreens are best used in conjunction with other sun protection measures and should not be used to prolong sun exposure.

Adapted from: American Academy of Dermatology. (2009). *Facts about sunscreens*. Retrieved March 20, 2009, from http://www.aad.org/media/background/factsheets/fact_sunscreen.htm; Guenther, L., Barankin, B., & Powell, J. (2007). *Sunburn*. Retrieved March 20, 2009, from http://emedicine.medscape.com/article/911358-print.

Planning and Implementation

The nursing management of children with sunburn focuses on promoting healing of the injured skin, enhancing the child's comfort, and educating the child and caregivers regarding sun protection. Since sunburn is typically managed by the caregivers at home, nursing care focuses primarily on family education. This education should be provided prophylactically as well as after sunburn occurs. If nurses work in a school or public health setting, they may foster protection from ultraviolet radiation through the development of educational programs.

Evaluation

The child and caregivers are able to utilize strategies to promote comfort and healing following the sunburn. Consequently, the child will experience relief from pain and resolution of the sunburn. Caregivers, and when appropriate the affected child, will be able to convey understanding of the factors that increase the risk of sun-related skin damage. They will be able to describe and successfully implement appropriate sun protection measures to avoid sunburn in the future.

FAMILY TEACHING

The family teaching for children with sunburn and their caregivers should include education about the over-the-counter and prescription medication to promote comfort and healing such as cool compresses or baths, moisturizers, pramoxine lotion, and topical corticosteroids, as well as the use of acetaminophen, aspirin, or ibuprofen if needed for pain relief. If blisters are present, nurses should advise that they should be left intact to protect against secondary infection.

Family teaching should also focus on educating the child and caregivers about methods to reduce exposure to ultraviolet radiation in the future. This education should include information about the long-term consequences of ultraviolet radiation exposure such as skin cancer and photoaging. The child and caregivers should also be made aware that even tan skin that does not burn is damaged skin that can lead to undesirable consequences. Specific ultraviolet protection strategies should be discussed (see Box 30-12) as well as the proper use of sunscreens (see Box 30-13) and tips on selecting the appropriate sunscreen (see Box 30-14). Caregivers should also be taught about the UV index and encouraged to watch the local weather forecast for UV Index ratings (Guenther et al., 2007).

IN THE REAL WORLD

When I first started working in dermatology, I met a 14-year-old boy with acne. He made an impression on me because he was so challenging to talk to. He had long hair that he wore down over his face and he looked at his shoes most of the time we were together. Even when he was prodded by his mom, he would not make eye contact with me and he answered my questions with as few words as possible. I figured that he did not really want to be in our office and had just come in because his mom made him. Still, I did what I could to help him understand more about acne and what he could do to treat it. As he came back for follow-up visits, I was surprised to see that he had listened and was seeing improvement in his acne. His hair was still long, but after a few visits he was tucking it behind his ears and looking me in the eye as we talked. He started to open up and it turns out that he had a really fun personality. It was so amazing to see what a dramatic effect having clear skin had on his attitude and self-esteem! I was also so grateful that I did not discount him the first time we met. It would have been tragic if I did not try very hard to help him because of my misperception that his withdrawn attitude meant he did not care. As it turns out, his behaviors were just an indication that he was one of the people who needed my help the most.

Because infants and young children are dependent on their caregivers to provide them with adequate sun protection, teaching for this age group should be aimed at the caregiver. Older children and adolescents are generally able to assume greater self-care responsibilities, so education for this population should be directed toward the child as well as the caregivers. Educational interventions should be initiated as soon as possible, because interventions for younger children are often more successful than those for adolescents (Boe & Tillotson, 2006). Furthermore, the use of ultraviolet protection behaviors by caregivers should be encouraged as well since research has shown that caregiver vigilance and the caregiver's own sun protection behaviors are related to greater sun protection practices and reduced likelihood of sunburn in their children (Boe & Tillotson, 2006; Cokkinides et al., 2006).

KEY CONCEPTS

- The skin consists of three distinct layers: the epidermis, the dermis, and the subcutaneous tissue.
- The integumentary system provides a protective barrier against infectious organisms, external agents, and mechanical trauma.

- Although integumentary disorders are rarely life-threatening, they can have a major impact on the child's comfort and social functioning.
- Impetigo is a highly contagious, superficial bacterial skin infection that can manifest in a bullous or nonbullous form.
- Cellulitis is an acute, spreading inflammation of the skin and subcutaneous tissue that is characterized by a painful area of warm, swollen erythema.
- Candidiasis commonly presents during infancy in the oral cavity or diaper area, though other anatomic locations and age groups may be affected.
- Tinea capitis is a fungal infection of the scalp and hair shaft that is associated with scaling, pruritus, and hair loss.
- Tinea corporis is a superficial fungal infection that can appear as a ring shaped eruption on most areas of the body.
- Tinea pedis and tinea unguium are fungal infections of the feet and nails that often require the implementation of measures to prevent recurrence of the infection.
- Verrucae and molluscum contagiosum are superficial cutaneous viral infections that result in the formation of single or multiple benign epidermal lesions.
- Herpes simplex virus type I (HSV-1) is an incurable viral infection that can cause primary and recurrent oral lesions in infected children.
- Pediculosis capitis and scabies are cutaneous conditions caused by ectoparasites that can cause pruritus as well as embarrassment, depression, or social stigma.
- Atopic dermatitis is a chronic, pruritic, inflammatory skin condition characterized by disease remissions and flares that can have a significant impact on the quality of life of the affected child and his/her caregivers.
- Contact dermatitis can occur as a local, nonimmunologic reaction to an irritant or as an immune-mediated hypersensitivity response to a contact allergen.
- Diaper dermatitis is an irritant contact dermatitis that is often managed by implementing hygienic measures.
- Seborrheic dermatitis may manifest as a self-limiting inflammatory condition on the scalp of infants or among adolescents as an often chronic eruption characterized by flaking, erythema, and pruritus.
- Acne is a chronic cutaneous disorder that is caused by underlying physiologic dysfunction and is commonly associated with scarring, emotional distress, and poor adherence to treatment.
- Animal bites can inflict extensive damage and introduce polymicrobial infection, particularly among young children.
- Arthropod bites and stings can transfer serious diseases or cause potentially fatal allergic reactions.
- Sunburns, as well as tanned skin, are manifestations of sun damage that indicate the need to utilize ultraviolet protection measures in order to reduce the occurrence of skin cancer.

REVIEW ACTIVITIES

1. What are the various functions of the skin?
2. How do racial and age-based skin differences influence nursing care?
3. How does the clinical presentation and management of impetigo differ from that of cellulitis?
4. What treatment options are available for infants with cradle cap?
5. What steps can children and caregivers take to prevent the spread and recurrence of various tinea infections?
6. What are the advantages and disadvantages of different treatment alternatives for warts and molluscum contagiosum?
7. What are the factors that have been implicated in the reactivation of herpes simplex virus type I infections?
8. How should caregivers clean the home environment after a child has been diagnosed with head lice or scabies?
9. What strategies can children and caregivers utilize to avoid common atopic dermatitis triggers?
10. How does the pathophysiology of allergic contact dermatitis differ from that of irritant dermatitis?
11. How can nurses distinguish between irritant diaper dermatitis and diaper dermatitis caused by *Candida albicans*?
12. How can nurses encourage acne treatment adherence among adolescents?
13. What measures can children and caregivers take to avoid injuries from dog bites?
14. What guidelines should nurses share with caregivers about the use of DEET insect repellents in children?
15. What are the recommended measures for reducing ultraviolet radiation exposure among children?

STUDY QUESTIONS

1. Which of the following has no bearing on a child's risk for developing candidiasis? The one who:
   a. Is taking oral antibiotics.
   b. Is a female.
   c. Is immunocompromised.
   d. Uses a steroid inhaler.
2. When assessing a child for tinea capitis, what would be a clinical manifestation of an uncomplicated case?
   a. Hair loss
   b. Scaling
   c. Honey-colored crusts
   d. Pustules
3. When teaching a mother about head lice treatments, which product should the nurse recommend as a first-line option for children?
   a. Petroleum jelly
   b. Permethrin
   c. Lindane
   d. Trimethoprim/sulfamethoxazole
4. Which of the following is not one of the four factors involved in the pathophysiology of acne?
   a. Proliferation of *Staphylococcus aureus*
   b. The body's inflammatory response
   c. Sebum production
   d. Abnormal epithelial keratinization
5. When educating children and caregivers about sunscreen application, which one of the following instructions is accurate?
   a. Use a broad spectrum product with at least SPF 45 or higher.
   b. Reapply the sunscreen every three hours.
   c. Sweat-resistant products last longer than waterproof products.
   d. Reapply sooner than recommended if swimming, perspiring heavily, or toweling dry.
6. When educating caregivers about preventing irritant diaper dermatitis, which one of the following instructions should be included?
   a. Use barrier creams such as zinc oxide to protect the skin.
   b. Use cloth diapers because they have natural fibers.
   c. Minimize the frequency of diaper changes to prevent irritation.
   d. Use baby wipes with alcohol to keep the area dry.
7. Which pathogen is the least likely to cause pediatric impetigo and cellulitis?
   a. *Staphylococcus aureus*
   b. *Pseudomonas aeruginosa*
   c. *Streptococcus pyogenes.*
   d. Community-acquired methicillin-resistant *Staphylococcus aureus*
8. When teaching parents, the nurse counsels them that which infection may recur because it remains dormant in the dorsal root ganglia of the nervous system?
   a. Tinea unguium
   b. Molluscum contagiosum
   c. Herpes simplex
   d. Candidiasis
9. When treating children with atopic dermatitis, which one of the following is not a treatment priority?
   a. Repairing and maintaining the stratum corneum
   b. Eradicating *S. aureus* colonization
   c. Reducing inflammation
   d. Stopping the itch-scratch cycle
10. What is the primary medical therapy for children who experience anaphylaxis from a bee sting?
    a. Oral corticosteroid (Prednisone)
    b. Pramoxine
    c. Diphenhydramine (Benadryl)
    d. Epinephrine

REFERENCES

Ali, S., Graham, T. A., & Forgie, S. E. (2007). The assessment and management of tinea capitis in children. *Pediatric Emergency Care, 23*(9), 662–665.

Allen, P. L. (2006). Leaves of three, let them be: If it were only that easy! *Dermatology Nursing, 18*(3), 236–242.

Alter, S. (2007). *Herpes simplex virus infection.* Retrieved March 20, 2009, from http://emedicine.medscape.com/article/964866-print.

American Academy of Dermatology. (2009). *Facts about sunscreens.* Retrieved March 20, 2009, from http://www.aad.org/media/background/factsheets/fact_sunscreen.htm.

Amin, K., Riddle, C. C., Aires, D. J., & Schweiger, E. S. (2007). Common and alternate oral antibiotic therapies for acne vulgaris: A review. *Journal of Drugs in Dermatology, 6*(9), 873–880.

Bernard, P. (2008). Management of common bacterial infections of the skin. *Current Opinion on Infectious Diseases, 21*(2), 122–128.

Bieber, T. (2008). Atopic dermatitis. *New England Journal of Medicine, 358*(14), 1483–1494.

Blumberg, M., Kantor, G. R., & Ratz, J. (2007). *Onychomycosis.* Retrieved March 20, 2009, from http://emedicine.medscape.com/article/1105828-print.

Boe, K., & Tillotson, E. A. (2006). Encouraging sun safety for children and adolescents. *Journal of School Nursing, 22*(3), 136–141.

Boschert, S. (2008). Pros and cons of pediatric wart therapy weighed. *Skin & Allergy News, 39*(9), 46–47.

Buys, L. M. (2007). Treatment options for atopic dermatitis. *American Family Physician, 75*(4), 523–528.

Centers for Disease Control and Prevention. (2007). Compendium of animal rabies prevention and control, 2007. *Morbidity & Mortality Weekly Report, 56*(22), 1–8.

Centers for Disease Control and Prevention. (2008a). *Head lice treatment.* Retrieved March 20, 2009, from http://www.cdc.gov/lice/head/treatment.html.

Centers for Disease Control and Prevention. (2008b). *Dog bite prevention.* Retrieved March 20, 2009, from http://www.cdc.gov/HomeandRecreationalSafety/Dog-Bites/biteprevention.html.

Chayavichitsilp, P., & Barrio, V. (2007). Choosing the best treatment to eradicate lice infestations. *Practical Dermatology, 4*(11), 43–47.

Chosidow, O. (2006). Scabies. *New England Journal of Medicine, 354,* 1718–1727.

Cokkinides, V., Weinstock, M., Glanz, K., Albano, J., Ward, E., & Thun, M. (2006). Trends in sunburns, sun protection practices, and attitudes toward sun exposure protection and tanning among US adolescents, 1998–2004. *Pediatrics, 118*(3), 853–864.

Collier, C. N., Harper, J. C., Cantrell, W. C., Wang, W., Foster, K. W., & Elewski, B. E. (2008). The prevalence of acne in adults 20 years and older. *Journal of the American Academy of Dermatology, 58*(1), 56–59.

Crawford, F., & Hollis, S. (2007). Topical treatments for fungal infections of the skin and nails of the foot. *Cochrane Database of Systematic Reviews,* 3(CD001434).

Dawson, T. L. (2006) Malassezia and seborrheic dermatitis: Etiology and treatment. *Journal of Cosmetic Science, 57*(2), 181–182.

Dohil, M. A., Lin, P., Lee, J., Lucky, A. W., Paller, A. S., & Eichenfield, L. F. (2006). The epidemiology of molluscum contagiosum in children. *Journal of the American Academy of Dermatology, 54,* 47–54.

Drugge, J. M., & Allen, P. J. (2008). A nurse practitioner's guide to the management of herpes simplex virus-1 in children. *Dermatology Nursing, 20*(6), 455–466.

Dupuy, A., Dehen, L., Bourrat, E., Lacroix, C. Benderdouche, M., Dubertret, L., Morel, P., Feuilhade de Chauvin, M., & Petit, A. (2007). Accuracy of standard dermoscopy for diagnosing scabies. *Journal of the American Academy of Dermatology. 56*(1), 53–62.

Elish, D., & Silverberg, N. B. (2006). Infantile seborrheic dermatitis. *Cutis, 77*(5), 297–300.

Elston, D. M. (2007a). Community-acquired methicillin-resistant Staphylococcus aureus. *Journal of the American Academy of Dermatology, 56,* 1–16.

Elston, D. M. (2007b). *Insect bites.* Retrieved March 20, 2009, from http://emedicine.medscape.com/article/1088253-print.

Fatahzadeh, M., & Schwartz, R. A. (2007). Human herpes simplex virus infections: Epidemiology, pathogenesis, symptomatology, diagnosis and management. *Journal of the American Academy of Dermatology, 57,* 737–763.

Fitzpatrick, T. B. (1988). The validity and practicality of sun-reactive skin types I through IV. *Archives of Dermatology, 124,* 86–871.

Fleischer, A. B. (2008). Diagnosis and management of common dermatoses in children: Atopic, seborrheic, and contact dermatitis. *Clinical Pediatrics, 47*(4), 332–346.

Gabillot-Carre, M., & Roujeau, J. C. (2007). Acute bacterial skin infections and cellulitis. *Current Opinion on Infectious Diseases, 20*(2), 118–123.

Gawkrodger, D. J. (2008). *Dermatology: An illustrated colour text* (4th ed.). Philadelphia, PA: Elsevier.

Gibbs, S., & Harvey, I. (2009). Topical treatments for cutaneous warts. *Cochrane Database of Systematic Reviews,* 3(CD001781).

Gonzalez, U., Seaton, T., Bergus, G., Jacobson, J., & Martinez-Monzon, C. (2007). Systemic antifungal therapy for tinea capitis in children. *Cochrane Database of Systematic Reviews,* 4(CD004685).

Grimalt, R. (2007). A practical guide to scalp disorders. *Journal of Investigative Dermatology Symposium Proceedings, 12*(2), 10–14 (ISSN: 1087-0024).

Guenther, L., Barankin, B., & Powell, J. (2007). *Sunburn.* Retrieved March 20, 2009, from http://emedicine.medscape.com/article/911358-print.

Hanifin, J. M., & Rajka, G. (1980). Diagnostic features of atopic dermatitis. *Acta Dermatovenerology, 92*(Suppl.), 44–47.

Hanna, D., Hatami, A., Powell, J., Marcoux, D., Maari, C., Savard, P. et al. (2006). A prospective randomized trial comparing the efficacy and adverse effects of four recognized treatments of molluscum contagiosum in children. *Pediatric Dermatology, 23*(6), 574–579.

Hernandez, R. G., & Cohen, B. A. (2006). Insect bite-induced hypersensitivity and the SCRATCH principles: A new approach to papular urticaria. *Pediatrics, 118*(1), e189–196.

Heukelbach, J., & Feldmeier, H. (2006) Scabies. *Lancet, 367*(9524), 1767–1774.

Hirschmann, J. V. (2007). Antimicrobial therapy for skin infections. *Cutis, 79*(Supp. 6), 26–36.

Hughes, R., Ward, D., Tobin, A. M., Keegan, K., & Kirby, B. (2007). The use of alternative medicine in pediatric patients with atopic dermatitis. *Pediatric Dermatology, 24*(2), 118–120.

Humphrey, S., Bergman, J. N., & Au, S. (2006). Practical management strategies for diaper dermatitis. *Skin Therapy Letter, 11*(7), 1–6.

Jacobson, C. C., & Abel, E. A. (2007). Parasitic infestations. *Journal of the American Academy of Dermatology, 56,* 1026–1043.

James, W. D., Berger, T. G., & Elston, D. M. (2006). *Andrew's diseases of the skin: Clinical dermatology* (10th ed.). Philadelphia, PA: Elsevier.

Jancin, B. (2007). Pediatric skin diseases strongly affect life quality. *Skin & Allergy News, 38*(5), 51.

Johnston, G., & Mansouri, Y. (2007). Common rashes in children. *British Journal of Hospital Medicine, 68*(8), M130–M132.

Kalyoussef, S., Tolan, R. W., & Greenberg, M. E. (2008). *Candidiasis.* Retrieved March 20, 2009, from http://emedicine.medscape.com/article/962300-print.

Katz, T. M., Miller, J. H., & Herbert, A. A. (2008). Insect repellents: Historical perspectives and new developments. *Journal of the American Academy of Dermatology, 58*(5), 865–871.

Kiken, D. A., & Silverberg, N. B. (2006a). Atopic dermatitis in children, Part 1: Epidemiology, clinical features, and complications. *Cutis, 78,* 241–247.

Kiken, D. A., & Silverberg, N. B. (2006b). Atopic dermatitis in children, Part 2: Treatment options. *Cutis, 78,* 401–406.

Krakowski, A. C., Eichenfield, L. F., & Dohil, M. A. (2008). Management of atopic dermatitis in the pediatric population. *Pediatrics, 122,* 812–824.

Kyle, T., & Kyle, T. (2007). *Essentials of pediatric nursing.* Philadelphia, PA: Lippincott Williams & Wilkins.

Lawton, S. (2006a). Anatomy and function of the skin, part 2. *Nursing Times, 102*(32), 28–29.

Lawton, S. (2006b). Anatomy and function of the skin, part 3. *Nursing Times, 102*(33), 26–27.

Lawton, S. (2006c). Anatomy and function of the skin, part 4. *Nursing Times, 102*(34), 26–27.

Lebwohl, M., Clark, L., & Levitt, J. (2007). Therapy for head lice based on life cycle, resistance, and safety considerations. *Pediatrics, 119*(5), 965–974.

Leone, P. A. (2007). Scabies and pediculosis pubis: An update of treatment regimens and general review. *Clinical Infectious Diseases, 44*(Supp. 3), S153–S159.

Leung, D. Y. M., Bogunmiewicz, M., Howell, M. D., Nomura, I., & Hamid, Q. A. (2004). New insights into atopic dermatitis. *Journal of Clinical Investigation, 113,* 651–657.

Lewis, F. S., & Smith, L. J. (2007). What's eating you? Bees, part 1: Characteristics, reactions, and management. *Cutis, 79,* 439–444.

Lim, H. W., & Wang, S. Q. (2007). The skin cancer foundation's guide to sunscreens. *The Melanoma Letter, 25*(2), 1–5.

Lott, M. E., Zember, G., & Lesher, J. L. (2008). *Tinea corporis.* Retrieved March 20, 2009, from http://emedicine.medscape.com/article/1091473-print

Magin, P., Adams, J., Heading, G., Pond, D., & Smith, W. (2006). The causes of acne: A qualitative study of patient perceptions of acne causation and their implications for acne care. *Dermatology Nursing, 18*(4), 344–349, 370.

Mansouri, Y., & Johnston, G. (2007). Common rashes in children: 2. *British Journal of Hospital Medicine, 68*(9), M166–M168.

McNamara, D. (2008a). Consider patient when choosing molluscum tx. *Skin & Allergy News, 39*(4), 26.

McNamara, D. (2008b). Answering parents' questions about DEET, "natural" repellents. *Skin & Allergy News, 39*(4), 36.

Meurer, L. N., & Jamieson, B. (2006). What is the appropriate use of sunscreens for infants and children? *The Journal of Family Practice, 55*(5), 437, 440, 444.

Micali, G., Dhawan, V. K., & Nasca, M. R. (2009). *Cellulitis.* Retrieved March 20, 2009, from http://emedicine.medscape.com/article/1053686-print.

Militello, G., Jacob, S. E., & Crawford, G. H. (2006). Allergic contact dermatitis in children. *Current Opinion in Pediatrics, 8*(4), 385–390.

Muirhead, G. (2007). Take a culture to confirm pediatric tinea capitis. *Skin & Allergy News, 38*(10), 33.

Nelson, K. C., & Morrell, D. S. (2007). Spreading bumps: Molluscum contagiosum in the pediatric population. *Pediatric Annals, 36*(12), 814–818.

Neumann, B. (2009). Management of dog and cat bites. *Advance for Nurse Practitioners, 17*(3), 53–54.

Nield, L. S., & Kamat, D. (2007). Prevention, diagnosis, and management of diaper dermatitis. *Clinical Pediatrics, 46*(6), 480–486.

Nijhawan, R. I., Matiz, C., & Jacob, S. E. (2009). Contact dermatitis: From basics to allergodromes. *Pediatric Annals, 38*(2), 99–108.

Page, T. L., Eiff, P., & Judkins, D. Z. (2007). When should you treat scabies empirically? *The Journal of Family Practice, 56*(7), 570–572.

Peterson, J. D., & Chan, L. S. (2006). A comprehensive management guide for atopic dermatitis. *Dermatology Nursing, 18*(6), 531–542.

Pleacher, M. D., & Dexter, W. W. (2007). Cutaneous fungal and viral infections in athletes. *Clinical Journal of Sport Medicine, 26*(3), 397–411.

Rawlings, A. V. (2006). Ethnic skin types: Are there differences in skin structure and function? *International Journal of Cosmetic Science, 28*(2), 79–93.

Robbins, C. M., & Elewski, B. E. (2008). *Tinea pedis.* Retrieved March 20, 2009, from http://emedicine.medscape.com/article/1091684-print.

Roebuck, H. L. (2006). Acne: Intervene early. *Nurse Practitioner, 31*(10), 24–43.

Ross, K. (2008). Head lice, resistance, and malathion. *Pediatrics, 121*(1), 222–223.

Rudy, S. J. (2007). Pediatric dermatology: Fungal/yeast infections, viral infections, acne, and hemangiomas. *Dermatology Nursing, 19*(5), 507–508.

Sarabi, K., & Khachemoune, A. (2007). Tinea capitis: A review. *Dermatology Nursing, 19*(6), 525–529.

Schalamon, J., Ainoedhofer, H., Singer, G., Petnehazy, T., Mayr, J., Kiss, K., et al. (2006). Analysis of dog bites in children who are younger than 17 years. *Pediatrics, 117*(3), e374–e379.

Schwartz, R. A., Janusz, C. A., & Janniger, C. K. (2006). Seborrheic dermatitis: An overview. *American Family Physician, 74*(1), 125–130.

Sciscione, P., & Krause-Parello, C. A. (2008). No-nit policies in schools: Time for change. *Journal of School Nursing, 23*(1), 13–20.

Serota, J. A. (2006). A bite in the night. *Journal of Pediatric Health Care, 20*(6): 407, 431–432.

Sethi, A., & Antaya, R. (2006). Systemic antifungal therapy for cutaneous infections in children. *Pediatric Infectious Disease Journal, 25*(7), 643–644.

Sheffield, R. C., & Wright, S. T. (2007). What's the best treatment for cradle cap? *Journal of Family Practice, 56*(3), 232–233.

Sicherer, S. H., & Simons, F. E. (2007). Self-injectable epinephrine for first-aid management of anaphylaxis. *Pediatrics, 119*(3), 638–646.

Sidbury, R., & Poorsattar, S. (2006). Pediatric atopic dermatitis: Should we treat it differently? *Dermatologic Therapy, 19*(2), 83–90.

Silva, L., Alencar, R., & Madeira, N. G. (2008). Survey assessment of parental perceptions regarding head lice. *International Journal of Dermatology, 47*(3), 249–255.

Spanierman, C. S. (2008). *Animal bites.* Retrieved March 20, 2009, from http://emedicine.medscape.com/article/925827-print.

Strauss, J. S., Krowchuk, D. P., Leyden, J. J., Lucky, A. W., Shalita, A. R., Siegfried, E. C., et al. (2007). Guidelines of care for acne vulgaris management. *Journal of the American Academy of Dermatology, 56,* 651–663.

Strong, M., & Johnstone, P. (2007). Interventions for treating scabies. *Cochrane Database of Systematic Reviews,* 3(CD000320).

Swanson, D. S. (2006). Methicillin-resistant Staphylococcus aureus infections in children. *Missouri Medicine, 103*(1), 77–80.

Theos, A. (2007). Diagnosis and management of superficial cutaneous fungal infections in children. *Pediatric Annals, 36*(1), 46–54.

Trovato, M. J., Schwartz, R. A., & Janniger, C. K. (2006). Tinea capitis: Current concepts in clinical practice. *Cutis, 77,* 93–99.

Vankawala, H. H., & Park, R. (2008). *Bee and hymenoptera stings.* Retrieved March 20, 2009, from http://emedicine.medscape.com/article/768764-print.

Webster, G. F. (2008). Commentary: Diet and acne. *Journal of the American Academy of Dermatology, 58*(5), 794–795.

Webster, G. F. (2009). Acne: Tips and tricks for the pediatrician. *Pediatric Annals, 38*(2), 80–83.

Wenner, R., Askari, S. K., Cham, P. M., Kedrowski, D. A., Liu, A., & Warshaw, E. M. (2007). Duct tape for the treatment of common warts in adults. *Archives of Dermatology, 143,* 309–313.

Wyndham, M. (2008). Head lice. *Community Practitioner, 81*(2), 33.

Xu, F., Lee, F. K., Morrow, R. A., Sternberg, M. R., Luther, K. E., Dubin, G., et al. (2007). Seroprevalence of herpes simplex virus type 1 in children in the United States. *Journal of Pediatrics, 51*(4), 374–377.

Zaenglein, A. L., & Thiboutot, D. M. (2006). Expert committee recommendations for acne management. *Pediatrics, 118,* 1188–1199.

SUGGESTED READINGS

Andresen, K., & McCarthy, A. M. (2009). A policy change strategy for head lice management. *Journal of School Nursing, 25*(6), 407–416.

Andrews, R. M., McCarthy, J., Carapetis, J. R., & Currie, B. J. (2009). Skin disorders, including pyoderma, scabies and tinea infections. *Pediatric Clinics of North America, 56*(6), 1421–1440.

Cercato, M. C., Nagore, E., Ramazzotti, V., Guillén, C., Terranoto, I., Villena, J., Lomuscio, M., Natali, P. G., & Schünemann, H. J. (2008). Self and parent-assessed skin cancer risk factors in school-age children. *Preventive Medicine, 47*(1), 133–135.

de Haen, M., Spigt, M. G., van Uden, C. J. T., van Neer, P., Feron, F. J. M., & Knottnerus, A. (2006). Efficacy of duct tape vs placebo in the treatment of verruca vulgaris (warts) in primary school children. *Archives of Pediatric & Adolescent Medicine, 160*(11), 1121–1125.

Eichenfield, L. F. (2009). Atopic dermatitis update. *Dermatology Nursing, 21*(5), 299–300.

Friedlander, S. F., Eichenfield, L. F., Leyden, J., Shu, J., & Spellman, M. C. (2009). Diaper dermatitis—appropriate evaluation & optimal management strategies. *Contemporary Pediatrics*, 2–14s.

Martel, M. J., Beauschesne, M. F., Malo, J. L., Rey, E., Perreault, S., Forget, A., & Blais, L. (2009). Maternal asthma, its control and severity in pregnancy, and the incidence of atopic dermatitis and allergic rhinitis in the offspring. *Journal of Pediatrics, 155*(5), 707–713.

RESOURCES

Refer to the online student StudyWARE for Potts & Mandleco at http://www.CengageBrain.com for additional content and study aids.

Organization: **American Academy of Dermatology**
Description: An organization of dermatologists that provides education for health care providers and patients. They are also active in promoting public interest in dermatology topics as well as advocating for public policy changes relevant to dermatology. The website offers information regarding practice management, government/advocacy, guidelines, and research.
Website/Resource: http://www.aad.org
Patient education website: http://www.skincarephysicians.com

Organization: **American Contact Dermatitis Society**
A society of health care providers that provides professional education about allergic contact dermatitis. They also have a Contact Allergen Replacement Database (CARD) that can be helpful when educating patients about specific contact allergens. The website also offers access to information regarding meetings and journal articles.
Website/Resource: http://www.contactderm.org

Organization: **DermIS**
A European based website that offers a large variety of information on dermatology topics. The brief overviews provided are focused on laypersons. The site also has an extensive atlas of dermatology images and case reports.
Website/Resource: http://www.dermis.net

Organization: **EMedicine**
An educational website focused on providing up-to-date medical information for health care professionals. Their dermatology page offers numerous articles on dermatology topics that can be viewed free of charge.
Website/Resource: http://emedicine.medscape.com

Organization: **Inflammatory Skin Disease Institute**
An institute that endeavors to promote public awareness of inflammatory skin diseases. In addition to providing patient advocacy, they provide education for health care providers and patients for issues ranging from treatment options to lifestyle issues. They also facilitate patient support groups.
Website/Resource: http://www.isdionline.org

Organization: **National Eczema Association**
An association that is committed to improving the health and quality of life of those with eczema. They provide education for health care providers and patients as well as support groups and patient conferences.
Website/Resource: http://www.nationaleczema.org

Organization: **National Pediculosis Association**
An association focused on encouraging the adoption of standardized head lice management programs as well as keeping children in school and protecting children from the misuse and abuse of potentially harmful pesticidal treatments. They provide educational resources for adults who are involved in the care of children as well as activities for children.
Website/Resource: http://www.headlice.org

Organization: **New Zealand Dermatological Society**
A professional organization for health care providers in New Zealand that also endeavors to provide accurate information for both consumers and health care professionals around the world. Their website provides educational overviews on a large variety of dermatology topics.
Website/Resource: http://www.dermnetnz.org

Organization: **Skin Cancer Foundation**
A foundation that aims to increase awareness and provide education about skin cancer. Both public and medical education efforts focus on promoting sun protection as well as the need for early detection and prompt, effective treatment.
Website/Resource: http://www.skincancer.org

Organization: **The Society for Pediatric Dermatology**
A society of health care providers focused on improving the care that is provided to children with dermatologic diseases. They provide education to health care providers as well as advocate for public and government awareness of pediatric skin disease.
Website/Resource: http://www.pedsderm.net

Organization: **U.S. National Library of Medicine and National Institutes of Health**
An American website that contains a variety of educational information for both patients and health care professionals. Within their section on skin condition, covered topics include general dermatology information, statistics, disease specific information, and clinical photographs.
Website/Resource: http://www.nlm.nih.gov

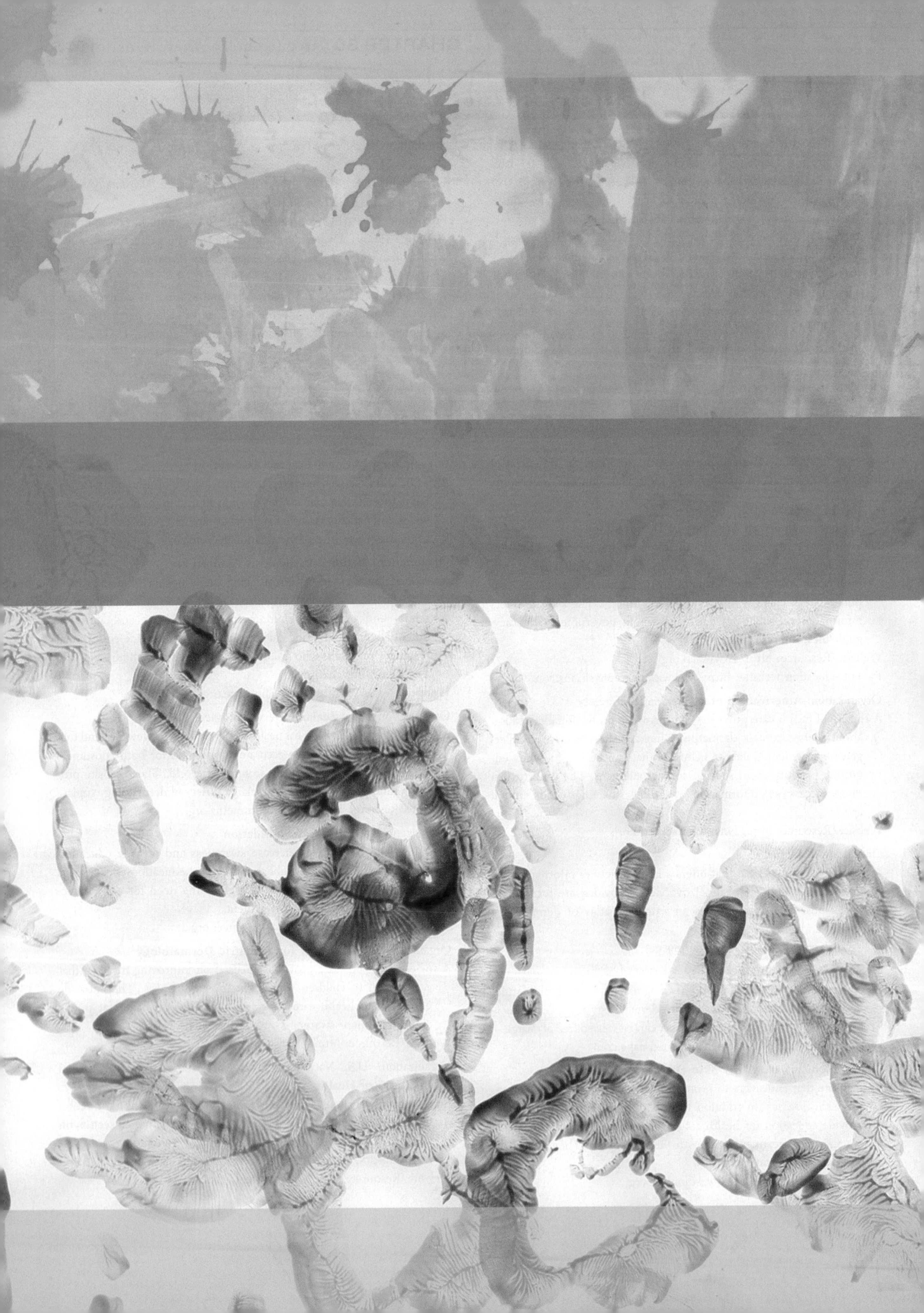

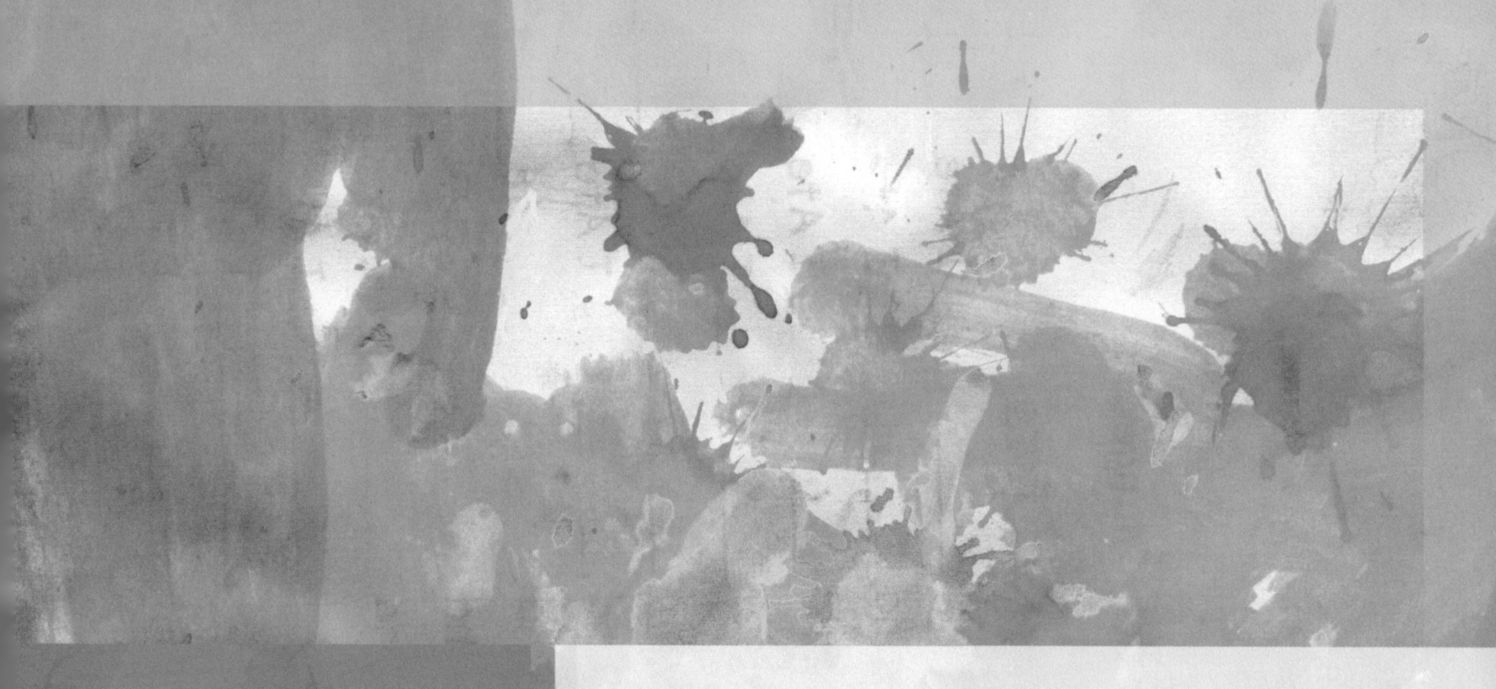

UNIT 7 Alterations in Sensorimotor Function

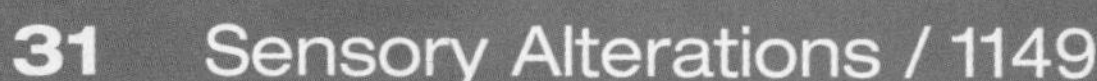

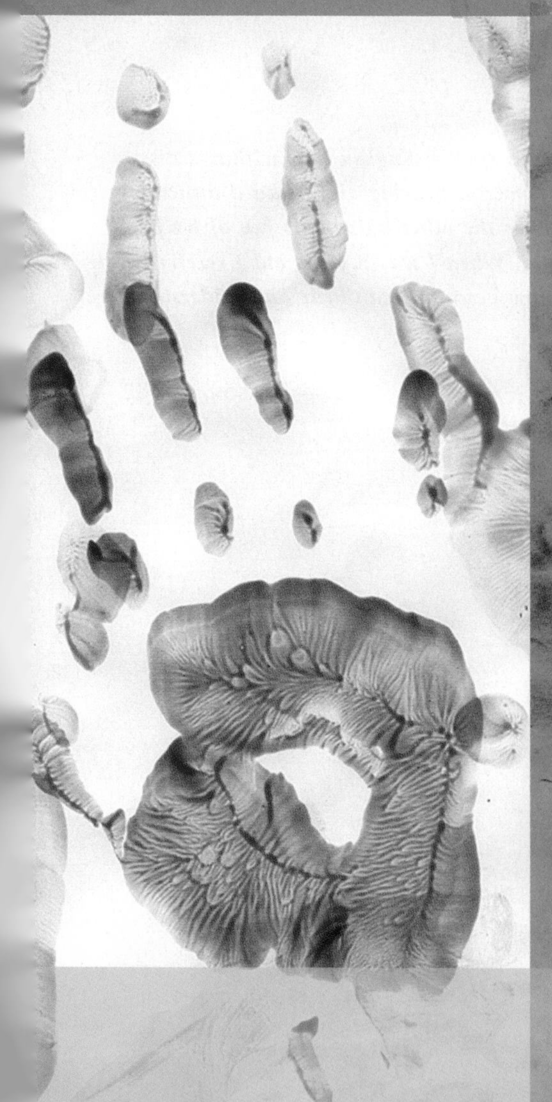

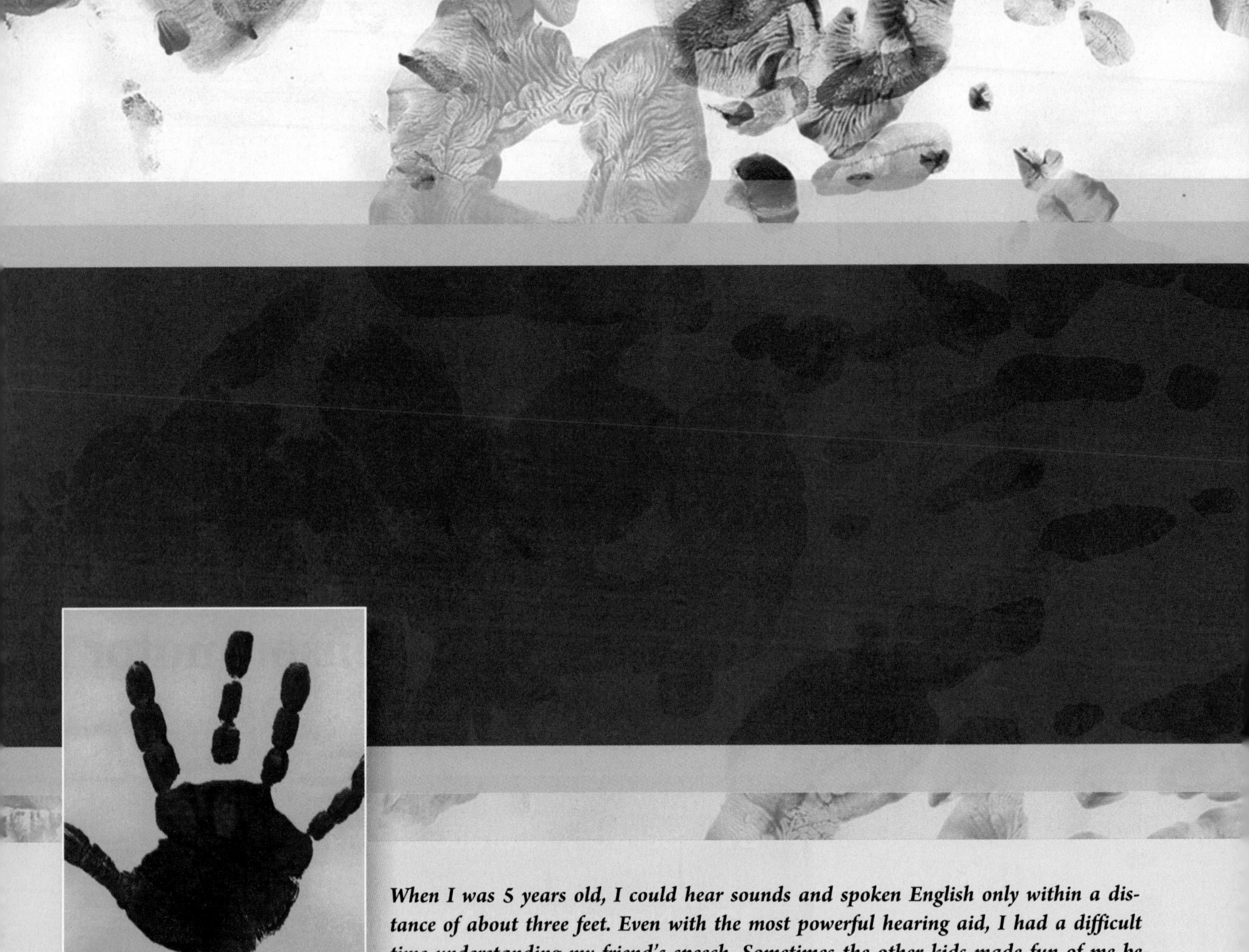

When I was 5 years old, I could hear sounds and spoken English only within a distance of about three feet. Even with the most powerful hearing aid, I had a difficult time understanding my friend's speech. Sometimes the other kids made fun of me because I couldn't hear; they thought I was stupid. When I was 8 years old I received a cochlear implant. My whole life has changed now because I can hear and understand my friends. Now my friends think I am smart.

—Jackson, Age 12

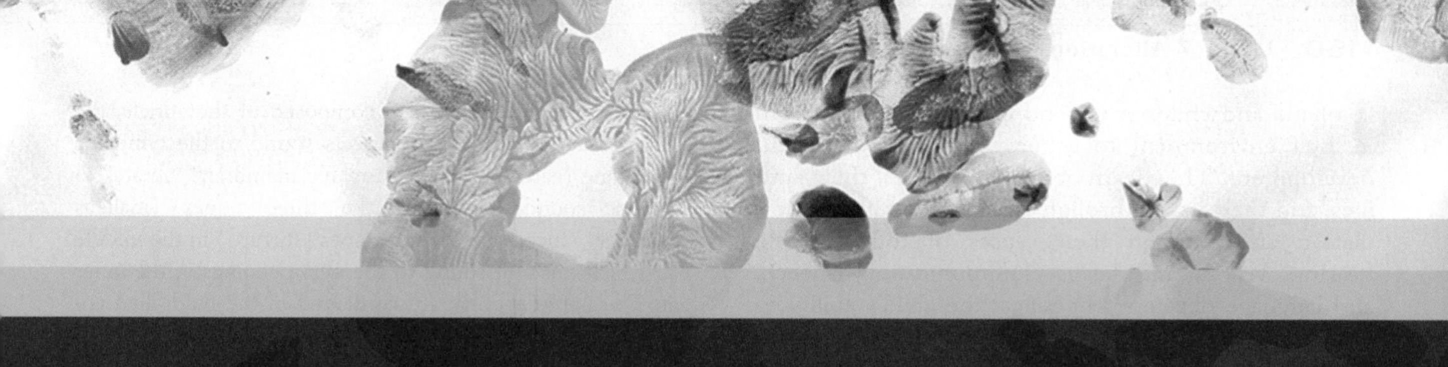

CHAPTER 31
Sensory Alterations

Debra Ann Mills, RN, MS

COMPETENCIES

Upon completion of this chapter, the reader will be able to:

- Identify how eye and ear structures differ between infants or children and adults.
- Describe the etiology of common childhood vision, hearing, and communication disorders.
- Describe why it is sometimes difficult to identify children with language disorders.
- Describe childhood language and speech disorders as they relate to sensory alterations.
- Describe current screening tests available to identify common hearing and vision impairments in children.
- Identify common hearing and vision impairments experienced by children.
- Describe the roles of the nurse and other interdisciplinary health care team members in the prevention, identification, and management of sensory disorders in children.
- Describe the nurse's role in promoting optimum development of children with sensory impairment.
- Discuss the nurse's role in providing support to families with children with sensory impairment.
- Identify prevention strategies useful in promoting safety of the eyes and ears.
- Successfully complete the games and activities in the online student StudyWARE.

Infants and children depend on sensory input from their environment to achieve normal growth and development. They learn about themselves, their families, and their world through visual and auditory stimulation and through their senses of touch, smell, hearing, vision, and taste. Communication, speech, and language development reflect the child's ability to interact with the outside environment in response to stimulation and sensations received. As members of the health care team, nurses have many opportunities to recognize sensory alterations and intervene early. Early intervention assists the child and families create an environment where optimal growth and development may be achieved. This chapter focuses on the nurse's role in caring for children with sensory impairments. Nursing management includes providing support and education for the child and family, education regarding prevention and treatment of traumatic injuries to sensory organs, and information regarding resources to support the child and family at home and in the community.

ANATOMY AND PHYSIOLOGY

The following discussion explains the anatomy of the ear and eye and discusses how structures differ between children and adults.

EAR

The ear has three main sections: the outer ear, the middle ear, and the inner ear (Figure 31-1) responsible not only for the sense of hearing, but also establishes the sense of equilibrium. The outer ear is composed of the auricle, the external auditory canal that directs sound to the tympanic membrane (eardrum). The tympanic membrane vibrates to conduct sound waves to the three bones (malleus [hammer], incus [anvil], and stapes [stirrup]) in the middle ear, which transmit sound to the nerve endings in the inner ear. The nerve endings are contained in the fluid-filled cochlea, which transmits the sound waves to the auditory nerve in the brain. The inner ear also contains the semicircular canal that maintains balance and body position. The Eustachian tube connects the middle ear with the nasopharynx. It allows fluid to drain into the nasopharynx and equalizes pressure between the outer and middle ear. Infants and young children have shorter, more horizontal, and more flaccid eustachian tubes than adults, predisposing them to middle ear infections.

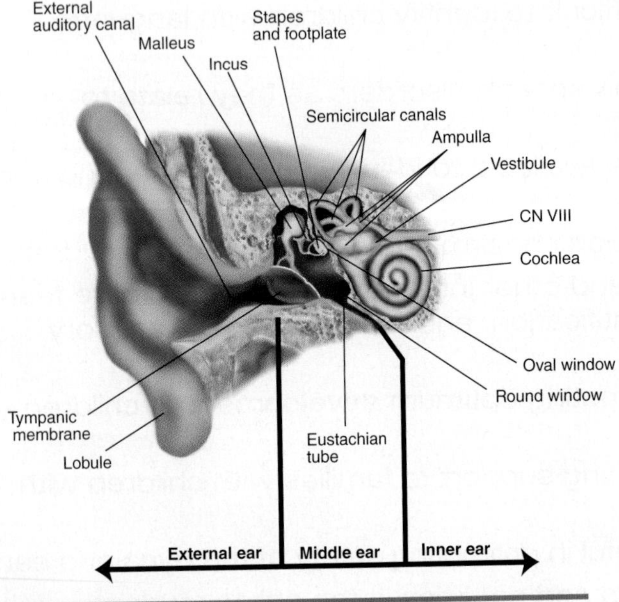

FIGURE 31-1 Cross-Section of the Ear (young child), Note short and flat Eustachian tube. DELMAR CENGAGE LEARNING.

EYE

The eye is composed of the external and internal eye. The external eye is composed of the eyelids, lacrimal glands, conjunctiva, and cornea. The internal eye is composed of the sclera, iris, pupil, lens, ciliary body, retina (containing rods and cones; the macula), and vitreous chamber. The eye is moved by six accessory muscles and affected by cranial nerves II, III, IV, V, and VI. Light enters the eye through the cornea and moves through the lens, whose shape is changed by the ciliary muscles to focus light on the retina. The rods and cones and the macula transmit light impulses via the optic nerve (cranial nerve II) to the brain. Although the eye is developed at birth, visual acuity is not well established. Binocularity (ability to fixate on one visual field with both eyes) occurs by 6 months of age. Visual acuity increases with age and physical development, reaching maturity by 5 years of age, with a visual acuity of 20/20. Tears are not present until the lacrimal gland begins to function, usually at 1–3 months of age (Chamley, Carson, Randall, & Sandwell, 2005; Olitsky, Hug, & Smith, 2007c).

SPEECH AND LANGUAGE

Speech involves the physical production of sound using the oral mechanism (tongue, teeth, oral cavity, and larynx). **Language** refers to the meaningful use of words, phrases, and gestures to transmit meaning from one person to another and is a reflection of expression as well as comprehension (Figure 31-2).

NORMAL LANGUAGE DEVELOPMENT

Children are born with the capacity to learn the complex system of language and speech. Optimal language development is influenced by cognitive ability, temperament, language environment, and intact auditory and visual senses.

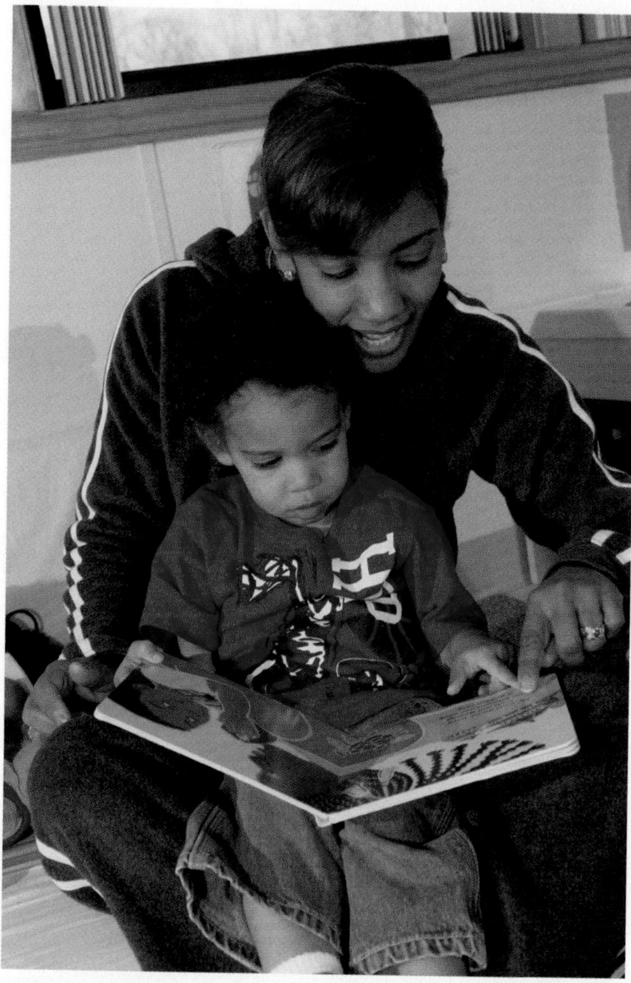

FIGURE 31-2 **Spoken and written words accompanied by colorful images enhance this child's language development.**
DELMAR CENGAGE LEARNING.

Communication is composed of speech and language. Language development involves two interrelated processes: *receptive language* (understanding what others say to you) and *expressive language* (the ability to speak verbally in a way that others can understand). The newborn will focus on the voice of an adult, by 3 months recognize the voice of a parent, and by 6 months visually seek for the source of sound. Children understand more than they can verbalize. By 8 months infants can point out objects, and by 9 months demonstrate comprehension by responding when their name is called. Cooing and babbling is apparent by 4–6 weeks of age and expressive language continues to expand over the next several months and years. When an infant reaches 9–10 months of age they are able to respond with specific words such as "mama." These few words expand to a minimum of 20 words by the time the child reaches 18–20 months of age. Typically the 3-year-old is able to use pronouns and simple verbs, speaking in short sentences. Five-year-olds are able to communicate similarly to an adult and can carry on a conversation (Simms & Schum, 2007).

SPEECH AND LANGUAGE DISORDERS

Communication, the ability to interact with and exchange thoughts, feelings, and information, involves both sensory receptive and expressive abilities. A communication disorder is any impairment in the ability to receive or process a symbol system, represent concepts or symbol systems, or transmit and use symbol systems. A communication disorder may involve speech, language, or hearing or any combination of these three functions. Communication impairment is commonly associated with children with developmental disabilities such as mental retardation and difficulties in motor development (Haapanen, Aro, & Isotalo, 2008). When impaired language and speech is not associated with developmental disabilities or other neurological conditions, the communication disorder is generally developmental in nature. That is, a child does not acquire language normally from the very beginning.

INCIDENCE AND ETIOLOGY

One of the challenges faced by nurses and health care providers is to determine if a child has an actual language disorder versus a developmental delay that can be overcome simply with time and further development. It is essential to identify children with delayed language skills and/or disorders in order to plan and provide appropriate early interventions to help children achieve optimal development. Family history of language delays/disorders and some perinatal risk factors (altered central nervous system [CNS] processing) may place a child at a higher risk for delayed language/language disorders. However there are other factors that may influence language development. These include age-appropriate mimicry or imitation, social and nonverbal communication skills, environmental deprivation, the degree of symbolic thinking and receptive language, hearing impairment, and anatomical abnormalities. Approximately 4% to 5% of children who may be identified as having a language delay/disorder at age 2 years continue to remain delayed. Between 5% and 10% of all children have language disorders (Grover, 2008). Language disorders in children are either a receptive disorder (failure to comprehend) or an expressive disorder (deviation or delay in speech or qualitative aspects of language). Early receptive language skills reflect the child's ability to hear and respond to sound. As developmental milestones are achieved, receptive language relates to the child's ability to understand spoken and written communication. Receptive disorders result from some type of central nervous system failure. Early expressive language skills reflect the child's ability to produce sounds and speech. As the child matures and develops, expressive language expands to using gestures, words, or written symbols to communicate with others (Figure 31-3). It is important to remember that at 3 years of age a child's speech should be understood and intelligible to strangers and not just family members (Grover, 2008). Expressive language disorders result when any of the elements that contribute to language development (cognitive ability, temperament, intact auditory or visual senses, and language environment) are impaired. Deviation or delay can occur in one or all three qualitative dimensions (syntax, semantics, and pragmatics) of language. Speech disorders may be caused by problems with voice, articulation, or fluency. Voice disorders can result from vocal cord polyps, chronic shouting or excessive talking, or medical conditions, such as cleft palate. Articulation disorders may be caused by neuromuscular disease, structural abnormalities, immaturity, or may be idiopathic. The most common cause of articulation disorders is idiopathic, and often may disappear as children mature. Nurses need to be alert to behaviors that might signal delayed language milestones (see Table 31-1) (Dale, Price, Bishop, & Plomin, 2003; Grover, 2008).

A fluency disorder can include impaired rate, rhythm, or general flow of speech (**dysfluency**). An example of a fluency disorder is stammering or stuttering. **Stuttering** is a speech impairment where an individual involuntarily repeats a sound or word, resulting in loss of speech fluency. Speech dysfluency is thought to be caused by neurological damage, genetic predisposition, and anxiety. Stuttering often begins at 3–4 years of age and occurs more often in males than females. Stuttering may be a result of impaired timing within the areas of the brain involved in language preparation and vocal execution of the words and/or phrases. Persistence of speech dysfluency beyond 5 years of age is considered significant and will require therapeutic intervention. It is important to teach parents about not placing the child under undue stress, criticizing, or reprimanding for stuttering. Speech therapy is most effective when begun during preschool years and includes behavioral feedback provided by parents (Simms & Schum, 2007).

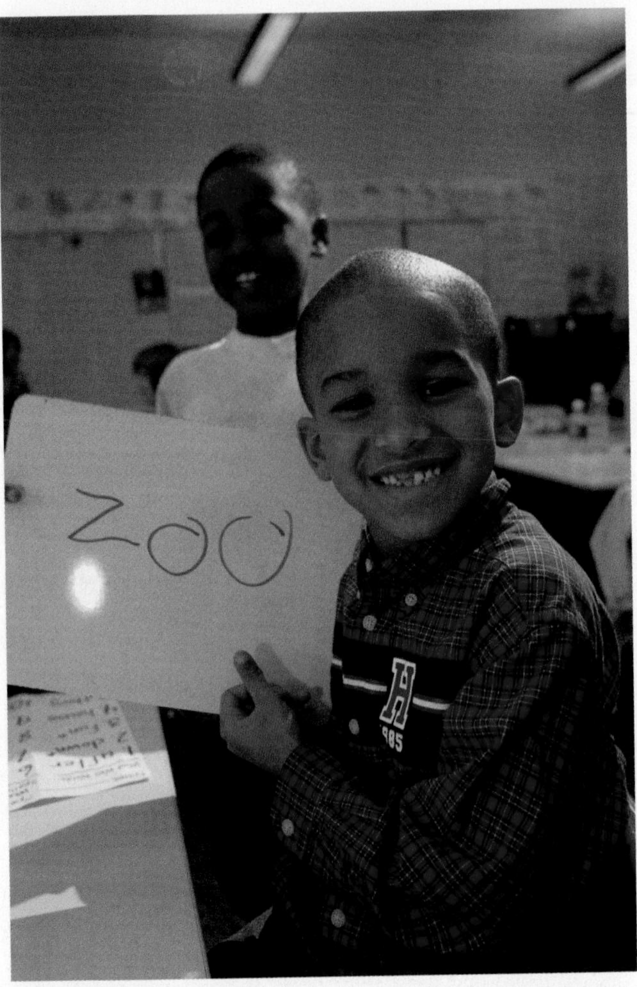

FIGURE 31-3 A child's expressive language is dependent on his ability to understand and process language input. DELMAR CENGAGE LEARNING.

CRITICAL THINKING

A Child with a Language Deficit

Mrs. Adams has brought Jerry and Jacob, 4-year-old twins, into the Family Clinic today. She has a 7-year-old daughter Camden who helps care for the twins. Mrs. Adams is worried because Jerry doesn't speak most of the time and when he does his words aren't understood by anyone, except Camden who sometimes "acts before he speaks" when Jerry wants something. He doesn't follow directions very well and sometimes seems distanced from even his twin brother. Mrs. Adams states that "Jacob is so different, he will 'read' aloud from his picture books and sometimes we can't get him to stop talking." As a pediatric nurse you know that it is important to recognize speech and language difficulties as they may adversely impact a child's development in several ways.

1. What are the behaviors that Jerry is demonstrating that would cause you to evaluate further for language delay/disorder?
2. Identify two nursing diagnoses with measurable outcomes for Jerry and his family.
3. What would be the overall nursing goal of early recognition of a child with a language delay/disorder?

CLINICAL MANIFESTATIONS

Signs of speech and language disorders can be subtle. Table 31-1 outlines the signs of problems in language and speech development. If a child displays any of these signs, a referral should be made immediately to a pediatrician and a speech-pathologist.

DIAGNOSIS

School-age children normally have well-developed communication systems; therefore, identification of a disorder in

TABLE 31-1 Signs Suggesting Speech and Language Disorders

COMMUNICATION	SIGNS
Language	6 mos: does not turn eyes and head to sound coming from behind or from side 10 mos: does not respond to own name 2 yrs: is not talking at all; does not respond to directions appropriately After 2 yrs: has excessive, inappropriate use of "jargon" 3 yrs: fails to use three or more word sentences; has speech that is not intelligible to strangers 5 yrs: exhibits noticeably impaired sentence structure
Articulation	After 3 yrs: uses vowels rather than consonants After 5 yrs: substitutes simpler sounds for difficult sounds According to developmental sequence, sounds appear more than a year late
Fluency	At 3 yrs: shows overt signs of tension when stuttering (i.e., grimacing, foot tapping) After 5 yrs: has dysfluent speech Has more than 10 speech dysfluencies per 100 words Excessive parental concern over the child's speech
Voice	Poor voice quality (monotone, loud, barely audible, or hoarse) Pitch is inappropriate for age

this population is a relatively simple task. However, language acquisition is a developmental process, so diagnosing irregularities in speech and language in infants, toddlers, or preschoolers is not as simple. Because of the importance of the preschool period in the child's language development it is very important to evaluate and assess for language acquisition during this period of time. The link between hearing loss and poor communication has been well-documented. The evaluation of any child for speech or language dysfunction should begin with a thorough physical examination to ascertain whether hearing ability is normal. Assessment of a child's speech and language can be accomplished both directly and indirectly. The nurse can directly observe a child's interaction by initiating a conversation that includes having a child describe an object or by having the child repeat words and short phrases. Parent reports of communication problems, a form of indirect assessment, are the most reliable pieces of data for the pediatric health care provider. However, it is important for the nurse to be aware of parents' knowledge or lack of knowledge or understanding of normal speech and language development. Parents may have expectations regarding their child's ability to communicate that is not realistic and may exaggerate the child's delay. The opposite may also be true when parents may not realize their child has a speech and language delay because of their ability to communicate with the child and their lack of realization regarding the child's impairment. If no abnormalities are noted on the physical examination, then a language-screening test should be administered. Table 31-2 lists the name and the appropriate age for administration of the most common language-screening instruments. These screening tests are administered and interpreted by appropriate language specialists (Figure 31-4).

TABLE 31-2 Language-Screening Instruments

NAME	APPROPRIATE AGE
Denver Articulation Screening Examination (DASE)	2 1/2 to 6 yrs
Early Language Milestone Scale (ELM)	2 to 3 yrs
Assessment of Children's Language Comprehension	3 to 6 yrs
Pre-School Language Scale	Birth to 3 yrs
Expressive One-Word Picture Vocabulary Test	2 to 12 yrs
Peabody Picture Vocabulary Test	2 1/2 to 18 yrs
Rockford Infant Developmental Evaluation Scale	Birth to 4 yrs
SKI-HI Language Development Scale	Birth to 5 yrs

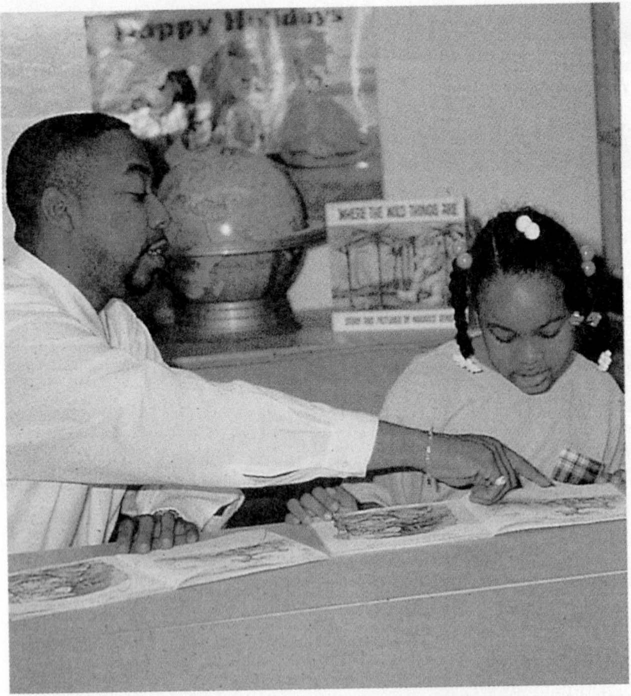

FIGURE 31-4 Speech therapists use a variety of techniques to help children with speech disorders, including having the child read aloud. DELMAR CENGAGE LEARNING.

TREATMENT

Children with expressive language disorders should receive speech therapy. Some clinicians advocate a wait-and-see position with the belief the problem is self-correcting for most children. Many, however, believe expressive disorders are not self-correcting, and therefore speech therapy should be instituted. Programs for stuttering utilize behavior modification of the child and education of parents as the treatment, as language disorders have a major impact on development and learning. An effective communication system is essential for children to integrate the phenomenon in the world around them. Because the ability to communicate is critical to academic learning, children with expressive language deficits have difficulty in school and are usually academically delayed. The earlier correction is accomplished the less learning delay will occur (Simms & Schum, 2007).

NURSING MANAGEMENT

The nurse's primary responsibilities when caring for children with communication impairments are assessment and family education. Assessment of abnormalities requires knowledge of normal language and speech development. Knowledge of normal milestones enables the nurse to distinguish when communication characteristics are normal and when there are deviations. During every well-child visit the nurse should assess the child's communication patterns and compare them to normal values for the age of the child. Box 31-1 suggests questions to ask the caregiver to assess the presence of communication impairment when there is a suspected problem.

BOX 31-1
QUESTIONS TO ASK WHEN TAKING A NURSING HISTORY RELATED TO COMMUNICATION DISORDERS

1. At what age did your child say his or her first words?
2. At what age did your child put two to three words together?
3. Does your child make mistakes in grammar? (For instance, "We goes home.")
4. Do directions need to be repeated?
5. Can your child follow two to three directions given at once? (For example, "Go upstairs, get your shirt, and put the shirt on.")
6. Can others understand your child's speech?
7. Does your child stutter?
8. Do you have any difficulty understanding your child's speech?
9. Has there been a recent change in your child's voice?

Social interactions and the development of interpersonal relationships are impaired when communication is not optimal. The frustration of not being able to express needs and ideas, and the embarrassment of impaired communication, influence the child's developing self-image and self-esteem. A behavior disorder may coexist with a communication disorder. Therefore, the nurse must assess each child, and intervene by assisting the child and family seek the appropriate professional resources to correct the communication disorder and thus diminish the impact on the child's development.

Nurses are in a pivotal position to recognize and initiate early intervention for infants or children who are at risk for communication disorders. These risks include inadequate environmental stimuli, impaired vision or hearing, impaired cognition, or behavioral problems. Other considerations should also include being alert to cultural and ethnic

NURSING ALERT

Early Identification of Communication Disorder

Early identification and intervention of a child with a communication disorder can prevent long-term detrimental effects on learning, development, and self-image. It is essential to conduct a thorough assessment and physical examination, make appropriate referrals, and encourage caregivers to follow through on therapy.

BOX 31-2
FAMILY TEACHING: GUIDELINES TO ENCOURAGE LANGUAGE ACQUISITION

- Talk to your child even when he or she cannot respond verbally; children learn through imitation.
- Use correct language; don't talk "baby talk."
- Describe daily activities as they occur.
- Build vocabulary by making new words part of the everyday activity.
- Do not respond to a child's gesture; encourage the child to say the word before fulfilling the request.
- Repeat the child's words using adult pronunciation.
- Look directly at the child's face when talking: 12 inches away from the newborn's face; increase the distance as the child grows.
- Initiate a play time each day when you talk to your child.
- Read to your child at a young age (under 12 months).
- Reinforce the child's attempt to use language with praise and affection.

differences as well as the implication of disparity on the child. Education and monitoring are essential tasks for the pediatric nurse when promoting health and intervening to prevent communication issues. Nurses can also assist family caregivers learn how to encourage language acquisition in their children as well as normal expectations of language. Strategies to assist caregivers in assisting children to acquire language can be found in Box 31-2.

Many children and their families are challenged when the child stutters. Nurses can assist these children and their families by offering support and education. Decreasing stress is most helpful in decreasing stuttering. Additional behaviors include: adopt a slow rate of speech; positively reinforce fluent speech; ask few direct questions and offer open-ended comments; and maintain eye contact. See the Nursing Tip box.

NURSING TIP
The Child Who Stutters

Teaching health promotion or other important health care principles to a child who stutters can be a challenge. Keep the following in mind: (1) Avoid completing the child's sentence when he or she "blocks." (2) Avoid doing anything that might emphasize the child's stuttering or speech skills. (3) Act in such a way as to convey that hesitancy is a normal developmental behavior. (4) Ensure an adequate amount of time for the child to respond, *be patient*. (5) Minimize stress.

CULTURAL CONSIDERATION
Communication Patterns

It is often difficult to identify communication impairment in children from other cultures, particularly children who have recently arrived in the United States. Nurses should be mindful of how communication may differ, pay particular attention to developmental milestones (they may vary from the established "norm"), observe communication patterns between family members, and consider possible environmental factors. What information would you need to gather from parents or family members to help you in identifying a risk for a communication impairment? How can you develop a cultural perspective with regards to possible communication impairment?

HEARING IMPAIRMENT

A child who has a hearing loss, even if it is mild, is significantly impacted. The first three to four years of childhood are the most important for speech and language development. A hearing deficit during this time can interfere with this process and can impact the child's cognitive, social, and emotional development (Figure 31-5). **Hearing impairment** can range in severity from mild to profound. Deafness is

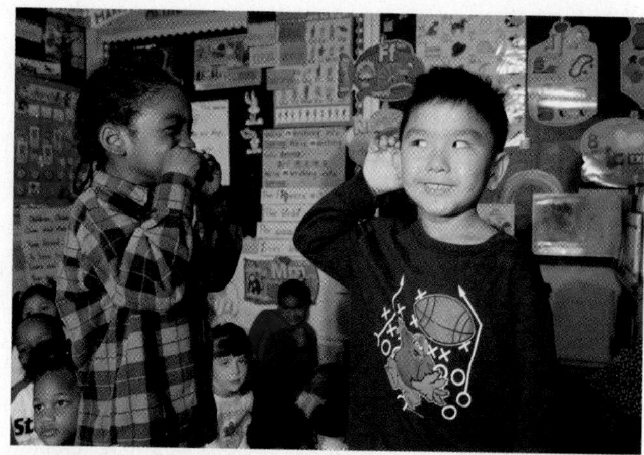

FIGURE 31-5 Listening and hearing are important to a child's social and cognitive development. DELMAR CENGAGE LEARNING.

defined as "a hearing impairment that is so severe that the child is impaired in processing linguistic information through hearing, with or without amplification" (National Information Center for Children and Youth with Disabilities [NICHCY], 1996). Children may be born with a hearing impairment or may develop various degrees of impairment during childhood.

NORMAL HEARING DEVELOPMENT

Table 31-3 summarizes the normal development of hearing from birth through 24 months of age.

HEARING LOSS

Hearing deficit may be present at birth (congenital deafness) or may develop anytime later in childhood (Haddad, 2007). This may be known as late-onset or progressive hearing loss (Nobel & Sifuentes, 2008). Being alert to the signs of hearing impairment early in the child's life enables the child to receive early intervention to prevent or reduce the effects of the disability on development.

Incidence and Etiology

The incidence of hearing loss in newborns is 1 in 1,000 to 2 in 1,000 and is one of the most common infant disabilities in the United States. There are approximately 1 million children who have some form of hearing impairment (Haddad, 2007; Moore, 2006; Yaeger et al., 2006). While 1% of children with hearing loss have severe to profound deafness, approximately 3 to 5 in 1,000 children are born with a mild to moderate hearing loss (Haddad, 2007; Nobel & Sifuentes, 2008). Approximately 90% of these children are born to hearing parents (National Institute on Deafness and Other Communication Disorders, 2007). It is estimated that an additional 20%–30% of children are diagnosed hearing impaired during childhood. These children who have acquired hearing impairment are most often identified by parents (Haddad, 2007; Nobel & Sifuentes, 2008).

Hearing loss is caused by a number of prenatal and postnatal conditions related to congenital or acquired factors (Haddad, 2007). About 50% of children with hearing loss can be attributed to a genetic link, while 25% are caused by environmental influences and the other 25% have no known cause (Weichbold, Nekahm-Heis, & Welzl-Mueller, 2006; Yaeger et al., 2006). However, there are some factors that may place an infant at a greater risk for hearing loss. These include documented family history of congenital hearing loss, presence of craniofacial deformities, very low birth weight, bacterial meningitis, and the presence of a syndrome that is known to be associated with hearing loss such as Pierre Robin Syndrome (Chu et al., 2003; Yaeger et al., 2006). Box 31-3 summarizes these etiologies. Environmental noise as an etiologic agent is increasing in two distinct age groups, the neonate and the adolescent. The noise level in neonatal intensive care units is producing hearing loss in newborns, especially in premature low birth weight babies, by damaging the stereocilia of

Table 31-3 Milestones of Normal Hearing Development

AGE	HEARING
Birth to 3 months	Soothed by parent's voice Gives a startled response to loud sudden noises
3 to 6 months	Looks to see where sounds come from Becomes frightened by an angry voice Smiles when spoken to Wakes up when spoken to or when a loud noise is made nearby
6 to 12 months	Stops for a minute when someone says "no-no," "bye-bye," and own name Looks at objects or pictures when someone talks about them Enjoys rattle and similar toys for their sounds
12 to 18 months	Sings and hums spontaneously Discriminates between sounds such as doorbell, telephone, barking dog, and so forth "Dances" and makes sounds to music
18 to 24 months	Brings objects to others when asked Hears and identifies sounds coming from another room

BOX 31-3
ETIOLOGY OF CHILDHOOD DEAFNESS

I. **Congenital**
   A. Genetic
      1. Family history of congenital hearing impairments
      2. Malformations of head and neck structures
      3. Down syndrome
      4. Tay-Sachs disease
      5. Arnold-Chiari Malformation
   B. Nongenetic
      1. Perinatal infection—maternal rubella, rubeola, cytomegalovirus, toxoplasmosis, herpes, syphilis, bacterial meningitis
      2. Metabolic disease
      3. Perinatal asphyxia
      4. Ototoxic drugs
      5. Rh incompatibility
      6. Radiation
      7. Anoxia and birth trauma
      8. Low birth weight

II. **Acquired**
   A. Infection—chickenpox, measles, mumps, otitis media, meningitis
   B. Ototoxic drugs
   C. Neoplastic disorders
   D. Trauma
   E. Metabolic disorders
   F. Loud noise

the cochlea directly and permanently. Sound levels over 80 decibels (dB) for a sustained amount of time have been shown to produce hearing loss in humans. The average NICU environment produces low-frequency sounds at the 50–80 dB level. Peak decibel levels for some equipment in the NICU fall within this range (incubator motor [51–71 dB], IV pump alarm [76 dB], opening a plastic incubator sleeve [76 dB]). In the adolescent group, the practice of listening to loud music on earphones (80 dB) (Figure 31-6) or at a concert and in blaring speakers in cars (120 dB), puts this group at risk for permanent sensorineural deafness.

Pathophysiology—Classification

Four types of hearing loss have been identified. They include conductive, sensorineural, mixed, and retrocochlear hearing loss (Haddad, 2007; Nobel & Sifuentes, 2008). **Conductive hearing loss** is a temporary or permanent hearing deficit resulting from any condition, such as fluids, that "affects the progress of sound into the ear canal or across the middle ear system" (NICHCY, 1996). The most

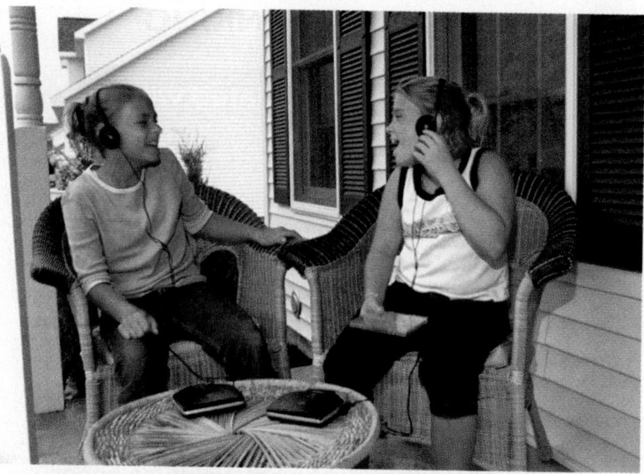

Figure 31-6 Listening to loud music through earphones can contribte to hearing loss. DELMAR CENGAGE LEARNING..

common causes are damage, inflammation, obstruction, or malformation of the outer or middle ear. **Sensorineural hearing loss** results from damage or malformation of the middle ear or auditory nerve. The most common causes are congenital defects, infection, exposure to loud noises or ototoxic drugs, and prematurity which causes damage to hair cells in the chochlea or along the auditory nerve. Sensorineural loss results are permanent. **Mixed hearing loss** occurs when both conductive and sensorineural damage results from interference with transmission of sound in the middle ear and along neural pathways, which produces problems with sound distortion and a reduction in the child's ability to hear sounds below a certain decibel level or loudness. The conductive component is reparable; however, the sensorineural effect is irreversible. A retrocochler hearing loss is caused by damage to the brain stem, cortex, or auditory nerve (Nobel & Sifuentes, 2008).

Hearing impairment is described in terms of loudness (intensity) and pitch (frequency) of sounds. Loudness is described in terms of decibel units, and pitch is described in terms of Hertz (Hz) units. Table 31-4 describes decibel levels of various sounds. The softest sound the normal human ear can hear is 0 dB. Sustained listening to sound is more than 140 dB will cause pain and permanent damage. Human beings can hear from a low pitch of 16 Hz to high pitch of 30,000 Hz. Normal speech tones generally fall between 45 and 55 dB and 500 and 2,000 Hz. Hearing impairment can be classified according to decibel level (as measured by an audiometer) and the degree to which it affects one's ability to hear speech. Table 31-5 describes the degree of hearing loss and its effect on speech and language. Because approximately 80% of language growth occurs by 3 years of age, early detection of hearing impairment is critical so that appropriate management can help to promote positive growth and development outcomes.

Clinical Manifestations

Early recognition of hearing loss is essential to control the level of developmental impact on the child. Infants and

CRITICAL THINKING

Hearing loss associated with low birth weight

Childhood hearing loss is a serious problem that not only impacts the child with the disability but also the family. Approximately 1-2 per thousand children have sensorineural hearing loss requiring hearing aids. Causes of sensorineural loss are not completely understood, but studies have found that the risk for hearing loss increased with low birth weight.

Knowing about the risk of hearing loss associated with low birth weight what would be important nursing actions to consider to prevent hearing loss in infants of families experiencing disparity issues?

Reference

Engdahl, B., & Eskild, A. (2007). Birthweight and the risk of childhood sensorineural hearing loss. *Paediatric and Perinatal Epidemiology*, *21*, 495–500.

children at risk, those with a family history of impairment, low birth weight, congenital prenatal infection, cranio-facial abnormalities, elevated bilirubin, asphyxia, low Apgar rating, meningitis, or administration of ototoxic drugs should be assessed very carefully. Children with hearing loss will show characteristic behavioral signs, described in Table 31-6 according to chronologic age. When any of these signs are present, a physical examination and tests of hearing function should be performed.

Table 31-4 Decibel Levels of Various Sounds

DECIBEL LEVEL	SOUND
0	Threshold of hearing
10	Heartbeat
45-55	Normal conversation
65	Telephone ringing
80	Loud music in earphones
120	Rock music concert, blaring car speakers
140	Jet airplane during departure
>140	Any sound at this level will cause pain and permanent damage

Table 31-5 Hearing Loss: Effect on Speech and Language

DEGREE OF LOSS	EFFECT ON HEARING	EFFECT ON SPEECH AND LANGUAGE
Slight loss 15–25 dB	No impairment	No significant speech and language delays
Mild loss 26–40 dB	Difficulty hearing faint or distant speech, some speech may be difficult to understand May benefit from hearing aid	Usually will not have school difficulty
Moderate loss 41–55 dB	Understands speaker face-to-face at 3–5 feet May need hearing aid	May miss 50% of class discussion if voices are faint or not within the line of sight May have problems pronouncing some speech sounds
Moderately severe loss 56–70 dB	Most "normal" conversation speech and sounds missed and to hear, conversation needs to be louder than 70 dB Will need hearing aid	Has increasing difficulty in classroom activities Probably has difficulty pronouncing some speech sounds May have deficiencies in language comprehension and usage
Severe Loss 71–90 dB	Normal speech sounds cannot be heard at a conversation level, many speech sounds may not be heard Can hear if using hearing aid	Speech and language development are delayed and will not develop spontaneously if loss present before 2 years of age
Deaf More than 90 dB	Deaf, no sounds heard	Severe speech and language delay

TABLE 31-6 Behavioral Signs Associated with Hearing Loss

AGE	BEHAVIORAL SIGNS
Birth to 6 months	• Does not startle, blink eyes, or change activity in response to a sudden loud noise • Does not awaken with loud environmental noise, only to touch • Is not soothed by mother's voice • Does not respond to voice • Does not imitate gurgling and cooing sounds or show response to noise-making toys • Does not turn eyes and head in direction of sound coming from the side or from behind
By 10 months	• Does not respond when name is called • Does not localize sound • Babbles only a little or not at all
By 12 months	• Does not respond to normal household sounds (dog barking, voice of a family member, etc.) • Engages in loud shrieking and sustained production of vowels • Tries to imitate speech sounds made by caregiver • Points to familiar objects when asked
15 months to 4–5 years	• Watches a speaker's face intently • May have difficulty following simple spoken instructions • Has poor social skills and interactions • Frequently says "huh" and "what" when spoken to • May appear developmentally delayed • Shows preference for high- or low-pitched sounds • Shows delayed acquisition of speech; speaks in monotone, unintelligibly, or not at all • Uses gestures rather than verbalization to get attention and objects
6 years to 16 years	• Answers questions inappropriately or not within context • Frequently asks speaker to repeat sentence • Poor school performance • May have abnormal speech, speaks in monotone

DIAGNOSIS

Congenital hearing loss causes major problems in a child's development. Early detection of impaired hearing or hearing loss is important in order to ensure appropriate help and support of the child and family, as well as to promote optimum development. Therefore all infants should undergo hearing screening by the time the infant is 1 month of age, an audiological evaluation by 3 months of age, and appropriate intervention for the infant with hearing impairment/loss begun by 6 months of age (Connolly, Carron, & Roark, 2007; McCracken, Young, & Tattersall, 2008; Windmill & Windmill, 2006). As a result of required newborn hearing screening tests the average age of diagnosis is 2 to 3 months (Nobel & Sifuentes, 2008).

The major screening tests for hearing are the automated auditory brain stem response (ABR) for newborns, Brainstem Auditory Evoked Response (BAER) and the Otoacoustic Emission Test (OAE) particularly of at-risk children. The ABR and the BAER are electrophysiological measurements that detect hearing loss from 1000–8000 Hz, reflects cochlea and 8th cranial nerve auditory brainstem pathway function. The OAE evaluates chochlear and hair cell function, measures low intensity sounds from the chochlea, but does not detect 8th cranial nerve function (Haddad, 2007; Nobel & Sifuentes, 2008). See Box 31-4.

The OAE used together with the BAER or the ABR provides a more complete picture of peripheral and brain stem functioning. These tests are performed by an audiologist to confirm suspected hearing impairment.

Other methods to assess hearing loss include a tympanogram, evaluating the ability of the middle ear to transmit sound, audiography testing the child's ability to hear various

EVIDENCE-BASED PRACTICE

Universal Newborn Hearing Screening: Parental Reflections on Very Early Audiological Management

CLINICAL PROBLEM

The implementation of universal newborn hearing screening (UNHS) presents several challenges for both parents and health care professionals. A major challenge is home audiological management of very young infants with hearing loss that promotes maximum achievement of developmental skills and abilities.

BEST CLINICAL PRACTICE

Early identification of hearing impairment/loss is critical to promote the infant's or child's optimum physical, cognitive, psychosocial, and emotional development.

IMPLICATIONS FOR NURSING

- Nurses must be observant of newborn and older infants' responses to sounds.
- Nurses must be alert to assessing hearing at each well child visit in the primary health care setting.
- Nurses need to ask parents if they have any concerns regarding their child's hearing. Nurses need to be alert to parents concern about their infant's or child's hearing.
- Nurses need to activate an interdisciplinary approach, involving pediatricians, audiologists, otolaryngologists, speech-language pathologists, teachers, and social workers.

Reference: McCracken, W., Young, A., & Tattersall, H. (2008). Universal newborn hearing screening: Parental reflections on very early audiological management. *Ear and Hearing, 29*, 54–64.

BOX 31-4
HEARING TESTS

ABR/BAER

Electrodes placed on forehead and mastoid process. A stimulus is presented and brain wave responses are recorded. Requires sleep; sedation may or may not be necessary. ABR used for newborns takes only about 10 minutes. The BAER is more comprehensive and takes up to 90 minutes.

OAE

As sound moves through the cochlea, thousands of hair cells vibrate and send a signal to the 8th cranial nerve to the brain. If the cochlea is functioning normally, the hair cells simultaneously emit an echo of sound back to the middle ear where a small sensitive microphone records the sound.

RESEARCH Highlight

Cochlear Implant Candidacy in the United States: Prevalence in Children 12 Months to 6 Years of Age

STUDY PURPOSE

To estimate the number of children with severe to profound hearing loss who could benefit from a cochlear implant.

To identify the number of projected children candidates to receive a cochlear implant.

METHODS

Using data gathered from the 2000 U.S. Census the number of children with severe to profound hearing loss, ages 12 months to 6 years, was calculated. Excluded from the calculations were children with absent 8th cranial nerves and those who were "neurologically devastated."

FINDINGS

Approximately 12,816 children were considered to be candidates for cochlear implantation. The number of children who presented with severe to profound hearing loss numbered 15,219. Using the information regarding the number of children who received implants in 2000, it is estimated that approximately 55% of the projected number of candidates received cochlear implants.

IMPLICATIONS

One of Healthy People 2010's goals is to increase the number of cochlear implants in people who are deaf or who have profound hearing loss. The results from this study indicate that many children who could benefit from a cochlear implant are not given the opportunity for this treatment option. Another challenge for nurses is the need to be mindful of the shortage of qualified providers, payment and reimbursement issues, and disparity amongst ethnic and socioeconomic status. Nurses need to be alert to the benefit of cochlear implants for children who are deaf or who have profound hearing loss. They also need to seek out appropriate resources and offer support to help meet the needs of these children and their families. This may be particularly important for the child and family who are faced with economic challenges and who desire to have the cochlear implant but due to economic issues are not able to have one.

REFERENCE

Bradham, T., & Jones, J. (2008). Cochlear implant candidacy in the United States: Prevalence in children 12 months to 6 years of age. *International Journal of Pediatric Otorhinolaryngology*, 72, 1023–1028.

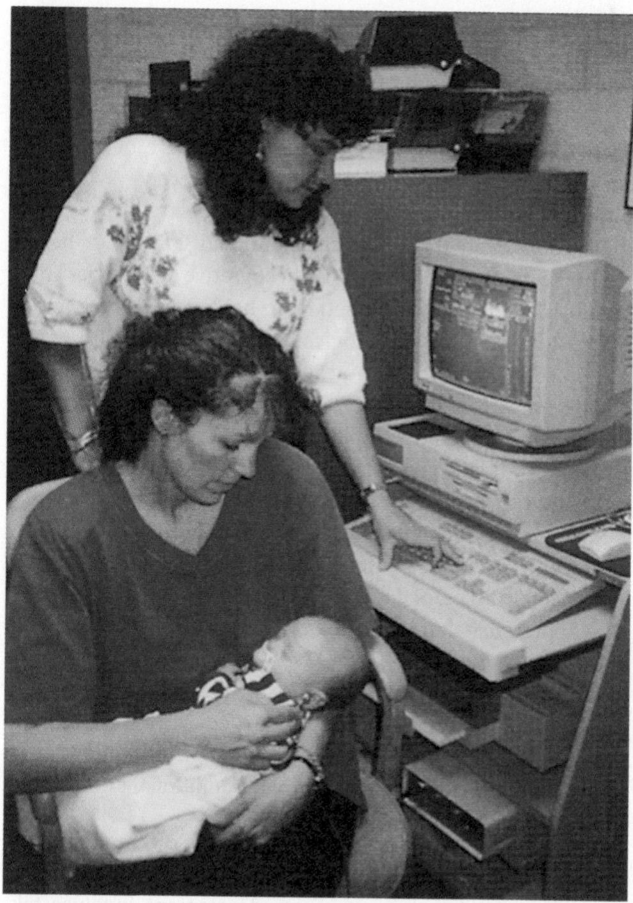

FIGURE 31-7A Infant Getting Hearing Tested. COURTESY OF AMERICAN ACADEMY OF AUDIOLOGY.

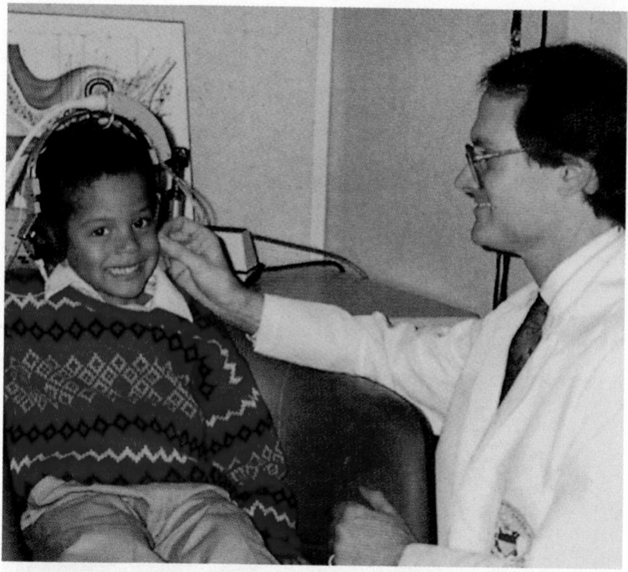

FIGURE 31-7B Preschooler Getting Hearing Tested. DELMAR CENGAGE LEARNING.

frequencies, the "whisper word" test, having the child repeat whispered words, and the Weber and Rinne test. Nurses must be alert to signs of hearing loss, be prepared and able to explain how these tests are done to caregivers, and help families learn about treatment options and access available resources (Figure 31-7).

TREATMENT

It is evident that the earlier treatment for hearing impairment is begun the greater chance the child will have to develop language skills close to a hearing infant. Interventions begun prior to 6 months of age result in infants able to accomplish language, social, and emotional skills appropriate for their age (Nobel & Sifuentes, 2008). Treatment of hearing loss depends on the type of hearing impairment. Conductive and sensineural loss can be improved with the use of a hearing aid to amplify sound. Sensorineural hearing loss is more challenging to treat. Some families are selecting cochlear implants to help children with sensorineural hearing loss.

To assist communication in the hearing-impaired child a number of techniques are utilized—hearing aids, lip reading, sign language, cued speech, and speech therapy. It will be very important to know how the child with a hearing loss compensates and what communication assistance is preferred. Hearing aid choice depends on the specific needs of the child. Hearing aids for pediatric clients can be worn behind the ear (postauricular), in the ear (in the ear canal or in the external ear canal), as a body aid, or as eyeglass aids. See Figure 31-8 for various types of hearing aids.

Cochlear implantation is a newer technique that can benefit some deaf children. The device has two major components, an internal and an external component. The internal component consists of an electrode implanted into or on the cochlea and an internal receiver embedded into the temporal bone behind the auricle. The external components consist of a microphone, external transmitter, and signal processor. The signal processor transforms the sound stimulus received from the microphone and sends it to the external transmitter and then to the internal receiver. The 8th cranial nerve is stimulated and the brain interprets the sound. The cochlear implant has proven to be both cost and beneficially effective for children who fit the candidacy requirements. Most children with implants show improved communication skills (Bradham & Jones, 2008; Nobel & Sifuentes, 2008). Healthy People 2010 has identified a goal of increasing the numbers of cochlear implants for those who meet the criteria (United States Department of Health and Human Resources, 2006). The child who receives a cochlear implant will require basic preoperative and postoperative surgical nursing care. Nursing care requires monitoring results of the procedure, integration of sound to the child, including identifying various methods of introducing sound to the child. The family should also be provided education about language and speech therapy, help in accessing community resources, including special education resources and parent support groups, and provided with appropriate Internet sites that may offer additional help and information. In addition it will be important to educate the family about the potential risk of bacterial meningitis associated with cochlear implants and emphasize the importance of immunizations (Nobel & Sifuentes, 2008; Wilson-Clark, Squires, & Deeks, 2006).

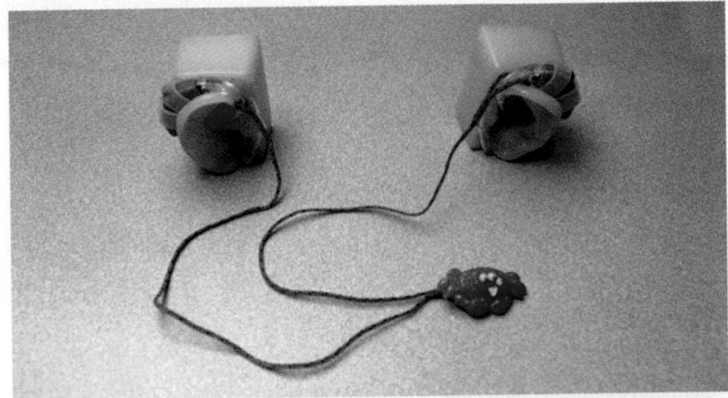

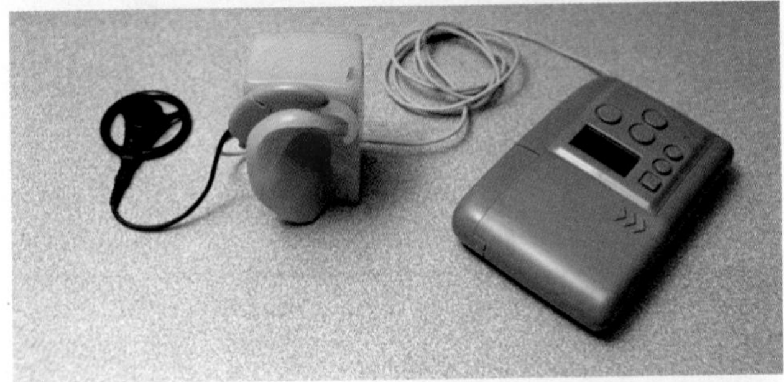

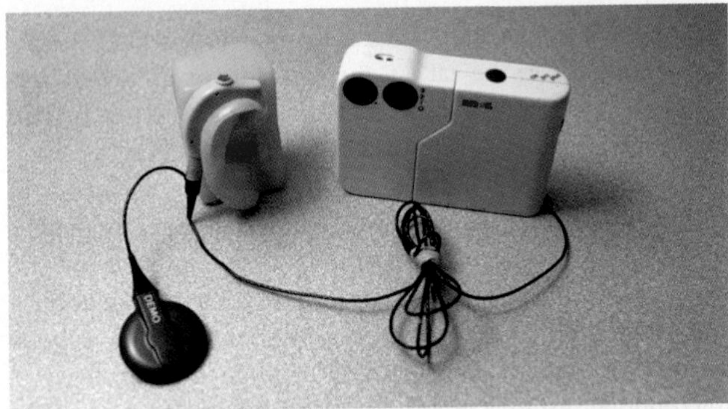

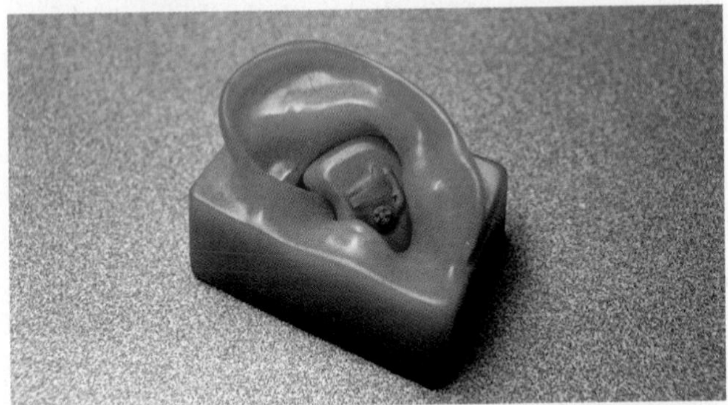

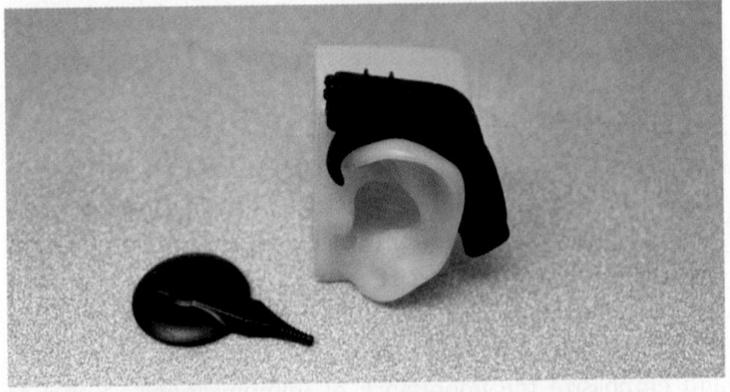

FIGURE 31-8 Various Types of Hearing Aids. DELMAR CENGAGE LEARNING.

The criterion for cochlear implantation has changed over the last few years. Previously to become a candidate for cochlear implantation a child needed to be at least 2 years of age. Now infants as young as 12 months are receiving cochlear implants. However, most children are between the ages of 2 to 6 years of age when they receive a cochlear implant. Another change involves children with cognitive disabilities. Even though cochlear implants may not be appropriate for some children with cognitive disabilities, they are not automatically excluded from being a candidate. However, if the child is neurologically devastated he/she would not be considered to fit the candidacy profile. The presence of bilateral 8th cranial nerve aplasia also excludes the child from having a cochlear implant. Other conditions that might exclude candidacy include the presence of other severe medical conditions, such as cancer or respiratory disorders, that would make the child medically fragile, and parental/family opposition (Bradham & Jones, 2008; Cochlear America, n.d.; National Institutes of Health [NIH], 2006; NIH, 2007).

Approximately 15,000 children have had cochlear implants in the United States (NIH, 2007). Nurses have many opportunities to assist these families. This includes advocating strong family support, providing appropriate education, performing routine follow-ups, and answering questions, in addition to identifying other resources that provide additional information.

Nursing Management

The nurse's most important role in caring for the child with hearing loss is early assessment to detect impairment. Assessment involves taking a careful nursing history to identify children who are at

CULTURAL CONSIDERATION

Supporting the Family's Decisions

As nurses we need to be aware of the perspective of many in the deaf community who view themselves as a distinct culture, much like an ethnic group, who share similar traditions, values, and life events. Because of this viewpoint, deaf parents of deaf children who meet the criteria for cochlear implants may elect not to have their child receive the implant. There are a variety of reasons for this decision, including financial cost, risks associated with the surgery, and the idea that the "world views our child as broken and they want to fix him/her." Because the benefit of the procedure is more impactful if done as early as possible, what is the concern when the parent denies the procedure for the child who is not old enough to make the decision? What are your thoughts about the ethical dilemma that this may present? Seek out information on this subject and reflect upon how you will support the child and family in choosing treatment options.

risk, screening all children during well-child visits, and observing the child's behavior. It is important to pay special attention if the caregiver reports behaviors indicating hearing loss described earlier in Table 31-6. The goal of early recognition and management of children with hearing impairment/loss is to lessen the impact of long term and persistent speech, language, and communication problems that most often lead to other developmental concerns, including lack of a positive self-image, academic failure, and a loss of a normal life (Jafari, Malayeri, & Ashayeri, 2007; Joint Commission on Infant Hearing, 2007; Weichbold, Nekahm-Heiss, & Welzl-Mueller, 2006).

Nursing Diagnosis

Nursing diagnoses include:

1. *Impaired verbal communication* related to impaired hearing.
2. *Impaired verbal communication* related to anxiety.
3. *Disturbed body image* related to impaired hearing.
4. *Delayed growth and development* related to impaired hearing.
5. *Interrupted family processes* related to the diagnosis of deafness of a child.

Outcome Identification

1. The child will achieve optimum communication.
2. The child will experience optimal growth, development, and socialization.
3. The child and caregivers will understand measures to be taken to prevent further hearing impairment.
4. The child and caregivers will understand the impact of the hearing impairment and incorporate support interventions into their daily lives to enable positive psychological adjustment.

Planning and Implementation

Initial nursing interventions to accomplish the goal of promoting communication must first address the impact of the child's hearing impairment on caregivers as they may feel disappointed and need to be assisted to accept and adapt to the impairment. However, caregivers must go through the stages of a grieving process before they can adapt and begin to deal with the challenges of a hearing-impaired child. Depression and anger, especially toward medical staff, are normal stages in the grieving process. The nurse may refer caregivers to a support group for help.

The nurse should remember the family is an integrated system and therefore *all* are influenced by the birth of the hearing-impaired child. Siblings may experience the same feelings of sadness, anger, fear, and guilt caregivers experience. Because much time and energy is devoted to the hearing-impaired child, the sibling may react to the inequity of attention by feeling jealousy and resentment. Each sibling's reaction will vary depending on age and developmental level, and often reflects the attitudes caregivers have expressed both by example and direct communication. Research, however, indicates siblings of children with disabilities appear to be much more positively, rather than negatively, affected by living with a child with a hearing loss.

Nurses play a critical role in educating the public on how to prevent hearing loss. For families where impairment deviations that include hearing loss are common, genetic counseling should be encouraged. During pregnancy, steps should be taken to prevent the effects of any Rh incompatibility and birth trauma, and to avoid infection and ototoxic drugs. Mothers who are at risk for early delivery should be monitored closely and steps taken to prevent premature delivery. Babies identified as having low birth weight need to have their hearing evaluated as soon as possible. After birth, all infants and children should have ear infections treated promptly. Protection of the neonate in the NICU must be instituted to provide a quieter environment in order to protect against iatrogenic hearing loss. As technology has advanced so too has the noise level. Preventive education must be undertaken with school-age children and adolescents who expose themselves to loud music via earphones and car speakers to alert them to the potential damage to hearing ability. Educating children and adolescents about the implications of listening to loud music with or without earphones is a very important role for the school nurse and should be a part of yearly educational plans (Chung, Des Roches, Meunier, & Eavey, 2006; Weichbold & Zorowka, 2007).

How does the nurse communicate with the hearing-impaired child? The nurse must know what method (hearing aid, lip reading, sign language) the child uses to communicate, and make an effort to continue these methods in the health care setting. Box 31-5 lists practices enhancing the communication process between nurse and child.

> **NURSING TIP**
>
> **Detecting Hearing Loss**
>
> **Remember, caregivers know their children well and notice subtle behaviors that may escape the attention of medical personnel. Listen to their comments carefully. If their input, together with a nursing assessment, indicates a possible hearing loss, the child must be referred to an audiologist and an ear, nose, and throat specialist for further evaluation.**

Family Teaching

From birth, communication interchange is altered between caregiver and infant. Caregivers should be advised deaf infants babble until approximately 6 months of age and then stop because of lack of auditory feedback (Lederberg & Everhart, 1998). Methods to enhance communication between child and caregivers should begin immediately upon detection of impairment. They must be taught how to use the various aids to hearing so they can manage and support the child's rehabilitation.

The nurse and caregivers must also learn to care for the hearing aid. All hearing aids must be fitted properly by the audiologist, and as the child grows, a new aid will be needed. For children under 4 years old, the aid must be changed every 3–6 months. After 4 years of age, the aid will need replacement yearly. All hearing aids have a volume control

CASE STUDY / CARE PLAN

A CHILD WITH A HEARING LOSS

Four-month-old Madison is brought to the community clinic for her immunizations by her mother. Madison is Sarah's first baby and Sarah has questions. You begin to escort them back to a room when a large box falls with a loud sound. Other infants and small children immediately begin to cry and look for what made the "scary noise." However, you note Madison did not cry and she is undisturbed by all the other infants' and children's cries and stressful sounds. When talking to Sarah you notice Madison does not respond to your voice or to Sarah's when trying to illicit visual focus and interaction. One of Sarah's questions has to do with Madison failing to look at her mother's face when Sarah speaks to her and seeming overly startled when someone approaches from out of Madison's field of view. Sarah is a single parent and is concerned because she has no one to help her.

NURSING CARE PLAN

ASSESSMENT

Vital signs are normal and afebrile. Madison was delivered at home. She was not ill nor has she been. She eats well and has wet and "dirty" diapers. She is not cuddly and her eyes wander from spot to spot. Madison fails to respond to a variety of auditory stimuli.

NURSING DIAGNOSIS 1

Disturbed sensory perception and risk for impaired verbal communication related to hearing impairment.

EXPECTED OUTCOMES

1. Infant is fitted with proper hearing aid and wears it as recommended.
2. Infant does not ingest hearing aid batteries.

NOC: Communication: Expressive, Receptive

NIC: Communication Enhancement: Hearing Deficit, Speech Deficit

INTERVENTIONS/*RATIONALES*

1. Discuss with mother possible types of hearing aids and their proper care to ensure maximum benefit. *To ensure maximum benefit of using hearing aid.*
2. Educate mother regarding proper care of batteries to prevent aspiration or ingestion of batteries. *To prevent infant's aspiration or ingestion of batteries.*
3. Refer Madison and her mother to appropriate speech and language therapists to begin early communication intervention. *Sign language (or other language) assists in developing speech development, verbal communication, and promotes normal development of the infant (and child).*
4. Encourage Sarah to look and touch Madison when speaking to her, to assist in establishing a trusting relationship. *To facilitate attainment of appropriate developmental levels.*

EVALUATION

Madison uses and interprets speech cues.

Sarah uses touch and other communication aids, and establishes a trusting relationship.

NURSING DIAGNOSIS 2

Delayed growth and development related to inability to hear verbal communication secondary to hearing impairment.

(Continues)

CASE STUDY / CARE PLAN (Continued)

EXPECTED OUTCOMES

1. Infant demonstrates appropriate levels of development.
2. Infant demonstrates social interaction with mom and others.

NOC: Child Development 4 Months

NIC: Developmental Care; Developmental Enhancement: Infant

INTERVENTIONS/*RATIONALES*

1. Provide visual motor activities (e.g., grasping objects such as toys, rattles). *To promote optimum development.*
2. Assist family in enrolling child in special programs for the deaf as soon as possible. *To facilitate child's acquisition of skills that promote independence.*
3. Assist mother in developing child-rearing practices. *To promote optimum development.*
4. Provide education and support regarding developmental levels that can be attained. *To promote optimal development.*

EVALUATION

Child engages in appropriate activities for level of development.

NURSING DIAGNOSIS 3

Ineffective coping: need for adjustment related to infant's newly diagnosed hearing loss and of local support systems.

EXPECTED OUTCOMES

1. Mother will adjust to infant's hearing loss.
2. Mother demonstrates coping skills.
3. Mother identifies and uses community resources.

NOC: Coping; Caregiver Stressors; Caregiver Lifestyle Disruption

NIC: Caregiver Support; Normalization Promotion; Support Group

INTERVENTIONS/*RATIONALES*

1. Anticipate grief reaction as part of adjusting to loss. *Grief reaction is an important part of adjusting to loss. Expression of feelings and concerns enhances coping and promotes adjustment to loss.*
2. Provide opportunities for mother to express feelings and concerns to promote adjustment. *To assist in coping with situation.*
3. Help mother identify available community resources for assistance to ensure overall needs are met. *Use of community resources is valuable in receiving emotional peer support, can aid in making informed decisions, and provide continuing/additional support and help.*
4. Identify support group for mother. *To assist in coping with situation.*

EVALUATION

Mother uses new strategies to communicate with infant.

Mother expresses her grief regarding loss of "normal" infant and other concerns.

Mother uses available support systems, resources, and coping mechanisms to adjust to infant's hearing impairment diagnosis.

BOX 31-5

PRACTICES TO ENHANCE COMMUNICATION WITH THE CHILD WHO IS HEARING-IMPAIRED

1. Encourage use of hearing aid.
2. Look directly into child's face—be on same level as child—get child's attention before speaking.
3. Speak slowly with normal volume and simple sentence structure.
4. Eliminate background noise and visual distractions.
5. Use visual aids such as pictures, objects, hand gestures.
6. Utilize a sign language interpreter.
7. When talking, use normal body gestures and facial expressions.
8. Check comprehension by asking simple questions.
9. Write notes.
10. Avoid restraining child's hands.
11. Avoid darkened room; light should be on face rather than behind speaker's head.

KIDS WANT TO KNOW

What do I say when other kids make fun of my hearing aid?

- Explain the hearing aid allows you to hear what they are saying to you.
- If they were listening to the radio and could not hear the music, they would turn up the volume. The hearing aid "turns up the volume" for you.

and an on-off switch. The ear mold is the only part that can be cleaned with pipe cleaners or toothbrushes. Heat and moisture damage the aid. Batteries that last 100–150 hours must be handled carefully, replaced when worn, and turned off when not in use to preserve battery life. Hearing aids amplify background noise as well as the speaker's voice, which can be annoying and confusing to a child. A whistling sound, termed **acoustic feedback**, is caused by improper fit into the ear or by too high a volume. To eliminate whistle, caregivers should be taught to clean the ear mold, reinsert the aid into the ear making sure no hair is caught between the ear mold and canal, and turn down the volume. Hearing aids should be removed before any medical procedures involving radiation because radiation damages the device.

There are two basic communication approaches the child can learn: lip reading or speech reading, and sign language. A third form that is less common is termed cued speech. When utilizing *lip reading* or *speech reading* only 40% of the spoken word is understood because during speaking, the tongue moves inside the mouth and is not visible. Therefore, the nurse or caregiver should speak clearly and slowly but without exaggeration, as exaggeration alters rhythm and decreases comprehension. Comprehension is further reduced if the speaker has a beard or an accent. The nurse or caregivers can refer to the suggestions in Box 31-5 to enhance comprehension.

Sign language has three forms: American Sign Language (ASL), Signed Exact English (SEE), and British Sign Language (BSL). Sign language is a visual-gestural language that uses hand signals corresponding to words in the English language. The caregivers and child should learn sign language as an adjunct to lip reading. *Cued speech* is a method of communication that uses eight configurations and four positions of the hand to supplement lip reading when words look alike when formed by the lips (e.g., "sin," "tin"). Other aids for hearing are lights wired to flash when the telephone and doorbell ring, trained dogs to alert one to sounds, closed captioning on TV that provides subtitles to translate the audio portion of the program, or telecommunications devices for the deaf, such as a typewriter that transmits the typed message over telephone lines to a monitor so people with hearing impairment can communicate with each other.

Children with hearing loss can learn to communicate effectively if the proper training is instituted early. Nurses should teach caregivers children learn with their eyes first, so stimulation is essential to development. Encouraging the child to speak by expecting speech and allowing time to try to speak no matter how the speech syllables sound is important. Techniques for handling behavior in hearing-impaired children are the same as for children with normal hearing. A feeling of adequacy and self-confidence is established in children if they learn to play with other children, especially hearing children. Educational opportunities for deaf children should be the same as for other children. Appropriate accommodations must be made in the educational setting for the hearing-impaired child.

NURSING ALERT

Battery Safety

Emphasize the importance of storing the batteries in a place where young children cannot reach for and swallow them. If this occurs, seek medical attention immediately.

Early Intervention Programs

The education that can take place in specialized or public school is essential to optimal development. The key element is that this education occurs as early as possible in the child's life, hence, early intervention program involvement. The Education for All Handicapped Children Act of 1975 (P.L. 94-142) was enacted to assure appropriate education for children with disabilities. In 1986, Public Law 99-457 reaffirmed P.L. 94-142 and amended it to include mandatory special education for children. It also funded early intervention

EVIDENCE-BASED PRACTICE

Negative Consequences of Uncorrected Hearing Loss—A Review

CLINICAL PROBLEM

Hearing impairment has many potential negative consequences including lack of or poor communication with family members, friends, teachers, and others in the child's environment. Children and their families may or may not be aware of the barriers or difficulties hearing impairment may cause. Studies have shown uncorrected hearing loss may result in poorer quality of life, lack of social activities, feelings of exclusion or isolation, and even possibly depression.

BEST CLINICAL PRACTICE

- Recognition of high-risk factors in the neonate and infant for hearing impairment is critical.
- Assessment of infants and children for hearing impairment is a critical nursing responsibility.
- Establishment of a screening program to determine auditory function is essential for children who exhibit behaviors indicative of a hearing loss.
- Therapeutic management of hearing loss depends on the cause and type of hearing impairment.
- Parents need extensive support, education, and resource information to adjust to having an infant or child with a hearing loss.

IMPLICATIONS FOR NURSING

- Be knowledgeable about infants and children who are at risk for having or developing hearing impairment (e.g., ototoxic drugs, birth anoxia or trauma, low birth weight, infections such as chickenpox, measles, mumps, or chronic otitis media).
- Play an important role in the early detection of hearing impairment (within the first 6 to 12 months) to prevent social, physical, and psychological delays in the child.
- Promote communication processes (e.g., hearing aids, lip reading, cued speech, sign language, speech therapy).
- Provide emotional support to the infant or child and family when a diagnosis of hearing impairment is made.
- Be aware of how to prevent hearing impairment (e.g., a child with a history of frequent otitis media or respiratory illnesses needs to receive periodic auditory testing, and adolescents need to be educated about noise pollution).

Reference: Harlor, A. D. (2009). Hearing assessment in infants and children: recommendations beyond neonatal screening. *Pediatrics, 124*(4), 1252–1263.

services for young children (birth to 3 years) with disabilities and changed the focus to include families. In 1990, P.L. 101-476 reauthorized the Education of the Handicapped Act (P.L. 94-142) and changed its name to the "Individuals with Disabilities Education Act" (IDEA). Revisions to Part H of P.L. 99-457 were made in P.L. 102-119 making the "case manager" a "family service coordinator" and also developing a system of services for infants and toddlers with developmental delay or disabilities. Under P.L. 94-142, the focus was on the individual with the IEP (Individual Education Plan). Under P.L. 102-119 the focus of services is on the family IFSP (Individual Family Service Plan).

This change in focus addresses the needs of the child within the dynamic of the family system. Nurses play a central position in delivering family-centered care and are a pivotal member of the early intervention team, which must learn to be culturally competent in order to deliver appropriate care. Behaviors demonstrating cultural sensitivity include: respects individuals from other cultures, makes sincere attempts to understand the world from others' points of view, has a sense of humor, tolerates ambiguity well, and approaches others with a desire to learn. The delivery of services by the multidisciplinary team (including the nurse) coordinates the care and education of the child with a disability so optimal development occurs (Figure 31-9).

REFLECTIVE THINKING

Self-Induced Hearing Loss

In recent years there is increasing concern over sensorineural deafness induced by frequent exposure to loud music. Studies have discovered sound levels over 80 dB can produce hearing loss in adults. The sound from rock concerts, car stereos, and home speakers can easily exceed the 80 dB level. Availability of high-intensity speakers and personal earphones have put adolescents at risk because adolescents consider loud music part of their lifestyle. The absorption in loud music is an escape from daily living, and is consistent with the normal developmental task of adolescents of achieving independence and developing identity. What can the nurse do to change this behavior? What can caregivers do to change this behavior?

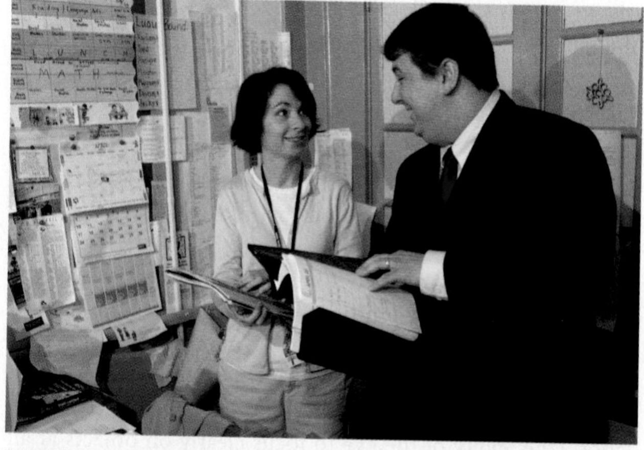

FIGURE 31-9 Nurses often consult with therapists in other specialties when caring for a child with sensory alterations.
DELMAR CENGAGE LEARNING.

Reflections from Families

I never realized how dangerous it was for my son Henry to listen to his music. He loves to have the volume up as high as it can go, to "make the car shake"! But one day sitting in the park he realized he couldn't hear the conversation between his two friends who were sitting a short distance away. He got scared and so did I. I took him to the doctor right away; he has a partial hearing loss in his right ear. The doctor said it might have started as a result of having frequent ear infections when he was little, but he has been fine all this time. Now I feel so guilty that I didn't set some ground rules or know myself about the danger of listening to music so loudly or being around other loud noises. So I have decided to work with the Parent Teachers' Group and try to educate the kids in my son's school.

VISION IMPAIRMENT

Vision is also an important sense for normal child development. From the moment of birth, the child begins to bond with parents and learn about the world using sight. Through sight, the child learns to read, move about the environment, and interact with the world. Impaired vision requires early assessment and intervention to ensure the child's optimal development.

NORMAL DEVELOPMENT

The eyes begin to develop at about 22 days of gestation. Development of the eye is not complete at birth; it is about 75% the size of an adult's eye. Pediatric differences include a lens that is more spherical, limiting the ability of the eye to accommodate, an optic nerve that is less mylinated, decreasing the ability to distinguish color and details, slowed papillary response, and uncoordinated rectus muscles. Other differences include a thinner, more translucent sclera and a cornea that occupies a larger portion of the orbit (O'Connor, Wilson, & Fielder, 2007; Olitsky, Hug, & Smith, 2007a). However, the newborn is able to focus on an object at a distance of 3 feet. Sensitivity to brightness develops rapidly in the first 2 months of life, and the infant displays the blink reflex. Tears begin to secrete within the first 2 weeks of birth. Secretion in relation to emotion occurs between 6 and 12 weeks. By 3 months of age the eyes should move in a coordinated manner. By 4 to 6 months of age infants show preference for bright colors such as red and yellow, are able to reach for familiar objects, and have visual accommodation (the ability of the eye to focus clearly on objects at all distances) equal to an adult (see Box 31-6 for information about color blindness). **Binocularity** (fixation of two ocular images into one cerebral picture, i.e., fusion) is established by 6 months of age. **Visual acuity** (clearness or sharpness of the image) changes with age from 20/50 at 18 months to 20/20 at 4 years of age. At birth, the iris appears blue or light gray in

BOX 31-6
COLOR BLINDNESS

Color blindness (color deficiency or color vision deficit) occurs in about 8% of the general population. It is seen more frequently in males (more often in Caucasian males) than females (Huether, 2010; Subramanian, 2007). It tends to be inherited as a sex-linked disorder and affects the ability to distinguish red from green or blue from yellow colors. There is no cure for the condition and it is detected by use of the Ishihara color plates, which have numbers of a particular color hidden within them. Children who are color blind cannot see the numbers and just see colored dots. Children who are not color blind are able to see the numbers within the plates. Nursing care involves helping children and families learn other ways to discriminate colors, for example, learning the order of lights on traffic signals, or to be observant for warning signs that may have a flashing light associated with them (railroad crossing, school crossing walk). Other implications involve helping children match their clothes according to ways other than coloring, by organizing, labeling, purchasing clothes that can be worn together, or making sure teachers are aware of the condition, so children are not assigned color identification or discrimination tasks.

color in light-skinned newborns, and brown in darker-skinned newborns. An indication of eventual color can be seen at 6 months of age. However, permanent eye color may not appear until 1 year of age.

VISUAL IMPAIRMENT

There are several common eye disorders that may cause vision impairment at various degrees of severity and seriousness. The United States Preventative Services Task Force (2005) estimates that approximately 5% to 10% of preschoolers have a vision impairment such as amblyopia, strabismus, or a refractive error. Approximately 2.5 per 100,000 children have severe visual impairment or blindness. These infants or children are more often from developing countries or are considered low birth weight. Most often they are diagnosed during the first twelve months (Olisky, Hug, & Smith, 2007b). Loss of vision is described in terms of its legal-medical, educational, and functional implications. The *legal-medical* definition emphasizes the clearness of vision at various distances (visual acuity). The *educational* definition emphasizes the extent to which vision can be used for reading and learning. The *functional* definition describes what a person actually can see. These definitions are important for determining eligibility for special services such as special types of schools, financial aid, etc. Box 31-7 summarizes these definitions. It is important for the pediatric nurse to participate in early detection, referral for prompt treatment, and educate communities about prevention strategies for eye health.

BOX 31-7
DEFINITIONS OF VISION IMPAIRMENTS

The Legal-Medical Definitions

Blind = Visual activity of 210/200 or less in the better eye, with correction; a visual field which subtends to an angle of not greater than 20 degrees. (Federal Regulations, P.L. 94-142, 1975)

Sighted Partially = Visual activity between 20/200 and 20/70 in the better eye with correction (Federal Regulations, P.L. 94-142, 1975)

The Educational Definitions

Blind = Visual loss is severe enough so child cannot read print

Partially Sighted = Residual vision is sufficient to allow child to read large print (for visually impaired) for educational purposes

The Functional Definitions

Blind = Vision allows only light perception

Low Vision = Can see if objects are a few inches to a maximum of 2 feet away

Limited Vision = Visual defects are correctable with lenses or surgery so child functions as a normally sighted person

INCIDENCE, ETIOLOGY, AND PATHOPHYSIOLOGY

The three underlying reasons for visual impairment are: the eyeball may be proportioned incorrectly, making it hard to focus on objects; there may be damage to one or more parts of the eye essential to vision that interferes with the way the eye receives or processes visual information; and the part of the brain processing visual information may not function properly, resulting in the brain not being able to analyze and interpret visual information. A visual impairment may be congenital (75%) or acquired (25%). Very low birth weight (VLBW) infants have significantly increased incidence of ocular muscle weakness. Research continues to determine if fluorescent lights are the cause of blindness observed in retinopathy of prematurity (ROP) in premature babies in the NICU. Approximately 5% to 10% of children have some form of impaired vision. Refractive errors (5% to 7%), such as myopia (near-sightedness), hyperopia (far-sightedness), amblyopia (1% to 4%), strabismus, glaucoma, and cataracts, are the most common type of visual impairments in children (Braverman, 2007; Hartmann et al., 2006). Approximately 2.5% of children have some form of visual impairment or blindness. Vision impairment rates increase in certain ethnic groups, 3.6% for Hispanic children and 2.6% of African-American children (MMWR, 2005).

CLINICAL MANIFESTATIONS

Some infants and children may not show any obvious clinical manifestations which would indicate a visual impairment. Others may demonstrate behaviors that would alert the nurse to a possible visual disorder. Total blindness can usually be identified during the first year of life. Partial vision loss often goes unnoticed until the child

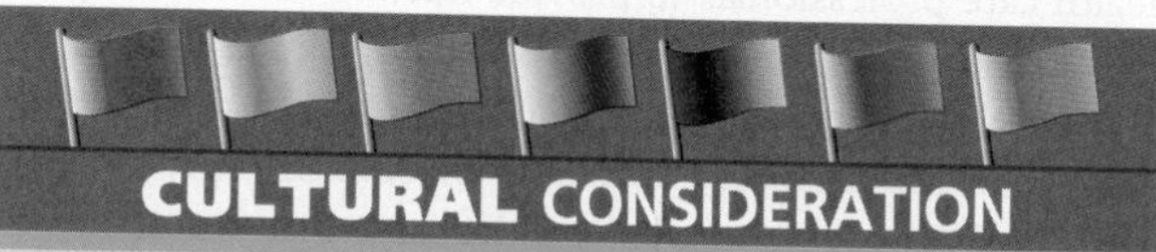

CULTURAL CONSIDERATION

Treatment of Visual Alterations

Consider the statistics regarding the higher numbers of Hispanic and African-American children who have vision impairments and their likelihood of economic disparity. Think about the potential outcomes for these children when screening and/or treatment does not occur or occurs late. What can you do to help promote early detection, treatment referral, and education for these children and their families?

BOX 31-8

CLINICAL MANIFESTATIONS OF VISUAL LOSS BASED ON AGE

Infants

- Pupils do not react to light.
- Eyes may appear misaligned.
- Does not gaze or stare at surroundings.
- Does not follow a moving object with eyes.
- Cloudy lens.
- Corneal clouding.
- Corneal light reflex or distorted red reflex.

Toddlers or Preschoolers

- Rubs eyes frequently.
- Squints or tilts head to see.
- Frequently bumps into objects.
- Moves hesitantly or walks close to the wall.
- Holds books or toys close to face.
- Shows difficulty in identifying faces or numbers that designate rooms or floors.
- Complains of headaches, dizziness, nausea, or vomiting.
- May have similar manifestations noted above in the infant category.

enters school and has functional difficulty. See Box 31-8 for a list of clinical manifestations based on age.

Diagnosis

It is important for early detection and treatment of vision abnormalities to help prevent loss of visual acuity or further visual impairment. The nurse is key as a partner in identifying eye problems, referring the child and family to the appropriate health care provider, and collaborating with other health care professionals to provide nursing care to the child with a visual impairment. Visual screening should take place not only during well-child care visits but also at birth. Preschool examination, as a part of reducing preventable vision loss, is recommended by the American Academy of Ophthalmology (Olisky, Hu, & Smith, 2007c; Ottar-Pfeifer, 2005). Visual acuity can only be assessed indirectly in children less than 3 years old. The nurse can accomplish this by using the cover-uncover test and examining the red reflex with an ophthalmoscope. Assessing vision in the infant includes observing an active blink reflex when a light shines across the eyes. Each eye is tested separately and the results compared. Pupillary light response (pupil constricts and the eye blinks closed) should occur equally. In early childhood or with developmentally delayed children, visual acuity can be tested with:

- Allen cards—seven black and white pictures of familiar objects (horse, house, etc.)—where the child is asked to name the objects
- Blackbird Preschool Vision Test—six cards, each with varying sizes of blackbirds—child indicates direction the bird is flying
- Snellen—child indicates which way the legs of the letter E point
- Denver Eye Screening Test (DEST)—a single E card—child indicates which way E is pointing
- STYCAR test—Chart with letters T, H, V, and O, and four individual cards with these same letters—child must match letter on chart with the appropriate letter on the card (American Academy of Pediatrics, 1996)

The Snellen Alphabet chart is used for older children who can identify letters (Figures 31-10 and 31-11). The numerical fraction, for example, 20/40, describes visual acuity. The numerator indicates the distance the child is from the chart. The denominator indicates the distance at which a person with normal vision can read the same letters. School nurses play an important role in planning and carrying out visual acuity screening. Planned screening is usually scheduled at the kindergarten level with additional times per state and local policies.

VISION DISORDERS

A variety of disorders can affect a child's vision. The disorders can be classified into four groups: visual acuity (how clearly the child sees); muscular efficiency (how well the two

CRITICAL THINKING

Healthy People 2010 Goals

In 2006 the United States Department of Health and Human Services completed a midcourse review of Healthy People 2010. As part of their review they identified several goals regarding childhood vision. Two of these goals include: (1) reducing blindness and vision impairment in children and adolescents 17 years old and under; (2) increasing the use of appropriate eyewear during physical and recreational activities.

1. **Identify two nursing interventions for each goal.**
2. **Identify the implications of health disparity and cultural ethnic factors for success in meeting these goals.**

Reference

U.S. Department of Health and Human Services. (2006). *Healthy People 2010: Midterm Review*. Washington, D.C.

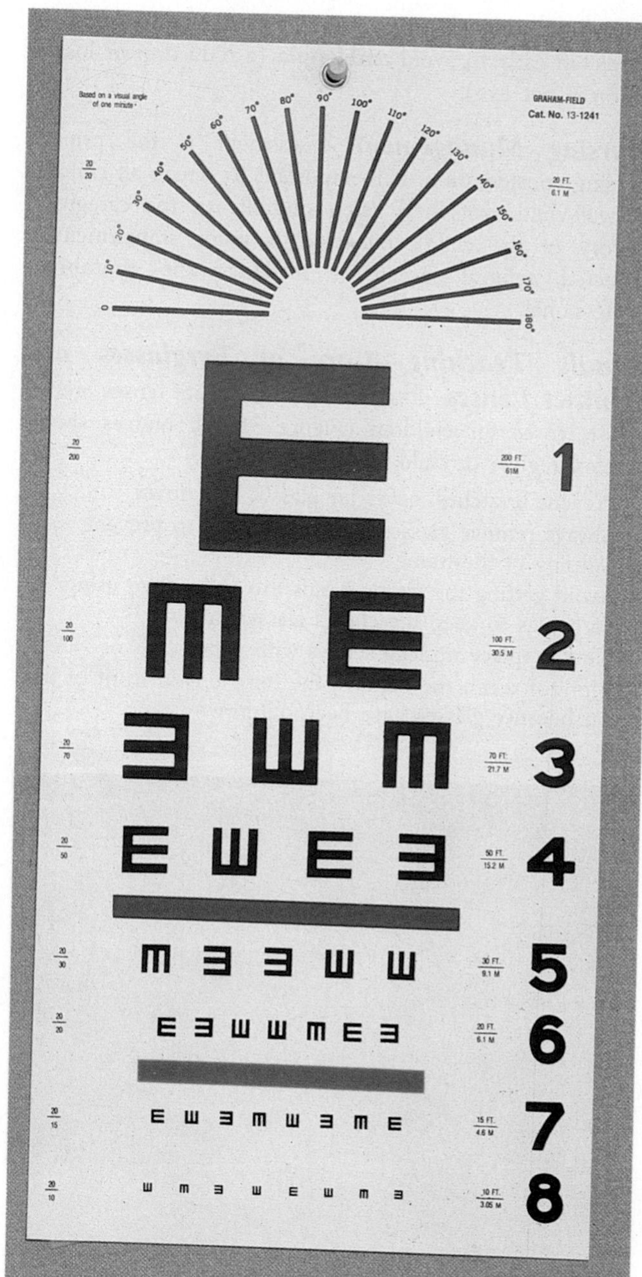

FIGURE 31-10 Snellen "E" or "Big E" Chart for Testing Distance Visual Acuity of children. DELMAR CENGAGE LEARNING.

eyes work together to focus on objects and to produce binocular vision); physical integrity (how intact and structurally normal are the physical mechanisms of the eye); and eye infections.

IMPAIRMENT OF VISUAL ACUITY

Detection and correction of disorders that cause impaired visual acuity in children are important for two reasons: to prevent irreversible vision loss, and to eliminate any visual impairment diminishing the child's normal development.

Refractive Disorders Refractive disorders include **myopia** (nearsightedness), **hyperopia** (farsightedness), and

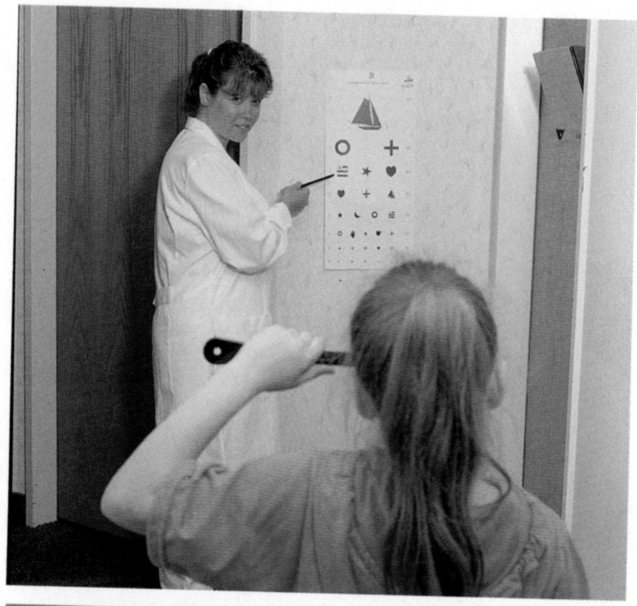

FIGURE 31-11 Measuring Distance Visual Acuity of a Child Using a Kindergarten Vision Screening Chart. DELMAR CENGAGE LEARNING.

astigmatism (blurred vision). A discussion of the three disorders follows.

Incidence and Etiology Refractive disorders are the most common type of visual disorders in children. **Refraction** refers to the process by which the cornea and lens of the eye bend light rays to focus on the retina. When the bending of the rays and the length of the eyeball are uncoordinated, the image does not fall on a single point on the retina. The three types of refractive disorders are illustrated in Figure 31-12. Theories on the etiology of myopia include it being inherited as a recessive gene, prolonged use of eyes on close work resulting in excessive tension on ciliary muscles, or vitamin deficiencies. Astigmatism is primarily caused by inheritance.

Pathophysiology Myopia occurs when the eyeball is too long, causing light rays to focus in front of the retina, resulting in difficulty with distance vision. Hyperopia occurs when the eyeball is too short, causing light to focus behind the retina resulting in difficulty with near vision. This is the most common refractive disorder in children. Astigmatism occurs when there is uneven curvature of the cornea or lens, preventing light rays from focusing correctly on the

NURSING ALERT

Possible Impaired Vision

The pediatric nurse should consider the possibility of impaired vision in the absence of a blink reflex or absence of pupillary constriction in the infant.

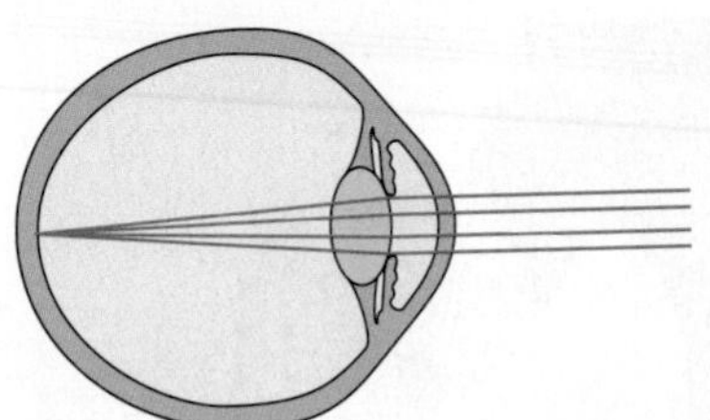

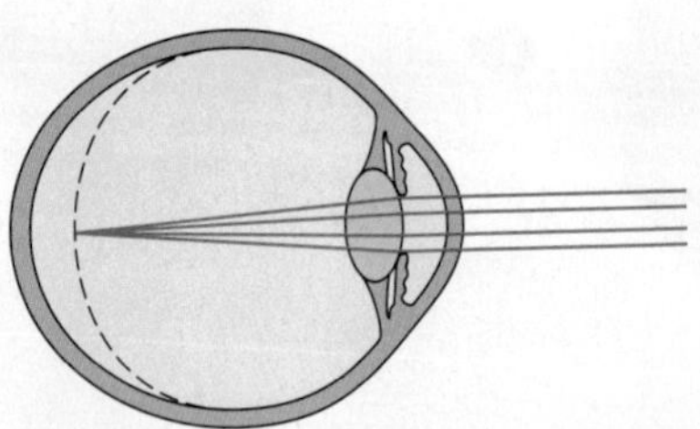

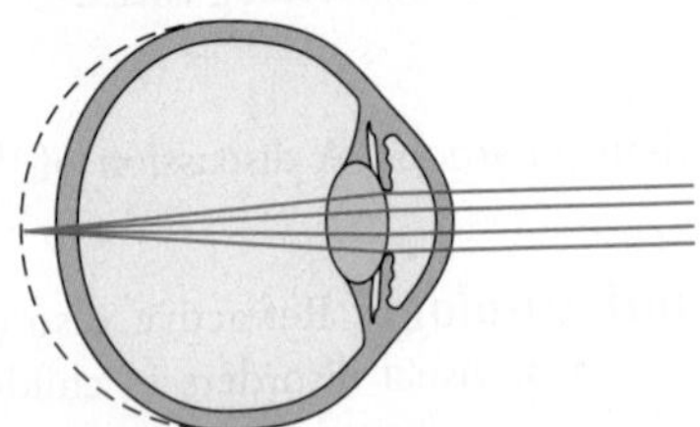

FIGURE 31-12 Eye Refraction. DELMAR CENGAGE LEARNING.

retina. Because normal refraction does not develop until the age of 4 1/2 years, diagnosis of refractive errors occurs after this age. Children who have experienced eye injuries or ptosis that result in an irregular corneal shape are at higher risk for astigmatism and amblyopia (Olitsky, Hug, & Smith, 2007d).

Clinical Manifestations Each impairment results in poor visual acuity. Associated symptoms may include headache, irritated eyes, nausea, eyestrain, and irritability. Classic complaints of children are difficulty reading or seeing things at a distance, such as on the blackboard.

Diagnosis Visual screening tests are routinely administered by nurses in various practice settings such as elementary schools, Head Start centers, or well-child visits.

Treatment Myopia is treated with biconcave lenses to improve distance vision. The child may need new lenses every year or two as he or she grows. Photorefractive keratectomy laser surgery is used to correct myopia, but most young children need no correction for hyperopia because their ability to accommodate overcomes their hyperopia as they grow. Astigmatism is treated with special lenses to correct unequal curvatures. High astigmatism must be corrected early to avoid **amblyopia** (a reduction or loss of vision in one eye).

Nursing Management Assessment is the primary nursing consideration. It is important to screen all children at well-child visits and listen carefully to the caregiver's history of the child's behavior. If vision impairment is detected, referral should be made to the appropriate professional.

Family Teaching—Care of Eyeglasses and Contact Lenses Plastic or polycarbonate lenses are the safest lenses for children (Figure 31-13). Nurses should teach caregiver or child to:

- Prevent scratches, never lay glasses lens down
- Always remove glasses with both hands to prevent warping of the frame
- Avoid getting the elastic bands too tight when using harnesses to keep the child's glasses in place
- Never replace missing screws with paper clips or wires
- Monitor when the bend of the temple is in front of the ear because glasses have been outgrown

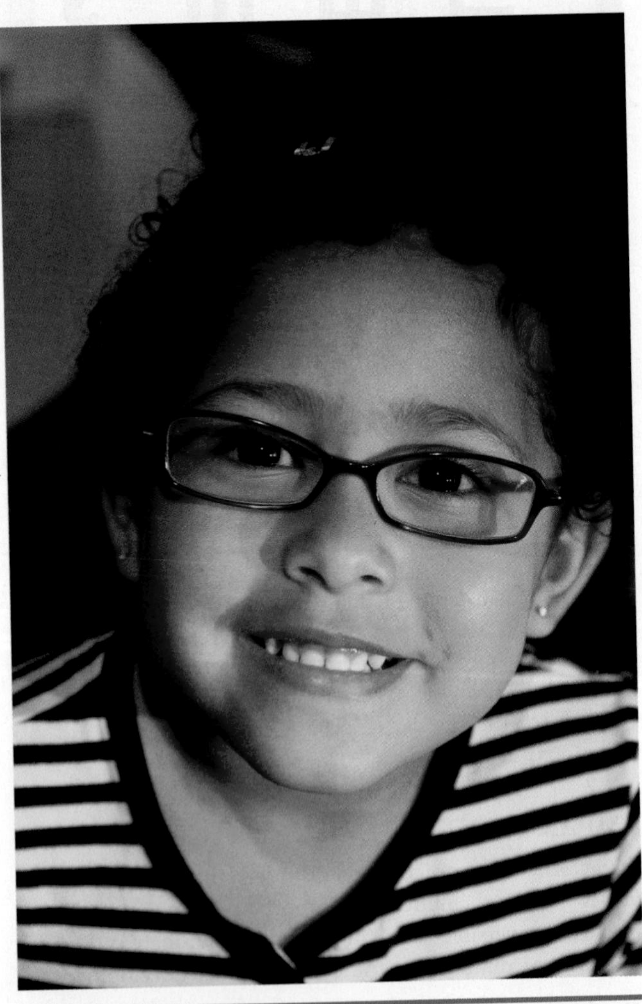

FIGURE 31-13 Children can learn proper care and maintenance of their eyeglasses. DELMAR CENGAGE LEARNING.

Contact lenses should not be prescribed until the child is able to care for them independently. Some suggestions for family teaching include:

- Safer for children engaged in active sports
- Allergic reactions to the lenses themselves or to the cleaning solutions may occur (symptoms include red eyes, discomfort, itching, burning)
- Complications are more likely to occur if lenses are worn on an extended basis (greater than 24 hours)
- Care and cleansing directions must be followed explicitly in order to avoid complications, such as corneal damage
- Improved body image—especially important for adolescents

Impairment of Muscular Efficiency

Eye movement, controlled by six small muscles and innervated by cranial nerves III, IV, and VI (Huether, 2010), should be smooth and coordinated. When the movement of these muscles becomes impaired, vision is compromised.

Strabismus

Incidence and Etiology **Strabismus** is a condition where the visual lines of each eye do not simultaneously focus on the same object in space because of a lack of muscle coordination, resulting in a crossed-eye appearance. Strabismus (Figure 31-14) occurs in approximately 3% of all children and is considered to be one of the most common childhood eye problems. Approximately half of these children have a positive family history for the defect, and as many as 75% of infants may have transient intermittent strabismus until 3 months of age (Olitsky, Hug, & Smith, 2007e; Rosales, 2008). **Pseudostrabismus** is a condition that makes a child appear crossed-eyed because of prominent epicanthic folds and a flat nasal bridge and disappears as the child grows. However, true strabismus is not outgrown.

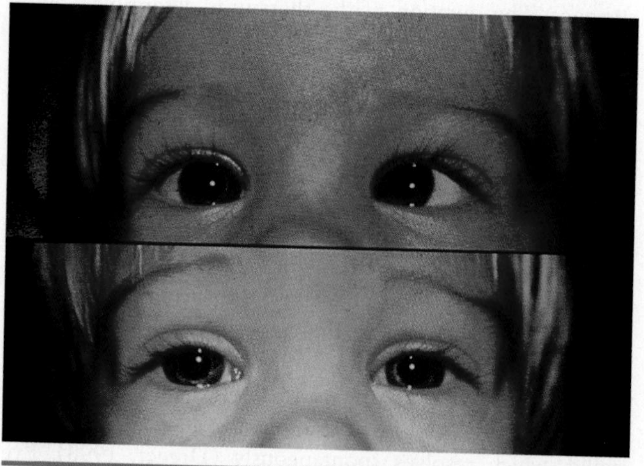

Figure 31-14 Child with Strabismus Before and After Corrective Treatment. COURTESY OF THE NATIONAL EYE INSTITUTE, NIH.

Pathophysiology When the extraocular muscles move the eyes in unison, the visual image falls on the fovea of each eye and the images fuse to form a single image. When one eye deviates (moves up, down, inward, or outward), the brain is unable to fuse the dissimilar images and double vision results. The brain will learn to suppress the image from the deviated eye (amblyopia) to allow clear sight in the straight eye. The earlier suppression begins and the longer it is allowed to continue, the more permanent the loss of vision. Strabismus may be nonparalytic (comitant) or paralytic (noncomitant). In nonparalytic strabismus, the most common type of strabismus, the extraocular muscles and controlling nerves are normal. Other refractive disorders, such as cataracts, may cause this type of strabismus. In paralytic strabismus, one or more of the extraocular muscles is paralyzed resulting in muscle imbalance. Paralytic strabismus may be congenital or acquired during infancy or childhood. Congenital strabismus is associated with neurodevelopmental disorders such as cerebral palsy or may result from birth trauma, congenital infections, or abnormal development of the optic cranial nerve (Olitsky et al., 2007e; Rosales, 2008).

Clinical Manifestations Because of CNS immaturity eye alignment in infants may vary from normal to intermittent exotropia or estropia. However, if these deviations continue after 4 months of age the infant should be referred to an ophthalmologist for evaluation and treatment (Rosales, 2008). Double vision in the older child causes the child to appear clumsy and to stumble or have difficulty picking up objects. The child may also squint to get a better image. Persistent crossing of the eyes is always abnormal regardless of the age of the client. Because of the potential loss of vision in the deviated eye, evaluation and treatment should begin as soon as possible, even as young as 3 months of age. If correction is not instituted before 6 years of age, reversal of the suppression of the image is difficult.

Diagnosis Screening should begin at 3–6 months of age to prevent loss of vision from strabismus. There are two major screening tests to detect strabismus: the Hirschberg Corneal Light Reflex Test and the cover test. To perform the Hirschberg test, a light is held in front of the child's face as the child stares straight ahead. The light should reflect off the cornea symmetrically, just medially to the center of the pupil. The cover test is more sensitive than the light reflex test but requires the child's cooperation. As the child looks at a toy, the examiner covers one of the child's eyes. If the uncovered eye moves, then it can be assumed it was not fixed on the target simultaneously with the other eye, and, therefore, the child has strabismus. Strabismus is classified into three primary types as illustrated in Figure 31-15.

RESEARCH Highlight

Refractive Error Study in Children: Sampling and Measurement Methods for a Multi-County Survey

STUDY PURPOSE

To assess the prevalence of refractive error and vision impairment in ethnic and culturally diverse pediatric populations.

METHODS

Ophthalmological examinations were conducted on cross-sectional samples of children, ages 5–15 years of age, of different ethnic and cultural settings.

FINDINGS

Outcome measure for evaluation included presenting uncorrected, and best-corrected visual acuity, along with refractive error under cycloplegia. Amblyopia and other uncorrectable vision impairments were identified. It was found current age-specific and sex-specific refractive errors can be determined and the methods used can be applied to children of different ethnic origins and cultural settings.

IMPLICATIONS

Prevention of visual impairment and blindness is an international concern. Nurses have the responsibility to be familiar with infants and children at risk for vision impairment (low birthweight, prematurity, retinopathy, other disabilities) and to encourage children and their families to seek routine ophthalmology exams to promote early identification and intervention.

REFERENCE

Negrel, A. D., Maul, E., Pokharel, G. P., Zhao, J. L., & Ellwein, L. B. (2000). Refractive error study in children: Sampling and measurement methods for a multi-county survey. *American Journal of Ophthalmology*, *129*, 421–426.

CORNEAL LIGHT REFLEX

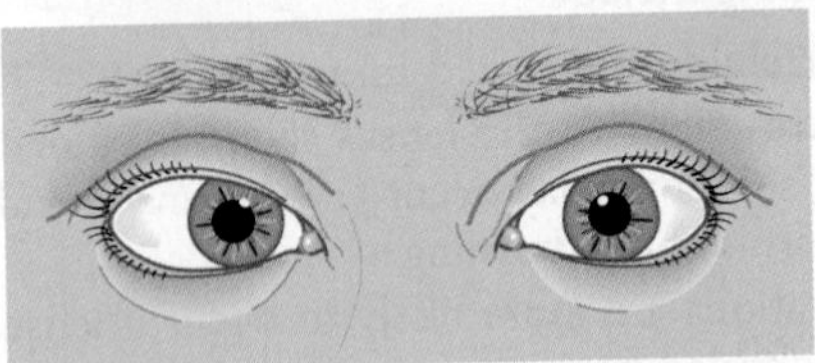

A. Right esotropia

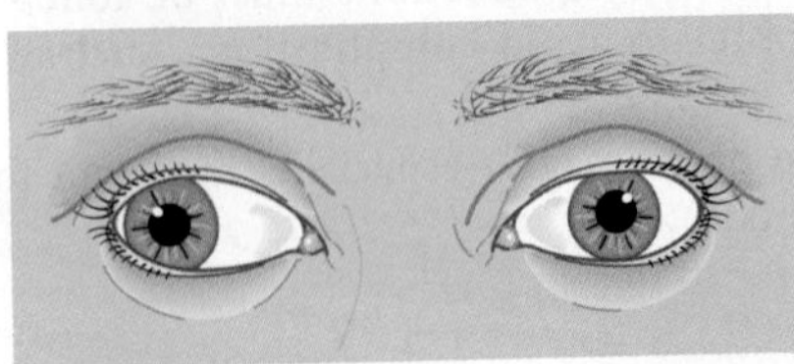

B. Right exotropia

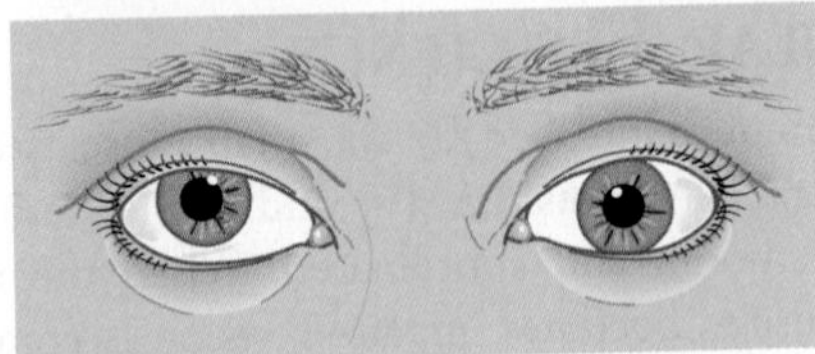

C. Hypertropia

FIGURE 31-15 (A) Right Esotropia. (B) Right Exotropia. (C) Hypertropia. DELMAR CENGAGE LEARNING.

Esotropia (convergent) occurs when the eye turns toward the midline.

Exotropia (divergent) occurs when the eye turns outward or away from the midline.

Hypertropia occurs when the eyes are out of vertical alignment. One pupil appears higher than the other.

Treatment The goal of treatment is to reduce or eliminate the deviation as much as possible and to attain the best possible vision in each eye while also attaining binocular vision. The type of treatment varies with the age of the child and the type of strabismus. Treatment can be medical or surgical. The medical approach may utilize occlusion therapy (eye patching) (refer to Figure 31-16), glasses, pharmacologic therapy, or eye exercises. Surgical correction is typically utilized for infants less than 12–18 months of age when glasses and pharmocologic therapy do not work. Eye patching is used prior to surgery to stimulate the noninvolved eye to function. Parents will need education about the need for continued monitoring as there is a risk that the child may redevelop strabismus or may develop amblyopia (Olitsky et al., 2007e; Rosales, 2008).

Patching the good eye is a common method of treatment. The stronger eye is covered to allow the weaker eye to work alone for all or part of each day, so it may become stronger. The duration of the therapy is determined by an ophthalmologist. Patching is most successful when done during the preschool years (American Academy of Ophthalmology, 1994). Eyeglasses with covered lenses are another method of occlusion. Pharmacologic therapy may utilize miotics (drugs that act on the ciliary muscle) to make accommodation easier. Another therapy is botulinum toxin (Botox, Oculinum), approved by the U.S. Food and Drug Administration in 1989 as an alternative to surgery. The toxin is injected into the eye muscle to produce temporary paralysis. This allows the muscles opposite the paralyzed muscle to straighten the eye. When the medication wears off in about 2 months the correction will be successful in 50% of clients. The most common side effect is a drooping eyelid, which resolves spontaneously (Dreger, 1998). Eye exercises may be prescribed in conjunction with patching and pharmacologic therapy.

Nursing Management

Assessment The most important nursing responsibility is early identification of the child with strabismus. Children should be assessed during well-child visits and referred immediately if needed. The nurse must support the family in managing the prescribed therapy. If the child is in school, the treatment plan should be explained to the school nurse.

Nursing Diagnosis

1. *Delayed growth and development* related to impaired visual perception.
2. *Anxiety* related to lack of knowledge about treatments used for strabismus.
3. *Parent education regarding the need for continued monitoring and evaluation for possible amblyopia or reoccurring strabismus.*

Outcome Identification

1. The child does not experience any impairment of growth and development.
2. The child wears patching as instructed.
3. Caregivers report diminished anxiety related to the child's treatment.
4. Caregivers are able to identify a schedule for follow-up examinations on a yearly basis.

Planning and Implementation Education of the caregivers is essential if the prescribed therapy is to be successful as they must understand why patching or corrective lenses are necessary. The nurse must stress the importance of compliance in promoting normal visual development. Caregivers need help and support in order to ensure the child's compliance. If the child is going to have surgery, the nurse must prepare the family. Caregivers need to know surgery may correct alignment, but not vision. Families must also be prepared for the possibility the surgery may not be successful and subsequent surgery may be necessary.

Evaluation As a result of the consistent use of prescribed therapy the strabismus will resolve. If surgery is required, then the family will understand the potential outcomes of the surgery and incorporate postsurgical care into their daily lives until instructed otherwise.

Family Teaching Children need to be taught how to take proper care of glasses. Caregivers and children must be provided with information about dressing changes, eye drops, corrective lenses, eye patches, and restraints.

Amblyopia

Amblyopia is the chief cause of preventable visual loss in children. Early detection and referral to the ophthalmologist can avert permanent disability. Amblyopia is a potential complication of strabismus that was not corrected in a timely manner or as a secondary disorder related to surgically corrected strabismus.

Incidence and Etiology **Amblyopia** ("lazy eye") is a reduction or loss of vision in one eye unrelated to an organic cause. Amblyopia occurs when the normal formation of retinal imaging is adversely impacted during the critical period of eye development, the first ten years of life (Olitsky et al., 2007b). Approximately 2% to 3% of the population has amblyopia in the preschool years. The most common cause is strabismus, where the brain suppresses the vision in the deviated eye to avoid the double image it is receiving. Eventually, sight is lost from the deviated eye. Additional causes of amblyopia are congenital cataracts, corneal opacity, or prolonged patching of the eye to correct strabismus, and refractive amblyopia, which occurs when there is asymmetric refractive error in each eye. When both eyes are not equally hyperopic, the brain receives one clear image and one blurred image. Just as in strabismus, the image from the eye with the greater hyperopia will be suppressed (Rosales, 2008).

Pathophysiology During the first 6 months of life, the infant develops the ability to clearly perceive images seen through both eyes. The normal infant's brain merges the images from the two eyes, enabling binocular vision (i.e., two eyes seeing a single image). If the brain suppresses the vision in one eye, the lack of stimulation to the portion of the brain associated with the affected eye does not develop. The critical period for the visual center in the brain to develop is up until 6 to 7 years of age. The longer visual suppression is present, the less reversible it becomes. If detected after the age of 7 years, restoration of sight in the suppressed eye is unlikely (Kelsey, 1998).

Clinical Manifestations Infants and young children with amblyopia often do not display any symptoms. However, they may occasionally develop a tendency to overreach for an object. Amblyopia is only detected by screening. Because of the lack of symptoms, and because amblyopia develops before the age of 7 years, tests for visual acuity should be part of each well-child visit for all young children.

Diagnosis Unless strabismus with the obvious sign of crossed eyes is present to alert the professional, amblyopia is largely asymptomatic because the good eye assumes the burden of vision and the child is unaware there is a problem. Therefore, it is essential a child's eyes be examined periodically before the age of 7. If any difference in visual acuity between the two eyes is detected during routine screening, referral to an ophthalmologist for a detailed examination should be made as early detection is the key to treatment.

Treatment The method of treatment is determined by the underlying cause. The underlying cause is always treated first, except when strabismus requires surgery, in which case the amblyopia is treated first (Kelsey, 1998). If cataracts are the cause, removal of cataracts and appropriate treatment are instituted. Refractive amblyopia is treated by correcting the refractive error with corrective lenses. Treatment may begin with removing any media opacity or by using appropriately prescribed glasses, to help the retinal image to focus well in both eyes. Occlusion therapy is then used for the sound eye. Occlusion of the good eye (occlusion therapy)

NURSING TIP

Care of Eye Patches

Suggest the following measures to maintain the treatment of eye patching:

- Apply tincture of benzoin around the eye where the sticky part of the patch goes to improve adhesion.
- If patch does not stay on, apply tape from the forehead to the cheek.
- Another method to keep the patch on is to apply tincture of benzoin to the tape as well.
- Wrap a bandage around the entire head and secure.
- Encourage children to pretend they are pirates or monsters to encourage compliance.
- When all else fails, restrict the child's ability to remove the patch by taping mittens on the hands of a young child. In older children, use cardboard tubes secured with gauze longitudinally around the elbows.
- Remove the eye patch for two hours per day to minimize the risk of occlusion amblyopia in the good eye. Patches can be put on one hour after the child awakens and removed one hour before bedtime.
- When child keeps patch on, use rewards, such as a trip to the park, to reinforce compliance.
- If all methods to keep patch on fail, glasses with opaque lens may be utilized.

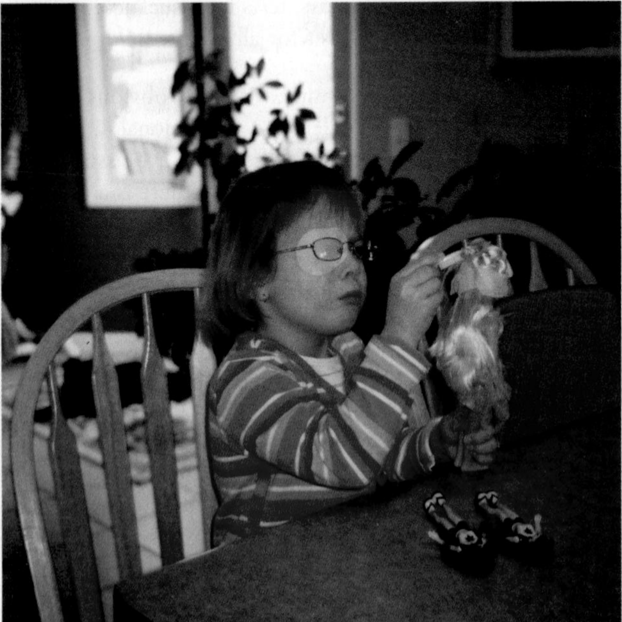

FIGURE 31-16 Even though this preschooler is wearing a patch for amblyopia, she is still able to participate in everyday activities. DELMAR CENGAGE LEARNING.

or blurring or penalization therapy (with glasses or drops) stimulates proper development of the affected eye, and forces vision in the "lazy eye" (see Figure 31-16). It is important to note that if the underlying cause of amblyopia is not corrected by age 7, the child may have permanent vision loss (Olitsky et al., 2007b; Rosales, 2008).

Nursing Management The screening of visual acuity to detect deficits during well-child visits in children younger than 7 years of age is the primary nursing responsibility. The nurse should understand how to administer screening tests and be cognizant of physical signs and symptoms of the disorder.

PHYSICAL INTEGRITY

Physical integrity problems occur when an alteration interferes with a child's vision. Cataracts and glaucoma are examples of such alterations.

Cataract

A **cataract** is an opacity (clouding) of the crystalline lens of the eye. Because light cannot pass through the opacity, vision is obscured.

Incidence and Etiology Approximately 2 out of 10,000 infants have infantile cataracts. Fifty to sixty percent of these are isolated cases of cataracts not associated with other defects or syndromes. However, 20% to 25% are related to congenital syndromes. Children with low birth weight are at higher risk for congenital cataracts (Olitsky, Hug, & Smith, 2007f). Worldwide about 200,000 children are blind because of cataracts. As the statistics continue to climb, Global Vision 2020 efforts are focused on early detection and treatment. The major cause of blindness associated with cataracts is deprivation amblyopia (Lloyd, Ashworth, Biswas & Abadi, 2007). Cataracts can be complete (entire lens is opaque) or incomplete (only part of the lens is opaque), bilateral or unilateral, or acquired or congenital. Acquired cataracts are caused by maternal infection during pregnancy, trauma, systemic disease, factors secondary to other eye malformations or diseases, or idiopathic factors. Congenital cataracts can be inherited as an autosomal dominant trait, caused by prenatal trauma, anoxia, maternal systemic disease, or acquired through prenatal infection (Olitsky et al., 2007f).

Pathophysiology The lens capsule forms during the fourth and fifth weeks of fetal development. It is normally a clear membrane allowing light rays to enter the eye and refract the rays for a clear image on the retina. When an organism or other factors interfere with lens development, it becomes milky white and cloudy, obscuring light rays and thus vision. Figure 31-17 illustrates the appearance of a cataract.

Clinical Manifestations The cloudiness of the lens is often visible to the naked eye. While checking pupils, an absent or abnormal reflex during a routine newborn examination is obtained. Caregivers might also notice their infant lacks visual attention to the environment or seems distressed in bright light. **Nystagmus** (oscillating movement of the eye) is a late sign.

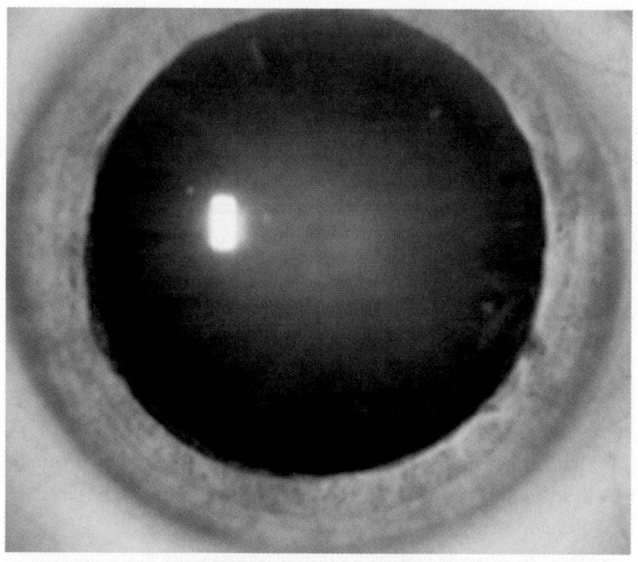

FIGURE 31-17 Cataract. COURTESY OF SALIM I. BUTRUS, M.D., SENIOR ATTENDING, DEPARTMENT OF OPHTHALMOLOGY, WASHINGTON HOSPITAL CENTER, WASHINGTON, DC & ASSOCIATE CLINICAL PROFESSOR, GEORGETOWN UNIVERSITY MEDICAL CENTER, WASHINGTON, DC.

Diagnosis Infants with a family or prenatal history placing them at risk for cataracts should be assessed as soon after birth as possible. The cloudiness of the lens usually can be seen by the caregiver or the nurse with the naked eye, or when the nurse is checking pupils with a penlight and notices a white pupillary reflex and an absent or abnormal red reflex. Early identification is essential to prevent the suppression of development of the visual cortex in the brain, which occurs during the first two months of life.

Treatment Referral to a pediatric ophthalmologist is necessary. The definitive treatment is surgical removal of the cataract from the affected eye. Timing of surgery is crucial to prognosis. If cataracts are visually present at birth, surgery must take place before 8 weeks of age to prevent an irreversible lack of vision development. After removal of the lens, the infant is considered aphakic or without lens and will need a corrective lens or contact lens to focus light on the retina. Intraocular lens implants have been used on some infants, but the long-term effects of permanent lens implants have not been established for infants. Because the developing eye will need frequent changes in corrective lenses, use of intraocular implants is not advised.

Nursing Management

Assessment The nurse must assess the child and family's responses to the diagnosis and identified preoperative treatment. The nurse must also assess the caregiver's knowledge regarding the postoperative follow-up care (patching, eye medications, etc.) required.

Nursing Diagnosis

1. *Anxiety* related to the surgical procedure and the surgical outcome.
2. *Deficient knowledge* related to the postsurgical care.

Outcome Identification

1. Child maintains a safe intraocular pressure.
2. Child does not develop an infection in the eyes.
3. Caregivers administer eye drops safely.
4. Caregiver demonstrates aptitude in postsurgical care.

Planning and Implementation In order to prevent an increase in intraocular pressure, the nurse must prevent the child from coughing, straining, or vomiting, with appropriate pain medication and comfort measures. The risk of infection can be minimized by using aseptic technique when handling dressings and closely monitoring for signs of local or systemic infection. The nurse must instill the appropriate eye drops per the ordered schedule in order to prevent the complications of increased intraocular pressure, infection, and glaucoma. Care must be taken to not put pressure on the globe of the eye when instilling drops. To prevent edema and pressure on the eye, the nurse should not place the child with the affected eye in a dependent body position.

Family Teaching Caregivers must be taught to safely perform the following postoperative care:

- Instillation of ordered eye drops
- Check for signs and symptoms of infection (drainage, redness, edema, itching)
- Check for signs and symptoms of increasing intraocular pressure (pain, bulging of eye)
- Care, purpose, and methods of maintaining eye patching

Glaucoma Glaucoma is a rare but serious visual impairment that, if untreated, can potentially end in blindness. Glaucoma is classified according to the age of the child at

NURSING ALERT

Postoperative Complications; Cataract Surgery

Acquired glaucoma is well-documented in infants and children following cataract surgery. It may occur shortly after surgery during the postoperative period or several years later. This has implications for the nurse working with infants and children who undergo surgical management of cataracts and their families including answering any questions families might have about postoperative care, potential postoperative risks, and how to prevent increased ocular pressure. Families should also be informed about follow-up assessment, evaluation, and vision care, including the prevention of eye injuries.

Reference

Lloyd, I. C., Ashworth, J., Biswas, S., & Abadi R. V. (2007). Advances in the management of congenital and infantile cataract. *Eye, 21,* 1301–1309.

diagnosis and the presence of other ocular or systemic conditions/disorders.

Incidence and Etiology Infantile (congenital) glaucoma occurs in children under 3 years of age, and although it can manifest itself in a child several months old, it is usually present at birth. Juvenile glaucoma affects children older than 3 years of age and is usually secondary to some other disease process (Olitsky, Hug, & Smith, 2007g). The signs and symptoms are essentially the same for the two forms of glaucoma. Because juvenile glaucoma is similar to the adult form, the remainder of this discussion refers to infantile glaucoma. Infantile glaucoma is a disease where the intraocular fluid pressure of the eye is increased because of a defect in the drainage system of the eye. This is usually caused by a developmental anomaly of the iridocorneal angle of the eye (also called trabeculodysgenesis). Glaucoma is also linked to congenital cataracts. Other causes of glaucoma in the pediatric population include trauma, ocular inflammatory disease, intraocular hemorrhage, and intraocular tumors. Glaucoma is also associated with some systemic disorders and syndromes such as Sturge-Weber syndrome and Marfan syndrome (Olitsky et al., 2007g).

Pathophysiology **Infantile glaucoma** results from a defective development of the trabecular meshwork, which does not allow a sufficient amount of aqueous humor to drain out of the intraocular space. When the aqueous humor accumulates in the anterior chamber of the eye, increased intraocular pressure results, causing damage to the ganglion cells of the retina, and leading to ischemia and necrosis of the optic disc, which may cause blindness. Glaucoma may occur in about 25% of children who have a history of cataracts and have undergone cataract surgery very early in life (Olitsky et al., 2007g).

Clinical Manifestations Clinical signs of glaucoma include excessive tearing (**epiphora**), involuntary closing of the eyelid, light sensitivity (**photophobia**), enlargement of the eyeball (**buphthalmos**), haziness or clouding of the cornea, and pain.

Diagnosis Diagnosis of glaucoma is made when the presenting clinical manifestations are recognized. Previously the measurement of intraocular pressure (IOP) was used to help in the diagnostic process, but is no longer a vital part of making the diagnosis. It does continue to be helpful in monitoring treatment and response (Olitsky et al., 2007g). Assessment of corneal diameter and clarity, and an examination of the retina to assess for optic nerve cupping (damage reflecting pressure), should also be done by the pediatric ophthalmologist. Treatment should begin immediately.

Treatment The definitive treatment is surgery (**goniotomy** or **trabeculotomy**) to open the outflow of the aqueous humor from the anterior chamber of the eye. It is essential to reduce the intraocular pressure as soon as possible (hours to days) in order to avoid cupping of the optic nerve. More than one surgical procedure is often necessary (Olitsky et al., 2007g). Medications may temporarily improve the drainage pre- and post-operatively. However, topical antiglaucoma drugs have been found to be generally ineffective in children.

EVIDENCE-BASED PRACTICE

Common Visual Defects and Peer Victimization in Children

CLINICAL PROBLEM

Many children who wear glasses or eye patches are victims of bullying in school and community settings.

BEST CLINICAL PRACTICE

- Nurses have a role and professional responsibility to advocate for children in various communities.
- Increasing violence is a factor in children's lives which can lead to adverse social, physical, cognitive, and psychosocial development.
- For effective correction of vision impairment disorders it is essential that children continue to wear their glasses and eye patch as prescribed by their health care provider. Failing to do so can lead to academic as well as safety issues.

IMPLICATIONS FOR NURSING

- Nurses need to ask children questions about their daily wearing of glasses or eye patches to determine if the child is following the recommended treatment plan.
- Nurses need to be alert to the risk of bullying victimization. If this is a possible situation, strategies should be developed and put into place to help decrease the child's vulnerability.

Reference: Horwood, J., Waylen, A., Herrick, D., et al. (2005). Common visual defects and peer victimization in children. *Investigative Ophthalmology and Visual Science, 46*, 1177–1181.

Nursing Management and Family Teaching

The major postoperative nursing goals are management of intraocular pressure, management of pain, reducing fear and anxiety, and teaching the caregivers to manage care at home. Measures to prevent an increase in intraocular pressure are instituted (prevention of straining, crying, startling). Bilateral eye patches increase anxiety. Therefore, measures to decrease anxiety and encourage caregiver involvement are helpful. The nurse must teach the caregivers how to manage care at home after surgery. Elements to include are:

- Management of eye patches
- Check for signs of increasing intraocular pressure

- How to prevent increase in intraocular pressure
- How to instill eye drops
- Check for signs of infection
- Need for follow-up care and monitoring

INFECTIONS

Conjunctivitis

Conjunctivitis ("pinkeye") is an inflammation of the conjunctiva. There are various causes of inflammation, viral or bacterial agents, allergens, irritants, or toxins. Inflammation in and around the eye of infants and children is irritating to the child and can be frightening to the caregiver. This condition always requires attention and prompt treatment.

Incidence and Etiology There are two types of conjunctivitis: neonatal conjunctivitis or ophthalmia neonatorium and childhood conjunctivitis. Neonatal conjunctivitis is caused by chemical irritation or infection. The incidence of neonatal conjunctivitis due to maternal chlamydial infection is 8 in 1,000 live births (Olitsky, Hug, & Smith, 2007h). Childhood conjunctivitis is caused by allergy or infection by bacterial or viral agents. The most common bacterial causes are *Haemophilus influenzae* and *Streptococcus pneumonia*.

Pathophysiology In neonatal conjunctivitis, chlamydia and gonnococci are spread to the newborn during passage through the birth canal. In childhood conjunctivitis, the child can be infected by either a bacteria or virus. Bacterial or viral conjunctivitis is highly contagious through contact with drainage from the eyes. Allergic conjunctivitis may arise in response to an allergen.

Clinical Manifestations Signs and symptoms of conjunctivitis may include itching eyelids, burning, light sensitivity (photophobia), redness, edema, and discharge. The appearance of the discharge from the eye can assist in identifying the etiologic agent. When an allergy is the cause, the drainage is stringy, clear, and usually bilateral. Bacterial drainage tends to be sticky and mucopurulent, and the child will often awaken with the eye "glued" shut; viral drainage is watery. Itching most often identifies the cause as an allergic response.

Diagnosis Diagnosis is made primarily on the presentation of the clinical manifestations. A culture may be obtained on the drainage to confirm the diagnosis.

Treatment In both neonatal or childhood conjunctivitis, identification of the etiologic agent is necessary to determine appropriate therapy. Antibiotic eye drops or ointments are the common treatment of infectious conjunctivitis. Both are self-limiting conditions lasting approximately one to two weeks. In allergic conjunctivitis, treatment is symptomatic. Cool eye compresses, oral antihistamines, and Crolom ophthalmic solution will bring some comfort (Rosales, 2007b).

Nursing Management If the conjunctivitis is allergic or viral in origin, the nursing management is primarily comfort measures, such as cold compresses on the eyes, reduced lighting, preventing rubbing of the eye, acetominophen for discomfort, and Crolom before allergy season (no effect on active inflammation). Conjunctivitis caused by bacterial agents is treated with appropriate antibiotic eye drops or ointments applied from the inner to the outer canthus, the use of baby shampoo to soften and remove crusting, or the use of dark glasses for photophobia (Rosales, 2007b).

Family Teaching Caregivers must be taught how to prevent transferring the extremely contagious drainage by following some simple steps:

- Use good hand washing before and after touching the eye.
- Use a separate towel, washcloth, sheets, and pillowcases.
- Don't allow the medicine dropper to touch the child's eyelid during medication administration.
- Use elbow restraints (infants or young children) to prevent rubbing of the eyes.
- Use Kleenex on each individual eye to wipe drainage and discard after use.
- Discard old contact lenses and use new ones after the infection resolves (if bacterial or viral).
- Discard old eye makeup; utilize new containers after the infection resolves.

The child will be excluded from school or day care until the drainage clears, even though the child is not communicable after 24 to 48 hours of treatment.

Periorbital Cellulitis

Periorbital cellulitis is an infection of the eyelid and soft tissues of the orbit of the eye.

Etiology Periorbital cellulitis can be caused by extension of infection from the sinuses or face, otitis media, upper respiratory infections, insect bites, or trauma (Nageswaran, Woods, Benjamin, & Shetty, 2006).

Pathophysiology Most often precipitated by organisms from wounds or infections elsewhere in the body, the most common causative organisms are *Staphylococcus aureus, Escherichia coli, group B streptococci, H. influenzae,* and *Staphylococcus pneumoniae* (Rosales, 2007b).

Clinical Manifestations Many of the same symptoms of conjunctivitis are exhibited in periorbital cellulitis, such as edema, warmth, and tenderness of the eyelid. Other symptoms that may be present are malaise, fever, elevated WBC count, decreased vision, and painful and reduced movement of the eyeball.

Diagnosis Diagnosis is made by close inspection and a culture of the drainage. Because sinusitis may be present, CT scan is also recommended to visualize the sinuses.

Treatment Intravenous antibiotics are usually the treatment of choice. The antibiotic used depends on the causative organism. Broad-spectrum antibiotics such as Ceftriazone (Rocephin) or Naficillin (Nafcil) are utilized for a 10-day period. It is important to treat the cellulitis, because if untreated, the infection can spread to the optic nerve or the brain, causing meningitis. Analgesics may be given for the pain (Olitsky, Hug, & Smith, 2007i; Rosales, 2007b).

Nursing Management The nurse monitors the administration of the intravenous antibiotics and analgesics. Warm soaks to the eyes three to four times per day may increase comfort. The cellulitis usually resolves without complication after antibiotic therapy is completed.

Sensorineural Blindness

The inability of a child to see presents a great challenge in achieving normal growth and development milestones. An interdisciplinary team and early intervention are necessary to ensure a child attains his or her maximum potential.

Incidence and Etiology A child is considered **blind** when other senses (hearing and touch) are relied upon as a chief means of task performance and learning. The overall incidence of children with severe visual impairment (vision when corrected less than 6/60 or blind) is 2.5 per 100,000 (Olitsky et al., 2007b). Legal blindness is defined as visual acuity of 20/200 or less with correction, or peripheral fields narrowed to an angle of 20 degrees or less. The legal definition must be verified by physical examination and determines eligibility for many rehabilitation programs. Blindness can result from any of the hereditary and acquired disorders noted in previous sections. Severe visual impairment or blindness is most often due to prenatal or perinatal causes. These may include genetic disorders (chromosomal syndromes, autosomal recessive, autosomal dominant, or X-linked) or hypoxia. Perinatal causes may include retinopathy of prematurity, infection, or hypoxia-ischemia. Older children may develop severe visual impairment or blindness as a result of tumors, injuries, infections, or juvenile idiopathic rheumatitis (Olitsky et al., 2007b; Olitsky et al., 2007j).

Pathophysiology Damage to the optic nerve or the visual center of the brain prevents the child from using vision to explore the world.

Clinical Manifestations Blind children have lost one of their most essential senses and must learn alternative ways to interact with their environment. Blindness may have an impact on every area of development, such as attachment, motor ability, mobility, language, learning, play, socialization, independence, self-concept, perception of space, and body image.

Diagnosis Visual acuity tests, neurological tests, and other diagnostic tests appropriate for specific etiologies are utilized to diagnose sensorineural blindness.

Treatment The blind child will require the assistance of a multitude of specially trained individuals in order to develop normally. Specialized training and adaptation of the early environment are essential to alter the impact of blindness in all areas of development. Special technologies are now available to help the blind child adapt to the environment. Technologies such as Braille (a system of raised dots that represent numbers and letters) to assist in reading a message, and a Braillewriter to write a message are useful. A tape recorder or a computer with a voice synthesizer can be used when the person being communicated with does not understand Braille. The tape recorder can also be used for note taking and listening to books on tape. With the visually impaired child, devices such as corrective lenses, magnifiers, large print books, magnified video projection systems, and tape recorders may also be helpful.

Families also need to understand the process of developing attachment to blind children and may require some adaptation in parenting behavior. When a child is blind, the usual facial interplay conveying emotion and communication between caregiver and child is impaired. The blind infant can develop attachment but usually does so more slowly (Moller, 1993). Fraiberg (1975) described a program that teaches caregivers to look for cues (other than visual) that suggest the infant is responding to them, for example, blinking of eyes, hand movements, and changes in activity level. Caregivers are also encouraged to show affection through nonvisual means, such as talking, cuddling, rocking, and so forth.

Since self-initiated mobility is delayed about 4 months in blind infants, and the blind infant does not have the stimulus of reaching to encourage mobility, the child must be stimulated by the use of sound. Delay will still occur as sound is not as strong a stimulus as sight. Although the child is physically ready to be mobile, the functional delay causes frustration, which results in some children exhibiting physical signs of frustration termed "**blindisms**" (for example, rocking and swaying) until the task is mastered. As a blind child becomes mobile, caregivers must make the environment safe as mobility is essential to later independence. Children are usually taught to walk by professionals known as orientation and mobility instructors. As the child becomes mobile, play takes on a new dimension. Blind children do not learn to play by imitation or active exploration, so they must be stimulated (especially by touch) and taught to play. Caregivers will need assistance in selecting toys and methods to teach the child how to play in order to develop gross and fine motor skills. Socialization needs of blind children are the same as for other children.

Promoting independence in activities of daily living is also important so the child will develop a positive self-concept. Caregivers need to be patient and persistent when teaching activities of daily living, and focus on the child's abilities, not the child's disabilities. Guidelines for caregivers and nurses include:

- When describing the environment, use words that are familiar to the child.
- Call the child by name and identify yourself before touching child.
- Keep objects in the environment in the same location, that is furniture, toys, and so forth.
- Utilize natural environmental cues to orient the child to associated event—for example, keys mean time to go for ride, water running means time for a bath.

CASE STUDY / CARE PLAN

VISUAL IMPAIRMENT

Karl is a 5-year-old child with sensorineural blindness admitted to the hospital for a hernia repair. Karl is legally blind and has had specialized training to adapt to his visual limitation. His growth and development are delayed. The family reports they are having some difficulty assisting Karl to integrate into the family and meet developmental tasks. You are the nurse admitting him to the pediatric unit. The nursing care plan is limited only to his visual impairment.

NURSING CARE PLAN

ASSESSMENT

The nurse should identify what difficulties the family is having integrating Karl into the family and the feelings both Karl and his family have. Information as to where Karl is developmentally must also be obtained.

NURSING DIAGNOSIS 1

Risk for injury related to visual perceptual alteration.

EXPECTED OUTCOMES

1. Karl moves confidently within his environment.
2. Karl does not experience any injuries when ambulating independently.

NOC: Risk Control: Visual Impairment

NIC: Environmental Management: Safety

INTERVENTIONS/*RATIONALES*

1. Describe the environment in words familiar to Karl. *The child needs orientation to the layout of the room to navigate safely.*
2. Keep objects in the environment in the same location. *Enables child to move within room independently.*
3. Call Karl by name and identify yourself before touching. *This avoids frightening Karl and gives him a chance to control his own environment.*
4. Encourage the family to re-enroll Karl in special programs for the blind as soon as possible. *Enables Karl to learn skills to ambulate safely.*

EVALUATION

Caregivers talk about their concern for Karl's safety and development. Karl moves confidently through his environment without injury.

NURSING DIAGNOSIS 2

Delayed growth and development related to visual perceptual alteration.

EXPECTED OUTCOMES

1. Karl maintains or increases his level of development through play activities.
2. Karl displays acceptable behavior and tolerates frustration.

NOC: Growth; Child Development

NIC: Developmental Care; Development Enhancement

(Continues)

CASE STUDY / CARE PLAN (Continued)

INTERVENTIONS/*RATIONALES*

1. Explain the day's activities early in morning. *Enables Karl to anticipate which activities will require assistance and which can be managed independently.*
2. Offer Karl choices and ask for his help in arranging the day's schedule. *Allows Karl to have some control and promote self-reliance.*
3. Anticipate that all tasks will take more time for Karl. *Karl needs detailed description of how to perform new activities and must move slowly to remain safe.*
4. Guide the family to select play material and activities suitable for visually impaired children. *Select activities that stimulate motor development and stimulate the senses of hearing and touch.*
5. Discuss the importance of consistent limit-setting. *To assist learning acceptable behavior and tolerating frustration.*
6. Encourage Karl to play with other children on unit. *This will encourage socialization.*

EVALUATION

Karl receives adequate stimulation to keep his growth and development moving in an acceptable direction.

NURSING DIAGNOSIS 3

Interrupted family processes related to Karl's visual alteration.

EXPECTED OUTCOMES

1. Caregivers express their feelings regarding Karl's impaired vision.
2. Caregivers express an understanding of Karl's unique abilities and special needs.
3. Karl expresses feelings regarding his sight.
4. Caregiver and Karl exhibit a positive relationship

NOC: Family Normalization

NIC: Caregiver Support; Family Integrity Promotion

INTERVENTIONS/*RATIONALES*

1. Assist the family gain a realistic concept of Karl's abilities. *Enables caregivers to encourage Karl to attain optimum level of development.*
2. Be available to the family for assistance. *Family will express problems and seek help when needed.*
3. Encourage and reinforce rehabilitation efforts for Karl. *Assists Karl gain optimal level of independence.*
4. Demonstrate Karl's acceptance by example. *Assists the family accept Karl in a positive manner.*
5. Encourage Karl and siblings to discuss their feelings regarding the disability. *Assists in positive reinforcement.*
6. Discuss the importance of grief and of chronic sorrow. *Helps them function in a healthier fashion.*

EVALUATION

The family feels comfortable and confident in accepting Karl's blindness and fosters his confidence and positive self-esteem.

- Do not overprotect the child; allow the child to gain self-confidence.
- A multidisciplinary team, together with the family, must collaborate to assist the child gain optimum independence.

EYE TRAUMA

Children are more likely than adults to sustain eye trauma, and males more often than females aged 11 to 15 years. Therefore, it is important to institute every possible measure to prevent injury that may cause transient or permanent loss of vision.

Incidence and Etiology

Trauma is the leading cause of blindness in children, with boys being twice as likely to sustain injury as girls. Approximately 21,000 eye injuries related to sports and recreation activities occur annually (American Academy of Pediatrics Committee on Sports Medicine and Fitness, 2004). Trauma is the cause of approximately 50% of the cases of blindness (Olitsky et al., 2007j).

Injuries to the eyeball and adjacent structures are classified as penetrating and nonpenetrating. Penetrating injuries are usually the result of sharp objects such as scissors, forks, sticks, knives, screwdrivers, pencils, and BBs (Olitsky et al., 2007j).

Nonpenetrating injuries are usually caused by foreign objects, such as blows from a blunt object (ball, fist, airbag), or thermal or chemical burns (Olitsky et al., 2007j). A blow from the hand or foot of another child is the most frequent cause of traumatic injury to the eye. The baseball continues to be a common cause of sports-related eye injuries. **Hyphema**, a hemorrhage into the anterior chamber of the eye, is a major complication of a blow to the eye. Chemical burns of the cornea are among the most serious eye injuries; alkali burns are more destructive than acid burns because alkali damages cell membranes and allows continuing penetration of alkali into the eye. Foreign bodies in the eye need to be removed carefully to avoid corneal abrasions and danger of an infection. Exposure to ultraviolet rays from the sun can cause solar retinopathy, cataracts, and age-related macular degeneration. Light-colored eyes are more sensitive than dark-colored eyes.

Use of Protective Eyewear in U.S. Children: Result from the National Health Interview Survey

STUDY PURPOSE

To assess the frequency of use of protective eyewear in children who participate in sports and recreational activities that can cause eye injury.

METHODS

The National Health Interview Survey (NHIS) was administered in 2002. Data from this survey were used to evaluate and analyze the use of protective eyewear by children while participating in sports and recreational activities that are prone to causing eye injuries. NHIS data are collected through a personal interview that is computer assisted. The survey was given to all members of households ages 17 years and older who were at home at the time of the interview. Data about household members not at home were provided by a knowledgeable adult family member. The 2002 sample consisted of 36,161 households and 93,386 people. Overall response rate was 89.6%. Data were obtained for children in the household who were 6 to 17 years of age, including demographic characteristics.

FINDINGS

A total of 8,256 children aged 6 to 17 years of age were included in the survey sample. Fifty percent of these children participated in sports and recreational activities that had potential for eye injury. While participating in these activities only 14.5% of children reported wearing protective eyewear. Children less than 12 years, males, and those children whose parents had some college or less than a high school education were more likely to wear protective eyewear. Females and children aged 12–17 years were less likely to wear protective eyewear. Results indicated parents' education, race/ethnicity, and region of residence were not significant factors in the use of protective eyewear.

IMPLICATIONS

- Nurses will need to develop and implement educational programs to inform children and parents about dangers when protective eyewear is not worn during sports, recreational activities, or hazardous home activities.
- The educational program offered to communities should include information about appropriate protection, how injuries can be prevented, and be given access to the protection or resources that may help to provide protective eyewear.

REFERENCE

Matter, K. C., Sinclair, S. A., & Xiang, H. (2007). Use of protective eyewear in U.S. children: Results from the National Health Interview Survey. *Ophthalmic Epidemiology*, *14*, 37–43.

NURSING ALERT

Eye Abrasions

Failure to treat an abrasion may result in corneal ulceration, infection, or permanent scarring and loss of visual acuity.

Topical anesthetics should never be used because they can retard healing and may mask painful symptoms of an infected abrasion.

Emergency Treatment

All treatment is focused on preventing further damage to the eye as a complication of the traumatic injury. Immediate and appropriate treatment at the scene can make a critical difference in the extent and permanence of the injury. Although the goal of treatment remains the same, once the child arrives at the hospital, the primary responsibility for care is in the hands of the ophthalmologist or eye surgeon. Nurses should understand and assist with treatment. See Box 31-9 and Box 31-10 for further information.

BOX 31-9

CARE OF PENETRATING EYE INJURIES

At the Scene

- Do not remove object.
- Secure the object with tape as appropriate to prevent movement.
- Cover uninjured eye to limit eye movement.
- Caution child against rubbing the eye.
- Transport child to the emergency room.

At the Hospital

- Sedate child.
- Remove object using aseptic technique (physician).
- Observe for aqueous or vitreous leaks, hemorrhage, prolapsed iris (not perfectly circular), pupils (shape, equality, and reaction to light), intraocular pressure, emphysema (air within orbit).
- Administer prophylactic antibiotics.
- Place an eye patch over the eye.
- Elevate head 30 degrees.
- Check immunization status of child, give tetanus if prescribed.

BOX 31-10

CARE OF NONPENETRATING EYE INJURIES

Foreign Body

At the scene

- Evert upper eyelid to look for foreign body; remove object with wet corner of a cotton swab.
- Caution child against rubbing the eye.
- If the eye irritation continues (continued blinking and tearing, pain, photophobia), take child to emergency room.

At the hospital

- Observe and treat hemorrhage or corneal abrasion (see below).

Corneal Abrasion

At the scene

- Attempt to remove foreign object from eye (as above).

At the hospital

- Physician will carefully examine eye for any abrasion (scraping of the cornea), using a fluorescein dye and visualizing injury under a blue filtered light (Wood's lamp or slit lamp).
- If the abrasion is small, instillation of antibiotic ointment four times per day is sufficient. If the abrasion is large, patching the eye for 24 hours, followed by instillation of antibiotic drops, will be necessary (Wingate, 1999).

Hyphema

At the scene

- Place eye patch over injured eye.
- Caution child not to move the head.
- Transport child to the emergency room.

At the hospital

- Determine amount of bleeding into the anterior chamber and intraocular pressure.
- Both eyes should be patched and the child placed on bedrest in the hospital with the head elevated 30 degrees to reduce mobility. (This will control further bleeding into the eye and prevent increase in intraocular pressure.)
- Cycloplegic (causing paralysis of the ciliary muscles of the eye) medications are administered to prevent movement of eye and to assist in reabsorption of blood.
- Close monitoring of the child to ensure bleeding does not recur and intraocular pressure does not increase is essential.

(Continues)

BOX 31-10
CARE OF NONPENETRATING EYE INJURIES (*Continued*)

Chemical Burns

At the scene

- Irrigate eye with water or saline from the inner to outer canthus.
- Transport immediately to the emergency room.

At the hospital

- Continue irrigation for 30 minutes if minor and 2 to 4 hours if severe.
- If chemical is unknown, use pH paper to determine if it is an acid or alkali. (pH paper also can be used after irrigation to check if it is normal.)
- Administer cycloplegic drugs as prescribed (will decrease eye movement and pain).
- Patch eye (will decrease eye movement and pain).
- Administer antibiotic drops.
- Monitor for inflammatory response and intraocular pressure readings.

Ultraviolet Rays

At the scene

- If skin is burned, close and patch the eyes, secure eye patches with a bandage wrapped around the head.
- Transport to the emergency room.

At the hospital

- Cold compresses can be applied to eyelids to decrease swelling.
- Eyes must be examined to ascertain whether damage is more than just to the skin of eyelids.

Nursing Management

The primary goals after injury are to institute immediate treatment for an eye injury in order to prevent further damage to the eye (at the scene), to continually monitor the injured child to detect complications after initial treatment (at the hospital), to support the frightened child and family, and to teach management of injury and prevention of future injuries.

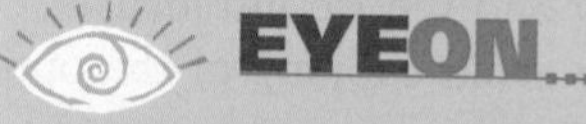

Traditional Methods of Maintaining Health

A traditional Chinese practice is to prepare amulets (a charm with an idol or Chinese character painted in red or black ink and written on a strip of yellow paper) to prevent evil spirits from causing them harm in the belief that children are kept safe with charms. Be sure whenever caring for a child who is wearing an amulet you acknowledge its importance and integrate its use into practice.

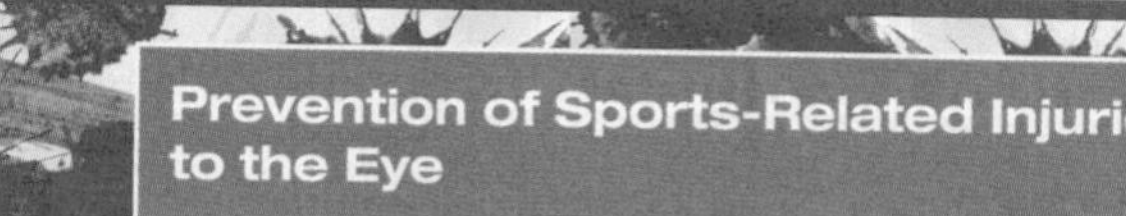

Prevention of Sports-Related Injuries to the Eye

Although sports injuries occur in all age groups, far more children and adolescents incur eye injuries than adults. The greater number of children participating in high-risk sports, their athletic immaturity, and the practice of wearing inadequate or no eye protection puts children and adolescents at greater risk for sports-related eye injuries. Although suitable eye protection exists for high-risk sports such as baseball, hockey, lacrosse, and racquet sports, children typically do not wear protective eyewear. Most of the traumatic eye injuries resulting in pain, decreased visual acuity, or permanent loss of vision could be prevented.

- What do you think are the reasons these preventive measures are not taken?
- What can you as a nurse or as a caregiver do to change this dangerous practice?
- Can professional athletes, for example, Karem Abdul Jabbar, serve as role models for children?

Eye injury statistics reveal a great need to educate caregivers, teachers, and coaches on the methods of prevention. Family and community education are a primary nursing role. As children grow and become mobile, the environment must be assessed for potential dangers and the child safeguarded. Chemicals such as cleaning and gardening products should be kept away from young children. Small objects that can be inserted into the nose, ear, and eye must be kept from the infant and toddler. If children play with sharp objects (such as scissors) and toys, they must be developmentally ready and supervised. Caregivers should be reminded of the dangers of glass (windows, doors, drinking) in the household.

In addition, many sports injuries can be avoided by the use of safety equipment (MMWR, 2005). High-risk sports (those where no eye protection can be worn such as boxing, wrestling, martial arts), those using a rapidly moving ball or puck (baseball, basketball, hockey, racquet sports), or those involving aggressive body contact (football) are especially dangerous. The highest percentage of injuries occurs in the sports of baseball and basketball. To prevent some injuries, polycarbonate goggles should be worn in sports that do not require a helmet or face mask; goggles should be worn under helmets for the hockey goalie and the baseball batter.

BOX 31-11
SUNGLASS GUIDELINES

- Labeled with "99% UV protection" or "meets ANSI UV requirements"
- Labeled with "100% UV protection" or "absorption up to 400 nm"
- Polarization reduces glare but has no relation to UV absorption
- Darkness of lens has no relation to protective capacity

Exposure to ultraviolet rays from the sun has caused solar retinopathy, cataracts, and age-related macular degeneration. Caregivers should be encouraged to have their children use sunglasses when exposed to the sun long enough to get a tan or a sunburn, or when in increased UV exposure situations such as beaches, snowfields, or high altitudes. Some guidelines for selection of effective sunglasses are found in Box 31-11.

All sensory alterations have an impact on growth, development, and learning to some degree. The nurse can alter the degree of impact by accurate and timely assessment and appropriate referral to other disciplines for intervention that will enhance the child's and the family's adaptation and enable the attainment of optimal growth and development.

IN THE REAL WORLD

My experiences with Helen helped me realize each client requires critical thinking on my part to recognize his or her needs and individualize his or her care. Nurses must gather information about client history, diagnosis, and present illness and then incorporate (organize, analyze) it into meaningful care. Because of her extensive medical experience, Lydia (mother) required far less general teaching and far more precise information. As nurses then, we need to adapt to schedules already established rather than trying to create our own for them. We need to be flexible and creative and help make the hospital environment as normal as possible for the child and family. (Written in response to caring for a child diagnosed at an early age with sensorineural blindness and hearing loss who had been admitted to the hospital frequently for treatment and surgery.)

KEY CONCEPTS

- Any alteration in a child's sensory perception or communication will affect growth and development.
- Early identification and intervention can prevent some detrimental effects of sensory alterations and promote growth and development.
- Optimal language development is influenced by cognitive ability, temperament, language, environment, and intact auditory and visual senses.
- Language disorders can be either receptive or expressive.
- Speech disorders may be caused by problems with voice, articulation, or fluency.
- Stuttering is the most common speech disorder. It may disappear as children mature.
- Hearing disorders may be classified as conductive, sensorineural, mixed, or retrocochlear.
- Prevention of hearing loss includes genetic counseling, prenatal care, prompt treatment of infection, immunizations, cautious use of ototoxic drugs, auditory screening, and protection from excessive decibel levels.
- Refractive errors are the most common type of visual disorders in children.
- Strabismus is the most common cause of amblyopia.
- Cataracts must be surgically removed no later than 17 weeks of age to prevent an irreversible lack of vision development.
- It is essential to identify and reduce intraocular pressure immediately to avoid cupping of the optic nerve in a child with infantile glaucoma.
- Trauma is the leading cause of blindness in children.
- Nursing goals include early detection of impairment, assisting the child and family to adjust to the impairment, promoting parent-child attachment, referring to specialized training personnel, providing parent education and the opportunity for play and socialization, and fostering optimum development.

REVIEW ACTIVITIES

1. What would you include in a teaching plan to assist caregivers enhance normal language acquisition?
2. What are the signs of visual and hearing impairment in children (infancy through adolescence)?
3. What are the leading causes of visual and hearing impairment in children?
4. What are the guidelines caregivers and nurses can utilize to enhance independence in daily living for blind children?
5. What is the most important role of the nurse in relation to hearing and visual loss?
6. What behaviors and actions will the nurse need to make to develop a trusting relationship with a child of ethnic diversity who has a hearing or vision impairment?

STUDY QUESTIONS

1. Rebecca, an 8-year-old with a severe hearing impairment, was hit by a car while riding her bicycle. Although she was wearing a helmet she was unconscious and has been admitted to the emergency department. She is now awake and somewhat agitated. What should be your first priority?
   a. Determine what her level of consciousness is and prepare her for a CAT scan.
   b. Establish communication with her using eye contact, touch, and correctly placing her hearing aids.
   c. Assign a patient care technician to stay at her side to help restrain her and to prevent her from injury.
   d. Assess her for any additional injuries that are likely to co-exist in an auto-bicycle accident, such as a fractured leg.
2. Which of the following statements would be most indicative of a language disorder?
   a. A 2-year-old child unable to carry on a conversation using at least 30 words.
   b. A 3-year-old child who has not spoken in a completed sentence.
   c. An 18-month-old who uses short, one- to two-word phrases.
   d. A 3-year-old who occasionally stutters, particularly when stressed.
3. Parents of a child who stutters should be encouraged to:
   a. Request that the child begin to speak again but more slowly.
   b. Reward the child when proper speech is used instead of stuttering.
   c. Complete the child's sentence while showing unconcern.
   d. Be patient and give the child time to complete thought and sentence.
4. Sarah, age 3 years, has recently been diagnosed with a hearing impairment. What would your major immediate goal be for Sarah?
   a. Prepare Sarah and her parents for a cochlear implant.
   b. Develop a teaching plan on how to use a hearing aid.
   c. Facilitate communication with Sarah.
   d. Provide Sarah's parents with a community resource guide.
5. Mario, born at 28 weeks, is deaf and blind. He is now 2 years old. To help Mario establish communication skills his parents will most likely:
   a. Place Mario in the same place in the room to help him identify his surroundings.
   b. Keep communication clues to him and received from him to a limited number.
   c. Limit his environmental stimuli to help him feel safe and secure.
   d. Select and consistently use the same clue to help him discriminate one person from another.
6. As the school nurse you are concerned about preventative eye care and sports. Which of the following statements would be considered when developing educational programs?
   a. Children who wear glasses may need to select noncontact sports.
   b. Protective eyewear should be required for sports such as baseball and volleyball.
   c. Children should be educated about the value of wearing contact lenses for improved visual acuity during sports.
   d. It is not a challenge to get children and adolescents to agree to wear their protective eyewear for sports activities.

7. Which of the following describes amblyopia?
   a. Increased intraocular pressure
   b. Squint or cross-eye; malalignment of one or both eyes
   c. Lazy eye; reduced visual acuity in one eye
   d. Different refractive strengths in one eye
8. Conductive hearing loss in infants and children is most often caused by:
   a. Recurrent otitis media that causes scarring and interferes with sound transmission.
   b. Antibiotics such as gentamicin or tobramycin which damages the eighth cranial nerve.
   c. Other disorders such as kernicterus.
   d. Frequent exposure to high decibel levels in the NICU as a premature infant.
9. Which of the following circumstances would need evaluation?
   a. A newborn who lacks binocularity
   b. A toddler whose mother expresses concern over his "cross-eyed" appearance
   c. A 6-year-old child with hyperopia
   d. The presence of a red reflex in an eight-year-old
10. As the nurse working with Henry, a 5-year-old newly diagnosed with moderate hearing loss, you identify altered growth and development related to impaired communication as a nursing diagnosis. To achieve the goal of optimum independence for age you will exclude which of the following nursing interventions?
    a. Encourage family to attend the local rehabilitation program.
    b. Discuss with family the importance of discipline and limit-setting.
    c. Provide opportunities for the child to express his feelings and concerns.
    d. Discuss advantages and disadvantages of amplifying devices.

REFERENCES

American Academy of Ophthalmology. (1994). Strabismus: Etiology, diagnosis, and treatment. *Journal of Ophthalmic Nursing and Technology, 13,* 121–123.

American Academy of Pediatrics, Committee on Practice of Ambulatory Medicine, Section on Ophthalmology. (1996). Eye examination and vision screening in infants, children, and young adults. *Pediatrics, 98,* 153–157.

American Academy of Pediatrics, Committee on Sports Medicine and Fitness: Protective eyewear for young athletes. (2004). *Pediatrics, 113,* 619–622.

Bradham, T., & Jones, J. (2008). Cochlear implant candidacy in the United States: Prevalence in children 12 months to 6 years of age. *International Journal of Pediatric Otorhinolaryngology, 72,* 1023–1028.

Braverman, R. (2007). Diagnosis and treatment of refractive errors in the pediatric population. *Current Opinion in Ophthalmology, 18,* 379–383.

Chamley, C. A., Carson, P., Randall, D., & Sandwell, M. (2005). *Developmental anatomy and physiology of children.* St. Louis, MO: Elsevier.

Chu, K., Elimian, A., Barbera, J., Ogbnutn, P., Spitzer, A., & Quirk, J. G. (2003). Antecedents of newborn hearing loss. *Obstretrics and Gynecology, 101,* 584–588.

Chung, J. H., Des Roches, C. M., Meunier, J., & Eavey, R. D. (2006). Evaluation of noise-induced hearing loss in young people using a web-based survey technique. *Pediatrics, 17,* 248–249.

Cochlear America, The cochlear experience: Candidacy criteria. Retrieved March 18, 2010, from http://www.cochlearamericas.com/378.asp.

Connolly, J. L., Carron, J. D., & Roark, S. D (2005). Universal newborn screening: Are we achieving the Joint Committee on Infant (JCIH) objectives? *Laryngoscope, 115,* 232–236.

Dale, P., Price, T., Bishop, D., & Plomin, R. (2003). Outcomes of early language delay: 1. Predicting persistent and transient language difficulties at 3 and 4 years. *Journal of Speech, Language, and Hearing Research, 46,* 544–560. doi:10.1044/1092-4388 (2003/044).

Dreger, V. (1998). Detection and treatment of strabismus. *Insight, 23,* 95–101.

Engdahl, B., & Eskild, A. (2007). Birth weight and the risk of childhood sensorineural hearing loss. *Paediatric and Perinatal Epidemiology, 21,* 495–500.

Fraiberg, S. (1975). Intervention in infancy: A program for blind infant. In B. Z. Friedlander, G. M. Sterritt, & G. E. Kirk (Eds.). *Exceptional infant, 3: Assessment and intervention.* New York: Brunner/Mazel, pp. 940–962.

Grover, G. (2008). Language development: Speech and hearing assessment. In C. D. Berkowitz (2008). *Pediatrics: A primary care approach* (3rd ed.). Elk Grove Village, IL: American Academy of Pediatrics, pp. 95–100.

Haapanen, M. L., Aro, T., & Isotalo, E. (2008). SPEEDY babies: A putative new behavioral syndrome of unbalanced motor-speech development. *Neuropsychiatric Disease and Treatment, 6,* 1225–1233.

Haddad, J. (2007). Hearing loss. In R. M. Kliegman, R. E. Behrman, H. B. Jenson, & B. F. Stanton (Eds.). *Nelson textbook of pediatrics* (18th ed.). Philadelphia, PA: Saunders, pp. 2620–2628.

Harlor, A. D. (2009). Hearing assessment in infants and children: Recommendations beyond neonatal screening. *Pediatrics, 124*(4), 1252–1263.

Hartmann, E. E., Bradford, G. E., Chaplin, P. K. N., Johnson, T., Kemper, A. R., Kim. S., et al. (2006). Project universal preschool vision screening: A demonstration project. *International Journal of Pediatric Otorhinolaryngology, 71,* 1429–1438.

Horwood, J., Waylen, A., Herrick, D., et al. (2005). Common visual defects and peer victimization in children. *Investigative Ophthalmology & Visual Science, 46,* 1177–1181.

Huether, S. (2010). Pain, temperature regulation, sleep, and sensory function. In K. McCance, & S. Huether (Eds.). *Pathophysiology: The biologic basis for disease in adults and children* (6th ed.). St. Louis, MO: Mosby. pp. 481–524.

Jafari, A., Malayeri, S., & Ashayeri, H. (2007). The ages of suspicion, diagnosis, amplification, and interventions in deaf children. *International Journal of Pediatric Otorhinolaryngology, 71,* 35–40.

Joint Commission on Infant Hearing. (2007). Year 2007 position statement: Principles and guidelines for early hearing detection and intervention programs. *Pediatrics, 120,* 898–921.

Kelsey, A. (1998). Amblyopia: The condition, the challenge, and the cure. *Journal of Ophthalmic Nursing and Intervention, 17,* 227–229.

Lederberg, A., & Everhart, V. (1998). Communication between deaf children and their hearing mothers. The role of language gesture and vocalization. *Journal of Speech, Language, and Hearing Research, 41,* 887–899.

Lloyd, I. C., Ashworth, J., Biswas, S., & Abadi, R. V. (2007). Advances in the management of congenital and infantile cataract. *Eye, 21,* 1301–1309.

Matter, K. C., Sinclair, S. A., & Xiang, H. (2007). Use of protective eyewear in U.S. children: Results from the National Health Interview Survey. *Ophthalmic Epidemiology, 14,* 37–43.

McCracken, W., Young, A., & Tattersall, H. (2008). Universal newborn hearing screening: Parental reflections on very early audiological management. *Ear and Hearing, 29,* 54–64.

Moeller, M. (1993). Working with visually impaired children and their families. *Pediatric Clinics of North America,, 40,* 881–889.

Morbidity and Mortality Weekly Report (MMWR). (2005). Visual impairment and use of eye-care services and protective eyewear among children—United States 2002. *Morbidity and Mortality Weekly Report, 54,* 425–429.

Moore, J. (2006). Pediatricians need greater awareness of hearing disorders. *Infectious Diseases in Children, 19,* 53–54.

Nageswaran, S., Woods, C. R., Benjamin, D. K., & Shetty, L. (2006). Orbital cellulitis in children. *Pediatric Infectious Disease Journal, 25,* 695–699.

National Information Center for Children and Youth with Disabilities. (1996). *Deafness and hearing loss* (Special Education Programs Publication No. H030A30003). Washington, DC: U.S. Government Printing Office.

National Institute on Deafness and Other Communication Disorders. (2007). *Healthy People 2010: Hearing health progress report.* Retrieved June 1, 2009, from http://www.nidcd.nih.gov/health/healthyhearing/what_hh/progress_review_04.asp, 2004.

National Institutes of Health (NIH). (2006). *Cochlear implants fact sheet.* Washington, D.C.: Author.

National Institutes of Health (NIH). (2007). *Cochlear implants.* Washington, D.C.: Author.

Negrel, A. D., Maul, E., Pokharel, G. P., Zhao, J. L., & Ellwein, L. B. (2000). Refractive error study in children: Sampling and measurement methods for a multi-county survey. *American Journal of Ophthalmology, 129,* 421–426.

Nobel, J. E., & Sifuentes, M. (2008). Hearing impairments. In Berkowitz, C. D. (2008). *Pediatrics: A primary care approach* (3rd ed.). Elk Grove Village, IL: American Academy of Pediatrics, pp. 341–346.

O'Connor, A. R., Wilson, C. M., & Fielder, A. R. (2007). Ophthalmological problems associated with preterm birth. *Eye, 21,* 1254–1260.

Olitsky, S. E., Hug, D., & Smith, L. P. (2007a). Growth and development. In R. M. Kliegman, R. E. Behrman, H. B. Jenson, & B. F. Stanton (Eds.). *Nelson textbook of pediatrics* (18th ed.). Philadelphia, PA: Saunders, pp. 2569–2572.

Olitsky, S. E., Hug, D., & Smith, L. P. (2007b). Disorders of vision. In R. M. Kliegman, R. E. Behrman, H. B. Jenson, & B. F. Stanton (Eds.). *Nelson textbook of pediatrics* (18th ed.). Philadelphia, PA: Saunders, pp. 2573–2576.

Olitsky, S. E., Hug, D., & Smith, L. P. (2007c). Examination of the eye. In R. M. Kliegman, R. E. Behrman, H. B. Jenson, & B. F. Stanton (Eds.). *Nelson textbook of pediatrics* (18th ed.). Philadelphia, PA: Saunders, pp. 2569–2572.

Olitsky, S. E., Hug, D., & Smith, L. P. (2007d). Abnormalities of refraction and accommodation. In R. M. Kliegman, R. E. Behrman, H. B. Jenson, & B. F. Stanton (Eds.). *Nelson textbook of pediatrics* (18th ed.). Philadelphia, PA: Saunders, pp. 2572–2573.

Olitsky, S. E., Hug, D., & Smith, L. P. (2007e). Disorders of eye movement and alignment. In R. M. Kliegman, R. E. Behrman, H. B. Jenson, & B. F. Stanton (Eds.). *Nelson textbook of pediatrics* (18th ed.). Philadelphia, PA: Saunders, pp. 2578–2582.

Olitsky, S. E., Hug, D., & Smith, L. P. (2007f). Abnormalities of the lens. In R. M. Kliegman, R. E. Behrman, H. B. Jenson, & B. F. Stanton (Eds.). *Nelson textbook of pediatrics* (18th ed.). Philadelphia, PA: Saunders, pp. 2593–2597.

Olitsky, S. E., Hug, D., & Smith, L. P. (2007g). Childhood glaucoma. In R. M. Kliegman, R. E. Behrman, H. B. Jenson, & B. F. Stanton (Eds.). *Nelson textbook of pediatrics* (18th ed.). Philadelphia, PA: Saunders, pp. 2608–2610, 2615.

Olitsky, S. E., Hug, D., & Smith, L. P. (2007h). Disorders of the conjunctiva. In R. M. Kliegman, R. E. Behrman, H. B. Jenson, & B. F. Stanton (Eds.). *Nelson textbook of pediatrics* (18th ed.). Philadelphia, PA: Saunders, pp. 2588–2591.

Olitsky, S. E., Hug, D., & Smith, L. P. (2007i). Orbital infections. In R. M. Kliegman, R. E. Behrman, H. B. Jenson, & B. F. Stanton (Eds.). *Nelson textbook of pediatrics* (18th ed.). Philadelphia, PA: Saunders, pp. 2611–2612.

Olitsky, S. E., Hug, D., & Smith, L. P. (2007j). Injuries to the eye. In R. M. Kliegman, R. E. Behrman, H. B. Jenson, & B. F. Stanton (Eds.). *Nelson textbook of pediatrics* (18th ed.). Philadelphia, PA: Saunders, pp. 2612–2615.

Ottar-Pfeifer, W. (2005). When should children have their eyes checked? *Insight: Journal of the American Society of Ophthalmic Registered Nurses, 30,* 17–22.

Rosales, T. (2008). Strabismus. In Berkowitz, C. D. (2008). *Pediatrics: A primary care approach* (3rd ed.). Elk Grove Village, IL: American Academy of Pediatrics, pp. 361–365.

Simms, M. D., & Schum, R. L. (2007). Language development and communication disorders. In R. M. Kliegman, R. E. Behrman, H. B. Jenson, & B. F. Stanton (Eds.). *Nelson textbook of pediatrics* (18th ed.). Philadelphia, PA: Saunders, pp. 152–161.

Subramanian, M. (2007). *Color blindness.* Retrieved May 31, 2009, from http://www.nlm.nih.gov/medlineplus/ency/article/001002.htm.

United States Department of Health and Human Services. (2006). *Healthy People 2010: Midcourse Review,* Washington, D.C.

United States Preventative Services Task Forces: Screening for visual impairments in children younger than five years: Recommendation statement. (2005). *American Family Physician, 27,* 333–336.

Weichbold, V., Nekahm-Heis, D., & Welzl-Mueller, K. (2006). Universal newborn hearing screening and postnatal hearing loss. *Pediatrics, 117,* 3631–3636.

Weichbold, V., & Zorowka, P. (2007). Can a hearing education campaign for adolescents change their music listening behavior? *International Journal of Audiology, 46,* 128–133.

Wilson-Clark, S. D., Squires, S., & Deeks, S. (2006). Bacterial meningitis among cochlear implant recipients—Canada, 2002. *Morbidity and Mortality Weekly Report, 55*(Supp01): 20–24.

Windmill, S., & Windmill, I. M. (2006). The status of diagnostic testing following referral from universal newborn hearing screening. *Journal of the American Academy of Audiology, 17,* 367–378.

Wingate, S. (1999). Treating corneal abrasions. *Nurse Practitioner, 24,* 53–60.

Yaeger, D., McCallum, J., Lewis, K., Soslow, L., Shah, U., Potsie, W. et al. (2006). Outcomes of clinical examination and genetic testing of 500 individuals with hearing loss evaluated through a genetics of hearing loss clinic. *International Journal of Audiology, 140,* 827–836.

SUGGESTED READINGS

Advanced Bionics Corporation, Package insert: HiResolution TM Bioic Ear System. Retrieved June 1, 2009, from http://www.bionicear.com/printables/HiRes90K.HelixPkgInsert.pdf,

American Academy of Pediatrics, Committee on Practice and Ambulatory Medicine, Section on Ophthalmology. (2002). Use of photoscreening for children's vision screening. *Pediatrics, 109*, 524–525.

Hunter, L. L., Davey, C. S., Kohtz, A., & Daly, K. A. (2007). Hearing screening and middle ear measure in American Indian infants and toddlers. *International Journal of Pediatric Otorhinolaryngology, 71*, 1429–1438.

Hyde, M., & Power, D. (2006). Some ethical dimensions of cochlear implantation for deaf children and their families. *Journal of Deaf Students and Deaf Education, 11*, 102–111.

Noyes-Grosser, D. M., Holland, J. P., Lyons, D., Holland, C. L., Romanczyk, R. G., & Gillis, J. M. (2005). Rationale and methodology for developing guidelines for early intervention services for young children with developmental disabilities. *Infants and Young Children, 18*(2), 119–135.

Wald, E. R. (2004). Periorbital and orbital infections. *Pediatrics in Review, 25*, 312–320.

RESOURCES

Refer to the online student StudyWARE for Potts & Mandleco at http://www.CengageBrain.com for additional content and study aids.

Organization: **Alexander Graham Bell Association for the Deaf & Hard of Hearing**
Description: Offers a wealth of information including specific links for parents, professionals, and deaf/hard of Hearing adults.
Website/Resource: http://www.agbell.org

Organization: **American Academy of Audiology**
Description: Offers users information about professional development for audiologists, practice management, advocacy, education/research, and publications.
Website/Resource: http://www.audiology.org

Organization: **American Deafness and Rehabilitation Association**
Description: Offers users information about membership, state chapters, special interest groups, legislation publications, and continuing education.
Webste/Resource: http://www.adara.org

Organization: **American Foundation for the Blind Information Center**
Description: Offers links to helpful resources including information about program blogs, education, and Braille for the Blind.
Website/Resource: http://www.afb.org

Organization: **American Printing House for the Blind**
Description: Offers access to products for the blind, a tactile visual graphics library, software, and research information.
Website/Resource: http://www.aph.org

Organization: **American Speech-Language-Hearing Association**
Description: Offers users information regarding speech-language-hearing careers, certification, publications, events, advocacy, continuing education, practice management, and research.
Website/Resource: http://www.asha.org

Organization: **Laurent Clerc/National Deaf Education Center**
Description: Provides information/training/technical assistance for professionals meeting needs of children who are deaf/hard of hearing; information about Gallaudet University; links to helpful resources.
Website/Resource: http://clerccenter.gallaudet.edu

Organization: **National Association for Parents of Children with Visual Impairments (NAPVI)**
Description: Provides information/resources for parents of children who are blind/visually impaired; offers information regarding conference dates, NAPVI chapters, publications, and a parents directory.
Website/Resource: http://www.spedex.com/napvi

Organization: **National Association of the Deaf (NAD)**
Description: Offers information about NAD issues/resources, news/events, youth leadership, and community contacts.
Website/Resource: http://www.nad.org

Organization: **National Easter Seal Society**
Description: Offers information about different programs focuses, services, and expert connections for people living with autism and other disabilities.
Website/Resource: http://www.easterseals.com

Organization: **National Eye Institute**
Description: Offers information related to news/events, research funding, educational programs, and training about blinding eye diseases, visual disorders, mechanisms of visual function, preservation of sight, and special health problems/requirements of the blind.
Website/Resource: http://www.nei.nih.gov

Organization: **National Federation of the Blind**
Description: Offers information about vision loss, program research/publications, and helpful technology/products.
Website/Resource: http://www.nfb.org

Organization: **National Institute on Deafness and Other Communication Disorders (NIDCD)**
Description: Offers information about research, news/events, and basic health information related to disorders of hearing, balance, smell, taste, voice, speech, and language.
Website/Resource: http://www.nidcd.nih.gov

Organization: **Self Help for Hard of Hearing People**
Description: Offers information regarding advocacy, the academy, convention dates, and local chapters for people with hearing loss and their families.
Website/Resource: http://www.shhh.org

Organization: **Stuttering Foundation of America**
Description: Offers users facts on stuttering, access to parent resources, and links for age groups.
Website/Resource: http://www.stuttersfa.org

Organization: **The Blind Children's Center**
Description: Offers information regarding news, special events, the annual report, and research publications related to young children with visual impairments.
Website/Resource: http://www.blindchildrenscenter.org

Organization: **The Foundation Fighting Blindness**
Description: Offers information about eye conditions, professionals/researchers, resources, community news, and upcoming news/events.
Website/Resource: http://www.blindness.org

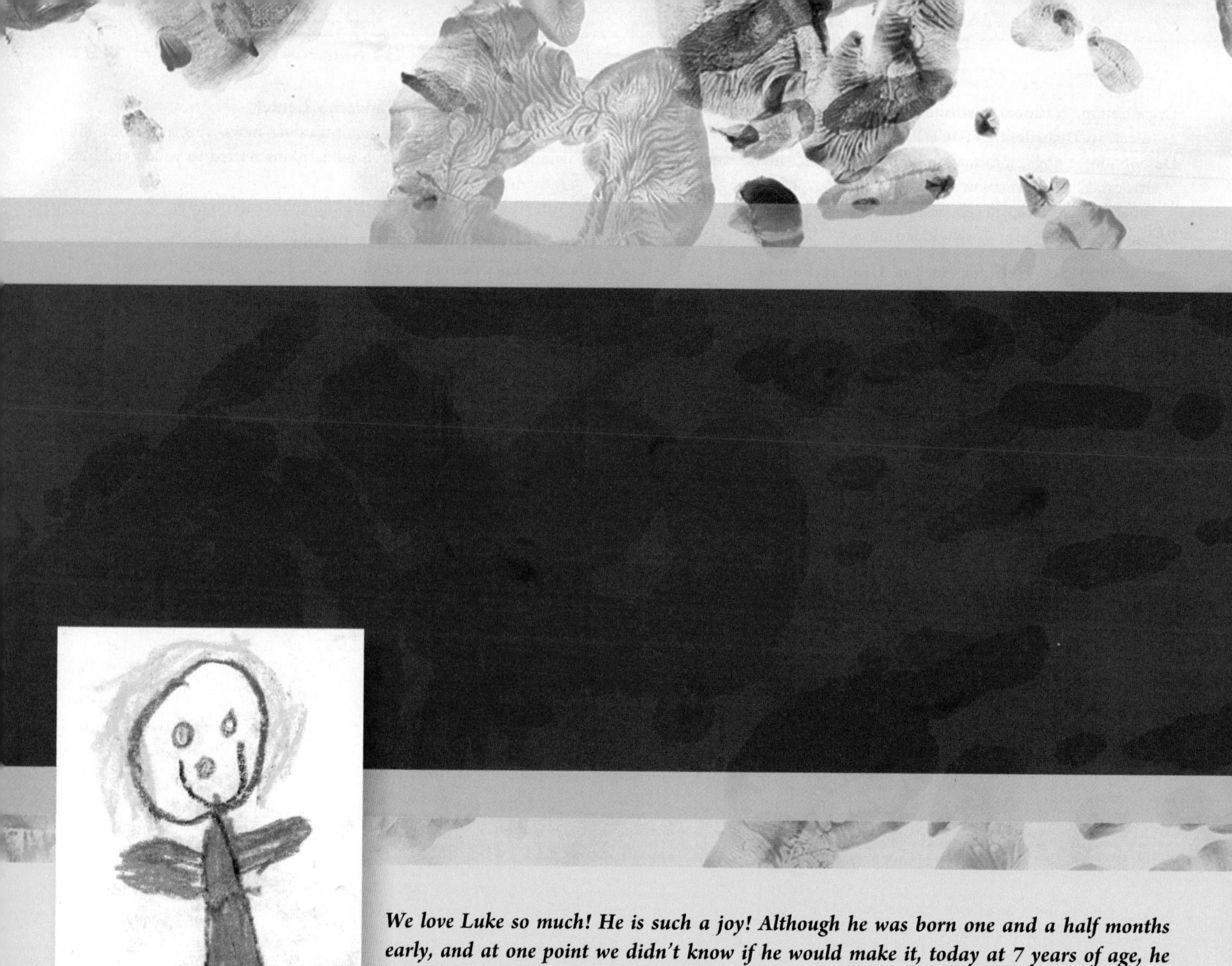

We love Luke so much! He is such a joy! Although he was born one and a half months early, and at one point we didn't know if he would make it, today at 7 years of age, he is doing so well! He wears glasses because of his nystagmus and uses a cane to help him walk. He is in second grade now and able to read at the level of most of his friends. The doctors say that as he gets older his motor control may get better and his speech may improve. We just hope he will remain the happy-go-lucky child he is and be able to be independent as an adult.

—Adrienne, Mother of a Child with Cerebral Palsy.

CHAPTER 32
Neurological Alterations

DONNA FREEBORN, FNP, CNM, PhD
BARBARAL L. MANDLECO, RN, PhD

COMPETENCIES

Upon completion of this chapter, the reader will be able to:

- Explain the anatomy and physiology of the nervous system
- Describe the differences in nervous system anatomy and physiology between children and adults.
- Describe the different types of seizures seen in children and demonstrate the appropriate nursing interventions.
- Discuss the etiology, signs and symptoms, and nursing management of hydrocephalus, craniosynostosis, and arteriovenous malformation.
- Describe the various types of neural tube defects and discuss appropriate pre- and post-operative nursing interventions.
- Discuss the etiology, signs, symptoms, and nursing care of a child with meningitis, encephalitis, or Reye's syndrome.
- Discuss the etiology, pathophysiology, and nursing care of a child with a head injury or a spinal cord injury.
- Explain the various types of drowning and the associated pathophysiology.
- Discuss the etiology, signs and symptoms, and nursing management of the various types of cerebral palsy.
- Discuss the etiology, pathophysiology, and clinical manifestations on nursing care of a child with a headache.
- Describe interventions needed to help families cope with a child who has alterations in neurological functioning.
- Successfully complete the games and activities in the online student StudyWARE.

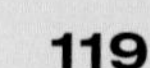

Neurological alterations seen in infants and children can be structural, infectious, or caused by an injury. Most often, pediatric alterations can be classified as either acquired or congenital. In some instances, however, these delineations are not as clear. For example, seizure and hydrocephalus may be present at birth or shortly thereafter, but also may occur later in infancy or childhood from infection, trauma, or neoplasm. In addition, although cerebral palsy does not manifest itself until many months, or even years after birth it can be attributed to prenatal, perinatal, and postnatal causes (Odding, Roebroeck, & Stam, 2006). A discussion of a variety of neurological alterations seen in infants, children, and adolescents follows.

ANATOMY AND PHYSIOLOGY

The nervous system consists of the brain, spinal cord, and nerves. A review of the anatomy and physiology of these components sets the stage for gaining an understanding of the alterations of the neurological system.

HEAD

The scalp is composed of five layers: the skin, the vascular subcutaneous tissue, the loose fitting galea or aponeurosis, the areolar tissue, and the periosteum. The skull is made up of the cranial vault and the calvarium or base. The outer surface of the skull is smooth, whereas the inner surface is rough and irregular, especially at the base. There are three membranes covering the brain called the **meninges** (Figure 32-1). The **dura mater** adheres to the inner surface of the skull, covering the meningeal arteries and veins. Below that is the thin, transparent **arachnoid mater** under which the cerebrospinal fluid flows. The third layer, the **pia mater**, is attached to the brain itself (Estes, 2010).

The **cerebrum** is the largest portion of the brain and consists of two hemispheres and several lobes. The frontal lobe controls personality, emotion, complex intellectual function, and voluntary movement. The parietal lobes, which are on the lateral and medial surfaces of the brain, are where sensory input such as pain, pressure, proprioception, and temperature are interpreted. Taste, smell, hearing, speech, and language are deciphered in the temporal lobes, whereas the vision center is in the occipital area, located at the back of the brain. The **cerebellum**, which is in the posterior fossa, controls motor coordination, posture, and equilibrium. The brain stem, which sits under the cerebellum, controls the vital centers. The **brain stem** is composed of three parts: the **midbrain**, which manages visual reflexes, tracking, and cranial nerves III and IV; the **pons**, which controls respiratory function and cranial nerves V, VI, VII, and VIII; and the **medulla oblongata**, which regulates the respiratory, cardiac, vasoconstrictor, sneeze, cough, and vomiting reflexes as well as cranial nerves IX, X, XI, and XII (Estes, 2010) (Figure 32-2).

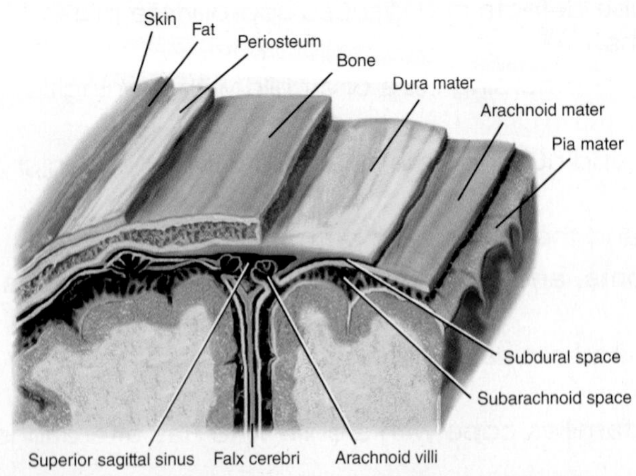

FIGURE 32-1 **Brain Coverings.** DELMAR CENGAGE LEARNING.

CEREBROSPINAL FLUID

Cerebrospinal fluid (CSF), which acts as a cushion to help protect the brain, is composed of choroid plexus secretions and interstitial brain fluid, and is produced at a rate of approximately 20 mL/hr in children. The normal volume of CSF ranges from 50 mL in infants to 150 mL in adults. Figure 32-3 illustrates the normal flow of CSF. This process works if the production rate of fluid is equal to the absorption rate and there is free flow within the ventricular system (Kinsman & Johnston, 2007).

CEREBRAL BLOOD FLOW

Cerebral blood flow (CBF) must be maintained in order to meet the metabolic needs of the brain. In the adult and older child, flow is thought to be 45–50 milliliters per gram of brain tissue per minute; it is less in younger children, although exact parameters are unknown. When CBF falls below 18 to 20 milliliters per gram of brain tissue per minute, ischemia will occur. Cerebral blood flow, measured by monitoring systemic arterial pressure, should remain between 60 and 150 millimeters of mercury. Flow may be influenced by changes in systemic blood pressure, arterial blood gas levels, metabolic demands of the brain, and intracranial pressure.

INTRACRANIAL PRESSURE

Intracranial pressure (ICP) is the force exerted by the brain, blood, and cerebrospinal fluid within the cranial vault. Natural variations and elevations of the ICP caused by activities that trigger the Valsalva maneuver are readily accommodated in healthy children. To compensate for increasing pressure in a rigid space, the body will first shunt cerebrospinal fluid through the subarachnoid space into the spinal canal, compress parenchymal tissue, and finally reduce blood flow to the brain, which affects cerebral blood flow and

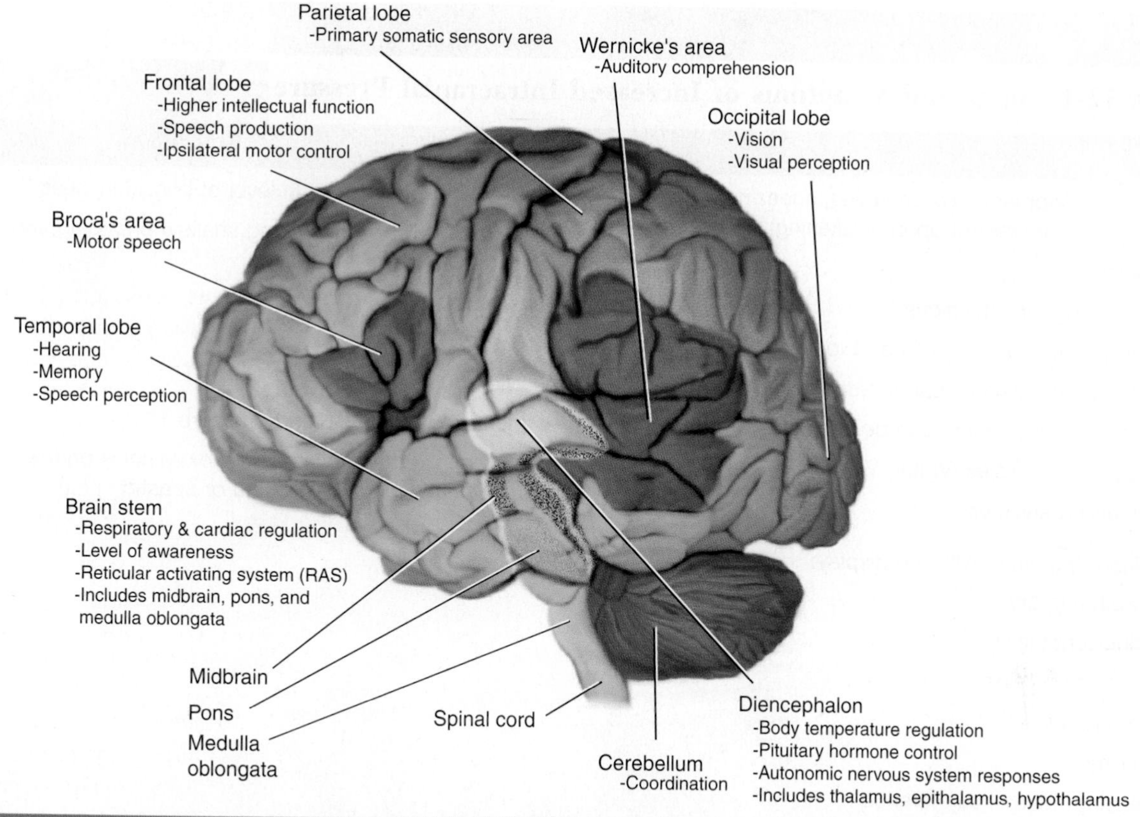

FIGURE 32-2 The Locations and Functions of the Cerebral Lobes, Brain Stem, and Cerebellum. DELMAR CENGAGE LEARNING.

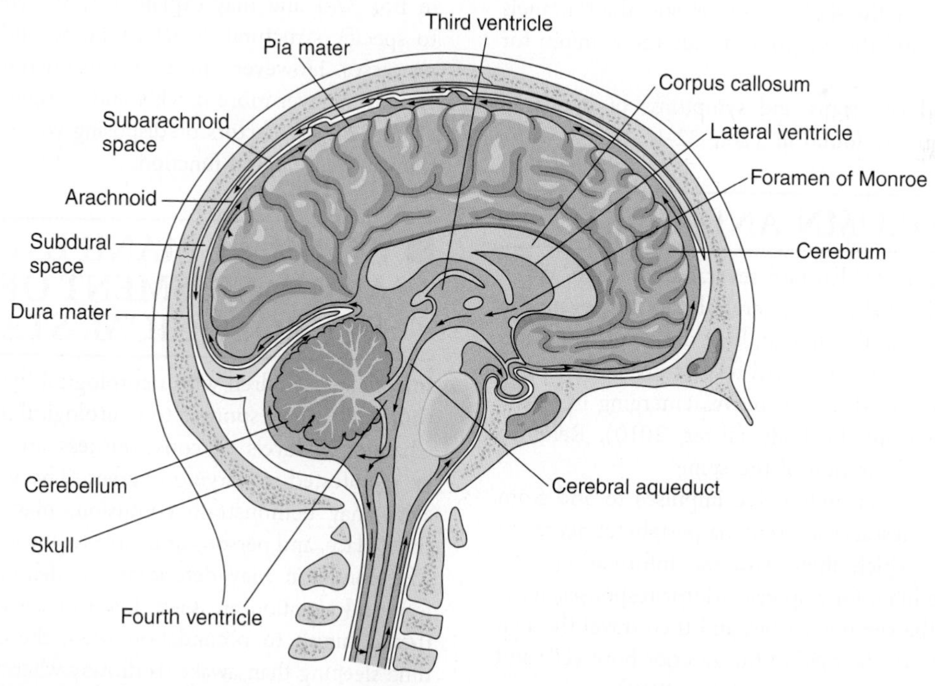

FIGURE 32-3 The Flow Pattern of the Cerebrospinal Fluid. DELMAR CENGAGE LEARNING.

cerebral perfusion pressure. If increased intracranial pressure persists, or more volume is added, brain tissue will be forced downward, past the tentorium, and through the foramen magnum (Mansfield, 2007).

Normal intracranial pressure is between 0 and 12 millimeters of mercury, although the body can adapt to 20 millimeters of mercury without detrimental effects. The infant is better able to accommodate higher pressure than

Table 32-1 Signs and Symptoms of Increased Intracranial Pressure

EARLY SIGNS	LATE SIGNS

• Headache (worsened by coughing, sneezing, lying down, or present upon awakening)
• Vomiting
• Slight change in vital signs
• Slight alteration in level of consciousness
• Pupils not as symmetrical or responsive
• Sunsetting eyes (sclera can be seen above the iris)
• Cranial nerve palsies (VI and VII)
• Generalized seizures
In addition, the infant will also display:
• High-pitched cry
• Bulging fontanelle
• Dilated scalp veins
• Wide sutures
• Irritability
• Increasing head circumference
	• Significant deterioration in level of consciousness
	• Respiratory distress including shallow breathing and Cheyne-Stokes respirations
	• Cushing's triad
	  • Bradycardia
	  • Wide pulse pressure
	  • Increased systolic blood pressure
	• One pupil fixed and dilated with extremities on the contralateral side either flaccid or spastic
	• Papilledem

an older child because the skull is more elastic, the fontanels are not yet closed, and there is room inside the cranium for brain growth.

The early and late signs and symptoms of increased intracranial pressure are found in Table 32-1.

SPINAL COLUMN AND CORD

The spinal column is divided into several areas, each with a specific number of vertebrae: the cervical area has seven; the thoracic region, twelve; the lumbar, five; the sacral, one; and the coccygeal, one. The spinal cord resides inside the spinal column, and there are 31 sets of nerves emerging from the spinal cord to enervate the body (Estes, 2010). Refer to Figure 32-4 for an illustration of the spine.

The spinal cord transmits nerve impulses to and from the brain. Sensory messages are sent via peripheral nerves to the spinal nerves, which then send the information to a specific area of the brain for response. Motor responses, however, originate in the cerebral cortex, and then travel through the medulla and down the cord to the anterior horn cells and muscle fibers to initiate movement (Estes, 2010).

DIFFERENCES IN CHILDREN AND ADULTS

The anatomy and physiology of a child's nervous system is different from an adult. These differences are summarized in Box 32-1 and may explain why the child is more prone to specific structural defects, injuries, and other pathologic processes. However, these very distinctions also enable the child to recover more quickly and completely than the adult. Table 32-2 lists factors predisposing young children to alterations in neurological function.

CLINICAL MANIFESTATIONS AND ASSESSMENT OF ALTERED NEUROLOGICAL STATUS

Infants and children with neurological dysfunction display a wide variety of responses to neurological injuries or illnesses. Changes in levels of consciousness are common and can be manifested in varying degrees. The youngster, although alert, may demonstrate confusion; may be disoriented to time, place, and person; or unable to answer simple questions. The condition may deteriorate to delirium, where anxiety, fear, and agitation are seen. Level of consciousness may further diminish to obtundation when the child spends more time sleeping than awake, is drowsy when awake, shows little interest in the environment, and exhibits a slow response to stimulation. The next level of decreased consciousness is **stupor** when the child is in an unresponsive state, reacts only to vigorous stimulation, and then returns to the original state once the insult is removed. **Coma**, the most severe form of depressed consciousness, is defined as no response to intense painful stimuli (Estes, 2010; Lehman & Mink, 2008).

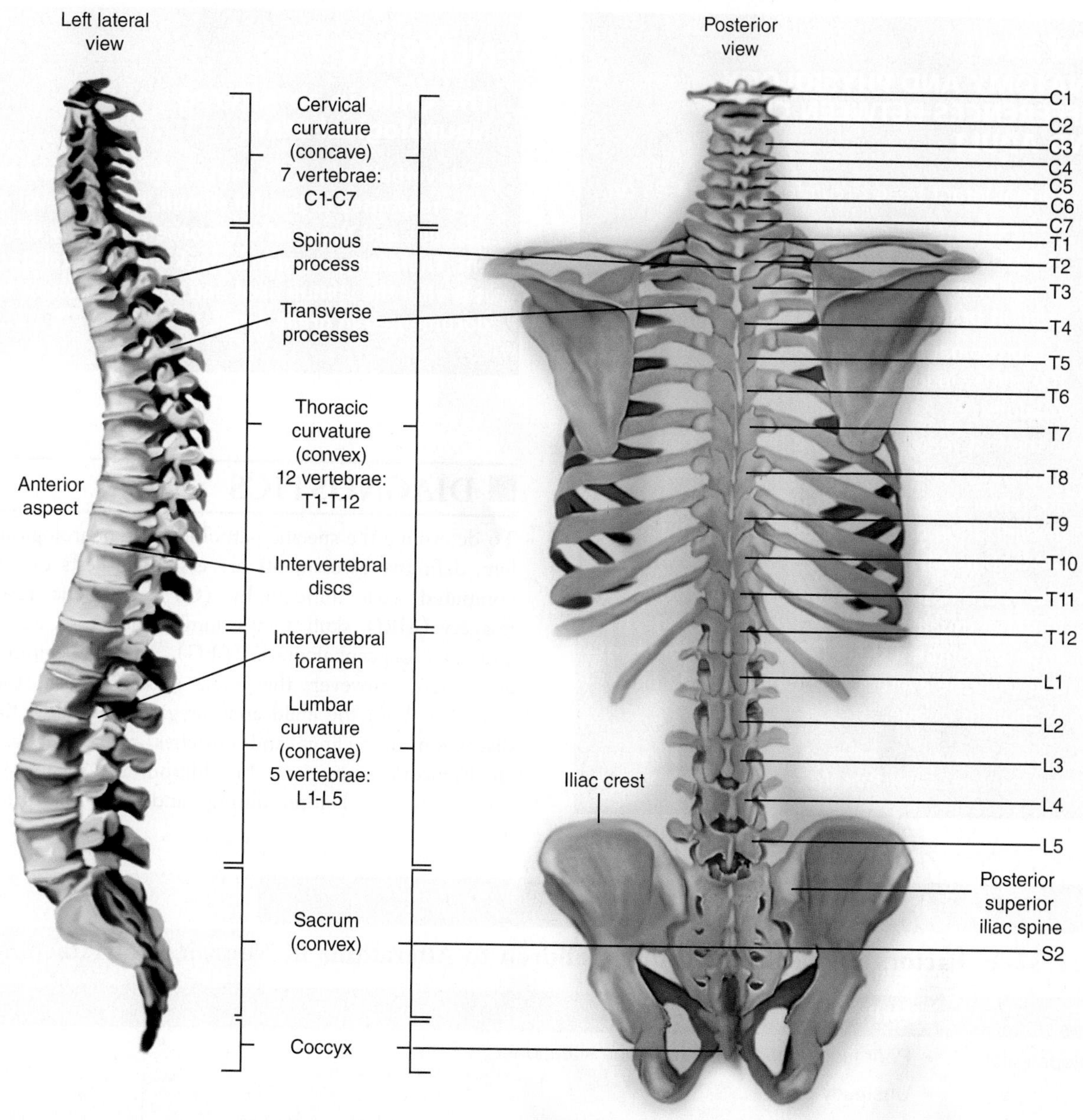

FIGURE 32-4 The Anatomy of the Spine. DELMAR CENGAGE LEARNING.

The child's level of consciousness may be evaluated several ways. "AVPU" is commonly utilized (refer to Box 32-2); however, it is necessary to state the exact stimulus and reaction elicited when used. For example, if assessing a painful response, the catalyst (pressure on a nail bed, a vigorous sternal rub) should be mentioned. The child's response should be specific: was the stimulus removed by request or did the child just moan or do nothing at all?

A second way to assess level of consciousness is a neurological assessment that includes the Glasgow Coma Scale (Table 32-3). However, the child's chronological age must be taken into account when using this scale. For example, a toddler may keep the eyes closed so what is happening in the environment will not be seen, whereas a 5-year-old may not verbally respond to the nurse because caregivers have told the child never to talk to strangers.

The presence or absence of posturing is another important indicator of level of consciousness (Figure 32-5). **Decorticate** or flexor posturing is associated with bilateral cerebral hemisphere injury. **Decerebrate** or rigid extensor posturing is secondary to trauma to the midbrain or pons; it is associated with poor prognosis (Estes, 2010). **Flaccid areflexia** or absence of response is indicative of severe brain stem injury and is evident most frequently in terminal coma or brain death. Asymmetry of tone or movement may be secondary to structural lesions, masses, or stroke (Lehman & Mink 2008).

BOX 32-1

ANATOMY AND PHYSIOLOGY DIFFERENCES BETWEEN CHILD AND ADULT

- Normal infant head circumference = 34–35 cm, by 1 year = 47 cm.
- At birth, brain weight is two-thirds of an adult. By age 6, the brain weighs approximately 90% of adult brain.
- Cerebrospinal fluid is produced at a rate of 100 ml/day in infants as compared to 500 ml/day in adults.
- In the first year, the neurons become completely myelinated and primitive motor reflexes are replaced by purposeful movement; myelinization occurs cephalocaudally and proximodistally.
- The infant has open fontanels; the posterior fontanel usually closes by 3 months of age; the anterior fontanel should close by 19 months of age with the average being between 12 and 18 months of age.

Adapted from Estes, M. E. Z. (2010). *Health assessment & physical examination* (4th ed.). Clifton Park, NY: Delmar Cengage Learning.

NURSING TIP

The Child in an Altered Neurological State

Both verbalizations ("it hurts") and moans are positive responses to painful stimuli, but the level of stimulus and the child's response are vastly different. Therefore, in order to track neurological status, it is vital the stimuli used and client responses are documented in great detail.

DIAGNOSTICS

To determine the specific pathology of a neurological problem, definitive assessments are essential. Tests can include computed axial tomography (CT), magnetic resonance imagery (MRI), skull X-rays, lumbar puncture, angiogram, and electroencephalogram (EEG). Before beginning the assessment, however, the nurse should explain the procedure to both the child and caregiver and allow time for discussion of feelings and anxieties concerning any and all diagnostic evaluations. In addition, any specific nursing actions needed before, during, and after the procedure

TABLE 32-2 Factors Predisposing Young Children to Alterations in Neurological Function

LEVEL	COMPONENTS
Developmental	• Poor judgment about dangerous situations • Unsteady gait • Immature immune system leads to increased susceptibility to infection
Cellular	• Fragile neurons • Nerve cells not completely myelinated

Structural	• Top-heavy: head large in relation to rest of the body
	• Neck muscles not very strong; may not be able to adequately support head
	• Cranium not well developed; thin and prone to fracture, especially temporal bones
	• Small subarachnoid space; decreases cerebrospinal fluid cushion
	• Dura: firmly attached to inner surface of skull, but can easily peel away with hemorrhage or hematoma
	• Brain: very vascular and prone to hemorrhage
	• Excessive spinal mobility caused by:
	  • Immature muscles, joints, and ligaments of the cervical spine
	  • Wedge-shaped cartilaginous vertebral bodies
	  • Incomplete ossification of vertebral bodies

Cognitive	• Has not yet learned hazards of the environment
Physical	• Fine or gross motor coordination not yet mastered

BOX 32-2
AVPU

A = Alert and Awake
V = Responsive to Verbal stimuli
P = Responsive to Painful stimuli
U = Unresponsive

should be taken to ensure the health, comfort, and safety of the child.

GENERAL NURSING ISSUES

The nurse caring for the child with alterations in neurological function must meet identified needs. This begins with a basic assessment of the child's physical condition using ABCDEs. Refer to Box 32-3 for the ABCDEs.

Once the nurse is assured the youngster's ABCDEs are stable, neurological status evaluation continues and should include:

TABLE 32-3 Glasgow Coma Scale Modified for Infants and Children

I. Eye opening	Points
a. Spontaneous	4
b. To command	3
c. With pain	2
d. No response	1
II. Verbal response	
a. Coos and babbles	5
b. Irritable cry	4
c. Cries to pain	3
d. Moans to pain	2
e. None	1
III. Motor response	
a. Normal spontaneous movement	6
b. Withdraws to touch	5
c. Withdraws to pain	4
d. Abnormal flexion	3
e. Abnormal extension	2
f. None	1
Maximum score	15

Adapted from Huff, K. (2008). Increased intracranial pressure in C. Berkowitz, (Ed.) *Pediatrics: A primary care approach* (3rd ed.). Elk Grove Village, IL: American Academy of Pediatrics. pps, 287–282

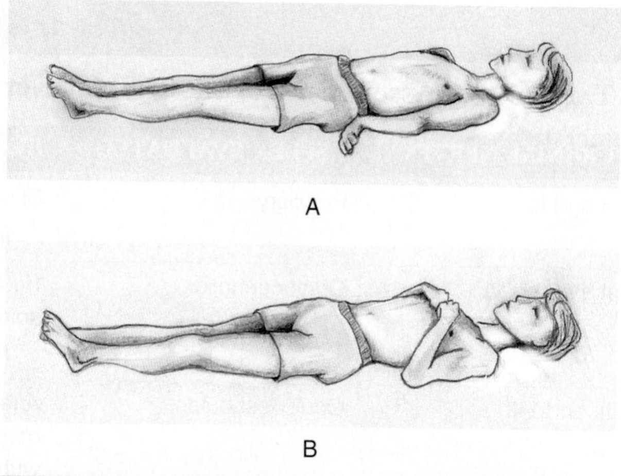

FIGURE 32-5 Motor System Dysfunction. A. Decerebrate Rigidity. B. Decorticate Rigidity. DELMAR CENGAGE LEARNING.

- Level of consciousness, which can be assessed using AVPU or the Glasgow Coma Scale.
- Motor responses including strength, symmetry, spontaneity, and posturing.
- Sensory evaluation including responses to temperature (hot versus cold), pressure (mild, moderate, or severe), pain (sharp versus dull), and **proprioception** (aware of posture, movement, and changes in equilibrium and knowledge of position, weight, and resistance of objects in relation to the body (Venes, 2009).
- Reflexes, noting presence, absence, symmetry, and strength of cranial nerves, as well as the Babinski, biceps, triceps, patellar, and ankle reflexes (refer to Table 32-4 for methods of assessing cranial nerves in an unconscious child).
- Physical abilities compromised by the illness or injury. In addition, any sequelae associated with immobility such as contractures, muscle atrophy, or skin breakdown should be noted.

The nurse should then determine the care the child requires, including physical, intellectual, social, and emotional needs, in order to encourage optimal development.

BOX 32-3
ASSESSMENT USING THE ABCDEs

A = Airway
B = Breathing
C = Circulation
D = Disability or neurological status
E = Exposure of body

Evaluation always follows the ABCDE progression, only moving to the next step once the area assessed is determined to be stable. If not, appropriate interventions are initiated before moving on. For example, if an airway cannot be determined as patent, intubation should occur immediately. Once the airway is secure, the remaining assessment can be addressed.

TABLE 32-4 Assessment of the Cranial Nerves in the Unconscious Child

CRANIAL NERVES	REFLEX EVALUATED	EVALUATION
II and III	Pupillary	Shine light source directly into eye. ***Intact response***: pupils will immediately constrict.
II, IV, and VI	Oculocephalic	Hold eyes open and turn head from side to side only *after* cervical spine has been cleared of injury. ***Intact response***: eyes should be gazing upward.
III and VIII	Oculovestibular	*After* cervical spine has been cleared of injury and tympanic membrane has been determined to be intact, place head in midline with child's head elevated. Inject ice water into the ear canal. ***Intact response***: eyes will deviate toward irrigated ear.
V and VII	Corneal	Gently swab cornea with sterile cotton-tipped applicator. ***Intact response***: Blink.
IX and X	Gag	Irritate pharynx with tongue depressor or cotton swab. ***Intact response***: Gag.

SEIZURES

Seizures are caused by uncontrolled electrical brain activity that results in an abrupt change in sensory perception or motor activity. Seizures are classified as partial, generalized, and unclassified, and can range from simple to complex.

INCIDENCE AND ETIOLOGY

An estimated 10% of children will experience some type of seizure during childhood. Seizures can be caused by fevers, infections, cardiac anomalies, trauma, hypoxia, ingestion of toxic substances, breath-holding spells, gastroesophageal reflux, epilepsy, genetic factors, or idiopathic causes. The incidence of febrile seizures in young children is 3–4% while the lifetime incidence of epilepsy is 3% (Johnston, 2007a).

Seizures can also be acquired, resulting from traumatic brain injury, central nervous system infection, hypoglycemia or other endocrine dysfunction, toxic ingestion or exposure, or intracranial lesion or vascular malformation. Typically, infants develop seizures because of birth injury, anoxic episodes, infection, intraventricular hemorrhage, or a congenital brain anomaly. Seizures in older children occur most often secondary to trauma or infection. In addition, changes in diet or hydration status, fatigue, or not taking prescribed medications may precipitate seizure activity. The various types of seizures as well as their etiology are found in Table 32-5. Refer to Box 32-4 for a description of infantile spasms. Prognosis depends on the etiology, the type, and the age of initial onset.

Febrile seizures are brief, clonic, or tonic/clonic in nature and can be simple or complex. They usually occur early in an illness with a high fever but can develop with temperatures as low as 37.8°C (100°F). Simple febrile seizures usually last less than 15 minutes, usually only a few seconds, and don't recur within a 24-hour period (see Box 32-5). However, complex febrile seizures can have focal attributes, recur on the same day, and last longer than 15 minutes. Febrile seizures rarely occur before 9 months or after 5 years of age. Children who have their first febrile seizure under the age of 12 months, with a relatively low fever, have a complex seizure, or have a family history of febrile seizures are at increased risk for recurrent seizures. These factors and a history of developmental delays or neurologic disorders also increase the child's risk of developing epilepsy later in life (Johnston, 2007a).

Unprovoked first seizure is a seizure that occurs without a known cause, such as a fever. Less than 50% of these children will have a second seizure. An in-depth history, including family history and developmental history, may indicate the likelihood of recurrent seizures. Laboratory testing is based on clinical presentation and may include glucose, electrolytes, toxicology screening, or metabolic testing. A lumbar puncture is only considered if meningeal signs, such as stiffneck or headache, are present. An EEG may be helpful in determining the presence of focal abnormalities (Johnston, 2007a).

Epileptic seizures are defined as the presence of more than one unprovoked seizure that are at least 24 hours apart. Childhood epilepsy is usually considered a benign condition that is attributed to CNS immaturity. More than one-third of children who experience epileptic seizures will be free of seizure activity and no longer require medication by 23 years of age. Factors that contribute to a poorer prognosis include onset of seizures in infancy or adolescence, difficulty in

TABLE 32-5 Common Seizure Etiologies

TYPE OF SEIZURE	COMMON ETIOLOGIES
Partial	
Complex	• Intracranial lesions, tumors, cysts • Birth or other traumatic injury • Arteriovenous malformations • Prolonged febrile seizures
Simple	• Tumors or other lesions • Focal damage to the brain • Arteriovenous malformation • Brain abscess
Generalized	
Tonic/clonic	• Cerebral damage secondary to birth injury or trauma • Metabolic or neuromuscular degenerative disorders • Fever • Unknown
Absence	• Possible genetic link
Myoclonic	• Prenatal or perinatal encephalopathy • Tuberous sclerosis • Microcephaly
Myoclonic and akinetic	• Gray matter degenerative disorders • Subacute sclerosing panencephalitis • Unknown

managing seizure activity, and presence of a developmental disorder such as cerebral palsy.

PATHOPHYSIOLOGY

Seizures are the result of a spontaneous electrical discharge of hyperexcited brain cells in an area called the **epileptogenic focus**. These cells can be triggered by either environmental or physiological stimuli such as emotional stress, anxiety, fatigue, infection, or metabolic disturbances. The exact location of the epileptogenic foci and the number involved determines the nature of the seizure. If a small area of the brain is affected, a focal (localized) seizure may occur. However, if the electrical discharge continues, it may become generalized. A generalized seizure will also occur if the epileptogenic focus is located in the brain stem, midbrain, or reticular formation.

Status epilepticus is a prolonged seizure or series of convulsions where loss of consciousness occurs for at least 30 minutes. **Refractory seizures** last more than 60 minutes.

BOX 32-4
INFANTILE SPASMS

Infantile spasms begin between the ages of 4 and 8 months. Spasm types are flexor, extensor, or mixed, and affect the neck, arms, legs, or trunk. During the seizure, this infant's head may suddenly drop forward while both arms and legs are flexed. The eyes may roll upward or downward, and the infant may cry out and turn pale, cyanotic, or flushed. There may be a loss of consciousness or awareness. Most infantile spasms occur during sleep or upon awakening, while the child is still drowsy. Benign infantile seizures affect approximately 10–20% of infants who experience spasms. These children have normal prenatal, antenatal, postnatal, and developmental histories, and seldom experience any long-term complications. The majority of children with this disorder, however, are affected by a more serious form of seizures known as West's syndrome. These children suffered from gestational difficulties, are developmentally delayed, or have other neurological abnormalities. These children may suffer infantile spasms up to 5 years of age, after which they will develop partial or generalized seizures (Johnston, 2007a: Ropper & Brown, 2005).

BOX 32-5
FEBRILE SEIZURES

Febrile seizures are a type of tonic/clonic seizure usually associated with rapid rise in temperature that reaches a minimum of 39°C (102.2°F). These episodes usually occur in children between 6 months and 5 years of age. There is often a positive family history of febrile seizures and they frequently accompany infectious processes such as upper respiratory infections, pneumonia, pharyngitis, shigella, urinary tract infections, otitis media, roseola, and meningitis. The seizures are usually self-limiting and have a postictal period lasting for less than 15 minutes (Johnston, 2007a).

Epilepsy refers to a chronic seizure disorder often associated with central nervous system pathology.

CLINICAL MANIFESTATIONS

Clinical manifestations depend on the specific type of seizure. **Partial seizures**, which arise from abnormal electrical activity in a small area of the brain, most often the temporal, frontal, or parietal lobes of the cerebral cortex, will have symptoms associated with the area of the brain affected. However, **generalized**

seizures, secondary to diffuse electrical activity throughout the cortex and into the brain stem, will cause the child to lose consciousness as well as demonstrate uncontrolled motor involvement with movements and spasms bilateral and symmetrical in nature (Blosser & Burns, 2004; Johnston, 2007a).

Partial seizures are characterized by local motor, sensory, psychic, and somatic manifestations. Partial seizures differ from generalized seizures in how they are manifested and how they affect consciousness. During partial seizures, movements are asynchronous and tend to involve only the face, neck, or extremities. Consciousness is usually maintained and patients may be able to talk through the seizure. In complex partial seizures, consciousness may be impaired or lost.

There are two types of partial seizures: simple and complex. **Simple partial seizures** or focal seizures can be manifested at any age. An **aura**, such as chest pain or headache, may occur. Most often, the symptoms seen are motor or sensory in nature. Movements may involve one extremity, or a part of that extremity, or the head and eyes will twist in the opposite direction of the extremities. The arm toward which the head is turned is abducted and extended with the fingers clenched. There may be numbness, tingling, or painful sensations as well that begin in one area of the body and spread out to others. Alterations in sensory perception may also be present. The child may have visual hallucinations and report seeing images or light flashes. In addition, a buzzing sound may be heard, unusual odors identified, or an odd taste experienced. The child may also report feeling emotional or anxious (Blosser & Burns, 2004; Johnston, 2007a).

Simple partial seizures may have unique features. Seizures that begin in a very specific area (fingers of one hand, toes of one foot, one side of the face, etc) progress, or "march" up adjacent muscles to include a much larger area of the affected extremity or side of the body. This phenomenon was formerly referred to as a "Jacksonian march" or Jacksonian seizure. Other patients will experience a localized paresis after a partial seizure that affects the same area affected by the seizure. This paresis can last for minutes to hours and is referred to as Todd's paralysis. Rarely, partial seizures will persist for hours or days. Known as epilepsia partalis, these seizures are often unresponsive to medical interventions (Lowenstein, 2008).

Complex partial seizures are also known as partial psychomotor or temporal lobe episodes. They can be manifested from age 3 years through adolescence. Just before the event, the child may have an aura. In addition, the youngster may have feelings of anxiety, fear, or deja vu, the sense an event has occurred before, or complain of abdominal pain, having an unusual taste in the mouth, smelling an odd odor, or visual or auditory hallucinations.

Consciousness is not completely lost during complex partial seizures. Rather, the child will appear confused or dazed, especially at the onset. When the seizure begins, the child stops the activity he or she is involved in and begins purposeless behaviors such as staring into space or assuming an unusual posture. The child may also perform **automatisms**, or repeated nonpurposeful actions, such as lip smacking, chewing, sucking, or uttering the same word over and over, wander aimlessly, or remove clothing. Violent acts or rages are rare. A postictal period follows this type of seizure when the child will be drowsy, confused, aphasic, or display sensory or motor impairments. Children usually do not remember the behaviors displayed (Johnston, 2007a; Lowenstein, 2008).

Generalized seizures, arising from both cerebral hemispheres, can occur at any time and last from several seconds to hours. There is no aura, but some children describe a prodrome of vague symptoms leading up to the seizure. There is always loss of consciousness. Generalized seizures appearing in children under 4 years of age are frequently associated with developmental delays, learning disabilities, and behavior disorders. There are four types of generalized seizures: tonic/clonic, absence, myoclonic, and akinetic.

Tonic/clonic seizures formerly referred to as grand mal seizures, can occur at any age. Onset is usually abrupt and begins when the child loses consciousness and falls to the ground. The initial phase is tonic when there are intense muscle contractions. The jaw clenches shut; the abdomen and chest become rigid; and often the child emits a cry or grunt as exhaled air is forced out because of the taut diaphragm. Pallor or cyanosis may occur as oxygenation and ventilation are impaired. The airway is compromised due to increased salivation the child cannot manage because of muscular contractions as well as the diminished mental status. The neck and legs are also extended while the arms are flexed or contracted. The eyes roll upward or deviate to one side, the pupils dilate, and there may also be bladder or bowel incontinence. The tonic phase of the seizure usually persists for 10 to 30 seconds. During the clonic phase, jerking movements are produced as a result of contraction and relaxation of the muscles. Excessive salivation can cause breathing difficulty and partial airway obstruction. Bladder and bowel incontinence are not uncommon. Clonic spasms dissipate as the seizure ends, and can last from 30 seconds to 30 minutes after onset of the seizure (Johnston, 2007a; Lowenstein, 2008).

Reflections from Families

Rylin just had a cold and fever. All of a sudden, I heard a cry and I ran in to see her shaking all over. Her face was pale and her eyes rolled back into her head. This seemed to last forever. I called 911 and by the time the paramedics got there, the shaking stopped and Rylin just slept. I was never so scared in my life. What was it caused by? Will it happen again?

A postictal or postconvulsive state follows a tonic/clonic seizure. Consciousness returns gradually over minutes to hours, and the child will appear confused, be combative, or complain of headache, fatigue, or muscle aches. The child may have no memory of the event and will often be hypertensive and diaphoretic. Nausea, vomiting, poor coordination, slurred speech, or visual disturbances may follow.

Absence seizures, which used to be called petit mal seizures, most often begin in early childhood (ages 4 to 8), but may begin in adolescence. They are characterized by a transient loss of consciousness, which may appear as cessation of current activity. The child seems to stare into space or the eyes may roll upward with ptosis or fluttering of the lids. There also may be lip smacking or a loss of muscle tone causing the head to droop or any objects in the hands to be dropped. These events usually last from 5 to 10 seconds and can occur hundreds of times per day. Children with this type of seizure are often accused of daydreaming and being inattentive in school. Absence seizures respond well to medication and usually spontaneously resolve during adolescence (Johnston, 2007a; Lowenstein, 2008). **Myoclonic seizures** are sudden repeated contractures of the muscles of the head, extremities, or torso. Benign, typical, and juvenile myoclonic seizures have good outcomes. These seizures can begin as young as 6 months, in early childhood, or adolescence, and occur when the child is drowsy and just falling asleep, or just waking up. There is usually no loss of consciousness, there is no postictal period, and the child recovers quickly. Complex and progressive myoclonic epilepsies have poor outcomes. They can result in cognitive and development delays, and can be difficult to control (Johnston, 2007a; Lowenstein, 2008).

Atonic or astatic-akinetic seizures (drop attacks) occur between ages 2 and 5 years, and are manifested by sudden loss of muscle tone with the head dropping forward for a few seconds. For seizures that last only 1 to 2 seconds, the child may exhibit only a head drop or nod. More significant events occur when the youngster loses consciousness and falls to the ground, most often face down. In either case, amnesia follows. These seizures often cause repetitive head injuries if the child is not protected by wearing a football or hockey helmet. Many have underlying brain abnormalities and are mentally retarded (Lowenstein, 2008).

DIAGNOSIS

The objectives of diagnosis are threefold: to ascertain whether the child truly had a seizure, to determine the cause of the episode, and to classify the type of seizure. This process begins with obtaining a thorough history from the caregivers or witnesses. In addition, a complete medical history must be obtained, noting any illnesses, medications, hospitalizations, or toxic exposures the child may have had as well as if previous episodes occurred. Family history is also important because of genetic predisposition to some types of seizures. Often the diagnosis is based solely on the history since the physical examination and laboratory studies may be normal (Johnston, 2007a; Lowenstein, 2008).

The history should also include an exploration of risk factors: fever, head trauma, illnesses, stroke, tumors, ingestion of toxin or poison, or chemical exposure. Other precipitating factors, such as sleep deprivation, systemic diseases, medications, alcohol or drugs, should be determined. Finally, the presence or absence of an aura should be determined (Lowenstein, 2008).

Once the history is obtained, a complete physical examination must be performed. This includes identifying signs of infection and a complete neurological evaluation, including checking the level of consciousness, reflexes, and sensory and motor responses. The child's developmental stage should also be determined.

A complete blood count can determine the presence or absence of infection such as meningitis or encephalitis, and serum electrolytes should be analyzed to rule out metabolic disturbances, particularly hypoglycemia. A lumbar puncture may also be performed to investigate for infectious processes or bloody cerebrospinal fluid. If a toxic ingestion is suspected, both urine and blood can be checked for its presence.

Radiologic imaging such as CT or MRI may be performed to note any structural abnormality while angiography would pinpoint vascular irregularities. In addition, an electroencephalogram (EEG) might be indicated to assess the brain's electrical activity while the child is asleep, awake, or receiving noxious stimuli, and a positron emission tomography (PET) scan done to highlight areas of brain abnormality (Deblaere & Achten, 2008; Lowenstein, 2008).

TREATMENT

The child with tonic/clonic seizures must be managed quickly. The airway must be assured; a short-term method is to perform the jaw thrust. Nothing, including a tongue blade, should ever be placed in the child's mouth. The

NURSING TIP

Obtain the Following Information if a Seizure Is Suspected

- Suffered a loss of consciousness or awareness?
- Did the seizure begin as a partial or generalized seizure?
- How long did the seizure last?
- Became pale, cyanotic, or flushed?
- Displayed any unusual movements, especially tonic/clonic actions, repeated muscle spasms, or head drops?
- Had dilated pupils or eyes rolled upward or deviated to one side?
- Was incontinent of urine or stool?
- Behavior after the episode? Was there a postictal period? If so, describe it.
- How soon after the event did the child's behavior return to normal?

CULTURAL CONSIDERATION

Neurological Tests and Procedures

In many Asian cultures, the head is sacred and considered to be the carrier of the soul. Therefore, when teaching family members about a CT scan and the child's need for the examination, you should be careful not to touch the child's head. It would be better for you to use a drawing of a child's head, or point to your own head instead.

child may then be placed on his or her side if the airway is patent to help prevent secretions from pooling in the mouth, and suction should be readily available. Because of thoracic and diaphragmatic muscle rigidity, air ventilation may be impaired and hypoxia may result. Therefore, children having tonic/clonic seizures should receive oxygen during the event either by a clear face mask or assisted ventilations. Many seizures are self-limiting and last less than five minutes; these require no further management other than airway management and oxygen administration. When a child is at risk for seizures, preparations include padded bed rails and the immediate availability of suction equipment and medications.

If the seizure does not resolve spontaneously, the hospitalized child will need intravenous medications. The benzodiazepines (diazepam [Valium] or lorazepam [Atavan]) are usually administered first, and if seizures continue, phenytoin (Dilantin) or fosphenytoin (Cerebyx) are administered next. Phenobarbital (Luminal) may also be given, but it takes 30 minutes before onset. It is important to place the child on a cardiorespiratory monitor during medication administration as an apneic response may follow administration of the benzodiazepines. There is also the risk of hypotension or cardiac dysrhythmias when phenytoin is administered, especially via a fast IV. Once the seizure is over, the child should be closely monitored during the postictal period. If the episode is a first-time event, diagnostics should begin after recovery (Johnston, 2007a).

Once the diagnosis and the type and cause of the seizure are identified, more definite treatment can begin. If the cause were infectious, a toxic exposure, metabolic abnormality, an intracranial lesion, or a vascular malformation, that particular cause would be treated. When a seizure is febrile in nature, the parents should be reassured of its benign nature. Early treatment of fevers has not been found to prevent febrile seizures. For the child with recurring convulsions caused by nonstructural pathology, anticonvulsant medications would be prescribed, and the child followed by neurologists who carefully monitor drug serum levels to ensure therapeutic ranges. If episodes continue, medications could be changed or added to the child's current regimen. Refer to Table 32-6 for commonly drugs used to treat seizures by type.

Over the last several years, the **Ketogenic Diet** has gained popularity in treating absence, akinetic, and myoclonic seizures that are pharmacoresistant. The diet severely limits the intake of proteins and carbohydrates, thereby forcing the body to use fats for fuel resulting in the creation of ketones. The amount of protein in the diet is regulated so that 90% of the calories are derived from fat, and the fat to carbohydrate ratio is 4:1. How the diet affects seizures is not clearly understood, however some evidence attributes an anticonvulsive effect to the ketone bodies released by ketosis (Johnston, 2007a; Moe, Benke, Bernard, & Levisohn, 2009).

The diet is especially useful in young children with infantile spasms, myoclonic, or atonic-kinetic seizures and those with mixed seizures of Lennox-Gastaut Syndrome when side effects to medications are intolerable or when allergies preclude administration. For infants and children under 2 years of age, the diet can be especially successful. For older children, adherence to the very restrictive, sometimes unpalatable diet can be challenging. Adherence to the diet is improved when seizures are controlled. Side effects of the diet include acidosis, hypoglycemia, and renal stones. Valproic acid is contraindicated for children on the diet (Johnston, 2007a; Moe et al., 2009).

Recent technological advances have led to the use of vagal nerve stimulation to prevent or interrupt seizures. A device is surgically implanted below the left clavicle and attached to the vagus nerve. Cyclic stimulation of the vagus nerve has been shown to reduce seizure activity by 50% in over half of children treated. In addition to the preset cyclic stimulation, a magnet can be used to trigger the stimulator to interrupt seizure activity (Johnston, 2007a; Moe et al., 2009).

When seizures are intractable, surgery may be the last hope for control. For children with focal seizures, the epileptogenic focus may be removed if there are no critical structures involved. Temporal lobectomy or a hemispherectomy could be performed on the client with unrelenting partial seizures with widespread hemispheric origin. Oftentimes, these youngsters will also display preexisting motor, cognitive, and sensory deficits. The goal of surgery is not only to decrease seizure activity, but also to improve the child's behavior and intellectual status. Surgery successfully eliminates seizures in 80% or more of cases (Johnston, 2007a; Moe et al., 2009).

NURSING MANAGEMENT

The nurse caring for the child with seizures has multiple responsibilities. If the child is actively convulsing, a patent airway and adequate oxygenation must be assured. Prescribed medications need to be administered in a safe and efficient manner, noting the specific rates of delivery, need for cardiorespiratory monitoring, and watching for potential adverse reactions. Once the episode is controlled, the nurse must document the event in detail, including the onset of any aura to resolution.

TABLE 32-6 Drugs Useful for Treating Seizures

SEIZURE TYPE	TOXIC SYMPTOMS
Absence seizures	
Ethosuximide (Zarontin)	Sedation, GI upset
Valproic acid (Depokene, Depakote)	Tremors, sedation
Lamotrigine (Lamictal)	Ataxia, diplopia
Generalized seizures	
Valproic acid	Tremors, sedation
Felbamate (Felbatol)	Insomnia, anorexia
Topiramate (Topamax)	Somnolence, speech disturbance
Lamotrigine (Lamictal)	Ataxia, diplopia
Carbamazepine (Tetrazol, Tegretol)	Vertigo, diplopia
Infantile spasms	
Adrenocorticotropic hormone	Increased appetite, acne
Valproic acid	Tremors, sedation
Vigabatrin	Drowsiness, behavioral disturbances
Myoclonic seizures	
Clonazepam (Klonopin)	Drowsiness, ataxia
Neonatal seizures	
Phenobarbital (Luminal)	Lethargy, irritability
Partial seizures	
Carbamazepine (Tetrazol, Tegretol)	Vertigo, diplopia
Gabapentin (Neurontin)	Somnolence, irritability
Oxcarbazepine (Trileptal)	Hepatitis, somnolence
Phenytoin (Dilantin)	Ataxia, nystagmus
Primidone (Mysoline)	Drowsiness, ataxia

Adapted from W. W. Hay, Jr., M. J. Levin, J. M. Sondheimer & R. R. Deterding (Eds.), (2009). *Current diagnosis & treatment pediatrics* (19th ed.). New York: McGraw-Hill Professional.

Nurses should provide a safe environment for the child with seizures to ensure injury will not occur. Suction and oxygen should be at hand and bed rails padded. If the event occurs when the child is in a chair or standing, the child should gently be helped to the ground, placed on one side, and any nearby objects moved out of the way. Children with atonic or recurrent seizures may wear helmets to protect their heads during falls.

The nurse must also care for the emotional needs of the child and family as seizures can often have a negative stigma, making the victim as well as caregivers and siblings uncomfortable or ashamed. The child may resent feeling different from peers and taking medications several times per day, or fear having a seizure in front of friends. The nurse should encourage the child to talk about these feelings and provide help so the condition can be accepted.

FAMILY TEACHING

The nurse must work with the family as well. Some caregivers feel guilty, especially if the episodes are a result of trauma or genetic predisposition. The nurse should allow these family members to express their feelings and frustrations. Caregivers may also worry about the financial aspects of having a youngster with a chronic condition, requiring daily medications, visits to the neurologist, and frequent drug serum monitoring. The nurse can arrange for caregivers to speak with social services for assistance in working out these issues.

Caregivers must also be taught how to give medications, and the importance of not missing doses. They also need to know drug serum levels should be checked periodically as the child grows. School-age children should be encouraged

EVIDENCE-BASED PRACTICE

Epilepsy and Quality of Life

CLINICAL PROBLEM

How can we help children and adolescents with epilepsy adjust to their diagnosis?

BEST CLINICAL PRACTICE

- Childhood and adolescent epilepsy is a distressing condition often accompanied by depression and learning problems. Stigma and discrimination may persist after treatment.
- After seizures are controlled, children or adolescents with epilepsy and their parents need information and counseling.

IMPLICATIONS FOR NURSING

- Education should include medical and psychosocial aspects of epilepsy.
- Medical aspects of epilepsy include types and definitions of seizures, medication management, alternative treatments, first-aid, and prognosis.
- Psychosocial aspects of epilepsy include fears, anxiety, depression, family dynamics (overprotective parents, parental guilt), school implications, and stigma.
- Written materials and handouts have limited value. Interactive structured educational programs are most beneficial.
- Internet sites, such as http://www.epilepsy.com, will provide children, siblings, parents, and educators with valuable information and support.

References: Adapted from: Shore, C. P., Perkins, S. M., & Austin, J. K. (2007). The Seizures and Epilepsy Education (SEE) Program for families of children with epilepsy: A preliminary study. *Epilepsy & Behavior, 12*(1), 157–164.

to accept responsibility for taking their own medications as this gives them feelings of control over their illness.

Safety is another issue to discuss with the child, caregivers, teachers, babysitters, and family members. All should know what to do when a seizure occurs and when to call emergency medical services. The child should wear a Medic Alert bracelet or necklace, and people caring for this youngster should be aware of activities that can and should not be encouraged. While most play is acceptable, contact sports are ill-advised. In addition, the child with a seizure disorder must be carefully watched at all times during a bath or if involved in any water activities such as swimming or boating. Instruct what to do if child seizes and when to call 911 for help. It will also be helpful to teach parents and caregivers CPR. Provide teachers, classroom assistants, school nurses or health aides, and administrative staff with information on what to do if the child has a seizure in school. If the school nurse or health aide must give a medication during the day, provide information about the drug. If the child and caregiver agree, talk to the children in the class at school about the child's condition as well as what a seizure is and what it looks like in order to reduce fears and anxieties about their classmate. Refer the family and child to groups offering support to families whose child has a seizure disorder.

STRUCTURAL ABNORMALITIES

Structural abnormalities discussed include hydrocephalus, spina bifida, craniosynostosis, and arteriovenous malformation.

HYDROCEPHALUS

Hydrocephalus is caused by impaired absorption, a block in the flow of CSF, or, rarely, increased CSF production, that results in an excessive amount of cerebral spinal fluid within the cerebral ventricles (Kinsman & Johnston, 2007).

INCIDENCE

Since there is no national registry or database, incidence and prevalence data are difficult to establish. However, 1 in 500 children are thought to be affected by the condition, and more than half of all cases are congenital. In addition, as many as 75% of children with the condition have some kind of motor disability (HyFi, n.d.; NINDS, n.d.d.).

ETIOLOGY AND PATHOPHYSIOLOGY

Hydrocephalus may be an acquired congenital disorder or of unknown etiology. There are two types of hydrocephalus: communicating and noncommunicating. In **communicating hydrocephalus**, there is an obstruction outside the ventricular system causing decreased absorption of cerebrospinal fluid in the subarachnoid space at the subarachnoid villi. This type of hydrocephalus most commonly occurs in premature infants after a subarachnoid hemorrhage, or is caused by an infection.

Noncommunicating or obstructive hydrocephalus is caused by an impediment of cerebrospinal fluid flow within the ventricular system. Most often, this is secondary to congenital malformation such as **aqueductal stenosis**, a hereditary deformity, **meningomyelocele** (MMC) (where the meninges protrude through an opening of the skull or spinal column), **Dandy-Walker syndrome** (an obstruction in the foramina of Luschka and Magendie) usually evident by age 2 years, or **Arnold-Chiari malformation** (ACM), a brain defect in the posterior fossa where there is herniation of the cerebellum, medulla, pons, and fourth ventricle into the cervical spinal canal through an enlarged foramen magnum (Beers, Porter, Jones, Kaplan & Berkwits, 2006; Kinsman & Johnston, 2007).

During the neonatal period and early infancy, hydrocephalus is regarded as a primary dysfunction caused by either intraventricular hemorrhage associated with prematurity, gram-negative meningitis, or a structural defect such as aqueductal stenosis, ACM, or meningomyelocele. The child and

CASE STUDY / CARE PLAN

CHILD WITH IDIOPATHIC SEIZURE DISORDER

Hans, a 3-year-old of German descent, was in apparent good health until one afternoon when he was playing with his siblings. He suddenly cried out, fell to the floor, and began shaking violently. In a panic state, his mother, who witnessed the event, grabbed him, put him in the car, and drove him to the hospital just a few blocks away.

When they got to the emergency room, Hans was having tonic/clonic movements. His skin was pale; his eyes rolled upward. His mother told the staff the episode began about 15 minutes before her arrival. She denied trauma, infection, fever, toxic exposure, or family history. This was the first such episode Hans had exhibited.

The nurse performed a jaw thrust to keep Hans' airway patent. She administered oxygen via face mask. An intravenous line was started and diazepam administered slowly. The convulsive activity ceased; however, within 5 minutes, the spasms began again. A second dose of diazepam was given with only short-term resolution. Next, phenytoin was pushed through the intravenous catheter and the seizure finally dissipated. Hans then slept for over an hour. When he awoke, he said his head, arms, and legs hurt; he did not remember what happened. A complete physical assessment was done: No pathology consistent with seizures was discovered, and Hans was referred to a neurologist for follow-up on an outpatient basis.

The neurologist saw Hans the next day and ordered more extensive evaluations. Again, no definitive pathology was noted.

NURSING CARE PLAN

ASSESSMENT

Hans's vital signs are normal. He has no other seizures other than the one he experienced yesterday. His parents will need education about seizures, including what to do if he has a seizure and the kinds of medications he will be on. They may also have several questions that will need to be answered.

NURSING DIAGNOSIS 1

Ineffective breathing patterns as evidenced during tonic/clonic motions.

EXPECTED OUTCOME

Hans's seizures do not compromise his respiratory effort.

NOC: Seizure Control

NIC: Seizure Management

INTERVENTIONS/*RATIONALES*

1. Perform jaw thrust as needed; administer oxygen either by face mask or assisted ventilations. The positioning will help maintain a patent airway during the seizure. *Oxygen is administered to any patient with tonic/clonic seizure activity for two reasons: first, the rigidity of the diaphragm as well as thoracic and abdominal muscles impede adequate air exchange; and second, the convulsing elevates body metabolism, thus increasing oxygen demand to the tissues.*
2. Suction as necessary. *Clients who are experiencing generalized seizures often have increased secretions which they cannot manage because of their diminished level of consciousness. These secretions may pool in the hypopharynx and occlude the airway or pose a risk for aspiration.*
3. Time the event. *Most seizures are self-limiting and last less than five minutes. If they are longer, however, interventions will need to be instituted to curtail the activity. Medications may be delivered, starting with benzodiazepins and followed by anticonvulsants as indicated.*
4. Assist with intubation. *The child who is having a prolonged seizure will need to have his airway protected; therefore, he will need to be intubated.*

(Continues)

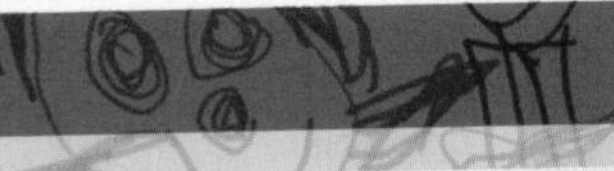

CASE STUDY / CARE PLAN (Continued)

EVALUATION

Hans's breathing patterns are not compromised.

NURSING DIAGNOSIS 2

High risk for injury secondary to tonic/clonic movements as well as diminished level of consciousness.

EXPECTED OUTCOME

Hans will not be injured during the seizure.

NOC: Seizure Control

NIC: Seizure Management

INTERVENTIONS/*RATIONALES*

1. Pad bed side rails and ensure no objects are in the bed. *The child having tonic/clonic convulsions must have a safe environment in which to move during the episode.*
2. Have seizure precaution equipment at the bedside. *Suction and a ventilation bag and mask may be needed for prolonged activity. It is more prudent to have them at hand than to find them during an emergent situation.*
3. If Hans begins to convulse when standing or sitting, gently ease him to the ground and remove any furniture or objects nearby that may be hazardous. *Helping to ease the child down will prevent a fall and possible trauma. The floor is a safe place for the youngster as long as there is nothing in the area on which he can be injured.*
4. Place Hans on his side during the event. *Putting the youngster on his side will help prevent aspiration of secretions and emesis if he vomits.*

EVALUATION

Hans is not injured during the tonic/clonic event.

NURSING DIAGNOSIS 3

High risk for injury related to medication administration during the acute episode.

EXPECTED OUTCOME

Hans will not have adverse reactions to medications.

NOC: Seizure Control

NIC: Seizure Management

INTERVENTIONS/*RATIONALES*

1. Administer benzodiazepines slowly; place Hans's on a monitor while giving them. *Clients are at risk for respiratory depression or apnea if these medications are delivered too quickly.*
2. Administer phenytoin very slowly using only normal saline as the fluid to flush the line. Place Hans on a cardiac monitor with rhythm recording capabilities. Also measure blood pressure frequently. Check intravenous catheter site often. *Phenytoin is an alkalotic compound which is incompatible with all intravenous solutions except normal saline; others will cause it to precipitate. This drug must be administered at a rate no greater than 0.5 to one milligram per kilogram per minute. Cardiac dysrhythmias and/or hypotension are not uncommon during delivery. In addition, the site may become red or extravasated.*

EVALUATION

Hans experienced no adverse reactions to the medications.

(Continues)

CASE STUDY / CARE PLAN (Continued)

NURSING DIAGNOSIS 4

Interrupted family dynamics related to caring for a child with a chronic condition.

EXPECTED OUTCOME

Hans's chronic condition will have minimal effects on family dynamics.

NOC: Caregiver Home Care Readiness; Caregiver Lifestyle Disruption

NIC: Caregiver Support; Family Support; Teaching Disease Process

INTERVENTIONS/*RATIONALES*

1. Work with the family on accepting the diagnosis. Facilitate caregiving and acceptance of responsibilities. *Giving the family control of their child's well-being will empower them and make them less angry and frustrated by their child's condition.*
2. Stress the actions and activities Hans can participate in rather than dwelling on what cannot or should not be done. *Be positive with the family and encourage them to treat Hans as normally as possible. Also, encourage them not to make Hans their "special" child at the expense of the other siblings. These actions will facilitate optional development.*

EVALUATION

The family will be able to accept Hans's special needs.

adolescent, however, develop hydrocephalus most often from intracranial tumors such as medulloblastoma, craniopharyngioma, ependymoma, or astrocytoma; infection such as meningitis; or head injury (NINDS, n.d.d.).

Prognosis depends on the cause of the obstruction. If the child has a neoplasm, the outcome will be based on the state and dissemination of the tumor. However, if the disorder is secondary to trauma, infection, or hemorrhage, the prognosis is based on the amount of brain damage incurred before treatment. Children who have shunts placed soon after diagnosis have a better survival rate, although some will display ataxia, decreased fine-motor coordination, spasticity, diplegia, perceptual deficits, or developmental delays. Clients with additional diagnoses, such as meningomyelocele, have more complications and disabilities (Kinsman & Johnston, 2007).

Clinical Manifestations

The signs and symptoms of hydrocephalus are generally caused by large ventricles (Figure 32-6) resulting from the

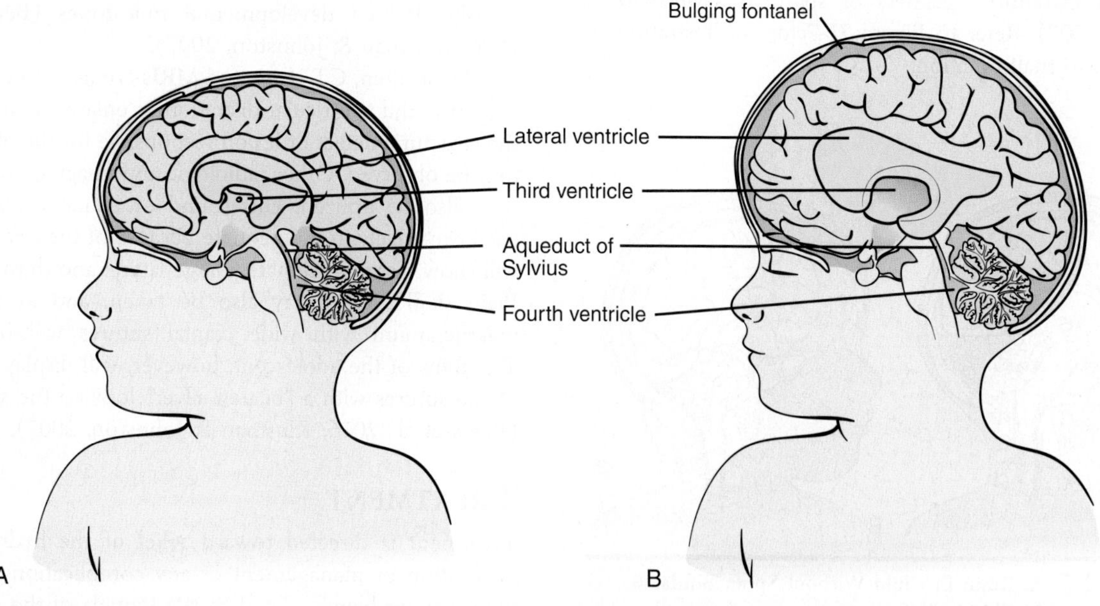

Figure 32-6 Comparison of A. Normal Size Ventricles and B. Enlarged Ventricles Associated with Hydrocephalus. DELMAR CENGAGE LEARNING.

trapped cerebrospinal fluid leading to compression of the brain parenchyma against the inner table of the skull and increased intracranial pressure. Infants will present with irritability, bulging fontanelles, and a high-pitched cry. Other symptoms include lethargy, vomiting, and strabismus. Older children may complain of headaches or decreased visual acuity (Beers et al., 2006; Kinsman & Johnston, 2007).

During the neonatal period, hydrocephalus is common with a meningomyelocele at the thoracolumbar junction or above. If a structural defect is not immediately apparent, however, the only sign of the disorder may be a rapidly increasing head circumference. In fact, within the first two to four weeks of life, the measurement may be as much as one to two standard deviations above normal (Beers et al., 2006; Kinsman & Johnston, 2007).

The head of the infant with hydrocephalus will be disproportionately large when compared to the face. In addition, there will be protrusion of the frontal region, translucent skin covering the forehead, prominent scalp veins, and wide palpable suture lines. The eyes may have a wide bridge between them and visible sclera above the iris (sunsetting sign). The anterior fontanelle may be bulging or tense. Other anatomic and physiologic abnormalities include a thin cerebral cortex; less dense cranium; and a positive **Macewen's sign** (a hollow or "cracked-pot" sound produced on percussion of the skull). Neurologically, the infant may be fussy, restless, irritable, apathetic, or have an altered or diminished level of consciousness accompanied by sluggish pupillary response to light, posturing, atypical reflex reaction, and lower extremity spasticity. In addition, the infant may feed poorly because of difficulties in proper positioning or swallowing, and the cry may be high-pitched and cat-like. In extreme cases, cardiopulmonary depression may occur (Beers et al., 2006; Kinsman & Johnston, 2007).

The infant with Arnold-Chiari malformation displays cranial nerve dysfunction caused by brain stem compression. In addition, there may be difficulties swallowing, stridor, apnea, respiratory distress, diminished or absent gag reflex, and upper extremity weakness or spasticity (Kinsman & Johnston, 2007). Refer to Figure 32-7 for an illustration of Arnold-Chiari malformation.

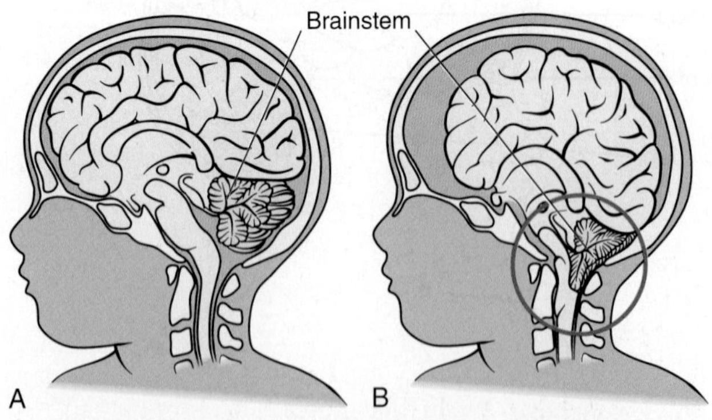

FIGURE 32-7 A. Brain in Child Without Spina Bifida. B. Brain with Arnold-Chiari Malformation. DELMAR CENGAGE LEARNING.

Dandy-Walker syndrome occurs when the roof of the fourth ventricle fails to form, allowing the ventricle to form a large cyst. Infants with Dandy-Walker syndrome exhibit rapid increase of their head circumference and a prominent occiput. The face will appear small as compared to the head, and nystagmus, cranial nerve palsies, and ataxia will be present (Kinsman & Johnston, 2007).

The hydrocephalic older child and adolescent display no enlargement of the head. Instead, most signs and symptoms are consistent with those of increased intracranial pressure. Upon awakening in the morning, the child may have a headache, often accompanied by nausea and vomiting. In addition, irritability, lethargy, apathy, or confusion may be reported. Judgment and reasoning skills may be impaired, and the child may become incoherent. There will also be a change in motor abilities (ataxia, spasticity). Further examination may reveal papilledema, strabismus, or decrease in visual acuity secondary to compression of the optic nerve. Other manifestations will be focal in nature resulting from the location of the space-occupying lesion (Kinsman & Johnston, 2007).

DIAGNOSIS

The advent of high-quality diagnostic prenatal ultrasounds has resulted in the diagnosis of hydrocephalus prenatally. After birth, hydrocephalus should be suspected when the infant has an enlarged head circumference or large, bulging fontanels. In many cases, rapid head enlargement is the first indication of hydrocephalus; therefore, daily measurement of cranial circumference is critical. Awareness of the clinical manifestations displayed by all age groups will also help in diagnosis. Newborns and young infants may exhibit facial structural manifestations including a broad forehead or eyes that are deviated downward. They may also have brisk tendon reflexes, spastisity, and clonus. Older children will exhibit irritability, lethargy, anorexia, and vomiting. They may also have personality changes and deterioration of previously attained developmental milestones (Beers et al., 2006; Kinsman & Johnston, 2007).

Most often, CT scans and MRIs are used to confirm the diagnosis and ventricular dilatation or enlargement, as well as the structural defect or lesion responsible for the obstruction, may be observed. Other radiologic and imaging examinations may also be utilized. Ultrasound or echoencephalography, used exclusively in the neonate because of the open fontanel, will show disproportionately large lateral and third ventricles. Plain skull X-rays may also be taken, and in the infant, macrocranium with wide cranial sutures will be evident. The films of the adolescent, however, will display a splitting of the sutures with a "beaten silver" look to the skull bones (Beers et al., 2006; Kinsman & Johnston, 2007).

TREATMENT

Treatment is directed toward relief of the hydrocephalus, prevention or management of any complications, and handling any problems related to the sequela of the underlying pathology. With few exceptions, treatment is surgical: the removal of any space-occupying lesion and the insertion of a shunt. The shunt system, made of radio-opaque plastic material, has a ventricular catheter, a unidirectional pressure valve and pumping chamber and a distal catheter that work together to direct the flow of cerebrospinal fluid from the ventricles to other areas of the body for absorption. In pediatrics, shunts are placed to manage progressive ventricular enlargement and increased intracranial pressure in the presence of the large ventricles. Most often, they are ventriculoperitoneal, from the ventricle to the peritoneum (Figure 32-8), or ventriculoatrial (from the ventricle to the left atrium). The first is more commonly used in infants and children as the peritoneal cavity provides both an adequate blood supply to ensure cerebrospinal fluid reabsorption and a large space to accommodate the coiled catheter tubing.

In clients with congenital hydrocephalus, shunts are typically placed as soon as the diagnosis is made, and modifications to handle physical growth are planned at regular intervals. Unexpected revisions, however, may occur at any time. The most serious complication associated with shunt placement is infection, which most often occurs within two months of the surgery. The causative agents are usually *Staph epidermidis* and *Staph aureus.* Children under 3 months of age and those infants who have had an intraventricular hemorrhage or central nervous system infection are at particular risk for shunt infection (Beers et al., 2006; Kinsman & Johnston, 2007).

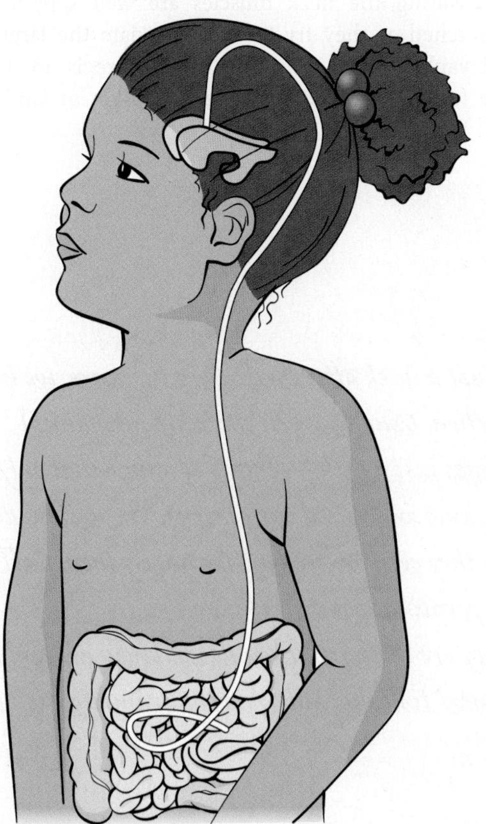

FIGURE 32-8 Ventriculoperitoneal Shunt. DELMAR CENGAGE LEARNING.

NURSING TIP

Other Types of Shunting Systems Used for Children

- Lumboperitoneal: diverts cerebrospinal fluid from the lumbar subarachnoid space to the peritoneum
- Ventricular plural: diverts fluid to the pleural cavity; it is used for children over age 5 years
- Ventricular bypass: intracranial channels are created in older children with obstructive hydrocephalus secondary to aqueductal stenosis or posterior fossa mass

Conservative treatment for shunt infection is administration of antibiotics. The medication used, however, will depend on the pathogen as well as the ability of the drug to cross the blood-brain barrier. After 48 hours of therapy, repeat cultures are taken. If there is still evidence of infection, an external ventricular drainage (EVD) device may be necessary (Beers et al., 2006; Kinsman & Johnston, 2007).

NURSING ALERT

Signs of a Shunt Infection

- Ventriculitis with a low-grade fever, malaise, nausea, and headache.
- Blood cultures may be negative, although there will be an increase in serum leukocytes.
- Cerebrospinal fluid will have an increase in white blood cell count and protein, a decrease in glucose, and the pathogen seen in cultures or Gram stain.
- Sepsis with a modest fever and weakness; laboratory tests reveal positive blood and cerebrospinal fluid cultures, leukocytosis, and anemia.

NURSING ALERT

Signs and Symptoms of Overdraining Ventricles When Using an External Drainage Device

- Change in blood pressure
- Decreased heart rate
- Apnea or change in respiratory pattern
- Severe headache
- Nausea and vomiting
- Lethargy, drowsiness, or irritability
- Seizures

Shunt malfunction, the other major complication, is caused by mechanical problems such as kinking, plugging, migrating, or separating of the tubing. Signs and symptoms mimic those of increased intracranial pressure as the CSF fluid is not draining effectively from the ventricles. Most often, surgical repair is needed.

Nursing Management

Assessment Preoperatively, the nurse must assess the child carefully by measuring head circumference daily, watching for signs and symptoms of increased intracranial pressure, assessing respiratory status, measuring intake and output, and monitoring nutritional status. Postoperatively, the nurse must assess vital signs and perform neurological checks every 2 hours. Baseline behaviors should be used to evaluate interactions with people and the environment, sleep patterns, and developmental capabilities. Intake and output, skin integrity, bowel sounds, and signs of infection should be monitored. The nurse must also watch for evidence of increased intracranial pressure.

Nursing Diagnosis

Preoperatively:

1. *Risk for injury to neck muscles* related to enlarged head and large, heavy cranial vault.
2. *Risk for impaired skin integrity* related to thin skin.
3. *Imbalanced nutrition: less than body requirements* related to potential for vomiting and need for proper positioning when feeding.
4. *Excess fluid volume* related to alteration in CSF flow.
5. *Decrease intracranial adaptive capacity* related to alteration in CSF flow.

Postoperatively:

1. *Risk for imbalanced fluid volume* related to cerebrospinal fluid draining too quickly.
2. *Risk for excess fluid volume* related to surgery.
3. *Risk for impaired skin integrity* related to thin skin.
4. *Risk for infection* related to surgical site.
5. *Decrease intracranial adaptive capacity* related to alteration in CSF flow prior to surgery.

Outcome Identification

Preoperatively:

1. The child's neck muscles will not show signs of strain.
2. The child will not show signs of skin breakdown.
3. The child will have proper intake of nutrition and exhibit normal weight gain.
4. The child will not have increased fluid volume prior to operation.

Postoperatively:

1. The child will not suffer from CSF drainage and pressure on valves.
2. The child will not show signs of intracranial pressure.
3. The child will not show signs of skin breakdown.
4. The child will not develop an infection.

Planning and Implementation Preoperatively, the nurse must take particular care when positioning the child, assuring the neck muscles are well supported and not stretched as they try to accommodate the large, heavy cranial vault. As the skin is so thin, there is an increased chance for breakdown; therefore, sheepskin or lamb's wool

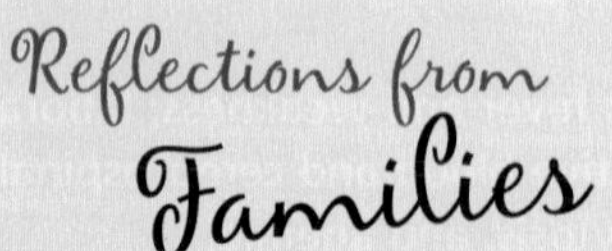

My son Carl is 10 years old and had his first V-P shunt placed just a week after birth. Over the years, we had some problems with malfunctions and once he even had an infection. Usually, when there are mechanical problems with the shunt, I know about them. His behavior changes just a little—this is so subtle that only his Dad and I are aware of it. I wish that when we went to the clinic and voiced our concerns the doctors and nurses would listen to us. Last time, we made three trips before they even ordered a CT scan. By then, Carl's ICP started to build up and he had to be literally rushed to the operating room.

My plea is simple: Please pay attention to parents and what they are telling you. You do not know my son, I do. When something is "not right" I can tell immediately. Perhaps, next time, we can avoid the dramatic rush to fix something that could have been taken care of quite simply.

should be placed under the head, and the position changed frequently. Special attention must be paid to the nutritional status of the infant as well. Holding to feed may prove a challenge because of the large head. Because the infant is prone to vomiting, the nurse should offer small, frequent feedings with intermittent burping.

Postoperatively, the child will be placed in a flat position on the unoperated side to prevent rapid CSF drainage and pressure on the valves. Gradually, the head of the bed will be elevated. If cerebrospinal fluid is drained too quickly, the child is at risk for a subdural hematoma caused by tears in the vessels secondary to the cerebral cortex pulling away from the dura.

The child should be monitored closely with vital signs and neurological checks taken frequently. Level of consciousness as well as evidence of irritability or restlessness should also be evaluated. Baseline behaviors should be used to evaluate interactions with people and the environment, sleep patterns, and developmental capabilities. Head circumference must be measured as should intake and output, especially as fluids may be restricted during the first 24 hours postoperatively. In addition, bowel sounds must be evaluated and reappear before oral hydration is started. Meticulous skin care should also continue. The child must be observed for signs of infection, such as fever, increased heart and respiratory rates, poor feeding or vomiting, altered mental status, seizures, and focal symptoms such as redness or cerebrospinal fluid leakage at the surgical site or erythema along the shunt tract. The nurse must also watch for evidence of increased intracranial pressure.

Evaluation The child will not show signs of strained neck muscles or skin breakdown. The child will take a normal amount of nutrition and will maintain current levels of fluid retention prior to the operation. Postoperatively, the child will experience proper CSF drainage. The child will exhibit normal vital signs, bowel sounds will be heard, skin integrity will be maintained, and the child will not exhibit signs of infection or increased intracranial pressure.

Family Teaching

The child's caregivers need support. If the disorder is diagnosed in the neonatal period or early infancy, the family will fear the obstruction sequelae or the surgical procedure itself. They are most often afraid of brain damage, mental retardation, or other developmental difficulties. However, if the hydrocephalus is secondary to neoplasm, the caregivers' anxieties are compounded by their child's potentially life-threatening illness. In either case, it is prudent to provide support and allow them to discuss their concerns.

The caregivers will also need explanations about the anatomy and physiology of hydrocephalus, how it affects the child, surgical procedures, and nursing care. Since much of the information may seem confusing or overwhelming, it is helpful to use photographs and illustrations. Once there is a clear understanding of what will initially happen, the nurse should begin teaching the caregivers how to care for their child. This will foster feelings of control and mastery of the situation and help them become members of the health care team.

Before discharge, the nurse should speak with the family about caring for the child with a shunt. They will need to know this is a lifelong condition requiring frequent follow-up consultation, and to be taught the signs and symptoms of shunt infection and failure as well as what to do if they suspect either is present.

Most children with shunts lead normal lives. They go to school and interact with peers: they should not be overprotected, but should avoid contact sports and, in general, be allowed to grow and develop as typically as their friends.

NEURAL TUBE DEFECTS

Spina bifida is a neural tube defect where there is an incomplete closure of the vertebrae and neural tube.

Incidence

Spina bifida develops during the first 28 days of gestation. It is a common developmental anomaly of the central nervous system, occurring in approximately 1 in every 2,000 births in the United States each year. Incidence is higher in families with Hispanic ancestry and whites of European ancestry. If other family members are affected, the chance of another infant having the defect is higher (Beers et al., 2006; Kinsman & Johnston, 2007; March of Dimes, n.d.).

Etiology and Pathophysiology

Spina bifida, which can occur anywhere along the spine, may be due to failure of the neural tube to close completely during the fourth week of gestation, or to a fissure resulting from increased cerebrospinal fluid pressure.

The exact cause of spina bifida is unclear. However, many factors are known to interfere with the normal development of the spinal cord. These factors include chemical exposure, medications, hyperthermia, maternal obesity or malnutrition, diabetes, genetics, and folic acid deficiency. The identification of low maternal folic acid levels prompted the American Academy of Pediatrics, in 1993, to recommend all women take 0.4 milligrams of folic acid per day at least 1 month before conception, a dose found in most vitamin preparations. For those women with a family history of spina bifida, the dosage is raised to four milligrams of folic acid each day beginning at least 1 month before conception and continuing through the first trimester (AAP, 1999). In the late 1990s, many countries mandated the fortification of grains products with folic acid. These measures have resulted in the reduction of neural tube defects by as much as 78% in some countries. A link between inadequate vitamin B12 intake and neural tube defects has prompted the recommendation that women planning pregnancies be tested to verify that they have vitamin B12 level >300 ng/L (Molloy et al., 2009). Prognosis depends on the type and level of the defect, the presence of other congenital anomalies, and whether or not there are additional complicating factors, such as hydrocephalus.

Clinical Manifestations

Spina bifida can occur anywhere along the spinal cord with varying pathologies. The most common defects include:

- **Ancephaly**: absence of the cranial vault with cerebral hemispheres either completely missing or greatly reduced in size. At times, the brain stem will be intact and vital functions can be maintained for weeks or even months. Death is usually caused by respiratory failure.
- **Cranioschisis**: a skull defect through which neural tissue protrudes.
- **Exencephaly**: a malformation where the brain is totally exposed or herniated through a skull defect.
- **Encephalocele** (Figure 32-9): a protrusion of the brain and meninges into a fluid-filled sac through a skull defect. This often occurs with other congenital anomalies.
- **Spina bifida occulta**: failure of the posterior vertebral arches to fuse, most often at the fifth lumbar or first sacral vertebrae; there is no herniation of the spinal cord or meninges. This defect is not usually visible externally, although a dimple or small depression may be noted. It can, however, be seen on X-ray. Initial suspicion that a problem may be present is not usually detected until toddlerhood. When the child begins to walk, there may be an abnormal gait with foot weakness or deformity. Later on, when toilet training is attempted, there may be disturbances in controlling either or both the bladder or bowel.
- **Rachischisis**: fissure in the vertebral column exposing the meninges and spinal cord.

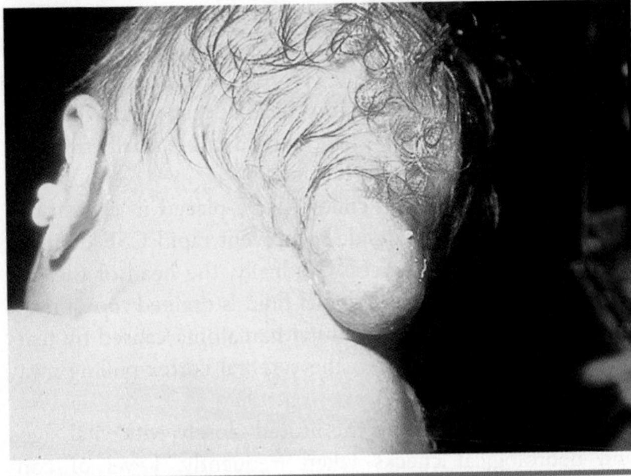

Figure 32-9 Encephalocele. DELMAR CENGAGE LEARNING.

- **Spina bifida cystica**: a defect in the closure of the posterior vertebral arch resulting in one of the following two anomalies:
  - **Meningocele**: a sac-like herniation through the bony malformation containing the meninges and cerebrospinal fluid. The sac covering may be thin and translucent or membranous (Figure 32-10).
  - **Meningomyelocele**: a sac-like extrusion through the bony defect containing the meninges, cerebrospinal fluid, and a portion of the spinal cord (myelo) or nerve roots. This lesion is poorly covered so there may be cerebrospinal fluid leakage at the site. It occurs most often at the lumbar or lumbosacral areas of the vertebrae (Figure 32-11).

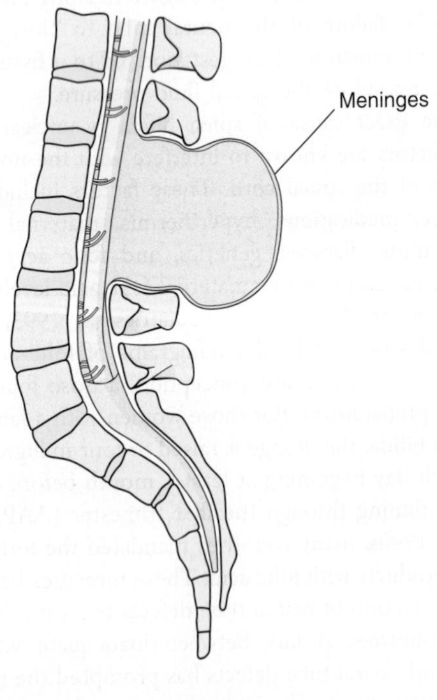

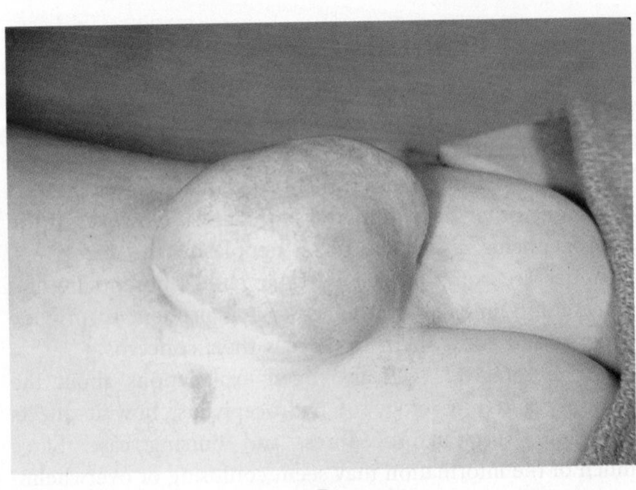

Figure 32-10 A. Illustration of Meningocele. B. Meningocele. DELMAR CENGAGE LEARNING.

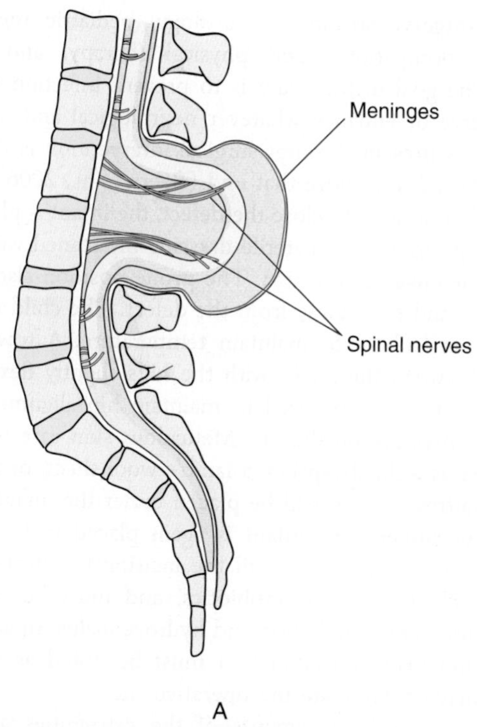

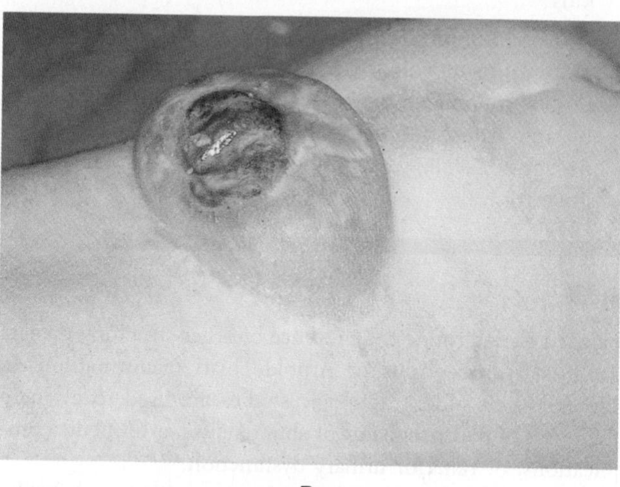

FIGURE 32-11 A. Illustration of Meningomyelocele, B. Meningomyelocele. DELMAR CENGAGE LEARNING.

Spina bifida, the generic term used to describe meningomyelocele, is noted at birth with the sac-like protrusion on the neonate's back. The clinical manifestations depend on the location of the lesion: the higher the deformity, the more neurological deficits will be present. The lower extremities may be partially or completely paralyzed and the bowel and bladder may or may not be affected. In addition, there may be renal impairment secondary to faulty kidney innervation. Orthopedic complications such as flexion or extension contractures, talipes valgus, or varus contractures may also be present at birth. Approximately 90% of infants with the most severe form of spina bifida also develop hydrocephalus (Kinsman & Johnston, 2007; March of Dimes, n.d.).

Infants and children with spina bifida may develop signs and symptoms of complications associated with the defect, the most common being urinary tract infections. Orthopedic problems are also seen in children with spina bifida. Although only 10% of the children with thoracic lesions are born with **kyphosis**, an abnormal curvature of the spine occurring in the thoracic region, its likelihood increases during the rapid growth of adolescence (Rowe & Jadhav, 2008). This deformity is not merely a cosmetic problem as it can lead to back pain, respiratory distress, recurrent skin breakdown, and difficulty ambulating. Scoliosis is also frequently seen, especially in adolescents, but lordosis (forward curvature of the spine) occurs less frequently. Tethering (abnormal adhesion to a bony structure causing traction) of the spinal cord because of adhesions may cause difficulties in older children and adolescents as well, resulting in back pain, increased spasticity, and decreased urinary control.

Because loss of sensation is secondary to interrupted nerve pathways, trauma to the lower extremities may occur without the infant's or child's knowledge and skin breakdown frequently is seen over bony prominences. In addition, these children are more susceptible to burns from water and the sun as well as idiopathic fracture because their bones are brittle. Finally, infants and children who have had shunts placed may develop shunt failure or infection.

DIAGNOSIS

Some neural tube defects may be diagnosed prenatally by ultrasound. Routine prenatal screening of maternal AFP levels performed between 16 to 18 weeks gestation may indicate elevated AFP levels, which identify an increased risk for spina bifida. Further testing, including an ultrasound and an amniocentesis test, may reveal an increase in alpha-fetoprotein, a fetal specific gamma-1 globulin in the amniotic fluid that indicates the presence of meningomyelocele, and support the diagnosis of a neural tube defect. Prenatal diagnosis of spina bifida can assist the parents and health providers determine the safest method of delivery for the baby (Beers et al., 2006).

Diagnosis after birth is made during the neonatal examination. If a lesion is noted, it can be evaluated using several techniques. **Transillumination** (shining a light through the sac) may be utilized to determine the structures in the sac. If the sac becomes translucent when the light source is held to it, it is a meningocele; if the sac does not become translucent, it is a meningomyelocele. Radiologic studies may also be performed. CT scans and MRIs as well as flat-plate films of the spinal column may be used to determine bony deformities and tissue herniation. In addition, neuroimaging may

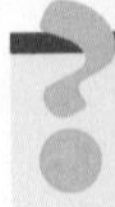

KIDS WANT TO KNOW

A Brother with Meningomyelocele

What's wrong with Ronnie? (newborn brother) Will he ever be normal? Can he run and play like other kids?

Answer: Ronnie has a defect in his back called a meningomyelocele. At this point we do not know if he will be able to walk independently, but he may be able to use a brace, crutches, or a cane. Even if he doesn't walk, you and he will be able to play and have fun.

be used to determine the presence of other structural defects such as hydrocephalus or Arnold-Chiari malformation. As the child gets older, radiologic studies are used to evaluate the onset of hydrocephalus or shunt failure, orthopedic complications, or renal or urinary dysfunction.

Neurological examination of the extremities must also be performed. Motor response and strength, sensory reaction to specific stimuli, and reflexes should be evaluated on an ongoing basis. In addition, routine developmental assessments are necessary to note delays. If milestones are not reached at the appropriate time, additional therapies may be added to the established regimen to encourage optimal development.

TREATMENT

Once the diagnosis is confirmed, treatment is begun using a multidisciplinary approach with input from neurosurgery, plastic surgery, orthopedics, urology, pediatric medicine, nursing, occupational and physical therapy, and social work. The goal of this team is to prevent infection as well as preserve or enhance whatever neurological and urologic function is present. Prompt surgical intervention is the first method used to achieve that end (Beers et al., 2006).

Before surgery to close the defect, the infant is placed in a prone position with a sterile dressing moistened with normal saline covering the area. The prone position also keeps the urine and feces away from the defect. The child may be kept in an isolette to maintain temperature. A towel roll, placed between the knees with the hips slightly flexed and legs abducted, can be used to maintain hip alignment and decrease pressure on the sac. Meticulous skin care must be provided as well; sheepskin, a lamb's wool sheet, or an egg-crate mattress pad should be placed under the infant.

After surgery, the infant is again placed in the prone position for several days until the incision has healed. The infant will also receive antibiotics, and must be watched closely for signs of infection and hydrocephalus. In addition, bowel and bladder dysfunction must be noted as incontinence may contaminate the operative site.

Neurological assessments of the extremities assist in planning the therapeutic regimen, as management of any orthopedic malformations often begins just after birth. Positioning, casting, splinting, bracing, traction, and surgeries are performed as soon as possible to enhance the chance for ambulation and decrease the risk of complications. Walkers, crutches, canes, and lightweight braces may be used with lesions at L-2 to L-5 while customized wheelchairs can be used with a high-level deformity, usually at L-2 or above.

Infants and children with neural tube defects often have neurogenic (neurologically dysfunctional) bladder and, therefore, are prone to urinary retention and frequent infection. Intermittent catheterization along with medications to enhance bladder storage and continence are utilized to help manage this problem. A vesicostomy where a stoma is created by bringing the anterior wall of the bladder to the abdominal wall is a surgical option for some children (Wilson & Clayton, 2009). To maintain bowel control, stool softeners and diets high in fiber have proven to be valuable.

NURSING ALERT

Latex Allergy

Infants, children, and adolescents with spina bifida are 41% more likely to have latex allergy than the general public. Signs and symptoms include:

- urticaria
- wheezing
- watery eyes
- rash
- anaphylaxis, in extreme cases

Equipment such as tourniquets, intravenous tubing, urinary and intravenous catheters, and tapes are now available latex-free; therefore, the nurse must ensure all products be checked before they are brought into client rooms and not used if they contain latex.

NURSING MANAGEMENT

The neonate diagnosed with spina bifida must be carefully observed. Preoperatively, the sac must be watched closely and its integrity maintained. The risk for infection is high and the nurse must be aware of the symptoms associated with it, including fever, irritability or lethargy, nuchal rigidity, and the signs of increased intracranial pressure. In addition, as hydrocephalus is a common adjunct to the deformity; nurses must be aware of its clinical manifestations. In both cases, the neurosurgery department must be notified as soon as possible when these conditions appear since immediate intervention is indicated.

Because providing comfort may be difficult, tactile stimulation such as touching, rubbing, and stroking are important. If held, the infant should be placed prone on a pillow on the nurse or caregiver's lap. Feeding in the prone position can be challenging. Therefore, the infant should be fed with the head turned to one side. Because breastfeeding may be contraindicated before surgery, mothers should be encouraged to pump their breasts and begin breastfeeding later.

Before surgery, a neurological assessment should be performed. Absence or presence of extremity movement must be observed as should any evidence of flaccidity or spasticity. In addition, dribbling urine or continuous stooling should be noted.

Postoperatively, the neonate should be monitored carefully and vital signs taken frequently. In addition, the infant must be observed for any signs of local or systemic infection, meningitis, hydrocephalus, or increased intracranial pressure. Also, the surgical site must be watched for cerebrospinal fluid leakage. The neonate's position now can be prone, side-lying, or upright while leaning against someone's chest. After the incision has healed, the infant may be held in a normal fashion for feeding either from the breast or bottle.

Because most problems associated with spina bifida are related to motor or sensory impairments, skin integrity must be maintained. To reduce the chance of breakdown, bony prominences should be protected, gentle massage provided, and linen changed frequently.

Orthopedic sequelae are common as well. For most children, range of motion exercises and other physical therapy maneuvers should be initiated early to prevent muscle atrophy and contractures.

Because urinary and bowel sequelae occur, the nurse should watch for retention difficulties or infection. In addition, hydrocephalus may emerge at any time, so any change in neurological status must be investigated.

The child with spina bifida has needs beyond those of the neonate and infant. Development must be assessed carefully, and it is critical the child be treated according to cognitive rather than motor capabilities. Independence should be encouraged and opportunities for choices provided. The physical, emotional, and intellectual environment must be

REFLECTIVE THINKING

Moms Have Special Needs, Too

It is important to remember during the neonatal period, that the mother has special needs. Not only is she dealing with the grief associated with not having a "normal" child and the medical, social, and intellectual implications associated with spina bifida, but she is going through the postpartum period and may be extremely emotional and vulnerable. Put yourself in her shoes. Can you imagine what your responses would be?

NURSING TIP

Monitor Height

Many children with spina bifida do not reach normal heights. Recombinant human growth hormone has been administered to some children with success as it improves both their growth rate and length, and assists these children to attain near normal adult heights (Rotenstein & Bass, 2004).

RESEARCH Highlight

Sibling Relationships in Families of Youths with Spina Bifida

STUDY PURPOSE

To delineate key individual, family, and peer factors associated with the quality of sibling relationships in families of youths with spina bifida.

METHODS

Two hundred and twenty-four sibling-parent dyads participated in the study. Siblings were between the ages of 11 and 18, had no current health concerns, and had a sibling with spina bifida. Self-reported sibling measures included attitude toward spina bifida, satisfaction with family functioning, peer support, warmth and conflict in the sibling relationship. Parent reported measure was the severity and level of the spina bifida lesion.

FINDINGS

Sibling relationships were generally positive in nature but emotional intimacy was restricted. Family functioning was the strongest factor associated with both warmth and conflict in sibling relationships, while peer support was the weakest factor.

IMPLICATIONS

Interventions should be targeted toward improving family functioning. For instance, adolescent siblings responded to their brothers and sisters with spina bifida in positive, warm ways when their own needs were met, they were included in family activities, they were free to express themselves, and they were a valued member of the family. By targeting family functioning, positive sibling interactions can be developed.

REFERENCE

Bellin, M. H., & Rice, K. M. (2009). Individual, family, and peer factors associated with the quality of sibling relationships in families of youths with spina bifida. *Journal of Family Psychology, 23*(1), 39–47.

EVIDENCE-BASED PRACTICE

Spina Bifida and Pain

CLINICAL PROBLEM

Do children and adolescents with spina bifida have pain?

BEST CLINICAL PRACTICE

Most children and adolescents with spina bifida have pain at least once a week. Pain occurs in the head, back, abdomen, shoulders, neck, hands, and legs. The severity of pain is directly correlated with the frequency of pain.

- Children with spina bifida also report pain associated with treatments, such as physical therapy.
- Frequency and severity of pain were inversely related to quality of life scores.
- Frequency and severity of pain are implicated in higher depression levels among youth with spina bifida

IMPLICATIONS FOR NURSING

- Children and adolescents who have spina bifida frequently report significant pain. However, it often is unrecognized and therefore untreated.
- Parents need to be made aware of the fact that children and adolescents with spina bifida often have pain.
- Parents and health care providers need to appropriately manage pain in children or adolescents with spina bifida and watch, listen to, and believe complaints of pain in this population.

References: Oddson, B. E., Clancy, C. A., & McGrath, P. J. (2006). The role of pain in reduced quality of life and depressive symptomology in children with spina bifida. *The Clinical Journal of Pain, 22*(9), 784–789.

stimulating, yet not frustrating. Because the adolescent may have concerns about physical disabilities (how they affect peer relations, sexual identity, career), sensitivity, respect, and referral to appropriate staff may be necessary.

At the time of diagnosis, the family has tremendous needs coping with a child who will have lifelong challenges and needs. The initial facts are usually overwhelming, especially as they make decisions relative to surgeries and treatments. The nurse might become the central figure to help caregivers sort out their feelings and learn about useful resources. Clergy or social workers might also be helpful in answering nonmedical questions such as how bills will be paid and in arranging for care of the other children at home.

Before the infant is discharged, the nurse should help the family contact needed community resources. Local and online support groups, such as http://www.sbafsc.org, can be helpful to families. In addition, home care services should be arranged so all clinic appointments, therapy sessions, and in-hospital teaching can be reinforced and coordinated. Also,

REFLECTIVE THINKING

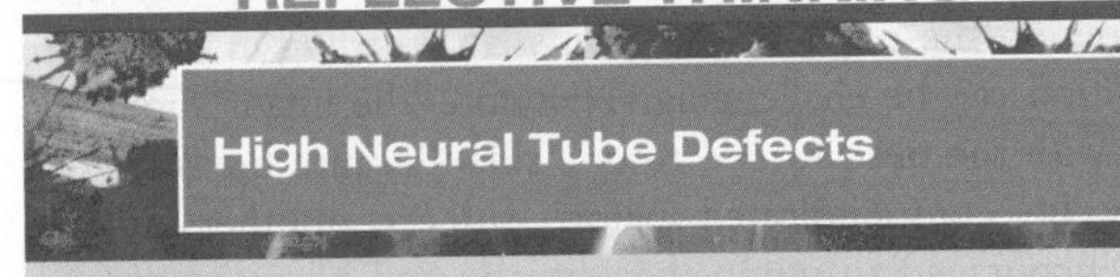

Neonates and infants with ancephaly are most often provided with comfort measures and palliative care. There is the ethical dilemma, however, about providing aggressive management of respiratory failure of these infants and the need for resuscitation following an arrest.

At least one case went to court where the mother of such an infant demanded her child receive the maximum care and most aggressive treatments available, while the hospital medical staff argued that was a futile and painful effort for a child with no chance for long-term survival. The court decided in favor of the mother.

Think about how you would feel if you had to work with a parent if your personal feelings differed.

any special equipment must be ordered and in place before the infant goes home.

FAMILY TEACHING

The infant will have special needs in terms of positioning, feeding techniques, skin care, intermittent catheterization, exercises, and special equipment such as braces or splints. Physical therapists, nutrition specialists, and nurses should teach caregivers how to care for the infant at home. In addition, caregivers need to realize the importance of follow-up care by the many specialists working with the child.

The family must not only learn the signs of hydrocephalus, idiopathic fractures, and urinary dysfunction or infection, but also what to do if these manifestations appear. They also need to understand while some symptoms are not life-threatening, others, such as shunt failure are, and require immediate medical attention.

CRANIOSYNOSTOSIS

Craniosynostosis is the premature closing of one or more cranial sutures (Figure 32-12).

INCIDENCE

Although rare, occurring in approximately 1 in 2,000 births, craniosynostosis is often a complex problem. There does not appear to be a racial predilection. Although recent genetic research has identified several different mutations responsible for craniosynostosis, in the majority of cases the cause is unknown (Morriss-Kay & Wilkie, 2005). Premature fusion of the sagittal sutures is the most common type with the incidence in the population being 1 in 4,200 births. Males are more commonly affected (3:1) (Plastic & Craniofacial

Normocephaly

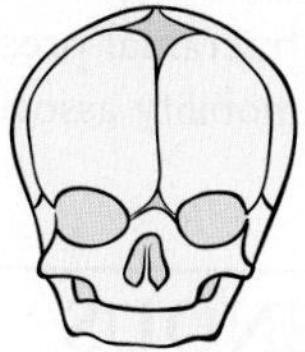
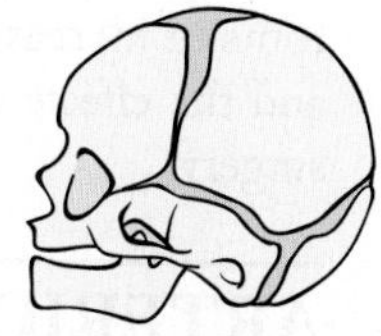
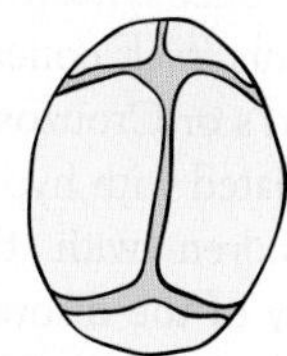

Scaphocephaly (dolichocephaly)

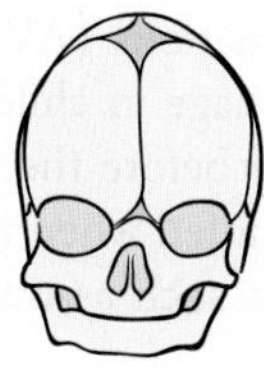
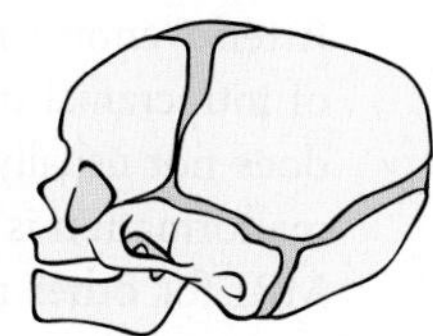
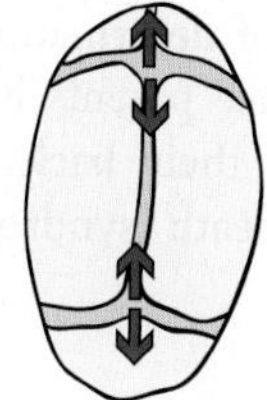

Plagiocephaly

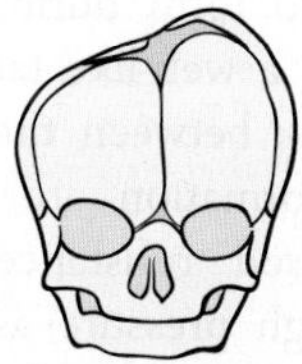
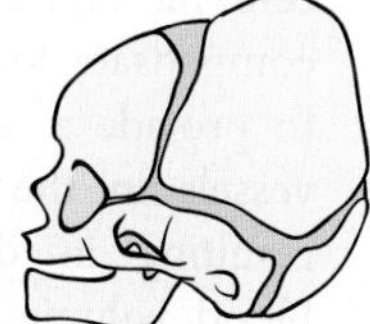
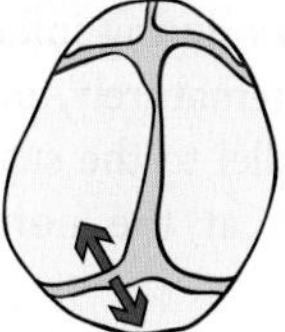
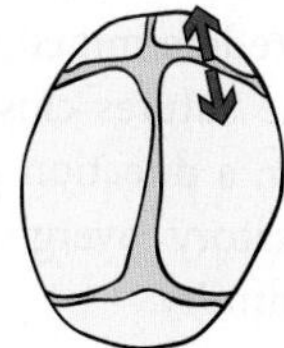

Brachycephaly

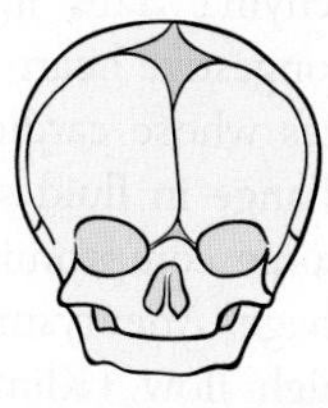
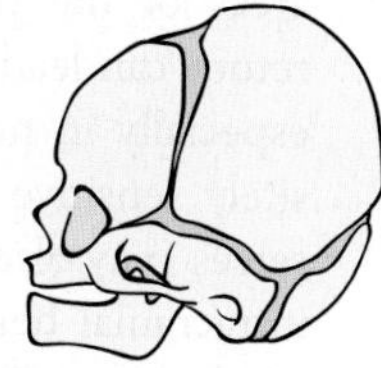
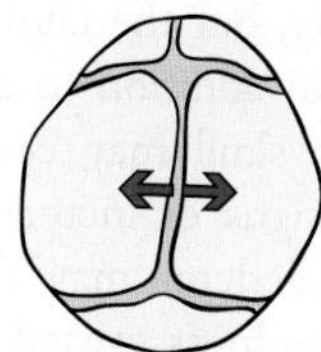

Oxycephaly

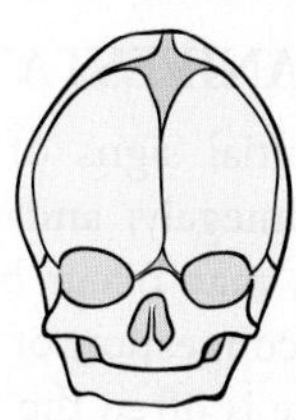
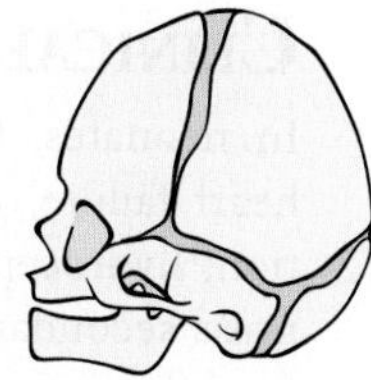
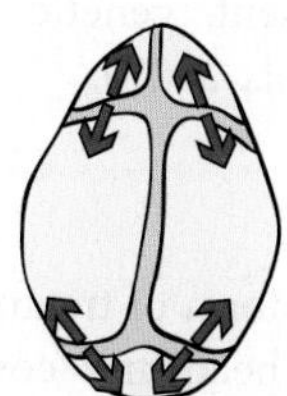

Trigonocephaly

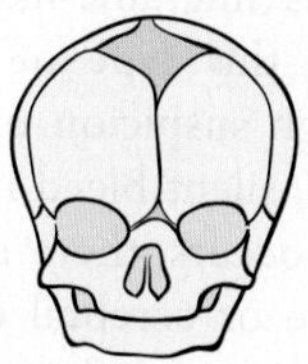
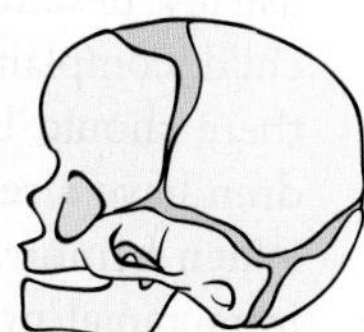
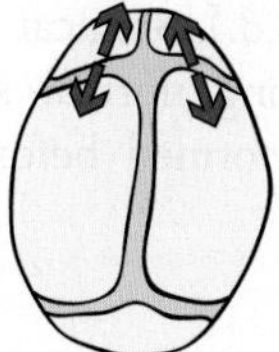

FIGURE 32-12 Craniosynostosis. DELMAR CENGAGE LEARNING.

Surgery for Infants & Children, n.d.). Twenty to twenty-five percent of cases are unilateral or bilateral coronal synostosis. In as many as 10–20% of the cases, it presents itself concurrently with inherited syndromes such as Apert's or Crouzon's. Craniosynostosis has occasionally been associated with hyperthyroidism or hypophospatasia. Most children with this abnormality, however, have no family history of the disorder (Kimonis, Gold, Hoffman, Panchal & Boyadjiev, 2007; Moe et al., 2009).

Carniosynostosis differs from deformational plagiocephaly, a flattening or misshapen head often due to an infant lying in the same position. The incidence of deformational plagiocephaly has increased dramatically since parents have been instructed to have babies sleep on their backs to reduce the incidence of sudden infant death syndrome (Tomlinson & Breidahl, 2007).

Etiology and Pathophysiology

The cause of craniosynostosis is unknown. Usually, bone growth occurs perpendicular to the suture lines, and normal suture closure occurs at predetermined times during infancy and early childhood. If the sutures close prematurely, bone growth will continue but in a direction parallel to the suture line, leading to compensatory overgrowth at the normal suture lines and skull deformity.

Clinical Manifestations and Diagnosis

The predominant feature is skull deformity, but the clinical picture depends on the sutures affected. In addition to the structural defect, the small or misshapen skull may cause problems with brain growth. Therefore, signs of increased intracranial pressure may be evident. Papilledema may also occur, and if left untreated may lead to blindness caused by atrophy of the optic nerve. Diagnosis is made by clinical appearance, skull X-rays, CT, and MRI. If development delays or other anomalies are also present, genetic syndromes must be considered (Kimonis et al., 2007).

Treatment

Surgical intervention is the most common form of treatment in order to reduce pressure within the head and correct deformities of the bone. The procedure is usually a linear craniotomy parallel to the fused sutures. Polyethylene film is inserted over the cut bony surface to delay closure (Children's Hospital and Health System, n.d.). Surgical outcomes are aimed at preserving or creating normal skull shape and are most successful when performed before 6 months of age (Moe et al., 2009).

Nursing Management

The nurse must support the family, as the appearance of their child can be a concern. Referral to social workers or support groups can often be beneficial. The nurse should also be able to manage the postoperative course of treatment for the child, including watching for signs and symptoms of increased intracranial pressure, infection, bleeding, and the effects of immobility associated with any intracranial surgery.

ARTERIOVENOUS MALFORMATION

Incidence

Arteriovenous malformations (AVMs) are a common cause of intracranial hemorrhage in children. Clinical presentation does not usually occur before the age of 10; oftentimes, the malformation is only noted when the child has a head CT or MRI for other reasons such as trauma.

Etiology and Pathophysiology

An **arteriovenous malformation** is caused by the failure of cerebral capillaries to form during fetal development. To compensate for this, a web-like tangle of vessels is created to provide a network between the arteries and veins. The vessels in the malformation are dilated and thin-walled, resulting in decreased resistance that causes increased blood volume at high pressure as blood moves from the artery involved to the vein. Initially, blood is shunted toward the malformation because of the low resistance, leading to "stealing" of cerebral blood with resulting ischemia in other areas of the parenchyma. This increased cerebral venous return can lead to congestive heart failure and cardiomegaly, especially in neonates whose cardiovascular status is exquisitely sensitive to change in fluid status. The vessels themselves may also become compromised and rupture, causing intracranial hemorrhage. Aneurysms can also form because of the incredibly high flow (Klimo, Rao, & Brockmeyer, 2007; NINDS, n.d.a.).

Clinical Manifestations

In neonates, the initial signs of an AVM are congestive heart failure, cardiomegaly, and a cerebral bruit. In addition, hydrocephalus may occur because of aqueductal stenosis secondary to congestion of the dilated vein of Galen. In children, a seizure is often the first sign of a neurological problem. The convulsion may be focal, Jacksonian (localized motor), or generalized. Headache may also occur, usually described as migraine-like in nature. In fact, if a child complains of this type of pain and has a seizure, there should be high suspicion of an AVM. Half the children have a remote, silent bleed before hospital admission. When hemorrhage occurs, there may be signs of increased intracranial pressure or cerebral edema, syncope, fainting, vertigo, dizziness, sensory deficits, tingling of extremities or motor weakness, aphasia, dysarthria, visual impairments such as hemianopia (blindness in half of the normal visual field), and confusion. In severe cases, there may be a profound decrease in the level of consciousness or coma (NINDS, n.d.a.).

Diagnosis

Cerebral angiography is used in diagnosis as the defect can be well visualized. In addition, CT with contrast, MRI, and skull films may be used. An EEG may be done; however, abnormal waves might be a reflection of brain ischemia rather than the vascular deformity. A lumbar puncture may be used to assess for subarachnoid bleeding, but it should not be performed until after CT has ruled out other structural pathology or intracranial shifts. Cerebral blood flow studies may also be performed, and chest X-ray may reveal cardiomegaly.

Treatment

Medical management involves close observation of the child using "AVM precautions" such as bed rest, sedation, a quiet environment, and decreased activity and stimulation. Invasive techniques can also be used to treat the malformation. Surgical intervention to excise the web is the ideal therapy but often impossible because of its location. When this is deemed the treatment of choice, the child must be medically stable for at least two to three weeks post initial bleed.

Flow-directed embolization is also used, especially with malformations in critical areas of the brain. Here, a catheter is introduced into the femoral artery and advanced to the defect. At that point, occlusive materials are introduced and carried to the malformation by direct blood flow. These materials, in essence, cause an occlusion to the deformity and divert blood flow through more normal channels (NINDS, n.d.a.; Zadeh et al., 2007).

For those children where surgery or embolization is not an option, radiotherapy using stereotaxic techniques may be utilized. The major disadvantage to this therapy is time as it may take up to two years before the treatment is completed.

Nursing Management

The nurse should manage the child with an AVM as any other client with a fragile neurological status. The ABCDEs, vital signs, and intracranial pressure should be closely monitored. Pupils should be checked and the Glasgow Coma Score calculated. "AVM precautions" must be strictly adhered to in order to maximize the child's recovery.

In addition, the nurse should watch for the sequelae of the treatment protocol chosen for the child whether it be surgical or radiological. The child who undergoes a craniotomy must be treated as all clients with intracranial surgery. However, the child who has embolization needs to be kept immobilized with pressure on the groin area to prevent arterial bleeding, and pedal pulses routinely checked. Families need information about the deformity and management options. The nurse should explain procedures as well as the post-treatment course for the child.

INFECTIONS

Infections of the neurological system discussed include meningitis (bacterial and viral), Reye's syndrome, and encephalitis.

MENINGITIS

Meningitis is an inflammation of the meninges that develops as a result of infection from either bacterial or viral agents. The causative organism is often age-dependent. Neonates develop meningitis as a result of *Escherichia coli*; *Haemophilus influenzae*, type B; Group B *Streptococcus*; *Neisseria meningitidis*; *Streptococcus pneumoniae*; *Listeria monocytogenes*; and *herpes*. Infants and children are susceptible to *Haemophilus influenzae*, type B; *Neisseria meningitidis*; *Streptococcus pneumoniae*; enterovirus; adenovirus; and the mumps virus. However, adolescents are at risk from exposure to *Neisseria meningitidis*; *Streptococcus pneumoniae*; *herpes*; adenovirus; and arbovirus (Prober, 2007).

Bacterial Meningitis

Incidence and Etiology

Bacterial or pyogenic meningitis affects many infants, children, and teenagers in the United States each year; most cases affect children under 5 years of age. The mortality rate is significant, even with appropriate antibiotic therapy (8% *H. influenzae;* 15% meningococcal; 25% pneumococcal). The infant/young child is at great risk for bacterial infection with males being affected more often than females (Prober, 2007). The most common pathogens have a seasonal pattern: *Haemophilus influenzae*, type B, occurs most frequently in the autumn and early winter although with the administration of the Hib vaccine, the rate of infection has fallen. *Neisseria meningitidis* and *Streptococcus pneumoniae* are prevalent in the later winter and early spring. Meningitis can also follow penetrating trauma or neurosurgical intervention, but it is usually a secondary response to a primary infection such as otitis media, sinusitis, pharyngitis, cellulitis, pneumonia, septic arthritis, or dental caries.

Pathophysiology

The bacteria enter the blood supply and are disseminated throughout the body, including the meninges. There, they are seeded into the cerebrospinal fluid and spread throughout the subarachnoid space. An inflammatory response follows, and white blood cells accumulate over the surface of the brain with a thick, purulent exudate. *Neisseria meningitidis* tends to cover the parietal, occipital, and cerebellar regions of the brain while *Streptococcus pneumoniae* spreads over the anterior lobes. In either case, the brain becomes hyperemic and edematous, resulting in increased intracranial pressure. Hydrocephalus may occur if the ventricles become infected and obstructed, or if the flow of cerebrospinal fluid within the subarachnoid space is impeded.

Prognosis depends on age, the organism, how quickly antibiotics and other medical interventions are initiated, and if there are complicating factors such as hydrocephalus, cerebritis, or disseminated intravascular coagulopathy. Sequelae such as hearing loss, blindness, paresis of facial muscles, and intellectual impairments are not uncommon (Prober, 2007).

Risk Factors Infants and children are at particular risk for meningitis because they lack immunity to many causative pathogens. Other risk factors include close contact with infected persons (crowded living conditions, daycare, college dormitories, military barracks), poverty, African-American or Native-American race, and male gender (Prober, 2007).

Clinical Manifestations Manifestations depend on age and the pathogen. The infant less than 3 months of age may have subtle signs and symptoms, including being lethargic, fussy, irritable, or displaying paradoxic irritability, a state in which activities that normally soothe a baby, such as rocking or cuddling, aggravate the infant further. Fever may or may not be present; hypothermia is a possibility. In addition, alterations in feeding or sleep patterns or vomiting or diarrhea with or without weight loss may be seen. The infant will usually have a bulging anterior fontanelle unless dehydration is present. The infant who is further compromised may seize, show diminished level of consciousness, and have a depressed respiratory state where apneic episodes are not uncommon (Prober, 2007).

The infant over 3 months of age and the toddler will show many of the same manifestations, with usually a gradual onset of symptoms and change in activity level, fever, or irritability. The child over age 2 years may have gastrointestinal upset and cold-like prodromal signs. Later, chills and fever will develop. The extent of the inflammatory process determines many other symptoms. When there is cortical involvement, the child may become irritable, agitated, confused, delirious, or lethargic and somnolent. In addition, there may be nausea and projectile vomiting. If the cranial nerves are involved, the youngster will suffer from photophobia (extreme light sensitivity), diplopia (double vision), and tinnitus. If the cervical nerves are irritated, the child will have nuchal rigidity. If this is the case, an opisthotonic position may be assumed, whereby the head and neck are hyperextended (Figure 32-13). This child may also complain of headache, most often frontal; myalgias; joint pain; and malaise.

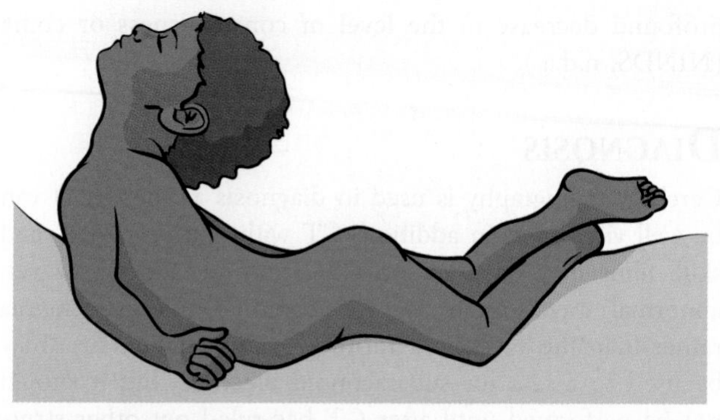

FIGURE 32-13 **Opisthotonic Position.** DELMAR CENGAGE LEARNING.

The onset of meningitis can be acute and dramatic. The child becomes seriously compromised, with signs of shock including poor perfusion with delayed capillary refill time, elevated heart rate, normal or low blood pressure, cool and pale extremities, and diminished level of consciousness. In addition, signs of increased intracranial pressure may be noted. A rash may also be present; if it is petechial, purpura-like, or ecchymotic, the child may have meningococcemia and need immediate medical intervention. Without intervention, coma or death may occur within 24 hours (Prober, 2007).

On further examination, the child with meningitis may have hyper-reactive reflexes. In addition, positive Kernig and Brudzinski's responses may be seen. **Kernig's sign** (Figure 32-14) is tested by having the child lie supine with hips and knees flexed. If meningitis is present, the child

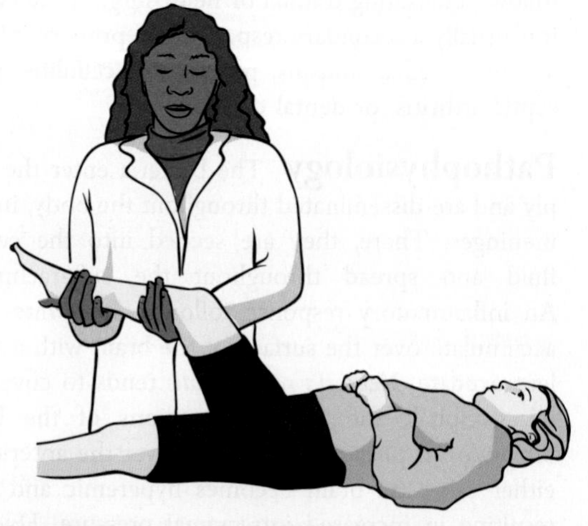

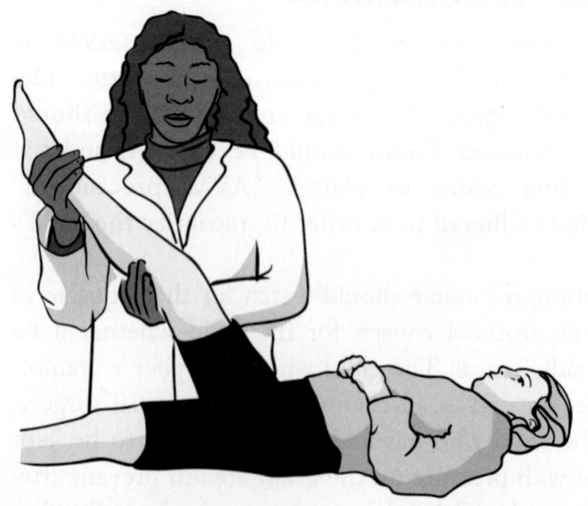

FIGURE 32-14 **Kernig's Sign.** DELMAR CENGAGE LEARNING.

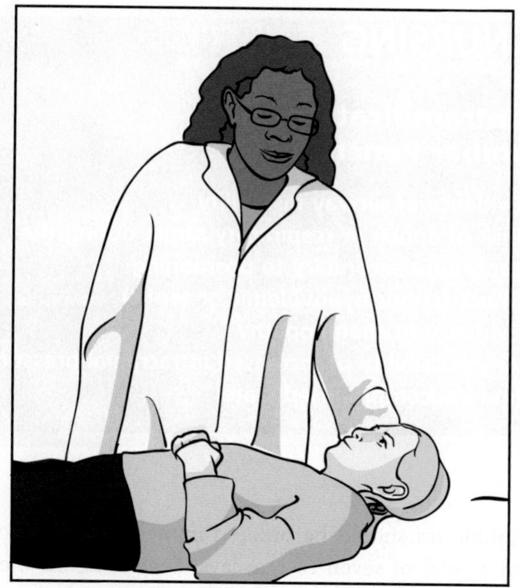

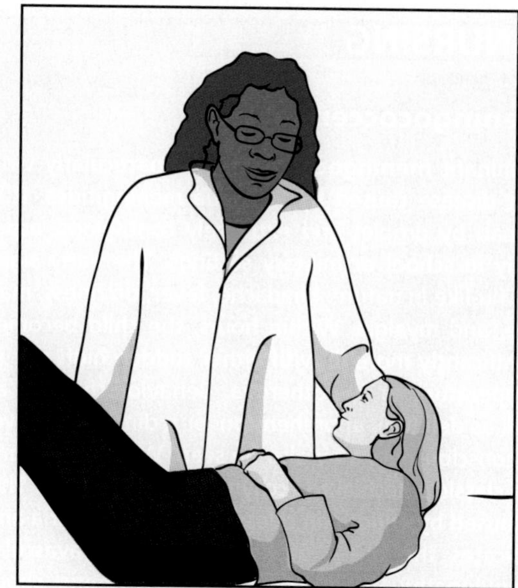

FIGURE 32-15 **Brudzinski's Sign.** DELMAR CENGAGE LEARNING.

will either resist the examiner's attempts to extend the knee or complain about pain on extension. **Brudzinski's sign** (Figure 32-15) is evoked when the youngster is supine. If there is meningeal irritation when the child's head is flexed forward, the child will automatically flex the hips and knees (Prober, 2007).

The meningitic infant or child is at risk for numerous complications, including sepsis, seizures, subdural effusions, brain abscess, or hydrocephalus, all of which will increase intracranial pressure. This child is also at risk for developing syndrome of idiopathic antidiuretic hormone secretion (SIADH) as well as disseminated intravascular coagulopathy (DIC). Refer to Chapter 26 for information about DIC and Chapter 28 for information about SIADH.

Diagnosis A detailed history is important, especially regarding the child's contact with other ill individuals, the duration of those illnesses, and their symptoms. The caregivers should also be asked if the youngster has developed a rash, had a seizure, or appears pale. In addition, they should be questioned about any changes in behavior, feeding, or sleeping patterns.

Laboratory tests include microscopic examination of blood, cerebrospinal fluid, and urine. A complete blood count will indicate if infection is present and whether or not it is bacterial. A culture of the CSF will identify the pathogen. Serum electrolytes and osmolarity should be checked to monitor hydration and note any signs of SIADH (headache, drowsiness, lethargy, confusion, diminished reflex response, hyponatremia, increased urine sodium, or urine specific gravity). In addition, clotting studies should be performed to determine if DIC is present.

Lumbar punctures should be performed on all children suspected of having bacterial meningitis, except in the presence (other than a bulging fontanel) of increased intracranial pressure (Prober, 2007). This assessment not only provides fluid samples, but also opening pressure measurements as well. The normal opening pressure value for the infant who is not crying is 50 millimeters of water; for the child, 85 millimeters of water. If the value exceeds 180 millimeters of water, meningitis should be suspected. Cerebrospinal fluid must also be examined microscopically, and the presence of white blood cells greater than 100 per cubic millimeter indicates meningitis. Fluid will appear cloudy to purulent depending on the number of neutrophils, and with meningitis, glucose will be decreased and protein increased (Prober, 2007). To identify the pathogen, culture and Gram stain should be performed.

Urine should be analyzed for culture, specific gravity, and osmolarity. Latex agglutination should also be done to rapidly identify the bacterial antigen. Chest X-ray is usually performed in conjunction with the septic work-up as a silent pneumonia may be present. In addition, a CT or MRI may be needed to confirm a subdural effusion, cerebral edema, or hydrocephalus.

Treatment The child with meningitis may be critically ill. Although intubation may not be needed, the child should be placed on a cardiorespiratory monitor until stable. In addition, this client may need supplemental oxygen as the illness will increase metabolism, thus raising oxygen consumption. It is not uncommon for infants and children with meningitis to be poorly perfused during the initial stages of this illness as vomiting and anorexia are often present. If signs of shock appear, the child may need fluid boluses or inotropic support. Signs of petechiae or purpura may indicate meningococcemia, DIC, or both, which need emergent management including intubation, fluid boluses, inotrope administration, blood or blood product infusions, and measures to control bleeding.

Seizure activity, generalized or focal, may also be present. If the episode is self-limiting or lasts less than five

NURSING ALERT

Meningococcemia

Fulminant **meningococcemia** is a particularly virulent disease caused by Neisseria meningitides. It is spread by droplet and extremely contagious, especially in school or military settings. The early signs are flu-like in nature: headache, fever, dizziness, malaise, and myalgia. Within hours, the child becomes significantly more ill with either sudden high rise in temperature or hypothermia. Behavior changes as well as delirium, apprehension, or a diminished level of consciousness may also be seen. Within 12 hours, the classic petechial to ecchymotic rash appears. This is caused by endotoxin release from the bacteria and indicates the onset of disseminated intravascular coagulopathy. In addition, signs of septic shock with alteration in vital signs, cyanosis, oliguria, and further depression of mental status may be seen.

As fulminating meningococcemia progresses the child goes into septic shock, with disseminated intravascular coagulopathy and bilateral adrenal hemorrhage. Immediate medical interventions are needed. The airway must be protected by intubation. Poor perfusion is treated with fluid bolus administration as well as inotropic support. Antibiotics are given as soon as possible; however, further deterioration may occur as antibiotic lysis releases an overwhelming amount of endotoxin, further compromising the client and possibly causing death. Family members as well as others who come into close contact with children who have meningococcemia must be treated prophylactically with rifampin (Wetzler, 2008).

minutes, a jaw thrust and oxygen administration will be the only interventions necessary. However, if status epilepticus is evident, benzodiazepine will be given as the first drug of choice; phenytoin may be needed as well if seizure activity remains uncontrolled. Generally speaking, seizures do not continue past the acute phase of the illness unless there is accompanying parenchymal damage.

CRITICAL THINKING

Signs and Symptoms of Meningitis

There are numerous signs and symptoms of meningitis that are neurological in nature: bulging fontanel, irritability, photophobia, nuchal rigidity, opisthotonic position, nausea, and vomiting. Discuss why these manifestations occur.

NURSING ALERT

Contraindications to a Lumbar Puncture

- Evidence of airway instability
- Risk of apnea or respiratory arrest during the procedure secondary to positioning
- Shock (either hypovolemic or septic)
- Evidence of coagulopathy
- Any possibility of increased intracranial pressure
- Immunocompromised state

Antibiotics should be ordered immediately and continued for a total of seven to ten days, depending on the bacteria and the child's clinical response. Dexamethasone may be administered as an adjunct with the first dose and may continue for the first four days of treatment to help decrease the inflammatory response to lysis of the bacterial cell walls (Prober, 2007). The antibiotics are usually given intravenously, the dosages are generally quite high, and peak and trough serum blood levels of the antibiotic are frequently obtained.

Complications must be quickly managed. Serum electrolytes and urine osmolarity should be checked daily during the acute phase to monitor trends toward SIADH. In addition, if septic joints appear, they should be treated vigorously with antibiotics. Subdural effusions or hydrocephalus should be treated in consultation with neurosurgery. Hearing loss or other sensory or motor deficits must be handled using a multidisciplinary approach.

Nursing Management Before entering the room, the nurse caring for the child with bacterial meningitis must don appropriate protective attire, which includes a gown, gloves, and mask. These items should be used for at least 24 hours after the antibiotics have been started. The nurse is also responsible for ensuring visitors adhere to these precautions. Furthermore, the family members or other individuals who have had recent close contact with the child should be encouraged to speak with their health care provider to assess their need for prophylactic antibiotics.

The nurse should check vital signs frequently. Tachycardia may be a sign associated with fever or septic shock. The child's blood pressure and capillary refill time should also be monitored, and the skin evaluated carefully for signs of petechiae or purpura. A neurological evaluation should be performed. Although it is common for this child to be fussy or irritable, level of consciousness should be assessed frequently as alteration in mental state may be caused by a myriad of potential complications associated with the disease such as subdural effusion, cerebral edema, or increased intracranial pressure. The infant's fontanel must be frequently palpated for bulging (common in meningitis) or depression (a result of dehydration), and head circumference measured daily as rapid enlargement may be secondary to development of hydrocephalus. The nurse should also observe for any seizure activity and notify the health care provider at once if it appears.

Antibiotics should be administered as prescribed. The nurse must try to maintain normothermia as elevated fever will increase metabolism and oxygen consumption. Either acetaminophen or ibuprofen can be administered to reduce fever, but if it persists, a hypothermia blanket may be utilized. In addition, the nurse should measure input and output along with urine specific gravity to watch for the signs associated with the SIADH.

Comfort measures include keeping the environment quiet and dark (the child may have photophobia) and allowing the child to assume a comfortable position. Pain should be managed using acetaminophen or a nonsteroidal anti-inflammatory preparation. Furthermore, the nurse caring for the child with meningitis should be on the alert for sequelae that may appear at any time. Changes in neurological status or urine output may become evident, and a warm, red, swollen joint may indicate the bacteria have spread, creating a septic arthritis.

The nurse should also address developmental and social needs. Family members should be encouraged to visit and bring toys or music from home to make the hospital a more familiar and less frightening environment. Once the child's condition is stable, the nurse should enlist the assistance of the youngster's primary caregivers in helping with bathing, feeding, and dressing. This activity not only makes the client feel more comfortable and secure, it also empowers the family members as they are providing care their child needs to become healthy again.

The child with meningitis may have deficits as a result of the infection such as cognitive changes or hearing impairment. Therefore, the nurse should enlist the assistance of the rehabilitation team within the hospital to begin working with the child and family and begin discharge planning with community resources if these complications occur.

Family Teaching The family should first be educated about the Hib vaccine to ensure this child and other children in the home are not at risk for *Haemophilus influenzae*, type B. A copy of the immunization protocol for children should be provided and referrals made to a clinic or health care provider for follow-up testing and treatment of any sequelae. If the child has sequelae, the caregivers will need to learn how to manage the problems at home. If the child has seizures or hydrocephalus, extensive teaching will be required. Learning or hearing difficulties will need special education, speech therapy, hearing aids, or classes in sign language or lip reading. The nurse may initiate treatment and education and arrange for community support.

Viral (Aseptic) Meningitis

Incidence and Etiology Aseptic or viral meningitis is an inflammatory response of the leptomeninges. Eighty-five percent of cases of viral meningitis are caused by the nonpolio enterovirus. Most cases occur in the summer or fall, and many are the result of inappropriately or partially treated bacterial disease (Prober, 2007; Roos & Tyler, 2008).

Pathophysiology Although many pathogens are not identified, adolescents are usually more at risk for viral meningitis than infants and toddlers. The pathogens include herpes, adenovirus, and arbovirus. Some cases may also be caused by mycoplasma, chlamydia, various protozoa, and fungi.

Clinical Manifestations The child with aseptic meningitis does not appear to be as ill as the child with bacterial infection. The onset may be gradual or abrupt, and the youngster irritable or lethargic. General malaise compounded by myalgia; headache; photophobia; anorexia, nausea, or vomiting; upper respiratory symptoms such as sore throat or chest pain; and a maculopapular rash may be seen. In addition, signs associated with meningeal irritation: nuchal rigidity, back pain, and positive Kernig's and Brudzinski's reflexes may occur. Fever is usually present, but rarely over 40°C (104°F). If seizures occur, they are associated with hyperthermia rather than the meningitis. Signs and symptoms subside within three to ten days (Prober, 2007; Roos & Tyler, 2008).

Diagnosis A septic work-up is needed, as meningitis must be confirmed as either bacterial or viral in nature. Analysis of cerebrospinal fluid will confirm the diagnosis: there will be less than 500 white blood cells per cubic millimeter; most will be leukocytes. Glucose will be greater than 40 milligrams per deciliter and protein decreased. Gram stain and culture will be negative. Initially, based on symptoms, it may be difficult to distinguish between bacterial and viral meningitis. Therefore, a second spinal tap should be performed within six to eight hours for reexamination of the fluid.

Treatment Until aseptic meningitis is verified, the child is treated as if the cause is bacterial, and antibiotics started. Once the diagnosis is determined to be viral, management usually becomes more palliative and supportive in nature.

Nursing Management The nurse caring for this child should concentrate on comfort measures. The room should be kept quiet with the lights dim, fluids given intravenously or orally, and medications administered to control fever, headache, and myalgias.

Family Teaching The nurse should help the caregivers prepare for managing their child at home as hospitalization will be brief, and provide the name of community resources for follow-up appointments and evaluations. Although viral meningitis is generally considered a benign disease where most children recover quickly and without incident, there may be sequelae. Many children complain

CASE STUDY / CARE PLAN

ADOLESCENT WITH BACTERIAL MENINGITIS

Henry, a 16-year-old of Japanese and European descent, was in apparent good health until one afternoon while shooting baskets at home with his friends. Henry, an easygoing young man who is excellent at making three-point shots, suddenly couldn't make a basket. He started complaining that the sun was shining in his eyes. As he tried to shield his eyes from the sun, Henry noticed that his neck was very stiff. Henry told his friends to go home and he went in to his bedroom, where he fell asleep. When Henry's mother came home from work, she was surprised to find the house so quiet and went to Henry's room to see if he were at home. She found him asleep and was about to leave his room when she noticed he appeared sweaty and flushed. Worried, she woke him, felt his forehead and found it very hot. Henry immediately complained that his neck was stiff and it was very painful to bend his neck. Henry was also very agitated, which was very unusual for him.

Henry's mother realized Henry was very ill and told him she was going to take him to the hospital. She was surprised that he didn't object, which frightened her even more. When they get to the emergency room, a lumbar puncture is performed, showing opaque, cloudy fluid. Analysis of the CSF reveals an elevated WBC, decreased glucose level, and increased protein level. The diagnosis of bacterial meningitis was made and Henry was admitted to the hospital.

NURSING CARE PLAN

ASSESSMENT

After admittance to an isolation room, Henry becomes disoriented. As the nurse is unable to understand what he is saying, Henry becomes agitated and thrashes around in his bed. He seems particularly upset by the self-protective gear the nurse is wearing. After the nurse talks quietly to Henry, he begins to calm down enough for an assessment. Henry's temperature is 104F. He has dry, cracked lips, and small petechiae on his trunk. He has a positive Kernig's sign. A broad-spectrum antibiotic is ordered.

NURSING DIAGNOSIS 1

Hyperthermia, as evidenced by abnormal temperature.

EXPECTED OUTCOME

NOC: Thermoregulation

NIC: Temperature Regulation

INTERVENTIONS/*RATIONALES*

1. Monitor vital signs every two hours. *Thermoregulation requires tracking of temperature changes. Dysrhythmias and blood pressure changes may indicate electrolyte imbalances or dehydration caused by hyperthermia.*
2. Provide oral care every four hours. *Hyperthermia and dehydration can cause dry mucous membranes, cracked lips, and oral discomfort. Oral care will promote oral health and patient comfort.*
3. Measure and compare intake and output every two hours. *Dehydration can occur secondarily to elevated temperature. Accurate I & O monitoring can indicate the presence of dehydration.*
4. Administer prescribed intravenous antibiotics. *Management of the underlying infection will promote thermoregulation and return to health.*

EVALUATION

Henry's temperature will return to normal.

NURSING DIAGNOSIS 2

Disturbed thought processes secondary to intracranial infection.

(Continues)

CASE STUDY / CARE PLAN (Continued)

EXPECTED OUTCOME

Henry will not be injured due to his agitation.

NOC: Cognitive Orientation

NIC: Environmental Management: Safety

INTERVENTIONS/*RATIONALES*

1. Keep bed in low position with side rails elevated. *The child who is agitated due to disturbed thought processes must be in a safe environment.*
2. Perform neurologic assessments every two to four hours. *The child who exhibits disturbed thought processes due to intracranial infection is at risk for deterioration of level of consciousness. Routine evaluation will reveal early indications of a deteriorating condition.*
3. Monitor for and report seizure activity. *The child with an intracranial infection is at risk for seizure activity. This must be monitored and reported ASAP.*

EVALUATION

Henry is not injured. Seizures do not occur.

NURSING DIAGNOSIS 3

Interrupted family processes related to hospitalization of an adolescent with life-threatening illness.

EXPECTED OUTCOME

Henry's family will participate in Henry's care during hospitalization.

NOC: Family Participation in Professional Care

NIC: Family Involvement Promotion; Teaching Disease Process

INTERVENTIONS/*RATIONALES*

1. Work with the family on understanding the diagnosis. *Educate parents on the disease processes, medications, treatments, and prognosis. As parents understand the disease process they can support their child through the illness and maintain their relationship.*
2. Promote normal family roles during hospitalization. *Allowing parents to continue their parental roles in the hospital setting will reduce stress and promote the continuation of family processes.*

EVALUATION

The family will feel reduced stress during Henry's hospitalization and will be prepared for his discharge.

NURSING DIAGNOSIS 4

Knowledge deficient related to disease treatment and hospital procedures.

EXPECTED OUTCOME

Henry will understand medications, treatments, and procedures he will undergo.

NOC: Knowledge: Illness Care; Knowledge: Treatment Procedures

NIC: Teaching: Disease Process; Teaching: Procedure/Treatment

INTERVENTIONS/*RATIONALES*

1. Facilitate Henry's understanding of meningitis by explaining its cause and disease course. *Educate Henry about meningitis, infectious diseases, medications, and treatments. Explain the purpose and need for self-protective gear and the isolation room.*
2. Encourage cooperation for treatments and procedures. *Explain procedures prior to their initiation to assist Henry the child in understanding their needs. Increased understanding will promote cooperation.*

EVALUATION

Henry will be able to demonstrate a basic understanding of meningitis. He will cooperate with procedures and treatments.

of fatigue, weakness, irritability, uncoordination, or muscle pain or spasms for several weeks postinfection. In addition, they are at risk for hearing loss, altered language development, or other learning deficits. Caregivers should be taught comfort measures and fever control as well as signs of any complications that need immediate medical attention such as change in mental status or development of seizures.

REYE'S SYNDROME

Reye's syndrome, first described in 1963, is an acute life-threatening nonicteric hepatic encephalopathy with accompanying microvascular fatty deposits in the liver and kidney (Johnston, 2007b; NINDS, n.d.h.; Ropper & Brown, 2005).

INCIDENCE AND ETIOLOGY

The incidence of Reye's syndrome in the United States has been steadily falling since its peak in 1980. The disease primarily affects children between the ages of 2 and 16 years with European Americans under 5 years of age who live in urban and suburban areas the most vulnerable.

The etiology of Reye's is unclear although there is consensus that it follows a mild viral illness such as varicella, influenza B, influenza A, Epstein-Barr, adenovirus, or coxsackievirus. Links between aspirin use with the original illness and Reye's have been suspected for some time, even though no definitive data have ever been produced to either confirm or deny this hypothesis. However, since caregivers have been advised to use acetaminophen rather than salicylates (aspirin) for their children, incidence rates of Reye's syndrome have declined (NINDS, n.d.; Ropper & Brown, 2005).

Even though mortality from Reye's has dropped dramatically in the last few years, many children do suffer from residual effects such as attention disorders, speech and language delays, fine or gross motor impairments, diminished visual acuity or coordination, and intellectual deficits.

PATHOPHYSIOLOGY

The liver becomes enlarged and assumes a yellow hue caused by fatty deposits in its microvasculature, which precipitate depletion of glucose stores, reduction in enzymes to convert ammonia to urea, and abnormalities in liver enzymes. At the same time cerebral edema with accompanying increased intracranial pressure becomes evident (Johnston, 2007b; Ropper & Brown, 2005).

CLINICAL MANIFESTATIONS

Initially, the child has symptoms of a mild viral infection, and signs of recovery may be noted; however, within 24 to 48 hours, the child's condition worsens. Vomiting with or without fever may be present, and when vomiting diminishes, there will be a marked change in the child's behavior, with confusion, fear, irritability, anxiety, or a flat affect apparent. Speech patterns may change and the level of consciousness deteriorates into a coma-like state, interrupted by periods of screaming, ranting, and raving. One or both pupils will be dilated and either exquisitely sensitive to light, or the child may lose vision entirely. Within 24 hours, the child slips into a deeper coma and demonstrates either decorticate or decerebrate posturing. Cranial nerve reflexes may be lost. Death from Reye's usually occurs within two to three days of onset, although the downward progression of the illness may stop abruptly at any time.

DIAGNOSIS

A complete blood count; chemistries; blood urea nitrogen; amylase; liver function tests; clotting times; and urine analysis should be done. Arterial blood should also be sampled to evaluate pH as well as for signs of acidosis, alkalosis, and respiratory sufficiency. Cerebrospinal fluid should be examined if there are no signs of inflammation; if there are less than eight leukocytes per cubic millimeter with normal glucose and protein concentrations, Reye's is the diagnosis. The lumbar puncture, however, may not be a safe procedure to perform during the acute phase of the illness as the increased intracranial pressure associated with cerebral edema may precipitate brain herniation. CT may be done to confirm the presence of cerebral edema. A liver biopsy will also be done as it is the only test to confirm Reye's (Johnston, 2007b; Ropper & Brown, 2005).

TREATMENT

Because children are acutely ill and at risk for rapid deterioration, they should be placed in an intensive care unit and intubated. Neuromuscular blocking agents, sedatives, and analgesics are administered to protect the airway, provide for adequate ventilation, correct any respiratory acidosis or alkalosis, and decrease intracranial pressure. As blood gases and other serum assessments are frequently measured, an arterial catheter is inserted. Electrolytes and glucose levels should be monitored often with replacements administered intravenously as needed. If clotting times are abnormal, vitamin K or fresh frozen plasma may be given. To reduce elevated ammonia levels, neomycin may be provided through a nasogastric tube. Once prothrombin levels are normal, neurosurgeons may place an intraventricular catheter to monitor intracranial pressure. If pressures remain elevated despite ventilatory interventions, mannitol, a hyperosmotic diuretic, may be administered to decrease the edema. Although fluid restriction is no longer recommended, strict measurement of intake and output is warranted; therefore, an indwelling urinary catheter should be placed. Seizures should be controlled with benzodiazepines and phenytoin.

NURSING MANAGEMENT

The child requires intensive care by the nurse, including frequent monitoring of vital signs, respiratory effort, neurological status, and laboratory values. The nurse also needs to observe for responses to the interventions performed and

FAMILY TEACHING

Salicylates and viral illness

Families should be educated about avoiding the use of salicylates in children with viral illnesses, given a list of over-the-counter medicines to avoid (see Nursing Alert Box), and shown where to find ingredients on all over-the-counter preparations, thereby avoiding any exposure.

NURSING ALERT

Over-the-Counter Medications Containing Aspirin

- Alka-Seltzer
- Anacin
- Anacin Maximum Strength
- Aspergum
- Bufferin
- Bufferin Extra-Strength
- Coricidin
- Coricidin Demilets
- Dristan Tablets
- Excedrin
- 4-Way Cold Tablets
- Medilets
- Pepto Bismol
- Triaminicin

medications administered. Once the child is past the acute phase, emotional support, appropriate play activities, and interactions with others should be provided.

Family Teaching

The family needs to be prepared for the sequelae associated with Reye's, and the nurse should work with them and community resources to ensure special needs are met upon discharge. In addition, the importance of childhood vaccines should be stressed.

ENCEPHALITIS

Encephalitis is an inflammation of the brain that can be diffuse or localized.

Incidence and Etiology

Encephalitis can be caused by bacteria, viruses, fungi, or protozoa, although most are caused by viruses. Table 32-7 lists the causes of encephalitis. The most common cause beyond the neonatal period is herpes type I, *herpes simplex*. The arboviruses, caused by arthropod bites to humans, are usually endemic to specific regional areas. Some children will develop encephalitis following vaccines for tetanus, measles, rubella, diphtheria, or pertussis; however, these cases are rare. More commonly, though, cases of encephalitis occur in immunosuppressed children, especially those with AIDS (Prober, 2007; Roos & Tyler, 2008).

Pathophysiology

Primary encephalitis is a result of the invasion of the pathogen into the central nervous system resulting in cerebral or cerebellar dysfunction. Postinfectious or parainfectious encephalitis occurs with other illnesses or following the administration of a vaccine or other substance. During the initial or nonneural stage, the child suffers from an acute febrile illness secondary to ingestion or vector bite. The neuronal phase occurs when the infection is seeded from the point of origin to the central nervous system.

Clinical Manifestations

The manifestations depend on the invading organism as well as the location of the infection within the brain. The disease has an acute onset with a strong neurological component. At first, the child may have an intense headache, signs of respiratory infection, nausea, or vomiting. Meningeal irritation (nuchal rigidity, photophobia, positive Kernig's and Brudzinski's signs), disorientation, confusion, personality and behavior changes, hemiplegia, ataxia, weakness, or slurred speech may also be seen. Alterations in cranial nerve and other reflex responses may be present as well as generalized or focal seizure activity with intermittent periods of screaming, hallucinating, or moving in bizarre fashions. Lastly, the child's level of consciousness may deteriorate from stupor to coma (NINDS, n.d.h.; Roos & Tyler, 2008).

Generally speaking, the younger the patient, the more devastating the sequelae. Although some children will recover completely, many have motor, intellectual, visual, and auditory deficits. The cardiovascular system, liver, and lungs may also be adversely affected by the pathogen.

Diagnosis

Diagnosis of encephalitis occurs when other pathologies such as mass lesions, metabolic disturbances, and other infectious processes have been ruled out. To confirm encephalitis, several procedures must be performed, including a complete history and physical examination. Laboratory analysis of blood, cerebrospinal fluid, and urine should be obtained. Initially, the CSF values may be within normal limits, but within 2 days, there is an increase in the number of leukocytes (most often monocytes). There also may be an elevation in protein. Stool and nasopharyngeal swabs should be taken to check for the presence of enteroviruses. Serologic assays can be done to detect Epstein-Barr virus. Brain biopsy is the only way to confirm *herpes simplex*. Noninvasive

Table 32-7 Causes of Encephalitis

Viruses	Enteroviruses: Poliovirus, echovirus, coxsackievirus
	Adenoviruses or herpesviruses: Herpes type I, herpes type II, varicella, herpes zoster, Epstein-Barr, cytomegalovirus
	Arboviruses: California virus, Western Equine, St. Louis, Colorado tick, West Nile, LaCrosse
	Measles
	Mumps
	Rubella
	Rabies
	Hepatitis B
Bacteria	*Haemophilus influenzas*
	Neisseria meningitidis
	Streptococcus pneumonias
	Cat scratch fever
Other	*Chlamydia pneumoniae*
	Rickettsial infections
	Rocky Mountain spotted fever
	Lyme disease
	Fungi
	Protozoa
	Drugs: Trimethoprim

measures (CT, MRI) can be utilized to assess for cerebral edema, ventricular compression, or temporal lobe necrosis associated with herpes simplex. Electroencephalography may show slight diffuse slowing.

Treatment

Supportive care is needed and antibiotics are administered to all children until bacterial infection is ruled out. Youngsters with viral infections should be given antiviral agents (NINDS, n.d.c.). There is an increased risk for seizures, respiratory failure, and increased intracranial pressure; therefore, during the acute phase of illness, close monitoring in intensive care units is important as the children may need to be intubated, mechanically ventilated, oxygenated, and treated for cerebral edema. Nutrition is supported either through intravenous supplementation or gastric tube placement. Meticulous skin care must occur if the child is in a coma (Prober, 2007; Roos & Tyler, 2008).

Nursing Management

Continual assessment of vital signs and paying special attention to the airway and respiratory function is critical. A complete neurological assessment should include pupil checks and Glasgow Coma Score evaluations to note possible increases in intracranial pressure. Being aware of seizure activity, and completing passive range of motion exercises, maintaining good skin integrity, and providing for adequate nutrition are other areas of nursing intervention. Caregivers should be involved in the child's care as appropriate.

Family Teaching

The family should always receive education about the causes of encephalitis, as well as procedures the child will undergo and any treatment needed. If the child has sequelae, caregivers will need to learn how to manage the problems at home. Sequelae involving any learning or hearing difficulties will require special education, speech therapy, hearing aids, or classes in sign language or lip reading. Caregivers will also need to become aware of governmental and private community agencies that can be helpful if their child has any residual problem.

■ NEUROLOGICAL INJURIES

Injuries discussed in this section include head trauma, spinal cord injury, and submersion (drowning).

HEAD TRAUMA

Head trauma or injury, defined as any pathologic process occurring to the scalp, skull, or brain parenchyma resulting from mechanical force, is a major cause of pediatric mortality. Head injuries can be either open or closed. Disabilities that result from a traumatic brain injury (TBI) depend on the location and severity of the injury as well as the age and health of the child-adolescent (NINDS, n.d.g.).

Incidence and Etiology

Brain injury is the leading cause of death for those under age 35. Half of all deaths due to head injuries occur in children under 15 years of age (Blosser & Burns, 2004). TBI is the leading cause of death in children, and severe TBI, present in 5–8% of children treated in hospitals, will produce a residual neurological deficit in 50% of those children (Ewing-Cobbs, Barnes & Fletcher, 2003). Of the nearly 5 million children sustaining a head injury every year, around 200,000 are hospitalized. More frequent in males than females, the causes may be varied: falls, bicycling, abuse, competitive sports, or motor vehicle accidents (Ewing-Cobbs et al., 2003). Traumatic brain injury is the largest source of intellectual impairment, seizures, and physical disability in children. The outcome of a TBI varies with the injury severity and can include death, persistent vegetative state, or various cognitive and physical sequelae. Injury severity frequently is based on the Glasgow Coma Scale, which evaluates motor response, verbal response, and eye opening (Ewing-Cobbs et al., 2003).

Children are prone to head injury because of their physical immaturity (refer back to Table 32-2), as well as their high activity level, immature developmental skills, and increased head to body mass ratio. In addition, developmentally they are at great risk for trauma, as infants, toddlers, and preschoolers are not aware of the dangers in their environments and cannot take precautions to avoid them. Once faced with a dilemma, young children do not have the experience or cognitive ability to quickly problem solve.

Age determines the type of head trauma seen in children. Infants who are not carefully attended often fall from high surfaces such as dressing tables, bed, sofas, and stairways. However, child abuse is the most prevalent cause of head injury in this age group. Shaken baby syndrome occurs when the infant is shaken violently or hit against a hard surface such as a wall or mattress. Refer to Chapter 36 for more information about shaken baby syndrome.

Toddlers and school-age children are often injured in motor vehicle crashes (MVCs) either as passengers, pedestrians, bike-riders, or skateboarders. The adolescent, however, is typically involved in a vehicle crash as either a passenger or driver, or injured during sports activities. Furthermore, in our violent society, more and more teens fall victim to penetrating trauma from firearms or sharp weapons. Skull fractures, which are often accompanied by underlying hematomas and brain injury, are common. Furthermore, the secondary effects of trauma, including cerebral edema, increased intracranial pressure or cerebral hypertension, and malignant brain edema (hyperemia) may occur.

Pathophysiology

Head injuries are categorized as either primary or secondary in nature (Mami & Nance, 2008). Primary injury, which occurs at the moment of impact, is when initial cellular damage occurs. The mechanism of injury (Figure 32-16), or

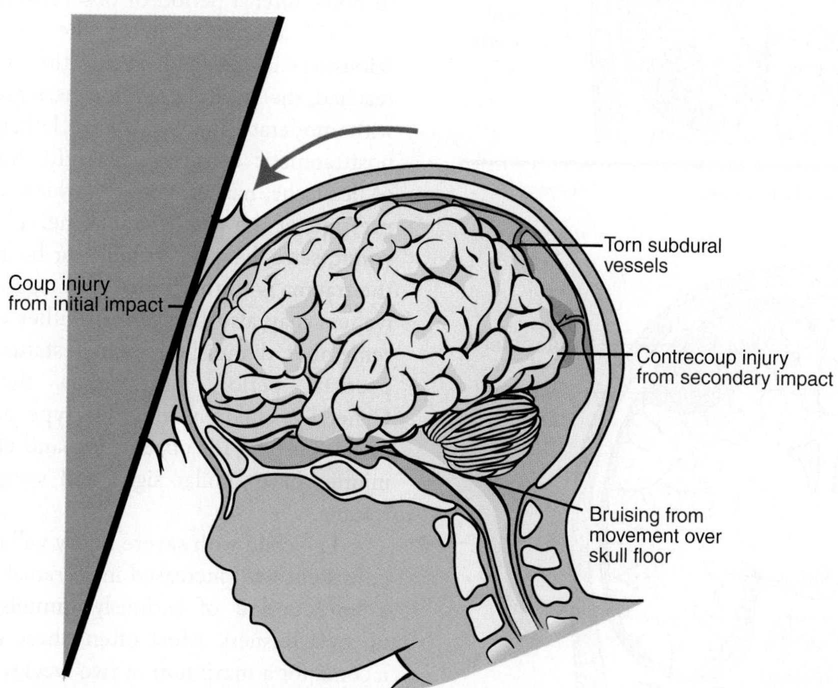

Figure 32-16 Coup-Contrecoup Injury. DELMAR CENGAGE LEARNING.

external force to the head or neck, may be a result of a direct blow to the head (such as being hit with a baseball bat) producing a coup injury. However, acceleration or deceleration movement of the brain within the skull causes a coup-contrecoup injury in which there are two points of trauma within the cranial vault (such as hitting the head on the windshield of a car when hit from behind). One is at the initial or coup site while the other is a result of the moving brain hitting the opposite side of the cranium. There may be shearing of the small veins and arteries that travel from the cerebral surface to the dural sinuses as well as diffuse axial injury. Regardless of the mechanism, at the time of impact, there is an increase both in arterial and intracranial pressures, bradycardia, hypertension, and alteration in level of consciousness. Table 32-8 presents information relative to the various forms of head trauma related to the specific type of injury received. Figures 32-17 and 32-18 provide illustrations of epidural and subdural hematomas which can occur due to head trauma.

Secondary injury involves both the brain and the body's response to the trauma, and is evident immediately after impact or several minutes, hours, days, weeks, or months later. Usually it is a result of brain tissue destruction secondary to hypoxia, hemorrhage, space-occupying lesions, hypotension, edema, or change in the blood-brain barrier. Whatever the cause, however, the end result is increased intracranial pressure, which if left unresolved will lead to irreversible brain damage and death.

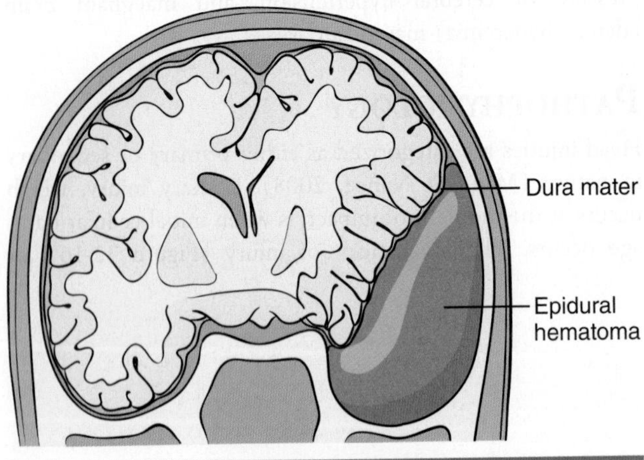

FIGURE 32-17 Epidural Hematoma. DELMAR CENGAGE LEARNING.

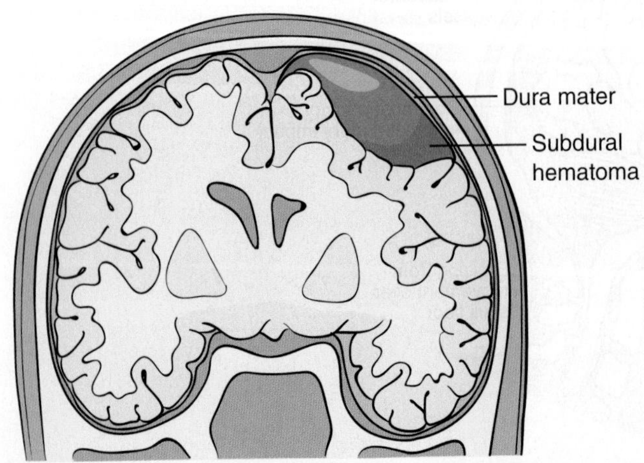

FIGURE 32-18 Subdural Hematoma. DELMAR CENGAGE LEARNING.

Two forms of secondary injury (cerebral edema and malignant brain edema) are particularly devastating to children. **Cerebral edema**, an increase in intracellular fluid in the brain resulting from anoxia, vasodilation, vessel damage, or vascular stasis, may not be seen for the first day or two post-injury (Frankel, 2007). Cerebral edema leads to an increased extravascular volume which in turn precipitates a rise in intracranial pressure. As autoregulation becomes impaired, edema continues to build and pressure rises further, causing compression of the ventricles, small cisterns, and a midline shift.

Malignant brain edema or cerebral hyperemia is unique to children. Rather than an edematous response to trauma, there is a hyperemic or vascular reaction because of the disruption in the blood-brain barrier. In addition, the mechanism to control cerebrospinal fluid absorption is impaired.

CLINICAL MANIFESTATIONS

Children with head injuries display a variety of symptoms depending on the specific pathology as well as its severity. The child with a mild injury or concussion may have no loss of consciousness or a very short episode (less than two minutes), and may or may not have amnesia of the event. In addition, headaches, nausea, or vomiting may occur. Behavior initially is within normal limits, and the child is discharged from the emergency room or urgent care center to home after a period of observation.

With a moderate injury, the child will have loss of consciousness in the field; by the time the emergency room is reached, the level of consciousness may improve. The infant with moderate injury may be lethargic, vomit, or have a posttraumatic seizure. The child, however, may complain of headache, nausea, vertigo (which may be caused by compression of the eighth cranial nerve), and fatigue, and may vomit, seize, become irritable, or be amnesic of the event. If the trauma is to the frontal area, aggressiveness and combativeness may also be seen. In either case, it is important to remember diminished mental status may be caused by a postictal period rather than the head injury itself. Generally, children with this type of trauma are admitted to the hospital for observation and close evaluation as their injuries have similar signs and symptoms of more severe trauma.

The child with severe injury will demonstrate symptoms consistent with increased intracranial pressure, and will have a long period of seriously diminished mental status or unconsciousness. Most often, these children will remain in a coma for a maximum of two weeks; beyond that time, they will either begin to show subtle signs of improvement or deteriorate further and be declared brain dead.

TABLE 32-8 Forms of Head Trauma, Pathology, Manifestation, Treatment, and Nursing Issues

INJURY	PATHOLOGY	CLINICAL MANIFESTATIONS	TREATMENT	NURSING ISSUES
Scalp injury	• Laceration to scalp which can be very vascular	• Copious bleeding at site • Hypovolemia if large vessel or small infant	• Irrigation with normal saline • Sutures	• Provide comfort to child
Concussive injuries *Concussion*	• Usually secondary to blunt injury • Caused by the stretching, compression, or tearing of nerve fibers near the brain stem without accompanying gross structural damage	• Transient alteration in mental status with loss of awareness or responsiveness • Soft neurological signs such as headache, nausea with or without vomiting, vertigo or dizziness, amnesia	• Palliative	• Observe closely for several hours as clinical manifestations seen mimic those of more serious injury
Pediatric concussive syndrome	• Results from insult to brain stem • Occurs most often in children under 3 years of age	• At time of injury, appears stunned • Later on, clammy, pale, lethargic, frequent episodes of vomiting	• IV hydration	• Observe closely for signs of more serious injury
Skull fractures *Linear*	• Account for 75% of cranial trauma • Results from impact to large area of the skull • Most benign unless middle meningeal artery is nicked, then epidural hematoma is formed	• No focal signs • Headache and tenderness at site	• Palliative	• Watch for signs of complications: • Subgaleal hematoma, a soft boggy mass at the site, which may be seen two to three days postinjury • Growing fracture in which the dura is trapped in the healing fracture line forming a lepto-meningeal cyst
Depressed	• Rare in children under 3 years as skull bones are soft; instead an indentation forms in the cranium at the point of impact causing a "ping-pong" appearance • Break in the integrity of the skull, shattering it into fragments that may be depressed into the brain tissue with a hematoma forming on top	• Pain and tenderness at the site • Visible or palpated depression of the skull • Seizures	• Surgical elevation of any bony fragment depressed more than the thickness of the skull or 5 millimeters • Antibiotics and tetanus prophylaxis	

(Continues)

TABLE 32-8 Forms of Head Trauma, Pathology, Manifestation, Treatment, and Nursing Issues (*Continued*)

INJURY	PATHOLOGY	CLINICAL MANIFESTATIONS	TREATMENT	NURSING ISSUES
Compound	• Combination of a scalp laceration and depressed skull fracture	• Same as above	• Same as above	• Same as above
Basilar	• Occurs in the inferior, posterior portion of the skull and involves the frontal, ethmoid, sphenoid, temporal, or occipital bones with or without dural tear	• CSF leakage from the nose or ears • Periorbital ecchymosis and Battle's sign or mastoid bruising	• Palliative • Dural repair for persistent CSF leak	• Check for presence of CSF in draining fluid • Test fluid present for glucose • Assure an NG tube is *never* placed as it may migrate through the fracture site into the cranial vault and into the brain itself • Watch for signs of cranial nerve injury, a common sequela, involving nerves I, II, III, VII, or VIII
Diastatic	• Separation of the sutures of the skull secondary to trauma • Most common site: lambdoid • Occur most often in children under 4 years of age	• Pain at the site	• Palliative	
Diffuse brain injury	• Results from tearing of the anterior bridging veins, petechial hemorrhage of white matter, shearing of myelin and axons, or contusion of the corpus callosum • May be secondary to increased ICP or subarachnoid hemorrhage • In infants, secondary to abuse; in older children, associated with other trauma such as cerebral contusion or laceration, cerebral edema, cortical trauma, or scattered intracranial hemorrhage	• No external signs of injury • Deep coma with decorticate posturing or flaccid areflexia • Fixed and dilated pupils • May be periods of apnea and bradycardia	• Dependent on concurrent trauma • Airway and ventilatory support as indicated	• Watch for change in neurological status • Observe for alterations in respiratory or cardiovascular systems

TABLE 32-8 Forms of Head Trauma, Pathology, Manifestation, Treatment, and Nursing Issues (*Continued*)

INJURY	PATHOLOGY	CLINICAL MANIFESTATIONS	TREATMENT	NURSING ISSUES
Cerebral contusion or laceration	• Bruising or pulping of brain tissue along with tears to vessels and petechial hemorrhage • Parenchymal and vessel injury causes brain necrosis and infarction	• Focal signs based on the area of the brain injured • Level of consciousness can range from confusion to deep and prolonged diminished mental state • Signs of increased ICP	• Rarely surgical • Management of any rise in ICP • Palliative	• Observe for change in neurological status
Intracranial hematomas and hemorrhages *Epidural*	• Rare in children, but may occur with linear skull fractures • Temporal and parietal areas most common site • After trauma, blood accumulates between the dura and skull (epidural hematoma, see Figure 32-17) forcing tissue downward and inward, as hematoma forms and expands, displacing brain parenchyma under tentorium, and precipitating herniation through foramen magnum • Pressure placed on cranial nerves and vessels • May be either arterial (rapid onset of symptoms) or venous in nature	• Diminished level of consciousness • Cushing's triad with wide pulse pressure, increased systolic blood pressure and bradycardia • Increased ICP • Respiratory depression • Fixed and dilated pupil with contralateral extremity spasticity or flaccidity • Paresis of cranial nerves III and VI • Papilledema	• Management of increased ICP • Surgical evacuation of hematoma	• Be aware pediatric presentation is different from adult: • Adults: period of unconsciousness caused by primary injury, then lucid period as concussive effects diminish, then degeneration of consciousness caused by expanding hematoma • Children: one-third present like adults, one-third have no initial loss of consciousness, one-third have immediate loss of consciousness not followed by lucid period
Subdural	• Occur most frequently under 6 months of age as a result of shaken baby syndrome • Results from damage to bridging veins, and spreads over both hemispheres (subdural hematoma, see Figure 32-18) until it reaches the tentorium and solidifies into a hematoma placing widespread pressure on the brain	• Altered mental status ranging from confusion and agitation to lethargy to stupor • Increased ICP • Retinal hemorrhage • Papilledema • General: vomiting, fever, seizures, irritability • Infant also: full fontanelle, increase in head circumference	• Surgical evacuation of hematoma if large and causing neurological or systemic compromise • Subdural taps in infant in which CSF is removed through a catheter placed into the ventricles	• Watch for change in neurological status • Help family accept child's changed state as many have neurological sequelae such as seizures and developmental regression

(Continues)

TABLE 32-8 Forms of Head Trauma, Pathology, Manifestation, Treatment, and Nursing Issues *(Continued)*

INJURY	PATHOLOGY	CLINICAL MANIFESTATIONS	TREATMENT	NURSING ISSUES
	• May occur with and without skull fracture • May be acute with signs and symptoms appearing within 72 hours postinjury or chronic in which manifestations are not seen for weeks or months	• Older child: headache with nausea, unsteady gait		
Subarachnoid	• Associated with severe head trauma and often accompany other intracranial injuries	• Those associated with concurrent injury • Signs of meningeal irritation from bloody CSF such as nuchal rigidity, diplopia, photophobia, and headache	• Manage concurrent trauma • Manage increased ICP • Palliative for meningeal irritation	• Observe for signs of severe concurrent injury • Comfort measures
Intracerebral	• Deep contusion or laceration of brain tissue most often as a result of penetrating injury • Result in diffuse bleeding within the parenchyma and formation of hematoma associated with the many small hemorrhages	• Focal signs dependent upon area of the brain injured • Increased ICP	• Manage increased ICP • Usually surgery not indicated because of diffuse nature of injury	• Monitor neurological status
Penetrating injury *Impalement*	• Foreign body traumatically entering the skull and brain	• Hemorrhage at site • Focal signs dependent upon area injured	• Removal of object in the operating room • Antibiotics and tetanus prophylaxis	• *Never* remove object, but stabilize until child gets to the operating room
Gunshot wounds	• Low velocity bullets enter the skull and ricochet within it causing multiple tracks of destruction of parenchyma and vessels • High-velocity bullets create immediate shattering of bone, tissue, and vessels	• Immediate loss of consciousness • Hemorrhage • Focal signs dependent upon area injured	• Surgical debridement of the track as well as removal of bony and bullet fragments	• Prepare family as children who survive often have seizures and multiple focal deficits

The child's vital signs will reflect the seriousness of the injury. Changes in respiratory effort or periods of apnea can occur because of hypovolemic shock, injury to the spinal cord above C-4, metabolic disturbances, or damage to or pressure on the medulla. In addition, the increased intracranial pressure will produce a pattern where respiratory rate is increased, decreased, again increased, and then becomes Cheyne-Stokes in nature. Heart rate is an index of brain stem function. Bradycardia is frequently associated with increased intracranial pressure. However, tachycardia (sign of blood or fluid loss, hypovolemic shock, hypoxia, anxiety, or pain) following bradycardia is a grave, preterminal sign in the head-injured child. Blood pressure also reflects the seriousness of injury. Hypotension is rare with isolated injury except as a terminal event; therefore, the child with low pressure should be evaluated for concurrent trauma and shock. Increased systolic pressure with a wide pulse pressure are classic signs of increased intracranial pressure. Hypertension alone may indicate pain, anxiety, or a preexisting condition.

Pathologic neurological changes may also be seen in the severely injured child, with signs of either extreme irritability or restlessness. Both can be attributed to increased intracranial pressure, an enlarging intracranial mass, cerebral edema, malignant brain edema, or hypoxia. Reflexes may become either hyporesponsive, hyperresponsive, or nonexistent and motor responses may deteriorate. In addition, the child might assume either a decorticate, decerebrate, or flaccid posture. Pupils may be sluggish in reacting to light or unequal in size. The child with one dilated pupil and contralateral spasticity or flaccidity displays the classic signs of intensely high intracranial pressure and is at risk for brain herniation if measures to mediate the pressure are not initiated immediately (Ewing-Cobbs et al., 2003; Frankel, 2007).

Diagnosis

Identification of the type and severity of head injury involves obtaining a history of the trauma, past medical history, observation, assessment, and evaluation. The first issue is to ascertain exactly what happened, the victim's initial response to the trauma, and how the status has changed. A thorough medical history must also be obtained to learn if the child has any congenital or acquired conditions that might have an impact on the head trauma or the response to it, such as previous head trauma, seizures, hydrocephalus, cranial surgery, or hemophilia. Furthermore, the child's baseline abilities and behavior should be ascertained, as intellectual or motor deficiencies, attention deficit disorder, or autistic or pervasive developmental disorder traits. Also, information should be obtained from caregivers relative to the child's reactions to stressful situations, especially with strangers, as what might be called abusive or combative behavior in one child might be considered normal in another.

Neurological evaluation, rather than a single assessment, is a continual series of observations and examinations that indicate the child's clinical improvement or deterioration. Generally speaking, maximum depression should occur just after the incident with some improvement beginning to show shortly thereafter. If this does not occur, serious brain injury may be diagnosed.

Two common tools for evaluation of neurological status are the Glasgow Coma Scale and AVPU. Refer back to Box 32-2 and Table 32-3. For them to be meaningful, however, they must be used frequently with results compared so trends in improvement or deterioration can be noted. Generally speaking, Glasgow scores can be used to help in the classification of head injury (Box 32-6).

Cranial nerves should also be assessed. The conscious child is asked to perform a variety of activities such as opening and closing the eyes, moving the mouth, and sticking out the tongue to evaluate nerves. In the unconscious child, however, other methods must be employed. Refer back to Table 32-4 for methods of assessing the cranial nerves in an unconscious child.

Pupils must also be assessed frequently. A unilateral fixed and dilated pupil implies pressure on the third cranial nerve, usually resulting from increased intracranial pressure, one of the classic signs of impending herniation. The eyes should also be carefully evaluated. It is crucial retinal hemorrhage be identified as it is frequently associated with subdural hematoma, an injury most often secondary to abuse. In addition, papilla edema, a late sign of increased intracranial pressure, may be present.

Examination of the head is critical. The face and scalp should be inspected for hematomas, abrasions, or lacerations. If the latter are present, the wound should be checked for debris as well as a dural tear or bony fragments. The cranium should be palpated for depressions or signs of crepitus. In addition, the ears and nose should be evaluated for blood or cerebrospinal fluid leakage.

Radiologic examinations are performed to determine specific pathologies. Most often, the first X-ray is the lateral cervical spine. Most victims of head injury are multiple-injured; therefore, this assessment must be done to rule out spinal trauma. Other plain films may be done to confirm simple skull fractures. The most widely used tool in the diagnosis of head injury is computerized axial tomography (CT), which is performed on all infants and children with altered level of consciousness, suspected basilar or depressed skull fracture, penetrating injury, or neurological or focal

BOX 32-6

CLASSIFICATION OF HEAD INJURY BASED ON GLASGOW COMA SCALE

Total Glasgow Score from 13 to 15 or motor score of 6: mild head injury

Total Glasgow Score from 9 to 12 or motor score from 4 to 5: moderate head injury

Total Glasgow Score less than 7 or motor score of 1, 2, or 3: severe head injury

deficits. Structural injuries such as hematomas, hemorrhages, contusions, or fractures can usually be visualized clearly. There may be times, however, when a CT appears normal despite a severely depressed sensorium. If the child shows signs of improvement after a short period of time, the injury may have been concussive in nature; however, if there is no change in client status or if deterioration begins, another series of films should be obtained to determine if venous hemorrhage has occurred. Magnetic resonance imaging (MRI) is an excellent adjunct to CT as subtle injury can be clearly detected. It is nearly impossible for this equipment to be used with the unstable child, however, as the process is slow, sometimes lasting 45 minutes.

Laboratory tests for the child with head injury involve complete blood count, chemistries, urine assays, and clotting times. If the child is intubated or hyperventilated, arterial blood gases will need to be checked frequently to ensure PaO_2 is kept at 100 while $PaCO_2$ is between 30 and 32. An electroencephalogram may be performed if the child seizes to determine the area of the brain involved and the type of convulsion occurring.

TREATMENT

The primary goals of care are to maintain ventilation, oxygenation, and perfusion while achieving an intracranial pressure that is safe; and prevent secondary injuries. To provide this, severely injured children should be in pediatric intensive care units with both invasive and noninvasive monitoring of their vital signs and pressures. About half of clients with severe head injuries will need surgery to repair or remove hematomas or contusions (NINDS, n.d.g.).

The child with a diminished level of consciousness or Glasgow Coma Score less than eight must be intubated, and arterial blood gases and pulse oximetry frequently monitored. To help control intracranial pressure, most intubated, head-injured children are sedated and chemically paralyzed, and oxygen and carbon dioxide levels frequently monitored. ICP can be reduced by producing mild hypocarbia (Frankel, 2007). The child who is not intubated must also be observed carefully for changes in respiratory status (apnea, Cheyne-Stokes), which might indicate neurological deterioration and the need to receive manual ventilation.

Perfusion must be maintained to ensure adequate cerebral perfusion pressure, and signs of hypovolemia aggressively treated with crystalloids. Response to fluid administration can be assessed by evaluating heart rate, blood pressure, capillary refill time, and the level of consciousness. Urine output can be measured by an indwelling catheter. If perfusion is not adequate despite aggressive fluid resuscitation or if signs of cerebral edema appear, inotropes such as dopamine or dobutamine will need to be administered. Until adequate cerebral perfusion pressure is ensured, the bed should be kept flat to promote blood flow to the head.

Increased intracranial pressure must be treated. Only during the initial phase is hyperventilation performed.

> **BOX 32-7**
> **MEASURING BRAIN OXYGENATION**
>
> The Licox tisssue probe is a reliable and sensitive diagnostic method to measure oxygen levels of the brain following head trauma. The risks of placing the intraparenchymal sensor are minimal. (Integra, n.d.)

Mannitol, a potent diuretic, may also be administered to shrink brain volume. It should be given slowly while watching for signs of tachycardia and low blood pressure. In some children, there may be a rebound effect with mannitol as it may increase cerebral blood flow. If that occurs, the signs of increased intracranial pressure will reappear with more intensity than originally noted, and the neurosurgery department must be called at once so other modalities to control the pressure can be initiated. Neurological status is difficult, if not impossible, to assess during this time. Therefore, intracranial monitoring will be needed. Steroids do not have a place in the acute management of head trauma.

Managing the environment may help keep intracranial pressure under control. The room should be kept quiet and minimal invasive procedures performed. If suctioning needs to be done, administering endotracheal lidocaine may help block the gag and cough reflexes, which intensify intracranial pressure. In addition, once cerebral perfusion pressure is adequate, the head of the bed should be elevated about 30 degrees. The child's head should be kept in the midline to promote venous drainage and the hips and knees should not be hyperflexed. Pain should initially be managed with acetaminophen, and if this is not effective, narcotics should be given and neurological assessments made with invasive ICP monitoring equipment. The room temperature should be kept comfortable; if the room is too hot, cerebral metabolism will increase; if the room is too cold, the child will shiver, and again raise cerebral metabolism.

Intracranial monitoring catheters may be placed in the epidural or subdural spaces; however, the standard at this

> **KIDS WANT TO KNOW**
>
> **When can I go back to school?**
>
> Ten-year-old Barbara was hit by a car and suffers from right-sided hemiplegia. There are no other neurological problems. She wonders when she can return to school.
>
> Explain that she needs to finish up inpatient rehab, but will return to school. In the meantime, encourage visits from schoolmates while Barbara is in the rehab unit. Reassure her that if she needs any special help while at school, it will be provided.

time is the intraventricular probe. This equipment has several advantages: it measures intracranial pressure and it also allows for withdrawal of fluid. In children, removing just 30 milliliters of cerebrospinal fluid may create enough room inside the skull to mediate the high pressure inside. There will be times when increased intracranial pressure will need to be managed surgically. Burr holes or craniotomies may be needed to remove hematomas, bony fragments, or foreign bodies. Some studies have even indicated that a bony window be removed from the skull to allow more space for brain expansion and when the pressure is down, the flap replaced.

Complications of head trauma are listed in Table 32-9. Some complications must be treated aggressively and quickly while others may be handled through rehabilitation.

Nursing Management

Nursing management begins with assessing the head-injured client using the ABCDE approach. The nurse also evaluates the child's physical, developmental, and social needs and plans actions accordingly. Working with these children, however, requires a team approach with nursing, medicine, neurosurgery, rehabilitation experts, and social services collaborating to meet the needs of the child and family, because if the trauma is severe, their life will be different.

The nurse must assess the airway of the child and check endotracheal placement frequently. Arterial blood gases and pulse oximetry should be monitored, and if intubated, the child should be positioned comfortably and assessed for signs of pain or need for sedation.

The child's respiratory status must be evaluated whether intubated or not because respiratory deterioration is a risk from the unstable neurological condition. Tissue perfusion must also be assessed frequently, and if inotropes such as dopamine or dobutamine are administered, the nurse must be aware of the side effects (tachycardia, increased blood pressure, cardiac dysrhythmias). Frequent monitoring for signs of increased intracranial pressure and being aware of the modalities used to treat increased ICP are also important.

If neurological sequelae are present, the nurse must work with the child in accepting the disability. The older child and adolescent can be challenging if they feel they

NURSING TIP

Assessing for Pain in the Chemically Paralyzed Child

- Tachycardia
- Pallor
- Increased blood pressure
- Tears

Table 32-9 Common Complications of Head Injury

COMPLICATION	MANAGEMENT
Seizures	
• Immediate: usually occur within seconds of injury; not precursor of long-term epilepsy	• Assure patent airway and provide oxygen
• Early: occur within first week post-injury but most often within first 24 hours; are associated with minor trauma or focal injury	• If occurring 30 minutes after injury, may administer benzodiazepines • If still seizing after benzodiazepins, may give phenytoin
• Late: occur one week after trauma; secondary to cortical scarring	• Give benzodiazepins and phenytoin initially • Since there is a high incidence of recurrent or permanent epilepsy, may be placed on oral anticonvulsants and then weaned off medication after six seizure-free months
Alterations in fluid homeostasis: either SIADH or diabetes insipidus (DI)	• Monitor electrolytes and fluid status • For DI, administer medications such as DDAVP
Postconcussive syndrome: may occur any time after the event; signs and symptoms include dizziness, vertigo, nausea, vomiting, photophobia, headache, trouble concentrating, changes in memory, and alterations in behavior such as aggression, regression, withdrawal, and emotional lability	• Provide palliative treatment • Refer to special education, rehabilitation, counseling for child as well as caregivers
Intellectual impairment, focal deficits, sensory disturbances, communication dysfunctions, motor abnormalities, or chronic alteration in mental status	• Refer to special education, rehabilitation, counseling for child as well as caregivers

have lost control of their lives and bodies and are different from their peers. The nurse can work with these children by encouraging them to vent their frustrations, providing positive feedback, and working with families and peers to ensure needed support is available.

Physical, occupational, and speech therapists should begin working with traumatic brain-injured children as soon as possible. The nurse, even in the intensive care unit, should reinforce the regimens and encourage family members to participate in therapeutic exercises as well.

If the child's injuries lead to a diminished level of consciousness or a vegetative state, the nurse should work with the family in collaboration with social workers, psychologists, and clergy. Caregivers should be encouraged to bring in favorite toys and tapes of music or the family speaking so the child can hear the familiar voices often during the day. When performing the daily assessments, all lacerations, abrasions, and hematomas should be examined to evaluate how well they are healing. Dressings, surgical incisions, and the child's temperature should also be assessed to determine their status.

Discharge planning needs to begin as soon as the child enters the hospital. The rehabilitation unit and social workers should help determine the services needed and how the family can arrange for them. Planning might include transfer to another center for therapy, making physical adjustments to the family home to accommodate a hospital bed or wheelchair, or securing appliances such as walkers or braces. The nurse should also arrange for follow-up with the multidisciplinary team members caring for the child during the acute phase of his recovery.

Family Teaching

Families with head-injured children have had their lives changed in seconds, and often come into emergency departments fearing the worst and hoping for the best, not really knowing what lies ahead. Most caregivers are ill-prepared for dealing with intensive care stays, surgical interventions, and long-term therapies, including acute care hospitalizations as well as rehabilitation in inpatient and ambulatory settings. They usually go through highs and lows emotionally as their child improves, plateaus, and/or deteriorates. The nurse can help by supporting and educating caregivers about the recovery process of brain injury, and enlist the help of other professionals as well as encourage the family to seek out peer groups and national foundations.

Furthermore, the nurse should act as liaison for the child, the family, and the resources needed for rehabilitation. This can begin in the hospital setting when caregivers can be taught various therapeutic techniques to perform. In addition, family members should be encouraged to bring in toys and books based on the child's new level of functioning. Finally, the nurse must be an advocate for injury prevention. It is important to talk with families about safety issues emphasizing that bike helmets and proper utilization of car seats and seatbelts can eliminate most head trauma.

SPINAL CORD INJURY

Spinal cord injury includes damage to the cervical, thoracolumbar, and lumbar regions. Behavioral and anatomic differences between children and adults lead to variation in injury type and severity; young children are more prone to high cervical injuries whereas older children (8–10) demonstrate an injury pattern similar to an adult (Haslam, 2007). Damage starts at the time of injury when the spinal tissue is bruised or torn by displaced bone fragments, ligaments, or disc material (NINDS, n.d.f.).

Incidence and Etiology

Spinal cord injury without radiologic abnormality (**SCIWORA**) occurs primarily in children; however, a high incidence of complete cord injuries reported in children 9 years and younger is associated with SCIWORA. Certain anatomic and biomechanical characteristics of younger children's spine predispose them to SCIWORA. These include poorly developed uncinate processes, increased elasticity of the spine relative to a less flexible spinal cord, anterior wedging of the vertebral bodies, shallow and horizontally oriented facet joint, and vulnerability of the growth zone of vertebral end plates. The incidence of SCIWORA in children under 10 is 60%, and 20% in older children and adolescents (Haslam, 2007).

Between 3% and 5% of spinal cord injuries (SCI) occurring every year in the United States are in individuals under 15 years of age; about 20% occur in individuals under 20 years of age (Vogel & Anderson, 2003). SCI occurs more commonly in females (2.5–3.0:1) but 80% of males with SCI are between 18 and 25 years of age (Schreiber, 2004). The category and level of SCI varies according to age, with younger children more likely than older children or adolescents to have complete injury or paraplegia.

Most spinal injuries are the result of motor vehicle crashes. In young children, the mechanism is either pedestrian-vehicle, bike-vehicle, or passenger-related, whereas in adolescence, passenger- and driver-related injuries account for most cord trauma. Violence is also a significant cause of SCI, especially among Hispanics and African Americans in all but the youngest age groups. Other unique etiologies seen in the pediatric age groups include child abuse, transverse mylelitis, lap belt injuries, and subluxation due to tonsillopharyngitis. Children with Down syndrome, juvenile rheumatoid arthritis, and skeletal dysplasias are susceptible to cervical SCI. Sports and medical surgical complications account for more SCIs in teens than adults (Haslam, 2007).

Pathophysiology

Children suffer from different types of injury than adults because of their physical and developmental immaturity. Because of these characteristics, children under 8 years of age are more likely to suffer upper cervical injuries but less likely to have C-4–C-6 injuries than older children. The

NURSING ALERT

Lap-Belt Syndrome

"Lap-belt syndrome" is often seen in children under age 13 years who are passengers in motor vehicle crashes and wearing two- or three-point restraints. However, because of their anatomic immaturity, children are not protected from injury by these belts. The seat belts, which normally sit on the pelvic girdle of adult passengers, lie on the abdomen of the child. When a crash occurs, the child is extremely hyperflexed over the belt, which acts as a fulcrum, and then snaps back upright. This impact directly hits the abdominal area with the force continuing posteriorly to the spinal column and cord.

Signs and symptoms include bruising across the pelvis and hematuria. Injuries include:

- lumbar or sacral fracture or subluxation, most commonly at L-1 or L-2
- lumbar or sacral cord injury, either complete or incomplete, most commonly at L-1 or L-2
- abdominal injury to hollow or solid organs
- perforated intestinal viscera
- bladder hematoma or rupture
- mild to moderate head injury

reason for younger children being at higher risk for experiencing an upper cervical injury is related to their underdeveloped neck musculature and proportionally larger head size (Vogel & Anderson, 2003). The second most common area is the thoracolumbar region, probably because of improperly placed seat belts. Lap-belt injuries occur most often in children weighing between 18 and 27 kg whose lap belt was positioned above the pelvic brim, causing flexion or distraction forces in the mid-lumbar spine. If children between 4 and 8 years of age are restrained in approved belt-positioning booster seats, the incidence decreases (Vogel & Anderson, 2003). Between ages 8 and 14 years, 60% of injury is cervical, 20% thoracolumbar, and the remaining solely lumbar.

Most spinal cord injuries resulting in permanent loss of movement or sensation are not caused by complete transection, but rather by contusion, compression, vascular damage, or hemorrhage. Life expectancy for children and adolescents with SCI, a function of the category of injury and the neurological level, is less than the general population. In addition, young children with cervical injuries are more likely to die than older children (Carreon, Glassman, & Campbell, 2004).

Clinical Manifestations

The clinical manifestations depend on whether concurrent injuries are present, the level of the trauma, and if the lesion is complete or incomplete. As the child is usually a victim of multiple traumas, the presenting picture is complex. However, another unique characteristic of pediatric onset SCI is that in 25–50% of children presenting with SCI, there can be a delay of from 30 minutes to 4 days in the onset of neurological abnormalities. Rather, these children may experience subtle and transient neurological symptoms such as parasthesia (Vogel & Anderson, 2003). Refer to Table 32-10 for manifestations of neurogenic and spinal shock and Table 32-11 for the symptoms according to the level of injury.

Diagnosis

All children with multisystem injury must be treated as if spinal cord injury is present until it has definitively been ruled out. Diagnosis of injury can be made either clinically or radiologically.

Treatment

The goals of the initial phase of managing the child with a spinal cord injury are to do no further harm and prevent further damage. Immobilization, the first step, is started where the trauma occurred by the prehospital providers and carried through to the hospital. Airway patency must be assured. Breathing will need to be evaluated and if high injury is present, the child must be intubated. If mechanical ventilation is a long-term possibility (clients with trauma above C-4) a tracheostomy should be performed. Proper perfusion and hydration must be ensured. Heart rate and blood pressure should be monitored by using electronic equipment, and any pathologic changes need to be treated quickly. The injuries to the vertebral column or spinal cord must be managed aggressively. Surgical management may be necessary to prevent further injury and promote healing. Debridement and decompression should take place as soon as possible after the injury; eight hours should be the maximum delay time. To stabilize the vertebrae, a spinal fusion may be performed using bone from other areas of the body. After this type of surgery, a body brace or shell is usually worn for six weeks for protection and alignment. If extensive trauma to the column has occurred, internal fixation devices may be required. To decrease the neurological sequelae associated with cord damage, methylprednisolone is administered to those clients with motor deficits. It *must* be started within eight hours of the injury, although it is prudent to begin the infusion as soon as possible.

Rehabilitation should begin early in the treatment regimen. Simple range of motion and other passive exercises may prevent contractures and muscle wasting as well as promote healing. Basic equipment such as footboards and splints should also be used to promote proper position in the initial stages of recovery. Later on, the physical and occupational therapists will work with the child in adaptive behaviors and use of equipment such as braces, crutches, walkers, or wheelchairs. In addition, if the youngster is mechanically

TABLE 32-10 Comparison of Neurogenic and Spinal Shock

NEUROGENIC SHOCK	SPINAL SHOCK

Neurogenic shock is a form of distributive shock that accompanies complete high spinal cord injury. It is caused by interruption of sympathetic impulses from the spinal cord in the cervical or thoracic region.
The hallmark signs include:
• Vasodilation
• Hypotension
• Bradycardia
• Warm flushed skin
• Inability to perspire
• Hypothermia
	Spinal shock is the complete loss of all reflex activity after spinal cord injury. This is a transient event that often occurs shortly after the trauma and can persist for as long as 7 to 10 days.
	Signs include:
	• Below the level of the lesion
	  • Flaccid, areflexic extremities
	  • Loss of deep tendon reflexes
	  • No sensory response
	• Autonomic dysfunction
	  • Hypotension
	  • Bradycardia
	  • Decreased peripheral vascular resistance
	  • Impaired temperature control
	  • Warm, flushed, dry skin
	• Loss of sphincter control with urinary retention
	• Priapism

TABLE 32-11 Deficits Displayed Secondary to Level of Lesion

LEVEL	DEFICITS
C-1 to C-2	• Quadriplegia with total loss of respiratory function • Flaccid paralysis
C-2 to C-4	• Quadriplegia with loss of phrenic innervation to diaphragm
C-4 to C-5	• Quadriplegia with possible phrenic nerve involvement caused by edema resulting in loss of respiratory function
C-5 to C-6	• Quadriplegia but with gross arm movements • Diaphragmatic breathing • No intercostal respirations
C-6 to C-7	• Quadriplegia but with biceps intact • Diaphragmatic breathing • Complete loss of shoulder movement
C-7 to C-8	• Quadriplegia with biceps and triceps intact • Diaphragmatic breathing • No function of intrinsic hand muscles
T-1 to T-2	• Paraplegia with loss of leg, bowel, bladder, and sexual function • Some loss of intercostal muscles • Arm function intact
T-2 to L-2	• Paraplegia with loss of varying degrees of intercostal and abdominal muscles
Below L-2	• Varying amounts of motor and sensory loss
Cauda Equina	• Bowel and bladder dysfunction

NURSING ALERT

Autonomic Dysreflexia

After spinal shock has resolved and reflex activity has returned, children with high cervical or thoracic lesions may react to a noxious stimulus such as a distended bladder, constipation, or fecal impaction with a potential life-threatening sympathetic nervous system response. Spasms of the pelvic viscera and arterioles produce vasoconstriction below the lesion, resulting in hypertension and superficial vasodilation, flushing, piloerection, and perfuse perspiration above the injury. To compensate for the increased blood pressure, the heart rate is slowed via vagal stimulation; however, because of the trauma to the cord, this impulse cannot be sent to areas below the damage. Without rapid reversal of these symptoms, which is typically accomplished by the removal of the stimulant, strokes, seizures, or death may result.

ventilated, team members from respiratory and pulmonary will be able to assist in ensuring portable ventilators are available.

The emotional needs of the client must also be addressed, and opportunities provided to express anger, frustrations, and expectations. Working with psychologists, psychiatrists, social workers, or clergy may prove very beneficial.

Nursing Management

Initially after SCI, the nurse's primary responsibility is to ensure adequate oxygenation, ventilation, and perfusion by carefully monitoring vital signs and respiratory status. Bony prominences must be checked often for breakdown although skin integrity can be maintained with proper alignment, positioning, and use of lotions, egg crates, or sheepskin. If external devices are used to maintain immobility, pin or screw care is important, and all surgical sites should be watched carefully for signs of leakage, inflammation, or infection.

Providing adequate nutrition can be challenging. The child with a lower lesion can chew and swallow regular food without problem; however, the youngster who is quadriplegic may need gastrostomy tube placement. If this occurs, skin care must be provided.

Bowel and bladder control may be difficult to achieve. The child may have an indwelling urinary catheter early in the course of recovery; but later on, training can begin with intermittent catheterization as the goal. Bowel and bladder management for children who receive a SCI before 3 or 4 years of age is different than those injured at older ages. Intermittent catheterization, the standard management for bladder control in pediatric SCI patients, is usually not initiated until the child reaches the age most children are toilet trained (3–4 years of age). However, if the child has obstructive uropathy or experiences recurrent urinary tract infections, intermittent catheterization may be started earlier. Usually children are able and willing to perform self-catheterization by 5–8 years of age (Vogel & Anderson, 2003). Credé's method, where pressure is placed over the symphysis pubis to expel the urine, is not advised if the bladder is full as it may rupture with pressure. Bowel training involves a diet high in fiber and use of stool softeners. The nurse should work with the rehabilitation specialists and reinforce all the exercises and skills learned during the sessions, and utilize any equipment specially adapted to the child's needs. Rehabilitative or habilitative care of children with pediatric onset SCI needs to be developmentally appropriate and change as the child becomes an adolescent and then an adult.

Perhaps the most difficult issue for the nurse working with these children is the emotional aspect of care. The lives of these youngsters change in an instant, and the nurse must provide the support needed in adapting to their different body function and image. It is important to avoid being

NURSING ALERT

SCIWORA

SCIWORA, spinal cord injury without radiologic abnormality, accounts for as much as one-quarter of all pediatric spinal cord traumas. The child may initially experience brief sensory or motor deficits; however, these symptoms are usually gone by the time the victim reaches the emergency room and are often not reported. Initial X-rays or CT show no bony abnormality. Therefore, based on the clinical and radiologic evidence, it is determined that the youngster has no spinal cord injury.

Onset of neurological symptoms can appear as late as four days posttrauma. Usually, signs of neurological deterioration are noted along with characteristics of either complete transection or partial cord syndromes.

Approximately two-thirds of the victims are under age eight years. Half the injuries are complete and thoracic in nature while the remaining 50% are incomplete and involve the cervical and lumbar regions.

This injury occurs as a result of the spinal column's cartilaginous structure and flexibility. It can withstand up to two inches of stretch without disruption. The cord, however, can rupture with only a quarter-inch elongation. Thus, on traditional X ray, the vertebrae will appear normal. MRI will be needed to appreciate the cord injury.

too solicitous or overprotective, yet at the same time encourage the children to meet small, short-term goals that will offer them as much independence as possible. The nurse should also provide an environment where the child is able to speak freely about frustrations, anxieties, and fears. Finally, as much normal activity as possible should be provided, while at the same time not presenting challenges that are too difficult to meet. In-house school or tutors may help meet educational needs and allow the school-age child and adolescent to keep up with classmates.

Family Teaching

The family of the child with a cord injury often goes from a state of shock and disbelief to one of unresolved grief, and may need professional help. The family needs to be involved with the multidisciplinary team and learn how to work with their youngster in the normal activities of living such as dressing, feeding, and mobility. Because of the central role parents and family play in the child's or adolescent's life, they will also need to learn exercises and various therapeutic techniques. Once these skills are mastered family members will feel they have gained some control over their lives.

Discharge planning should begin early, and most often a rehabilitation center is the next step for these children as it helps them achieve their maximum potential physically, emotionally, and intellectually. The family will decide if the child is treated as an inpatient or as an outpatient. The financial burdens associated with having a spinal cord injured child are phenomenal. Social workers can be helpful in securing funds for training, special appliances, and alterations that may need to be made to the home.

DROWNING

Drowning is defined as death from a submersion incident in a liquid medium within the first 24 hours postinjury. **Near-drowning** refers to an immersion episode of such severity that it warrants medical attention and may lead to death and morbidity. It also refers to survival for more than 24 hours regardless of the final outcome. **Secondary drowning** refers to the rapid deterioration of respiratory function from several hours to days after successful resuscitation.

Incidence and Etiology

Drowning is one of the most preventable causes of childhood morbidity and mortality. Claiming around 2,000 victims per year, it is second only to transportation injuries as the most common cause of unintentional injury in the pediatric population. Almost half the children are under 4 years of age, with the peak incidence between 1 and 3 years of age, and then again during adolescence. The rate for boys is higher than for girls. However, bathtub drowning is more common in girls and those under 1 year of age. Residential swimming pool drownings are most common in the preschool-age groups, and 70% of these drowning cases occur because gates are left open in fenced-in pools. Adolescents and young adults most commonly drown in lakes, rivers, ponds, and oceans (Brayden, Bunik, Brown, & Daley, 2009; Kallas, 2007; Shepherd & Martin, 2005).

Over 90% of all submersion injuries occur in fresh water; 50% of those are in swimming pools. Ninety percent are residential pools. Drownings most often occur between 4:00pm and 6:00pm when family members are busy preparing dinner. Caregivers suspect something is wrong when the child is missing, usually for less than five minutes. Interestingly, splashes, screams, or cries for help are rarely heard.

Bathtubs account for about 7% of all drownings; most often from either poor supervision or intentional trauma. Hot tubs and spas cause 10% of the drowning deaths of toddlers between ages 10 and 23 months by entrapping their hair or extremities in the mechanical suction devices. As these tubs and spas are filled with warm or hot water that is often laden with *Pseudomonas aeruginosa,* survivors of this type of submersion have a recovery complicated by infection. Three- to five-gallon buckets can also be hazardous, especially to toddlers as they are too top-heavy and uncoordinated to lift themselves out of the pail if they fall in head first. Only a very small number of submersion injuries are a result of boating or diving mishaps.

Children with convulsive disorders are high risk for submersion. Although swimming and water activities are not ill-advised for these youngsters, they must be carefully supervised in pools, tubs, or boats at all times.

Pathophysiology

There are two types of drowning. **Wet drowning** is caused by the aspiration of fluid into the lungs; it is the most common form, especially for infants and toddlers. **Dry drowning,** which only occurs 10–15% of the time, is secondary to hypoxemia resulting from intense laryngospasm. In these cases, fluid has not entered the lungs.

Cold water victims have a better chance of recovery than warm water victims because either the reduced body temperature slows cerebral metabolism enough to protect the brain and heart, or the child undergoes a diver's reflex where blood is diverted to the vital organs. Most often, children whose body temperatures are lower than 28°C (82.4°F) have the best survival rates and outcomes.

The sequences occurring with drowning are that first, the child who is trapped in the water panics, struggles, and attempts to move using swimming-like motions. The breath is then held before some water is swallowed. Vomiting, and then aspiration of the vomit, and laryngospasms, lasting less than two minutes, follow. The child then panics, hypoxia follows, and then the child swallows even more fluid. If this is a dry drowning, profound laryngospasms then occur, and the child becomes severely hypoxic, seizes, and dies. If it is a wet drowning, the child will become unconscious. Laryngospasms lessen as reflexes are lost and large amounts of fluid passively enter the airway and stomach.

The major insult associated with submersion is hypoxemia, and, initially, the body will try to compensate for this by shunting blood to the lungs to increase circulating oxygen. This fluid shift results in pulmonary edema, which when combined with the aspirated liquid causes decreased lung compliance. This is further complicated by the inactivation of pulmonary surfactant.

Hypoxia and acidosis lead to the complications associated with submersion. Cardiac dysrhythmias such as asystole, bradycardia, and ventricular fibrillation are frequently manifested. Other common pathologies seen include neurological dysfunction and renal failure. Hypothermia may also occur with submersion as youngsters tend to lose heat rapidly as their surface area is large and their fat stores do not provide enough insulation. Although extreme hypothermia may prove advantageous, a milder form may precipitate decreased coordination, increased muscle rigidity, decreased breath holding time, and deterioration in the level of consciousness.

Clinical Manifestations

The clinical presentation depends on the length of time underwater, the temperature of the fluid, the child's response to the event, and the initial maneuvers or treatments done at the scene, first by bystanders and then by the prehospital providers. Refer to Table 32-12 for the signs and symptoms.

The child submerged for a short period of time and those needing no immediate interventions will present with the least symptomatology, and may show few, if any, signs of neurological dysfunction; display minimal respiratory distress; have normal or almost normal blood gases and chest X-rays; and be mildly hypothermic. Most often, there are no concurrent injuries. This child usually recovers without complication. However, the child with a longer submersion will display more pathology; if cardiopulmonary resuscitation was required at the scene, symptoms will be more devastating. There will be a diminished level of consciousness, ranging from stupor to coma, and there may or may not be appropriate reactions to painful stimuli. Reflex responses may or may not be intact, and decorticate, decerebrate, or areflexive posturing may be present. If the victim was also hypothermic, cardiac dysrhythmias commonly associated with hypoxia and acidosis may be exacerbated.

The child's clinical picture may change within the first 24 hours after the event. Cerebral edema may occur, leading to the classic signs of increased intracranial pressure as well as seizures. Respiratory function may also be affected as pulmonary edema, bronchospasm, and irregularities in breathing pattern such as Cheyne-Stokes, periodic breathing, or apnea may occur. In addition, chest X-ray may show marked abnormalities. Signs and symptoms of concurrent injuries may be manifested at this time as well, and the child may be hypovolemic, neurogenic, or exhibit spinal shock. Furthermore, the victim of a wet drowning may be a prime candidate for pneumonia. Other complications such as clotting abnormalities, electrolyte imbalances, and renal disturbances may also be seen.

Recovery from a submersion incident is painfully slow. Some children will survive intact, while others will have neurological sequelae such as cerebral palsy, intellectual deficits, and emotional lability. Still other victims will remain in a chronic vegetative state.

Diagnosis

The first step in making the diagnosis of drowning or near-drowning is getting an accurate history from any witnesses at the scene as well as the prehospital providers. It is vital to ascertain the following information:

- Amount of time the child was submerged
- Temperature of the fluid
- What the fluid was: salt or fresh water, from a hot tub or spa, or a cleaning solution in a bucket
- If the mechanism (inability to swim versus diving into a shallow pool) was conducive to causing other trauma such as head or spinal cord injury
- Victim's initial response after the rescue:
  - If there were spontaneous respirations or heart beats
  - If the child was awake, semiconscious, or totally unresponsive
- Actions taken by the bystanders, including CPR, and the child's response to them
- Time the prehospital providers arrived
- Interventions performed by the paramedics and the victim's reaction
- Child's status during transport to the hospital

The child must have a thorough physical assessment with evaluation of the airway, ventilatory status, and circulation occurring immediately. If signs of shock are present, causes should be quickly determined as either from hypovolemia or neurological injury. Temperature must be monitored to rule out hypothermia. In addition, level of consciousness should be measured and pupils checked for both size and reaction to light. Arterial blood gases should be drawn to note pathologic changes in carbon dioxide or oxygen levels; pulse oximetry may not be a useful tool initially because of poor perfusion or hypothermia. Other laboratory assessments should include serum chemistries; blood, urea, nitrogen; creatinine; and clotting factors as well as cultures of blood, urine, and tracheal aspirate if the drowning occurred in a pond, spa, hot tub, or other source of potential infection. The radiologic examinations performed are chest X-ray to note the presence of an infiltrate, and a head CT to observe for intracranial or skull injury or cerebral edema. If concurrent injury is suspected, other films such as lateral cervical spine and pelvis are also taken.

Treatment

Treatment of the submersion victim must begin at the scene with immediate initiation of ventilations, compressions, and rewarming as indicated. If the airway is unstable, gas exchange poor, breathing effort minimal at best, and level of consciousness diminished (Glasgow Coma Score of 8 or less), the child must be intubated. A nasogastric or

Table 32-12 Manifestations of Near-Drowning by Category

CATEGORY	SIGNS AND SYMPTOMS
A	• Awake, alert, and oriented with Glasgow Coma Score of 14 to 15 • Minimal, if any, concurrent injury • Mild, if any, hypothermia • Minimal, if any, changes on chest X-ray • Slight signs of acidosis on arterial blood gas • May develop characteristics of neurological or pulmonary deterioration in 24 hours
B	• Alteration in neurological status ranging from stupor to coma with Glasgow Coma Score between 8 and 13; intact pupil and pain responses • Moderate concurrent injury • Mild to moderate hypothermia • Alteration in respiratory pattern • Abnormal chest X-ray and arterial blood gas
C	• Comatose with nonpurposeful response to pain and reflex responses, which may or may not be intact • Seizures • Compromised cardiovascular system with dysrhythmias, signs of shock, and DIC • Alteration in pulmonary function ranging from slight respiratory distress to failure • Abnormal chest X-ray • Arterial blood gas with a metabolic acidosis • Electrolyte imbalance such as hyperkalemia and hyperglycemia
C-1	As in "C" plus • Decorticate posturing • Cheyne-Stokes respirations
C-2	As in "C" plus • Decerebrate posturing • Central hyperventilation
C-3	As in "C" plus • Flaccid posturing • Apneustic breathing
C-4	As in "C" plus • Flaccid posturing • Apneic • No detectable circulation

Adapted from Wellington, M. C & Wayner, R. F. (1995). *Alterations in neurologic function*. In J. Ball & R. Bindler (eds.), *Pediatric nursing: Caring for children*. Norwalk, CT: Appleton and Lange.

orogastric tube should then be placed both to empty the stomach to prevent emesis and the threat of aspiration as well as to relieve gastric distention and enhance ventilation. Furthermore, if the respiratory status is compromised by pulmonary edema and aspiration, positive end expiratory pressure will need to be delivered. If the victim has a stable airway and normal ventilation, he should receive oxygen by mask. In either case, bronchodilators may be delivered by either intravenous route or aerosol to control bronchospasm.

Circulation and perfusion must be maintained. Fluid boluses should be given in the amount of 20 milliliters per kilogram for signs of hypovolemic shock. If the condition does not improve after two infusions or if signs of pulmonary edema occur, inotropic support should be initiated. Cardiac rhythms must be closely monitored. If severe hypothermia is present; that is, the child's core body temperature is less than 28°C (82.4°F), rewarming must be accomplished before treatments are initiated as they are ineffective in the cold victim.

Hypothermia accompanies many submersion injuries. Warming should begin at the scene by removing wet clothing and covering the victim with blankets and heat packs. In the hospital, it is vital to continue rewarming. Body surfaces can be warmed using heat lamps or warm blankets. However, internal methods such as providing humidified oxygen at a temperature between 42° and 46°C (107.6–114.8°F) through the endotracheal tube; administering intravenous fluids and blood warmed to 43°C (109.4°F); performing peritoneal or gastric lavage with fluids heated to 43°C (109.4°F); or utilizing extracorporeal rewarming technologies are far more successful. These modalities begin in the emergency department and may need to be continued after admission to the intensive care unit. It is important to remember that a drowning victim cannot be pronounced dead if extremely hypothermic; rewarming must take place first, even if the outcome is certain.

Neurological dysfunction will be managed after the victim's airway, breathing, and circulation have been stabilized. Neurological involvement may range from not being affected at all to being severely obtunded and in a coma. If signs of increased intracranial pressure are evident just after the event, head injury should be suspected as cerebral edema usually does not manifest itself until 24 hours later. Signs and symptoms must be quickly recognized as interventions should begin at once. First, the child should be hyperventilated to achieve a PaCO2 level between 30 and 32, by intubation, sedation, and chemical paralysis. If there is no clinical or radiologic indication of spinal injury, the head of the bed should be elevated at least 30° keeping the child's head in the midline. If there is still no response, administration of mannitol should be considered. Any seizure activity should be controlled initially giving benzodiazepines. If, however, convulsions continue, anticonvulsants such as phenytoin or phenobarbital should be administered. If despite aggressive measures, intracranial pressure is still not reduced to below 30 millimeters of mercury and cerebral perfusion pressures remain below the normal 50 to 60, the prognosis for the child's survival is dismal. If the victim shows any signs of infection, aggressive treatment with antibiotics is essential.

Nursing Management

Assessment

The nursing management of the near-drowning victim depends on the degree of injury. Assessment and monitoring of the minimally involved child is important as well as close observation for late developing sequelae. The more impaired child, however, will need intensive care for continual monitoring of respiratory, cardiac, and neurological status. In addition, the nurse will need to monitor for increased intracranial pressure, cardiac dysrhythmias, electrolyte imbalances, clotting abnormalities, and closely watch for changes in laboratory values.

Nursing Diagnosis

1. *Impaired communication* related to altered state of consciousness.
2. *Impaired mobility* related to altered state of consciousness.
3. *Decreased cardiac output* related to near-drowning sequelae.
4. *Decreased intracranial adaptive capacity* related to brain anoxia.
5. *Impaired skin integrity* related to inability to control movements.
6. *Compromised family coping* related to feelings of guilt.
7. *Interrupted family processes* related to hospital stay and subsequent sequelae.

Outcome Identification

1. The child will feel comfort and less isolated through touch and listening to the nurse and family members.
2. The child will not suffer from contractures and muscle atrophy.
3. The child will maintain acceptable cardiac output.
4. The child will maintain acceptable intracranial pressure.
5. The child will not exhibit signs of skin breakdown.
6. The family will work through feelings of guilt.
7. The family will adapt to the child's disabilities.

Planning and Implementation

Care for the child with a severely diminished level of consciousness means providing a safe, comfortable environment where attention is paid to skin care, positioning, and communication. Furthermore, arrangements should be made for occupational and physical therapies to begin to prevent contractures and muscle atrophy that may occur from immobility. Ideally, plans for and initiation of rehabilitation must begin in the intensive care unit just after admission.

The nurse must work with the family. Often, they are tormented by feelings of guilt; therefore, the nurse should provide a nonthreatening, nonjudgmental environment where they can vent frustrations, anxieties, and fears. Most often, caregivers of a near-drowning victim are faced with an unknown prognosis, but most have hope of recovery. At other times, however, when family members realize the outcome for their child is dismal, they may wish for the end of suffering and death. In either case, the nurse should support the caregivers through the crisis with the assistance of social workers, clergy, friends, or other family members. It is also important to remember the siblings and ensure their emotional needs are met.

Evaluation The hope is that the child will fully recover and receive appropriate care, and the family who loses a child will effectively recover from their loss.

Family Teaching

If the child survives with minor deficits, home care and special education can be arranged before discharge. Follow-up visits with physicians at the hospital or in the community can also be scheduled. The child who is more impaired may also be discharged home. Those children with severe hypoxic responses may need special appliances such as wheelchairs. Even children in a coma can be managed in their residences with home care nurses assisting family members. Caregivers of these children will need to learn how to work with any equipment, handle their child, and meet special needs. They should also be informed about caregiver support groups as well as government or private facilities that may be helpful.

Prevention is the best education for these families. It is up to the nurse to make all families aware children must be carefully supervised when near any body of water, including bath tubs, hot tubs, buckets of water, and spas; residential pools must be surrounded by a four-sided, locked barrier at least 4–5 feet tall. Children should also be taught to check water for depth and objects before diving. In addition, the nurse should advise families the American Academy of Pediatrics states children under the age of 3 years are too young to learn to swim. Therefore, caregivers of toddlers who have attended swimming lessons should not allow their children to be near water without an adult close by. Furthermore, life jackets on boats and watercraft must be the correct size; if not, children will come out of them when in the water. Finally, the nurse should emphasize learning CPR so, if tragedy occurs despite all these efforts, interventions can begin immediately to enhance the child's chance of survival.

CEREBRAL PALSY

Cerebral palsy (CP) is a chronic nonprogressive motor dysfunction caused by damage to the motor areas of the brain during antepartal, intrapartal, or neonatal periods. CP refers to a heterogenous group of disabilities which include spastic, athetoid, and mixed physical manifestations (Johnston, 2007b).

INCIDENCE AND ETIOLOGY

Causes of cerebral palsy include prenatal factors (maternal vaginal bleeding, toxemia, preeclampsia, intrauterine drug exposure or infections, breech presentation, low Apgar scores, multiple fetuses, and prematurity). Low birth weight infants are 100 times more likely to develop CP than infants of normal birth weight (NINDS, n.d.b.). Congenital cerebral malformations and head trauma (shaken baby syndrome, abuse, falls, accidents, meningitis, encephalitis) are other causes. However, 25–50% of cases have an unknown etiology (Odding et al., 2006).

The incidence, estimated to be 7 per 1,000 live births per year, may in fact be increasing because many very low birth weight infants are now surviving. Low birth weight newborns now account for half of all cases of CP (Odding et al., 2006). Many persons with CP have accompanying disabilities such as cognitive and language delays, which range from mild to severe.

PATHOPHYSIOLOGY

Congenital malformation of or injury to the brain, or anoxia of the brain, at any time before, during, or after birth may contribute to the development of CP (Johnston, 2007b; NINDS, n.d.b.). Table 32-13 lists the various factors contributing to cerebral palsy.

Prognosis for infants and children diagnosed with CP depends on the level of physical involvement as well as concurrent medical problems. Many children with hemiplegia and ataxia show improvement with therapy and are eventually able to ambulate independently. However, if a toddler does not sit independently by 2 years of age, there is almost no chance of walking, even with intense therapy and the use of braces, crutches, or a walker.

Table 32-13 Factors Contributing to Cerebral Palsy

TIME PERIOD	FACTORS
Prenatal	• Genetic or chromosomal abnormalities • Brain malformation • Exposure to teratogens • Multiple fetuses • Intrauterine infection • Ineffective placenta causing insufficient nutrition and oxygen delivery to fetus
Birth	• Preeclampsia • Complicated labor and delivery • Birth injury caused by direct head trauma • Asphyxia secondary to cord collapse or strangulation
Perinatal	• Central nervous system infection or sepsis • Kernicterus (hyperbilirubinemia of the newborn)
Childhood	• Head trauma • Meningitis • Toxic ingestion or inhalation

CLINICAL MANIFESTATIONS

Cerebral palsy is an abnormality of muscle tone and movement. Tables 32-14 and 32-15 present the characteristics of cerebral palsy according to the muscle response seen and the area of the body involved.

Infants and children with cerebral palsy display a wide range of clinical manifestations. Alterations in muscle tone such as abnormal posturing and movements, and continued primitive reflex responses make reaching normal developmental milestones almost unattainable. There is usually delay in gross motor skills such as sitting, crawling, cruising,

TABLE 32-14 Characteristics of CP According to Muscle Response

DESCRIPTOR	CHARACTERISTICS
Hypotonia	• Floppiness • Increased range of motion of the joints • Diminished reflex responses
Hypertonia	• Rigidity; muscles are extremely tense or tight • Spasticity; movements are uncoordinated, awkward, and stiff • Scissoring or crossing of the lower extremities • Reflex reactions (Babinski, deep tendon) are exaggerated • Affects 70–80% of clients
Athetosis (dyskinetic)	• Constant involuntary writhing motions; affect entire body but more severe distally • Movements increase during emotional stress and disappear during sleep; may have difficulty coordinating muscle movements needed for speech (dysarthria); affects 10–20% of clients
Ataxia	• Irregularity in muscle action or coordination; may have intention tremors • Wide-based gait • Affects 5–10% of clients
Mixed	• Symptoms of more than one form described above

TABLE 32-15 Characteristics of CP According to the Body's Topographic Response

TYPE OF CP	CHARACTERISTICS
Hemiplegia	• Involvement of one side of the body with the upper extremities more dysfunctional than lower extremities • Sensory deficits • Asymmetric postures or positions • Atypical reflex responses on affected side • Alteration in muscle tone, most often spastic
Diplegia	• Involvement of similar parts of both sides of the body such as the arms or legs • Lower extremity dysfunction greater than upper extremity function • Alteration in muscle tone (hypertonicity or spasticity) • Delay in meeting gross motor developmental milestones such as sitting, standing, or walking • Achievement of fine motor hand skills usually at normal pace
Quadriplegia	• Involvement of all four extremities with equal involvement although arms are usually flexed while legs are extended • Delay in attaining developmental milestones dependent on motor ability • Speech dysfunction; swallowing may be impaired • Emotional lability not uncommon

or walking. In addition, fine motor coordination may be affected, hampering the ability to perform activities of daily living including self-feeding and dressing. Furthermore, many infants and children have other deficits such as poor vision, strabismus or nystagmus, hearing loss, cognitive impairments, speech or language delays, swallowing/sucking difficulties, seizures, and growth problems.

DIAGNOSIS

Diagnosis is based on clinical findings. However, a definitive diagnosis may not be possible until the child is between 18 months and 2 years of age as many infants displaying delayed development may improve with maturation. Table 32-16 presents the early warning signs of cerebral palsy.

TABLE 32-16 Early Warning Signs of Cerebral Palsy

AGE	WARNING SIGNS
Neonate	• Weak or absent sucking or swallowing difficulties
	• Periods of apnea or bradycardia
	• Encephalopathic cry (high pitched)
	• Extreme fussiness and irritability
	• Poor muscle tone
	• Twitching of an arm or leg
	• Not moving extremities normally
	• Absent or weak primitive reflex responses
3 months	• Feeding difficulties; may be caused by tongue thrust or poor swallowing
	• Irritability or listlessness
	• Hypotonia, but may have head control in prone position
	• One or both hands in fisted position
	• Strabismus
	• Presence of primitive reflexes
	• Brisk tendon reflex response
6 months	• Delay in reaching developmental milestones (motor, speech)
	• Continued primitive reflexes
	• Hands remain clenched; one hand becomes dominant
	• Hypertonia
	• Arching or tendency to stand when held up
	• Lack of interest in people or toys
	• Unaware of or indifferent to stimuli in environment
	• Little if any spontaneous actions
9 months	• Persistent delay in motor milestones
	• Reach may be atypical as fingers are extended and arms tremble with purposeful movement
	• Arms flexed
12 months	• Inability to sit alone
	• Scissoring of lower extremities
	• Toe walking while held, but unable to stand alone
	• Crawl, if present, may be abnormal as only arms may be used
	• Athetoid (irregular, twisting) movement
	• Poor articulation or lack of speech

Infants and children suspected of having cerebral palsy must be carefully and continually evaluated to determine if and when specific motor milestones are met, such as holding onto an object or sitting without support. In addition, if primitive postures or reflexes are present or last beyond normal parameters, if feeding or swallowing difficulties remain, if other central nervous system dysfunctions are present, or if the neurologic abnormalities seem static or are progressively worse, the child should be referred for further evaluation.

> **NURSING TIP**
>
> **Use of Botulism Toxin**
>
> A new and relatively innovative therapeutic intervention for children with cerebral palsy is to use botulism toxin A to manage their spasticity. Children receiving this therapy have had significant improvement in muscle tone, range of motion, and functional motor status (NINDS, n.d.b.).

TREATMENT

There is no cure for cerebral palsy. Therefore, interventions enable the infant or child to achieve the best movement, locomotion, and communication skills possible as well as encourage as much self-sufficiency as he or she is able to achieve.

Many toddlers and children are fitted with technical aids such as braces and walkers, enabling them to ambulate independently. Others must use customized wheelchairs powered either manually or with special electronic devices. Physical and occupational therapies are provided to enhance the child's motor potential and prevent contractures or other complications associated with immobility. Speech therapy is also available to help with feeding as well as language and communication skills. For those unable to verbalize clearly, computers and voice synthesizers may be utilized.

Some children, especially those with spastic CP, may need surgical interventions to reduce the effects of hypertonic muscles. The Achilles tendon may be lengthened to increase the range of motion of the ankle and allow the heel to touch the floor. Hamstrings can be released to correct knee flexion. Other procedures may be needed to prevent hip contractures or adduction, or improve the foot positioning. To reduce muscle spasms or improve muscle tone, a selective dorsal root **rhizotomy**, a procedure where surgeons locate and sever overactivated nerves that control leg muscles, may be performed. Other surgical procedures which are experimental include chronic cerebellar stimulation, where electrodes are implanted in the cerebellar surface and then used to stimulate certain cerebellar areas, and stereotaxic thalamotomy, where precise parts of the thalamus are cut. Results of both procedures are mixed (NINDS, n.d.b.).

Medication administration is usually reserved for the older child or adolescent. Muscle relaxers may be used to decrease contractures and can be given orally, intravenously, or intrathecally. Antianxiety drugs may reduce the excessive motions associated with athetosis.

NURSING MANAGEMENT

The nurse should ensure the infant's or child's body is in the best possible alignment, using pillows and bolsters as supports. Special care should be taken to protect bony prominences as they are prone to breakdown. Handling and moving the child can be challenging. For example, the floppy infant will need extra head and body support, the spastic child's extended legs may scissor when lifted, and the athetoid patient will writhe constantly. Caregivers as well as therapists may assist the nurse in determining the best way to handle and move these children. Feeding may prove challenging as chewing and swallowing problems are common. Techniques such as stroking the throat may help; however, the nurse should turn again to the family for guidance.

If the infant or child is hospitalized, the at-home regime should be followed as much as possible, and physical, occupational, and speech therapy departments should be contacted so therapy sessions can be scheduled. Care for the older child or adolescent can be challenging since many are mentally competent but physically limited. Therefore, respect and dignity need to be integrated into all interventions.

FAMILY TEACHING

Nurses must work with the families, providing them with support and resources to meet their child's needs. As soon as a diagnosis is confirmed, caregivers should be referred to a developmental clinic or center. These agencies will often have peer support groups for family members including siblings, as well as financial advisors.

Because the child will need a wide range of therapeutic services, family members will have to learn how to do the exercises and follow the techniques used by the rehabilitation specialists so their child receives consistent therapy at home. They may also need to learn about braces or walkers, and purchase adaptive feeding equipment. Support and education provided by early intervention programs help families adjust to their lifestyle changes.

HEADACHES

Headaches in children may be either acute or chronic and be vascular (migraine), cluster (muscle contraction), tension or chronic, and low grade. The prevalence of vascular headaches (migraine) is 2.5% in children under 7 years, 5% in puberty and post puberty (males), and 10% in post pubertal females. More common in females (3:2 ratio), 90% of patients have a positive family history of both parents having

EVIDENCE-BASED PRACTICE

Headaches in Children

CLINICAL PROBLEM

What role do menstrual cycles play in adolescent girls' headaches?

BEST CLINICAL PRACTICE

- Over 50% of adolescent girls with headaches have menstrual-related headaches.
- Menstrual-related headaches are most likely migraine-type headaches.
- Menstrual-related headaches begin between two days before onset of menstruation to three days after onset.
- Menstrual-related headaches are described as unilateral headaches, pulsating pain, constant pain, and pressure, and often include photophobia, phonophobia, and nausea.
- Premenstrual girls report headaches that occur monthly, which may indicate that menstrual-related headaches will persist after menarche.

IMPLICATIONS FOR NURSING

- Cyclic headaches should be investigated as menstrual-related headaches.
- The diagnosis of menstrual-related headaches promotes the use of intermittent prophylaxis for prevention.
- Parents should be taught that headaches beginning before or at menarche may be menstrually related.

References: Crawford, M. J., Lehman, L., Slater, S., Kabbouche, M. A., LeCates, S. L., Segers, A. et al. (2009). Menstrual migraine in adolescents. *Headache: The Journal of Head and Face Pain*, *49*(3), 341–347.

had the condition. Cluster headaches are uncommon in children, occur more often in females over 10 years of age, and there is no positive family history. Tension headaches occur in both genders, during all ages, and there is a positive family history with onset during childhood. Chronic, low-grade headaches are the most common type, and have a positive history of caffeine use or nonprescription pain relievers. By age 7 years, 37% of children will have had a headache. By mid-adolescence, this percentage has risen to 69% (Moe et al., 2009; NINDS, n.d.e.).

ETIOLOGY AND PATHOPHYSIOLOGY

Few cranial structures are capable of producing pain. However, the walls of the large intracranial blood vessels are lined by pain fibers. These large blood vessels are found in the sinuses, meninges, periosteum, and muscles around the jaw area, eyes, scalp, neck, and head. Inflammation and vasodilatation stimulate these pain-sensitive blood vessels. Traction and displacement of these blood vessels, by intracranial pressure, can also result in pain. Another explanation of how headache occur are temporary increases in dopamine levels as well as low serotonin levels. Other structures that are pain-producing include the scalp, dural sinuses, and falx cerebri (Goadsby & Raskin, 2008; NINDS, n.d.e.).

CLINICAL MANIFESTATIONS

Symptoms of a migraine include nausea, vomiting, abdominal pain, unilateral and pulsating pain, an aura, visual changes, and relief with sleep. Infants and toddlers may present with pallor, sleepiness, and irritability. Stress, head trauma, hunger, noise, cold weather exercise, or the menstrual cycle are triggers. Cluster headaches manifest unilaterally and recur daily over a four- to eight-week period with one- to two-years between occurrences. Typically occurring in the spring, the pain bursts may last 30–90 minutes and be repeated several times a day. There is no nausea or vomiting, but it hurts to lie down and there is constant, throbbing pain. The scalp may be tender, and the conjunctiva infected and tearing. Tension headaches rarely are accompanied by nausea or vomiting and there usually is no prodrome. The pain is bifrontal or occipital and dull. Although they can last for days, tension headaches usually do not interfere with activities. Psychosocial stress may be a major factor in precipitation, and a tension headache can occur at the same time as a migraine. A chronic, low-grade headache presents with generalized pain that has low intensity and is accompanied with a dull ache (Goadsby & Raskin, 2008; NINDS, n.d.e.).

DIAGNOSIS

Differential diagnoses include hypertension, sinusitis, eye strain, sleep disorder, or an intracranial mass. If a brain tumor is the cause of the headache, 95% of children will have reported the headache for less than four months. Headaches may also serve as warning signs for more serious disorders, especially those caused by inflammation, meningitis, or diseases of the spine, neck, ears, and teeth. Imaging studies are not usually indicated unless the child's or adolescent's history suggests symptoms of increased intracranial pressure. Usually a good history and physical examination help determine the diagnosis.

TREATMENT

Preventative treatment is recommended when headaches occur three or more times a month. Management usually includes prophylactic medications to reduce or prevent the severity and frequency of acute attacks, or general pain medications during the headache. Prophylactic therapy may be considered if the headaches cause the child to miss school more than once a month. If the child has seizure disorders, anticonvulsants are used. Specific medications used for pain management include acetaminophen, ibuprofen, naproxen, or ergot for acute pain; promethazine for nausea or vomiting; and cold compresses. Propanalol and amitriptyline are used for prophylaxis. Massage, relaxation techniques, and biofeedback may also help prevent the episodes, as does regular exercise such as vigorous walking or swimming. Sumatriptan is commonly used for migraine pain and methysergide maleate, which counteracts blood vessel constriction, helps prevent migraines. Ergotamine tartrate, a vasoconstrictor that helps counteract the painful dilation stage of the headache; propanalol hydrochloride, which reduces the severity and frequency; and verapamil, a calcium channel blocker; are also helpful (Goadsby & Raskin, 2008; NINDS, n.d.e.).

NURSING MANAGEMENT

When there is no organic cause (i.e., tumor, structural cause) children and their families will need reassurance. Pain relief, biofeedback, relaxation exercises, and stress management techniques, as well as avoiding triggers, may be helpful. Watching for side effects and therapeutic results if medications are prescribed is important. If headaches cause the child to miss school, activities should be restricted to bed and the child allowed to do homework. If headache pain diminishes during a school day, the child should return to school.

FAMILY TEACHING

The family should initially be educated about headaches, their cause, and treatment. If prophylactic therapy is prescribed, nurses should help families learn how to successfully carry out those therapies and be willing to clarify or assist as needed. Finally, nurses should help families explain the child's condition to teachers if school is missed frequently.

IN THE REAL WORLD

As a student nurse I wondered how I would care for a child who suffered from severe neurological injuries. When youngsters get sick, I think that is something out of their control, but serious neurological injuries can often be prevented. It makes me angry parents do not put their children in car seats or use bike helmets. I spoke with some of the nurses on the floor and in the emergency department about this. They advised me to concentrate on the child's needs; care should be my first priority. When I questioned how to approach "negligent" parents, they told me mothers and fathers sometimes just do not have the correct or up-to-date information to make informed decisions about their child's care and I should be nonjudgmental when dealing with them. If they do have all the information, however, and choose the path of least resistance (such as not using a car seat because the restraints make the child cry), they will probably feel extremely guilty about the incident and I should allow them to vent those feelings. In addition, when the time seems right, I should present information to them on injury prevention.

KEY CONCEPTS

- Differences in the anatomy and physiology of the nervous system from infant to adult include head circumferences, brain weight, cerebrospinal fluid production, myelinization of neurons, and open or closed fontanelles.
- Different types of seizures include partial: complex and simple; generalized: tonic/clonic, absence, myoclonic, and akinetic.
- Management of seizure activity includes maintaining a patent airway and oxygenation, providing a safe environment, and medication administration as indicated.
- Hydrocephalus, an increased amount of CSF within the ventricles, is most often treated with a shunt. Nurses must be aware of the signs and symptoms of shunt infection or failure.
- Neural tube defects range in severity from simple spina bifida occulta to complex meningomyelocele. The defect's type and location determine the level of dysfunction, treatment, and care required.
- Initial signs of arteriovenous malformation include congestive heart failure, cardiomegaly, and a cerebral bruit.
- Meningitis can have a viral or bacterial cause. Signs and symptoms include change in level of consciousness or feeding, irritability, bulging fontanelle (infants), or headache, nuchal rigidity, photophobia, and malaise (child).
- Reye's syndrome usually follows a viral illness, and even though there is a rapid deterioration in patient condition, many survive because of prompt

ventilatory and circulatory support in intensive care settings.

- Head injury is a common cause of childhood morbidity and mortality. Management depends on the particular trauma as well as the child's response.
- Many spinal cord injuries in children do not manifest themselves on radiologic exam.
- The major insult associated with near-drowning is hypoxemia.
- Cerebral palsy is a nonprogressive motor dysfunction caused by damage in the motor areas of the brain. It is most commonly associated with prematurity but it can be caused by other kinds of neurologic trauma as well. Rehabilitation should begin as soon as diagnosis is made, as early therapy promotes improvement in both fine and gross motor skills.
- Families must be closely involved in the planning and management of their neurologically impaired child.
- Headaches, occurring in childhood or adolescence, may be acute or chronic, and manifest as migraine, cluster, or tension.

REVIEW ACTIVITIES

1. Describe a neurologic assessment based on a child's developmental age.
2. Define increased intracranial pressure. List the signs and symptoms associated with it.
3. Differentiate between partial and generalized seizures. Identify the characteristics of each.
4. Explain how the signs and symptoms of hydrocephalus are related to its pathology.
5. Describe the preoperative and postoperative care of the infant with spina bifida.
6. Describe the nursing assessments and interventions for an infant with bacterial meningitis.
7. Discuss the early signs and symptoms of Reye's syndrome.
8. Describe the ABCDE assessment of a neurologically injured child.
9. Explain the initial management of a child with a severely diminished level of consciousness secondary to head trauma.
10. Describe the difference between incomplete and complete spinal cord lesions.
11. Identify the signs and symptoms of a child with a cervical, thoracic, or lumbar cord lesion.
12. Explain the difference between drowning and near-drowning.
13. Describe the processes of both wet and dry drowning.
14. Discuss several characteristics displayed by infants who should be assessed for cerebral palsy.
15. Describe how neurologic pathology may have been averted by using preventive techniques.
16. Describe cluster, migraine, and tension headaches.

STUDY QUESTIONS

1. Which of the following is not an early sign of increased intracranial pressure?
   a. Asymmetrical paralysis
   b. Headache worsened by coughing
   c. Seizures
   d. Sunsetting
2. Which of the following is an incorrect expression of the acronym AVPU?
   a. A = Alert and Awake
   b. V = Visual changes
   c. P = Responsive to painful stimuli
   d. U = Unresponsive
3. When parents report that their child daydreams and is inattentive at school, the nurse recognizes that the child may be experiencing:
   a. Absence seizures
   b. Atonic seizures
   c. Cluster headaches
   d. Migraine headaches
4. The family of a child with frequent seizures asks the nurse about the Ketogenic Diet. The nurse should explain that the Ketogenic diet:
   a. Is unproven and should be avoided.
   b. Can eliminate the need for medication.
   c. May be unpalatable for older children.
   d. Has few side effects.
5. Your patient with hydrocephalus has a shunt in place. You become concerned about a shunt infection when:

a. The child's blood pressure decreases.
b. The child begins vomiting.
c. The child becomes lethargic and has a low grade fever.
d. The child has seizure activity.

6. A child with a meningomyelocele is most likely also to have:
a. Bowel and bladder incontinence.
b. Hydrocephalus.
c. Kyphosis.
d. Scoliosis.

7. Which group of children is most at risk for meningitis?
a. Premature infants in a neonatal care unit
b. Children under the age of 5
c. School-age children
d. Adolescents

8. The most common cause of traumatic head injuries in infants is:
a. Birth injury.
b. Child abuse.
c. Falls.
d. Motor vehicle accidents.

9. Accidental drowning of young children is most likely to occur in:
a. Bath tub
b. Hot tub
c. Ocean
d. Swimming pool

10. The greatest risk factor for developing cerebral palsy is:
a. Birth trauma.
b. Genetics.
c. Low APGAR scores.
d. Prematurity.

REFERENCES

American Academy of Pediatrics Committee on Genetics. (1999). Folic acid for the prevention of neural tube defect (RE9834). *Pediatrics, 104*(2), 325–327.

Beers, M. H., Porter, R. S., Jones, T. V., Kaplan, J. L., & Berkwits, M. (Eds.). (2006). *Merck manual of diagnosis and therapy* (18th ed.). Whitehouse Station, NJ: Merck Research Laboratories.

Bellin, M. H., & Rice, K. M. (2009). Individual, family, and peer factors associated with the quality of sibling relationships in families of youths with spina bifida. *Journal of Family Psychology, 23*(1), 39–47.

Blosser, C. G., & Burns, C. E. (2004). Neurologic disorders. In C. E. Burns, A. M. Dunn, M. A. Brady, N. B. Starr, & C. G. Blosser (Eds.), *Pediatric primary care*. St. Louis: Saunders, pp. 673–705.

Brayden, R. M., Bunik, M., Brown, J. M., & Daley, M. F. (2009). Ambulatory & community pediatrics. In W. W. Hay, Jr., M. J. Levin, J. M. Sondheimer, & R. R. Deterding (Eds.). *Current diagnosis & treatment pediatrics* (19th ed.). New York: McGraw-Hill Professional.

Carreon, L. Y., Glassman, S. D., & Campbell, M. J. (2004). Pediatric spine fractures—A review of 137 hospital admissions. *Journal of Spinal Disorders & Techniques, 17*(6), 477–482.

Children's Hospital and Health System. (n.d.). Pediatric Health Information. *Craniosynostosis*. Retrieved December 21, 2009, from http://www.chw.org/display/PPF/DocID/21810/router.asp.

Crawford, M. J., Lehman, L., Slater, S., Kabbouche, M. A., LeCates, S. L., Segers, A. et al. (2009). Menstrual migraine in adolescents. *Headache: The Journal of Head and Face Pain, 49*(3), 341–347.

Deblaere, K., & Achten, E. (2008). Structural magnetic resonance imaging in epilepsy. *Eur Radiol, 18*, 119–129.

Estes, M. (2010). *Health assessment & physical examination* (4th ed.). Clifton Park, NY: Delmar Cengage Learning.

Ewing-Cobbs, L., Barnes, M. A., & Fletcher, J. M. (2003). Early brain injury in children: Development and reorganization of cognitive function. *Developmental Neuropsychology, 24*(2 & 3), 669–704.

Frankel, L. R. (2007). Neurologic emergencies and stabilization. In R. M. Kliegman, R. E. Behrman, H. B. Jenson, & B. F. Stanton (Eds.), *Nelson textbook of pediatrics* (18th ed.). Philadelphia, PA: Saunders.

Goadsby, P. J., & Raskin, N. H. (2008). Headache. In A. S. Fauci, D. L. Kasper, D. L. Longo, E. Braunwald, S. L. Hauser, J. L. Jameson, & J. Loscalzo (Eds.). *Harrison's principles of internal medicine* (17th ed.). New York: McGraw-Hill Professional.

Haslam, R. H. A. (2007). Spinal cord disorders. In R. M. Kliegman, R. E. Behrman, H. B. Jenson, & B. F. Stanton (Eds.), *Nelson textbook of pediatrics* (18th ed.). Philadelphia, PA: Saunders.

Hay, W. W. Jr., Levin, M. J., Sondheimer, J. M., & Deterding, R. R. (Eds.). (2007). *Current diagnosis & treatment pediatrics* (19th ed.). New York: McGraw-Hill Professional.

HiFY. Hydrocephalus Foundation. (n.d.). *What is hydrocephalus?* Retrieved December 18, 2010, from http://www.hydrocephalus.org/facts/.htm.

Huff, K. (2008). Increased intracranial pressure in C. Berkowitz, (Ed.) Pediatrics: *A primary care approach* (3rd ed.). Elk Grove Village, IL: American Academy of Pediatrics. pp. 287–292.

Integra, *Licox*. (n.d.). Retrieved April 29, 2005, from http://www.integra-ls.com/products/?product548.

Johnston, M. V. (2007a). Seizures in childhood. In R. M. Kliegman, R. E. Behrman, H. B. Jenson, & B. F. Stanton (Eds.). *Nelson textbook of pediatrics* (18th ed.). Philadelphia, PA: Saunders.

Johnston, M. V. (2007b). Enchepalopathies. In R. M. Kliegman, R. E. Behrman, H. B. Jenson, & B. F. Stanton (Eds.), *Nelson textbook of pediatrics* (18th ed.). Philadelphia, PA: Saunders.

Kallas, H. J. (2007). Drowning and submersion injury. In R. M. Kliegman, R. E. Behrman, H. B. Jenson, & B. F. Stanton (Eds.). *Nelson textbook of pediatrics* (18th ed.). Philadelphia, PA: Saunders.

Kimonis, V., Gold, J. A., Hoffman, T. L., Panchal, J., & Boyadjiev, S. A. (2007). Genetics of craniosynostosis. *Seminars in Pediatric Neurology, 14*, 150–161.

Kinsman, S. L., & Johnston, M. (2007). Congenital anomalies of the central nervous system. In R. M. Kliegman, R. E. Behrman, H. B. Jenson, & B. F. Stanton (Eds.). *Nelson textbook of pediatrics* (18th ed.). Philadelphia, PA: Saunders.

Klimo, P., Jr., Rao, G., & Brockmeyer, D. (2007). Pediatric arteriovenous malformations: A 15-year experience with an emphasis on residual and recurrent lesions. *Child's Nervous System, 23*, 31–37.

Lehman, R. K., & Mink, J. (2008). Altered mental status. *Clinical Pediatric Emergency Medicine, 9*(3), 68–75.

Lowenstein, D. H. (2008). Seizures and epilepsy. In A. S. Fauci, D. L. Kasper, D. L. Longo, E. Braunwald, S. L. Hauser, J. L. Jameson & J. Loscalzo (Eds.), *Harrison's principles of internal medicine* (17th ed.). New York: McGraw-Hill Professional.

Mami, A. G., & Nance, M. L. (2008). Management of mild head injury in the pediatric patient. *Advances in Pediatrics, 55*, 385–394.

Mansfield, R. T. (2007). Severe traumatic brain injuries in children. *Clinical Pediatric Emergency Medicine, 8*(3), 156–164.

March of Dimes. (n.d.). *Spina bifida.* Retrieved December 21, 2009, from http://www.marchofdimes.com/pnhec/4439_1224.asp.

Moe, P. G., Benke, T. A., Bernard, T. J., & Levisohn, P. (2009). Neurologic & muscular disorders. In W. W. Hay, Jr., M. J. Levin, J. M. Sondheimer, & R. R. Deterding (Eds.), *Current diagnosis & treatment pediatrics* (19th ed.). New York: McGraw Hill Professional.

Molloy, A. M., Kirke, P. N., Troendle, J. F., Burke, H., Sutton, M., & Brody, L. C. (2009). Maternal vitamin B12 status and risk of neural tube defects in a population with high neural tube defect prevalence and no folic acid fortification. *Pediatrics, 123*(3), 917–923.

Morriss-Kay, G. M., & Wilkie, A. O. M. (2005). Growth of the normal skull vault and its alteration in craniosynostosis: Insights from human genetics and experimental studies. *Journal of Anatomy, 207*, 637–653.

National Institute of Neurological Disorders and Stroke. (n.d.a). *Arteriovenous malformations and other vascular lesions of the central nervous system fact sheet.* Retrieved December 18, 2010, from http://www.ninds.nih.gov/disorders/avms/detail_avms.htm.

National Institute of Neurological Disorders and Stroke. (n.d.b). *NINDS cerebral palsy information page.* Retrieved December 21, 2009, from http://www.ninds.nih.gov/disorders/cerebral_palsy/cerebral_palsy.htm.

National Institute of Neurological Disorders and Stroke. (n.d.c). *NINDS encephalitis and meningitis information page.* Retrieved December 18, 2010, from http://www.ninds.nih.gov/disorders/encephalitis_meningitis/encephalitis_meningitis.htm.

National Institute of Neurological Disorders and Stroke. (n.d.d). *NINDS hydrocephalus information page.* Retrieved December 18, 2010, http://www.ninds.nih.gov/disorders/hydrocephalus/hydrocephalus.htm.

National Institute of Neurological Disorders and Stroke. (n.d.e). *NINDS Headache information page.* Retrieved December 18, 2010, from http://www.ninds.nih.gov/disorders/headache/headache.htm.

National Institute of Neurological Disorders and Stroke. (n.d.f). *NINDS Spinal cord injury information page.* Retrieved December 18, 2010, from http://www.ninds.nih.gov/disorders/sci/sci.htm.

National Institute of Neurological Disorders and Stroke. (n.d.g). *NINDS Traumatic brain injury information page.* Retrieved December 18, 2010, from http://www.ninds.nih.gov/disorders/tbi/tbi.htm.

National Institute of Neurological Disorders and Stroke. (n.d.h). *Reye's Syndrome Information Page.* Retrieved December 18, 2010, from http://www. ninds.nih.gov/disorders/reyes_syndrome/reyes_syndrome.htm.

Odding, E., Roebroeck, M. E., & Stam, H. J. (2006). The epidemiology of cerebral palsy: Incidence, impairments and risk factors. *Disability & Rehabilitation, 28*(4), 183–191.

Oddson, B. E., Clancy, C. A., & McGrath, P. J. (2006). The role of pain in reduced quality of life and depressive symptomology in children with spina bifida. *Clinical Journal of Pain, 22*(9), 784–789.

Plastic & Craniofacial Surgery for Infants & Children. (n.d.). *Craniosynostosis.* Retrieved April 15, 2009, from http://www.kidsplastsurg.com/skull.cfm.

Prober, C. G. (2007). Central nervous system infections. In R. M. Kliegman, R. E. Behrman, H. B. Jenson, & B. F. Stanton (Eds.), *Nelson textbook of pediatrics* (18th ed.). Philadelphia, PA: Saunders.

Roos, K. L., & Tyler, K. L. (2008). Meningitis, encephalitis, brain abscess, and emphysema. In A. S. Fauci, D. L. Kasper, D. L. Longo, E. Braunwald, S. L. Hauser, J. L. Jameson & J. Loscalzo (Eds.), *Harrison's principles of internal medicine* (17th ed.), New York: McGraw-Hill Professional.

Ropper, A. H., & Brown, R. H. (2005). *Adams and Victor's principles of neurology* (8th ed.). New York: McGraw-Hill.

Rotenstein, D., & Bass, A. N. (2004). Treatment to near adult stature of patients with myelomeningocele with recombinant human growth hormone. *Pediatric Endocrinology & Metabolism, 17*(9), 1195–2000.

Rowe, D. E., & Jadhav, A. L. (2008). Care of the adolescent with spina bifida. *Pediatric Clinics of North America, 55*(6), 1359–1374.

Schreiber, D. (2004). *Spinal cord injuries.* Retrieved December 21, 2009, from http://www.emedicine.com/EMERG/topic553.htm.

Shepherd, S., & Martin, J. (2005). *Submersion injury, near drowning.* Retrieved April 29, 2005, from http://www.emedicine.com/emerg/topic744.htm.

Shore, C. P., Perkins, S. M., & Austin, J. K. (2007). The Seizures and Epilepsy Education (SEE) Program for families of children with epilepsy: A preliminary study. *Epilepsy & Behavior, 12*(1), 157–164.

Tomlinson, J. K., & Breidahl, A. F. (2007). Anterior fontanelle morphology in unilateral coronal synostosis: A clear clinical (nonradiographic) sign for the diagnosis of frontal plagiocephaly. *Plastic and Reconstructive Surgery, 19*(6), 1882–1888.

Venes, D. (Ed.). (2009). *Taber's cyclopedic medical dictionary* (21st ed.). Philadelphia: FA Davis.

Vogel, L., & Anderson, C. (2003). Spinal cord injuries in children and adolescents: A review. *Journal of Spinal Cord Medicine, 26*, 193–203.

Wellington, M. C., & Wayner, R. F. (1995). Alterations in neurologic function. In J. Ball & R. Bindler (Eds.), *Pediatric nursing: Caring for children.* Norwalk, CT: Appleton and Lange.

Wetzler, L. M. (2008). Meningococcal infections. In A. S. Fauci, D. L. Kasper, D. L. Longo, E. Braunwald, S. L. Hauser, J. L. Jameson & J. Loscalzo (Eds.), *Harrison's principles of internal medicine* (17th ed.). New York: McGraw-Hill Professional.

Wilson, P. E., & Clayton, G. H. (2009). Rehabilitation medicine. In W. W. Hay, Jr., M. J. Levin, J. M. Sondheimer, & R. R. Deterding (Eds.), *Current diagnosis & treatment pediatrics* (19th ed.). New York: McGraw Hill Professional.

Zadeh, G., Andrade-Souza, Y. M., Tsao, M. N., Scora, D., Armstrong, D., Humphreys, R. et al. (2007). Pediatric arteriovenous malformation: University of Toronto experience using sterotactic radiosurgery. *Childs Nervous System, 23*, 195–199.

SUGGESTED READINGS

Anderson, V. A., Catroppa, C., Dudgeon, P., Morse, S. A., Haritou, F., Rosenfeld, J. V. (2006). Understanding predictors of functional recovery and outcome 30 months following early childhood head injury. *Neuropsychology, 20*(1), 42–57.

Araki, T., Drake, J. M., Rutka, J. T., Dirks, P. B., Yokota, H., & Yamamoto, Y. (2006). Clinical diagnosis and treatment of pediatric head trauma. *Neurological Surgery, 34*(2), 135–146.

Awaad, Y. M. (2007). Safety and efficacy of high doses of botox in the treatment of cerebral palsy. *European Journal of Neurology, 14,* 152.

Bayona, C. L. (2006). School-based occupational therapy for children with fine motor difficulties: Evaluating functional outcomes and fidelity of services. *Physical & Occupational Therapy in Pediatrics, 26*(3), 89–110.

Bello, D. (2007). Hypothermia. *Family Safety & Health, 66*(4), 28–29.

Bjornson, K., Hays, R., Graubert, C., Price, R., Won, F., McLaughlin, J. F. et al. (2007). Botulinum toxin for spasticity in children with cerebral palsy: A comprehensive evaluation. *Pediatrics, 120*(1), 49–58.

Bulechek, G. M., Butcher, H. K., & Dochterman, J. M. (2008). *Nursing Interventions Classification (NIC)* (5th ed.). St. Louis, MO: Mosby.

Coley, B. D., & Kosnik, E. J. (2006). Abdominal complications of ventriculoperitoneal shunts in children. *Seminars in Ultrasound, CT, and MRI, 27*(2), 152–160.

Dalen, K., Bruaroy, S., Wentzel-Larsen, T., Nygaard, M., & Laegreid, L. M. (2006). Non-verbal learning disabilities in children with infantile hydrocephalus, aged 4–7 years: A population-based, controlled study. *Neuropediatrics, 37*(1), 1–5.

Dennis, M., Edelstein, K., Hetherington, R., Copeland, K., Frederick, J., Blaser, S. E. et al. (2004). Neurobiology of perceptual and motor timing in children with spina bifida in relation to cerebellar volume. *Brain, 127*(6), 1292–1301.

Dumas, H. M., Haley, S. M., Ludlow, L. H., & Carey, T. M. (2004). Recovery of ambulation during inpatient rehabilitation: Physical therapist prognosis for children and adolescents with traumatic brain injury. *Physical Therapy, 84*(3), 232–242.

Elgamal, E. A., Elwatidy, S., Zakaria, A. M., & Abdel-Raouf, A. A. (2008). Spinal cord injury without radiological abnormality (SCIWORA): A diagnosis that is missed in unconscious children. *Neurosciences, 13*(4), 437–440.

Eliasson, A., Krumlinde-Sundholm, L., Shaw, K., & Wang, C. (2005). Effects of constraint-induced movement therapy in young children with hemiplegic cerebral palsy: An adapted model. *Developmental Medicine & Child Neurology, 47,* 266–275.

Fenichel, G. M. (2005). *Clinical pediatric neurology: A signs and symptoms approach* (5th ed.). Philadelphia: W. B. Saunders.

Gibson, C. S., Maclennan, A. H., Goldwater, P. N., & Dekker, G. A. (2008). The antenatal causes of cerebral palsy? Genetic and viral associations. *Fetal & Maternal Medicine Review, 19*(3), 181–201.

Gupta, N., Park, J., Solomon, C., Kranz, D. A., Wrensch, M., & Wu, Y. W. (2007). Long-term outcomes in patients with treated childhood hydrocephalus. *Journal of Neurosurgery, 106*(5), 334–339.

Haley, S. M., Dumas, H. M., Rabin, J. P., & Ni, P. (2003). Early recovery of walking in children and youths after traumatic brain injury. *Developmental Medicine & Child Neurology, 45,* 671–675.

Hammar, G. R. (2009). Body image in adolescents with cerebral palsy. *Journal of Child Health, 13*(1), 19–29.

Hurlbert, R. J. (2008). Methylprednisolone for acute spinal cord injury: 5-year practice reversal. *Canadian Journal of Neurological Sciences, 35*(1), 41–45.

Hwang, H., & Kim, K. J. (2008). New antiepileptic drugs in pediatric epilepsy. *Brain & Development, 30*(9), 549–555.

Ibsen, L. M., & Koch, T. (2002). Submersion and asphyxial injury. *Critical Care Medicine, 30*(11), S402–S408.

Jackson, A. P., & Vessey, J. (2004). *Primary care of the child with a chronic condition* (4th ed.). St. Louis, MO: Mosby.

Johnson, K. A., & Klaas, S. J. (2007). The changing nature of play: Implications for pediatric spinal cord injury. *Journal of Spinal Cord Medicine, 30,* S71–S75.

Kamienski, M. C. (2003). Reye syndrome. *The American Journal of Nursing, 103*(7), 54–57.

Lee, P., & DiPatri, A. J. (2008). Evaluation of suspected cerebrospinal fluid shunt complications in children. *Clinical Pediatric Emergency Medicine, 9*(2), 76–82.

Lomax-Bream, L. E., Taylor, H. B., Landry, S. H., Barnes, M. A., Fletcher, J. M., & Swank, P. (2007). Role of early parenting and motor skills on development in children with spina bifida. *Journal of Applied Developmental Psychology, 8*(3), 250–263.

Lukban, M. B., Rosales, R. L., Dressler D. (2009). Effectiveness of botulinum toxin A for upper and lower limb spasticity in children with cerebral palsy: A summary of evidence. *Journal of Neural Transmission, 116*(3), 319–331.

Mackway-Jones, K. (2008). Dexamethasone in meningitis. *Emergency Medical Journal, 25*(1), 39–40.

Maltais, D. B., Pierrynowski, M. R., Galea, V. A., Matsuzaka, A. & Bar-Or, O. (2005). Habitual physical activity levels are associated with biomechanical walking economy in children with cerebral palsy. *American Journal of Physical Medicine & Rehabilitation, 84,* 36–45.

Mammarella, M., Cornoldi, C., & Donadello, E. (2003). Visual but not spatial working memory deficit in children with spina bifida. *Brain and Cognition, 53,* 311–314.

Meinecke, L., Breitbach-Faller, N., Bartz, C., Damen, R., Rau, G., & Disselhorst-Klug, C. (2006). Movement analysis in the early detection of newborns at risk for developing spasticity due to infantile cerebral palsy. *Human Movement Science, 25*(2), 125–144.

Menkes, J., & Sarnat, H. (2005). *Child neurology* (7th ed.). Philadelphia: Lippincott Williams & Wilkins.

Montouris, G. D., Pellock, J. M., & Schachter, S. C. (2007). Epilepsy on our terms: Stories by children with seizures and their parents. New York: Oxford University Press.

Moorhead, S., Johnson, M., Maas, M., & Swanson, E. (2008). *Nursing Outcomes Classification (NOC)* (4th ed.). St. Louis, MO: Mosby.

Nadeau, L. (2009). Social adjustment at school: Are children with cerebral palsy perceived more negatively by their peers than other at-risk children? *Disability & Rehabilitation, 31*(4), 302–308.

NANDA International, (2009). *Nursing diagnoses: Definitions and classifications 2009–2011.* New Jersey: Wiley-Blackwell.

National Institute of Neurological Disorders and Stroke. (n.d.). *NINDS Reye's syndrome information page.* Retrieved April 15, 2009, from http://www.ninds.nih.gov/disorders/reyes_syndrome/reyes_syndrome.htm.

Neal, E. G., Chaffe, H., Schwartz, R. H., Lawson, M. S., Edwards, N. Fitzsimmons, G. et al. (2008). The ketogenic diet for the treatment of childhood epilepsy: A randomised controlled trial. *The Lancet Neurology, 7*(6), 471–472.

Nield, L. S., Brunner, M. D., & Kamat, D. (2007). The infant with a misshapen head. *Clinical Pediatrics, 46*(4), 292–298.

Nordmark, E., Josenby, A. L., Lagergren, J., Andersson, G., Stromblad, L. G., & Westbom, L. (2008). Long-term outcomes five years after selective dorsal rhizotomy. *BMC Pediatrics, 8*(540).

Platenkamp, M., Hanlo, P. W., Fischer, K., & Gooskens, R. H. (2007). Outcome in pediatric hydrocephalus: A comparison between previously used outcome measures and the Hydrocephalus Outcome Questionnaire. *Journal of Neurosurgery, 107*(1), 26–31.

Pollard, A. J., Nadel, S., Ninis, N., Faust, S. N., & Levin, M. (2007). Emergency management of meningococcal disease: Eight years on. *Archives of Disease in Childhood, 92*(4), 283–286.

Proctor, M. R. (2002). Spinal cord injury. *Critical Care Medicine, 30* (11), S489–S499 Suppl. S.

Rey, E., Bulteau, C., Motte, J., Tran, A., Sturm, Y., D'Souza, J., et al. (2004). Oxcarbazepine pharmacokinetics and tolerability in children with inadequately controlled epilepsy. *Journal of Clinical Pharmacology, 44*, 1290–1300.

Rosenblum, R. K. (2005). Brain stem glioma: Two case studies. *Journal of Pediatric Oncology Nursing, 22*, 114–118.

Rosenbaum, P. (2009). A randomized controlled trial of the impact of therapeutic horse riding on the quality of life, health, and function of children with cerebral palsy. *Developmental Medicine & Child Neurology, 51*(2), 111–119.

Schaan, M., Jaksche, H., & Boszczyk, B. (2002). Predictors of outcome in head injury: Proposal of a new scaling system. *Journal of Trauma, 52*(4), 667–674.

Schoenmakers, M., Gulmans, V., Gooskens, R., & Helders, P. (2004). Spina bifida at the sacral level: More than minor gait disturbances. *Clinical Rehabilitation, 18*, 178–185.

Shavelle, R. M., DeVivo, M. J., Paculdo, D. R., Vogel, L. C., & Strauss, D. J. (2007). Long-term survival after childhood spinal cord injury. *Journal of Spinal Cord Medicine, 30*, S48–S54.

Van Empelen, R., Jennekens-Schinkel, A., Van Rijen, P. C., Helders, P. M. M., & Van Nieuwenhuizen, O. (2005). Health-related quality of life and self-perceived competence of children assessed before and up to two years after epilepsy surgery. *Epilepsia, 46*(2), 258–271.

Vargus-Adams, J. (2009). Quality of life for adolescents with cerebral palsy: Perspectives of adolescents and parents. *Developmental Medicine & Child Neurology, 51*(3), 169–170.

Vogel, L. C. (2007). Ambulation in children and youth with spinal cord injuries. *Journal of Spinal Cord Medicine, 30*, S158–S164 Suppl. 1.

Wu, K. N., Lieber, E., Siddarth, P., Smith, K., Sankar, R., Caplan, R. (2008). Dealing with epilepsy: Parents speak up. *Epilepsy & Behavior, 13*(1), 131–138.

Yuceer, N., & Semra, K. (2008). Ventriculosubgaleal shunt in a premature infant with posthemorrhagic hydrocephalus. *Journal of Pediatric Neurology, 6*(1), 65–68.

Zickler, C. F., & Richardson, V. (2004). Achieving continence in children with neurogenic bowel and bladder. *Journal of Pediatric Health Care, 18*(6), 276–283.

Zuckerbraun, N. S., & Saladino, R. A. (2005). Pediatric drowning: Current management strategies for immediate care. *Clinical Pediatric Emergency Medicine, 6*(1), 49–56.

RESOURCES

Refer to the online student StudyWARE for Potts & Mandleco at http://www.CengageBrain.com for additional content and study aids.

Organization: **American Liver Foundation**
Description: Offers information about organization divisions, educational resources, and events as well as specific information for parents/families and health care professionals.
Website/Resource: http://www.liverfoundation.org

Organization: **Brain Injury Association of America**
Description: Offers information about brain injuries, state offices, media/events, policy/legislation, and research.
Website/Resource: http://www.biausa.org

Organization: **Brain Trauma Foundation**
Description: Offers information regarding news, education, and helpful resources related to brain trauma.
Website/Resource: http://www.braintrauma.org

Organization: **Christopher Reeve Paralysis Foundation**
Description: Offers access to information regarding community forums, educational videos, and research regarding spinal injuries/paralysis.
Website/Resource: http://www.christopherreeve.org

Organization: **Epilepsy Foundation**
Description: Offers information regarding research and advocacy as well as basic data about seizures and life with epilepsy.
Website/Resource: http://www.epilepsyfoundation.org

Organization: **March of Dimes**
Description: Provides information regarding March of Dimes professionals/researchers, and pregnancy/newborn conditions.
Website/Resource: http://www.marchofdimes.com

Organization: **Meningitis Foundation of America**
Description: Helps support families/sufferers of meningitis; educates public/medical professionals about meningitis; supports vaccines development/other methods of preventing meningitis; offers information about support, resources, contributions, forums, and news/media.
Website/Resource: http://www.musa.org

Organization: **National Easter Seals Society**
Description: Offers information about different programs focuses, services, and expert connections for people living with autism and other disabilities.
Website/Resource: http://www.easterseals.com

Organization: **National Headache Foundation**

Description: The National Headache Foundation exists to enhance the health of headache sufferers. The website offers users information about programs, blogs, clinical trials, and headache education.

Website/Resource: http://www.headaches.org

Organization: **National Hydrocephalus Foundation**

Description: Offers information about treatment, articles, stories, and survey results about/for hydrocephalus.

Website/Resource: http://www.nhfonline.org

Organization: **National Dissemination Center for Children with Disabilities**

Description: Offers information about child disabilities for families/communities, early intervention providers, school/administration, and state agencies.

Website/Resource: http://www.nichcy.org

Organization: **National Institute of Neurological Disorders and Stroke**

Description: Offers information about neurological disorders as well as institute news, research funding, and training/career awards.

Website/Resource: http://www.ninds.nih.gov

Organization: **National Spinal Cord Injury Association (NSCIA)**

Description: Offers access to an online store, forums, association news, and membership information for people with spinal cord injuries and diseases (SCI/D).

Website/Resource: http://www.spinalcord.org

Organization: **Safe Kids**

Description: Offers information regarding public policy, programs, research, and safety tips as well as access to an online media center.

Website/Resource: http://www.safekids.org

Organization: **Spina Bifida Association of America (SBAA)**

Description: Offers information regarding SBAA programs/services/events, and chapters as well as access to an online marketplace.

Website/Resource: http://www.sbaa.org

Organization: **United Cerebral Palsy**

Description: Offers information about disability education, employment, housing, sports/leisure, products/services, and transportation related to people with cerebral palsy.

Website/Resource: http://www.ucp.org

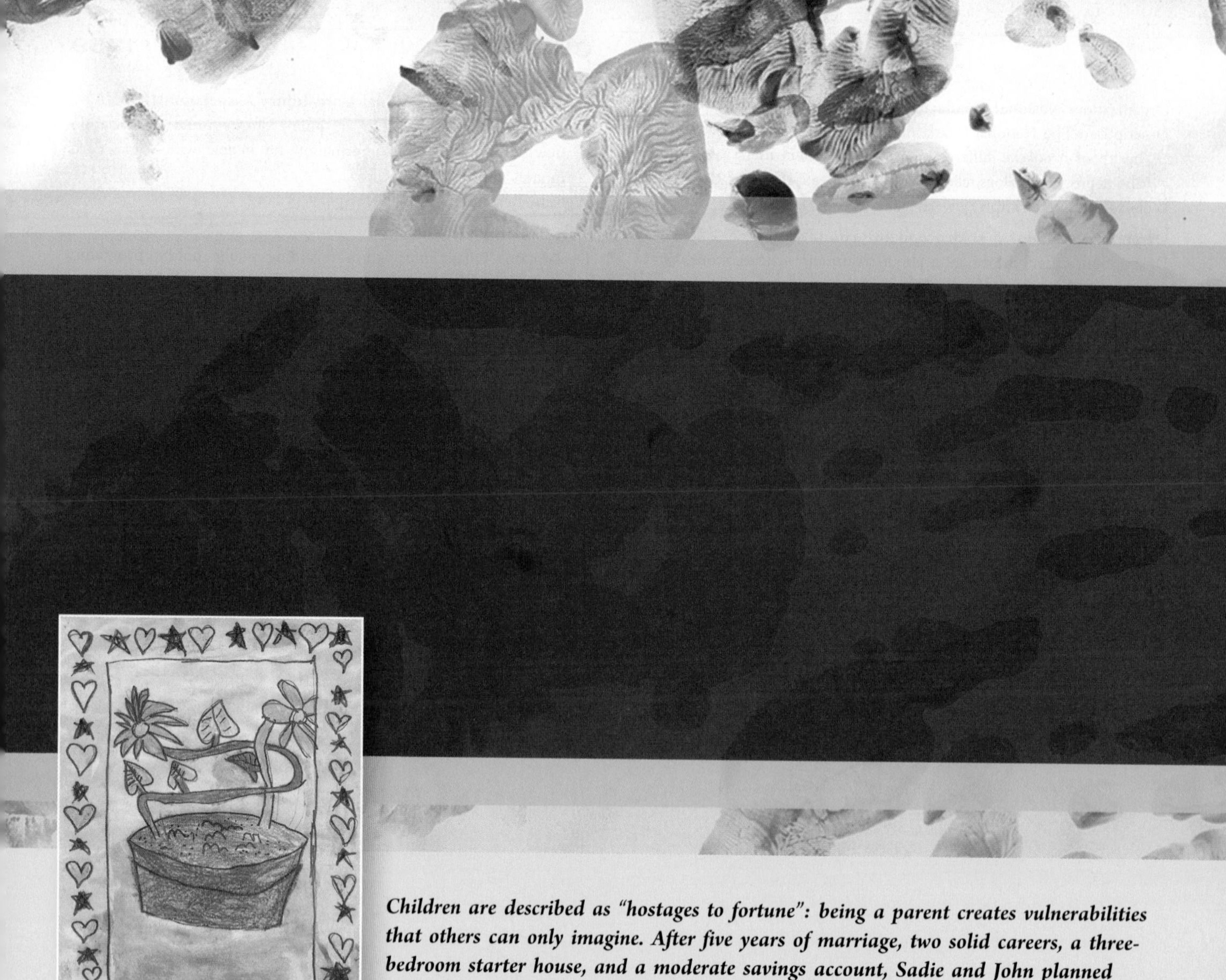

Children are described as "hostages to fortune": being a parent creates vulnerabilities that others can only imagine. After five years of marriage, two solid careers, a three-bedroom starter house, and a moderate savings account, Sadie and John planned their eldest child's birth for early spring. When Sadie was pregnant with the third and last baby, their 3-year-old Philip was diagnosed with mental retardation. Guilt, questions about how this was caused, concern for their subsequent children's health, and worry soon gave way to digging in, doing their utmost for all of their children, and making family life the best it could be.

Now in her late 60s, Sadie explains, "Having a mentally retarded child changed our dreams, changed the size of, and plans for, our family, and made us experts at something we never planned to understand. Despite the work of raising Philip, at age 28 he has a vulnerable sweetness that others cannot touch, and in many ways he remains the dearest of our children."

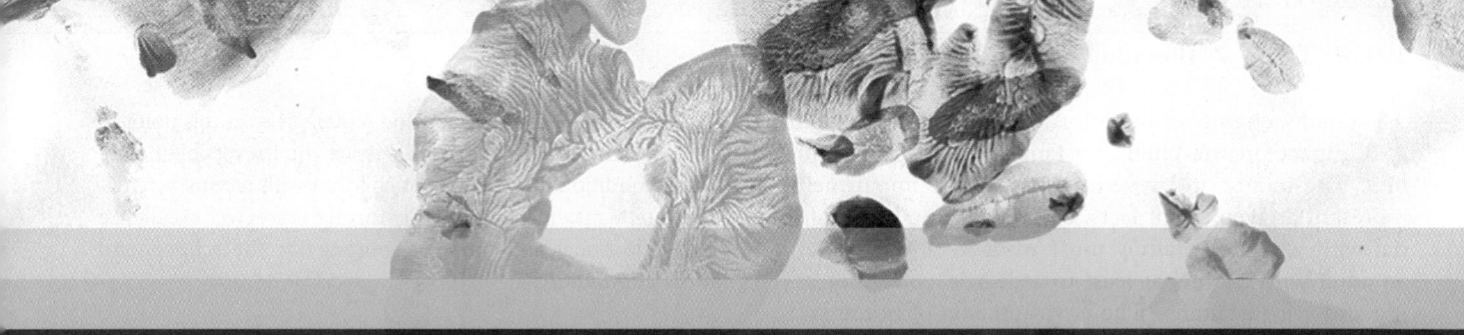

CHAPTER 33
Cognitive Alterations

SUZANNE SUTHERLAND, RN, PhD

COMPETENCIES

Upon completion of this chapter, the reader will be able to:

- Discuss the various causes of mental retardation.
- Describe the characteristics of a child with mental retardation.
- Discuss at least three commonly used tests for evaluating the presence and extent of mental retardation.
- Describe the appearance and behaviors of a child with Down syndrome, a child with fragile X syndrome, and a child with autism.
- Discuss the family's reaction to having a child with a cognitive alteration and the anticipated grieving process.
- Formulate a plan of care for the family and the child with a cognitive alteration.
- Successfully complete the games and activities in the online student StudyWARE.

A child's cognitive alteration or impairment has an impact on the child, the family, and the community. The nature and severity of a specific impairment represent a given set of facts, embodying the raw material with which the family must work in order to craft an adult who can be, at least to a degree, communicating and self-sustaining. The environments of home and school then become the variables, the factors that can be altered in order to maximize the child's ability to eventually function in the adult world.

This chapter presents an overview of mental retardation and the manner in which it is identified and quantified in children. Down syndrome, fragile X syndrome, and fetal alcohol syndrome, the three most prevalent syndromes associated with mental retardation, are presented. The symptom cluster autism is described, with its probable causation and most common treatment modality.

MENTAL RETARDATION

Mental retardation is defined as significantly subaverage general intellectual functioning manifested before age 18, with limited adaptive skills in at least two or more areas of functioning: communication, self-care, home living, social or interpersonal skills, use of community resources, self-direction, functional academic skills, health and safety, work, and leisure (American Psychiatric Association, 2000). It is, at this point in time, an unalterable condition. Despite the irreversible nature of the condition, the abilities of children with mental retardation can be maximized, primarily through caregiver excellence and educational and training programs in the schools and in the community.

> **REFLECTIVE THINKING**
>
> **Valuing Cognitively Impaired Children**
>
> Cognitive alterations in children produce effects upon the child, the family, and the whole of society. Humans revel in their ability to conceptualize. Some of their richest delight is grounded in their own cleverness. Like peacocks, they are possessed of an array of gifts that they confidently flaunt for purposes of befriending, courtship, or dominance. Unlike peacocks, whose brains are a disappointing contrast to their stunning green and blue plumage, humans are, at turns, witty, creative, amusing, cynical, or profound. They draw others to them, using their scintillating mental attributes as coin.
>
> How then do humans as a society value a person with a cognitive alteration? How can we bright and educated humans reevaluate our self-serving stance of "brighter is better" to embrace humans on a multifaceted basis of worth that is grounded in philosophical and spiritual beliefs, as well as in the egotism of our own cognitive endowments? How can we value the child who is cognitively impaired and transmit wholly and sincerely to the caregivers that the child is indeed respected and unique, and of inestimable worth?

INCIDENCE AND ETIOLOGY

The incidence of mental retardation is estimated to be about 2.5% in the general population (Schwartz, 2005; Shapiro & Batshaw, 2007). This percentage is greater than the number of children actually identified as mentally retarded, possibly because of reluctance to identify children as mildly affected because that "labels" them. It may exist in isolation or in a **syndrome** (a named condition characterized by a group of findings or attributes), such as Down syndrome or fetal alcohol syndrome. Identifiable causes of mental retardation can be categorized as genetic, prenatal, perinatal, or postnatal. Genetic causes may be purely genetic or a combination of genetic and environmental. Prenatal causes may be environmental, chemical, or infectious. Perinatal causes may be environmental, perfusion-related, oxygen-related, chemical, traumatic, or infectious. Postnatal causes may be perfusion-related, oxygen-related, chemical, traumatic, or infectious. Table 33-1 lists categories and examples of etiologies of mental retardation.

PATHOPHYSIOLOGY

In general, mental retardation is associated either with syndromes in which genetic or structural differences in the brain affect its physiology, or with damaged or absent cerebral structures. The former case is found in infants who are born with genetic variants or intracranial lesions. The latter case is typical of children who have suffered hypoxic brain damage resulting from perinatal mishap or from accidents in the developmental years.

Plasticity refers to the ability of neural cells in a certain area of the brain to assume the functions of a different area, or to the ability of the brain to act as a computer does in rerouting signals around a nonfunctioning piece of circuitry (Tranquillo, 2008). Because the brain of the neonate displays considerable anatomic plasticity, portions of an infant's brain are able to assume functions not ordinarily performed in those areas and substitute for those lost through a hypoxic incident or to develop complementary abilities that compensate for deficits (Kolb & Fantie, 2009). The older child's brain relies most heavily upon rerouting around injured areas made possible because of the child's or adolescent's "extra" synapses that can serve in a reserve capacity (Kolb & Fantie, 2009).

CLINICAL MANIFESTATIONS

Clinical manifestations vary according to the severity of mental retardation, which can be classified as mild, moderate, severe, and profound (American Psychiatric Association

Table 33-1 Categories and Examples of Causes of Mental Retardation

CAUSE	EXAMPLE
Genetic	
Entirely genetic	Down syndrome
Combination of genetic and environmental	Anencephaly
Prenatal	
Environmental	Profound maternal acid-base balance disorder
Chemical	Maternal ingestion of drugs and alcohol
Infectious	Maternal rubella
Perinatal	
Environmental	Maternal exposure to a powerful toxin, low birth weight, prematurity
Perfusion-related	Premature placental separation
	Umbilical cord kinking
Oxygen-related	Maternal asphyxia
Chemical	Maternal overdose
Traumatic	Intrapartal brain injury
Infectious	Maternal cytomegalovirus
Postnatal	
Perfusion-related	Severe shock
Oxygen-related	Aspiration of a foreign object
	Drowning
Chemical	Poisoning
Traumatic	Cranial injury, especially motor vehicle accidents and child abuse
Infectious	Meningitis, encephalitis

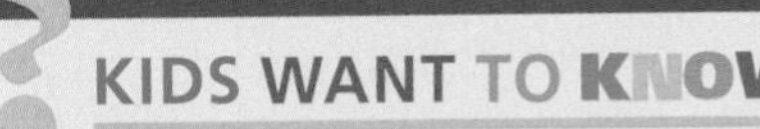

Will my kids be mentally retarded?

I'm Kenny. My sister Joellen is mentally retarded. I'm 18 and my girlfriend Carrie and I are getting married some day. I want to know if we'll have retarded children, or if we should just skip having a family.

Answer: Kenny, we all dream about our futures, and we need to do this. Of course, you're wondering what life with Carrie would be like. You need to find out more about why your sister Joellen is mentally retarded. A few causes of mental retardation run in families but most do not. If you can talk to your parents, you can let them know this is worrying you. Your family physician or nurse practitioner, or a geneticist recommended by them, will be able to explain Joellen's type of mental retardation and what the chances are that you and Carrie could have a baby with the same type of impairment.

[APA], 2000). Mild mental retardation is the most common type. Infants with mild degrees of mental retardation are often not identified as mentally retarded by observers. However, during infancy and early childhood, the caregiver may note **developmental delays** (achievement of developmental milestones later than expected) in language acquisition, social development, and motor skills. Many children with mild mental retardation remain undiagnosed until primary grades, when they manifest delays in academic cognates such as reading or arithmetic. Eventually with special education, they can acquire these skills at a third- to sixth-grade level, and can learn the rules that govern social exchanges. In adulthood, many persons with mild mental retardation live independently, working in the community.

Children with moderate mental retardation display obvious delays in motor development and speech; yet, they can learn self-help activities. During the school-age years, they can learn simple methods to communicate, basic health and safety habits, and simple manual skills. They may benefit from vocational training, but seldom progress academically beyond the second-grade level. As adults, persons with moderate mental retardation are usually able to work, and most live in supervised settings.

With severe mental retardation, children typically acquire little if any communicative speech during preschool years, but may learn some language in school years. Education focuses on the basics of independent living skills, such as toileting, bathing, simple communication, self-feeding, and rules of behavior. Severely mentally retarded children usually walk if no other disability is present. Some understanding of speech eventually develops, and they may profit from learning to sight-read words such as *stop, don't walk, quiet, men, women,* and their own names.

Most children with profound mental retardation also have an identified syndrome that limits their abilities, both motor and sensory. They need a highly structured setting with constant monitoring and supervision. Delays are obvious in all developmental areas. Children with profound retardation may display basic emotional responses and may respond to training in using their legs, hands, and muscles of eating, and speech.

NURSING TIP

Sibling Sensitivity

Sisters and brothers of a child with mental retardation are aware that their sibling is different and are changed by the experience. Perhaps as early as the preschool years, but certainly by school age, they experience both protective affection and resentment of the sibling. They begin to feel different from their peers and sometimes even isolated, especially during late school age and adolescence. They may feel reluctant to let new friends and acquaintances know about the sibling. When they meet new people, they often don't know how to bring the subject up. Teenagers can feel very embarrassed by even an average-intelligence sibling's "uncool" mannerisms or appearance; imagine how much greater this can be for the siblings of a child with mental retardation. The nurse should take opportunities to allow the siblings to discuss their feelings.

DIAGNOSIS

The diagnosis of mental retardation is based on the following: (1) a thorough physical examination and history; (2) routine developmental assessments; and finally (3) standardized tests of intellectual and adaptive functioning. These correspond roughly to, "Is this child physically within normal range?" "Is a delay present?" and "How far from average are the child's cognitive functioning and behavior?" The most frequently used developmental assessment tool in the United States is the *Denver Developmental Screening Test II* (DDST-II) (Frankenburg, Dodds, Archer, Shapiro, & Bresnick, 1992). The *Denver II,* designed for screening the child from birth through 6 years, identifies a broad range of ages at which achievement of certain verbal, motor, and social skills is expected. Failure to meet these milestones by the designated age range is labeled a delay. A child who is delayed is screened again in a week or two. If the delay persists, referrals are initiated. Following identification of a persistent delay, various tests may be performed in order to diagnose mental retardation (Table 33-2).

Several scales are used to identify and quantify mental retardation in infants and young children. They are more useful for determining whether severe mental retardation exists. The most commonly used are the Bayley Scales of Infant Development (BSD-II) (Bayley, 1969) and the Wechsler Preschool and Primary Scale of Intelligence-Revised (WPSSI-R) (Wechsler, 1989). The Bayley Scales are designed to be used up to 30 months of age and provide an actual score that corresponds to intelligence. The "Wechsler," used until 7 years of age, also produces a quantification of intelligence. There is a Wechsler scale for children 6 years and older as well (Wechsler, 1991). Testing for children with language and hearing impairments is accomplished with the Peabody picture vocabulary test (Dunn &

TABLE 33-2 Common Tests for the Diagnosis of Mental Retardation

TEST	AGE RANGE	SPECIAL CONSIDERATIONS
Bayley Scales of Infant Development (Bayley, 1969)	1 month to 30 months	Provides scores with a mean of 100
Stanford-Binet Intelligence Scale (4th ed.)	2 years to adulthood	Provides scores with a mean of 100
Wechsler Preschool and Primary Scale of Intelligence—Revised (WPPSI-R)	3 years to 7 years	Provides scores with a mean of 100
Wechsler Intelligence Scale for Children (3rd ed.) (WISC-III)	6 years to 16 years, 11 months	Same as WPPSI-R—scores on this are quite close to scores children obtain years earlier on the WPPSI-R
Peabody Picture Vocabulary Test—Revised	2.5 through 18 years	Designed for the physically or linguistically handicapped—Gives scores with mean of 100
Leiter International Performance Scale—Revised	2 years to 20 years	For hearing-impaired children—Provides scores with a mean of 100
Vineland Adaptive Behavior Scales	Birth to 18 years, also delayed adults	Provides checklist information related to behavior and self-care skills
AAMR Adaptive Behavior Scale	Any age	Provides checklist information related to behavior and self-care skills

Dunn, 1981) or with the Leiter International Performance Scale (Leiter, 1969).

General intellectual functioning is assessed with a standardized test of intelligence quotient (IQ), such as the *Stanford-Binet Intelligence Scale* (Terman & Merrill, 1973). The **intelligence quotient** is the child's functional age on the intelligence test divided by the chronological age and then multiplied by 100. All this yields is a number. A child with a measured IQ that is confirmed as less than 70 on the *Stanford-Binet* (Terman & Merrill, 1973), corroborated by other tests as necessary, is classified as mentally retarded (American Psychiatric Association, 2000).

Examples of tests that assess adaptive skills are the American Association on Mental Retardation's (AAMR) *Adaptive Behavior Scale* (Nihira, Foster, Shellhaas, & Leland, 1975) and the *Vineland Behavior Scale* (Sparrow, Balla, & Cicchette, 1984). The Vineland Adaptive Behavior Scale, which is not an IQ test, is widely used for assessing ability in the four functional areas of communication, socialization, gross motor, and daily living skills. It is useful for infants, children, and delayed adults.

Children's performance on all tests can fluctuate according to mood, sleep, wellness, attention level, arousal, and many other factors. Because of this, and because the diagnosis of mental retardation is so traumatic for a family, repeated testing before definitive diagnosis is mandatory.

TREATMENT

There is no standard medical treatment of mental retardation; however, an interdisciplinary approach is frequently used. Management is directed toward maintaining the child's health and intervening early to improve the degree of adaptive functioning. Specialized educational and therapeutic services are central elements in the treatment of children with mental retardation. Functionally speaking, however, the child will need more than an average child—extra attention in school, extra time to master some concepts, extra vigilance by caregivers, and extra options by society in order to learn safely how to survive and to reach maximum potential. Educationally, this may include infant stimulation programs, preschools with a low teacher-to-pupil ratio, special education programs in school years, and special work-training programs in secondary and postsecondary education.

FAMILY TEACHING

Teaching is a vital part of planning and implementation. Although this can take the form of teaching actual psychomotor skills to caregivers, the nurse also often functions as interpreter, clarifying for them information from professionals on the interdisciplinary team. The child with mental retardation may not differ at all from an average child, except in delay of developmental milestones. Caregivers may need assistance in teaching the child self-care skills such as self-feeding. If a physical impairment prevents the child from using cups, plates, and utensils, specially designed ones can be obtained (Figure 33-1).

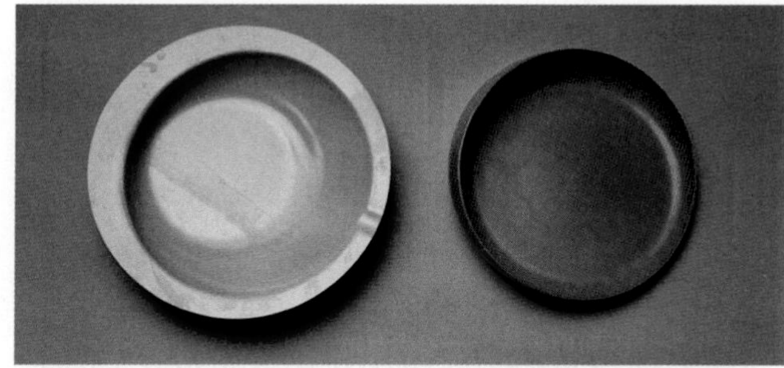

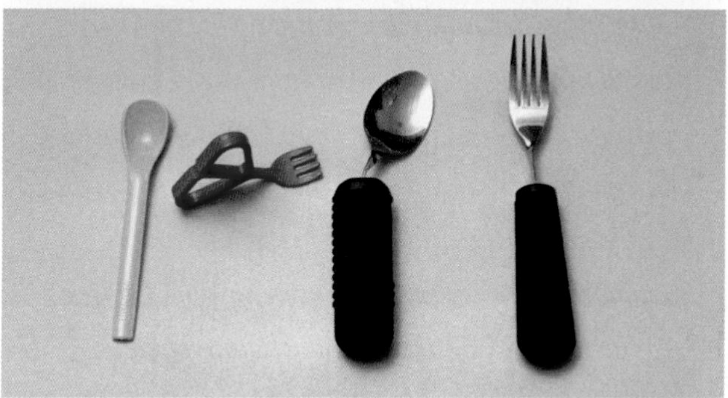

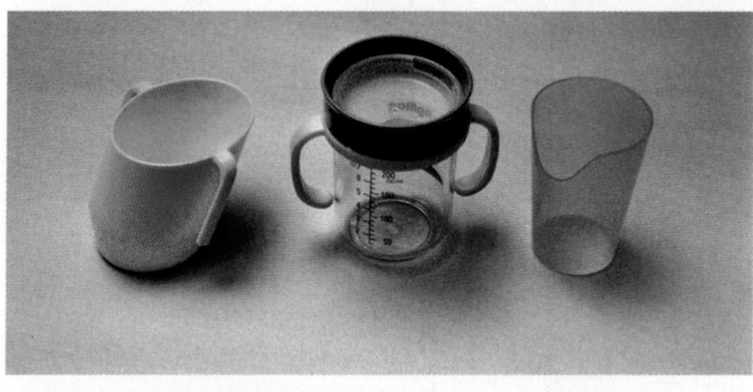

FIGURE 33-1 Several self-care aids are available commercially for the child who displays motor delays in addition to mental retardation. DELMAR CENGAGE LEARNING.

It is important to remember, though, that the caregiver is also a solace person and comforter, not a therapist. The tendency for a caregiver to work at skills for all the child's waking hours should be discouraged. A well-rounded child, whatever his or her IQ, requires singing, cuddling, field trips to malls or zoos, tickling, pretending, visits to playgrounds, laughing, water play, games, and silliness. These activities are almost as important for caregivers as for children.

The nurse needs to decide what bits of knowledge are essential and which are optional. Then the nurse must communicate this real-world knowledge to the caregiver. Sometimes all the caregiver can do is try to get through the next day without mishaps. The nurse has a responsibility to ask whether the caregiver would like to know something and then to prioritize teaching intelligently.

Parents of a child who is mentally retarded may seek genetic counseling in order to make decisions about having subsequent children. (This is more commonly performed when mental retardation exists within an identifiable syndrome or when the child has physical impairments as well.) The nurse can be enormously helpful to the parents,

Reflections from Families

Paul is severely mentally retarded. His brother Vernon is not. In fact, Vern was tested as very mentally gifted at the age of 5, with an IQ of 160, as were his sister and other brother. One day Vern asked me, "Mom, if all three of us gave Paul our extra brains, we'd still be smart enough. Would it be enough to make him normal?" I was so touched by his generosity and by his graciously and magically creative notion that brains, like water to the thirsty, might be siphoned among all the children of the family, for the common good.

both as moral support before counseling and as a person able to remember, clarify, and define medical terms after the process.

THE FAMILY'S RESPONSE TO HAVING A CHILD WITH MENTAL RETARDATION

Imagine for a moment what it is like for caregivers to learn their child will be mentally retarded; developmental milestones will be achieved later than they expected, and they will have to worry about keeping the child safe in a world filled with taunts and exclusions. They will have to endure stares and questions. They will put on their "public face" when they take the child out in the world, uncertain of the degree of warmth or rejection they will encounter. Words like *retard* and *dummy* will burn their ears. They will feel at once defensive on their child's behalf and guilty, feeling in some way responsible.

Many caregivers react with significant grief when they learn that their child is mentally retarded. Ken Moses (Moses and Kearney, 1995) described caregivers' adaptation

Reflections from Families

Mrs. Anderson used to work in the neonatal intensive care unit years ago when my youngest son was born. Peter arrived on the planet, far tinier than my other children, with a complete bilateral cleft lip and palate and hypotonia. He was a very difficult feeder and spent 12 days in the hospital. He would grow up to be deaf, mentally retarded, and autistic, with slight cerebral palsy. But when Peter was an infant, 40 years ago, I didn't know that. In fact, I didn't even know what hypotonia was. I just knew he wasn't as strong as my other children.

Mrs. Anderson took care of him all the days that she worked. She held him carefully. She held my concerns and my heart just as carefully, as she taught me how to feed my little baby with a cross-cut preemie nipple and how to keep him safe. She smiled at him. She beamed at him. She told me, without a word, that he was precious, and decent, and just as lovable as any baby in her nursery. She sent us home and told me to bring him back to see her and she meant it.

For about a year after he was born, every month or so, I would drive over to the hospital and bring Peter to see Mrs. Anderson. I would call up to the nursery and she would come down to see him. She would smile at him, laughing when he finally learned to smile back. She would comment on how big he was getting. After his repair surgeries for the clefts, she would remark on what a good repair he had had. Her approval set the stage for me to value him. Her approval of me made me proud of the good job I did. She did such a beautiful job of supporting my evolving relationship with my son that I never realized that it was part of her job, until years later when I became a nurse.

CASE STUDY / CARE PLAN

A CHILD WITH MENTAL RETARDATION

Amanda was identified at birth with Down syndrome. Her caregivers register her for kindergarten at the local elementary school, and they speak with the school nurse on that day, as well, eliciting her support. The nurse generates a working care plan, based on assessments of Amanda and her family.

NURSING CARE PLAN

ASSESSMENT

School nurses often care for children who have been previously diagnosed with mental retardation but may also be instrumental in identification of children with delays. In the latter case, teachers often speak with the nurse when a child seems unable to keep up with academic work, triggering developmental screening by the school nurse, as well as vision screening, hearing testing, and observations of social behaviors in the classroom and on the playground. History-taking and observation are both appropriate for prevention and health maintenance for children with and without previous diagnoses of mental retardation. For children without defined diagnoses, history-taking must be tactful and nonaccusatory, since questions may include prenatal maternal infection, substance abuse, or trauma. Nurses in office settings may identify infants who exhibit poor tone, decreased responsiveness to environment, poor interaction during feedings, or altered responsiveness to caregivers. These variances should stimulate complete physical and sensory examination to rule out correctable causes. Social and emotional causes are possible but not encountered as frequently.

The rationale for earliest possible assessment, identification, and intervention is the plasticity of the central nervous system and the possibility for decreasing the impact of mental retardation through early childhood enrichment, caregiver support, and preventive care. Whether mental retardation has been previously identified or not, ongoing assessment of the child's caregivers is often overlooked. The child has an effect on the caregivers, and a child with a delay can stimulate both normal and abnormal grieving in them and in the siblings. The caregivers' ability and willingness to provide as much independence as possible will optimize the child's development and progress.

NURSING DIAGNOSIS 1

Impaired social interaction related to developmental delay.

EXPECTED OUTCOME

Child will display adequate social interaction skills, interfacing appropriately with peers, engaging in play, forming friendships, and participating in group activities.

NOC: Social Involvement

NIC: Socialization Enhancement; Teaching: Individual

INTERVENTIONS/*RATIONALES*

1. Remind the caregivers to encourage use of "the golden words" please and thank you. *Use of gracious language acknowledges the goodness of others.*
2. Encourage caregivers to spend time in the classroom, especially during the first few days of school. *Presence of a familiar person provides a feeling of security for the child.*
3. Provide caregivers with information about neighborhood programs that promote peer relationships with the same peers that the child will encounter in the classroom, such as Boy or Girl Scouts, YMCA Guides, and area sports activities of swimming and soccer. *Inclusion in the same activities that the peer group enjoys reinforces social ties.*

(Continues)

CASE STUDY / CARE PLAN (Continued)

4. Give caregivers information about after-school recreational programs sponsored by the school. *Further socialization with the peer group is supported.*
5. Encourage caregivers to volunteer as class tutors, "room parents," or field trip helpers. *The presence of a caregiver helps model acceptance and warmth toward the child and demonstrates that the child is valued and cared for. There is status in having one's caregiver be a class helper, especially in the primary grades.*

EVALUATION

The child begins to display adequate social interaction skills, begins to form friendships, and engages in group activities.

NURSING DIAGNOSIS 2

Grieving related to raising a child with mental retardation.

EXPECTED OUTCOME

The family will proceed through the normal stages of grieving, with support, resolving their issues over time.

NOC: Family Coping; Grief Resolution

NIC: Grief Work Facilitation

INTERVENTIONS/*RATIONALES*

1. Get to know the members of the family, if possible. *Expression of feelings is more likely with a health care professional one knows.*
2. Encourage family members to express fear, guilt, frustrations, and hopes about the child. *Family members talk about the aspects of the grieving process through which they are currently passing. Talking with a trusted person can speed satisfactory process through the various stages of grieving.*
3. If the family is interested, provide bridges to other families also experiencing grieving (children with mental retardation or physical illness). *Sharing can be beneficial, but some families need their privacy and experience peer support as an intrusion.*
4. Provide referrals for family members who appear "stuck" in one certain part of the grieving process (extreme anger, depression, anxiety) and who would benefit by therapeutic assistance. *The anonymity of a therapeutic relationship can be beneficial when the grieving process does not proceed in the usual way.*
5. Provide acceptance of the family's normal stages of grieving through listening and reflecting. *Having an emotion acknowledged is sometimes all that a family member needs in order to feel understood and supported.*

EVALUATION

Caregivers express feelings related to the grieving process, relative to raising a child with mental retardation. They contact and use external resources, if needed. Grieving proceeds along the normal course.

NURSING DIAGNOSIS 3

Delayed growth and development related to cognitive impairment.

EXPECTED OUTCOME

Child will be able to master average academic tasks for kindergarten completion, such as letter and number recognition and copying, simple word recognition, counting, and simple sums.

(Continues)

CASE STUDY / CARE PLAN (Continued)

NOC: Child Development; Knowledge: Parenting

NIC: Developmental Enhancement: Child

INTERVENTIONS/*RATIONALES*

1. Suggest conferences with the teacher at bimonthly intervals during the school year and more frequently as needed. *Caregivers need up-to-date information about the child's academic progress.*
2. If possible, provide at-home materials that duplicate or resemble school books and workbooks. *After-school or evening reading can review materials used in school, reinforcing learning.*
3. Provide the caregivers information about tutors and summer school programs, if they so desire, and if the child appears to benefit by extra coaching. *Some children benefit by extra teaching time, but others do not. Also, the caregivers' priorities might include other enrichments instead.*
4. Teach the caregivers to expect academic success. *Most children with Down syndrome learn to read and write.*

EVALUATION

The child demonstrates steady progress toward mastering academic tasks.

after the birth of a child with an impairment of any kind, for instance mental retardation, club foot, or missing fingers. The grieving process is composed of six principal stages: denial, anxiety, fear, depression, guilt, and anger (Moses & Kearney, 1995) (Box 33-1).

According to Ken Moses (Moses & Kearney, 1995), denial serves the purpose of buying time, delaying the impact of the purported diagnosis until parents can brace themselves and gather strength. Denial can be total denial: denial of the impact upon one's own life, denial of the permanency of the impairment, denial of its extent or seriousness, or denial of the steps one must take in order to create possibilities for oneself and the child. Anxiety serves the purpose of alerting one's family and friends that there is something amiss. It also has the added benefit of contributing energy to the equation. It is almost as if one's unconscious mind declares, "There's an appalling amount of work to do here and I'm going to have to do it!" Parents have experienced the worst thing that they can know: loss of their genetic future, their healthy, perfect child. They are bound to be fearful of what else is in store for them. They may feel depressed and guilty, as they search for reasons, because any cause is better than no identifiable one for such a life-changing event. They feel anger because they have done their best to be healthy during the pregnancy, to diminish risks, to seek prenatal care, and what happened? Despite all their efforts, their dream was crushed, and it just isn't fair.

As Ken Moses explains, the normal grieving process runs its course, and new dreams are generated in the process. Ideally, a mentally retarded baby's smile and sunny disposition become an unforeseen joy. The caregivers come to see the child as unique, important, and irreplaceable. And hopes for the future, new dreams, are crafted by them. Counseling may be helpful for some families so that they can be reassured that their feelings are normal. It may also help families who are immobilized in one stage or another to work through this and subsequent stages. However, with or without counseling, families will eventually progress toward some resolution of their grief.

Nurses can act as sounding boards for families who are grieving. During all phases of grieving over a child's

BOX 33-1

THE GRIEVING PROCESS FOR CAREGIVERS OF A CHILD WITH AN IMPAIRMENT (MOSES & KEARNEY, 1995)

Denial—denial of reality or of one of its aspects; denial of the importance of the reality in one's child's life or in one's own.

Anxiety—a state of chronic uneasiness, often accompanied by physiological symptoms such as hyperventilation, nervousness, or hyperactivity.

Fear—a state of dread, apprehension, or trepidation related to the future.

Depression—overwhelming, heavy, deep sadness or sorrow; the inability to see a clear and positive future.

Guilt—the taking upon oneself of responsibility for a past event.

Anger—rage, indignation, or hostility, born of pain and injury.

impairment, family members can benefit by telling their story, with its feeling and emotion, to someone who listens and cares. For example, parents may be in denial, but they can hear themselves talking about the very issues they are denying when a nurse takes the time to listen. They can, little by little, summon their inner resources, edging close enough to the end of their denial to ask, "What if my daughter really is mentally retarded? What will I do then? What can I do then? How will I act? What can I do for her?"

Nurses frequently interact with individuals with mental retardation, on the job and in private life. The tone that they set in acceptance, in daily living as well as on the job, serves as a role model for members of the community and the health care profession. Nurses have the responsibility and the privilege of being central figures in the growing emancipation and acceptance of individuals with mental retardation and other cognitive alterations.

REFLECTIVE THINKING

Placement When Caregivers Can No Longer Care for Their Child

Ephraim Smith is mentally retarded. He lives at home with his parents, is 18 years old, goes to work at a fast-food restaurant four days a week for five hours each day, eats lunch there, and then goes to a group day care facility. In the evenings he goes home. His life is routine, predictable, and happy. He talks about the events of his day to his mother and father every evening, looks forward to trips and family outings, and is proud to have a job. He collects little plastic animals; teddy bears are his favorite. He has 41 little plastic teddy bears, which are arranged on display stands along the west wall of his room.

Ephraim has an older brother Lee, who has been married and divorced a number of times. He is a very successful attorney, and despite alimony and child care payments, is extremely wealthy. He is in his forties, is a chronic alcoholic, with a tendency to overuse sedatives, and has attempted suicide twice in the past three years. He lives in the same town as Ephraim. Lee wants their parents to make a will stating Ephraim will live with him in case anything happens to them. They are in excellent health now, but are in their late sixties. Lee assures them Ephraim will have everything he wants. The brothers love each other and seem to enjoy one another's company. There are also three sisters; none of them thinks she would be able to take Ephraim at this time, although they are open to the possibility later when their own children are older. What should Ephraim's caregivers do? Should they make a will? Can they trust Lee? What is your opinion about Ephraim's future?

INSTITUTIONALIZATION AND OUT-OF-HOME PLACEMENT

Parents and other caregivers make the difficult decision about whether or not their child with mental retardation will live with them, in their home, not once but many times. Most attempt to raise their children in their homes or nearby, visiting with them when they are able. Those who raise their children at home may do so because it is easier or because they experience less guilt with this arrangement. They make such choices based on what they were taught in their formative years, what their families and friends believe, how their extended families feel, what other children in the home desire, the availability of safe out-of-home placement, the number of other caregivers who are able to share raising of the child, and many other variables about which they are not even aware. Not all parents and caregivers can bear the scenario of trusting their dependent child to others. For them, institutionalization and out-of-home placement are to be avoided at all costs. When placement becomes inevitable, it must be complete, because every brief visit with the child brings back the pain of the original decision.

It is never the nurse's responsibility to make the decision regarding placement. It is, however, the nurse's responsibility to offer information about options. Information about out-of-home placement is usually provided when the caregiver requests it, but it is not inappropriate to broach the subject when the child has achieved certain developmental milestones, such as the end of high school. Caregivers will invariably have thought about placement on their own, and their first reply will be that they are not interested. A wise nurse replies, "Of course you're not. But if you are interested, some day, I will be happy to tell you more."

CRITICAL THINKING

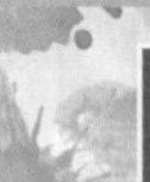

How to Support Caregivers Who Have Been Told Their Child Has a Developmental Delay

You are a school nurse. Alice, the parent of a first grader at your school, comes to your office with her toddler and tells you that the 26-month-old boy Tony has just been identified as developmentally delayed. The pediatrician has referred the child for further "testing" and the worried mother doesn't understand what is wrong and how she can best help her child. Alice has brought a copy of Tony's *Denver Developmental Screening Test II* (DDST-II) with her. What can you do to help her?

SPECIAL OLYMPICS

The Special Olympics organization provides both training and formal athletic events for children and adults with mental retardation. The Special Olympics effort is truly international; the organization has officially sanctioned programs in more than 150 countries. Within the United States and many other countries, schools serve as centers of athletic programs that lead to the Special Olympics competition. The object is to allow participation and competition with people of similar age and ability. Each participant is welcomed as he or she completes an event by a person designated to recognize the effort. These designees bestow a handshake or a hug, sometimes both, upon the contestant. Competitions in the United States and elsewhere boast an array of well-known celebrity, sports, and entertainment figures. The Special Olympics oath further underscores the importance of competition: Let me win. But if I cannot win, let me be brave in the attempt.

DOWN SYNDROME

Down syndrome is a congenital chromosomal disorder and is characterized by varied degrees of mental retardation and a characteristic appearance. Years ago, children with Down syndrome were called mongoloids (or, worse, mongoloid idiots) because their eyes have the epicanthic fold seen in Asian racial groups.

INCIDENCE AND ETIOLOGY

Down syndrome, the most common chromosomal disorder, is usually caused by the presence of an extra chromosome 21 (resulting in three instead of two), hence the name trisomy 21. It occurs in 1 in every 660–800 live births (Descartes & Carroll, 2007; Schwartz, 2005). The incidence has increased somewhat in the United States within the past half century, as more women are postponing childbearing until after 35 years of age. The exact cause of Down syndrome is not known; however, the incidence increases as the mother's age increases. The incidence of Down syndrome for women over 30 years of age is 1 in 1,500, and it increases in women over 40 years to 1 in 100 live births (Schwartz, 2005).

PATHOPHYSIOLOGY

In most children with Down syndrome, every cell of the body contains extra chromosomal material. An extra chromosome in each cell causes the dozens of changes associated with the syndrome. Many of these changes affect musculature or connective tissue. Several changes represent pathophysiological conditions. For example, defects that involve valves or chambers of the heart are common, with 50% of children with Down syndrome having congenital heart disease (Johns Hopkins Hospital et al., 2008).

NURSING ALERT

Cardiac Defects in Neonates with Down Syndrome

Early detection of cardiac defects in neonates with Down syndrome can vastly improve both the duration and the quality of their lives. Defects that produce cyanosis and a heart murmur are almost always detected. However, many heart murmurs are difficult to hear in a newborn, and some cardiac defects do not produce cyanosis. Consequently, major medical centers routinely perform echocardiograms for neonates with Down syndrome. If an infant with Down syndrome in the nurse's care has not received an echocardiogram, it is imperative to obtain an order for this noninvasive screening procedure.

By microscopic examination during chromosome analysis, 4% to 10% of individuals with Down syndrome appear to have 46 chromosomes (Descartes & Carroll, 2007); however, upon closer scrutiny, the genetic material for an extra cell is found attached or translocated onto another chromosome. Rarer still, about 1% of children have some cells with 46 chromosomes and some with 47. Like people with one blue eye and one brown one, they possess two different genetic strains. The presence of two different cell lines in an individual or an organism is called **mosaicism** (Descartes & Carroll, 2007). Children with Down syndrome who have this cellular mosaicism are less severely affected than are children in whom all the cells have 47 chromosomes.

CLINICAL MANIFESTATIONS

Common features of Down syndrome include:

- Muscle weakness and hypotonia
- Oblique palpebral fissures, and an upward slant to the eyes
- A small nose and a depressed nasal bridge
- A large tongue in a small mouth
- A high arched palate
- Square hands with short fifth finger, and a simian (single transverse) crease across the palm of the hand
- A wide space between the great and second toe
- Epicanthic folds (small skin folds at the inner corners of the eyes)

Some children may have only a few of these distinguishing features while others may have many (Figures 33-2 and 33-3). There are numerous physical conditions associated with Down syndrome. Congenital heart defects (especially septal defects) are common. Respiratory tract infections and chronic otitis media occur with greater frequency among children with Down syndrome because of

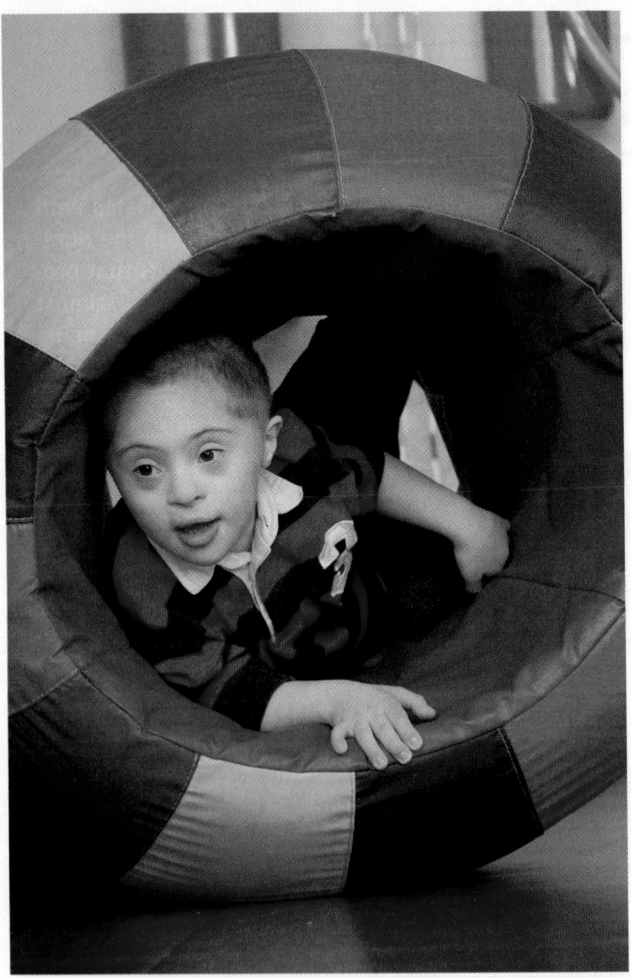

FIGURE 33-2 **Young Boy with Down Syndrome.** DELMAR CENGAGE LEARNING.

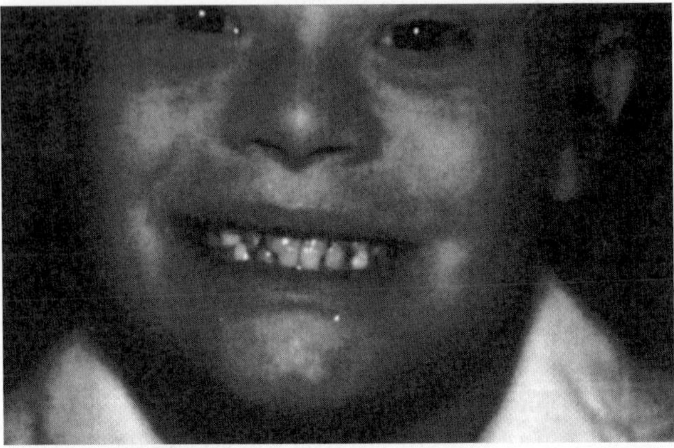

FIGURE 33-3 **Wide Spacing of the Teeth in a Child with Down Syndrome.** DELMAR CENGAGE LEARNING.

hypotonicity of the chest and abdominal muscles, altered immune system, and anatomical differences of the ears (narrow and short eustachian tube). Other problems include gastrointestinal conditions (Hirschsprung's megacolon, tracheoesophageal fistula), hypothyroidism, ocular cataract, **atlantoaxial deformity** (a spinal deformity resulting in instability of the upper cervical spine), leukemia, and Alzheimer's disease after the age of 30 (Descartes & Carroll, 2007; Chen, 2006). The teeth are abnormally aligned and eruption is delayed.

DIAGNOSIS

The presumptive diagnosis of Down syndrome is usually based on the characteristic features alone. Definitive diagnosis is based on **karyotyping**, or identification of the chromosomes' appearance, performed by growing cells from a blood or tissue sample, staining them during the metaphase stage of replication, and scanning them with a microscope. Chromosomes are examined, revealing extra genetic material.

TREATMENT

There is no cure for Down syndrome. However, several physical problems may be present that must be addressed in order to assure the best health possible. The visible stigmata of Down syndrome, the uptilting almond-shaped eyes, enlarged tongue, and flat bridge of the nose can be altered with plastic surgery. This is a highly personal choice and is controversial.

Treatment includes monitoring of growth and development; special growth charts developed for the child with Down syndrome, who tend to be shorter than the average child, can be used. These growth charts are available at http://www.growthcharts.com. In the neonatal period, assessment of cardiac structural integrity is imperative, as are tests of thyroid function, assessment for ocular cataract, and screening of vision and hearing. Symptoms of Hirschsprung's megacolon should be evaluated. Constipation should be addressed with stool softeners and the possibility of Hirschsprung's reevaluated if problems persist. Failure to thrive is a distinct possibility, especially if a heart defect is present. Recurrent otitis media should be referred to an otorhinolaryngologist. The child or adolescent should have a thyroid function test at yearly intervals. Atlantoaxial instability should be frequently assessed.

Early intervention programs include enrichment during the infant, toddler, and preschool years, either within an infant-stimulation or preschool-stimulation program, or with one-on-one time in the home. Modern wisdom stresses the importance of early enrichment programs because of the belief that transneuronal synapses in all babies are profuse but that they extinguish with disuse. Some communities educate children with Down syndrome exclusively in the "mainstream" setting of the public school system. Others maintain special needs schools, in which children are provided academic and social education. Caregivers' beliefs and attitudes, the child's aptitudes, and the community's resources all contribute to the decision about which educational services the family chooses.

Reflections from Families

As I look back on it now, my first recollection of our Theodore, kind of like a snapshot, was when he was just seconds old. The nurse midwife held him up so I could see him and touch him. I wasn't allowed to hold him for the first few minutes, though, because he was pale and blotchy, and a little blue. The nurse rubbed him with a towel and put him under a warmer. I saw that he was pretty floppy, compared with our older girls. Right after birth, their bodies had tended to go back into that egg-shaped newborn roundedness, curling up like Alice's hedgehog. The nurse midwife told me what a beautiful baby boy he was, but then she said she wanted a pediatrician to look at him right away because she was concerned. So then, of course, I was concerned, too. Really, those first hours were like an overcast day, with skies the color of uncertainty. The pediatrician confirmed the nurse midwife's suspicions—here was a little fellow who had a heart defect and who probably had Down syndrome. The pediatrician was honest with me, uncovering Theodore for a more complete physical exam—his skin became even more blotchy when he was chilly. After the exam, I bundled him up. He was very floppy, with noodle-like muscles. Yet all the time we were fussing over him, he never cried but looked placidly at me with his lovely almond eyes.

NURSING MANAGEMENT

The nurse's role in the care of a child with Down syndrome is much the same as that discussed in the section on mental retardation, but it also includes follow-up to confirm that periodic screening is performed for the specific anomalies and malfunctions for which the Down syndrome child is at increased risk. Caregivers of infants need to be aware of the increased likelihood of respiratory infection. If a cardiac defect is present, they must learn about its medical or surgical treatment. If hypothyroidism is present, they need to know how to administer thyroid replacement hormone.

Parents of children with Down syndrome routinely receive genetic counseling and are informed of their relative risk of having subsequent children who also have Down syndrome. But before genetic counseling can be initiated, the family suffers the huge jolt of learning that their infant has a chromosomal disorder. The initial impact upon a family may be immense. Definitive prenatal prediction of Down syndrome involves amniocentesis or chorionic villus sampling (CVS). However, before this invasive and occasionally spontaneous-abortion-inducing procedure is performed, relative risk assessment is arithmetically calculated at the end of the first trimester of pregnancy. Various tests may be used, but common ones include maternal blood testing for serum-alphafetoprotein, unconjugated estriol, human chorionic gonadotropin, pregnancy-induced plasma protein A, and inhibin-A, as well as ultrasound examination of the cervical region of the fetus. Maternal age is also figured into the equation. The resultant decimal provides the relative risk. The decision to perform amniocentesis or chorionic villus sampling is made by the mother, based on this relative risk (Sharpe & Carter, 2006). Use of four blood tests, referred to as the quadruple test, is common practice, and its sensitivity for detecting Down syndrome is 85%, with a false-positive rate of 6.8% (Jacques et al., 2006). Testing may be performed early in the second trimester. With modern gene marker techniques, a one-day result can usually be obtained, followed by confirmation with cell analysis. **Chorionic villus sampling** is a procedure for obtaining prenatal evaluation data in early pregnancy by withdrawing a chorionic villus sample from fetal membranes. Even after a woman is confirmed as carrying a child with Down syndrome, she must then choose whether or not to have an abortion. This is a highly personal choice based on religious and personal beliefs, personal experience, duration of pregnancy, and individual circumstances. The sensitive nurse can provide accurate information and support. The decision must rest with the woman herself, since she will be affected for the rest of her life, regardless of which course she follows.

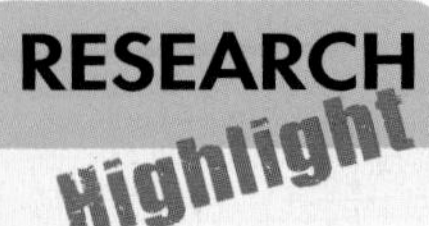

Predictors of Depressive Symptoms in Primary Caregivers of Young Children With or at Risk for Developmental Delay

STUDY PURPOSE

To clarify the relative contributions of child characteristics, parental resources, parental self-efficacy, and potential mediating and moderating influences between caregiver distress and child problems.

METHODS

A variety of instruments were completed in the homes of 178 caregivers of 194 2-year-old children with developmental delay. Trained interviewers administered the instruments and clarified caregivers' questions. Instruments completed included the Family Information Questionnaire, the Beck Depression Inventory, the Ways of Coping Questionnaire—Revised, the Interpersonal Support Evaluation List, the Child Behavior Management Survey, the Vineland Adaptive Behavior Scale, and the Child Behavior Check List for ages 2 to 3. Data were analyzed using the ANOVA, the ANCOVA, and hierarchical multiple regression. Explained variance R^2 was only 40%.

FINDINGS

Of the parents in the sample, 20% were clinically depressed, based on the Beck Depression Inventory, which substantially exceeds that of the general population, but is less than the 29% of parents of developmentally delayed children previously reported in the literature. In addition, child behavior problems were more severe if caregivers were depressed. Parents with good social support were, understandably, less likely to be depressed.

IMPLICATIONS

These findings are a strong indication for assessment of depression in parents of 2-year-olds with developmental delay. In addition, the findings almost mandate assessment for parents of 2-year-olds with behavioral problems, since the problems are exacerbated in the presence of depression.

Depression isn't necessarily a binary entity; there are many gradations of depression that occur before a person arrives at a severe clinical depression. Consequently, nurses who interface with parents who have developmentally delayed toddlers should be prepared to listen empathically and verify that parents' stated emotional states are both plausible and valid. Referrals should be made if there is a suspicion of depression.

REFERENCE

Feldman, M., McDonald, L., Serbin, L., Stack, D., Secco, M. L., & Yu, C. T. (2007). Predictors of depressive symptoms in primary caregivers of young children with or at risk for developmental delay. *Journal of Intellectual Disability Research*, *51*(8), 606–619.

SOCIETY'S RESPONSE TO CHILDREN WITH DOWN SYNDROME

With all its cleverness and research and innovation, society has not yet devised a way to perform microsurgery on every cell in the body of a child with Down syndrome, thus altering such societally important variables as intelligence, independent living capability, earning capacity, and ability to create and raise children. Consequently, based on the values of the 19th and early 20th centuries, society's efforts toward Down syndrome have been either eugenic or compensatory in nature: either abort the fetus based on prenatal diagnosis, or attempt to improve intelligence, independent living capability, and earning capacity.

Since the middle of the century, a peculiar tendency has been noted. The measured intelligence quotient and the expected life span for people with Down syndrome in the United States have both increased markedly. Concurrently, there are more school-age children with Down syndrome today than there were 50 years ago.

In the 1940s, many considered the child with Down syndrome "hardly human" (Spock, 1949). Since the 1960s, social patterns have changed. In the first half of the century, Down syndrome neonates and other babies with birth anomalies were often relegated to the back rows of the hospital nursery in bassinets with signs that read, "Do not feed!" They were kept warm, bundled in blankets, but were allowed to die from dehydration. In 1975, 77% of pediatric surgeons in this country favored withholding food and medical treatment from newborns with Down syndrome (Colson & Pearcey, 1997). Others were placed in institutions or in foster homes from birth. Mothers were told of a child who would not be able to learn and might not even be able to speak. Families were told that the children would surely need institutionalization in a few years and that it was easier on the caregivers, the siblings, and the infant to opt for institutionalization at birth. The measured IQ of persons with Down syndrome has risen from the profoundly

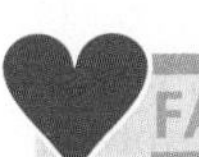

FAMILY**TEACHING**

Respiratory Infections in Children with Down Syndrome

The following topics are important to teach:

- the increased incidence and severity of both upper and lower respiratory infections
- symptoms of a respiratory illness, such as elevated temperature, foul-smelling nasal discharge, or a rattling, frequent cough, which should be reported to the health care provider
- minimizing exposure to cigarette smoke
- clarifying that school personnel must notify caregivers if the child displays symptoms of respiratory illness
- coordination of administration of medications with the school
- referral to an allergist, pulmonologist, or otorhinolaryngologist if respiratory infections are severe

retarded range observed at the middle of the 20th century to the current range of 25 – 55 at the beginning of the 21st century (Tsao & Kindelberger, 2009), probably due to a combination of early intervention, inclusion in public education programs, and prevalence of home placement rather than institutional.

A generation ago, life expectancy for infants with Down syndrome who were raised in institutions was only 9 years (Yang, Rasmussen, & Friedman, 2002). In the 1960s there was a growing consciousness of developmental slowness as a normal variant of the human race and not a shameful condition. Soon thereafter, legal mandates were enacted that protected infants and children from lack of medical intervention based solely upon their impairments. Additionally, it became more socially acceptable for families to keep their mentally retarded children at home for an extended period of time instead of institutionalizing them at birth. Individuals with Down syndrome live longer and experience better health than their cohorts did half a century ago. With adequate care, it turns out that life expectancy in the United States is now in the late 50s, and in Australia is approximately 60 years (Vis et al., 2009).

THE AUTISTIC SPECTRUM DISORDERS

The five autistic spectrum disorders are sometimes called the pervasive developmental disorders: (1) autism; (2) Asperger's disorder/syndrome; (3) childhood disintegrative disorder; (4) Rett syndrome; and (5) pervasive developmental disorder not otherwise specified (PDD-NOS) (American Psychiatric Association, 2000; Menkes, Sarnat, & Maria, 2006; Volkmar & Klin, 2005). All are characterized by impaired communication abilities and patterns, inadequate social skills, and some degree of obsessiveness. As such, they severely limit a child's ability to function in peer settings and in traditional classroom activities.

Autism is a neurodevelopmental disorder and the most widely recognized of the autistic spectrum disorders. Autism is characterized by extreme difficulty communicating with and relating to the environment, especially the social environment of other humans. It is manifested by bizarre behavior, delayed language acquisition, poor social relations, impairment of self-care skills, and altered sensory responses. Kanner (1943), a psychiatrist at Johns Hopkins University, initially described autism in children exhibiting relationship impairment before age 30 months, language impairment, and a combination of ritualism and obsessiveness. These children were self-absorbed, aloof, and indifferent to others. They made little eye contact and demonstrated lack of imaginative or pretend play (Chawarska & Volkmar, 2006). Autism was initially classified as a type of schizophrenia (Creak, 1961).

INCIDENCE AND ETIOLOGY

The worldwide incidence of all five autistic spectrum disorders combined is between 5 and 10 per 1,000 (Fombonne, 2009). The incidence of autism only is estimated to between 1.3 in 1,000 (Fombonne, 2006) and 2 in 1,000 (Shah, Dalton, & Boris, 2007). Autism is increasing in incidence (Fombonne, 2006). Autism is now the third most prevalent pediatric developmental disorder, after mental retardation and cerebral palsy. Although some of this increase is explained by better and earlier diagnostics, there is a substantial actual increase in incidence as well (Fombonne, 2009; Shah, Dalton, & Boris, 2007). Boys are afflicted with autism more often than are girls, by a ratio of three or four to one. It is also more common in siblings of affected children. The exact cause of autism is unknown; however, like most other behavioral syndromes, it seems multifactorial. Genetic studies indicate a greater likelihood that monozygotic (i.e., identical) twins will share autism than dizygotic (i.e., fraternal) twins. As is true of all five spectrum disorders, autism is multifactorial in that its cause appears to have both genetic and environmental contributions: a genetic predisposition plus a prenatal or postnatal environmental trigger.

Autism is sometimes associated with other syndromes or diseases. Somewhat fewer than 5% of children with autism test positive for fragile X syndrome (Rutter, 2006). Tourette's syndrome is present in as many as 8% of autistic children. Some children with chromosomal disorders also exhibit autism, as do a few blind, hearing impaired, and mentally retarded children. About 75% of children with autism test as mentally retarded, but if one includes all children with autistic spectrum disorders, including a large number of children with Asperger's syndrome and PDD-NOS, the figure is estimated to be between 15% and 25% (Shea & Mesibov, 2006). An association has been reported between autism and unfavorable events in pregnancy, delivery, and the neonatal phase. Examples of these factors or events include breech presentation (Bilder,

Pinborough-Zimmerman, Miller, & McMahon, 2009), prematurity (Johnson & Marlow, 2009), and hyperbilirubinemia (Jangaard, Fell, Dodds & Allen, 2008).

Historically, autism was described as a result of altered mothering, and mothers were described as cold and unloving (the "refrigerator mother theory") (Bettelheim, 1967). Autistic children's mothers were observed to touch and interact socially with their children in a different way than did those of children without autism. Then it was realized that the child-caregiver dyad is a complex feedback system. A caregiver responds to a child's cues; a child responds to a caregiver's cues. A child who responds in a negative way to traditional cues stimulates different behavior in the caregiver: for instance, if a child does not present a positive response when touched or hugged, the caregiver will show approval or affection in different ways. This pattern was initially confusing to the observers of autistic children and their mothers. It was later noted that autistic children frequently developed seizure disorders in adolescence (Rutter, 1970). The occurrence of seizures in 33% to 75% of autistic children indicated that the disorder was rooted in abnormalities of brain chemistry. Therefore, it was a neurodevelopmental disorder, not a result of abnormal parenting.

PATHOPHYSIOLOGY

Although the etiology of autism remains unclear, there is strong support for a genetic model of inheritance (Shah, Dalton, & Boris, 2007; Smith, 2006). There is an occurrence rate of over 5% in siblings of autistic children (Filipek, 2006). Identical twins demonstrate concordance rates ranging from 36% to 91%, whereas fraternal twins' concordance rate is about 5%, the same as for nontwin siblings (Bohm & Stewart, 2009; Muhle, Trentacoste, & Rapin, 2004). Bohm and Stewart (2009) posed an elegant mathematical explanation of the huge range in concordance for identical twins, suggesting that since the ratio of monochorionic to dichorionic identical twins is 2:1, and the average concordance for identical twins is very close to 2:1, the varying differences in incidence may be due to studies failing to include the variable of monochorionic versus dichorionic in their analysis. The authors hypothesized that the existence of a separate chorion may provide a level of protection during the first trimester between twins. This suggests exposure of one twin by unspecified means. It is possible that substances carried by the maternal bloodstream, or even some forms of radiation, could provide exposure to one twin, but not the other.

Current research has focused on locating the genes associated with autism. Genes on the second, third, seventh, fifteenth, sixteenth, and seventeenth chromosomes, and the sex chromosomes, have been identified as potentially significant in autism inheritance (Muhle, Trentacoste, & Rapin, 2004; Shah, Dalton, & Boris, 2007). However, with the exception of Rett syndrome and fragile X syndrome, which are both single-gene defects (Hagerman, 2002; Rutter, 2006), the genetics of the remaining three autistic spectrum disorders remain elusive. It was originally speculated that autism was a result of three to ten genes working in concert; now it is thought that as many as 100 different genes may be involved, and that different phenotypes of autism, with shared appearance and behavior, may each have a distinct genetic basis.

Because of the differences between identical and fraternal twins' concordance rates, the hypothesis of a genetic mode of inheritance acted upon by an environmental trigger is also promising. Historically, in studies of identical twins, the one with autism had the more difficult delivery, but abnormalities of the affected twin could have accounted for difficulty during the delivery process (Bilder et al., 2009). Presumably, differences in brain chemistry and in the stress response could precipitate changes in measurements of vital signs, tone, and neonatal responses. Other triggers may be infections such as congenital rubella or influenza, maternal smoking, metals, pollutants, pesticides (Hertz-Picciotto et al., 2006), or agricultural pesticides in conjunction with iodine deficiency (Roberts et al., 2007). Caregivers of an autistic child with documented allergies commonly continue to refuse routine immunizations for their subsequent children, especially the MMR, believing that it could represent the trigger if genes for autism are present. Despite the fact that the 1998 publication posing this connection has been discredited (Rutter, 2006), there remains support within a minority of the academic community for the possible trigger of thiomersol, a mercury preservative used in vaccines (Downing, 2007).

CLINICAL MANIFESTATIONS

Delayed and impaired social skill development is one hallmark for autistic disorder. Autistic children have poor communication, unusual forms of play, bizarre body movements, repetitive actions, withdrawal, absent eye contact, an aversion to some or all physical contact, unusual hand movements, sensitivity to tactile stimuli, unresponsiveness to auditory stimuli, altered responses to pain, and a resistance to usual teaching and learning methods. The play, or behaviors, of an autistic child will typically involve solitary activities. These are repeated, apparently meaningless activities that the child finds essentially important and seems compelled to repeat in sequence. One or more objects or toys are of great importance in these behavioristic rituals or play activities (American Psychiatric Association, 2000). Obsessive behaviors concerning eating, dressing, moving, and the physical environment, including the people in it, are often present.

Some of the bizarre body movements seen in autistic children are stiff gestures, awkward gait, rocking, and waving or flipping the hands back and forth. If repeated, these body movements are often accompanied by repetitious sounds. Sensitivity to tactile stimulation is usually demonstrated as aversion to being touched. It can also include seeking contact with the hands or head by slapping an object or banging the head into it, or as extreme delight in touching or holding certain objects. Autistic children's altered response to pain usually takes the form of impassivity to mild or moderate pain, but can also be observed as loud howling in response

Reflections from Families

Thinking back on it, four years later, the most awful thing about that first couple of years was the exhaustion. Babies are supposed to be asleep most of the time, right? Here we were with this new baby, our first, and even though we weren't experienced at this sort of thing, it seemed suspiciously as if this was that dreaded entity we'd read about called The Difficult Child pattern. Matthew never slept. Never.

OK, so he slept, but it wasn't enough, and it wasn't nearly enough for my wife Martha. At a year, Matt was sleeping for an hour or two every afternoon and about 6 hours at night. That was it. Martha was so tired that all she had to do was sit down and she'd nod off. I have pictures (and he displays a picture of a very tired-looking woman sprawled in an easy chair), and the lack of sleep wasn't all of it. Matt insisted on breastfeeding, making Martha even more tired. Matt was never still. He walked well before a year: he was into everything. He was exploring, but in a way that wasn't like other kids. He was relentless in checking out one thing and then moving on to something else, climbing, reaching, climbing, checking doors, opening cupboards. He seemed to be on a mission from God. Supervising him was a full-time stand-up job, and injury—he was absolutely fearless. You know how other children are timid about this and that, how they won't go near the furnace because it makes a loud noise? He had no fear. He didn't climb the furniture—he swarmed up it, absolutely swarmed. He had no rubber band. (What's a rubber band?) That's the invisible cord that goes between a toddler and his mother—the kid gets just so far and then is uncomfortable with the amount of physical distance between them. Matt didn't have one. Consequently, all our doors have two-handed locks up by the ceiling, but it's just a matter of time before he figures that out, too. He can already scale six foot fences. At 4, he has finally begun to sleep—to sleep at predictable times and to stay asleep. We used to have to tiptoe but he'd wake too often anyhow. Thank Heaven he's sleeping. After a few years, I wasn't sure whether we'd all make it through as a family, whether we'd all be living together, whether we'd all be left standing. That's the thing that causes institutionalization faster than anything else, you know, the inability to survive the sleeplessness.

to insignificant injuries. An autistic child will often put one hand on an adult's wrist or forearm and advance it toward a desired object to signal wanting that object, in a kind of proxy reach.

The root of these odd behaviors seems to be the impaired ability of autistic children to assign meaning to the same objects and events that others find meaningful, including customary modes of communication. Behaviors may also reflect the compulsion for sameness and ritual in objects and events that others fail to grasp (Szatmari, 2004). The child who is autistic may begin life as a normal infant or may display abnormal signs in infancy, including an unusual response to auditory stimuli, a severe sleep disorder, a feeding disorder, or lack of normal eye contact, with a lack of interaction. The classic picture is the toddler who has apparently begun to use language and then loses most or all of it. Subsequently, the child develops abnormal behaviors, hyperfocusing on some objects and ignoring others. An autistic child typically is hyperfearful of some situations, does not indicate wants by pointing, seems to have a hearing deficit, does not exhibit "pretend" activities, and does not interact voluntarily with others. He, for most autistic children are boys, may show extreme food preferences, exaggerated attachments to key possessions, complete lack of stranger anxiety, no desire when in strange environments to maintain closeness to caregivers, lack of spontaneous language, **echolalia** (repeating the last word or words heard, sometimes initially mistaken for real speech), and extreme difficulty in toilet training.

DIAGNOSIS

The diagnosis of autism is based mainly on clinical manifestations and begins by ruling out other disorders like deafness. Interviews, observations, and autism-specific assessment instruments are used to formulate the diagnosis. Correct diagnosis depends on accurate developmental history focused on types of behavior typical of autism, and on evaluation of current social skills. A developmental history can reveal mental retardation and social skills significantly below global level of functioning. Social skills significantly delayed relative to overall developmental functioning, especially communication, constitute one of the most important criteria for the diagnosis of autism.

Because early diagnosis fosters earlier intervention, the American Academy of Pediatrics and the Centers for Disease Control and Prevention recommend that all children be screened for autistic spectrum disorders by 18 to 24 months of age, and be rescreened at intervals (Centers for Disease Control & Prevention, 2009; Council on Children with Disabilities, 2006; Zwaigenbaum et al., 2009). This is because the diagnosis of autism can often be made reliably by 24 months, since symptoms are clear in 90% of autistic children by that age (Volkmar & Klin, 2005), whereas diagnosis of Asperger's syndrome and PDD-NOS may not be able to be made until school age, since language does not vary as far from average.

REFLECTIVE THINKING

I'm the Child's Parent. Why Won't You Believe Me?

Your 14-month-old child babbled and said about four words at 1 year of age. Now he says only one word, and that is infrequent. You know something is wrong. Your heart is cold with fear because you used to live next door to a little boy who was autistic, and you are beginning to see commonalities, one by one, week by frightening week. This loss of speech in your child is the saddest and cruelest thing you have known. You make an appointment and take him to the pediatrician. You tell the physician that you think your child is autistic. He tells you that many children are late to talk and that you shouldn't worry. You ask for a referral for hearing evaluation. The pediatrician is reluctant to make one because you had told him previously that the child was a light sleeper and woke to every little noise. You insist and get your referral. The physician tells you that your child looks fine to him. It seems as if you are being patronized. How would you feel about this whole experience?

Standardized autism-specific assessment instruments exist to aid in making the diagnosis of autism. The first widely-used instrument specific to autism was the *Childhood Autism Rating Scale* (CARS) (Schopler, Reichler, & Renner, 1988). With this instrument, the child is evaluated in 14 areas of behavior such as listening response, verbal communication, activity level, relating to people, object use, and imitation. The examiner gains an overall impression of whether the behavior in general seems autistic. The scale was designed for use with children 2 years and older and requires training in order to administer. The reliability of the diagnosis of autism in children under 3 years of age has been supported (Beauchesne & Kelley, 2004; Szatmari, 2004). Subsequently, the Checklist for Autism in Toddlers (CHAT) (Baird & Charman, 2000), which screens for protodeclarative pointing, gaze-monitoring, and pretend play, all of which are conspicuously present in children by 14 months but absent in autism, proved useful for autism screening, but the test was criticized for its low sensitivity (tendency to underdiagnose) (Nadel & Poss, 2007). In order to address this problem, the M-CHAT (Robins, Fein, Barton, & Green, 2001) was developed and has proven to demonstrate increased sensitivity, without loss of specificity (Nadel & Poss, 2007). Early diagnosis is best for both child and caregivers, for purposes of early intervention.

TREATMENT

Although there is no cure for autism, various treatment modalities have been used. Many of these have focused on behavior modification and have involved the family as well, so that the child's behavioral reinforcements continue around the clock. The Committee on Educational Interventions for Children with Autism of the National Research Council (Lord et al., 2001) generated consensus guidelines for children with autism, supporting a comprehensive intervention program that should begin immediately after diagnosis and specifying that the program should be tailored to individual children's specific deficits and include a family component. Further, the guidelines mandated a formal program of 20 to 25 hours per week, with a high teacher-to-student ratio. There is a growing body of evidence that intensive early intervention services for children diagnosed with autism before the age of 5 years may lead to better overall outcomes, especially if begun before age 3.

The first controlled study of early intensive interventions with young children was conducted by Ivar Lovaas (Lovaas, 1987). This study has received significant attention because of its remarkable results. Children in the experimental group were treated with an intensive program of behavioral training on a one-to-one basis for 40 hours per week for two years. The operant conditioning program focused on acquisition of language, compliance behavior, imitation activities, and integration with peers. Caregivers adhered to the same treatment regimen during the remainder of the child's waking hours. After two years of therapy almost 50% of the children were functioning typically for their age in intellectual and academic areas. However, the intervention group was self-selected and there are no replications that use random assignment to confirm Lovaas's findings. As a parent of an autistic son explained ten years ago, "It's not scientific proof, but behavioral therapy is my kid's best shot at a normal life." Although very little of it is experimental, additional research conducted since 1987 lends support to Lovaas's findings.

Various developmental, behavioral, and educational strategies have been developed for the treatment of autism during the last 25 years. Generally, the goals of treatment are to improve the overall functional status of the child by teaching communication and social, adaptive, and academic skills; decreasing unacceptable behaviors through behavioral interventions; and helping the family manage the stress associated with raising a child with autism. As long as intensive education and behavior management are used, it matters little what the particular variants of each treatment are. Buddying with an unaffected child (Stahmer & Ingersoll, 2004) and structured play (Whiteford, 2000) are two interventions yielding positive results.

Providing a highly structured environment with as much one-on-one instruction as possible is very important in the management of autism. These interventions are designed to stimulate the child's communication skills, stressing expressive and receptive speech, and to promote emergence and mastery of other developmental tasks including eye contact, play skills, repetitive pattern recognition, and social interactions. Because negative behavior patterns can emerge and become ingrained in a very short time, common undesired behaviors that are developmentally normal, such as hitting or biting, are predicted, immediately identified, and redirected by use of supervision, vigilance, and consistent response. The caregivers are partners in the treatment plan and are educated in the delivery of behavioral reinforcers and systematic responses to the child's behavior so that desired behaviors can be reinforced at all times of day.

Several comprehensive educational curricula have been developed specifically for children with autism, including the most well known, *Treatment and Education of Autistic and Communication Handicapped Children* (TEACCH) (Schopler, 1997), which is used worldwide and has been demonstrated to be effective across cultures (Panerai et al., 2009; Tsang, Skek, Lam, Tang, & Cheung, 2007). In such programs, the educational approach is tailored to the child's particular preferences, the caregivers' ability to be involved, and the child's functional level. The basic elements of the TEACCH philosophy include the following (Schopler, 1997):

1. Collaboration between caregiver and professional.
2. Individualized treatments based on comprehensive assessments of the child.
3. Highly structured and holistic teaching.
4. Improved adaptation by teaching new skills and environmental accommodations.
5. Lifelong and community-based services.

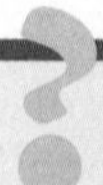

KIDS WANT TO KNOW

How should I feel about my autistic brother?

"My brother Joe is 4 and he's autistic. I'm 7 and I think he's really a pest. He gets into my dolls and my play horses and my games. He makes a mess of everything that isn't locked up, and sometimes I forget to lock my room door. It's like being a prisoner in my own house. What I want to know is this—Joe's my brother and all, but do I have to like him?"

You can reply: "How frustrating for you to have to be so careful every time you leave your room. Having a little brother who is autistic is almost always harder than having a little brother who is not. You have to take special care to protect your toys and treasures, because Joe isn't good at following directions and staying in the rooms he's supposed to be in. What is really sad is that he may not ever learn this, so locking your room might be something you always have to do. He's probably pretty crafty at getting into your room quickly before your mom even knows he's in there. It sounds as if Joe would be hard for any big sister to like, and it's especially hard for you when he bothers your stuff. While we are supposed to love and respect our family members, there's nothing that says that we have to like them all the time. The way you feel is the way you feel, and it's OK to love him and at the same time not like him much when he doesn't behave."

NURSING MANAGEMENT

ASSESSMENT

When a child with autism is hospitalized, it is essential for the nurse to obtain information from the caregivers about the child's routines, likes and dislikes, and rituals. The nurse needs to evaluate as well as ask the caregivers about the child's skills and abilities regarding self-care, such as feeding, dressing, bathing, and toileting. Assessment should also include the child's communication skills, interactive patterns, and response to others. The nurse should inquire about the method the caregivers use to give the child medications, as well as ask about the family's support system.

NURSING DIAGNOSIS

Nursing diagnoses that may be appropriate for the child and family include:

1. *Risk for injury* related to lack of average caution and sensory deficits.
2. *Impaired verbal communication* related to limited language skills.

3. *Impaired social interaction* related to inability to develop and maintain social relationships and lack of social or emotional reciprocity.
4. *Caregiver role strain* related to child's need for constant care or supervision, limited ability to relate to caregivers, and increased stress.

Outcome Identification

1. The child will not sustain major accidental injury.
2. The child will develop a means of communicating needs and wants to others.
3. The child will acknowledge others in the environment and attempt to initiate interaction with them.
4. The caregivers will discuss their need for respite care and their feelings related to the frustrations and stress of caring for a child with autism.

Planning and Implementation

Children with autism lack organic disturbances that would bring them into contact with health care providers more frequently than the average child, yet nurses will occasionally encounter them in the health care setting, either for wellness care or for treatment of childhood illnesses. Each autistic child is an individual, often with strong, even violent, preferences and aversions.

Incorporation of the caregivers in the care of these children is absolutely essential. In the school setting, roles of teachers and nurses may overlap, especially around problem issues such as nutrition, communication, and undesirable behaviors. Nurses, as well as educators, bring specialized background knowledge related to normal nutritional needs, the range of communication patterns in the growing child, and limit-setting. The specialized role of the nurse as the child's advocate is of utmost importance throughout planning meetings and daily work with the individual. Additionally, the nurse may be called upon to administer medication during the school day. This should not be attempted until the caregivers have clarified their at-home strategies and a cooperative plan has been devised. It is important to maintain consistency for medication administration, especially for children with oral aversion.

Everything the caregivers know about the child may be helpful to the nurse who is planning care. This is especially true in the hospital setting, especially if the caregivers have other responsibilities and must leave the child for a period of time. Regardless of the hospital policies on visitation, caregivers need to have 24-hour access to the autistic child or, more important, vice versa. Caregivers can be extremely valuable in calming the child, explaining the environment, supervising the child in areas that would not present hazard to an average child, and assisting with procedures. They need to be acknowledged by nursing staff as the experts. Caregivers' detailed knowledge about their autistic child is golden.

However, caregivers do not come by this expert knowledge of their autistic child benignly. Often their lives are a

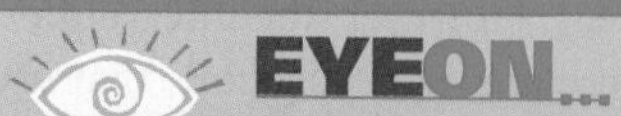

Alternative Therapies for Children with Autism

Because autism is a chronic, lifelong condition for which there is no cure, it has become the focus of several nontraditional, alternative treatments. Several nutritional supplements have been used such as high-dose pyroxine (vitamin B_6) and magnesium (Nye & Brice, 2005), ascorbic acid (vitamin C), and dimethylglycine (DMG) (Montgomery, 2006). Food allergies and intolerance are beginning to receive much attention as possible contributors to autistic behaviors. It is proposed that the body is unable to break down certain ingested proteins into amino acids. Therefore, some families have eliminated certain foods from their children's diets such as those containing gluten (e.g., wheat and barley) and casein (found in milk).

Many children with autism have strong food preferences and aversions, and many have gastrointestinal symptoms. Campbell et al. (2009) have demonstrated that one amino acid receptor may be lacking in some autistic persons. It is known that many autistic children experience gastrointestinal inflammation (Baron-Cohen et al., 2006). In the face of pain or discomfort of the gastrointestinal system, autistic children with poor verbal skills tend to develop exaggerated behaviors that include writhing, moaning, insomnia, increased hyperactivity, increased regurgitation, and food aversion. Increase in undesired behaviors may be a reasonable indication for gastrointestinal referral and evaluation, since so many autistic children are affected.

Another controversial alternative therapy for children with autism is the administration of synthetic human secretin hormone. However, recent research failed to demonstrate significant improvement in autistic behaviors (Matson & Minshawi, 2006). Controversial, nontraditional therapies will continue to gain local and national attention because of the caregivers' desire to pursue anything that might help their child and furnish hope for a cure. Some treatments are detailed in journals, others on the Internet, and caregivers often have accessed and used them, so nurses must be familiar with them. In the area of alternative medicine for autism, physicians, in general, support the use of vitamins, probiotics, fatty acids, and melatonin, while discouraging secretin, chelation, and anti-infectives (Golnik & Ireland, 2009).

Because the incidence of autism in much higher in boys than in girls, research has investigated the correlation between fetal testosterone levels and subsequent autistic traits, and found that they are positively associated, and that this finding occurs not only in male fetuses but across genders (Auyeung et al., 2009). Subsequent research in this area is anticipated.

symphony of sleep deprivation, misinformation, cognitive dissonance, and lulls in motivation. The misinformation that they accrue from various sources ranges from laughable to discriminatory. It includes a stereotypic view of all autistic children ("Oh, he's just like the Rain Man!"), the assumption that autistic children are all savants; the expectation that autistic adults can never survive independently; a lingering perception by some that autistics are created, not born; and a reluctance of funding agencies to support what they consider excessively expensive experimental behavioral programs.

The cognitive dissonance that caregivers of autistic children experience emanates from the gap between their own knowledge and the expectations of the health care community, the school system, and society in general. On one hand, the health care community sets itself up as expert in matters of medication; however, the caregivers of an autistic child may be told only to administer a medication to their orally aversive toddler, not *how* to administer it. School systems, the experts on children's education, may offer no publicly funded toddler or preschool programs for autistic children, despite the knowledge that intervention is best instituted early. Programs that do exist can be expensive, inadequately staffed, or of inadequate duration to produce behavioral change.

Diminished motivation is experienced by all caregivers, regardless of whether their children are average or have special needs. However, caregivers of autistic children experience motivational dips because of three unrelated factors: first, the gap between their own instinctive and self-acquired knowledge and the world's knowledge; second, the enormous time and energy expenditure between the initiation of the intervention program and any lasting behavioral change; and third, their chronic sleep deprivation. It is very difficult to feel optimistic implementing a program that experts consider experimental, when there is no end in sight and no real improvement in any behavior for months at a time.

In the community setting, the nurse may encounter children with mild rather than severe forms of autism in the public school system or in special needs classrooms within larger schools. However, siblings of autistic children attend public schools and the nurse may be called upon to provide information and referrals. It is important to recognize the large extent to which these siblings are expected to be responsible for themselves, physically, socially, and emotionally, because of the caregiver's expenditure of time with the affected sibling. The nurse's role here includes provision of support as well as formal teaching. Caregivers can be experts in autism and yet have difficulty perceiving the effects it has on their families.

EVALUATION

Questions for evaluating nursing interventions may include:

- Have the interventions directed toward supervision, monitoring, and limit-setting been effective in protecting the child from injury?
- Has the child established a way to communicate needs and wants?
- Have all self-care needs been met?
- Has the child acknowledged others in the environment and attempted to interact with them?
- Has eye contact improved?
- Have the caregivers expressed their feelings and needs with the nurse?

NURSING TIP

Ideas for Medicating an Autistic Child

It is almost impossible to administer a disagreeable oral medication to an autistic child. If a health care provider orders a new medication for an autistic child, the nurse should perform the following actions:

- **Urge the provider to talk with the caregivers before selecting the medication, the route, and the amount.**
- **Suggest prescribing double-doses if the child is likely to spit the medication.**
- **Inform the caregivers of a child who is intensely oral-aversive that acetaminophen, for example, is available in rectal suppositories, which may be accepted better than the oral form.**
- **Clarify alternatives for the caregivers.**

FAMILY TEACHING

Teaching the family of a child who is autistic is a delicate matter. The typical caregiver raising a child with autism is far more knowledgeable about the care of that child than is the average nurse. Consequently, the critical cluster of things for the nurse to remember is to listen, to learn, to respect, and to remember. The nurse needs to understand each particular caregiver's knowledge base and beliefs about autism, its cause, its treatment, its prognosis and, most important, the individual hopes and concerns the caregiver holds for this child. Will the caregiver be able to keep him at home, at least for his childhood? Will he speak? Will he be able to coexist peacefully with siblings he may have? Will he learn to read? Will he be able to live independently?

In general, the school nurse will be the person who is close enough to the caregiver to be entrusted with specific hopes for the child's future. Alternatively, a nurse or nurse practitioner in a primary care setting might develop such a relationship with the caregiver over time. Occasionally, a community health nurse would be in this privileged position of trust. Then, within the framework of caregiver beliefs and hopes, the nurse can proceed with teaching. The first focus is routine health care. The caregiver needs to know about healthy practices that encompass all children. For instance, a nurse may have information about a strategy or product that may improve general safety, such as a new brand of

EVIDENCE-BASED PRACTICE

Early Intensive Behavioral Intervention (EIBI)

CLINICAL PROBLEM

Even though anecdotal, and later quasi-experimental data have existed for decades in support of early intensive behavioral intervention (EIBI) for autism spectrum disorders, reports of the only two controlled experimental studies were published in 2000 and in 2005 (Sallows & Graupner, 2005; Smith, Groen, & Wynn, 2000). Practitioners may not be aware that evidence from the first experimental trial has finally been replicated, conferring definitive support for EIBI.

BEST CLINICAL PRACTICE

In their comprehensive synthesis, consisting of descriptive statistics and a meta-analysis, as well as detailed analyses of effect size and methodology across studies, Reichow and Wolery (2009) have summarized thirteen research results, two experimental and eleven quasi-experimental in design, supporting the best clinical practice of EIBI in the field of education for children diagnosed with autism, PDD, and PDD-NOS. EIBI, according to previously published protocols (Lord et al., 2001), should be initiated as soon as the child is diagnosed and provided for at least 25 hours per week, year-round, with low student-to-teacher ratios, as well as training and participation by family members so that the intervention continues evenings, nights, and weekends. Almost all of the programs described in the research studies analyzed by Reichow and Wolery (2009) provided between 20 and 39 hours per week of EIBI and continued for one to three years. Results in all programs were overwhelmingly positive, both for fostering change in autistic symptoms and for increasing measured IQ.

IMPLICATIONS FOR NURSING

The findings of the article supported the use of the effectiveness of EIBI for children with autistic spectrum disorders, in general, but noted that it is not effective for each individual child. School nurses should be aware of this fact and be prepared for questions by families who are considering EIBI for their children or who already have children in programs. In addition, progress should be seen within a year but it may not be discernible in a short period of time, and nurses should also be aware of this.

Regional centers that support optimal treatment for autism possess limited funds, especially as the incidence of autism spectrum disorders increases and, more recently, economic recession impacts service budgets. The fiscally-mediated response to cut hours for one-to-one behavioral training, while preserving some services for all children with autism and providing training for all parents, has not been supported by activist parent groups, who maintain that Lovaas's (1987) original recommendation, 40 hours a week of EIBI for three years, is the gold standard. As a matter of fact, Reichow and Wolery's (2009) analysis demonstrated a trend, although it was not statistically significant, that programs with more hours per week fostered more progress for the children who attended them. Understandably, conflicts have resulted from this issue, since parents want the best for their children, rather than adequate services for all of the children of the community with autism spectrum disorders. Many parents interpret "the best" as 40 hours per week.

Reference: Reichow, B., & Wolery, M. (2009). Comprehensive synthesis of early intensive behavioral interventions for young children with autism based on the UCLA Young Autism Project model. *Journal of Autism and Developmental Disorders, 39* 23–41.

childproof doorknob covers, or be able to suggest an unusual but especially nutritious food or food product, such as tofu, that other children with strong food preferences have tolerated. Caregivers of autistic children may be so busy with other issues that they forget simple routines, such as initiating dental visits during toddlerhood.

Another teaching focus is caregiver emotional health. This again is individualized. Because many children with autism have sleep disturbances, caregivers may be too exhausted to cognitively realize that they are tired. Initiating a referral for respite care, so the caregiver can get some much needed sleep, may be the most important thing the nurse can offer. Caregivers may be deep within the grieving process and have a wealth of anger displayed inappropriately, or they may be very depressed and in need of someone to hear about how they feel. If caregivers will accept a referral for supportive counseling, that can be initiated. However, most caregivers realize this is not a "fix-it" problem, and their time is very much at a premium. Consequently, the nurse must be familiar with the grieving process and be prepared to listen empathetically to caregivers' stories (Moses & Kearney, 1995).

Parents who originally planned to have other children may seek genetic counseling when their toddler is diagnosed as autistic. At present, although a genetic contribution is suspected, and although the incidence of autism is higher in families where other autistic individuals are found (Rutter, 2006), no genes causing autism have been positively identified. Siblings are certainly affected by having to adapt to living with someone who is autistic, and their feelings must also be expressed and heard. Caregivers may consciously or unconsciously treat the siblings of the autistic child as cocaregivers, as small adults sharing a common task. Caregivers need to be encouraged to see the siblings' achievements, tasks, sorrows, and needs, and to acknowledge important milestones in their lives. An autistic child is reared predominantly for a protected, circumscribed, and sheltered adulthood; the siblings need to be raised for full inclusion in the wide world that is both their heritage and their burden.

RESEARCH Highlight

The First Year Inventory: Retrospective Parent Responses to a Questionnaire Designed to Identify 1-Year-Olds at Risk for Autism

STUDY PURPOSE

To discover whether retrospective scores on the First Year Inventory (FYI), an autism screening tool, are significantly higher for children with autism, as compared with unaffected children and with children diagnosed with other developmental disorders. (This is the second part of a research series that will eventually put the FYI in place for screening all 12-month-old children.)

METHODS

Parents of three groups of preschoolers were recruited: 38 with autism, 15 with other developmental delays, and 40 with typical development. They were asked to complete the FYI retrospectively, reflecting their children's behaviors at one year of age. In addition, both children and parents completed various other assessments related to stages of development, adaptive behavior, and intelligence.

FINDINGS

Children with autism scored much higher on the FYI than did children with developmental delay or unaffected children.

IMPLICATIONS

The FYI may be a valuable clinical tool for the early identification of autism spectrum disorders. It is becoming accepted practice for physicians to perform periodic developmental assessments of children up to 3 years of age, because of the increased incidence of the autism spectrum disorders and because of the value of early identification and intervention. The nurse is free to ask about a 12-month-old's usual behaviors, paying attention to answers that imply that the child has unusual patterns of communication, interaction, language development, eye contact, sleep patterns, and types of play, and making referrals if indicated.

REFERENCE

Watson, L. R., Baranek, G. T., Crais, E. R., Reznick, J. S., Dykstra, J., & Perryman, T. (2007). The first year inventory: retrospective parent responses to a questionnaire designed to identify one-year-olds at risk for autism. *Journal of Autism and Developmental Disorders*, *37*(1), 49–61.

FRAGILE X SYNDROME

Fragile X syndrome is a commonly inherited cause of mental retardation. In 1991, the genetic code of the fragile X mental retardation 1 gene (FMR1) located on the X chromosome was determined (Sherman, 2002).

INCIDENCE AND ETIOLOGY

Fragile X syndrome occurs in 0.25–0.8 per 1,000 live male births (Johns Hopkins Hospital et al., 2008). The occurrence in females is 1 to 3 per 10,000, and they are less severely affected than males (Hagerman, 2002). Approximately 7% of mild mental retardation in females is caused by fragile X. About 30% of families with an X-linked pattern of inheritance of mental retardation are those with fragile X syndrome (Hagerman, 2002). It has been described in all races and ethnic groups.

PATHOPHYSIOLOGY

The gene mutation in fragile X syndrome is a nucleic acid repeat on the X chromosome. When this nucleic acid occurs more than 200 times, an individual is said to have the "full mutation" and fragile X syndrome. If the nucleic acid repetition occurs fewer than 200 times, the individual is unaffected or less severely affected. This is said to be the premutation, and the individual is identified as a carrier (Sherman, 2002). The disorder transmits from a mother with the premutation to a son with either the premutation or the full mutation, and occasionally from a father with the premutation or the full mutation to a daughter. Because of shortening of the nucleic acid repeat in gamete production, affected individuals can produce children with the premutation (Robin, 2007; Sherman, 2002).

CLINICAL MANIFESTATIONS

The more severe manifestations of fragile X syndrome are seen very infrequently in girls, because they have two X chromosomes and usually only one is affected. However, boys with fragile X syndrome have large ears, cupping of the ears, velvet-like skin, a slim build, broad and somewhat squinting eyes, large testes, hyperextensible joints, and mental retardation (Figure 33-4) (Hagerman, 2002; Robin, 2007). The degree of mental retardation is in the moderate to severe range, with IQ scores of about 20 to 50. Many are autistic, with a 15% to 30% occurrence rate (Harvard Mental Health Letter, 2009). In fact, Clifford et al. (2007) found that among individuals with the full mutation, 67% of males and 23% of females demonstrated one of the autism spectrum disorders. Children also may have a high, arched palate, flat feet, large heads, a transverse palmar crease, and prominent ears. In adulthood, a defined jaw line develops and the face becomes longer. Adults are often shy and

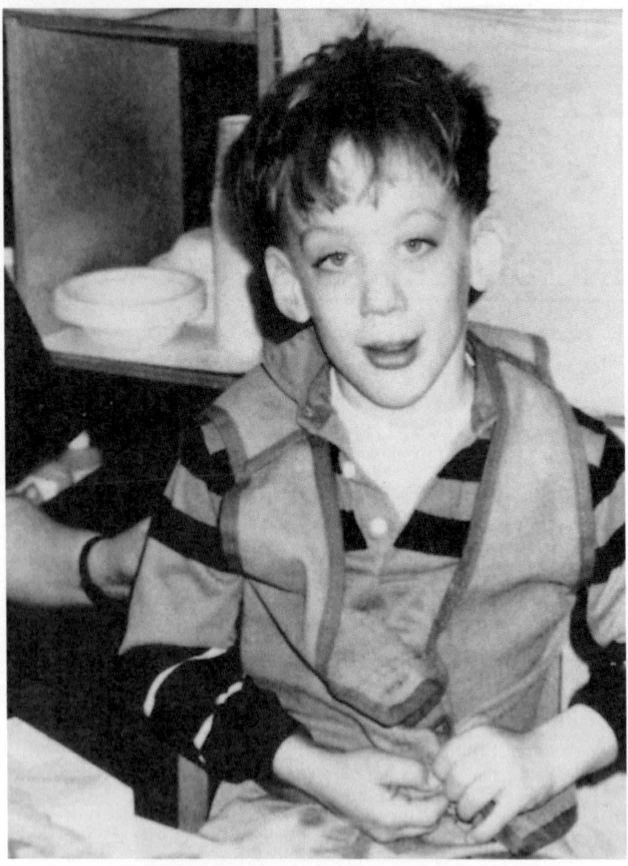

FIGURE 33-4 **Young Boy with Fragile X Syndrome.** DELMAR CENGAGE LEARNING.

hyperactive, have a short attention span, exhibit hand-biting and hand-flapping, but have a fairly good ability to relate to other people (Hagerman, 2002). Speech is typically delayed in both acquisition of language and complexity of sentence structure. In the school years, children with fragile X syndrome have problems with mathematics. They have poor auditory memory skills but good visual memory (Hagerman, 2002). Behaviorally, children may also display mood instability, poor eye contact, and a tendency to chew on their clothes (Hagerman, 2002). A very good example of some of the behaviors of a teenaged boy with fragile X syndrome is in the movie "What's Eating Gilbert Grape?" Although the movie is not a presentation of mental retardation, it provides an example of some of the stressors the sibling of an adolescent with fragile X syndrome experiences.

There appears to be a "developmental decline" in IQ, a decrease as boys with fragile X syndrome pass from preschool years to adulthood (Bennetto & Pennington, 2002). Although preschool-age boys display normal or borderline IQ 44% of the time, studies of adults reflect deterioration in IQ, with only 13% of men high-functioning. As is true in Down syndrome, children who are mosaics display higher levels of functioning (Bennetto & Pennington, 2002). In families in which fragile X syndrome occurs over subsequent generations, there seems to be increased severity with each generation (Hagerman, 2002). Boys and girls with the premutation are not necessarily unaffected, however. Individuals with a greater number of gene repeats demonstrate more severe symptoms. They may display anxiety and obsessional thinking (Hagerman, 2002), depression (Grossman et al., 2003), learning disabilities especially surrounding mathematics (Murphy & Mazzocco, 2008), autism, tremor ataxia (Jacquemont et al., 2003), and attention-deficit disorder (ADD) (Hagerman, 2002).

DIAGNOSIS

Diagnosis of fragile X syndrome is made by karyotyping. Although prenatal diagnosis through amniocentesis is possible, testing for fragile X syndrome is not routinely performed, unless there is a positive family history. As with Down syndrome, amniocentesis can be performed promptly in order to allow an early second trimester abortion, should the mother decide upon this choice.

TREATMENT

Most persons with fragile X syndrome require special education and therapeutic services. Unfortunately little research has systematically examined the effectiveness of various treatments or interventions. Generally treatment resembles that for other developmentally delayed children. Suggestions include providing a structured, predictable environment, eliminating distractions, and maintaining clear communication of expectations and feedback. Diagnosis is often not made until the child is past toddler age. At that time, enrollment in a preschool is valuable for the acquisition of social skills and for caregiver support and respite. The majority of children with fragile X syndrome manifest hyperactivity and are typically treated with a combination of medication and behavior modification. Medically, children with fragile X syndrome are prone to otitis media from early childhood and are also at risk for mitral valve prolapse and for gastroesophageal reflux (Hagerman, 2002).

NURSING MANAGEMENT

It is rare for a child with fragile X syndrome to be identified in the first year of life. Occasionally children with fragile X syndrome will be hospitalized for reasons unrelated to this diagnosis. Nurses involved in wellness care of children with fragile X syndrome need to be aware of their more frequent health complications. Aside from mitral valve prolapse, gastroesophageal reflux, and otitis media, there appears to be an increased incidence of visual problems, sinus problems, seizure disorders, and hearing loss associated with otitis. Special precautions in caring for the child with fragile X syndrome are related to these deficits.

Caregivers can be extremely helpful providing information as to preferences, level of supervision required, and aversive stimuli. They will need information about the nature of the genetic impairment and their child's expected development. Genetic counseling is advised if other children are planned. Although the syndrome can be identified through amniocentesis, counseling is also required in order to inform caregivers about the differing manifestations of the full mutation in boys and girls. Siblings may have the same difficulties as those of any mentally retarded child. If autism is present, siblings may also encounter the stresses of living with an autistic brother or sister.

ADDITIONAL COGNITIVE ALTERATIONS

FETAL ALCOHOL SYNDROME

Fetal alcohol syndrome (FAS) is a cluster of physical, behavioral, and cognitive abnormalities associated with a history of maternal alcohol exposure, either as substantial regular intake or as heavy episodic drinking. FAS is the leading cause of mental retardation worldwide and more importantly, it is the single most preventable cause of neurobehavioral and developmental abnormalities (Murthy, Kudlur, George & Mathew, 2009). FAS occurrence ranges from 0.3 to 5 per 1,000 live births (Stoll, 2007), and the incidence in the United States is increasing, despite prominent warnings on alcohol containers and in public places where alcohol is served. The exact amount of maternal alcohol ingestion that causes FAS is not known; however, the harm to the fetus is greater with large amounts of maternal alcohol intake compared with smaller amounts. Although damage can occur at any time, the fetus is most vulnerable during early pregnancy (Stoll, 2007).

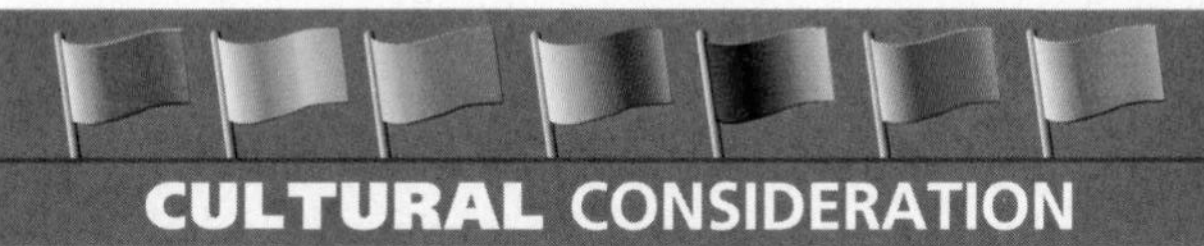

CULTURAL CONSIDERATION

Ethnic Disparities and FAS

Substantially higher rates of fetal alcohol syndrome have been demonstrated among low socioeconomic and minority groups. Using data gathered from 22 states participating in the Pregnancy Risk Assessment Monitoring System from 2001 to 2005, a recent study investigated the likelihood that women of different racial and ethnic groups would reduce their alcohol consumption during pregnancy. Overall, Black, Asian/Pacific Islander, and Hispanic women were all significantly less likely than White women to reduce their heavy drinking after becoming pregnant. American Indian/Alaskan Native women who were moderate drinkers before conception were over 2 times more likely than White women to reduce drinking after becoming pregnant. Among those who binge drank in the months before pregnancy, compared to White women, Black, Hispanic, American Indian/Alaskan Native, and Asian/Pacific Islander women were all less likely to quit binge drinking while pregnant. Significant racial differences in pregnancy-related drinking reduction are evident, and may help explain racial disparities in FAS (Tenkku, Morris, Salas, & Xaverius, 2009).

Clinical Manifestations

Characteristic features seen in the infant with FAS include:

- Prenatal or postnatal growth retardation—height, weight, and head circumference below the tenth percentile; decreased adipose tissue
- Central nervous system neurodevelopmental abnormalities of varying severity—developmental delay, intellectual impairment, language delays, poor abstract reasoning, poor math skills, mental retardation, abnormal cognitive functioning (learning and attention difficulties), behavioral problems (infant irritability, child hyperactivity, oppositional behavior)
- Facial dysmorphology—short palpebral fissures, smooth philtrum, ptosis and thin upper lip; microcephaly, abnormally small eyes, epicanthic folds, maxillary hypoplasia, and micrognathia may also be present (Figure 33-5)
- Other abnormalities such as cardiac, skeletal, or ocular defects and renal anomalies

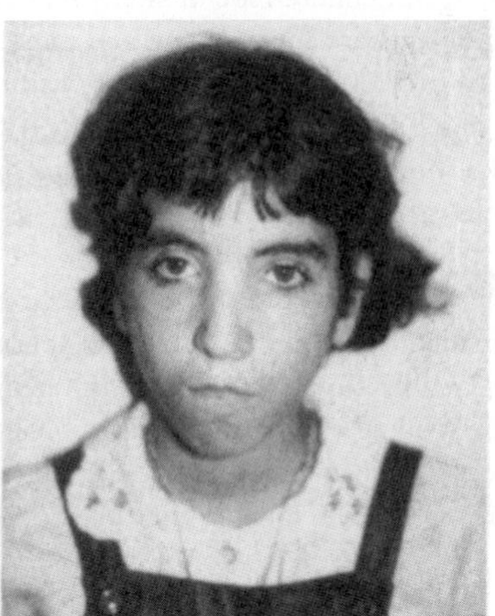

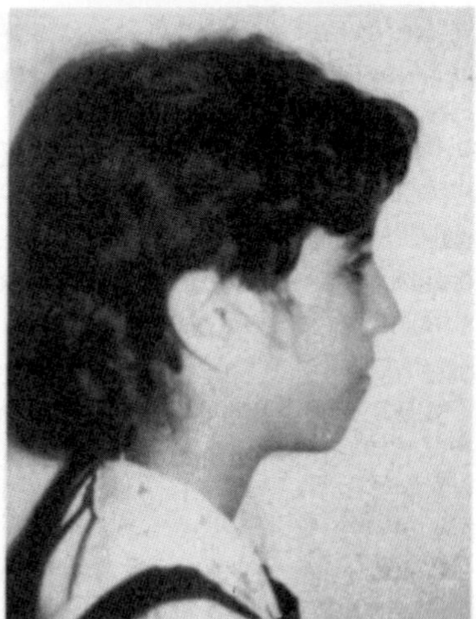

FIGURE 33-5 Young Girl with Fetal Alcohol Effects Whose Mother Drank Heavily Only During the Last Trimester. DELMAR CENGAGE LEARNING.

IN THE REAL WORLD

When I was between college semesters, I spent some time volunteering at various agencies. The volunteer coordinator scheduled me for two days at a school for mentally retarded preschoolers and primary grade children. I told her I just wanted to do one day but, no, she insisted that I would do a Friday and a Monday. She told me that volunteers tended not to want to go back unless they had 2 days at the school, because it took some desensitization. I did my two days and subsequently did many more. After that first Friday, though, I remember thinking that if I hadn't promised to go back on Monday I wouldn't have done it. Now I teach pediatric nursing. I schedule some of my students into school experiences with mentally retarded children. At first I scheduled them for two half-days. One semester, I acceded to their requests for longer experiences and less travel, and scheduled some of them for a whole school day, expecting negative reactions. Maybe times have changed in the intervening years. Maybe our young adults have been introduced to mentally retarded people all their lives and are less squeamish. However, my nursing students are so mature, so less apt to shrink from children with deficits than I was. Almost all enjoyed their school day, learning something about remedial reading or language development or special equipment or physical therapy or the role of the school nurse. In fact, one nursing student, a young man, had to schedule a two-hour experience to make up for missing part of a clinical day. Faced with many choices, he asked, "Can't I just go back to that school that has the mentally retarded children? There was a kid there named Arthur who asked me at the end of my day, 'Are you coming back to play with me tomorrow?' and it just broke my heart to say no."

A percentage of children are mentally retarded, but their most striking deficits are in reasoning and attention. IQ ranged from 40 to over 100 in a recent study, with a mean near 90 (Sayal et al., 2009). IQ is dependent upon the mother's alcohol intake, her patterns of drinking, and total time of exposure (Schwartz, 2005).

Treatment

FAS is permanent and irreversible but not degenerative. Treatment is mainly supportive during the neonatal period. Because poor feeding is common, nutritional intervention may be necessary. Strategies include monitoring weight gain, optimizing caloric intake, and promoting suck and swallow patterns. Infants and children who are suspected to have FAS should be evaluated at an early age. For those with the disorder, referral to early intervention and education agencies should be made. Caregivers, especially the mother, should receive support services such as alcohol treatment for the child's sake. Many previously accepted behavioral effects of FAS, such as depression and ADD, have been demonstrated to be due to continued alcohol use by mothers after pregnancy, not to FAS itself (Coles, Kable, Drews-Botsch, & Falek, 2000). There is no known "safe" amount of alcohol consumption during pregnancy. Health care providers should caution pregnant women and those planning pregnancy to abstain from alcohol use.

KEY CONCEPTS

- Two to three percent of the human population is mentally retarded. There is no treatment or cure.
- A mentally retarded person has subaverage general intellectual functioning existing concurrently with deficits in adaptive behavior.
- Diagnosis of mental retardation is made on the basis of history and physical examination, developmental assessments, and tests of intellectual and adaptive functioning.
- Siblings of mentally retarded children may have to exhibit extra patience and assume added responsibility. This may affect their lives both positively and adversely.
- Caregivers and siblings of mentally retarded children undergo a grieving process related to their separation from a significant dream.
- Down syndrome is the most frequent and most widely recognized chromosome disorder of humans.

- Health problems associated with Down syndrome include cardiac defects, hypothyroidism, ocular cataract, atlantoaxial deformities, frequent respiratory infections ranging from pneumonia to chronic sinusitis, hearing deficit, and Down-associated Alzheimer's syndrome after the age of 30.
- Autism is a genetic developmental disorder, characterized by extreme difficulty communicating with and relating to the environment, and manifested by bizarre behavior, delayed language acquisition, poor social relations, impairment of self-care skills, and altered sensory responses.
- Because of behavior disturbances and disordered sleep patterns, caregivers of autistic children experience substantial stress.
- Individuals with fragile X syndrome have large ears, velvet-like skin, a slim build, broad and somewhat squinting eyes, large testes, and mental retardation. Some are autistic.

REVIEW ACTIVITIES

1. By percentage, how many children are mentally retarded?
2. Describe the appearance of a child with Down syndrome.
3. Explain the importance of knowing whether or not an echocardiogram was performed for a neonate with Down syndrome.
4. Give two reasons why the age span of Down syndrome children has increased over the past 50 years.
5. List the behavioral manifestations of an autistic child.
6. Explain why the care plan for the autistic child should include the diagnosis potential for injury.
7. Explain why genetic counseling may or may not be important for the parents of an autistic child if they are planning on subsequent children.
8. Describe the appearance of a boy with fragile X syndrome.

STUDY QUESTIONS

1. Why is early identification of autism important?
   a. Parents of autistic children need support.
   b. Early intervention fosters better outcomes.
   c. Prevention of subsequent pregnancies is essential.
   d. Cure is possible only if diagnosed by 18 months.
2. Down syndrome is definitively diagnosed by which of the following?
   a. The quadruple screen
   b. Amniocentesis
   c. Karyotyping
   d. Presence of eight or more clinical features
3. Fragile X syndrome often co-exists with:
   a. Autism.
   b. Fetal alcohol syndrome.
   c. Down syndrome.
   d. Childhood schizophrenia.
4. Which of the following has the highest prevalence among children?
   a. Down syndrome
   b. Mental retardation
   c. Fragile X syndrome
   d. Autism spectrum disorder
5. Why is periodic radiographic examination of the neck essential for children's health in Down syndrome?
   a. Webbing can be minimized through treatment.
   b. Adenoidal hypertrophy can obstruct the airway.
   c. Chronic sinusitis affects hearing and speech.
   d. Atlantoaxial stabilization can prevent quadriplegia.
6. What is the Denver Developmental Screening Test II (DDST-II)?
   a. A rule-out examination for mental retardation
   b. An age-scaled IQ test used up until school age
   c. A measure of healthy normal pediatric adaptation
   d. A measurement of the child's abilities across four spectra
7. What is the general purpose of counseling for parents of mentally retarded children?
   a. It teaches parents things they need to know to maximize children's outcomes.
   b. It educates parents about ways that they can prevent mental retardation in subsequent children.

c. It allows parents to recognize their feelings and assures them that those feelings are normal.
d. It teaches parents how to grieve effectively, so as to achieve resolution.

8. What is the probable cause of autism?
a. Aloof, "refrigerator" mothers who cannot relate to their children
b. A single recessive gene
c. An interaction between genetics and environment
d. Reaction to the MMR vaccination

9. Which behavior is NOT commonly found in autistic children?
a. Savant or unusual aptitude
b. Communication impairment
c. Abnormal social skill development
d. Preference for sameness

10. Of the causes of mental retardation, which are most preventable?
a. Prenatal
b. Genetic
c. Perinatal
d. Postnatal

REFERENCES

American Psychiatric Association. (2000). *Diagnostic and statistical manual of mental disorders* (4th ed.). (Text revision, *DSM-IV-TR*). Washington, DC: Author.

Auyeung, B., Baron-Cohen, S., Ashwin, E., Knickmeyer, R., Taylor, K., & Hackett, G. (2009). Fetal testosterone and autistic traits. *British Journal of Psychology, 100*(1), 1–22.

Baird, G., & Charman, T. (2000). A screening instrument for autism at 18 months of age: A 6-year follow-up study. *Journal of the American Academy of Child and Adolescent Psychiatry, 39*(6), 694–702.

Baron-Cohen, S., Wheelwright, S., Lawson, J., Griffin, R., Ashwin, C., Billington, J., & Chakrabarti, B. (2006). Empathizing and systemizing in autism spectrum conditions. In F. R. Volkmar, R. Paul, A. Klin, & D. Cohen, *Handbook of autism and pervasive developmental disorders* (3rd ed.). Hoboken, N.J.: John Wiley & Sons.

Bayley, N. (1969). *Bayley scales of infant development.* New York: Psychological Corporation.

Beauchesne, M. A., & Kelley, B. R. (2004). Evidence to support parental concerns as an early indicator of autism in children. *Pediatric Nursing, 30*(1), 57–67.

Bennetto, L., & Pennington, B. F. (2002). Neuropsychology. In R. J. Hagerman & P. J. Hagerman (Eds.). *Fragile X syndrome: Diagnosis, treatment and research* (3rd ed.). Baltimore, MD: The Johns Hopkins University Press, pp. 206–248.

Bettelheim, B. (1967). *The empty fortress: Infantile autism and the birth of self.* New York: Free Press.

Bilder, D., Pinborough-Zimmerman, J., Miller, J., & McMahon, W. (2009). Prenatal, perinatal, and neonatal factors associated with autism spectrum disorders. *Pediatrics, 123*(5), 1293–1300.

Bohm, H. V., & Stewart, M. G. (2009). Brief report: On the concordance percentages for autistic spectrum disorder of twins. *Journal of Autism and Developmental Disorders, 39*, 806–808.

Campbell, D. B., Buie, T. M., Winter, H., Bauman, M., Sutcliffe, J. S., Perrin, J. M., & Levitt, P. (2009). Distinct genetic risk based on association of MET in families with co-occurring autism and gastrointestinal conditions. *Pediatrics, 123*(3), 1018–1024.

Centers for Disease Control and Prevention. (2009). Learn the Signs. Act Early. Early Identification of Children with Autism or other Developmental Disorders Awareness Campaign. Retrieved June 30, 2009, from http://www.cdc.gov/ncbddd/actearly/index.html.

Chawarska, K., & Volkmar, F. R. (2006). Autism in infancy and early childhood In F. R. Volkmar, R. Paul, A. Klin, & D. Cohen, *Handbook of autism and pervasive developmental disorders* (3rd ed.). Hoboken, N.J.: John Wiley & Sons.

Chen, H. (2006). Atlas of genetic diagnosis and counseling [electronic resource on CD-ROM]. Totowa: N.J.: Humana Press.

Clifford, S., Dissanayake, C., Bui, Q. M., Huggins, R., Taylor, A. K., & Loesch, D. Z. (2007). Autism spectrum phenotype in males and females with fragile X full mutation and premutation. *Journal of Autism and Developmental Disorders, 37*(4), 738–747.

Coles, C. D., Kable, J. A., Drews-Botsch, C., & Falek, A. (2000). Early identification of risk for effects of prenatal alcohol exposure. *Journal of Studies on Alcohol, 61*(4), 607–616.

Colson, C., & Pearcey, N. (1997). Why Max deserves a life. *Christianity Today, 41*(7), 80.

Council on Children with Disabilities (2006). Identifying infants and young children with developmental disorders in the medical home: An algorithm for developmental surveillance and screening. *Pediatrics, 118*, 405–420.

Creak, M. (1961). Schizophrenic syndrome in childhood: Progress report of a working party. *Cerebral Palsy Bulletin, 3*, 501–504.

Descartes, M., & Carroll, A. J. (2007). Cytogenetics. In R. M. Kliegman, R. E. Behrman, H. B. Jenson, & F. B. Stanton, *Nelson textbook of pediatrics* (18th ed.). Saunders: Philadelphia, PA.

Downing, D. (2007). Autism: Are we entering the final straight? In memory of Bernard Rimland. *Journal of Nutritional and Environmental Medicine, 16*(3–4), 173–180.

Dunn, L. M., & Dunn, L. M. (1981). *Peabody picture vocabulary test – revised.* Circle Pines, NM: American Guidance Services.

Feldman, M., McDonald, L., Serbin, L., Stack, D., Secco, M. L., & Yu, C. T. (2007). Predictors of depressive symptoms in primary caregivers of young children with or at risk for developmental delay. *Journal of Intellectual Disability Research, 51*(8), 606–619.

Filipek, P. A. (2006). Medical aspects of autism In F. R. Volkmar, R. Paul, A. Klin, & D. Cohen, *Handbook of autism and pervasive developmental disorders* (3rd ed.). Hoboken, N.J.: John Wiley & Sons.

Fombonne, E. (2006). Epidemiological studies of pervasive developmental disorders. In F. R. Volkmar, R. Paul, A. Klin, & D. Cohen, *Handbook of autism and pervasive developmental disorders* (3rd ed.). Hoboken, N.J.: John Wiley & Sons.

Fombonne, E. (2009). A wrinkle in time. *Journal of the Academy of Child and Adolescent Psychiatry, 48*(5), 463–464.

Frankenburg, W. K., Dodds, J. B., Archer, P., Shapiro, H., & Bresnick, B. (1992). The Denver II: A major revision and restandardization of the Denver Developmental Screening Test. *Pediatrics, 89*(1), 91–97.

Golnik, A. E., & Ireland, M. (2009). Complementary alternative medicine for children with autism: A physician survey. *Journal of Autism and Developmental Disorders, 39*, 996–1005.

Grossman, A. W., Churchill, J. D., McKinney, B. C., Kodish, I. M., Otte, S. L., & Greenough, W. T. (2003). Experience effects on brain development: Possible contributions to psychopathology. *Journal of Child Psychology and Psychiatry and Allied Disciplines, 44*(1), 33–63.

Hagerman, R. J. (2002). Physical and behavioral phenotype. In R. J. Hagerman & P. J. Hagerman (Eds.), *Fragile X syndrome: Diagnosis, treatment and research* (3rd ed.). Baltimore: Johns Hopkins University Press, pp. 3–109.

Harvard Mental Health Letter, 2009. Rare diseases offer insights into autism spectrum disorders: Preliminary laboratory studies suggest new biological targets for intervention. 25(10), 3.

Hertz-Picciotto, I., Croen, L. A., Hansen, R., Jones, C. R., van de Water, J., & Pessah, I. N. (2006). The CHARGE study: An epidemiologic investigation of genetic and environmental factors contributing to autism. *Environmental Health Perspectives, 114*(7), 1119–1125.

Jacquemont, S., Hagerman, R. J., Leehey, M., Grigsby, J., Zhang, L., Brunberg, J. A., Greco, C., Des Portes, V., Jardini, T., Levine, R., Berry-Kravis, E., Brown, W. T., Schaeffer, S., Kissel, J., Massone, F., & Hagerman, P. J. (2003). Fragile X premutation tremor/ataxia syndrome: Molecular, clinical and neuroimaging correlates. *American Journal of Human Genetics, 72*(4), 869–878.

Jacques, A. M., Collins, V. R., Haynes, K., Sheffield, L. J., Francis, I., Forbes, R., & Halliday, J. L. (2006). Using record linkage and manual follow-up to evaluate the Victorian maternal serum screening quadruple test for Down's syndrome, trisomy 18 and neural tube defects. *Journal of Medical Screening 13*(1), 8–13.

Jangaard, K. A., Dell, D. B., Dodds, L., & Allen, A. C. (2008). Outcomes in a population of healthy term and near-term infants with serum bilirubin levels of ≥ 325 μmol/L (≥19 mg/dL) who were born in Nova Scotia, Canada, between 1994 and 2000. *Pediatrics, 122*(1), 119–124.

Johnson, S., & Marlow, N. (2009). Positive screening results on the modified checklist for autism in toddlers: Implications for very preterm populations. *Journal of Pediatrics, 154*(4), 478–480.

Kanner, L. (1943). Autistic disturbances of affective contact. *Nervous Child, 2*, 217–250.

Kolb, B., & Fantie, B. D. (2009). Development of the child's brain and behavior. In C. R. Reynolds & E. Fletcher-Janzen (Eds.) *Handbook of clinical child neuropsychology* (3rd ed.). New York: Springer.

Leiter, R. G. (1969). *The Leiter International Performance Scale.* California: Western Psychological Services.

Lord, C., Bristol-Power, M., Cafiero, J. M., Filipek, P. A., Gallagher, J. J., Harris, S. L. (2001). Educating children with autism. Washington, DC: National Academy Press.

Lovaas, M. (1987). Behavioral treatment and normal educational and intellectual functioning in young autistic children. *Journal of Consulting and Clinical Psychology, 55*, 3–9.

Matson, J. L., & Minshawi, N. F. (2006). *Early intervention for autism spectrum disorders.* Kidlington, Oxford, UK: Elsevier.

Menkes, J. H., Sarnat, H. B., & Maria, B. L. (Eds.). (2006). *Child neurology* (7th ed.). Philadelphia: Lippincott, Williams & Wilkins.

Montgomery, A. (2006). Dimethylglycine and people with autism. *Learning Disability Practice, 92*, 34–36.

Moses, K., & Kearney, R. (1995). *Transition therapy: An existential approach to facilitating growth in the light of loss.* Evanston, IL: Resource Networks, Inc.

Muhle, R., Trentacoste, S. V., & Rapin, I. (2004). The genetics of autism. *Pediatrics, 113*(5), 472–486.

Murphy, M. M., & Mazzocco, M. M. (2008). Mathematics learning disabilities in girls with fragile X or Turner syndrome during late elementary school. *Journal of Learning Disabilities, 41*(1), 29–46.

Murthy, P., Kudlur, S., George, S., & Mathew, G. (2009). A clinical overview of fetal alcohol syndrome. *Addictive Disorders & Their Treatment, 8*(1), 1–12.

Nadel, S., & Poss, J. E. (2007). Early detection of autism spectrum disorders: Screening between 12 and 24 months of age. *Journal of the American Academy of Nurse Practitioners, 19*(8), 408–417.

Nihira, K., Foster, R., Shellhaas, M., & Leland, H. (1975). *AAMR adaptive behavior scale.* Washington, DC: American Association on Mental Retardation.

Nye, C., & Brice, A. (2005). Combined vitamin B6-magnesium treatment in autism spectrum disorder. Cochrane Database of Systematic Reviews [electronic resource].

Panerai, S., Zingale, M., Trubia, G., Finocchiaro, M., Zuccarello, R., Ferrri, R., & Elia, M. (2009). *Journal of Autism and Developmental Disorders, 39*, 874–882.

Reichow, B., & Wolery, M. (2009). Comprehensive synthesis of early intensive behavioral interventions for young children with autism based on the UCLA Young Autism Project model. *Journal of Autism and Developmental Disorders, 39*, 23–41.

Roberts, E. M., English, P. B., Grether, J. K., Windham, G. C., Somberg, L., & Wolff, C. (2007). Maternal residence near agricultural pesticide applications and autism spectrum disorders among children in the California Central Valley. *Environmental Health Perspectives, 115*, 1482–1489.

Johns Hopkins Hospital, Custer, J., Rau, R., & Lee, C. (2008). *The Harriet Lane handbook* (18th ed.). Philadelphia: Elsevier.

Robin, N. H. (2007). Patterns of genetic transmission. In F. R. Volkmar, R. Paul, A. Klin, & D. Cohen, *Handbook of autism and pervasive developmental disorders* (3rd ed.). Hoboken, N.J.: John Wiley & Sons.

Robins, D. L., Fein, D., Barton, M. L., & Green, J. A. (2001). The modified checklist for autism in toddlers: An initial study investigating the early detection of autism and pervasive developmental disorders. *Journal of Autism and Developmental Disorders, 31*, 131–144.

Rutter, M. (1970). Autistic children: Infancy to adulthood. *Seminars in Psychiatry, 2*, 435–450.

Rutter, M. (2006). Genetic influences and autism In F. R. Volkmar, R. Paul, A. Klin, & D. Cohen, *Handbook of autism and pervasive developmental disorders* (3rd ed.). Hoboken, N.J.: John Wiley & Sons.

Sallows, G. O., & Graupner, T. D. (2005). Intensive behavioral treatment for children with autism: Four-year outcome and predictors. *American Journal on Mental Retardation, 110*, 417–438.

Sayal, K., Heron, J., Golding, J., Alati, R., Smith, G. D., Gray, R., & Emond, A. (2009). Binge pattern of alcohol consumption during pregnancy and childhood mental health outcomes: Longitudinal population-based study. *Pediatrics, 123*, e289–e296.

Schopler, E. (1997). Implementation of TEACCH philosophy. In D. J. Cohen & F. R. Volkmar (Eds.), *Handbook of autism and pervasive developmental disorders* (2nd ed.). New York: Wiley & Sons, pp. 767–795.

Schopler, E., Reichler, R. J., & Renner, B. R. (1988). *The childhood autism rating scale.* Los Angeles: Western Psychological Services.

Schwartz, M. W. (Ed.) (2005). *The 5-minute pediatric consult* (4th ed.). Philadelphia: Lippincott, Williams & Wilkins.

Shah, P. E., Dalton, R., & Boris, N. W. (2007). Pervasive developmental disorders and childhood psychosis. In R. M. Kliegman, R. E. Behrman, H. B. Jenson, & B. F. Stanton (Eds.). *Nelson textbook of pediatrics* (18th ed.). Philadelphia, PA: Saunders.

Shapiro, B. K., & Batshaw, M. L. (2007). Mental retardation (intellectual disability). In R. M. Kliegman, R. E. Behrman, H. B. Jenson, & B. F. Stanton (Eds.). *Nelson textbook of pediatrics* (18th ed.). Philadelphia, PA: Saunders.

Sharpe, N. F., & Carter, R. F. (2006). *Genetic testing: Care, consent and liability.* Hoboken, N.J.: John Wiley & Sons.

Shea, V., & Mesibov, G. (2006). Adolescents and adults with autism In F. R. Volkmar, R. Paul, A. Klin, & D. Cohen, *Handbook of autism and pervasive developmental disorders* (3rd ed.). Hoboken, N.J.: John Wiley & Sons.

Sherman, S. (2002). Epidemiology. In R. J. Hagerman & P. J. Hagerman (Eds.), *Fragile X syndrome: Diagnosis, treatment and research* (3rd ed.). Baltimore: The Johns Hopkins University Press, pp. 136–168.

Smith, M. (2006). *Mental retardation and developmental delay.* Oxford: Oxford University Press.

Smith, T., Groen, A. D., & Wynn, J. W. (2000). Randomized trial of intensive early intervention for children with pervasive developmental disorder. *American Journal on Mental Retardation, 105,* 269–285.

Sparrow, S. S., Balla, D. A., & Cicchette, D. V. (1984). *Vineland adaptive behavior scales.* Circle Pines, MN: American Guidance Service.

Spock, B. (1949). *The pocket book of baby and child care.* New York: Pocket Books.

Stahmer, A. C., & Ingersoll, B. (2004). Inclusive programming for toddlers with autism spectrum disorders: Outcomes from the children's toddler school. *Journal of Positive Behavior Interventions, 6*(2), 67–80.

Stoll, B. J. (2007). Metabolic disturbances. In R. M. Kliegman, R. E. Behrman, H. B. Jenson, & B. F. Stanton (Eds.). *Nelson textbook of pediatrics* (18th ed.). Philadelphia, PA: Saunders.

Szatmari, P. (2004). *A mind apart.* New York: The Guilford Press.

Tenkku, L. E., Morris, D. S., Salas, J., Xaverius, PK. (2009). Racial disparities in pregnancy-related drinking reduction. *Journal of Maternal Child Health. 13*(5), 604–613.

Terman, L., & Merrill, M. (1973). *Stanford-Binet intelligence scale.* Boston: Houghton Mifflin.

Tranquillo, J. V. (2008). *Quantitative neurophysiology* [electronic resource]. San Rafael, CA: Morgan & Claypool Publishers.

Tsang, S. K., Shek, D. T. L., Lam, L. L., Tang, F. L. Y., & Cheung, P. M. P. (2007). *Journal of Autism and Developmental Disorders, 37,* 390–396.

Tsao, R., & Kindelberger, C. (2009). Variability of cognitive development in children with Down syndrome: Relevance of good reasons for using the cluster procedure. *Research in Developmental Disabilities, 30*(3), 426–432.

Vis, J. C., Duffels, M. G. J., Winter, M. M., Weijerman, M. E., Cobben, J. M., Huisman, S. A., & Mulder, B. J. M. (2009). Down syndrome: A cardiovascular perspective. *Journal of Intellectual Disability Research, 53*(5), 419–425.

Volkmar, F. R., & Klin, A. (2005). Issues in the classification of autism and related conditions In F. R. Volkmar, R. Paul, A. Klin, & D. Cohen, *Handbook of autism and pervasive developmental disorders* (3rd ed.). Hoboken, N.J.: John Wiley & Sons.

Watson, L. R., Baranek, G. T., Crais, E. R., Reznick, J. S., Dykstra, J., & Perryman, T. (2007). The first year inventory: Retrospective parent responses to a questionnaire designed to identify one-year-olds at risk for autism. *Journal of Autism and Developmental Disorders, 37*(1), 49–61.

Wechsler, D. (1989). *Wechsler preschool and primary scale of intelligence – revised.* New York: Psychological Corporation.

Wechsler, D. (1991). *Wechsler intelligence scale for children – III.* New York: Psychological Corporation.

Whiteford, H. (2000). Early intervention programs for children with autism: Conceptual frameworks for implementation. *American Journal of Orthopsychiatry, 70*(1), 82–94.

Yang, Q., Rasmussen, S. A., & Friedman, J. M. (2002). Mortality associated with Down's syndrome in the U.S. from 1983 to 1997: A population-based study. *The Lancet, 359*(9311), 1019.

Zwaigenbaum, L., Bryson, S., Lord, C., Rogers, S., Carter, A., Carver, L., Chawarska, K., Constantino, J., Dawson, G., Dobkins, K., Fein, D., Iverson, J., Klin, A., Landa, R., Messinger, D., Ozonoff, S., Sigman, M., Stone, W., Tager-Flusberg, H., & Yirmiya, N. (2009) Clinical assessment and management of toddlers with suspected autism spectrum disorder: Insights from studies of high-risk infants. *Pediatrics 123*(5), 1383–1391.

SUGGESTED READINGS

American Academy of Pediatrics, Committee on Genetics. (2001). Health supervision for children with Down syndrome. *Pediatrics, 107*(2), 442–449.

Bosch, J., & Ringdahl, J. (2001). Functional analysis of problem behavior in children with mental retardation: What is it, and why should pediatric nurses care? *Maternal and Child Nursing, 26*(6), 307–311.

Centers for Disease Control and Prevention. (2002). Delayed diagnosis of fragile X syndrome—United States, 1990–1999. *Morbidity and Mortality Weekly Report, 51*(33), 740–742.

Dales, L., Hammer, S. J., & Smith, N. J. (2001). Time trends in autism and in MMR immunization coverage in California. *Journal of the American Medical Association, 258*(9), 1183–1185.

Rutter, M. (1999). The Emmanuel Miller Memorial Lecture 1998. Autism: Two-way interplay between research and clinical work. *Journal of Child Psychology and Psychiatry, 40*(2), 169–188.

Schall, C. (2000). Family perspectives on raising a child with autism. *Journal of Child and Family Studies, 9*(4), 409–423.

Sivberg, B. (2003). Parents' detection of early signs in their children having an autism spectrum disorder. *Journal of Pediatric Nursing, 18*(6), 433–440.

Van Riper, M. (2003). A change of plans: The birth of a child with Down syndrome doesn't have to be a negative experience. *American Journal of Nursing, 103*(6), 71–74.

RESOURCES

Refer to the online student StudyWARE for Potts & Mandleco at http://www.CengageBrain.com for additional content and study aids.

Organization: **The Arc of the United States**
Description: The Arc of the United States advocates for the rights and full participation of all children and adults with intellectual and developmental disabilities. Their network of members and affiliated chapters improves systems of supports and services, connects families, inspires communities, and influences public policy. The website provides information about chapters and public policies.
Website/Resource: http://www.thearc.org

Organization: **Association for Children with Down Syndrome**
Description: Based in Long Island, New York, ACDS is Long Island's service provider for children and adults with Down syndrome, and provides year-round programs for all ages. The website provides information regarding services, careers, and events.
Website/Resource: http://www.acds.org

Organization: **Autism Society of America**
Description: The Autism Society, co-founded by Dr. Bernard Rimland, increases public awareness, advocates for people with autistic spectrum disorders, and provides information about the day-to-day issues faced by people on the autism spectrum.
Website/Resource: http://www.autism-society.org

Organization: **California Department of Developmental Services**
Description: This site offers an overview of services available to persons in California with developmental disabilities.
Website/Resource: http://www.dds.cahwnet.gov

Organization: **Center for the Study of Autism**
Description: The Center for the Study of Autism focuses on parent-associated research initiatives. The website provides links to numerous autism organizations.
Website/Resource: http://www.autism.org

Organization: **Families for Early Autism Treatment**
Description: FEAT is a non-profit organization begun by parents in the Sacramento, California area. They are politically active in implementation of best practices and research support, mostly in conjunction with The Mind Institute in Sacramento, and maintain a newsletter for information.
Website/Resource: http://www.feat.org

Organization: **FRAXA Research Foundation**
Description: Founded by parents of three children with fragile X, FRAXA research foundation funds grants and fellowships for research. The website provides general information concerning fragile X as well as research projects.
Website/Resource: http://www.fraxa.org

Organization: **Growth Charts for Children with Down Syndrome**
Description: Provides growth grids for children with Down syndrome
Website/Resource: http://www.growthcharts.com

Organization: **National Association for Down Syndrome**
Description: Based in Chicago, NADS provides services for children and adults with Down syndrome in the Chicago area. The website provides access to resources and contact information.
Website/Resource: http://www.nads.org

Organization: **National Down Syndrome Congress**
Description: It is the purpose of the National Down Syndrome Congress to create a national climate in which all people will recognize and embrace the value and dignity of people with Down syndrome. The website offers users access to affiliates, self-advocates, and informational resources.
Website/Resource: http://www.ndsccenter.org

Organization: **National Fragile X Foundation**
Description: Based in San Francisco, the National Fragile X Foundation provides education and support for families. In addition, it supports ongoing research about fragile X syndrome. The website provides information regarding fragile X issues.
Website/Resource: http://www.fragilex.org

Organization: **National Organization on Fetal Alcohol Syndrome**
Description: Based in Washington, D.C., NOFAS provides information and political impetus for legislation to prevent and treat fetal alcohol syndrome. The website provides information regarding legislation, issues/priorities, and policy statements.
Website/Resource: http://nofas.org

Organization: **New York Families for Autistic Children**
Description: Based in New York City, NYFAC provides support and services for children and adults with autism and for their families. The website has photographs and links to other websites about autism.
Website/Resource: http://www.nyfac.org

Organization: **Special Olympics**
Description: Based in Washington, D.C., for the past 40 years Special Olympics has provided sports competition activities worldwide for persons who are mentally retarded. The website is a wealth of information regarding athletes, involvement, and regional sites.
Website/Resource: http://www.specialolympics.org

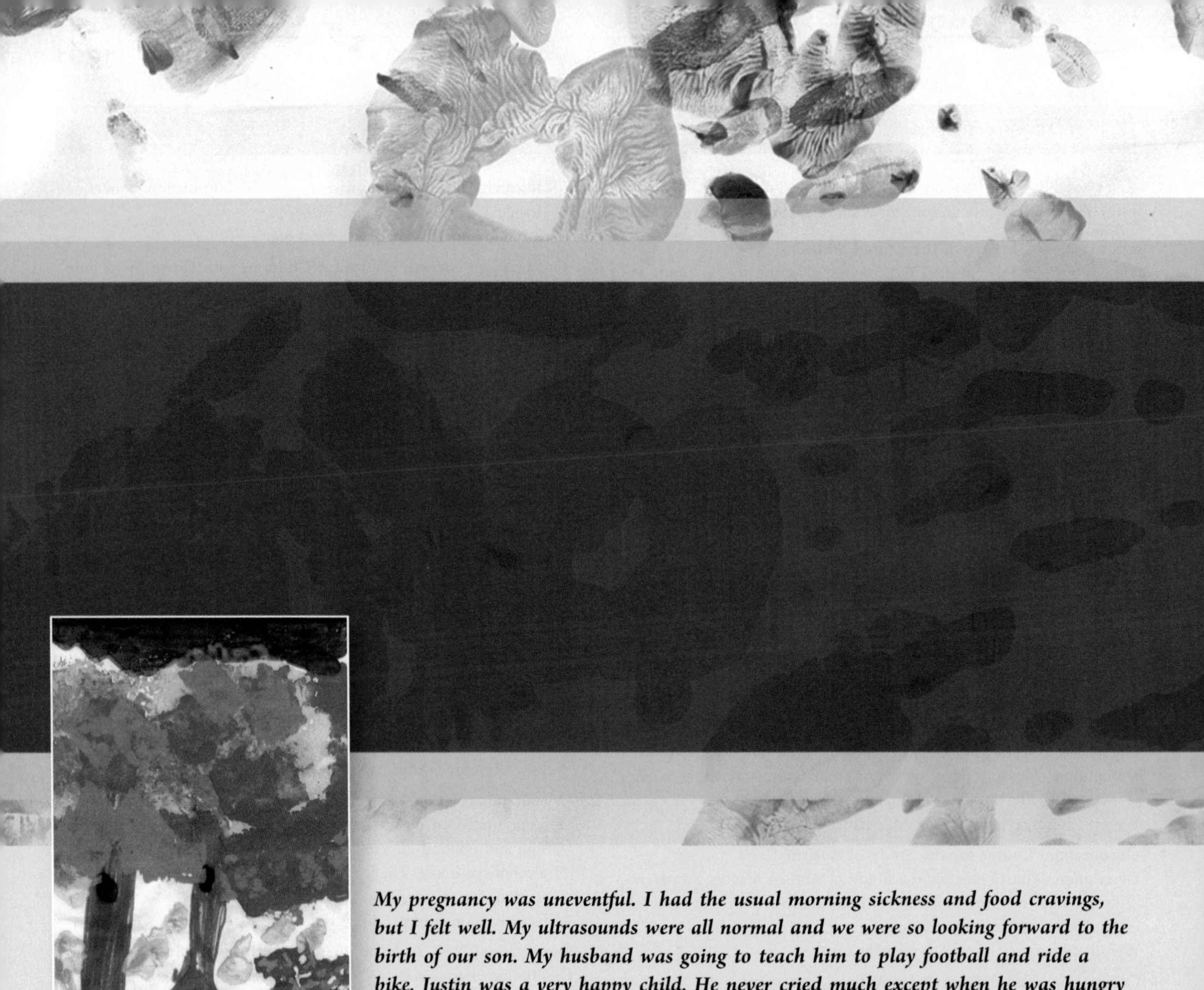

My pregnancy was uneventful. I had the usual morning sickness and food cravings, but I felt well. My ultrasounds were all normal and we were so looking forward to the birth of our son. My husband was going to teach him to play football and ride a bike. Justin was a very happy child. He never cried much except when he was hungry or wanted attention. We were never really worried when at 12 months he wasn't walking yet. Justin was just slow in walking, but when he did walk, he would walk on his toes. He had difficulty standing up. He would get in a position like he was going to crawl, pull his hands in close to his feet, and raise himself up by placing his hands on his knees and thighs. When Justin was about 2½ years old, we enrolled him in a day care center so I could go back to work. Justin had problems in the day care center keeping up physically with the other children.

Justin could not walk up the three steps to the slide during play time. A teacher became concerned when Justin kept falling down all the time and called my husband and me to express her concerns. We took Justin to the pediatrician. The doctor did a range of tests on him. After three weeks we were given the news: Justin has Duchenne muscular dystrophy. If we're lucky he'll live to be 20 years old, but he will be confined to a wheelchair. Our only hope is that a cure is found. Maybe then our Justin will have a chance at a semi-normal life.

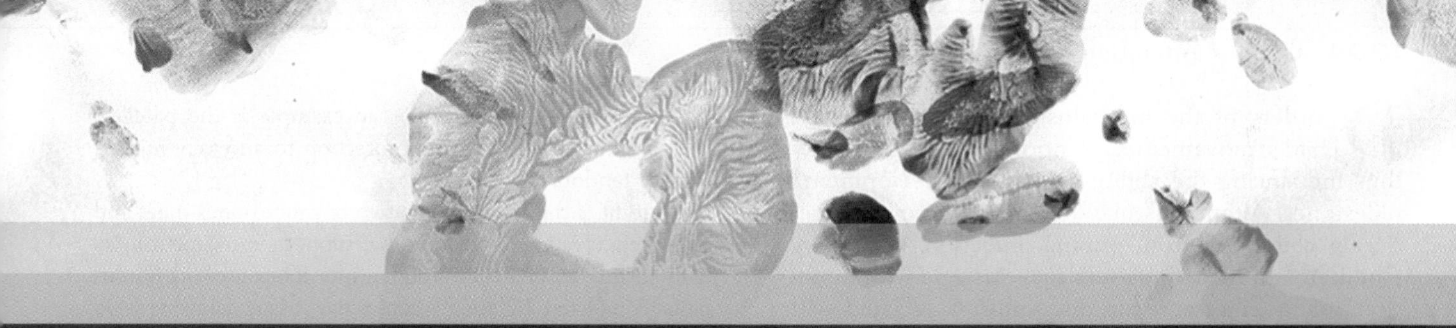

CHAPTER 34
Musculoskeletal Alterations

Nicki L. Potts, RN, PhD

COMPETENCIES

Upon completion of this chapter, the reader will be able to:

- Describe the anatomy and physiology of, and differences between, the musculoskeletal systems of the developing child and an adult.
- Describe various acute musculoskeletal injuries that may occur in children, including sprains, strains, contusions, dislocations, and fractures.
- List and identify different types of fractures.
- Explain the use of slings, braces, splints, casts, external and internal fixation.
- Be familiar with current interventions and treatments in the pediatric population.
- Discuss the importance of identifying an injury of the epiphyseal growth plate, and how best to proceed when suspected.
- Identify the inflammatory and infectious disorders that can affect the pediatric musculoskeletal system.
- Describe congenital musculoskeletal disorders common to children and adolescents.
- Describe the nursing management associated with various growth-related disorders.
- Identify the education needs of the families of children with musculoskeletal alterations.
- Successfully complete the games and activities in the online student StudyWARE.

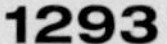

Disorders of the musculoskeletal system affect a child's movement and normal physical activity, thus influencing the ability to achieve developmental milestones. Alterations may be congenital or acquired during childhood from trauma, infection, or disease. Children and their caregivers may struggle with limitations of mobility and the discomfort associated with treatment of musculoskeletal disorders. This chapter highlights the most common musculoskeletal alterations experienced during childhood and is organized into the following categories: (1) injuries; (2) inflammatory and infectious disorders; (3) congenital disorders; and (4) disorders related to growth. This chapter also focuses on the nurse's role in supporting children and their caregivers during assessment, diagnosis, treatment, and evaluation of musculoskeletal alterations.

In the United States, a rising number of children and adolescents will experience musculoskeletal injuries. Injury is the leading cause of death and disability for the pediatric population. Top causes are automobile crashes and falls (Agran, Winn, Anderson, Trent, & Walton-Haynes, 2001). The trauma of high energy automobile accidents and even the nonspectacular fall in the schoolyard from playground equipment directly affect the health and well-being of children and adolescents. Musculoskeletal injuries are one of the most frequently encountered problems in pediatric practice (Hart, Albright, Rebello, & Grottkau, 2006).

ANATOMY AND PHYSIOLOGY

The musculoskeletal system is composed of more than 200 bones and over 600 muscles, joints, and supportive connective tissues (cartilage, tendons and ligaments) that maintain form and perform specific functions of the body. This system provides protection for the internal organs (including heat production and breathing) and allows for movement. The skeletal system manufactures red blood cells, white blood cells, and other blood elements in the bone marrow and provides storage for minerals such as calcium and phosphorus (Judge, 2007). Bone is unique as a tissue and an organ because it is a rigid and variable structure, and it can heal and replace itself with normal tissue without scarring.

Bones are typically classified as long bones, short bones, irregular bones, flat bones, or sesamoid bones. Long bones have greater length than width, and act as levers for large movements of the body. These bones are moved by the pull of contracting muscles (examples are the femur, tibia, humerus and radius). Short bones are often irregular in shape and measure approximately the same in length and width. Movement of the short bones is limited (examples are carpal and tarsal). Irregular bones are essentially those that do not fit any of the other four classifications, such as facial bones and the vertebrae. Flat bones are generally curved but thin, and serve a protective function and provide large spaces for muscle attachments (examples are the ribs and scapula). The sesamoid bones are small and found where a tendon passes over the joint of a long bone (an example is the patella). The sesamoid bones provide protection to an easily injured joint or tendon.

A joint is the site at which two or more bones meet and are united, creating a structure that supports movement in its many forms. Three major groupings for joints are: (a) fibrous joints connected by tough connective tissue allowing very little movement (examples are sutures in the skull); (b) cartilaginous joints connected by a plate of hyaline cartilage or fibrous cartilage and allowing some or slight movement (examples are the pelvic symphysis or vertebral bodies); and, (c) synovial joints that contain a synovial cavity, an articular capsule, and a synovial membrane, and are filled with synovial fluid.

The synovial joints are of seven types and enable extensive range of movement (examples are the hip and shoulder joints). The seven types of synovial joints are: (1) ball and socket (hip); (2) ellipsoid (occipital joint); (3) "plane" or gliding joint (vertebrae); (4) hinge (elbow); (5) condyloid (metacarpophalangeal joint); (6) saddle (thumb); and (7) pivot (radius and ulna) (Judge, 2007).

There are many differences in the musculoskeletal system of a child in comparison to an adult. The bones of children contain large amounts of cartilage making them more flexible and more porous, thus, allowing them to bend and buckle rather than break. The periosteum of the immature bone is thicker, more vascular, and is stronger and tougher. These qualities account for children's bones being able to absorb more energy before breaking and when they do break, they are more resistant to disruption. The periosteum (the thin, tough layer on the outside of the bone) is more metabolically active, and leads to more rapid healing and remodeling. Another major difference is that children have an epiphyseal growth plate at the end of the long bones. A fracture that disrupts or transects this plate may interfere with the growth of the bone and lead to serious complications such as limb length disparity or cessation of growth in height. Musculoskeletal injuries in children also differ significantly from those of adults. Soft-tissue attachments are stronger in children; hence bony injury especially at the growth plate is more common than sprains. Sprains are more frequently seen in adolescents and adults than children. The child's tissues also heal at a much faster rate, allowing quicker resumption of activity.

As shown in Figure 34-1 each bone consists of a diaphysis, epiphysis, and the metaphysis. The **diaphysis** is the shaft of the long bone; the epiphysis is the proximal and distal ends of the long bone. The **epiphysis** is considered the ossification center of the bone. Muscles are attached to the proximal and distal epiphysis. The **metaphysis**, a section of the long bone in which the diaphysis and epiphysis converge, is responsible for growth until the child's adult height is attained. The metaphysis contains cartilage and produces bone. The medullary cavity is the interior of the bone, which contains red and yellow marrow. Hematopoiesis (production of blood cells) occurs in the red marrow. The yellow marrow is the site for fat storage.

Bone formation begins in the second month of life and ossification is nearly complete at birth. Bone growth is more

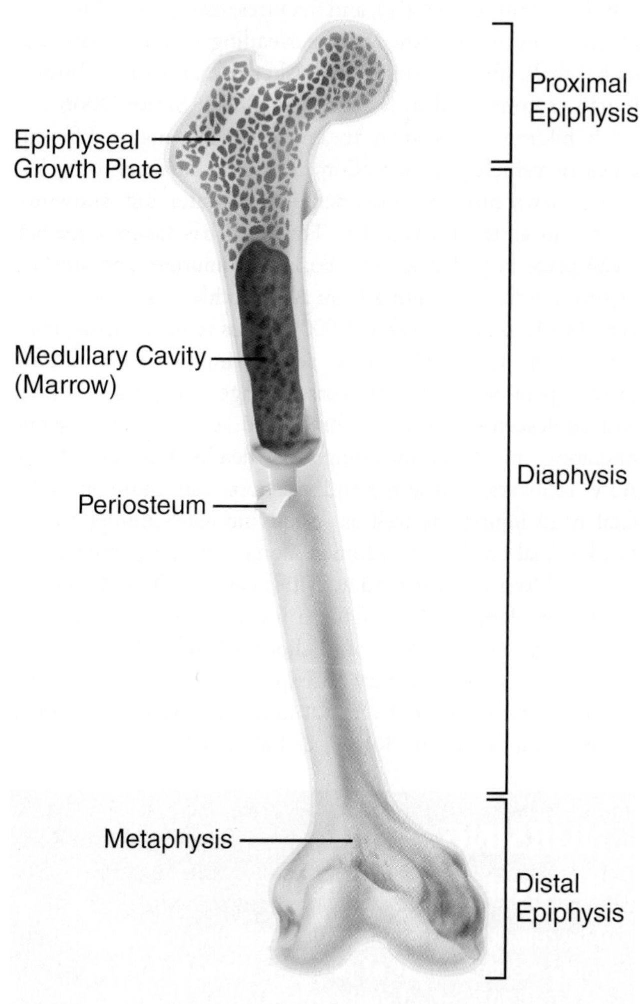

FIGURE 34-1 **Structure of a Long Bone.** DELMAR CENGAGE LEARNING.

complicated than adding length or girth. The bone formation process is known as endochondral ossification. Most long bones add layers on the outside of the bone (subperiostal apposition), at the same time removing layers on the inside (endosteal resorption, i.e., breaking down and reabsorbing material). However, the majority of skull bones and the clavicle are formed directly from an embryonic tissue (mesenchyme) using a process called intramembraneous ossification. All other bones are formed via endochondral ossification. The **epiphyseal growth plate** or physis is a thin layer of cartilage located between the metaphysis and the epiphysis at the end of the long bones. This growth plate controls long bone growth and is a vascular area of active cell division. New cartilage is laid down on the epiphyseal end of the plate. It is converted to bone at the metaphyseal end of the growth plate. The growing cells of the epiphysis are sensitive to nutrition and hormonal changes. Growth hormone, secreted by the anterior lobe of the pituitary gland, is responsible for increasing bone length. Maturation and bone modeling continues until 21 years of age. The skull is not rigid during infancy and fusing of the posterior fontanel occurs at 2 to 3 months of age. The anterior fontanel closes at approximately 16 to 18 months of age. This allows for growth of the brain and skull. Increased intracranial pressure prior to fontanel closure leads to separation of the sutures, causing the infant's head to enlarge.

All muscles are present at birth, and as the child grows, their length and circumference increases. Muscle tissue is of two types, striated and smooth. Striated muscle is the predominant type, which enables movement, maintains the body's posture, generates heat, and accounts for about half the body's weight (Knight, Matthew, & Muir, 2005). Smooth muscle is responsible for, among other things, gastrointestinal peristalsis. Muscle actions are controlled through sensory mechanisms, reflexes, and the nervous system.

MUSCULOSKELETAL INJURIES

Although all children old enough to walk can suffer musculoskeletal injuries, older preadolescents and adolescents are most at risk because of their higher level of athletic activity and greater body mass. Accidents and injuries may be caused by immature cognitive development, increased mobility, and immature or underdeveloped motor skills. They often occur during play and during participation in sports and recreation activities. Trauma is a frequent cause of injuries, especially fractures. Musculoskeletal injuries are among the most commonly occurring causes for visits to the school nurse, the clinic, the doctor's office or the emergency room. Nearly 20% of all musculoskeletal injuries will involve fractures (Hart, Albright, Rebello, & Grottkau, 2006).

An understanding of growth and development is helpful whether assessing, planning interventions, or evaluating care of the child with injuries. Nurses can teach children and caregivers preventive and safety measures, not only in health care settings, but also in schools and after-school activities, such as scouting, and in the community. Common musculoskeletal injuries that are discussed will include sports and recreation injuries, soft tissue injuries (sprains, strains and contusions), dislocations, and fractures.

SPORTS AND RECREATION INJURIES

Sports and recreation activities generate approximately 40,000 hospitalizations each year in the United States. About half involve fractures, while the rest are soft tissue injuries and dislocations. Half of these hospitalizations were males aged 15 and 18, and males account for 87% overall (Yang et al., 2007).

Sports injuries involve an increasingly wide range of organized activities: baseball, football, basketball, ice hockey have been joined by soccer, softball, volleyball, rugby, lacrosse, field hockey, gymnastics, wrestling, cheerleading, and dance teams. Most school districts and private/parochial schools sponsor male and female participation. However, as we have seen above, boys are six times more likely than girls to be hospitalized for sports injuries.

Comparing injury rates among the competitive team sports has generally measured baseball, soccer, softball and football. Contusions were the most common injury. Contact with equipment was the most frequent cause (hit by baseball, for example), except in football, where contact with another player was the most likely cause. In baseball, 3% of reported injuries were considered serious (dislocations, fractures, concussion); in soccer, 1%, and football, 14%. Competitive events increased the risk for injury. The most unexpected result was those participants aged 8 to 10 were injured more frequently than those younger or those older (Lawson, Comstock, & Smith, 2009).

Blunt trauma to the chest wall (commotio cordis) resulting in sudden death is the second leading cause of death in youth athletics (ages 7 to 16 years of age). These events almost always involve a projectile striking the chest, such as a baseball, lacrosse ball, or hockey puck (Weinstock et al., 2006).

A comparison of skating injuries (ice skating, roller skating, in-line skating) reveals falls as the most common cause (83.1%), resulting in higher rates of head injuries, including concussions and facial injuries. Ice skating is associated with three times more head injuries when compared to roller skating (Knox, Comstock, McGeehan, & Smith, 2006). Females are equally represented with males in skating injuries.

"Heeling" or "street gliders" have emerged as a skate-like recreational activity and have emerged as a cause for orthopedic injuries among children. In general, these have a roller in the heel, built-in or strapped on to a sports shoe, allowing the kids to go from walking to rolling by shifting their body weight. First appearing in the United States in 2000, millions have been sold in 75 countries around the world. These "heelers" have a very steep learning curve, as the child must learn to shift their weight backward over their heels (often resulting in falling backward). Fully 20% of all injuries reported are the first time the child has tried "heeling," and another 36% occur during the next four attempts. Injuries are highest among females (Vioreanu et al., 2007).

Gymnastics generates about 30,000 emergency department visits annually in the United States, at a rate of 4.8 injuries per 1,000 participants per year. Those aged 12 to 17 years have over two times more injuries than those from 6 to 11. Most injuries are strains/sprains (44.5%), followed by fractures/dislocations (30.4%), and abrasions/contusions (15.6%) (Singh, Smith, Fields, & McKenzie, 2008).

Skateboarding, roller skating, and scooter riding are prevalent recreational activities enjoyed by a large number of children and adolescents, mostly without adult supervision. One study in Southern California found that these three activities accounted for almost 14% of all fractures among children. Skateboarding was involved in over half of the fractures, while the other two activities split the difference (Zalavras, Nikolopoulou, Essin, Manjra, & Zionts, 2005).

ER visits attributable to cheerleading in the United States have more than doubled over the last decade, resulting in injury to almost 20,000 girls each year. Almost all are treated and released: most injuries are strains/sprains (52.4%), soft tissue injuries (18.4%), and fractures/dislocations (16.4%). Overall, the injury rate for cheerleading is about half that of baseball, about a third for basketball, and only about a fourth as compared to football (Shields & Smith, 2006).

Children are known to enjoy driving many different types of vehicles as recreation, including cars, motorcycles, ride-on lawn mowers, tractors, personal watercraft, snowmobiles, and all-terrain vehicles. The ATV has taken a special, awful place in pediatric musculoskeletal injuries. The number of severe injuries resulting from ATV accidents is rising (Altizer, 2008). In 2004, over 136,000 injuries required emergency department visits. The most serious injuries were among those operators under 16 years of age. In 2004, children and adolescents accounted for 45,000 serious injuries while operating an ATV, including 103 deaths (Atlizer, 2008). ATV rollovers, collisions, and ejections can cause instantly fatal head injuries as well as serious nonfatal injuries to the head, spinal cord, and abdomen along with many fractures.

Children's playground activities generate 40,000 injuries each year. Almost 90% of these involve falls from monkey bars, jungle gyms, swings, and slides. Most of these injuries involve fractures. Contrary to expectations, the surface below the play equipment did not influence the type of injury (Waltzman, Shannon, Bowen, & Bailey, 1999).

NURSING TIP

Referral to Specialist

Musculoskeletal medicine is becoming an increasingly essential part of pediatric primary care as at least 20% of all visits to the nurse practitioner or family physician involve musculoskeletal complaints. When should a referral to a pediatric/orthopedic specialist be automatic?

1. **infants with serious malformations of limbs (examples, idiopathic clubfoot, congenital limb deficiency)**
2. **children or adolescents with significant limb deformity secondary to metabolic bone disease or growth arrest**
3. **infants and children with developmental dysplasia of the hip**
4. **infants and children with bone or joint infection (osteomyelitis or septic arthritis)**
5. **children with Legg-Calve-Perthes disease**
6. **children with slipped capital femoral epiphysis**
7. **children with severe scoliosis (over 40 degrees) or limb length discrepancy**
8. **children with deformity of gait abnormality secondary to neuromuscular conditions (examples, cerebral palsy, muscular dystrophy)**
9. **children with complex fractures and dislocations**

Reference: Reeder, B. M., Lyne, E. D., Patel, D. R. & Cucos, D. R. (2004). Referral patterns to a pediatric orthopedic clinic: implications for education and practice. *Pediatrics, 113*(3 Pt 1), e163–7.

Most sports injuries in children and adolescents are caused by organized and nonorganized sports activities. Winter sports injuries are prevalent in children under age 15. Snowboarding causes the majority of winter injuries with about 55,000 injuries annually. Skiing is the second most common type of winter injury, causing about 45,000 injuries annually. Sledding, hockey, and ice-skating also contribute to winter injuries in children.

In the spring and summer about 4.8 million children between 5–14 years of age participate in baseball or softball. Injuries from baseball and softball usually peak at 12 years of age. Most injuries due to baseball or softball are fractures, contusions, and abrasions. Other injuries include sprains, strains, dental injuries, and concussions. Life-threatening and fatal injuries in baseball are due to direct contact with the bat or ball. Deaths occur from intracranial bleeding and blunt chest trauma that leads to asystole (the heart ceases to beat) and ventricular fibrillation (the heart vibrates, but does not pump). Children ages 5–15 are particularly susceptible to blunt trauma due to the fact that their thoracic structure is elastic and, therefore, more easily compressed.

Given the large number of youth involved in organized sports activities starting at ever younger ages, overuse injuries, overtraining, and burnout are growing problems (Brenner & the Council on Sports Medicine, 2007). Although inactivity and obesity represent a growing challenge for the United States, each year the number of children and adolescents participating in organized athletic activities continues to expand. It is estimated that 30 to 45 million youth from 6 to 18 years of age participate in some form of organized athletics. The range of activities has expanded from the basic sports of baseball, football, basketball, and volleyball to include soccer, lacrosse, field hockey, rugby, cheerleading and dance, and each activity has their own list of sports medicine concerns.

An overuse injury is microtraumatic damage to a bone, a muscle, or a tendon that has been repetitively used without allowing sufficient time to heal or repair itself (Brenner & the Council on Sports Medicine, 2007). Up to 50% of all athletic injuries may be due to overuse. Overuse injuries can be classified in four basic stages: (1) pain after physical exertion; (2) pain during physical exertion, which does not restrict performance; (3) pain during performance which does diminish performance; and, (4) chronic, unremitting pain even at rest.

The risks of overuse are more serious in the youthful athlete for several reasons. First, the immature and growing bones cannot endure as much stress as mature bones. Second, the youthful athlete has not always learned the best mechanics and techniques which can reduce overuse injuries. Finally, the young athlete is not as quick to recognize the vague symptoms of fatigue or poor performance as early signs of injury.

Compartment syndrome is a potential complication of musculoskeletal injury and surgery. Muscles, nerves, blood vessels, and bone are surrounded and protected by a tough, inelastic fibrous tissue called fascia. Fascia creates "compartments" around muscles. These compartments do not tolerate increases in volume or pressure resulting from pooling of fluids after soft tissue injury or trauma. As the compartment "fills," further vascular compromise occurs. Sports injuries and trauma are one of the three prime causes for "compartment syndrome" in children and adolescents (Grottkau, 2005). Hence, the nurse must be alert to any change or impairment of neurovascular status in athletic injuries.

Prevention of sports injuries involves understanding risk factors, knowledgeable coaching and supervision, use of protective equipment when appropriate, and safe playing conditions. Risk factors are related to the type of sport and level of training intensity. Individual activities with continual and repetitive training, such as skating or dancing, have a greater risk for overuse injury. While team sports are generally considered safer, sports involving running, blocking, or cutting increase the risks of acute injuries. Inadequate conditioning is a major factor in both types of injuries as muscles are tighter and susceptible to injury without warm-up periods.

Readiness to participate in sports is related not only to chronological age but the individual's physical and emotional readiness. The smaller child who is placed on a team with bigger, more skeletally mature children is at greater risk for injury. Children of the same chronological age may have different levels of cognitive maturity, and their understanding of the concepts of position or a role on a team may be different. Placing children on a team is best determined by several factors including age, size, and emotional, social, and cognitive maturity.

Warm-ups and cool-downs help, and the use of proper protective equipment protects against and prevents some sprains and strains. Conditioning before beginning an intensive sports season is also critical. All equipment should be well-fitting and specific to the sport. Helmets, protective eye gear, footwear, chest protection, and facemasks are types of protective gear available for different sports.

School nurses as well as pediatric nurses should educate children against the use of anabolic steroids for muscle enhancement and body building. Nurses should be aware of visible signs and symptoms of anabolic steroid use which include temper tantrums, personality changes, decreasing body fat, and increasing acne. Other adverse effects include stunted growth, decreased sperm production, irreversible breast enlargement in males, an increase in low density lipoproteins (LDL), a decrease in high density lipoproteins (HDL), and an increased probability of strokes and heart attacks in the teenage years. Table 34-1 summarizes strategies for preventing sports injuries.

SOFT-TISSUE INJURIES

Most sports injuries in older children and adolescents are not skeletal (fractures) but rather are injuries to soft tissues, including sprains, strains, and muscle contusions. In young children sprains and strains are very uncommon because the growth plates or physes are weaker than the ligaments and will usually separate before a ligament will tear.

Pelvic avulsion fractures are a relatively common injury in adolescents where the tendon pulls a fragment of bone (at the epiphyseal growth plate) away from the immature pelvis.

Table 34-1 Prevention of Sports Injuries

SPORT	STRATEGY
Baseball or softball	Ensure adequate training of the sport, and teach sportsmanship. Ensure players have helmets, mouth and face guards, and cups. Ensure clear area before bat swinging.
Bicycle riding	Teach safety issues: wear helmet, knee, and elbow pads; teach safety issues, like riding on the sidewalk; make sure children ride in the daytime, in groups or pairs, and stay away from deserted areas; and make sure tires have plenty of air.
Football	Ensure adequate training of the sport, and teach sportsmanship. Make sure players have helmets, pads, cup, and mouth guards.
Playground	Supervise children on the playground. Do not allow children to play on wet or slippery equipment.
Skateboard or scooter	Ensure children or adolescents using a skateboard or scooter are wearing protective equipment, such as a helmet, knee, and elbow pads. Skateboards and scooters should be used by adolescents age 15 or over. Adolescents should be of a mature level so as not to give in to peer pressure.
Overuse	Condition body parts by stretching, drink plenty of fluids, and participate in moderate temperatures.

The most common is at the ischial tuberosity (hamstring) and is seen most frequently among boys ages 12 to 14 (Hart, Albright, Rebello & Grottkau, 2006).

A **sprain** is the stretching or tearing of a ligament from injury to a joint. A **strain** is the stretching or tearing of either a muscle or a tendon from overuse, overstretching, or misuse. A **contusion** occurs when there is damage to soft tissues, subcutaneous structures, small vessels, and muscles, yet the integrity of the skin is not disrupted. Contusions are the most common of all sports injuries.

Incidence and Etiology

Sprains usually occur during forceful sports activities such as football, wrestling, or from a fall. Common sites include the knee, ankle, wrist, shoulder, and elbow. Strains are related to excessive physical activity or effort such as high action sports or from lifting heavy objects. Muscle contusions are common in contact and collision-type sports such as football and are caused by a blow to the body. The quadriceps muscle is the most common site of a contusion.

Pathophysiology and Clinical Manifestations

A sprain is the result of a twisting or turning injury to a joint in which the ligaments are stretched or torn. Strains are caused by excessive stretching of a muscle-tendon unit from an antagonist muscle group, an external object, or active muscle contraction. Sprains and strains are graded according to the severity of the injury. With a mild sprain there is microscopic tearing of the ligament with local tenderness and minimal swelling with no instability of the affected joint. A moderate sprain involves partial tearing of the ligament, partial joint instability, immediate pain, a moderate amount of swelling, and **ecchymosis** (black and blue discoloration of an area of skin caused by extravasation of blood into subcutaneous tissue as a result of trauma). A severe sprain is associated with less pain than a moderate one because the pain fibers are not being stretched. However, other manifestations of a severe sprain are markedly diffuse swelling, severe ecchymosis that develops rapidly, complete tearing of a ligament, joint instability, and loss of function.

The clinical manifestations of strains vary depending on whether the muscle or tendon is injured and the severity of the injury. Mild muscle strains are associated with microscopic tears in the muscle, local tenderness, and minimal swelling and ecchymosis. With a moderate strain a larger number of muscle fibers are torn, a "pop" is felt by the individual, and a small defect can be palpated. In severe muscle strains there is a popping or snapping sound complete with rupture of the muscle, severe pain, marked ecchymosis, and loss of function. Because tendons are relatively avascular, injuries involving them swell and are painful but do not bleed.

In a contusion, tearing of the soft tissues and small blood vessels occurs, leading to an inflammatory response. Hemorrhaging into the damaged tissues causes ecchymosis. The injured body part is painful to move.

Diagnosis

Soft-tissue injuries are diagnosed based on the clinical manifestations. Radiographic studies may be obtained to rule out a fracture; however, they are routinely negative if the injury resulted in a sprain, strain, or contusion.

Treatment

Treatment of sprains and strains involves the RICE treatment: **R**est, **I**ce, **C**ompression, and **E**levation immediately after the injury. The treatment for a contusion mirrors that of sprains and strains. During the first 24–48 hours, apply ice to the bruise at least three times a day for 30 minutes (off 15 minutes between 30 minute intervals), elevate the affected extremity higher than the heart, and wrap the contused area with an elastic or Ace bandage. Box 34-1 includes a description of the acronym RICE (Box 34-1).

Analgesics, such as acetaminophen (Tylenol) or ibuprofen (Advil), are usually adequate to achieve pain control. Further treatment for mild sprains includes supporting the injured area with elastic bandages or splints. For moderate and severe sprains in which ligaments are torn, casting or bracing for several weeks is usually required. Severe sprains with complete tearing of ligaments may also be treated surgically. Healing time is determined by the extent of the injury. As the pain decreases, weight bearing is increased, moving from partial to full weight bearing as tolerated. Stretching and strengthening exercises may be helpful when resuming weight bearing. Physical therapy referrals may be necessary if the exercise regimen is long-term or complex.

Nursing Management

Determining the severity of a soft-tissue injury as well as the presence of fractures is the major function of the nurse's assessment. Range of motion, neurovascular involvement, localized tenderness of the joint, and limited joint movement are also considered. Goals for management include keeping the child as pain-free as possible and helping the individual to return to normal activity level as the soft-tissue injury heals. Nursing interventions include monitoring the neurovascular status of the child. Skin color should be pink with brisk capillary refill; skin temperature should be warm, and motion and pulses of the distal extremity should be present. Elevation of the affected limb will reduce swelling. If elastic wraps are used they should not be wrapped too tightly as this may impair neurovascular status. Activity restriction may be necessary in the effective management of the child's pain.

BOX 34-1

TREATMENT FOR SOFT-TISSUE INJURIES (RICE)

Rest—Staying off the injury for several hours to several days depending on the severity.
Ice—On for 30 minutes, off for 15 minutes, at least 3 times per day.
Compression—Use of an elastic wrap.
Elevation—Elevation of the injured part at a level with or above the level of the heart.

Family Teaching

Family teaching focuses on the need for rest, elevation of the affected extremity, and the use of ice. Teaching crutch-walking principles is necessary if the child requires the use of crutches. Activity restrictions pose a challenge for caregivers if the child has been active in sports. Stressing the importance of activity restriction is essential. Follow-up appointments and further sports restrictions need to be adhered to until the injury is fully healed.

DISLOCATIONS

A **dislocation** is a displacement of two bone ends or of a bone from its articulation with a joint. **Subluxation** is an incomplete or partial dislocation of the articular surfaces of a joint.

Incidence and Etiology

Areas of dislocation commonly seen in children are the fingers and elbows. Dislocation of the elbow, known as **nursemaid's elbow** or subluxation of the radial head, typically occurs in children younger than 5 years of age. This type of injury results when a child's hand is suddenly jerked by an adult to prevent a fall or when a child is forcibly lifted by the hand. Dislocation of the shoulder is uncommon in children but increases in frequency during adolescence as a result of participation in sports. Dislocation occurs when the force of stress on the ligament is so great as to displace a bone from its normal articulation within a joint.

Pathophysiology and Clinical Manifestations

A dislocation is associated with severe damage to the ligaments and joint capsule. Typical manifestations include pain, immobility, and change in the normal contour of the joint or length of the extremity.

Diagnosis

Observation and physical assessment also are used to determine the presence of a dislocation. Radiographs are used to diagnose the dislocation. They frequently reveal an associated fracture.

Treatment

Dislocations are treated with closed manual reduction with the child under conscious sedation or general anesthesia. Following reduction the joint is immobilized with a splint, sling, or cast for at least three weeks. Mobilization of the joint with active range of motion should begin after the immobilization period.

Nursing Management and Family Teaching

Nursing interventions include pain management and assessment of neurovascular status. The family needs to be instructed on caring for equipment such as slings or support devices and prevention of reinjury. The nurse also needs to provide information for appropriate school personnel about resumption of activity and participation in sports.

FRACTURES

Musculoskeletal injuries are very common among children, and fractures occur with surprising frequency (Hart, Albright, Rebello & Grottkau, 2006). Children have many falls and mishaps. A fracture is a break or disruption in the structure of the bone when subjected to more energy than it can absorb. Ligaments and tendons are stronger than immature bone. As a consequence, fractures are more common than strains in young children. Nearly 20% of injured children will present with a fracture. It is generally estimated that almost 50% of males and 30% of females will sustain a fracture during childhood (Beaty & Kasser, 2010). Fractures can lead to serious and life-threatening complications; therefore, early diagnosis and appropriate treatment and nursing management are essential.

Incidence and Etiology

Among the pediatric population, fractures may be classified as upper extremity or lower extremity fractures. Fractures of the upper extremities are much more common among younger children, while fractures of the lower extremities become more typical among older children and adolescents.

Upper Extremity Fractures The most common fractures of the upper body are: (a) finger/hand; (b) clavicle; (c) proximal humerus; (d) elbow; (e) supracondylar fractures of the humerus; (f) distal radius fracture.

The hand is the most frequent site of fracture in children and adolescents, and occurs 3 to 1 among males as compared to females. Sports and direct trauma (crush injuries) were the most common causes among both males and females. The peak age of incidence is between 11 and 14 years of age. Generally, hand fractures involve the growth plate (Hart, Grottkau, Rebello, & Albright, 2006).

Clavicle (collarbone) fractures are also common in children, and affect even neonates. Most of these fractures will heal spontaneously and without complication, and many may never be treated. When treated, the child will wear an arm sling for two to three weeks, while the infant can be treated by pinning the sleeve to their shirt (with the elbow bent at 90 degrees).

The proximal humerus fracture site (near the shoulder socket) often occurs with shoulder injuries among children ages 9 to 15 years of age. This fracture also may be seen as a birth-related injury among newborns.

Elbow fractures account for 10–12% of all childhood fractures. The immature pediatric elbow is almost entirely composed of cartilage, and these structures slowly ossify until age 11 in most children. This unique anatomy makes these fractures more complex, and most require precise, often surgical reduction.

Between 60% and 80% of elbow fractures will occur at the bottom of the humerus, supracondylar fractures. Given the complexity of the elbow, the supracondylar fracture has the highest complication rate of any pediatric fracture. This fracture peaks among children aged 5 to 7 years of age (Hart, Grottkau, Rebello, & Albright, 2006). This fracture often involves malunion or displacement, and neurovascular injuries are to be expected. Several important nerves and vessels surround the elbow, and they may sustain injury from contact with sharp edges of fracture or fracture fragments. The possibility for compartment syndrome must be assessed immediately and continuously (Grottkau, 2005).

The distal radius fracture is the most common long bone fracture in children and adolescents (Beaty & Kasser, 2010). The mechanism of fracture is frequently a fall on an outstretched wrist/hand as they attempt to break their fall. These fractures have increased significantly over the last several decades with the increase in sports and recreational activities. Salter-Harris (Figure 34-2) classifies fractures of the distal radius as: (1) plastic deformation (bowing/bending); (2) buckle (torus); (3) greenstick; (4) complete (transverse); (5) comminuted (multiple fragments or pieces); or 6) physeal (across the epiphyseal growth plate). The distal radial physis is the most commonly injured physis in the body (Hart, Grottkau, Rebello, & Albright, 2006).

Lower Extremity Fractures The most common fractures of the lower extremities are: (a) pelvic and tibial eminence avulsion fractures; (b) femoral shaft; (c) metatarsal/phalanx; (d) tibia fractures; (e) ankle; (f) femoral neck.

Pelvic avulsion and tibial eminence avulsion fractures involve ligature attachments which tear away small fragments of bone from the epiphyseal growth plate (pelvis or the knee). These fractures are seen commonly in athletes. The tibial eminence fracture is rare while the pelvic avulsion is common. Both are more generally seen among males ages 10 to 14 years of age. The tibial eminence fracture is the more serious injury, often requiring a cast and surgical repair. The pelvic avulsion fracture is treated conservatively by resting the involved tendon, usually for a minimum of 2 to 3 months.

The femoral shaft (diaphysis) fracture is one of the most common fractures in children (Rewers et al., 2005) and is the fracture which most frequently requires hospitalization (Wright et al., 2005). The injury is the most common fracture treated by orthopedic surgeons. In general, younger and small children (< 80 pounds) are treated with closed reduction and spica casting or Pavlik harness. Larger children and adolescents are treated with flexible/rigid intermedullary nailing (Anglen & Choi, 2005).

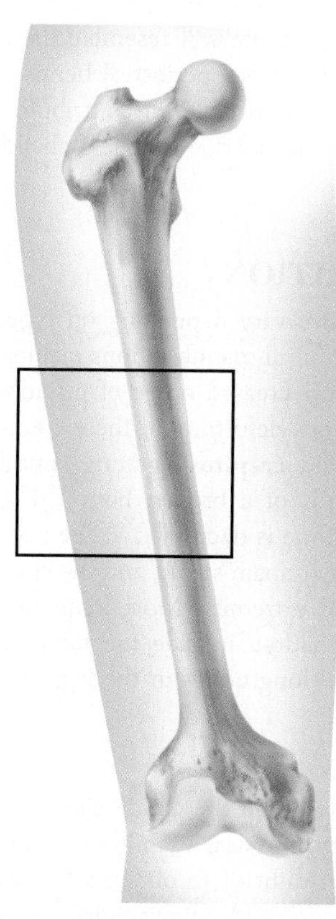

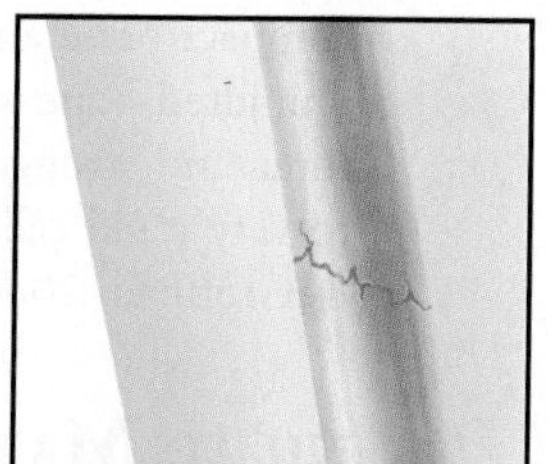

In a closed or simple fracture, the skin over the broken bone remains intact.

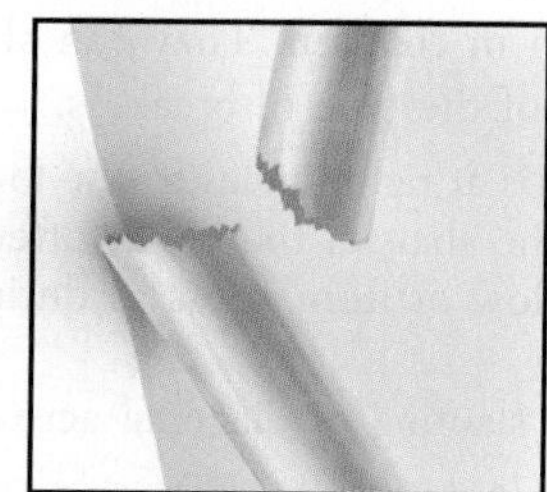

In an open or compound fracture, the broken bone protrudes through the skin.

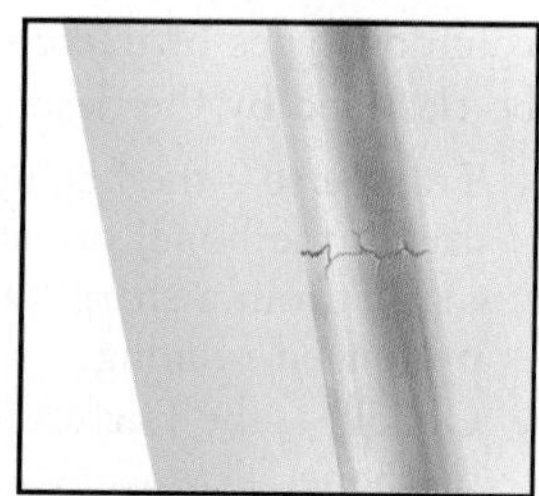

A transverse fracture occurs at a right angle to the long axis of the bone.

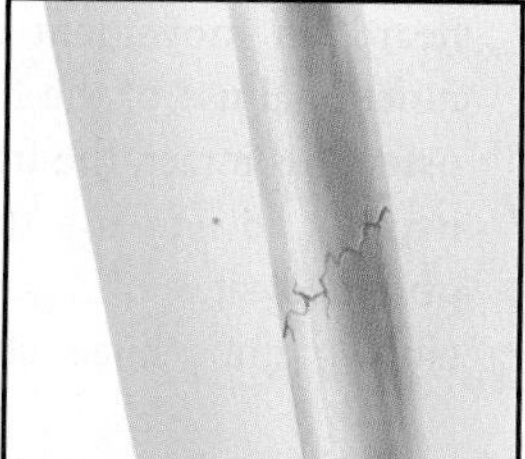

An oblique fracture is a slanting or diagonal break across the bone.

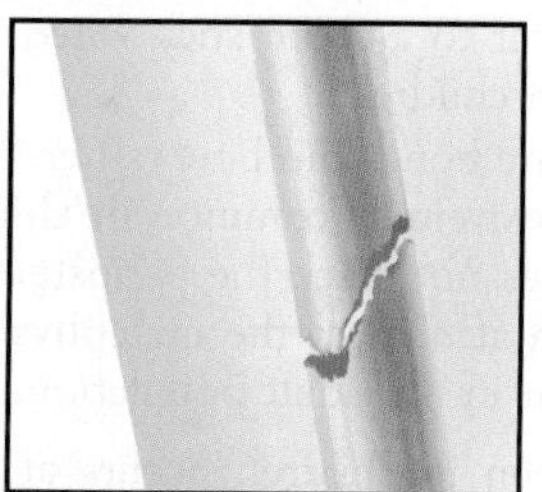

A spiral fracture is circular and twists around the bone shaft.

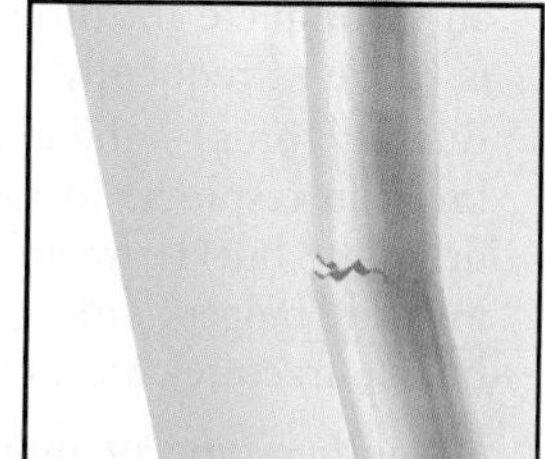

A greenstick fracture is a break through the periosteum and bone on one side while the other side only bends.

FIGURE 34-2 **Common Childhood Fractures.** DELMAR CENGAGE LEARNING.

Fractures of the foot represent 6% of all fractures seen in children. About half of these occur at the metatarsals. The fifth metatarsal (outside edge of the foot) is most commonly fractured followed by the first metatarsal (behind the great toe). Forefoot and toe injuries are usually caused by crushing or stubbing the toes.

Tibia fractures account for 15% of all fractures in children. These fractures can occur in relatively minor trauma. Motor vehicle crashes or other significant trauma will present displaced, open, or comminuted (fragmented) fractures, whereas a simple fall may explain a fractured tibia. About half (50%) of tibial fractures occur at and above the ankle, and about 39% occur midshaft. Common causes of tibia fractures are falls, pedestrian-car accidents, motor vehicle crashes, and sporting injuries (especially skiing and football).

Proximal tibia fractures are fewer in number but often present the greatest problems. These fractures most often are seen in children between 3 and 6 years of age. Typically, the proximal tibia fracture is an incomplete (greenstick) fracture, and easily treated by cast. On occasion, the tibial fracture involves the fibula. Most diaphyseal (mid shaft) tibia fractures in children under 5 to 6 years of age are nondisplaced or minimally displaced (spiral or oblique) fractures (Hart, Luther, & Grottkau, 2006). Indications for operative treatment include open fractures, fractures that have failed casting, child with multiple fractures, and the child with irreducible fractures (Setter & Palomino, 2006).

Distal fibula physeal injuries are the second most common growth plate fracture and are the most common pediatric ankle injury (Hart, Luther, & Grottkau, 2006). The physeal fractures as the ligament pulls at the growing bone. The fractures above the ankle are at a specific interval (ages 12 to 14) as the growth plate begins to transition from "open" to "closed." This fracture often involves multiple fragments and may include a fractured fibula.

Femoral neck fractures are uncommon in children (about 1%). This fracture is usually associated with high-energy trauma. Falls from heights (not the sofa or bed), motor vehicle crash, ATV accident, falls from a bike at high speed, or pedestrian versus motor vehicle accidents are the most typical causes. Other injuries to the chest, head, or abdomen should be expected and must be assessed. Other disease processes may be involved. Nonaccidental trauma (NAT or child abuse) should be considered if the history is not consistent with the expected high-energy causes.

PATHOPHYSIOLOGY

Fractures are described as simple (closed) or compound (open). In a simple or closed fracture, the skin surface over the broken bone remains intact. In a compound or open fracture, the broken bone protrudes through the skin, causing an external wound and the potential for infection and significant blood loss. Figure 34-2 illustrates the most common types of fractures seen in children. They can also be classified by the description of the type of break as:

- Transverse—the fracture line is at right angles to the long axis of the bone; occurs on the shaft of the bone; often results from a sharp, direct blow or from stress as during prolonged running.
- Oblique—the fracture line is slanting or diagonal across the bone.
- Spiral—the fracture line is circular and twists around the bone shaft; produced by a twisting force; commonly seen in child abuse.
- Greenstick—a break through the periosteum and bone on one side while the other side only bends, resulting in an incomplete fracture; similar to a green stick when it is broken; frequently seen in children.
- Buckle (torus)—the immature bones can bow rather than break in response to force; extremely common in children, the buckle fracture does not crack the periosteum, instead "bulges" (most often at or near the metaphysis); buckle fractures are not seen in the adult population.

Another type of injury seen in children occurs at the epiphyseal growth plate, which is vulnerable because it is the weakest part of the long bone. These fractures (also called Salter fractures) can be serious because they can cause growth disruption, arrest, or uneven growth. Injuries of the growth plate can be classified with the Salter-Harris system (Figure 34-3). Salter I and II injuries generally have the best prognosis for normal growth, whereas Salter III and IV will be more problematic, causing a higher incidence of growth alteration (Hart, Albright, Rebello & Grottkau, 2006).

After a fracture occurs several physiologic processes take place:

1. Inflammatory—Blood vessels inside the bone and surrounding soft tissues tear and bleed, forming a hematoma. The bleeding causes a decrease of perfusion (blood flow) to the bone tissue. Without adequate perfusion, bone tissue becomes necrotic and leads to an inflammatory response, which includes vasodilation and swelling around the fracture site. White blood cells arrive at the site. Fracture healing initiates very shortly after the injury occurs.
2. Reparative—**Callus** is tissue mass that forms at the fracture site in order to join and stabilize the two ends of the fracture. Fibroblasts and new capillaries form at the site in order to begin repair. The hematoma disappears and macrophage phagocytosis (eating away) of the cellular debris occurs. **Osteoblasts** (cells which form new bone) migrate to the area, forming collagen which leads to the callus formation at the fracture site.
3. Bony callus formation or ossification—The callus is now replaced with spongy woven, cancellous bone (also called spongy bone) made up of calcium and mineral salts. This mass of woven bone acts like a bridge to the fracture ends, stabilizing the fracture.
4. Bone remodeling—Osteoblasts are continually forming new bone, while osteoclasts remodel the fracture site. The fracture site will eventually be made up of compact bone and the injured site will resemble the uninjured bone section. Greater subperiosteal hematoma and stronger periosteum in children contribute to very rapid callus formation (Hart, Albright, Rebello & Grottkau, 2006).

Clinical Manifestations

Signs and symptoms of a fracture vary depending on type, location, and cause. The usual clinical manifestations include pain or tenderness, edema, and decreased range of motion. Others that may occur are obvious deformity of the extremity, bruising, muscle spasms, and **crepitus** (grating sound heard on movement of the ends of a broken bone). The functional use of the fractured bone is decreased. If the periosteum is intact, the fracture may remain stable, and the child may be able to use the affected extremity. Most frequently observed sites of fractures in children include the forearm, elbow, femur, knee, clavicle, and long bones in the leg.

Diagnosis

The diagnosis of a fracture is based on the child's signs and symptoms, history of the injury, physical examination, and standard radiographs. It is often difficult to obtain a history of the trauma from the very young child. The caregivers may be able to provide information if they were present; however, the best informant is usually someone who witnessed the events leading to the injury. Radiographs are the most reliable method of determining if a bone is fractured as well as the type of fracture. However, for elbow fractures, the predominance of cartilage until age 10 or 11 may require Ultrasound, CT, or MRI as standard radiographs will often not produce useful images.

Treatment

The vast majority of pediatric fractures can be treated without surgery (Hart, Albright, Rebello, & Grottkau, 2006). The goals of treatment are to promote bone healing, restore function and appearance, and return the child to his or her normal lifestyle as soon as possible. For bone union to occur the fragments should be in approximation and alignment

NURSING ALERT

Damage to the Epiphyseal Growth Plate

Damage to the epiphyseal growth plate (a physeal fracture) disrupts the growth process of the child who has not reached skeletal maturity and is still growing. Preserving normal growth is essential; therefore, injuries to this area should be evaluated as soon as possible.

Type I

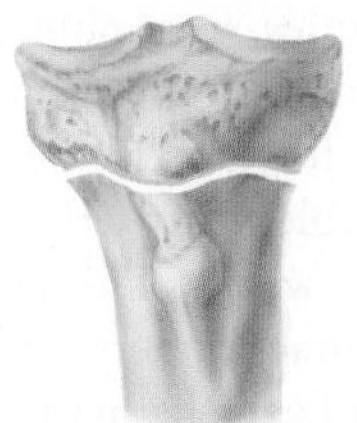

Separation of the epiphysis from the metaphysis. Usually does not affect growth. No fracture of the bone.

Type II

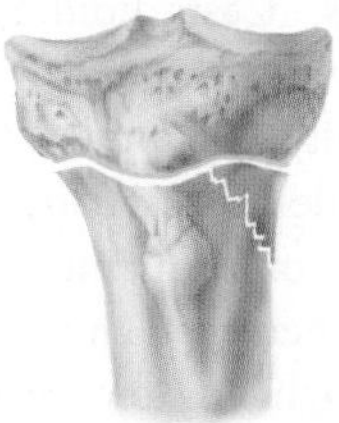

Separation of the epiphyseal growth plate and fracture of the metaphysis. Usually does not affect growth.

Type III

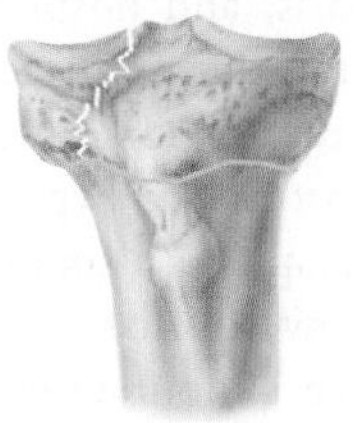

Fracture of the epiphysis extends into the joint. If reduced properly, does not usually affect growth.

Type IV

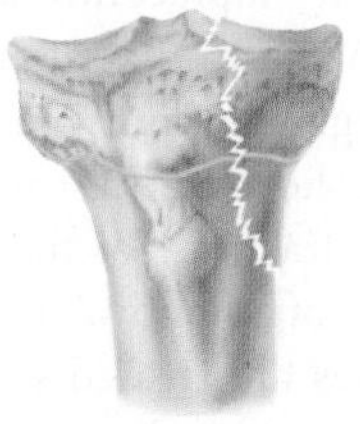

Fracture of growth plate, epiphysis, and metaphysis. Open reduction and internal fixation usually necessary to prevent growth disturbance.

Type V

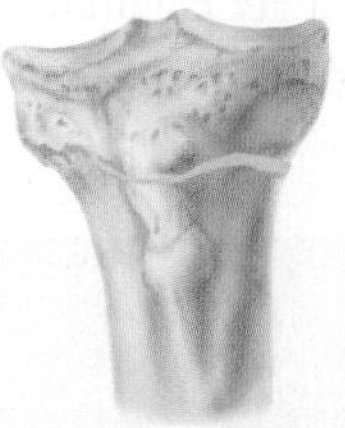

Crushing injury of the epiphyseal growth plate. Results in premature closure of the plate on one side with growth arrest.

FIGURE 34-3 Epiphyseal Injuries. ADAPTED FROM SALTER, R. B., & HARRIS, R. (1963). INJURIES INVOLVING THE EPIPHYSEAL PLATE. *THE JOURNAL OF BONE & JOINT SURGERY*, 45-A(3), 587–622.

and must be held relatively immobile during the period of healing. Closed or open reduction and casting are the usual treatment methods. **Closed reduction** is the alignment of the bone by manual manipulation or traction. **Open reduction** is surgical alignment of the bone using wires, pins, bone screws, or plates (internal fixation). External fixation has been added as a means for "portable traction." The majority of fractures in children can be managed by closed reduction. Immobilization following reduction is necessary to reduce pain, to prevent rotation at the fracture site, to maintain the position by preventing displacement or angulation until bony union occurs, and to allow free movement of uninvolved joints.

Slings, Braces, and Splints Given the rapid healing of pediatric fractures and the fact that there is a higher incidence of incomplete breaks, slings and braces are in common use. Often, the brace, sling, or splint will be used before casting to give the swelling at or around the fracture site time to subside. In addition, casting a break

NURSING ALERT

Can the Fracture Be Due to Physical Abuse (Nonaccidental Trauma)?

You should be aware of:

1. A fracture that is the result of a reported "accident" when the injury was unlikely to occur due to developmental age (Can a 1-month-old infant fall down?)
2. Multiple fractures in differing stages of healing
3. Femur fractures in preambulatory children less than 12 to 14 months of age
4. Sternal or rib fractures
5. Scapula fractures or ulna "nightstick" fractures
6. The caregiver's explanation of how the injury occurred is inconsistent with the injury
7. Skull, nose, or facial fractures
8. Spiral fractures or "chip" fractures around the knee

Reference: Jenny, C. (2006). Committee on Child Abuse and Neglect. Evaluating infants and young children with multiple fractures. *Pediatrics, 118*(3): 1299–1303.

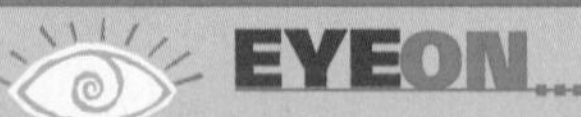

Need for Calcium in African-American Children with a Fracture

Foods high in calcium are important for children for the growth of bones. When a child sustains a fracture, the need for calcium may be increased. A major source of calcium is dairy products. Many African Americans have a lactose intolerance in which they are unable to digest lactose, and ingestion of dairy foods causes abdominal bloating, diarrhea, and excessive flatus. Therefore, when they experience a fracture, they may need to obtain calcium from other food sources such as green leafy vegetables, broccoli, cauliflower, and cabbage. If they do consume dairy products, they may need to take a commercially available lactose preparation such as Lact-Aid or Dairy-Ease.

immediately increases the probability of "compartment syndrome." Delayed union or nonunion are rare occurrences in children (exception is other underlying disease processes). Fractures of the clavicle are treated with a sling for two to three weeks or until comfortable. For newborns with clavicle fractures, the sleeve of the infant's shirt may be pinned (Onsie-style) with the elbow held in a 90 degree angle. Proximal humerus fractures use the simple sling, but for three to four weeks. In closed or simple fractures of the upper extremities, a combination of slings, splints, or braces are frequently the option of choice for immobilization. A buckle fracture of the distal radius may be treated with a removable volar wrist splint or a short-arm cast for three to four weeks. The permanent cast is often preferred by many practitioners and caregivers as it often proves difficult to keep the active child from discarding or not using the removable splint.

Casts Casts hold bones immobile and offer protection after reduction of a fracture or may be used to correct a deformity (Figure 34-4). Immobilization casts are most often made of plaster or a synthetic material such as fiberglass. Plaster conforms more readily to the body part but deteriorates when wet and is relatively heavy. Synthetic casts are lightweight, water resistant, available in colors and dry quickly (15 minutes); yet, they are more expensive than plaster (Figure 34-5). Most casts are applied on an outpatient basis, and hospitalization is not required. The nurse needs to educate the caregivers about caring for the child with a cast at home (see Box 34-2).

Most Salter Type I (separation of the epiphysis from the metaphysis) supracondylar fractures (humerus above the elbow) can be treated nonsurgically in a long-arm cast for three to four weeks. Salter Type II (separation of the epiphyseal growth plate and fracture of the metaphysis) and Salter Type III (fracture of the epiphysis extends into the joint) supracondylar fractures of the elbow will be placed in a long-arm cast after closed reduction and percutaneous (through the skin) pin placement.

A short-arm cast may be used for a fracture (including a buckle fracture) of the distal-radius (wrist above the hand) instead of a removable splint. Most pediatric hand and finger fractures are treated with closed reduction and immobilization in a cast whereas splints are used with adults.

The spica cast (see Figure 34-11) is used with infants and younger children to treat femoral neck and femoral shaft fractures.

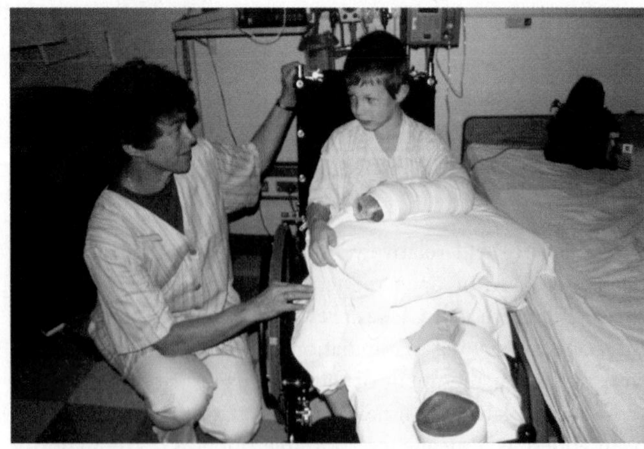

FIGURE 34-4 This child has a short leg cast for a fracture of the distal tibia and an arm cylinder cast for a dislocated elbow.
DELMAR CENGAGE LEARNING.

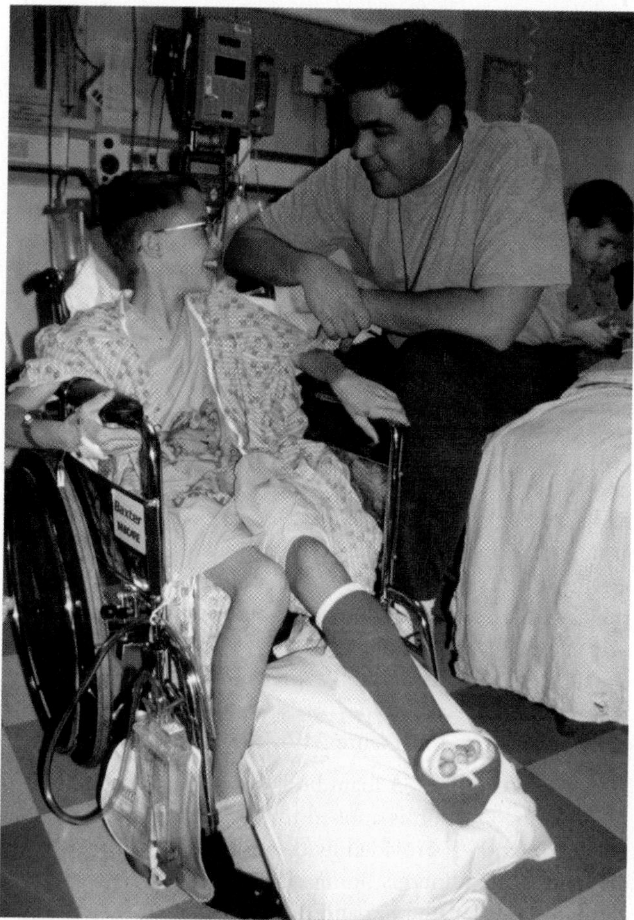

FIGURE 34-5 **A Short Leg Fiberglass Cast. Advantages of fiberglass casts include the availability of a wide variety of colors, fast drying time, and their light weight.** DELMAR CENGAGE LEARNING.

Nondisplaced (Salter Type I) tibial eminence fractures (physeal growth plate at the top of the tibia at the knee) are usually treated conservatively, using closed reduction and long-leg casting. Proximal (top) tibia fractures are almost always treated with closed reduction and the long-leg cast with a small knee flexion (Setter & Palomino, 2006) for four to six weeks.

Distal fibula (ankle) physeal fractures (growth plate, second most common growth plate injury and most common ankle fracture) are treated using closed reduction and casting. Fractures of the foot in children and adolescents are most often treated with closed reduction with a short-leg walking cast for three to four weeks.

BOX 34-2

HOME CARE FOR THE CHILD WITH A CAST

1. After application of a plaster cast, let it dry thoroughly. This will take from 24 to 48 hours. Handle the cast gently. Use the palms of the hands to pick up the cast to prevent dents. Use of a fan or cool-air hair dryer will facilitate drying.
2. Elevate the cast on a pillow above the level of the heart to reduce swelling and improve circulation.
3. Do not hit or bang the cast as this may damage the cast or cause reinjury.
4. Avoid getting plaster casts wet. Plastic wrap or a plastic bag can be used to protect the cast from moisture during bathing.
5. "Petal" the edges with moleskin or adhesive tape to protect the child's skin from rough and irritating edges. The edges are rounded with scissors, and each of these "petals" is placed over the edge of the cast, with each slightly overlapping the previous one to form a smooth, finished edge. "Petaling" the cast around the edges, especially the groin and perineum, will protect it from urine and stool.
6. Do not allow the child to push small or sharp objects under the cast, such as a pencil, pen, or small game piece, as these may injure the skin.
7. Assess neurovascular status frequently on the extremity distal to the cast.
8. For itching, a hair dryer set on a cool setting can be used to blow air into the cast. An antihistamine can be used if the itching is bothersome.
9. Report any foul smelling odors, excessive swelling, bleeding, or excessive pain to the health care provider. The odor may indicate infection or skin breakdown. Bleeding, excessive pain, or swelling indicate problems and are not to be ignored.
10. Report any slippage, cracking, softness, or looseness of the cast to the health care provider.

External Fixation Sometimes referred to as "portable traction," external fixation has displaced in-hospital and at home use of traction. External fixation is primarily used for femoral shaft fractures, allowing the patient to go home, hence reducing the length of the hospital stay. External fixation is used when flexible intermedullary nailing is not appropriate (based upon the fracture pattern or type), for example with open fractures, fractures involving severe soft tissue injury, and multiple trauma or head injury. Most orthopedic surgeons use a stable unilateral fixator along the lateral aspect (outer) of the leg. Pins are attached to the parts of the bone through the skin. Pin site care with half-strength hydrogen peroxide commences on the second postoperative day. Studies have found a high incidence (72.6%) of pin tract infection (Hart, Luther, & Grottkau, 2006).

Internal Fixation Almost all pediatric femoral neck fractures are treated in the operating room under general anesthesia and fluoroscopic guidance. Following closed or open reduction of the fracture, the surgeon often needs to place internal fixation (nails) to retain and maintain reduction while the bone heals and remodels. The exception to this rule is among younger children. For these patients, the surgeon will use smooth pins for fixation and then apply a spica body cast (Figure 34-11) for six to eight weeks. Smooth pins can cross the physis (epiphyseal growth plate) with a lower risk to growth arrest or interruption.

Typically, Salter Type II and III tibial eminence fractures (top of the tibia at the knee) are open or orthoscopic manual reduction with internal fixation.

Percutaneous Pin Fixation, Smooth Pins, and Intramedullary Nailing

Salter Type II and III supracondylar fractures of the elbow are currently treated with closed reduction and percutaneous pin fixation (Kirchner wires). Smooth pins are often used in fractures which cross or intersect an epiphyseal growth plate. Intramedullary (through the bone) nails, flexible or rigid types, are frequently used in femoral shaft fractures. The choice to use flexible nailing is determined by age (6 to 12 years of age, immature skeleton). Rigid nails are used in skeletally mature children (closed physes). Flexible nails are less likely to result in osteonecrosis or avascular necrosis. Unstable fractures of the tibia and fibula may require operative reduction and stabilization (percutaneous pins, flexible nails, external fixation, or plates and screws). Recently, there is an increased reliance upon the flexible nailing of tibia fractures. A comparison of flexible nailing to external fixation produced better results: faster healing, decreased scarring, decreased infection, and decreased incidence of re-fracture (Kubiak et al., 2005).

Traction

Traction has been used for more than 3,000 years to maintain fracture alignment, relieve pain and decrease muscle spasms. Traction can promote exercise or rest and can relieve pressure on the musculoskeletal system. In addition, traction may be used to correct, lessen, or prevent deformities, or to expand spaces between fractured bone ends prior to surgery. Traction is the application of pulling force to a body part against a countertraction pull exerted in the opposite direction. Think of Newton's third law of motion: for every action there must be an equal and opposite reaction. The process is used to treat a variety of injuries such as of the spine, long bones of the upper and lower extremities, and pelvis. In straight traction the child's body weight serves as the countertraction. In balanced or suspended traction the body part is suspended by a sling, and the countertraction as well as the primary pull is accomplished by pulleys and weights. The angle of the involved joint and the angle formed by placement of the pulley on the bed determine the direction of the pull or force. The primary purposes of traction are to immobilize the fracture, realign the proximal and distal ends of the bone while healing takes place, decrease muscle spasms, and prevent further soft-tissue damage. The two types of traction are skin and skeletal.

Observed as early as 1995 in nursing journals, trends in orthopedic care were reducing the use of traction in the hospital and after the hospital (Nichol, 1995). Insurance companies and Diagnostic Related Groups Panels have greatly curtailed the reimbursements for certain tractions, and have generally relegated traction to home use and other skilled nursing facilities.

A comparative analysis, for example, for treating a pediatric femoral shaft fracture revealed that external fixation and early mobilization of the patient had a 280% lower cost when compared to in-hospital traction until the fracture was fully healed (Hedin, Borgquist, & Larsson, 2004). However, traction has not disappeared entirely in the United States, and consequently the 21st century nurse needs to be familiar with the primary theory underlying its application and use.

Skin Traction

Skin traction is applied directly to the skin and exerts force on the body surface. It is easy to use, noninvasive, and does not require anesthesia. A variety of materials such as Ace bandages, boots, or belts are secured around a body part and attached to weights. The amount of weight used as a pulling force is limited to prevent injury to the skin. Skin traction should not be used if the child has a skin infection or breakdown, open wound, or extensive tissue damage. Frequent skin and neurovascular assessments are required. Several types of skin traction are discussed and are illustrated in Figure 34-6.

Buck Extension A foam boot or circular wrap is applied to the skin. Traction is applied to the boot or the wrap, and countertraction is provided by the child's body. It is used for short-term, continuous immobilization such as preoperatively for a dislocated hip and to treat contractures and muscle spasm prior to surgery. It is important to keep the ropes and pulleys hanging freely for this type of traction to be effective. The usual weights are between 5 and 10 pounds.

Bryant Traction The child is in a supine position with both legs flexed slightly less than 90 degrees. The child's buttocks should be lifted off the mattress. Bryant traction is a continuous skin traction used to treat developmental hip dysplasia and fractured femurs in children younger than 2–3 years of age or weighing less than 30 pounds. Countertraction is provided by the child's weight; therefore, the child needs to remain supine. Both legs are always suspended, even if just one is broken. Bilateral traction allows better stability, prevents body rotation, and promotes equal growth of the long bones. This type of traction must be used with caution as it is possible to create a tourniquet effect with the bandages and traction leading to vasospasms and avascular necrosis. Check for color, movement, pulse, and temperature at the extremities. Note if edema is present.

Russell Traction Russell traction is similar to Buck's except a sling under the knee suspends the affected leg. It is a continuous skin traction used to reduce and immobilize hip fractures, fractures of the tibial plateau, and femur. The traction pulls from two directions, from the knee sling and from the foot. Elevating the foot of the bed provides countertraction. The sling is often sheepskin. Sling placement needs to be checked frequently to maintain the desired amount of flexion and to prevent damage to the nerve under

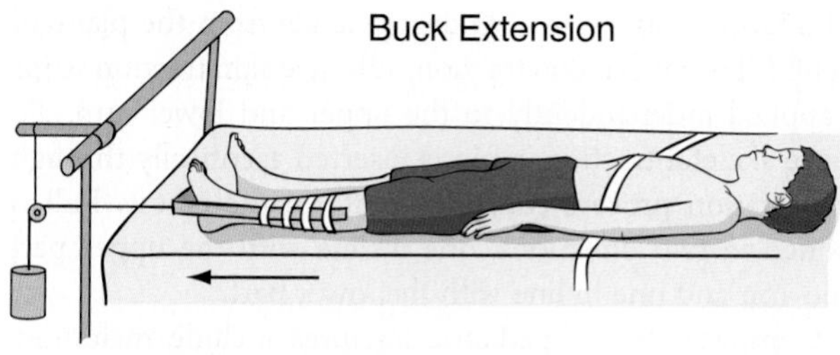

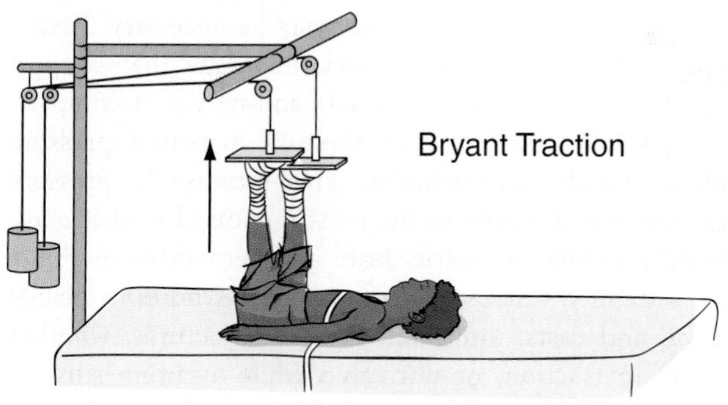

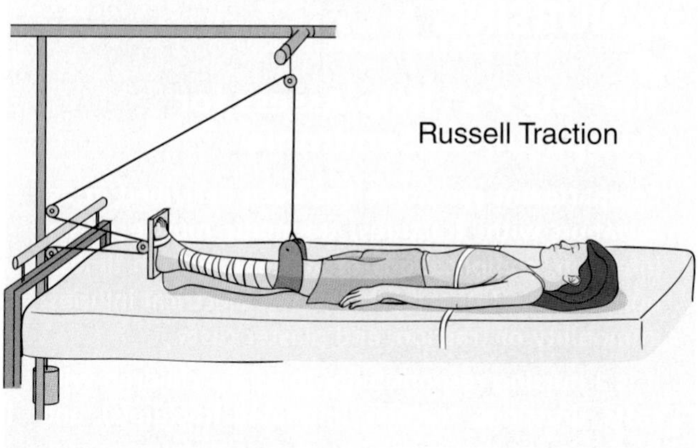

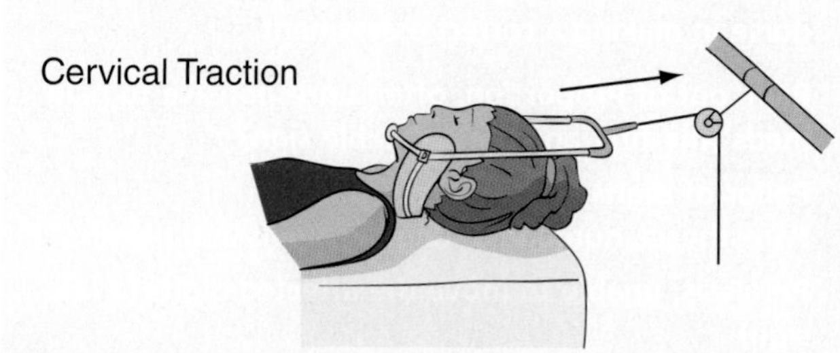

FIGURE 34-6 **Types of Skin Traction.** DELMAR CENGAGE LEARNING.

the knee, thus preventing footdrop. Check the skin routinely and assess for arterial compression. Follow physician orders precisely, and make changes only after consulting with the physician.

Cervical Skin Traction Cervical skin traction provides traction to the cervical spine and uses a head halter and weight to maintain the head in extension. A front strap fits under the chin and a rear strap rests at the base of the skull. It is used to treat mild cervical trauma without spinal cord injury, cervical strains and sprains, whiplash, spastic contractions of the neck, degenerative spine and disc disorders, arthritis, and subluxations. The head of the bed is elevated 20 to 30 degrees for proper alignment. It is usually short-term and intermittent. This type of traction is becoming more prevalent outside the hospital, at home and skilled nursing facilities.

Skeletal Traction Skeletal traction uses pins, wires, tongs, or other special apparatus that have been surgically placed through the distal end of the bone to apply direct pull to the bone. Weights are attached to the pins, wires, or thongs using rope, pulleys, and spreader bars. This allows the use of longer traction time and heavier weights. It is used to ensure correct alignment of the bony fragments and proper healing. Skeletal traction is used for management of humeral, cervical, and femoral fractures. Without traction, muscle contractions cause overriding and displacement of bone fragments and may result in improper healing. Skeletal traction provides a continuous pull and is used for unstable and fragmented fractures, fractures requiring greater than 10 pounds to reduce the fracture or to overcome muscle spasms, for control of rotation, and for fractures requiring long terms. A discussion of several types of skeletal traction follows; these are illustrated in Figure 34-7.

Skeletal (Crutchfield or Gardner-Wells) Tong Tongs are used to stabilize fractures or displaced vertebrae in the cervical and high thoracic areas of the spine. Crutchfield tongs are inserted into either side of the scalp through burr holes in the skull, while Gardner-Wells tongs require no incision or drilling. No flexion of the neck should ever occur, and the tongs should be checked frequently for displacement or looseness. Special beds are often used with cervical skeletal traction to assist with repositioning the patient and to guard against flexion of the neck.

Balanced Suspension Balanced suspension may be used with skeletal or skin traction for fractures of the femur, hip, and tibia. The Thomas ring splint fits around the upper leg and provides support of the hip. The Pearson attachment is connected with the ring at the knee and supports and provides flexion of the lower leg. Canvas slings may be used to further support the lower leg. The child is able to move, and the suspension apparatus adjusts without disturbing the traction pull. A footplate is used to prevent foot drop. The bed should be maintained in a flat position to reduce flexion contracture of the hip. This type of traction may be used with an older, heavier child, especially if much lifting is anticipated in the child's care as it allows the patient more movement.

90/90 Femoral Traction This type of traction is the most commonly used traction for complicated fractures of the femur. The lower part of the leg is in a boot cast, and a skeletal Steinmann pin or Kirschner wire is placed in the distal fragment of the femur. Traction ropes are applied on the boot cast and at the pin site to maintain a 90-degree flexion of the hip and knee.

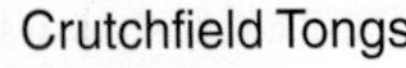

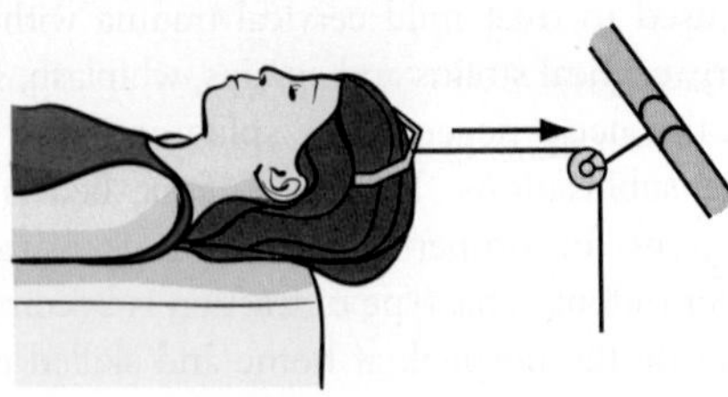

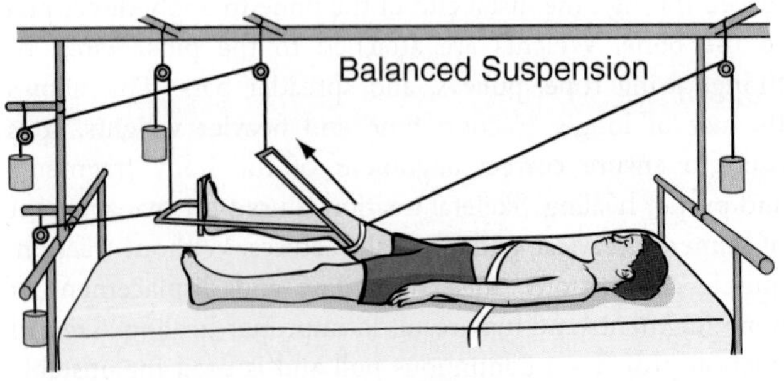

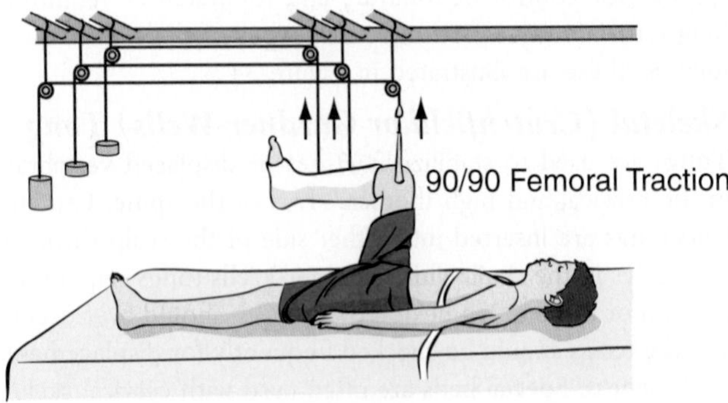

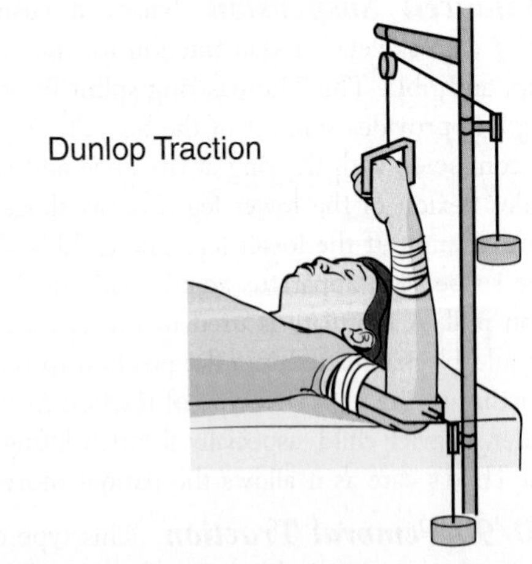

FIGURE 34-7 **Types of Skeletal Traction.** DELMAR CENGAGE LEARNING.

Dunlop or Sidearm Traction Dunlop traction can use either skeletal or skin traction for supracondylar fractures of the humerus (fractured elbow), and dislocations of the elbow, humerus, and shoulder. The upper arm is abducted and the forearm is placed in a 90-degree angle from the plane of the child. To achieve skin traction, adhesive skin traction strips are applied independently to the upper and lower arm. To achieve skeletal traction, a pin is inserted aseptically through the olecranon process (outside point) of the elbow. Pull is obtained in two directions, one in line with the upper part of the arm and one in line with the lower part.

Complications of pediatric fractures include malunion, compartment syndrome, and growth disturbances. Malunion or growth of the fracture into an incomplete or faulty position may occur even with the use of traction or casting. If malunion is severe, surgical repair may be necessary. Fascial compartments are sheaths of inelastic tissue that support and partition muscles, blood vessels, and nerves. A compartment syndrome occurs when there is increased pressure within a muscle compartment. This increase in pressure blocks the blood supply to the muscle encased in that compartment, leading to muscle death and permanent disability to the extremity. Causes of a compartment syndrome include dressing and casts, infiltrated IVs, and fractures, whether splinted, in traction, or untreated while awaiting surgical repair. The compartments involved are usually the forearm and the lower leg. The child complains of severe, unrelenting

NURSING ALERT

The "Six P's" Help Assess for Compartment Syndrome

Compartment syndrome has been described in association with: fractures, traumatic muscle strain, infection, complications of surgery, system illness, burns, snake bites, crush injuries, electrical injuries, immobility or traction, and plaster casts.

It is a nursing responsibility to assess children with casts, dressings, traction, untreated fracture(s), and IV fluids for the possibility of a compartment syndrome. Knowing the "Six P's" should assist the nurse in making a correct assessment.

Pain, out of Proportion, often unresponsive to pain meds (the first and most reliable sign)

Pallor of digits on the affected limb
Paresthesia, numbness, tingling, "pins and needles"

Paralysis, unable to move the affected digits (a late sign)

Pulselessness, the last sign (amputation may be necessary)

The digits may feel cold as compared to other limbs. An untreated compartment syndrome can lead to permanent disability of the affected extremity or even amputation. Compartment pressure often requires surgery.

Reference: Wright, E. (2009). Neurovascular impairment and compartment syndrome. *Paediatric Nursing*, 21(3), 26–9.

pain distal to the injury site that is unrelieved by analgesics. Severe swelling and **paresthesia** (numbness or tingling sensation) are noted of the digits below the affected compartment. Treatment involves immediate relief of the pressure, by splitting of the cast if present. In some cases, surgical intervention is required. The surgical procedure is a fasciotomy in which an incision is made along the outside of the compartment, thus relieving the pressure and allowing for adequate perfusion. Growth disturbances, another complication of fractures, are a result of shortening of a fractured extremity as a result of injury to the growth plate.

Nursing Management

Immediately following a musculoskeletal injury, immobilization with splints or sandbags may be necessary to avoid further trauma and reduce pain. Assessment of neurovascular status is performed to monitor for injury to the blood vessels and nerves after application of an immobilization device (cast, traction) and after surgery. Swelling or compression can interfere with blood flow, damage nerves beyond repair, and cause permanent disability or loss of limb. A neurovascular assessment includes evaluation of the following seven areas: pain, skin color, pulses, sensation, motion, skin temperature, and capillary refill (Table 34-2). It is important that nurses be cognizant of changes in a child's neurovascular and pain status. Therefore, a rule of thumb in nursing is to assess the neurovascular status of a child at risk for a compartment syndrome at least every 30–60 minutes for the first 48 hours. A compartment syndrome can occur at any time, so vigilance must be continued after the initial 24–48 hours, with an assessment done at least every four hours.

Musculoskeletal pain associated with soft-tissue damage, fractures, muscle spasms, surgical procedures, and immobilization devices is one of the most severe types of pain that can be experienced. The child often has pain for a prolonged period of time, making management and control difficult. It is important to remember that an initial sign of compartment syndrome is often sudden inability of the medications to relieve pain.

CRITICAL THINKING

Child in External Fixation

Four-year-old Juan was hit by a car while riding his bicycle and sustained a fractured left femur. The surgeon utilized the Ilizarov external fixator three weeks earlier. His mother tells you he has been impatient and demanding with her. She says Juan is always on the go, never sits still, and is bored and frustrated with being in bed for so long. How would you respond to her concerns? What suggestions would you make to help alleviate his boredom and frustration?

Immobilization is the usual method for treating musculoskeletal disorders, yet it can cause physiological and psychosocial complications. No body system is immune from the effects of immobility. The greater the extent and longer the duration of immobility, the more pronounced the consequences. Table 34-3 presents the physiological effects of immobilization and nursing interventions.

The nurse caring for a child who is immobile needs to recognize that a variety of psychological responses are possible. The child may become angry, uncooperative, or engage in aggressive behaviors (especially toward caregivers), or may become withdrawn, passive, and submissive. It is important to reassure caregivers that if their child lashes out at them, they should not take it personally. The child is displacing anger about the loss of physical mobility, and they are safer "targets" than the nurses and other health care providers. Immobilizing a young child for an extended period of time may result in regressive behaviors. For example, a toddler who was drinking from a cup and feeding himself or herself may demand a bottle and to be fed by the caregiver or nurse. Again caregivers need to be told that disruptions in development (regression) are temporary. The immobilized toddler who is striving for autonomy and independence may feel angry about losing autonomy and enforced dependence. To encourage a sense of autonomy, allow the child to make choices (e.g., food, daily schedule, clothes, and activities). If the child is school-age, it is important to continue with schoolwork via tutoring. This allows the child to participate in age-appropriate activities and alleviates some of the social isolation.

NURSING TIP

Cast Removal

Cast removal is very frightening for most children. The cast cutter creates vibrations and generates heat and a "tickling" feeling on the skin. Removing the cast is noisy, and many children are afraid that their skin will be cut. Demonstration of how the cast cutter works may relieve some of the child's fears. Therapeutic play, such as allowing the child to hold the cast cutter, even remove a cast from a doll with supervision, can be helpful. Caregivers should be allowed to stay with the child during the procedure. After removal of the cast, good skin care is essential as the skin under the cast may be flaky and yellow or brown because of the accumulation of dead skin. Some muscle atrophy may have occurred if the extremity has been immobile for a period of time. The extremity may also be stiff. Reassure the child and caregivers that muscle mass will return soon with normal use and movement.

Table 34-2 Assessment of Neurovascular Status

TECHNIQUE	NORMAL	ABNORMAL
Pain		
Assess using behavioral and physiological cues and age-appropriate rating scales	Some pain is normal after an injury or surgery	Excessive or increasing pain especially with passive motion or unrelieved with analgesia may indicate neurovascular compromise
Skin Color		
Inspect area distal to the injury	No change in color compared with unaffected extremity	Pallor, cyanotic, or dusky
Pulses		
Palpate pulses distal to the injury or immobilizing device if possible	Pulses are strong; no difference in affected and unaffected extremity	Weak or absent pulse (pulselessness)
Sensation		
Ask child if numbness or tingling is present	No difference in sensation in both extremities	Numbness or tingling (paresthesia); decreased sensation
Touch fingers or toes of affected and unaffected extremity especially the web space between thumb and index finger and between first and second toes		
Motion		
Ask child to move fingers or toes of affected extremity	Able to move fingers or toes of affected extremity	Unable to move fingers or toes of affected extremity; paralysis
Skin Temperature		
Palpate extremity (the back of the hand is most sensitive to temperature)	Skin is warm or comparable to unaffected extremity	Cool or cold (may be caused by cool environment; if so, apply blanket to extremity, then reassess)
Capillary Refill		
Press each nail bed and note the time until color returns	Returns to usual color in less than 3 seconds	Returns to usual color in more than 3 seconds

Additionally, children whose mobility is restricted and who are confined in a hospital room often experience sensory deprivation and social isolation. Promoting mobility as soon as allowed by the health care provider's orders and the child's recovery will ameliorate some of these effects. Use of crutches, walkers, beds, wheelchairs, wagons, and carts provides means of transporting children out of their rooms and increasing their environmental stimulation. The nurse needs to encourage the child and family members to invite peers and relatives to visit. Caregiver participation helps to channel energies in positive directions and provides the child with a measure of security and safety.

Family Teaching

Initially, family teaching focuses on the hospital routine, casts, traction devices, and mobility restrictions. Before discharge the nurse must teach caregivers cast care and review restrictions on mobility and activities of daily living. Nurses should help caregivers identify any modifications they need to make in the home or school environment, and refer them to social services and physical therapy for special services and equipment that may be needed in the home, school, or community. Child and caregiver education may be necessary about the use of safety equipment during sports activities. All equipment should be well-fitting and in good repair.

Table 34-3 Physiological Effects of Immobilization and Nursing Interventions

BODY SYSTEM	CLINICAL MANIFESTATIONS	NURSING INTERVENTIONS
Respiratory	• Decreased lung expansion • Weakness of respiratory muscles • Stasis of secretions • Increased potential for pneumonia and atelectasis	• Frequent repositioning • Turn, cough, and deep breathing • Incentive spirometer
Cardiovascular	• Increased venous stasis • Decreased cardiac output and circulatory fluid volume • Formation of thrombus • Potential for pulmonary emboli	• Passive and active range of motion exercises • Antiembolism stockings
Musculoskeletal	• Decreased muscle strength and mass • Atrophy of muscle • Decreased bone density • Joint contractures • Foot drop	• Passive and active range of motion exercises • Foot support
Gastrointestinal	• Constipation • Anorexia	• Increased intake of fiber and fluids • Stool softeners and rectal suppositories as ordered • Small frequent meals • Encourage family to bring child's favorite foods
Urinary	• Decreased urine output • Increased urine concentration • Retention of urine • Renal calculi • Urinary tract infection	• Increased fluid intake • Maintain acidic urine with cranberry juice • Monitor intake and output • Monitor urine concentration
Integumentary	• Skin breakdown • Pressure ulcers	• Frequent repositioning • Keep skin clean and dry • Use pressure reducing devices, such as sheepskin
Psychosocial	• Crying • Anger • Regression	• Provide activities the child enjoys • Provide "surprise" activities daily • Allow the child to ventilate fears or concerns • Allow friends to spend as much time as possible • Allow family to stay overnight • Allow as much independence as feasible • Allow child to participate in some decision making • Explain all procedures in terms the child understands

CRITICAL THINKING

Care of the Child with an Orthopedic Problem

Caitlin, age 8, is admitted to your unit at 8:30 P.M. after a softball injury. Her diagnosis is a fractured right fibula. She is currently in a long leg cast until an open reduction and internal fixation will be performed the next day. Caitlin arrives on your unit crying in pain. Her mother asks if you can give her something for pain. You check the orders and find one for Demerol 10–15 mg IV PRN every 3–4 hours. According to the nurse's notes, Caitlin was last given 15 mg of Demerol IM at 6:30 P.M. in the emergency room. Caitlin is also complaining of tingling in her right foot.

1. **What would you include in your initial assessment of Caitlin?**
2. **What areas are assessed in a neurovascular assessment?**
3. **What would you do regarding Caitlin's pain status, as it is too soon to administer the pain medication?**

NURSING ALERT

Calcium Loss Caused by Immobility

Loss of calcium is a response to immobility and indicates an imbalance between bone formation and breakdown. The lack of pressure (e.g., weight-bearing) on bones triggers calcium loss. Bone demineralization occurs as early as two to three days after the onset of immobility; therefore, the nurse needs to perform or encourage passive and active range of motion exercises for the child.

EVIDENCE-BASED PRACTICE

Pin Site Care in Injured Children

CLINICAL PROBLEM

What is the best method of performing pin care for children who have had external fixation of a fracture?

BEST CLINICAL PRACTICE

- There is no one single protocol or policy for performing pin care. However, the site should be inspected for signs of infection and cleaning should be done with a type of cleaning agent.
- Half-strength hydrogen peroxide is usually started on the second postoperative day.
- Showering is allowed once the wound is stable and there is no communication between the pin and the fracture hematoma.
- There is good evidence that pin sites should be inspected for signs of infection (some studies have found over 70% incidence of at least one pin tract infection).
- External fixation is being used much less frequently due to continued advances of flexible intramedullary nailing.

IMPLICATIONS FOR NURSING

- Assess for infection (redness, swelling, elevated temperature, drainage, odor, and complaints of pain) at the pin site every shift and document findings.
- Follow the facility's protocol for pin tract care.
- Monitor WBC's for any elevation.
- Obtain a culture if the site has any drainage.
- Educate the caregivers about pin site care and how to identify early symptoms of infection (drainage, redness, increased pain).

Reference: Hart, E. S., Luther, B. & Grottkau, B. E. (2006). Broken bones: Common pediatric lower extremity fractures—Part III. *Orthopedic Nursing, 25*(6), 390–407.

INFECTIOUS DISORDERS

The most prevalent infectious disorders of the bones and joints are osteomyelitis and septic arthritis. Both disorders present as a limping child and require immediate attention as a limp can be a sign of serious and life-threatening conditions (Sawyer & Kapoor, 2009). If infections of the bones and joints are not diagnosed and treated quickly and adequately, permanent damage as well as alterations in growth may result.

OSTEOMYELITIS

Osteomyelitis is defined as infection in the bone. Progressive destruction of bone and the formation of sequestra (fragments of dead bone partially detached) are characteristics of this disease (Pineda, Vargas, & Rodriguez, 2006). Microorganisms, usually bacterial but maybe viral or fungal, are the cause of the infection and may infect the entire bone (periosteum, medullary cavity, and marrow).

Incidence and Etiology

In children, osteomyelitis occurs in 0.2 per 1,000 children. Neonates have a higher incidence with 1 out of 1,000 contracting the infection. Osteomyelitis is one of the most common invasive bacterial infections in children that result in hospitalization and prolonged antimicrobial administration (Pineda, Vargas, & Rodriguez, 2006). Males have a higher ratio than females by about 2:1. Children acquire osteomyelitis by the following routes:

1. Hematogenous—more common, due to microorganisms spreading to the bone through the bloodstream from an infection elsewhere. Hematogenous osteomyelitis is most commonly seen in the femur, tibia, and humerus.
2. Exogenous—caused by invasion of the bone from the outside such as penetrating wounds, open fractures, contamination during surgery, or trauma.

Hematogenous osteomyelitis primarily affects children and adults over 50 (Zeller, Burke, & Glass, 2008). Exogenous osteomyelitis is more common in adolescents associated with injuries and trauma. The causes of hematogenous osteomyelitis are usually age specific (Table 34-4).

Pathophysiology

Pathogenic organisms from the site of an infection travel to the small end arteries in the bone metaphysis, where inflammation with hyperemia and edema occur. The infectious process leads to local bone destruction and abscess formation. Edema, pus, and vascular congestion are the result of the body's inflammatory response to the infection. Pressure increases as the pus collects and is confined within the rigid bone, contributing to vascular occlusion, ischemia, and eventually bone necrosis.

Biofilm bacteria such as Staphylococcus aureus (the most common cause for osteomyelitis), Staphylococcus epidermidis, Group A Strep, and pseudomonas aeruginosa are among the key culprits in osteomyelitis. These biofilm bacteria can adhere to inert surfaces such as the outside and inside of the long bones. As a consequence, these bacteria become far less susceptible to serum-based antimicrobial eradication (Ziran, 2007).

Increasing pressure within the bone expands through the periosteum into adjacent soft tissues. Elevation (bump) of the periosteum is prominent in infants and children (immature skeleton), but is not as observable in older adolescents and adults (Pineda, Vargas, & Rodriguez, 2006). The soft tissues surrounding the bone infection will swell, feel warm to the touch, be very painful, and may appear red.

Clinical Manifestations

Osteomyelitis in the neonate and the infant is often clinically silent. In infants, the manifestations may be subtle, presenting as irritability, diarrhea, or poor feeding. Toddlers may present with pseudoparalysis, pain on passive movement, or limping (Sawyer & Kapoor, 2009). In older children the manifestations are more striking, with bone pain that is constant, localized, and increases with movement or palpation. There may also be restricted movement, swelling, heat, red skin, and fever, with the temperature usually above 101°F (38.3°C). The parent may report night sweats, weight loss, and anorexia. Further assessment may reveal a systemic infection.

Diagnosis

Delay in the treatment of osteomyelitis significantly diminishes the cure rate and increases both the risks of complications and morbidity (Pineda, Vargas, & Rodriguez, 2006). Though difficult, early diagnosis is critical. However, early diagnosis is often missed, and it remains challenging. A very focused and thorough history obtained from the child and the parents is the best starting point. The history should be structured to determine the presence and nature of the pain, any history of trauma, and to identify associated systemic signs. The presence of systemic symptoms, fever, weight loss, night sweats, and loss of appetite is correlated with infection, but also may indicate inflammation or malignancy (Sawyer & Kapoor, 2009). Without a history of trauma or overuse, and presenting with systemic symptoms,

Table 34-4 Organisms Causing Hematogenous Osteomyelitis

AGE	ORGANISMS
Newborns less than 4 months	Staphylococcus aureus, Enterobacter species, Group A & B Streptococcus series, Candida
4 months–4 years	Staphylococcus aureus, Group A Streptococcus series, (Haemophilus influenzas*), Enterobacter series, Kingella kingae, Escherichia coli, Pseudomonas aeruginosa, (Streptococcus pneumoniae)*
4 years and older	Staphylococcus aureus, (Haemophilus influenzae)*, Enterobacter species, Escherichia coli, Pseudomonas aeruginosa, (Streptococcus pneumoniae)*

*The incidence of infection by Haemophilus influenzae and Streptococcus pneumoniae has declined dramatically because of widespread immunizations for HIB and S pneumoniae. However, this might be providing a niche for Kingella kingae.

Reference: Kiang, K. M. Ogunmodede, F., Juni, B. A., Boxrud, D. J. & Glennen, A. (2005). Outbreak of osteomyelitis/septic arthritis caused by kingella kingae among child care center attendees. *Pediatrics*, 116, 206–213.

a battery of tests and procedures are required. No single test can reliably confirm the diagnosis of osteomyelitis (Zeller, Burke, & Glass, 2008). Typically, conventional radiographs are ordered, although the sequestra or osseous lesions may not be visible until 10 to 21 days after onset (conventional radiographs require a 30% to 50% reduction in bone density before osteomyelitis may be visible) (Pineda, Vargas, & Rodriguez, 2006). Laboratory tests include complete blood count with differential and measurement of erythrocyte sedimentation rate (ESR), C-reactive protein, and blood cultures when infection is suspected. ESR and C-reactive protein tests are typically elevated. The white blood cell count (WBC) is usually elevated, although blood tests may be normal in some patients (Zeller et al., 2008).

Before the initiation of antibiotic therapy, bone cultures are required to accurately identify the causative organism. Ultrasonagraphy may be useful to identify displacement of the soft tissue adjacent to the bone secondary to an elevated periosteum or bone necrosis, and though subtle, may be visible within three days after bacterial contamination (Pineda, Vargas, & Rodriguez, 2006). Bone necrosis appears between the tenth and fourteenth days following the onset of osteomyelitis and is visible on a standard radiograph. Optionally, bone scintigraphy (bone scanning) may be used to image the entire skeleton quickly, allowing for a quick check for other sites potentially infected (Sawyer & Kapoor, 2009). Though sensitive, bone scan imaging lacks specificity. CT is used for cortical bone (mineralized) and MRI is especially useful for making treatment decisions.

Diagnosis of osteomyelitis is confirmed by extensive microbial investigation using blood cultures and bone cultures (Girschick et al., 2005). These lab tests utilize standard culture techniques to detect fungi and microbes. A confirmed diagnosis of osteomyelitis requires at least two of the following findings: (1) pus on aspiration from the infection site(s); (2) positive bacterial culture from bone or blood; (3) presence of classic signs, i.e., localized pain, swelling, increased skin temperature, limited mobility of the adjacent joint; and, (4) a positive imaging study (radiography, scintigraphy, CT, or MRI).

Treatment

Treatment options are: cure the offending infection or suppress it; attempt surgical ablations (excision, removal, amputation); drainage of the infected area; and surgical procedures to improve or restore blood flow (Ziran, 2007).

Treatment for osteomyelitis begins with culturing the tissue surrounding the infected bone as well as blood cultures and is begun based on the clinical signs and symptoms. The treatment regimen for hematogenous osteomyelitis includes penicillin and a third-generation cephalosporin. Vancomycin and clindamycin accompanied by a third generation cephalosporin may be used, as well as ciprofloxin.

Initially, antibiotics are always given intravenously in order to obtain and maintain high concentrations of the drug in the serum. If the initial treatment is positive, antibiotics are changed from the intravenous to the oral route. Recent studies have demonstrated the efficacy of an earlier transition from IV to oral antimicrobial therapy, thereby avoiding catheter-associated complications (Zaoutis et al., 2009). Splinting of the limb minimizes pain and decreases the spread of infection by lymph channels. The splint should be removed periodically to allow movement and to prevent stiffening and muscle atrophy. Surgery may be necessary if the infection fails to respond to antibiotics or an abscess is present. Drainage and surgical debridement cleans and removes dead bone and soft tissue and improves blood supply to the underlying bone.

Nursing Management

Health history and assessment are necessary to establish the onset of pain, restricted movement, or loss of mobility. Information from the caregivers helps to determine the source of infection; therefore, the nurse asks if the site was traumatized, or if the child had a recent infection. Soft-tissue swelling at the site may indicate elevation of the loosely attached overlying periosteum by purulent effusion within the subperiosteum. The nurse administers analgesics as prescribed and monitors their effectiveness. Splints or traction may be ordered for comfort. The nurse should help the client maintain proper alignment and move the limb cautiously to avoid further injury to the bone. As the child is able to bear weight, participation in activities of daily living can increase. Crutches, wheelchair, or walker may be necessary for a short while. Because multiple antibiotics are frequently used, thorough knowledge of side effects, therapeutic blood levels, and incompatibility problems is necessary. Maintaining adequate blood level of antibiotics is a critical component of successful therapy. Neurovascular and skin assessments are performed at least once every shift.

Family Teaching

Because antibiotics are continued at home, family teaching relevant to administration of oral or intravenous medications is necessary. Since many of the antibiotics used in treating osteomyelitis have adverse audiologic side effects, caregivers need to be taught to watch for hearing loss and to report this to their health care provider. The family should be instructed in the importance of administering all of the medication prescribed.

SEPTIC ARTHRITIS

Septic arthritis is an infection of a joint that usually develops through the hematogenous route (bloodstream) from another site of infection.

Incidence and Etiology

One study of children presenting to the emergency department for an acute atraumatic limp reported a rate of 1.8 per 1000 children younger than 14 years, a male-to-female ratio of 1.7:1, with a median age of 4.4 years (Fischer & Beattie, 1999). Septic arthritis represents approximately 25% of these cases and usually affects weight-bearing joints. In children it is most prevalent in the knee, ankle, or hip (Butbul-Aviel, Koren, Halevy, & Sakran, 2005). The incidence of joint infection in infancy is equal between males and females, but in adolescence it occurs predominantly in males. Haemophilus influenzae type b is a common pathogen accounting for 20% to 50% of cases in children ages 2 months to 5 years. Staphylococcus aureus is the most common organism in neonates and in children older than 5 years of age. Other organisms include pyrogenic Streptococcus and Streptococcus pneumonia. Staph A and Streptococcus pyogenes account for 60% culture confirmed pediatric skeletal infections (Kiang, Ogunmodede, Juni, Boxrud, & Glennen, 2005).

Pathophysiology

Inflammation begins in the synovial membrane, and as pus forms, the synovial fluid thickens. The purulent effusion destroys the articular cartilage within hours after the bacteria enter the joint. Cartilage disintegration may be followed by osteomyelitis in the underlying bone. Scar tissue replaces the cartilage and eventually the mobility of the joint is impaired. The seriousness of these risks demands speedy and accurate action by all members of the health profession team.

Clinical Manifestations

Nonweight bearing on the affected side, painful limitation of range of motion, overlying warmth or redness, fever, a toxic appearance (look sickly), and a swelling of the joint are present (Sawyer & Kapoor, 2009). An elevated white blood cell count is present and helps to differentiate septic arthritis from transient synovitis. **Transient synovitis** is an acute, nonpurulent inflammation of the synovial membrane of a joint, is benign, and occurs most commonly in the hip joint (Caird et al., 2006).

Transient synovitis is often mistaken for septic arthritis, presenting as approximately 25% of limping children, and must be considered and eliminated. The child with transient synovitis will have less acute pain and less range-of-motion restriction, and will appear nontoxic (not sickly looking) (Sawyer & Kapoor, 2009). Clinicians can discriminate between transient synovitis and septic arthritis using history and physical examination without resorting to needle aspiration (Caird et al., 2006). The child presenting with a slight limp of recent onset should be monitored for septic arthritis, but these symptoms are most typical of transient synovitis.

Another study seems promising. The study found that plasma procalcitonin (PCT) may be a useful bedside test for differentiating among osteomyelitis, septic arthritis, and transient synovitis. Blood cultures or cultures obtained by diagnostic puncture (aspiration) require time to reveal the presence of the offending microbe (if any). As a consequence, treatment may be initiated without certainty of the causative agent or may be delayed. Plasma procalcitonin (PCT) increases rapidly during bacterial infections but remains low in viral infections or other inflammatory processes. On admission, the study found all children had a fever greater than 100.4° F (38° C). Diagnosed osteomyelitis patients had fever for a longer period prior to admission. The PCT level was higher than 0.5 n/mL in 58.3% of children later diagnosed with osteomyelitis and only 27.2% in confirmed cases of septic arthritis. The advantage of this test is it can be done at the bedside and results are available in a half hour (Butbul-Aviel, Koren, Halevy, & Sakran, 2005). More research is required.

RESEARCH Highlight

Distinguishing Septic Arthritis from Transient Synovitis in Children

STUDY PURPOSE

To identify presenting symptoms which most accurately distinguish septic arthritis from transient synovitis.

METHODS

Prospectively data were collected on 53 children who underwent hip aspiration because of a suspicion of septic arthritis. Diagnoses of septic arthritis and transient synovitis were determined on the basis of the results of Gram staining, culture, and a cell count of the hip aspirate.

FINDINGS

The study used the following clinical features to differentiate septic arthritis and transient synovitis: (1) oral temperature > 101.3° F (38.5° C); (2) refusal to bear weight on the affected limb; (3) ESR > 40 mm per hour; (4) peripheral WBC > 12,000 cells per mm^3; (5) C-reactive protein level > 2.0 mg per dL. With one of these signs, the probability of septic arthritis was 37%; with two, 63%; with three, 83%; with four, 93%, and with all five, 98%.

IMPLICATIONS

The study concluded that fever (>38.5° C or 101.3° F) was the single best predictor of septic arthritis. Unlike transient synovitis, septic arthritis requires early intervention including intravenous antibiotics, operative irrigation and debridement to avoid unfavorable outcome. The pediatric nurse can use fever as a key finding along with the hip pain and the limping to guide action.

REFERENCE

Caird, M. S., Flynn, J. M., Leung, Y. L., Millman, J. E., D'Italia, J. G., & Dormans, J. P. (2006). Factors distinguishing septic arthritis from transient synovitis of the hip in children. *Journal of Bone and Joint Surgery*, *88*-A(6), 1251–1257.

Diagnosis

Suspecting septic arthritis, a complete blood count with differential and measurement of the erythrocyte sedimentation rate (ESR) and C-reactive protein (CRP) are ordered. All will be elevated including the white blood cell count (WBC). Based upon these tests, the test of choice for rapid diagnosis of septic arthritis is aspiration of joint fluid, "the gold standard" (Frick, 2006).

Normal synovial fluid is clear, colorless, or straw-colored. Turbid, purulent, cloudy fluid with a WBC >50,000 to 100,000 indicates the presence of an infection. The aspirated fluid is cultured to identify the causative organism. If septic arthritis, the synovial fluid culture will be Gram positive, whereas in transient synovitis, the culture would be Gram negative (Sawyer & Kapoor, 2009). Plain radiography, ultrasound, and bone scan aid in the diagnosis. Ultrasonography is highly sensitive for detecting effusion in the hip joint, and is also used to guide aspiration.

Treatment

Treatment for septic arthritis requires early intervention including intravenous antibiotics and operative irrigation and debridement (Caird et al., 2006). Initial treatment includes needle aspiration or open surgical drainage of the joint, administration of intravenous antibiotics after wound cultures have been obtained, immobilization of the joint, and pain relief. The length of antibiotic therapy is based on the type of causative organism; however, usually four to six weeks is required. Intravenous antibiotic therapy is administered initially, followed by oral medications.

Nursing Management

The nurse focuses on maintaining comfort, administering antibiotics, and avoiding complications of impaired mobility. (See nursing management for the child with osteomyelitis.)

Family Teaching

Education for the family and child is similar to that of the child with osteomyelitis. If the infection is in a superficial joint, it may be swollen and intensely painful; therefore, extreme care must be used when moving or handling it. Caregiver reliability in oral antibiotic administration is important because the usual course of therapy is several weeks long. Caregivers need to notify the health care provider if the child vomits or has diarrhea while on the antibiotics. If bedrest is necessary because of a painful joint, caregivers need to support and enforce this restriction.

CONGENITAL DISORDERS

Congenital disorders include clubfoot, developmental dysplasia of the hip, and muscular dystrophy.

CLUBFOOT

Clubfoot, also known as talipes equinovarus, is a congenital anomaly of the foot and the entire lower leg involving abnormalities of bony architecture and soft tissue. Clubfoot is classified as a minor birth defect (does not produce significant health consequences) (Romitti, 2007). Although not life-threatening, the birth of a child with a clubfoot has a significant impact on the family (Figure 34-8). Congenital talipes equinovarus deformity is probably the most common orthopedic condition requiring intensive treatment (El-Sayed, Correll, & Pholig, 2008).

Incidence and Etiology

The incidence of clubfoot is 0.6 cases per 1,000 live births in the United States with a higher occurrence in males of 3:1 (Morcuende, Dolan, Dietz, & Ponseti, 2004; Ponseti, 1996), while the incidence is 1.5 in 1,000 live births in England (Patel, Jeer, & Cornell, 2007). The exact cause of clubfoot is unknown; however, several theories have been postulated. It may be caused by arrested fetal development in utero during the first trimester when the foot is formed or by neuromuscular abnormalities. There is a genetic predisposition for clubfoot as seen in the increased incidence in first-degree relatives (parents, siblings). Recent studies have linked maternal smoking, even secondhand smoke, with clubfoot (Honein, Lindstrom, & Sweder, 2007; Skelly, Holt, Mosca, & Alderman, 2002). Clubfoot deformities are also seen in conjunction with congenital abnormalities such as cerebral palsy.

Pathophysiology and Clinical Manifestations

Clubfoot can affect one foot or both feet (bilateral in 41% of the cases in a Canadian study) (Templeton et al., 2006). The affected foot points downward with the toes turned inward and the bottom of the foot also twisted inward. If both feet are clubbed, the toes turn inward facing one another.

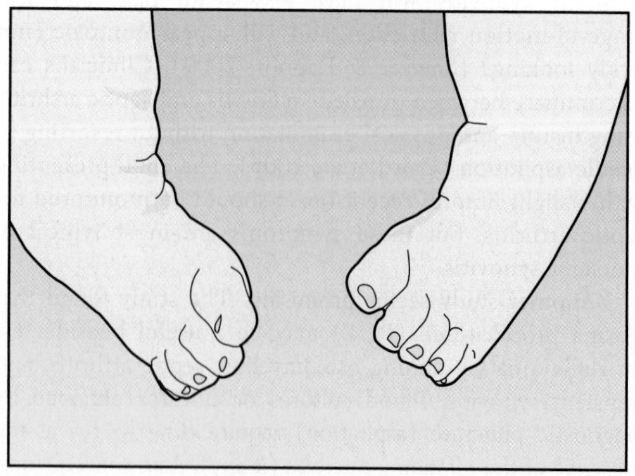

Figure 34-8 Bilateral Clubfoot. DELMAR CENGAGE LEARNING.

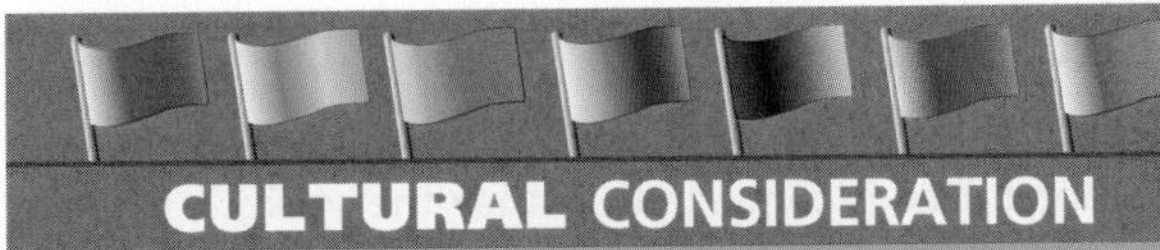

CULTURAL CONSIDERATION

Incidence of Clubfoot

The incidence of clubfoot varies among ethnic populations, with Caucasians and Asians having the lowest. The incidence is higher in Mexican and South African groups; the condition is most commonly found in Hawaiian Polynesians.

Clubfoot may also affect the bones and ankle joints, as well as the tendons and ligaments. Because the heel cord is so tight, the foot will not be in the normal position without medical intervention. Clubfoot is painless and does not present a problem until the child begins to stand or walk. Left untreated, the ankle remains in the twisted position and the foot is unable to move up or down, leading to an abnormal, awkward gait. If both feet are affected, which occurs in about 40% of the cases, the child will walk on the balls, sides, or top of the foot. This may lead to infection, calluses, and an inability of the leg to grow normally.

Diagnosis

Diagnosis is made at birth on the basis of visual inspection. Radiographs are used to confirm the degree and severity of the deformity. Magnetic resonance imaging (MRI) may be used in further diagnosis.

Treatment

Today there is almost universal agreement that initial treatment of idiopathic clubfoot is nonsurgical, regardless the severity of the deformity (El-Sayed et al., 2008). Treatment is begun as soon as possible after birth. Serial casting, the major method of nonsurgical treatment (the Ponseti method), consists of manipulation of the foot into the correct anatomic position and application of a series of casts (Ponseti, 1996). The cast is changed every week or so until complete correction has occurred, usually requiring two months or less. Braces have been developed to avoid the issues of taking care of infants in casts (Patel, Jeer, & Cornell, 2007), and also aimed at eliminating the need for surgery. Casting is also still widely used. When casting is used, about 90% of patients achieve satisfactory improvement with less than five casts. If neither braces nor casts achieve correction, surgical intervention is considered. The most common surgical approach is cutting the joint and tendons and restoring the bones to their normal positions. Realigned bones are held in place by pins. The surgery is followed by two to three months of casting. After the casts are removed, braces may be used to maintain the correction. Recent studies of surgical outcomes clearly demonstrate that better functional results will be realized if surgery is performed after the first six months after birth and before twelve months of age (Templeton et al., 2006).

Nursing Management

Nursing assessment begins at birth. Visual inspection and straightening the newborn's feet to the midline is part of the initial assessment to detect this defect. The nurse obtains a history that includes information about the birth and any genetic defects in other members of the family. Providing support and education for the caregivers about care of the infant with a cast is an important aspect of nursing. If surgery is required, postsurgical care includes neurovascular status checks, assessment for edema, and drainage. Ice bags applied to the casted area and elevation of the foot with a pillow help reduce swelling. Analgesia is administered as needed.

Emotional support for the family allows them the opportunity to explore and verbalize their feelings regarding their child with a physical deformity. Caregivers should participate in all aspects of the child's care, as this allows them to carry out the normal activities of parenting and reinforces their role as important. Promoting a healthy body image is essential as the prognosis for clubfoot is for the child's foot to become fully functional. Until the age of 1 year, there is a 25% chance of reoccurrence even after surgical intervention. Children born with clubfoot are usually followed until their late teens.

Family Teaching

Bathing, skin care, dressing, and safety are areas for the nurse to address with the caregivers. Since tub baths are not allowed while the child is in a cast, nurses should teach the

Reflections from Families

I was 35 years old when Juan was born. I had put off marriage until my career as an attorney was well established. I had two miscarriages before I became pregnant with Juan. My husband and I were so excited when this pregnancy did not end in a miscarriage. We both wanted a child so much. When Juan was born, he had bilateral clubfoot. We were so disappointed because we had waited so long for this event. Then our thoughts turned to the baby. We wondered if he would ever walk and run or if his feet would ever look like a normal child's.

caregivers how to give a sponge bath. Urinary and fecal incontinence in infancy increases the risk of soiling the casts, which cannot be adequately cleaned. As a consequence, parents often demand cast changes before they are scheduled. Domestic cling film (example, Saran Wrap) has proven an effective and inexpensive solution. Before changing the diaper, wrap the casts in the plastic film, discard the diapers inside the plastic film when done (Patel, Jeer, & Cornell, 2007). Teaching should include checking the skin around the cast edges for redness or irritation and assessing the neurovascular status of the foot. Other important areas to be covered include precautions for fresh casts and signs of infection. Clothing will need to be selected or adapted so it will fit over the cast. The nurse needs to discuss potential safety hazards when using various equipment. Caregivers need to check car seats, swings, and infant carriers to make sure the cast allows the safety belt, pads, and so forth to operate correctly. When using an infant seat on the floor or in a grocery cart, they need to make sure the additional weight of the cast does not overbalance it.

DEVELOPMENTAL DYSPLASIA OF THE HIP

Developmental dysplasia of the hip (DDH) is a congenital anomaly in which the head of the femur has an abnormal relationship with the acetabulum (hip socket). The head of the femur may slip in and out of the acetabulum or may be completely outside of the acetabulum. While hip dysplasia is commonly diagnosed in the newborn, it is also noted later in infancy. DDH may be found in older children, especially those with neuromuscular disorders such as spina bifida or cerebral palsy.

Incidence and Etiology

The true incidence of DDH can only be estimated as there is no "gold standard" for diagnosis (Gelfer & Kennedy, 2008). Most developed countries report an incidence of 1.5 to 20 cases per 1,000 live births (Shipman, Helfand, Moyer, & Yawn, 2006). It affects females more than males. DDH is noted in many cultures worldwide. In the United States, the prevalence in Native-American children is high, while the incidence is lower in populations of African descent (Phillips, 2008). The causes of DDH are multifactorial and include physiological, mechanical, and genetic factors. Ligamentous laxity plays an important role in predisposing the developing hip to mechanical forces that make the femoral head separable from the joint (Phillips, 2008). Other physiological factors are maternal hormone secretion and increased maternal pelvic laxity. Toward the end of pregnancy estrogen secretion is increased leading to greater pelvic laxity of the mother. This affects the fetal joints as well. Female infants have a greater reactivity to estrogen; thus, the predominance of DDH in girls. Mechanical factors include cesarean section that is often associated with abnormal intrauterine position, breech presentation, primigravida (first birth), and increased birth weight (>4000g). Genetic factors include a positive family history.

Pathophysiology

The spectrum of DDH includes hips that are: (1) dislocated (the femoral head is completely outside the socket); (2) subluxated (the femoral head is incompletely or partially displaced outside the socket); (3) dysplastic (the sockets at the hip are not completely formed); (4) dislocatable (the femoral head is in the socket but can be displaced with manipulation).

Dislocated hips are of two types: (1) teratologic dislocations (occur early in utero and are often associated with other problems, such as Larson syndrome, arthrogryposis [fibrous, stiffness of one or more joints], or spina bifida); and (2) typical dislocations (usually occur in healthy infants and may develop prenatally or postnatally) (Gelfer & Kennedy, 2008).

Clinical Manifestations

Clinical instability of the hip is the traditional hallmark (Shipman, Helfand, Moyer, & Yawn, 2006). Newborns present with hip instability, infants have limited hip abduction on examination, and children and adolescents present limping, with joint pain and osteoarthritis (Gelfer & Kennedy, 2008) (Figure 34-9). In the older child the physical signs are more obvious. Gait abnormalities such as toe walking or limping may be present, or the level of the pelvis may be unequal. The longer the disorder goes undiagnosed, and therefore untreated, the more severe the clinical manifestations.

Diagnosis

Repeated, frequent examination of infants from birth throughout the first year or until the child walks are the best means for early detection (AAP, 2000). Provocative tests include the Barlow or Ortolani maneuvers. In the Barlow maneuver, the examiner pushes an unstable femoral head out of the acetabulum by use of gentle lateral pressure of the lower trochanter. In the Ortolani maneuver, the examiner reduces the dislocated femoral head into the acetabulum by gentle abduction and external rotation. A distinctive "clunk" is heard and felt as the dislocated femoral head reduces into the acetabulum. By 8 to 12 weeks of age, these maneuvers lose reliability (Shipman, Helfand, Moyer, & Yawn, 2006). The disorder is usually, but not always, diagnosed at birth. Therefore examination of the hip is carried out at each well-child visit to detect late-onset dislocation.

After 3 months of age, limitation of abduction is the most reliable sign associated with DDH (Patel, 2001). Radiographic examination is used to confirm the diagnosis, but is not reliable in early infancy because ossification of the femoral head does not normally take place until the third to sixth month of life. In the first four to six months of life, ultrasound is more sensitive to immature bone, and may explain why there is an increase in the reported incidence of DDH (Shipman, Helfand, Moyer, & Yawn, 2006). Since female infants with positive family history of DDH (i.e., genetic cause) and females born in breech presentation have

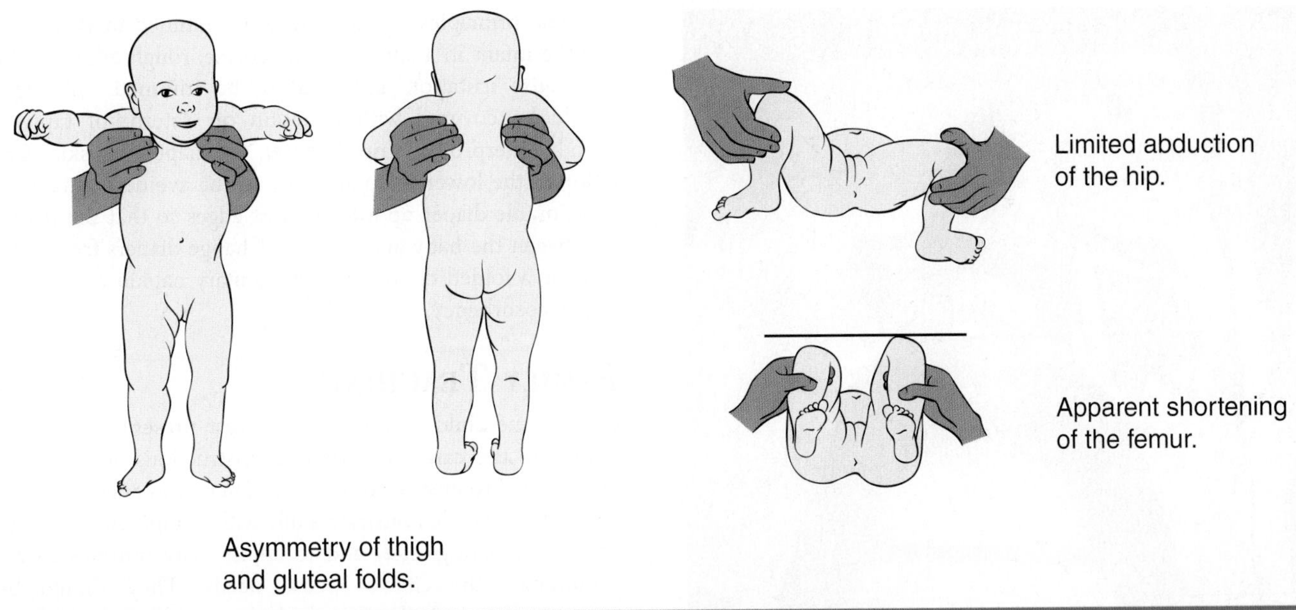

FIGURE 34-9 Signs of Developmental Dysplasia of the Hip. DELMAR CENGAGE LEARNING.

the highest risks of DDH (about 44/1000 and 120/1000 respectively), imaging with ultrasound or radiography is recommended for these infants (AAP, 2000).

TREATMENT

The treatment plan varies depending on the age of the child. For infants younger than 3 months an abduction device is the preferred method. The Pavlik harness is a commonly used device that seats the head of the femur in the acetabulum by keeping the knees and hips flexed and the hips abducted (Figure 34-10). It is worn 24 hours a day for three to four months. After this period the child is examined for a decreased laxity. Radiographs and ultrasounds will confirm improvement in position. Skin traction or surgery is used if the abduction device is not successful or if the child is older than 3 months. Traction stretches the soft tissue and moves the femoral head down to the level of the acetabulum. Achieving closed reduction without disruption of the blood supply to the femoral head is the goal. Surgery may be performed to reduce the dislocated hip. This procedure is followed by application of a hip spica cast (Figure 34-11).

Important to note, the US Preventive Services Task Force in reviewing the literature using a best evidence approach found inadequate evidence supporting nonsurgical (Pavlik harness) or surgical interventions. In all interventions for DDH, avascular necrosis of the femoral head is one disastrous outcome. Because of the high rate of an unpredictable nature of spontaneous resolution of DDH, net benefits of DDH screening are not clear (Shipman, Helfand, Moyer, & Yawn, 2006). However, the overall goal for all health care is prevention of late detection of DDH (Gelfer & Kennedy, 2008).

NURSING MANAGEMENT

Nurses are in a position to detect DDH in the newborn. During routine assessments, bathing, and diaper changes the hips can be inspected for any deviations from normal.

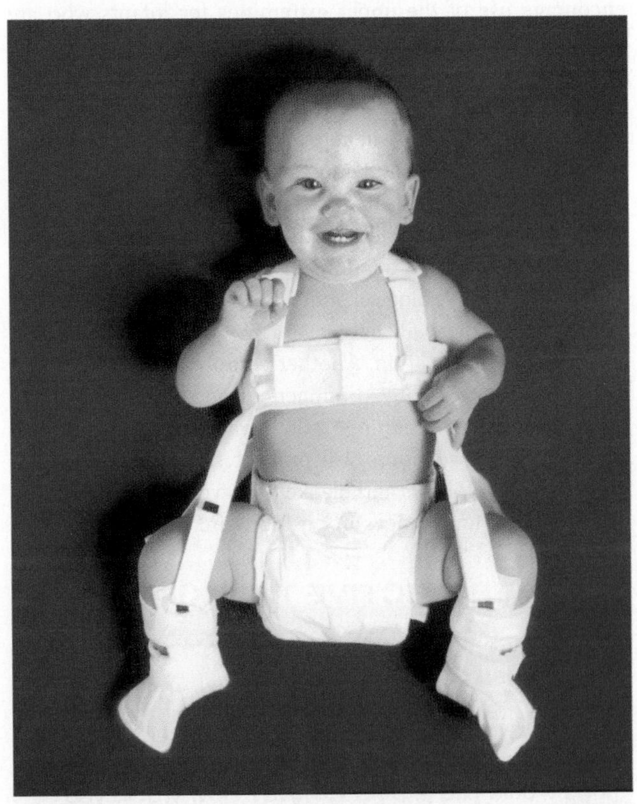

FIGURE 34-10 Infant with Developmental Dysplasia of the Hip in a Pavlik Harness. COURTESY OF WHEATON BRACE CO., CAROL STREAM, IL.

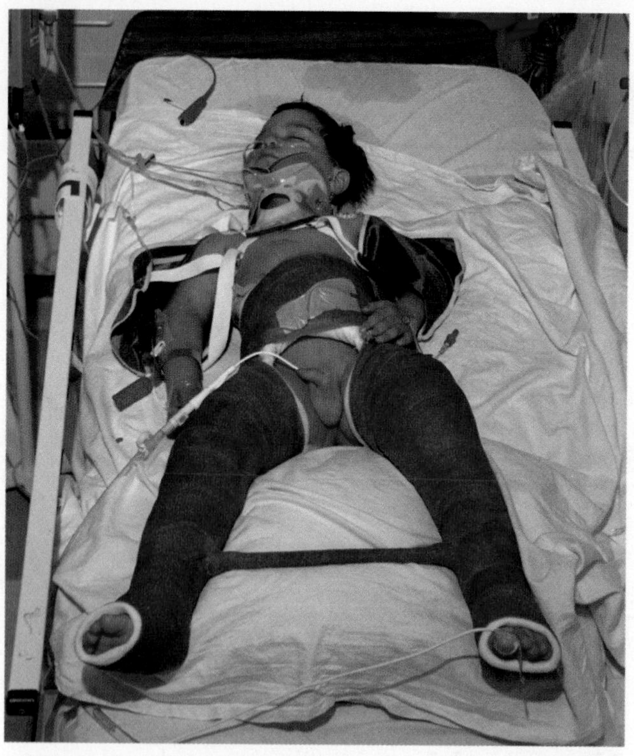

FIGURE 34-11 **Boy in a Hip Spica Cast.** DELMAR CENGAGE LEARNING.

Nursing management considers the normal growth and development of the infant or toddler. Reaching and pulling at toys or mobiles hung above the crib provide distraction and encourage use of the upper extremities for infants who are immobilized. Development of fine motor skills may be rapid while the child is immobilized, while development of gross motor skills may be delayed until after treatment is completed when the rate will return to normal. The child will use her or his arms and uncasted limb to aid in mobility. Nurses should reassure family members that the child will learn to maximize mobility in the cast or brace.

Immobility from traction, casts, or braces may lead to alterations in physiological functions. Use of bulk and bran in the child's diet will help maintain good bowel function and prevent constipation. Another complication of immobility is pressure on bony prominences and skin breakdown. Use of adequate padding, skin wrapping, and position changes every two hours will prevent skin breakdown and pressure sores. Pillows and blankets or even the floor may be used to allow for changes in position and diversion.

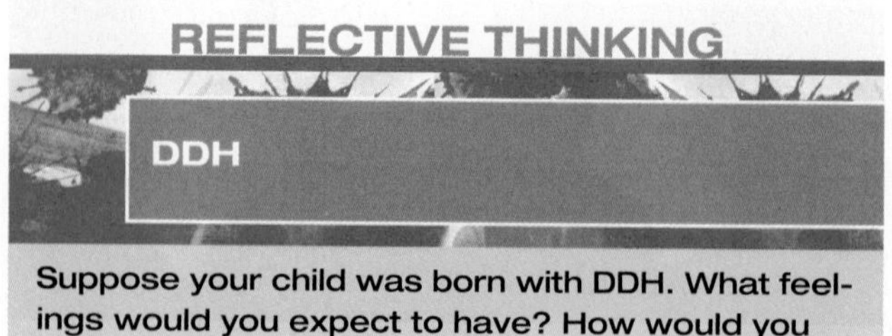

REFLECTIVE THINKING

DDH

Suppose your child was born with DDH. What feelings would you expect to have? How would you channel any negative feelings into positive ones?

The principles of cast care were outlined in Box 34-2. For the infant in a spica cast the coarse, rough edges of the cast cause irritation and need to be trimmed. All edges should be covered with moleskin or waterproof tape to form a waterproof barrier between the diaper and skin. Irritation of the lower torso and legs can be avoided by tucking a disposable diaper up into the cast edges so that the plastic is between the baby and the cast. Change diapers frequently and use a folded cloth diaper or sanitary napkin to increase diaper absorbency.

FAMILY TEACHING

Care of the child in traction or a cast presents significant change in the caregivers' routine. Instructions and support are essential to ensure compliance. They need adequate time to practice and demonstrate skills with equipment and procedures (toileting, etc.) and to adjust daily routines to accommodate the child's special needs. They should be encouraged to verbalize fears and concerns about the impact of treatment on the family's life.

Family members will need to be informed about cast care, including issues related to urinary and bowel elimination, bathing, and positioning. If skin traction is to be used, additional instructions will be required for skin care and traction application. Planning for nutritional requirements for the growing infant or toddler with restricted movement is necessary. An understanding of the age-appropriate developmental milestones will help the family members plan activities that will promote normal growth and development.

Caregivers need time to practice and demonstrate proper application of the Pavlik harness if used. They need to be taught how to diaper the child without removing the harness. Feeding is done in the upright position to maintain abduction of the hips. Wearing a cotton undershirt and cotton socks protects the skin by absorbing perspiration in warm weather and providing warmth in cold weather. Lotions, oils, or powder should not be used under the straps. Soothing and pacifying the infant or child may be a challenge. Caregivers need to be encouraged to hold the child despite a bulky harness or cast. They should bring experiences to the child because the child is unable to crawl or walk toward new and interesting objects in their surroundings.

MUSCULAR DYSTROPHY

Muscular dystrophy (MD) refers to a group of progressive degenerative inherited diseases causing wasting of the muscles. The word dystrophy, with Latin and Greek roots, means "faulty nutrition." Muscles waste away in this disease, and it was theorized that persons with muscular dystrophy were not being properly nourished. This has proved unfounded. There are various patterns of inheritance and age of onset. The most common type of muscular dystrophy of childhood is Duchenne muscular dystrophy (DMD); therefore, the following discussion relates to DMD. Table 34-5 describes the common types of MD seen in children and adolescents.

Table 34-5 Common Childhood Muscular Dystrophies

TYPE	ONSET AND PROGRESSION	INHERITANCE AND INCIDENCE	CLINICAL MANIFESTATIONS
Duchenne	Onset: 2–6 yr. Progression: Rapid	X-linked; males Most common childhood form Affects all races Incidence: 0.2 per 1,000 live births	Affects upper arms and legs and trunk muscles first; calves enlarged due to fatty infiltrates; child has difficulty getting up from a sitting or lying position; waddling gait; mental retardation in some cases; life expectancy: adolescence—early 20s
Becker	Onset: 2–16 yr. Progression: slow	X-linked; males Incidence: 0.05 per 1,000 live births	Similar to Duchenne but appears later and progresses more slowly; child is mobile until late adolescence; normal intelligence; longer life expectancy than Duchenne
Limb-girdle (LGMD)	Onset: Adolescence to early adulthood Progression: Usually slow	Autosomal recessive and dominant forms; males and females	Weakness begins in hips and moves to shoulders; progresses to include arms and legs
Facioscapulohumeral	Onset: Adolescence to early adulthood Progression: Slow, with long periods of stability interspersed with shorter periods of rapid muscle weakness	Autosomal dominant; males and females	Muscles of face and shoulder area are affected first; forward sloping shoulders, difficulty closing eyes, and lifting arms above head; progresses in following order: abdomen, feet, upper arms, pelvic area, and lower arms; half are able to walk for their entire life

Incidence and Etiology

Duchenne muscular dystrophy occurs in 1.0 in 3,000 live births (Daftary, Crisanti, Kalra, Wong, & Amin, 2007). It is inherited as an X-linked recessive disease; therefore, it affects males almost exclusively. Females may be carriers and pass the defect to their male children. A family history of MD is not present in as many as one-third of affected children.

Pathophysiology

In DMD there is an absence of the muscle protein dystrophin, which appears to play a role in supporting the structure of muscle fibers. The absence of dystrophin results in degeneration of skeletal or voluntary muscles that control movement. Fat and connective tissue replace the degenerated muscle fibers.

Clinical Manifestations

Duchenne muscular dystrophy is characterized by progressive loss of muscle function that eventually results in respiratory insufficiency and death frequently from respiratory failure (Daftary et al., 2007). Early motor development in DMD is usually normal or just minimally delayed; however, between 2 and 4 years of age, the pelvic muscles begin to weaken. Children have difficulty climbing stairs, running, and riding a bicycle. They develop a waddling gait and fall often. By 5 to 6 years of age, in order for the child to rise from a sitting to a standing position he must use a series of maneuvers and walks his hands up his legs. This is known as Gower's sign, and the maneuver is necessary because of weakness of the pelvic and trunk muscles (Figure 34-12).

Involvement of the shoulder girdle muscles usually occurs within three to five years after the onset of the disease, and the arms become weak. As muscles of the trunk atrophy, scoliosis frequently occurs. Enlargement of the calves and wasting of the thigh muscles are classic features. The calves appear large and strong, but they are weak because of infiltration of the muscles with fat and connective tissue. This abnormal enlargement of the muscles caused by an overgrowth of fatty and fibrous tissues is referred to as **pseudohypertrophy**. As the disease progresses, contractures develop usually in the ankles, knees, hips, and elbows. Between the ages of 9 and 12 years walking becomes impossible. In the later stages of the disease the auxiliary muscles of breathing and the diaphragm weaken, and respiratory function is poor. Respiratory infections become more common. The myocardium of the heart deteriorates and weakens resulting in

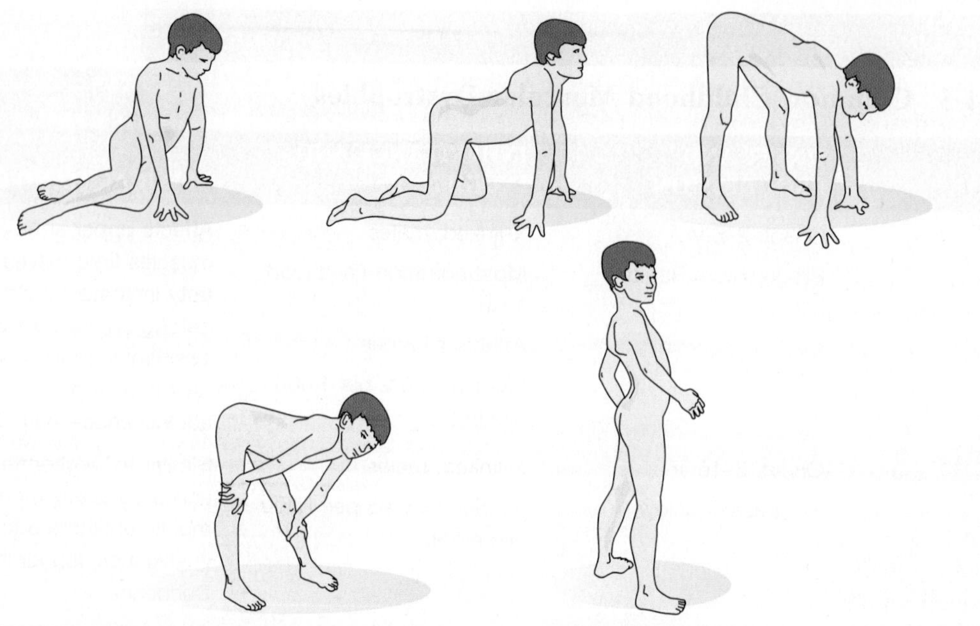

FIGURE 34-12 **Gower's Sign. Because of the weakness of the pelvic and trunk muscles, the child with muscular dystrophy must use a series of maneuvers to rise from a sitting or lying position.** DELMAR CENGAGE LEARNING.

cardiomyopathy. Eventually death results from respiratory infections or cardiac failure in the child's late teens or early twenties.

Diagnosis

The diagnosis is made by observation of clinical manifestations during physical examination and several tests. The most common diagnostic tests are muscle biopsy, electromyogram (EMG), nerve conduction velocity (NCV), and blood enzyme tests. With a muscle biopsy a small piece of muscle tissue is taken from an individual. If muscular dystrophy is present, the biopsy will reveal a replacement of normal muscle with connective and fatty tissue. An EMG involves placing a small electrode into the muscle to measure the electrical impulses, which are decreased in DMD. NCV involves sending electrical impulses down the nerves of the arms and legs. The speed of these impulses is measured with electrodes to determine whether the nerves are functioning normally. Because EMG and NCV are uncomfortable for most children, they will need adequate support during these tests. Blood enzyme tests are used to determine levels of the enzyme creatine kinase (CK). The CK level is elevated in many forms of muscular dystrophy because these enzymes leak from degenerating muscles.

Treatment

Treatment is supportive, as there is no cure for muscular dystrophy. A team approach, including the caregivers, health care provider, nurse, physical and occupational therapists, nutritionist, and social worker, is necessary. The goal of management is to provide support and prevent complications. Physical and occupational therapies help children achieve their maximum level of functioning and independence. Physical therapy helps the individual maintain strength and maximize range of motion, posture, and comfort. Muscle weakness can lead to contracture and shortening of muscle tissue. A child with DMD typically walks on the tips of the toes as the tendon shortens, which is the result of the muscle breakdown and fibrosis in calf muscles. A daily routine of stretching these muscles delays the deformities caused by the contracture. Physical therapies help the individual and the family members develop an individualized exercise program that includes the type and amount of activity best for each child. The goal of occupational therapy is to help the child compensate for physical limitations and learn to adapt to a new level of achievement in the activities of daily living at home and school. Adaptation of wheelchairs, seating systems, and computers to aid with writing are a few of the possibilities. Prolongation of survival has been demonstrated by cough augmentation and noninvasive ventilatory support (Bach, Ishikawa, & Heakyung, 1997). Additionally, steroid therapy has increased respiratory capacity, improving quality of life (Balaban, Matthews, Clayton, & Carry, 2005).

Surgery may be performed as contractures progress. One of the common procedures is a release of the heel cord, which relieves developing contractures and improves mobility. Surgery is performed on the hips and knees as they become contracted, thus allowing the child to sit in a wheelchair with an increased level of comfort.

Nursing Management

The care of the child with DMD is complex and requires cooperation among many health care providers and the child's caregivers. Monitoring of respiratory and cardiac status needs to be performed regularly. Proper nutrition and avoiding obesity are ongoing concerns. Activities such as swimming or water exercises are often recommended as a way to keep muscles toned and to promote mobility without causing undue stress on the muscles. As the child's stamina decreases, activities that involve less expenditure of energy can be suggested.

Members of the interdisciplinary team may need to meet with teachers and caregivers to evaluate the child's learning needs and functioning in the classroom. Reading books to the child, listening to tapes, and using the computer offer the child stimulation and promote normal development. It is important to provide good back support and posture by keeping the child's body in alignment when confined to a wheelchair.

In the later stages of DMD the child is unable to move himself and needs to be turned frequently to prevent skin breakdown. Adequate amounts of fluids must be encouraged to prevent urinary stasis. The combination of weak abdominal muscles and immobility can lead to severe constipation; therefore, the child's diet should be high in fluid, fiber, and fresh fruits and vegetables. A bowel regime including stool softeners and laxatives may be necessary to prevent stool retention and constipation. Respiratory therapy is needed to maintain pulmonary function for as long as possible. Modifications of the home to accommodate a wheelchair may be necessary. Supportive devices and lifts may be necessary to get the child in and out the bathtub without undue strain on the caregivers.

Genetic counseling and testing are recommended for females in the family of the affected child to determine if they are carriers of DMD. Accurate protein and DNA-based carrier detection tests are available. As gene and protein defects are identified, better diagnostic tests and understanding of the biological basis of a disease may lead to more effective treatment. Genetic counseling provides families with valuable information about current genetic testing methods.

Family Teaching

Mothers may deal with feelings of guilt since they are the carriers of DMD and passed the defective gene to their child. Nurses should encourage the family to discuss their feelings about the genetic aspect of the disease, the eventual fatal outcome, and how the disease is affecting all members and their lifestyle. Feelings of hopelessness are common as the child's disease progresses and he requires total care. Caregivers need to be taught how to assist with basic activities of daily living. Attention to the needs of siblings is important, as they may feel neglected because the child with DMD receives so much attention. If the child with muscular dystrophy needs a special diet, it is important to make mealtimes a family affair and to include that child despite his special diet. Use of an electric wheelchair, cellular phones, and other assistive devices decrease the risk for social isolation. Resources, such as the Muscular Dystrophy Association of America, can provide emotional support and arrange for special assistance as family energies are depleted.

GROWTH-RELATED DISORDERS

Growth-related disorders occur during periods of rapid growth of the musculoskeletal system before skeletal maturity is achieved. The disorders discussed in this section include scoliosis, kyphosis, lordosis, and Legg-Calve-Perthes disease. Scoliosis, kyphosis, and lordosis are deformities that affect the spine (Figure 34-13).

SCOLIOSIS

A normal spine viewed from the posterior is vertical or straight. Viewed from the side, the normal spine has a slightly rounded kyphotic contour (20–40 degrees) [Figure 34-13B] of the thoracic (upper) spine and a lordotic curve of the lumbar (Figure 34-13C) that faces the opposite direction, like a backward "C" (Napierkowski, 2007).

Scoliosis describes any lateral (sideways) deviation of the normal, straight, vertical line of the spine which exceeds 10 degrees. The severity of the scoliosis measures the extent of the curvature from the vertical plus the angle of trunk rotation (twist). The Cobb method is the standard technique for measurement of the curvature and spinal deformities. Curves between 10–25 degrees are considered mild. Most curves over 25 degrees are considered significant, with curves between 25–40 degrees treated with braces. If curvature progresses rapidly during growth spurts or exceeds 40 degrees, surgery is normally considered (Napierkowski, 2007).

Scoliosis is the lateral curvature ("S" shaped) of the spine with vertebral body rotation. As the spine curves, the vertebral column rotates around its long axis, pulling the ribs in the thoracic region along and causing them to become prominent on the convex side. The disorder can be structural (a primary deformity) or functional (a curve caused by a secondary problem). Figures 34-14A and B illustrate an adolescent girl with scoliosis.

Incidence and Etiology

Although scoliosis is fairly common, it is clinically significant in less than 1 in 1000 children aged 6 to 14 (Oxborrow, 2000). Mild curvatures (less than 20 degrees) occur equally in boys and girls, but curve progression beyond 20 degrees is 10 times more likely to occur in girls. For boys, the risk of progression is greater when a larger curvature exists at the time of diagnosis. Scoliosis is typically diagnosed before the age of 14 in boys, and before age 11 in girls. Girls requiring treatment is estimated to be 1%, while treatment in males is about 0.1% (Karol, Johnston, Browne, & Madison, 1993).

The etiology of scoliosis is unknown, but several theories have been postulated. These include growth disturbance in the paravertebral muscles or malfunctioning of the vestibular balancing system, genetic or hereditary patterns, muscular weakness or problems with coordination, collagen

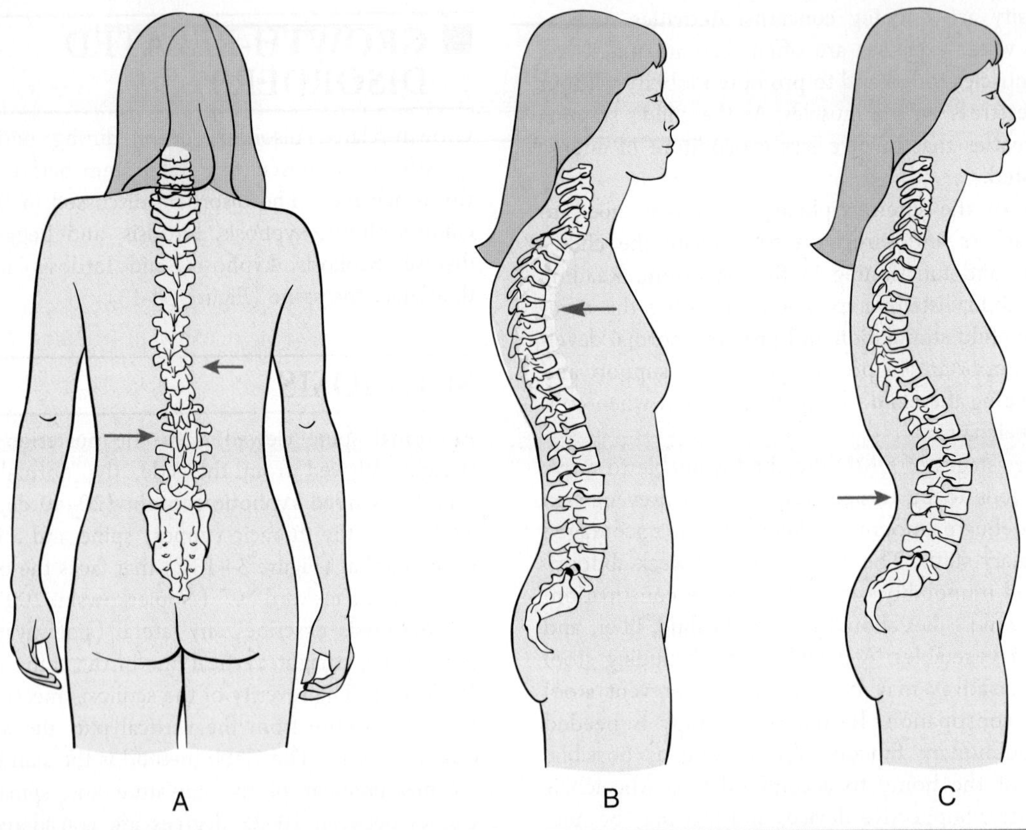

FIGURE 34-13 Spinal Deformities: (A) Scoliosis (B) Kyphosis (C) Lordosis. DELMAR CENGAGE LEARNING.

metabolism, and abnormalities in the central nervous system. In the majority of cases the cause is unknown, called idiopathic scoliosis (approximately 80% of cases). This type is further divided into three classes: infantile, juvenile, and adolescent. The age of the child at the time of the diagnosis determines the classification. The most common of all types of scoliosis is adolescent idiopathic. Other conditions known to cause spinal deformity are congenital spinal column abnormalities, neuromuscular disorders (muscular dystrophy, cerebral palsy, spina bifida), tumors, rheumatic disease, myelomingocele and spinal muscular atrophy, and radiation therapy (Napierkowski, 2007). Radiation often produces asymmetric growth in adjacent growth plates and soft tissues, leading to subsequent spinal deformity.

Pathophysiology

When the vertebral column begins to curve laterally, the spine and ribs rotate toward the convex portion of the curve. On the concave side, the muscles and ligaments are contracted and thickened, whereas on the convex side they become thin and atrophied. A compensatory curve results as the child attempts to maintain erect posture. The thoracic cavity also changes and becomes asymmetrical, resulting in respiratory problems.

Clinical Manifestations

In adolescent idiopathic scoliosis the time of highest risk for curve progression occurs around puberty when the growth rate is the fastest. Adolescents may notice that clothing does not fit right, and girls might notice an uneven hemline. The individuals may have unequal shoulder and hip level, prominence of one scapula or a curved spinal column, and truncal asymmetry. In normal children the elbow level falls above the iliac crest; in those with scoliosis one elbow will be closer to the iliac crest than the other. When the child bends over the rotation of the spine becomes more prominent. The scapula on one side becomes prominent, and the other side is hollow. Scoliosis curves occur in the thoracic, lumbar, or thoracolumbar sections of the spine, with the thoracic being the most common. They may complain of neck pain and headache. Other neurological signs may include sensory losses and absent unilateral superficial abdominal reflexes (Inoue et al., 2003). There may also be muscle weakness, gait defects or other abnormal or absent reflexes (Napierkowski, 2007).

Diagnosis

Scoliosis is frequently detected initially during routine physical examinations or school screenings. Screening is performed

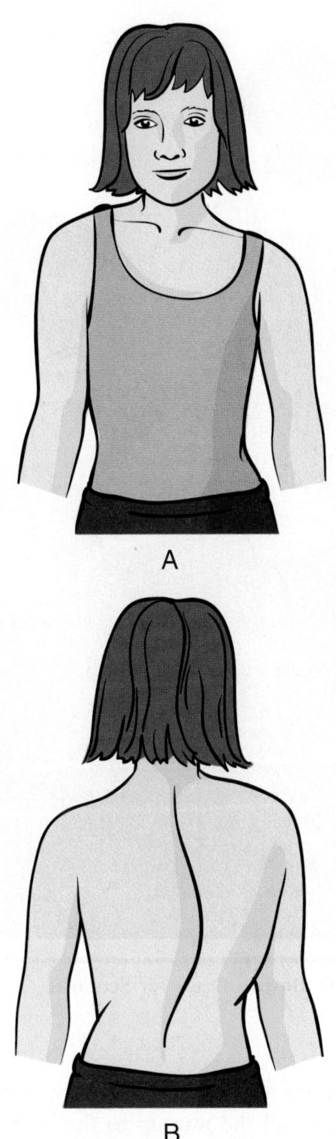

FIGURE 34-14 **Adolescent Girl with Scoliosis: (A) Frontal View (B) Posterior View.** DELMAR CENGAGE LEARNING.

during peak adolescent growth, and almost all significant curvatures can be found by about age 10 (Bunnell, 2005). Box 34-3 describes a procedure for a school screening. Radiographs confirm the diagnosis of scoliosis by applying the Cobb method.

Treatment

Scoliosis requires treatment when the curvature of the spine progresses to greater than 10 to 11 degrees. The treatment depends on the severity of the curvature and the age of the child and includes three options: (1) monitoring the child, (2) bracing, and (3) surgery.

Option 1—Monitoring If the curve does not progress and remains below 40 degrees, intervention may not be necessary. However, if the curve worsens and there is prominence of one scapula or unequal shoulder, breast, and hip level, treatment should be initiated.

Reflections from Families

When I was 15 years old, I was diagnosed with scoliosis and was told I would have to wear a Milwaukee brace for at least one year. When I saw pictures of the brace, I thought it was ugly, like something out of the Dark Ages. I was a sophomore in high school and was just beginning to like the attention I was receiving from boys. I was so angry about having to wear this awful brace. Even wearing blouses and shirts in bigger sizes couldn't conceal the head and chin rests. I was so worried that all the kids would stare at me. I didn't even want to go to school.

BOX 34-3
SCOLIOSIS SCREENING PROCEDURE

Using the Adam's Bend test (forward bend test), assess girls prior to age 10, assess boys at age 10 and repeat for boys again at age 14 years (Napierkowski, 2007):

1. Have the child bend forward at the waist dangling their arms toward the floor, with feet together and knees straight (Figure 34-15).
2. Visually inspect the back for any rotational asymmetry, observe the scapula for symmetry, or other irregularities.
3. Palpate progression of the spinal processes with the forefinger or first two to three fingers, starting at the cervical spine, proceeding toward the sacral spine.
4. Make sure each vertebrae is palpated for alignment.
5. Identify a lateral curve to one or another side, which may indicate scoliosis, estimate the degree of lateral deviation.

Adapted from Estes, *Health Assessment & Physical Examination*, 4th ed. 2010.

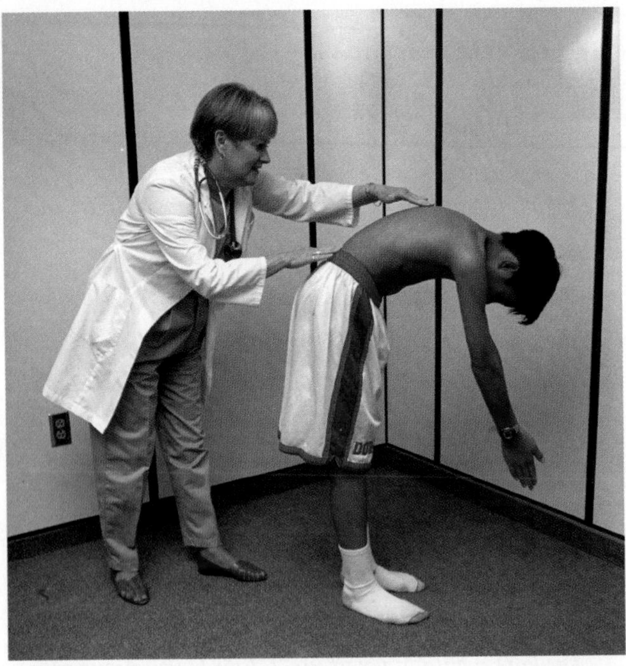

FIGURE 34-15 School Nurse Performing Scoliosis Screening. DELMAR CENGAGE LEARNING.

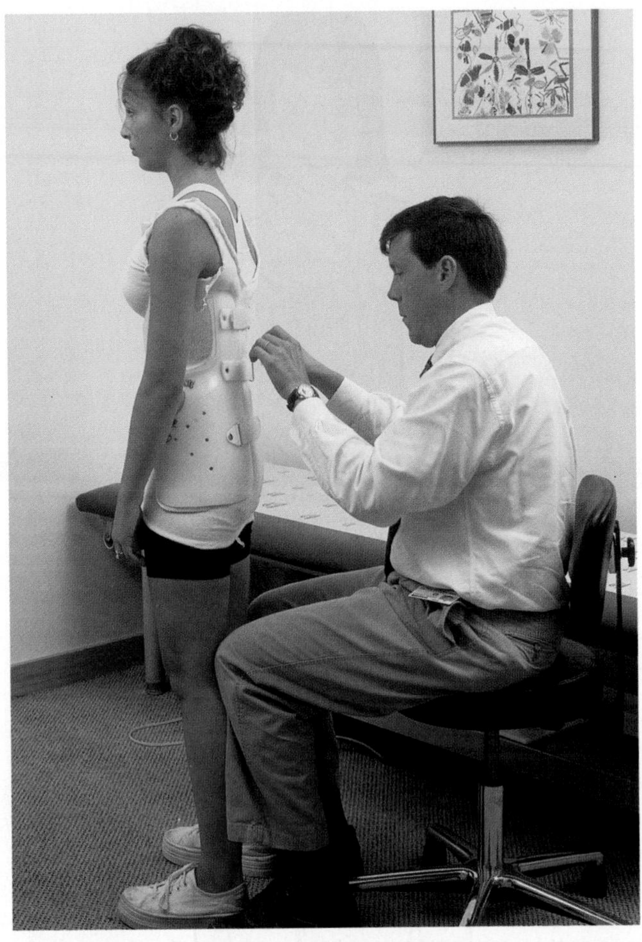

FIGURE 34-16 Boston Brace for Scoliosis. COURTESY OF BOSTON BRACE INTERNATIONAL.

Option 2—Bracing Bracing has been effective in preventing the curvature from worsening. Bracing is recommended to prevent further progression of moderate curves (24–40 degrees). It is important that children and caregivers understand that bracing will not correct a curvature, but will prevent it from worsening (Table 34-6). Three types of braces are used for scoliosis:

1. Boston or thoracolumbar sacral orthoses—The Boston brace is a molded brace used for mid-back or lower degrees of curvature. It comes up to the underarms and can be hidden under clothing. Studies have shown a 61% compliance with this type of brace (Figure 34-16).
2. Milwaukee brace—This is used for especially high curves. The Milwaukee brace has one wide flat bar in the front and two in the back that are attached to a bar that has rests for the chin and back of the head. The brace comes all the way up to the back. The Milwaukee brace must be worn for 23 hours a day, taken off only for bathing and exercises or sports. This type of brace cannot be hidden, so these children are prone to self-esteem issues. Compliance is poor; a recent study showed only 15% compliance with the Milwaukee brace (Figure 34-17).

TABLE 34-6 Bracing Therapy

FOR BRACING TO BE EFFECTIVE	BRACING WILL BE INEFFECTIVE
Brace should be started early, while the child is still growing	Child does not wear it for the prescribed amount of time—curve may not improve or may worsen
Spinal curve is between 24–40 degrees	Brace is irritating to the skin; treatments should be ordered
Brace should be a customized fit	Bracing is not comfortable
Child must wear the brace for the ordered amount of time	
Child must have a good support network	

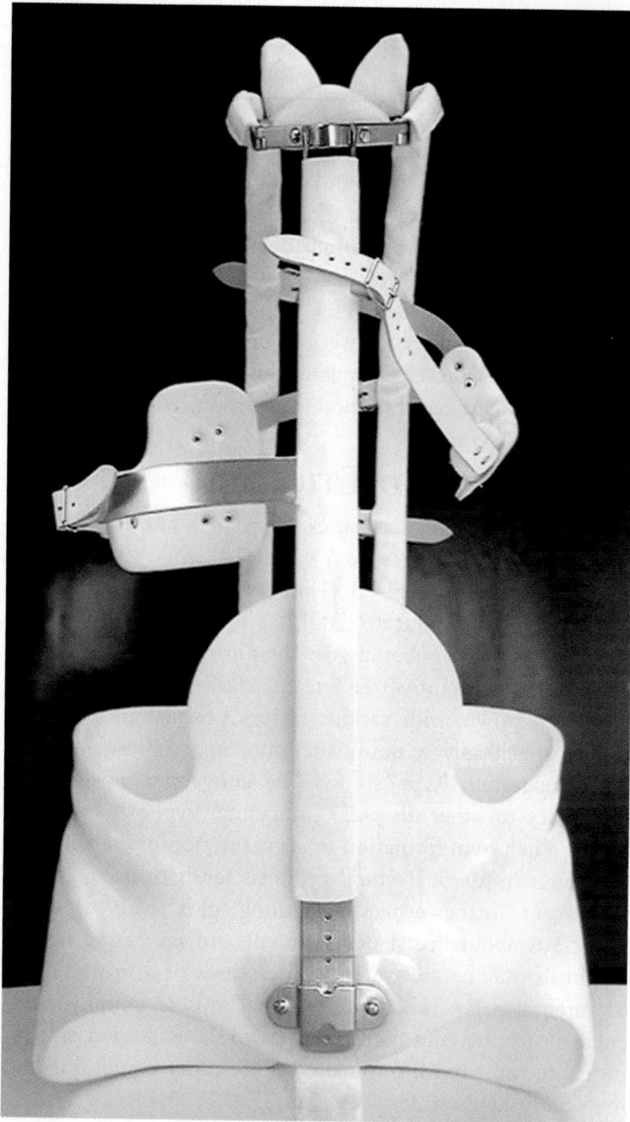

FIGURE 34-17 **The Milwaukee brace is used for high thoracic scoliosis curves.** COURTESY OF BERTIL HOLMBERG, MD, MALMOE, SWEDEN.

3. Charleston bending brace—This is worn only at night. This type of brace is appropriate for small, flexible curves. In a 2002 study, it was found that the Charleston bending brace was as effective as the Boston brace with a success rate of 56–66%.

Option 3—Surgery Surgery is usually performed on children and teenagers whose curve is greater than 45–50 degrees. A scoliotic curve greater than 40 degrees will potentially progress until the patient stops growing (LaMontaigne, Hepworth, Cohen, & Salisbury, 2004). If left untreated, scoliosis causes respiratory problems and chronic back pain as well as psychiatric problems for these patients. The goals of spinal surgery are to straighten the spine and balance the torso and pelvic areas (Napierkowski, 2007). It is important for the child and family to understand that surgery will not completely straighten the spine, but will improve the child's quality of life and prevent complications.

KIDS WANT TO KNOW

Do I really have to wear this Milwaukee brace when I go to school? I'll look like a freak!

I understand you're concerned about the appearance of the brace, but wearing loose, colorful shirts, blouses, sweaters, or sweatshirts will help. You'll also feel better about how you look if you continue using your makeup and keep your hair clean and stylish. Instead of waiting for others to ask about the brace, a better approach is for you to mention it first and explain why you're wearing it. I know many kids think not wearing the brace now is more important than preventing progression of the curve in the future. However, the curve will get worse and may cause you considerable pain and difficulty breathing. I can get you in touch with another girl your age that also has a Milwaukee brace so you can share your feelings and concerns. Would you like that?

NURSING ALERT

Spinal Cord Injury After Surgery for Scoliosis

During surgical intervention for scoliosis, spinal cord injury is a potential complication caused by compression or trauma. Therefore, all clients who will be undergoing surgery should be assessed for neurological impairment. Assessment includes numbness, sensation, motion, paresthesia in all extremities, and bowel and bladder function.

Surgical treatment for scoliosis is spinal fusion along the curve and support for the fused bones with various kinds of instrumentation. In a spinal fusion, the surgeon removes the vertebral processes in the curvature and replaces them with bone grafts that touch the adjoining vertebrae. The fusion process requires bone from other parts of the child's body, usually the hip or spine. This is called an **autogenous** (originating within the child's body) graft because the bone comes from the child, not from another person.

Various types of instrumentation are used. Various types of rods are used to permanently support the vertebrae. The most common types of rods are the Harrington and the Cotrel-Dubousset. Instrumentation is used to stabilize the spine and improve alignment in various sections of the curvature. The Harrington rod supports the fusion using hooks. Usually after 1–2 years the rod is not required for vertebral support, but is generally not removed. Correction of the curve is usually more than 50%, but studies have shown a loss of correction between 10–25% over time. One inherent complication with the Harrington procedure is called "flat back syndrome" which occurs because it eliminates the inward curve of the back.

The Cotrel-Dubousset procedure corrects the curve itself as well as correcting rotation, and does not cause the "flat back syndrome."

Other types of rods used to correct scoliosis include the Texas Scottish Rite Hospital instrumentation, the Luque instrumentation, the Wisconsin segmental spine instrumentation, the Halm-Zielke instrumentation, and the Dorsal Dynamic Spondylodesis system (DDS). With any surgery there are complications. Possible complications of back surgery include nerve damage, spinal cord damage, and lung problems. A potential complication for children who undergo a spinal fusion is the cessation of growth at the area where the fusion occurred.

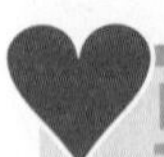

FAMILY**TEACHING**

The Child After Spinal Fusion for Scoliosis

- Instruct and demonstrate the correct technique for wound care.
- Instruct the child to avoid any extremes of bending, twisting, stooping, or lifting of heavy objects.
- Encourage caregivers to administer an iron supplement if the child is anemic because of blood loss during surgery.
- Explain that the diet should be well-balanced, especially with adequate protein, vitamin C, and calcium to promote healing.
- Discuss the potential for constipation caused by decreased motility and pain medication. Encourage increased fluid and fiber intake for prevention.
- Teach caregivers about appropriate medications for constipation, such as stool softeners.
- Make arrangements for child to contact someone who has undergone similar treatment for scoliosis as a support.
- Assist caregivers in obtaining home tutor until child returns to school, usually within 4–6 weeks after surgery.
- Provide appropriate school personnel (teachers, coaches, etc.) with instructions about activity restrictions, such as playing contact sports, diving in a pool, gymnastics, bicycle riding, ice skating, and horseback riding.
- Refer family to the National Scoliosis Foundation, for educational support materials and support groups.
- Provide referral to appropriate community agency for special equipment if needed such as a raised toilet seat, straight backed chair, and so forth.

KYPHOSIS

Kyphosis (humpback or round back deformity) is an excessive convex curvature at the thoracic level of the spine when viewed from the side. A certain degree of kyphosis (Figure 34-13B) is normal (20–45 degrees, Cobb's angle) but curvature greater than 45 degrees is generally considered excessive. Scheuermann kyphosis is defined as a structural deformity that presents in late childhood associated with thoracic wedged vertebral bodies (Fardon, 2002).

Incidence and Etiology

The reported incidence varies from 0.5% to 8%, and its male-female-ratio ranges from 1:2 to 7:1, while some suggest the male-female-ratio at 1:1 (Damborg, Engell, & Anderson, 2006; McIntosh & Sucato, 2007). The condition has its onset during the prepubertal growth spurt at around 10 to 12 years of age (McIntosh & Sucato, 2007). The etiology remains unknown, with various factors postulated. A genetic factor, specifically a dominant autosomal inheritance, has been suggested. Kyphosis may be congenital, postural, or secondary to other diseases. Congenital kyphosis is the result of a failure of formation or segmentation of the vertebral structures in utero. Postural kyphosis tends to occur in preadolescent years, especially among girls who are self-conscious about breast development and increasing height. Kyphosis may be associated with diseases or disorders, such as cerebral palsy, tuberculosis, spinal muscle atrophy, muscular dystrophy, and metabolic disorders. Radiation and tumor removal from the spinal cord are other conditions that may cause kyphosis.

Pathophysiology

With congenital kyphosis one side of the vertebrae either incompletely develops or fails to grow, resulting in narrowing of the vertebrae and the disks. The affected vertebrae rotate and cause physical changes in the spine. Spinal curvature occurs in postural kyphosis; however, there are no changes in the vertebrae. Kyphosis secondary to neuromuscular disorders results from an imbalance of the pull of muscles on either side of the spine.

Clinical Manifestations

Children with kyphosis have a hunchback or rounded appearance to their spine. Lumbar lordosis usually develops as a compensatory curve in children with postural kyphosis. Some children complain of mild pain in the back or shoulders. The pain is progressive low back pain which may keep them from play and sports activities. They may also complain of radiating pain into the buttocks and lower extremities. Some report that pain awakens them from sleep (McIntosh & Sucato, 2007).

CASE STUDY / CARE PLAN

THE CHILD UNDERGOING SURGERY FOR SCOLIOSIS

Clara, 14 years of age, has been followed for 3 years in the scoliosis clinic. Her spinal curve has progressed significantly over the past year. She has worn a Milwaukee brace for 1 year. Her older sister also had scoliosis and wore the same brace during her adolescence. Asymmetry of the shoulder, scapular prominence, and increase in pain are present. Radiographs, including anterior, posterior, and lateral, indicate a spinal curve of 50 degrees. Clara has no other health-related problems. Spinal fusion with Cotrel-Dubousset instrumentation is planned. Both an anterior and posterior approach will be used. Removal of the lower ribs is planned to allow better respiratory function. Rib bone will be used for autogenous graft for the spinal fusion.

NURSING CARE PLAN

ASSESSMENT

Preoperatively, the nurse should assess the child's and family's understanding of the diagnosis of scoliosis and ask about what treatments, if any, have been used in the past. It is also important to determine their understanding of the treatment plan, specifically bracing, which must be explained so they know the anticipated results. Education is essential to promote compliance with bracing. If noncompliance is detected early, other approaches to treatment can be considered before spinal curvature has time to worsen. The nurse must also assess the child's concerns about body image. Before surgery, an assessment of the child's and family's understanding of the surgical procedure and postoperative care is performed. Significant information to obtain includes plans to continue schoolwork and expectations for the recovery period at home. Postoperatively, it is important for the nurse to monitor for complications such as respiratory alterations, altered neurovascular status, hemorrhage, fluid imbalances, altered cardiac status, pain, and paralytic ileus.

PREOPERATIVE

NURSING DIAGNOSIS 1

Risk for impaired skin integrity related to bracing and other corrective therapies.

EXPECTED OUTCOMES

1. Clara will not experience skin irritation or breakdown.
2. Clara's brace will fit appropriately without skin irritation.

NOC: Tissue Integrity: Skin

NIC: Pressure Ulcer Prevention

INTERVENTIONS/*RATIONALES*

1. Gradually increase orthosis wearing time as comfort allows. *Protects the skin from breakdown or irritation.*
2. Develop goals with Clara to achieve optimal orthosis wearing time. *The likelihood of compliance improves if the individual is allowed to participate in planning increased orthosis wearing time.*
3. Assess skin for breakdown or irritation. *Orthosis wearing time is uninterrupted if skin irritation or breakdown is avoided. Decreases the risk of infection, and comfort is maintained.*
4. Assess orthosis for proper fit. *An improperly fitting brace can result in skin breakdown and pressure sores.*

EVALUATION

Clara's brace is properly fitted, and she wears it as prescribed. Her skin remains intact with no evidence of redness, irritation, or breakdown.

(Continues)

CASE STUDY / CARE PLAN (Continued)

NURSING DIAGNOSIS 2

Disturbed body image related to postural deformity presence of brace, and scar after surgery.

EXPECTED OUTCOMES

1. Clara will verbalize feelings about how the disorder and treatments affect her body image and self-esteem.
2. Clara will demonstrate a positive self-image and involvement with activities and support groups.

NOC: Body Image
NIC: Active Listening; Body Image Enhancement

INTERVENTIONS/*RATIONALES*

1. Assess and encourage verbalization of feelings about bracing, surgery, casting, and other procedures related to spinal deformity. *Assessment of her feelings and perceptions provides information to use in planning care. Verbalization provides an outlet for possible anger and resentment about disorder and its treatment.*
2. Encourage participation in activities of daily living as limitations allow (e.g., hair washing, grooming, and dressing in own clothing). *Promotes a positive self-image.*
3. Provide contact with other adolescents who have undergone treatment for scoliosis. *Support from others who have experienced the same treatments is often therapeutic.*

EVALUATION

Clara's grooming demonstrates that she feels positive about herself. She is able to emphasize her strengths. She becomes involved with others who have scoliosis.

NURSING DIAGNOSIS 3

Deficient Knowledge regarding condition, treatment, brace care, and surgical procedure related to lack of prior experience.

EXPECTED OUTCOMES

1. Clara and her family will verbalize an understanding of scoliosis, treatment aims, and surgery.
2. Clara and her family will ask appropriate questions about postoperative care.

NOC: Knowledge, Disease Process
NIC: Teaching: Disease Process/Treatment

INTERVENTIONS/*RATIONALES*

1. Teach the adolescent and family about scoliosis, its nonsurgical and surgical treatment, anticipated outcomes of both types of treatment, and follow-up care. *Education and knowledge increase comfort level and compliance with treatment, and decrease fears.*
2. Explain preoperative tests and routines to Clara and family members. *Understanding of procedures and tests increases compliance and decreases anxiety.*
3. Encourage questions and provide honest answers. Adolescent and family may be hesitant to ask questions. *An honest approach establishes a trusting relationship with the nurse.*
4. Provide explanations and rationale for surgical procedure and postoperative care. *Information about upcoming surgery decreases anxiety, and an understanding of the reasons for postoperative routines may increase client cooperation.*

EVALUATION

Clara and her caregivers express an understanding of the disorder, treatment plan, preoperative and postoperative care, and comply with treatment plan.

(Continues)

CASE STUDY / CARE PLAN (Continued)

POSTOPERATIVE

NURSING DIAGNOSIS 1

Ineffective breathing pattern related to bedrest, anesthesia, and immobility.

EXPECTED OUTCOME

Clara will maintain effective breathing pattern and avoid pulmonary complications (pneumonia, atelectasis).
NOC: Respiratory Status: Airway Patency
NIC: Respiratory Monitoring

INTERVENTIONS/*RATIONALES*

1. Reposition Clara every two hours. *Frequent position changes prevent pooling of secretions.*
2. Administer oxygen as needed. *Increases peripheral oxygen saturation.*
3. Provide respiratory care: coughing, deep breathing, and use of incentive spirometer every two hours for first 24 hours, then every four hours until ambulatory. *Promotes adequate pulmonary hygiene. Spirometry increases lung expansion and aeration of alveoli and prevents pooling of secretions and atelectasis.*
4. Monitor intake and output. Provide approximately 2,000–3,000 mL of fluid per 24 hours. *Ensures adequate hydration of the client, which helps to loosen lung secretions.*

EVALUATION

Clara achieves adequate ventilation and remains free of respiratory distress or infections. Lung sounds are clear bilaterally with no adventitious sounds.

NURSING DIAGNOSIS 2

Acute pain related to surgery, incision, donor site, and muscle stretching.

EXPECTED OUTCOME

Clara will demonstrate diminished pain.
NOC: Comfort Level
NIC: Pain Management

INTERVENTIONS/*RATIONALES*

1. Assess physiological, behavioral, and verbal indicators of pain. *Physiological manifestations and behavior provide clues to pain experience. Children and adolescents may be unwilling to express pain and to request medication because of fear of an injection.*
2. Use a pain assessment scale appropriate for developmental level to determine severity of pain. *A pain scale provides objective data about pain.*
3. Administer prescribed analgesics by patient-controlled analgesia (PCA), epidural, or intermittent IV "around the clock." *Optimal pain management allows client to be more cooperative with postoperative respiratory regimen and promotes faster healing and recovery. Postoperative pain is intense for 72 hours after a spinal fusion.*
4. Encourage use of nonpharmacological methods to manage pain such as therapeutic touch, music, relaxation, and guided imagery. *These techniques can be an effective adjunct to medication.*

EVALUATION

Clara experiences effective pain relief early in the postoperative period. She has no verbal complaints of pain and participates in conversations and diversional activities.

(Continues)

CASE STUDY / CARE PLAN (Continued)

NURSING DIAGNOSIS 3

Impaired physical mobility related to postsurgical restrictions.

EXPECTED OUTCOME

Clara will progress with physical activity as prescribed.
NOC: Ambulation
NIC: Exercise Therapy: Ambulation

INTERVENTIONS/*RATIONALES*

1. Reposition the child every two hours using the logrolling technique. Support the head and legs by using pillows. *Promotes circulation, increases comfort, and prevents skin breakdown. Proper positioning prevents injury to the spine.*
2. Perform passive and active range of motion exercises. *Exercises help maintain circulation, muscle tone, and strength, and prevent muscle atrophy.*
3. Dangle on the side of the bed when allowed per health care provider's order and gradually progress to unassisted ambulation. *Early mobilization decreases risk of thrombophlebitis and pulmonary emboli.*
4. Assist client with a return to normal activities and self-care as ordered and as client's condition allows. *Maintains circulation, muscle tone, and strength.*

EVALUATION

Clara resumes full ambulation without adverse complications.

NURSING DIAGNOSIS 4

Risk for injury related to altered neurovascular status secondary to circulatory or nerve damage during surgical instrumentation.

EXPECTED OUTCOME

Clara will not experience neurovascular injury as evident by intact sensation or motion of extremities, voluntary control over voiding and bowel evacuation, warm extremities, and capillary refill, 3 sec.
NOC: Immobility Consequences: Physiological
NIC: Circulatory Precautions

INTERVENTIONS/*RATIONALES*

1. Assess circulatory and nerve status of all extremities every two hours for the first 24 hours, then every four hours for the next 48 hours. *Altered neurovascular status, paralysis, and thrombus formation are complications of surgery for scoliosis secondary to injury and compression of the spine.*
2. Monitor intake and output and assess for bladder distention or bowel incontinence. *Loss of bowel and bladder control may indicate spinal cord injury.*
3. Maintain flat position if prescribed. Logroll every two hours. *Maintaining proper alignment prevents injury to the spine. Logrolling is necessary to prevent nerve damage.*

EVALUATION

Clara is free of neurovascular impairment and has full range of motion and sensation in lower extremities.

Diagnosis

The diagnosis is made by visualizing the spine and scapular area from the side with the child bending 90 degrees at the waist. A comprehensive orthopedic and neurologic evaluation may be performed to determine if the kyphosis is associated with other diseases or conditions.

Treatment

Treatment for kyphosis is dependent upon the severity of the deformity, as well as the amount of pain the child is having. Any curvature over 50 degrees is considered abnormal. If the curvature is not severe and the child experiences no pain, the treatment is conservative. An exercise regimen is developed, and the child is placed on anti-inflammatory agents. If the child is still growing, then a brace may be worn until the child reaches skeletal maturity (see Figure 34-18). If the curvature is greater than 75 degrees, surgery to straighten the spine with fusion of some segments may be required. Nursing management is similar to that discussed in the section on scoliosis.

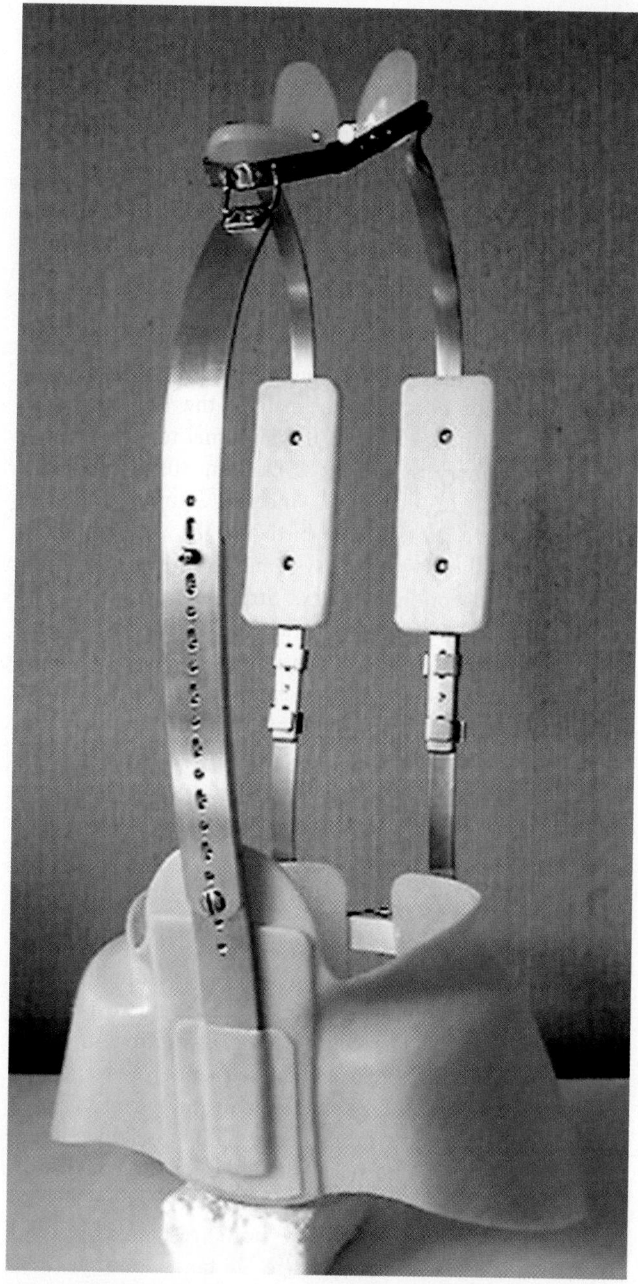

Figure 34-18 This brace is used in the treatment of kyphosis. COURTESY OF BERTIL HOLMBERG, MD, MALMOE, SWEDEN.

LORDOSIS

Lordosis is an excessive concave curvature of the lumbar spine. In the normal spine a mild concave curve exists in the lumbar region. Lordosis is an exaggeration of that normal curve.

Incidence and Etiology

Lordosis is a normal finding in toddlers that should disappear as the child grows in height, usually by school-age. It is often observed in adolescents, especially girls, during the growth spurt. However, in other children it may be associated with conditions such as obesity, flexion contractures of the hip, developmental dysplasia of the hip, and slipped femoral capital epiphysis.

Pathophysiology

With lordosis the muscles of the spine are unable to support an erect position. This results in straining of the ligaments, which causes lower back pain and fatigue.

Clinical Manifestations

The child with lordosis presents with a swayback and may exhibit a protruding chest and abdomen. Other clinical manifestations include complaints of lower back pain, hip pain, and fatigue.

Diagnosis

Lumbar lordosis is diagnosed by visualization of the spine and radiographs.

Treatment

One aspect of treatment is managing or correcting the associated etiological factor. Postural exercises are the usual form of treatment once the associated condition has been dealt with. Bracing and surgery are rarely needed. Nursing management is similar to that discussed in the section on scoliosis.

LEGG-CALVE-PERTHES DISEASE

Legg-Calve-Perthes (LCP) disease, is characterized by avascular necrosis of the femoral head with collapse and subsequent regeneration. It is a self-limiting disease. Most commonly, the disease called Legg-Perthes disease, LCPD, or Perthes is considered a vascular disease.

Incidence and Etiology

LCPD occurs between the ages of 2 and 12 years, most frequently from 4 to 8 years of age. The incidence is approximately 1 in 1,200, and males are 3 to 5 times more likely than females to be affected. Almost 5% of the diagnosed cases are bilateral (both hips). It is more common among first-born children and those with low birth weight. The cause is unknown, but it is known that bone death occurs in the ball of the hip due to an interruption in blood flow to the proximal femur (Bahmanyar, Montgomery, Rudiger, & Ekbom, 2008). Risk factors linked to LCPD include impaired and disproportionate growth, low birth weight, delayed skeletal maturity, short stature, systemic hormonal changes, and low socioeconomic index. Strangely, children who are extremely active are more at risk. According to the National Osteonecrosis Foundation, LCPD occurs more often in Asians, Eskimos, and whites, with a much lower incidence in Australian aboriginals, Native Americans, Polynesians, and African Americans. Exposure to secondhand smoke is correlated to LCPD, and recent studies are finding LCPD correlates with maternal smoking while pregnant (Aycicek & Ipek, 2008).

Pathophysiology

LCPD is due to an interruption of blood supply to the femoral capital epiphysis, leading to aseptic necrosis of the head of the femur. The cause of the disruption in blood supply is unknown, but a certain sequence of events occurs (Figure 34-19). LCPD has four distinctive stages: (1) femoral head becomes more dense with possible fracture of the supporting bone; (2) fragmentation and reabsorption of bone; (3) reossification when new bone has regrown; (4) healing, when new bone reshapes. Stage 1 takes two to six months, stage 2 takes one year or more, while stages 3 and 4 go on for many years. Without treatment the child will have changes in the epiphyseal growth plate and later in life is prone to osteoarthritis of the hip.

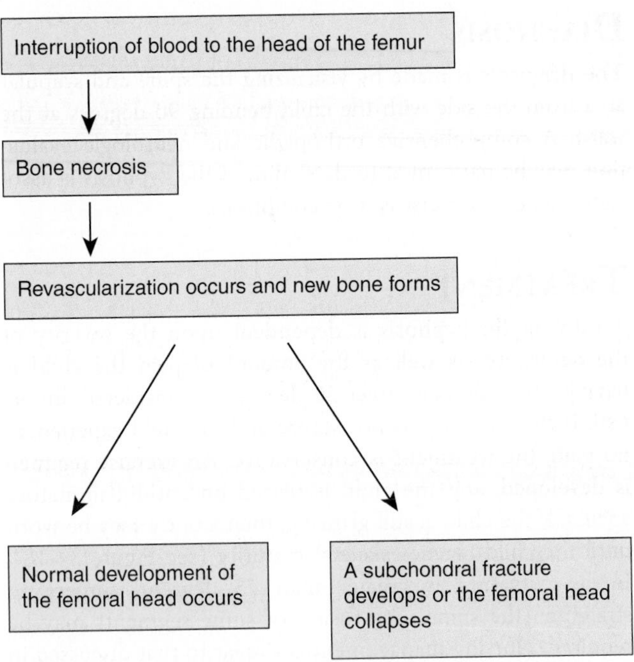

Figure 34-19 Pathophysiology of Legg-Calve-Perthes Disease. DELMAR CENGAGE LEARNING.

Clinical Manifestations

The onset of LCPD is insidious with a prolonged course of symptoms. Pain, present in the hip or only in the knee or groin (referred pain), may be worse with activity and relieved with rest. In some children a limp is present with or without pain. They cannot offer an explanation of how they might have hurt themselves. The child presents with an abnormal gait and limitations of hip range of motion, especially abduction and internal rotation. Inspection of the affected leg may show atrophy of the thigh muscles.

Diagnosis

LCPD is diagnosed and classified with use of radiograph. Occasionally a bone scan may be used to differentiate LCPD from toxic synovitis of the hip, septic arthritis, or osteomyelitis.

Treatment

Permanent deformity of the bone may also occur without treatment. The goals of treatment are to keep the femoral head in the acetabulum and as round as possible and to prevent deformity during the healing process with traction, casting, brace wearing, or surgery. Bed rest and the use of abduction traction will reduce pain and improve range of motion. A non-weight-bearing brace device, crutches, or harness may be used. Performing non-weight-bearing exercises prevents atrophy of the extremity during this time. Another approach is to allow weight bearing as long as the femoral head remains in the acetabulum; therefore, treatment may consist of a long leg cast with an abduction bar. Surgery is necessary in some cases to maintain the femoral head within the acetabulum.

Nursing Management

To prevent injury and complications it is necessary to assess and plan interventions to maintain neurovascular integrity. Ongoing assessment of the neurovascular system is important during therapy with traction or surgery throughout the course of treatment. Meticulous skin care is important to reduce friction between the skin and traction equipment, cast, or brace. Teaching the child to crutch walk during hospitalization reduces the risk of falls after discharge as does instructing caregivers to make the home environment safe. Rearranging furniture and removing loose rugs promote safe space for ambulating with either a brace or crutches.

Deficient knowledge related to home care is addressed early in the course of treatment. The child is usually in the hospital during the initial stages of treatment. During this time the nurse is able to work with the child and family to increase their understanding of the rationale for treatment and the correct use of the equipment. Other teaching includes the assessment of the skin and neurovascular status, signs of muscular atrophy, appropriate activities of daily living, and safety measures to be initiated in the home or school.

Family Teaching

Family teaching includes assessment skills of the skin and neurovascular system. The emphasis on safety and promoting a positive self-image of the child are two issues that involve ongoing recognition and support from the hospital and follow-up by the clinic staff. The child, between the ages of 4 and 8, is likely to associate disease and its accompanying restrictions with punishment; therefore, raising the caregivers' awareness of this developmental issue is critical. They are then better able to provide positive reinforcement for the child. It may be necessary to work with school personnel about adaptations to accommodate the child's limitations, such as safe hallways or an elevator for going up and down stairs.

ADDITIONAL MUSCULOSKELETAL DISORDERS

The following disorders are rare in children; therefore, they are discussed only briefly.

OSTEOGENESIS IMPERFECTA

Osteogenesis imperfecta (OI), known as brittle bone disease, is a heritable autosomal dominant disorder of collagen synthesis resulting in weak bones that are easily fractured and are often deformed (Tainmont, 2007). The disturbance in the synthesis of type 1 collagen results in osteoporosis, and can also involve the teeth, the sclerae (the tough outer layer of the eyeball), ligaments, blood vessels and the skin. Sillence described four types in 1979 (Sillence, Senn, & Danks, 1979). Type I is the dominantly inherited form with blue sclerae; Type II is the perinatal, lethal form; Type III is the progressively deforming kind with normal sclerae; and, Type IV is the dominantly inherited form with normal sclerae. Osteogenesis imperfecta has no predilection for race or gender. Type I is the most common, occurring approximately 1 in 28,500 live births. Type II is notable for its lethality and occurs 1 in 62,500 live births (Tainmont, 2007).

Clinical Manifestations

The major clinical manifestation is severe bone fragility with multiple fractures caused by poor collagen formation, often mistaken for child abuse (Jenny, 2006). Some children's bones are so fragile that fractures result not only from trauma, but also from normal activities of life such as walking. Other manifestations include associated deafness, dental deformities, blue sclera, hyperlaxity of ligaments, and short stature. The child may develop kyphosis or scoliosis if the vertebral bones are involved. Multiple fractures throughout childhood tend to cause limb and spinal column deformities that interfere with growth and bone alignment. Usually there is little pain at the site of the fracture; however, the older child may report tenderness. Soft-tissue damage may be minimal secondary to bone fragility. The child bruises easily and there is a tendency for frequent epistaxis. Dentition may be immature, and the teeth may break easily.

Treatment

Intervention is aimed at improving bone mass. Among the options, biophosphonates are used to decrease bone resorption and to increase bone formation. Intravenous pamidronate is effective in promoting bone growth and relieving chronic pain when given cyclically (every 4 to 6 months) (el-Sobky, Hanna, Basha, Tarraf, & Said, 2006). Treatment consists of early intervention of fractures and prevention of deformities using splints, braces, casts, and surgery. Insertion of rods into the long bones may prevent future fractures. Healing usually requires long periods of time to promote remineralization of the bones. Adequate nutrition with supplements of calcium, magnesium, and vitamins are used to strengthen the bony structure. A supportive, nonjudgmental approach is important for these families. Education of caregivers should include information about promoting normal development within the child's limitations and methods to protect the individual from injury.

SLIPPED CAPITAL FEMORAL EPIPHYSIS

Slipped capital femoral epiphysis (SCFE) is a misnomer. SCFE is actually the femoral neck metaphysis that displaces in relationship to the capital femoral epiphysis. However, SCFE is retained as the name for the disorder. SCFE is the most common adolescent acquired hip disorder. SCFE involves the displacement of the femoral head from the femoral neck occurring through an open femoral capital physis (growth plate). The femoral head remains seated in the acetabulum and the femoral neck moves upward and outward.

Incidence

SCFE affects 2 to 10 adolescents per 100,000 in the United States (Hart, Grottkau, & Albright, 2007). It usually occurs in early adolescence during rapid growth spurts, peaking at age 10 to 13 in females and 12 to 16 in males. The male-to-female ratio is 2 to 3:1. The incidence of SCFE among black children is almost 4 times greater than among white children, 2.5 times greater among Hispanics as compared to white children, and disproportionally affects Pacific Islanders (Gholve, Cameron, & Millis, 2009).

While the etiology of SCFE is unknown, most orthopedic surgeons agree it is multifactorial, likely a combination of biochemical and biomechanical factors. An endocrine basis has been suggested because it is frequently accompanied by growth disturbances. The weakening effect of elevated testosterone on the physis among boys likely explains why it is more commonly seen in boys (elevated estrogen may actually shield females) (Gholve et al., 2009). Obesity is a prominent factor with 81% of adolescents with SCFE reporting a body mass index (BMI) above the 95th percentile (Hart, Grottkau, & Albright, 2007). Increased BMI increases the shear stress across the physis causing weakness and slippage (Gholve et al., 2009). When slippage occurs, it is considered stable or unstable. Stable SCFE is preponderant with 80–90% of all cases diagnosed. Unfortunately, SCFE may effect both hips, some studies citing 25–40% bilateral involvement, but usually not at the same time (Hart, Grottkau, & Albright, 2007).

Clinical Manifestations

SCFE is the most common orthopedic hip condition affecting adolescents, but diagnosis is frequently delayed or missed due to the subtlety of signs and symptoms. The stable SCFE patient is able to bear weight on the affected limb, while unable to bear weight on an unstable SCFE. All patients with SCFE present with pain in the affected hip, the groin, thigh, or knee. It is critical to be aware of two keys to SCFE: (1) groin pulls are very rare in adolescents, and require the practitioner to rule out SCFE; (2) hip pain is often referred to the knee due to sensory distribution of the obturator and femoral nerves. Patients may vaguely recall an antecedent event or injury. Parents may report change in gait or limping. These symptoms for stable SCFE are subtle, often mild, but the out-toeing gait is very common, and limitation of hip internal rotation is nearly universal (Gholve et al., 2009).

Stable SCFE deteriorates and worsens without treatment. A patient with unstable SCFE will present much differently. These children will recall or report groin, thigh or medial knee pain. However, they will report a sudden exacerbation after a sports-related injury or a minor fall. These children will not be able to bear weight on the affected limb, with or without crutches (Hart, Grottkau, & Albright, 2007).

It is important to note that SCFE can occur in younger children, usually thin, and without classic risk factors. These individuals will almost always have bilateral SCFE, and must be evaluated for endocrine abnormalities (hypothyroidis, panhypopituitarism, and renal osteodystrophy (Hart, Grottkau, & Albright, 2007).

Diagnosis

The diagnosis of SCFE utilizes symptoms, physical examination and standard radiographic studies. The most important physical finding upon examination is in the hip range of motion. Limited internal rotation is universal with SCFE. Plain radiographs are sufficient for diagnosis, and given the likelihood of bilateral involvement, both hips should be visualized on X-ray (Gholve et al., 2009).

Treatment

The goal of treatment is to prevent further slippage and complications and involves surgery. For mild to moderate SCFE the surgical procedure is percutaneous placement of pins across the growth plate into the femoral head to hold the head in place until closure of the femoral physis is attained. A small incision is made, and the child is able to ambulate with crutches shortly after surgery. Open correction (**osteotomy**) may be performed for chronic cases of SCFE or severe degrees of displacement. In this procedure the bone is redesigned surgically to alter the alignment or weight-bearing stress areas. Since there is an increased likelihood of SCFE to occur in the opposite hip, nurses should make sure the child and family are aware of symptoms such as pain or decrease in range of motion.

IN THE REAL WORLD

I began working with a boy born with clubfeet. The degree of severity was significant. Over the years this child has endured countless casts and surgeries. He has spent many days in a wheelchair and had to ride the special bus to school, not easy things when one is growing up. At 13, he has visible scars on his feet and ankles, heels that need to be aligned, and abnormally thin calves. In some people these issues would be devastating. However, this child is a bright, energetic, wonderful young man. I credit his parents for his positive adjustment to the clubfeet. They never held him back from doing anything, promoted his self-esteem, and allowed him to voice his feelings. I am buoyed by the physical and mental outcome of this young man. When I asked him how he is doing, he replied, "I am great! Happy to be walking around on my own two feet." I often think of this statement as I work with families in similar situations. It encourages me to really emphasize the client-teaching part of my job. I know that my teachings can have a positive effect.

KEY CONCEPTS

- The differences in the musculoskeletal system of children as compared to adults includes the child having a large amount of cartilage, the periosteum being stronger and tougher, and the growth plates being not yet closed.
- A significant number of school-age children and adolescents experience musculoskeletal injuries related to sports and recreation, which account for substantial morbidity and cost.
- Most sports injuries in older children and adolescents affect the soft tissues rather than the bones. Examples of soft-tissue injuries include sprains, strains, and muscle contusions.
- Types of fractures include transverse, oblique, spiral, greenstick, and buckle.
- Splints, braces, slings, casts, external fixation, internal fixation are common current fracture treatment modalities, whereas casting is less common.
- Injury to the epiphyseal growth plates is very serious in skeletally immature children because they can cause growth disruption, arrest, or uneven growth.
- Many musculoskeletal injuries and treatment methods can result in neurovascular compromise. Therefore, continuous assessment of neurovascular status is a key nursing responsibility.
- Oral antibiotic treatment for osteomyelitis and septic arthritis is effective only if the caregivers are compliant with the treatment protocol.
- Clubfoot is treated with serial casting. Surgery is necessary if casting is not effective.
- Treatment for developmental dysplasia of the hip includes an external abduction device such as a Pavlik harness, which maintains the head of the femur in the acetabulum.
- Instructing caregivers in the general care, skin care, and handling and positioning methods for the infant in a Pavlik harness ensures infant safety and the benefits of maintaining the hips in flexion and abduction.
- Duchenne muscular dystrophy is the most common type of muscular dystrophy in childhood. It is rapidly progressive, resulting in loss of the ability to walk between 9 and 12 years of age and death by the early 20s.
- Scoliosis is treated with bracing or surgery, that is, spinal fusion with instrumentation.
- Legg-Calve-Perthes disease is characterized by avascular necrosis of the femoral head. The goal of treatment is to keep the femoral head in the acetabulum during the healing process with traction, casting, bracing, or surgery.

REVIEW ACTIVITIES

1. Discuss the nurse's role in preventing sports injuries.
2. Describe the differences between a sprain and a strain.
3. Discuss the treatment for a sprain.
4. What would be included in teaching caregivers about cast care?
5. List the different types of traction and explain each.
6. What important principles will the nurse use when caring for the child in traction?
7. What should be included in the assessment of the neurovascular status of a child who is immobilized?
8. Discuss the clinical manifestations of osteomyelitis, septic arthritis, and transient synovitis, what they have in common, how they are not alike.
9. How would the nurse plan for caregiver involvement following surgery on the child with a clubfoot?
10. How would the nurse prepare the caregivers for the child going home in a Pavlik harness?
11. How would the nurse provide emotional support for the child with Duchenne muscular dystrophy and for the family?
12. What initial and ongoing assessments would the nurse make for an adolescent after spinal surgery?
13. Describe the treatment for the child with Legg-Calve-Perthes disease.
14. Why would the nurse advise parents of genetic testing if their child was born with osteogenesis imperfecta?

STUDY QUESTIONS

1. The nurse evaluates the musculoskeletal systems of children to be different from adults in which of the following ways?
   a. Tendons and ligaments are weaker in children until puberty
   b. Periosteum is not as strong in children
   c. Bones of children are less porous and dense than adult bones
   d. Skull bones are not rigid or fused at birth
2. The immature bones differ from adult bones:
   a. Because adult bones bend and do not break.
   b. Because the bones continue to grow and have open epiphyseal growth plates.
   c. Because immature bones have a weaker, less resilient periosteum.
   d. Because they repair less rapidly.
3. The nurse completes an orthopedic assessment of a 6-year-old child who has a new cast applied for a fractured radius. Which of the following clinical manifestations is a priority for the nurse to report immediately to the physician?
   a. Skin around the cast is warm
   b. The child states that hand feels "asleep"
   c. Edema in fingers that lessens with elevation
   d. Capillary refill of three seconds in affected hand
4. Fractures in the pediatric population:
   a. Are relatively rare.
   b. Among preadolescents occur primarily in the lower extremities.
   c. Are a frequent occurrence in about one half of all visits to any healthcare provider.
   d. Include a "buckle fracture" that does not occur in the adult population.
5. The nurse is caring for a child with a new full-leg cast. Which of the following is an appropriate nursing intervention for this client?
   a. Avoid changing the child's position for 24 hours after application of the cast.
   b. Handle the cast with the tips of the fingers.
   c. Avoid elevating the casted extremity until the cast is completely dry.
   d. Make sure that all cast edges are smooth and free of irritating projections.
6. What do osteomyelitis, septic arthritis, and transient synovitis have in common?
   a. A limping child is a significant presenting symptom.
   b. The child presents with a high fever.
   c. The site of pain is also located by redness of skin.
   d. These three maladies always involve the hip joint.
7. What is the primary difference between septic arthritis and transient synovitis?
   a. A needle aspiration of the hip will produce clear synovial fluid in both cases.
   b. Septic arthritis is never in the hip joint.
   c. Transient synovitis is always benign.
   d. Neither transient synovitis nor septic arthritis present with systemic symptoms.
8. The nurse caring for a child with muscular dystrophy observes the child using the Gower maneuver while trying to:
   a. Sit.
   b. Walk.
   c. Stand.
   d. Bend over.
9. With an upright adolescent girl with scoliosis, viewed from the posterior, the spine:
   a. Will be straight as an arrow.
   b. Will form a hump near the base of the neck.
   c. Will form an "s-like" curve.
   d. Will bend at the waist with her shoulders toward you.
10. The nurse should assess a child admitted with a diagnosis of slipped capital femoral epiphysis for which of the following additional health problems?
    a. Emaciated appearance
    b. Nutritional anemia
    c. Developmental delays
    d. Obesity

REFERENCES

Agran, P. E., Winn, D., Anderson, C., Trent, R., & Walton-Haynes, L. (2001). Rates of pediatric and adolescent injuries by year of age. *Pediatrics, 108*(3), 45–51.

Altizer, L. L. (2008). All-terrain vehicle safety: A long-standing issue. *Orthopedic Nursing, 27*(4), 243–245.

Anglen, J., & Choi, L. (2005). Treatment options in pediatric femoral shaft fractures. *Journal of Pediatric Orthopedics, 19*, 724–733.

Aycicek, A., & Ipek, A. (2008). Maternal active or passive smoking causes oxidative stress in cord blood. *European Journal of Pediatrics, 167*(1), 81–85.

Bach, J. R., Ishikawa, Y., & Heakyung, K. (1997). Prevention of pulmonary morbidity for patients with Duchenne muscular dystrophy. *Chest, 112,* 1024–1028.

Bahmanyar, S., Montgomery, S. M., Rudiger, J. W., & Ekbom, A. (2008). Maternal smoking during pregnancy, other prenatal and perinatal factors, and the risk of Legg-Calve-Perthes disease. *Pediatrics, 122,* e459–e464.

Balaban, B., Matthews, D. J., Clayton, G. H., & Carry, T. (2005). Corticosteroid treatment and functional improvement in Duchenne muscular dystrophy: Long-term effect. *American Journal of Physical Medicine and Rehabilitation, 84,* 843–850.

Beaty, J. H., & Kasser, J. R. (Eds.). (2010). *Rockwood & Wilkins' fractures in children.* (7th ed.) Philadelphia: Lippincott, pp. 3–17.

Brenner, J. S., and the Council on Sports Medicine. (2007). Overuse injuries, overtraining, and burnout in child and adolescent athletes. *Pediatrics, 119,* 1242–1245.

Bunnell, W. (2005). Selective screening for scoliosis. *Clinical Orthopedics and Related Research, 434,* 40–45.

Butbul-Aviel, Y., Koren, A., Halevy, R., & Sakran, W. (2005). Procalcitonin as a diagnostic aid in osteomyelitis and septic arthritis. *Pediatric Emergency Care, 21*(12), 828–832.

Caird, M. S., Flynn, J. M., Leung, Y. L., Millman, J. E., D'Italia, J. G., & Dormans, J. P. (2006). Factors distinguishing septic arthritis from transient synovitis of the hip in children: A prospective study. *Journal of Bone and Joint Surgery (Am.), 88*(6), 1251–1257.

Daftary, A. S., Crisanti, M., Kalra, M., Wong, B., & Amin, R. (2007). Effect of long-term steroids on cough efficiency and respiratory muscle strength in patients with Duchenne muscular dystrophy. *Pediatrics, 119,* e320–e324.

Damborg, F., Engell, V., & Anderson, M. (2006). Prevalence, concordance, and heritability of Scheuermann kyphosis based on a study of twins. *Journal of Bone and Joint Surgery (Am.), 88*(10), 2133–2136.

El-Sayed, M. H., Correll, J., & Pholig, J. (2008). New promising brace for clubfoot management a new unilateral dynamic custom-made brace used after Ponseti manipulation for idopathic congenital talipes equinovarus deformity. *Journal of Orthopaedics, 5*(3), e10.

el-Sobky, M. A., Hanna, A. A., Basha, N. E., Tarraf, Y. N., & Said, M. H. (2006). Surgery versus surgery plus pamidronate in the management of osteogenesis imperfecta patients: A comparative study. *Journal of Pediatric Orthopedics B, 15*(3), 222–228.

Estes, M. E. Z. (2010). *Health assessment & physical examination* (4th ed.). Delmar Cengage Learning.

Fardon, D. F. (2002). *North American Spinal Society. Orthopaedic Knowledge Update. Spine 2.* (2nd ed.). Rosemont, IL: American Academy of Orthopaedic Surgeons.

Fischer, S. U., & Beattie, T. F. (1999). The limping child: Epidemiology, assessment and outcome. *Journal of Bone and Joint Surgery (Br.), 81*(6), 1029–1034.

Frick, S. L. (2006). Evaluation of the child who has hip pain. *Orthopedic Clinics of North America, 37*(2), 133–140.

Gelfer, P., & Kennedy, K. A. (2008). Developmental dysplasia of the hip. *Journal of Pediatric Health Care, 22*(5), 318–322.

Gholve, P. A., Cameron, D. B., & Millis, M. B. (2009). Slipped capital femoral epiphysis update. *Current Opinion in Pediatrics, 21*(1), 39–45.

Girschick, H. J., Raab, P., Surbaum, S., Trusen, A., Kirschner, S., Schneider, P., Papadopoulos, T., Muller-Hermelink, H. K., & Lipsky, P. E. (2005). Chronic non-bacterial osteomyelitis in children. *Annals of the Rheumatic Diseases, 64,* 279–285.

Grottkau, B. (2005) Compartment syndrome in children and adolescents. *Journal of Pediatric Surgery, 40*(4), 678–682.

Hart, E. S., Albright, M. B., Rebello, G. N., & Grottkau, B. E. (2006). Broken bones: Common pediatric fractures—Part I. *Orthopaedic Nursing, 25*(4), 251–256.

Hart, E. S., Grottkau, B. E, Rebello, G. N., & Albright, M. B. (2006). Broken bones: Common pediatric upper extremity fractures—Part II. *Orthopaedic Nursing, 25*(5), 311–323.

Hart, E. S., Luther, B., & Grottkau, B. E. (2006). Broken bones: Common pediatric lower extremity fractures—Part III. *Orthopaedic Nursing, 25*(6), 390–407.

Hart, E. S., Grottkau, B. E., & Albright, M. B. (2007). Slipped capital femoral epiphysis: Don't miss this pediatric hip disorder. *The Nurse Practitioner, 32*(3), 14–21.

Hedin, H., Borgquist, L., & Larsson, S. (2004). A cost analysis of three methods of treating femoral shaft fractures in children: A comparison of traction in hospital, traction in hospital/home, and external fixation. *Acta Orthopaedica Scandinavica, 75*(3), 241–248.

Honein, M. A., Lindstrom, J. A., & Sweder, S. L. (2007). Can we assure the safe use of human teratogens? The iPLEDGE test case. *Drug Safety, 30,* 5–15.

Inoue, M., Nakata, Y., Minami, S., Kitahara, H., Otsuku, Y., & Isobe, K. (2003). Idiopathic scoliosis as a presenting sign of familial neurologic abnormalities. *Spine, 28*(1), 40–45.

Jenny, C. (2006). Committee on Child Abuse and Neglect. Evaluating infants and young children with multiple fractures. *Pediatrics, 118*(3), 1299–1303.

Judge, N. L. (2007). Assessing and managing patients with musculoskeletal conditions. *Nursing Standard, 22*(1), 51–57.

Karol, L., Johnston, C., Browne, R., & Madison, M. (1993). Progression of the curve in boys who have idiopathic scoliosis. *The Journal of Bone & Joint Surgery, 75A*(12), 1804–1810.

Kiang, K. M., Ogunmodede, F., Juni, B. A., Boxrud, D. J., & Glennen, A. (2005). Outbreak of osteomyelitis/septic arthritis caused by kingella kingae among child care center attendees. *Pediatrics, 116,* 206–213.

Knight, C., Matthew, A., & Muir, J. (2005). The locomotor system. In J. Kneale & P. Kneale Davis (Eds.). *Orthopaedic and Trauma Nursing* (2nd ed.). Edinburgh: Churchill Livingstone. pp. 47–75.

Knox, C. L., Comstock, D., McGeehan, J., & Smith, G. A. (2006). Differences in risk associated with head injury for pediatric ice skaters, roller skaters, and in-line skaters. *Pediatrics, 118,* 549–554.

Kubiak, E. N., Egol, K. A., Scher, D., Wassermann, B., Feldman, D., & Koval, K. (2005). Operative treatment of tibial fractures in children: Are elastic stable intramedullary nails and improvement over external fixation? *Journal of Bone and Joint Surgery, 87,* 1761–1768.

LaMontaigne, L., Hepworth, J., Cohen, F., & Salisbury, M. (2004). Adolescent scoliosis: Effects of corrective surgery, cognitive-behavioral interventions, and age on activity outcomes. *Applied Nursing Research, 17*(3), 168–177.

Lawson, B. R., Comstock, D., & Smith, G. A. (2009). Baseball-related injuries to children treated in hospital emergency departments in the United States, 1994–2006. *Pediatrics, 123*(6), 1028–1034.

McIntosh, A. L., & Sucato, D. J. (2007). Scheuermann's kyphosis. *Current Opinion in Orthopedics, 18,* 536–543.

Morcuende, J. A., Dolan, L. A., Dietz, F. R., & Ponseti, I. V. (2004). Radical reduction in the rate of extensive corrective surgery for clubfoot using the Ponseti method. *Pediatrics, 113,* 376–380.

Napierkowski, D. B. (2007). Scoliosis: A case study in an adolescent boy. *Orthopaedic Nursing, 26*(3), 147–154.

Nichol, D. (1995). Understanding the principles of traction. *Nursing Standard, 9*(46), 25–28.

Oxborrow, N. J. (2000). Assessing the child with scoliosis: The role of surface topography. *Archives of the Diseased Child, 83,* 453–455.

Patel, H. (2001). Canadian Task Force on Preventive Health Care, Update: Screening and management of developmental dysplasia of the hip in the newborn. *Canadian Medical Association Journal, 164,* 1669–1677.

Patel, N. K., Jeer, P. J. S., & Cornell, M. S. (2007). Using "cling film" to protect lower limb plaster casts in babies with clubfoot. *British Journal of Nursing, 16*(18), 1140–1142.

Phillips, W. needs year Developmental dysplasia of the hip. *UpToDate.* Retrieved January 10, 2008, from www.utdol.com.

Pineda, C., Vargas, A., & Rodriguez, A. V. (2006). Imaging of osteomyelitis: Current concepts. *Infectious Disease Clinics of North America, 20,* 789–825.

Ponseti, I. V. (1996). *Congenital clubfoot: Fundamentals of treatment.* New York: Oxford University Press.

Reeder, B. M., Lyne, E. D., Patel, D. R., & Cucos, D. R. (2004). Referral patterns to a pediatric orthopedic clinic: Implications for education and practice. *Pediatrics, 113*e: 163–167.

Rewers, A., Hedegaard, H., Lezotte, D., Meng, K., Battan, K., & Emery, K. (2005). Childhood femur fractures, associated injuries, and sociodemographic risk factors: A population-based study. *Pediatrics,* 5(115), 543–553.

Romitti, P. A. (2007). Utility of family history reports of major defects as a public health strategy. *Pediatrics, 120(Supplement)*: S71–S77.

Salter, R. B., & Harris, W. R. (1963). Injuries involving the epiphyseal plate. *The Journal of Bone & Joint Surgery,* 45-A(3), 587–622.

Sawyer, J. R., & Kapoor, M. (2009) The limping child: A systematic approach to diagnosis. *American Family Physician, 79*(3), 215–224.

Setter, K. J., & Palomino, K. E. (2006). Pediatric tibia fractures: Current concepts. *Current Opinion in Pediatrics, 18*(1), 30–35.

Shields, B. J., & Smith, G. A. (2006). Cheerleading-related injuries to children 5 to 18 years of age, United States, 1990–2002. *Pediatrics, 117,* 122–129.

Shipman, S., Helfand, M., Moyer, V. A., & Yawn, B. P. (2006). Screening for developmental dysplasia of the hip: A systemic literature review for the U.S. Preventive Services Task Force. *Pediatrics, 117*(3), e557–e576.

Sillence, D. O., Senn, A., & Danks, D. M. (1979). Genetic heterogeneity in osteogenesis imperfecta. *Journal of Medical Genetics, 16*(2), 101–116.

Singh, S., Smith, G. A., Fields, S. K., & McKenzie, L. B. (2008). Gymnastics-related injuries to children treated in emergency departments in the United States, 1990–2005. *Pediatrics, 121,* 954–960.

Skelly, A. C., Holt, V. L., Mosca, V. S., & Alderman, B. W. (2002). Talipes equinovarus and maternal smoking: A population-based study in Washington State. *Teratology,* 66: 91–100.

Tainmont, J. (2007). History of osteogenesis imperfecta or brittle bone disease: A few stops on a road 3000 years long. *B-ENT.,* 3 (3), 157–173.

Templeton, P. A., Flowers, M. J., Latz, K. H., Stephens, D., Williams, G. C., & Wright, J. G. (2006). Factors predicting the outcome of primary clubfoot surgery. *Canadian Journal of Surgery, 49*(2), 123–126.

Vioreanu, M., Sheehan, E., Glynn, A., Casidy, N., Stephens, M., & McCormack, D. (2007). Heelys and street gliders injuries: A new type of pediatric injury. *Pediatrics, 119,* 1294–1298.

Waltzman, M. L., Shannon, M., Bowen, A. P., & Bailey, M. C. (1999). *Pediatrics, 103,* e58.

Weinstock, J., Maron, B. J., Song, C., Mane, P. P., Estes, M., III, & Link, M. (2006). Failure of commercially available chest wall protectors to prevent sudden cardiac death induced by chest wall blows in an experimental model of commotio cordis. *Pediatrics, 117,* 656–662.

Wright, E. (2009). Neurovascular impairment and compartment syndrome. *Paediatric Nursing, 21*(3), 26–29.

Wright, J., Wang, E., Owen, J., Stephens, D., Hanlon, N., Nattrass, G., & Reynolds, R. (2005). Treatment for paediatric femoral fractures: A randomized trial. *Lancet, 365,* 1153–1159.

Yang, J., Peek-Asa, C., Allareddy, V., Phillips, G., Zhang, Y., & Cheng, G. (2007). Patient and hospital characteristics associated with length of stay and hospital charges for pediatric sports-related injury hospitalizations in the United States, 2000–2003. *Pediatrics, 119,* 813–820.

Zalavras, C., Nikolopoulou, G., Essin, D., Manjra, N., & Zionts, L. E. (2005). Pediatric fractures during skate-boarding, roller skating, and scooter riding. (2005). *American Journal of Sports Medicine,* 33(4), 568–573.

Zaoutis, T., Localio, A. R., Leckerman, K., Saddlemire, S., Bertoch, D., & Kelen, R. (2009) Prolonged intravenous therapy versus early transition to oral antimicrobial therapy for acute osteomyelitis in children. *Pediatrics, 123*(2), 636–642.

Zeller, J. L., Burke, A. E., & Glass, R. M. (2008). Osteomyelitis. *Journal of the American Medical Association, 299*(7), 857–858.

Ziran, B. H. Osteomyelitis. (2007). *Journal of Trauma, 62*(6), S59–S60.

SUGGESTED READINGS

Bulechek, G. M. Butcher, H. K., & Dochterman, J. M. (2008). *Nursing interventions classification (NIC)* (5th ed.). St. Louis: Mosby.

Halfon, N., Regalado, M., Sareen, H., Inkelas, M., Reuland, C., Glascoe, F., & Olson, L. (2004). Assessing development in the pediatric office. *Pediatrics, 113*(6), 1926–1933.

Magee, D. (2002). *Orthopedic physical assessment* (4th ed.). Philadelphia: W. B. Saunders.

Moorhead, S., Johnson, M., Maas, M., & Swanson, E. (2008). *Nursing outcomes classification (NOC)* (4th ed.). St. Louis: Mosby.

RESOURCES

Refer to the online student StudyWARE for Potts & Mandleco at http://www.CengageBrain.com for additional content and study aids.

Organization: **Muscular Dystrophy Association of America**
Description: MDA is the nonprofit health agency dedicated to curing muscular dystrophy, ALS, and related diseases by funding worldwide research. The Association also provides comprehensive health care and support services, advocacy, and education. The website offers users information regarding diseases, researchers, and sponsors.
Website/Resource: http://www.mdausa.org

Organization: **National Institute of Arthritis and Musculoskeletal and Skin Diseases (NIAMS)**
Description: The National Institute of Arthritis and Musculoskeletal Skin and Diseases is a subset of the National Institutes of Health and the Department of Health and Human Services. Its mission is to support research into the causes, treatment, and prevention of arthritis and musculoskeletal and skin diseases, the training of basic and clinical scientists to carry out this research, and the dissemination of information on research progress in these diseases. The website offers users information regarding listed diseases, research, and funding.
Website/Resource: http://www.niams.nih.org

Organization: **National Osteonecrosis Foundation**
Description: The goal of the National Osteonecrosis Foundation is to provide the much needed funding for medical research and education of patients, physicians, and other health professionals investigating osteonecrosis and Perthes' Disease. The website provides basic information regarding these diseases as well as links to other related websites.
Website/Resource: http://www.nonf.org

Organization: **National Scoliosis Foundation**
Description: The National Scoliosis Foundation (NSF) is a patient-led nonprofit organization dedicated to helping children, parents, adults, and health-care providers to understand the complexities of spinal deformities such as scoliosis. The website provides users with information regarding various spinal deformities and links to helpful resources.
Website/Resource: http://www.scoliosis.org

Organization: **Osteogenesis Imperfecta Foundation, Inc.**
Description: The Osteogenesis Imperfecta Foundation, Inc. (OI Foundation) is the only voluntary national health organization dedicated to helping people cope with the problems associated with osteogenesis imperfecta. The Foundation's mission is to improve the quality of life for people affected by OI through research to find treatments and a cure, education, awareness, and mutual support. The website provides users with information regarding support networks and current research studies.
Website/Resource: http://www.oif.org

Organization: **Scoliosis Association, Inc.**
Description: The Scoliosis Association is a tax-exempt, nonprofit organization founded by scoliosis patients and their families. Among its goals is the education of the public about spinal deviations. The website provides users with information regarding scoliosis and local chapters.
Website/Resource: http://www.scoliosis-assoc.org

Organization: **Scoliosis Research Society**
Description: The Scoliosis Research Society (SRS) has gained recognition as one of the world's premier spine societies. The SRS has maintained a commitment to research and education in the field of spinal deformities. Strict membership criteria ensure that the individual Fellows support that commitment. Current membership includes over 1,000 of the world's leading spine surgeons, researchers, physician assistants, and orthotists who are involved in research and treatment of spinal deformities. The website provides users with information regarding upcoming meetings and research proposals.
Website/Resource: http://www.srs.org

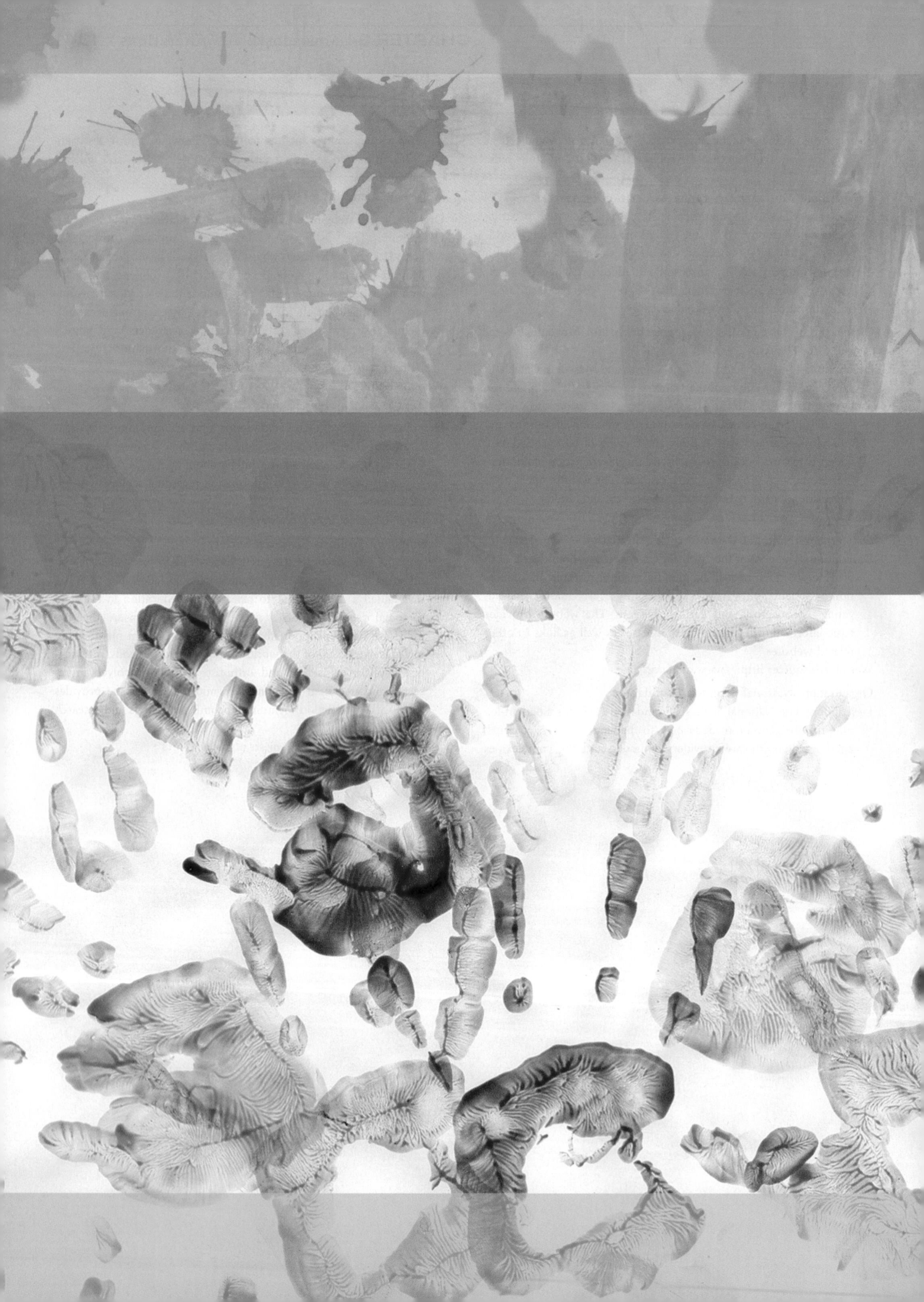

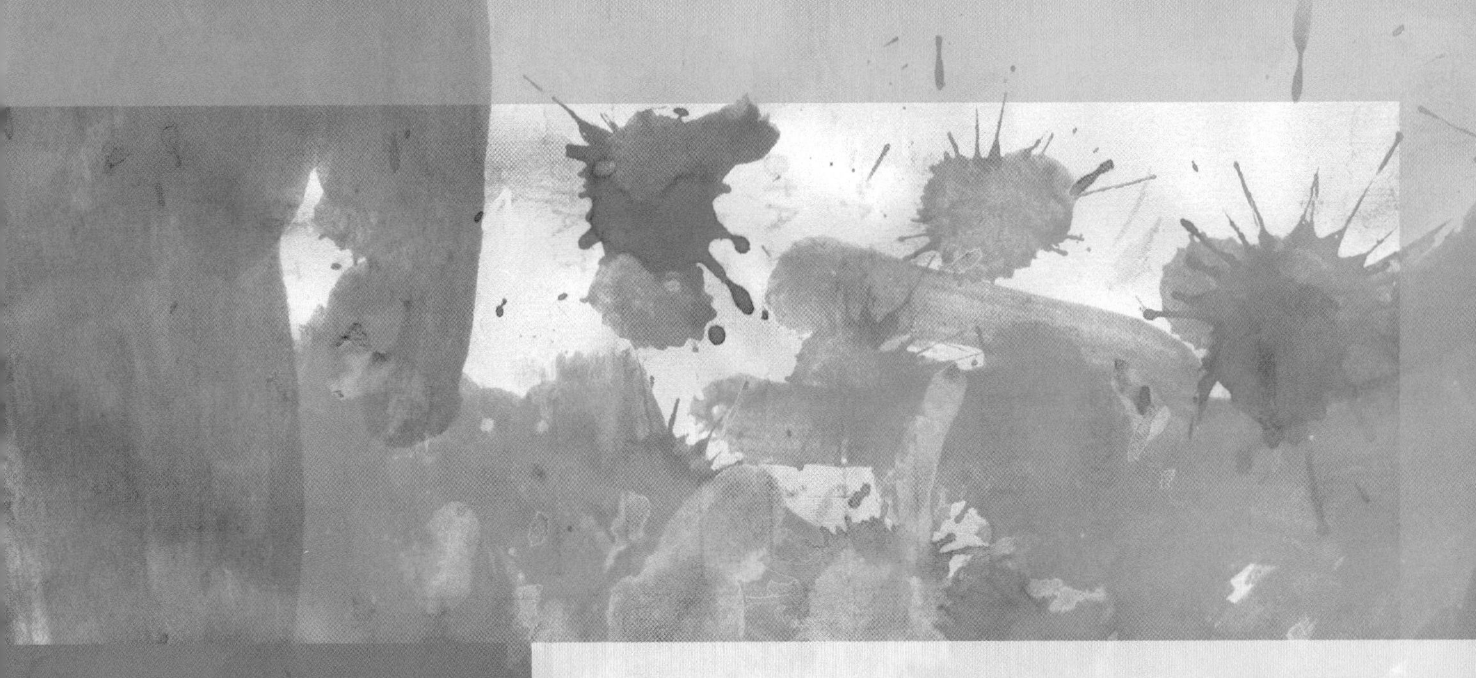

UNIT 8 Other Alterations to Children's Health

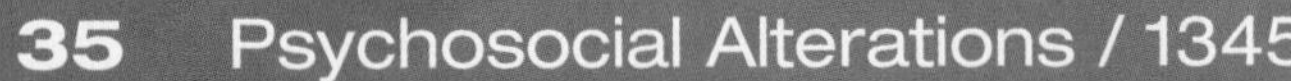

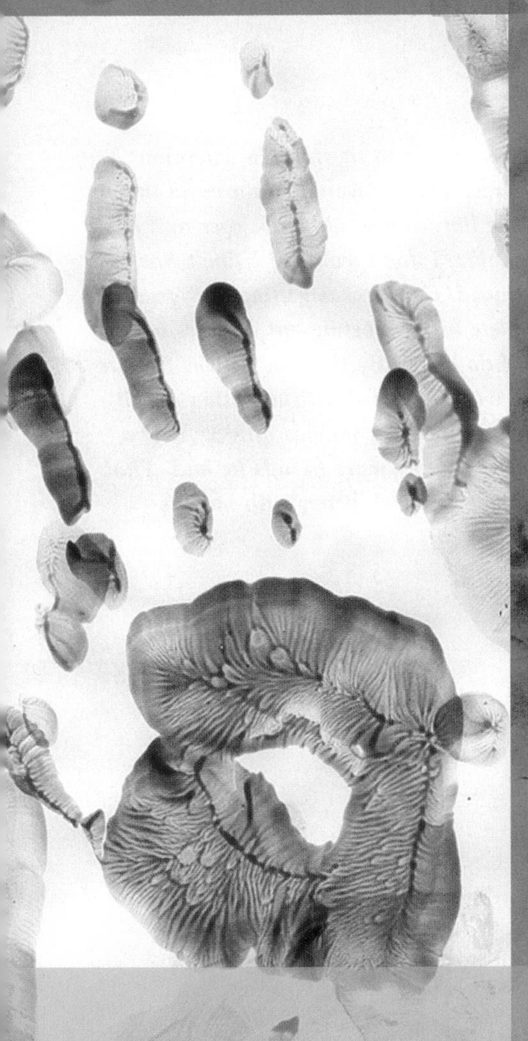

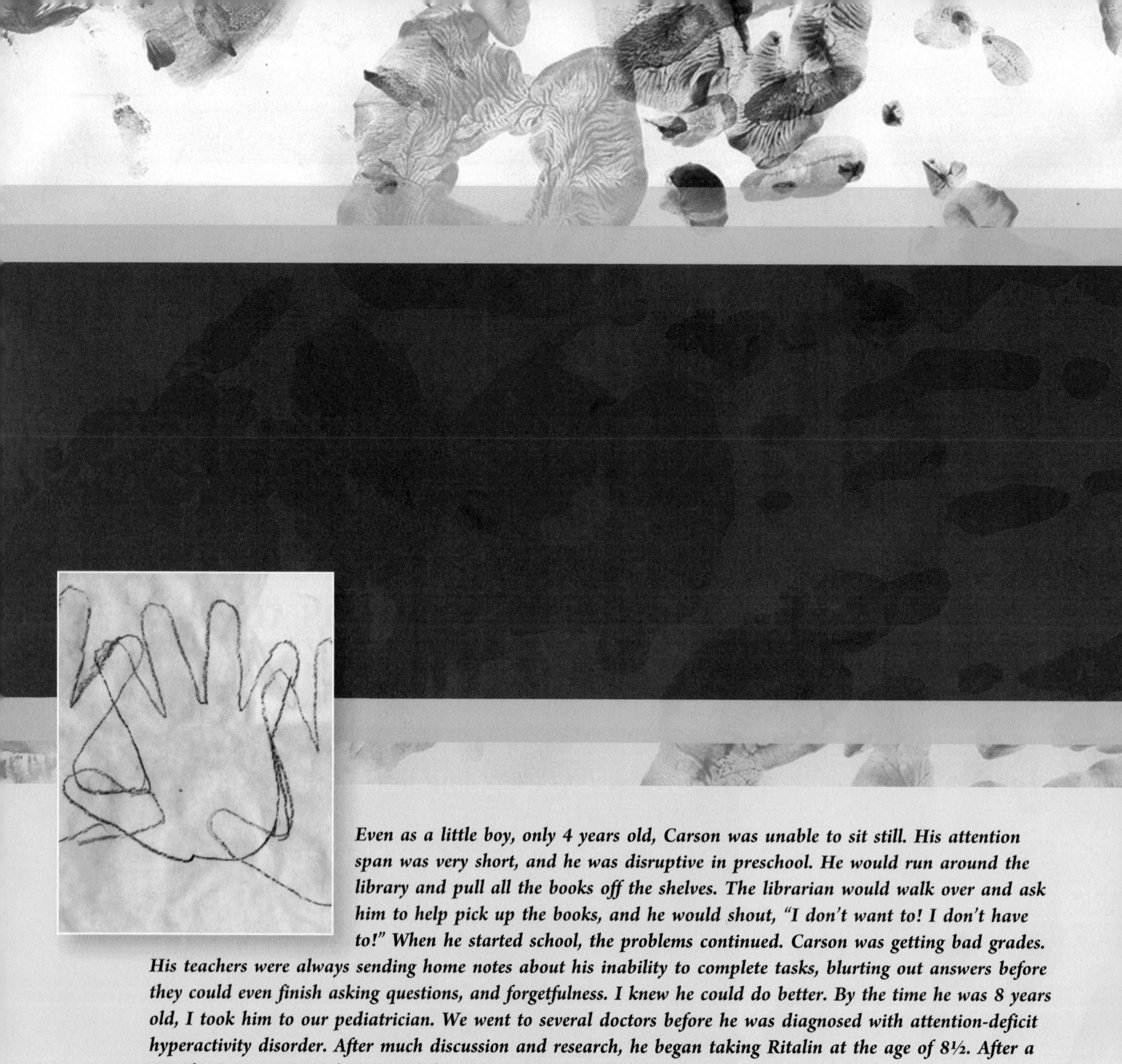

Even as a little boy, only 4 years old, Carson was unable to sit still. His attention span was very short, and he was disruptive in preschool. He would run around the library and pull all the books off the shelves. The librarian would walk over and ask him to help pick up the books, and he would shout, "I don't want to! I don't have to!" When he started school, the problems continued. Carson was getting bad grades. His teachers were always sending home notes about his inability to complete tasks, blurting out answers before they could even finish asking questions, and forgetfulness. I knew he could do better. By the time he was 8 years old, I took him to our pediatrician. We went to several doctors before he was diagnosed with attention-deficit hyperactivity disorder. After much discussion and research, he began taking Ritalin at the age of 8½. After a month, Carson was so happy with how much better his grades were and how many more friends he had. That was about 4 years ago. If Carson takes the medicine every day, he gets along so much better with me, his father, his brother, Sammy, and his friends, and he gets good grades.

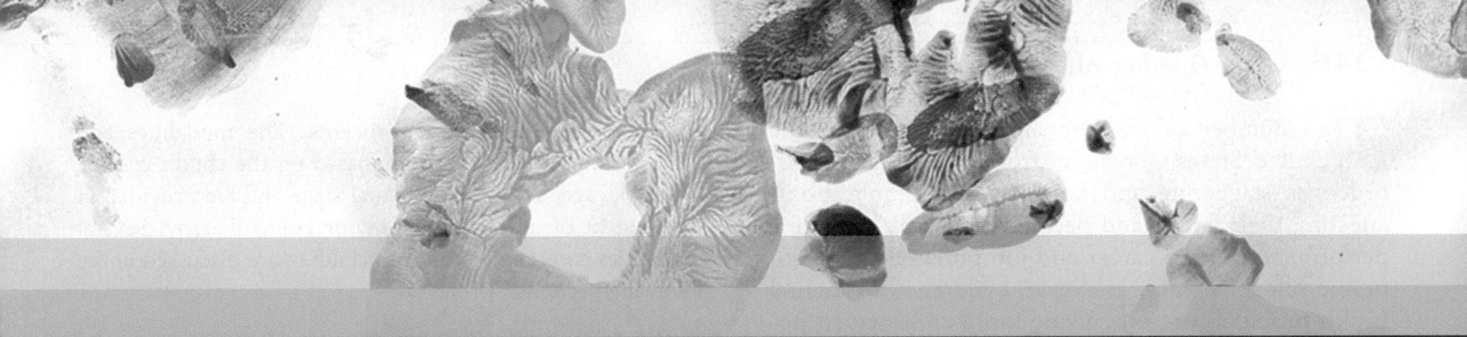

CHAPTER 35

Psychosocial Alterations

Barbara A. Caldwell, APRN-BC, PhD
Nicki L. Potts, RN, PhD

COMPETENCIES

Upon completion of this chapter, the reader will be able to:

- Discuss various treatment modalities for children and adolescents with psychosocial alterations. Identify the primary clinical manifestations of attention-deficit hyperactivity disorder (ADHD). Develop a nursing care plan for a child with ADHD and the family.
- Differentiate between major depressive disorder and dysthymic disorder.
- Explain the conditions and circumstances that make an individual at high risk for suicide.
- Describe a means for assessing suicide potential in a child or adolescent.
- Define and describe the major anxiety disorders of childhood (separation anxiety disorder, school phobia or refusal, generalized anxiety disorder, social phobia, obsessive-compulsive disorder, and post-traumatic stress disorder).
- Describe the sleep disorders common in children and adolescents.
- List the types of substances subject to abuse by children and adolescents.
- Plan nursing care for individuals with eating disorders, including nutritional rehabilitation and psychotherapy.
- Successfully complete the games and activities in the online student StudyWARE.

The number of children and adolescents in the United States who suffer from mental health disorders is staggering and has long-term implications, affecting their family and peer relationships, academic performance, future career and job potential, and economic self-sufficiency. However, children with mental health problems are one of the most underserved populations in the health care system. Inadequate distribution of services continues to compound the lack of availability of mental health services for children in rural and some urban areas.

Children and adolescents with psychosocial alterations or disorders are primarily treated in ambulatory and community settings. The nurse's role focuses on assessment, identification, referral, education, and support of the child and family, and working collaboratively with other disciplines in their therapy programs. The alterations included in this chapter include attention-deficit hyperactivity disorder, mood or depressive disorders, suicide, anxiety disorders, substance abuse, eating disorders, and failure to thrive.

TREATMENT MODALITIES

Through therapy, improved communication skills, and self-knowledge, children and their families gain hope and the ability to see their current situation in a new light, focusing on their strengths and abilities. They may be able to develop new patterns of behavior and more effective methods of coping with problems and concerns. The modalities and types of interventions used are based on the child's specific diagnosis, age, and developmental stage and are provided in the context of individual, family, or group therapy. Several modalities commonly used with children are discussed in the following sections.

REFLECTIVE THINKING

The Politically Active Nurse

A large percentage of children require mental health services. Among youth between the ages of 10 and 24, suicide is the leading cause of death, with approximately 4500 deaths per year (National Center for Injury Prevention and Control, 2008). Each year, approximately 149,000 youth between the ages of 10 and 24 receive medical services for self-inflicted injuries in emergency departments in the United States (National Center for Injury Prevention and Control, 2008). Even children with serious emotional disturbances appear to be greatly underserved. There is a need for effective systems of care in which agencies work collaboratively, and in which service delivery and financing are viewed comprehensively. A proactive voice from professionals will be necessary to improve the availability of mental health services for children. How can you become politically active as a proponent of improved availability, access, and funding of mental health services for children and adolescents?

INDIVIDUAL THERAPY

Individual therapy involves the child or adolescent and a therapist and is usually used in conjunction with other treatment modalities. The focus is on the child's behavioral, developmental, and psychological issues and problems. The age, developmental level, and psychosocial alteration of the child determine the therapeutic interventions used. Caregivers are not in the session during individual therapy, but they are an important part of a comprehensive treatment program. The therapist and the child determine what will be shared with the caregivers. Older children may request that caregivers be denied access to their records.

FAMILY THERAPY

The focus of **family therapy** is the relationships and communication patterns among family members. The therapist looks at the child's symptoms or problems as a reflection of the family's problems. Family therapy may include the child, the primary caregivers, siblings, and other people from the extended family, for example, grandparents, ex-partners, and step siblings. The goal of therapy is to change family interactions, improve communication, and help each member achieve autonomy, independence, and self-effectiveness.

GROUP THERAPY

Group therapy involves a group of children or adolescents, usually 6 to 10 in number, with a focus on interpersonal relationships. The socialization process occurs among group members, and feedback and support come from peers rather than the therapist alone. This treatment modality is powerful and effective for the school-age child and the adolescent because of the importance of peers for these age groups. Children learn to improve their social and communication skills through role modeling, group socialization, reality testing, feedback, and practice (Malekoff, 2006).

PLAY THERAPY

Play is the child's means of expression and often is called the work of childhood. As the child moves through each developmental stage, he or she learns to explore and communicate feelings and needs through play. One of the ways the child is prepared for more complex cognitive tasks of problem solving and abstract thought is through play. A child can also learn self-control and self-mastery, thereby increasing self-esteem. The focus of **play therapy** is to help the child reveal emotions,

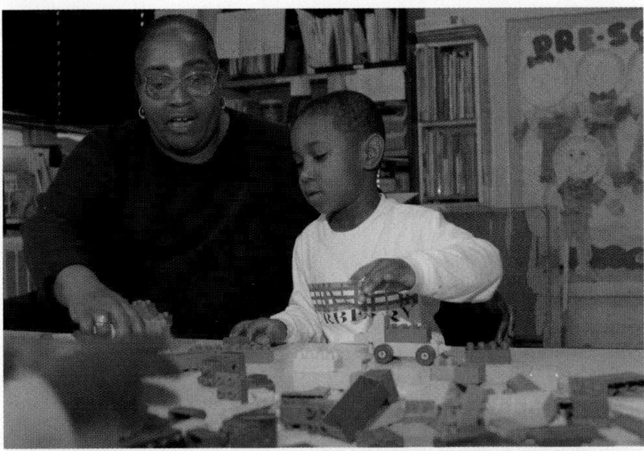

FIGURE 35-1 **Through play therapy, a child's fears and emotions may be revealed.** DELMAR CENGAGE LEARNING.

feelings, and problems. Toys, dolls, blocks, cars, or other play objects are used in the sessions (Figure 35-1). The process of being with the therapist, toy selection, and interaction during the therapy session are part of the therapeutic process. Anger, sadness, fear, and stress may be revealed, consciously or unconsciously, through play. The therapist is available to help the child understand her or his emotions and response to these emotions. Play therapy is usually individual but may be conducted in a group setting.

The initial stage of this type of therapy allows the therapist to assess the child and build a therapeutic relationship. In the middle stage, the child attempts to resolve conflicts and problems and work toward healthy personality change. During the termination, feelings of separation and rejection are worked through, and the therapist summarizes what changes have occurred for the child.

ART THERAPY

In **art therapy** drawings and other art objects are used to help the therapist gain information about the child, her or his behaviors, concerns, and problems. The child is encouraged to use drawing as a means to express feelings and issues that are difficult to verbalize. Drawings provide information about relevant situations and problems that are complex and remain hidden from the child's immediate level of consciousness.

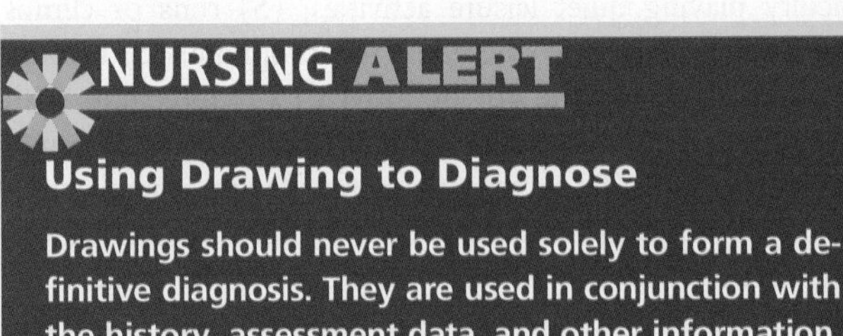

NURSING ALERT

Using Drawing to Diagnose

Drawings should never be used solely to form a definitive diagnosis. They are used in conjunction with the history, assessment data, and other information.

ATTENTION-DEFICIT HYPERACTIVITY DISORDER

Attention-deficit hyperactivity disorder (ADHD) is characterized by inattention, hyperactivity, and impulsivity. It is the most commonly encountered neurobehavioral disorder of childhood (Biederman, 2005) and among the most prevalent chronic health conditions of school-age children (American Academy of Child and Adolescent Psychiatry, 2007). The basic impairment in ADHD is a deficit with inhibiting behavior that interferes with the process of learning self-regulation behaviors. This deficiency of internal self-regulation typically results in school difficulties, academic underachievement, low self-esteem, and difficulties with family and social relationships. ADHD is now seen as a chronic disorder that may persist into adulthood. There are three subtypes:

1. Inattentive only (formerly known as attention-deficit disorder)—Children with this type are not overly active. Their symptoms may not be noticed because they do not disrupt the classroom or other activities. Girls with ADHD most commonly have this form, as well as 30–40% of all children with ADHD.
2. Hyperactive or impulsive—this subtype accounts for only 10% of children with ADHD. These children exhibit hyperactive and impulsive behaviors; however, they can pay attention.
3. Combined inattentive, hyperactive and impulsive—this is the most common type of ADHD, accounting for 50–60% of children with the disorder. These children have all three symptoms (American Psychiatric Association, 2000).

INCIDENCE, ETIOLOGY, AND PATHOPHYSIOLOGY

ADHD affects approximately 5%–10% of all children and is more common in boys than girls at a ratio ranging from 3-6:1 (Faraone, Seargent, Gillberg, & Biederman, 2003). The disorder is found in all cultures, although incidences differ. Whether these differences reflect real biological and psychological variation or merely variable diagnostic criteria is unclear. ADHD is frequently associated with other disorders such as conduct disorder, oppositional defiant disorder, depression, anxiety disorders, and many developmental disorders (speech and language delays and learning disabilities) (Biederman, 2005).

Etiology of ADHD is unknown, but the following factors have been suggested: genetic, neurophysiological, dietary, and environmental. The disorder is more common in first-degree relatives of the affected child than in the general population. Between 10% and 35% of these children have a first-degree relative with past or present ADHD (Swanson et al., 2001). In fact, many of the parents of these children go through childhood and early adulthood with undiagnosed ADHD only to discover their own diagnosis when their child's symptoms bring him or her to clinical attention (Biederman, 2005). Twin studies have shown that when ADHD is present in one twin, it is significantly more likely to occur in the other twin if the relationship is identical (monozygotic) rather than fraternal (dizygotic).

A deficiency in the neurotransmitter dopamine has also been implicated in ADHD. Dopamine plays a key role in initiating purposive movement, increasing alertness and motivation, reducing appetite, and inducing insomnia.

Numerous environmental factors have been proposed as potential causes. These include perinatal insult, head injury, lead poisoning, cigarette and alcohol exposure, maternal smoking during pregnancy, low birth weight, and diet (i.e., food allergies or sensitivity to food additives). Although these hypotheses may explain some cases, none alone is likely to account for a significant portion of children with ADHD. The claim that food additives or allergies cause ADHD has very limited data to support it (Biederman, 2005).

NURSING TIP

Conditions Producing Behaviors Similar to ADHD

Children with other conditions can exhibit behaviors similar to those seen with ADHD:

- Underachievement at school because of a learning disability
- Attention lapses caused by absence seizures
- Intermittent hearing problems caused by otitis media
- Disruptive or unresponsive behavior caused by anxiety or depression
- Psychological trauma such as severe physical, sexual, or psychological abuse

CLINICAL MANIFESTATIONS

The primary clinical manifestations of ADHD are dependent on the subtype and include inattention, hyperactivity, and impulsivity. Inattention is the inability to sustain concentration for an appropriate period of time, and to disregard attending to external stimuli. Associated problems are related to poor organization, time management and planning (Abikoff et al., 2009). There are several functional areas that impact a child's daily behavior and vary depending on the age, and social and psychological status. Children with the symptom of inattention have difficulties with executive functioning located in the frontal lobe of the neurocortex. These children manifest problems such as paying attention, excessive shifting of attention, distractibility, and screening out unimportant information. As a result they almost always have problems in school and are often mistakenly thought by teachers and caregivers to ignore instructions or assigned tasks or chores purposefully. Inattentive children have problems keeping their concentration on one idea; therefore, they may not listen, remember, or complete tasks. Time management problems lead to procrastination and incomplete assignments. Because of these behaviors, they may underachieve in school and become frustrated or even depressed. Recent research reports note that ADHD children are at higher risk for comorbid depression (Blackman, Ostrander, & Herman, 2005).

Hyperactive or overactive children tend to fidget or squirm, are disruptive in the classroom by frequently getting out of their seat, and interfere with teaching activities for other students. These behaviors often result in negative social consequences for the child with ADHD and interfere with peer relationships. Children exhibiting impulsivity may appear socially immature because they tend to interrupt and have difficulty delaying responses such as volunteering answers to class questions without being called on by the teacher. These behaviors are unpopular not only with fellow students but also with teachers. Impulsive children act before they think and are impatient.

DIAGNOSIS

Distinguishing between normal and ADHD behaviors is often difficult in the young child because developmental changes occur rapidly. Caregivers often wonder whether the child is just going through a stage, such as the "terrible twos," or whether the behaviors are early signs of ADHD. No one test or instrument is able to diagnose a child as having ADHD. Multiple data sources are used over a period of time to make the diagnosis and include: a complete health history; physical examination; behavior rating scales completed by teachers and caregivers; psychoeducational tests to identify learning disabilities, cognitive, language, and visual-spatial-motor problems; and the *DSM-IV-TR* criteria.

In order to be diagnosed with ADHD the child must have six or more of the following symptoms of *inattention:* (1) fails to attend to details or makes careless mistakes in schoolwork, work, or other activities; (2) has difficulty sustaining attention with tasks or play activities; (3) is easily distracted; (4) does not follow instructions and complete what is started; (5) has difficulty with organization; (6) avoids or is reluctant to perform tasks that require sustained mental effort; (7) loses things needed for schoolwork or play activities; (8) does not seem to listen; and (9) is often forgetful. Additionally, six or more of the following symptoms of *hyperactivity or impulsivity* must also be present: (1) fidgets with hands or feet and squirms in seat; (2) leaves seat when remaining seated is expected; (3) talks excessively; (4) has difficulty playing quiet leisure activities; (5) runs or climbs excessively in situations where it is inappropriate; (6) is often characterized as "on the go" or "driven"; (7) interrupts with answers before the question is completed; (8) has difficulty taking turns; and (9) interrupts or intrudes in others' activities. The symptoms must have been present before the age of 7; occurred in two or more settings (home, school, or work); persisted for 6 or more months; and adversely affected functioning in school, work, or social situations (APA, 2000).

TREATMENT

Treatment includes pharmacotherapy, behavior management, educational interventions, and family education. Stimulant medications, including methylphenidate (Ritalin), dextroamphetamine (Dexedrine), pemoline, and a mixture of amphetamine salts (Adderall), consistently improve the symptoms of ADHD in the majority of children (Biederman & Faraone, 2005). These drugs increase the availability of dopamine and norepinephrine in the neural synapses, thus improving concentration and attention, and reducing the child's activity level. Common side effects of these medications include anorexia, weight loss, abdominal pain, headache, insomnia, tachycardia, and hypertension. The minimal dose to treat the core symptoms of ADHD is critical to minimize the frequency or severity of sleep problems (Faraone et al., 2009). If stimulants are ineffective or produce adverse side effects that are unacceptable to the child or caregivers, other medications may be used.

Antihypertensive medications, such as clonidine (Catapres) and guanfacine (Tenex), may also be used to treat ADHD. These medications decrease impulsivity, hyperactivity, and aggression. Antidepressants (bupropion [Wellbutrin] or tricyclic antidepressants) may also be considered. In 2002 the Food and Drug Administration approved atomoxetine (Strattera) for ADHD in children older than 6 years of age. It is a selective norepinephrine reuptake inhibitor and the first nonstimulant approved for this disorder. One advantage of Strattera is that it is not a controlled substance, does not appear to be habit forming, and apparently cannot be used as a drug of abuse. The FDA in 2009 issued a warning that Strattera can cause serious liver damage (USDHHS, 2009). Serious symptoms include the development of jaundice, pruritis, dark urine, upper right quadrant tenderness, and unexplained flu-like symptoms (Biederman & Faraone, 2005).

Stimulant drugs can be abused, forcing strict prescription rules. Although Strattera has not been shown to be superior to the current standard of care, it remains an alternative for children who are intolerant or unresponsive to stimulant medications (Biederman & Faraone, 2005).

Behavior management includes assisting the child to follow rules, complete tasks, improve self-control, and providing positive feedback for appropriate behavior. Other techniques are clearly defining acceptable and unacceptable behaviors and the accompanying consequences and rewards, and periodically changing or varying them to motivate the child. Research has demonstrated that a 12 week parental group training program enhances the effectiveness of treatment of children with ADHD, particularly by decreasing behavioral and internalizing problems (van Den Hoofdakker et al., 2007).

ADHD is regarded as a developmental disability. According to federal law, The Education for All Handicapped Children Act (Public Law 94-142), these children must receive free public education in the least restrictive environment. For this reason, many children with ADHD are "mainstreamed" in regular classrooms with their peers. When disruptive behavior is severe, special education or resource placement where the setting is smaller and more controlled may be recommended. Children with ADHD are often placed in classes with individuals who have serious

EVIDENCE-BASED PRACTICE

Treatment of Attention-Deficit Disorder with Stimulant Medications

CLINICAL PROBLEM

Do children become addicted to stimulants when used for the treatment of ADHD?

BEST CLINICAL PRACTICE

- Early medication treatment with stimulants for ADHD in childhood significantly reduces the risk for subsequent substance use disorders (SUD).
- There is compelling evidence that pharmacotherapy with stimulants for ADHD in childhood does not lead to SUD. Instead it is associated with a reduction in the risk for subsequent drug and alcohol use disorders.
- There is growing evidence that children with ADHD-combined type are at greater risk for co-occurring psychiatric illness, such as depression and anxiety than children without ADHD (Baldwin & Dadds, 2008; Blackman et al., 2005; Daviss, 2008).
- ADHD without a comorbid externalizing problem is not associated with the risk of drug abuse. ADHD with a comorbid externalizing problem such as oppositional defiant disorder is associated with an increased risk of drug abuse (August et al., 2006).

IMPLICATIONS FOR NURSING

- Stimulant medications, when used with medical supervision, are considered quite safe.
- Nurses need to educate and reassure parents that their children will not become addicted to the medications.
- Children with ADHD should be routinely assessed for signs and symptoms of anxiety and depression.
- Caretakers should be educated to observe their child for signs and symptoms of anxiety and depression.
- Nurses need to provide prevention programs on the hazards of substance abuse to children and adolescents with ADHD and their caretakers.

References: Baldwin, J., & Dadds, M. (2008). Examining alternative explanations of the covariation of ADHD and anxiety symptoms in children: a community study. *Journal of Abnormal Child Psychology, 36*(1), 67–79.

Daviss, W. B. (2008). A review of co-morbid depression in pediatric ADHD: etiology, phenomenology, and treatment. *Journal of Child and Adolescent Psychopharmacology, 18*(6), 565–571.

psychiatric morbidity. Many caregivers are hesitant to agree to such placements out of concern for their child's emotional development and safety. Family education should provide information about the disorder, address concerns, and emphasize the child's and family's strengths. Caregivers should be reminded that they are not at fault for their child's situation and should be referred to and encouraged to seek ADHD support groups.

Many controversial treatments for ADHD have been proposed and used by caregivers who are eager to help their child. These alternative methods have been successful for some children but are not standard therapeutic treatments. There is no scientific evidence of improved behavioral or cognitive symptoms. Some of these controversial therapies include restricted diets, EEG biofeedback, megavitamins and mineral supplements, and chiropractic adjustment and bone realignment.

NURSING MANAGEMENT

Assessment

Assessment incorporates information from the child, caregivers, and teachers. The nurse may interview the child to gain information from his or her perspective. Direct observations of the child within the home and school will provide valuable data to assess the degree of inattention, impulsivity, motor hyperactivity, and behavioral problems.

Caregivers are an essential part of the assessment interview as their perceptions of the child's behaviors help determine the diagnosis. They can provide a detailed family and developmental history. They are also able to share information about the child's hyperactivity, attention deficits, and moods in the home. Standardized behavior rating scales are available for them to complete as part of the assessment process. Teachers' reports are also a part of the clinical assessment. Developmental age, language, and conceptual ability must be assessed to ensure an appropriate treatment plan is instituted. A physical examination should be performed to rule out any medical problems.

Nursing Diagnosis

The following diagnoses are relevant for the child with ADHD:

1. *Impaired social interaction* related to poor impulse control, short attention span, and aggressive behavior.
2. *Risk for injury* related to impulsivity and inability to perceive harm.
3. *Chronic low self-esteem* related to lack of satisfactory peer relationships and positive feedback, and academic underachievement.
4. *Compromised family coping* related to the child's disruptive and intrusive behaviors, hyperactivity, and inability to heed directions.

Outcome Identification

1. The child will demonstrate acceptable social skills and improved ability to interact with peers.
2. The child will be free of injury or unnecessary risks.
3. The child will demonstrate increased feelings of self-worth by verbalizing positive statements about himself or herself.
4. The family will identify coping strategies for managing disruptive and intrusive behaviors.
5. The caregivers will set appropriate limits and structure the environment to facilitate the child's developing increased control over own behavior.

Planning and Implementation

Because pharmacotherapy is a major aspect of the treatment for the child with ADHD, education of the caregivers about the medication regimen is vital. The nurse teaches them about the importance of the regimen and about the side effects. The nurse works with the family to encourage compliance and explores their feelings and concerns that might impede this. Do they fear they are "drugging" their child by giving the medication? Are they concerned that giving their child a stimulant medication will lead to drug addiction later in life? Weight, height, and blood pressure are frequently monitored if the child is taking stimulant medication. Growth rate may be decreased, and weight loss is common during the first few months of treatment because of appetite suppression. Appetite may return to normal with long-term use. "Drug holidays" may be used every few months to determine if therapy is still necessary. Signs and symptoms of anxiety and depression need to be routinely assessed by both caregivers and nurses.

Caregivers need to be well educated about ADHD because of their involvement in implementing a behavioral management program at home. They often have to educate others, such as school personnel, about the needs of their child. The nurse should provide them with information about strategies for implementing the treatment regimen at home (see Box 35-1).

Family support is necessary initially to help caregivers understand the complexity of the disorder and to deal with their feelings of possible guilt and shock. Support groups for families are helpful and may offer understanding and expertise in managing daily problems of living with the child with ADHD.

Evaluation

The nurse acts as a liaison between health care providers, the home, and school to coordinate referrals and to promote ongoing evaluation of intervention strategies. Indications that the interventions are effective include an increase in the child's ability to concentrate, fewer disruptive and intrusive behaviors, improvement in academic performance, and more positive social relationships. An evaluation of the

BOX 35-1
HOME INTERVENTIONS FOR THE CHILD WITH ADHD

1. Develop specific time periods for waking, bedtime, chores, homework, playtime, TV, and meals. Maintain consistency in the child's routine. Explain any changes in routine ahead of time so that the child understands and can anticipate the changes.
2. Establish clear and concise rules of acceptable and appropriate behavior for the child. Rules, as well as consequences and rewards for appropriate behavior, can be written down and posted in a prominent place.
3. Give instructions as simply and clearly as possible, demonstrating if necessary. Ask the child to repeat them back to you. Then praise the individual when responding correctly.
4. Do not give more than one or two instructions at a time. If a task is difficult, break it into smaller parts and teach each separately.
5. Provide the child time with his or her own "special" quiet spot without distractions in which to do school work.
6. Allow the child choices within the limits you have set.
7. Help the child find avenues of self-expression that will help him or her express wants in acceptable, useful ways.
8. Provide positive feedback and praise for appropriate behaviors and tasks completed.
9. Help child with social skills development, especially related to peers and age-related physical activities.
10. Encourage activities that feed the child's sense of success to improve self-esteem.
11. Sleep schedules should be established to ensure that the child is feeling rested in the mornings.

EYE ON...

Controversy Regarding Ritalin

There has been concern from the public regarding the overdiagnosis of ADHD and the overprescribed use of Ritalin (AAP, 2000). There are many opinions circulating. It is important for the caregivers to understand that they are just opinions. What is right for their child can only come from consultation with qualified individuals and thorough diagnostic testing.

interventions for the caregivers and other family members focuses on their acceptance of the diagnosis, understanding of the disorder and treatment regimen, compliance with the medication administration, and provision of a safe and supportive home environment. Nurses must continue to remember that as the child develops both socially, academically and psychologically, assessment will be ongoing and adaptations may be needed in the types of intervention strategies.

FAMILY TEACHING

Caregivers will monitor medication administration for the younger child; therefore, awareness of side effects is essential. Education for the caregivers, child, and siblings regarding characteristics and interventions for ADHD is essential. Children with ADHD need to understand that they have a manageable illness, and that there are many resources such as support groups, medication therapy, and organizational strategies available to help them. The caregivers are to be educated that as the child develops, there may need to be alterations in both the dosages and a constant reexamination of the types of educational and home supports a child may require.

MOOD DISORDERS

Mood disorders, also referred to as depressive disorders, are common among children and adolescents, but are frequently unrecognized. The American Academy of Child and Adolescent Psychiatry reports that 5% to 10% of children and adolescents have symptoms of depression that do not meet full diagnostic criteria (AACAP, 2007). Only recently have mood disorders come to be recognized and treated in this population. In the past it was believed that this age group lacked the psychological and cognitive structure necessary to experience these problems. Previously children could spend years in severe depression without their symptoms being recognized, diagnosed, or treated. However, a growing body of evidence has confirmed that they not only experience the whole spectrum of mood disorders, but also suffer from the significant morbidity and mortality (from suicide) associated with them (AACAP, 2007).

There are two types of mood disorders: bipolar disorder and depressive disorder. Depressive disorder has two subtypes: major depressive disorder (MDD) and dysthymic disorder (DD). Bipolar disorder is characterized by episodes of depression alternating with episodes of mania. MDD is marked by a single episode or recurrent episodes of depression, whereas DD involves a chronic disturbance of mood.

INCIDENCE, ETIOLOGY, AND PATHOPHYSIOLOGY

The incidence of MDD is estimated to be approximately 0.3% in preschoolers, 2% in school-age children, and 5–8% in adolescents. The ratio of boys and girls is equal in prepubertal children but increases to a 2:1 female-to-male ratio in adolescents. The incidence of depression appears to be increasing with each successive generation, and depressive disorders are being recognized at a younger age. DD has an incidence of 0.6–1.7% in prepubertal children and 1.6–8% in adolescents (AACAP, 2007; Dulcan, Martini, & Lake, 2003).

Many theories about the etiology of depression have been proposed, such as genetic, biological, and psychosocial ones; however, the exact cause is not known, partly because less research has been conducted with children. Children with at least one depressed parent are three times more likely to have a lifetime episode of MDD than children with nondepressed parents. Biological theory proposes that the lack or excess of one or more neurotransmitters, specifically, serotonin, and endocrine dysfunction may contribute to the development of depression. Further, brain alterations occur with smaller hippocampal volume and prefrontal cortex volume (Dopheide, 2006).

Psychosocial factors include family dysfunction, personality dynamics, and exposure to negative or adverse life events. Children who were physically abused or were exposed to multiple types of abuse are at higher risk for mood disorders (Widom, DuMont, & Czaja, 2007). Family interactions characterized by conflict, child maltreatment, rejection, and lack of expression of affection and support may be risk factors. Caregivers of depressed children have high rates of psychiatric disorders, including anxiety, substance abuse, and personality (antisocial) disorders. Personality dynamics such as unrealistic, overly harsh, internal judgment of the child's own impulses, thoughts, and mood may contribute to the development of depression. These dynamics contribute to low self-esteem, self-blame, and shame, which are prominent in MDD. A child's style of coping with stress contributes to thinking patterns that are inflexible and rigid. Depressed children report having experienced significantly more adverse or negative life events in areas of school, relationships with friends or caregivers, health, and work than their non-depressed counterparts. Exposure to the loss of a caregiver through death, separation, or divorce also raises the risk. Children may also have a medical disorder that precipitates depressive symptoms such as hypothyroidism, mononucleosis, anemia, and autoimmune disorders. In addition, medications such as stimulants, corticosteroids, or contraceptives may induce depressive symptoms in children.

CLINICAL MANIFESTATIONS

The clinical manifestations of MDD in children and adolescents are similar to those seen in adults and include one or more major depressive episodes lasting on average from 7 to 9 months. In order to be diagnosed with MDD, the child must experience five or more of the following symptoms: (1) depressed or irritable mood; (2) markedly diminished interest or pleasure in previously enjoyed activities (**anhedonia**); (3) changes in eating habits indicated by weight loss or gain; (4) psychomotor agitation or inactivity; (5) feelings of worthlessness or inappropriate guilt; (6) diminished ability to think or concentrate; (7) fatigue or energy loss; (8) insomnia or hypersomnia; and (9) recurrent thoughts of death and suicidal ideation. The symptoms must cause clinically significant distress or impairment in social, school, or other important areas of functioning (APA, 2000). The distinction between the depressed child and the unhappy child is made by determining the duration of the sad mood. A child with MDD experiences a depressed mood that persists for most of the day, nearly every day for least 2 consecutive weeks (APA, 2000) (Figure 35-2).

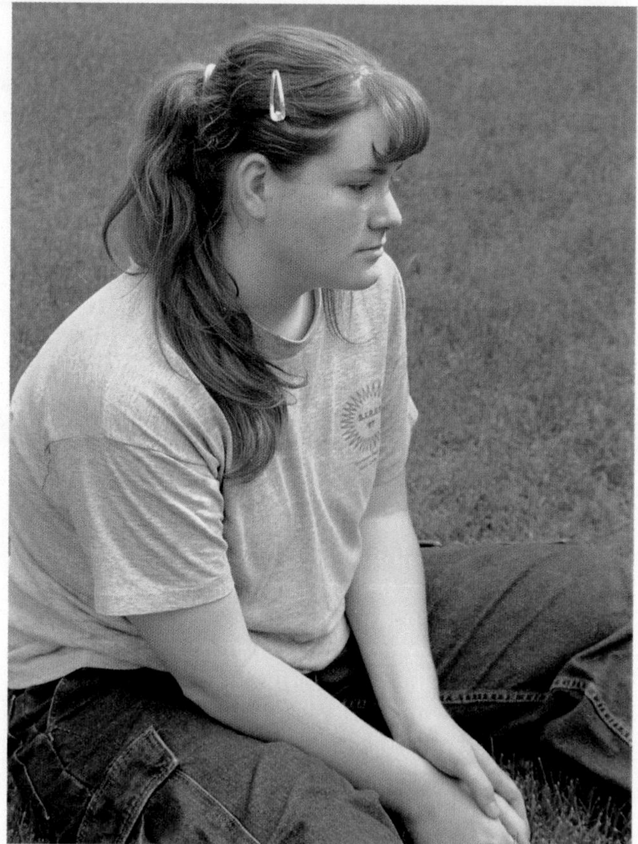

FIGURE 35-2 Loneliness and depression may be seen in some adolescents. DELMAR CENGAGE LEARNING.

Compared to adults, depressed children are often irritable, are more likely to express symptoms of anxiety (such as school or social phobia), and have more somatic complaints, such as stomachaches and headaches. Further, children have more severe mood swings, low frustration tolerance, temper tantrums, and have problems with academic performance. The presentation of MDD in adolescents is manifested by more impairment in functioning than younger children, and more behavioral problems than adults. Forty to seventy percent of children and adolescents with MDD also have other psychiatric disorders including anxiety disorders, disruptive disorders (conduct disorder, ADHD), substance abuse, and personality disorders (AACAP, 2007).

DD consists of a persistent long-term depressed mood that is less intense but more chaotic than MDD. The affected child has a depressed or irritable mood for most of the day, on most days, for a period of 1 year. Other manifestations

NURSING ALERT

Family Stigma & Denial Associated with Children Experiencing a Depressive Disorder

A caretaker may not have the necessary education or believe that their child can be experiencing a depressed mood. They may feel that their child is going through a "phase" and will outgrow the feelings of sadness and other associated behaviors. Only a small fraction of children who need treatment are receiving services due to denial or stigma. The role of the nurse is to advocate for children's need for assessment and interventions in all types of service agencies.

Reference: Fritz, G. (2007). Stigma and childhood mental illness: can advocates turn the tide? *The Brown University Child and Adolescent Behavior Letter*. (November, 2007).

of DD are poor appetite or overeating, low energy or fatigue, poor concentration, difficulty making decisions, and feelings of hopelessness. Because the development of DD is one of the major pathways to recurrent depressive disorders, early identification and treatment are critical.

DIAGNOSIS

The most useful tool in diagnosing depressive disorders is a comprehensive evaluation, including interviews with the child, caregivers, teachers, and social services professionals, if appropriate. Clinician-completed rating scales and self-report instruments may also be used. The following instruments are used in pediatrics: (1) Children's Depression Inventory; and (2) Children's Depression Rating Scale. A thorough physical evaluation is necessary as a number of medical disorders can mimic depression, such as mononucleosis, seizure disorder, hypo- and hyperthyroidism, drug abuse and withdrawal, and other psychiatric disorders. Lastly, a developmental history, a family history of psychiatric disorders, an assessment of home and school environments, and potential stressors are obtained. The history and physical examination can help determine which laboratory tests may be appropriate.

TREATMENT

Treatment is usually psychotherapy and psychotropic medication. Psychotherapy encompasses a multitude of approaches including play therapy; individual, family, and group therapy; and **cognitive behavioral therapy** (CBT). CBT is a behavioral modification using stimulus and response to alter inappropriate behavior. Appropriate behavior is reinforced while inappropriate behavior is extinguished and replaced with a more desirable one. CBT is based on the premise that individuals with depression have cognitive distortions in how they view themselves, the world, and the future that contribute to their depression. CBT teaches them to identify and change these negative cognitions into more positive thoughts. It is important to determine the child's developmental and cognitive level in deciding the most appropriate approach. For example, play therapy would be appropriate for the preschool-age child with depression, while individual, group, and CBT would be more appropriate for older children and adolescents (Dopheide, 2006). Group therapy is effective for adolescents because of the importance of the peer group and is most effective if individuals in the group have a variety of diagnoses, as the depressed adolescent is often quiet, withdrawn, and non-interactive. Within the group the adolescent learns interpersonal and communication skills and expression of affect. Role-playing and social interaction skills are used in the group setting (Malekoff, 2006).

Antidepressants may be prescribed. Research in children and adolescents has failed to demonstrate the effectiveness of tricyclic antidepressants, including imipramine (Tofranil) and amitriptyline (Elavil). However, the selective serotonin reuptake inhibitors (SSRIs) such as fluoxetine (Prozac), sertraline hydrochloride (Zoloft), and paroxetine (Paxil) appear to have efficacy and safety. The SSRIs dominate the pharmacotherapy of depression because of their relatively safe side effect profile, very low lethality after overdose, and easy administration (once a day). The only FDA-approved antidepressant for children 8 years or older is Prozac; however, the other SSRIs are used to treat depression. Sleep problems may accompany depressed mood in children and adolescents and contribute to exacerbation in symptoms. Sleep hygiene education for the caretaker and child should be integrated into a treatment plan (Box 35-2).

Hospitalization is based on the seriousness of the mood disorder as determined by assessment and observation of the child. The hospital provides a safe and controlled environment and has strategies for protecting the child with suicidal

CULTURAL CONSIDERATION

Ethnic and Cultural Factors and Depression

It is imperative for the health care provider to be alert to ethnic and cultural factors that may influence the assessment of depressive disorder. Children from many cultures or ethnic groups are encouraged to be silent and to avoid direct eye contact when in the presence of authority figures. These behaviors easily can be misinterpreted as indicators of depression, and the child may be misdiagnosed with MDD or DD.

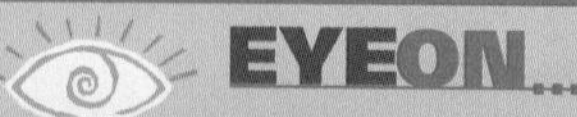

Complementary Alternative Therapy for the Child with Depression

Complementary alternative medicine (CAM) may be used in the treatment of depression. Many herbal remedies have been effective for some individuals. Knowledge about the side effects and efficacy of CAM for treating depression is important, but research with herbs is limited in children. The research that has been performed has used adults as subjects. You should query caregivers and the child as to herbal use.

NURSING TIP

Social Anxiety Can Lead to Depression

Social anxiety is considered a risk factor for depression in children and adolescents. Children with social anxiety may be shy and have deficit social skills to effectively interact with their environment, especially in school and with their interactions with peers. A child's self-esteem can be impacted by not engaging in activities and age-appropriate behaviors that reinforce self-confidence and pride. Caretakers need education and counseling related to intervention strategies and when the social anxiety interferes with psychological or academic functioning, referral for evaluation is warranted.

Reference: Beesdo, K., Bittner, A., Pine, D. S., Stein, M. B., Höfler, M., Lieb, R. & Wittchen, H. U. (2007). Incidence of social anxiety disorder and the consistent risk for secondary depression in the first three decades of life. *Archives of General Psychiatry, 64*(8), 903–912.

behaviors or ideation. These measures include restrictions or precautions that limit the child's movements and activities in the hospital setting.

NURSING MANAGEMENT

Assessment

A thorough history from the child and caregivers is important in the nurse's assessment. When asking children about the feelings of depression, a variety of words such as sad, depressed, blue, down, and very unhappy should be used. Depending on the child's developmental and cognitive level, information about sleep problems, somatic complaints, worries and stressors, feelings of worthlessness, and suicide ideation should be obtained. Caregivers can provide information about the duration of depressed mood, observable behaviors, sleep disturbances, somatic complaints, self-deprecatory remarks, and recent family stressful events (moving, death of family member or pet, loss of a job). A thorough family history should also be obtained. Teachers need to be asked about changes in the child's academic performance and peer relationships.

Nursing Diagnosis

Nursing diagnoses for a child with depression may include the following:

1. *Low self-esteem* related to cognitive distortions, negative view of self, feelings of worthlessness.
2. *Impaired social interaction* related to low self-esteem, withdrawn behavior, and feelings of worthlessness.
3. *Disturbed sleep pattern* related to biochemical alterations (decreased serotonin), lack of activity, and anxiety.
4. *Risk for injury: self-directed,* related to depressed mood, feelings of worthlessness and hopelessness, and verbalization of suicidal ideation or plan. Further, making small superficial cuts in wrists is also a cause for concern.
5. *Risk for use of drugs or alcohol* related to attempts to modulate mood.

Outcome Identification

1. The child will express positive feelings about self and will display more self-confidence.
2. The child will interact appropriately with others.
3. The child will demonstrate less withdrawn behavior and will be less socially isolated.
4. The child will verbalize improved sleep patterns and will be free of signs of sleep deprivation (irritability, lethargy).
5. The child will remain safe, free from self-inflicted harm, and will not engage in high risk activities.

Planning and Implementation

A major focus for nursing intervention is education of the child and family about the disorder and treatment. This not only enhances their understanding but can also improve compliance with therapy. Because mood disorders do increase the risk of suicide, any suicidal ideation or behavior should be taken seriously and appropriate action taken. Caretakers will need to be educated on the signs and symptoms of suicide and ensure that they are aware of the actions to be taken should the child become more symptomatic. Because medication does not work immediately, children will need to be closely observed and monitored in the home setting. Because of the high incidence of depressive disorders in first-degree relatives of the child with MDD, family education can be an integral component of improving the individual's environment and support structure by allowing for the treatment of the whole family. This education should occur within the child's community as well, especially the school, to provide improved support in all settings.

Caregivers need to know that SSRIs usually take several weeks before the child will feel less depressed. The nurse instructs the child and caregivers about the possible side effects such as agitation, nausea, increased anxiety, insomnia, and changes in appetite. Depression in children and adolescents is often unrecognized and unnoticed; therefore, an important nursing function is the recognition of depression and suicidal ideation.

EVALUATION

Evaluation of nursing interventions for the depressed child may be facilitated by gathering information using the following types of questions: Is the child able to express being less sad? Does the child express positive aspects of self and feelings of worthiness? Does the child resume normal sleeping patterns? Does the child seem interested in others? Is the child seeking out interaction with others? Has self-harm to the child been avoided? Has the child's academic performance improved?

BOX 35-2
SLEEP HYGIENE AND DEPRESSION

Since sleep problems occur with depression in children and adolescents, caretakers need to understand how to support sleep.

1. Use the bedroom and bed for sleeping only: do not watch TV or play video games.
2. Limit caffeine and soft drinks during the day and excessive fluids before bedtime.
3. Do not try to catch up with a night of lost sleep by putting a child to sleep earlier the next night.
4. Have a regularly scheduled sleep routine including preparation for bed with bathing, showering, calming the environment, and settling into bed on time.
5. A small glass of warm milk helps to promote sleep.
6. Regular daily physical exercise helps promote sleep.
7. Try to avoid napping during the day so that the child is tired at bedtime.
8. Ensure that adolescents are getting enough sleep and not staying awake after the rest of the family is asleep.
9. Alert the health care practitioner that sleep problems are persisting and may need further intervention.

Perlis, M. L., Jungquist, C., Smith, N. T., & Posner, D. (2008) *Cognitive behavioral treatment for insomnia*. New York: Springer.

FAMILY TEACHING

Depression is an illness, not a weakness and has its origin in both genetic and environmental factors. Caretakers need to be educated to recognize signs and symptoms of depression. Family dysfunction is a risk factor for depression; therefore, the nurse works with the family to improve their overall functioning. Interventions with the family focus on their willingness to participate in therapy and the importance of following planned interventions in the home. The family needs to be able to assess the child's risk to himself or herself and take appropriate action to ensure that the child is safe. The cultural and ethnic backgrounds of the family need to be considered in the intervention strategies and may need additional resources to ensure that the child is safe.

SUICIDE

Suicide is the intentional or purposeful taking of one's own life. It is the ultimate act of self-destruction. Suicide may be completed, attempted, or **suicidal ideation** (thoughts about killing oneself). Because mood disorders increase the risk of suicide, any suicidal behavior is a matter of serious concern.

INCIDENCE, ETIOLOGY, AND PATHOPHYSIOLOGY

While completed suicide is relatively rare in children, the incidence of suicide attempts reaches a peak during mid-adolescent years. Mortality from suicide, which increases steadily through the teens, is the third leading cause of death in 10- to 19-year-olds. The suicide rate among US youth younger than 20 years increased by 18% from 2003 to 2004 (the largest change in the past 15 years) (Centers for Disease Control and Prevention, 2007). Suicide represents 4500 lives lost each year. In a nationwide survey of grades 9 to 12 in the US, 15% of students reported seriously considering suicide, 11% reported having a plan to carry out the event, and 7% reported that they tried to take their own life in the previous 12 months (CDC, 2008). The Center for Disease Control and Prevention (2007) reports that an average of 11.3 suicide deaths per day occurs in youth 15 to 24 years of age. The methods of suicide changed substantially. Suicides by firearms declined, whereas deaths by suffocation (mostly hanging) increased (CDC, 2008).

Suicide affects adolescents of all races and socioeconomic groups, yet some groups have higher rates than others. Native American males have the highest rates; African American females have the lowest. Gay and bisexual individuals have rates of attempting suicide three times higher than other adolescents. Females are three times as likely to attempt suicide, whereas males are three times as likely to succeed in their attempts. Firearms are the leading cause of death for males and females committing suicide and are used in more than

67% of all suicides. Firearms are the most common method used among those who attempt suicide (CDC, 2007),

Stresses related to psychosocial, psychosexual, and physiological issues have been identified as causes for the increasing number of suicides. Alcohol use, access to firearms, influence of the internet, higher rates of untreated depression and adolescents serving in the military are all possible causes of the increase (Bridge, Greenhouse, Weldon, Campo, & Kelleher, 2008). Children and adolescents at higher risk for suicide typically have a history of depression, have previous suicide attempts, a family history of psychiatric disorders (depression and suicidal behavior), family disruption, substance abuse, a chronic or debilitating physical disorder, history of physical or sexual abuse, a recent relationship breakup, and gender identity issues (Greydanus & Calles, 2007). A significant increase in suicides is being observed among adolescents suffering from asthma (Katon et al., 2007).

DIAGNOSIS

The suicide-risk diagnosis is made when certain warning signs are present (Box 35-3). Many suicidal children and adolescents have experienced the warning signs for at least a month before the suicide or attempt. Days or weeks of loneliness usually precede the attempt due to the loss of the few remaining relationships.

NURSING TIP

Interviewing an Adolescent

Many times adolescents will not share their feelings directly with caretakers or other professionals especially when it relates to hurting themselves. Nurses must assess adolescents who appear depressed or irritable, or display other behaviors that would place then at risk for suicide. The best method to assess for suicidal ideation is to directly ask the adolescent, "Have you ever thought about killing yourself or wished you were dead"? The best place to ask the question is in the middle or end of a list of questions about feeling depressed. Regardless of the answer to the first question, the second question should be, "Have you ever done anything on purpose to hurt or kill yourself?' If the response to either of these questions is yes, the adolescent needs to be referred for an immediate mental health evaluation. Options for an immediate evaluation include hospitalization, transfer to the emergency department, or an appointment with a mental health professional that same day.

Reference: Shain, B., and the Committee on Adolescents. (2007). Suicide and suicide attempts in adolescents. *Pediatrics*, *120*(3), 669–676.

BOX 35-3
WARNING SIGNS OF SUICIDE

- Major life changes such as death of a family member or friend (especially by suicide), separation or divorce, and loss of financial security
- Serious conflict with caretakers
- Suicidal clues (giving away possessions, writing or talking about death, suicide, or self-harm)
- Decreased performance in school or work
- Accident proneness
- Mood swings
- Withdrawal from family and friends
- Increase in alcohol or drug use
- Change in appetite
- Loss of interest in personal appearance

TREATMENT

Children and adolescents who are at high risk for suicide have a well-thought-out plan that includes the method, place, time, clear intent, and no rescue plan. The degree of intent is related to the lethality of the method. Use of a firearm has a high degree of lethality, whereas taking pills in the presence of friends is considered a low risk because there is a good chance of rescue. For those who are at high risk or have previously attempted suicide, evaluation by a mental health professional should be performed immediately. This can be obtained in a hospital, an emergency department, or via an appointment the same day with a professional. The safest course of action is hospitalization in which a safe, protected environment can be provided (Box 35-4). The individual can have a thorough medical and psychiatric evaluation, and therapy can be initiated. Those who are not at high risk should be followed up closely or referred for a psychological or mental health evaluation.

NURSING ALERT

The Decision to Commit Suicide

A sudden change in affect for the better or a dramatic lifting of depression may be an indication that the individual has resolved the ambivalence about living or dying and has made the decision to commit suicide. Increased energy and the ability to concentrate and plan facilitate the suicidal actions.

NURSING MANAGEMENT

Assessment of clients at risk for suicide includes gathering information about individual and family history of depression and suicide attempts, mood changes, cognitive changes including suicidal ideation, expression of feelings of despondency and hopelessness, and behavioral or social changes. Obtaining information from caregivers and significant others in the child's social and support systems is essential. Physical assessment for health problems and changes in sleeping and eating patterns are also part of the assessment. Children and adolescents with high risk behaviors and high risk factors should be asked about suicide. Inquiring about suicide does not precipitate the behavior, as is commonly believed. In fact, most individuals are relieved that someone has heard and recognized their cry for help. One approach to this process is to ask a general question such as "Have you ever been so depressed or sad that you thought about killing yourself or wished you were dead?" (Shain & Committee on Adolescents, 2007). If the answer is yes, the nurse should ask about the suicide plan (method, time, and place), availability of the means (gun, rope, and medication), lethality of the means, the individual's support system, and coping resources. Younger children are also at risk for self-harm behaviors and may exhibit behaviors such as somatic complaints (stomach aches, headaches).

Nursing management focuses on the safety of the child and all family members. Threats or gestures to hurt oneself are always taken seriously regardless of the child's developmental age. Interventions are on the primary, secondary, or tertiary level. The focus of the interventions is to keep the child safe and provide the least restrictive setting possible.

Primary interventions include activities that provide support, information, and education. At the primary level the nurse can offer educational programs for children and their caregivers that focus on parenting, development of coping skills, normal growth and development, and risk factors. Caregivers need to be taught to identify risk factors and symptoms of depression. The school nurse and counselor can be instrumental in the development of programs that focus on strengthening children's awareness of their feelings,

RESEARCH Highlight

Suicide and Access to Firearms

STUDY PURPOSE

To determine whether there was a difference in an adolescent's household access to firearms between those who did commit suicide and those who did not.

METHODS

A case-control design was used to compare 36 adolescents who committed suicide using firearms with an equal number of adolescents matched for age and sex. Controls were randomly selected from the same schools attended by the adolescents who committed suicide. Study participants were an average of 15 years of age, and 75% were males. Data were collected by telephone interview with caregivers of both groups.

FINDINGS

The majority (67%) of those who committed suicide used a gun (handgun 42%; rifle 46%) obtained from their homes. The majority of these guns were not in locked storage. Those who committed suicide were significantly more likely than controls not to attend school and to be the only child in the family. Past mental health problems and conduct disorder were found as independent risk factors associated with those who committed suicide with guns.

IMPLICATIONS

Findings from this research suggest that public health interventions should be instituted to limit household access to firearms and to identify those at risk for this type of suicide. Although previous suicide attempts were not measured in this study, it is important for nurses and health care providers working in emergency departments to discuss access to firearms with caregivers of any adolescent treated for attempted suicide. It is also important for school nurses to follow up by implementing suicide prevention with adolescents who have a history of mental health problems or conduct disorder.

REFERENCE

Shain, B., and the Committee on Adolescents (2007). Suicide and suicide attempts in adolescents. *Pediatrics*, *120*(3), 669–676.

Grossman et al. (2005). Gun storage practices and risk of youth suicide and unintentional firearm injuries. *Journal of the American Medical Association*, *293*(6), 707–714.

BOX 35-4
REASONS FOR HOSPITALIZING A CHILD OR ADOLESCENT FOR SUICIDAL BEHAVIORS

- Inadequate home care and supervision
- Agitated behaviors or history of aggressive behaviors
- Mania
- Intoxicated state or substance use
- Actively psychotic
- Positive family history for a completed suicide
- Male gender
- Prior attempts

Greydanus, D. E., and Calles, Jr., J. (2007). Suicide in children and adolescents. *Primary Care: Clinics in Office Practice*, *34*(2), 259–273.

building self-esteem, and enhancing coping skills. Secondary interventions involve the treatment of the actual suicidal crisis. Key elements in the success of any treatment modality include: establishing a personal relationship with the suicidal child or adolescent; encouraging more realistic problem-solving behavior; and reaffirming hope for the individual.

Tertiary interventions are provided for the child or adolescent after a suicide attempt or for the family and friends of a person who has committed suicide. Self-help groups have been beneficial for the survivors of the youth who has committed suicide. Nurses working with clients who successfully commit suicide need the opportunity to work through their own feelings of self-blame, grief, and guilt. Debriefing sessions and support groups may be a routine part of work environments to support nurses after a client successfully commits suicide.

FAMILY TEACHING

Caregivers' ability to identify behaviors associated with depression and anxiety disorders decreases the risk of a successful suicide for the child. Therefore, educational programs focusing on suicide and risk factors can be part of family educational programs offered by community-based nurses. Family dysfunction is correlated with depression and suicide. Social service programs that improve family functioning for the at-risk family will improve the outlook for the at-risk child.

Caretakers must also be aware that children and adolescents can engage in self-harming behaviors such as self-mutilation. Self-mutilation behavior, such as self-cutting, is associated with an indication of psychological distress and sexual risk taking behaviors. Self-cutting may represent a child and adolescent's difficulty with managing their strong emotions. Self-cutting is a mechanism used to reduce tension or anxiety, helps with expressing their distress or directs their impulsive behaviors. Adolescents may select to self-cut in private and others engage in these behaviors with friends. Research has indicated that these adolescents may be at risk for HIV infection because they may share cutting instruments (Brown, Houck, Grossman, Lescano, & Frenkel, 2008).

ANXIETY DISORDERS

The child growing up in today's world deals with complex and rapidly changing norms. Anxiety is unavoidable and can be useful in promoting growth and helping the child adapt to new experiences. However, if anxiety is overwhelming, it can result in psychosocial alterations. Anxiety is a sense of apprehension or uneasiness caused by uncertain, nonspecific danger or threat. The child may cope with anxiety or fear by becoming overly dependent, avoiding problems, or withdrawing. Anxiety disorders are one of the prevalent categories of child and adolescent psychopathology. Included in the category of anxiety disorders are separation anxiety disorder, school phobia or refusal, generalized anxiety disorder, social phobia, obsessive-compulsive disorder, and post-traumatic stress disorder.

Separation anxiety disorder (SAD) is defined as excessive anxiety that occurs when a child is separated from home or from significant attachment figures. Such anxiety occurs as part of normal development in infants at approximately 8–12 months of age and disappears by 2 years of age. However, when symptoms have an onset later during childhood, and they become excessive to the point of impairing functioning, a disorder is diagnosed.

A form of separation anxiety is school phobia or refusal, which is defined as difficulty attending or remaining in school for an entire day, associated with emotional distress, especially anxiety and depression (Khalid-Khan, Santibanez, McMicken, & Rynn, 2007). Children who refuse to attend school are generally suffering from separation anxiety rather than a true phobia. The caregivers often have ambivalent feelings about their child's attendance, which contributes to their ineffectiveness in helping to return the child to school.

Generalized anxiety disorder (GAD), is characterized by excessive worry and anxiety about future events, such as academic or athletic performance, being on time, or natural disasters (hurricanes, earthquakes). These children and adolescents worry even when school and social successes demonstrate that they have nothing substantive to be concerned about. They are often labeled as "worriers." These children are often perfectionists and seek constant reassurance that they have done well.

Children with social phobia either avoid or endure with significant distress social or performance situations in which they anticipate scrutiny by others, embarrassment, and humiliation (Khalid-Khan et al., 2007). For some children anxiety can be provoked by nonjudgmental situations such as simple conversation or even eating in public. These children have fear of participating in classroom activities, engaging in a conversation with peers and adults and participating in normal types of social and school activities.

Obsessive-compulsive disorder (OCD) is characterized by recurrent, intrusive, unwanted thoughts called obsessions (e.g., fears of contamination) or compulsive behaviors or rituals such as repetitive handwashing, finger or hair picking. These thoughts or behaviors are acknowledged as unreasonable and are accompanied by distress. The child may have either obsessions or compulsions, although most have both. It is considered a chronic and debilitating condition that can co-exist with other psychological problems such as Tourette disorder, body image problems and impulse control disorders. Family studies have found that there is greater risk for anxiety and depression among these children (Barrett, Farrell, Pina, Peris, & Piacentini, 2008).

INCIDENCE, ETIOLOGY, AND PATHOPHYSIOLOGY

The prevalence of GAD ranges from 10% to 20% (Costello, Egger, & Angold, 2004) and the disorder manifests at anytime from 5 to 16 years of age, with a mean age of 9 years. The incidence decreases with age. School refusal occurs in approximately 5% of all school-age children, tends to be equally common in boys and girls, and can occur throughout the entire range of school years. However, the disorder peaks at certain ages (between 5–6 years and 10–11 years) and certain transition points in the child's life. The onset of social phobia most commonly occurs in early to mid-adolescence, and similar numbers of males and females develop the disorder. Individuals with social phobia have a high incidence of concurrent anxiety and mood disorders. Social phobia is more prevalent in girls than boys and in Caucasian children from middle- and upper-class families. Five per 1,000 children are affected by OCD. The etiology is unknown. Hypotheses suggest it may be the result of an interaction between the amygdala and the prefrontal cortex and the processing of sensory information. There is also evidence of the dysfunction of the HPA axis, altering cortisol levels and changes in the neurotransmitter, glutamate levels in the brain (Matthew, Price, & Charney, 2008).

The cause of anxiety disorders is not known. Environmental as well as biological factors have been suggested. More research is needed to determine the exact cause. Some researchers have suggested that between the ages of 6 and 8 children should be watched for signs of anxiety disorders because at this age they are usually less fearful of the dark and imaginary images, but may become fearful of school, social situations, and relationships.

CLINICAL MANIFESTATIONS

A child with separation anxiety disorder may exhibit complaints of stomachaches, headaches, nausea, vomiting, and low-grade fevers that occur without any underlying physiologic cause. Older children experience symptoms such as vertigo, palpitations, and faintness. These symptoms usually improve gradually as the day progresses.

School refusal behavior is a serious problem because it is often associated with significant short- and long-term consequences. Short-term problems include poor academic performance, family difficulties, and peer relationship problems. Long-term sequelae may include fewer opportunities to attend institutions of higher learning, employment problems, social difficulties, and increased risk for later psychiatric illnesses (Khalid-Khan et al., 2007). Clinical manifestations may also include frequent somatic complaints in the absence of a physical condition (stomachache, headache, dizziness, and fatigue), sleep difficulties, morning tantrums, and marked distress on school days.

In addition to excessive worry and anxiety about future events, the clinical manifestations of generalized anxiety disorder include:

- Restlessness
- Fatigue
- Difficulty concentrating
- Irritability
- Sleep disturbances
- Muscle tension

Children with social phobia experience feelings of anxiety, which can often produce physical reactions such as tremors, palpitations, sweating, diarrhea, and blushing. They may exhibit their fears by crying or staying in close proximity to familiar adults. They often appear very shy and often are found to be on the periphery of social situations, for example, not participating at birthday parties. The symptoms may interfere with class performance and social activities. If the onset is in childhood, it may lead to a failure to achieve, and adolescents may experience a decline in functioning.

Table 35-1 Common OCD Behaviors

COMMON OBSESSIONS	COMMON COMPULSIONS
Contamination/cleanliness thoughts	Washing
Aggressive thoughts	Repeating
Thoughts of harm coming to self or others	Checking, counting, ordering
Urges for symmetry	Touching

The clinical manifestations of OCD include obsessions (recurrent, persistent thoughts) characterized by four criteria: (1) they are experienced as intrusive and inappropriate and cause marked anxiety and distress; (2) they are not simply worries about real-life problems; (3) attempts are made to ignore obsessions or neutralize them with some other thought or actions; (4) the person recognizes the obsession as a product of his or her own mind, rather than imposed from outside as in thought insertion.

The compulsive behaviors take place in response to obsessions or rigid rules. Compulsive behaviors are aimed at reducing distress or preventing a dreaded event. They are clearly excessive or unconnected in a realistic way with the event they are trying to neutralize (Table 35-1).

DIAGNOSIS

The diagnosis is made if excessive anxiety or worry dominates the child's thoughts and begins to interfere with the ability to function and perform regular activities. Inquiry about anxiety symptoms should be a standard part of a diagnostic interview regardless of the presenting problem. Often these symptoms will not be elicited unless specifically asked about. Caregivers should be asked about the child's verbal expressions of fear or worry and signs of anxiety such as sweating, hyperventilation, and somatic complaints. A family history of anxiety and mood disorders and other psychiatric conditions should be obtained. The developmental and social history needs to be detailed enough to give the examiner a sense of the child's usual style of coping with stress in general and anxiety provoking situations in particular. The caregivers' coping styles should also be assessed.

TREATMENT

The broad goals of treatment are: (1) to reduce the symptoms and relieve distress; (2) to minimize the disability associated with the disorder; and (3) to enhance the developmental potential of the child or adolescent. Although anxiety disorders are relatively common in children and adolescents, there has been little definitive research on the efficacy of psychotherapy. The treatment usually involves a variety of approaches, including education of the individual and caregivers about the disorder, consultation with school personnel, cognitive behavioral interventions, individual and family psychotherapy, and pharmacological therapy. Treatment approaches are individualized for the child and the specific disorder. Family therapy allows the family to gain insight into the dynamics of the disorder. Cognitive, supportive, and behavioral psychotherapy have been used with varying degrees of success. Individual therapy is used to address the specific problems the child or adolescent experiences. For the child with school refusal the goal of therapy is to return the child to school as soon as possible. Cognitive techniques such as desensitization and operant conditioning are treatment methods used for this purpose.

Psychotropic drugs should not be used as a sole intervention, but as an adjunct to psychotherapeutic interventions. Commonly used medications include the antidepressants (tricyclics and SSRIs) and the benzodiazepines or antianxiety drugs. The benzodiazepines such as lorazepam (Atavan) or diazepam (Valium) may be used on a short-term basis for the anxiety symptoms or sleep disturbances (Khalid-Khan et al., 2007).

NURSING MANAGEMENT

Assessment

A school nurse may be the person who identifies patterns of absenteeism or tardiness in attendance. Calling caregivers to inform them and discuss the patterns may give them an opportunity to discuss their concerns about the child's fear of school. A child with school phobia or refusal will present with frequent complaints of illness, especially of stomachaches early in the morning, which go away as the day progresses. Well-child visits to the care providers are another avenue where the nurse may be available to listen to a caregiver's concerns about the child's anxiety about school or other anxious situations.

Nursing Diagnosis

Nursing diagnoses for children experiencing anxiety disorders may include the following:

1. *Fear* related to separation from caregiver and social or performance situations.
2. *Impaired social interaction* related to inability to interact with unfamiliar people and insufficient contact with peers.
3. *Ineffective individual coping* related to perception of the situation and changes in personal and family life.

Outcome Identification

1. The child will be able to experience normal developmental situations (staying overnight at a friend's house, attending camp) with minimal anxiety.
2. The child will attend school and experience minimal or no anxiety.
3. The child will initiate social interactions with peers.
4. The child will cope effectively with anxiety.
5. The child will use relaxation, deep breathing techniques, and self-talk to control anxiety.

Planning and Implementation

The family of the child with an anxiety disorder should be included in every aspect of the care. Caregivers provide important historical information about the child and give insight into the working of the family unit. They are involved in the implementation of the treatment plan; therefore, compliance depends on their cooperation. The nurse can assist the child in identifying sources of anxiety and tensions, and environmental factors that create a feeling of anxiety. Nurses should teach caregivers to recognize that a change in school performance may indicate anxiety. The child should be helped to identify alternative outlets for anxiety such as sports, running, climbing, and group games. Stress reduction, imagery, and deep breathing are other strategies to integrate into the intervention plan. The nurse can assist caregivers in exploring ways in which they reinforce dependent behavior in the child and in adopting alternative patterns of behavior. Teaching the child and caregivers to monitor the effectiveness and side effects of psychotropic drugs is also an important part of the nurse's role.

Evaluation

Is the child able to attend school and be successful in academic and social activities during school hours? Does the child participate in social activities, such as visits to a friend's home, "sleepovers," and camp? Is the child able to recognize feelings of anxiety and use techniques that help control the feelings? Are caregivers knowledgeable about normal developmental milestones and are their expectations of the child realistic? Can caregivers provide support and implement cognitive strategies to support their child's success both socially and academically?

FAMILY TEACHING

Changing family structure and contemporary culture contribute to the stress of childhood, and caregivers serve as protectors and teachers for their children. Parenting skills that reinforce adaptive behaviors and provide positive role models for children are critical. Limit-setting skills are complex, and even the most skilled caregivers need guidance. They also need to learn functional coping behaviors if they hope to guide and influence their children positively.

POST-TRAUMATIC STRESS DISORDER

Post-traumatic stress disorder (PTSD) is an anxiety disorder characterized by a constellation of symptoms and psychological reactions that follows an extreme or life-threatening traumatic event. The trauma can be the result of a single event that is abrupt, often lasting a few minutes and as long as a few hours, or chronic, repeated, and ongoing events such as physical and sexual child abuse.

INCIDENCE AND ETIOLOGY

The incidence rates of PTSD for children are reported as 1–2%. Traumatic events capable of causing PTSD fall into three categories:

1. Natural disasters—tornadoes, floods, hurricanes, earthquakes
2. Accidental disasters—automobile, train, and airplane accidents, fires, explosions, nuclear plant accidents
3. Intentional human-made disasters—combat, bombings, rape, armed robbery, assault, physical and sexual abuse (Kessler, 2000)

CLINICAL MANIFESTATIONS

The hallmark symptoms of PTSD are re-experiencing the trauma, avoidance of stimuli associated with the event and numbing of general responsiveness, and increased states of arousal. Re-experiencing symptoms include recurrent, intrusive, unwanted thoughts, dreams, and nightmares related to the traumatic experience. In young children this symptom may be manifested by repetitive play in which the traumatic themes occur. Avoidance symptoms involve physical avoidance of situations that resemble the traumatic event, efforts to avoid thoughts, feelings, or conversations associated with the trauma, and numbing of responsiveness to the outside world (diminished interest in normal activities, restriction of emotions). Increased arousal states are exemplified by hypervigilance, an exaggerated startle response, sleep difficulties, and irritable or angry outbursts. These symptoms must be present for more than one month and cause significant impairment in daily functioning.

DIAGNOSIS

A comprehensive clinical interview with the child and caregivers is a primary assessment tool in the evaluation of PTSD. Both the child and caregivers should be asked directly about the traumatic event and re-experiencing, avoidant, and hyperarousal symptoms. Teachers should also be questioned about behavior changes in the child and the time these changes began. Although there are several questionnaires and semi-structured interviews that purport to measure this disorder, there is no single instrument accepted as a "gold standard" in making the diagnosis.

TREATMENT

The cornerstone of treatment for PTSD is the education of the child and family regarding the nature of the disorder so that the child's symptoms are not mistakenly viewed as "crazy" or "manipulative." Essential components of treatment include: (1) direct exploration of the trauma; (2) use of stress management techniques; (3) exploration and correction of inaccurate attributions regarding the event; and (4) inclusion of caregivers. Direct exploration of the traumatic experience and its meaning to and impact on the child is crucial. Stress management techniques such as muscle relaxation, positive imagery, and deep breathing frequently are used in conjunction with direct discussion of the event. This intervention enables the child to gain a sense of control over thoughts and feelings instead of being overwhelmed by them. The child can then directly discuss the trauma with diminished hyperarousal and negative feelings states through relaxation and desensitization procedures. The third element of treatment is exploration of attributional distortions such as "It was my fault," or "Nothing is safe anymore." These attributions should be challenged by step-by-step logical analysis of the child's cognitive distortions during therapy. Caregivers should be included in treatment because they can provide support, monitor the child's symptoms, and learn appropriate behavioral management techniques.

Despite a lack of systematic research of pharmacologic therapy for children with PTSD, clinicians have prescribed a variety of medications. However, medications should be considered as an adjunct to treatment, not the sole mode of therapy. SSRIs are generally used as the first-line drugs when medication is required. Medication should be considered when symptoms are severe, functioning is very impaired, or when symptoms persist despite active psychotherapy.

NURSING MANAGEMENT

It is important for the nurse to establish a trusting relationship with the child, to offer reassurance of safety and security, and to explain that the symptoms are not uncommon following a trauma of the magnitude she or he has experienced. Resolution of the post-trauma response is largely dependent on the effectiveness of the coping strategies and social support. Therefore, the nurse should discuss with the child coping strategies used in response to the trauma, as well as those used during stressful situations in the past, and together determine the most helpful. Guilt at having survived a trauma in which others have died is common.

The child needs to discuss these feelings and recognize that he or she is not responsible for what happened. It is important to assess the impact of the trauma on the child's ability to resume activities of daily living. The child should be assessed for self-destructive ideas and behavior as the trauma may result in feelings of hopelessness and worthlessness, leading to high risk for suicide. The child and family may need to be referred to community resources such as support groups for victims of trauma during the recovery process.

SUBSTANCE ABUSE

Substance use is a precursor to dependence or abuse, and regular use increases the risk of developing a substance use disorder (SUD). SUD encompasses both substance abuse and substance dependence. **Substance abuse** is a maladaptive pattern of substance use leading to significant distress or impairment (APA, 2000). In children and adolescents the impairment is usually in psychosocial and academic functioning. Substance abuse is further manifested by recurrent substance use in situations in which it is physically hazardous (driving an automobile while impaired); recurrent substance-related legal problems; and continued substance use although the individual is having persistent social or interpersonal problems. **Substance dependence** involves a substantial degree of involvement with a substance, including withdrawal (adverse physical symptoms due to cessation of or reduction in prolonged and heavy substance use); tolerance (a need for increased amounts of the substance to achieve the desired effect); and loss of control over use (efforts to cut down use are unsuccessful) (APA, 2000). Substances that are used and abused by preadolescents and adolescents include alcohol, tobacco, marijuana, opiates, cocaine, amphetamines, barbiturates, hallucinogens, and inhalants (Box 35-5).

BOX 35-5
ECSTASY

Methylenedioxymethamphetamine (MDMA) is the drug known as Ecstasy, also referred to as *XTC, Adam,* and *the love drug.* MDMA is both a CNS stimulant and hallucinogenic. According to users, MDMA replaces anxiety and depression with feelings of pleasure. According to the Partnership for a Drug-Free America, MDMA use has doubled among the teenage population since 1995, and one in 10 adolescents has experimented with the drug. It is often used in combination with LSD. The rate of emergency room visits for complications of use and overdose of this drug is on the rise.

Adapted from Broyles, B., Reiss, B., & Evans, M. (2007). *Pharmacological aspects of nursing care* (7th ed.). Clifton Park, NY: Delmar Cengage learning.

RESEARCH Highlight

Prospective Study of Adolescent Drug Use among Community Samples of ADHD and Non-ADHD Participants

STUDY PURPOSE

To describe the late adolescent drug use outcomes from a relatively large, community-identified sample of children with attention-deficit hyperactivity disorder (ADHD) who have been assessed longitudinally from childhood through late adolescence.

METHODS

Adolescent drug use outcomes were compared between ADHD-only (n = 27), ADHD externalizing (mostly oppositional defiant disorder) (n = 82), and normal control (n = 91) groups.

FINDINGS

The ADHD externalizing group revealed significantly worse drug use outcomes (drug use frequency and substance use disorders) compared to the other two groups, and the ADHD-only group showed outcomes comparable to the community control group. The present prospective longitudinal study found increased rates of drug use among a community-derived sample of children diagnosed with childhood ADHD and followed into the late adolescent years compared with a sample of community controls. These findings were true regardless of whether the drug use outcomes were assessed as categorical or continuous variables. However, increased rates were found only in children in whom ADHD was comorbid with another early-onset externalizing disorder (ODD/CD). No differences were observed between a group with childhood ADHD-only and controls.

IMPLICATIONS

The ADHD-externalizing group showed elevated rates of alcohol use disorder, marijuana use disorder, two or more SUDs, and tobacco use (measured in terms of ever used or frequency of use). The data suggest that there is a relationship between adolescents with ADHD and other behavioral problems such as oppositional defiant disorders and conduct disorders and substance use. Adolescents who meet these criteria should be carefully screened and treatment for behavioral problems initiated.

REFERENCE

August, G. J. et al. (2006). Prospective study of adolescent drug use among community samples of ADHD and non-ADHD participants. *Journal of American Academy of Child & Adolescent Psychiatry, 45*(7), 824–832.

INCIDENCE AND ETIOLOGY

There are two national surveys conducted by agencies of the federal government that provide regularly updated data on substance abuse in youth. One is the National Institute on Drug Abuse (NIDA)-sponsored *Monitoring the Future* survey, an ongoing study of the behaviors, attitudes, and values of American secondary school students, college students, and young adults (Johnston, O'Malley, & Bachman, 2003). Each year, approximately 50,000 8th-, 10th-, and 12th-grade students are surveyed. The second survey is the National Household Survey on Drug Abuse (NHSDA) conducted by the Substance Abuse and Mental Health Services Administration (SAMHSA, 2008). It uses an interactive, computer-based questionnaire to provide annual reports on the prevalence, patterns, and consequences of drug and alcohol use and abuse in the general U.S. civilian population ages 12 years and older.

In 2007, rates of past month illicit drug use varied with age. Through the adolescent years (12 to 17), the rates of current illicit drug use increased from 3.3% at ages 12–13 to 8.9% at ages 14–15 to 16.0% at ages 16–17. From 2002 to 2007, however, the rate of current illicit drug use among 12 to 17 year olds decreased from 11.6 to 9.5%. In 2007, 9.5% of youths aged 12 to 17 were current illicit drug users. Among this cohort (12 to 17), 6.7% used marijuana, 3.3% engaged in nonmedical use of prescription-type psychotherapeutics, 1.2% used inhalants, 0.7% used hallucinogens, and 0.4% used cocaine (SAMSHA, 2008). More than half of American young people have tried an illicit drug (marijuana/hashish, cocaine, crack, heroin, hallucinogens, inhalants, or prescription type psychotherapeutics). The use of alcohol and nicotine is even more common. Cigarette smoking and inhalant use have continued to decline since the late 1990s. Use of alcohol and marijuana remain relatively constant. The use of heroin has begun to decline after years of increase, due largely to the use by smoking or snorting rather than injection.

There are multiple theories concerning causes of substance abuse and SUD that include (Shain & the Committee on Adolescents, 2007):

- Genetic factors—twin and adoption studies point to the probable contribution of genetic or constitutional factors to the risk for SUDs.
- Family factors—caregiver substance use; their beliefs, attitudes, and tolerance of substance use; dysfunctional family relationships (e.g., lack of closeness, neglect, lack of supervision); poor parenting skills.
- Peer influence—peer network substance use; peer pressure; peer attitudes; desire to be "in the mainstream"; feeling inadequate because of social or cultural group.
- Individual factors—early antisocial behavior; poor academic performance and school failure; ineffective coping skills; psychiatric conditions (e.g., ADHD, depression, conduct disorder); low self-esteem.
- Community or neighborhood factors—low socioeconomic status; high crime; high population density; gang opportunities.
- Media factors—advertising that links drinking and drug use with highly valued personal attributes.

CLINICAL MANIFESTATIONS AND PATHOPHYSIOLOGY

Generally all drugs involve alterations in sensorium as well as other physiological and psychological alterations that become more significant as the amount and frequency of usage increases. Clinical manifestations will vary depending on the type of substance used and the age and weight of the child.

Central nervous system depressants such as alcohol, barbiturates, and nonbarbiturate sedatives produce states that range from calmness and drowsiness to delirium and coma. Physiological alterations include cardiac and respiratory depression, hyperthermia, coma, and death. Alcohol decreases inhibitions and causes relaxation and slurred speech. Toxicity leads to lack of coordination, impaired judgment, accidents, respiratory depression, coma, and death. Opiates create a feeling of euphoria or analgesia. Toxicity leads to respiratory depression, cerebral edema, and death.

Central nervous system stimulants such as amphetamines create a feeling of well-being or euphoria. Toxicity leads to hypertension, hyperthermia, convulsions, cardiovascular shock, and death. Hallucinogens alter perceptions, thoughts, and feelings. Side effects include convulsions and cardiovascular collapse. Suicide, fatal accidents, and homicide often occur secondary to paranoid delusions, hallucinations, psychosis, and flashbacks. Effects of marijuana include

KIDS WANT TO KNOW

How intoxicating are different types of alcohol?

I overheard my older brother and his friends talking about alcohol yesterday. By the way, he is in college. They were saying that beer has less alcohol than wine or "hard" liquor like vodka or bourbon, so you can drink more of it before you get "drunk." Is this true?

You should explain that a 12-ounce can or bottle of beer, an 8-ounce glass of wine, and a 1.5-ounce glass of liquor all have about the same alcohol content. When a person drinks one of any of these, it is enough to impair judgment and reflexes and interfere with driving.

feelings of unreality, distorted sense of time, and perceptual distortions. Side effects range from hallucinations to tachycardia, decreased motor skills, impaired memory, and chronic bronchitis. Inhalants create feelings of euphoria and excitement. Side effects include ataxia, stupor, seizures, and cardiac and respiratory arrest.

TREATMENT

Treatment varies depending on the substance being abused, the willingness of the child and family to cooperate with treatment, the age of the client, and the availability of treatment modalities. Broad treatment goals include the elimination of substance abuse and any accompanying undesirable behaviors and restoration of the child to a healthy functional status. Individuals with substance abuse should be treated in the least restrictive setting that is safe and effective. Treatment settings can range from inpatient (hospital-based or free-standing rehabilitation center); residential; partial-hospitalization or day treatment; and outpatient. Children who require inpatient treatment include: (1) those with severe psychiatric disorders, symptoms, or behaviors (acute psychosis, suicidal, homicidal, or other acutely dangerous behavior); (2) those with a history of treatment failure in less restrictive programs; and (3) those at risk for substance use withdrawal or with a history of withdrawal problems. Because family dysfunction is frequently a factor in the etiology of the problem, family-based treatment programs and family participation are essential.

Pharmacotherapy may also be used for treating withdrawal effects and other psychiatric disorders. Although significant symptoms of withdrawal from substances are rare in children, the treatment should proceed as for adults.

Self-help or peer-support groups such as Alcoholics Anonymous (AA) and Narcotics Anonymous (NA) are important adjuncts to the treatment program. These groups are thought to be an essential element in the recovery process and help prevent relapse. Members meet and support each other in dealing with their substance abuse problems. The programs offer suggestions for a way of living without the use of substances. Both AA and NA are nonprofessional, multicultural, nondenominational, and apolitical and are located in communities throughout the world. Several reports conclude that AA or NA have a high success rate secondary to group support and one-on-one interactions between the sponsor and the affected individual.

DIAGNOSIS

The first goal of assessment for suspected substance abuse is to determine whether a problem of using substances exists. A physical examination is performed to identify signs and symptoms that may indicate a substance use problem, such as bloodshot eyes, weight loss, nasal irritation, slurred speech, abnormal pupil constriction or dilation, and increase in accidents and injuries. Because of the covert nature of substance abuse, information should be gathered from a variety of sources, such as the child or adolescent, caregivers, other family members, peers, and school personnel. A comprehensive developmental, social, academic, and medical history is part of a complete assessment. Information is gathered about the child or adolescent's substance use behavior. The health care provider needs to determine the effect of the substance use on various areas of the individual's life and psychosocial functioning. It is also essential to ascertain if associated problems, such as mood disorders or antisocial behavior, are present and what family and environmental stressors exist. Substance abuse is differentiated from social drinking or nonpathological substance use by the presence of compulsive use, craving, or substance related problems.

NURSING MANAGEMENT

Assessment of risk factors is important in identifying individuals who may be using or abusing substances. Nurses may suspect substance abuse when they observe irrational behavior; preoccupation with the occult; frequent absences from school and decline in academic performance; disinhibition, lethargy, hyperactivity or agitation, and hypervigilance; changes in personality, friends, activities, or appearance; difficulty communicating; rebelliousness; mental or physiological deterioration; unexplained loss of money; and actual substances or paraphernalia.

Substance abuse can occur in any socioeconomic family system. Children with low self-esteem, family history of substance abuse, and peer pressure often use drugs to "be cool" or to cope with social pressures; therefore, nursing management focuses on the causes of the substance abuse. Long-term counseling may be necessary to support changes in lifestyle and behaviors and address and resolve underlying issues of self-esteem and family history of abuse. The nurse must identify the precipitating problems and plan interventions to help the child or adolescent cope with these. The nurse focuses on social skills such as problem solving, self-esteem building, and values clarification.

Another important role for nurses is prevention of substance abuse, which focuses on drug education, self-awareness, decision-making abilities, and clarification of values and beliefs about substances. Prevention programs may begin as early as elementary school and include education and family involvement. Children are taught to make knowledgeable and value-based choices, ways to resist social and peer pressure, methods of improving communication with caregivers, and alternative ways to feel good about oneself without using substances. Strategies can be small group discussions and role-playing.

Interventions focus on support and reassurance for the child and the family. Changes in lifestyle and new patterns of coping with stress need to be reinforced. Self-help and

Reflections from Families

January: My family. On the outside we seem perfect. Big house, nice cars, best schools, vacations every year. On the inside, that is a different story. My mom drinks through the day, my dad avoids her at all cost and spends most of his time at work. Me? I drink alcohol and do drugs. The release I feel from my problems is tremendous. After snorting some cocaine, I feel invincible. Ecstasy helps me dance the night away.

January, one year later: My family. My mom still drinks. I am not sure what Dad does. Me? I am in jail pending conviction of running a child over while DWI. How I wish I could bring that child back. How I wish I could rewind my life and get the counseling I needed to stop my drug abuse.

support groups encourage abstinence through a framework for lifestyle and personal change. They also provide a place to learn social skills and interact with successful role models. Other nursing interventions include individual, family, and group therapy. After a short time in individual therapy, the older child is often moved to a group therapy setting because this is an excellent place to learn new behaviors and interact with others who are struggling with similar problems. Substance abuse is often a coping mechanism for living in a dysfunctional family; therefore, the interventions must focus on resolving the family problems or treatment for the substance abuse will not be successful.

EATING DISORDERS

Eating disorders such as **anorexia nervosa** (AN) and **bulimia nervosa** (BN) are common disorders encountered in children, especially adolescents. These disorders are affecting adolescents with increasing frequency and continue to be associated with serious physical complications and significant morbidity and mortality. Anorexia nervosa tends to have a chronic course and carries a high risk of mortality (Hudson, Hiripi, Pope, & Kessler, 2007).

ANOREXIA NERVOSA

Anorexia Nervosa is characterized by voluntary refusal to eat, significant weight loss, an intense fear of becoming overweight, and a pronounced disturbance of body image. The individual with AN may exclusively restrict dietary intake (restrictive subtype), or may regularly engage in binge eating or purging behaviors (i.e., self-induced vomiting or misuse of laxatives, diuretics, or enemas), binge eating, or purging subtype (APA, 2000).

INCIDENCE AND ETIOLOGY

The prevalence rates for AN is approximately 0.5–1% of adolescent females (Keel & Haedt, 2008) and 5–10% of all cases occur in males. The highest incidence is for females aged 10 through 19 years; thus, the first occurrence takes place almost exclusively during adolescence (Lewinsohn, Striegel-Moore, & Seeley, 2000).

While the exact etiology of AN is unknown, several theories offer insight into the complex nature of the disorder. Biological theory suggests that anorexic individuals suffer a disturbance in levels of neurotransmitters in the brain. Norepinephrine and its metabolites have been found to be low, but they increase to normal levels as weight is restored. However, it is not clear whether these biochemical changes are the cause or the effect of the disorder.

The psychodynamic theory suggests that deficits in ego development may predispose the young woman to AN. Appropriate ego development is necessary for the child to function separately from the family. Without encouragement for independence during the individuation-separation phase, the child does not develop autonomy and the ability to make decisions (Bruch, 1982).

Family systems theory suggests that AN is caused by intrafamilial conflicts and dysfunctional family patterns. The adolescent's eating behavior allows the family to focus on the problem of the sick child, rather than on the conflicts among the adult partners and other family members. Alliances are formed, and the child is encouraged to side with one caregiver against the other. Subsequently, this behavior allows the child some degree of control in the family.

CRITICAL THINKING

Cultural Trends and Eating Disorders

Cultural ideals of beauty have always been reflected in fashion for women. The trend in fashion since the 1960s has been increasingly toward thinness. With the media as the vehicle, adolescents are bombarded with images of the thin, fit, "perfect" woman, an ideal unattainable for most of them. Very few women have a natural body type that matches the ideal, leading most to believe that their normal, healthy shape is too fat. Many resort to excessive and unhealthy dieting to achieve this ideal body, which may lead to an eating disorder in some individuals. As a school nurse in a junior high school, what can you do to prevent adolescents from developing an eating disorder?

Clinical Manifestations and Pathophysiology

The clinical manifestations of AN include the following:

- Extreme weight loss
- Refusal to maintain body weight at or above the minimum recommended weight for age and height (weight less than 85% of that expected)
- Intense and irrational fear of gaining weight or becoming fat, although underweight
- Denial of the seriousness of the current low weight
- Distorted body image, weight, or shape, that is, seeing oneself as fat when emaciated
- Physical manifestations (amenorrhea or absence of at least three consecutive menstrual cycles, hypothermia, muscle wasting, growth of lanugo, cardiac dysrhythmias, hypotension, dry skin, brittle nails, and cold intolerance).

Diagnosis

Criteria for the diagnosis of AN includes: refusal to maintain body weight at or above a minimally normal weight for age and height; weight loss leading to maintenance of body weight at less than 85% of expected weight; intense fear of gaining weight; in the postmenarcheal female absence of at least three consecutive menstrual cycles; altered perceptions of how the body looks; and denial of the seriousness of the current body weight (APA, 2000).

Treatment

The initial goals for managing the individual with AN are overall improvement of body weight, normalization of eating patterns, and the restoration of physical health through weight gain. Until this goal is achieved, disordered thinking caused by malnutrition may inhibit the success of other therapies (Fairburn, Cooper, Shafran, & Wilson, 2008). Because the real issue is not food, but rather issues such as poor self-esteem, a need to be in control, a need for perfection and a belief in the myth of thinness and dieting, effective treatment is complex and long-term. Other goals for treatment include correction of medical complications such as fluid, electrolyte, and nutritional imbalances; improvement in personal and social functioning; improvement of family dynamics; and treatment of additional conditions (e.g., depression). Because of the limited number of studies providing evidence-based support, family therapy is the preferred course of treatment in adolescents with AN (Keel & Haedt, 2008).

Currently, hospitalization is limited to brief, acute weight restoration and refeeding for severe cases. Weight should not be regained too quickly as it is medically unsafe and may lead to cardiac overload and death. An appropriate target goal weight should be within 10% of the individual's ideal body weight. Referral to a dietician, education related to healthy eating habits, and a balanced diet with sufficient calories to allow weight gain are all part of the treatment plan. Once malnutrition is reversed and normal nutrition is obtained, treatment goals involve: (1) individual therapy to correct distortions and deficits in psychological thinking and functioning; and (2) family therapy to correct disturbed patterns of interaction and resolve the adolescent's incomplete individuation-separation issues.

Numerous medications have been studied for treatment of AN: antidepressants, hormones, antipsychotics, and gastric motility enhancers. Most have shown inconsistent benefits. However, the antidepressants, selective serotonin reuptake inhibitors, have been effective in the treatment of AN.

Nursing Management

During the nutritional rehabilitation phase the priority is to establish nutrition adequate to stop and reverse the malnutrition and starvation. The nurse may need to promote the individual's physical well-being by monitoring food intake and weight gain. Once an appropriate eating pattern is established, the adolescent should focus on psychotherapy. Most anorectics experience a significant amount of fear and anxiety as they begin to gain weight. The nurse needs to adopt a kind, nurturing yet firm manner in managing the care of the individual. Interventions that increase self-esteem and self-worth are helpful as the individual learns to like herself, learns to trust, and develops an identity beyond her thin body.

BULIMIA NERVOSA

Whereas the prominent features of AN are the caloric restriction and resulting weight loss, the major elements of BN are episodes of binge eating (large amounts of food with a lack of control) followed by various compensatory behaviors (e.g., self-induced vomiting) to control weight gain. The individual usually suffers painful guilt and remorse after such behaviors but is unable to control the impulse to repeat the cycle of binge-purge.

CASE STUDY / CARE PLAN

AN ADOLESCENT WITH BULIMIA NERVOSA

Cara is a 17-year-old senior in high school diagnosed with bulimia nervosa. She is 5 feet 5 inches tall and weighs 95 pounds. Her mother and father are considering divorce and there is considerable conflict in the home. Her father is an executive at a major corporation and travels every week and is home during the weekend. Her mother is a stay at home mom and is currently using alcohol for the past 5 years. She is drunk most days of the week. Cara describes her family as close but says her mother and father hardly speak and fight when they are together over the weekends. Her grades in school had been all A's and she has made the honor roll for the past 3 years. During the past year Cara has lost 35 pounds (from 130 to 95 pounds). A friend went to the school counselor and told him that Cara was vomiting every day and had been doing so for over a year. She has also been running 5 miles a day to lose weight. The counselor notified Cara's mother.

NURSING CARE PLAN

ASSESSMENT

Assessment data includes: Cara states she felt "really good" when she began to lose weight. Cara has motivation for working hard and doing well in school. Social interactions consist of watching television, talking on the phone, and shopping. Her mother's history includes lifelong dieting and sexual abuse as a child. Her father's history includes substance abuse and suicide in his family of origin. Cara's own history includes experimentation with alcohol and marijuana. She has felt depressed over the family conflict and at times, has thoughts of hurting herself but reports that she would never act on them. Cara reports that she cannot sleep most nights and lies awake for several hours each night. She feels isolated from her family members and friends and has no one with whom to share her feelings. She spends approximately 4 hours per day on the internet after exercising. Cara was encouraged to take ballet and modeling lessons as a young girl.

NURSING DIAGNOSIS 1

Imbalanced nutrition: Less than body requirements, related to purging and inadequate food intake.

EXPECTED OUTCOMES

1. Cara will regain 20% of weight lost (20% of 35 pounds = 7 pounds) within the next two months.
2. Cara will demonstrate nutritionally adequate eating pattern without binging or purging.
3. Cara will verbalize an understanding of her nutritional needs.
4. Cara will reduce energy expenditure.

NOC: Nutritional Status

NIC: Eating Disorders Management

INTERVENTIONS/*RATIONALES*

1. Implement nutritionally balanced diet as prescribed. *To allow gradual weight gain. Malnutrition is a mood altering condition affecting cognitive functioning and decision making. Improving nutrition enhances thinking ability and therapeutic work can begin.*
2. With a nutritionist, Cara, and her caregivers, selects a balanced diet with gradual increase in calories and allowing Cara choices as much as possible. *Allows client to have some control over diet plan, encourages compliance, and avoids cardiac overload from rapid weight gain.*
3. Provide supervision of Cara after meals and snacks to prevent purging. *As weight is gained, the bulimic experiences severe anxiety and fear and may resort to purging.*
4. Supervise selection and performance of activity. Watch for secretive exercising. *Client may use excessive exercising as weight loss strategy.*

(Continues)

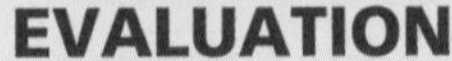

CASE STUDY / CARE PLAN (Continued)

EVALUATION

Cara will be within 10% of ideal body weight. She will understand and demonstrate positive eating habits and engage in normal levels of exercise activity.

NURSING DIAGNOSIS 2

Disturbed body image related to inaccurate perception of body size and shape.

EXPECTED OUTCOMES

1. Cara will develop realistic attitudes and perception of body size and shape.
2. Cara will display evidence of developing a positive self-image.
3. Cara will express feelings and concerns.

NOC: Body Image

NIC: Body Image Enhancement: Self-Esteem Enhancement

INTERVENTIONS/*RATIONALES*

1. Discuss misconceptions of body image. *Provides opportunity to discuss client's perception of self and body image and realities of her own body.*
2. Encourage identification and expression of feelings. *Learning to express feelings and having a sense of internal control helps the client deal with emotions in ways other than binging and purging. Bulimics are often not aware of unpleasant or unacceptable feelings such as anger and resort to binge eating to control anxiety associated with such feelings.*
3. Provide positive support and encouragement for accurate perceptions of body. *To reinforce new and appropriate behaviors.*
4. Teach assertion skills and identify strengths. *Lack of control and feeling ineffective are common problems for the bulimic. Enables client to focus on inner strengths rather than physical appearance.*

EVALUATION

Cara will express fewer negative comments about her body size and image, and adopt one coping strategy for handling anger or stress.

NURSING DIAGNOSIS 3

Anxiety related to family conflict and mother's use of alcohol.

EXPECTED OUTCOMES

1. Cara will report improved feelings of pleasure and improved sleep patterns.
2. Cara will display improved interactions with her peers in face to face activities.
3. Cara will express feelings and concerns about her family.

NOC: Depressed Mood

NIC: Elevated Mood

INTERVENTIONS/*RATIONALES*

1. Discuss depressed feelings. *Provides opportunity to discuss client's perception of her depressed mood and realities of her family life.*
2. Encourage identification and expression of feelings. *Learning to express feelings and having a sense of internal control helps the client cope with emotions of sadness and depression. Bulimics have co-occurring mood disorders and may not aware of unpleasant or unacceptable feelings such as anger and resort to binge eating.*

(Continues)

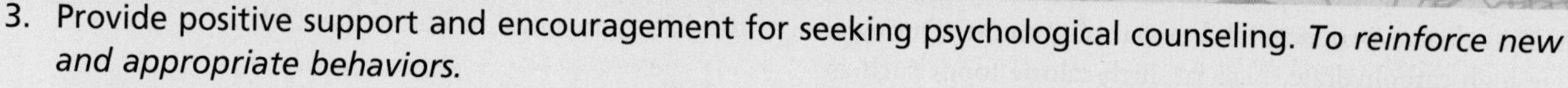

CASE STUDY / CARE PLAN (Continued)

3. Provide positive support and encouragement for seeking psychological counseling. *To reinforce new and appropriate behaviors.*
4. Teach skills related to stress reduction and ways to increase pleasurable activities in her life. *Lack of control and feeling ineffective are common mood problems for the bulimic. Enables client to focus on inner strengths rather than physical appearance.*
5. Encourage parents to participate in counseling *to improve family functioning and become aware of Cara's need to express her feelings in a safe and nurturing environment.*

EVALUATION

Does Cara have an understanding of the origin of her depressed mood? Does she know where to seek support for obtaining individual counseling and family support? Does she understand the co-occurring problems associated with depressed mood and seek assistance?

NURSING DIAGNOSIS 4

Compromised family coping related to issues of control and dysfunctional dynamics.

EXPECTED OUTCOMES

1. Family members will learn about dysfunctional family dynamics that contribute to eating disorders.
2. Family members will establish boundaries that are clearly defined.
3. Family members will demonstrate effective communication patterns.

NOC: Family Coping

NIC: Family Integrity Promotion: Family Therapy

INTERVENTIONS/*RATIONALES*

1. Educate the family about healthy boundaries and normal separation and individuation versus overprotection and family enmeshment. Interact with family members to help increase their awareness of dysfunctional patterns of interaction. *An enmeshed or overprotective family often is not aware of the dysfunctional dynamics. To help the family relinquish unnecessary controls. To promote mutually satisfying interpersonal relationships among family members.*
2. Encourage caregivers to recognize the importance of their relationship as a couple. *Caregivers need to improve their relationship and restore balance in their lives, thus moving the focus off the bulimic's illness. Attention directed toward the bulimic often serves to protect the caregivers from dealing with their own issues.*
3. Help arrange referrals for family therapy. *Family therapy is directed toward redirection of malfunctioning process in the family.*

EVALUATION

Have family members begun to alter interaction patterns and improve dynamics of the family? Does every family member communicate in a healthy manner? Do the family members understand the psychological needs of a teenage daughter?

Incidence and Etiology

Incidence of BN is higher than AN and occurs in about 1% to 1.5% of females with lower rates in males. The client with BN is typically between the ages of 15 and 30 with a peak in later adolescence, at about 18 to 19 years of age (Dunn, 2000). BN is found in all socioeconomic and ethnic groups. Individuals most at risk for developing this disorder are those who are involved in a career or sport requiring low body weight or frequent "weigh-ins" (e.g., ballet, wrestling); who have been sexually abused; and who have a family history of depressive disorders, substance abuse, and eating disorders.

Clinical Manifestations and Pathophysiology

The individual with bulimia may be unable to express feelings accurately. Low self-esteem, feelings of ineffectiveness, depression, and substance abuse are frequently seen. The bulimic typically has an intense fear of getting fat, is very sensitive to weight gain, and fears she is constantly at risk for getting fat because she lacks impulse control.

Binge eating usually occurs in secret and stops when the individual experiences abdominal discomfort. During a binge high-carbohydrate, high-fat, high-calorie foods such as sweets, ice cream, and pastries are usually consumed. Insulin production is increased during the binge. When vomiting occurs, the extra insulin stimulates hunger and eating, and the binge-purge cycle begins again. Following the binge the adolescent feels out of control, depressed, guilty, and anxious. Purging behaviors, commonly self-induced vomiting and laxative abuse, decrease the anxiety, abdominal discomfort, and bloating. The binge-purge cycle is practiced many times a day, and the bulimic loses the ability to respond to normal cues of hunger and satiety. Vomiting and laxative misuse result in complications such as dehydration, abdominal distension, fluid and electrolyte imbalances, esophagitis, and esophageal lacerations. Erosion of tooth enamel, increased dental caries, and tooth discoloration are present secondary to regurgitation of gastric acids. Frequent vomiting also may result in parotid gland enlargement. Cardiovascular symptoms may include hypotension, arrhythmias, and cardiomyopathy.

DIAGNOSIS

Criteria for the diagnosis of BN include the following: recurrent episodes of binge-eating; a sense of lack of control over eating; recurrent inappropriate compensatory behavior to prevent weight gain, such as self-induced vomiting, misuse of laxatives, diuretics, or other medications; fasting; or excessive exercise (APA, 2000).

TREATMENT

Therapeutic interventions for the person with BN include individual, family, and group therapy, and pharmacologic interventions. Behavioral modification is used to control the binge eating and purging. Cognitive therapy may be used after the client's weight has stabilized. Most individuals with BN, as well as AN, demonstrate distorted thoughts and beliefs related to food, weight, body image, and self-concept. The goals of cognitive therapy include: developing an initial sense of self and an understanding of the underlying conflicts; developing a realistic perception of one's body; and enhancing self-esteem and self-concept. Other interventions are psychoeducational groups, dietary counseling, and psychotropic drugs. SSRIs have been effective in reducing the urge to binge and in treating depression. Hospitalization may be necessary for an individual with severe symptoms such as dehydration and fluid and electrolyte imbalances.

FAILURE TO THRIVE

Failure to thrive (FTT) is a term used to describe a child with inadequate growth, usually weight, on standardized growth charts. There is no clear consensus regarding the definition of FTT; however, the term usually describes a child whose weight is below the third to fifth percentile or falls more than two major percentile groups (i.e., from above the 75th percentile to below the 25th).

INCIDENCE AND ETIOLOGY

The incidence of FTT has been reported as 1–5% of hospitalized children under 1 year of age and 5% to 10% of children in a primary care setting (APA, 2006). The causes of FTT can be classified as organic (OFTT), caused by a physical problem or non-organic (NOFTT), caused by psychosocial factors, or mixed failure, caused by a combination of organic and non-organic factors. Most cases of FTT are non-organic in origin. Organic causes vary widely, with the most common being gastrointestinal, such as gastroesophageal reflux, celiac disease, and pyloric stenosis. Other causes of OFTT are increased metabolic demands (e.g., congenital heart disease, chronic infections, and very low birth weight), central nervous system abnormalities, and endocrine disorders (e.g., diabetes mellitus, growth hormone deficiency). Several environmental and psychological factors have been identified as the cause of NOFTT. These include:

- Poverty
- Insufficient social support
- Family stress
- Inadequate caregiver nutritional information
- Errors in formula preparation
- Inadequate breast milk
- Difficulties in the maternal-child attachment
- Maternal psychopathology (affective, anxiety, psychotic, and substance abuse disorders)

CLINICAL MANIFESTATIONS AND PATHOPHYSIOLOGY

The clinical manifestations of FTT include:

- Growth failure—weight for age is less than the 10th percentile & height for age is less than the 5th percentile (Olsen, 2006)
- Failure to maintain previously established growth trajectory
- Loss of subcutaneous fat
- Reduced muscle mass
- Developmental delays
- Apathy and listlessness
- Flattened occiput from lying in one position
- Infrequent and scanty (low bulk) stools
- Signs of neglect: poor hygiene such as dirty body, clothes, fingernails, and extensive diaper rash
- Avoidance of eye contact
- Expressionless face

REFLECTIVE THINKING

Failure to Thrive

You have been assigned to work with a caregiver whose child is suffering from non-organic failure to thrive. Assuming you have not met with the child and caregiver yet, what are your initial feelings toward this caregiver?

Long-term effects of failure to thrive include developmental delays, secondary immune dysfunction, and growth delays.

DIAGNOSIS

To rule out an organic cause of FTT, dietary interventions including provision of nutrients and nurturing should be implemented. If the infant or child gains the expected amount of weight, a diagnosis of NOFTT is appropriate. The history should include past and present medical histories of the child and family members, a social history to obtain information about economic resources and social supports of the family, and a detailed dietary and feeding assessment. The dietary history can be used to determine whether the child's diet is appropriate for age. The caregiver-child feeding interaction observation is another essential aspect of the FTT assessment. Other diagnostic tests are used only to rule out organic problems.

TREATMENT

The primary goal of treatment is to provide sufficient calories and nutrition for the child to attain **"catch-up" growth** (a rate of growth greater than the expected rate for age). These children need to receive 150% of their recommended daily caloric intake, based on their expected, not actual, weight. In infants, this increased calorie intake may be accomplished by concentrating formula or adding rice cereal to pureed foods. Toddlers can receive more calories by adding taste-pleasing fats such as cheese, sour cream, butter, and peanut butter to their foods. Additionally, other medical and psychosocial problems must be addressed. One critical factor contributing to success with management of FTT is to use a multidisciplinary team approach (nurse, health care provider, dietician, social worker, occupational or physical therapist, mental health professional) as the problems are complex. Any underlying organic conditions should also be treated.

NURSING MANAGEMENT

Nursing care focuses on observation of the caregiver-child interactions during feeding and when not feeding. A feeding schedule should be developed and taught to the caregivers. Education is provided about appropriate feeding techniques, for example, how to hold the infant, the importance of eye contact, cues from the infant about satiety, and desire to feed more. The nurse monitors weight gain, intake, and plots weights and lengths or heights on grids to monitor growth. It is important for the nurse to role model appropriate caregiver-child interactions. The nurse can role model feeding behaviors, can talk to the infant or child, and initiate playful interactions. Caregivers may need to see that the nurse views it as appropriate to talk to an infant or young child and that the child can respond.

Success in this educational process depends on building a trusting relationship between the family and the professionals. A supportive, nonblaming approach is essential. By adopting the attitude that the caregivers have not had the opportunity to learn healthy parenting behaviors rather than assuming their behavior is willful, a trusting relationship can be established. Another nursing intervention is providing emotional support for the caregivers. The nurse can help them increase their self-esteem through positive parenting skills. The nurse should praise and encourage them for displaying any such skills, and encourage as much caregiver participation in care as is practical. Another significant nursing role is to emphasize the importance of frequent health visits to monitor weight gain and developmental progress. A home health referral may be appropriate in some situations so these parameters can be assessed on a regular basis.

IN THE REAL WORLD

Her mother cried, "If I only knew the signs!" Her father said through tears, "Why didn't we see?" Her grandmother was too distraught for words. Her brother said, "What could have been so bad?" These are words or feelings expressed in the hospital emergency room reacting to news that 15-year-old Elizabeth had committed suicide.

As a nurse who has had opportunities to counsel children who have tried to commit suicide and their families, the suicide risk signs are almost always apparent. It just doesn't happen out of the blue. We must as nurses strive to observe for these signs in our clients and to encourage caregivers, school officials and teachers, coaches, and the general public to take notice of these signs and be proactive. Working together we might just save a life.

KEY CONCEPTS

- Individual, family, group, play, and art therapy are the various types of therapy used to treat the pediatric client with psychosocial alterations. The modalities and types of interventions are based on a child's diagnosis, age, and developmental stage.
- Children with attention-deficit hyperactivity disorder have difficulty inhibiting behavior, which interferes with the process of learning self-regulation behaviors.
- Nursing management of attention-deficit hyperactivity disorder includes pharmacological education, providing family support, and acting as a liaison with health care providers, caregivers, school, and other members of the interdisciplinary team.
- Nursing management of mood disorders includes assessing the child physically; talking with the child and family about their feelings and concerns; and educating the family about the disorder and treatment. The nurse should work with the family to improve intrafamily communication and resolution of dysfunctional family patterns.
- The incidence of suicide is rising in the adolescent age group. The nurse should be active in promoting the signs of suicide risk including identification of potential stressors.
- Nursing interventions for attempted suicide include primary, secondary, and tertiary levels of intervention.
- Anxiety disorders include separation anxiety disorder, school phobia or refusal, generalized anxiety disorder, social phobia, obsessive-compulsive disorder, and post-traumatic stress disorder.
- Nurse interventions for anxiety disorders include pharmacologic teaching, encouraging identification of sources of anxiety, teaching caregivers to recognize signs of anxiety, and methods for diffusing the anxiety.
- Nursing interventions for substance abuse include support and reassurance for the client and family, encouraging positive changes in lifestyle, and referral to support groups.
- The mortality rate for anorexia nervosa and bulimia nervosa are the highest of any of the major psychiatric disorders.
- Causes of non-organic failure to thrive include poverty, insufficient social support, family stress, inadequate caregiver information, difficulty in maternal-child attachment, and maternal psychopathology.

REVIEW ACTIVITIES

1. Explain why you would use play therapy for one child and art therapy for another.
2. What are the clinical manifestations of ADHD?
3. Explain the difference between major depressive disorder and dysthymic disorder.
4. What interventions would you include in a primary prevention education program related to suicide?
5. What are the goals for the caregivers of a child with school refusal?
6. Compare anorexia nervosa symptoms and nursing interventions with those of bulimia nervosa.
7. What information would you include in a class you planned to teach junior high students about substance abuse?
8. List three to five risk factors for the development of substance abuse and substance abuse disorder.
9. List three factors identified as causes of non-organic failure to thrive.

STUDY QUESTIONS

1. ADHD symptoms, associated with the hyperactivity type, can include interrupting, fidgeting, excessive talking, and inattention. Which of the following choices will not produce behaviors similar to ADHD?
   a. Absence seizures
   b. Intermittent otitis media
   c. Depression
   d. Diabetes
2. There is growing evidence that ADHD can be associated with a greater risk of which psychiatric illness?
   a. Anxiety
   b. Enuresis
   c. Hypersomnia
   d. Asperger's disorder
3. Which of the following would not be a clinical manifestation of Major Depressive Disorder in children?
   a. Irritable mood
   b. Memory problems
   c. Trembling
   d. Hypersomnia
4. The following statement best describes a child who is experiencing Generalized Anxiety Disorder:
   a. Child blames self for poor school performance
   b. Child is overly concerned about above average school performance
   c. Child is careless in their homework and school work
   d. Child is satisfied with their grades of Cs and Ds
5. In providing clinical care to a 7-year-old child who just witnessed the death his parents in a car accident, the following support by the nurse would be appropriate:
   a. Explore the child's reaction to the accident
   b. Explore the child's feelings of being the only survivor
   c. Explore who in the family the child will be living with
   d. Explore the child's thinking about feeling responsible for the event
6. Adolescents with ADHD who are at higher risk for substance abuse are more likely to have which behavioral problem?
   a. PTSD
   b. Oppositional Defiant Disorder (ODD)
   c. Anxiety
   d. Sleep problems
7. Anorexia Nervosa is a serious disorder in adolescents and treatment involves monitoring the patient's body weight and addressing issues related to body image. Which of the following statements highlights a female who has AN and her thinking of her body?
   a. An adolescent thinks that she needs to be perfect in all areas of life and her body must be thin.
   b. An adolescent feels that she has the power to change her weight by eating if she needs to gain weight.
   c. An adolescent feels that her thin body is really not that much of a problem for her but does not mind if others are concerned about her weight.
   d. An adolescent compares herself to others and feels that she needs to look like her "thin" friends.
8. Working with a caretaker who has a child diagnosed with "Failure to Thrive" can be challenging. One of the important goals for nursing management is to ensure that:
   a. The nurse models appropriate child interactions for the caretaker.
   b. The nurse holds the caretaker responsible for the child's health.
   c. The nurse educates the caretaker in the hospital of nutritional requirements but does not allow the caretaker to feed the child.
   d. The child and caretaker have private time during most of the hospitalization.
9. Obsessive Compulsive Disorder in children has a set of behaviors that involves reduction or prevention of a dreaded event. Common compulsive behaviors that are manifested would be:
   a. Frequent hand washing.
   b. Frequent aggressive thoughts.
   c. Frequent thoughts of hurting others.
   d. Frequent imagining that the worse will happen.
10. Select one of the following statements that best characterizes depression in children:
    a. Depression is not genetically based.
    b. Family dynamics do not contribute to a child's depression.
    c. Child's coping styles can contribute to depressed thinking.
    d. Child's thinking patterns are not a contributory factor.

REFERENCES

Abikoff, H., Nissley-Tsiopinis, J., Gallagher, R., Zambenedetti, M., Seyffert, M., Boorady, R., McCarthy, J. (2009). Effects of MPH-OROS on the organizational, time management, and planning behaviors of children with ADHD. *Journal of the American Academy of Child & Adolescent Psychiatry, 48*(2), 166–175.

American Academy of Child and Adolescent Psychiatry. (2007a). Practice parameter for the assessment and treatment of children and adolescents with Attention-Deficit Hyperactivity Disorder. *Journal of the American Academy of Child and Adolescent Psychiatry, 46*(7), 894–921.

American Academy of Child and Adolescent Psychiatry. (2007b). Practice parameter for the assessment and treatment of children and adolescents with anxiety disorders. *Journal of the American Academy of Child and Adolescent Psychiatry, 46*(2), 267–283.

American Psychiatric Association. (2000). *Diagnostic and statistical manual of mental disorders* (4th ed. rev.) *(DSM-IV-TR)*. Washington, DC: Author.

American Psychiatric Association Working Group on Eating Disorders. (2006). Practice guidelines for the treatment of patients with eating disorders. Retrieved December 20, 2010, from http://www.psych.org

August, G. J., Winters, K. C., Realmuto, G., Fahnhorst, T., Botzet, A., & Lee, S. et al. (2006). Prospective study of adolescent drug use among community samples of ADHD and non-ADHD participants. *Journal of American Academy of Child & Adolescent Psychiatry, 45*(7), 824–832.

Baldwin, J., & Dadds, M. (2008). Examining alternative explanations of the covariation of ADHD and anxiety symptoms in children: A community study. *Journal of Abnormal Child Psychology, 36*(1), 67–79.

Barrett, P., Farrell, L., Pina, A., Peris, T., & Piacentini, J. (2008). Evidenced-based psychosocial treatment for child and adolescent obsessive-compulsive disorder. *Journal of Clinical Child & Adolescent Psychology, 37*(1), 131–155.

Beesdo, K., Bittner, A., Pine, D. S., Stein, M. B., Höfler, M., Lieb, R., & Wittchen, H. U. (2007). Incidence of social anxiety disorder and the consistent risk for secondary depression in the first three decades of life. *Archives of General Psychiatry, 64*(8), 903–912.

Biederman, J. (2005). Attention-deficit hyperactivity disorder: A selective overview. *Biological Psychiatry, 57*(11), 1215–1220.

Biederman, J., & Faraone, S. V. (2005). Attention-deficit hyperactivity disorder. *Lancet, 366*(9481), 237–248.

Blackman, G., Ostrander, R., & Herman, K. (2005). Children with ADHD and depression: A multisource, multimethod assessment of clinical, social, and academic functioning. *Journal of Attention Disorders, 8*(4), 195–207.

Bridge, J., Greenhouse, J., Weldon, A., Campo, J., & Kelleher, K. (2008). Suicide trends among youths aged 10 to 19 years in the United States, 1996–2005. *Journal of the American Medical Association, 300*(9), 1025–1026.

Brown, L. K., Houck, C., Grossman, C., Lescano, C., & Frenkel, J. (2008). Frequency of adolescent self-cutting as a predictor of HIV risk. *Journal of Developmental and Behavioral Pediatrics, 29*, 161–165.

Broyles, B., Reiss, B., & Evans, M. (2007). *Pharmacological aspects of nursing care* (7th ed.). Clifton Park, NY: Delmar Cengage Learning.

Bruch, H. (1982). *The golden cage: The enigma of anorexia nervosa.* Cambridge, MA: Harvard University Press.

Centers for Disease Control and Prevention (CDC). (2007). Suicide trends among youths and young adults aged 10–24 years: United States, 1990–2004. *Morbidity and Mortality Weekly Report, 56*(35), 902–908.

Centers for Disease Control and Prevention (CDC). (2008). Suicide Prevention. Retrieved December 20, 2010, from http://www.cdc.gov/ncipc/dvp/Suicide/youthsuicide.htm.

Costello, E. J., Egger, H. L., & Angold, A. (2004). *Developmental epidemiology of adolescents.* New York: Oxford University Press.

Daviss, W. B. (2008). A review of co-morbid depression in pediatric ADHD: Etiology, phenomenology, and treatment. *Journal of Child and Adolescent Psychopharmacology, 18*(6), 565–571.

Dopheide, J. A. (2006). Recognizing and treating depression in children and adolescents. *American Journal of Health Systems Pharmacy, 63*(3), 233–243.

Dulcan, M., Martini, D., & Lake, M. (2003). *Concise guide to child and adolescent psychiatry* (3rd ed.). Arlington, VA: American Psychiatric Publishing, Inc., pp. 129–131.

Dunn, A. (2000). Nutrition. In C. Burns, M. Brady, A. Dunn, & N. Starr (Eds.). *Pediatric primary care: A handbook for nurse practitioners* (2nd ed.). Philadelphia: W. B. Saunders, pp. 243–302.

Fairburn, C. G., Cooper, A., Shafran, R., & Wilson, T. (2008). Eating disorders: A transdiagnostic protocol. In D. H. Barlow, *Clinical handbook of psychological disorders* (4th ed.). New York: Guilford Publications, pp. 578–614.

Faraone, S. V., Glatt, S. J., Bukstein, O. G., Lopez, F. A., Arnold, L. E., & Findling, R. L. (2009). Effects of once-daily oral and transdermal methylphenidate on sleep behavior of children with ADHD. *Journal of Attention Disorders, 12*(4), 308–315.

Faraone, S. V., Sergeant, J., Gillberg, C., & Biederman, J. (2003). The worldwide prevalence of ADHD: Is it an American condition? *World Psychiatry, 2*, 104–113.

Fritz, G. (2007). Stigma and childhood mental illness: Can advocates turn the tide? *The Brown University Child and Adolescent Behavior Letter* (November, 2007).

Greydanus, D. E., & Calles Jr., J. (2007). Suicide in children and adolescents. *Primary Care: Clinics in Office Practice, 34*(2), 259–273.

Grossman, D., Mueller, B., Riedy, C., Dowd, M., Villaveces, A., Prodzinski, J., Nakagawara, J., Howard, J., Thiersch, N., & Harruff, R.

(2005). Gun storage practices and risk of youth suicide and unintentional firearm injuries. *Journal of the American Medical Association, 293*(6), 707–714.

Hudson, J. I., Hiripi, E., Pope, H. G., & Kessler, R. C. (2007). The prevalence and correlates of eating disorders in the National Comorbidity Survey Replication. *Biological Psychiatry, 61*, 348–358.

Johnston, L., O'Malley, P., & Bachman, J. (2003). *Monitoring the future national results on adolescent drug use: Overview Of key findings, 2001* (NIH Publication No. 03-5374). Bethesda, MD: National Institute on Drug Abuse.

Katon, W., Lozano, P., Russo, J., McCauley, E., Richardson, L., & Bush, T. (2007). The prevalence of DSM-IV anxiety and depressive disorders in youth with asthma compared with controls. *Journal of Adolescent Health. 41*, 455–463.

Keel, P., & Haedt, A. (2008). Evidenced based psychosocial treatments for eating problems and eating disorders. *Journal of Clinical Child and Adolescent Psychology, 37*(1), 39–61.

Kessler, R. (2000). Post-traumatic stress disorder. *Journal of Clinical Psychiatry, 61*(Supp. 15): 4–12.

Khalid-Khan, S., Santibanez, M. P., McMicken, C., & Rynn, M. (2007). Social anxiety disorder in children and adolescents: Epidemiology, diagnosis, and treatment. *Pediatric Drugs, 9*(4), 227–237.

Lewinsohn, P., Striegel-Moore, R., & Seeley, J. (2000). Epidemiology and natural course of eating disorders in young women from adolescence to young adulthood. *Journal of the American Academy of Child and Adolescent Psychiatry, 39*, 1284–1292.

Malekoff, A. (2006). *Group work with adolescents: Principles and practices.* New York: Guilford Press.

Matthew, S., Price, R., & Charney, D. (2008). Recent advances in the neurobiology of anxiety disorders. *American Journal of Medical Genetics Part C, 148C*: 89–98.

National Center for Injury Prevention and Control, Division of Violence Prevention. Youth Suicide, (2008). Retrieved March 6, 2009, from www.cdc.gov/ncipc/dvp/Suicide/youthsuicide.htm.

Olsen, E. M. (2006). Failure to thrive: Still a problem of definition. *Clinical Pediatrics, 45*, 1–6.

Perlis, M. L., Jungquist, C., Smith, N. T., & Posner, D. (2008). *Cognitive behavioral treatment for insomnia.* New York: Springer.

Shain, B., & the Committee on Adolescents. (2007). Suicide and suicide attempts in adolescents. *American Academy of Pediatrics, 120*(3), 669–675.

Substance Abuse and Mental Health Services Administration. (2008). Results from the 2007 National Survey on Drug Use and Health: National Findings (Office of Applied Studies, NSDUH Series H-34, DHHS Publication No. SMA 08-4343). Rockville, MD.

Swanson, J., Posne, M., Fusella, J., Wasdell, M., Sommer, T., & Fan, J. (2001). Genes and attention-deficit hyperactivity disorder. *Current Psychiatry Report, 3*(2), 92–100.

van Den Hoofdakker, B. J., van der Veen-Mulders, L., Sytema, S., Emuelkamp, P., Minderra, R., & Nauta, M. H. (2007). Effectiveness of behavioral parent training for children with ADHD in routine clinical practice: A randomized control study. *Journal of the American Academy of Child and Adolescent Psychiatry, 46*, 1263–1271.

U.S. Food and Drug Administration. Atomoxetine (Marketed as Strattera): Serious liver injury. Retrieved April 4, 2009, from http://www.fda.gov/Drugs/DrugSafety/DrugSafetyNewsletter/ucm110235.htm.

Widom, C., DuMont, K., & Czaja, S. (2007). A prospective investigation of major depressive disorder and comorbidity in abused and neglected children grown up. *Archives of General Psychiatry, 64*, 49–56.

SUGGESTED READINGS

Andrist, L. C. (2003). Media images, body dissatisfaction, and disordered eating in adolescent women. *MCN, 28*(2), 119–123.

Breiner, S. (2003). An evidence-based eating disorder program. *Journal of Pediatric Nursing, 18*(1), 75–80.

Bulechek, G., Butcher, H., & Dochterman, J. (2008). *Nursing Interventions Classification (NIC)* (5th ed.). St. Louis, MO: Mosby.

Grunbaum, J., Kann, L., Kinchen, S., Williams, B., Ross, J., Lowry, R., and Kolbe, L. (2002). Youth risk behavior surveillance—United States, 2001. In *Surveillance Summaries, Morbidity and Mortality Reports, 51*(No. SS-4), 1–66.

Harrison, L. (2001). Understanding the differences in youth drug prevalence rates produced by the MTF, NHSDA, and YRBS studies. *Journal of Drug Issues, 31*, 665–694.

Khan, A., Khan, S., Kolts, R., & Brown, W. (2003). Suicide rates in clinical trials of SSRIs, other antidepressants and placebo: Analysis of FDA reports. *American Journal of Psychiatry, 160*, 790–792.

Moorhead, S., Johnson, M., Maas, M., & Swanson, E. (2008). Nursing Outcomes Classification *(NOC)* (4th ed.). St. Louis, MO: Mosby.

Parsons, C. (2002). The client with attention-deficit disorder. In D. Antai-Otong (Ed.). *Psychiatric nursing: Biological and behavioral concepts.* Clifton Park, NY: Delmar Cengage Learning, pp. 447–479.

Scahill, L., & Schwab-Stone, M. (2000). Epidemiology of ADHD in school-age children. *Child and adolescent psychiatric clinics of North America, 9*(3), 541–555.

Schiffman, R. (2004). Drug and substance use in adolescents. *MCN, 29*(1), 21–27.

Seidenfeld, M., & Rickert, V. (2001). Impact of anorexia, bulimia and obesity on the gynecologic health of adolescents. *American Family Physician, 64*(4), 445–454.

RESOURCES

Refer to the online student StudyWARE for Potts & Mandleco at http://www.CengageBrain.com for additional content and study aids.

Organization: **Al-Anon and Alateen**

Description: The Al-Anon Family Groups are a fellowship of relatives and friends of alcoholics who share their experience, strength, and hope in order to solve their common problems. Al-Anon and Alateen believe alcoholism is a family illness and that changed attitudes can aid recovery. The website provides users with information regarding publications, media, and podcasts.

Website/Resource: http://www.al-anon.alateen.org

Organization: **Alcoholics Anonymous**

Description: Alcoholics Anonymous® is a fellowship of men and women who share their experience, strength, and hope with each other that they may solve their common problem and help others to recover from alcoholism. The only requirement for membership is a desire to stop drinking. There are no dues or fees for AA membership. The website provides access to local meetings.

Website/Resource: http://www.aa.org

Organization: **American Academy of Child and Adolescent Psychiatry (AACAP)**

Description: The AACAP is the leading national professional medical association dedicated to treating and improving the quality of life for children, adolescents, and families affected by mental, behavioral, or developmental disorders. The AACAP website provides information regarding the understanding of mental illnesses and removing the stigma associated with them. In addition, the website provides data concerning efforts in the prevention of mental illnesses and how to seek proper treatment, and offers access to services for children and adolescents.

Website/Resource: http://www.aacap.org

Organization: **American Association of Suicidology**

Description: American Association of Suicidology is a membership organization for all those involved in suicide prevention and intervention, or touched by suicide. AAS is a leader in the advancement of scientific and programmatic efforts in suicide prevention through research, education and training, the development of standards and resources, and survivor support services. The website provides users with statistics and research regarding suicide.

Website/Resource: http://www.suicidology.org

Organization: **Attention Deficit Disorder Association**

Description: The Attention Deficit Disorder Association (ADDA) is the world's leading adult ADHD organization. ADDA's mission is to provide information, resources, and networking opportunities to help adults with attention-deficit hyperactivity disorder (AD/HD) lead better lives. The website helps facilitate support groups, provides access to resources, and announces upcoming events and conferences.

Website/Resource: http://www.add.org

Organization: **Children and Adults with Attention-Deficit Hyperactivity Disorder**

Description: Children and Adults with Attention-Deficit Hyperactivity Disorder is the nation's leading non-profit organization serving individuals with AD/HD and their families. CHADD has over 16,000 members in 200 local chapters throughout the U.S. Chapters offer support for individuals, parents, teachers, professionals, and others. The website offers access to upcoming conferences, training sessions, and membership information.

Website/Resource: http://www.chadd.org

Organization: **Mothers Against Drunk Driving (MADD)**

Description: The mission of Mothers Against Drunk Driving (MADD) is to stop drunk driving, support the victims of this violent crime, and prevent underage drinking. The website provides information regarding victim services, underage drinking, and law enforcement.

Website/Resource: http://www.madd.org

Organization: **National Association of Anorexia Nervosa and Associated Disorders**

Description: The National Association of Anorexia Nervosa and Associated Disorders (ANAD) is the oldest non-profit in the country dedicated to alleviating and preventing eating disorders. The website provides links to contact therapists, support groups, and treatment programs.

Website/Resource: http://www.anad.org

Organization: **National Clearing House for Drug and Alcohol Information**

Description: The National Clearing House for Drug and Alcohol Information is a subset of the U.S. Department of Health and Human Services and the SAMHSA's National Clearinghouse. The website offers readers general information regarding many classes of drugs, drug/alcohol issues, and recent publications.

Website/Resource: http://www.ncadi.samhsa.gov

Organization: **National Mental Health Association**

Description: Mental Health America (formerly known as the National Mental Health Association) is the country's leading nonprofit dedicated to helping all people live mentally healthier lives. With more than 320 affiliates nationwide, Mental Health America represents a growing movement of Americans who promote mental wellness for the health and well-being of the nation—every day and in times of crisis. The website provides information regarding health information, action, and affiliates.

Website/Resource: http://www.nmha.org

Organization: **National Sleep Foundation**

Description: Alerting the public, health care providers, and policymakers to the life-and-death importance of adequate sleep is central to the mission of the National Sleep Foundation (NSF). NSF is dedicated to improving the quality of life for Americans who suffer from sleep problems and disorders. This means helping the public better understand the importance of sleep and the benefits of good sleep habits, and recognizing the signs of sleep problems so that they can be properly diagnosed and treated. The website provides access to NSF's online community as well as links that help locate sleep professionals.

Website/Resource: http://www.sleepfoundation.org

Organization: **Students Against Drunk Driving (SADD)**

Description: The mission of Students Against Drunk Driving (SADD) is to provide students with the best prevention tools possible to deal with the issues of underage drinking, other drug use, impaired driving, and other destructive decisions. The website offers users access to information regarding events and chapters.

Website/Resource: http://www.sadd.org

Organization: **Substance Abuse and Mental Health Services Administration (SAMHSA)**

Description: The mission of the Substance Abuse and Mental Health Services Administration (SAMHSA) is to reduce the impact of substance abuse and mental illness on America's communities. The Agency was established in 1992 and directed by Congress to target substance abuse and mental health services to the people most in need and to translate research in these areas more and more rapidly into the general health care system. The website offers readers a wealth of information regarding publications, statistics, programs, and much more.

Website/Resource: http://www.samhsa.gov

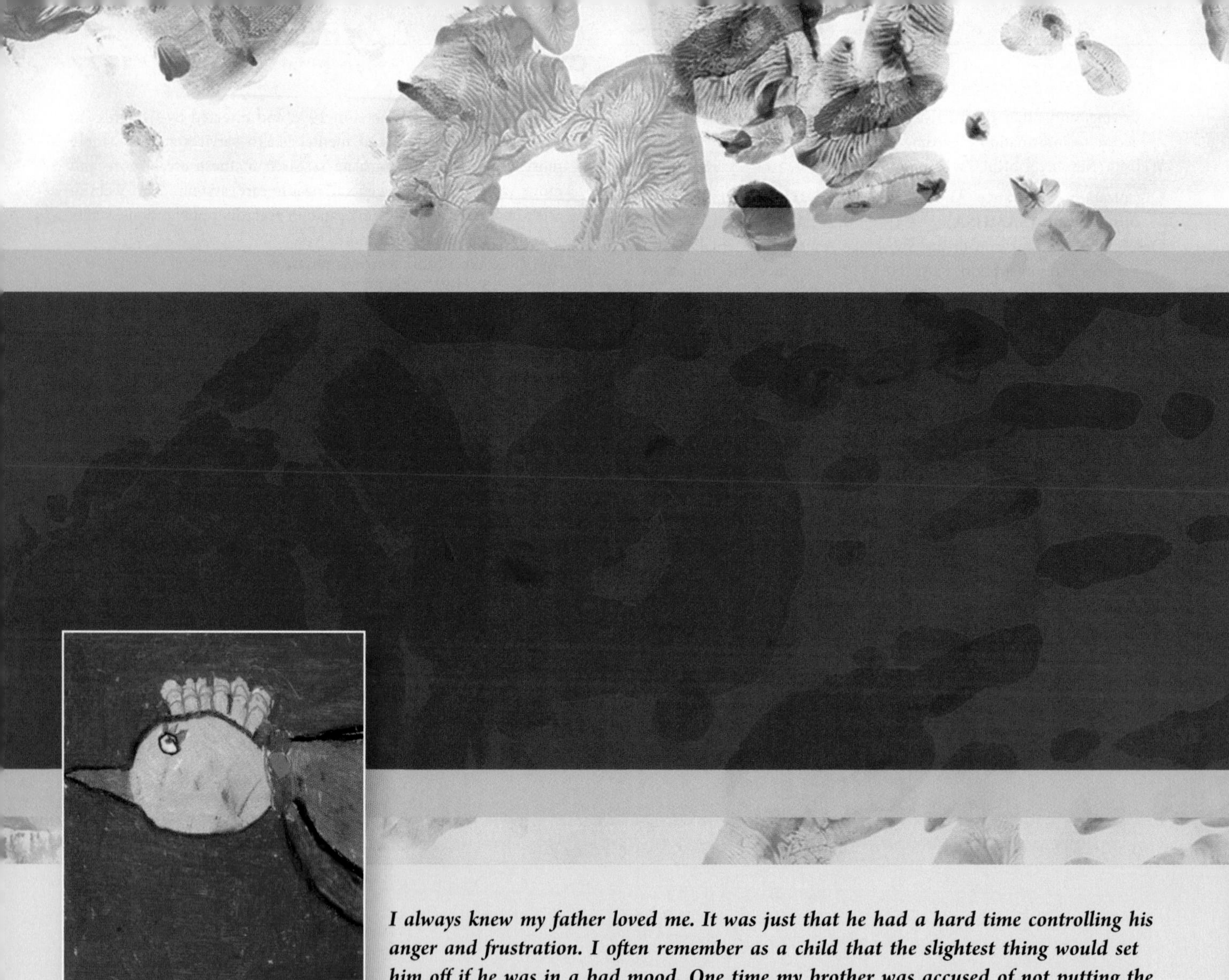

I always knew my father loved me. It was just that he had a hard time controlling his anger and frustration. I often remember as a child that the slightest thing would set him off if he was in a bad mood. One time my brother was accused of not putting the tools back in the right place on the wall in the garage. Wally said he had put them back but they were not there. I know Wally used them to work on a friend's bicycle and had left them at the neighbor's house. When dad came home and couldn't find them, he got really angry and started to yell. He grabbed Wally by the arm and Wally started to cry and said he had put the tools back. I knew that unless Dad had the tools, his anger would just get worse and soon he would start hitting me and my sisters. So, I went to the neighbor's house, got the tools, and brought them to my Dad. He was furious that I had "borrowed" the tools and not returned them (even though it was Wally who borrowed the tools). My punishment was six lashings with his belt. I can still remember the pain. Wally never did fess up that he was the one who borrowed the tools. He was just happy he did not get spanked with the belt.

—Carl, Age 26, who was abused by his Father as a Child

CHAPTER 36
Child Abuse and Neglect

Barbara A. Caldwell, APRN-BC, PhD

COMPETENCIES

Upon completion of this chapter, the reader will be able to:

- Compare child abuse and neglect.
- Describe the incidence and prevalence of child abuse and neglect in the United States.
- Explain the theoretical origins of family violence in the United States.
- Describe components of a nursing assessment for a child who has been abused or neglected.
- Describe the clinical manifestations of physical, psychological, and sexual abuse.
- Identify nursing interventions related to child abuse and neglect.
- Understand and explain the nurses' legal and ethical roles and responsibilities in assessing child abuse and neglect.
- Successfully complete the games and activities in the online student StudyWARE.

Child maltreatment, a major public health crisis, encompasses abuse and neglect, and has a significant impact on the child's physical, psychological, cognitive, and social development. Further, the child who experiences maltreatment is at serious risk for becoming an abusive parent (Taylor, Guteman, Lee, & Rathouz, 2009). The family clearly provides part of the intergenerational transmission of violence, as some children witness the abuse of their mother, father, or caregiver. These experiences influence how individuals resolve problems and cope with difficult situations. Unfortunately, the occurrence and continuation of physical abuse seems to be supported among the U.S. culture since the government has been reluctant to interfere with parents' rights to raise their children (Hines & Malley-Morrison, 2005). Nurses have an integral role in preventing child abuse and family violence through educating the public and in national, state, and community health policy and advocacy efforts supporting family health and mental health initiatives.

Child abuse and neglect include physical, emotional, and sexual abuse. Children of any age, race, gender, religion, and socioeconomic group can be victims (Figure 36-1). Therefore, it is imperative the nurse utilize skills, knowledge, and intuition to ensure a child is safe and not in an abusive environment. The following pages not only define and discuss child abuse and neglect, but also provide information regarding the nursing care of these children.

Child maltreatment is the intentional injury of a child. **Child neglect** is harmful, malicious, or ignorant withholding of physical, nutritional, or health care, or emotional and educational necessities that provide a foundation for healthy childhood development. **Child abuse** includes a range of intentional behaviors by a parent or caregiver that can involve neglect, or physical, emotional, or sexual abuse. **Physical abuse**, the most commonly reported type of abuse, represents bodily injury to a child that appears to have been inflicted by other than accidental means. The type of physical injuries a child receives may include damage to skin, as bruises, burns, bite marks, and lacerations; damage to the head, including scalp hematomas, lacerations, bruises, brain injuries, or shaken baby syndrome; damage to the internal organs (chest, abdomen, liver, pancreas, spleen, kidney, bladder); or damage to the skeleton (fractures) (Kellogg & the Committee on Child Abuse and Neglect, 2007). **Psychological** or **emotional abuse** results from habitual lack of attention to the child's needs and includes lack of affection, emotional support, or supervision. Emotional abuse may also occur when a caregiver refuses to accept recommended treatment or services by school officials or medical personnel.

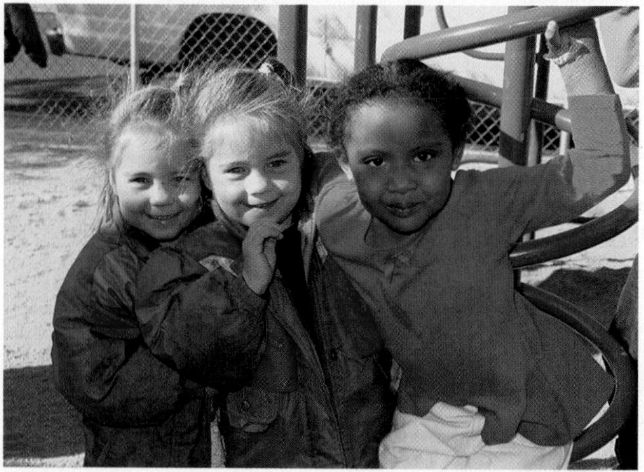

FIGURE 36-1 Child abuse occurs in any family regardless of race, income bracket, religious background, neighborhood, or sexual orientation. DELMAR CENGAGE LEARNING.

All types of abuse have profound implications on a child's growth and development; some effects are short-lived and others are lifelong. Therefore, understanding the incidence, etiology, clinical manifestations, and nursing management of child abuse is important and can affect the course of the child's developmental trajectories.

In 2007, an estimated 3.5 million children were referred to state Child Protective Service (CPS) agencies as suspected victims of abuse and neglect. Over 60% of the victims (physical abuse, neglect, sexual abuse, psychological abuse, and other abuses) received postinvestigation services and more than 20% were placed in foster care as a result of the CPS investigation (U.S. Department of Health and Human Services, Administration on Children, Youth, and Families, 2009). During 2006, an estimated 905,000 children were identified to be victims of abuse or neglect (Child Welfare Information Gateway, 2008).

Children in the age group of birth to 1 year had the highest rate of victimization at 24.4 per 1,000 children of the same age group in the national population. More than one-half of the child victims were girls (51.5%) and 48.2% were boys; and approximately one-half of all victims were White (48.8%); one-quarter (22.8%) were African-American; and 18.4% were Hispanic. Based on the 2006 statistics, 64.2% of child victims were identified as being neglected, 16.0% were physically abused, 8.8% were sexually abused, and 6.6% were emotionally or psychologically maltreated. For 2006, a nationally estimated 1,530 children died of abuse or neglect at a rate of 2.04 children per 100,000 in the national population. More than three-quarters (78%) of the child fatality victims were younger than 4 years. Infant boys (younger than 1 year) had the highest rate of fatalities, at 18.5 deaths per 100,000 of boys in the of the same age in the national population (Child Welfare Information Gateway, 2008).

Each state has its own definitions of child abuse and neglect based on standards set by federal law. Federal legislation provides a foundation for states by identifying a minimum set of acts or behaviors that defines child abuse and neglect. The federal Child Abuse Prevention and Treatment Act (CAPTA), 42 U.S.C.A. §5106g, as amended by the Keeping Children and Families Safe Act of 2003, defines child abuse and neglect as: "Any recent act or failure to act on the part of a parent or caretaker which results in death, serious physical or emotional harm, sexual abuse or exploitation; or an act or failure to act which presents an imminent risk of serious harm."

African-American children, American Indian or Alaska Native children, and children of mixed races had the highest rates of victimization at 16.7, 14.2, and 14.0 per 1,000 children of the same race or ethnicity, respectively. White children and Hispanic children had rates of approximately 10.3 and 9.1 per 1,000 children of the same race or ethnicity, respectively. Asian children had the lowest rate of 2.4 per 1,000 children of the same race or ethnicity. Nearly one-half of all victims were white (46.1%), one-fifth (21.7%) were African-American, and one-fifth (20.8%) were Hispanic. For all racial categories except Native Hawaiian and Pacific Islander, the largest percentage of victims suffered from neglect (U.S. Department of Health and Human Services, Administration on Children, Youth and Families, 2009).

Recurrence was defined as a second substantiated or indicated maltreatment occurring within a six-month period. The statistics found that there were three results that indicated the risk for a recurrence:

- Children who had been prior victims of maltreatment were 96% more likely to experience a recurrence than those who were not prior victims.
- Child victims who were reported with a disability were 52% more likely to experience recurrence than children without a disability.
- The oldest victims (16–21 years of age) were the least likely to experience a recurrence, and were 51% less likely than were infants (younger than age 1).

THEORETICAL APPROACHES TO CHILD ABUSE AND NEGLECT

Three theoretical models explain the phenomena of child abuse and neglect: the sociological model, the social-interactional systemic perspective model, and the attachment model.

SOCIOLOGICAL MODEL

The sociological model of family violence helps the professional understand how social structures affect people and their behavior (Straus & Gelles, 1989). Here, child abuse and neglect are seen as isolated events in a family system, and family violence is a pattern of behavior passed from generation to generation. Although the form of abuse may change, the pattern continues; for example, physical abuse in one generation changing to sexual abuse in the next generation.

Gelles (1987) described nine risk factors that make families less nurturing and more prone to hurtful, violent behavior. They are found in Table 36-1.

SOCIAL-INTERACTIONAL SYSTEMIC PERSPECTIVE MODEL

The social-interactional systemic perspective model suggests society contains the attitudes, values, and beliefs that legitimize violence in the family (Gelles, 1997). For example, violent acts, interactions, and roles are part of society, and television programs, movies, and videos demonstrate and illustrate the value society places on violence. In this model, the family selects behaviors that maintain, escalate, or reduce the level of violence tolerated by its members. The behaviors selected by family members best suit the psychological disposition, cultural background, and coping strategies used to resolve conflict within the family. Unfortunately, social norms also expose individuals to violent methods of resolving problems, resulting in impulsive and violent acts toward family members.

According to this perspective, four factors place family members at risk for abuse and family violence. These risk factors include the (a) family itself, (b) the caregiver, (c) the child, and (d) the presence of a family crisis. The first factor is the family. The family's economic resources that are at risk due to unemployment or welfare recipients are at risk (Berger & Brooks-Gunn, 2005). Poverty can be associated with parental childrearing practices and lead to increased caregiver strain and mental health problems. The environment in which the family lives can contribute to social isolation, low levels of social support, high local unemployment rates, and high population density (Elliott, Cunningham, Linder, Colangelo, & Gross, 2005). Living in a high-poverty community is a risk factor for maltreatment above and beyond the effects of family poverty.

Caregivers are the second factor, and they can be at risk for maltreating their children if they have experienced physical abuse as a child or witnessed abuse in their past (Lounds, Borkowski, & Whitman, 2006). Researchers (Kemp et al., 2008) found that evidence of the intergenerational cycle of child maltreatment, specifically, being a parent under 21 years of age, having a history of mental illness or depression, and living with a violent adult partially explained the relationship between parental history of child maltreatment and parental maltreatment of one's own children.

Further, caretaker qualities such as poor impulse control anger or management, conflict, and problems solved by blaming or hurting others also contribute to family violence. Caregivers who have a history of domestic violence are also at risk for harming their children, as are children who are born into family systems that lack the financial or psychological resources to create healthy nurturing environments for their individual personalities (Romano, Zoccolillo, & Paquette, 2006).

Caregivers who abuse their children tend to be young. Many are single mothers struggling with poverty, role strain, lack of education, and limited personal resources. Many are unprepared for their role in childrearing, immature,

TABLE 36-1 Risk Factors for Abuse

FACTORS	RATIONALE	EXAMPLE
Stress	Families who spend increased time together under stressful conditions may not have appropriate social supports.	Poor environment, poverty, unemployment, lower educational level.
Intolerance for normal development	Caregivers may not know normal development and have inappropriate expectations.	Hostility toward the very young child who asks many questions or is very active.
Intensity of involvement	Communication patterns expose mutual antagonism, higher levels of criticism, threatening behaviors or conflict.	Belittling adolescent for attempting to dress differently; criticizing a school-age child for failing to make a goal at a soccer game.
Coercive actions	Deficient parenting skills related to age-appropriate discipline techniques, and use of coercive tactics and physical punishment to maintain control of family members.	Physically punishing a child rather than using time-out strategies or a behavioral chart.
Right to influence	Abusive caregivers are either very authoritarian and punitive to the child's developmental needs or neglectful of emotional needs. The child has little power to negotiate or claim a safe space in such a family system.	The caregiver directs and supervises clothes shopping for a 17-year-old daughter, or in contrast, punishes the daughter when she interacts with peers in after-school activities.
Characteristics of perpetrator	Often, the perpetrator is a young adult in his/her mid-20s. The perpetrator many times does not have a high school diploma, is depressed, may have trouble coping with stressful situations, and lives at or below the poverty level. Many times, the perpetrator has experienced violence first-hand. Even though mothers are most often responsible for deaths resulting from child neglect, fathers or other male caretakers are responsible for most fatalities (National Clearinghouse on Child Abuse and Neglect Information, 2006).	Family violence occurring within patriarchal and matriarchal dominated systems.
Patterns of abuse	Intergenerational patterns of violence are passed down from generation to generation.	Caregivers will construct similar abusive relationships with their own children based on their own experiences of having violent caregivers. Mothers and fathers abused as children sometimes do not know any other method of disciplining than what they experienced as children.
Privacy of the home	Rules for appropriate punishment and discipline can grow and become extreme in a family system that has little contact with community groups such as school, church, or recreational programs. These rules may give rise to abnormal, inappropriate, harmful, and secretive practices that can destroy the self-worth of a child or family member.	Children are not involved in after-school programs or activities or not allowed to play with other neighborhood children.
Difficult transitions	Family transition periods (births, deaths, separations, loss, unemployment, and illness) create stressful conditions, and when abuse is present, these transitions can be particularly problematic and sources of violent and hurtful acts.	Alcohol use may increase during stressful periods for at-risk families and can precipitate violent behaviors.

Adapted from Gelles, R. J. (1997). *Intimate violence in the family.* Thousand Oaks, CA: Sage.

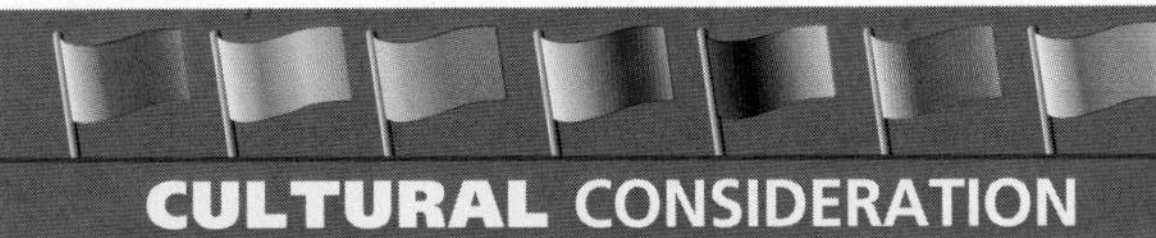

CULTURAL CONSIDERATION

Child Maltreatment among Asian Americans

Systematic reviews found that Asian and Pacific Islander children had the lowest rate of maltreatment among all racial groups at 3.5 per 1,000 children (Children's Bureau, 2006). Physical abuse, however, was the most prevalent, but Asian-American victims appear to be older. Asian boys tend to have been exposed to more frequent but less severe physical abuse than girls, and the average age was 7.3 in 2004 (Children's Bureau, 2006). In Los Angeles, it was reported that the average child victim in Korean immigrant families was 8.8 years. Further, male relatives were found to be the most common perpetrators, mostly biological fathers. The authors present an explanatory framework that examines the influence of Confucian philosophy and emphasizes hierarchical social structures, patriarchal authority, submissiveness, obedience, and loyalty as shaping childrearing practices, and focuses on children' obedience, loyalty, reverence, and duties to their parents. Family harmony and stoicism must be maintained, and there are high expectations of children to bring great success, wealth, and achievement to the family. Asian parents are more likely to believe that physical punishment is a legitimate form of discipline and that the resolution of problems must be kept within the family rather than seeking outside resources.

Source: Zhai, F., & Gao, Q. (2008). Child maltreatment among Asian Americans. *Child Maltreatment*, *20*(10), 1–17.

impulsive, and have low self-esteem. Caregivers who are physically abusive may not only have been abused as children, but also have poor role models and weak social supports.

Another characteristic of caregivers at risk for abusing children is a lack of knowledge, skills, and emotional maturity in understanding and meeting the needs of their child in developmentally appropriate ways as well as inappropriate expectations for their children's behavior. In this situation, the child also often assumes a caregiver role toward the caregiver, as when a 5-year-old consoles the unemployed parent. Termed "role-reversal," this commonly occurs in abusive families. A depressed caregiver is also at risk for physically or emotionally abusing children. Such an individual may be irritable or withdrawn from family members, not have the emotional energy to manage the demanding developmental needs of a child, or become provoked and use harsher punishment than necessary or appropriate.

Intimate partner violence increases the likelihood of child maltreatment in the home and if present, both partners were aggressive toward their children (Taylor et al., 2009). Caregivers who abuse substances are more likely to utilize severe punishment and be unable to tolerate a child's normal developmental behaviors (Edwards, Holden, Felitti, & Anda, 2003).

The third factor is the characteristics of individual infants that can place a family at risk for maltreatment. An infant who is born with a "fussy" or difficult temperament, and is not easily soothed or calmed, can be at risk for abuse. One caregiver may become frustrated and short-tempered with such an infant, whereas another caregiver may have the skills or patience to comfort the infant. Fussy, overactive, and unsoothable infants are also more likely to resist a caregiver's attempt at comforting, placing them at greater risk for abuse. Premature birth and low birth weight may also place an infant at risk for abuse and neglect (Sidebotham & Heron, 2006). Young children with hyperactivity and chronic health issues such as cerebral palsy and mental retardation are at an elevated risk. Prolonged hospitalization by either the child or caregiver can also interfere with establishing

EVIDENCE-BASED PRACTICE

Mothers with Methamphetamine Abuse

CLINICAL PROBLEM

What are the nursing interventions for mothers who abuse methamphetamines?

BEST CLINICAL PRACTICE

Methamphetamine abuse is now a national problem in the United States and poses significant problems for child's development, welfare, and health. The risk of child physical and sexual abuse is two times greater if parental substance abuse is present.

IMPLICATIONS FOR NURSING

Since nurses have involvement with caretakers and their children in diverse service delivery settings, nurses should be observing caretakers for signs and symptoms of drugs, in particular methamphetamine:

1. Recognize the signs and symptoms of methamphetamine abuse: cognitive changes, myocardial infarction, stroke, significant dental decay, euphoria, decreased sleeping and appetite, anxiety, irritability, unpredictability, paranoia, auditory and visual hallucinations, compulsive behaviors, labile mood, rages, and difficulty processing information.
2. Intervene immediately to protect the children involved and assess for abuse and neglect.
3. Consider the collection and testing of urine to evaluate if a child is being exposed to methamphetamine.

Reference: McGinness, T. M., & Pollack, D. (2008). Parental methamphetamine abuse and children. *Journal of Pediatric Health Care*, *22*(3), 152–158.

a nurturing bond or appropriate attachment behaviors. Weak attachment bonds from chronic hospitalization can result in a caregiver viewing the child as an "imperfect child" and place the child at risk for abuse. In particular, studies have demonstrated children with disabilities were found to be maltreated multiple times and in multiple ways. All types of disabilities, including mental retardation, speech or language impairments, emotional disabilities, learning disabilities, and physical disabilities, show high prevalence rates of abuse and neglect (Hibbard & Desch, 2007).

The fourth factor that places a family at risk for maltreatment and violence is when a family member is in situational crises (sudden or prolonged unemployment, illness of family members, residential changes, a caregiver's separation or possible divorce) that precipitates child abuse (Hibbard & Desch, 2007). Minor misbehavior can precipitate an abusive interaction, especially when caregivers have exhausted their ability to cope effectively with everyday hassles. In addition, families experiencing constant and chronic stress (financial, physical, mental health problems) are more susceptible to being physically or emotionally abusive. Finally, extra-marital affairs, which can create situations where the caregiver is angry and burdened with additional childrearing responsibilities, may result in child abuse and neglect.

ATTACHMENT MODEL

Attachment between a young child and the caregiver involves emotional availability, nurturance, warmth, protection, and the provision of comfort on the part of the caregiver. In return, the young child will demonstrate a sense of security, trust, balanced emotional regulation, and comfort-seeking behaviors (Zeanah & Boris, 2000). Bowlby (1969) considered attachment behavior a preprogrammed set of behavior patterns designed to keep the mother or caregiver close to the infant. Four attachment styles assist in understanding how infants and children are emotionally connected to their caregiver. These attachment patterns are listed in Box 36-1.

BOX 36-1
PATTERNS OF ATTACHMENT

Secure Attachment

The caregiver meets physical, developmental, and psychological needs, and the infant is able to balance proximity to the caregiver with exploration prior to separation. When an infant is distressed during separation, contact with the caregiver is sought, who then soothes the infant.

Avoidant Attachment

Infant realizes the caregiver will not always be available to provide comfort. The infant exhibits "independent" behavior without acknowledging the caregiver prior to separation, exhibits minimal distress during separation, and avoids emotional support offered by the caregiver upon reunion.

Ambivalent Attachment

The infant understands the caregiver is not reliable in meeting physiological and psychological needs and remains close before separation, is distressed during separation, demonstrates a combination of contact-seeking behaviors with temper tantrums during reunion, and may display indifference when comforted by the caregiver.

Disorganized Attachment

The infant is confused and cannot understand how to get physiological and psychological needs met by the caregiver. This infant may be rejected or comforted by the caregiver. Children with this type of attachment display no organized strategy toward the attachment figure.

Adapted from Cassidy, J., & Shaver, P. (2008). *Handbook of attachment: Theory, research, and clinical applications* (2nd ed.). New York: Guilford Press.

EYE ON...
Distinguishing Child Abuse from Cultural Practices

The cultural background of the family must be considered because some folk medicine practices resemble abuse. For instance, **cao gao**, practiced by Southeast Asians to treat minor ailments, involves rubbing a coin or a spoon heated in oil on an ill child's neck, spine, and ribs, that may create a burn or abrasion. **Cupping** (ventosos), practiced by Latin American and Russian cultures to treat headaches or abdominal pain, occurs by creating a vacuum under a cup or glass when a small amount of burning material is placed on the skin. The child may then present with first- or second-degree burns.

NURSING ALERT
Signs of Abuse

- **Unusual ecchymotic areas such as at the base of the skull or the face, buttocks, breasts, or abdomen should warrant a high index of suspicion of abuse.**
- **Burns, belt marks, or whip marks should always be investigated.**
- **The explanation of the injury doesn't seem consistent with the injury or the child's ability.**

CRITICAL THINKING

Suspecting Child Abuse

Mary, a young mother of five children, brings her 2-year-old, Helen, into the emergency department. The child has been vomiting for the past 24 hours, and appears dehydrated, weak, and smells of urine and feces. Upon examination, you notice six circular 3 mm areas on the lower back thigh areas that appear to be healing burns. There is erythema and tissue damage surrounding each of the borders. Mary appears angry at having to be in the emergency department and curses at Helen several times. Helen is lying on the stretcher in a fetal position with no eye contact and a sad and withdrawn affect.

1. **How does a child receive this type of injury to the back of the legs?**
2. **How would you proceed with the assessment process? What are the questions that you need to focus on with the mother?**

The attachment model suggests children demonstrating avoidant, ambivalent, and disorganized attachment are at risk for being abused.

TYPES OF CHILD ABUSE

Child abuse includes physical abuse, psychological abuse, sexual abuse, and abandonment and neglect.

PHYSICAL ABUSE

Physical abuse should always be suspected when there is an injury that cannot be explained or if the explanation is not supported by the facts: when the history provided is incongruent with the physical findings; the child's history is inconsistent or does not explain the injury; or the child's developmental level does not support the physical findings. Suspicion should also be aroused when the caregiver claims the injury was self-inflicted or inflicted by a sibling, or when there is a delay in seeking medical services.

Clinical Manifestations: Physical

Physical abuse indicators include unexplained bruises, scars, or welts that appear in various stages of healing; bruises on the mouth, lips, or eyes; an unexplained swollen extremity; bite marks, especially around the genitals or buttocks; bruises the shape of recognizable objects (hand, belt, electric cord), or injuries in locations a child cannot reach. Burns may be visible on the face, hands, legs, or feet, or appear as hot water scalding marks (an even line across the skin, usually on the legs or buttocks). Limited range of motion and complaints of tenderness may suggest skeletal injuries the result of direct blows, twisting forces, shaking, or squeezing. Figures 36-2 and 36-3 show marks and burns caused by commonly used objects. Figure 36-4 provides five examples of physical abuse.

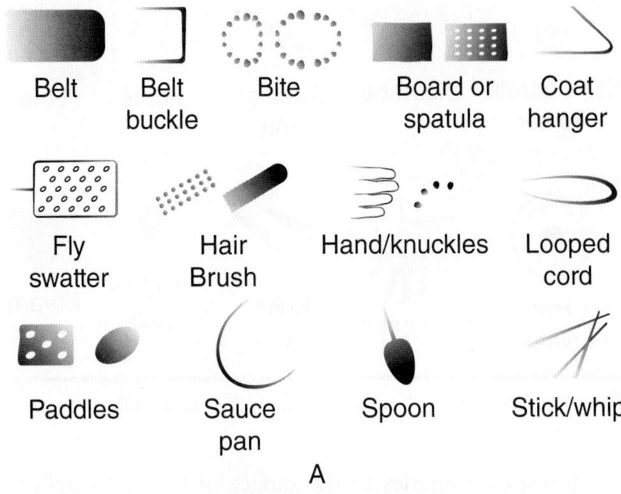

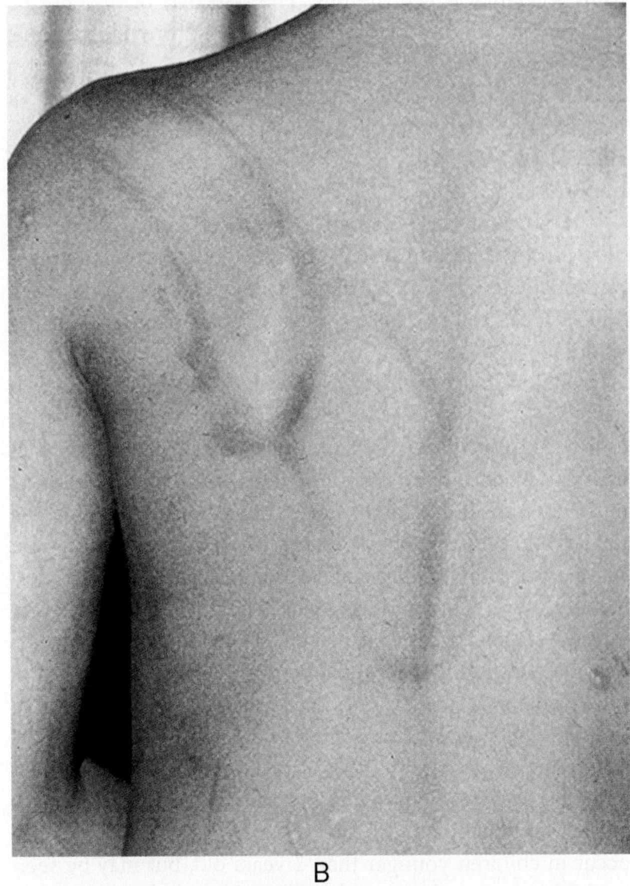

FIGURE 36-2 (A) Marks on skin left by objects. (B) Bruising in specific patterns, such as the loop of a strap, often is an indicator of child abuse. PHOTO COURTESY OF EMERGENCY MEDICAL SERVICES FOR CHILDREN, NERA, TORRANCE, CA.

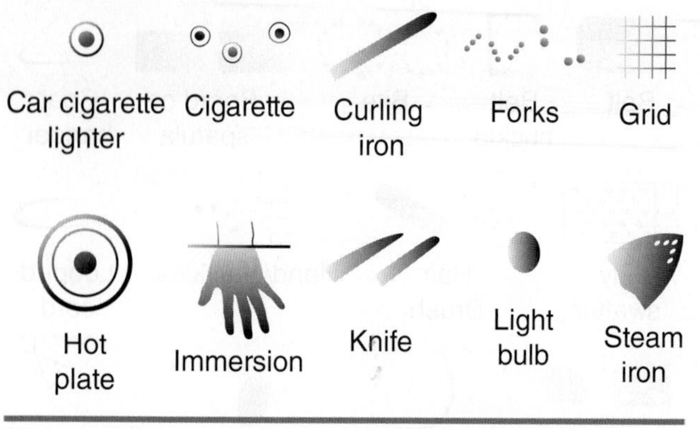

FIGURE 36-3 **Burns on Skin Left by Common Objects.** DELMAR CENGAGE LEARNING.

Bruises are injuries to the surface of the skin resulting from accidental falls or bumps. The skin may or may not be broken, and will be discolored. Table 36-2 provides a guide for assessing the characteristics and timeframe for bruising in children. Because young children may have a number of bruises as a result of their normal activities, nurses must be able to talk with children and caregivers about the origins of the bruises.

Head trauma in children is the most common cause of death from child abuse and involves skull fractures and intracranial hemorrhage (Tang, Buzney, Lashkari, & Weiter, 2008). Head injury can also lead to brain damage with developmental delays.

Shaken baby syndrome (SBS), first described by Caffey in 1946, is a type of head injury affecting 50,000 children each year (Epilepsy Association of Central Florida, n.d.). It happens when a baby is violently shaken. A baby has weak neck muscles and a large, heavy head. Shaking makes the fragile brain bounce back and forth inside the skull and causes bruising, swelling, and bleeding that can lead to permanent, severe brain damage or death. The characteristic injuries of shaken baby syndrome are subdural hemorrhages (bleeding in the brain), retinal hemorrhages (bleeding in the retina), damage to the spinal cord and neck, and fractures of the ribs and bones. These injuries may not be immediately noticeable. Symptoms of SBS include extreme irritability, lethargy, poor feeding, breathing problems, convulsions, vomiting, and pale or bluish skin. Shaken baby injuries usually occur in children younger than 2 years old, but may be seen in children up to the age of 5 (NINDS, 2009).

In the United States, an estimated 1,300 infants are hospitalized or die each year from shaken baby syndrome. One in four babies will die as a result of their injuries, and among those who survive, approximately 80% will suffer brain injury, blindness and deafness, fractures, paralysis, cognitive and learning disabilities, or cerebral palsy (NINDS, 2009). The infant is usually held around the trunk, impeding venous return and causing a pooling of blood in the larger vessels, especially of the head. The shaking motion causes tearing of the large vessels within the head, and the increased blood volume because of impeded venous return contributes to rupture of the blood vessels (Rangarajan & Shams, 2006). The development of imaging technology, in particular computed tomography (CT) scans and magnetic resonance imaging, has resulted in better identification and diagnosis of SBS. In the past, injuries associated with SBS may have been attributed to sudden infant death syndrome or unusual or mysterious neurological disorders. Shaken baby syndrome can go unattended, undetected, and unreported because there often are no outward symptoms. In addition, caregivers are not always willing to acknowledge they were responsible for shaking a baby. It is estimated that 70% of the perpetrators are male (father or mother's live-in boyfried) and have reported that they made attempts to respond to the infant's crying that escalated out of control (Russell, Trudeau, & Britner, 2008).

According to Fiske & Hall (2008), shaken baby syndrome is more than a mere act of abuse. The authors believe that the action should be relabeled as "inflicted childhood neurotrauma" (ICN) and is based on a breach of human rights of children and the violation of the ethic to provide due care to infants and children. They believe that parental rights as protective of children cannot exist; an "ownership" quality that the perpetrator was "provoked" by the infant to respond with violence cannot be tolerated. The primary ethic of a "child's rights" over the rights of the parents must be upheld.

Infants and children should be suspected of SBS with any signs as noted in Box 36-2. An ophthalmologic examination assists in confirming a diagnosis of SBS: one classic sign is retinal hemorrhage, usually bilaterally with subdural or subarachnoid hemorrhages (Tang et al., 2008). It is also important for the nurse to be alert to significant alterations in neurological symptoms of a child even when a family member claims no apparent reason for the acute neurological symptoms.

SBS should be managed by a multidisciplinary team, and includes a neurological evaluation, ophthalmologic examination, CAT scan, ultrasound, radiography, and careful history of the injury or illness. Birth trauma, meningitis, severe accidental trauma, infection, severe coagulopathy (hemophilia, von Willebrand's disease, and vitamin K deficiency), seizure disorders, and metabolic disorders should be ruled out before the diagnosis of SBS is determined. Retinal hemorrhages were more likely to be bilateral and extend to the periphery of the retina in SBS (Bechtel, Stoessel, Leventhal, & Duncan, 2005).

Risk factors for SBS include caregivers' gender as well as those experiencing stressful life events such as social, physical, or financial problems. Men are responsible for 70% of the physical abuse and physical abuse deaths attributed to SBS. A mother's partner or boyfriend, as well as babysitters, have also been implicated (Stirling & the Committee on Child Abuse and Neglect, 2007).

Health care professionals in all settings are in a unique position to assess for families that are at high risk and infants that may exhibit characteristics signs and symptoms. History taking, physical assessment, and accurate documentation are important to the evaluation and referral to child protective services.

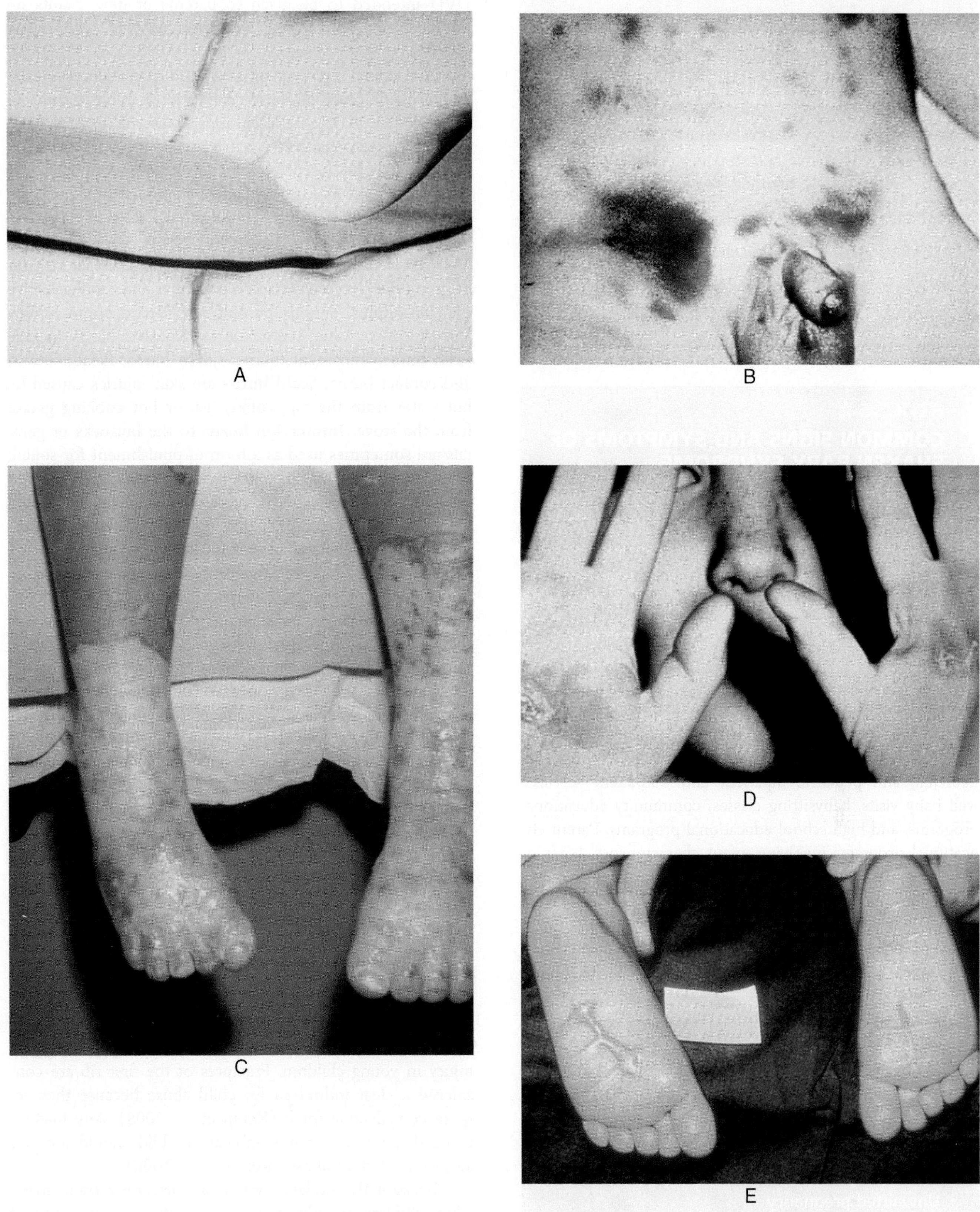

FIGURE 36-4 Photos of Child Abuse. (A) Bruises that encircle the extremities may indicate the child has been bound. (B) Bruises in various stages of healing may indicate a child is being abused. (C) Circumferential bums (stocking or glove bums) to the extremities may indicate the child was intentionally held in scalding water. (D) Cigarette Bums. (E) Bums that have specific shapes and patterns, called branding, may be an indicator of abuse. ALL PHOTOS COURTESY OF EMERGENCY MEDICAL SERVICES FOR CHILDREN, NERA, TORRANCE, CA.

TABLE 36-2 Date Estimation of Bruising in the Abused Child

TIME ELAPSED	CHARACTERISTICS
Less than 1 day	Reddish-blue to purple with margins
1 to 2 days	Bluish-brown to dark purple
3 to 5 days	Yellowish-green to brown
5 to 7 days	Yellow-fading
Past 1 week	Yellow-brown-fading

BOX 36-2

COMMON SIGNS AND SYMPTOMS OF SHAKEN BABY SYNDROME

Lethargy/loss of muscle tone/poor sucking or swallowing/inability to lift head/trouble moving arms or legs

Extreme irritability/rigidity/posturing/problems breathing

Vomiting without other signs of illness

Seizures/bulging fontanelles/pupils not same size

Redness in the eye/ecchymotic areas around the eye or face

Prevention programs should be available on obstetric, neonatal, and pediatric inpatient and outpatient services, well baby visits, babysitting classes, community educational programs, and high school educational programs. Parent educational programs involving infant characteristics, types of temperaments, and coping with crying and fussy infants are especially important. Another helpful program, *The Period of PURPLE Crying Program,* is an SBS prevention program from the National Center on Shaken Baby Syndromes. It includes a full-color 11-page booklet and a 10-minute DVD intended to be given to parents of new infants on the problems and coping strategies involved with crying infants.

NURSING ALERT

Infants at Greater Risk for SBS

- Crying and colicky babies
- Difficult temperaments
- Prematurity
- Unwanted pregnancy
- Special needs baby
- Low birth weight
- Congenital defects
- Experiencing drug or alcohol withdrawal

Abdominal injuries rank second to neurological injuries as the major cause of abuse-related death. Blunt trauma to the abdomen may cause lacerations to internal organs (liver, bladder, spleen, pancreas, bowel) resulting in distension. Bruising may be absent or minimal. If an abdominal injury is suspected, the child should also be examined for puncture wounds and the hematocrit monitored because of possible internal hemorrhage.

Children between 1 and 5 years of age are at risk for burn injuries because their skin is thinner and more sensitive than an adult's. Serious burning also occurs more rapidly and at lower water temperatures. Abusive burns include scald burns, immersion burns, splash burns, flexion burns, and contact burns. **Scald burns** are skin injuries caused by hot water from the tap, coffee, tea, or hot cooking grease from the stove. **Immersion burns** to the buttocks or genitals are sometimes used as a form of punishment for soiling or problem behaviors in toilet training, and create an even line across the legs, buttocks, or hands. They are caused either by an accidental fall into hot bath water or by purposefully placing the child in a tub of hot water.

"Stocking or glove" type **burns** represent attempts by the child to prevent and protect himself or herself from being immersed in hot scalding tub water; the burn has the appearance of a glove or stocking with an even edge. **Splash burns** occur when the caregiver pours hot liquid on the child, and usually involve the back, lateral side of the face, or shoulder. The direction the hot liquid flows down the child's body assists in diagnosis. **Flexion burns** occur when caregivers purposefully immerse a child in hot liquids and the body part immersed is held in a flexed position so that a "zebra" pattern occurs. For example, a child who has hot coffee thrown on his arm may flex the arm so that only the top parts of the forearm and upper arm are burned, and the inside of the arm is protected by flexion in response to the oncoming hot liquid. **Contact burns** involve certain implements such as curling irons, steam irons, cigarette lighters, matches, hot pots, space heaters, or radiators. Old burn marks should give additional cues to nurses that an abusive pattern may exist in the family.

Skeletal trauma is another common manifestation of abuse. The metaphyseal fracture is considered an inflicted injury in young children. Fractures of the first rib are considered a clear indication for child abuse because they require considerable force (Kemp et al., 2008). Any fracture being diagnosed in a nonambulatory child should increase suspicion of child abuse (Kemp et al., 2008).

Because the skeletal system is commonly traumatized when children are physically abused, all extremities should be examined for swelling, crepitus, or hematomas. Pulse, color, sensitivity, and function of all limbs are also part of the assessment. Suspicious fractures include chip fractures of the metaphysic, spiral fractures resulting from twisting of the limb, epiphysis separations, and fractures in unusual places

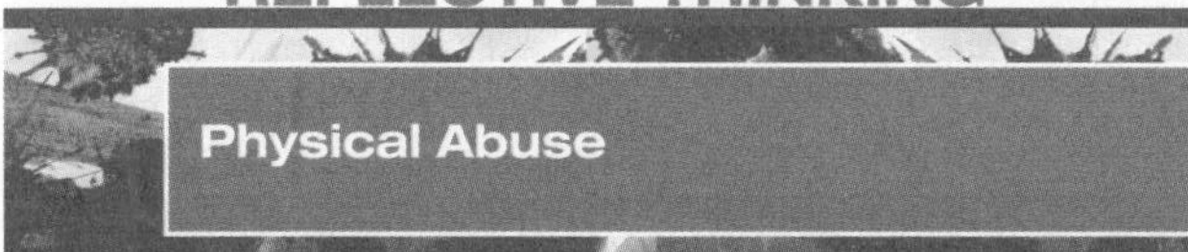

REFLECTIVE THINKING

Physical Abuse

As a new pediatric intensive care unit nurse, you are assigned to care for a child with second-degree burns on her buttocks and legs. According to Tena, her mother, Emily had been placed in a tub of scalding water by accident. Now Emily requires 24-hour intensive care but each time care is provided, one had to wonder how such an "accident" could have occurred. The family was referred to Child Protective Services.

1. How does your attitude influence the care you provide an abused and neglected child like Emily and her caregiver?
2. What responsibility do you have to ensure the care provided to Emily and Tena is nonjudgmental and still professional?

such as the ribs, vertebrae, scapula, sternum, or metacarpal bones (Kemp et al., 2008). Children with two or more injury-related ED visits in one year are more likely to be reported for child maltreatment and to have a substantiated report (Spivey, Schnitzer, Kruse, Slusher, & Jaffe, 2009). Figure 36-5 depicts spiral fracture in a young child.

Clinical Manifestations: Psychological

Physically abused children may also exhibit passive behaviors such as withdrawal, depression, or a sad mood. Other behaviors can include anger, hostility, or being frightened when approached. Children who have been physically abused may also harm their siblings, peers, pets, or neighborhood animals. Box 36-3 lists other behavioral indicators of abuse.

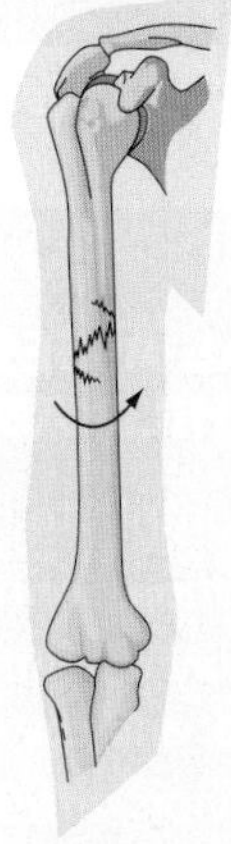

Figure 36-5 Spiral fractures of long bones are caused by twisting forces. DELMAR CENGAGE LEARNING.

BOX 36-3
BEHAVIORAL INDICATORS OF PHYSICAL ABUSE

- Frightened stance when adults approach
- Hyper-alert when caregivers give directions
- Anxiety and distress when hearing other children cry
- Fear of returning home
- Increased startle reflex
- Over eagerness to please
- Lack of ability to attach to caregiver
- Extremes of behavior: aggressive, or passive and withdrawn
- Frequent daydreams or staring into space
- Detached stance toward others

Diagnosis

The diagnosis of physical abuse is based on a complete nursing history and assessment, medical examination, and laboratory tests. X-rays or CT scans may also be ordered to confirm the diagnosis.

Treatment

Treatment may vary depending on the severity of abuse. Extreme physical abuse including internal hemorrhage or organ injury will likely require admission to a pediatric intensive care unit. Neurological evaluation and monitoring may be necessary if a head injury is suspected. Consultation with specialists such as orthopedists or neurologists may also be required. The child will often need counseling and the caregiver will need education related to parenting skills, anger management, and normal human development so the abuse is not repeated. Table 36-3 lists some measures of assessment of parental care. In some cases, removal of the child from the abuser's care will be mandated.

Nursing Management

The nursing assessment for a child suspected of being physically abused should include a comprehensive evaluation, photographs, and written documentation of the body systems affected by using a body chart and careful descriptions (Box 36-4). It is also important to obtain height and weight measurements to determine whether or not they are within the normal range for age. The integumentary system, including the skin, scalp, bottoms of the feet, and the complete trunk and genital areas, should be carefully examined. All bruises, scars, burns, and discoloration of the skin should be noted and in some institutions photographs taken to document the injuries. The musculoskeletal system should be assessed for painful muscles, swollen ribs, or past

Table 36-3 Measures for Assessing Parental Care

MEASURE	RESPONDENTS	AUTHORS
Adolescent Abuse Inventory	Adolescents who are parents	Sebes, 1983
Psychological Maltreatment Scale	Administered by a trained observer	Taylor, Underwood, Thomas, and Franklin, 1988
Home Observation for Measurement of the Environment (HOME) Inventory	Administered by a trained observer	Caldwell and Bradley, 1984
Parenting Stress Index	Caretaker of a child, administered by a trained observer	Abidin, 1990

fractures. The urinary-genital system will also need to be evaluated, and the presence of blood or protein in the urine, along with past urinary tract infections, noted. Finally, the child's psychological status and interpersonal skills should be assessed utilizing the information listed in Box 36-5 and Box 36-6.

Relevant information about a family's history of or experience with abuse can be obtained from conversations with the caregivers and the child. Because nurses are professionals perceived as helpful and caring, caregivers and children may be more open and honest in sharing information with the nurse about how discipline is practiced and how problems in the family are handled. Box 36-7 and Box 36-8 provide guidelines to use when talking with both the child and caregiver.

Munchausen Syndrome

Munchausen Syndrome is considered a separate form of physical abuse, and was coined by Asher (1951) to designate patients who traveled from hospital to hospital presenting with illnesses and receiving treatments that at times included surgery. The condition was named after Baron Karl Friedrich Hieronymus Freiherr van Munchausen (1720–1797), a German cavalry officer, who was also a world-class liar.

BOX 36-4
HISTORY AND PHYSICAL ASSESSMENT CATEGORIES—CHILD ABUSE

- Location, color, size, shape of any injury recorded on body chart
- Specific characteristics of bruise, including an outline and the depth of injury
- Pain or tenderness associated with injury
- Complete assessment of all body systems
- General level of hygiene
- Exact date, time, and place of event
- Chronological account of injury
- Witnesses present at time of injury
- Exact quotations by child and caregiver of how the injury occurred

BOX 36-5
PSYCHOLOGICAL ASSESSMENT CATEGORIES—CHILD ABUSE

- Appearance
- Mood (feelings, lability, fluctuations, appropriateness, ease in displaying feelings)
- Manner of relating to examiner
- Modes of thinking and intellectual skills
- Play (capacity, fantasy, amount, quality of involvement, use of materials, themes, spontaneity, and interaction with examiner)
- Sensorimotor development (fine and gross motor activities, symmetry of movement, eye-hand coordination)
- Speech and language skills; the capacity to communicate with examiner

BOX 36-6
INTERPERSONAL ASSESSMENT: CAREGIVER—CHILD ABUSE

- Willingness to contribute information
- Level of cooperation during interview
- Capacity to display empathy, support, and care toward the child, and the child's response
- Nonverbal behaviors, affect, and level of cooperation (eye contact, posture)
- Quality of child-caregiver relationship (fearful, anxious, hostile, indifferent, close)

BOX 36-7
INTERVIEWING THE CHILD

- Interview privately without interruptions.
- Reassure child is not "in trouble" nor has done anything wrong. (Because children often assume they are to blame for the caregiver's actions, it is important to remind them the injuries are not their fault.)
- Assure child the conversation is confidential; if the information provided needs to be shared with others, inform the child.
- Consider the child's developmental level when talking about the incident. Use the child's own words when documenting the incident (they become part of the legal record).
- Allow talking at own pace; use a supportive matter-of-fact attitude.
- Encourage the child to show injuries.
- Utilize therapeutic play, drawings, puppet play, or story time to share thoughts and feelings if the child does not have verbal skills to talk openly about experiences.
- Inform child it is okay to talk to the caregiver about conversations; if the authorities are to be notified, both child and caregivers need to be informed.

BOX 36-8
INTERVIEWING THE CAREGIVERS

- Allow caregivers to feel comfortable; conduct interview privately.
- Be professional, honest, direct, and avoid showing anger or hostility.
- Establish a supportive relationship.
- Be aware of the role Child Protective Services will play in the situation so accurate information is to be provided; explain how Child Protective Services will provide support and assistance.
- Inform caregivers not to punish the child for sharing information.

The label **Munchausen syndrome by proxy** refers to caregivers who fabricate signs and symptoms of disease, expose their child to harmful medical interventions, or cause illness in their child which leads to painful invasive procedures. The perpetrator denies the etiology of the child's illness. The individual parent or caregiver (usually the mother) who injures children in this manner is recognized as a child abuser. The *Diagnostic and Statistical Manual of Mental Disorders* classifies Munchausen syndrome by proxy as a Fictitious Disorder Not Otherwise Specified. The criteria for a caregiver to meet the diagnosis of the Munchausen Syndrome include: (1) intentional production or feigning of psychological or physical signs or symptoms in a person who is under the individual's care; (2) external incentives for the behavior causing illness or injury are absent; (3) motivation for the behavior is to assume a sick role by proxy; (4) the behavior is not accounted for by another mental disorder (APA, 2000).

The adult abuser receives this diagnosis rather than the child, and uses the disease to escape from marital, physical, or emotional problems, or poor self-esteem (Forsyth, 2002). By attending to the supposed needs of the child, the caregiver escapes the reality of his or her problems. Many times there is also a history of psychiatric problems and treatment, and there usually is a poor emotional relationship between the child's parents. Frequently the caregiver has had some exposure to the medical field and is quickly accepted as competent by professionals caring for the child.

Children are often brought to the hospital or emergency room with a variety of suspected problems including infections, electrolyte imbalances, nonaccidental poisonings, apnea, hemorrhage, seizures, or respiratory illnesses. Assessment includes videotaping the child-caregiver interaction when Munchausen syndrome by proxy is suspected. The warning signs of the disease in a child are found in Box 36-9.

Nursing Management

Nursing management includes establishing a trusting relationship with caregivers, accurately assessing family dynamics, patterns of illness, and quality of relationships; carefully documenting all caregiver-child interactions and behaviors; corroborating all histories with appropriate professionals and reporting inconsistencies; reviewing suspected cases of Munchausen syndrome by proxy with the multidisciplinary teams; and following up as indicated to the appropriate child

BOX 36-9
WARNING SIGNS OF MUNCHAUSEN SYNDROME BY PROXY

- Prolonged, unexpected, or extraordinary illness; extensive history provided by caregiver (usually the mother)
- Inappropriate signs and symptoms with no relationship to the history provided
- Several prior medical contacts and evaluations, with negative diagnostic findings
- Appropriate treatment is poorly tolerated and ineffective
- Past family history of serious childhood disorders and possibly unexplained sibling deaths and an already known abused sibling

REFLECTIVE THINKING

Beliefs and Values about Child Abuse

1. What is your personal understanding of why child abuse occurs?
2. How can you advocate for a child in spite of caregivers' protests or denials?
3. How do you feel about disciplining a child with physical force?

Reflections from Families

Chad has not been doing well in preschool. He hits and punches the other children, has been having terrible temper tantrums, and is sent home from school at least once a week. The program director has advised me to place him in a therapeutic nursery program. During that time, I began to realize the many times I have spanked and hit Chad with my belt have caused him to want to hurt other children. At first I could not believe this, because this is how my mother raised me. I know I need to discipline differently to stop Chad from hurting others. I am now seeking assistance from a nurse who works in the preschool program.

protection agencies and mental health services. Admission to an inpatient hospital unit where the child's actual signs and symptoms can be documented and reported is very important to see if the parent is exaggerating the child's physical problems (Stirling & the Committee on Child Abuse and Neglect, 2007).

CHILDHOOD ABANDONMENT AND NEGLECT

Child abandonment is, in many states, a form of neglect. The child is considered abandoned when the parent's identify or whereabouts are unknown, the child has been left alone in circumstances where the child suffers serious harm, or the parent fails to maintain contact with the child or provide reasonable support for a specified period (Child Welfare Information Gateway, 2008). Table 36-4 identifies the categories of various forms of neglect in children.

Child neglect occurs when a child experiences predictable injury or impairment because of caregiver inattention. Neglect is often suspected in children who are not of normal height and weight for age. In addition, neglectful caregivers may not have kept up with yearly child health assessments, or acted on school recommendations for such services as speech, language, or physical therapy evaluations. Other signs of child neglect appear in Box 36-10.

Nursing Management

Nursing interventions for child neglect are similar to those of physical abuse. In addition, the nurse should understand the child's attachment to the caregiver even though the caregiver is neglectful. The nurse should provide a safe, positive, trusting, and nurturing environment, where the child is allowed to interact with other children and receive adult attention in a caring and warm manner. The child may need an explanation regarding why the caregiver may not be allowed to visit or why the child is placed in foster care. Additional services needed for families of neglected children or foster families include visiting nurse service, homemaker services, parenting classes, parent support groups, follow-up programs with school systems, and parent hotline telephone numbers when feelings of anger or frustration are building within the family setting.

Psychological Abuse

Psychological abuse is defined as acts of omission (willfully not attending a child's graduation or award ceremony) or commission (a child is told that he or she is ugly) deemed psychologically damaging. It also involves the presence of hostile behavior as well as the absence of positive parenting behaviors. Psychologically damaging or abusive acts are acts where caregivers engage in behavior that has a pattern of sustained and repetitive quality. Messages like "Nothing you do is of any value or good enough," or "You are no-good and worthless" have serious consequences when it comes from a significant caregiver or attachment figure during childhood. Caregivers can be aware or unaware of the hurt and emotional pain their words cause, and often are repeating experiences they had with their own caregivers relative to discipline and guidance, without considering the effects and meaning they have on their child's psychological growth (Dubowitz, Feigelman, Lane, & Kim, 2009). Refer to Box 36-11 for a list of behaviors seen in adults who psychologically abuse children.

The intergenerational potential for emotional abuse stems from an unavailable or psychologically neglectful caregiver who has unmet emotional needs coupled with low levels of social support. Many times caregivers did not experience caring, warm, and comforting parenting styles that taught them how to nurture their children. Psychiatric

CASE STUDY / CARE PLAN

THE PHYSICALLY ABUSED CHILD

Kamdin, a 4-year-old female, was admitted for vomiting and diarrhea for the past several days. When she was assessed by the nurse, Kamdin was found to have small round burn marks on her upper back and behind her legs. The caregiver is her 19-year-old mother, Veronica, who also has three other children less than 5 years of age. Currently she is living in a one-room apartment with her partner, Jonah, who just was released from jail for selling cocaine. Veronica indicated that both she and her partner smoke cigarettes but has little money to provide regular meals for her children. Veronica appeared somewhat numb to her children, who were crying and asking to be picked up and held. When asked about the marks on Kamdin's back, she indicated that her partner, Jonah, was responsible for the cigarette marks. She said she also got beaten after trying to stop him from hurting her children.

NURSING CARE PLAN

ASSESSMENT

Kamdin has been abused, probably by her mother's partner Jonah. Veronica needs to receive information on appropriate parenting and discipline, as well as on behaviors to expect from her young children. She may also need a supportive network to help her learn how to interact more appropriately with her children, and a referral should be made to child protective services. Because of Jonah's past history of drug use, he may be using drugs and his behavior may again become violent and harsh.

NURSING DIAGNOSIS 1

Interrupted family process caused by disrupted attachment, lack of nurturing qualities, or past abusive parenting experiences.

EXPECTED OUTCOMES

1. Kamdin will begin to feel safe with Veronica.
2. Veronica will begin to model appropriate nurturing behaviors toward Kamdin.

NOC: Family Support during Treatment

NIC: Family Involvement Promotion

INTERVENTIONS/*RATIONALES*

1. Teach nurturing behaviors to Veronica. *Caregivers need to be taught normal human development and the role of nurturing in facilitating development.*
2. Focus on the ability to comfort Kamdin, provide age-appropriate discipline, engage in age-appropriate activities, and understand Kamdin's needs based on normal growth and development. *Positive attachment behaviors provide the foundation for nurturing caregiver roles.*
3. Explore with Veronica behavior that may interfere with the ability to nurture. *Caregivers may have personal problems that impact their caregiving ability.*
4. Teach and engage in role-modeling behaviors with Veronica. *Intergenerational transmission of violence is common.*
5. Provide time during hospitalization where Kamdin and Veronica can participate in age-appropriate, nurturing activities. *Caregivers may not have had nurturing experiences during their childhood years and need support and acknowledgment for their caring efforts and information about how to nurture.*
6. Be supportive and nurturing to Veronica when attempting to change her behavior. *Caregivers need opportunities to engage in play activities with their child and practice supportive behaviors.*

(Continues)

CASE STUDY / CARE PLAN (Continued)

7. Provide referral for counseling and in-home supportive resources if needed. *Caregivers may need ongoing in-home support from community agencies.*
8. Discuss with Veronica need to secure social services for safe home away from her partner who has been abusive not only to her but also to her children. *Caregivers and their children may need support from social service agencies.*
9. Discuss need for a social service consultation to secure a restraining order to prevent her partner from entering her home and harming her children. *Caregivers and their children may need to seek help to prevent harm from abusive partners through the courts.*

EVALUATION

Kamdin is more comfortable around her mother. Veronica will demonstrate nurturing attachment behaviors toward Kamdin, and will acknowledge past problems and willingness to accept support.

NURSING DIAGNOSIS 2

Risk for trauma related to evidence of physical abuse, physical neglect, and an unsafe environment.

EXPECTED OUTCOMES

1. Kamdin will remain safe within the family system: no evidence of physical abuse or neglect.
2. The family will be involved in ongoing counseling to eliminate abusive behaviors.
3. Veronica will be open and responsive to supportive interventions.

NOC: Abuse Recovery

NIC: Abuse Protection Support

INTERVENTIONS/*RATIONALES*

1. Assess Kamdin's physical and emotional status; intervene as indicated in Nursing Diagnosis. Refer to appropriate counseling and support. *An emotional status assessment may reflect signs of posttraumatic stress disorder from repeated abusive episodes. Interventions listed previously will help prevent further abuse.*
2. Assess the other children for signs of abuse and neglect. *Other family members may be at risk for the same problems as Kamdin.*
3. Refer family to appropriate counseling and explain importance of obtaining ongoing counseling. *Ongoing counseling will decrease abuse and increase parenting skills.*
4. Schedule Kamdin and her mother for child therapy such as play therapy *so that she can begin to deal with her anger and feelings,*
5. Approach Veronica in a supportive and nonjudgmental manner. *The child's safety rests on ensuring that caregivers stay in the health care system and utilize services.*
6. Provide Veronica education in age-appropriate and safe discipline, time-out methods; age-appropriate growth and development; Kamdin's need for psychological and social support; nutrition; self-care activities; care of a sick child; and enhancement of nurturing behaviors. *Teaching normal development behavior and discipline practices helps improve interactions.*

EVALUATION

1. Veronica will accept teaching and resources offered; Kamdin and her siblings will remain free from further injury.
2. Veronica will be able to accept her partner as a victimizer and distance herself from him so that she can protect her children and herself.
3. Veronica will attend counseling and integrate information into her behavior with her children.
4. Veronica will understand the value of attending or participating in counseling and integrate information taught into her interactions with her children.

(Continues)

CASE STUDY / CARE PLAN (Continued)

NURSING DIAGNOSIS 3

Situational low self-esteem related to past physical abuse and neglect and unsafe environment.

EXPECTED OUTCOMES

1. Veronica will express feelings related to past abuse.
2. Veronica will regain a sense of control and positive self-regard.
3. Kamdin will be able to express feeling related to being abused and not protected by her mother.

NOC: Abuse Recovery: Emotional

NIC: Self-Esteem Enhancement

INTERVENTIONS/*RATIONALES*

1. Acknowledge to Kamdin that she is safe and loved; encourage talking and supporting child's attempts at talking about experiences. *Support builds trust and security.*
2. Encourage Kamdin to engage in self-care decisions, give praise and support to initiate the activities. *Positive experiences facilitate self-esteem and sense of control.*

EVALUATION

Veronica begins to feel more comfortable and begins talking about experiences related to abuse. Kamdin will be able to express positive feelings toward self, engage in age-appropriate activities, and demonstrate the ability to have control through choice of several aspects of daily activities. She will also be able to express her fears and report any additional abuse to other family members such as her grandmother or nursery school teacher.

TABLE 36-4 Types of Neglect and Their Manifestations

TYPES	MANIFESTATIONS
Physical neglect	Conspicuous inattention to avoidable hazards in the home; other forms of reckless disregard for the child's safety and welfare, such as driving while intoxicated and leaving a young child unattended in a motor vehicle
Medical neglect	
• Refusal of health care	Failure to provide or allow needed care in accordance with recommendations of a competent health care professional for a physical injury, illness, medical condition, or impairment
• Delay in health care	Failure to seek timely and appropriate medical care for a serious health problem that any reasonable layman would have recognized as needing professional medical attention
Custody-related neglect	
• Abandonment	Desertion of a child without arranging for reasonable care and supervision. This category includes cases in which children were not claimed within two days and when children were left by parents or substitutes who gave no (or false) information about their whereabouts
• Expulsion	Other blatant refusals of custody, such as permanent or indefinite expulsion of a child from the home without adequate arrangements for care by others, or refusal to accept custody of a returned runaway

(Continues)

Table 36-4 Types of Neglect and Their Manifestations (*Continued*)

TYPES	MANIFESTATIONS
• Inadequate supervision	Child left unsupervised or inadequately supervised for extended periods or allowed to remain away from home overnight without the parent or substitute knowing (or attempting to determine) the child's whereabouts
• Other custody issue	Custody-related forms of inattention to the child's needs other than those covered by abandonment or expulsion. For example, repeated shuttling of a child from one household to another because of apparent unwillingness to maintain custody, or chronically and repeatedly leaving a child with others for days or weeks at a time
Emotional neglect	
• Inadequate nurturance or affection	Marked inattention to the child's needs for affection, emotional support, attention competence
• Chronic or extreme abuse	Chronic or extreme spousal abuse or other domestic violence in the child's presence or domestic violence
• Permitted drug or alcohol abuse	Encouraging or permitting drug or alcohol use by the child; cases of the child's drug or alcohol use are included if it appears the parent or guardian had been informed of the problem and had not attempted to intervene
• Permitted other maladaptive behavior	Encouragement or permittance of other maladaptive behavior (e.g., severe assaultiveness, chronic delinquency) in circumstances in which the parent or guardian has reason to be aware of the existence and seriousness of the problem but does not attempt to intervene
• Refusal of psychological care	Refusal to allow needed and available treatment for a child's emotional or behavioral impairment or problem in accordance with competent professional recommendation
• Delay in psychological care	Failure to seek or provide needed treatment for a child's emotional or behavioral impairment or problem that any reasonable layman would have recognized as needing professional psychological attention (e.g., severe depression, suicide attempt)
• Other emotional neglect	Other inattention to the child's developmental or emotional needs not classifiable under any of the previous forms of emotional neglect (e.g., markedly overprotective restrictions that foster immaturity or emotional overdependence, chronically applying expectations clearly inappropriate in relation to the child's age or level of development)
Educational neglect	
• Permitted chronic truancy	Habitual truancy averaging at least five days a month is classifiable under this form of maltreatment if the parent or guardian has been informed of the problem and has not attempted to intervene
• Failure to enroll or other truancy	Failure to register or enroll a child of mandatory school age, causing the school-age child to remain at home for no legitimate reasons (e.g., to work, to care for siblings) an average of at least three days a month
• Inattention to special need	Refusal to allow or failure to obtain recommended remedial educational services, or education neglect in obtaining or following through with treatment for a child's diagnosed learning disorder or other special education need without reasonable cause

Adapted from Gaudin, J. M. (1993). *Child neglect: A guide for interventions.* Washington, DC: U.S. Department of Health and Human Services, Administration for Children and Families, Westover Consultants (Contract No. HHS-105-89-1730).

BOX 36-10
SIGNS OR SYMPTOMS OF NEGLECT

Inadequate Care (General)

- Inappropriate meals (serving cereal for breakfast, lunch, and nothing for dinner)
- Clothing that is old, dirty, inappropriate for age, or fits poorly
- Lack of personal hygiene
- Lack of health care maintenance (routine immunizations, yearly examinations)
- Poor supervision, inadequate limit setting (allowing a 5-year-old to play outside until 11 P.M.)
- Child welfare endangerment caused by caregiver dependency on chemicals or drugs

Inadequate Physical Environment

- Inadequate shelter (unheated rooms, lack of running water or proper plumbing)
- Inadequate sleeping conditions (having female child sleep with an older brother)
- Poor sanitary conditions (garbage in the home or play area)
- Structural, electrical, or fire hazards (unprotected electrical outlets)
- Chemicals or drugs not in locked cabinets or within child's reach
- Water temperature hazards (temperature too hot)

Inadequate Parenting

- Frequent school absences
- Inappropriate discipline (locked in a closet, physically punished)
- Emotional abandonment (never attending school conferences, not involved in caregiver-child school-related activities)
- Locked out of house
- Independent decisions made without setting parent limits
- Parent uncooperative when school supports child

illnesses such as depression or personality disorders are additional risk factors for psychological abuse. Finally, a caregiver's behavior may represent the recreation of patterns of psychological abuse experienced as a child or poor problem-solving ability. Refer to Box 36-12 for characteristics commonly seen in parents who abuse their children.

Indicators suggesting a child may experience psychological abuse are found in Box 36-13. Assessment scales that

BOX 36-11
BEHAVIORS OF ADULTS WHO PSYCHOLOGICALLY ABUSE CHILDREN

- Ignoring or degrading child and child's developmental, social, and psychological needs
- Rejecting child's value and requests
- Isolating child from the family or community
- Terrorizing or threatening child
- Corrupting or exploiting child
- Verbally assaulting child
- Pressuring child to mature and assume an older child's role than is appropriate
- Exposing child to family and community violence

identify children who are abused or caregivers who are at increased risk to maltreat infants and children are listed in Table 36-5.

A multidisciplinary team, composed of a nurse, physician, and social worker, needs to work collaboratively in assessing and diagnosing psychological abuse. Areas for assessment include the clinical manifestations listed earlier, as well as noting if the child has school-related problems such as poor grades or withdrawn behaviors.

Treatment may involve complete physical examination and X-rays to ensure physical or sexual abuse is not also present. Professionals who work with children suspected of being abused may also have interactions with the legal system and CPS workers for coordinated, multidisciplinary efforts. Treatment will be initiated by the legal and court system to protect children and will include ongoing supervision, family counseling, and resources such as parenting and anger management classes.

SEXUAL ABUSE

Sexual abuse is defined as inappropriately exposing or subjecting a child to sexual contact, activity, or behavior. Sexual abuse includes oral, anal, genital, buttock, and breast contact. It also includes the use of objects for vaginal or anal penetration, fondling, or sexual stimulation. Exploitation of a child for pornographic purposes or stimulating a child with inappropriate solicitation or erotic material is also considered sexual abuse (Prevent Child Abuse America, 2009). There are several forms of sexual abuse or maltreatment, including assault, incest, exploitation, exhibitionism, pedophilia, and child molestation.

Assault is an unlawful, sudden, violent attack on another person; **rape,** considered a type of assault, is sexual intercourse with force or a threat of force, and without a person's consent. **Statutory rape** is consensual sexual relations between a minor and an adult. **Date or acquaintance**

BOX 36-12

CHARACTERISTICS COMMON TO PSYCHOLOGICALLY ABUSIVE PARENTS

- Psychologically abused as a child
- Use of alcohol or drugs
- Stressed with few resources
- Inappropriate expectations of child
- Angry and hostile affect
- Poor parenting and coping skills
- Psychiatric illness such as depression, schizophrenia, or personality disorders
- Marital conflict with violence

BOX 36-13

INDICATORS OF PSYCHOLOGICAL ABUSE

- Poor self-esteem
- Poor academic performance
- Acting-out behaviors in school and community
- Fighting and hitting other children
- Lack of friends or peer group
- Lack of involvement in school and after-school activities
- Depression
- Little time spent at home
- Suicidal ideation
- Involvement in drugs or alcohol
- Problems with personal hygiene
- Self-defeating and self-mutilating behaviors
- Lack of trust in adults
- Speech disorder
- Failure to thrive
- Physical illness

rape is sexual intercourse with force or threat where the victim and perpetrator know one another either socially or professionally. Teenagers and college-age students are at most risk for this type of abuse. Reported cases of sexual abuse are three times more likely in girls than boys. Children in the poorest income category (less than $15,000/year) are 18 times more likely to be reported for sexual abuse than children whose parents earned more than $30,000 per year (Hines & Malley-Morrison, 2005; Prevent Child Abuse America, 2009).

Incest is sexual intercourse between closely related persons in a position of trust and authority over the child. Incest by fathers, stepfathers, and siblings has increased over the past 20 years. Characteristics of incestuous families include power imbalances in the family; fear of authority in the children; isolation from the community; denial; blurred and inappropriate boundaries or role confusion; highly sexualized or highly repressive atmosphere; history of multigenerational sexual or physical abuse, or alcoholism; lack of empathy; poor communication patterns; inadequate limit setting; and emotional deprivation (Herman, 2000).

Exploitation involves prostitution and child pornography. Exploitation can range from nudity, disrobing, and genital exposure by an adult in front of a child, to observing a child undress, bathe or use the toilet, intimate kissing, fondling, or masturbation. The child's emotional development is affected by this type of abuse, resulting in shame, guilt, depression, anxiety, psychosomatic disorder, substance abuse, attention-deficit hyperactive disorders, and conduct or oppositional disorders. **Exhibitionism** is exposing one's genitals to strangers. **Pedophilia** is when an adult directs his or her sexual interests primarily or exclusively toward children. **Child molestation** is sexual involvement (oral-genital contact, genital fondling and viewing, masturbation) involving a child.

Certain factors place children at risk for sexual assault or incest (Hines & Malley-Morrison, 2005). Those factors

TABLE 36-5 Scales to Use in Assessing Abused Children or Abusive Caregivers

MEASURE	DESCRIPTION
Maternal Attitude Scale (Cohler, Weiss, & Grunebaum, 1970)	Maternal beliefs about child needs and parenting practices
Family Stress Checklist (Murphy, Orkow, & Nicola, 1985)	Parental experiences of abuse, mental illness, psychological problems, and other risk factors
Home Observation for home environment (Caldwell & Bradley, 1984)	Measures the quality and quantity of support for development available in a child's Measurement of Environment

RESEARCH Highlight

The Legacy of Childhood Sexual Abuse and Family Adversity

STUDY PURPOSE

To describe the process by which childhood adversity influences the life course of survivors of childhood sexual abuse

METHODS

The current study involves 48 female and 40 male survivors of childhood sexual abuse and family adversity. Data were analyzed using the constant comparison method.

FINDINGS

Participants described their perceptions of a life of abuse and adversity. The theory representing the process labeled "Living a Family Legacy" included three major life patterns: (a) being stuck in the family legacy and continuing to live adult lives plagued by addictions, imprisonment, prostitution, poor health, family instability, and experiences of interpersonal violence, as a victim and perpetrator; (b) being plagued by the family legacy and having issues related to trust; and (c) rejecting the family legacy and creating a new one by finding new ways to live their adulthood.

IMPLICATIONS

Family legacies can have a profound impact on the life course of an individual who has been sexually assaulted and can influence the physical health, social and emotional development. Care must be taken to maintain clear boundaries with these individuals and foster trust through the use of supportive measures.

REFERENCE

Martsolf, D. S., & Draucker, C. B. (2008). The legacy of childhood sexual abuse and family adversity. *Journal of Nursing Scholarship, 40*(4), 333–340.

include the presence of a stepfather in the home; a caregiver and child who are not emotionally connected; a caregiver who never finished high school and is sexually punitive or repressive; and the child has two or fewer friends.

Many times children are raised by caregivers who were sexually or physically abused themselves. These caregivers either do not believe they were sexually assaulted or kept it a secret from their family members. Therefore, the caregivers fail to protect or teach their own children how to protect themselves from potentially unsafe situations. In addition, personal safety rules may not be discussed openly in the family. For example, a 12-year-old girl who allows a male friend of the family to visit the house while the caregiver is not present in the home, and is consequently raped, should

REFLECTIVE THINKING

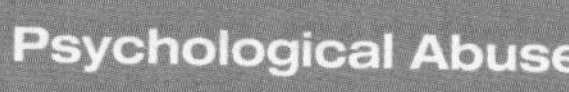

Psychological Abuse

Fourteen-year-old Ryan comes from an upper-middle-class family where both parents are employed. Ryan has developed suicidal ideation in response to ongoing verbal abuse and being either left at home alone or with neighbors most of the week. This is his father Ron's second marriage, and he spends most of his time with his new wife. Your nursing assessment reveals Ryan is depressed, withdrawn in school, and failing three major subjects. Ryan's teacher reports since the divorce he is "not the same." The teacher knows Ryan was very close to his mother but Ron was awarded custody. When you interview Ryan, he reports his father always tells him he is "worthless, just like his mother," he "always puts me down no matter what grades I bring home," and he "never allows me to leave the house to play with my friends after school."

1. What would you say to Ryan?
2. How would you handle the report of abuse from Ryan?

have been taught to never let anyone, even friends of the family, into the home while alone.

Finkelhor (1988) suggests four factors to describe the experience of sexually abused children, and the consequent effect they have on their growth and development. The factors are traumatic sexualization, stigmatization, betrayal, and powerlessness.

First, children can be rewarded for inappropriate and unsafe sexual behavior, and learn affection and love are equated with sex. Termed **traumatic sexualization**, the child is confused and becomes preoccupied with sexual behavior, demonstrates precocious sexual behaviors or prostitution, or becomes sexually aggressive toward peers and younger children. The children may also have flashbacks of past sexual assaults.

The second factor, stigmatization, occurs when abusers blame children for their sexual behaviors by telling them they (the children) asked to be touched or did not make the abuser stop after it started. The child is perceived as "spoiled goods," feels different from other children, and has a lowered sense of self-esteem. The secret of this abuse is maintained by coercion or threats related to personal and bodily safety.

In betrayal, a close family member or family friend victimizes the child who then experiences a breach of trust, care, and protection. The child is unable to tell anyone about the abuse because of being physically threatened or fearing retaliation. Manifestations include anxiety, depression, mistrust, anger, hostility, and clinging or aggressive behaviors.

Finally, the child experiences a sense of extreme powerlessness, vulnerability, fear, violation of bodily integrity, and

TABLE 36-6 Manifestations of Sexual Abuse in Children

INAPPROPRIATE COPING BEHAVIORS	MOOD REGULATION PROBLEMS	COGNITIVE PROBLEMS	SEXUAL PROBLEMS	PHYSICAL INDICATORS
• Substance use or abuse • Running away from home • Self-mutilation • Victimizing others • Eating disorders • Sleeping problems	• Depression • Anxiety • Hostility • Irritability • Phobias • Aggression	• Learning problems • Failing grades • Daydreaming • Dissociation • Nightmares • Low self-esteem	• Sexualized or promiscuous behaviors • Prostitution • Confusion about sexual identity • Masturbation	• Strong fear of examination • Presence of sexually transmitted diseases • Abnormal discharge or odor from genital area • Repeated urinary tract infections • Encopresis • Enuresis • Urethral irritation • Rectal or vaginal tears; bruising around the buttocks and hip areas; cuts, tears, or bleeding around the anal mucosa • A broken hymen (Estes, 2010)

the inability to control the assaults. Even though the child may tell an adult about the abuse, the adult often does not believe the child because the adult may have been sexually abused, is denying this abuse, or is unable to tolerate any thoughts and feelings related to past abuse. Table 36-6 lists other manifestations of sexual abuse in children.

Assessment of the physical signs of sexual abuse requires special care and attention. In addition to the physical indicators listed in Table 36-6, any venereal disease or diagnosis of pregnancy in a young adolescent is a strong indicator of sexual abuse and may require further investigation, interviewing, or referral. Refer to Box 36-14 and Box 36-15 for more information about suspected sexual abuse.

The Centers for Disease Control and Prevention (CDC) has published guidelines for the evaluation of sexually transmitted infections (STIs) in sexually abused children (CDC, 2006). Sexually transmitted infections are found in up to 5% of sexually abused children. In general, testing in prepubertal children is indicated when the victim is symptomatic (i.e., discharge), genital injury is present, a history of genital-to-genital contact is present, or if the perpetrator is known to have an STI. All adolescents should be tested given the higher prevalence of STIs in teenagers. A colposcopic examination of the genital and rectal areas by an expert in the field is often requested by law enforcement officials to determine if there is evidence of acute trauma or past injury (Adams et al., 2007). Any sexual abuse that involves oral, genital, rectal, or penile contact or penetration within 72 hours normally requires collection of appropriate forensics specimens and cultures for Neisseria gonorrhea, Chlamydia trachomatis, syphilis, HIV, hepatitis B, herpes

BOX 36-14
WHEN SEXUAL ABUSE IS SUSPECTED

Only an experienced member of the child abuse team should perform a genitalia examination. Adequate explanation, preparation, and possible sedation prior to examination are important, even though speculum examination of prepubescent females is often not required. The examination should be careful and complete, with accurate documentation of any bleeding, bruising, ligature, or teeth marks. Be sure to note the child's general appearance (including state of cleanliness) and demeanor and save all clothing in a sealed bag. Photograph any wound or injury. Use of a Wood's lamp can help in identifying semen.

Adams, J., Kaplan, R., Starling, S., Mehta, N., Finkel, M., Botash, A., Kellogg, N., & Shapiro, R. (2007). Guidelines for medical care of children who have been sexually abused. *Journal of Pediatric and Adolescent Gynecology*, *20*, 163–172.

BOX 36-15

QUESTIONS TO ASK IF SEXUAL ABUSE IS SUSPECTED (CAN BE ASKED OF EITHER CAREGIVER OR CHILD)

- How are beds arranged; do children sleep in parents' bed?
- Who bathes the children; are the doors open or closed during this time?
- Are the bedroom doors kept open or closed at night?
- Does either parent have trouble sleeping at night; if so, where does he or she go?
- Do the children and a parent have secrets from the other parent?
- Does the child engage in activities that the other parent is suspicious of?
- Do the children have a method for keeping themselves safe from being sexually abused?

simplex, bacterial vaginosis, human papillomavirus, and T. vaginitis (Adams et al., 2007).

The local forensic medical authority should be consulted prior to examination and a kit is often provided with written instructions regarding obtaining and preserving specimens. Specimens from the cervix, vagina, and rectum are needed to check for gonorrhea, motile sperm, acid phosphatase, or the presence of blood group antigens.

Other strategies for evaluating suspected sexual abuse in children include asking them to make a family drawing and then talking about the drawing. The child could also be asked who takes care of them, important things or activities they do together, or if family members engage in activities that scare or make the child sad. If a child begins to disclose sexual information during these conversations, be sure to seek additional staff, such as a physician or social worker, to validate and corroborate the statements.

KIDS WANT TO KNOW

Is it my fault that he hurt me this way?

Seven-year-old Gwyneth was admitted with a diagnosis of a gonococcus infection. While she was your client, she was evaluated by the pediatric psychologist for suspected sexual abuse. After she disclosed to the psychologist that her mother's boyfriend had sexually abused her, she states to you: "It was all my fault that he did this to me." The nurse responds: "It is never your fault for what happened. It is always the adult who is responsible for what happened and making you feel this way."

The child and nurse may also need to use a common set of terms to talk about sexualized behaviors. Having the child or caregiver give the usual names for body parts helps improve communication as families may have special names for breasts, penis, buttock, and so forth. An easy way to learn family terms is to have the child label body parts on a human figure drawing. Then the nurse can be more sensitive in interactions and if the child talks about inappropriate touching or abuse, the nurse will know what the child means.

Another way of eliciting information is through puppet play, which can facilitate a child's ability to talk about secrets surrounding sexual abuse. The child may be more likely to share a problem, or get permission from the nurse that it is "OK" to talk about other people touching his or her body parts during play activities. This also supports the child's attempt to deal with the shame and potential consequences of telling and talking about their own experiences.

Children suspected of being sexually abused should be referred to specialists in child and adolescent psychiatry, a clinical social worker, or a clinical psychologist specializing in sexual abuse. The nurse and other professionals can then work collaboratively to devise more effective ways to help the child deal with the powerlessness and guilt of the abuse. The nurse must follow facility protocol when suspecting child abuse.

Many children who have been sexually abused are diagnosed with post traumatic stress disorder (PTSD) (APA, 2000). Refer to Chapter 35 for additional information about PTSD.

Children who have experienced sexual abuse present with a wide range of symptoms and require complex intervention strategies. Immediate issues relate to ensuring a safe and protective place for the child and requiring all suspicious symptoms be reported to the proper authorities. If hospitalization is required, the child must be protected and all caregiver visitations supervised. During caregiver's visits, documentation of interactions as with all suspected cases of abuse is critical. If the child is depressed or anxious, the nurse should spend time alleviating fears and anxieties. Efforts to prepare the child for discharge to other family members or foster care will also need to be addressed.

Ongoing enrollment in individual and family treatment by teams specializing in sexual abuse treatment is essential. Cognitive changes in memory, academic functioning, and level of awareness are occurring. Therefore, caregivers need to understand children cannot remember what happened, and may begin failing in school and appear to daydream and stare. This behavior should not be considered uncooperative or acting out and should never be punished.

Teachers may need to be informed of the possibility of academic problems, the child provided with extra positive attention, and monitored in the school setting to ensure no further victimization occurs. Children may react violently to loud noises such as fire and police sirens. In addition, the child should not be exposed to any additional traumatic movie or television programs as this may stimulate memories and result in behavior problems. The child may have

FAMILY TEACHING

Ways for Caregivers to Protect Children from Sexual Abuse

1. Teach children to have a name for private parts of their body, such as calling their buttock a "butt or bottom."
2. Teach children to differentiate appropriate or safe touch (hugs, kisses on the cheek) from inappropriate touch such as touching private areas of body.
3. Teach children to shake hands with others so they feel safer.
4. Teach children to tell a trusted caregiver or a teacher immediately if anyone touches them inappropriately.
5. Teach children about good secrets (birthday parties) and bad secrets (if someone were to touch them inappropriately and ask them to keep it a secret).
6. Teach children the four basic feeling states (sad, angry, mad, and scared) and help them learn how to share feelings.
7. Empower children to maintain personal boundaries, not approach strangers or sit on adult laps, and verbalize feelings when certain children or adults touch them in ways that do not "feel" OK.
8. Supervise play, especially when children are of different ages. Do not allow children to play unsupervised or in bedrooms with the door shut.
9. Be alert to any changes in feelings or behaviors after a child returns from visiting friends or family members.
10. Become involved in school activities and support programs that teach personal safety skills.
11. Be aware of the National Committee to Prevent Child Abuse (NCPCA) materials used to help caregivers and children prevent sexual abuse. Contact information can be found in the Resources section of this chapter.

frequent nightmares and sleeping problems, and may need to have a night light or medications for sleep. Eating problems (overeating) may serve to soothe the child if the caregiver is unable to provide a safe and nurturing environment. Finally, the child may have angry and violent outbursts, which need to be acknowledged as anger directed to the perpetrator and handled within therapy.

LONG-TERM CONSEQUENCES OF CHILD ABUSE AND NEGLECT

Research provides evidence a child who was abused or neglected will experience higher rates of violence, psychiatric symptoms, and drug use (Prevent Child Abuse America,

CRITICAL THINKING

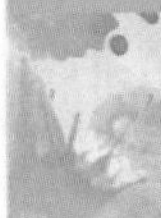

Identifying Sexual Abuse

You are caring for 6-year-old Sophia who has a diagnosis of chronic urinary tract infections. She has just been admitted and complains of pain in her abdomen. You go into her room to take her vital signs. She appears sad and withdrawn, and asks you to stay with her when her father visits because she does not want him to touch her "flower." You ask her to tell you what her "flower" is and she points to her vaginal area. You believe further assessment for possible sexual abuse is indicated. What interventions will need to be completed?

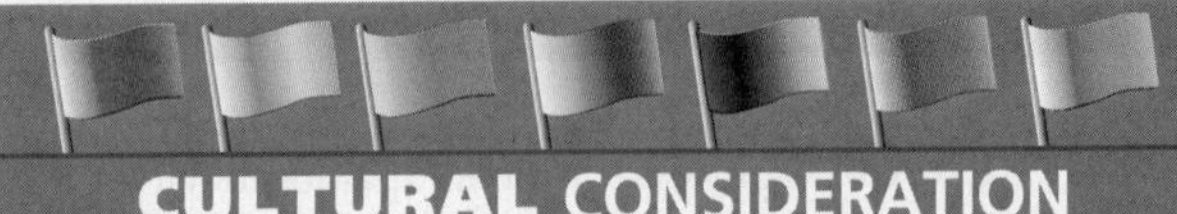

CULTURAL CONSIDERATION

Culturally Sensitive Community Interventions for Young Runaways

Minnesota Wheel of Public Health Nursing Interventions identifies coalition building and community organizing as effective approaches to address the growing problem of young Hmong girls who run away from home, are truant from school, and subsequently become sexually exploited. The Public Health Nurses outlined the steps in effective coalition building:

1. Deciding that the coalition approach was the best fit for the problem identified.
2. Outreach to bring in members from various professions and senior leaders in the Hmong organizations such as Hmong police, advocates and counselors.
3. Development of primary goals, objectives, and an action plan.
4. Leadership eventually arose from the District Attorney's office, which had connections to the school system.
5. Appreciation of cultural diverse backgrounds.
6. Identification of the barriers and challenges as the action plan was implemented.
7. Outcomes: Systems change at all levels, education and prevention programming, network relationships and improved communication, community supports and a research agenda.

From Saewyc, E., Solsvig, W., & Edinburgh, L. (2007). The Hmong youth task force: Evaluation of a coalition to address the sexual exploitation of youth runaways. *Public Health Nursing*, *25*(1), 69–76.

Reflections from Families

I just learned that my 13-year-old daughter, Ariana, was molested by her boyfriend at school today. She came home crying and initially went to her room and told me it was nothing serious. After a time, I realized she was still crying. I sat with her and she finally admitted that her new boyfriend, Michael, touched her breasts and would not stop so she had to hide in the girl's bathroom until he left school. I have always taught my daughters never to let anyone touch them without their permission. We are left wondering what to do. Do we bring it to the attention of the principal? Do we leave it alone? We need help in deciding our next steps.

2009). Two-thirds of abused adolescents had behavioral problems such as clinically deviant levels of aggression, anxiety, or depression; problems with law enforcement; running away from home, pregnancy, or impregnating someone; and gang membership. Prostitution was almost three times as likely in girls who had experienced childhood abuse or neglect. Maltreated children had lower academic achievement, lower attendance at school, and more placements in special education programs (Prevent Child Abuse American, 2009).

The Child Welfare Information Gateway (2008) reports the long-term consequences of childhood abuse and neglect. Victims of violence may also continue the cycle of violence. Physical violence effects neurological development and brain development with major impact on cognitive development, language acquisition, and academic abilities. Children who experience physical abuse were 1.9 times as likely to be arrested for violence; victims of neglect were 1.6 times more likely to be arrested for violence than control participants. Many individuals grow up with physical problems such as respiratory, cardiovascular, and gastrointestinal problems. The psychological consequences are enormous. Youths with histories of abuse are at risk for relationship-based difficulties. Children exposed to marital violence in childhood are at risk for engaging in dating violence as adolescents or young adults. Thirty percent of incarcerated adolescent boys, who were perpetrators of sexual assault, reported previous victimization. There are greater incidences of psychiatric problems such as panic disorders, dissociative disorders, attention deficit-hyperactivity disorder, depression, anxiety, anger management and posttraumatic stress disorder (Springer, Sheridan, Kuo, & Carnes, 2007). Behavioral consequences involve delinquency, Drug use is also higher in victims of abuse and neglect and abusive behaviors such as victimizing their own children.

PREVENTION OF CHILD ABUSE AND NEGLECT

Several strategies can reduce the occurrence of abuse. The first is directed at preventing maladaptive behaviors by providing help before the behavior occurs. Caregivers can assess their own family of origin and make informed choices regarding raising their children differently from how they were raised if abused. Nurses can facilitate this by providing parenting classes both in the community and health care settings where caregivers can be encouraged to teach their children respect for both genders, individual family role expectations, normal growth and development, and appropriate methods of communicating (verbal and nonverbal) that distinguish between nurturing affection and erotic contact. Children need to be able to discuss sexual issues, engage in family problem solving, receive accurate information, and have shared sexual values and attitudes (Hines & Malley-Morrison, 2005). Primary care services can identify early risk factors that may impact parental functioning and intervene. One such model, SEEK, used special training of health care provider, parent education, and social services resource availability to reduce the rates of abuse in low income clinics (Dubowitz et al., 2009). Consequently, the family atmosphere and experiences will be sexually age-appropriate, respectful of members' personal space, and demonstrate open and honest communication concerning sexual issues. Children will know about appropriate and safe touch between caregivers and siblings and any breach of this safe touch will immediately be reported to a responsible person for follow-up.

A second strategy focuses on high-risk communities. Even though child abuse occurs in all socioeconomic levels, identifying families at high risk is critical. Poverty, high community violence, substandard housing, high unemployment, and welfare-dependent communities are areas for special interventions. Support for a family's basic survival needs (economic and material) can contribute to a more stable home environment and improve the caregivers' capacity to rear children competently. Communities can assist by providing food pantries, secondhand clothing, and household supplies to supplement needy families at times of crisis.

This second strategy can also include parent competency enhancement programs developed by professionals who are knowledgeable about growth and development and share strategies for effective parenting. Local schools, community colleges, hospitals, and social service agencies normally provide these programs at low cost for caregivers. Pediatric and obstetric units can also be instrumental in combining resources to jointly offer such programs for new parents and caregivers. Formalized content can include growth and development across the life span, and specific issues related to each developmental stage, such as temper tantrums, toilet training, or assertive discipline. Other areas include how to play with your child, how to help your child learn, effective praise and encouragement, effective limit setting, and handling common misbehaviors (Hines & Malley-Morrison, 2005). In addition, caregivers may need to learn how to care for a sick child, how to take a temperature, how to deal with common childhood illnesses such as fever and colds, and when to seek medical services.

The third strategy focuses on a child's ability to recognize and resist assault. Here children are taught to: (1) recognize potentially abusive situations; (2) resist by saying "no" and removing themselves from the situation or perpetrator; (3) report previous or ongoing abuse to an authority figure; and (4) learn it is never their fault (Hines & Malley-Morrison, 2005). The children focus on the idea they are the "boss" of their bodies and can make rules to protect their bodies.

The fourth strategy focuses on reducing the long-term impact of physical and emotional abuse by providing a variety of support services to prevent continually abusive behaviors and situations. Specific interventions include the use of crisis hotlines and increased parent-child contact with supplemental in-home services such as a visiting nurse or parent aide. These services, often offered in conjunction with Child Protective Services as support for a family at risk, help caregivers learn new strategies for child discipline, anger and stress management, and healthy parenting practices. Caregiver involvement in religious affiliations can provide additional emotional and spiritual supports.

The fifth strategy focuses on maintaining or reducing the severity of the consequences of long-term abusive situations and occurs in general hospitals, psychiatric inpatient hospitals, group homes, or shelters where the person struggles with sequelae of violence. For instance, children may be referred to a day treatment facility specifically established for children experiencing serious mental illness as a result of prolonged abusive parenting. These children may be diagnosed with major depression, posttraumatic stress disorder, attachment disorders, or violent behaviors. Long-term family and individual counseling, medication management, parenting classes, social skills training, and other programs to overcome the impact of long-term abuse may be required. Refer to Box 36-16 for further information related to activities found to be helpful in preventing abuse, and Box 36-17 for protective factors associated with preventing child abuse.

BOX 36-16
COMMON ACTIVITIES FOR PREVENTION

1. Public awareness such as posters and brochures that promote child safety and parenting and how to report suspected child abuse cases.
2. Skills-based curriculum that teaches children safety and protection skills, especially with a focus on prevention of sexual abuse.
3. Parent education to help caretakers develop positive skills and decrease behaviors associated with child abuse and neglect.
4. Parent support groups where parents work together to strengthen their families and build social networks.
5. Home visitation that focuses on increasing child safety by helping pregnant women and new families learn about positive parenting and child development.
6. Respite and crisis care programs which offer temporary relief to caretakers in stressful situations by providing care for their children.
7. Family resource centers which work with community members to develop a variety of services to meet specific needs of families in surrounding neighborhoods.

BOX 36-17
PROTECTIVE FACTORS ASSOCIATED WITH PREVENTION OF CHILD ABUSE

1. Nurturing and strong attachment between caretaker and child
2. Knowledge of caretaking and of child and youth development by caretakers
3. Parental resilience and a positive attitude about challenges and problems, and less likely to use anger and frustration
4. Social connections to family friends and community to assist in daily challenges
5. Concrete supports for caretakers such as food banks, clothing, housing, transportation, and access to physical and psychological health services

Child Welfare Information Gateway. (2008). *Child Abuse and Neglect.* Washington, DC: Children's Bureau/Administration on Children, Youth and Families. Retrieved March 2, 2009, from www.childwelfare.gov.

LEGAL ISSUES RELATED TO CHILD ABUSE AND NEGLECT

Historically, children have experienced all types and severity of physical, psychological, and sexual abuse at the hands of their caregivers. Many children were removed from their homes and caregivers and placed in houses of refuge, or juvenile, orphan, or foundling asylums. These were religious or private organizations for abandoned or abused children. However, the 20th century awakened awareness on the part of the states and public social service agencies to take ultimate responsibility for protecting children.

The Child Abuse Prevention and Treatment Act (CAPTA) was enacted in 1974 to protect vulnerable children in the United States. CAPTA provides federal funding to the states to support prevention, assessment, investigation, prosecution, and treatment activities to public agencies and nonprofit organizations. They also provide funding for research, evaluation, and technical assistance and data collection activities. In 2003 it was amended and reauthorized by the Keeping Children and Families Safe Act of 2003 (P.L. 108-36) (Child Welfare Information Gateway, 2008).

Two legal doctrines have an impact on all judicial proceedings affecting abused and neglected children: *parens patriae,* where the state is vested with the power to set standards for the care and protection of children within its borders; and the state's responsibility to ensure that its actions are in the best interest of the child (Child Welfare Information Gateway, 2008). However, not until Kempe's (1962) landmark publication of *The Battered Child Syndrome* did efforts occur on a state level to address legislation related to child abuse (Kempe, Silverman, Steele, Droegemueller, & Silver, 1962).

Many state laws now define the grounds, set the limits, and establish procedures for limiting or severing the caregiver-child relationship. When abuse is suspected, child abuse and neglect reporting laws and welfare codes allow child protective and law enforcement agencies to investigate and intervene in family relationships (Child Welfare Information Gateway, 2008). The state's court systems authorize juvenile or family court involvement in such cases, and the prosecution of individuals found guilty of criminal acts against a child.

Even though caregivers do have the right of due process, their right to maintain connections with their child is not as important as a child's right to an environment that is free from physical and emotional violence. Unfortunately, the Child Protective System is not perfect and a child removed from the family may face many years in foster care, which in itself has serious consequences. Consequently, a critical balance must be maintained when considering removing a child from the home.

Each state has child abuse and neglect laws that require they prove "(1) one or more individuals named in the state law prohibiting child abuse, (2) have physically, sexually, mentally, or emotionally abused a child, or (3) have abandoned a child, or (4) have failed to provide a child with adequate food, clothing, shelter, or parental control or supervision, or (5) have medically or educationally neglected the child, or (6) have subjected a child to an immoral or criminal lifestyle" (Kramer, 1996, p. 13). If the caregiver was aware of the abuse but did not stop it, the state must prove that individual willfully permitted the abuse through indifference and inaction in order to prosecute the perpetrator for assault and battery.

Many states also have laws providing a legal defense to child abuse where **corporal punishment** (physical restraint or causing pain to the body by a person in authority) is inflicted by a caregiver. However, the punishment must be appropriate and reasonable to the child's misbehavior, so the force used is limited to what is believed necessary to maintain discipline, safeguard and promote the child's welfare, prevent or punish misconduct, or restrain or correct a child. Any act that exceeds reasonable bounds is considered child abuse.

Under the law, which may vary from state to state, the act of abandonment can also result in intervention by Child Protective Services. Abandonment occurs when a caregiver fails to visit a child who lives away from the caregiver, fails to display love or affection, or has no personal contact or concern for the child's personal welfare. If a caregiver demonstrates a reasonable degree of interest, concern, and responsibility, the child has not been abandoned.

The failure to provide food, clothing, shelter, care, or supervision is considered child neglect. These actions are often combined with failure to provide adequate medical care, education, and supervision. Some states (Delaware, Iowa, and Pennsylvania) include juvenile noncriminal behaviors (such as runaways who are endangering their own safety) under their neglect laws as well. Therefore in these states, caregivers of runaways or children who are endangering their own safety are considered neglectful.

However, emotional abuse does not constitute sufficient evidence to prove child abuse unless it occurs in conjunction with physical abuse. Only a few states make any attempt to define mental or emotional injury, and caregivers who neglect the educational needs of their children can be taken to court under the contribution to the delinquency of a minor complaint. Emotional abuse can also include failure on the part of the caregiver to provide an appropriate educational environment, such as enrolling a special needs child, or a child who is deaf, in a public school system.

REPORTING CHILD ABUSE

Each state has similar legal requirements for reporting child abuse. The central tenet of the reporting law designates certain persons as **mandated reporters** (individuals who are required to report to appropriate authorities' suspicions of child abuse or neglect). Most states specify who is required to report, and these individuals typically include physicians, nurses, school personnel, social workers, and law enforcement personnel. These reports are usually made by telephone to the child protective agency, and followed up by a written report. If a member of the staff at a hospital makes the report, the hospital is required to provide a medical record of the child.

Every state reporting law contains similar information that includes what must be reported (definitions and reportable areas), who must or may report, when a report must be made, procedures to follow, rules for protective custody, immunity for good faith reporters, privileged abrogation (to do away with) of communication rights, sanctions for failure to report, and information regarding the existence and operation of a central registry. Those reporting abuse in good faith are immune from any civil or criminal liability.

Each state also has a child protection system that primarily protects children and, secondarily, preserves the family unit whenever possible. Taking children from their home is the least desirable method of treating child abuse, and when children are removed, the first goal is to reunify the family. Child Protective Services receive reports of suspected abuse and neglect 24 hours per day, 7 days per week, and then must investigate and determine whether or not abuse or neglect has occurred. They also petition the court to protect children and mandate caregivers to take certain remedial steps or risk losing parental rights. Child Protective Services are also responsible for establishing resources that support families in the community including teaching and assisting caregivers with basic child rearing and household skills, and providing counseling services related to mental health, parenting, anger management, and vocational resources (Child Welfare Information Gateway, 2008).

Occasionally, individuals (parent, teacher, other adult) will be falsely accused of being abusive. This occurs most commonly during custody hearings associated with divorce proceedings, but may also occur when a child is telling a parent or an interviewer what the child thinks the adult wants to hear. Because Child Protective Services is legally charged with investigating any and all accusations of child abuse, even if they may not be true, it is important whenever interviewing a child that care be taken not to encourage the child to remember experiences that did not occur, or lead the child into making statements about events that did not occur.

NURSING TIP

Legal Issues and Child Abuse

Because nurses may be called as codefendants in lawsuits, they must practice in a professional and reasonably prudent manner at all times. Specific guidelines for the nurse to consider are:

- Document all client and caregiver interactions.
- Practice within the ethical code of nursing.
- Respect client and caregiver's confidentiality. If child abuse is suspected, confidentiality can (and must) be breached.
- Do not release information to other agencies other than protective services without specific family or caregiver permission; if a child is removed from the caregiver and the Child Protective Services has temporary custody, Child Protective Services must approve release of information.
- Respect a client's right to privacy.
- Respect a client's right to refuse treatment or assessments (document accordingly).
- Know your institution's policies and procedures related to all matters of child abuse.
- Know your state's Nurse Practice Act and practice within that scope.
- Always consult with your nurse manager, risk manager, and treatment team members when indicated (Adapted from Estes, 2010).

IN THE REAL WORLD

One of the most difficult children to care for is a child whose caregiver has been abusive or neglectful. Most people believe a child is a special gift to be loved and cherished. Unfortunately, some caregivers do not hold similar beliefs and engage in hurtful and harmful behaviors. As nurses, we are educated to understand abuse and neglect as symptoms of some larger problem in the caregiving family. Yet, we feel anger and frustration at caregivers who can take away a child's spirit, injure them physically, or leave a child with lifetime psychological and physical scars. As nurses, we must model caring and nurturing behaviors for abusive caregivers, coordinate resources for caregiver healing, and always are on guard to advocate and report any suspected abuse or neglect.

As professionals, nurses, physicians, police, and teachers have a legal obligation to report child abuse and neglect. In some states, any person who suspects abuse or neglect is legally required to report that abuse. Make sure you are vigilant and always aware of potential harm a child may be in. Remember, child abuse or neglect comes from all socioeconomic, ethnic, cultural, and religious backgrounds.

KEY CONCEPTS

- Child abuse includes intentional behaviors by a caregiver that can involve neglect, or physical, emotional, or sexual abuse. Neglect is harmful, malicious, or ignorant withholding of physical, nutrition and health care, or emotional and educational necessities that provide a foundation for healthy childhood development.
- Three models explaining child abuse and neglect are the Sociological Model, the Social-Interactional Systemic Model, and the Attachment Model.
- Clinical manifestations of physical abuse include bruises, fractures, burns, abdominal injuries, and neurological injuries.
- Children with an intracranial bleed (subdural or subarachnoid hemorrhages), retinal hemorrhage, and possibly long bone fractures should be suspected of having shaken baby syndrome.
- Munchausen syndrome by proxy is a pattern of behavior demonstrated by the caregiver to fabricate signs and symptoms of diseases and expose a child to harmful medical interventions and painful invasive procedures.
- Abandonment is defined as intentionally withholding from a child, without just cause or excuse, care, presence, love, protection, maintenance, and affection.
- Psychological abuse consists of acts of omission or commission (telling a child that he or she is ugly or worthless) deemed psychologically damaging, and involving hostile behavior or negative caregiving behaviors.
- Sexual abuse is an exploitive sexual act(s) imposed on a child who lacks the emotional, cognitive, or maturational development to deal with the actions.
- Nursing management of child abuse includes obtaining an accurate history and assessment, and intervening according to the type of abuse.
- The nurse is a mandatory reporter of child abuse.

REVIEW ACTIVITIES

1. Discuss the differences and similarities between child abuse and child neglect.
2. Describe the clinical manifestations of a child who has been physically abused.
3. Describe the process of transmission of violence in families.
4. Identify the nursing interventions for a child who has been abused.
5. Describe the legal issues related to reporting child abuse in your state.
6. Describe strategies for prevention of child abuse.

STUDY QUESTIONS

1. A 30-year-old mother was physically punished with a paddle as a child by her father. What statement conveys the most likely type of discipline she will use with her two daughters aged 2 and 5?
   a. The mother may continue the cycle of family violence and use a similar pattern of discipline.
   b. The mother would never use a similar pattern of discipline that she experienced as a child by her father.
   c. The mother's psychological problems may interfere with her capacity to discipline her children.
   d. If the mother marries a man who has not had the same kinds of discipline experiences she may change how she disciplines.
2. A parent who believes a "child should be seen and not heard" and does not understand the child's need to ask questions and challenge a parent's thinking about his or her environment may be at risk for which type of abuse?
   a. Physical abuse
   b. Sexual abuse
   c. Emotional abuse
   d. Physical neglect
3. Munchausen syndrome by proxy is known by the following warning signs:
   a. Caretaker(s) reports an extensive history of the child's illness but with inappropriate signs and symptoms of the illness.
   b. Caretaker(s) reports appropriate signs and symptoms and is very knowledgeable of the illness.

c. Caretaker(s) reports symptoms have not subsided but the symptoms do fit the diagnosis.
d. Caretaker(s) reports appropriate signs and symptoms but is not very knowledgeable about the illness.

4. Children who have experienced sexual abuse can manifest the following cognitive problems:
   a. Learning problems
   b. Self-mutilation
   c. Depression and anxiety
   d. Confused identity

5. An infant is brought to the emergency room with bradycardia, vomiting, and retinal hemorrhage. The parents' report that the baby fell off the changing table yesterday but seemed to have no further problems. This morning is when the child started vomiting. As a nurse who works in the Pediatric Emergency Department, you suspect which of the following problems?
   a. Shaken Baby Syndrome
   b. Pyloric stenosis
   c. Cardiac insufficiency
   d. Seasonal flu

6. Common injuries seen in children as a result of shaken baby syndrome include:
   a. Lacerations
   b. Burns
   c. Retinal bleeding
   d. Welt marks

7. A 4-year-old female child is being admitted by a nurse to the pediatric unit for a gastrointestinal disorder of unknown origin. The child is crying for no apparent reason while being held by the mother. The nurse notices that when the child is placed in the crib, the crying stops. In completing the assessment the nurse found several large bruises on the child's upper chest, and cigarette burns on her buttock. As a professional registered nurse, the nurse's first action should be to:
   a. Ask the mother about how the child acquired the bruises.
   b. Call Child Protective Services immediately.
   c. Consult your nurse manager immediately.
   d. Review policy on suspected child abuse.

8. There are a number of strategies that professional nurses can utilize to improve the quality of parenting in young families. The type of interventional plan that would have the greatest impact would be to:
   a. Develop a parent competency program as part of the obstetric Programs.
   b. Distribute materials to parents of children who are coming for immunizations at 1 year of age.
   c. Provide handouts to kindergarten children at the local schools.
   d. Offer sibling training programs.

9. You are a new elementary school nurse in an urban community. One of the most effective methods to teach children to prevent sexual abuse in this community would be to:
   a. Teach children to say "no" and remove themselves from the situation.
   b. Teach children never to talk to strangers.
   c. Teach children it is all right if someone touches them only once in their "private parts".
   d. Teach children to call police if threatened.

10. Children who have been sexually assaulted often engage in behavioral patterns that affect their growth and development. Which behavior would the nurse not expect to see in a child who has been sexually abused? The child:
    a. Believes love is equated with sex and may be precocious or engage in prostitution.
    b. Feels stigmatized.
    c. Feels betrayed by a family member.
    d. Feels powerful because she cannot trust anyone and have to rely on herself

REFERENCES

Abidin, R.R. (1990). Parenting Stress Index. Charlottesville, VA: Pediatric Psychology Press.

Adams, J. A., Kaplan, R. A., Starling, S. P., Mehta, N. H., Finkel, M. A., Botash, A. S., Kellogg, N. D., & Shapiro, R. A. (2007). Guidelines for medical care of children who may have been sexually abused. *Journal of Pediatric and Adolescent Gynecology, 2*, 163–172.

American Psychiatric Association. (2000). *Diagnostic and statistical manual of mental disorders* (4th ed.). Washington, DC: Author.

Asher, R. (1951). Munchausen's syndrome. *Lancet, 1*, 339–341.

Bechtel, K., Stoessel, K., Leventhal, J., Duncan, C. (2005). Retinal hemorrhages in accidental and nonaccidental injury: In reply. *Pediatrics, 115*(1), 192.

Berger, L. M., & Brooks-Gunn, J. (2005). Socioeconomic status, parenting knowledge and behaviors, and perceived maltreatment of young low-birth-weight children. *Social Service Review, 79*, 237–267.

Bowlby, J. (1969). *Attachment and loss.* New York: Basic Books.

Caldwell, B., & Bradley, R. (1984). *Home observation for measurement of the environment.* Little Rock: University of Arkansas.

Cassidy, J., & Shaver, P. (2008). *Handbook of attachment: Theory, research, and clinical applications* (2nd ed.). New York: Guilford Press.

Centers for Disease Control and Prevention (2006). 2006 guidelines for the treatment of sexually transmitted diseases. *Morbidity and Mortality Weekly Report, 55*(RR11), 1–94.

Child Welfare Information Gateway. (2008). *Child Abuse and Neglect.* Washington, DC: Children's Bureau/Administration on Children, Youth and Families. Retrieved March 2, 2009, from http://www.childwelfare.gov.

Children's Bureau. (2006). *Child maltreatment 2006* U.S. Department of Health and Human Services, Administration on Children, Youth and Families. Washington, DC: U.S. Government Printing Office.

Cohler, B. J., Weiss, J. L., & Grunebaum, H. U. (1970). Child-care attitudes and emotional disturbance among mothers of young children. *Genetic Psychology Monographs, 82*(1), 3–47.

Dubowitz, H., Feigelman, S., Lane, W., & Kim, J. (2009). Pediatric primary care to prevent child maltreatment: A safe environment for every kid (SEEK) model. *Pediatrics, 123,* 858–864.

Edwards, V., Holden, G., Felitti, V., & Anda, R. (2003). Relationship between multiple forms of childhood maltreatment and adult mental health in community respondents: Results from the adverse childhood experiences study. *American Journal of Psychiatry, 160,* 1453–1460.

Elliott, G. C., Cunningham, S. M., Linder, M., Colangelo, M., & Gross, M. (2005). Child physical abuse and self-perceived social isolation among adolescents. *Journal of Interpersonal Violence, 20*(12), 1663–1684.

Epilepsy Association of Central Florida. (n.d.). *Shaken baby syndrome.* Retrieved December 28, 2009, from http://www.aboutshakenbaby.com.

Estes, M. E. Z. (2010). *Health assessment & physical examination* (4th ed.). Clifton Park, NY: Delmar Cengage Learning.

Finkelhor, D. (1988). The trauma of child sexual abuse: Two models. In G. Wyatt & G. Povell (Eds.). *Lasting effects of child sexual abuse.* Newbury Park, CA: Sage, pp. 61–84.

Fiske, E., & Hall, J. (2008). Inflicted childhood neurotrauma. *Advances in Nursing Science, 31*(2), E1–E8.

Forsyth, B. W. (2002). Munchausen syndrome by Proxy. In M. Lewis, *Child and adolescent psychiatry: A comprehensive textbook.* Philadelphia: Lippincott, Williams & Wilkins, pp. 1224–1230.

Gaudin, J. (1993). *Child neglect: A guide for intervention.* Washington, DC: U.S. Department of Health and Human Services, Administration for Children and Families, Westover Consultants (Contract NO. HHS-105-89-1730).

Gelles, R. J. (1987). *Family violence* (2nd ed.). London: Sage.

Gelles, R. (1997). *Intimate violence in the family.* Thousand Oaks, CA: Sage.

Herman, J. (2000). *Father-daughter incest.* Cambridge, MA: Harvard University Press.

Hibbard, R. A., & Desch, L. W. (2007). Maltreatment of children with disabilities. *Pediatrics, 119*(5), 1018–1025.

Hines, D., & Malley-Morrison, K. (2005). Family violence in the United States: Defining, understanding and combating abuse. London: Sage Publications.

Keeping Children and Families Safe Act of 2003. Retrieved December 28, 2009, from http://www.acf.hhs.gov/programs/cb/laws_policies/policy/im/2003/im0304a.pdf.

Kellogg, N., & the Committee on Child Abuse and Neglect. (2007). Evaluation of suspected child physical abuse. *Pediatrics, 119*(6), 1232–1241.

Kemp, A. M., Dunstan, F., Harrison, S., Morris, S., Mann, M., Rolfe, K., Datta, S., Thomas, D. P., Sibert, J. R., & Maguire, S. (2008). Patterns of skeletal fractures in child abuse: Systematic review. *British Medical Journal, 337,* a1518.

Kempe, C. H., Silverman, F. N., Steele, B. F., Droegemueller, W., & Silver, H. K. (1962). The battered child syndrome. *Journal of the American Medical Association, 181,* 17–24.

Kramer, D. (1996). *Legal rights of children (vol. 2).* New York: Clark, Boardman & Callaghan.

Lounds, J., Borkowski, J. G., & Whitman, T. L. (2006). The potential for neglect: The case of adolescent mothers and their children. *Child Maltreatment, 11*(3), 281–294.

Martsolf, D., & Draucker, C. (2008). The legacy of childhood sexual abuse and family adversity. *Journal of Nursing Scholarship, 40*(4), 333–340.

McGinness, T., & Pollack, D. (2008). Parental methamphetamine abuse and children. *Journal of Pediatric Health, 22,* 152–158.

Murphy, S., Orkow, B., & Nicola, R. M. (1985). Prenatal prediction of child abuse and neglect: A prospective study. *Child Abuse and Neglect, 9*(2), 225–235.

National Clearinghouse on Child Abuse and Neglect Information. (2006). *Child Abuse and Neglect Fatalities: Statistics and Interventions.* Retrieved February 25, 2006, from http://nccanch.acf.hhs.gov/pubs/factsheets/fatality.cfm.

NINDS Shaken Baby Syndrome Information Page (2009). Retrieved December 23, 2009, from http://www.ninds.nih.gov/disorders/shakenbaby/shakenbaby.htm.

Rangarajan, N., & Shams, T. (2006). Correspondence: Shaken baby syndrome: A flawed biomechanical analysis. *Forensic Science International, 16*(2), 280–281.

Prevent Child Abuse America. (2009). Frequently Asked Questions. Accessed December 28, 2009, from http://www.preventchildabuse.org/about_us/faqs.shtml#abuse.

Romano, E., Zoccolillo, M., & Paquette, D. (2006). Histories of child maltreatment and psychological disorders in physical abuse. *Journal of the American Academy of Child and Adolescent Psychiatry, 45*(3), 329–336.

Russell, B., Trudeau, J., & Britner, P. (2008). Intervention type matters in primary prevention of abusive head injury: Event history analysis results. *Child Abuse and Neglect, 32,* 949–957.

Saewyc, E., Solsvig, W., & Edinburgh, L. (2007). The Hmong youth task force: Evaluation of a coalition to address the sexual exploitation of youth runaways. *Public Health Nursing, 25*(1), 69–76.

Sebes, J. M. (1983). *Determining risk for abuse in families with adolescents: The development of a criterion measure.* Unpublished doctoral dissertation, The Pennsylvania State University.

Sidebotham, P., & Heron, J. (2006). Child maltreatment in the "children in the nineties": A cohort study of risk factors. *Child Abuse and Neglect, 30*(5), 497–522.

Spivey, M. I., Schnitzer, P. G., Kruse, R. L., Slusher, P., & Jaffe, D. M. (2009). Association of injury visits in children and child maltreatment reports. *Journal of Emergency Medicine, 36*(2), 207–214.

Springer, K. W., Sheridan, J., Kuo, D., & Carnes, M. (2007). Long-term physical and mental health consequences of childhood physical abuse: Results from a large population-based sample of men and women. *Child Abuse & Neglect, 31,* 517–530.

Stirling, J., & the Committee on Child Abuse and Neglect. (2007). Beyond Munchausen Syndrome by Proxy: Identification and treatment of child abuse in medical settings. *Pediatrics, 119,* 1026–1030.

Straus, M., & Gelles, R. (1989). *Intimate Violence.* Clearwater, FL: Touchstone Books.

Tang, J., Buzney, S., Lashkari, K., & Weiter, J. (2008). Shaken baby syndrome. *International Ophthalmology Clinics, 48*(2), 237–246.

Taylor, C., Guteman, N., Lee, S., & Rathouz, P. (2009). Intimate partner violence, maternal stress, nativity, and risk for maternal maltreatment in young children. *American Journal of Public Health, 99*(1), 175–183.

Taylor, J., Underwood, C., Thomas, L., & Franklin, A. (1988). Measuring psychological maltreatment of infants and toddlers. In R. Jones (Ed.). *Tests and measures for Black populations.* Berkeley, CA: Cobb and Henry.

U.S. Department of Health and Human Services, Administration on Children, Youth and Families. (2009). *Child Maltreatment 2007.* Retrieved December 28, 2009, from http://www.acf.hhs.gov/programs/cb/pubs/cm07/chapter3.htm#subjects.

Zeanah, C. H., & Boris, N. (2000). Disturbances and disorders of attachment in early childhood. *Handbook of infant mental health* (2nd ed.). New York: Guildford Publications, pps. 353–368.

Zhai, F., & Gao, Q. (2008). Child maltreatment among Asian Americans. *Child Maltreatment, 20*(10), 1–17.

SUGGESTED READINGS

Altimier, L. (2008). Shaken baby syndrome. *Journal of Perinatal Nurisng, 22*(1), 68–76.

Angelo, P. G. (2009). Child maltreatment: Is the glass half full yet? *Journal of Forensic Nursing, 5*(1), 1–4.

Asawa, L. E., Hansen, D. J., & Flood, M. F. (2008). Early childhood intervention programs: Opportunities and challenges for preventing child maltreatment. *Education and Treatment of Children, 31*(1), 73–110.

Bottoms, B. L., & Quas, J. A. (2006). Recent advances and new challenges in child maltreatment research, practice, and policy: Previewing the issues. *Journal of Social Issues, 62*(4), 653–662.

Butchart, A., Harvey, A., Mian, M., & Furniss, T. (2006). *Preventing child maltreatment: A guide to taking action and generating evidence.* Geneva: World Health Organization.

Clemmons, J. C., Walsh, K., DiLillo, D., & Messman-Moore, T. L. (2007). Unique and combined contributions of multiple child abuse types and abuse severity to adult trauma symptomatology. *Child Maltreat, 12*(2), 172–181.

Crooks, C. V., Scott, K. L., Wolfe, D. A., Chiodo, D., & Killip, S. (2007). Understanding the link between childhood maltreatment and violent delinquency: What do schools have to add? *Child Maltreat, 12*(3), 269–280.

Duncan, D. F., Kum, H.-C., Caplick Weigensberg, E., Flair, K. A., & Stewart, C. J. (2008). Informing child welfare policy and practice: Using knowledge discovery and data mining technology via a dynamic web site. *Child Maltreat, 13*(4), 383–391.

Feldman, M. D., Light, M. J., Lasher, L. J., & Sheridan, M. S. (2007). Beyond Munchausen syndrome by proxy. *Pediatrics, 120*(5), 1217–1218.

Flaherty, E. G., Sege, R. D., & Hurley, B. (2008). Translating child abuse research into action. *Pediatrics, 122*(Suppl1): S1–5.

Gilbert, R., Kemp, A., Thoburn, J., Sidebotham, P., Radford, L., Glaser, D., & Macmillan, H. L. (2009). Recognising and responding to child maltreatment. *Lancet, 373*(9658), 167–180.

Greeley, C. S. (2009). The future of child maltreatment prevention. *Pediatrics, 123*(3), 904–905.

Hazen, A. L., Connelly, C. D., Roesch, S. C., Hough, R. L., & Landsverk, J. A. (2009). Child maltreatment profiles and adjustment problems in high-risk adolescents. *Journal of Interpersonal Violence, 24*(2), 361–378.

Herrenkohl, T., & Herrenkohl, R. (2007). Examining the overlap and prediction of multiple forms of child maltreatment, stressors, and socioeconomic status: A longitudinal analysis of youth outcomes. *Journal of Family Violence, 22*(7), 553–562.

Hui, C., Joughin, E., Goldstein, S., Cooper, N., Harder, J., Kiefer, G., Parsons, D., & Howard, J. (2008). Femoral fractures in children younger than three years: The role of nonaccidental injury. *Journal of Pediatric Orthopaedics, 28*(3), 297–302.

Kaplow, J. B., & Widom, C. S. (2007). Age of onset of child maltreatment predicts long-term mental health outcomes. *Journal of Abnormal Psychology, 116*(1), 176–187.

Kleinman, P. K. (2008). The Roentgen manifestations of unrecognized skeletal trauma in infants—A Commentary. *American Journal of Roentgenology, 190*(3), 559–560.

Klevens, J., & Whitaker, D. J. (2007). Primary prevention of child physical abuse and neglect: Gaps and promising directions. *Child Maltreat, 12*(4), 364–377.

Lane, W. G., & Dubowitz, H. (2007). What factors affect the identification and reporting of child abuse-related fractures? *Clinical Orthopaedics and Related Research, 461*, 219–225.

Lansford, J. E., Miller-Johnson, S., Berlin, L. J., Dodge, K. A., Bates, J. E., & Pettit, G. S. (2007). Early physical abuse and later violent delinquency: A prospective longitudinal study. *Child Maltreat, 12*(3), 233–245.

Leventhal, J. M., Larson, I. A., Abdoo, D., Singaracharlu, S., Takizawa, C., Miller, C., Goodman, T. R., Schwartz, D., Grasso, S., & Ellingson K. (2007). Are abusive fractures in young children becoming less common? Changes over 24 years. *Child Abuse & Neglect, 31*(3), 311–322.

Leventhal, J. M., Martin, K. D., & Asnes, A. G. (2008). Incidence of fractures attributable to abuse in young hospitalized children: Results from analysis of a United States database. *Pediatrics, 122*(3), 599–604.

MacMillan, H. L., Wathen, C. N., Barlow, J., Fergusson, D. M., Leventhal, J. M., & Taussig, H. N. (2009). Interventions to prevent child maltreatment and associated impairment. *Lancet, 373*(9659), 250–266.

Mersky, J. P., Berger, L. M., Reynolds, A. J., & Gromoske, A. N. (2009). Risk factors for child and adolescent maltreatment: A longitudinal investigation of a cohort of inner-city youth. *Child Maltreat, 14*(1), 73–88.

Murray-Close, D., Han, G., Cicchetti, D., Crick, N. R., & Rogosch, F. A. (2008). Neuroendocrine regulation and physical and relational aggression: The moderating roles of child maltreatment and gender. *Developmental Psychology, 44*(4), 1160–1176.

Olds, D. (2008). Preventing child maltreatment and crime with prenatal and infancy support of parents: The nurse-family partnership. *Journal of Scandinavian Studies in Criminology and Crime Prevention, 9*, 2–24.

Prinz, R. J., Sanders, M. R., Shapiro, C. J., Whitaker, D. J., & Lutzker, J. R. (2009). Population-based prevention of child maltreatment: The U.S. Triple P system population trial. *Prevention Science, 10*(1), 1–12.

Quas, J. A., Davis, E. L., Goodman, G. S., & Myers, J. E. B. (2007). Repeated questions, deception, and children's true and false reports of body touch. *Child Maltreat, 12*(1), 60–67.

Reynolds, A. J., Mathieson, L. C., & Topitzes, J. W. (2009). Do early childhood interventions prevent child maltreatment? A review of research. *Child Maltreat, 14*(2), 182–206.

Rhee, S., Chang, J., Weaver, D., & Wong, D. (2008). Child maltreatment among immigrant chinese families: Characteristics and patterns of placement. *Child Maltreat, 13*(3), 269–279.

Rodriguez, C. M., & Richardson, M. J. (2007). Stress and anger as contextual factors and preexisting cognitive schemas: Predicting parental child maltreatment risk. *Child Maltreat, 12*(4), 325–337.

Salzinger, S., Rosario, M., & Feldman, R. S. (2007). Physical child abuse and adolescent violent delinquency: The mediating and moderating roles of personal relationships. *Child Maltreat, 12*(3), 208–219.

Schnitzer, P. G., Covington, T. M., Wirtz, S. J., Verhoeck-Oftedahl, W., & Palusci, V. J. (2007). Public health surveillance of fatal child maltreatment: Analysis of three state programs. *American Journal of Public Health*, AJPH.2006.087783.

Shen, A. C. T. (2008). Self-esteem of young adults experiencing interparental violence and child physical maltreatment: Parental and peer relationships as mediators. *Journal of Interpersonal Violence*, 0886260508317188.

Starling, S. P., Sirotnak, A. P., Heisler, K. W., & Barnes-Eley, M. L. (2007). Inflicted skeletal trauma: The relationship of perpetrators to their victims. *Child Abuse & Neglect, 31*(9), 993–999.

Stith, S. M., Liu, T., Davies, L. C., Boykin, E. L., Alder, M. C., Harris, J. M. Som, A., McPherson, M., & Dees, J.E.M.E.G. (2009). Risk factors in child maltreatment: A meta-analytic review of the literature. *Aggression and Violent Behavior, 14*(1), 13–29.

Stotts, A. K. (2007). Orthopaedic aspects of child abuse. *Current Opinion in Orthopaedics, 18*(6), 550–554.

Thompson, R., & Wiley, T. R. (2009). Predictors of re-referral to child protective services: A longitudinal follow-up of an urban cohort maltreated as infants. *Child Maltreat, 14*(1), 89–99.

Turner, H. A., Finkelhor, D., & Ormrod, R. (2006). The effect of lifetime victimization on the mental health of children and adolescents. *Social Science & Medicine, 62*(1), 13–27.

Vranceanu, A.-M., Hobfoll, S. E., & Johnson, R. J. (2007). Child multi-type maltreatment and associated depression and PTSD symptoms: The role of social support and stress. *Child Abuse & Neglect, 31*(1), 71–84.

Wall, A. E., & Kohl, P. L. (2007). Substance use in maltreated youth: Findings from the national survey of child and adolescent well-being. *Child Maltreat, 12*(1), 20–30.

Waney, S. (2008). Shaken baby syndrome: The quest for evidence. *Developmental Medicine & Child Neurology, 50*(1), 10–14.

Westby, C. E. (2007). Child maltreatment: A global issue. *Language, Speech & Hearing Services in Schools, 38*(2), 140–148.

Wolfe, D. A. (2009). Child maltreatment, bullying, gender-based harassment, and adolescent dating violence: Making the connection. *Psychology of Women Quarterly, 33*(1), 21–24.

Wood, J. N., Christian, C. W., Adams, C. M., & Rubin, D. M. (2009). Skeletal surveys in infants with isolated skull fractures. *Pediatrics, 123*(2), e247–e252.

RESOURCES

Refer to the online student StudyWARE for Potts & Mandleco at http://www.CengageBrain.com for additional content and study aids.

Organization: **American Academy of Child and Adolescent Psychiatry (AACAP)**
Description: Provides information regarding mental illnesses, data concerning efforts to prevent mental illnesses, how to seek proper treatment, and access to services for children and adolescents.
Website/Resource: http://www.aacap.org

Organization: **American Academy of Family Physicians**
Description: Offers information regarding family physician careers, clinical research, advocacy, practice management, and recent news/publications.
Website/Resource: http://www.aafp.org

Organization: **American Academy of Pediatrics (AAP)**
Description: Offers general information related to child health, specific guidelines concerning many pediatric issues, information regarding AAP programs, activities, policies, guidelines, publications, and other child health resources.
Website/Resource: http://www.aap.org

Organization: **American Humane Association, Children's Division**
Description: Offers information regarding programs, research, advocacy, membership, and resources about the association.
Website/Resource: http://www.americanhumane.org

Organization: **American Professional Society on the Abuse of Children**
Description: Offers information regarding events/meetings, membership, publications, resources, and state chapters.
Website/Resource: http://www.apsac.org

Organization: **Center for Improvement of Child Caring**
Description: Offers information regarding parenting seminars, programs, books, kits, and partnerships.
Website/Resource: http://www.ciccparenting.org

Organization: **Childhelp USA**
Description: Exists to meet physical, emotional, educational, and spiritual needs of abused, neglected, or at-risk children; focuses on advocacy, prevention, treatment, and community outreach; offers information regarding programs, learning centers, and involvement opportunities.
Website/Resource: http://www.childhelpusa.org

Organization: **Every Person Influences Children (EPIC)**
Description: Offers links for parents, teachers, schools, and communities on how to raise responsible and academically successful children.
Website/Resource: http://www.epicforchildren.org

Organization: **Family Resources Coalition (FRC)**
Description: Offers information regarding annual conference; links to helpful resources about working with families of children and youth ages birth to 21 years with special health care needs.
Website/Resource: http://www.frc4kids.org

Organization: **Family Violence Prevention Center**

Description: Offers information regarding campaigns, programs, public policy and action centers to help prevent violence within the home and community, and offer resources for those affected by violence.

Website/Resource: http://www.endabuse.org

Organization: **Healthy Families America**

Description: Strives to provide expectant and new parents with the opportunity to receive education/support needed when their baby is born; offers information regarding network resources, advocacy, publications, and research.

Website/Resource: http://www.healthyfamiliesamerica.org

Organization: **Kempe Children's Center**

Description: Offers information regarding Kempe Center for the Prevention and Treatment of Child Abuse and Neglect events, programs, resources, news and volunteers.

Website/Resource: http://www.kempecenter.org

Organization: **National Center for Children Exposed to Violence (NCCEV)**

Description: Offers information concerning childhood violence, resource centers, and NCCEV initiatives.

Website/Resource: http://www.nccev.org

Organization: **National Center for Education in Maternal and Child Health**

Description: Offers access to publications, the Maternal Child Health library, and program information.

Website/Resource: http://www.ncemch.org

Organization: **National Clearinghouse on Child Abuse and Neglect Information**

Description: Provides information on preventing, identifying, and treating child abuse and neglect and related child welfare issues; maintains databases on child abuse, neglect, child welfare, and adoption.

Website/Resource: http://www.childwelfare.gov

Organization: **National Center on Shaken Baby Syndrome**

Description: Offers information regarding shaken baby syndrome as well as conferences, programs, online training, news, and advocacy.

Website/Resource: http://www.dontshake.com

Organization: **Prevent Child Abuse America (PCA America)**

Description: Offers information about upcoming child abuse conferences, research, advocacy, and publications.

Website/Resource: http://www.preventchildabuse.org

Organization: **SOS Help for Parents: A practical guide for handling common everyday behavior problems**

Description: Offers links to information regarding child behavior, DVD videos, free resources, and order forms.

Website/Resource: http://www.sosprograms.com

Organization: **U.S. Department of Health and Human Services (HHS)**

Description: Offers access to health information pertaining to family health, prevention, diseases, regulation, and preparedness.

Website/Resource: http://www.hhs.gov

Organization: **U.S. Department of Health and Human Services Children's Bureau**

Description: Offers information regarding services, policy/planning, and research/statistics offered by the US Department of HHS Children's Bureau.

Website/Resource: http://www.acf.hhs.gov

Organization: **The Shaken Baby Alliance**

Description: Offers information regarding family/professional support, prevention/awareness, and products related to shaken baby syndrome.

Website/Resource: http://www.shakenbaby.com

APPENDIX A The Friedman Family Assessment Model (Short Form)

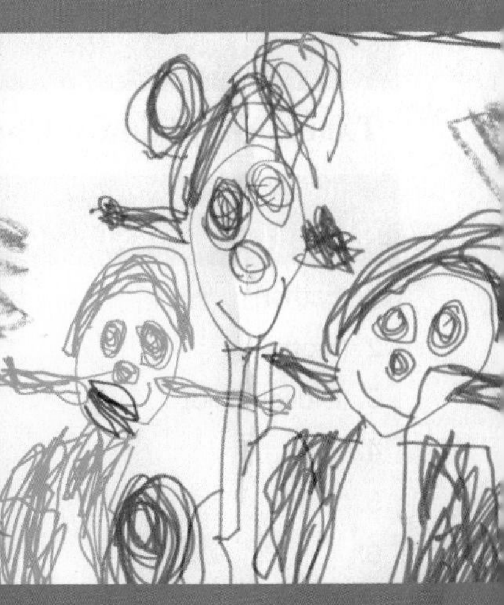

Before using the following guidelines in completing family assessments, two words of caution: First, not all areas included will be germane for every family. The guidelines are comprehensive and allow depth when probing is necessary. The student should not feel that every subarea needs to be covered when the broad area of inquiry poses no problems to the family or concern to the health care professional. Second, by virtue of the interdependence of the family system, one will find unavoidable redundancy. For the sake of efficiency, the assessor should try not to repeat data, but to refer the reader back to sections where this information has already been described.

IDENTIFYING DATA

1. **Family Name**
2. **Address and Phone**
3. **Family Composition**
   See Table A-1.
4. **Type of Family Form**
5. **Cultural (Ethnic) Background**
6. **Religious Identification**
7. **Social Class Status**
8. **Family's Recreational or Leisure Time Activities**

DEVELOPMENTAL STAGE AND HISTORY OF FAMILY

9. **Family's Present Developmental Stage**
10. **Extent of Family Developmental Tasks Fulfillment**
11. **Nuclear Family History**
12. **History of Family of Origin of Both Parents**

ENVIRONMENTAL DATA

13. **Characteristics of Home**
14. **Characteristics of Neighborhood and Larger Community**
15. **Family's Geographic Mobility**
16. **Family's Associations and Transactions with Community**
17. **Family's Social Support System or Network**
    Ecomap
    Family genogram

FAMILY STRUCTURE

18. **Communication Patterns**
    Extent of Functional and Dysfunctional Communication (types of recurring patterns)
    Extent of Emotional (Affective) Messages and How Expressed
    Characteristics of Communication Within Family Subsystems
    Extent of Congruent and Incongruent Messages
    Types of Dysfunctional Communication
    Processes Seen in Family
    Areas of Open and Closed Communication
    Familial and Contextual Variables Affecting Communication
19. **Power Structure**
    Power Outcomes
    Decision-Making Process
    Power Bases
    Variables Affecting Family Power
    Overall Family System and Subsystem Power (family power continuum placement)

TABLE A-1 Family Composition Form

NAME (LAST, FIRST)	GENDER	RELATIONSHIP	DATE AND PLACE OF BIRTH	OCCUPATION	EDUCATION
1. (Father)					
2. (Mother)					
3. (Oldest child)					
4.					
5.					
6.					
7.					
8.					

20. Role Structure

Formal Role Structure

Informal Role Structure

Analysis of Role Models (optional)

Variables Affecting Role Structure

21. Family Values

Compare the family with American or family's reference group values or identify important family values and their importance (priority) in family.

Congruence between the Family's Values and Values of the Family's Reference Group or Wider Community

Congruence Between the Family's Values and Family Members' Values

Variables Influencing Family Values

Values Consciously or Unconsciously Held

Presence of Value Conflicts in Family

Effect of the Above Values and Value Conflicts on Health Status of Family

FAMILY FUNCTIONS

22. Affective Function

Family Need-Response Patterns

Mutual Nurturance, Closeness, and Identification

Family attachment diagram

Separateness and Connectedness

23. Socialization Function

Family Child-Rearing Practices

Adaptability of Child-Rearing Practices for Family Form and Family's Situation

Who Is (Are) Socializing Agent(s) for Child(ren)?

Value of Children in Family

Cultural Beliefs That Influence Family's Child-Rearing Patterns

Social Class Influence on Child-Rearing Patterns

Estimation about Whether Family Is At Risk for Child-Rearing Problems and If So, Indication of High-Risk Factors

Adequacy of Home Environment for Children's Needs to Play

24. Health Care Function

Family's Health Beliefs, Values, and Behaviors

Family's Definitions of Health-Illness and Their Level of Knowledge

Family's Perceived Health Status and Illness Susceptibility

Family's Dietary Practices

Adequacy of family diet (recommended three-day food history record)

Function of mealtimes and attitudes toward food and mealtimes

Shopping (and its planning) practices

Person(s) responsible for planning, shopping, and preparation of meals

Sleep and Rest Habits

Physical Activity and Recreation Practices (not covered earlier)

Family's Drug Habits

Family's Role in Self-Care Practices

Medically Based Preventive Measures (physicals, eye and hearing tests, and immunizations)

Dental Health Practices

Family Health History (both general and specific diseases—environmentally and genetically related)

Health Care Services Received

Feelings and Perceptions Regarding Health Services

Emergency Health Services

Source of Payments for Health and Other Services

Logistics of Receiving Care

FAMILY STRESS AND COPING

25. **Short- and Long-Term Familial Stressors and Strengths**
26. **Extent of Family's Ability to Respond, Based on Objective Appraisal of Stress-Producing Situations**
27. **Coping Strategies Utilized (present and past)**
    Differences in Family Members' Ways of Coping
    Family's Inner Coping Strategies
    Family's External Coping Strategies
28. **Dysfunctional Adaptive Strategies Utilized (present and past; extent of usage)**

Appendix A lists the broad content areas recommended for family assessment. In-depth discussion of each of these content areas and related theoretical and research foundation, as well as relevant diagnoses and intervention guidelines, are included in the original Friedman text.

APPENDIX B
Physical Growth Charts

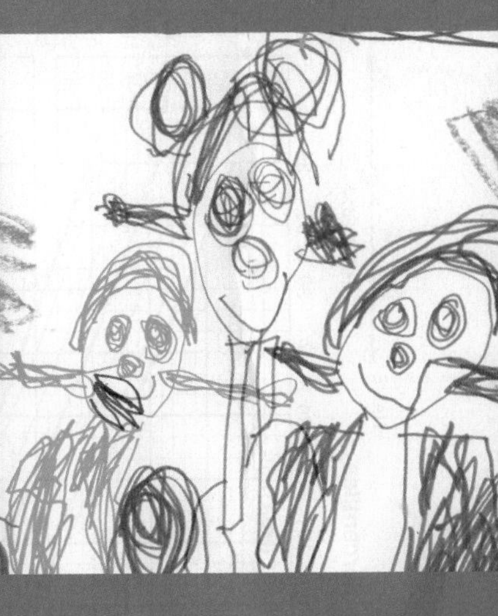

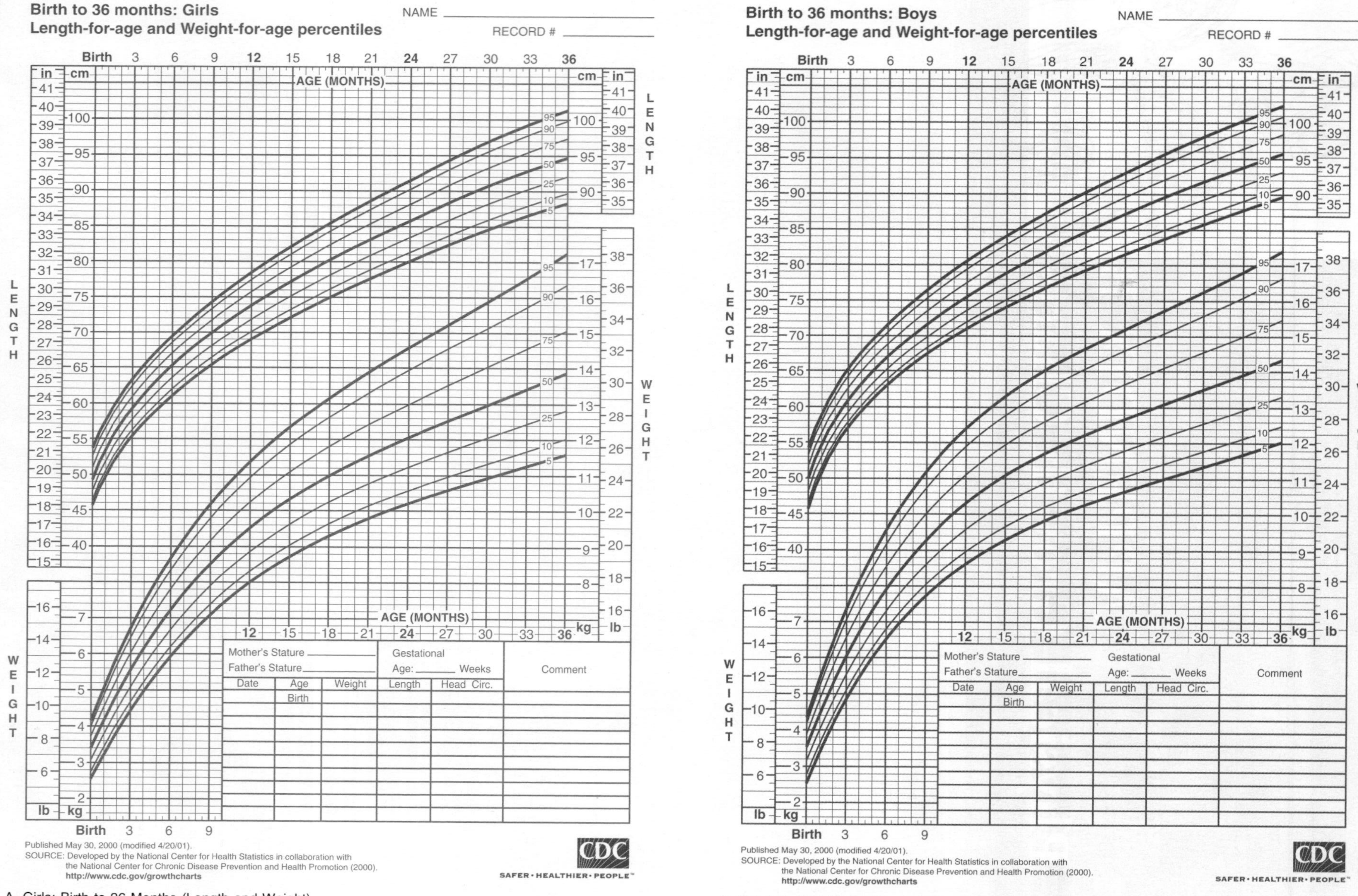

FIGURE B-1 Physical Growth Charts. COURTESY OF NATIONAL CENTER FOR HEALTH STATISTICS, U.S. CENTERS FOR DISEASE CONTROL AND PREVENTION, 2001.

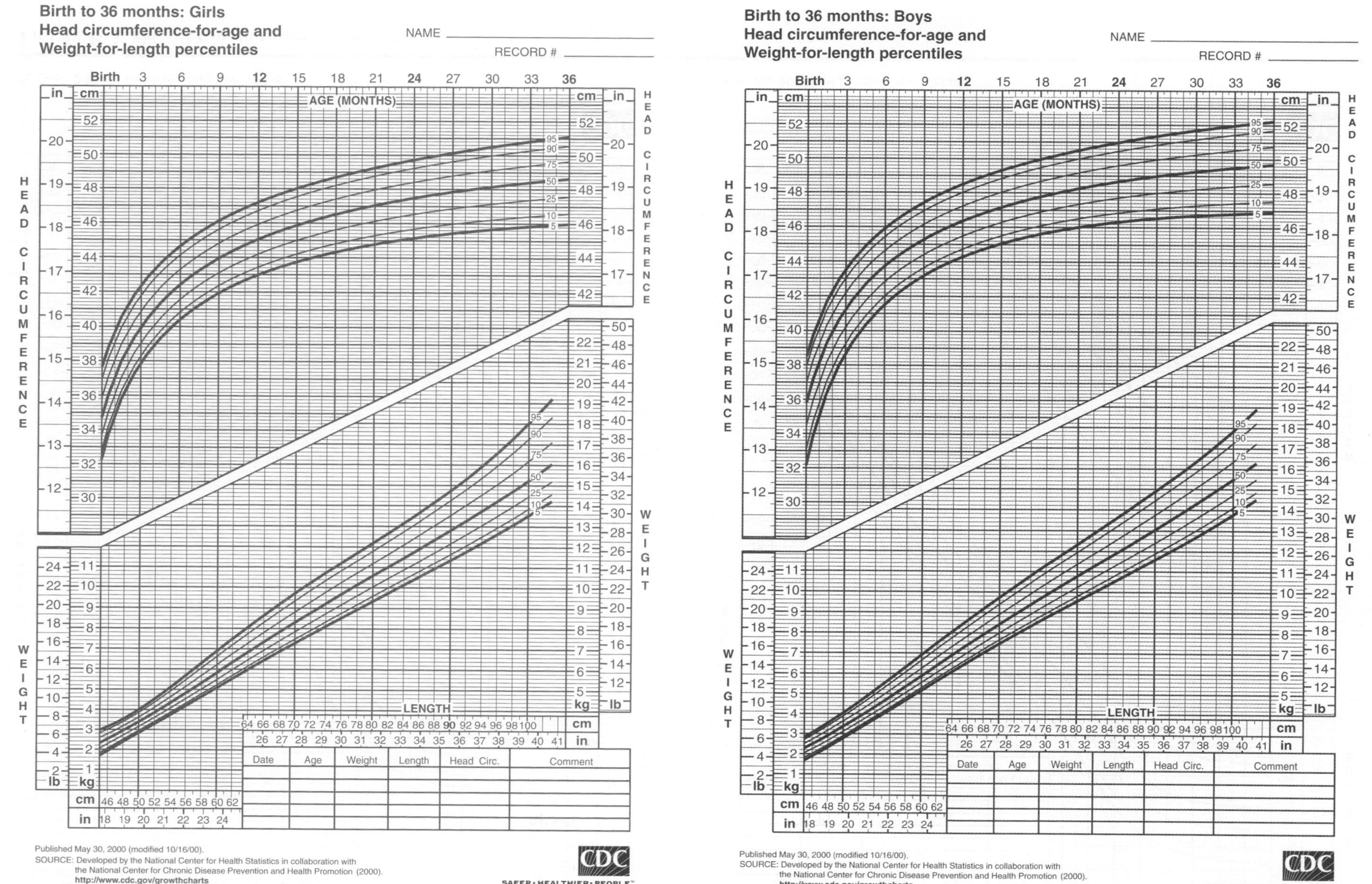

C. Girls: Birth to 36 Months (Head Circumference)

D. Boys: Birth to 36 Months (Head Circumference)

FIGURE B-1 Physical Growth Charts. *(Continued)*

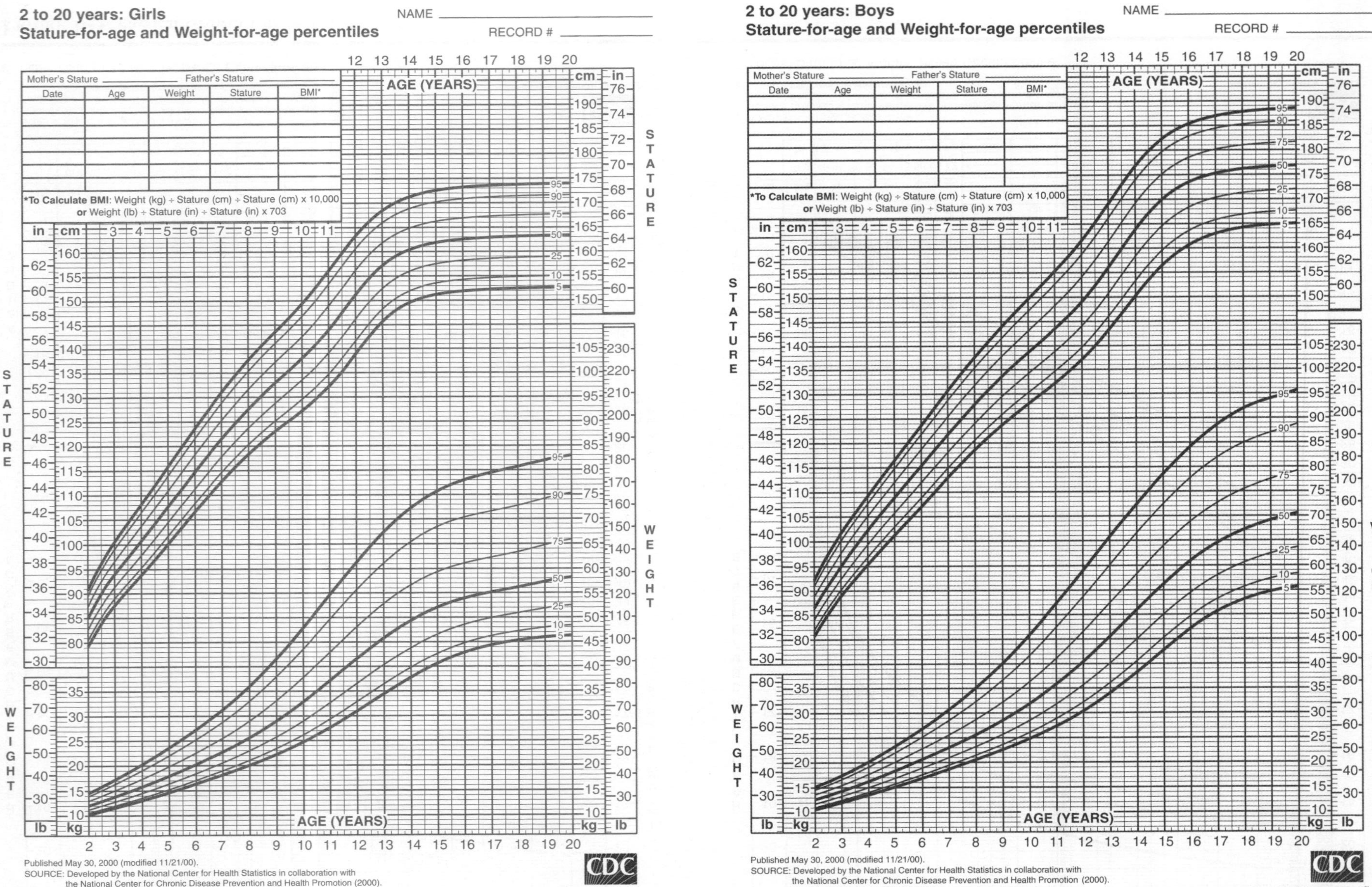

E. Girls: 2 to 20 Years (Stature and Weight)

F. Boys: 2 to 20 Years (Stature and Weight)

FIGURE B-1 Physical Growth Charts. *(Continued)*

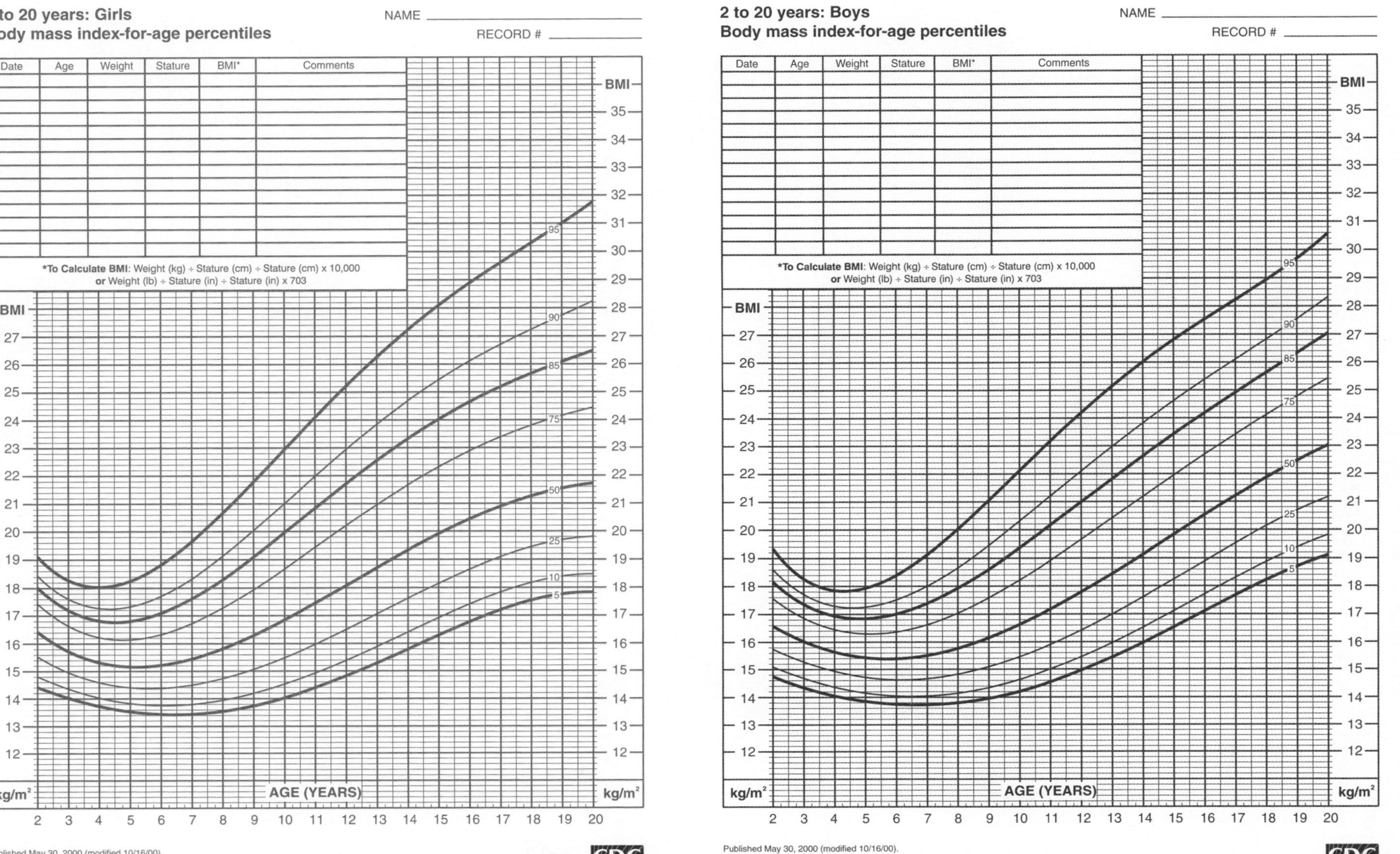

G. Girls: 2 to 20 Years (Body Mass Index for Age)

H. Boys: 2 to 20 Years (Body Mass Index for Age)

FIGURE B-1 Physical Growth Charts. *(Continued)*

APPENDIX C
Immunization Schedules

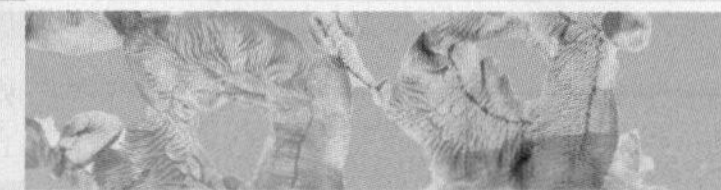

TABLE C-1 Recommended Immunization Schedule for Persons Aged 0 Through 6 Years—United States, 2010

Recommended Immunization Schedule for Persons Aged 0 Through 6 Years—United States • 2010

For those who fall behind or start late, see the catch-up schedule

Vaccine ▼ Age ►	Birth	1 month	2 months	4 months	6 months	12 months	15 months	18 months	19–23 months	2–3 years	4–6 years
Hepatitis B[1]	HepB	HepB			HepB						
Rotavirus[2]			RV	RV	RV[2]						
Diphtheria, Tetanus, Pertussis[3]			DTaP	DTaP	DTaP	see footnote[3]	DTaP				DTaP
Haemophilus influenzae type b[4]			Hib	Hib	Hib[4]	Hib					
Pneumococcal[5]			PCV	PCV	PCV	PCV				PPSV	
Inactivated Poliovirus[6]			IPV	IPV	IPV						IPV
Influenza[7]					Influenza (Yearly)						
Measles, Mumps, Rubella[8]						MMR		see footnote[8]			MMR
Varicella[9]						Varicella		see footnote[9]			Varicella
Hepatitis A[10]						HepA (2 doses)				HepA Series	
Meningococcal[11]										MCV	

Range of recommended ages for all children except certain high-risk groups

Range of recommended ages for certain high-risk groups

This schedule includes recommendations in effect as of December 15, 2009. Any dose not administered at the recommended age should be administered at a subsequent visit, when indicated and feasible. The use of a combination vaccine generally is preferred over separate injections of its equivalent component vaccines. Considerations should include provider assessment, patient preference, and the potential for adverse events. Providers should consult the relevant Advisory Committee on Immunization Practices statement for detailed recommendations: **http://www.cdc.gov/vaccines/pubs/acip-list.htm**. Clinically significant adverse events that follow immunization should be reported to the Vaccine Adverse Event Reporting System (VAERS) at **http://www.vaers.hhs.gov** or by telephone, **800-822-7967**.

1. **Hepatitis B vaccine (HepB).** (Minimum age: birth)
   At birth:
   - Administer monovalent HepB to all newborns before hospital discharge.
   - If mother is hepatitis B surface antigen (HBsAg)-positive, administer HepB and 0.5 mL of hepatitis B immune globulin (HBIG) within 12 hours of birth.
   - If mother's HBsAg status is unknown, administer HepB within 12 hours of birth. Determine mother's HBsAg status as soon as possible and, if HBsAg-positive, administer HBIG (no later than age 1 week).

   After the birth dose:
   - The HepB series should be completed with either monovalent HepB or a combination vaccine containing HepB. The second dose should be administered at age 1 or 2 months. Monovalent HepB vaccine should be used for doses administered before age 6 weeks. The final dose should be administered no earlier than age 24 weeks.
   - Infants born to HBsAg-positive mothers should be tested for HBsAg and antibody to HBsAg 1 to 2 months after completion of at least 3 doses of the HepB series, at age 9 through 18 months (generally at the next well-child visit).
   - Administration of 4 doses of HepB to infants is permissible when a combination vaccine containing HepB is administered after the birth dose. The fourth dose should be administered no earlier than age 24 weeks.
2. **Rotavirus vaccine (RV).** (Minimum age: 6 weeks)
   - Administer the first dose at age 6 through 14 weeks (maximum age: 14 weeks 6 days). Vaccination should not be initiated for infants aged 15 weeks 0 days or older.
   - The maximum age for the final dose in the series is 8 months 0 days
   - If Rotarix is administered at ages 2 and 4 months, a dose at 6 months is not indicated.
3. **Diphtheria and tetanus toxoids and acellular pertussis vaccine (DTaP).** (Minimum age: 6 weeks)
   - The fourth dose may be administered as early as age 12 months, provided at least 6 months have elapsed since the third dose.
   - Administer the final dose in the series at age 4 through 6 years.
4. ***Haemophilus influenzae* type b conjugate vaccine (Hib).** (Minimum age: 6 weeks)
   - If PRP-OMP (PedvaxHIB or Comvax [HepB-Hib]) is administered at ages 2 and 4 months, a dose at age 6 months is not indicated.
   - TriHiBit (DTaP/Hib) and Hiberix (PRP-T) should not be used for doses at ages 2, 4, or 6 months for the primary series but can be used as the final dose in children aged 12 months through 4 years.
5. **Pneumococcal vaccine.** (Minimum age: 6 weeks for pneumococcal conjugate vaccine [PCV]; 2 years for pneumococcal polysaccharide vaccine [PPSV])
   - PCV is recommended for all children aged younger than 5 years. Administer 1 dose of PCV to all healthy children aged 24 through 59 months who are not completely vaccinated for their age.
   - Administer PPSV 2 or more months after last dose of PCV to children aged 2 years or older with certain underlying medical conditions, including a cochlear implant. See *MMWR* 1997;46(No. RR-8).
6. **Inactivated poliovirus vaccine (IPV)** (Minimum age: 6 weeks)
   - The final dose in the series should be administered on or after the fourth birthday and at least 6 months following the previous dose.
   - If 4 doses are administered prior to age 4 years a fifth dose should be administered at age 4 through 6 years. See *MMWR* 2009;58(30):829–30.
7. **Influenza vaccine (seasonal).** (Minimum age: 6 months for trivalent inactivated influenza vaccine [TIV]; 2 years for live, attenuated influenza vaccine [LAIV])
   - Administer annually to children aged 6 months through 18 years.
   - For healthy children aged 2 through 6 years (i.e., those who do not have underlying medical conditions that predispose them to influenza complications), either LAIV or TIV may be used, except LAIV should not be given to children aged 2 through 4 years who have had wheezing in the past 12 months.
   - Children receiving TIV should receive 0.25 mL if aged 6 through 35 months or 0.5 mL if aged 3 years or older.
   - Administer 2 doses (separated by at least 4 weeks) to children aged younger than 9 years who are receiving influenza vaccine for the first time or who were vaccinated for the first time during the previous influenza season but only received 1 dose.
   - For recommendations for use of influenza A (H1N1) 2009 monovalent vaccine see *MMWR* 2009;58(No. RR-10).
8. **Measles, mumps, and rubella vaccine (MMR).** (Minimum age: 12 months)
   - Administer the second dose routinely at age 4 through 6 years. However, the second dose may be administered before age 4, provided at least 28 days have elapsed since the first dose.
9. **Varicella vaccine.** (Minimum age: 12 months)
   - Administer the second dose routinely at age 4 through 6 years. However, the second dose may be administered before age 4, provided at least 3 months have elapsed since the first dose.
   - For children aged 12 months through 12 years the minimum interval between doses is 3 months. However, if the second dose was administered at least 28 days after the first dose, it can be accepted as valid.
10. **Hepatitis A vaccine (HepA).** (Minimum age: 12 months)
    - Administer to all children aged 1 year (i.e., aged 12 through 23 months). Administer 2 doses at least 6 months apart.
    - Children not fully vaccinated by age 2 years can be vaccinated at subsequent visits
    - HepA also is recommended for older children who live in areas where vaccination programs target older children, who are at increased risk for infection, or for whom immunity against hepatitis A is desired.
11. **Meningococcal vaccine.** (Minimum age: 2 years for meningococcal conjugate vaccine [MCV4] and for meningococcal polysaccharide vaccine [MPSV4])
    - Administer MCV4 to children aged 2 through 10 years with persistent complement component deficiency, anatomic or functional asplenia, and certain other conditions placing tham at high risk.
    - Administer MCV4 to children previously vaccinated with MCV4 or MPSV4 after 3 years if first dose administered at age 2 through 6 years. See *MMWR* 2009;58:1042–3.

The Recommended Immunization Schedules for Persons Aged 0 through 18 Years are approved by the Advisory Committee on Immunization Practices (**http://www.cdc.gov/vaccines/recs/acip**), the American Academy of Pediatrics (**http://www.aap.org**), and the American Academy of Family Physicians (**http://www.aafp.org**).

Department of Health and Human Services • Centers for Disease Control and Prevention

CS207330-A

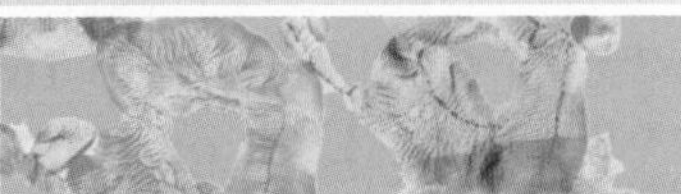

Table C-2 Recommended Immunization Schedule for Persons Aged 7 Through 18 Years—United States, 2010

Recommended Immunization Schedule for Persons Aged 7 Through 18 Years—United States • 2010

For those who fall behind or start late, see the schedule below and the catch-up schedule

Vaccine ▼ Age ►	7–10 years	11–12 years	13–18 years
Tetanus, Diphtheria, Pertussis[1]		Tdap	Tdap
Human Papillomavirus[2]	*see footnote 2*	HPV (3 doses)	HPV series
Meningococcal[3]	MCV	MCV	MCV
Influenza[4]	Influenza (Yearly)		
Pneumococcal[5]	PPSV		
Hepatitis A[6]	HepA Series		
Hepatitis B[7]	Hep B Series		
Inactivated Poliovirus[8]	IPV Series		
Measles, Mumps, Rubella[9]	MMR Series		
Varicella[10]	Varicella Series		

Range of recommended ages for all children except certain high-risk groups

Range of recommended ages for catch-up immunization

Range of recommended ages for certain high-risk groups

This schedule includes recommendations in effect as of December 15, 2009. Any dose not administered at the recommended age should be administered at a subsequent visit, when indicated and feasible. The use of a combination vaccine generally is preferred over separate injections of its equivalent component vaccines. Considerations should include provider assessment, patient preference, and the potential for adverse events. Providers should consult the relevant Advisory Committee on Immunization Practices statement for detailed recommendations: **http://www.cdc.gov/vaccines/pubs/acip-list.htm.** Clinically significant adverse events that follow immunization should be reported to the Vaccine Adverse Event Reporting System (VAERS) at **http://www.vaers.hhs.gov** or by telephone, **800-822-7967.**

1. **Tetanus and diphtheria toxoids and acellular pertussis vaccine (Tdap).** (Minimum age: 10 years for Boostrix and 11 years for Adacel)
   - Administer at age 11 or 12 years for those who have completed the recommended childhood DTP/DTaP vaccination series and have not received a tetanus and diphtheria toxoid (Td) booster dose.
   - Persons aged 13 through 18 years who have not received Tdap should receive a dose.
   - A 5-year interval from the last Td dose is encouraged when Tdap is used as a booster dose; however, a shorter interval may be used if pertussis immunity is needed.
2. **Human papillomavirus vaccine (HPV).** (Minimum age: 9 years)
   - Two HPV vaccines are licensed: a quadrivalent vaccine (HPV4) for the prevention of cervical, vaginal and vulvar cancers (in females) and genital warts (in females and males), and a bivalent vaccine (HPV2) for the prevention of cervical cancers in females.
   - HPV vaccines are most effective for both males and females when given before exposure to HPV through sexual contact.
   - HPV4 or HPV2 is recommended for the prevention of cervical precancers and cancers in females.
   - HPV4 is recommended for the prevention of cervical, vaginal and vulvar precancers and cancers and genital warts in females.
   - Administer the first dose to females at age 11 or 12 years.
   - Administer the second dose 1 to 2 months after the first dose and the third dose 6 months after the first dose (at least 24 weeks after the first dose).
   - Administer the series to females at age 13 through 18 years if not previously vaccinated.
   - HPV4 may be administered in a 3-dose series to males aged 9 through 18 years to reduce their likelihood of acquiring genital warts.
3. **Meningococcal conjugate vaccine (MCV4).**
   - Administer at age 11 or 12 years, or at age 13 through 18 years if not previously vaccinated.
   - Administer to previously unvaccinated college freshmen living in a dormitory.
   - Administer MCV4 to children aged 2 through 10 years with persistent complement component deficiency, anatomic or functional asplenia, or certain other conditions placing them at high risk.
   - Administer to children previously vaccinated with MCV4 or MPSV4 who remain at increased risk after 3 years (if first dose administered at age 2 through 6 years) or after 5 years (if first dose administered at age 7 years or older). Persons whose only risk factor is living in on-campus housing are not recommended to receive an additional dose. See *MMWR* 2009;58:1042–3.
4. **Influenza vaccine (seasonal).**
   - Administer annually to children aged 6 months through 18 years.
   - For healthy nonpregnant persons aged 7 through 18 years (i.e., those who do not have underlying medical conditions that predispose them to influenza complications), either LAIV or TIV may be used.
   - Administer 2 doses (separated by at least 4 weeks) to children aged younger than 9 years who are receiving influenza vaccine for the first time or who were vaccinated for the first time during the previous influenza season but only received 1 dose.
   - For recommendations for use of influenza A (H1N1) 2009 monovalent vaccine. See *MMWR* 2009;58(No. RR-10).
5. **Pneumococcal polysaccharide vaccine (PPSV).**
   - Administer to children with certain underlying medical conditions, including a cochlear implant. A single revaccination should be administered after 5 years to children with functional or anatomic asplenia or an immunocompromising condition. See *MMWR* 1997;46(No. RR-8).
6. **Hepatitis A vaccine (HepA).**
   - Administer 2 doses at least 6 months apart.
   - HepA is recommended for children aged older than 23 months who live in areas where vaccination programs target older children, who are at increased risk for infection, or for whom immunity against hepatitis A is desired.
7. **Hepatitis B vaccine (HepB).**
   - Administer the 3-dose series to those not previously vaccinated.
   - A 2-dose series (separated by at least 4 months) of adult formulation Recombivax HB is licensed for children aged 11 through 15 years.
8. **Inactivated poliovirus vaccine (IPV).**
   - The final dose in the series should be administered on or after the fourth birthday and at least 6 months following the previous dose.
   - If both OPV and IPV were administered as part of a series, a total of 4 doses should be administered, regardless of the child's current age.
9. **Measles, mumps, and rubella vaccine (MMR).**
   - If not previously vaccinated, administer 2 doses or the second dose for those who have received only 1 dose, with at least 28 days between doses.
10. **Varicella vaccine.**
    - For persons aged 7 through 18 years without evidence of immunity (see *MMWR* 2007;56[No. RR-4]), administer 2 doses if not previously vaccinated or the second dose if only 1 dose has been administered.
    - For persons aged 7 through 12 years, the minimum interval between doses is 3 months. However, if the second dose was administered at least 28 days after the first dose, it can be accepted as valid.
    - For persons aged 13 years and older, the minimum interval between doses is 28 days.

The Recommended Immunization Schedules for Persons Aged 0 through 18 Years are approved by the Advisory Committee on Immunization Practices (**http://www.cdc.gov/vaccines/recs/acip**), the American Academy of Pediatrics (**http://www.aap.org**), and the American Academy of Family Physicians (**http://www.aafp.org**).

Department of Health and Human Services • Centers for Disease Control and Prevention

CS207330-A

TABLE C-3 Catch-up Immunization Schedule for Persons Aged 4 Months Through 18 Years Who Start Late or Who Are More Than 1 Month Behind—United States, 2010

Catch-up Immunization Schedule for Persons Aged 4 Months Through 18 Years Who Start Late or Who Are More Than 1 Month Behind—United States • 2010

The table below provides catch-up schedules and minimum intervals between doses for children whose vaccinations have been delayed. A vaccine series does not need to be restarted, regardless of the time that has elapsed between doses. Use the section appropriate for the child's age.

Vaccine	Minimum Age for Dose 1	Minimum Interval Between Doses			
		Dose 1 to Dose 2	Dose 2 to Dose 3	Dose 3 to Dose 4	Dose 4 to Dose 5
PERSONS AGED 4 MONTHS THROUGH 6 YEARS					
Hepatitis B[1]	Birth	**4 weeks**	**8 weeks** (and at least 16 weeks after first dose)		
Rotavirus[2]	6 wks	**4 weeks**	**4 weeks**[2]		
Diphtheria, Tetanus, Pertussis[3]	6 wks	**4 weeks**	**4 weeks**	**6 months**	**6 months**[3]
Haemophilus influenzae type b[4]	6 wks	**4 weeks** if first dose administered at younger than age 12 months **8 weeks (as final dose)** if first dose administered at age 12–14 months **No further doses needed** if first dose administered at age 15 months or older	**4 weeks**[4] if current age is younger than 12 months **8 weeks (as final dose)**[4] if current age is 12 months or older and first dose administered at younger than age 12 months and second dose administered at younger than 15 months **No further doses needed** if previous dose administered at age 15 months or older	**8 weeks (as final dose)** This dose only necessary for children aged 12 months through 59 months who received 3 doses before age 12 months	
Pneumococcal[5]	6 wks	**4 weeks** if first dose administered at younger than age 12 months **8 weeks (as final dose for healthy children)** if first dose administered at age 12 months or older or current age 24 through 59 months **No further doses needed** for healthy children if first dose administered at age 24 months or older	**4 weeks** if current age is younger than 12 months **8 weeks (as final dose for healthy children)** if current age is 12 months or older **No further doses needed** for healthy children if previous dose administered at age 24 months or older	**8 weeks (as final dose)** This dose only necessary for children aged 12 months through 59 months who received 3 doses before age 12 months or for high-risk children who received 3 doses at any age	
Inactivated Poliovirus[6]	6 wks	**4 weeks**	**4 weeks**	**6 months**	
Measles,Mumps, Rubella[7]	12 mos	**4 weeks**			
Varicella[8]	12 mos	**3 months**			
Hepatitis A[9]	12 mos	**6 months**			
PERSONS AGED 7 THROUGH 18 YEARS					
Tetanus, Diphtheria/ Tetanus, Diphtheria, Pertussis[10]	7 yrs[10]	**4 weeks**	**4 weeks** if first dose administered at younger than age 12 months **6 months** if first dose administered at 12 months or older	**6 months** if first dose administered at younger than age 12 months	
Human Papillomavirus[11]	9 yrs	**Routine dosing intervals are recommended**[11]			
Hepatitis A[9]	12 mos	**6 months**			
Hepatitis B[1]	Birth	**4 weeks**	**8 weeks** (and at least 16 weeks after first dose)		
Inactivated Poliovirus[6]	6 wks	**4 weeks**	**4 weeks**	**6 months**	
Measles,Mumps, Rubella[7]	12 mos	**4 weeks**			
Varicella[8]	12 mos	**3 months** if person is younger than age 13 years **4 weeks** if person is aged 13 years or older			

1. **Hepatitis B vaccine (HepB).**
   - Administer the 3-dose series to those not previously vaccinated.
   - A 2-dose series (separated by at least 4 months) of adult formulation Recombivax HB is licensed for children aged 11 through 15 years.
2. **Rotavirus vaccine (RV).**
   - The maximum age for the first dose is 14 weeks 6 days. Vaccination should not be initiated for infants aged 15 weeks 0 days or older.
   - The maximum age for the final dose in the series is 8 months 0 days.
   - If Rotarix was administered for the first and second doses, a third dose is not indicated.
3. **Diphtheria and tetanus toxoids and acellular pertussis vaccine (DTaP).**
   - The fifth dose is not necessary if the fourth dose was administered at age 4 years or older.
4. ***Haemophilus influenzae* type b conjugate vaccine (Hib).**
   - Hib vaccine is not generally recommended for persons aged 5 years or older. No efficacy data are available on which to base a recommendation concerning use of Hib vaccine for older children and adults. However, studies suggest good immunogenicity in persons who have sickle cell disease, leukemia, or HIV infection, or who have had a splenectomy; administering 1 dose of Hib vaccine to these persons who have not previously received Hib vaccine is not contraindicated.
   - If the first 2 doses were PRP-OMP (PedvaxHIB or Comvax), and administered at age 11 months or younger, the third (and final) dose should be administered at age 12 through 15 months and at least 8 weeks after the second dose.
   - If the first dose was administered at age 7 through 11 months, administer the second dose at least 4 weeks later and a final dose at age 12 through 15 months.
5. **Pneumococcal vaccine.**
   - Administer 1 dose of pneumococcal conjugate vaccine (PCV) to all healthy children aged 24 through 59 months who have not received at least 1 dose of PCV on or after age 12 months.
   - For children aged 24 through 59 months with underlying medical conditions, administer 1 dose of PCV if 3 doses were received previously or administer 2 doses of PCV at least 8 weeks apart if fewer than 3 doses were received previously.
   - Administer pneumococcal polysaccharide vaccine (PPSV) to children aged 2 years or older with certain underlying medical conditions, including a cochlear implant, at least 8 weeks after the last dose of PCV. See *MMWR* 1997;46(No. RR-8).
6. **Inactivated poliovirus vaccine (IPV).**
   - The final dose in the series should be administered on or after the fourth birthday and at least 6 months following the previous dose.
   - A fourth dose is not necessary if the third dose was administered at age 4 years or older and at least 6 months following the previous dose.
   - In the first 6 months of life, minimum age and minimum intervals are only recommended if the person is at risk for imminent exposure to circulating poliovirus (i.e., travel to a polio-endemic region or during an outbreak).
7. **Measles, mumps, and rubella vaccine (MMR).**
   - Administer the second dose routinely at age 4 through 6 years. However, the second dose may be administered before age 4, provided at least 28 days have elapsed since the first dose.
   - If not previously vaccinated, administer 2 doses with at least 28 days between doses.
8. **Varicella vaccine.**
   - Administer the second dose routinely at age 4 through 6 years. However, the second dose may be administered before age 4, provided at least 3 months have elapsed since the first dose.
   - For persons aged 12 months through 12 years, the minimum interval between doses is 3 months. However, if the second dose was administered at least 28 days after the first dose, it can be accepted as valid.
   - For persons aged 13 years and older, the minimum interval between doses is 28 days.
9. **Hepatitis A vaccine (HepA).**
   - HepA is recommended for children aged older than 23 months who live in areas where vaccination programs target older children, who are at increased risk for infection, or for whom immunity against hepatitis A is desired.
10. **Tetanus and diphtheria toxoids vaccine (Td) and tetanus and diphtheria toxoids and acellular pertussis vaccine (Tdap).**
    - Doses of DTaP are counted as part of the Td/Tdap series
    - Tdap should be substituted for a single dose of Td in the catch-up series or as a booster for children aged 10 through 18 years; use Td for other doses.
11. **Human papillomavirus vaccine (HPV).**
    - Administer the series to females at age 13 through 18 years if not previously vaccinated.
    - Use recommended routine dosing intervals for series catch-up (i.e., the second and third doses should be administered at 1 to 2 and 6 months after the first dose). The minimum interval between the first and second doses is 4 weeks. The minimum interval between the second and third doses is 12 weeks, and the third dose should be administered at least 24 weeks after the first dose.

Information about reporting reactions after immunization is available online at **http://www.vaers.hhs.gov** or by telephone, **800-822-7967**. Suspected cases of vaccine-preventable diseases should be reported to the state or local health department. Additional information, including precautions and contraindications for immunization, is available from the National Center for Immunization and Respiratory Diseases at **http://www.cdc.gov/vaccines** or telephone, **800-CDC-INFO** (800-232-4636).

Department of Health and Human Services • Centers for Disease Control and Prevention

CS207330-A

APPENDIX D
Sexual Maturity Ratings (SMR)

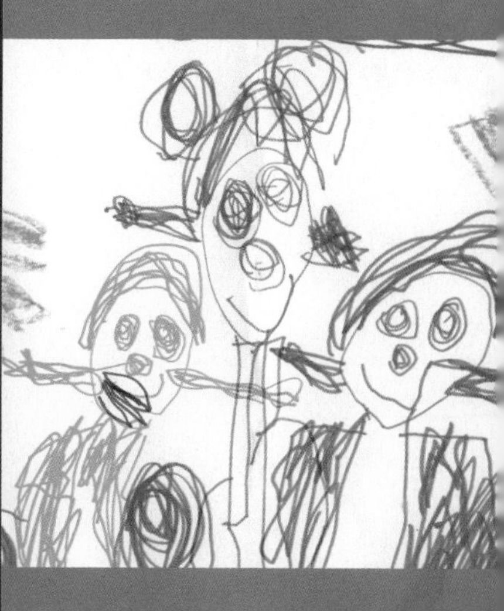

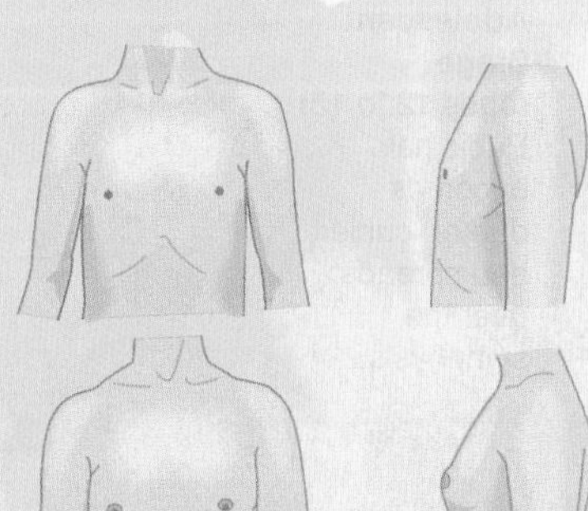

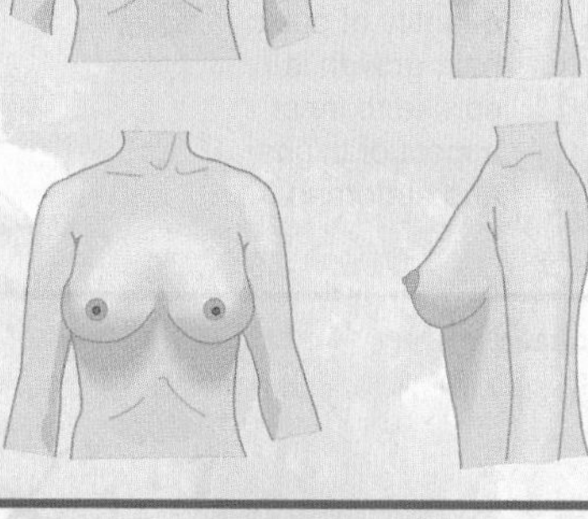

Developmental Stages

1. **Preadolescent Stage**
   (before age 8)
   Nipple is small, slightly raised.

2. **Early Adolescent Stage**
   Breast bud development (after age 8). Nipple and breast form a small mound. Areola enlarges. Height spurt begins.

3. **Adolescent Stage**
   (10-14 years)
   Nipple is flush with breast shape. Breast and areola enlarge. Menses begins. Height spurt peaks.

4. **Late Adolescent Stage**
   (14–17 years)
   Nipple and areola form a secondary mound over the breast. Height spurt ends.

5. **Adult Stage**
   Nipple protrudes; areola is flush with the breast shape.

FIGURE D-1 Sexual Maturity Rating (SMR) for Female Breast Development. ADAPTED FROM MARSHALL, W. A., & TANNER, J. M. (1969). VARIATIONS IN THE PATTERN OF PUBERTAL CHANGES IN GIRLS. *ARCHIVES OF DISEASE IN CHILDHOOD, 44,* 291–303; MARSHALL, W. A., & TANNER, J. M. (1970). VARIATIONS IN THE PATTERN OF PUBERTAL CHANGES IN BOYS. *ARCHIVES OF DISEASE IN CHILDHOOD, 45,* 13–23.

Stage 1

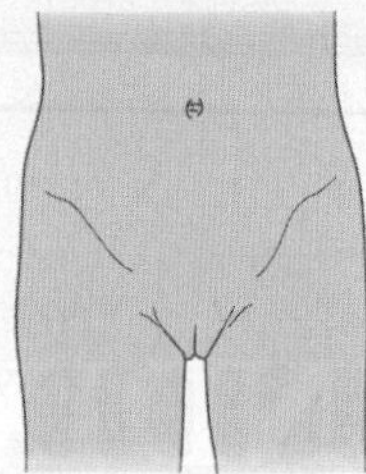

Preadolescent Stage
(before age 8)
No pubic hair, only body hair (vellus hair).

Stage 2

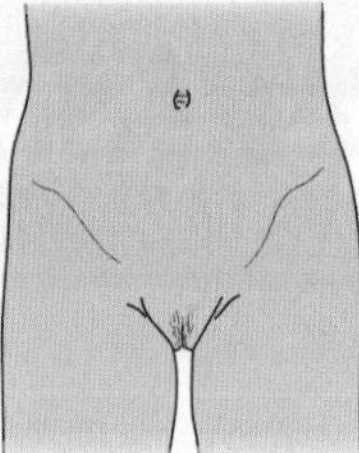

Early Adolescent Stage
(ages 8 to 12)
Sparse growth of long, slightly dark, fine pubic hair, slightly curly and located along the labia.

Stage 3

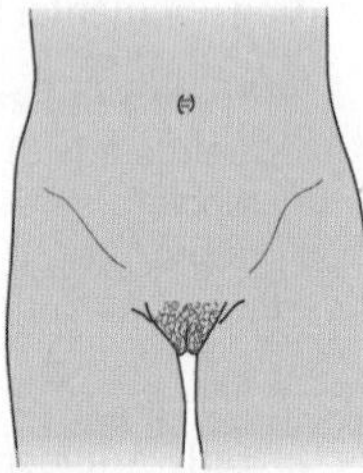

Adolescent Stage
(ages 12 to 13)
Pubic hair becomes darker, curlier, and spreads over the symphysis.

Stage 4

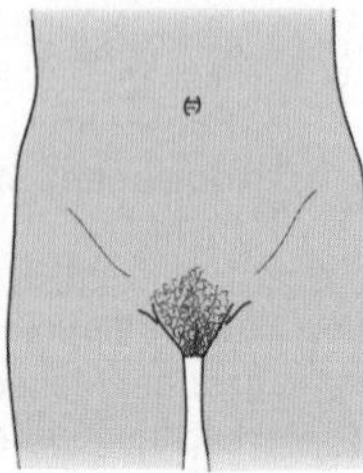

Late Adolescent Stage
(ages 13 to 15)
Texture and curl of pubic hair is similar to that of an adult but not spread to thighs.

Stage 5

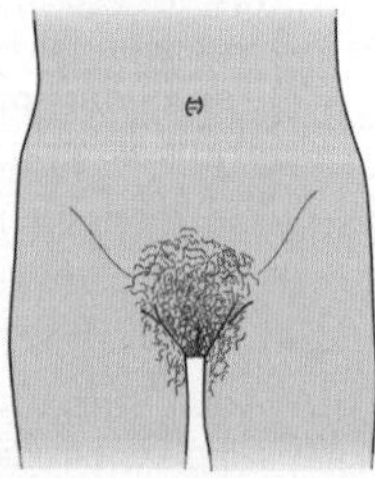

Adult Stage
Adult appearance in quality and quantity of pubic hair; growth is spread to inner aspect of thighs and abdomen.

FIGURE D-2 **Sexual Maturity Rating (SMR) for Female Genitalia.** ADAPTED FROM MARSHALL, W. A., & TANNER, J. M. (1969). VARIATIONS IN THE PATTERN OF PUBERTAL CHANGES IN GIRLS. *ARCHIVES OF DISEASE IN CHILDHOOD, 44,* 291–303; MARSHALL, W. A., & TANNER, J. M. (1970). VARIATIONS IN THE PATTERN OF PUBERTAL CHANGES IN BOYS. *ARCHIVES OF DISEASE IN CHILDHOOD, 45,* 13–23.

Developmental Stage	Pubic Hair	Penis	Testes
1. 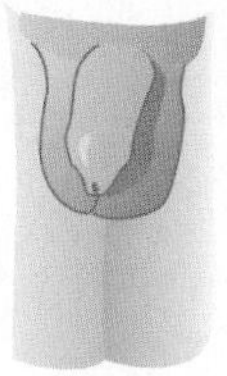	No pubic hair, only fine body hair (vellus hair)	Preadolescent; childhood size and proportion	Preadolescent; childhood size and proportion
2. 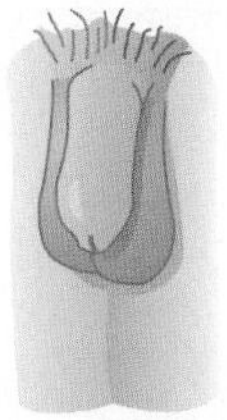	Sparse growth of long, slightly dark, straight hair	Slight or no growth	Growth in testes and scrotum; scrotum reddens and changes texture
3. 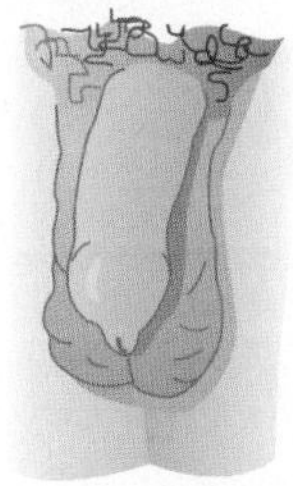	Becomes darker and coarser; slightly curled and spreads over symphysis	Growth, especially in length	Further growth
4. 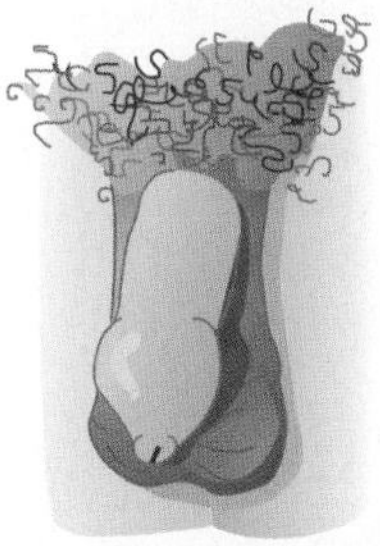	Texture and curl of pubic hair is similar to that of an adult but not spread to thighs	Further growth in length; diameter increases; development of glans	Further growth; scrotum darkens
5. 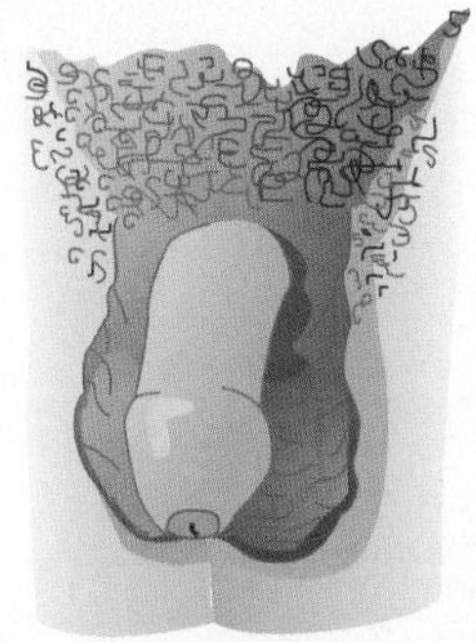	Adult appearance in quality and quantity of pubic hair; growth is spread to medial surface of thighs	Adult size and shape	Adult size and shape

FIGURE D-3 Sexual Maturity Rating (SMR) for Male Genitalia. ADAPTED FROM MARSHALL, W. A., & TANNER, J. M. (1969). VARIATIONS IN THE PATTERN OF PUBERTAL CHANGES IN GIRLS. *ARCHIVES OF DISEASE IN CHILDHOOD, 44,* 291–303; MARSHALL, W. A., & TANNER, J. M. (1970). VARIATIONS IN THE PATTERN OF PUBERTAL CHANGES IN BOYS. *ARCHIVES OF DISEASE IN CHILDHOOD, 45,* 13–23.

APPENDIX E
Common Laboratory Tests and Normal Values

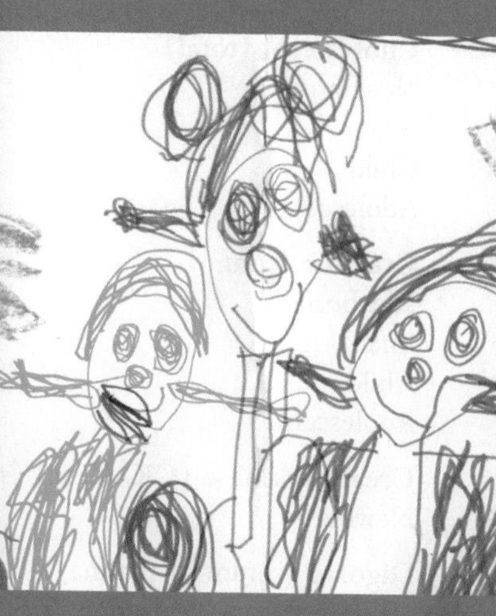

Acetaminophen (serum or plasma)

Therapeutic concentration	10–30 mcg/mL
Toxic concentration	>200 mcg/mL

Albumin (plasma)

Newborn	2.5–3.4 g/dl
< 5 yr	3.4–5.0 g/dl
5–19 yr	4.0–5.6 g/dl

Alkaline phosphatase (ALP) (serum)

1–9 yr	145–420 units/L
2–10 yr	100–320 units/L
11–18 yr male	100–390 units/L
11–18 yr female	100–320 units/L

Ammonia nitrogen (serum or plasma)

Newborn	90–150 mg/dl
Child	40–80 mg/dl

Amylase (serum)

1–19 yr	35–127 units/L

Antistreptolysin O titer (ASO titer) (serum)

2–4 yr	<166 Todd units
School-age	170–330 Todd units

Bicarbonate (HCO_3) (serum)

Infant (venous)	20–24 mEq/L
>2 years (venous)	22–29 mEq/L
>2 years (arterial)	21–28 mEq/L

Bilirubin (conjugated) (serum)

0.0–0.2 mEq/L

Bilirubin (total) (serum)

Premature Infant	
Cord blood	<2 mg/dl
0–1 day	<8 mg/dl
1–2 days	<12 mg/dl
2–5 days	<16 mg/dl
>5 days	<20 mg/dl
Full-term Infant	
Cord	<2.8 mg/dl
0–1 day	<2–6 mg/dl
1–2 days	<6–8 mg/dl
2–5 days	<4–6 mg/dl
>5 days	<10 mg/dl

Blood volume (whole blood)

Female	50–75 mL/kg
Male	52–83 mL/kg

C-reactive protein (CRP) (serum)

2–12 yr	67–1800 ng/mL

Calcium (Ca)—Total (serum)

Newborn	9.0–10.6 mg/dl
Child	8.8–10.8 mg/dl

Carbon dioxide

Partial pressure (PCO_2) (whole blood, arterial)

Newborn	27–40 mm Hg
Infant	27–41 mm Hg
Thereafter: Male	35–48 mm Hg
Female	32–45 mm Hg

Total (tCO_2) (serum or plasma)

Newborn	13–22 mmol/L
Infant	20–28 mmol/L
Child	20–28 mmol/L
Thereafter	23–30 mmol/L

Chloride (Cl) (serum)

Newborn	97–110 mmol/L
Thereafter	98–106 mmol/L

Chloride (sweat)

Normal	<40 mmol/L
Borderline	45–60 mmol/L
Cystic fibrosis	>60 mmol/L

Cholesterol (total)

Newborn	53–135 mg/dl
Infant	70–175 mg/dl
Child	120–200 mg/dl
Adolescent	<200 mg/dl

Creatine (serum)

Newborn	0.3–1.0 mg/dl
Infant	0.2–0.4 mg/dl
Child	0.3–0.7 mg/dl
Adolescent	0.5–1.0 mg/dl

Creatine kinase (CK, CPK) (serum)

Newborn	87–725 units/L

Digoxin (serum or plasma)

Therapeutic concentration	
Congestive heart failure (CHF)	0.8–1.5 ng/mL
Arrhythmias	1.5–2.0 ng/mL
Toxic concentration	>2.5 ng/mL

Erythrocyte (RBC) count (whole blood)

Newborn	4.8–7.1 million/mm^3
3–6 mo	3.1–4.5 million/mm^3
0.5–2 yr	3.7–5.3 million/mm^3
2–6 yr	3.9–5.3 million/mm^3
6–12 yr	4.0–5.2 million/mm^3
12–18 yr: Male	4.5–5.3 million/mm^3
Female	4.1–5.1 million/mm^3

Erythrocyte sedimentation rate (ESR) (whole blood)

Westergren (modified)	
Child	0–10 mm/hr
Wintrobe	
Child	0–13 mm/hr

Fibroginogen (plasma)

Newborn	125–300 mg/dl
Thereafter	200–400 mg/dl

Glucose (serum)

Newborn	50–90 mg/dl
Child	60–100 mg/dl
Thereafter	70–105 mg/dl

Growth hormone (hGH, somatotropin) (plasma, fasting)

Newborn	5–40 ng/mL
Child	0–10 ng/mL

Hematocrit (HCT, Hct) (whole blood)

Newborn	44–72%
2 mo	28–42%
6–12 yr	35–45%
12–18 yr: Male	37–49%
Female	36–46%

Hemoglobin (Hb) (whole blood)

Newborn	14–27 g/dl
2 mo	9–14 g/dl
6–12 yr	11.5–15.5 g/dl
12–18 yr: Male	13–16 g/dl
Female	12–16 g/dl

Iron (serum)

Newborn	100–250 mcg/dl
Infant	40–100 mcg/dl
Child	50–120 mcg/dl
Thereafter: Male	50–160 mcg/dl
Female	40–150 mcg/dl

Lead (whole blood)

Child	<10 mcg/dl

Leukocyte (WBC) Count (whole blood)

Newborn	9–30 × 1000 cells/mm^3
1–3 yr	6.0–17.5 × 1000 cells/mm^3
4–7 yr	5.5–15.5 × 1000 cells/mm^3
8–13 yr	4.5–13.5 × 1000 cells/mm^3
Adult	4.5–11.0 × 1000 cells/mm^3

Leukocyte differential count (whole blood)

Myelocytes	0%
Neutrophils—"bands"	3–5%
Neutrophils—"segs"	54–62%
Lymphocytes	25–33%
Monocytes	3–7%
Eosinophils	1–3%
Basophils	0–0.75%

Osmolality (serum)

Child, adult	275–295 mOsmol/kg H_2O

Oxygen, partial pressure (PO_2) (whole blood, arterial)

Birth	8–24 mm Hg
1 day	54–95 mm Hg
Thereafter (decreased with age)	83–108 mm Hg

Oxygen saturation (SaO_2) (whole blood, arterial)

Newborn	85–90%
Thereafter	95–99%

Partial thromboplastin time (PTT) (whole blood) (Na citrate)

Nonactivated	60–85 seconds (Platelin)
Activated	25–35 seconds (differs with methods)

Phenylalanine (serum)

Premature	2.0–7.5 mg/dl
Newborn	1.2–3.4 mg/dl
Thereafter	0.8–1.8 mg/dl

Plasma volume (plasma)

Male	25–43 mL/kg
Female	28–45 mL/kg

Platelet count (thrombocyte count) (whole blood)

Newborn (After 1 wk. same as adult)	84–478 × 10^3 mm^3
Adult	150–400 × 10^3 mm^3

Potassium (serum)

<2 yr	3.0–6.0 mmol/L
2–12 yr	3.5–7.0 mmol/L
>12 yr	3.5–5.0 mmol/L

Protein (serum, total)

Premature	4.3–7.5 g/dl
Newborn	4.6–7.4 g/dl
1–7 yr	6.1–7.9 g/dl
8–12 yr	6.4–8.1 g/dl
13–19 yr	6.6–8.2 g/dl

Prothrombin time (PT)

One-stage (Quick) (whole blood)

In general	11–15 seconds (varies with type of thromboplastin)
Newborn	Prolonged by 2–3 sec

Sodium (serum or plasma)

Newborn	136–146 mmol/L
Infant	139–146 mmol/L
Child	138–145 mmol/L
Thereafter	136–146 mmol/L

Specific gravity (urine)

Newborn	1.016–1.030
Infant	1.002–1.006
Thereafter	1.016–1.030

Thyrotropin (thyroid stimulating hormone [TSH])

Newborn	<25 mcIU/mL by day 3 of life
Thereafter	0.35–5.5 mcIU/mL, or <3 ng/mL

Thyroxine (T_4, T_4 total, T_4 RIA) (serum)

Newborn	9–18 mcg/dl
Infant	7–15 mcg/dl
1–5 yr	7.3–15 mcg/dl
5–10 yr	6.4–13.3 mcg/dl
Thereafter	5–12 mcg/dl

Triglycerides (TG) (serum) (after ≥12 hr fast)

	Male	**Female**
0–5 yr	30–86 mg/dl	32–99 mg/dl
6–11 yr	31–108 mg/dl	35–114 mg/dl
12–15 yr	36–138 mg/dl	41–138 mg/dl
16–19 yr	40–163 mg/dl	40–128 mg/dl

Triiodothyronine (T_3, T_3 total, T_3 RIA) (serum)

Newborn	72–260 ng/dl
1–5 yr	100–260 ng/dl
5–10 yr	90–240 ng/dl
10–15 yr	80–210 ng/dl
Thereafter	115–190 ng/dl

Urea nitrogen (serum or plasma)

Newborn	3–12 mg/dl
Infant or child	5–18 mg/dl
Thereafter	7–18 mg/dl

Urine volume (urine, 24 hr)

Newborn	50–300 mL/d
Infant	350–550 mL/d
Child	500–1000 mL/d
Adolescent	700–1400 mL/d
Thereafter: Male	800–1800 mL/d
Female	600–1600 mL/d (varies with intake and other factors)

Note: Normal lab values differ depending on lab used. Verify your facility's normal values.

Modified from *Nelson Textbook of Pediatrics* (18th ed.), by R. Kliegman, R. Behrman, H. Jenson, and B. Stanton. (2007). Philadelphia: W. B. Saunders; *A Manual of Laboratory and Diagnostic Tests* (8th ed.) by F. Fischbach. (2009). Philadelphia: Lippincott.

APPENDIX F
Temperature Equivalents and Pediatric Weight Conversion

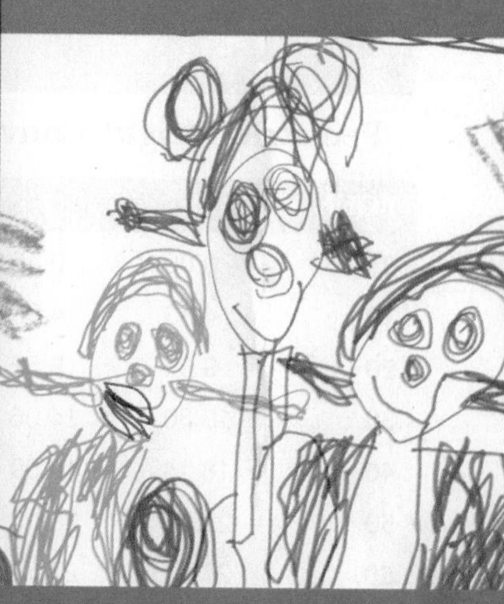

Celsius and Fahrenheit Temperature Equivalents

CELSIUS	FAHRENHEIT	CELSIUS	FAHRENHEIT
34.0	93.2	38.4	101.1
34.2	93.6	38.6	101.4
34.4	93.9	38.8	101.8
34.6	94.3	39.0	102.2
34.8	94.6	39.2	102.5
35.0	95.0	39.4	102.9
35.2	95.4	39.6	103.2
35.4	95.7	39.8	103.6
35.6	96.1	40.0	104.0
35.8	96.4	40.2	104.3
36.0	96.8	40.4	104.7
36.2	97.1	40.6	105.1
36.4	97.5	40.8	105.4
36.6	97.8	41.0	105.8
36.8	98.2	41.2	106.1
37.0	98.6	41.4	106.5
37.2	98.9	41.6	106.8
37.4	99.3	41.8	107.2
37.6	99.6	42.0	107.6
37.8	100.0	42.2	108.0
38.0	100.4	42.4	108.3
38.2	100.7	42.6	108.7
		42.8	109.0

Conversion formulas:

Fahrenheit to Celsius $(°F - 32) \times (\frac{5}{9}) = °C$

Celsius to Fahrenheit $(°C) \times (\frac{9}{5}) + 32 = °F$

Pediatric Weight Conversion (Pounds to Kilograms)

POUNDS	0	1	2	3	4	5	6	7	8	9
0	0.00	0.45	0.90	1.36	1.81	2.26	2.72	3.17	3.62	4.08
10	4.53	4.98	5.44	5.89	6.35	6.80	7.35	7.71	8.16	8.61
20	9.07	9.52	9.97	10.43	10.88	11.34	11.79	12.24	12.70	13.15
30	13.60	14.06	14.51	14.96	15.42	15.87	16.32	16.78	17.23	17.69
40	18.14	18.59	19.05	19.50	19.95	20.41	20.86	21.31	21.77	22.22
50	22.68	23.13	23.58	24.04	24.49	24.94	25.40	25.85	26.30	26.76
60	27.21	27.66	28.22	28.57	29.03	29.48	29.93	30.39	30.84	31.29
70	31.75	32.20	32.65	33.11	33.56	34.02	34.47	34.92	35.38	35.83
80	36.28	36.74	37.19	37.64	38.10	38.55	39.00	39.46	39.93	40.37
90	40.82	41.27	41.73	42.18	42.63	43.09	43.54	43.99	44.45	44.90
100	45.36	45.81	46.26	46.72	47.17	47.62	48.08	48.53	48.98	49.44
110	49.89	50.34	50.80	51.25	51.71	52.16	52.61	53.07	53.52	53.97
120	54.43	54.88	55.33	55.79	56.24	56.70	57.15	57.60	58.06	58.51
130	58.96	59.42	59.87	60.32	60.78	61.23	61.68	62.14	62.59	63.05
140	63.50	63.95	64.41	64.86	65.31	65.77	66.22	66.67	67.13	67.58
150	68.04	68.49	68.94	69.40	69.85	70.30	70.76	71.21	71.66	72.12
160	72.57	73.02	73.48	73.93	74.39	74.84	75.29	75.75	76.20	76.62
170	77.11	77.56	78.01	78.47	78.92	79.38	79.83	80.28	80.74	81.19
180	81.64	82.10	82.55	83.00	83.46	83.91	84.36	84.82	85.27	85.73
190	86.18	86.68	87.09	87.54	87.99	88.45	88.90	89.35	89.81	90.26
200	90.72	91.17	91.62	92.08	92.53	92.98	93.44	93.89	94.34	94.80

Example: To determine the kilogram equivalent of 43 pounds, read 40 pounds on the vertical scale, read 3 pounds on the horizontal scale, then add. 43 pounds equals 19.5 kilograms.

APPENDIX G Common NANDA Nursing Diagnoses for Children and Their Families

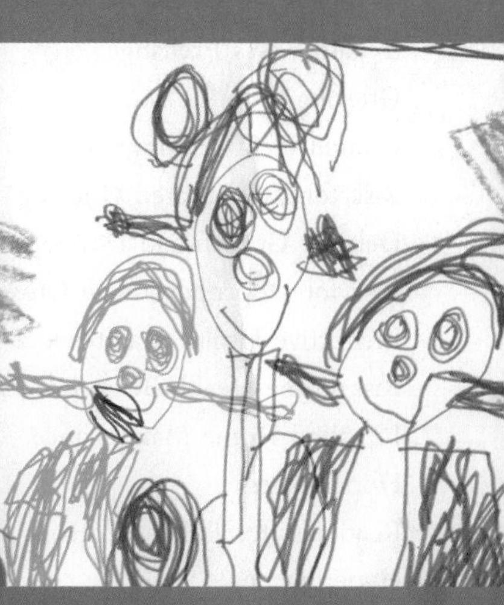

Activity Intolerance
Risk for **A**ctivity Intolerance
Ineffective **A**irway Clearance
Latex **A**llergy Response
Risk for Latex **A**llergy Response
Anxiety
Death **A**nxiety
Risk for **A**spiration
Risk for Impaired Parent, Infant, and Child **A**ttachment
Autonomic Dysreflexia
Risk for **A**utonomic Dysreflexia
Disturbed **B**ody Image
Risk for Imbalanced **B**ody Temperature
Bowel Incontinence
Effective **B**reastfeeding
Ineffective **B**reastfeeding
Interrupted **B**reastfeeding
Ineffective **B**reathing Pattern
Decreased **C**ardiac Output
Caregiver Role Strain
Risk for **C**aregiver Role Strain
Impaired Verbal **C**ommunication
Readiness for Enhanced **C**ommunication
Decisional **C**onflict (Specify)
Parental Role **C**onflict
Acute **C**onfusion
Chronic **C**onfusion
Constipation
Perceived **C**onstipation
Risk for **C**onstipation
Defensive **C**oping
Ineffective **C**oping
Readiness for Enhanced **C**oping
Ineffective Community **C**oping
Readiness for Enhanced Community **C**oping
Compromised Family **C**oping
Disabled Family **C**oping
Readiness for Enhanced Family **C**oping
Risk for Student Infant **D**eath Syndrome
Ineffective **D**enial
Impaired **D**entition
Risk for Delayed **D**evelopment
Diarrhea
Risk for **D**isuse Syndrome
Deficient **D**iversional Activity
Energy Balance
Disturbed **E**nergy Field
Impaired **E**nvironmental Interpretation Syndrome
Adult **F**ailure to Thrive
Risk for **F**alls
Dysfunctional **F**amily Processes
Interrupted **F**amily Processes
Readiness for Enhanced **F**amily Processes
Fatigue
Fear
Readiness for Enhanced **F**luid Balance
Deficient **F**luid Volume
Excess **F**luid Volume
Risk for Deficient **F**luid Volume
Risk for Imbalanced **F**luid Volume

Impaired **G**as Exchange
Grieving
Complicated **G**rieving
Risk for Complicated **G**rieving
Delayed **G**rowth and Development
Risk for Disproportionate **G**rowth
Ineffective **H**ealth Maintenance
Risk-Prone **H**ealth Behavior
Impaired **H**ome Maintenance
Hopelessness
Readiness for Enhanced **H**ope
Hyperthermia
Hypothermia
Disturbed Personal **I**dentity
Functional Urinary **I**ncontinence
Reflex Urinary **I**ncontinence
Stress Urinary **I**ncontinence
Total Urinary **I**ncontinence
Urge Urinary **I**ncontinence
Risk for Urge Urinary **I**ncontinence
Disorganized **I**nfant Behavior
Risk for Disorganized **I**nfant Behavior
Readiness for Enhanced Organized **I**nfant Behavior
Ineffective **I**nfant Feeding Pattern
Risk for **I**nfection
Risk for **I**njury
Risk for Perioperative-Positioning **I**njury
Decreased **I**ntracranial Adaptive Capacity
Deficient **K**nowledge
Readiness for Enhanced **K**nowledge (Specify)
Risk for **L**oneliness
Impaired **M**emory
Impaired Bed **M**obility
Impaired Physical **M**obility
Impaired Wheelchair **M**obility
Nausea
Unilateral **N**eglect
Noncompliance
Imbalanced **N**utrition: Less than Body Requirements
Imbalanced **N**utrition: More than Body Requirements
Readiness for Enhanced **N**utrition
Risk for Imbalanced **N**utrition: More than Body Requirements
Impaired **O**ral Mucous Membrane
Acute **P**ain
Chronic **P**ain
Readiness for Enhanced **P**arenting
Impaired **P**arenting
Risk for Impaired **P**arenting
Risk for **P**eripheral Neurovascular Dysfunction
Risk for **P**oisoning
Post-Trauma Syndrome
Risk for **P**ost-Trauma Syndrome
Powerlessness
Risk for **P**owerlessness
Ineffective **P**rotection
Rape-Trauma Syndrome
Rape-Trauma Syndrome: Compound Reaction
Rape-Trauma Syndrome: Silence Reaction
Impaired **R**eligiosity
Readiness for Enhanced **R**eligiosity
Risk for Impaired **R**eligiosity
Relocation Stress Syndrome
Risk for **R**elocation Stress Syndrome
Ineffective **R**ole Performance
Sedentary Lifestyle
Bathing **S**elf-Care Deficit
Dressing **S**elf-Care Deficit
Feeding **S**elf-Care Deficit
Toileting **S**elf-Care Deficit
Readiness for Enhanced **S**elf-Concept
Chronic Low **S**elf-Esteem
Situational Low **S**elf-Esteem
Risk for Situational Low **S**elf-Esteem
Self-Mutilation
Risk for **S**elf-Mutilation
Disturbed **S**ensory Perception (Specify: Visual, Auditory, Kinesthetic, Gustatory, Tactile, Olfactory)
Sexual Dysfunction
Ineffective **S**exuality Pattern
Impaired **S**kin Integrity
Risk for Impaired **S**kin Integrity
Sleep Deprivation
Disturbed **S**leep Pattern
Readiness for Enhanced **S**leep
Impaired **S**ocial Interaction
Social Isolation
Chronic **S**orrow
Spiritual Distress
Risk for **S**piritual Distress
Readiness for Enhanced **S**piritual Well-Being
Risk for **S**uffocation

Risk for **S**uicide
Delayed **S**urgical Recovery
Impaired **S**wallowing
Effective **T**herapeutic Regimen Management
Ineffective **T**herapeutic Regimen Management
Ineffective Community **T**herapeutic Regimen Management
Ineffective **T**hermoregulation
Disturbed **T**hought Processes
Impaired **T**issue Integrity
Ineffective Peripheral **T**issue Perfusion
Risk for Decreased Cardiac **T**issue Perfusion
Risk for Ineffective Cerebral **T**issue Perfusion
Impaired **T**ransfer Ability
Risk for **T**rauma
Impaired **U**rinary Elimination
Readiness for Enhanced **U**rinary Elimination
Urinary Retention
Impaired Spontaneous **V**entilation
Dysfunctional **V**entilatory Weaning Response
Risk for Other-Directed **V**iolence
Risk for Self-Directed **V**iolence
Impaired **W**alking
Wandering

APPENDIX H
Abbreviations

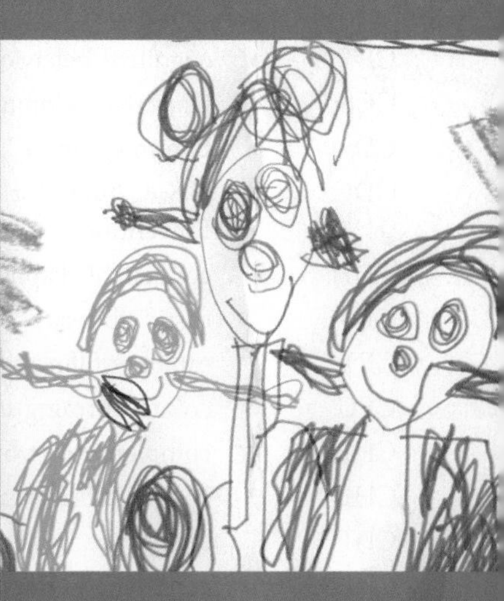

AA	Alcoholics Anonymous
AACAP	American Academy of Child and Adolescent Psychiatry
AAFP	American Academy of Family Physicians
AAMR	American Association of Mental Retardation
AAP	American Academy of Pediatrics
ABG	arterial blood gas
ACCH	Association for the Care of Children's Health
ACE	angiotensin-converting enzyme
ACHA	American College Health Association
ACIP	Advisory Committee on Immunization Practices
ACTH	adrenocorticotropic hormone
AD	atopic dermatitis
ADD	attention deficit disorder
ADH	antidiuretic hormone
ADHD	attention-deficit/hyperactivity disorder
ADL	activities of daily living
AFDC	Aid for Families with Dependent Children
AGA	appropriate for gestational age
AGN	acute glomerulonephritis
AGS	adolescent growth spurt
AHA	American Heart Association
AIDS	acquired immune deficiency syndrome
AN	anorexia nervosa
ANA	American Nurses Association
ANA	antinuclear antibody
AOM	acute otitis media
APA	American Psychiatric Association
APPT	Adolescent and Pediatric Pain Tool
APSGN	acute poststreptococcal glomerulonephritis
ARDS	acute (or adult) respiratory distress syndrome
ARF	acute renal failure
ARF	acute rheumatic fever
AS	aortic stenosis
ASD	atrial septal defect
ASHA	American School Health Association
ASHA	American Speech-Language-Hearing Association
ASL	American Sign Language
ASO	antistreptolysin O
ATG	antithymocyte antibodies
A-V or AV	atrioventricular, arteriovenous
AVC	atrioventricular canal
AZT	Zidovudine, also known as ZDV
BAER	Brainstem Auditory Evoked Response
BIA	Brain Injury Association
BID	twice a day (Latin *bis in die*)
BLL	blood lead level
BMI	body mass index
BMR	basal metabolic rate
BN	bulimia nervosa
BP	blood pressure
BPD	bronchopulmonary dysplasia
BRAT diet	bananas, rice, applesauce, and toast or tea
BSE	breast self-examination
BSL	British Sign Language
BT shunt	Blalock-Taussig shunt
BUN	blood urea nitrogen
CARS	Childhood Autism Rating Scale
CAV	continuous arteriovenous
CBC	complete blood cell count

CBT	cognitive behavioral therapy
CCSC	Children's Coping Strategies Checklist
CD	Crohn's disease
CDC	U.S. Centers for Disease Control and Prevention
CDH	congenital diaphragmatic hernia
CF	cystic fibrosis
CFT	capillary filling time
CFU	colony forming units
CHB	complete heart block
CHD	congenital heart defect
CHF	congestive heart failure
CI	confidence interval
CIC	clean intermittent catheterization
CK	creatine kinase
CL	cleft lip
CMS	U.S. Centers for Medicare & Medicaid Services
CMV	cytomegalovirus
CN	cranial nerve
CNS	central nervous system
CO	cardiac output
COA	coarctation of the aorta
CP	cerebral palsy
CP	cleft palate
CPB	cardiopulmonary bypass
CPS	Child Protective Service
CPT	chest physiotherapy
CRF	chronic renal failure
CRP	C-reactive protein
CSF	cerebrospinal fluid
CSHCN	Children with Special Health Care Needs (Title V program)
CT	computerized tomography
CVA	cerebral vascular accident
CVP	central venous pressure
CXR	chest radiograph
d4T	Stavudine, also known as Zerit
DASE	Denver Articulation Screening Examinations
dB	decibel
DD	dysthymic disorder
DDAVP	desmopressin acetate
ddC	Zalcitabine, also known as Hivid
DDH	developmental dysplasia of the hip
ddI	Didanosine, also known as Videx
DDST	Denver Developmental Screening Test
DEET	diethyltoluamide
DEST	Denver Eye Screening Test
DHHS	U.S. Department of Health and Human Services
DIC	disseminated intravascular coagulopathy
DIT	Defining Issues Test
dl	deciliter
DMD	Duchenne muscular dystrophy
DMG	dimethylglycine
DNA	deoxyribonucleic acid
DRG	diagnosis-related group
DS	Down syndrome
DSM-IV	*Diagnostic and Statistical Manual of Mental Disorders,* Fourth Edition
DTaP	diphtheria, tetanus toxoid, and acellular pertussis vaccine
DTP	diphtheria, tetanus toxoid, pertussis
DTwP	DT with whole-cell pertussis
DWI	driving while intoxicated
EA	esophageal atresia
EBV	Epstein-Barr virus
ECF	extracellular fluid
ECHO	echocardiogram
ECI	early childhood intervention
ED	emergency department
EIA	enzyme immunoassay
EKG	electrocardiogram
ELISA	enzyme linked immunosorbent assay
ELM	Early Language Milestone Scale
EMG	electromyogram
EMLA	eutectic mixture of local anesthetics
EMS	emergency medical service
EPA	U.S. Environmental Protection Agency
EPSDT	early and periodic screening, diagnosis, and treatment
ESR	erythrocyte sedimentation rate
ESRF	endstage renal failure
ESSR	"enlarge, stimulate, swallow, rest"
ET	enterostomal therapist
ETT	endotracheal tube
FA	Fanconi's anemia
FAS	fetal alcohol syndrome
FDA	U.S. Food and Drug Administration
FFT	failure to thrive
FSH	follicle-stimulating hormone
GABHS	group A beta-hemolytic streptococci
GAD	generalized anxiety disorder
GER	gastroesophageal reflux
GFR	glomerular filtration rate
GH	growth hormone

GHT	gentle human touch
GI	gastrointestinal
GPA	grade point average
HAART	highly active antiretroviral therapy
HAV	hepatitis A virus
Hb A	adult hemoglobin
Hb F	fetal hemoglobin
Hb S	sickle hemoglobin (hemoglobin S)
HBV	hepatitis B virus
HCFA	U.S. Health Care Financing Administration
HCG	human chorionic gonadotropin
HCl	hydrochloric acid
Hct	hematocrit
HCV	hepatitis C virus
HD	Hirschprung's disease
HDL	high-density lipoprotein
hep B	hepatitis B vaccine
H-flu	*Haemophilus influenzae*
HIB (Hib)	*Haemophilus influenzae* type B
HIV	human immunodeficiency virus
HLHS	hypoplastic left heart syndrome
HMO	health maintenance organization
HP	Healthy People [2010]
HPS	hypertrophic pyloric stenosis
HPV	human papilloma virus
HR	heart rate
HSV-1	herpes simplex virus type I
HUD	U.S. Department of Housing and Urban Development
HUS	hemolytic uremic syndrome
Hz	hertz
IBD	inflammatory bowel disease
ICF	intracellular fluid
ICU	intensive care unit
IDEA	Individuals with Disabilities Education Act
IE	infective endocarditis
IEP	Individualized Educational Plan
IFSP	Individual Family Service Plan
IgA	immunoglobulin A
IgD	immunoglobulin D
IgE	immunoglobulin E
IgG	immunoglobulin G
IgM	immunoglobulin M
IHP	Individual Health Plan
IM	intramuscular
IMR	infant mortality rate
INR	international normalized ratio
IPV	inactivated polio vaccine
IQ	intelligence quotient
IRB	institutional review board
ITP	immune thrombocytopenic purpura
IV	intravenous
IVIG	intravenous immune globulin
IVP	intravenous pyelogram
JA	juvenile arthritis
JCA	juvenile chronic arthritis
JRA	juvenile rheumatoid arthritis
KD	Kawasaki disease
KOH	potassium hydroxide
LA	left atrium
LBW	low birth weight
LGMD	Limb-Girdle muscular dystrophy
LCP	Legg-Calve-Perthes disease
LDL	low-density lipoprotein
LES	lower esophageal sphincter
LGA	large for gestational age
LH	luteinizing hormone
LIP	lymphoid interstitial pneumonia
LPD	lymphoproliferative disease
LSD	lysergic acid diethylamide
LTB	laryngotroacheobronchitis
LV	left ventricle
MCHC	mean corpuscular hemoglobin concentration
MCV	mean corpuscular volume
MD	muscular dystrophy
MDD	major depressive disorder
MDI	metered dose inhaler
MDMA	methylenedioxymethamphetamine
MHC	mean corpuscular hemoglobin
ml	milliliter
MMPI	Minnesota Multiphasic Personality Inventory
MMR	measles, mumps, rubella
MMWR	*Morbidity and Mortality Weekly Report*
MR	mental retardation
MRI	magnetic resonance imaging
NA	Narcotics Anonymous
NASN	National Association of School Nurses
NCPCA	National Committee to Prevent Child Abuse
NCV	nerve conduction velocity
NEC	necrotizing enterocolitis
NG	nasogastric
NHANES	National Health and Nutrition Examination Survey
NIAID	National Institute of Allergy and Infectious Disease

NICHCY	National Information Center for Children and Youth with Disabilities
NICU	neonatal intensive care unit
NIS-3	Third National Incidence Study of Child Abuse and Neglect
NJ	nasojejunal
NMDA	N-methyl-D-aspartate
NMPMC	nursing mutual participation model of care
NNRTI	non-nucleoside reverse transcriptase inhibitors
NOFTT	non-organic failure to thrive
NPA	National Pediculosis Association
NPO	nothing by mouth
NRTI	nucleoside reverse transcriptase inhibitor
NS	nephrotic syndrome
NS	normal saline
NSAIDs	nonsteroidal anti-inflammatory drugs
NVS	neurovascular status
OAE	otoacoustic emission test
OASPE	Office of the Assistant Secretary for Planning and Evaluation
OFFT	organic failure to thrive
OI	osteogenesis imperfecta
OM	otitis media
OME	otitis media with effusion
OPV	oral polio vaccine
ORS	oral rehydration solution
ORT	oral rehydration therapy
OSHA	U.S. Occupational Safety and Health Administration
PA	pulmonary artery
PCA	patient-controlled analgesia
PCC	Poison Control Center
PCR	polymerase chain reaction
PDA	patent ductus arteriosus
PERF	peak expiratory flow rate
PFO	patent foramen ovale
PGE	prostaglandin E
PHV	peak height velocity
PI	protease inhibitor
PICU	pediatric intensive care unit
PKU	phenylketonuria
PL	prolactin
PPD	purified protein derivative
PPI	parent-present induction
PPO	preferred provider organization
PQRST	mnemonic device for pain assessment format
PR	by rectum
prn (PRN)	as needed (pro re nata)
PS	pulmonary stenosis
PT	prothrombin time, also known as INR
PTSD	post-traumatic stress disorder
PTT	partial thromboplastin time
PVR	pulmonary vascular resistance
Q	every (quid)
QD	every day (quaque die)
RA	right atrium
RAPS	recurrent abdominal pain syndrome
RDI	recommended daily intake
RDS	respiratory distress syndrome
REM	rapid eye movement
RF	rheumatoid factor
RICE	rest, ice, compression, elevation
RL	Ringer's lactate
RLQ	right lower quadrant
ROP	retinopathy of prematurity
RR	respiratory rate
RSV	respiratory syncytial virus
RSV-IGIV	RSV immune globulin intravenous (RespiGam)
RV	right ventricle
SA	sinoatrial
SAARDs	slow-acting anti-rheumatic drugs
SAD	separation anxiety disorder
SaO_2	oxygen saturation
SBHC	school-based health center
SBS	shaken baby syndrome
SC	subcutaneous
SCA	sickle cell anemia
SCFE	slipped capital femoral epiphysis
SCHIP	State Children's Health Insurance Program
SCT	sickle cell trait
SEE	Signed Exact English
SGA	small for gestational age
SIDS	sudden infant death syndrome
SLE	systemic lupus erythematosus
SLHC	school-linked health center
SPF	sun protection factor
SSI	Supplemental Security Income
SSRI	selective serotonin reuptake inhibitor
STAIC	State-Trait Anxiety Inventory for Children
STD	sexually transmitted disease
STI	sexually transmitted infection
SUD	substance use disorder
SV	stroke volume
SVR	systemic vascular resistance
SVT	supraventricular tachycardia
TA	truncus arteriosus

TAC	tetracaine, adrenoline, cocaine
TB	tuberculosis
Td	tetanus and diphtheria
TEACCH	Treatment and Education of Autistic and Communication Handicapped Children
TEF	tracheoesophageal fistula
TEN	toxic epidermal necrolysis
TENS	transcutaneous electrical nerve stimulation
TGA	transposition of the great arteries
3TC	Lamivudine, also known as Epivir
TIBC	total iron binding capacity
TM	tympanic membrane
TOF	tetralogy of Fallot
TORCH	toxoplasmosis, other (e.g., hepatitis), rubella, cytomegalovirus, and herpes simplex
TPN	total parenteral nutrition
TSH	thyroid-stimulating hormone
UA	urinalysis
UAP	unlicensed assistive personnel
UC	ulcerative colitis
UDT	undescended testis, also known as cryptorchidism
UGI	upper gastrointestinal
URI	upper respiratory infection
Urine C&S	urine culture with sensitivity
UTI	urinary tract infection
UV	ultraviolet
UVA	ultraviolet A
UVB	ultraviolet B
VCUG	voiding cystourethrogram
VLBW	very low birth weight
VSD	ventricular septal defect
VUR	vesicoureteral reflux
vWF	von Willebrand's factor
WBC	white blood cell count
WIC	Women, Infants, and Children
WPPSI	Wechsler Preschool and Primary Scale of Intelligence
WPPSI-R	Wechsler Preschool and Primary Scale of Intelligence-Revised
ZDV	Zidovudine, also known as AZT
ZPD	zone of proximal development

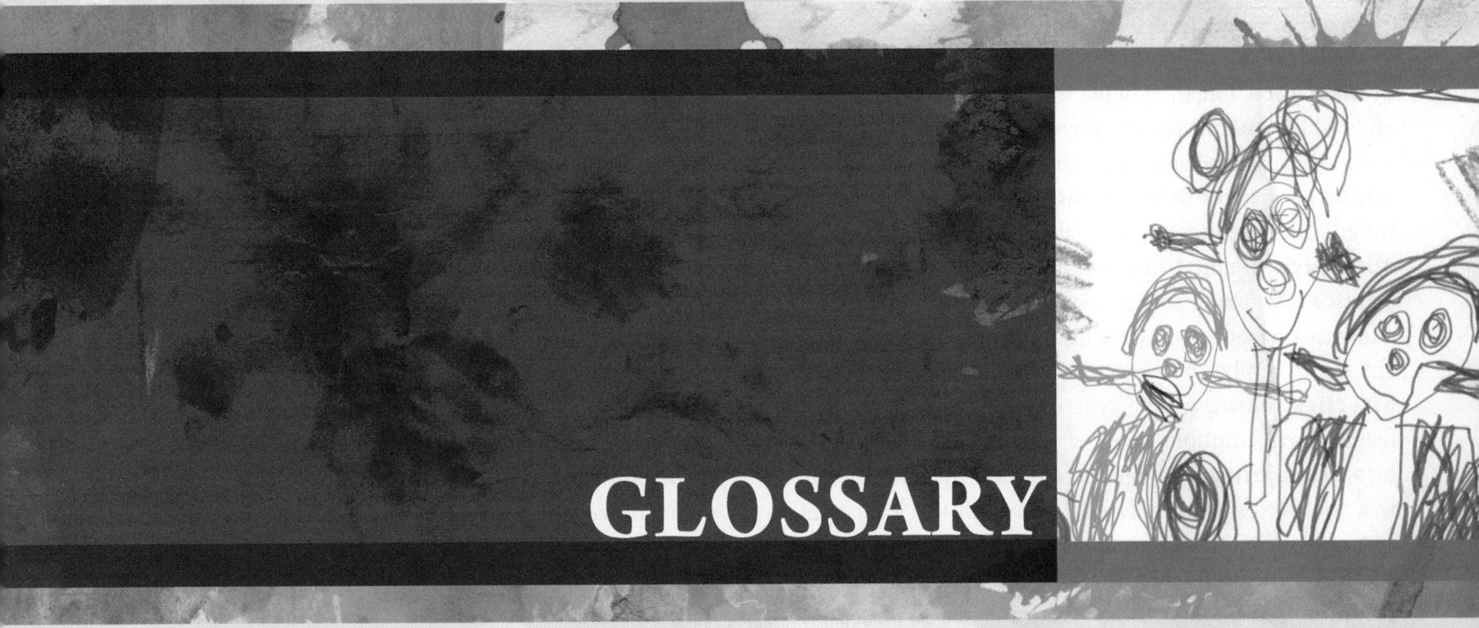

GLOSSARY

A

504 plan Refers to Section 504 of the Rehabilitation Act and the Americans with Disabilities Act which specifies that no one with a disability can be excluded from participating in federally funded programs or activities including elementary, secondary, or post secondary schooling.

ABC-X model of family stress Model that describes how families adjust to crisis.

absence seizures Characterized by a transient loss of consciousness that may appear as cessation of current activity; a type of generalized seizure.

absorption Process whereby a drug moves from site of administration into the bloodstream.

acceptance When the griever is consciously aware of what has happened or what is most likely to occur. Kubler-Ross's fifth stage of grief.

accessory muscles Muscles used to increase ventilation in individuals with labored breathing. Accessory muscles may include muscles in the neck, back, and abdomen.

accommodation Modification of behavior and mental structures as a result of new experiences; the process of modifying existing schema to adapt to or incorporate new experiences, Piagetian term; the ability of the eye to focus clearly on objects at all distances.

acidosis An acid-base imbalance indicated by a blood pH below 7.35.

acoustic feedback A whistling sound in a hearing aid caused by improper fit into the ear or too high a volume.

acquired immunity Specific immunity, triggered when a person has had a prior contact with a specific foreign agent.

acrocyanosis A condition characterized by blue discoloration, coldness, and sweating of the extremities, especially the hands.

acromion process The lateral extension of the spine of the scapula, forming the highest point of the shoulder and connecting with the clavicle at a small oval surface in the middle of the spine. It gives attachment to the deltoideus and trapezius muscles.

active euthanasia Giving a treatment that will directly and intentionally result in the death of a person.

active transport Movement of particles against a concentration gradient, a process requiring energy; the sodium-potassium pump is an example.

acute pain Pain generally lasting 3 to 5 days and attributed to a specific injury or cause.

adaptation Using resources, coping and problem solving strategies to manage stressor demands.

adaptation phase Stage of the resiliency model of family stress in which the family adjusts to the situation by making essential structural or systemic changes in functioning.

adjustment phase Stage of the resiliency model of family stress which reflects stress or crisis that is not a major hardship; the family makes only minor adjustments or changes in their established patterns.

adaptive immune system Produces a specific reaction to infectious agents, remembers that agent, and prevents a later infection by the same agent.

addiction Psychological and physiological need to use a medication for nonprescribed purposes.

A-delta nerve fibers Mylineated nerve fibers that fire rapidly.

adolescence The time of life that begins with puberty and ends when the individual is physically and psychologically mature and able to assume adult responsibilities.
adolescent growth spurt (AGS) Rapid acceleration in weight and height gain; lasts about 4.5 years.
adrenarche Pubic hair development.
advocate Nursing role involved in pleading causes for and assisting others in making informed decisions in the child and family's best interest.
affective learning One type of learning related to feelings and emotions.
age of majority The age, determined by state law, at which a person is considered to have all the legal rights and responsibilities of an adult.
AIDS A term used when the immune system has become compromised enough to allow advanced HIV disease to occur.
akinetic seizures Total lack of movement; child appears frozen in a position.
alkalosis An acid-base imbalance indicated by a blood pH above 7.45.
allergen Antigen responsible for clinical manifestations of allergy.
alopecia Hair loss.
alopecia areata The sudden onset of asymptomatic, noninflammatory, round bald patches. Traumatic alopecia, bald patches created by traction from braids, pony tails, corn rows.
amblyopia ("lazy eye") A reduction of vision in one eye. The most common cause is strabismus; the brain suppresses the vision in the deviated eye to avoid the double image that it is receiving.
amniocentesis The drawing out of a portion of amniotic fluid with a long aspirating needle for the purposes of direct examination, chemical testing, and cell culture.
anal stage Anal activities become primary ways of gratifying the sexual instinct; Freud's second stage of psychosexual development.
analgesia Pain control using medication or other interventions for relief.
anaphylaxis An acute, life-threatening reaction to an antigen.
anastomosis The surgical joining of two ducts, blood vessels, or bowel segments to allow flow from one to the other.
ancephaly Absence of cranial vault with cerebral hemispheres either completely missing or greatly reduced in size.
anemia Decrease in the hemoglobin content of the blood due to underlying disease or injury.
anencephaly Congenital absence of major portions of the brain and malformation of the brain stem.
anergy The inability to respond to infectious challenges.
anger Feeling of rage, envy, and resentment. Kubler-Ross's second stage of grief.
angioedema Swelling of the skin, subcutaneous, or submucosal tissue.
anhedonia Markedly diminished interest or pleasure in previously enjoyed activities.
animism Belief that inanimate objects have human qualities.
aniridia A congenital absence of the iris.
annular Ring shaped lesions with an erythematous, scaly border and central clearing.
anorexia nervosa A potentially life-threatening disorder characterized by voluntary refusal to eat and significant weight loss.
anthracycline Chemotherapeutic agent known to cause cardiac toxicity.
anthropometric measurements The science of measuring the human body as to height, weight, and size of component parts, including skinfolds, to study and compare the relative proportions under normal and abnormal conditions.
antigen A foreign substance capable of stimulating an immune response.
anuric Without urine output.
anxiety A subjective feeling of apprehension or uneasiness caused by uncertain, nonspecific danger or threat.
aplastic anemia A condition in which the bone marrow fails to produce adequate numbers of erythrocytes, leukocytes, and platelets because of injury to or abnormal expression of the stem cells.
aplastic crisis A type of sickle cell crisis characterized by a decrease in erythropoiesis.
apocrine glands Sweat glands concentrated in the axillae, scalp, face, abdomen, and genital area.
aqueduct of Sylvius Canal between the third and fourth ventricle through which CSF flows.
aqueductal stenosis Stenosis of the aqueduct of Silvius; a cause of hydrocephalus.
arachnoid mater The second meningeal membrane under which the cerebrospinal fluid flows.
Arnold-Chiari malformation (ACM) A brain defect in the posterior fossa that allows herniation of the cerebellum, medulla, pons, and fourth ventricle into the cervical spinal canal.
arrhythmia Abnormal heart rhythm, caused by electrical abnormalities of the heart.
art therapy Drawings and other art objects used to help the therapist gain information about the child, as well as her or his behaviors, concerns, and problems.
arteriovenous malformation A web-like tangle of vessels providing a network between the cerebral arteries and veins.

assault An unlawful, sudden, violent attack on another person; rape is considered a type of assault.
assent When a child is explained the process of a procedure or treatment and agrees to cooperate with it.
assimilation Incorporating new experiences into existing mental structures; Piagetian term.
astatic-akinetic seizures (see atonic seizures).
astigmatism Blurry vision caused by abnormal curvature of the cornea or the lens.
atelectasis Collapse of lung tissue.
atlantoaxial deformity A spinal deformity resulting in instability of the upper cervical spine (associated with Down syndrome).
atonic seizures Drop attacks; sudden loss of muscle tone with the head dropping forward for a few seconds.
atopy A heredity predisposition to develop allergic disease.
atraumatic care A philosophy of providing therapeutic care through the use of interventions that eliminate or minimize the psychological and physical distress experienced by children and families during hospitalization.
atresia Complete occlusion of or lack of normal opening in a body part.
atrial septostomy A procedure to enlarge the patent foramen ovale or to create an atrial septal defect. This allows mixing of blood at the atrial level.
attachment Reciprocal, enduring, emotional, and physical affiliation behaviors between a child and a caregiver.
attention-deficit hyperactive disorder (ADHD) The presence of impaired social interaction; impaired communication; and restricted repetitive and stereotyped patterns of behavior, interests, and activities.
aura A somatic, sensory, or psychic warning that a seizure will occur; premonition, usually lights or sounds, experienced prior to the onset of a migraine headache.
authority and social order maintaining orientation Laws should be obeyed because they are the laws; Kohlberg's fourth stage of moral development.
autism A genetic developmental disorder, characterized by extreme difficulty communicating with and relating to the environment; manifested by bizarre behavior, delayed language acquisition, poor social relations, impairment of self-care skills, and altered sensory responses.
autogenous Originating from within one's own body.
autoimmunity An inability of the body to distinguish self from nonself, causing the immune system to respond against itself.
autoinoculation Transfer of infection from one site to another on the same individual.
automatisms Repeated nonpurposeful actions such as lip smacking, chewing, sucking, or uttering the same word over and over.
autonomy The patient's ability to make his or her own decision, even if the nurse does not agree with that decision.
autonomy versus shame and doubt Psychosocial conflict where toddlers demonstrate independence and learn competencies related to self-care; Erikson's second stage of psychosocial development.
average for gestational age (AGA) Newborn lies between the 10th and 90th percentile of weight for gestational age.
avulsion The tearing away of tissue either accidentally or surgically.

B

B lymphocytes Lymphocytes produced in the bone marrow; differentiate into producers of one of five major classes of immunoglobulins.
Baby-Friendly Hospital Initiative (BFHI) An effort by the World Health Organization (WHO) and the United Nations Children's Fund (UNICEF) designed to help hospitals maximize their ability to help mothers breastfeed.
bacteremia Bacteria in the blood.
bacteriuria The presence of bacteria in the urine.
bad touch Any physical contact in which the child is told "not to tell anyone."
bargaining Attempt to postpone the occurrence of the event, by "making a deal." Kubler-Ross's third stage of grief.
barotrauma Physical injury sustained as a result of exposure to increased environmental air pressure.
behavioral perspective Posits that human actions and interactions come from learned responses to environmental stimuli.
behavioral therapy Behavioral modification that uses stimulus and response to alter inappropriate behaviors. Appropriate behavior is reinforced while inappropriate behavior is extinguished and replaced with a more desirable one.
beneficence Always doing the best for the patient.
bereavement The process of mourning; an adaptation to a loss. The behavior one exhibits after a loss.
beta-thalassemia major (Cooley's anemia) A type of thalassemia characterized by impaired beta hemoglobin synthesis that is associated with a life-threatening form of anemia.
bifid Split into two parts.
binocularity Fixation of two ocular images into one cerebral picture.
bioavailability The proportion or fraction of an administered drug that reaches general circulation and is available at site of action.
bioethics The application of ethics into the lives of individuals via the health care system.

biologic response modifiers (BRMs) Agents and therapies used to stimulate the body's immune system to destroy cancerous cells.
biotransformation (metabolism) Transformation or alteration of chemical structures from their original form.
blind Vision allows only light perception; other senses are relied upon as a chief means of learning.
blindisms Movements or behaviors that are repetitive and not purposeful, such as body rocking, eye rubbing, and head shaking. Used by blind children to compensate for inadequate stimulation.
body image A mental conception of one's physical appearance.
bonadaptation When families adapt well to crisis or stress, they are able to carry out their various functions (affective, health care, socialization) without compromising individual members; at the same time, they can also interact with the community appropriately.
bonadjustment Families adjust to stress or crisis by using their typical ways of functioning and make only minor changes.
bone age Calculation of skeletal maturation utilizing an X ray of the hand and wrist or knee.
bone marrow transplantation Replacement of hematopoietic stem cells into a person whose own bone marrow has been destroyed by disease or treatment for a malignant disease.
bottle-mouth caries (see nursing caries)
boundary workers Pediatric nurses practice across health care settings and are required to negotiate their responsibilities to children, families, members of the health care delivery team, and the institution in which they work.
bradyarrhythmia Abnormally slow heart rhythm.
brain stem Area of the brain that is below the cerebellum; controls the vital centers.
bronchiectasis A lung condition characterized by irreversible dilation and destruction of the bronchial walls.
brown fat Increases cellular metabolic rates and oxygen consumption, resulting in heat; found primarily in the subscapular, axillary, adrenal, and mediastinal regions.
Brudzinski's sign Sign of meningeal irritation; when child is supine, will automatically flex hips and knees if head is flexed forward.
buffer A substance that either releases or absorbs hydrogen ions in order to maintain a stable blood pH.
bulimia nervosa Characterized by episodes of binge eating followed by various methods of purging to control weight gain.
bullae Large blisters.
BUN The concentration of urea, an end-product of protein metabolism, formed in the liver and excreted by the kidney (as measured by blood urea nitrogen).
buphthalmos Enlargement of the eyeball.

C

callus Osseous material woven between the ends of a fractured bone that is ultimately replaced by new bone.
cancer Group of diseases in which there is out-of-control growth and malignant cells.
candidiasis Yeast infection caused by Candida species.
cao gao Practiced by Southeast Asians; involves rubbing a coin or a spoon heated in oil on an ill child's neck, spine, and ribs; may create a burn or abrasion.
caput succedaneum A localized pitting edema in the scalp of a fetus that may overlie sutures of the skull. It is usually formed during labor as a result of the circular pressure of the cervix on the fetal occiput.
carcinoma Cancer that originates from epithelial tissue that consists of cells from glands, hollow organs, and the outer layer of skin that lines the blood vessels.
cardiomegaly Enlarged heart.
cardiomyopathy Primary disease of the heart muscle caused by a multitude of etiologies (familial, infectious, ischemic) that results in poor pump function. There are three types: dilated, hypertrophic, and restrictive.
cardioversion A process whereby an abnormal heart rhythm is converted to normal sinus rhythm. This can be accomplished by electrical cardioversion via a defibrillator, or by medication.
carditis Inflammation of the heart.
caregiver Nursing role involved in delivering direct nursing care to children and their families that is based on the nursing process; also a parent, guardian, or other person responsible for the child.
caregiver burden The effect of the challenges and demands of caring for a child with a chronic condition.
care theory A major theoretical orientation that bases ethical decision making on the individual's needs or concerns.
carriers Persons who can harbor and spread the organism to others without becoming ill.
case management A practice model initially developed to minimize fragmentation of services and maximize individualization of care by using a systematic approach ensuring optimal client outcomes.
cataract Opacity (clouding) of the crystalline lens of the eye.
"catch-up" growth A rate of growth greater than the expected rate for age.
cat's eye reflex A whitish glow in the pupil, a sign of retinoblastoma.
causality The notion that death has an internal and external cause. These causes may be natural, unnatural, good or bad.

cavernous sinus thrombosis A syndrome caused by an infection of the eye that results in venous congestion of the eye and paralysis of the extraocular muscles.
ceiling dose Maximum dose of a medication thought to be effective; increasing the dose beyond this point will not increase the effectiveness.
cell mediated system T cells; they specifically recognize antigens and interact with the B cells and other components of the innate system to inactivate the immune challenge.
cellular elements The erythrocytes or red blood cells, the leukocytes or white blood cells, and the thrombocytes or platelets.
central hearing loss Damage that interrupts sound transmission between the brain stem and the cerebral cortex.
cephalhematoma Swelling caused by subcutaneous bleeding and accumulation of blood. It may begin to form in the scalp of a fetus during labor and enlarge slowly in the first few days after birth; subperiosteal bleeding over a cranial bone that is due to ruptured blood vessels from a traumatic delivery. The swelling does not cross suture lines.
cephalocaudal Principle that growth proceeds from the head downward.
cerebellum Found in the posterior fossa, controls motor coordination, posture, and equilibrium.
cerebral edema An increase in intracellular fluid in the brain.
cerebral palsy (CP) Nonprogressive motor dysfunction caused by damage in the motor areas of the brain.
cerebrum Largest area of the brain that controls thinking, speech, vision, and hearing.
channel The medium through which a message is transmitted; it may be visual, auditory, or kinesthetic.
chelating agent A drug used to either prevent or reverse the toxic effects of a heavy metal or to accelerate the elimination of the metal from the body.
child abandonment Caregiver's intentional withholding from a child, without just cause or excuse, the caregiver's care, presence, love, protection, maintenance, and opportunity for displaying affection for a child.
child abuse A range of intentional behaviors by a parent or caregiver that can include neglect, physical, emotional, or sexual abuse.
child life program An organized program conducted by child life staff in health care settings that are designed to promote optimum development of children and their families, to maintain normal living patterns, and to minimize psychological trauma. (Child Life Council. [1995]. *Child life position statement.* Rockville, MD: Author.)
child life staff Specialists with expertise in child growth and development who provide children with opportunities in gaining a sense of mastery, for play, for learning, for self-expression, for family involvement, and for peer interaction.
child maltreatment The intentional injury of a child.
child molestation Sexual involvement (oral-genital contact, genital fondling and viewing, masturbation) involving a child.
child neglect Caregiver inattention to the child's basic need for care, protection, or control, which results in the child experiencing serious injury or impairment.
chloromas Localized collections of malignant cells.
choanal atresia A congenital anomaly in which a bony or membraneous occlusion blocks the passageway between the nose and pharynx.
cholestasis Interruption in the flow of bile.
chordee Downward curvature of the penis.
chorea Abnormal uncontrollable, involuntary, purposeless movements of extremities and the trunk.
chorionic villus sampling A procedure for obtaining prenatal evaluation data in early pregnancy by withdrawing a chorionic villi sample from fetal membranes.
choroid plexus Area within the ventricle that secretes cerebrospinal fluid.
chronic (cyclic) sorrow Cyclical, never-ending grief response of caregivers of children with chronic conditions. Occurs at somewhat predictable times in the child's and family's life.
chronic condition A physical, psychological, or cognitive condition that places limitations on day-to-day functioning or requires reliance on special treatments and is expected to last for at least several months.
chronic pain Pain lasting for long periods of time or coming and going frequently over long periods of time.
Chvostek's sign Twitching of the facial muscles after gently tapping over the facial nerves near the parotid gland.
circumcision The surgical removal of the foreskin, the skin that covers the glans or head, of the penis.
classical conditioning Learning occurs when a response that is already part of the organism's normal activities can be reproduced by an associated stimulus that previously would not have produced it.
classification The ability to group items according to common characteristics.
clinical cure Resolution of signs and symptoms of infection.
clinical nurse specialist Usually a nurse with a master's degree who provides expert physical, social, and psychological support and care; consults with nursing staff and other health care personnel; educates clients and families in health care management; conducts practice outcome research; and serves as a role model for staff.
clinical pathways Plans of care designed to achieve specific client outcomes in a defined time frame.

clinical trials Carefully designed investigation of drug effects on human subjects.
cliques Three to nine "buddies" or "mates" who exhibit a strong sense of cohesion.
closed adoption An adoption where there is no contact between the birth and adoptive parents.
closed reduction The alignment of the bone by manual manipulation or traction.
C-nerve fibers Slow conducting, unmyelinated nerve fibers.
cognitive ability The capacity to understand and then use phenomena in the world around us.
cognitive behavioral therapy (CBT) Focuses on the interplay of maladaptive behavioral, emotional, and cognitive responses that characterize and perpetuate psychological disorders. CBT focuses on the modification of maladaptive patterns of thought, emotions, and behaviors.
cognitive learning One type of learning where describing or explaining something or answering questions occurs.
colic Recurrent episodes of unexplained crying and inability to be consoled occurring in infant less than 3 months of age.
collaborative Mutual sharing and working together to achieve common goals in such a way that all persons or groups are recognized and growth is enhanced.
collateral Extra vessels that are formed to supply blood if the normal vessels are stenotic or absent.
color blindess Color deficiency or color vision deficit.
coma The most severe form of depressed consciousness; no response to intense painful stimuli.
comedone Lesions associated with noninflammatory acne. Lesions may be closed (whiteheads) or open (blackheads).
communicable diseases Infectious illnesses that exhibit the potential to spread through the community.
communicating hydrocephalus Hydrocephalus caused by an obstruction outside the ventricular system leading to decreased absorption of cerebrospinal fluid in the subarachnoid space.
communication The process of creating common or shared meaning.
communitarianism The opposite of liberal individualism, focusing on communal values more than the rights and interests of the individual.
community acquired pneumonia (CAP) Pneumonia occurring in a previously healthy child with no underlying contributing disorder or disease, outside of the hospital setting.
community health nursing A synthesis of nursing and public health practice directed toward promoting, restoring, and preserving the health of a community or a total population.
compartment syndrome Condition caused by increased pressure within a compartment, leading to impairment of circulation.
compensation Body process used to restore blood pH to normal by changing the partial pressure of carbon dioxide (pCO_2) or the bicarbonic ion concentration.
complement Twenty different proteins that, when activated by an antigen-antibody contact, respond, amplify, and "complement" antibody activity.
complex partial seizures Partial psychomotor or temporal lobe episodes.
concrete operations The mental ability to group objects, actions, and events.
concrete operations stage Acquisition of logical operations and effective reasoning skills; Piaget's third stage of cognitive development; ages 7–11.
conductive hearing loss A temporary or permanent hearing deficit that occurs when something (such as fluid) affects the progress of sound into the ear canal or across the middle ear system.
confusion A form of depressed consciousness; although alert, disoriented to time, place, and person; unable to answer simple questions.
conjunctivitis ("pink eye") An inflammation of the conjunctiva.
conscious sedation Administration of central nervous system depressant drugs or analgesics which allows a child to be both pain-free and also sedated for a procedure.
conservation The ability to acknowledge that a change in shape does not mean a change in amount.
consolidation phase Second phase of leukemia therapy that aims at eradicating any residual leukemic cells.
contact burns Burns that are the result of certain implements such as curling irons, steam irons, cigarette lighters, matches, hot pots, space heaters, or radiators.
contact dermatitis Delayed hypersensitivity; occurs when an antigen is applied directly to the skin.
context specificity Suggests there are differences in children related to cultural values, beliefs, and experiences.
continuity Developmental change is orderly and built upon earlier experiences; a gradual and smooth process without abrupt shifts.
contusion An injury resulting in damage to soft tissues, subcutaneous structures, small vessels, and muscles without disrupting the skin.
conventional level According to Kohlberg's theory of moral development, the school-age child is at the conventional level of moral development. During this level the child's conscience develops an internal set of "rules" that must be followed in order to "be good."

conventional morality Societal values are internalized; moral judgments are based on a desire to uphold the law and social order or gain approval; Kohlberg's third level of moral development.

coordination of secondary schemes phase Infant understands concepts of space and object permanence, learns to direct actions toward an intended goal, and anticipates actions of others; Piaget's fourth phase of cognitive development.

cor pulmonale Right-sided heart failure caused by pulmonary disease.

corporal punishment Physical restraint or infliction of pain to the body by a person in authority.

crackles An adventitious lung sound caused when air passes over airway secretions or collapsed airways are suddenly opened.

cradle cap (seborrhea) A dry, scaly scalp condition.

cranioschisis Defect in the skull through which neural tissue protrudes.

craniosynostosis Premature ossification and closing of the sutures of the skull, often associated with other skeletal defects.

craniotabes Benign congenital thinness of the top and back of the skull of a newborn.

crawling Pulling self forward with abdomen on the floor.

creeping Moving on hands and knees with abdomen off floor.

cremasteric reflex A superficial neural reflex elicited by stroking the skin of the upper thigh in a male. This action results in a brisk retraction of the testis on the side of the stimulus.

crepitus Grating sound heard on movement of the ends of a broken bone.

cretinism Stunted physical growth and severe mental retardation caused by untreated thyroid deficiency.

critical orientation model A focus on environmental issues (physical and social) that tend to stigmatize and exclude individuals with chronic conditions.

critical period A limited time span when a child is biologically prepared to acquire certain behaviors, but needs the support of a suitably stimulating environment.

crowd An association of two to four cliques in which relations are less intimate than in the smaller groups.

cruising Walking sideways while holding onto furniture for support.

cryptorchidism A developmental defect characterized by failure of one or both of the testicles to descend into the scrotum. They are retained in the abdomen or inguinal canal.

crystalluria Crystals in the urine that may be a source of urinary irritation.

cultural relativism Differences in children are related to cultural values, beliefs, and experiences.

cultural sensitivity Having an awareness and appreciation of cultural influences in health care and being respectful of differences in cultural belief systems and values.

cupping (ventosos) Practiced by Latin American and Russian cultures; occurs by creating a vacuum under a cup or glass when a small amount of burning material is placed on the skin.

cystitis Inflammation of the bladder with symptoms including urinary frequency and dysuria, often accompanied by urgency and tenesmus.

cystogram Radiograph of the bladder that examines the bladder, urethra, and ureters.

cytokines Substances secreted by cells participating in the immune response.

cytoreduction Conditioning regimen for bone marrow transplant in which lethal doses of chemotherapy, often combined with radiation, are used to eradicate all malignant cells and to suppress the child's immune system to prevent rejection of the transplanted marrow.

cytotoxic or killer T lymphocytes Lymphocytes that attack infected or pathogenic cells.

D

dacrocystitis An infection of the lacrimal sac caused by obstruction of the nasolacrimal duct, characterized by tearing and discharge from the eye.

Dandy-Walker syndrome An obstruction in the foramina of Luschka and Magendie causing hydrocephalus.

date or acquaintance rape Sexual intercourse with force or threat of force where the victim and perpetrator know one another either socially or professionally.

dating scripts What is expected of dating partners.

debridement Removal of dead skin tissue from a burn site.

decerebrate Rigid extensor posturing secondary to trauma to the midbrain or pons; associated with poor prognosis.

deciduous teeth The first 20 teeth to develop and erupt in a child; also referred to as primary or baby teeth.

decontamination Decreasing absorption of an ingested poison from the GI tract.

decorticate Flexor posturing; associated with bilateral cerebral hemisphere injury.

deep partial-thickness burn Second degree burn which involves the epidermis and deeper dermis; sensation is usually diminished, and capillary refill is prolonged. Skin grafting is often needed for satisfactory healing.

deficit-orientation model Views of chronic conditions that depict them as pathological states with major negative consequences in most, if not all, aspects of life.

delayed hypersensitivity A cellular reaction involving T cells and macrophages; there is a longer duration between exposure and reaction.

delirium Condition where anxiety, fear, and agitation are seen.
denial Detachment; having lost hope for permanent reunion with caregiver. Third stage in adapting to hospitalization; when the grieving person does not accept the loss or believes it is true. Kubler-Ross's first stage of grief.
deontologic theory A major theoretical orientation focused on rules, obligation, and commitment.
depot injection An intramuscular injection of a medication that will be absorbed over a longer period of time.
depression A great sense of loss or sadness. Kubler-Ross's fourth stage of grief.
depressive disorder Disturbance in mood characterized by loss of interest or pleasure in normal activities.
dermatophytes Keratin-loving fungi that are parasitic upon the skin.
dermis The fibrous inner layer of skin just below the epidermis.
despair Withdrawal, refusal of food, diminished communication, and general loss of interest in the environment. Second stage in adapting to hospitalization.
desquamation Shedding of the outer layer of the epidermis.
devastating full-thickness burn Fourth degree burn which extends into the muscle, fascia, and bone; is lethal.
development Physiological, psychosocial, and cognitive changes occurring over one's life span due to growth, maturation, and learning.
developmental delay Achievement of developmental milestones later than expected.
dextrocardia The location of the heart in the right hemithorax, either as a result of displacement by disease or as a congenital defect.
diagnosis-related group (DRG) A classification system used to determine Medicare payments to hospitals and providers of medical services based on client diagnosis, procedures, age, and length of hospitalization.
dialysis Treatment that acts as a filtration system outside the body to rid the body of waste products.
diaphysis The shaft of the long bone.
diastasis recti The separation of the two rectus muscles along the median line of the abdominal wall.
differentiated practice A nursing practice model being implemented in some care settings, refers to a philosophy that delineates a nurse's role and functions according to experience, competence, and education.
diffusion The movement of a solute from an area of higher concentration to an area of lower concentration until an equilibrium is reached.
DiGeorge syndrome A congenital syndrome associated with hypoplasia or aplasia of the thymus and parathyroid gland; it is associated with congenital heart disease. There is lack of parathyroid with hypocalcemia, and deficits of cell-mediated immunity caused by hypoplasia of the thymus.
direct services Providing nursing care to individual clients.
disability A functional limitation that prevents or interferes with a person's ability to perform age-expected activities.
discontinuity Development is a series of discrete steps or stages that elevate the child to more advanced or higher levels of functioning with increased age.
dislocation A displacement of two bone ends or of a bone from its articulation with a joint.
disseminated intravascular coagulation (DIC) A coagulation disorder in which the stimulus for coagulation overwhelms the control mechanisms that normally confine coagulation to the area of bleeding.
distribution Process whereby a drug moves from blood to interstitial spaces of tissues and from there into cells.
diurnal cycle Sleeping through the night alternating with daytime wakefulness.
divorce decree Legal document approved by the court that grants divorce, divides marital property, and specifies child custody.
domestic mimicry One way of expressing an understanding of the differentiated sex-roles observed within the family or community. In imaginative play, the child enacts the role of "mommy," "daddy," and "baby."
double ABC-X model Model that explains the complexity of family life, situations, and accumulation of normative and non-normative events over time, that often cause families to be so stressed they are in crisis.
Down syndrome A congenital chromosomal disorder caused by an extra chromosome 21 characterized by varying degrees of mental retardation and a characteristic appearance.
downward comparisons Assuming another's situation is worse than one's own.
drowning Death from a submersion incident.
dry drowning Drowning secondary to hypoxemia resulting from intense laryngospasm; fluid has not entered the lungs.
ductus arteriosus Fetal connection between the aorta and pulmonary artery that closes shortly after birth.
ductus venosus A shunt in the fetus that carries oxygenated blood from the umbilical veins to the inferior vena cava.
dura mater The first meningeal membrane that adheres to the inner surface of the skull.
dysfluency Impaired rate, rhythm, or general flow of speech.

dyshormonogenesis Inborn error in the synthesis of a hormone.
dysmorphic Abnormal or unusual features, commonly associated with various genetic syndromes.
dyspnea Shortness of breath or difficulty in breathing.
dysuria Difficult or painful urination.

E

ecchymosis Black or blue discoloration of an area of skin caused by extravasation of blood into subcutaneous tissue as a result of trauma; bruise.
eccrine glands Sweat glands distributed across the body and responsible for thermoregulation.
echolalia Repeating the last word or words heard; sometimes initially mistaken for true speech.
ecological theory Bronfenbrenner's view suggesting developing individuals are embedded in a series of environmental systems.
ecomap A visual overview of the complex ecological system of a family, showing the family's organizational patterns and relationships.
ectasia Larger than normal.
ectoparasites Parasites living on the surface of the host's body.
educator Nursing role involved in providing information to clients, families, and staff as indicated and needed.
ego Freud's term for the rational component of the personality.
egocentrism Viewing the world only from one's own point of view. Cannot imagine that another may have a different perspective; when children and adolescents are unable to appropriately differentiate between themselves and the objects of their attention.
Electra complex Complex described by Freud where preschool female child has strong feelings of attraction for the caregiver of the opposite sex and thus feels that she must compete with the caregiver of the same sex.
electrolytes Charged particles that are found in body fluid. Most important body electrolytes are sodium (Na^+), potassium (K^+), calcium (Ca^{++}), and chloride (Cl^-).
electrophysiology Study and treatment of heart rate, rhythm, and electrical abnormalities.
elicitation phase Phase of a hypersensitivity reaction that occurs with reexposure to the antigen.
emancipation The legal recognition that a minor lives independently and is legally responsible for his or her own support and decision making.
emotional abuse (see psychological abuse)
empathy The ability to put one's self in the other person's shoes—to feel as well as to intellectually know what the other person is experiencing.
encephalitis Inflammation of the brain.
encephalocele Protrusion of the brain and meninges into a fluid-filled sac through a defect in the skull.
endocarditis Inflammation of the endocardial lining of the heart.
endocardium Serous inner membrane of the heart.
enterocolitis Inflammation of the small intestine and colon.
enucleation Surgical removal of the eye.
enuresis Urinary incontinence.
envenomation The poisonous effects caused by venom following a bite or sting such as that from a spider, insect, or snake.
epidermis The outermost layer of the skin.
epidural hematomas Space-occupying lesions in the brain usually secondary to rupture of the meningeal artery.
epilepsy A chronic seizure disorder often associated with central nervous system pathology.
epileptic seizures The presence of more than one unprovoked seizure that occurs at least 24 hours apart.
epileptogenic focus Area in the brain where seizures originate.
epiphora Excessive tearing.
epiphyseal growth plate Thin layer of cartilage located between the metaphysis and the epiphysis at the end of the long bones; controls long bone growth.
epiphysis The proximal and distal ends of the long bone.
epistaxis Nose bleed.
Epstein's pearls Small white pearl-like epithelial cysts that occur on both sides of the midline of the hard palate of a newborn.
equilibrium Harmonious relationships between thought processes (assimilation, accommodation, adaptation) and the environment; Piagetian term.
erythema marginatum Fine, pink rash.
erythema multiforme An erythematous, maculopapular, vesicular, urticarial rash; may include target lesions; 20% are caused by drugs.
erythema toxicum A transient newborn rash characterized by a red macular base with a white vesicular center.
erythematous Diffuse redness over the skin.
erythrocytosis Increase in red blood cell production in response to chronic hypoxemia.
erythropoiesis The production of red blood cells.
erythropoietin A hormone released by the kidneys that stimulates the bone marrow to produce red blood cells.
eschar Thick leather-like dead skin that forms as a result of a burn.
esotropia An inward turning of one eye relative to the other fixating eye.
esotropia (convergent) strabismus One or both eyes turn toward midline.

ethics The study of the nature and justification of principles that guide human behaviors and that are applied when moral problems arise.
ethnocentrism The tendency for all individuals and cultures to believe their values are the best and the most correct.
eutectic mixture of local anesthetics (EMLA) An anesthetic cream applied for one hour or more prior to procedures such as injections and venipunctures to minimize pain.
euthanasia Ending life by passive or active means.
euthyroid Normal thyroid hormone levels.
evulsed tooth Tooth that has been knocked out or removed from socket.
exancephaly Malformation where the brain is totally exposed or herniated through a defect in the skull.
excretion Process whereby a drug or its metabolites move from the tissues back into the circulation and then to the organs of elimination.
exhibitionism Exposing one's genitals to strangers.
exophthalmos Bulging of the eyeballs.
exosystem Bronfenbrenner's term for settings influencing individuals even though not experienced directly.
exotropia A visual disorder in which the deviating eye looks outward. The eye often is blind or has defective vision.
exotropia (divergent) strabismus One or both eyes turn away from midline.
exploitation A category of sexual abuse that involves prostitution and child pornography.
expressive language The ability to use gestures, words, and written symbols to communicate with others.
extensor surfaces Surfaces of an extremity that do not come into contact when the extremity is flexed.
extracellular fluid (ECF) Body fluid that is outside the cells and includes interstitial, intravascular, and lymphatic fluid; ECF contains large amounts of sodium, chloride, and bicarbonate.
extramedullary Outside the bone marrow.
extravasate The leaking out of the vein of a drug that is being administered.
exudate Fluids, cells, or other substances released from body.

F

family Two or more persons who are joined by bonds of sharing and emotional closeness and who identify themselves as members of the family.
family as client The family considered as a set of interacting parts; assessment of the dynamics among these parts renders the whole family the client.
family as context The family considered as the context within which individuals are assessed; emphasis is placed primarily on the individual, keeping in mind that she or he is part of a larger system.
family assessment The process of collecting data about the family structure; relationships, and interactions among individual members.
family-centered care A philosophy of care that recognizes the centrality of the family in the child's life and inclusion of the family's contribution and involvement in the plan for and the delivery of care.
family developmental theory A theory used to understand families that suggests families are social groups influenced by developmental processes. The theory is based on the premise that families evolve through predictable developmental stages, and experience growth and development in much the same way as individuals.
family therapy The therapist looks at the child's symptoms or problems as a reflection of the family's problems. Family therapy may include the child, the primary caregivers, siblings, and other people from the extended family, for example, grandparents, ex-partners, and step siblings.
Family Stress Theory A family theory that examines how families deal with normative and/or nonnormative stress.
Family Systems Theory A theory which views the family as a system where all family members interact interdependently with one another. The theory emphasizes family elements and the processes existing within and between families and their various environments.
Fanconi's anemia The inherited form of aplastic anemia in which the bone marrow fails to produce adequate numbers of erythrocytes, leukocytes, and platelets.
fantasy stage (of career development) Adolescents choose careers they are most impassioned about.
febrile seizures A type of tonic-clonic seizure usually associated with rapid rise in temperature that reaches a minimum of 39° centigrade (102.2° Fahrenheit).
fecalith A hard, impacted mass of feces in the colon.
feedback Information from the receiver about the message sent.
ferritin A stored form of iron.
fibrin The end result of the coagulation cascade and the primary protein from which clots are formed.
fibrosis The repair and replacement of injured or infected tissue with scar tissue.
fidelity Keeping one's promise or word.
filtration Movement of a solute based on the force exerted by the weight of the solution.
first-pass-effect Effect of biotransformation of a drug by the liver before reaching systemic circulation.

flaccid areflexia Absence of response; an indication of severe brain stem injury.
flexion burns Occur when caregivers purposefully immerse a child in hot liquids and the body part immersed is held in a flexed position so that a "zebra" pattern occurs.
flexural surfaces Surfaces of an extremity that come into direct contact when the extremity is flexed.
fomites Inanimate objects on which disease-causing organisms may be conveyed.
Fontan One of three staged palliative procedures for patients with single ventricle physiology. Goal of procedure is to connect inferior vena caval blood to the pulmonary artery.
fontanels Soft spots found at junctions of suture lines of skull bones; allow for adaptation to the pelvis shape during delivery and growth of the brain over the coming year.
foramen ovale Normal in utero communication between the right and left atrium that normally closes after birth. A patent foramen ovale is one that has not closed.
foreclosed Individuals who demonstrate a strong sense of commitment, but have not experienced a crisis or exploratory period to establish commitment.
formal communication Organized communication with a particular agenda.
formal operations stage Piaget's fourth and final stage of cognitive development; individuals from 11–12 and up begin thinking systematically and rationally about hypothetical events and abstract concepts.
fragile X syndrome A chromosomally caused syndrome that includes mental retardation, unusual behaviors, and a characteristic appearance.
friendship dyad The most fundamental peer relation, and the one most likely to be based on similar interests and emotional support.
full-thickness burn Third degree burn which involves the epidermis and the entire dermis and can extend into the subcutaneous tissue; may appear white, black, or brown.

G

gastric residuals Feeding retained in stomach following tube feeding.
gate control theory of pain Theory which explains how pain impulses travel and are interpreted in the body.
gender identity The way we think about ourselves as either male or female; a culmination of biological make-up, personal experiences, social expectations, and recommendations about how males and females should think and behave.
generalized seizures Tonic-clonic movements arising from both cerebral hemispheres; usually no aura, but always loss of consciousness.
genital stage Freud's fifth stage of psychosexual development (puberty and onward); sexual desires reemerge, but are more appropriately directed toward opposite-sex peers.
genogram A graph outlining a family's history over a period of time, usually over three generations.
Glenn shunt A prodecure where the superior vena cava (SVC), which normally carries unoxygenated blood back to the right atrium (RA), is disconnected from the RA and sutured directly to the right pulmonary artery.
glial cells Cells that provide the supporting structure of the brain.
glomerular filtration rate (GFR) The amount of fluid that is filtered by the glomeruli (a semi-permeable membrane).
gluconeogenesis Formation of glucose in the liver from fat and protein.
glycogenolysis Formation of glucose from glycogen.
goiter Enlargement of the thyroid gland.
goniotomy A surgical procedure for glaucoma. A linear incision is made into the trabecular meshwork to increase drainage of the aqueous humor from the anterior chamber of the eye, therefore controlling intraocular pressure.
good touch Any physical contact that helps the child in getting clean or taking care of bruises or abrasions and is done by the parent or a caregiver approved by the parent.
grief An individual's response to a loss. Thoughts and feelings associated with a loss.
group therapy Involves a group of children, usually 6 to 10, with a focus on interpersonal relationships. Socialization process occurs among group members whereby feedback and support come from peers rather than from the therapist alone.
growth A physiological increase in size through cell multiplication or differentiation.
grunting A sound produced by the premature closure of the glottis during early expiration. Grunting increases airway pressure and preserves or increases the functional residual volume.
guarding A rigid contraction of the abdominal wall muscles. It usually occurs as an involuntary reaction to pain such as when an examiner attempts to palpate inflamed areas or organs in the abdominal cavity.

H

habituation The ability to decrease responses to disturbing stimuli.
half-life Time required for 50% of a drug to be excreted from the body.
hand-foot syndrome A type of vaso-occlusive crisis in the bone marrow of the hands and feet that causes severe pain.

handicap A barrier imposed by society, the environment, or one's self in response to perceived differences.
health-orientation model View of chronic conditions that depicts them as a common variation in life and focuses on an individual's strengths.
health promotion Activities or interventions that identify risk factors related to disease; the lifestyle changes related to disease prevention; the process of enabling individuals and communities to increase control over and improve their health; these activities or strategies are directed toward developing the resources of clients to maintain or enhance their physical, social, emotional, or spiritual well-being.
health protection Activities designed to maintain the current level of health, actively prevent disease, detect disease early, thwart disease processes, or maintain functioning within constraints of disease.
hearing impairment Impairment in processing linguistic information through hearing, with or without amplification.
heave A lifting of the cardiac area secondary to an increased workload and force of the left ventricular contraction.
helper T cells Cells that stimulate B lymphocytes to divide and mature into plasma cells.
hemarthrosis A condition wherein bleeding occurs in the joints, causing pain and limited movement.
hematemesis Vomiting of blood.
hematogenous Originating or transported in the blood.
hematomas Pockets of blood under the skin that result from excessive bleeding into the space following trauma.
hematuria Presence of blood in the urine.
hemihypertrophy A relative increase in size of one half of the body as compared to the other.
hemisensory Loss or decrease of function of a sense organ on one side of the body.
hemodialysis A hemofiltration system that occurs outside the body. It requires an arteriovenous fistula or shunt placed in a large vessel.
hemofiltration A continuous form of dialysis by means of an arteriovenous or venovenous shunt. These shunts, like hemodialysis, require an extracorporeal circuit through which the blood flows into a filter system.
hemoglobin (Hb) A protein within red blood cells that enhances the cells' ability to transport oxygen to the tissues.
hemoglobin S (Hb S) An abnormal form of hemoglobin that undergoes sickling.
hemolysis The destruction of red blood cells.
hemophilia A The most common type of hemophilia, caused by a deficiency of factor VIII.
hemophilia B (Christmas disease) A type of hemophilia caused by a deficiency of factor IX (Christmas factor).
hemophilia C A type of hemophilia caused by a deficiency of factor XI.
hemophilias A group of bleeding disorders in which a factor in the first phase of coagulation is deficient.
hemoptysis Coughing up blood from the respiratory tract.
hemorrhagic cystitis An abnormal bleeding of the bladder.
hemosiderin An iron-rich pigment that is a product of red cell hemolysis. Iron is often stored in this form.
hemosiderosis A buildup of excess iron in the body, eventually causing organ failure and death.
hemostasis The control of bleeding in order to maintain blood volume, pressure, and flow through injured vessels.
hepatomegaly Liver enlargement.
herd immunity Reduction of the number of persons susceptible to a communicable disease by immunization, preventing the spread of disease in epidemic proportions.
highly active antiretroviral therapy (HAART) Antiretroviral drugs, such as zidovudine and epivir, used to treat HIV or AIDS; administered during pregnancy and delivery or during the neonatal period.
hirsutism Excessive body hair in a masculine distribution pattern.
HIV disease An illness continuum, from asymptomatic to death, with an acquired immunodeficiency syndrome (AIDS) diagnosis usually occurring in the latter part of the continuum.
HIV infection A multisystem disease known primarily for its effects on the immune system.
homeostasis Dynamic equilibrium of the body that is maintained by dynamic processes of feedback and regulation.
hormone A chemical substance produced by an endocrine gland that is secreted into the bloodstream and produces a specific effect on a target organ.
humoral system Consists of B lymphocytes.
hydrocele A collection of fluid between the parietal and visceral layers of the tunica vaginalis.
hydrocephalus An enlargement of the head without enlargement of the facial structures, due to an accumulation of CSF in the ventricles of the brain.
hydrolyze To cause a substance to break down into its component parts by adding water.
hydronephrosis Distension of the kidney caused by urine accumulating in the renal pelvis secondary to outflow obstruction.
hydrostatic pressure Pressure of blood against the capillary walls generated by the contraction of the heart; hydrostatic pressure within the capillary bed pushes fluid across capillary membranes into the interstitial space and is balanced by osmotic pressure.
hypercapnia An excess of carbon dioxide in the blood.

hypercyanotic spells Spells commonly associated with tetralogy of Fallot, precipitated by agitation; result in extreme cyanosis and distress.
hyperopia (farsightedness) Improper focusing of light on the retina; difficulty with near vision.
hyperplasia Abnormal proliferation of normal cells.
hyperpnea Deep, rapid respirations.
hypertonic dehydration State in which the water loss is greater than the sodium loss.
hypertonic fluid Fluid that is more concentrated (higher osmolality) than normal body fluid.
hypertrophy An increase in the size of a cell or a group of cells resulting in an increase in the size of an organ.
hypertropia Occurs when the eyes are out of vertical alignment.
hyphema A hemorrhage into the anterior chamber of the eye.
hypoalbuminemia Low levels of albumin in the blood.
hypoplastic Underdeveloped or incompletely developed organ or tissue.
hypotonic dehydration State in which the sodium loss is greater than the water loss.
hypotonic fluid Fluid that is less concentrated (lower osmolality) than normal body fluid.

I

iatrogenic A condition caused by treatment or diagnostic procedures.
id Freudian term for the inborn element of personality driven by selfish urges or instincts.
identity Adolescents' definition of who they are based on their cumulative understanding of their inherent motivations, personal belief systems, and previous experiences.
identity achievement Individuals who have experienced a crisis period and have achieved a sense of commitment to their resulting decisions.
identity diffusion Individuals who have not experienced an identity crisis or made a commitment to any ideologic or occupational direction.
identity versus role confusion Fifth stage of Erikson's psychosocial development whereby adolescents need to form a coherent self-definition or otherwise remain confused about life directions.
idiosyncratic Peculiar to an individual.
imaginary audience Adolescents' exaggerated sense that they are always on stage, the focus of others' attention.
immediate hypersensitivity A reaction to an antigen; has a short duration between exposure and reaction.
immersion burns Burns that are found on the arms, buttocks, or genitals that are sharply demarcated or circumferential due to either an accidental fall in hot bath water or from the child being held in hot water.
immune system Spleen, lymph nodes, lymphoid tissue, white blood cells, phagocytes; natural killer cells; skin, mucus secretions, cilia, sebaceous gland secretions, stomach acid, normal intestinal flora that protect the human from disease.
immune thrombocytopenic purpura (ITP) An autoimmune disorder characterized by low platelet counts and exaggerated bleeding.
immunity Processes used by the body to protect against harmful organisms.
immunoglobulins Chemicals that "tag" or identify an antigen or pathogen for destruction by other immune cells.
immunosuppression The reduction or prevention of the normally occurring reaction by the immune system to respond to antigenic stimuli.
immunotherapy The use of synthetic or natural elements to stimulate or suppress the body's immune response.
incarceration Strangulation of a portion of the bowel leading to circulation impairment and tissue necrosis.
incest Sexual intercourse between closely related persons.
indirect services Consulting with school and district to deliver services to meet a child's health needs.
individual health plan (IHP) A document, based on the health assessment of a child, that outlines special health needs, goals, and strategies necessary to improve and maintain the health of the child and allow full participation in school experiences.
individual therapy The focus is on the child's individual behavioral, developmental, and psychological issues and problems. The age, developmental level, and psychosocial alteration of the child determine the therapeutic interventions used.
individual education plan (IEP) A written plan, spelling out the type and duration of services needed for a particular child.
induction The initial phase of chemotherapy used to reduce the tumor burden to an undetectable level.
industry The ability to be useful and productive.
industry versus inferiority Erikson's fourth stage of psychosocial development whereby school-age children learn to master important social and cognitive skills or otherwise feel incompetent.
infant mortality rate The number of infant deaths during the first year of life per 1,000 live births.
Infantile glaucoma A defective development of the trabecular meshwork which does not allow a sufficient amount of aqueous humor to drain out of the intraocular space; if untreated, can lead to ischemia and necrosis of the optic disc, which may cause blindness
infantile spasms A type of seizure in which the head may suddenly drop forward while both arms and legs are

flexed; eyes may roll upward or downward; infant may cry out and turn pale, cyanotic, or flushed.

infectious disease One that can be transmitted from one person to another or from animal to human by either direct or indirect contact.

inflammation The protective response of body tissues to irritation or injury characterized by redness, heat, swelling, pain, and loss of function.

informal communication When communication has no particular agenda or protocol.

informed consent The duty of a health care provider to discuss the risk and benefits of a treatment or procedure with a client prior to giving care.

infratentorial In the posterior third of the brain, primarily in the cerebellum and brain stem and below the tentorium.

initiative versus guilt Erikson's third stage of psychosocial development whereby preschool-age children learn to initiate new activities or otherwise become self-critical.

injury Damage or harm to an individual resulting in destruction of health, disability, or death.

innate immune system The first line of defense against infections; includes biochemical and physical barriers.

innate immunity Physical barriers such as skin, mucous membranes, and cough reflex.

innate purity Doctrine that suggests children are inherently good and born without an intuitive sense of right and wrong.

inotropes Medications that increase the force of muscular contractions.

instrumental realistic orientation stage Rules are obeyed to gain rewards or satisfy personal objectives; Kohlberg's second stage of moral development.

insufflation Act of blowing air into a cavity.

intelligence quotient The individual's functional age on the intelligence test divided by the chronologic age and multiplied by 100.

interferons Chemicals that inhibit replication of many viruses; have anti-tumor effects; host specific rather than antigen specific; secreted by infected cells.

interleukins Chemical mediators or messengers; also termed cytokines.

interpersonal concordance orientation Behavior and decisions are evaluated on the basis of one's intent and concerns about others' reactions; Kohlberg's third stage of moral development.

interpersonal theory Sullivan's view suggesting self-concept development, the key to personality development, is impacted by the home environment.

interstitial fluid The portion of extracellular fluid that is between the cells and outside the blood and lymphatic vessels.

intertriginous Skin surfaces that are apposing or form folds such as the interdigital, axillary, cubital, popliteal, and inguinal areas.

intertrigo An erythematous skin eruption occurring on apposed skin surfaces.

intracellular fluid (ICF) Body fluid that is located inside the cells; ICF contains large amounts of potassium, phosphate, sulfate, and proteins.

intracranial pressure (ICP) The force exerted by the brain, blood, and cerebrospinal fluid within the cranial vault.

intrathecal Administration of medication directly into the spinal canal for diffusion throughout the spinal fluid.

intravascular fluid The portion of extracellular fluid that is in the blood vessels.

intravenous pyelogram (IVP) Radiographic examination of the entire urinary tract; also called excretory urography.

intuitive phase Characterized by sophisticated language, decreasing egocentrism, incessant questioning, reality-based play; Piaget's eighth phase of cognitive development.

iron deficiency anemia An anemia caused by insufficient amounts of iron for adequate hemoglobin synthesis.

irreversibility Knowledge that death is permanent.

isotonic dehydration State in which the loss of sodium and water are equal.

isotonic fluid Fluid that has the same concentration (osmolality) as normal body fluid.

J

Jacksonian seizures Motor episodes beginning with tonic contractions of either the fingers of one hand, toes of one foot, or one side of the face, which then progress into tonic-clonic movements that "march" up adjacent muscles of the affected extremity or side of the body.

jaundice The yellowish discoloration of the skin and eyes caused by excess bilirubin.

justice Making sure that all clients are cared for in the same manner regardless of their culture, religious faith, ethnicity, or socioeconomic status.

juvenile arthritis (JA); juvenile chronic arthritis (JCA); juvenile rheumatoid arthritis (JRA) Terms used for an inflammatory autoimmune disease causing many forms of arthritis in children.

K

karyotyping Identification of the chromosomes' appearance, performed by growing cells from a blood or tissue sample, staining them during the metaphase stage of replication, and scanning them with a microscope.

kernicturus A form of icterus neonatorum in which nuclear masses of the brain and spinal cord undergo pathologic changes accompanied by deposition of bile pigments within them.
Kernig's sign Sign of meningeal irritation; child resists attempts to extend flexed leg or complains of pain on extension.
ketogenic diet A diet used to treat absence, akinetic, and myoclonic seizures that severely limits the intake of proteins and carbohydrates, thereby forcing the body to use fats for fuel resulting in the creation of ketones.
killer T lymphocytes (see cytotoxic T lymphocytes)
kismaul respiration Abnormally slow, deep respiration characteristic of air hunger in acidotic states.
kyphosis An abnormal thoracic curvature of the spine.

L

language The meaningful use of words, phrases, and gestures to transmit meaning from one person to another.
lanugo hair Very fine hair present in utero and shed before or at birth.
large for gestational age (LGA) An infant at greater than the 90th percentile of weight for gestational age, or >4,000 grams.
latchkey children Children who are home alone after school for a period of time without adult supervision.
latency stage Freud's fourth stage of psychosexual development; sexual drives are submerged, appropriate gender roles are adopted, the Oedipal or Electra conflict is resolved.
liberal individualism Focuses on protecting basic human rights and interests of individuals but may neglect the rights of the community.
libido Freudian term for psychic energy of basic biological instincts.
lichenification Thickening and hardening of the skin with exaggeration of its normal markings.
limit setting The caregiver defines boundaries and expectations for the toddler by words, pictures, or role modeling. Setting boundaries requires consistency on the part of the caregiver in adhering to the limits set and following through on delivering consequences when the toddler exceeds the limits.
limited vision Visual defects which are correctable with lenses or surgery so child functions as a normally sighted person.
lipoatrophy Indentation or atrophy of subcutaneous fat.
lipohypertrophy Lumpiness or hypertrophy of subcutaneous fat.
lipolysis The hydrolysis of fat.
listening Providing verbal and nonverbal clues that communicate interest.
locomotion The ability to move from place to place without assistance.
lordosis Exaggerated curve of the lumbar spine, normal during the toddler years.
low birth weight Weight of less than 2,500 grams—or 5 pounds, 8 ounces—at birth.
lymphadenopathy Enlargement of the lymph nodes.
lymphatic fluid Thin, watery fluid originating in organs and tissues of the body that circulates throughout the lymphatic vessels and is filtered by the lymph nodes; comprised of chyle (emulsified fats from digestion), erythrocytes (red blood cells), and leukocytes (white blood cells); primary function is delivering these components into the vascular system.
lymphangitis Red streaks leading from the affected area to adjacent lympth nodes.
lymphoblasts Immature white cells, which when malignant are the leukemia cells that crowd out normal red cells, white cells, and platelets.
lymphokine A substance that prevents or contains the migration of antigens.

M

Macewen's sign A hollow or "cracked-pot" sound heard when percussing the head of a child with hydrocephalus.
macrosystem Bronfenbrenner's term for the larger cultural or subcultural context of development.
macules Small flat lesions.
maculopapular rashes The most common form of cutaneous reactions to an antigen; symmetric, characterized by macules or papules.
mainstreaming The placement of children with disabilities in a classroom with children without disabilities.
maintenance therapy Phase of chemotherapy that follows consolidation in order to destroy residual cancer cells.
maladaptation When families have difficulty adapting to stress or crisis, they may move back into a crisis situation.
maladjustment When faced with stress or crisis, the family moves into a crisis situation because minor changes do not adequately manage the stress or crisis.
maldistribution Abnormal distribution.
malignant brain edema (cerebral hyperemia) Unique to children; a hyperemic or vascular reaction to head trauma because of the disruption in the blood-brain barrier; the mechanism to control cerebrospinal fluid absorption also is impaired.
malocclusion An abnormality in the coming together of teeth, leaving the teeth uneven or crowded.
malpractice Professional negligence.
managed care A vehicle for cost-effective delivery of health care services.

manager or leader Nursing role involved in being responsible for a group of clients or a group of staff.
mandated reporters Individuals who are required to report to appropriate authorities suspicions of child abuse or neglect.
marginality A situation in which a condition is less visible to others resulting in ambiguity about whether an individual is different from or like others. This results at times in inappropriate expectations.
matching hypothesis Selection of a dating partner based on attractiveness.
maturation Changes that are due to genetic inheritance rather than life experiences, illness, or injury.
mature minor doctrine Some states have defined circumstances in which a child who has not reached the age of majority may make legal decisions, if that child can demonstrate adequate maturity.
meconium First feces of a neonate, greenish black in color, tarry, and almost odorless.
medical forensic examination An examination performed for the purpose of collecting medical evidence when the healthcare provider suspects the client may be the victim of a crime.
medically fragile children Children that are medically stable but require skilled nursing care, specialized therapy, or medical equipment and supplies to enhance or sustain their lives.
medulla oblongata Area of the brain stem that regulates the respiratory, cardiac, vasoconstrictor, sneeze, cough, and vomiting reflexes as well as cranial nerves IX, X, XI, and XII.
melanin Black or dark brown pigment that occurs naturally in the hair, skin, iris, choroid of the eye.
melanocytes Cells within the epidermis that produce melanin, which gives pigment to the skin.
melena Black or tarry stool indicating the presence of blood.
memory cells T cells that remember an immune response.
menarche The first menstrual period.
meninges The three membranes covering the brain.
meningitis Inflammation of the meninges.
meningocele A sac-like herniation through the bony malformation that contains the meninges and cerebrospinal fluid.
meningococcemia A particularly virulent and extremely contagious disease caused by Neisseria meningitides.
meningomyelocele A sac-like extrusion through the bony defect that contains the meninges, cerebrospinal fluid, and a portion of the spinal cord or nerve roots.
menorrhagia Abnormally long and heavy menstrual periods.
mental combinations phase One thinks before acting, uses memory for simple problem solving, imitates behavior of others, engages in symbolic, ritualistic play; Piaget's sixth phase of cognitive development.
mental retardation A disorder characterized by subaverage general intellectual functioning with deficits in adaptive behavior.
mesosystem Bronfenbrenner's term for the interrelationship between microsystems.
message A verbal or nonverbal stimulus produced by a sender and responded to by a receiver.
metaphysis A section of the long bone in which the diaphysis and epiphysis converge; it is responsible for growth until the child's adult height is attained.
microcephaly A congenital anomaly characterized by a small brain with a resultant small head and a mental deficit.
microsystem Bronfenbrenner's term for the immediate settings of a person's life (i.e., the family).
midbrain Area of the brain stem that manages visual reflexes, tracking, and cranial nerves III and IV.
milia A minute white cyst of the epidermis caused by obstruction of hair follicles and eccrine sweat glands. One variety is seen in newborns and disappears within a few weeks; small white papules on the nose, face, forehead, and upper torso caused by the plugging of the sebaceous gland.
Millennium Development Goals (MDGs) Time-bound and quantified targets for addressing extreme poverty across the world and including the United States and Canada.
minor A person who has not yet reached the age at which he or she is considered to have the rights and responsibilities of an adult.
mixed hearing loss Occurs when both conductive and sensorineural damage occur; results from interference with transmission of sound in the middle ear.
modulation The cascade of events that affect the firing of the pain nerve impulses or messages.
molding The natural process by which a baby's head is shaped during labor as it is squeezed through the birth passage by the forces of labor.
mongolian spot An irregularly dark pigmented area on the posterior lumbar region.
monokines Chemical mediators (messengers) produced by monocytes and macrophages.
moral behavior Behavior in accordance with custom or tradition that usually reflects personal or religious beliefs.
morality of care Gilligan's term for the dominant moral orientation of women; the individual emphasizes responsibility and concern for the welfare of others rather than abstract rights.
morality of justice Gilligan's term for the dominant moral orientation of men; moral dilemmas are seen as inevitable conflicts between the rights of two or more parties needing to be settled by laws.

moratorium Individuals experiencing an occupational or ideologic crisis that has not yet been resolved, delaying the establishment of an ideologic or occupational commitment.
mosaicism The presence of two differing cell lines in an individual or organism.
mourning The process an individual undergoes in order to adapt to a loss.
mucositis An inflammation of the oral mucosa ranging from mild redness to severe painful ulceration.
Munchausen syndrome by proxy Mental disorder that causes caregivers to fabricate signs and symptoms of disease or expose their child to harmful medical interventions and painful invasive procedures.
Mustard procedure Intra-atrial baffling performed for correction of transposition of the great vessels. This procedure has almost completely been replaced by the arterial switch procedure.
mycologic cure Cure defined as the absence of fungal species.
myelodysplasia Malformation of the neural tube during the first 28 days of gestation.
myelosuppression A transient decrease in blood cell production.
myocarditis Inflammation of the myocardium, or middle muscular layer of the heart.
myocardium The cardiac muscle, middle layer of the heart.
myoclonic seizures Sudden repeated contractures of muscles of the head, extremities, or torso.
myopia (nearsightedness) Improper focusing of light on the retina; difficulty with distance vision.

N

nadir The lowest point of myelosuppression.
nasal flaring The widening of nostrils during inspiration; indicates air hunger.
natural immunity (see innate immunity).
nature Belief that development is predetermined by genetic factors and not altered by the environment.
near-drowning Survival for more than 24 hours after a submersion episode.
negativism The toddler's quest for independence leads to rejection of the wishes and ideas of others.
negligence When a person owes a duty to another and through failure to fulfill that duty causes harm.
nephrogenesis Development or growth of the kidney.
neurogenic shock A form of distributive shock that accompanies complete high spinal cord injury; caused by interruption of sympathetic impulses from the spinal cord in the cervical or thoracic region.
neutropenia A decrease in the number of neutrophils, putting one at risk of life-threatening bacterial infections.
nevus flammeus (port wine stain) A hemangioma or vascular tumor that does not disappear with time.
N-methyl-D-aspartate (NMDA) receptors Chemical receptors that make spinal column nerve receptors more responsive.
nociceptors Nerve receptors specific to pain.
noncommunicating hydrocephalus Hydrocephalus caused by an impediment of cerebrospinal fluid flow within the ventricular system, also called obstructive hydrocephalus.
nonfunctionality All functions that make being alive stop, and there is no longer an ability to carry out functions needed to be alive.
nonmaleficence Making sure that nothing harmful happens to the patient.
nonverbal communication Communicating a message without using words.
normalization Cognitive and behavioral strategies used by a family of a child with a chronic condition in order to view itself as normal.
nursing caries Dental decay that occurs from frequent or prolonged exposure to the sugars present in milk, formula, or juice.
nursing interview Discussion with caregivers that provides an opportunity for the nurse to establish helping relationships while learning essential information about child and family.
nursing mutual participation model of care A collaborative approach used in nursing practice, based on the premise that optimal therapeutic interventions result from equal partnerships between nurses and caregivers.
nurture Belief that environmental influences affect development.
nystagmus An oscillating movement of the eye; it is a late sign of a cataract.

O

object permanence The ability to know that an object will continue to exist even when it cannot be seen.
obstructive hydrocephalus (see noncommunicating hydrocephalus).
Oedipal or Oedipus complex Complex described by Freud where male child has strong feelings of attraction for the caregiver of the opposite sex and thus feels that he must compete with the caregiver of the same sex.
olecranon process A proximal projection of the ulna that forms the point of the elbow and fits into the olecranon fossa of the humerus when the forearm is extended.
oligohydramnios An abnormally small amount or absence of amniotic fluid.
oligomenorrhea Abnormally light or a reduction in menstruation.

oliguria A decreased ability to form and excrete urine.
oncogene Gene that is capable of causing normal cells to transform to a malignant state.
oncotic pressure A force within the capillary beds that holds fluids in the capillaries and is caused by the amount of plasma proteins present in the vascular system.
on-demand feeds Feeding the newborn when hungry instead of according to a prearranged time schedule.
onycholysis Describes separation of the nail plate from the nail bed.
onychomycosis Term used to refer to fungal infections of the nail.
open adoption An adoption where there is contact between the birth and adoptive parents.
open reduction Surgical procedure for reducing a fracture or dislocation by exposing the skeletal parts involved using wires, pins, bone screws, or plates.
operation Mental action, according to Piagetian theory.
opisthotonus Severe spasm of back muscles, causing back to arch acutely and head to bend back on neck.
opportunistic infections Infections that take advantage of a suppressed immune system.
opportunistic organisms Any organism that acts as a pathogen when the resistance of the host is impaired and conditions favor its growth.
oral rehydration solution Solution of electrolytes and glucose used in oral rehydration therapy.
oral stage Freud's first stage of psychosexual development; children gratify the sex instinct by stimulating the lips, gums, teeth, and mouth.
ordinary model A health orientation model of chronic conditions in which awareness of the health condition follows a developmental sequence and is not central to identity and daily activities.
original sin Belief that children are inherently evil and selfish egotists who must be controlled by society.
osmolality The concentration of solute within a solution measured by the number of moles of particles per kilogram of water; used as a measure of fluid concentration.
osmolarity The concentration of solute within a solution measured by the number of moles per liter of water.
osmosis Movement of water across a semipermeable membrane from a solution that has a lower solute concentration to one that has a higher solute concentration.
osmotic pressure A force within the capillary beds that tends to pull fluid into the capillaries and serves to balance hydrostatic pressures.
osteoblasts Cells of mesodermal origin concerned with formation of bone.
osteoclastic Resorption of old bony tissue by osteoclasts in periods of growth or repair.
osteotomy Surgical procedure in which the bone is redesigned to alter the alignment or weight-bearing stress areas.
ovicidal Product that kills unhatched lice eggs.

P

palliative Therapies or procedures performed to relieve or reduce the intensity of uncomfortable symptoms but do not result in correction of a defect or a cure.
palpebral fissures The opening between the margins of the upper and lower eyelids.
palpitations Sensation of abnormal, forceful, or rapid heart beats.
pancarditis Inflammation of the entire heart.
pancytopenia A marked reduction in the number of RBCs, WBCs, and platelets.
papilledema An inflammation of the optic disk, evident by edema seen on funduscopic examination.
papules Small raised lesions.
parallel play The ability to play side-by-side, yet totally independent of other children. There may be close physical proximity, but seldom talking or sharing of toys.
paraverbal cues Tone, pitch, volume, inflection, and the speed of the voice used in communication; not considered language.
parenchyma The functional tissue of an organ as distinguished from supporting or connective tissue.
parens patrie A legal rule that allows the state to take the place of the caregivers when the actual caregivers are unable or unwilling to provide for the best interests of the child.
parentification The process of assuming the role of a caregiver (parent) such as caring for siblings, or organizing and performing household chores.
parenting A dynamic process that provides guidance and nurturing to a child.
paresthesia Numbness or tingling sensation.
paroxysmal Coughing that is severe in nature.
partial seizures Arise from abnormal electrical activity in a small area of the brain; symptoms seen are associated with the area of the brain affected.
partial-thickness burn Second degree burn, divided into *superficial partial-thickness,* involving the epidermis and superficial dermis, and *deep partial-thickness burns,* involving the epidermis and deeper dermis.
partially sighted Residual vision is sufficient to allow child to read large print (for visually impaired) for educational purposes.
passive immunity The passing or administration of preformed antibodies to a person without that antibody.
pathogens Organisms that invade the body and produce disease.

patient-controlled analgesia Means of delivering pain medication by client self-administration.
peak height velocity (PHV) The period of greatest growth in height during the adolescent growth spurt (AGS).
peak weight velocity (PWV) The period of greatest weight gain during the AGS.
pediatric nurse practitioner Usually a nurse with a master's degree who functions independently or under the guidance of a physician and focuses on disease prevention and minor disease management.
pediculocidal Product that kills live lice.
pedophilia An act by an adult where the adult directs his or her sexual interests primarily or exclusively toward children.
perception The cognitive awareness of pain experienced at the end of the physiological pain cascade.
pericardial effusion Abnormal collection of fluid in the pericardial sac; limits filling and decreases cardiac output.
pericarditis Inflammation of the pericardium.
pericardium Fluid-filled sac that encases the heart.
periorbital cellulitis An infection of the eyelid and soft tissues of the orbit of the eye.
peristalsis Coordinated, rhythmic, serial contraction of the smooth muscle of the GI tract.
peritoneal dialysis Requires the placement of a catheter into the peritoneal cavity for the purposes of removing excess fluids, solutes, and nitrogenous wastes. This placement may or may not require an open surgical procedure.
periungual Located around the fingernail or toenail.
personal fable Psychological state in which adolescents have an exaggerated notion of their own uniqueness.
petechiae Small, pinpoint, nonraised, perfectly round, purplish red spots that are a result of an intradermal or submucosal hemorrhage.
phagocytosis The ingestion and destruction of foreign particles by cells of natural immunity.
phallic stage Freud's third stage of psychosexual development; children gratify the sex instinct by developing an incestuous desire for the parent of the opposite gender, or fondling their own genitals.
phantom limb pain Pain perceived to be coming from the area of an amputated limb.
pharmacodynamics Biochemical and physiologic effects of drugs and their mechanisms of action within the body.
pharmacokinetics Movement of drugs throughout the body by the processes of absorption, distribution, biotransformation, and excretion.
pharyngitis Infection or inflammation of the pharynx.
photophobia Light sensitivity.
phototherapy The use of special high-intensity fluorescent lights to reduce serum bilirubin levels and prevent kernicterus.
physical abuse Bodily injury that appears to have been inflicted by other than accidental means.
physical dependence Physical adaptation to the presence of a drug in the bloodstream.
physiologic anorexia A decreased appetite and ritualistic interest in limited types of food; this usually accompanies a period of slowed physiological growth and is considered a normal occurrence of toddlerhood.
pia mater The third meningeal membrane, which is attached to the brain itself.
pilosebaceous unit Unit consists of hair follicle (pore), a hair shaft, and a sebaceous gland.
plasticity The ability of neural cells in a certain area of the brain to assume the functions of a different area.
platelets Disk-shaped cytoplasmic fragments that facilitate blood coagulation.
play therapy The child expresses him- or herself through the use of toys, dolls, blocks, cars, or other play objects. The process of being with the therapist, toy selection, and interaction during the therapy session are part of the therapeutic process.
pneumatosis intestinalis Air within the bowel wall.
pneumoperitoneum Free air in the peritoneal cavity.
pneumothorax A collection of air or gas in the pleural cavity.
polyarthritis Inflammation of many joints.
polydactyly A congenital anomaly characterized by the presence of more than the normal number of fingers or toes.
polydipsia Excessive thirst.
polyhydramnios An excess of amniotic fluid.
polymorphous Appearing in many forms.
polyphagia Excessive hunger.
polyuria Excretion of abnormally large quantity of urine.
pons Area of the brain stem that controls respiratory function and cranial nerves V, VI, VII, and VIII.
postconventional morality Kohlberg's term for the third level of moral reasoning; moral judgments are based on an abstract understanding of universal principles of justice.
postpubertal Late adolescence.
postvoid residual urine A measurement of the amount of urine remaining in the bladder after voiding.
preconceptual phase Increasing use of symbols, especially language, egocentric thought, symbolic play, mental imagery; Piaget's seventh phase of cognitive development.
preconventional morality Kohlberg's term for the first level of moral reasoning; societal rules are not yet internalized, judgments are based on reward or punishment.

preconventional or premoral stage Initial stage of moral development described by Kohlberg where right and wrong are determined by the rules that others place upon you; impulses rule behavior; unable to differentiate right from wrong.
precordium The part of the front of the chest that overlays the heart and the epigastrium.
preoperational stage Piagetian term for second stage of cognitive development; children between 2 and 7 years old think symbolically and have not mastered logical operations.
prepubertal Early adolescence.
prepuce Skin forming a hood over the glans, which is abnormally small ventrally and may be redundant dorsally.
primary circular reaction phase Infant performs complex, repetitive behaviors appearing to be responses to initial chance events centering on the infant's own body; Piaget's second phase of cognitive development.
primary prevention Involves interventions that promote health and prevent disease processes from developing.
processus vaginalis A fold of peritoneum that precedes the testicle as it descends through the inguinal canal into the scrotum.
prodrome The earliest phase or sign of a developing condition or disease.
professional boundaries The spaces between the nurse's power and the client's vulnerability. The power of the nurse comes from professional position and access to private -knowledge about the client. Establishing boundaries allows the nurse to control this power differential and allows a safe connection to meet the client's needs.
proprioception Awareness of posture, movement, and changes in equilibrium and knowledge of position, weight, and resistance of objects in relation to the body.
proptosis A protrusion or forward displacement of the eyeball.
prostaglandins A group of fatty acid substances present in many tissues. Extremely active biological substances responsible for a number of cellular interactions.
proteolysis The hydrolysis of protein to simpler and soluble products.
protest The first phase of Robertson's (1958) effect of separation on young children from their parents due to hospitalization. During this phase, the toddler cries loudly and desparately, making every effort to bring parents back. The toddlers are inconsolable and constantly look in the direction of where their parent departed.
proximodistal Growth proceeds from the inside out.
pseudohermaphrodism Ambiguous development of external genitalia.
pseudohypertrophy Abnormal enlargement of an organ or body structure caused by an overgrowth of fatty and fibrous tissues.
pseudomenstruation Blood observed on the diaper due to the withdrawal of the maternal hormones at the time of delivery.
pseudostrabismus An appearance of strabismus caused by a fold of skin of the lower eyelid, which narrows the visible width of the sclera medial to the iris.
psychological abuse Acts of omission or commission involving both the presence of hostile behavior as well as the absence of positive parenting behaviors.
psychomotor learning One type of learning concerned with physical skills.
psychosexual theory Freud's theoretical perspective emphasizing conflicts within the personality, unconscious motivations for behavior, and stages of development.
psychosocial theory Theoretical perspective advocated by Erikson; stresses the complexity of interrelationships existing between emotional and physical variables during one's lifetime.
ptosis A drooping of the eyelid.
pubertal Middle adolescence.
puberty The state of physical development when secondary sex characteristics begin to appear, sexual organs mature, reproduction first becomes possible, and the adolescent growth spurt starts.
pulse dosing The process of switching between periods when medications are administered in higher doses followed by drug-free intervals. This approach to medication dosing allows for greater individualization of therapy and higher rates of compliance.
pulsus paradoxus Excessive variation in forcefulnes of arterial pulse during respiration demonstrated by a systolic reduction of more than 10 mm Hg.
punishment and obedience orientation stage Behaviors, decisions, and conformity to rules are based on fear of punishment rather than respect for authority; Kohlberg's first stage of moral development.
pupil personnel team (service team) A team of professionals who work together with teachers to provide interventions for students having difficulties.
purpura Areas of blood underneath the skin or mucous membranes.
pyelonephritis An inflammation of the kidney(s).
pyloromyotomy Surgical procedure performed to relieve hypertrophic pyloric stenosis.
pyuria White blood cells in the urine (a sign of bacterial or nonbacterial infection of the urinary tract).

R

rachischisis Fissure in the vertebral column exposing the meninges and spinal cord.
radiation pneumonitis Acute reaction caused by the swelling and sloughing of the endothelial cells of the small vessels of the lung, which allows fluid to accumulate in the interstitial tissues.
rape Sexual intercourse with force or a threat of force, and without a person's consent.
rate of growth A calculation of the amount of growth over a specific period of time.
realistic stage (of career development) Young people begin to extensively explore and focus on available careers.
rebound tenderness Sign of inflammation of the peritoneum elicited by a sudden release of a hand pressing on the abdomen.
receiver The person intercepting the sender's message.
receptive language The ability to understand spoken and written communication.
red blood cells (RBCs) The blood cells whose primary function is to supply the tissues with oxygen.
reflexive phase Predictable, innate survival reflexes becoming more efficient and generalized; first phase of Piaget's cognitive development.
refraction The process by which the cornea and lens of the eye bend light rays so that they focus on the retina.
refractory seizures Seizures lasting more than 60 minutes.
regenerative family Displays hardiness (feelings of being in control, committed to each other, seeing stresses as challenges to be overcome) and coherence.
regression Returning to a previous level of function or action. Often occurs when the toddler's routine and security are threatened (e.g., hospitalization, new baby enters family).
renal scanning Examination of the urinary tract by ultrasound.
renal ultrasound Radiographic examination of the kidney utilizing sound waves above the range of human hearing to formulate a two-dimensional image.
researcher Nursing role involved in collecting, using, and evaluating evidence-based data in practice.
resiliency model of family stress, adjustment, and adaptation The model explores how families process stressful/threatening live events by evaluating and assessing the stressor and then reaching homeostasis by using problem solving and coping skills.
resilient family Demonstrates flexibility and emotional closeness.
respiratory distress syndrome (RDS) An inadequate production of surfactant in the lungs of premature infants, thereby reducing the surface tension of these surfaces, and interfering with the ability of the lungs to remain inflated during exhalation.
respite care Involves having a person who relieves the usual caregiver of caregiving responsibilities for a period of time.
retractions Inward motion of the muscles of the chest wall during inspiration; associated with increased respiratory effort.
retrograde Moving backward.
reverse attention Method of behavior management where attention is given to positive behaviors and negative behaviors are ignored.
reversibility The ability to recognize that actions can move in reverse order.
Reye's syndrome Acute, life-threatening, postinfectious encephalopathy.
rhizotomy A procedure used to treat cerebral palsy, where a small secction of the spinal cord is cut.
rhythmic family Focuses on family times and routines that help them cope with stress.
ritualism The repetition of sequences of occurrences, which produce structure and organization in the mind of a toddler. The repetition may involve a repeated action, phrase, or food or clothing choice and may continue for days or weeks.
rolandic or sylvian seizure Tonic-clonic movements of the face with increased salivation and arrested speech; commonly occurs during sleep.

S

sarcoma Cancer that originates in connective tissue.
scald burns Skin that is injured by hot water from the tap, coffee, tea, or hot cooking grease.
schema Patterns of thought used to interpret or make sense of experiences, Piagetian term; one's own mental or physical structure developed through assimilation of new experiences.
school-age The phase of development from 6 to 12 years.
school-based health clinics (SBHC) Health centers within a school building set up and staffed by health care professionals other than the school nurse.
school-linked health clinics (SLHC) Health centers set up and staffed by health care professionals to serve several schools, students, and other family members. May or may not be located within a school building.
SCIWORA Spinal cord injury without radiologic abnormality.
scoliosis A C-shaped or S-shaped curvature of the spine.
sebaceous glands Glands that open into the hair follicles and secrete sebum, which helps lubricate the skin.

sebum A complex lipid mixture produced by the sebaceous glands, which helps lubricate the skin.
secondary circular reaction phase Infant learns from intentional behavior and begins to show some understanding of objects; Piaget's third phase of cognitive development.
secondary drowning The rapid deterioration of respiratory function from several hours to days after successful resuscitation.
secondary prevention Aims to detect disease in the early stages before clinical signs and symptoms manifest in order to intervene with early diagnosis and treatment.
self-competency Adolescents' sense of how well they can function within a particular realm.
self-understanding Adolescents' cognitive representation about themselves.
self-worth The extent to which adolescents perceive themselves as individuals of worth.
sender Generator of a message.
sensitive period A time span that is optimal for certain capacities to emerge when the individual is especially receptive to environmental influences.
sensitization phase Phase of a hypersensitivity reaction in which initial exposure to the antigen occurs.
sensorimotor stage Piaget's first stage of cognitive development; during the first two years of life, the individual relies on motor behavior and senses to adapt to the world.
sensorineural hearing loss Permanent hearing impairment that results from damage or malformation of the middle ear or auditory nerve.
separation anxiety The behaviors demonstrated by an infant when separated from the caregiver.
sequestration crisis A type of sickle cell crisis characterized by excessive pooling of blood in the liver and spleen.
sexual abuse A sexual act, from fondling to vaginal or anal intercourse, imposed on a child who lacks the emotional, cognitive, or maturational development to deal with the actions.
shaken baby syndrome (SBS) Vigorous manual shaking of a child, usually less than 3 years of age, that results in a subdural hematoma of the brain, occult bone fractures, and retinal hemorrhages.
sibling rivalry Intense feelings of jealousy, envy, and stress toward a new infant sibling.
sickle cell anemia (SCA) An anemia caused by the sickling of red blood cells caused by the presence of hemoglobin S.
simple partial seizures Focal seizures characterized by local motor, sensory, psychic, and somatic manifestations.
sleep consolidation Fewer periods of sleep with longer durations.
small for gestational age (SGA) An infant who has a weight to gestational age ratio that is below the tenth percentile.
smegma A collection of cells that shed from the outer layer of skin and gather under the foreskin of the penis.
social contract legalistic orientation Just laws should be followed because they further human values and express the majority will; Kohlberg's fifth stage of moral development.
social learning theory Bandura's theory; the individual learns behavior by observing behaviors of others.
social perspective taking ability The understanding adolescents have about who they are in relation to those around them and their ability to understand the perspectives of others.
solute A substance that is dissolved in a solution.
somnambulism Sleepwalking.
somniloquy Sleep talking.
somnolence syndrome Subacute neurological toxicity seen 5–7 weeks postradiation therapy to the whole brain where drowsiness can be experienced up to 20 hours a day, and may be accompanied by fatigue, malaise, fever, dysphagia, ataxia, and transient papilledema.
span Measurement obtained from measuring fingertip to fingertip.
speech The physical production of sound using the oral mechanism (tongue, teeth, oral cavity, larynx).
spina bifida A congenital, neural tube defect in the walls of the spinal cord caused by a lack of union between the laminae of the vertebrae.
spina bifida cystica A defect in the closure of the posterior vertebral arch resulting in a protruding sac containing meninges (meningocele), spinal cord (myelocele), or both (meningomyelocele).
spina bifida occulta A type of spina bifida where there is no herniation of the spinal cord or meninges.
spinal shock Spinal shock is the complete loss of all reflex activity after spinal cord injury.
splash burns Occur when hot liquid is poured on a child; usually involves the back, lateral side of the face, or shoulder; the direction the hot liquid flows down the child's body assists in the diagnosis.
sprain A ligament that is stretched or torn from injury to a joint.
stage The amount of spread of a malignancy, rated from stage I (1), with only local disease in one area or organ, to stage IV (4), with disseminated metastatic disease.
standard of care Accepted action expected of an individual of a certain skill or knowledge level.
status epilepticus A prolonged seizure or series of convulsions; loss of consciousness that may last for at least 30 minutes.

statutory rape Consensual relations between a minor and an adult.

steatorrhea Greater-than-normal amounts of fat in the feces, characterized by frothy, foul-smelling fecal matter that floats.

Stevens-Johnson syndrome The most severe form of erythema multiforme caused by exposure to an antigen, usually a drug.

"stocking or glove" burns Represent attempts by a child to prevent and protect himself or herself from being immersed in hot scalding tub water; burn has the appearance of a glove or stocking with an even edge.

strabismus A condition in which each eye does not simultaneously focus on the same object in space because of lack of muscle coordination.

strain The stretching or tearing of either a muscle or tendon from overuse, overstretching, or misuse.

stranger anxiety The behaviors demonstrated by an infant with the appearance of a stranger and seen at approximately 8 to 12 months of age.

stratum corneum The outermost layer of the epidermis, which is composed of several layers of dead skin cells.

stridor A high-pitched sound produced by an obstruction of the trachea or larynx that can be heard during inspiration or expiration.

stupor An unresponsive state; only responds to vigorous stimulation, and then returns to the original state once the insult is removed.

stuttering A speech impairment in which an individual involuntarily repeats a sound or word, resulting in a loss of speech fluency.

subarachnoid villi Area of the brain that reabsorbs CSF.

subdural hematomas Space occupying lesions in the brain caused by rupture of the cortical veins bridging the subdural space.

subluxation Incomplete or partial dislocation of the articular surfaces of a joint.

substance abuse A maladaptive pattern of substance use manifested by recurrent and significant adverse consequences related to the repeated use of substance.

substance dependence Involves a substantial degree of involvement with a substance, including withdrawal (adverse physical symptoms due to cessation of or reduction in prolonged and heavy substance use); tolerance (a need for increased amounts of the substance to achieve the desired effect); and repetitious failure to control overuse (efforts to cut down use are unsuccessful).

substance P A neuropeptide that sensitizes nerve endings to fire more rapidly.

subungual hyperkeratosis An accumulation of keratin debris under the nail, yellowish nail discoloration, and thickening of the nail.

sudden infant death syndrome (SIDS) The sudden, unexplained death of an apparently normal and healthy infant under the age of 1 year even after a complete autopsy and review of history reveals no evidence of disease.

suicidal ideation Thoughts about killing oneself.

suicide The intentional or purposeful taking of one's own life. Suicide may be completed, attempted, or suicidal ideation.

sunblock A sun protection product that reflects and scatters ultraviolet A and ultraviolet B radiation.

sunscreen A sun protection product that absorbs the sun's rays. Protection against either or both ultraviolet A and ultraviolet B radiation may be provided.

superego Freudian term for personality component consisting of internalized moral standards (conscience).

superficial burn First degree burn which involves only the epidermis; typically is somewhat painful for 48 to 72 hours and heals spontaneously without scarring in 5 to 10 days.

superficial partial-thickness burn Second degree burn which involves the epidermis and superficial dermis; is erythematous, moist, and painful. Typically heals spontaneously without scarring in 1 to 3 weeks.

superior vena cava syndrome (SVC) Syndrome caused by obstruction of the superior vena cava, resulting in edema of the face, neck, and upper trunk.

suppressor cells T cells that reduce immunoglobulin production against a specific antigen.

suppurative Pus forming.

supratentorial A location in the anterior two-thirds of the brain, above the tentorium, primarily in the cerebrum.

synchronized cardioversion Cardioversion of an abnormal rhythm to a normal rhythm using electrical shock (via a defibrillator) that senses the QRS and applies the energy in an appropriately timed manner in synchrony with the client's own rhythm. Can only be used in hemodynamically stable clients with normally upright QRS.

syncope Fainting.

syndactylism Congenital anomaly characterized by the fusion of the fingers or toes.

syndrome A named condition characterized by a group of findings or attributes.

synovitis An acute, nonpurulent inflammation of the synovial membrane of a joint; occurs most commonly in the hip joint.

T

T lymphocytes The immune system's main defense against viruses; direct and regulate the immunologic response; secrete lymphokines; produced by the thymus gland.

tabula rasa Doctrine that suggests children enter the world as a blank slate.

tachyarrhythmia Abnormally fast heart rhythm.

tachypnea Rapid respirations.

tamponade An abnormal fluid collection around the heart in the mediastinal space that results in restricted filling of the heart and poor cardiac output. Can be life-threatening.

Tanner stages The five stages of development of secondary sexual characteristics for males and females.

teething The period of eruption of deciduous teeth.

telangiectatic nevi A common skin condition of neonates, characterized by flat, deep-pink localized areas of capillary dilation that occur predominantly on the back of the neck, lower occiput, upper eyelids, upper lip, and bridge of the nose. The areas disappear permanently by 2 years of age.

telegraphic speech Short sentences made up of only the key words.

teleologic theory A major theoretical orientation that judges the rightness of actions by the ends achieved.

temper tantrums An outward expression of the inner turmoil experienced by a toddler: openly angry and unpredictable. Usually disappears by preschool period.

temperament The way in which a child behaviorally interacts with the surrounding environment.

tentative stage (of career development) Adolescents begin to consider how they might fit in with the various career options they are considering.

tentorium The dura mater located between the cerebrum and cerebellum supporting the occipital lobes.

teratogen Any substance or process that interferes with normal prenatal development, causing developmental abnormalities in the fetus.

terminal hair Hair found on the scalp, eyebrows, eyelashes, beard, axillae and pubic areas.

tertiary circular reactions phase Characterized by interest in novelty and repetition, understanding causality, soliciting adult help, object permanence; Piaget's fifth phase of cognitive development.

tertiary prevention Prevention directed toward children with clinically apparent disease.

thalassemias A group of inherited autosomal recessive disorders, characterized by an impaired rate of hemoglobin chain synthesis.

therapeutic play An intervention used by nurses and child life specialists where supervised play helps ill and hospitalized children express and understand their thoughts, feelings, and motivations.

thrill A fine vibration, felt by an examiner's hand on a client's body over the site of an aneurysm or on the precordium, the result of turmoil in the flow of blood, indicating the presence of an organic murmur of grade 4 or greater intensity.

thrombocytopenia A decrease in the platelet count below 150,000/mL.

tidal volume The amount of air inhaled or exhaled with each breath.

time-out A discipline strategy in which reinforcement for unacceptable behavior is removed to interrupt a pattern of negative behavior; a defined period of time in which the child is removed from activities and social interactions.

titration Delivery of small doses of medication to achieve desired effect.

tolerance Need to use increasing doses of a substance over time to achieve desired effect.

tonic-clonic seizures Onset is usually abrupt and begins when the child loses consciousness and falls to the ground.

toxic epidermal necrolysis An acute illness of fever, epidermal loss of more than 30% of the body surface area; 30–40% mortality rate caused by visceral involvement.

trabeculotomy A surgical procedure for glaucoma; a direct opening between the canal of Schlemm and the anterior chamber of the eye, which controls intraocular pressure.

trajectory The expected course of a health care alteration.

transduction Beginning of the pain sensation when stimulus provokes electrical activity in pain receptors.

transductive reasoning Unrelated events are linked to determine a reason for a particular event.

transferrin An iron-transport molecule within the bloodstream.

transillumination The use of a light to determine what structures are in the meningomyelocele.

transmission Movement of impulses from peripheral site to terminals in spinal column dorsal horn.

traumatic sexualization Children have learned that affection and love are equated with sex that is inappropriate and unsafe.

trigone A small triangular area at the base of the bladder where the ureters normally join the bladder.

trismus Difficulty opening the mouth.

trisomy The presence of three instead of two of a given chromosome.
tropic hormone A hormone that causes a target organ to produce its hormone.
Trousseau's sign Spasms of the carpals after pressure is applied to the upper arm nerves. Carpal spasms occur when the fingers contract and the individual is unable to open the hand. This is a sign of hypocalcemia.
trust versus mistrust Erikson's first stage of psychosocial development; infants must learn to trust others to meet their needs so they learn to trust themselves.
tumor lysis syndrome Complication of initial cancer treatment; when tumor cells are killed by chemotherapy, purines are released from the lysed tumor cells, causing elevation of uric acid that can lead to renal failure.
tympanostomy Surgical incision in the tympanic membrane for draining fluid.

U

uncertainty Situations in which there is ambiguity about what can be expected. Typically results in stress.
unintentional injury Injuries that occur without intent of harm.
universal ethical principle orientation Right and wrong are defined on universal, comprehensive, consistent, yet personal ethical principles; Kohlberg's sixth stage of moral development.
universality Belief that death is all inclusive, comes to every living thing; death is inevitable.
unlicensed assistive personnel (UAP) Individuals who perform services for clients, such as first aid, medication administration, tube feedings, and catheterizations under the supervision of a registered nurse.
unprovoked first seizure A seizure that occurs without a known cause, such as a fever.
upper or lower body ratio A ratio calculated from a measurement from the top of the head to the top of the synthesis pubis and from the synthesis pubis to the bottom of the feet.
uremia A condition where excessive amounts of nitrogenous waste products, blood urea, and creatinine exist in the blood.
ureteropelvic obstruction An obstruction at the junction of the ureters into the renal pelvis.
ureterovesical obstruction An obstruction at the junction of the ureters into the bladder.
ureterovesical or vesicoureteral junction Site where the ureter enters the bladder.
urethritis Infection of the urethra.
urticaria Wheal-like skin lesions seen in response to an antigen, often a drug; resolve fairly rapidly after discontinuing the drug.
utilitarianism To carry out an action based on the benefits versus its cost.

V

values Constructs that give meaning to our lives.
valvotomy An incision into a cardiac valve to correct a defect.
valvulitis Inflammation of the cardiac valves.
valvuloplasty Procedure involving a balloon-tipped catheter used to dilate a cardiac valve.
vasculitis Inflammation of blood vessels, including arteries or veins.
vaso-occlusive crisis A type of sickle cell crisis characterized by the aggregation of sickled cells within a vessel, causing obstruction and infarction of the distal tissues.
vectors Animals or insects that carry the infectious organism from one host to another.
vegetations Abnormal growths inside body organs. In the heart they usually develop on heart valves.
vellus hair Short, fine, often inconspicuous hair distributed across the body.
venous access device Implanted device to facilitate the delivery of drugs, blood sampling and blood product administration, and the simultaneous administration of multiple drugs and intravenous fluids.
ventilation/perfusion (V/Q) ratio The ratio of alveolar ventilation to capillary perfusion.
veracity When the health care provider always gives and uses the facts when caring for children and families.
verbal communication Messages using words and language.
vernix caseosa A thick, cheesy, protective, integumentary deposit that consists of sebum and shed epithelial cells present on the newborn's skin.
verrucae Benign epidermal tumors caused by the human papilloma virus, also known as cutaneous warts.
vertical transmission The process of transmitting a disease from one generation to another.
vesicant A chemotherapy agent that is a skin irritant and can cause discomfort, burning, and inflammation, if leaked outside the vein.
vesicles Thin roofed blisters.
violent crime Murder, forcible rape, robbery, and aggravated assault.
virilize To develop sexual characteristics of a male. For example, a clitoris that is virilized will have the appearance of a penis.

virtue theory A major theoretical orientation that focuses on the moral agent's intent, such as the virtue of truthfulness.
virulence The degree or power of microorganisms to cause disease.
visual acuity Clearness or sharpness of the image seen by the eye.
voiding cystourethrogram (VCUG) Radiograph of bladder, urethra, and ureters during voiding.
von Willebrand's disease A mild, congenital bleeding disorder caused by a deficiency of von Willebrand's factor.
von Willebrand's factor (vWF) A protein that facilitates adhesion between platelets and injured vessel walls.

W

Waterhouse-Friderichsen syndrome Fulminant meningococcemia.
weaning A process of giving up one method of feeding for another.
wet drowning Drowning caused by the aspiration of fluid into the lungs.
wheezing A high-pitched musical sound produced by air flow through a narrowed airway.
white blood cells (WBCs) The blood cells responsible for defending against invading microorganisms and removing debris.
windshield survey A systematic assessment performed while the nurse travels through the community.

X

xanthelasma Creamy, yellow plaque on eyelid due to hyper-cholesterolemia.
xanthomas Slightly elevated yellow nodules that develop in the subcutaneous layer of skin.
xerosis Dry skin as a result of impaired skin barrier functions.
xerostomia Dryness of the mouth, which occurs from decreased or arrested production of salivary secretions.

Z

zone of proximal development (ZPD) Tasks that are too difficult for individuals to master alone but that can be mastered with the guidance and assistance of adults or more skilled adolescents.

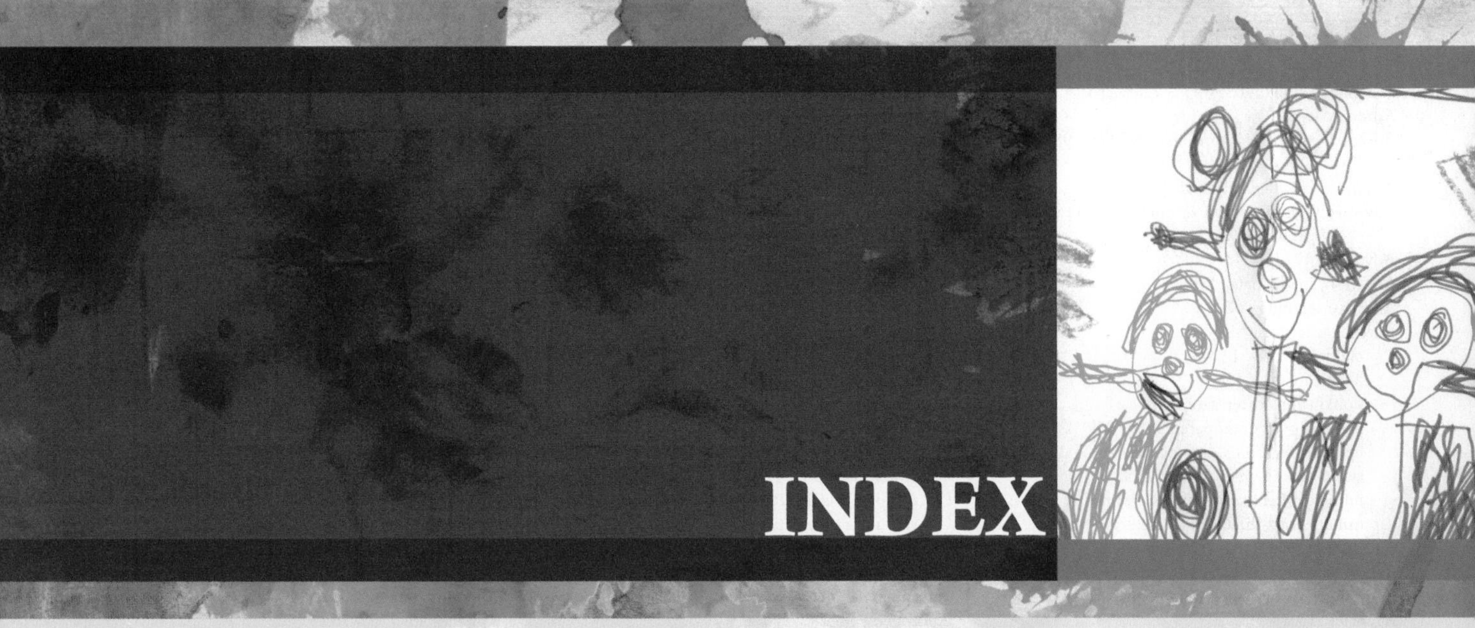

INDEX

Note: Page numbers followed by an *f* refer to figures. Page numbers followed by a *b* refer to boxes. Page numbers followed by a *t* refer to tables.

A

B

C

D

E

G

H

I

J

K

L

M

Q

R

S

T

U